The Essential Guide to Prescription Drugs

The Essential Guide to Prescription Drugs

1990 EDITION

James W. Long, M.D.

PERENNIAL LIBRARY

Harper & Row, Publishers, New York
Grand Rapids, Philadelphia, St. Louis, San Francisco
London, Singapore, Sydney, Tokyo, Toronto

Designed by C. Linda Dingler

Library of Congress Catalog Card Number 87-657561
ISSN 0894-7058
ISBN 0-06-055171-2   90 91 92 93 HC 10 9 8 7 6 5 4 3
ISBN 0-06-096394-8 (pbk.)   90 91 92 93 HC 10 9 8 7 6 5 4

Quality Printing by:
Haddon Craftsmen, Inc.
Bloomsburg Plant
4411 Old Berwick Road
Bloomsburg, PA 17815, U.S.A.

Contents

SECTION SIX:
Tables of Drug Information

Author's Note for the 1990 Edition

Upon reflection on significant changes in health care services and public awareness that have occurred during the last decade, it seems prudent to rethink the mission of this book and the nature of the information it should provide. Several forces signal the need for change: the rapid increase in the introduction of new and more powerful drugs that require greater knowledge and vigilance by both physician and patient; the expanding emphasis on multiple-drug regimens for treating serious disorders; and the growing tendency of more informed individuals to assume an active role (some would say "take charge") in the management of their drug therapy. Changes of progress always require appropriate adjustments.

This new edition of the Guide will enhance its character as a responsible "bridge text" that can better facilitate the exchange of information between health care providers (physicians, dentists, nurses, pharmacists) and consumers. The drugs included for presentation (always limited by the size of the book) will be confined to those of major importance. They will be selected primarily on the basis of the seriousness of the disorder being treated and the complexity of the drug's actions and usage. The scope of information presented for each drug will provide the breadth and depth of detail required to achieve optimal therapeutic benefit with minimal risk and harm—in language suitable for the reading public. Drugs of minor and fading importance (though used widely) will be omitted to allow the inclusion of the major drugs in current use. Information regarding drug advantage and choice will attempt to reflect medical consensus at the time of writing.

While some readers may be disappointed that "their drug" is not presented in a given edition, it is the author's opinion that the overriding need is for information in depth that relates to those drugs and disorders that impact most significantly on the health and well-being of the public at large.

Newly added features of this edition include: (1) a separate information category in each Drug Profile detailing the drug's effect on sexual function; (2) ten new Drug Profiles of major drugs, eight of them introduced (or soon to be introduced) for use in the United States since publication of the last edition; (3) expansion of the information categories dealing with *New Drugs in Development, Current Controversies in Drug Management, Possible Advantages of This Drug*, and *Drug of Choice* designations; (4) the provision of names, addresses and telephone numbers of national organizations that provide helpful information and guidance to those with the major disorders presented in Section Two.

As noted in each previous edition, no claim is made that all known actions, side-effects, adverse effects, precautions, interactions, etc., for a drug are included in the information provided in the six sections that comprise this book. While diligent care was taken to ensure the accuracy of the information provided during the preparation of this revision, the continued accuracy and currentness are ever subject to change relative to the dissemination of new information derived from drug research, development and general usage.

1

HOW TO USE THIS BOOK

2

GUIDELINES FOR SAFE AND EFFECTIVE DRUG USE

1

How to Use This Book

Your physician has advised you to take a drug (or drugs), or you have been directed to administer a drug (or drugs) to someone under your care. The kind and amount of information you have been given about how to use these drugs, and what to expect from them, will vary tremendously. In many instances it will not be practical or possible for the physician to provide you with *all* the information that could be considered appropriate and useful, or it will be difficult for you to remember it. From time to time you will find it desirable—even necessary—to seek clarification and guidance about some aspect of drug action or drug use. The aim of this book is to give you the kind of information you may need to supplement the direction and guidance you receive from your physician.

The book consists of six sections. The first section will give you the orientation and insight necessary to appreciate the complexities of modern drug therapy and help you to make the best use of the information contained in Sections Two through Six.

Section Two presents useful information regarding the role of drugs in treating 25 common chronic disorders that require long-term drug therapy. A synopsis of each disorder is followed by information categories that cover drug selection, the goals of drug treatment and an overview of drug management during the period of therapy. A list of the disorders reviewed is found in the introduction to the section.

Section Three is a compilation of Drug Profiles covering 220 prescription (and several nonprescription) drugs used widely in the United States and Canada. The selection of each drug was based upon three considerations: the extent of its use; the urgency of the conditions for which it is prescribed; the volume and complexity of the information essential to its proper utilization. The Drug Profiles are arranged alphabetically by generic name. (Some generic names have spellings similar to other generic names; be careful not to confuse one with another.)

The Profile of each drug is presented in a uniform sequence of information categories. (When you become familiar with the format, you will be able to find quickly specific items of information on any drug, without having to read the entire Profile.) Each Drug Profile contains 42 (or more) separate categories of information. The principal categories include the following.

Year Introduced

This tells you how long the drug has been in general use. The older the drug, the more likely its full spectrum of actions is known and the less likely its continued use will produce new surprises. The date given represents the year the drug was introduced for human use anywhere in the world.

Drug Class

This identifies the principal therapeutic class(es) to which the drug belongs. When appropriate, the chemical and/or pharmacological class designations are also given. You will find it helpful to recognize the class of the drug you are taking because many actions, reactions and interactions with other drugs are often shared by drugs of the same class. Throughout this book (and in most literature on drug information) you will find reference to drugs by their class designation. (Section Four provides alphabetically arranged listings of the classes of drugs referred to in this guide.)

Prescription Required

This indicates whether a drug is a prescription or a nonprescription (over-the-counter) purchase. Because there are significant differences in prescription requirements between the United States and Canada, the designation for each country is given when appropriate.

Controlled Drug

Drugs subject to regulation under the Controlled Substances Act of 1970 (those with potential for abuse) are so designated by the particular schedule that governs their dispensing in the United States. A corresponding schedule is also given for Canada when applicable.

A description of the Schedules of Controlled Drugs is found inside the back cover of this guide.

Available for Purchase by Generic Name

Increasing interest in the availability of prescription drugs for purchase by their generic names has been prompted by two issues of major significance. The first is concerned with the cost of prescription drugs. The comparison shopper realizes that in general the cost of prescription medication is significantly less when a generic equivalent of a brand name product is purchased. The second issue relates to what is termed "bioavailability and bioequivalence"—the comparative composition, quality and effectiveness of the generic versus the brand name drug product. Further discussion of bioavailability and bioequivalence of drug products will be found in the Glossary, Section Five.

Brand Names

These are provided to confirm that you are consulting the correct Drug Profile. They may also help you to recognize a brand name that identifies this drug as one that produced in you an unfavorable reaction on previous use. Brand names are listed for the United States and for Canada (✦). A combination drug (a drug product with more than one active ingredient) is identified by [CD] following the brand name.

In a few instances a particular brand name in current use in both the United States and Canada will represent entirely different generic drugs (in a single drug product), or a significantly different mixture of generic ingredients (in a combination drug product). The generic composition of such brand name products is identified by country in the index. Travelers between the two countries who obtain their medications by brand name in either country are advised to ascertain that they are being provided the intended generic drug(s) in every instance.

Benefits versus Risks

A deliberate attempt is made here to crystallize the "pros" and "cons" for each drug. The format adopted for this category utilizes capital letters to give weight (emphasis) to the drug's principal benefits and risks, and lower case letters are used for benefits and risks of lesser significance. A glance reveals the comparative "weights" of the two columns and provides an initial and tentative impression as to whether a drug's benefits exceed its risks, or vice versa, or whether its benefits and risks seem to be roughly equivalent.

This presentation is not intended to be the principal basis for decision on whether or not to use the drug. Its purpose is to enjoin the reader to be more circumspect and discriminating in his or her use of drugs. The failure to give adequate attention to the individualization of drug selection and dosage is perhaps the greatest weakness seen in the current management of drug therapy.

Principal Uses

A drug may be available as a single drug product or in combination with other drugs. In this section of the Profile under the designation As a Single Drug Product, you will find the primary use(s) of the drug when used alone. Under the designation As a Combination Drug Product [CD], you will find the primary use(s) when combined with other active drugs within the same tablet, capsule, etc. The uses stated are those determined by consensus within the medical community and substantiated by current scientific study. Combination drugs have been developed because some conditions that warrant drug therapy have more than one cause, are characterized by a variety of symptoms or may be treated in more than one way. Where appropriate, in this guide, the logic for combining certain drugs to enhance their therapeutic value is explained. When you find the designation for Combination Drugs [CD] in the Brand Name list at the beginning of the Drug Profile, read under the Principal Uses section to learn more about the drug's use in combination products.

How This Drug Works

This simplified explanation is limited to consideration of how the drug acts to produce its principal (intended) therapeutic effect(s). If a specific method of action has not been established, the currently held theory is given.

Available Dosage Forms and Strengths

This represents a composite of available manufacturers' dosage forms (tablets, capsules, elixirs, etc.) and strengths, without company identification. Included are those dosage forms appropriate for use by outpatients and in extended care facilities and nursing homes. Dosage forms limited to hospital use are not included. Refer to Dosage Forms and Strengths in the Glossary for an explanation of those few abbreviations used to designate the strengths of each dosage form.

Usual Adult Dosage Range

The dosage information given represents a carefully derived consensus by appropriate authorities and is the currently recommended standard. It is provided as a guide that indicates the amount of the drug that is reasonably expected to be both effective and safe when properly used for its intended purpose. Under certain circumstances, your physician may elect to modify this "standard" dosage scheme. Adhere strictly to his or her prescribed dosages and schedules.

Dosing Instructions

Specific guidance is given here regarding the timing of oral medication with regard to food intake. In addition, there are occasions when an individual finds it difficult or impossible to swallow a tablet or a capsule, and the drug to be taken is not available in a liquid dosage form. On those occasions when the patient's condition urgently requires the medication, one may wish to crush the tablet or open the capsule and mix the contents with a palatable food or beverage for administration. Many of today's drugs are available in a bewildering array of solid dosage forms, some of which should *not* be altered to accommodate administration. This information category identifies those dosage forms of each drug that may be and those that should not be altered for administration. In addition, your pharmacist can provide appropriate guidance if you should need it.

Usual Duration of Use

Many factors influence the period of time required for any drug to exert beneficial effects. Among them are the nature and severity of the symptoms being treated, the formulation and strength of the drug, the presence or absence of food in the stomach, the ability of the patient to respond and the concurrent use of other drugs. The information in this category is helpful in preventing premature termination of medication in treatment situations where improvement may seem to you to be unreasonably delayed. Where appropriate, limitations in the duration of use are given.

This Drug Should Not Be Taken If

This category consists of the *absolute* contraindications to the use of the drug (see Contraindications in Glossary). It is most important that you alert your physician or dentist if any information in this category applies to you.

Inform Your Physician Before Taking This Drug If

This category lists the *relative* contraindications to the use of the drug. Here again, it is important that you communicate all relevant information to your physician or dentist.

Possible Side-Effects

This category describes the natural, expected and usually unavoidable actions of the drug—the normal and anticipated consequences of taking it. It is important that you maintain a realistic perspective that balances properly the occurrence of side-effects and the goals of treatment. Consult your physician for guidance whenever side-effects are troublesome or distressing, so that appropriate adjustments of your treatment program can be made.

Possible Adverse Effects

This category includes those unusual, unexpected and infrequent drug effects that are commonly referred to as adverse drug reactions. For the sake of evaluation, adverse effects are classified as mild or serious in nature. It is always wise to inform your physician as soon as you have reason to suspect you may be experiencing an adverse drug effect. Serious adverse reactions usually announce their development initially in the form of mild, unthreatening symptoms. It is important that you remain alert to significant changes in your well-being when you are taking a drug that is known to be capable of producing a serious adverse effect. It is also possible to experience an adverse reaction that has not yet been reported. Do not discount the possibility of an adverse effect just because it is not listed in this category. Following standard practice, some adverse reactions (and interactions) of certain drugs are listed, as a precaution, because these reactions are associated with the use of a particular class of drugs. Although the literature may not document such reactions in connection with the use of an individual drug within that class, the possibility of their occurrence must be considered.

A word of caution is appropriate here. You have consulted your physician for medical evaluation and management. He or she has advised you to take a drug (or administer it to someone else). It is important that you recognize and understand that *in the vast majority of instances a properly selected drug has a comparatively small chance of producing serious harm.* Most of the drugs included in this book produce serious adverse effects rarely. Knowledge that a drug is capable of causing a serious adverse reaction should not deter you from using it when it has been properly selected and its use will be carefully supervised.

Possible Effects on Sexual Function

The growing interest and concern of the medical community and the general public regarding the potential effects of many drugs on sexual function justify this designated category for the provision of relevant information. This aspect of drug performance has not received the professional scrutiny or public disclosure commensurate with its importance. Currently available information (often inadequate and vague) from all reliable sources is presented for consideration. In the interest of compliance and effective management, both physician and patient are well advised to discuss frankly the full significance of any potential effect that proposed drug therapy could have on all aspects of sexual expression.

Adverse Effects That May Appear Similar to Natural Diseases or Disorders

The failure to recognize that a given symptom or disorder is actually drug induced occurs with surprising frequency. Quite often this inadvertent error is compounded by the administration of yet another drug to relieve the "symptoms" (unrecognized manifestations) of a drug being taken on a regular basis. For milder symptoms (*e.g.*, the nasal congestion and diarrhea caused by reserpine), the oversight may not be too serious. But in the case of parkinsonlike effects of some drugs, the mistake can be devastating. This category can alert you to this common flaw in the management of drug therapy.

Natural Diseases or Disorders That May Be Activated by This Drug

Similar to the situation described in the previous category, many drugs in common use are capable of "activating" latent disorders that may not be recognized as drug induced. The development of a new and seemingly unrelated disorder during the course of any treatment program should arouse suspicion that it may be drug related.

Caution

This category provides information on certain aspects of drug action and/or drug use that require special emphasis. Occasionally these warnings may relate to information provided in other categories.

When included here, such entries are of sufficient importance to warrant repetition.

Precautions for Use by Infants and Children

In addition to mandatory adjustments of drug dosage for infants and children under twelve years of age, some drugs and/or treatment situations call for special precautions. This category provides such information for selected drugs. When administering *any* drug (whether prescription or over-the-counter drug), it is advisable to ask the attending physician about precautions to observe or procedures to follow.

Precautions for Use by Those over 60 Years of Age

Changes in body composition and function occur naturally as part of normal aging. As would be expected, there is enormous individual variation in the speed with which such changes occur and the degree of these changes. With regard to medical management—and to drug therapy in particular—the assessment of one's "age" must be based upon the individual's mental and physical condition and never upon years alone. In general, however, it should be recognized that changes that accompany aging may affect the actions of the body on the drug, as well as the actions of the drug on the body. Appropriate precautions are outlined in this category.

Advisability of Use During Pregnancy: Pregnancy Category

Information regarding the safe use of a particular drug during pregnancy was one of the most forceful concerns that led to the formal petitioning of the Food and Drug Administration in 1975 for the provision of such guidance to the public. Most category designations are labeled "tentative" at this time in recognition of the fact that data not readily available now may be advanced by pharmaceutical manufacturers as they negotiate with the FDA to eventually determine final category assignments. The FDA definitions of the five Pregnancy Categories are listed inside the back cover of the book. It should be noted that the FDA does not make the initial category assignment; this is the responsibility of the manufacturer that markets the drug. The initial designation is then subject to review and modification by the FDA as deemed appropriate. The Pregnancy Category designations presented in each Profile were determined by the author after thorough review of pertinent literature and consultation with appropriate authorities. They are offered at this time for initial guidance only. They are in no sense "official" and do not have the endorsement of either the manufacturer or the FDA.

Advisability of Use If Breast-Feeding

Information presented here includes what could be ascertained regarding the effects of the drug on milk production, the presence of the drug in human milk and the possible effects of the drug on the nursing infant. Prudent recommendations are given where appropriate.

Suggested Periodic Examinations While Taking This Drug

This category lists those examinations your physician may recommend you undergo while taking the drug(s) he or she has prescribed, in order to monitor your reaction to them and the course of your condition. You should remember that the advisability of performing such examinations varies greatly from one situation to another, and is best left to the judgment of your physician. The selection and timing of examinations are based on many variables, including your past and present medical history, the nature of the condition under treatment, the dosage and anticipated duration of drug use and your physician's observations of your response to treatment. There may be many occasions when he or she will feel no examinations are necessary.

To assure optimal results from drug treatment, it is important that you keep your physician informed of all developments you think may be drug related.

While Taking This Drug, Observe the Following:
Marijuana Smoking

The widespread "social" use of marijuana by virtually all age groups has led to inquiries regarding the possibility of interactions between the pharmacologically active chemicals in marijuana smoke and medicinal drugs in common use. Currently available literature on the health aspects of marijuana use contains very little practical information concerning the potential for drug interactions. The limited information presented in this category of selected Drug Profiles represents those *possible interactions* that are considered likely to occur in view of the known pharmacological effects of the principal components of marijuana and of the medicinal drug reviewed in the Profile. In most instances, the interaction statements are not based on documented evidence since very little is available. However, the conclusions stated—derived by logical inductive reasoning—represent the concurrence of authorities with expertise in this field.

While Taking This Drug, Observe the Following: Other Drugs

For clarification of this confusing and often controversial area of drug information, this category is divided into five subcategories of possible interactions between drugs. Observe carefully the wording of each subcategory heading (see also Interaction in Glossary). Some of the drugs listed as possible interactants do not have a representative Profile in Section Three. If you are using one of these drugs, consult your physician or pharmacist for guidance regarding potential interactions. A brand name (or names) that follows the generic name of an interacting drug is given for purposes of illustration only. It is not intended to mean that the particular brand(s) named have interactions that are different from other brands of the same generic drug. If you are taking the generic drug, *all* brand names under which it is marketed are to be considered as possible interactants.

Driving, Hazardous Activities

In addition to driving motor vehicles, the information in this category applies to any activity of a dangerous nature such as operating machinery, working on ladders, using power tools and handling weapons.

Aviation Note

Until the publication of Dr. Stanley Mohler's *Medication and Flying: A Pilot's Drug Guide* in 1982, there was no authoritative source of current drug information written specifically to serve the needs of civil aviation. The military airman enjoys the expert guidance and surveillance provided by the flight surgeon, but no tightly structured control system exists for his civilian counterpart. However, the need for practical information regarding the possible effects of medicinal drugs on flight performance is the same for pilots in all settings. This category is designed to inform the civilian pilot how a particular drug may affect his or her eligibility to fly and when it is advisable or necessary to consult a designated Aviation Medical Examiner or an FAA medical officer.

Occurrence of Unrelated Illness

This category relates to those drugs that require careful regulation of daily doses to maintain a constant drug effect within critical limits. Anticoagulants, antidiabetic medication and digitalis are examples of such drugs. Emphasis is given to those interim illnesses, separate from the condition for which the drug has been prescribed, that might affect the established schedule of drug use.

Discontinuation

This aspect of drug use is often overlooked when a plan of drug therapy is first discussed. However, for some drugs it is mandatory that the patient be fully informed on *when* to discontinue, when *not* to discontinue and precisely *how* to discontinue use of the drug.

Another consideration in discontinuation is the need to adjust the dosage schedules of other drugs being taken concurrently. The physician who is primarily responsible for your overall management must be kept informed of *all* the drugs you are taking at a given time.

The remaining information categories in the Drug Profile are self-explanatory.

Section Four is a presentation of Drug Classes arranged alphabetically according to their chemical or therapeutic class designation. The drugs within each class are listed alphabetically by their generic names. Because of their chemical composition and biological activities, some drugs will appear in two or more classes. For example, the drug product with the brand name Diuril will be represented by its generic name, chlorothiazide, in three drug classes: the Thiazide Diuretics (a chemical classification), the Diuretics (a drug action classification) and the Antihypertensives (a disease-oriented classification).

Frequently in the Drug Profiles in Section Three you are advised to "See (a particular) Drug Class." This alerts you to a possible contraindication for drug use, or to possible interactions with certain foods, alcohol or other drugs. In each case, you can determine the more readily recognized brand names for each drug listed generically within a drug class by consulting the appropriate Drug Profile. Timely use of these references will enable you to avoid many possible hazards of medication.

Section Five is a glossary of drug-related terms used throughout the book. The preferred use of each term is explained. Frequent references to the Glossary are made in the Drug Profiles. Use of the Glossary will increase your understanding of how to recognize and interpret significant drug effects.

Section Six consists of tables of drug information. The title and introductory material explain the content and purpose of each table. The information in the tables is drawn from certain information categories in the Profiles and is rearranged to emphasize pertinent aspects of drug behavior. The tables are intended to provide another source of ready reference.

The index of Brand and Generic Names in the back of the book is a single alphabetical listing that provides page references to the appropriate Drug Profile(s) for all drugs found in this book. Its usefulness will be enhanced if you read first the introductory explanation of the special features of this combined index.

2

Guidelines for Safe and Effective Drug Use

DO NOT

- pressure your physician to prescribe drugs that, in his or her judgment, you do not need.
- take prescription drugs on your own or on the advice of friends and neighbors because your symptoms are "just like theirs."
- offer drugs prescribed for you to anyone else without a physician's guidance.
- change the dose or timing of any drug without the advice of your physician (except when the drug appears to be causing adverse effects).
- continue to take a drug that you feel is causing adverse effects, until you are able to reach your physician for clarification.
- take *any* drug (prescription or nonprescription) while pregnant or nursing an infant until you are assured by your physician that no harmful effects will occur to either mother or child.
- take any more medicines than are absolutely necessary. (The greater the number of drugs taken simultaneously, the greater the likelihood of adverse effects.)
- withhold from your physician important information about previous drug experiences. He or she will want to know both beneficial and undesirable drug effects you have experienced in the past.
- take any drug in the dark. Identify every dose of medicine carefully in adequate light to be certain you are taking the drug intended.

- keep drugs on a bedside table. Drugs for emergency use, such as nitroglycerin, are an exception. It is advisable to have only one such drug at the bedside for use during the night.

DO

- know the name (and correct spelling) of the drug(s) you are taking. It is advisable to know both the brand name and the generic name.
- read the package labels of all nonprescription drugs to become familiar with the contents of the product.
- follow your physician's instructions regarding dosage schedules as closely as possible. Notify him or her if it becomes necessary to make major changes in your treatment routine.
- thoroughly shake all liquid suspensions of drugs to ensure uniform distribution of ingredients.
- use a standardized measuring device for giving liquid medications by mouth. The household "teaspoon" varies greatly in size.
- follow your physician's instruction on dietary and other treatment measures designed to augment the actions of the drugs prescribed. This makes it possible to achieve desired drug effects with smaller doses. (A familiar example is the reduction of salt intake during drug treatment for high blood pressure.)
- keep your personal physician informed of all drugs prescribed for you by someone else. Consult him or her regarding nonprescription drugs you intend to take on your own initiative at the same time that you are taking drugs prescribed by him or her.
- inform your anesthesiologist, surgeon and dentist of *all* drugs you are taking, prior to any surgery.
- inform your physician if you become pregnant while you are taking any drugs from any source.
- keep a written record of *all* drugs (and vaccines) you take during your entire pregnancy—name, dose, dates taken and reasons for use.
- keep a written record of *all* drugs (and vaccines) to which you become allergic or experience an adverse reaction. This should be done for each member of the family, especially the elderly and infirm.
- keep a written record of *all* drugs (and vaccines) to which *your children* become allergic or experience an adverse reaction.
- inform your physician of all known or suspected allergies, especially allergies to drugs. Be certain that this information is included in your medical record. (Allergic individuals are four times more prone to drug reactions than those who are free of allergy).

- inform your physician promptly if you think you are experiencing an overdose, a side-effect or an adverse effect from a drug.
- determine if it is safe to drive a car, operate machinery or engage in other hazardous activities while taking the drug(s) prescribed.
- determine if it is safe to drink alcoholic beverages while taking the drug(s) prescribed.
- determine if any particular foods, beverages or other drugs should be avoided while taking the drug(s) prescribed.
- keep all appointments for follow-up examinations to determine the effects of the drugs and the course of your illness.
- ask for clarification of any point that is confusing or difficult to understand, at the time the drug(s) are prescribed or later if you have forgotten. Request information in writing if circumstances justify it.
- discard all outdated prescription drugs. This will prevent the use of drugs that have deteriorated with time.
- store all drugs to be retained for intermittent use out of the reach of children to prevent accidental poisoning.

PREVENTING ADVERSE DRUG REACTIONS

Our knowledge of the mechanisms of adverse reactions is very limited. For the most part, we cannot identify with certainty the person who is at greater risk of experiencing a true adverse effect. Available tests for the early detection of toxicity are of definite value, but they do not provide as full a measure of protection as we could wish.

As our understanding of drug actions and reactions expands, it becomes more apparent that there *is* a sizable proportion of adverse effects that are, to some extent, predictable and preventable. The exact percentage of preventable reactions is yet to be determined, but several contributing factors are now well recognized, and specific recommendations are available to guide both physician and patient. These fall into eleven categories of consideration.

Previous Adverse Reaction to a Drug

There is evidence to indicate that an individual who has experienced an adverse drug reaction in the past is more likely to have adverse reactions to other drugs, even though the drugs are unrelated. This suggests that some individuals may have a genetic (inborn) predisposition to unusual and abnormal drug responses. *The patient should inform the physician of any history of prior adverse drug experiences.*

Allergies

Individuals who are allergic by nature (hayfever, asthma, eczema, hives) are more likely to develop allergies to drugs than are non-allergic individuals. The allergic patient must be observed very closely for the earliest indication of a developing hypersensitivity to any drug. Known drug allergies must be noted in the medical record. The patient must inform every physician and dentist consulted that he or she is allergic by nature and is allergic to specific drugs by name. *The patient should provide this information without waiting to be asked.* The physician will then be able to avoid those drugs that could provoke an allergic reaction, as well as those related drugs to which the patient may have developed a cross-sensitivity.

Contraindications

Both patient and physician must strictly observe all known contraindications to any drug under consideration. *Absolute contraindications* include those conditions and situations that prohibit the use of the drug for any reason. *Relative contraindications* include those conditions that, in the judgment of the physician, do not preclude the use of the drug altogether, but make it essential that special considerations be given to its use to prevent the intensification of preexisting disease or the development of new disease. Such conditions and situations usually require adjustment of dosage, additional supportive measures and close supervision.

Precautions in Use

The patient should know about any special precautions to observe while taking the drug. This includes the advisability of use during pregnancy or while nursing an infant; precautions regarding exposure to the sun (or ultraviolet lamps); the avoidance of extreme heat or cold, heavy physical exertion, etc.

Dosage

The patient must adhere to the prescribed dosage schedule as closely as possible. *This is most important with those drugs that have narrow margins of safety.* Circumstances that interfere with taking the drug as prescribed (nausea, vomiting, diarrhea) must be reported to the physician so that appropriate adjustments can be made.

Interactions

Much is known today about how some drugs can interact unfavorably with certain foods, alcohol and other drugs to produce serious adverse effects. *The patient must be informed regarding all likely interactants* that could alter the action of the drug he or she is using. If, during the course of treatment, the patient has reason to feel he or she has discovered a new interaction of importance, the physician should be informed so that its full significance can be determined. (It is through such observations that much of our understanding of drug interactions has come.)

Warning Symptoms

Experience has shown that many drugs will produce symptoms that are actually early indications of a developing adverse effect. Examples include the appearance of severe headaches and visual disturbances *before* the onset of a stroke in a woman taking oral contraceptives; the development of acid indigestion and stomach distress *before* the activation of a bleeding peptic ulcer in a man taking phenylbutazone (Butazolidin) for shoulder bursitis. *It is imperative that the patient be familar with those symptoms and signs that could be early indicators of impending adverse reactions.* With this knowledge he or she can act in his or her own behalf by discontinuing the drug and consulting the physician for additional guidance.

Examinations to Monitor Drug Effects

Certain drugs (less than half of those in common use) are capable of damaging vital body tissues (bone marrow, liver, kidney, eye structures, etc.)—especially when these drugs are used over an extended period. Such adverse effects are relatively rare, and many of them are not discovered until the drug has been in wide use for a long time. As our knowledge of such effects accumulates, we learn which kinds of drugs (that is, which chemical structures) are most likely to produce such tissue reactions. Hence, we know those drugs that should be monitored periodically to detect as early as possible any evidence of tissue injury resulting from their use. *The patient should cooperate fully with the physician in the performance of periodic examinations for evidence of adverse drug effects.*

Advanced Age and Debility

The altered functional capacity of vital organs that accompanies advancing age and debilitating disease can greatly influence the body's response to drugs. Such patients tend not to tolerate drugs with inherent toxic potential well; it is usually necessary for them to use smaller doses at longer intervals. *The effects of drugs on the elderly and severely ill are often unpredictable.* The frequent need for dosage adjustments or change in drug selection requires continuous observation of these patients if adverse effects are to be prevented or minimized.

Appropriate Drug Choice

The drug(s) selected to treat any condition should be the most appropriate of those available. Many adverse reactions can be prevented if both physician and patient exercise good judgment and restraint. *The wise patient will not demand overtreatment.* He or she will cooperate with the physician's attempt to balance properly the seriousness of the illness and the hazard of the drug.

Polypharmacy

This term refers to the concurrent use by an individual of several drugs prescribed separately by two (or more) physicians for different disorders—often without appropriate communication between patient and prescriber. This frequent practice is conducive to potentially serious drug/drug interactions. *The patient should routinely inform each physican (and dentist) consulted of all the drugs— prescription and nonprescription—that he or she may be taking at the time.* It is mandatory that each physician have this information before prescribing additional drugs.

DRUGS AND THE ELDERLY

Advancing age brings changes in body structure and function that may alter significantly the action of drugs. An impaired digestive system may interfere with drug absorption. Reduced capacity of the liver and kidneys to metabolize and eliminate drugs may result in the accumulation of drugs in the body to toxic levels. By impairing the body's ability to maintain a "steady state" (homeostasis), the aging process may increase the sensitivity of many tissues to the actions of drugs, thereby altering greatly the responsiveness of the nervous and circulatory systems to standard drug doses. If aging should cause deterioration of understanding, memory, vision or physical coordination, people with such impairments may not always use drugs safely and effectively.

Adverse reactions to drugs occur three times more frequently in the older population. An unwanted drug response can render a functioning and independent older person whose health and reserves are at marginal levels, confused, incompetent or helpless. For these reasons, drug treatment in the elderly must always be accompanied by the most careful consideration of the individual's health and tolerances, the selection of drugs and dosage schedules and the possible need for assistance in treatment routines.

Guidelines for the Use of Drugs by the Elderly

- Be certain that drug treatment is necessary. Many health problems of the elderly can be managed without the use of drugs.
- Avoid if possible the use of many drugs at one time. It is advisable to use not more than three drugs concurrently.
- Dosage schedules should be as uncomplicated as possible. When feasible, a single daily dose of each drug is preferable.
- In order to establish individual tolerance, treatment with most drugs is usually best begun by using smaller than standard doses. Maintenance doses should also be determined carefully. A maintenance dose is often smaller for persons over 60 years of age than for younger persons.
- Avoid large tablets and capsules if other dosage forms are available. Liquid preparations are easier for the elderly or debilitated to swallow.
- Have all drug containers labeled with the drug name and directions for use in large, easy-to-read letters.
- Ask the pharmacist to package drugs in easy-to-open containers. Avoid "child-proof" caps and stoppers.
- Do not take any drug in the dark. Identify each dose of medicine carefully in adequate light to be certain you are taking the drug intended.
- To avoid taking the wrong drug or an extra dose, do not keep drugs on a bedside table. Drugs for emergency use, such as nitroglycerin, are an exception. It is advisable to have only one such drug at the bedside for use during the night.
- Drug use by older persons may require supervision. Observe drug effects continuously to ensure safe and effective use.
- Remember the adage: "Start low, go slow and (when appropriate) learn to say no."

Drugs Best Avoided by the Elderly Because of Increased Possibility of Adverse Reactions

antacids (high sodium)*   cyclophosphamide
barbiturates*   diethylstilbestrol

*See Drug Class, Section Four.

estrogens
indomethacin
monoamine oxidase inhibitors
   (MAOI's)* type A
oxyphenbutazone
phenacetin
phenylbutazone
tetracyclines*

Drugs That Should Be Used by the Elderly in Reduced Dosages Until Full Effect Has Been Determined

anticoagulants (oral)*
antidepressants*
antidiabetic drugs*
antihistamines*
antihypertensives*
anti-inflammatory drugs*
barbiturates*
beta-blockers*
colchicine
cortisonelike drugs*
digitalis preparations*
diuretics* (all types)
ephedrine
epinephrine
haloperidol
isoetharine
nalidixic acid
narcotic drugs
prazosin
pseudoephedrine
quinidine
sleep inducers (hypnotics)*
terbutaline
thyroid preparations

Drugs That May Cause Confusion and Behavioral Disturbances in the Elderly

amantadine
antidepressants*
antidiabetic drugs*
antihistamines*
anti-inflammatory drugs*
atropine* (and drugs containing
   belladonna)
barbiturates*
benzodiazepines*
carbamazepine
cimetidine
digitalis preparations*
diuretics*
ergoloid mesylates
levodopa
meprobamate
methocarbamol
methyldopa
narcotic drugs
pentazocine
phenytoin
primidone
reserpine
sedatives
sleep inducers (hypnotics)*
thiothixene
tranquilizers (mild)*
trihexyphenidyl

Drugs That May Cause Orthostatic Hypotension in the Elderly

antidepressants*
antihypertensives*
diuretics* (all types)
phenothiazines*
sedatives
tranquilizers (mild)*
vasodilators*

*See Drug Class, Section Four.

Drugs That May Cause Constipation and/or Retention of Urine in the Elderly

amantadine

androgens

antidepressants*

antiparkinsonism drugs*

atropinelike drugs*

epinephrine

ergoloid mesylates

isoetharine

narcotic drugs

phenothiazines*

terbutaline

Drugs That May Cause Loss of Bladder Control (Urinary Incontinence) in the Elderly

diuretics* (all types)

sedatives

sleep inducers (hypnotics)*

tranquilizers (mild)*

THERAPEUTIC DRUG MONITORING
(Measuring Drug Levels in Blood)

The routine use of measuring drug levels in blood as an aid in managing drug therapy has evolved gradually over the past 20 years. Because individuals vary so greatly in the nature and degree of their responses to drugs, it became apparent that greater precision in determining optimal dosage for the individual was needed. For many drugs, the responses observed by the physician (clinical changes) clearly indicate that the drug is working as intended and that the dosage scheme is satisfactory. However, for some drugs—especially those with narrow safety margins—the toxic reactions closely resemble the symptoms of the disorder for which the drugs are prescribed. In many instances the patient's response is not in keeping with his or her clinical condition or program of drug therapy. By measuring the blood levels of certain drugs at appropriate times, the physician can adjust dosage schedules more accurately, predict drug response more precisely, reduce the risk of toxicity and achieve greater benefit.

The timing of the blood samples is an important consideration. As a general rule, the best time for sampling is just before the next scheduled dose of the drug to be measured (the "trough" level). Sampling should be avoided during the two hours following oral administration; during this absorption period, blood levels do not represent tissue levels of the drug.

*See Drug Class, Section Four.

The following drugs are those most suitable for therapeutic drug monitoring. If you are using any of these on a regular basis, consult your physician regarding the advisability or need for periodic measurement of drug levels in your blood.

Generic Name	Brand Name(s)
acetaminophen	Datril, Tylenol, etc.
amikacin	Amikin
amitriptyline	Amitril, Elavil, Endep, etc.
aspirin (other salicylates)	Bufferin, Ecotrin, etc.
carbamazepine	Tegretol
chloramphenicol	Chloromycetin
chlorpromazine	Thorazine
ciprofloxacin	Cipro
clonazepam	Clonopin
desipramine	Norpramin, Pertofrane
digitoxin	Crystodigin
digoxin	Lanoxin
disopyramide	Norpace
doxepin	Adapin, Sinequan
dyphylline	Brophylline, Neothylline, etc.
ethosuximide	Zarontin
ethotoin	Peganone
gentamicin	Garamycin
gold salts	Auranofin, Myochrisine, etc.
imipramine	Imavate, Tofranil, etc.
isoniazid	INH, Niconyl, etc.
kanamycin	Kantrex
lidocaine	Xylocaine, etc.
lithium	Lithobid, Lithotabs, etc.
mephenytoin	Mesantoin
mephobarbital	Mebaral
methotrexate	Mexate
methsuximide	Celontin
nortriptyline	Aventyl, Pamelor
paramethadione	Paradione
phenobarbital	Luminal, etc.
phensuximide	Milontin
phenytoin	Dilantin
primidone	Mysoline
procainamide	Pronestyl
propranolol	Inderal
protriptyline	Vivactil
quinidine	Cardioquin, Quinaglute, etc.

theophylline	Aminophylline, Theo-Dur, etc.
thioridazine	Mellaril
tobramycin	Nebcin
trimethadione	Tridione
valproic acid	Depakene

THE USE
OF DRUGS IN TREATING
CHRONIC DISORDERS

Chronic Disorders Reviewed in This Section

Acne
Alzheimer's Disease
Angina Pectoris
Asthma
Cholesterol Disorders
Congestive Heart Failure
Crohn's Disease
Depression
Diabetes
Epilepsy
Glaucoma
Gout
Hypertension (High Blood Pressure)
Hypothyroidism
Menopause
Migraine Headache
Myasthenia Gravis
Osteoarthritis
Osteoporosis
Parkinson's Disease
Peptic Ulcer
Psoriasis
Rheumatoid Arthritis
Schizophrenia
Ulcerative Colitis

INTRODUCTION

Of the 200 drugs prescribed most frequently by physicians in the United States in 1988, 130 (65%) are used in the treatment of chronic disorders. This section provides an overview of the management of some of the more common disorders that require drug therapy for long periods of time, some of them for life. As you read this section, you will become familiar with important principles in the use of selected drugs and will gain perspectives that can help you to understand what your physician is attempting to accomplish with the therapy recommended. Since the lack of reasonable compliance by the patient is one of the major causes of failure in today's use of drugs, your greater understanding will encourage you to cooperate fully with your physician's instructions so that together you can achieve the greatest benefit with the least risk from the drugs prescribed.

Although drugs are essential to the rational treatment of most chronic disorders, proper attention must also be given to other treatment procedures, of equal importance. Examples include adherence to the appropriate diet in the management of diabetes, cessation of smoking in the treatment of angina (coronary artery disease), weight control in the treatment of high blood pressure (hypertension) and the use of "allergy shots" (immunotherapy) in the management of asthma. The intelligent use of drugs can make a significant contribution, but it must be recognized that drugs have their limitations and should be looked upon as but one part of a comprehensive and integrated treatment program.

WARNING: Each physician develops his or her own favored approach to the use of drugs. This is based upon knowledge of the drug's characteristics plus personal experience and observation of drug performance. The treatment program recommended by your physician may vary somewhat from the guidelines provided in this book. It is important that you follow your physician's instructions precisely as given—that you comply fully. If you question any aspect of drug selection, dosage schedule, drug effects, etc., consult your physician before attempting any modification of your drug treatment program on your own. *Under no circumstances should you attempt to initiate prescription drug therapy for yourself or others without the full knowledge and guidance of a qualified physician.*

ACNE

Other Name: Acne vulgaris

Prevalence in USA: Approximately 4.6 million cases: 2.4% of the population under 18 years of age; 3% of the population 18 to 44 years of age.

Age Group: Most common in adolescents and young adults. Usually begins at puberty (9 to 12 years of age) and subsides at 18 to 20 years of age. A small percentage of cases will persist into the twenties and thirties.

Male to Female Ratio: Slightly more common in women.

Principal Features: Common acne is a disorder of the hair follicles and sebaceous (oil-producing) glands of the skin. It is characterized by the formation of open comedones (blackheads), closed comedones (whiteheads), inflamed papules (pimples) and pustules in the superficial layers of the skin. The deep form of acne includes the formation of inflamed nodules and pus-filled cysts. These skin changes occur most commonly on the face, but are also found on the neck, chest, shoulders and upper back. The degree of inflammation will vary from mild to severe throughout the course of the disorder. It is often worse in the winter and better during the summer, probably due to the beneficial effects of sun exposure.

Causes: Acne is primarily due to overactivity of the oil-producing sebaceous glands. This usually begins with the changes of puberty when the associated increase in sex hormones (principally androgens) stimulates the growth and production of the glands. The opening of the gland becomes plugged with a mixture of dead skin cells, oils and bacteria, resulting in a comedo; this progresses to the formation of fatty acids within the gland that causes inflammation, swelling and eventual rupture into the skin. Contributing causes include familial predisposition, excessive heat and humidity, poor personal hygiene, the use of oil-based cosmetics and exposure to industrial oils and tars.

Drugs That Can Cause This Disorder: The following drugs can initiate
acne or aggravate existing acne:
androgens (male hormonelike drugs)
cortisonelike drugs
cytotoxic drugs (those used to treat various types of cancer)
methotrexate
oral contraceptives that contain norethindrone or norgestrel (Brevicon, Loestrin, Lo/Ovral, Micronor, Modicon, Norinyl, Norlestrin,
Norlutin, Nor-Qd, Ortho-Novum, Ovcon, Ovral, Ovrette)
progesterone
The following drugs can cause acnelike eruptions but do not cause true
comedo formation:
bromides
disulfiram
iodides
isoniazid
lithium
phenobarbital
phenytoin
quinine
thiouracil
trimethadione
vitamin B-12

Drugs Used to Treat This Disorder
Locally (Topically)
  • benzoyl peroxide (Benoxyl, Clearasil, Epi-Clear, Topex, etc.).
  • tretinoin (retinoic acid preparations, Retin-A).
  • antibiotic lotions.
  • metronidazole gel (MetroGel).
Internally (Systemically)
  • tetracycline (see Drug Profile).
  • erythromycin (see Drug Profile).
  • isotretinoin (see Drug Profile).
  • prednisone (see Drug Profile).
  • ibuprofen (see Drug Profile).

Goals of Drug Treatment
Improvement and control are the primary objectives; cure is not pos-
sible.
Prevention of new blemishes.
Prevention of scarring.
Note: Appropriate treatment, conscientiously followed, is beneficial in
95% of all cases.

Drug Management
Local (Topical) Drug Treatment
Often sufficient to control superficial acne with mild to moderate in-
flammation.

May be used concurrently with internal (systemic) treatment for control of deep acne with severe inflammation, nodule and cyst formation.

Start treatment slowly; determine tolerance by applying small amounts of low-concentration products to small areas of skin.

Limit applications to once or twice daily.

Apply to *dry* skin, one-half hour after washing.

Use soap and water to remove skin oils; wash skin no more than twice daily.

Avoid abrasive preparations.

Irritation from topical drugs is common; true allergy is uncommon.

Use of Benzoyl Peroxide

1. This is the single most effective drug for the topical treatment of acne. Many preparations are available without prescription.
2. Its principal action is anti-infective; its primary use is treating superficial, inflammatory, papulo-pustular acne.
3. Start with a 5% preparation; apply once daily—in the morning.
4. This drug inactivates tretinoin (retinoic acid); do not apply these two drugs at the same time.

Use of Tretinoin (Retinoic Acid)

1. This is the only practical drug available for the topical management of comedones. It does require a prescription.
2. It is used in all forms of acne to facilitate the removal of existing comedones and to prevent the formation of new ones.
3. Start with the 0.01% gel; increase the strength of the preparation as needed and tolerated.
4. Apply once daily—in the evening or at bedtime.
5. This drug may require continual use for up to 12 weeks to obtain initial benefit; continued control will require maintenance treatment for months or years.
6. Drying and irritation of the skin are common. However, deliberate irritation and peeling are not necessary for benefit.
7. This drug may increase skin sensitivity to sunlight; use sun screen preparations if necessary, but avoid them if possible.

Use of Topical Antibiotics

1. Erythromycin is the drug of choice; tetracycline and clindamycin preparations are also used.
2. These anti-infective drugs are used primarily to treat inflammatory acne; they do not clear existing lesions but do prevent the development of new ones.
3. May be used concurrently with benzoyl peroxide or tretinoin.
4. Apply twice daily—morning and evening.
5. These drugs may require continual use for 3 to 4 weeks to obtain significant improvement.

Internal (Systemic) Drug Treatment

Required for control of moderate to severe deep acne (inflammatory nodules, cysts, abscesses) and to reduce permanent scarring.

A firm commitment to conscientious treatment for many months or years is often required to accomplish desired results.

Use of Tetracycline
1. Generally considered to be the drug of choice for long-term use. (See Drug Profile for complete description.)
2. May be used alone or concurrently with benzoyl peroxide or tretinoin.
3. Begin treatment with 500 mg to 1000 mg daily for 4 weeks or until a satisfactory result is obtained. Then reduce gradually to the smallest effective dose for long-term maintenance; this may be as low as 250 mg every 1 to 3 days.
4. This is best taken on an empty stomach, 1 hour before or 2 hours after eating.
5. Continual use for 3 months may be required to obtain optimal benefit.
6. If tetracycline is not effective or cannot be tolerated, erythromycin is the next drug of choice.

Use of Isotretinoin
1. This drug is reserved for the treatment of severe acne that has not responded to conventional management. (See Drug Profile for complete description.)
2. Its primary action is to inhibit the production of sebum (a mix of sebaceous oils and skin cell debris). This reduces the source of fatty acids that cause inflammatory reaction.
3. ***Do not use this drug during pregnancy. Use effective birth control measures while taking it.***
4. Continual use for 20 or more weeks is usually required to produce significant benefit.
5. Monitor triglyceride blood levels during use; if level exceeds 400 mg, reduce the dose; if level exceeds 600 mg, discontinue this drug.
6. Use this drug with caution in those with type I diabetes or inflammatory bowel disease (Crohn's disease, ulcerative colitis).

Use of Prednisone
1. Cortisonelike drugs may induce acne in some individuals. However, it may be useful for some with extensive, severe inflammatory acne that is unresponsive to other treatments.
2. Initiate treatment with 30 mg to 45 mg of prednisone daily, gradually reducing this dose within 1 month. Low-dose maintenance using 2.5 mg each evening may extend control. (See Drug Profile for complete description.)

Use of Ibuprofen
1. This anti-inflammatory drug may enhance the beneficial effects of systemic tetracyline. (See Drug Profile of Ibuprofen for complete description.)
2. A trial of 600 mg 4 times per day is warranted for those with severe inflammatory acne that has shown limited benefit from standard drug therapy.

Use of Oral Contraceptives
1. High-estrogen birth control pills that contain a nonandrogenic progestin (ethynodrel, norethisterone, norethynodrel) are sometimes
   used to treat severe acne.
2. The beneficial action of these preparations is the reduction of sebum formation.
3. Because of the inherent risks, this use of oral contraceptives is
   generally not recommended. (See Drug Profile for complete description.)

Ancillary Drug Treatment (as required)

Condition	Drug Treatment
For candidiasis (yeast infection of genital or anal region, a complication of long-term antibiotic or oral contraceptive use):	clotrimazole (Lotrimin) nystatin (Mycostatin)

Note: Drug selection, dosage and administration schedule must be determined
by the physician for each patient individually.

Resource for Additional Information and Services

Acne Research Institute
1587 Monrovia Avenue
Newport Beach, CA 92663
Phone: (714) 722-1805

Telecommunications services: 1-800-235-2263 (outside CA); 1-800-225-
2263 (inside CA)
Publications available.

ALZHEIMER'S DISEASE

Other Names: Alzheimer's presenile and senile dementia, senile dementia
(Alzheimer type)

Prevalence in USA: Approximately 2.5 million; more than 7% of the American population aged over 65 years; the cause of 50% of all progressive
dementias.

Age Group: Occurs occasionally under 50 years of age; uncommon before
65 years; the majority occurs over 65 years: mild dementia in 5% and
moderate to severe in 10–20%. Moderate to severe dementia occurs
in 20% of all over 80.

Male to Female Ratio: More common in women.

Principal Features

Insidious onset leading to progressive and permanent decline of all intellectual functions.

Mood changes: apathy, depression, irritability, anxiety, paranoia.

Loss of recent memory, inability to recall facts of common knowledge, disorientation, confusion, all worse at night.

Impaired attention, understanding, judgment. Loss of ability to think abstractly, to use language correctly, to calculate.

Eventual gait disturbances, incoordination of movements.

Social skills may be retained until late in course of disease.

Course is from 3 to 20 years, with mean duration of 7 years.

Causes: Degeneration of nerve cells in the areas of the brain that control intellectual functions. Actual cause of degeneration is unknown. Genetic predisposition appears probable; Alzheimer type dementia is four times more frequent among family members than in the general population. There is a history of previous head injury in 15% to 20% of cases. One common feature is a marked deficiency of the nerve transmitter acetylcholine.

Drugs That Can Cause This Disorder: No drugs cause true Alzheimer's dementia. However, 3% of all dementias are drug induced. The following drugs can cause symptoms in the elderly that resemble Alzheimer's disease (see Drug Classes, Section Four):

antidepressants

atropinelike drugs

barbiturates

benzodiazepines

butyrophenones

cortisonelike drugs

digitalis preparations

MAO inhibitors

Drugs Used to Treat This Disorder

No specific or truly effective drug treatment is available at this time.

Ergoloid mesylates (Deapril-ST, Hydergine) are tried during the early stages to relieve symptoms; benefits are infrequent, negligible and fleeting. (See Drug Profile, Section Three.)

Experimental drugs: choline, lecithin, physostigmine (none are curative or significantly beneficial).

Goals of Drug Treatment

Temporary improvement of alertness and memory.

Relief of confusion, depression and behavioral disturbances.

Drug Management

Keep all medications to a minimum.

If any drug is used, start treatment with small doses, increase the dosage cautiously and monitor the response very closely.

Avoid drugs with strong atropinelike effects and strong sedative effects.

Ergoloid mesylates may act as a mild antidepressant and may improve mood. If it is tolerated well, a trial of 6 months is justified.

Lecithin may increase the acetylcholine content of brain tissue and temporarily improve memory in some individuals. It is available in health food stores without prescription. It is safe to try. Ask your physician for guidance.

Use antipsychotics (Haldol, Mellaril, etc.) and sedatives (chloral hydrate, Benadryl, etc.) only when clearly needed. Use the smallest dose that proves to be effective.

Ancillary Drug Treatment (as required)

Condition	*Drug Treatment*
For agitation, confusion:	haloperidol (Haldol)
	thioridazine (Mellaril)
	thiothixene (Navane)
For insomnia:	chloral hydrate (Noctec, Somnos, etc.)
	diphenhydramine (Benadryl)
For depression:	trazodone (Desyrel)
For constipation:	docusate (Colace, Doxinate, Surfak, etc.)

Note: Drug selection, dosage and administration schedule must be determined by the physician for each patient individually.

Resource for Additional Information and Services

Alzheimer's Disease and Related Disorders Association
70 East Lake Street, Suite 600
Chicago, IL 60601
Phone: 1-800-621-0379; (312) 853-3060

Available 24 hours a day, 7 days a week.
Sends packet of information; offers information by phone.
National network of 180 chapters and 1200 support groups.

ANGINA PECTORIS

Other Names: Coronary artery insufficiency, coronary artery disease, coronary heart disease, ischemic heart disease

Prevalence in USA: Approximately 6 million; coronary artery disease is the leading cause of death in the USA.

Age Group: Under 45 years—0.2% of population; 45 to 64 years—6.5% of population; over 65 years—11% of population.

Male to Female Ratio: Under 45 years—1.5 to 1; 45 to 64 years—3 to 1; 65 to 74 years—1.8 to 1; over 75 years—1 to 1.

Principal Features

Classical Angina-of-Effort (Exertional Angina): A moderate to severe discomfort (pain, pressure, tightness, fullness, squeezing or burning sensation) usually located deeply behind the breastbone (but may be felt in the jaw, neck, shoulder, arms, upper back or pit of the stomach). It is characteristically brought on by physical exertion, a large meal, emotional stress or exposure to cold; it usually lasts 1 to 3 minutes and disappears with rest.

Variant (Prinzmetal's) Angina: Usually occurs at rest, and is unpredictable and unrelated to the situations that provoke effort angina. It often occurs between midnight and 8 a.m. The two types of angina can coexist. Acute anginal pain may be accompanied by weakness, sweating, shortness of breath or nausea.

Causes

Exertional Angina: Due to atherosclerosis (thickening and hardening) of segments of coronary arteries. Contributory causes of these arterial changes include heredity (genetic susceptibility), hypertension, high blood cholesterol, diabetes and smoking.

Variant (Prinzmetal's) Angina: Due to spontaneous spasm of segments of coronary arteries; the cause of the spasm is not known. Anemia, hyperthyroidism, aortic valve disease and heart rhythm disorders predispose to angina.

Drugs That Can Cause This Disorder: The following drugs do not cause coronary artery disease per se, but they can affect heart function adversely and induce or intensify angina in susceptible individuals:

amphetamines	isoproterenol
beta blocker drugs (abrupt withdrawal)	metaproterenol
	methysergide
bromocriptine	nifedipine (first dose)
cocaine	nylidrin
epinephrine	oral contraceptives
ergot preparations	phenylpropanolamine
5-fluouracil	prazosin
hydralazine	terbutaline
indomethacin	thyroid
isoetharine	

Drugs Used to Treat This Disorder

Nitrate Preparations
- nitroglycerin lingual aerosol (Nitrolingual Spray).
- nitroglycerin sublingual tablets (Nitrostat).
- nitroglycerin buccal tablets (Susadrin).
- nitroglycerin prolonged-action forms (Nitro-Bid, etc.).
- nitroglycerin ointment (Nitrol, etc.).
- nitroglycerin patches (Nitrodisc, Nitro-Dur, etc.).
- isosorbide dinitrate (Isordil, Sorbitrate).

- erythrityl tetranitrate (Cardilate).
- pentaerythritol tetranitrate (Peritrate).

Beta Blocker Drugs
- atenolol (Tenormin).
- labetalol (Normodyne, Trandate).
- metoprolol (Lopressor).
- nadolol (Corgard).
- propranolol (Inderal).

Other beta blockers are used but have not yet been approved by the FDA for specific use in the management of angina.

Calcium Blocker Drugs
- nicardipine (Cardene).
- nifedipine (Adalat, Procardia).
- diltiazem (Cardizem).
- verapamil (Calan, Isoptin).

Others
- aspirin (for its antiplatelet action).
- dipyridamole (Persantine). Antianginal effect is questionable and under review.

Goals of Drug Treatment

Prompt relief of acute anginal attack.

Prevention of anticipated angina by use of nitroglyerin just before physical activity.

Long-term prevention of angina; reduced frequency, severity and duration of recurrent anginal episodes.

Prevention of heart rhythm disturbances.

Prevention of heart attack (myocardial infarction).

Drug Management

For Stable Exertional Angina

Frequency and severity of angina-of-effort remain at a constant level.

Nitroglycerin spray or sublingual tablet for relief of acute attacks.

Long-acting nitrates and/or a beta blocker.

If control is not adequate, add a calcium blocker.

For Unstable Angina

Frequency and severity of angina increase over time; angina occurs with exertion and at rest, is less responsive to treatment.

Hospitalization in coronary care unit.

Mild sedation with benzodiazepines (Valium, etc.).

Combined use of nitrates, beta blocker and calcium blocker.

Aspirin, for antiplatelet effect.

For Variant (Prinzmetal's) Angina

Anginal attacks primarily at rest.

Nitroglycerin spray or sublingual tablets.

Long-acting nitrates.

Calcium blocker.

Avoid beta blockers (unless it is established that both types of angina are present).

Use of Nitroglycerin

1. Nitroglycerin is the mainstay of managing angina. Always have a supply of fresh, active tablets available. Keep them in the original dark glass bottle, tightly closed, no cotton added. Do not transfer them to a metal or plastic container.
2. The sublingual tablet will produce a mild stinging sensation under the tongue, flushing of the face and throbbing in the head. These reactions are normal and indicate that the drug is active and you are having a good response.
3. Use nitrolycerin promptly and as often as necessary, no matter how often. Unless instructed otherwise, do not consciously keep count of the tablets used.
4. If the lingual spray or sublingual tablet causes weakness, dizziness or faintness, sit down or lie down until the sensation passes.
5. Use the spray or tablet to prevent an attack by taking it just before starting a specific physical activity that is known to induce angina.
6. If anginal pain persists after taking 3 successive sublingual tablets (1 tablet at 3-to-5-minute intervals for 3 doses), consult your physician immediately or seek assistance at the nearest hospital emergency room.
7. Nitroglycerin ointment may be used at bedtime to prevent angina during sleep. Follow the instructions for application carefully. Do not use your fingers. Do not rub the ointment into the skin.
8. Nitroglycerin patches (discs) may induce tolerance to the drug and cause it to be less effective with continuous use. The intermittent use of oral dosage forms may be more effective for long-term treatment. Ask your physician for guidance.
9. If you have glaucoma, consult your physician regarding the periodic measurement of your internal eye pressures while using long-term nitrates for angina.
10. Following long-term use, nitrates should be discontinued gradually to prevent symptoms of withdrawal.

Use of Beta Blocker Drugs

1. Do not use this type of drug without your physician's knowledge and guidance.
2. Beta blockers are not recommended for mild angina that is well controlled by nitrates. Their use is generally reserved for severe and unstable angina.
3. Beta blockers are not recommended for variant (Prinzmetal's) vasospastic angina.
4. If your angina worsens with the use of a beta blocker drug, notify your physician promptly.
5. Atenolol (Tenormin) and metoprolol (Lopressor) are preferred for individuals with asthma, emphysema, diabetes or peripheral circulatory disorders.
6. Atenolol (Tenormin) and nadolol (Corgard) are effective with once-daily dosage and tend to cause less depression and insomnia.

7. Beta blocker drugs must not be discontinued suddenly. Abrupt withdrawal can cause severe angina and increase the risk of heart attack (myocardial infarction).

Use of Calcium Blocker Drugs

1. A calcium blocker is the drug of choice for treating variant (Prinzmetal's) angina.
2. Nifedipine (Adalat, Procardia) is the most potent antianginal calcium blocker. However, angina may worsen if the heart rate increases excessively.
3. Verapamil (Calan, Isoptin) can delay the excretion of digoxin and increase the risk of digoxin toxicity. Dosage adjustments may be necessary.
4. These drugs can be used initially by individuals who should not use beta blockers.

Current Controversies in Drug Management

The nitrate drugs are well established as effective therapeutic agents for the management of angina and congestive heart failure, two conditions that require long-term drug therapy. Recent studies have shown that the "standard" practice of continuous administration of nitrates can lead to the development of tolerance (see Glossary) and loss of effectiveness. Tolerance is most likely to occur with frequent dosing and the use of prolonged-action capsules or tablets and the use of transdermal nitroglycerin patches. Continuous treatment with nitrates produces tolerance within 24 hours of the first dose and complete loss of effect when continued for one week or more. The intermittent use of nitrates ("pulse" dosing) causes only partial tolerance and is more effective for long-term protection. Intermittent rather than continuous nitrate dosing is now recommended for treating angina and congestive heart failure.

Comments: Current guidelines for the optimal use of nitrates include the following recommendations.

- Take isosorbide dinitrate (Isordil, short-acting form) 2 or 3 (but not 4) times daily; take at 8:00 a.m. and 1:00 or 3:00 p.m., or at 8:00 a.m., 1:00 p.m. and 5:00 p.m.; no dosing again until the following 8:00 a.m.
- Take the prolonged-action dosage forms of isosorbide dinitrate at 8:00 a.m., only once daily.
- Use the nitroglycerin patch for only 12 hours daily, from 8:00 a.m. to 8:00 p.m.; leave it off during the night.
- Long nitrate-free intervals appear to preserve responsiveness to the drug.

Ancillary Drug Treatment (as required)

Condition	*Drug Treatment*
For anxiety:	benzodiazepines (Valium, etc.) (See Drug Class, Section Four.)
For hypertension:	see Profile of Hypertension in this section
For congestive heart failure:	see Profile of Congestive Heart Failure in this section
For hyperthyroidism:	methimazole (Tapazole) propylthiouracil propranolol (Inderal)
For anemia:	iron preparations

Note: Drug selection, dosage and administration schedule must be determined by the physician for each patient individually.

Resource for Additional Information and Services

Heartlife (Heart Disease Heart Line)
P.O. Box 54305
Atlanta, GA 30308
Phone: 1-800-241-6993; (404) 523-0826

Available 9:00 a.m.–4:00 p.m. EST, M–F; Spanish-speaking counselor available.
Publications available.

ASTHMA

Other Names: Bronchial asthma, reversible airway disease, reversible obstructive airway disease

Prevalence in USA: Approximately 7 million, 3% of population (includes 1.5 million school-age children).

Age Group: Under 18 years—2.5 million; 18 to 44 years—2.7 million; 45 to 64 years—1.6 million; 65 to 74 years—726,000; 75 years and over—308,000.

Male to Female Ratio: About equal.

Principal Features: Recurring acute attacks of shortness of breath, wheezing (labored breathing), a sensation of tightness in the chest and cough, with symptom-free intervals between attacks. Episodes of active asthma may last an hour to several days. The acute attack begins with tightening of muscles in the walls of bronchial tubes (airways), which causes constriction and reduced air flow. This is followed by swelling of the lining of bronchial tubes and the excessive production of mucus, both of which cause additional narrowing of the airways, forced breathing and coughing. Severe asthma may be accompanied by sweating, insomnia and bluish discoloration of the face and extremities (cyanosis). Asthma that begins in infancy (under 2 years of age) may persist into adulthood. With onset after 2 years, 50% of asthma cases will "outgrow" the disorder by 16 years. Asthma with onset in adulthood is often severe and persistent.

Causes

Extrinsic (Allergic) Asthma: Due to a true allergy (allergen-antibody reaction); hereditary susceptibility to the development of allergies. Common allergens are house dust (and mites in house dust), pollens, animal danders, feathers, wool, molds.

Intrinsic (Idiosyncratic) Asthma: Due to an unusual individual sensitivity (not a true allergy). Onset usually 35 to 45 years of age; 10% to 15% are sensitive to aspirin and have nasal polyps.

Exercise-induced Asthma: Usually in children and young adults; occurs alone or with other types of asthma; often worse 15 minutes after exercise.

Asthma "Triggers": Cold air, smoke, cooking odors, respiratory infections, emotional stress.

Drugs That Can Cause This Disorder

acetaminophen
aspirin (and substitutes)
beta blocker drugs
erythromycin
griseofulvin
hydralazine
ibuprofen
indomethacin
ketoprofen
mefenamic acid
monoamine oxidase inhibitors

naproxen
nitrofurantoin
oral contraceptives
penicillin
pentazocine
phenothiazines
phenylbutazone
procainamide
propoxyphene
reserpine
tartrazine dye

Drugs Used to Treat This Disorder

Xanthine Preparations
- aminophylline (Aminophyllin, Aminodur, etc.).
- oxtriphylline (Brondecon, Choledyl).
- theophylline (Bronkodyl, Slo-bid, Theo-Dur, etc.).

Beta-Adrenergic Drugs
- albuterol (Proventil, Ventolin).
- terbutaline (Brethine, Bricanyl).
- metaproterenol (Alupent, Metaprel).
- isoetharine (Bronkometer, Bronkosol).
- isoproterenol (Isuprel, Medihaler-Iso, etc.).

Cortisonelike Steroids
- beclomethasone aerosol (Beclovent, Vanceril).
- prednisolone (Delta-Cortef, Sterane, etc.).
- prednisone (Deltasone, Meticorten, etc.).

Others
- cromolyn (Intal).
- ipratropium (Atrovent).
- oxygen.

Goals of Drug Treatment

Prompt relief of acute asthmatic attacks.

Prevention of recurrent acute attacks.

Stabilization of lung function: freedom from asthma to the greatest degree possible, with a minimal use of drugs.

Prevention of later complications: bronchiectasis, emphysema, heart disease (cor pulmonale).

Drug Management

For Extrinsic (Allergic) Asthma

For occasional and predictable acute attacks, start treatment with beta-adrenergic inhalers.

For attacks of increasing frequency and duration, add albuterol or terbutaline tablets or a long-acting oral theophylline preparation.

For severe acute attacks or aggravation of chronic asthma, add beclomethasone aerosol inhaler.

If control is not adequate, use albuterol (or terbutaline) tablets and a theophylline preparation concurrently.

If control is still inadequate, add cromolyn on a regular basis.

If an adequate trial of all of the above fails to produce satisfactory relief and control, add cortisonelike steroids (tablets by mouth).

For Intrinsic (Idiosyncratic, Late-Onset) Asthma

Attacks may be less responsive to the use of the bronchodilators (beta-adrenergics and theophylline) as outlined above.

Earlier control may require the use of cromolyn and steroid preparations on a regular schedule.

For Exercise-induced Asthma

Try cromolyn on a regular schedule for prevention of attacks that follow exercise.

Use albuterol or terbutaline inhalation 5 to 10 minutes before exercise and following exercise for prevention.

Long-acting theophylline preparations may be effective in children for prevention.

Use of Theophylline Preparations

1. Theophylline elixir and uncoated tablets are used for prompt relief of acute asthma.
2. Theophylline sustained-release forms (Slo-bid, Slo-phyllin, Theo-Dur) are used for smooth maintenance therapy of chronic asthma. Theophylline blood levels are helpful in determining optimal dosage schedules.

3. Theophylline potentiates beta-adrenergic bronchodilators and increases their effectiveness.
4. See the Drug Profile of Theophylline in Section Three for important drug interactions.

Use of Beta-Adrenergic Bronchodilators

1. These presssurized inhalers are potent drugs that must be used cautiously. Avoid excessive use; follow dosage schedules precisely.
2. They are most effective at the beginning of an asthmatic attack and before exercise that induces asthma.
3. For the most effective use of aerosol bronchodilators, learn the correct procedure: exhale through the mouth to empty lungs; squirt and inhale the first dose at the same time; hold your breath and count to 10, then exhale. If necessary, use a second inhalation in 10 to 15 minutes.
4. Limit inhalations to 1 or 2 at a time, and at least 3 to 4 hours apart.
5. Do not use isoproterenol (Isuprel) aerosol and epinephrine (Adrenalin) aerosol concurrently.

Use of Cortisonelike Steroids

1. Steroids are not bronchodilators; they will not relieve acute asthma. This includes beclomethasone.
2. Their use should be restricted to the treatment of severe acute and chronic asthma that is not controlled by conventional drugs.
3. Steroids should never be used as the sole drug for managing asthma.
4. For short-term use: when an acute attack is prolonged and fails to respond to bronchodilators; steroids are very effective when used for 7 to 10 days of a "burst and taper" schedule—high initial dose followed by gradual dose reduction and withdrawal.
5. For long-term use: when asthma becomes severe and continuous and cannot be controlled by other drugs; a trial period of 2 to 4 weeks of steroids will determine effectiveness. The optimal long-term use consists of a relatively large single dose of prednisone (or prednisolone) every other morning (alternate-day schedule). This provides adequate asthma control with minimal adverse effects of long-term steroid use.
6. The steroid beclomethasone, inhaled in aerosol form, is used to control asthma as steroid tablets are withdrawn.

Use of Cromolyn

1. Cromolyn is not a bronchodilator; it will not relieve acute asthma.
2. It is used only by inhalation; powder and liquid aerosol forms are available.
3. A trial of cromolyn (as an asthma preventive) should begin while you are free of asthma, before acute attacks occur.
4. When used on a regular schedule, cromolyn is 70% to 75% effective in preventing recurrences of acute asthma.

5. It is most effective in preventing extrinsic (allergic) asthma, and least effective in preventing intrinsic (idiosyncratic) asthma. It may or may not prevent exercise-induced asthma but is worth a trial.
6. Cromolyn should be used on a regular basis for 8 to 10 weeks to evaluate its protective benefit.
7. For best results, a beta-adrenergic aerosol should be used 10 minutes before inhaling cromolyn.

Ancillary Drug Treatment (as required)

Condition	*Drug Treatment*
For anxiety:	promethazine (Phenergan). Note: Avoid *all* sedatives in active asthma.
For pain, mild to moderate:	acetaminophen (Tylenol, etc.)
For pain, severe:	methotrimeprazine (Levoprome). This does not depress respiration.
For bacterial infection of respiratory tract (complicating asthma):	ampicillin amoxicillin trimethoprim and sulfamethoxazole tetracycline (avoid during pregnancy and under 8 years of age)
For viral infection of respiratory tract (triggering asthma):	steroids: prednisone and methylprednisolone

Note: Drug selection, dosage and administration schedule must be determined by the physician for each patient individually.

Resources for Additional Information and Services

Asthma and Allergy Foundation of America
1717 Massachusetts Avenue, N.W., Suite 305
Washington, DC 20036
Phone: (202) 265-0265

Publications available.

National Asthma Center
3800 East Colfax Avenue
Denver, CO 80206
Phone: 1-800-222-5864

Available 8:00 a.m.–5:00 p.m. MST, M–F
Publications available.

National Foundation for Asthma
P.O. Box 30069
Tucson, AZ 85751
Phone: (602) 323-6046
Publications available.

CHOLESTEROL DISORDERS

Other Names: Dyslipidemia, hypercholesterolemia, hyperlipidemia, hyperlipoproteinemia, hypertriglyceridemia, lipid transport disorder, lipoprotein disorder

Prevalence in USA: An estimated 25% of adults are thought to have a total cholesterol level in the "too high" range: 200 to 240 mg (current standard). 0.1% of the population has congenital (familial) hypercholesterolemia. 1.0% of the population has congenital (familial) hypertriglyceridemia.

Age Group: In the USA, the low-density lipoprotein (LDL) cholesterol begins to rise after adolescence and continues to rise for 30 years. Significant elevations of LDL cholesterol levels are found in the 20-to-50-year age group.

Male to Female Ratio: 25 to 54 years of age: men show moderately higher levels of total cholesterol and LDL cholesterol; 55 years and older: women show moderately higher levels of total cholesterol and LDL cholesterol.

Principal Features

The principal blood fats (lipids)—notably cholesterol and triglycerides—are combined in the liver with proteins (to form lipoproteins) that facilitate their transport to body tissues. There are normally 3 major classes of lipoproteins: very low-density lipoproteins (VLDL), low-density lipoproteins (LDL) and high-density lipoproteins (HDL). Each class contains differing proportions of fat and protein. VLDL consists of five-sixths triglycerides and one-sixth cholesterol. While circulating in the blood, VLDL is transformed first to intermediate-density lipoprotein (IDL), which is 30% cholesterol and 40% triglyceride, and then to low-density lipoprotein (LDL), which carries from 60% to 75% of the total blood cholesterol. High levels of LDL cholesterol are associated *statistically* with an increased risk of coronary heart disease—the higher the level, the higher the risk. HDL carries less than 25% of the total blood cholesterol. It is thought to assist with the removal of LDL cholesterol from the blood and body tissues. High levels of HDL cholesterol appear to be protective against coronary heart disease—the higher the HDL level, the lower the risk.

The principal cholesterol disorders are classified into 5 major types according to the nature of the lipoprotein abnormality and associated clinical features. Types I and V are not associated with the development of atherosclerosis. Types II, III and IV are associated with the atherosclerotic process that causes coronary heart disease and peripheral vascular disorders. The lipoprotein features of these classes are as follows:

Type IIa: increased total cholesterol and LDL cholesterol; normal triglycerides.

Type IIb: increased total cholesterol, LDL cholesterol and VLDL; moderately increased triglycerides.

Type III: increased IDL cholesterol (abnormal form); increased triglycerides.

Type IV: normal total cholesterol, increased VLDL, decreased HDL cholesterol; increased triglycerides.

Causes: The major cholesterol disorders are primarily hereditary (familial) and therefore genetically determined. Secondary causes can contribute to congenital lipid disorders or can independently account for abnormalities of blood lipid metabolism. Among the secondary causes are the following conditions: Hypothyroidism, biliary cirrhosis, nephrosis, anorexia nervosa and acute intermittent porphyria can cause significant increases in blood cholesterol levels. Diabetes, chronic alcoholism, chronic kidney failure and acute hepatitis can cause significant increases in blood triglyceride levels. However, the most apparent secondary cause of lipid disorders is the high dietary cholesterol and fat content consumed by the American public.

Drugs That Can Cause This Disorder: The following drugs have been reported to cause abnormal increases in cholesterol blood levels: anabolic (male-hormonelike) steroids, chenodiol, disopyramide, thiazide diuretics (see Drug Class, Section Four), trimeprazine. The following drugs have been reported to cause abnormal increases in triglyceride blood levels: cortisonelike drugs (see Drug Class, Section Four), estrogens, isotretinoin, oral contraceptives, thiazide diuretics (see Drug Class, Section Four), timolol.

Drugs Used to Treat This Disorder

Drugs that inhibit synthesis of cholesterol and lipoprotein: lovastatin (Mevacor), niacin (nicotinic acid, Nicobid, Nicotinex, etc.).

Drugs that hasten the clearance of lipoproteins in the bloodstream: clofibrate (Atromid-S), gemfibrozil (Lopid).

Drugs that accelerate breakdown and elimination of lipoproteins: cholestyramine (Questran), colestipol (Colestid), probucol (Lorelco).

Other drugs used less often: dextrothyroxine (Choloxin), neomycin.

New Drugs in Development for Treating This Disorder

Drugs of the lovastatin class: mevastatin (Compactin), pravastatin (Eptastatin), simvastatin (Synvinolin). These drugs, for the most part,

significantly reduce total and LDL cholesterol and raise HDL cholesterol. They may prove to be effective in lower dosage and therefore
less likely to cause adverse effects.

Drugs of the fibric acid class: fenofibrate. This drug (in use in Europe
for several years) effectively reduces LDL cholesterol and triglycerides, raises HDL cholesterol and is well tolerated.

Goals of Drug Treatment

Normalization of blood lipid levels to currently accepted standards:
total cholesterol of less than 200 mg; LDL cholesterol of less than 130
mg; triglycerides of less than 250 mg (in the absence of other significant lipid abnormalities).

Avoidance or reduction of adverse drug effects.

Prevention, retardation or reversal of atherosclerotic arterial changes
throughout the body to reduce the risk of coronary heart disease,
peripheral vascular disease and stroke.

Note: The following values reflect the evolving opinion regarding the
"normalcy" of blood lipids over the past 15 years:

Normal Upper Limit	1975	1980	1989
Total cholesterol	300	280	200
LDL cholesterol		180	130
Triglycerides	200	165	150

A "normal" HDL cholesterol range is 40 to 80.

Drug Management

Introduction

Our present understanding of how cholesterol disorders are causally
related to the development of atherosclerosis (coronary and peripheral vascular disease) is incomplete and controversial. While large
population studies have demonstrated that high cholesterol blood levels are associated statistically with an increased incidence of atherosclerosis, cholesterol values alone have low predictability for the actual development of coronary heart disease on an individual basis.
The somewhat exaggerated emphasis on "statistical significance" has
resulted in the creation of unrealistic risk ratios based on minor
changes in blood lipid levels that are meaningless in the light of wide
individual variability and the unreproducibility of laboratory test results as currently obtained. Determination of isolated blood lipid levels provides at best an incomplete appraisal of an individual's status
regarding an inclination to develop atherosclerosis. They represent
only one aspect of a disease process in which many other causative
factors are involved. An understanding of the complex interactions of
the numerous cholesterol-triglyceride-apoprotein linkages (lipoprotein fractions) is the key to learning which components and what
concentrations can be relied upon to predicate an increased risk for
the consequent development of atherosclerosis. For example, high levels of apolipoproteins (a), AI and B are much stronger predictors than

cholesterol values for identifying those at high risk for atherosclerotic heart disease. Anyone who has reason to be concerned about a possible cholesterol disorder is well advised to reduce dietary fat and cholesterol intake. The majority of individuals with elevated blood lipid values do not require drug therapy to manage their disorder. Before starting a long-term, expensive and somewhat risky program of drug treatment, the concerned individual should first seek a detailed evaluation at a reputable lipid research center, either in person or by submission of appropriate blood samples and medical information.

Determining the Need for Treatment

Observe the following procedures for the measurement of blood lipid values:

1. Do not alter your regular diet in preparation for testing. You should not be on a reducing diet.
2. You should be free of any kind of infection.
3. Avoid all alcoholic beverages for 24 hours prior to testing.
4. Fast for 12 to 16 hours prior to testing.
5. Your blood samples should be examined by a reliable laboratory that has established a record for providing accurate, precise and reproducible test results.
6. For proper evaluation, a blood lipid profile should include values for total cholesterol, LDL and HDL cholesterol fractions and triglycerides.
7. Obtain blood lipid measurements on at least 2 separate occasions (3 if in doubt) and use the average of the test results.

When to Treat

Current recommendations regarding initiation of treatment are based on the following guidelines. Either diet therapy alone or diet plus drug therapy is recommended when the blood lipid values exceed those stated in the table.

| | **DIET ALONE** | | **DIET AND DRUGS** | |
Age Group	*Cholesterol*	*LDL*	*Cholesterol*	*LDL*
20–29	200	140	220	160
30–39	220	155	240	175
Over 40	240	160	260	185

How to Treat

1. Diet modification is the primary treatment for all individuals with elevated blood lipid levels. The total caloric intake should be designed to achieve ideal body weight. The initial diet should restrict saturated fats to 10% of the total calories and restrict cholesterol to less than 300 mg daily. This low-fat, low-cholesterol diet should be adhered to for 4 to 6 months to fully evaluate its effectiveness. Individuals with severe blood lipid disorders may require the guidance of a registered dietitian.

2. If an adequate trial of dietary therapy fails to lower blood lipid values to acceptable levels, consideration may be given to adding a trial of drug therapy while dietary modification continues. No single drug is appropriate for treating all blood lipid disorders. The choice of the initial drug depends upon the specific nature of the lipoprotein abnormality. Begin with an adequate trial of a single drug. If the response is insufficient, substitute another drug or add a second drug as appropriate. Measure blood lipid levels 4 to 6 weeks after starting drug treatment and at 3-month intervals until a stable response is obtained.

3. To reduce LDL cholesterol (the most common form of cholesterol disorder in the USA):
   weight reduction if necessary
   diet low in saturated fats and cholesterol
   effective drugs:
      cholestyramine (Questran)
      colestipol (Colestid)
      lovastatin (Mevicor)
      niacin (nicotinic acid)

4. To reduce VLDL triglycerides:
   weight reduction
   diet low in saturated fats and cholesterol
   alcohol restriction
   effective drugs:
      niacin (nicotinic acid)
      gemfibrozil (Lopid)

5. To reduce IDL (abnormal lipoprotein):
   weight reduction
   diet low in saturated fats and cholesterol
   effective drugs:
      niacin (nicotinic acid)
      gemfibrozil (Lopid)
      clofibrate (Atromid-S), not recommended due to serious adverse drug effects

6. To raise HDL cholesterol:
   weight reduction
   smoking cessation
   regular exercise
   modest use of alcohol (no more than 1 to 2 drinks daily)
   avoidance of progestin-containing contraceptives
   no specific drug recommended currently

Notes on Specific Lipid-Lowering Drugs

(See the respective Drug Profiles in Section Three for a complete discussion.)

Lovastatin (Mevacor)

The prototype of a new and most promising class of drugs

Recent studies show it to be more effective and better tolerated than cholestyramine.

Can reduce total cholesterol 22% to 33%

Can reduce LDL cholesterol 32% to 42%

Can reduce triglycerides 8% to 27%

Can raise HDL cholesterol slightly

More effective in women than in men

Most effective when used in combination with cholestyramine or colestipol

Infrequent adverse drug effects: indigestion, localized muscle pain

Cholestyramine (Questran) and colestipol (Colestid)

Have demonstrated effectiveness in reducing the development of coronary heart disease

Currently the drugs of choice for treating Type IIa hyperlipidemia

Can reduce total cholesterol 20%

Can reduce LDL cholesterol 23% to 27%

Can raise HDL cholesterol slightly

Triglycerides unchanged or increased

Cause severe constipation in 20% of users

Cause decreased absorption of many other drugs (due to binding)

Large doses cause deficiencies of vitamins A, D, E and K; calcium;
iron

Niacin (nicotinic acid)

Used to treat Types IIa, IIb, III and IV hyperlipidemia

Can reduce total cholesterol 25%

Can reduce LDL cholesterol 35%

Can reduce triglycerides 26%

Can raise HDL cholesterol 20%

Not well tolerated by many users

Advise use of timed-release dosage form; increase dose slowly over 2
to 3 months; take with meals; take one adult aspirin tablet 30 minutes before each dose to reduce skin flushing

Significant adverse effects: liver toxicity, reduced sugar tolerance, increased blood uric acid levels, stomach irritation

Gemfibrozil (Lopid)

Used primarily to treat Types IIb, III, IV and V hyperlipidemia

Can reduce total cholesterol 10%

Can reduce LDL cholesterol 11%

Can reduce triglycerides 35%

Can raise HDL cholesterol 11%

Significant adverse effects: reduced sugar tolerance, decreased white
blood cell counts, doubled risk for gall stone formation, reduced
libido in 12% of men

Should be discontinued if not beneficial after 3 months of treatment

Probucol (Lorelco)

Used primarily to treat Type IIa hyperlipidemia

Can reduce total cholesterol 10% to 15%

Can reduce LDL cholesterol 8%

Can reduce HDL cholesterol 23% (possibly undesirable)

Triglycerides unchanged or raised

Significant adverse effects: anemia, diarrhea
Of limited usefulness due to reduction of HDL cholesterol
May be used in combination with more effective drugs

Current Controversies in Drug Management

1. Should individuals with "moderate" elevations of cholesterol be treated initially with diet modification alone or with combined dietary and drug treatment?

   Comments

   Dietary reduction of saturated fats and cholesterol usually reduces blood cholesterol levels by no more than 10% to 20%; no significant benefit in morbidity or mortality has been demonstrated.

   Cholestyramine drug therapy reduces blood cholesterol levels by 25% with an associated 50% reduction in the risk of developing coronary heart disease.

   Generalizations are not always appropriate or applicable in therapeutic decisions. *Individual* assessment of benefit versus risk (and cost) must be made jointly by patient and physician. The early introduction of drug therapy is justified when there is a family history of premature coronary heart disease (before age 60), recent coronary bypass surgery or other risk factors, such as obesity, high blood pressure, diabetes or heavy use of tobacco.

2. Should individuals with "moderate" elevations of triglycerides (primarily) be treated with diet modification only or with combined dietary and drug treatment?

   Comments

   Not all forms of triglycerides are associated with increased risk for atherosclerosis. A detailed lipoprotein profile is necessary for specific recommendations. The triglycerides found primarily in chylomicrons (Types I and V disorders) are not atherogenic and drug therapy is not indicated. The triglycerides associated with IDL (Type III disorder) are atherogenic and require drug treatment.

Ancillary Drug Treatment (as required)

Condition	*Drug Treatment*
For constipation (due to cholestyramine or colestipol):	docusate (Colace, Dialose, Doxidan, Surfak, etc.)
	Citrucel
	Metamucil
For diarrhea (due to probucol):	diphenoxylate (Lomotil) loperamide (Imodium)
For associated diabetes mellitus:	see Profile of Diabetes in this section
For associated hypertension:	see Profile of Hypertension in this section

For associated hypothyroidism: see Profile of Hypothyroidism in this section

Note: Drug selection, dosage and administration schedule must be determined by the physician for each patient individually.

Resource for Additional Information and Services

Council on Arteriosclerosis of the American Heart Association
c/o The American Heart Association
7320 Greenville Avenue
Dallas, TX 75231
Phone: (214) 750-5431

Publications available.

CONGESTIVE HEART FAILURE

Other Names: Chronic heart failure, cardiac decompensation, myocardial decompensation

Prevalence in USA: 2.3 million; 400,000 new cases annually.

Age Group: 45 to 54 years—2.6/1000 population; 55 to 64 years—7/1000 population; 65 to 74 years—15/1000 population.

Male to Female Ratio: 1.5 to 1.

Principal Features: The designation "congestive heart failure" refers to a condition in which the heart is unable to pump enough blood to satisfy the needs of the body. Diseased heart muscle loses its contracting power, allowing increased filling pressures inside the heart chambers (ventricles); further stretching and weakening of muscle tissue leads to muscle exhaustion and reduced pumping capacity; the forward flow of blood is impaired and excessive volumes of blood accumulate in vital areas throughout the body, producing congestion. Resulting symptoms include shortness of breath (dyspnea), first with exertion and later at rest; inability to breathe comfortably while lying down (orthopnea); fatigue and weakness, especially in the legs; a dry cough; night urination; swelling of the feet and ankles at the end of the day; and vague discomfort in the chest and abdomen.

Causes: Primary causes of heart disease that ultimately lead to congestive heart failure:

hypertension (75%)	myocarditis
coronary heart disease (10%)	diabetes (16%)
valvular heart disease (10%)	emphysema
congenital heart disease	

Precipitating causes in predisposed individuals: reduction of therapy (most common), heart rhythm disorders, severe infections, obesity, pregnancy, anemia, hyperthyroidism, excessive heat and humidity.

Drugs That Can Cause This Disorder: In individuals with borderline heart function, the following drugs can precipitate congestive heart failure:
amantadine (Symmetrel)
beta-adrenergic-blocking drugs (see Drug Class, Section Four)
cortisonelike steroids (see Drug Class, Section Four)
disopyramide (Norpace)
nonsteroidal anti-inflammatory drugs (see Drug Class, Section Four)

Drugs Used to Treat This Disorder
- digitalis preparations: digitoxin, digoxin.
- diuretics (see Drug Class, Section Four).
- vasodilators: arterial dilators—hydralazine, prazosin; venous dilators—isosorbide dinitrate, nitroglycerin.
- calcium channel-blocking drugs: ditiazem, nifedipine, verapamil.
- ACE inhibitors: captopril, enalapril, lisinopril.
- milrinone (investigational only).
- oxygen.

New Drugs in Development for Treating This Disorder: Xamoterol (Carwin), a new heart muscle stimulant under study in Europe and in the US, has been shown to be significantly better than digoxin in treating chronic heart failure. This drug is not yet available for general use.

Goals of Drug Treatment
Improvement of the heart's pumping performance by the use of digitalis.
Reduction of the heart's workload by the use of arterial and venous vasodilators.
Removal of excess salt and water from the body by the use of diuretics.
Relief of symptoms—fatigue, shortness of breath, ankle swelling, etc.—by means of the above procedures.

Drug Management
For Early, Mild Congestive Heart Failure
Two variations of initial treatment are used widely:
1. Treatment is started with digitalis (digoxin or digitoxin). This may be the only drug used if response is satisfactory. If necessary, a thiazide diuretic (or equivalent) is added.
2. Treatment is started with a thiazide diuretic (or equivalent), given alone. This may give a very adequate response, especially in the elderly. If necessary, digoxin (or digitoxin) is added.
For Moderate to Severe Congestive Heart Failure
Digoxin (or digitoxin) and thiazide diuretics are used in maximal tolerated dosage.
As necessary, a stronger diuretic, such as furosemide or ethacrynic acid, is added.

If the response is inadequate, vasodilators are started: isosorbide dinitrate or nitroglycerin patches for venous dilation; hydralazine for arterial dilation.

If additional improvement is sought, captopril (or enalapril) may be tried as a replacement for the nitrates (isosorbide dinitrate or nitroglycerin).

For long-term maintenance, a combination of hydralazine and nitrates or hydralazine and captropril may be tried.

For congestive heart failure with angina and/or hypertension, a trial of nifedipine is justified.

Use of Digitalis

1. Should be started only when there is a firm diagnosis of heart failure. Periodic reassessment is necessary to determine continued need. Maintenance digitalis may not be necessary for life. Following correction of congestive heart failure, stable heart function may be achieved by using only diuretics and vasodilators.
2. Digoxin is the form of digitalis most frequently used. Because digoxin products vary in their absorbability, refill your prescriptions with the same brand to ensure uniform drug effects.
3. Take the exact dose at the same time each day.
4. Learn to count your pulse and check its regularity. Notify your physician if your pulse rate is below 60 beats/minute or your pulse rhythm changes significantly.
5. The elderly and individuals with hypothyroidism often have a reduced tolerance for digitalis; smaller doses are advisable.
6. Digitalis toxicity (overdosage) occurs in 20% of users; it is more common in the elderly. The earliest indications of toxicity are usually loss of appetite, nausea and vomiting; other indications include headache, facial pains, blurred vision, seeing "snowflakes" or yellowish-green halos, fatigue, weakness and disturbances of heart rhythm. The elderly may show confusion; rarely, seizures may occur.
7. Periodic blood levels can help to determine optimal dosage, especially if kidney function is impaired. The blood sample should be taken no less than 6 hours after the last dose.
8. See the Drug Profile of Digoxin in Section Three for important drug interactions.

Use of Diuretics ("Water Pills")

1. Thiazide (or equivalent) diuretics may suffice as the only drug treatment for mild heart failure in many elderly patients.
2. When possible, diuretics should be taken in the morning to minimize nighttime urination.
3. If your diuretic is one that increases the excretion of potassium in the urine, it is important that your blood level of potassium be checked periodically. An abnormally low potassium level can increase the risk of digitalis toxicity. Consult your physician regarding the advisability of omitting your diuretic every third day to minimize the loss of potassium.

4. If your diuretic is one that does not increase the excretion of potassium (amiloride, spironolactone, triamterene), you should not take a potassium supplement or eat excessive amounts of high-potassium foods.
5. If you use diuretics on a regular basis, consult your physician regarding the degree of salt restriction he or she recommends for you.
6. Many salt substitutes have a high potassium content. Ask your physician for guidance regarding the selection and use of commercially available salt substitutes.
7. In advanced congestive heart failure, you may be advised to use a thiazide diuretic concurrently with furosemide (or ethacrynic acid) and a potassium-saving diuretic; the combined actions of the three types of drugs give a maximal diuretic effect.

Use of Vasodilators
1. These are generally used when heart failure does not respond adequately to digitalis and diuretics.
2. These may be used earlier for those who cannot tolerate digitalis, and for those who need a vasodilator to treat hypertension (hydralazine) or angina (nifedipine).
3. Nitrate vasodilators (primarily venous dilators) contribute to the relief of shortness of breath.
4. Hydralazine (primarily an arterial dilator) contributes to the relief of fatigue and weakness.
5. Isosorbide dinitrate (venous) and hydralazine (arterial) vasodilators can be used concurrently to advantage; they are quite effective in the majority of cases of chronic congestive failure.
6. Prazosin (both an arterial and a venous dilator) is an alternative choice. However it causes fluid retention and requires increasing doses and additional diuretics with continued use.

Use of Oxygen
1. Oxygen must be properly humidified to prevent drying of tissues of the respiratory tract.
2. Administer by nasal prongs; avoid a mask.

Current Controversies in Drug Management

With the advent of new drugs and improved understanding of the altered physiology associated with congestive heart failure, controversy regarding drug selection for its treatment has increased. A consensus has emerged indicating that diuretics should now be considered the first-line drugs of choice, replacing digoxin.

Controversy continues, however, as to which drug should be added next if diuretics are inadequate. Some authorities favor digoxin as the second drug; others favor vasodilators (see above). Current evidence seems to favor vasodilators as the second drug, with digoxin added as a third drug when required. New studies show that angiotensin-converting enzyme (ACE) inhibitors (see above) can enhance treatment and prolong survival. Further experience and detailed analysis of drug performance are required to resolve current controversies.

Drug choices at this time will remain a matter of individual physician preference.

Ancillary Drug Treatment (as required)

Condition	*Drug Treatment*
For anxiety:	diazepam (only as needed)
For insomnia:	chloral hydrate (Noctec, Somnos)
For anemia:	iron preparations
For hypertension:	see Profile of Hypertension in this section

Note: Drug selection, dosage and administration schedule must be determined by the physician for each patient individually.

Resources for Additional Information and Services

Heartlife (Heart Disease Heart Line)
P.O. Box 54305
Atlanta, GA 30308
Phone: 1-800-241-6993; (404) 523-0826

Available 9:00 a.m.–4:00 p.m. EST, M–F; Spanish-speaking counselor available.
Publications available.

American Heart Association
7320 Greenville Avenue
Dallas, TX 75231
Phone: (214) 373-6300

Publications available.

CROHN'S DISEASE

Other Names: Regional enteritis, regional ileitis, granulomatous colitis, inflammatory bowel disease

Prevalence in USA: 1 million (includes 100,000 children); 15,000 new cases annually.

Age Group: Onset from infancy to 25 years of age; 15% to 30% have onset before puberty. Peak incidence is from 10 to 25 years of age.

Male to Female Ratio: Slightly more common in females.

Principal Features: An intermittent to chronic disorder of the small intestine and colon; one third of cases occur in the lower segment of the small intestine (the ileum), one third in the colon and one third in both. Less than 50% of cases involve the rectum. The onset is usually insidious, but may be rapid and resemble acute appendicitis. Symptoms include loss of appetite, fatigue, fever, loss of weight, abdominal cramps and pain after eating, nausea, vomiting, diarrhea (occasionally bloody), anal sores and retarded growth in children. There may also be inflammatory disorders in the skin, eyes, mouth and large joints. Children may experience fever and joint pains before any indications of disease in the intestine or colon. Adults may have a higher incidence of gallstones or kidney stones. This disorder often recurs throughout life.

Caution: The early manifestations of Crohn's disease may vary. Loss of appetite and weight may lead to the mistaken diagnosis of anorexia nervosa.

Causes: The primary cause is unknown. There is a familial clustering in 15% to 20% of cases. It is thought that an inherited susceptibility may predispose to unknown environmental factors capable of inducing the disorder.

Drugs That Can Cause This Disorder: By altering the normal balance of bacteria in the intestine, several antibiotics can cause a form of enteritis that might resemble Crohn's disease. These include some of the tetracyclines, penicillin and chloramphenicol. Antibiotic-induced enteritis is transient and easily corrected; no permanent damage occurs. The vitamin A derivative etretinate (Tegison) has been reported to cause Crohn's disease.

Drugs Used to Treat This Disorder
- sulfasalazine (Azulfidine).
- cortisonelike steroids, principally prednisone.
- azathioprine (Imuran); 6-mercaptopurine (Purinethol).
- metronidazole (Flagyl).
- antidiarrheals: diphenoxylate (Lomotil), loperamide (Imodium).
- antispasmodics: belladonna (Donnatal), dicyclomine (Bentyl).
- antibiotics: ampicillin (Amcill, etc.), tetracycline (Achromycin, etc.); used when appropriate for bacterial infections of intestine.

Goals of Drug Treatment
Induction of a remission (return to normal) during the active phase of the disease.
Relief of symptoms.
Protection of bowel, avoidance of complications.
Maintenance of general nutrition.

Drug Management
General Principles
For initial treatment of mild disease: sulfasalazine.
For moderate to severe disease: prednisone, used concurrently with sulfasalazine.
For acute recurrences: prednisone.

For long-term maintenance: sulfasalazine; avoid use of cortisonelike steroids (prednisone).

For active disease that fails to respond to combined use of sulfasalazine and prednisone: (1) a trial of metronidazole as replacement for sulfasalazine; (2) a trial of azathioprine or 6-mercaptopurine added to sulfasalazine and prednisone programs.

Use of Sulfasalazine

1. Used to initiate treatment in active disease.
2. About 50% effective when used with prednisone.
3. Most beneficial in treating Crohn's disease of the colon.
4. Usually not effective in preventing recurrences; however, it may be tried for long-term maintenance until a better treatment is developed.
5. Common adverse effects are headache, nausea and vomiting; take with or immediately following food.

Use of Cortisonelike Steroids (Prednisone, etc.)

1. Usually 60% to 70% effective during first 6 months of treatment; if use is extended to 12 months, only 20% to 30% remain in remission.
2. Good initial response in treating Crohn's disease of the colon, but the majority relapse within 1 year.
3. Long-term use for mild disease or to prevent recurrences is usually ineffective and is not advised.
4. Use primarily to control worsening symptoms and to suppress acute flare-ups. Continue use until a sustained improvement is established. Try to use the lowest effective dose.
5. When possible, an alternate-day dosing schedule is recommended: a single morning dose every 48 hours.
6. When appropriate, taper dose very slowly over a period of 4 to 12 months.
7. Repeated intermittent short courses are preferable to continual long-term use.
8. Crohn's disease of the rectum should be treated with steroid suppositories and retention enemas.

Use of Antidiarrheals

1. Use very cautiously and as sparingly as possible.
2. Excessive use can induce two complications: (1) paralytic (adynamic) ileus, a paralysis of the small intestine that results in a functional obstruction; (2) toxic megacolon, a marked distention of the colon with air, and a danger of perforation.

Use of Adsorbents

1. Cholestyramine (Questran) and aluminum hydroxide (Amphojel) can adsorb bile in the intestine and reduce bile-induced diarrhea.
2. These adsorbents can also adsorb other drugs being used concurrently. Schedule all dosages to ensure maximal effectiveness—adequate spacing between adsorbents and other active drugs.

Use of Immunosuppressants
1. Azathioprine (Imuran) and 6-mercaptopurine (Purinethol) may be tried when sulfasalazine and prednisone have failed to control the disease after an adequate trial.
2. Either one may be tried as an adjunct to the established treatment program.
3. A trial of 4 to 6 months of treatment is often necessary to determine effectiveness.
4. These drugs make it possible to reduce the dose of steroids or withdraw them completely in some individuals.

Use of Antibiotics
1. Appropriately selected antibiotics may be used to treat a diarrhea due to specific bacterial overgrowth (superinfection).
2. Antibiotics should not be taken concurrently with sulfasalazine.

Ancillary Drug Treatment (as required)

Condition	Drug Treatment
For anemia (common):	iron preparations, vitamin B-12, folic acid (as required)
For malnutrition:	multiple vitamins and the minerals calcium, magnesium, zinc
For depression:	see Profile of Depression in this section

Note: Drug selection, dosage and administration schedule must be determined by the physician for each patient individually.

Resource for Additional Information and Services

American Digestive Disease Society
7720 Wisconsin Avenue
Bethesda, MD 20814
Phone: (301) 652-9293

Telecommunications services: Gutline, available to the public every Tuesday evening from 7:30 to 9:00 p.m.
Publications available.

DEPRESSION

Other Names: Depressive reaction (reactive depression, secondary depression), depressive illness (biologic depression, major depressive disorder), affective disorder: depressive phase of manic-depressive disorder

Prevalence in USA: Approximately 30 million; 5% to 8% of general population. One third of all depressions are severe enough to require medical treatment.

Age Group: Can occur at any age. Peak occurrence is between 25 and 44 years of age.

Male to Female Ratio: 1 male to 2 females; 25% of women and 10% of men will experience depression during their lifetime.

Principal Features
  Depressive Reaction: A situational (exogenous) reactive depression that represents an understandable adaptive response to a significant loss or stressful life situation; a sense of despondency and distress, comparatively mild to moderate, usually self-limiting with a duration of 2 weeks to 6 months.
  Depressive Illness: A spontaneous (endogenous) unexplained and seemingly unprovoked depression of moderate to severe degree; characterized by (1) a depressed mood—sadness, dejection, hopelessness, despair; (2) reduced energy level—loss of interest, fatigue, inability to function effectively; (3) negative self-image—sense of inferiority, incompetence, exaggerated guilt. Common features include loss of appetite, broken sleep, early morning awakening, constipation. Often clears spontaneously in 6 to 12 months, even without treatment.

Causes: Depressive reactions are normal mood responses to the stresses and strains of daily life. The primary cause of major depressive illness is unknown. Research indicates that in many cases there appears to be a genetic (constitutional) predisposition to depression. The actual onset of depressive illness is attributed to a deficiency of certain brain chemicals—the neurotransmitters norepinephrine, dopamine and/or serotonin. What initiates the deficiency is not known.

Drugs That Can Cause This Disorder: Drug-induced depressions are more likely to occur in those who are genetically susceptible to depression. The following drugs are known to cause depression:

benzodiazepines (in excess)	levodopa
certain beta-blocking drugs	methyldopa
clonidine	oral contraceptives
cortisonelike steroids	some phenothiazines
digitalis (toxicity)	reserpine (and related drugs)
indomethacin	

Drugs Used to Treat This Disorder
  Bicyclic Antidepressant
   • fluoxetine (Prozac).
  Tricyclic Antidepressants (TCA's)
   • amitriptyline (Elavil, Endep).
   • amoxapine (Asendin).
   • desipramine (Norpramin, Pertofrane).
   • doxepin (Adapin, Sinequan).
   • imipramine (Imavate, Presamine, Tofranil).

- nortriptyline (Aventyl, Pamelor).
- protriptyline (Vivactil).

Tetracyclic Antidepressant
- maprotiline (Ludiomil).

Monoamine Oxidase Inhibitors (MAOI's) Type A
- phenelzine (Nardil).
- tranylcypromine (Parnate).

Other Drugs
- alprazolam (Xanax)
- lithium (Eskalith, Lithane, Lithobid, Lithotab)
- methylphenidate (Ritalin)
- trazodone (Desyrel)

Goals of Drug Treatment

Alleviation of symptoms.

Termination of depression, restoration of normal mood.

Prevention of recurrence.

Prevention of swing from depression to manic psychosis (in manic-depressive disorder).

Drug Management

For Depressive Reactions: Reactive depressions are often mild and self-limiting; they usually respond well to supportive psychotherapy. Drug treatment is not necessary for everyone who is depressed. If this type of depression becomes severe or is unreasonably prolonged, a tricyclic antidepressant (or a new generation equivalent) may be tried for 1 month to determine its effectiveness.

For Depressive Illness: Major endogenous depressions are usually very responsive to an appropriate and adequate trial of antidepressant drug therapy. Spontaneous remissions often occur within 6 to 12 months, but recovery can be initiated earlier and greatly accelerated by proper medication. Adequate dosage and a sufficient period of treatment are essential to a successful outcome.

Treatment is usually started with a tricyclic antidepressant or one of the newer equivalents. If response is inadequate after a reasonable trial, another tricyclic or similar antidepressant should be tried. If this fails, a monoamine oxidase inhibitor may be considered. Some cyclic depressions respond better to lithium than to tricyclic antidepressants.

Not all depressions are recurrent. For a first episode, the antidepressant drug may be gradually reduced and discontinued after 3 to 6 months of a stable mood, free of depression.

For the 50% of depressions that are recurrent, the optimal maintenance dose of the most effective drug should be determined and continued indefinitely.

Use of Tricyclic Antidepressants (TCA's)
1. These are the drugs of choice when drug treatment is deemed necessary.

2. They are 60% to 75% effective in treating major endogenous depressive illness. They may also be effective in treating severe reactive depressions.

3. Continual use on a regular schedule for 2 to 5 weeks is necessary to determine a drug's effectiveness in relieving depression.

4. Treatment with all antidepressants is necessarily empirical; a period of trial and error is unavoidable for both the selection of the best drug and the determination of optimal dosage.

5. If one TCA (or equivalent) shows no significant benefit after 3 weeks of adequate dosage, it is advisable to try another drug of the same or similar class.

6. During drug trials, and during maintenance treatment later, stay with the same brand (manufacturer) to ensure uniform results.

7. Periodic measurement of blood levels of the drug can be helpful in determining optimal dosage. (See Therapeutic Drug Monitoring in Section One.)

8. Most drugs of this class cause drowsiness, especially during the first several weeks of use. Avoid alcoholic beverages and use extreme caution in driving and engaging in all hazardous activities.

9. When the correct total daily dose has been determined, it can usually be taken as a single dose at bedtime.

10. Use these drugs cautiously if you have glaucoma, prostatism or a heart rhythm disorder.

11. Avoid rapid withdrawal of TCA's; abrupt discontinuation may cause restlessness, headache, anxiety, insomnia, muscle aches, nausea. Withdraw gradually over a period of 10 to 14 days.

12. See the Drug Profiles of respective TCA's in Section Three for important drug interactions.

Use of Newer ("Second Generation") Antidepressants

1. Maprotiline (Ludiomil) may act more rapidly than TCA's; it is quite sedating. Avoid if you have a seizure disorder.

2. Alprazolam (Xanax) is sedating. After long-term use, withdraw gradually to avoid possible seizures.

3. Amoxapine (Asendin) is less sedating. It can cause parkinsonlike symptoms, restlessness and tardive dyskinesia (rarely). Do not use longer than 3 to 4 months.

4. Trazodone (Desyrel) is also sedating, but it has little or no atropinelike effects. It is very useful in the elderly and for those with glaucoma or prostatism.

Use of Monoamine Oxidase Inhibitors (MAOI's) Type A

1. Used to treat biologic endogenous depressions that do not respond to TCA's.

2. Also useful for treating "atypical" and neurotic depressions that are characterized by marked anxiety, phobias, hypochondriasis, excessive eating and excessive sleeping.

3. Continual use on a regular schedule for 2 to 5 weeks is necessary to determine effectiveness in relieving depression.

4. Avoid concurrent use of over-the-counter diet pills, nose drops and cold and allergy preparations.
5. Avoid foods and beverages that contain tyramine and similar compounds. (See Tyramine in Glossary.)
6. If switching from a TCA to a MAOI, allow a "washout" period of 7 to 10 days before starting the MAOI. If switching from a MAOI to a TCA, allow a "washout" period of 14 days before starting the TCA.
7. MAOI's can cause low blood pressure, overstimulation, insomnia, confusion, nausea, vomiting, diarrhea and fluid retention.
8. MAOI's can provoke an abrupt swing from depression to manic psychosis in manic-depressive disorder.
9. MAOI's can activate psychosis in those with schizophrenia.
10. Do not discontinue these drugs suddenly. A rebound depression can follow abrupt withdrawal.
11. See the Drug Profiles of respective MAOI's in Section Three for important drug interactions.

Use of Lithium

1. Can be 70% effective in stabilizing mood, especially in bipolar manic-depressive illness; reduces the frequency and severity of attacks of both mania and depression.
2. Often effective in preventing recurrences of depression in unipolar (depression only) disorders.
3. Must be taken in divided doses to avoid stomach irritation and excessively high (toxic) blood levels.
4. When lithium proves to be effective in preventing recurrence of depression, it is very important to continue maintenance treatment when feeling well and free of depression.
5. Periodic measurements of blood levels are mandatory to maintain effective concentrations and to prevent toxicity. Blood samples should be taken 12 hours after the last dose.
6. Mild side-effects (not toxicity) include loss of appetite, metallic taste, indigestion, nausea, thirst, fatigue, tremor, fluid retention, acne.
7. Early toxic effects include vomiting, dizziness, unsteadiness, weakness, slurred speech, muscle twitching, confusion.
8. While taking lithium, maintain a high liquid intake, but avoid excessive coffee, tea and cola drinks.
9. Do not restrict your salt intake.
10. Use lithium cautiously if you have heart disease, kidney disease or a thyroid disorder.
11. Check thyroid and kidney functions before and during lithium therapy.

Use of Other Antidepressant Drugs

1. Methylphenidate (Ritalin) may be tried for long-term treatment of selected elderly persons with depression.
2. Alprazolam (Xanax), a benzodiazepine tranquilizer, may be useful for short-term treatment of minor depression.

Ancillary Drug Treatment (as required)

Condition	*Drug Treatment*
For mild anxiety:	alprazolam (Xanax)
For severe anxiety and agitation:	thioridazine (Mellaril) thiothixene (Navane)
For psychosis:	amitriptyline and perphenazine (Etrafon, Triavil)
For constipation:	docusate (Colace, Doxinate, etc.)

Note: Drug selection, dosage and administration schedule must be determined by the physician for each patient individually.

Resources for Additional Information and Services

Depressives Anonymous: Recovery From Depression
329 East 62nd Street
New York, NY 10021
Phone: (212) 689-2600

Publications available.

Emotions Anonymous
P.O. Box 4245
St. Paul, MN 55104
Phone: (612) 647-9712

Telecommunications services: Telephone referrals to local chapters.
Publications available.

National Depressive and Manic Depressive Association
222 South Riverside Plaza
Chicago, IL 60606
Phone: (312) 993-0066

Telecommunications services: Offers information, one-to-one support, referrals.
Publications available.

DIABETES

Other Names: Diabetes mellitus; insulin-dependent diabetes mellitus (IDDM), type I; non-insulin-dependent diabetes mellitus (NIDDM), type II

Prevalence in USA: Approximately 10 million: 6 million known, 4 million undiagnosed; 2% to 4% of the population, with a 6% increase (new cases) annually.

Age Group: Under 18 years—90,000; 18 to 44 years—880,000; 45 to 64 years—2.6 million; 65 to 74 years—1.6 million; 75 years and over—800,000.

Male to Female Ratio: Type I—same incidence in men and women. Type II—greater incidence in women.

Principal Features: A disorder of carbohydrate, protein and fat metabolism that renders the body unable to convert foods properly into energy for vital functions.

Type I (10% to 15% of All Diabetes): Occurs most commonly in children and adolescents, with peak onset from 11 to 14 years; can begin at any age. Individuals are usually thin or normal weight (nonobese). Requires lifelong insulin for control of blood sugar and prevention of acidosis.

Type II (85% to 90% of All Diabetes): Most common after 40 years of age, with peak onset from 45 to 64 years. Up to 90% of individuals are obese. Does not require lifelong insulin for control; not prone to development of acidosis.

Characteristic symptoms include excessive hunger and thirst, excessive urination, unexplained weight loss, blurred vision, fatigue, itching of skin, anal and vaginal yeast infections and delayed healing of wounds.

Causes: Primary causes are unknown, but a genetic (hereditary) predisposition appears certain for both types of diabetes. In addition, some individuals who develop type I diabetes may have a genetic susceptibility to viral infection of the pancreas that initiates destruction of the tissue cells that produce insulin. In type I diabetes the pancreas produces very little or no insulin. In type II diabetes insulin production may be normal or partially reduced, but not absent; the diabetes is due to insulin resistance in body tissues.

Drugs That Can Cause This Disorder: In susceptible individuals and those with latent diabetes, the following drugs may induce diabetic manifestations; these are usually mild in nature and reversible:

cortisonelike steroids	phenothiazines
ethacrynic acid	phenytoin
furosemide	propranolol
indomethacin	thiazide diuretics
lithium	tricyclic antidepressants
oral contraceptives	

Drugs Used to Treat This Disorder

The Insulins: See Drug Profile of Insulin in Section Three.

The Sulfonylureas (Oral Hypoglycemic Drugs)

- acetohexamide (Dymelor).
- chlorpropamide (Diabinese).
- glipizide (Glucotrol).
- glyburide (Diabeta, Micronase).

- tolazamide (Tolinase).
- tolbutamide (Orinase).

New Drugs in Development for Treating This Disorder: Nazlin, a nasal insulin product, is now in clinical trials to evaluate its effectiveness and determine proper dosage. This dosage form will be absorbed through the nose, providing rapid absorption that more closely resembles the body's natural release of insulin.

Goals of Drug Treatment

Normalization of carbohydrate, protein and fat metabolism insofar as possible; control of blood sugar; elimination of acidosis.

Elimination of symptoms; restoration of well-being.

Prevention of hypoglycemia (insulin "shock").

Prevention of recurrent acidosis.

Promotion of normal growth and development in diabetic children.

Prevention or minimization of late complications.

Achievement of normal life expectancy.

Drug Management

General Principles

"Good control" consists of the optimal balance of properly selected foods, exercise and drugs—either insulin or a sulfonylurea in correct dosage. The degree of control is estimated by periodic measurement of blood-sugar levels or urine sugar content.

"Tight control" consists of maintaining a fasting blood sugar between 100 and 140 mg, and a 2-hour (after eating) blood sugar betweeen 100 and 200 mg. Consideration must be given to the possible benefits of "tight control" versus the possible risks of inducing hypoglycemia.

"Tight control" is appropriate for the young diabetic who is otherwise healthy, free of coronary artery and cerebral circulatory disease, capable of excellent self-care and not living alone. It is not appropriate for the elderly, those with circulatory disorders of the brain or heart, those with established complications of long-standing diabetes and those with other serious disorders.

Although more expensive and inconvenient, the home monitoring of blood-sugar levels is the method of choice for managing diabetic control. The blood-sugar strips Chemstrip bG and Visidex II are recommended for this purpose.

The use of urine-testing strips for the detection of urine sugar and ketones is a useful and practical alternative to the use of blood-sugar strips. Regular testing of urine before meals and at bedtime provides adequate information for the proper adjustment of insulin dosage schedules and the prevention of hypoglycemia and acidosis. Accuracy is improved when the bladder is first emptied and the urine for testing is collected 30 minutes later; the sugar content of this second voiding is more representative of the current blood-sugar level.

If urine testing reveals the repeated presence of ketones, consult your physician promptly.

The following drugs can cause a *false positive* test result for urine sugar when using Clinitest: aspirin (with doses larger than 2400 mg/day), ascorbic acid (vitamin C), cephalosporins, chloral hydrate, chloramphenicol, isoniazid, levodopa, methyldopa, nalidixic acid, penicillin G, probenecid, streptomycin.

The following drugs can cause a *false negative* test result for urine sugar when using Diastix or Testape: aspirin (with doses larger than 2400 mg/day), ascorbic acid (vitamin C), levodopa, methyldopa.

The following drugs can cause a *false positive* test result for urine ketones when using Acetest or Ketostix: aspirin (in moderate to high doses), levodopa, phenazopyridine (Ketostix only).

Learn to recognize the early indications of hypoglycemia and what to do to correct it. Signs that warn of a developing insulin reaction include hunger, sweating, headache, dizziness, nervousness, trembling, blurred vision, drowsiness, confusion, inability to think, sense of inebriation. At the first indication of impending hypoglycemia, take sugar immediately: 5 small sugar cubes; or 2 teaspoonsful or 2 packets of granulated sugar; or ½ to 1 cup of fruit juice; or 1 candy bar. An alternative treatment is the injection of 1 mg of glucagon, repeated in 5 to 10 minutes if necessary. Glucagon is a pancreatic hormone that increases the level of blood sugar.

Learn to recognize the early indications of acidosis. These include the slow development of increasing thirst, excessive urination, drowsiness, fatigue, nausea, vomiting, stomach pain.

The use of beta-blocking drugs (especially in high doses) may predispose to hypoglycemia and mask its symptoms.

For Type I, IDDM

Insulin is a lifelong requirement for control. Sulfonylureas (oral hypoglycemics) are not effective and should not be used.

Insulin requirements will vary continually throughout a lifetime. Therefore, you must learn how to manage your diabetes on a day-by-day basis, modifying insulin types and dosage schedules as necessary, according to the results of regular blood- or urine sugar testing.

For the newly diagnosed diabetic who is not acutely ill and is without complications, the usual American procedure for initiating treatment is to give a single morning dose of 15 to 30 units of an intermediate-acting insulin (NPH or Lente) before breakfast; the dose is then increased by 5 units every 48 hours as required to achieve normal blood-sugar levels. The British method is to start with 6 to 10 units of an intermediate-acting insulin given twice daily, before the morning and evening meals. Either method will relieve most symptoms in 90% of cases within 4 days.

The optimal schedule of insulin injections for regulating the disordered metabolism is determined by periodic monitoring of blood-sugar levels at appropriate times during the 24-hour day. In this way individual patterns of blood-sugar fluctuation and response to insulin can be studied so that the most appropriate types and doses of insulin are given in proper relationship to eating.

A most effective and practical method of providing adequate insulin for the average diabetic is to give a mixture (1 injection) of a rapid-acting insulin (Regular) and an intermediate-acting insulin (NPH or Lente) 20 to 30 minutes before the morning and evening meals, just 2 injections daily. This scheme provides for easy modification of doses of each type of insulin as necessary to obtain smooth control throughout 24 hours.

During periods of stress—infections, injuries, surgery—insulin requirements will increase. Consult your physician for guidance if you have difficulty in making the necessary adjustments of insulin dosage, food intake, etc.

Even during periods of fasting, small amounts of insulin are necessary to control blood sugar and prevent acidosis.

For Type II, NIDDM

Diet is of primary importance and should be tried diligently before starting drugs. Dietary goals are reduction of blood sugar and correction of obesity. Seventy-five percent of cases of Type II diabetes can be controlled by diet alone.

If an adequate trial of dietary management fails, either sulfonylurea drugs (oral hypoglycemics) or insulin may be added to the treatment program. If the blood sugar is only moderately above normal, a sulfonylurea may be tried. If the blood sugar is quite high and the individual is thin, it is best to initiate drug treatment with insulin. After the blood sugar has been stabilized for 3 to 4 weeks, the insulin may be withdrawn and a sulfonylurea may be started to determine its effectiveness.

The major reaction to sulfonylureas is hypoglycemia. It is most likely to occur in the elderly, in alcoholics and in those with significant impairment of liver or kidney function. Hypoglycemic reactions occur most frequently with the use of chlorpropamide (Diabinese), the longest acting sulfonylurea.

If you experience a primary failure (on initial trial) or a secondary failure (after a temporary period of effectiveness) on attempting control with a sulfonylurea, you may need insulin to manage your diabetes successfully.

Insulin is used primarily to control the levels of blood sugar. It is not required to prevent acidosis except under stressful conditions, such as infections, trauma or surgery.

Type II diabetes is often well controlled with a single daily dose of an intermediate-acting insulin. Some individuals with a high degree of insulin resistance may require unusually high doses of insulin to achieve satisfactory control.

Use of Insulins

1. Twenty percent of all diabetics require insulin for satisfactory control.
2. Available insulins differ in their times of peak action and duration of action. An understanding of these differences is necessary for planning an insulin schedule and adjusting it to control your in-

Type of insulin	Peak action (hours)	Duration (hours)	Hypoglycemia most likely to occur
Short-acting			
Regular	2–4	5–7	Before lunch
Semilente	2–8	12–16	Before lunch
Actrapid	2.5–5	8	Before lunch
Semitard	7	9	Early afternoon
Velosulin	2–5	8	Before lunch
Humulin R	2–5	6–8	Before lunch
Intermediate-acting			
Lente	8–12	18–28	Late afternoon
NPH	6–12	18–28	Late afternoon
Monotard	7–15	18–24	Late afternoon
Lentard	8–12	16–24	Late afternoon
Insulatard	4–12	16–24	Mid-afternoon
Humulin N	6–12	14–24	Late afternoon
Novolin N	4–12	18–24	Mid-afternoon
Long-acting			
Protamine Zinc	14–24	24–36	During night–early morning
Ultralente	18–24	32–36	During night–early morning
Ultratard	10–28	24–36	During night–early morning

dividual pattern of blood-sugar fluctuations during each 24-hour day. The accompanying table illustrates the characteristics of the three principal types of insulin.

3. The peak action times and the duration of action vary greatly from person to person. Each individual will show variations of absorption from one injection site to another and from day to day. Insulin programs must be tailored to each person individually based on response to trials. All insulin schedules need adjustment from time to time.

4. Most insulin-dependent diabetics require from 20 to 60 units of insulin daily. If the requirement reaches 200 units/day, a marked degree of insulin resistance has developed. This is best treated with highly purified pork insulin or human insulin.

5. Most of the time satisfactory control can be achieved with an intermediate-acting insulin, or with the addition of a short-acting insulin. Regular insulin can be mixed with either Lente or NPH in the same syringe and given as a single injection. The mixture retains the short and intermediate characteristics of action.

6. Long-acting insulins are rarely necessary and are seldom used.

7. Hypoglycemia that occurs during the night (excessive insulin effect) causes a "rebound" hyperglycemia that is detected by blood- or urine sugar testing the next morning. This is known as the Somogyi effect. The proper adjustment is to reduce the dose of the long-

acting insulin taken in the morning or the dose of the intermediate-acting insulin taken before the evening meal; this will prevent the nocturnal hypoglycemia that causes the confusing high blood or urine sugar on arising.

8. If a true allergy to insulin develops, or if the fatty tissue under the skin at the sites of insulin injection should disappear (lipoatrophy), change to highly purified pork or human insulin.

9. If insulin use is to be intermittent (as in some cases of type II diabetes), it is best to use human insulin to reduce the possibility of developing insulin antibodies that cause insulin resistance.

10. Insulin pumps using either Regular or Ultralente insulin have been developed for use in selected individuals. While they are capable of providing excellent control, their use is quite complex and demanding. They are suitable only for the highly motivated and educated individual who needs and is dedicated to achieving "tight control."

Use of Sulfonylureas (Oral Hypoglycemic Drugs)

1. These drugs are used only for the treatment of type II, NIDDM, in those whose diabetes is not adequately controlled by diet and exercise and who cannot or will not take insulin.

2. The best candidates for a trial of sulfonylureas
   - are over 50 years old.
   - are otherwise healthy.
   - are not allergic to "sulfa" drugs.
   - have no tendency to develop acidosis.
   - have an insulin requirement of less than 30 units/day.
   - prefer tablets by mouth to injections.

3. Sulfonylureas are not suitable for treating
   - type I, insulin-dependent diabetes.
   - the acutely ill diabetic with acidosis.
   - the diabetic with infection or with injury, or undergoing surgery.
   - the diabetic using long-term cortisonelike steroids.
   - the pregnant diabetic.
   - the diabetic whose blood sugar is over 300 mg.

4. Sulfonylureas should be used with caution in treating
   - the very old.
   - alcoholics.
   - those taking multiple drugs.
   - those with significantly impaired liver or kidney function.
   - those who comply poorly with recommendations.

5. Recommended dosage schedules:

Short-acting	Duration	Doses/day
tolbutamide	6–12 hrs.	2–3

Intermediate-acting

acetohexamide	12–24 hrs.	1–2
glipizide	18–30 hrs.	1–2
glyburide	10–30 hrs.	1–2
tolazamide	10–18 hrs.	1–2

Long-acting

chlorpropamide	60 hrs.	1

6. All sulfonylureas can cause hypoglycemia. Because of its accumulative effects and long period of action, chlorpropamide requires the greatest caution in use; any hypoglycemic reaction is apt to be quite prolonged.
7. Sulfonylureas as a group have a high rate of primary failure (40%). A primary failure is an inability to control hyperglycemia after 3 months of continual treatment with adequate dosage. Secondary failures (25% to 30%) occur when a sulfonylurea drug loses its effectiveness after an initial period of demonstrated ability to control hyperglycemia.
8. During apparently successful long-term use of a sulfonylurea, it is prudent to periodically reduce the dosage and gradually withdraw the drug to determine if its continued use is justified. The success rate of adequate control by long-term use of sulfonylureas is no more than 20% to 30%.
9. There appears to be no general support for the concurrent use of sulfonylureas and insulin. If it is found that insulin is necessary for adequate control, the customary practice is to discontinue the sulfonylurea.

Ancillary Drug Treatment (as required)

Condition	*Drug Treatment*
For yeast infections of skin:	ciclopirox (Loprox)
	clotrimazole (Lotrimin)
	haloprogin (Halotex)
	miconazole (Micatin)
	nystatin (Mycostatin)
For yeast infections of the vagina:	clotrimazole (Gyne-Lotrimin, Mycelex-G)
	miconazole (Monistat)
For diabetic diarrhea:	diphenoxylate (Lomotil)
	loperamide (Imodium)
For peripheral neuritis:	carbamazepine (Tegretol) and amitriptyline (Elavil) concurrently
For neurogenic bladder:	bethanechol (Urecholine)
For high blood pressure:	see Profile of Hypertension in this section

Note: Drug selection, dosage and administration schedule must be determined by the physician for each patient individually.

Resources for Additional Information and Services

American Diabetes Association
National Service Center
P.O. Box 25757
1660 Duke Street
Alexandria, VA 22313
Phone: 1-800-232-3472; (703) 549-1500

Publications available.

Joslin Diabetes Center
One Joslin Place
Boston, MA 02215
Phone: 1-800-223-1138; (617) 732-2400

Available 9:00 a.m.–5:00 p.m. EST, M–F. Spanish-speaking counselors available. Offers public information on specific diabetic needs.
Publications available.

Juvenile Diabetes Foundation
432 Park Avenue South, 16th Floor
New York, NY 10016
Phone: 1-800-223-1138; (212) 889-7575

Publications, films, tapes available.

EPILEPSY

Other Names: Seizure disorders, convulsive disorders

Prevalence in USA: Approximately 2 million, 1% of the population.

Age Group: 24% of epileptics are under 18 years of age; 53% are 18 to 44 years; 18% are 45 to 64 years; 4% are 65 to 74 years; 1% is 75 years and older.

Male to Female Ratio: About equal.

Principal Features: True epilepsy is a chronic disorder characterized by recurring seizures lasting from a few seconds to several minutes and requiring specific medication for prevention and control. Sixty-six percent of epileptic patients require lifelong drug therapy. The principal types of epilepsy include:

Tonic-Clonic Seizures (Grand Mal): Sudden attacks that begin with an involuntary cry, followed by a loss of consciousness and falling, violent convulsive movements of the head, trunk and extremities, excessive salivation and sometimes loss of bladder and/or rectal control. The seizure lasts from 1 to 3 minutes. The individual awakens spontaneously, is dazed, confused and exhausted, and usually falls into a deep sleep that lasts several hours. The subject cannot remember the episode.

Absence Seizures (Petit Mal): These begin between 2 and 12 years of age; 90% cease by 20 years; 50% go on to develop tonic-clonic seizures by 20 years. The seizure consists of a sudden, momentary lapse of consciousness lasting several seconds (30 at the most), during which the subject has a blank stare and is oblivious of surroundings; there is no actual loss of consciousness, no fall and no convulsion; there may be a minor twitching of an eyelid or facial muscle, chewing movements or a jerk of a hand or arm. Such episodes may recur more than 100 times a day. Following each seizure, the subject resumes normal functioning as though nothing had happened; the attack is not remembered.

Complex Partial Seizures (Psychomotor or Temporal Lobe Epilepsy): This type comprises 40% of all epilepsies. It consists of sudden alterations of behavior that involve speech, hearing, memory and emotional response. Some episodes begin with an "aura" that may take the form of distorted vision, unpleasant odors, visual and auditory hallucinations and bizarre illusions; the subject may walk about aimlessly, talk irrationally, laugh, engage in purposeless and inappropriate actions, such as striking at walls in anger or fear. When the seizure ends, the subject is confused and does not recall what has happened.

Causes: The actual epileptic seizure is due to a sudden, abnormal and excessive electrical discharge within the brain. Normal electrical impulses of 80/second are suddenly increased to 500/second. In primary epilepsy the basic cause is unknown; there is usually a familial (genetic) predisposition. Secondary epilepsy can be a complication following head injuries, bacterial meningitis and malaria; it is often associated with cerebral palsy, mental retardation, brain tumors and cysts and hydrocephalus.

Drugs That Can Cause This Disorder: The following drugs have been reported to cause seizures or to aggravate existing epileptic disorders:

amphetamines	monoamine oxidase inhibitors
antihistamines	(MAOI's)
chloroquine	nalidixic acid
cimetidine (with large doses in	oral contraceptives
the elderly)	phenothiazines
cycloserine	tricyclic antidepressants
isoniazid	vincristine
metronidazole	

Drugs Used to Treat This Disorder (in order of preference)
Generalized Tonic-Clonic Seizures (Grand Mal)
- phenytoin (Dilantin).
- phenobarbital (Luminal).
- carbamazepine (Tegretol).
- primidone (Mysoline).

Absence Seizures (Petit Mal)
- ethosuximide (Zarontin).
- valproic acid (Depakene).
- trimethadione (Tridione).
- clonazepam (Clonopin).

Complex Partial Seizures (Psychomotor, Temporal Lobe)
- carbamazepine (Tegretol).
- phenytoin (Dilantin).
- primidone (Mysoline).
- clonazepam (Clonopin).
- valproic acid (Depakene).

Goals of Drug Treatment
Complete prevention of seizures if possible (or marked reduction in frequency), with no (or minimal) adverse drug effects.

Restoration of ability to function independently.

Promotion of participation in school, employment and societal activities.

Drug Management
General Principles

Each individual who is subject to epilepsy experiences a pattern of seizures that is unique; the onset, frequency, severity and specific type (or types) of seizures are never exactly the same as those experienced by someone else.

The drugs used to control epilepsy are selected according to the specific type(s) of seizures the patient experiences.

Antiepileptic drugs are not curative; they are used to control seizures—to reduce their frequency and severity. Seizures should be prevented whenever possible; repeated, uncontrolled convulsions can cause significant brain damage.

When the drug of choice is used in adequate dosage to manage a correctly diagnosed type of epilepsy, seizures can be controlled completely in 60% of patients and substantially reduced in another 20%.

In every case a period of trial and error is necessary to find the most effective drug, the optimal dose and the correct timing of use.

Complete control of seizures with one drug is the ideal; this is possible in 85% of cases. If one drug does not give adequate control, a second drug may be added. The first drug may be continued or gradually withdrawn, depending upon individual response.

Dosage schedules are adjusted gradually to achieve the maximum of seizure control with the minimum of drug side-effects.

Because of the wide variation in drug absorption and elimination from person to person, the periodic measurement of drug levels in blood is necessary to determine the optimal dosage for each drug. An attempt is made to establish for each individual that drug level which will ensure freedom from seizures without toxic drug effects. Blood samples for measurement are usually taken just before the morning dose. (See Therapeutic Drug Monitoring in Section One.)

All antiepileptic drugs have toxic effects when taken in large doses; dosage adjustments are often necessary to prevent toxicity. However, the controllable risks of proper use do not justify withholding treatment in view of the much greater risks resulting from uncontrolled repeated seizures.

Birth defects are two to three times higher in children whose parents (father or mother) are using antiepileptic drugs, especially phenytoin, trimethadione and valproic acid. Consult your physician regarding the best course of action for you in managing your epilepsy during pregnancy.

Do not discontinue any antiepileptic drug suddenly unless advised to do so by your physician. Normally the dosage should be reduced gradually over a period of several weeks. Abrupt withdrawal can cause status epilepticus—a prolonged period of continual seizures without interruption.

Any consideration of discontinuing antiepileptic medications permanently should be made jointly with your physician. Such consideration can be made for absence seizures (petit mal) after a period of 2 to 3 years without a seizure. For other types of epilepsy, a period of 3 to 5 years is advisable. Seizures tend to return in 20% to 50% of cases after stopping medication. Any attempt to withdraw medication must be done very gradually over a period of several months.

Use of Phenytoin

1. Used to control all types of epilepsy except absence seizures.
2. A drug blood level within the therapeutic range correlates well with a decrease in seizure frequency and relative freedom from toxic effects.
3. Due to variation of absorbability among available products, it is advisable to stay with the same brand to gain and maintain control.
4. When the daily maintenance requirement has been established, it may be taken in a single dose.
5. Possible adverse effects include a measleslike rash within the first 2 weeks, excessive growth of hair (5%) and enlargement of the gums (30%).
6. Indications of early toxicity include rapid involuntary eye movements (nystagmus), dizziness, unsteadiness, lethargy and slurred speech.
7. If another drug is added for concurrent use, any significant interaction will occur within 6 weeks.

Use of Phenobarbital

1. Used to control all types of epilepsy except absence seizures.
2. Use with caution if liver or kidney function is impaired.
3. Should be taken twice a day with the largest dose at bedtime.
4. More sedative than phenytoin and carbamazepine, but relatively free of long-term adverse effects.
5. Indications of early toxicity include drowsiness, unsteadiness and impaired thinking.

Use of Primidone
1. Closely related to phenobarbital. Used to control all types of epilepsy except absence seizures.
2. Must be taken in divided doses because of its sedative effect.
3. Indications of early toxicity are the same of those for phenobarbital.

Use of Ethosuximide
1. Used to control absence seizures and some myoclonic seizures. About 75% effective in reducing the frequency of absence seizures when used in adequate dosage.
2. Indications of early toxicity include headache, drowsiness and dizziness.

Use of Valproic Acid
1. Used primarily to control both simple and complex absence seizures. Also used adjunctively to control all other types of epilepsy. It may control both absence and tonic-clonic seizures in the same individual.
2. Multiple doses are necessary to maintain 24-hour control.
3. Avoid use in presence of liver disease.
4. A possible side-effect is weight gain.
5. Monitor for indications of liver toxicity.
6. If used concurrently with other antiepileptic drugs, the periodic measurement of blood levels of all drugs being used is necessary to ensure adequate dosage and prevent toxicity.

Use of Carbamazepine
1. Used to control both tonic-clonic seizures and partial complex seizures (psychomotor epilepsy).
2. Should be taken with food to improve absorption.
3. Avoid use in presence of liver disease or impaired function.
4. Indications of early toxicity include double vision, blurred vision, dizziness, unsteadiness and tremor.
5. Routine, periodic, complete blood counts are mandatory to detect early bone marrow toxicity.

Ancillary Drug Treatment (as required)

Condition	*Drug Treatment*
For increased seizures before or after menstruation:	acetazolamide (Diamox)
For anxiety:	benzodiazepines (Tranxene, Valium, etc.)
For depression:	see Profile of Depression in this section

Note: Drug selection, dosage and administration schedule must be determined by the physician for each patient individually.

Resources for Additional Information and Services

American Epilepsy Society
179 Allyn Street, #304

Hartford, CT 06103
Phone: (203) 246-6566

Publications available.

Epilepsy Concern Service Group
1282 Wynnewood Drive
West Palm Beach, FL 33409
Phone: (305) 586-4804

Promotes formation of self-help groups.
Publications and telephone referrals available.

Epilepsy Foundation of America
4351 Garden City Drive, Suite 406
Landover, MD 20785
Phone: 1-800-EFA-1000 (outside MD); (301) 459-3700

Provides a low-cost pharmacy program for members.
Publications and audiovisual materials available.

GLAUCOMA

Other Names: Primary glaucoma, secondary glaucoma

Prevalence in USA: 1.7 million known, an estimated 1 million undiagnosed; 2% of the population over 40 years of age.

Age Group: Under 18 years—13,000; 18 to 44 years—124,000; 45 to 64
years—513,000; 65 to 74 years—534,000; 75 years and over—527,000.

Male to Female Ratio: Under 45 years—same incidence in men and
women; 45 to 64 years—more common in men; 65 years and over—
more common in women.

Principal Features: A chronic disorder characterized by abnormally high
internal eye pressure that destroys the optic nerve and causes partial
to complete loss of vision. Principal types include
Chronic Open-Angle (Simple, Wide-Angle) Glaucoma: The most common
type, a primary glaucoma that is rare in children and young adults;
usually begins after 30. The rise in intraocular pressure is gradual;
the loss of vision is insidious and slowly progressive. Usually both
eyes are affected. Characteristic symptoms include blurring of vision,
frequent need for change of glasses, occasional headache, colored
halos seen around electric lights and impaired visual adaptation to
the dark.
Acute/Chronic Angle-Closure (Narrow-Angle, Closed-Angle) Glaucoma: A primary glaucoma that usually occurs after 60. The acute glaucoma attack begins in one eye; the rise in intraocular pressure is sudden and
dramatic. Within a few hours the patient experiences severe head-

ache, throbbing eye pain, blurred vision, halos around lights, tearing, swollen eyelids, nausea and vomiting. Initially the episode may be misdiagnosed as an acute abdominal disorder, such as gallbladder disease. Attacks of lesser severity can recur in chronic fashion.

Secondary Glaucoma: The rise in intraocular pressure is a consequence of a preexistent condition, such as infection (uveitis), eye tumor, enlarged cataract or long-term treatment with cortisonelike drugs. Headache, halos and blurred vision occur in proportion to the degree and duration of increased pressure.

Causes: Increased intraocular pressure is due to an imbalance between production and drainage of the liquid (aqueous humor) in the front portion of the eye; obstruction to normal drainage is the main mechanism. The primary types of glaucoma occur in individuals with hereditary predisposition, but specific initiating causes responsible for the rise in pressure are not known. Secondary types of glaucoma are associated with other eye disorders: uveitis, tumors, cataracts, hemorrhage, injury. "Steroid responders" develop increased pressure after 1 to 8 weeks of using cortisonelike steroids.

Drugs That Can Cause This Disorder: The following drugs do not cause true, permanent glaucoma, but they can increase intraocular pressure and thereby precipitate an attack of acute angle-closure glaucoma or aggravate chronic open-angle glaucoma:

amyl nitrite	nitroglycerin
atropine and atropinelike drugs	phenylephrine
cortisonelike drugs	tolazoline
epinephrine	tricyclic antidepressants
isosorbide dinitrate	

Drugs Used to Treat This Disorder

Eye Drops/Inserts (for Local Effects)
- carbachol (Carbacel, Isopto Carbachol).
- demecarium (Humorsol).
- dipivefrin (DPE, Propine).
- echothiopate (Phospholine).
- epinephrine (Epifrin, Epitrate, Glaucon, Lyophrin).
- phenylephrine (Neo-Synephrine, Ocusol).
- pilocarpine solution (Almocarpine, Isoptocarpine, etc.).
- pilocarpine inserts (Ocuserts Pilo-20, Pilo-40).
- timolol (Timoptic).

Internal Medications (for Systemic Effects)
- acetazolamide (Diamox).
- glycerine (Glyrol, Osmoglyn).

Goals of Drug Treatment

Prompt reduction of intraocular pressure in acute angle-closure glaucoma; stabilization of eye status in preparation for corrective eye surgery.

Gradual reduction and long-term normalization of intraocular pressure in chronic, simple, open-angle glaucoma.

Prevention of optic nerve damage; preservation of vision.

Drug Management
General Principles
Drug treatment cannot cure but can control glaucoma.

Factors that can increase intraocular pressure and reduce the effectiveness of drugs include emotional stress (anger, fear, worry); heavy physical exertion; straining with defecation; tight collars, belts and girdles; upper respiratory infections.

Periodic measurement of intraocular pressure is most advisable during long-term use of cortisonelike steroid drugs, especially eye drops and ointments.

Soft contact lens can act as a drug reservoir for pilocarpine (when administered in eye-drop solutions).

Some individuals cannot use pilocarpine Ocuserts successfully; some cannot retain them in the eye, and the loss may be unnoticed; some cannot tolerate the foreign-body sensation.

Pilocarpine is the pupil-constricting (miotic) drug of choice for use in the elderly. The stinging sensation felt on initial use usually disappears with continued application. Some blurring of distant vision is unavoidable.

Timolol (a beta blocker) is as effective as pilocarpine in treating open-angle and secondary glaucoma; twice daily dosage (every 12 hours) is usually sufficient; it should be used very cautiously in those with asthma, slow heart rates or borderline congestive heart failure.

Epinephrine may be used concurrently with pilocarpine (or other miotic drugs) for greater effectiveness in reducing intraocular pressure; it is important that the pilocarpine be used first and be allowed to act for 5 minutes before using epinephrine. Avoid use in presence of high blood pressure (hypertension). Do not use discolored solutions of epinephrine.

Acetazolamide is usually reserved for glaucoma that is unresponsive to eye drops alone. Effectiveness is improved when both are used concurrently.

For Chronic Open-Angle Glaucoma
Eye drops: pilocarpine, timolol, carbachol, epinephrine, dipivefrin, demecarium.

Internal medications: acetazolamide.

Most cases are controlled by eye drops alone.

Treatment is started with the weakest strength; the most effective strength and dosage schedule are determined by trial and error.

Acetazolamide is not used routinely; it is added after an adequate trial of eye drops fails to maintain normal intraocular pressure.

For Acute Angle-Closure Glaucoma (Acute Attack)
Eye drops: pilocarpine, timolol.

Internal medications: glycerine and water mixture, acetazolamide.

The initial treatment is designed to lower intraocular pressure as rapidly as possible to prevent irreversible damage to the optic nerve. Eye drops and internal medications are used concurrently. The combination can reduce the pressure rapidly and abort the acute attack. The ultimate treatment for this condition is surgical.

For Chronic, Recurrent Episodes of Subacute Angle-Closure Glaucoma
Eye drops: pilocarpine and timolol concurrently.
Internal medications: glycerine and water; acetazolamide is used only during the acute phase, not long-term.
The ultimate treatment is surgical.

For Secondary Glaucoma
Eye drops: atropine, cortisonelike steroids.
Internal medications: cortisonelike steroids, acetazolamide.
When appropriate, corrective treatment is directed at the primary eye disorder that is causing increased intraocular pressure.

For Cortisone-Induced Glaucoma
Discontinue all cortisonelike steroids if possible.
Eye drops: pilocarpine, timolol, demecarium.
Internal medications: acetazolamide.

Ancillary Drug Treatment (as required)

Condition	*Drug Treatment*
For itching, burning, redness of eyes:	naphazoline (Naphcon, Privine, Vasoclear) tetrahydralazine (Visine)

Note: Drug selection, dosage and administration schedule must be determined by the physician for each patient individually.

Resources for Additional Information and Services

Foundation for Glaucoma Research
490 Post Street, Suite 1042
San Francisco, CA 94102
Phone: (415) 986-3162

Publications available.

National Society to Prevent Blindness
National Center for Sight
500 East Remington Road
Schaumburg, IL 60173
Phone: 1-800-221-3004; (312) 843-2020

Available 9:00 a.m.–4:00 p.m. CST, M–F.
Answers questions about vision problems.
Provides publications and films on specific problems and conditions.

GOUT

Other Names: Gouty arthritis, podagra (gouty arthritis of the big toe), hyperuricemia (abnormally high blood uric acid)

Prevalence in USA: Approximately 2.3 million, 2.8% of males in middle age. Hyperuricemia occurs in 5% to 10% of the population; 1% to 2% will have gout manifestations during a lifetime.

Age Group: Under 18 years—12,000; 18 to 44 years—316,000; 45 to 64 years—1.01 million; 65 to 74 years—494,000; 75 years and over—396,000.

Male to Female Ratio: Approximately 95% in men, 5% in women.

Principal Features: Gout consists of a group of related disorders having a single underlying feature—abnormally high blood levels of uric acid; this is referred to as hyperuricemia and implies a blood level of more than 7.0 mg of uric acid per 100 ml of blood. (The normal ranges generally recognized are 2.5 to 8.0 mg for men and 1.5 to 7.0 mg for women.) During the early years of primary (genetic) gout, hyperuricemia may exist without any symptoms to indicate its presence. During a lifetime, a small minority of these individuals will experience recurrent acute attacks of severe joint pain with tender swelling (usually one joint in an upper or lower limb), episodes of kidney stones, serious impairment of kidney function or the development of tophi—localized deposits of uric acid salts in the skin, on earlobes, on tendons and bones in and around joints (tophaceous gout).

Causes: Primary gout is due to an inherited defect in the metabolism of purines—end products of protein digestion. In approximately 10% of cases the defect results in an overproduction of uric acid; in 90% the defect is responsible for decreased excretion of uric acid by the kidneys. Either defect causes hyperuricemia. When tissue fluids cannot dissolve excessive levels of uric acid (due to saturation), uric acid crystals are deposited in joints (acute arthritis), kidneys (kidney damage and stone formation) and in soft tissue (tophi).

Drugs That Can Cause This Disorder: The following drugs can raise the blood level of uric acid and precipitate acute gouty arthritis in susceptible individuals:

acetazolamide	furosemide
alcohol	levodopa
antineoplastic drugs	nicotinic acid
aspirin (less than 2 grams/day)	pyrazinamide
ethacrynic acid	thiazide diuretics
ethambutol	triamterene

Drugs Used to Treat This Disorder

For Reducing Blood and Tissue Levels of Uric Acid
- allopurinol (Lopurin, Zyloprim).
- probenecid (Benemid).
- sulfinpyrazone (Anturane).

For Treating and Preventing Acute Attacks of Arthritis
- colchicine.
- fenoprofen (Nalfon).
- ibuprofen (Advil, Motrin, Nuprin, Rufen).
- indomethacin (Indocin).
- naproxen (Naprosyn).
- oxyphenbutazone (Oxalid).
- phenylbutazone (Azolid, Butazolidin).
- piroxicam (Feldene).
- prednisone (Deltasone, Meticorten, Orasone, etc.).
- sulindac (Clinoril).
- tolmetin (Tolectin).

Goals of Drug Treatment

Prompt relief of symptoms of acute attack of gouty arthritis.

Maintenance of blood uric acid level below 6 mg/100 ml. (Prevention of recurrent attacks of acute arthritis, kidney stone formation, kidney damage and tophi formation.)

Dissolution of existing tophi.

Drug Management

General Principles

Only 20% of individuals with hyperuricemia will develop manifestations of gout during their lifetime. At present there is no way of identifying those who will.

Gouty arthritis is the most responsive to treatment and the most easily controlled of all types of arthritis.

The patient and physician together should determine by trial and error which drug is most effective and acceptable for treating acute attacks of gouty arthritis.

After the acute attack of arthritis has subsided, minor symptoms may persist for 2 to 3 months. If maintenance treatment with antigout drugs is started, it is advisable to use low-dose colchicine concurrently to prevent recurrent flare-ups.

Measurement of the amount of uric acid in a 24-hour collection of urine can identify the overproducer of uric acid (greater than 800 mg) and the underexcretor (less than 800 mg). The overproducer is best treated with allopurinol; the underexcretor is best treated with probenecid or sulfinpyrazone.

Authorities differ on whether and when to initiate long-term treatment for hyperuricemia. Conservative opinion: initiate drug therapy only after 2 or more episodes of gouty arthritis or kidney stone within a year. Many first attacks are not followed by recurrent episodes. Withholding long-term treatment avoids the risks of adverse drug reactions. Aggressive opinion: initiate drug therapy after the first episode of gouty arthritis or kidney stone to prevent recurrent attacks and reduce the risks of kidney damage and tophi formation. Hyperuricemia is often present for 20 years or more before the first attack; bone, cartilage and kidney damage may already have occured. The risks of untreated hyperuricemia are thought to exceed the risks of long-term drug therapy. The prudent physician will consider the pros and cons of each case individually and make the decision jointly with the patient.

Once long-term treatment is started with allopurinol and/or probenecid or sulfinpyrazone, it should be maintained for life. Start-stop treatment has no lasting benefit and may precipitate acute attacks. Low-dose colchicine should be taken preventively until the uric acid blood level is stabilized below 6.0 mg/100ml and there have been no acute attacks for 6 to 12 months.

Acute attacks of gouty arthritis can be precipitated by injury, surgery, systemic infections and severe medical illnesses. Colchicine may be used preventively to minimize acute episodes of arthritis when such events occur.

Patients with kidney stones should use allopurinol to treat hyperuricemia; probenecid and sulfinpyrazone should be avoided because they increase the uric acid content of urine.

Do not take aspirin (or other salicylates) in doses of less than 2 grams while taking probenecid or sulfinpyrazone. It abolishes the effectiveness of these drugs and raises the blood level of uric acid.

Avoid fasting to lose weight; fasting can raise the blood level of uric acid. Treat obesity by long-term reduction of food intake and gradual loss of weight.

While taking antigout drugs on a regular basis, drink 2 to 3 quarts of liquids daily to ensure a copious flow of dilute urine.

Use of Allopurinol

1. Used to lower the blood level of uric acid by reducing its formation. Of no value in treating the acute attack, and should not be started until all symptoms of acute arthritis have subsided.
2. The drug of choice for individuals who
   - are overproducers of uric acid (more than 800 mg/24-hour urine excretion).
   - are over 60 years of age.
   - have impaired kidney function.
   - are subject to kidney stones.
   - have tophi formations.
   - are allergic or overly sensitive to probenecid or sulfinpyrazone.
3. The total daily requirement may be taken in a single dose.
4. Once started, a commitment should be made to a lifetime of continual use.
5. May be combined with all other antigout drugs as appropriate for increased effectiveness.

6. Recommended for use prior to and during chemotherapy or irradiation therapy for selected cancers to counteract resulting hyperuricemia.
7. Serious toxicity is extremely rare.

Use of Colchicine
1. Used to treat acute attacks of gouty arthritis. It does not lower the blood level of uric acid.
2. For the quickest response and best results, treatment should be started as soon as possible after the onset of symptoms. If started within the first 12 hours, colchicine gives effective relief of acute arthritis in 90% of cases.
3. The long-term use of low-dose colchicine is very effective in preventing recurrent acute attacks of gouty arthritis.
4. Its use is recommended during the early months of maintenance therapy with allopurinol and/or probenecid or sulfinpyrazone to prevent flare-ups of acute arthritis.
5. Use with caution and reduce the dose in the presence of liver disease or impaired liver function.
6. Colchicine is destroyed by exposure to light. Be sure your supply is fresh and fully effective.

Use of Indomethacin (and Other Nonsteroidal Anti-inflammatory Drugs)
1. Now considered by many authorities to be the drug(s) of choice for treating acute attacks of gouty arthritis. They relieve pain and inflammation, but do not lower the blood level of uric acid.
2. When given promptly and in adequate dosage, these drugs usually provide relief within 6 to 12 hours and complete recovery in 3 days.
3. Take with food to prevent stomach irritation and indigestion.
4. Avoid in the presence of active peptic ulcer disease. Use with caution in hypertension and congestive heart failure.

Use of Phenylbutazone or Oxyphenbutazone
1. Used to provide prompt relief of acute gouty arthritis. It reduces pain and inflammation effectively, but does not lower the blood level of uric acid.
2. Because of its rare but very serious potential for causing bone marrow depression, this drug should never be used for long-term treatment. Treatment courses of no more than 5 to 7 days are advised.
3. This drug should not be used by the elderly (over 60 years of age).

Use of Prednisone (or Similar Cortisonelike Steroids)
1. Used to abort acute attacks of gouty arthritis. Relieves inflammation, swelling and pain, but does not lower the blood level of uric acid.
2. Should be used only after adequate trials of all other appropriate drugs have failed to relieve the acute attack.
3. "Rebound" attacks are common following withdrawal of steroid medications.
4. Not recommended for frequently repeated or long-term use.

Use of Probenecid or Sulfinpyrazone
1. Used to lower the blood level of uric acid by increasing its excretion in the urine. Of no value in treating the acute attack, and should not be started until acute arthritis has subsided.
2. Best suited for individuals who
   - are underexcretors of uric acid (less than 800 mg/24-hour urine excretion).
   - are under 60 years of age.
   - have good kidney function.
   - have no history of kidney stones.
3. Should not be used by those who
   - are overproducers of uric acid (more than 800 mg/24-hour urine excretion).
   - have impaired kidney function and low urine volume.
   - are subject to kidney stones.
4. Begin treatment with small doses to avoid precipitating an acute attack of arthritis.
5. Must be taken in 2 to 4 doses/day.
6. If the tolerance of either drug is limited, the two drugs can be taken concurrently in reduced dosage.
7. Ensure a high intake of liquids (up to 3 quarts daily). Effectiveness is improved by the concurrent use of sodium bicarbonate or potassium citrate.

Ancillary Drug Treatment (as required)

Condition	*Drug Treatment*
For mild pain:	acetaminophen (Tylenol, etc.). Do not use aspirin or other salicylates.
For severe pain:	codeine or meperidine (Demerol)
For diarrhea due to colchicine:	paregoric or loperimide (Imodium)
For high blood pressure:	see Profile of Hypertension in this section
For "secondary" gout due to chemotherapy for leukemia, lymphoma, multiple myeloma, polycythemia:	allopurinol (Zyloprim)

Note: Drug selection, dosage and administration schedule must be determined by the physician for each patient individually.

Resources for Additional Information and Services

Arthritis Foundation
1314 Spring Street, N.W.

Atlanta, GA 30309
Phone: (404) 872-7100
Publications available.

Association for People With Arthritis
P.O. Box 954
6 Commercial Street
Hicksville, NY 11802
Phone: 1-800-323-2243
Publications available.

HYPERTENSION

Other Names: Arterial hypertension, essential hypertension, primary hypertension, secondary hypertension high blood pressure

Prevalence in USA: 26.5 million—15% of adult white population; 25% of adult black population.

Age Group: Under 18 years—184,000; 18 to 44 years—5.6 million; 45 to 64 years—10.8 million; 65 to 74 years—6 million; 75 years and over—3.8 million.

Male to Female Ratio: Under 45 years—same incidence in men and women; 45 to 64 years—slightly more common in women; 65 years and over—more common in women (2 to 1).

Principal Features: During the early years of high blood pressure there are usually no symptoms. Brief periods of sudden elevation of blood pressure above usual levels may cause throbbing headaches and/or dizziness. After years of untreated high blood pressure, manifestations of "target organ" disease include stroke (blood clot or hemorrhage in the brain), impaired vision (retinal hemorrhage and deterioration), heart attack (myocardial infarction), congestive heart failure and kidney failure (uremia).

Causes: In primary (essential) hypertension (95% of all hypertension), no specific cause is apparent. There is a definite hereditary predisposition; 80% of hypertensive individuals have a close relative with high blood pressure. In those who are genetically susceptible, obesity and high salt intake contribute significantly to the development of hypertension. Secondary hypertension (5% of all hypertension) is due to a demonstrable (and sometimes curable) cause: narrowing of the main artery to one or both kidneys, chronic kidney disease, adrenalin or renin producing tumors, coarctation of the aorta.

Drugs That Can Cause This Disorder: The following drugs (or drug combinations) can cause significant elevations of blood pressure:

amphetamines and related drugs
carbenoxolone
ephedrine
ergot preparations
licorice
oral contraceptives
phenylephrine
phenylpropanolamine
pseudoephedrine
tricyclic antidepressants taken
 concurrently with appetite
 suppressants, decongestants
 or antihistamines

Drugs Used to Treat This Disorder
Diuretics
- thiazides (see Drug Class, Section Four).
- chlorthalidone (Hygroton).
- quinethazone (Hydromox).
- metolazone (Diulo, Zaroxolyn).
- indapamide (Lozol).
- bumetanide (Bumex).
- furosemide (Lasix).
- *potassium-saving diuretics:* amiloride (Midamor); spironolactone (Aldactone); triamterene (Dyrenium).

Drugs Acting on the Sympathetic Nervous System
Beta-Adrenergic-Blocking Drugs
- acebutolol (Sectral).
- atenolol (Tenormin).
- labetalol (Normodyne, Trandate).
- metoprolol (Lopressor).
- nadolol (Corgard).
- penbutolol (Levatol).
- pindolol (Visken).
- propranolol (Inderal).
- timolol (Blocadren).

Alpha-Adrenergic-Blocking Drugs
- prazosin (Minipres).
- terazosin (Hytrin).

Centrally Acting Drugs (in the Brain)
- clonidine (Catapres).
- guanabenz (Wytensin).
- guanfacine (Tenex).
- methyldopa (Aldomet).

Peripherally Acting Drugs (in Peripheral Blood Vessels)
- guanadrel (Hylorel).
- guanethidine (Ismelin).
- reserpine (Serpasil).

Direct Vasodilators
- hydralazine (Apresoline).
- minoxidil (Loniten).

Calcium Channel-Blocking Drugs
- diltiazem (Cardizem).
- nicardipine (Cardene).
- nifedipine (Procardia).
- verapamil (Calan, Isoptin).

Angiotensin Converting Enzyme (ACE) Inhibitors
- captopril (Capoten).
- enalapril (Vasotec).
- lisinopril (Prinivil, Zestril).

Goals of Drug Treatment

Maintenance of blood pressure below 140/90, or as close as possible to this level with an acceptable program of drug therapy (minimal drug side-effects and expense).

Prevention or postponement of "target organ" disease in the brain, retina (eye), heart, major blood vessels and kidneys.

Drug Management

General Principles

Although hypertension is difficult to define precisely, blood pressure is considered to be abnormally high if the systolic level is 140 or above or the diastolic level is 90 or above.

Hypertension may be classified as follows:

Diastolic pressure less than 85—normal
Diastolic pressure of 85 to 89—high normal
Diastolic pressure of 90 to 104—mild hypertension
Diastolic pressure of 105 to 114—moderate hypertension
Diastolic pressure of 115 or above—severe hypertension
Systolic pressure less than 140—normal
Systolic pressure of 140 to 159—borderline systolic hypertension
Systolic pressure of 160 or above—systolic hypertension

Most men who develop primary hypertension will have a diastolic pressure of 90 or above by age 35, most women by age 40 to 45.

An adequate program of drug therapy for hypertension will postpone serious disability and death for most hypertensive individuals.

The selection of antihypertensive drugs for initial treatment is based upon the range of the abnormally high pressures recorded on repeated measurements *and* the status of the "target organs" (brain, heart, kidneys and blood vessels) at the time hypertension is discovered.

One practical and effective approach to drug therapy for hypertension initiates treatment with a single drug and adds stronger drugs in stepwise fashion as needed to control blood pressure:

Step 1 begin treatment with — either a diuretic or a beta blocker drug.

Step 2 if necessary, add — clonidine, methyldopa or prazosin (or a diuretic or a beta blocker if not used in Step 1)

Step 3 if necessary, add   hydralazine, a calcium channel
                                blocker or an ACE inhibitor
Step 4 if necessary, add   guanethidine or minoxidil

For most individuals, the initial drug treatment will normalize blood
pressure within the first 2 months. Up to 60% of cases are controlled
with a diuretic alone; 50% can be controlled with a beta blocker
alone. From 70% to 80% of all hypertensive individuals will achieve
satisfactory blood pressure control by compliance with Step 1 or Step
2 drug therapy. The majority of the remainder can be controlled by
Steps 3 and 4.

Tranquilizers and sedatives are not effective for lowering elevated blood
pressure and should not be relied upon as primary treatment for hypertension.

Obtain a blood pressure measuring instrument (preferably an aneroid
manometer, arm cuff and stethoscope) and ask your physician to
teach you how to take your own blood pressure. Measurements of
blood pressure made at home (or at work) are far more representative
of your actual day-by-day pressures than are readings made in the
physician's office. By taking your own blood pressure at home, at
work and at varying times and under different circumstances, you
can create a record that clearly reflects your response to the antihypertensive drugs prescribed for you.

Read the Drug Profiles (Section Three) of the drugs you are taking. If
you think you may be experiencing any of the side-effects or adverse
effects listed in the Profile, discuss this with your physician so appropriate adjustments can be made. It is to your benefit to work along
with your physician until a satisfactory selection of drugs is reached.

Avoid isometric exercises—body building, weight lifting, push-ups;
these raise the blood pressure significantly. Consult your physician
regarding the advisability of isotonic exercises—walking, bicycling,
swimming.

Consumption of more than 2 ounces of alcohol daily can raise the blood
pressure. One ounce of alcohol is present in 2 ounces of 100-proof
whiskey, in 8 ounces of wine, or in 24 ounces of beer.

Five percent of oral contraceptive users will develop a diastolic blood
pressure of over 90. If this occurs, the contraceptive pill should be
discontinued for 6 months and the blood pressure monitored. Women
with this sensitivity should use an alternative method of contraception.

The elderly individual with hypertension must approach antihypertensive drug therapy very cautiously. Goals of drug treatment
are more liberal; reduction of pressures to 140–160/95–100 are usually adequate. This can usually be achieved with small doses of a
diuretic. If a Step 2 drug is needed, methyldopa is better tolerated
than the other choices. However, the response to all drugs must be
observed closely. Drugs that cause emotional depression in the young
individual can cause symptoms in the elderly that closely resemble
senile dementia.

In type I diabetes, thiazides are well tolerated, but beta blockers may mask the symptoms of hypoglycemia. In type II diabetes, thiazides are best avoided; small doses of furosemide or spironolactone are preferable. Beta blockers can impair insulin release.

After blood pressure has been well controlled for a year, consideration may be given to a "step-down" reduction of both drug dosage and the number of drugs used. The blood pressure response to the gradual withdrawal of drugs must be monitored very carefully. A recent study showed that 28% of the group of hypertensives studied had normal blood pressure one year after discontinuing all antihypertensive medication. Your physician can determine if and when you meet the criteria for attempting to discontinue your program of drug treatment.

Treatment of Hypertension According to Severity

For Borderline Hypertension (120–160/90–94)

- Reduce excessive weight.
- Reduce salt intake moderately.
- Reduce stress in daily living.
- Avoid excessive consumption of alcohol.
- Stop smoking.
- Avoid isometric exercise.
- Increase isotonic exercise.
- Defer drug treatment for 3 to 6 months to determine effectiveness of above measures.

For Mild Hypertension (140–160/95–104) (80% of All Hypertensives)

- Urge all of the above measures.
- Begin Step 1 drug treatment: Use a single drug—currently a thiazide diuretic or a beta blocker. Some authorities are now advocating a trial of a calcium channel blocker or an ACE inhibitor for initiating treatment.

For Moderate Hypertension (140–180/105–114)

- Begin with Step 2 drug treatment; it is not likely that a single drug will control this degree of hypertension.
- A diuretic will enhance the effectiveness of a beta blocker, a calcium channel blocker, or a centrally acting drug.

For Severe Hypertension (160+/115+)

- Adequate control may require Step 3 or Step 4 drug treatment. When multiple drugs are used, smaller doses of individual drugs are often effective and better tolerated. A trial-and-error approach is often necessary to determine the most effective and acceptable combination of drugs.

For Isolated Systolic Hypertension (160+/85–90)

- This is usually found in the elderly. Cautious and conservative drug treatment is recommended for those under age 70.
- Calcium channel-blocking drugs may be very effective for this type of hypertension.
- If a diuretic is used, avoid dehydration and potassium loss.
- If methyldopa is used, monitor for any tendency to depression or dementia.

Use of Diuretics

1. Used as Step 1 or Step 2 drugs, diuretics are most appropriate for treating hypertensives who are black or elderly, those with congestive heart failure or kidney failure and those who cannot use a beta blocker drug.
2. A thiazide diuretic is the initial drug tried in the majority of cases. It is effective in a single dose taken in the morning.
3. While using thiazide diuretics, observe for loss of potassium (10% of users), increased blood level of uric acid (66% of users) and increased blood-sugar level.
4. Spironolactone and triamterene are as effective as thiazides in reducing blood pressure; they are used to prevent potassium loss.
5. The more potent diuretics furosemide and ethacrynic acid are no more effective than the thiazides for reducing blood pressure.
6. The most practical and reliable way to prevent a significant decline in the potassium blood level is to use a potassium-saving diuretic— amiloride, spironolactone or triamterene. The use of high-potassium foods is often unreliable. Compliance with the long-term use of oral potassium supplements is very poor.
7. It is advisable to discontinue the use of diuretics gradually to prevent fluid retention (edema) after withdrawal.

Use of Beta-Adrenergic-Blocking Drugs

1. Used as Step 1 or Step 2 drugs, beta blockers are most appropriate for treating hypertensives who are young, those who have an overactive heart (fast rate, palpitation, premature beats) and those with gout, migraine headaches and angina (coronary artery disease).
2. Avoid beta blockers if you have asthma, emphysema or a history of heart block or congestive heart failure.
3. These drugs characteristically cause fatigue and lethargy. Propranolol and metoprolol can cause emotional depression.
4. When propranolol is used alone, 10% of users can experience an increase in blood pressure. It is advisable to use a diuretic prior to starting propranolol in sensitive individuals.
5. Avoid sudden discontinuation of beta blockers, especially in the presence of coronary artery disease. Abrupt withdrawal can cause rapid heart rate, palpitation and intensification of angina; myocardial infarction has been reported.

Use of Labetalol (an Alpha- and Beta-Adrenergic Blocker)

1. This drug may be effective when the beta blockers have failed to control blood pressure.
2. Functions primarily as a vasodilator in the elderly, with no significant alteration of heart function.
3. Avoid in presence of asthma, emphysema, heart block and congestive heart failure.

Use of Clonidine

1. Characteristically causes drowsiness, fatigue and dry mouth. Is capable of causing depression.

2. Do not discontinue this drug abruptly; sudden withdrawal can cause a severe rebound hypertension with higher blood pressure than prior to treatment. Withdraw over 2 to 4 days.
3. After discontinuation of clonidine, delay the start of a beta blocker drug for 48 hours.

Use of Methyldopa

1. Usually causes lethargy and fatigue at beginning of treatment; these often subside with continued use. Is also capable of causing depression.
2. This drug causes salt and water retention; a diuretic should be taken concurrently.
3. Discontinue this drug if any of the following develop: emotional depression, drug fever, breast enlargement, milk production, indications of liver toxicity (loss of appetite, nausea, jaundice).
4. Sudden discontinuation of this drug can cause agitation, insomnia, rapid heart rate and intensification of angina.

Use of Prazosin

1. In 10% of users, this drug can provoke an idiosyncratic reaction that results in a sudden extreme drop in blood pressure following the first dose. It is advisable to begin treatment with a bedtime dose and a warning to arise cautiously the next morning in anticipation of possible orthostatic hypotension (see Glossary).
2. This drug can cause fluid retention and can aggravate angina. It is best used in conjunction with a diuretic and a beta blocker.
3. Do not use this drug concurrently with hydralazine or guanethidine because of the potential for additive postural hypotension.
4. A rapid loss of effectiveness can limit this drug's long-term usefulness.

Use of Hydralazine

1. This drug is rarely used alone. It can cause fluid retention and should be used concurrently with a diuretic.
2. This drug characteristically increases heart activity, which can be counteracted by the concurrent use of a beta blocker drug.
3. Use cautiously in the presence of angina (coronary artery disease).
4. Monitor for possible development of a lupuslike drug reaction.

Use of Reserpine

1. Limit the daily dose to 0.25 mg or less.
2. Avoid completely if you have a history of depression.
3. This drug can cause salt and water retention; a diuretic should be used concurrently.
4. Do not use this drug concurrently with methyldopa; the combination can cause marked sedation, excessive dreaming and sexual impotence.
5. Observe for the following possible adverse effects: drowsiness, lethargy, depression (can be very insidious), nightmares, nasal congestion, acid indigestion (possible ulcer), diarrhea, impotence, parkinsonlike syndrome.

Use of Guanethidine
1. This is the most potent antihypertensive drug in general use. It is usually reserved to treat the most severe cases of hypertension and those that have been difficult to control.
2. It causes marked orthostatic hypotension. Users should avoid prolonged sitting (without moving the legs) and prolonged standing (without walking around); these are conducive to excessive drops in blood pressure and resultant fainting. Users should also arise cautiously in the morning to avoid fainting shortly after getting out of bed.
3. This drug causes salt and water retention and should be taken concurrently with a diuretic.
4. Tricyclic antidepressants can reduce this drug's antihypertensive effectiveness.

Use of Minoxidil
1. This drug is a potent, long-acting vasodilator. Its use is usually restricted to treating those whose blood pressure cannot be controlled by conventional treatment with other drugs.
2. It is generally used concurrently with a diuretic and a beta blocker drug.
3. Observe for excessive growth of hair.

Use of Calcium Channel-Blocking Drugs
1. These drugs are approved by the U.S. Food and Drug Administration only for use in the management of angina (coronary artery disease). However, they are effective antihypertensives and are being used as such by many physicians.
2. They may be used as Step 1, 2, or 3 drugs in the management of hypertension.
3. They are especially useful in treating the elderly individual with isolated systolic hypertension.
4. Use these drugs with caution if a beta blocker drug is being used concurrently.
5. A dosage of 3 to 4 times daily is required.
6. Observe for fluid retention. Effectiveness is improved if a thiazide diuretic is taken concurrently.

Use of Angiotensin Converting Enzyme (ACE) Inhibitors
1. These may be used as Step 1, 2, 3, or 4 drugs in the management of hypertension.
2. To prevent an excessive drop in blood pressure, any diuretic in use should be discontinued 5 to 7 days before starting an ACE inhibitor. After the dose is stabilized, a diuretic may be resumed if necessary.
3. Captopril should be taken 1 hour before eating, 2 to 3 times daily, for maximal effectiveness. Enalapril may be taken once or twice daily without regard to eating.
4. Full effectiveness of these drugs may not be apparent until after several weeks of continual use.

5. These drugs may increase the blood potassium level. Do not use any commercial salt substitute (most of which contain potassium) without first consulting your physician.

Current Controversies in Drug Management

The standard "stepped-care" approach to treating hypertension usually recommends the use of a thiazide diuretic as the drug of choice to initiate therapy. If an adequate trial with thiazide therapy fails to lower the blood pressure sufficiently, other drugs of the various classes listed above are *added* in a somewhat arbitrary and rigid fashion. While the guidelines provided by a standardized approach were beneficial in promoting rational therapy, new information about the older drugs and the availability of many new and more effective drugs call for a reappraisal of drug selection for managing hypertension.

Recent review of thiazide drug performance discloses that (1) while they are effective in mild hypertension, they have not decreased the incidence of heart attacks; (2) they can cause loss of potassium and/or magnesium and thereby contribute to the development of dangerous heart rhythm disorders; and (3) they cause a 10% increase in LDL cholesterol blood levels and may increase the risk of coronary artery disease. Some authorities no longer consider thiazides to be the drugs of choice for initiating treatment; they also recommend that thiazides be used in the lowest effective dose to reduce the potential risks of long-term therapy.

Current recommendations call for a greater emphasis on individualization of drug management; this includes wider flexibility in selecting drugs for starting treatment and in substituting and deleting drugs as individual monitoring dictates. Several drug classes are admirably suited for initiating treatment and provide a broad spectrum of features that permit tailoring the drug to the individual characteristics of the patient.

Ancillary Drug Treatment (as required)

Condition	*Drug Treatment*
For thiazide-induced gout:	allopurinol (Zyloprim)
	probenecid (Benemid)
For drug-induced fluid retention:	bumetanide (Bumex)
For guanethidine-induced diarrhea:	diphenoxylate (Lomotil)
For tension headache:	acetaminophen (Tylenol, etc.)
For migraine headache (short-term use):	ibuprofen (Motrin, Advil, Nuprin)
	oxycodone (Percodan)
	Avoid ergotamine preparations.

For musculo-skeletal
pain, arthritis (long-
term use):   sulindac (Clinoril)

Note: Drug selection, dosage and administration schedule must be determined by the physician for each patient individually.

Resources for Additional Information and Services

Citizens for the Treatment of High Blood Pressure
888 17th Street, N.W., Suite 904
Washington, DC 20006
Phone: (202) 466-4553

Publications available.

The Joint National Committee on Detection, Evaluation and Treatment of High Blood Pressure
National Heart, Lung and Blood Institute
National Institutes of Health
Box 120/80
Bethesda, MD 20892
Phone: (301) 496-4000

Publication: *The 1988 Report of the Joint National Committee.*

National Institute of Hypertension Studies
13217 Livernois
Detroit, MI 48238
Phone: (313) 931-3427

Publications available.

HYPOTHYROIDISM

Other Names: Hypometabolism, myxedema, primary hypothyroidism, secondary hypothyroidism

Prevalence in USA: 1.9 million—0.8% of the general population; 1 in 5000 newborn infants has hypothyroidism (cretinism).

Age Group: Juvenile hypothyroidism: under 18 years—2% of total incidence. Adult hypothyroidism: percentage of total incidence by age: 18 to 44 years—34%; 45 to 64 years—40%; 65 years and over—24%.

Male to Female Ratio: More common in women—8 to 1.

Principal Features: Hypothyroidism spans a wide spectrum from very mild thyroid hormone deficiency (hypometabolism) with few nonspecific symptoms to severe deficiency (myxedema) that can be fatal if not treated adequately. The most common form of hypothyroidism is the mild to moderate hormone deficiency seen primarily in women age 20 to 65. The onset is usually insidious and the early symptoms are so vague that medical attention is rarely sought. With progression of the deficiency, the subject gradually becomes aware of lethargy, fatigability, intolerance of cold, weight gain (with no increased food intake), loss of hair, vague muscle and joint pains, and irregular menstruation. The skin may become dry and scaly, the face may appear puffy (fluid retention), the speech slows, the voice becomes hoarse and the pattern of activity becomes sluggish. Hypothyroidism in the elderly can cause mental changes, confusion, paranoia, depression and dementia.

Causes: Primary hypothyroidism can be due to (1) a congenital defect in thyroid gland development or function; (2) an "autoimmune" impairment of thyroid hormone production (45% of cases); (3) a lack of iodine in the food or water supply; or (4) intentional thyroid gland suppression by the administration of radioactive iodine or by surgical removal of thyroid tissue (35% of cases). Secondary hypothyroidism is due to inadequate stimulation of thyroid gland function from the hypothalamus (in the brain) or from the pituitary gland (the "master" gland that regulates most hormone-producing glands).

Drugs That Can Cause This Disorder: The following drugs can impair the normal production of thyroid hormones and induce varying degrees of hypothyroidism (see Drug Classes, Section Four):

amiodarone

cyclophosphamide

disulfiram (?)

ethionamide

iodine compounds (iodides)

lithium

methimazole

pentazocine

phenylbutazone

propylthiouracil

sulfonylurea antidiabetic drugs

Drugs Used to Treat This Disorder
- synthetic thyroxine (T-4) (Synthroid, Levothroid).
- synthetic liothyronine (T-3) (Cytomel).
- synthetic liotrix (combinations of T-4 and T-3) (Euthroid, Thyrolar).
- thyroid extract (animal origin) (Dessicated thyroid Armour).
- thyroglobulin (animal origin) (Proloid).

Goals of Drug Treatment

Adequate replacement of thyroxine; restoration of normal blood levels of T-4, T-3 and the Thyroid Stimulating Hormone (TSH).

Relief of symptoms associated with deficiency of thyroid hormones (hypothyroidism, cretinism, myxedema).

Drug Management

General Principles

Primary hypothyroidism is diagnosed by finding the blood level of the principal thyroid hormone—thyroxine (T-4)—below the normal range and the blood level of the pituitary hormone—Thyroid Stimulating Hormone (TSH)—above the normal range.

Once the diagnosis of true primary hypothyroidism is established, treatment for life is generally thought to be necessary. However, periodic evaluation is advisable to determine the need for continual thyroid hormone replacement.

Individuals taking replacement thyroid hormones should be monitored every 6 to 12 months by measurements of T-4 and TSH along with evaluation of general well-being.

Until thyroid deficiency is adequately corrected, the subject may be overly sensitive to drugs that depress brain function—sedatives, tranquilizers, hypnotics, narcotic analgesics.

In treating hypothyroidism of infancy, avoid formula feedings that contain soybean extract; they can prevent the absorption of thyroxine and perpetuate cretinism.

Anxious, thin individuals usually require smaller doses of maintenance thyroxine than lethargic, obese individuals require. Significant reduction in weight (correction of obesity) is usually followed by a reduction in the daily requirement of maintenance thyroxine.

The use of thyroid hormones for weight reduction in the presence of normal thyroid function (no hormone deficiency) is unjustified and dangerous.

Hypothyroidism causes an increase in bone mass. Thyroid replacement therapy can result in a significant loss of bone (osteoporosis) in the lumbar vertebrae (spine). Consult your physician regarding the advisability of taking supplements of calcium and vitamin D during thyroid hormone replacement. (See Profile of Osteoporosis in this section.)

Use of Thyroxine

1. Hypothyroidism is best treated with a synthetic preparation of thyroxine (see Drug Profile, Section Three). This provides replacement that approximates most closely the normal status of thyroid hormones in circulating blood.

2. Young, basically healthy individuals with hypothyroidism may take thyroxine in full dosage—1 microgram per pound of body weight daily. This usually achieves normal blood levels of T-4 and TSH.

3. Older individuals, with incipient or established heart disease, should initiate thyroxine treatment with small doses that can be increased gradually over 2 to 3 months. This reduces the risk of precipitating disturbances of heart function, such as angina and abnormal rhythm.

4. Thyroxine should be taken in the morning on an empty stomach to ensure maximal absorption and uniform effectiveness.

5. Cholestyramine and colestipol can prevent absorption of thyroxine and liothyronine; for best results, take thyroxine (and/or liothyronine) first (preferably in the morning, fasting), 2 to 3 hours before the first daily dose of either cholestyramine or colestipol.

6. Observe for possible seasonal variation in your response to thyroxine replacement therapy. Some individuals may need less in warm months and more in cold months. If the winter dose of thyroxine is somewhat excessive for summer requirements, you may develop nervousness, insomnia, headaches, intolerance of heat and loss of weight. Consult your physician if you think dosage adjustment is necessary.

7. Long-term thyroxine therapy may lead to premature bone loss in the upper femur (thigh bone) in women. Periodic monitoring of thyroxine blood levels is advised to detect excessive dosage.

8. Do not purchase thyroxine tablets in large quantities (such as 500 to 1000). Thyroxine products can lose up to 6% of their potency per year. It is advisable to obtain a 3 to 6 months' supply (100 to 200 tablets) to ensure full-strength medication.

Ancillary Drug Treatment (as required)

Condition	*Drug Treatment*
For anemia:	iron preparations
	vitamin B-12 (if appropriate for type of anemia)
For constipation:	docusate (Colace, Doxinate, etc.)
	docusate with casanthranol (Peri-Colace, etc.)
For muscle or joint ache/ pain:	aspirin
	acetaminophen (Tylenol, Panadol, etc.)
	ibuprofen (Advil, Nuprin, etc.)

Note: Drug selection, dosage and administration schedule must be determined by the physician for each patient individually.

Resource for Additional Information and Services

American Thyroid Association
Mayo Clinic
200 First Street, S.W.
Rochester, MN 55905
Phone: (507) 284-4738

Maintains professional membership directory for geographical referrals.

MENOPAUSE

Other Names: Menopausal syndrome, estrogen withdrawal syndrome, female climacteric, change of life

Prevalence in USA: 12.8 million women (candidates for menopause).

Age Group: 45 to 55 years; the mean age of natural menopause is 50 years.

Principal Features: The term "menopause" refers to the permanent cessation of menstruation. This occurs naturally in most women between 45 and 55 years of age. The characteristic indication of the "change"—altered menstrual pattern with eventual cessation of menstrual periods—usually lasts from 6 to 18 months. The majority of women (85%) experience some physical effects of progressive estrogen withdrawal: recurring hot flushes, episodic sweating, shrinkage of breast tissue, reduction of vaginal secretions and a variety of nervous and emotional symptoms—anxiety, depression, insomnia, headaches, dizziness, nausea. For approximately 25%, the symptoms are of sufficient intensity to warrant a trial of estrogen replacement therapy. Up to 35% of menopausal women experience hot flushes for 5 or more years.

Causes: Natural menopause occurs spontaneously to terminate reproductive capability. Therapeutic menopause follows surgical removal of the uterus or ovaries and irradiation or removal of the pituitary gland.

Drugs That Can Cause This Disorder: The following drugs can cause cessation of menstruation for varying periods of time, sometimes permanently: busulfan, chlorambucil, cyclophosphamide, mechlorethamine, oral contraceptives and vincristine. The antiestrogen drug tamoxifen, used for the treatment of breast cancer, can cause hot flushes, dizziness and menstrual irregularities typical of the menopausal syndrome.

Drugs Used to Treat This Disorder
"Natural-type" estrogens are preferred:
- conjugated estrogens (Genisis, Premarin).
- esterified estrogens (Evex, Menest).
- estradiol cypionate (Depo-Estradiol, injection).
- estradiol valerate (Delestrogen, injection).
- estriol (Hormonin, a mixture of estriol, estradiol, and estrone).
- piperazine estrone sulfate (Ogen).
- micronized 17-B estradiol (Estrace).
- transdermal estradiol skin patch (Estraderm-50 and 100).

Goals of Drug Treatment
Reduction in the frequency and severity of hot flushes and night sweats with attendant insomnia.
Relief of nervous and emotional symptoms.
Prevention or relief of atrophic changes of the vulva, vagina and urethra.
Prevention of thinning of the skin.
Prevention of osteoporosis (long-term treatment).

Drug Management

General Principles

It is now generally held that for the well-informed menopausal woman who has obvious symptoms of estrogen deficiency and does not have any contraindications to its use, the benefits of estrogen replacement therapy outweigh the possible risks. The use of estrogen is considered effective and safe when prescribed appropriately and monitored properly.

As each women reaches the menopausal years (45 to 55), she should assess her own status and perceived needs. Next she should familiarize herself with the benefits and possible risks of estrogen replacement therapy. (See the Drug Profile of Estrogen, Section Three.) If she thinks she needs medical guidance and/or treatment, she should discuss all aspects of her situation with her physician and share in the decision regarding the use of hormones.

A clear indication for the use of estrogen should exist. It should not be given routinely to the menopausal woman, but should be reserved to treat those with symptoms of estrogen deficiency. Estrogen does not retard the natural progression of general aging; it should not be used for the sole purpose of "preserving femininity."

Before estrogen therapy is started, appropriate examinations should be performed and due consideration given to the following possible contraindications to the use of estrogen:

1. Pregnancy
2. History of deep venous thrombosis or pulmonary embolism
3. Present or previous cancer of the breast
4. Cancer of the uterus
5. Strong family history of breast or uterine cancer
6. Current liver disease or previous drug-induced jaundice
7. Chronic gallbladder disease, with or without stones
8. Abnormal elevation of blood fats (cholesterol, triglycerides, etc.)
9. History of porphyria
10. Large uterine fibroid tumors
11. Any estrogen-dependent tumor
12. Combination of obesity, varicose veins and cigarette smoking
13. Diabetes mellitus
14. Severe hypertension

In the young woman experiencing premature menopause (destruction or removal of both ovaries), the *long-term* use of estrogen replacement is justified, provided appropriate precautions are observed (see Guidelines below).

In the menopausal woman experiencing hot flushes and/or atrophic vaginitis, the *short-term* use of estrogen therapy is generally felt to be acceptable with appropriate supervision and guidance. Estrogen replacement therapy provides symptomatic relief; it is not a permanent cure for hot flushes. *Long-term* estrogen therapy for *all* women after the menopause cannot be justified. Treatment must be carefully individualized (see Guidelines below).

It is generally recommended that estrogens be taken cyclically. The customary schedule is from the 1st through the 25th day of each month, with no estrogen during the remaining days of the month. After 6 to 12 months of continuous use, the estrogen dose should be gradually reduced over a period of 2 to 3 months and then discontinued to assess the individual's need for resumption of use.

The lowest effective daily dose of estrogen should be determined and maintained for the duration of the treatment.

Vaginal cream preparations of estrogen may be considered instead of orally administered estrogen if the only indication is atrophic vaginitis. However, it should be noted that these preparations allow rapid absorption of estrogen into the systemic circulation, and do not permit accurate control of dosage. They should be used intermittently and only as needed to correct the symptoms of atrophic vaginitis. (Note: The estrogen in vaginal creams can be absorbed through the skin of the penis and cause tenderness of the breast in men.)

The unnecessary prolongation of estrogen therapy should be avoided. It is advisable to use estrogens in the lowest effective dose and for only as long as necessary to relieve symptoms.

Guidelines for the Use of Estrogens in Specific Deficiency States

I. The young woman (under 45 years of age) with both ovaries and uterus removed:
   1. Choice of estrogen: a conjugated "natural" estrogen (see list of estrogen preparations).
      The lowest effective dose should be used.*
   2. Dosage schedule: once daily from the 1st through the 25th day of each month.
      Note: If the uterus is present, it is advisable to add a progestin (medroxyprogesterone), 4 to 10 mg daily during the last 7 to 10 days of the estrogen course.**
   3. Duration of use: if well tolerated, until 50 years of age, when assessment of continued need is made individually.
   4. Periodic examinations:
      Base-line mammogram (low-radiation-dose xeroradiography); mammogram should be repeated only as necessary to evaluate possible breast tumor (American Cancer Society guideline).
      Self-examination of breasts monthly.
      Physician examination of breasts (and uterus if present) every 6 to 12 months.
      Measurement of blood pressure.

---

*The lowest effective dose is determined by keeping a daily "flush count" to ascertain the lowest daily dose that will reduce the frequency and severity of flushes to an acceptable level.
**The use of a supplemental progestin during the last 7 to 10 days of estrogen administration is still controversial. A possible benefit is the reduced potential for uterine cancer; a possible risk is the increased potential for coronary artery disease; a possible inconvenience is withdrawal bleeding (induced menstruation). The risks of this form of long-term progestin therapy are not known.

II. The woman experiencing the "menopausal syndrome" of hot flushes and sweating (usually 45 to 55 years of age):

A. Uterus not removed

1. Choice of hormones and recommended dosage range:

Estrogen: conjugated equine estrogens—0.3 to 0.625 mg daily. (See list of alternative estrogen preparations.)

Progestin: medroxyprogesterone—5 to 10 mg daily.

The lowest effective dose of estrogen should be used.*

2. Dosage schedule:

Estrogen: once daily from the 1st through the 25th day of each month.

Progestin: once daily during the last 7 to 10 days of the estrogen course.**

3. Duration of use: 6 to 12 months, followed by gradual reduction of dose over a period of 2 to 3 months, and then discontinuation to assess the need for continued use. Treatment should be resumed only if symptoms require it. An attempt should be made to discontinue all hormones after 2 to 3 years of continual use, unless a clear need for continuation is apparent.

4. Periodic examinations:

Base-line mammogram (low-radiation-dose xeroradiography).

Low-dose mammogram annually (over 50 years of age) during continuous use of estrogen (American Cancer Society guideline).

Self-examination of breasts monthly.

Physician examination of breasts every 6 to 12 months.

Cervical cytology and endometrial biopsy (aspiration curettage) annually.

Blood pressure measurement every 3 to 6 months.

Two-hour blood sugar assay annually.

B. Uterus removed

1. Choice of estrogen and dose: conjugated equine estrogens—0.3 to 0.625 mg daily.

The lowest effective dose should be used.*

2. Dosage schedule: once daily from the 1st through the 25th day of each month.

---

*The lowest effective dose is determined by keeping a daily "flush count" to ascertain the lowest daily dose that will reduce the frequency and severity of flushes to an acceptable level.

**The use of a supplemental progestin during the last 7 to 10 days of estrogen administration is still controversial. A possible benefit is the reduced potential for uterine cancer; a possible risk is the increased potential for coronary artery disease; a possible inconvenience is withdrawal bleeding (induced menstruation). The risks of this form of long-term progestin therapy are not known.

3. Duration of use: 6 to 12 months, followed by gradual reduction of dose over a period of 2 to 3 months, and then discontinuation to assess the need for continued use. Treatment should be resumed only if symptoms require it. An attempt should be made to discontinue all hormones after 2 to 3 years of continual use.

4. Periodic examinations:

Base-line mammogram (low-radiation-dose xeroradiography).

Low-dose mammogram annually (over 50 years of age) during continuous use of estrogen (American Cancer Society guideline).

Self-examination of breasts monthly.

Physician examination of breasts every 6 to 12 months.

Blood pressure measurement every 3 to 6 months.

Two-hour blood sugar assay annually.

III. The woman in the "post-menopausal" period (usually over 55 years of age): treatment should be individualized as follows:

1. If there are no specific symptoms of estrogen deficiency (hot flushes or atrophic vaginitis), estrogen should not be given.

2. If specific symptoms of estrogen deficiency persist to a degree requiring subjective relief, the recommendations in category II apply. However, in addition to limiting courses of estrogen to 6 to 12 months followed by gradual withdrawal, dosage might be limited to 3 times weekly on a trial basis. Estrogen should be discontinued altogether as soon as possible. If only flushes persist beyond 60 years of age, all estrogen should be discontinued. Nonhormonal drugs such as clonidine, ergot preparations and certain sedatives may be substituted for the relief of hot flushes.

3. Although we do not yet have accurate and reliable predictive indicators, an attempt should be made to identify the woman who may be at high risk for the development of osteoporosis. The following features suggest the possibility of increased risk:

(1) slender build, light-boned, white or Oriental race

(2) a sedentary life style or restricted physical activity

(3) a family history (mother or sister) of osteoporosis (reported by some investigators)

(4) a low-sodium diet (also likely to be a low-calcium diet)

(5) heavy smoking

(6) excessive use of antacids that contain aluminum

(7) long-term use of cortisone-related drugs

(8) habitual use of carbonated beverages (reported by some investigators)

(9) excessive consumption of alcohol

(10) increased urinary excretion of calcium

For the woman thought to be at increased risk for the development of osteoporosis, estrogen treatment should be started within 3 years after menstruation ceases. The following schedule of estrogen therapy may be recommended for prevention: conjugated equine estrogens— 0.625 mg daily or 3 times weekly, for the first 3 weeks of each month.

Periodic examinations as outlined in category II above should be performed. Estrogen replacement therapy may continue indefinitely, always with appropriate supervision.

In addition to the prudent use of estrogen, regular exercise and a daily intake of 1500 mg of calcium and 400 units of vitamin D are generally thought to be beneficial in slowing the development of osteoporosis.

Ancillary Drug Treatment (as required)

Condition	*Drug Treatment*
For anxiety and/or depression:	alprazolam (Xanax), for intermittent, short-term use
For insomnia:	doxylamine (Unisom), available OTC diphenhydramine (Benadryl)
For headache:	aspirin acetaminophen (Tylenol, Panadol, etc.) ibuprofen (Advil, Nuprin, etc.)
For atrophic vaginitis and painful intercourse:	estrogen creams (Dienestrol, Estrace, Premarin)

Note: Drug selection, dosage and administration schedule must be determined by the physician for each patient individually.

Resource for Additional Information and Services

WARM (Women's Association for Research in Menopause)
128 East 56th Street
New York, NY 10022
Phone: (212) 418-0610

Operates support groups; gathers and disseminates information on menopause.

MIGRAINE HEADACHE

Other Names: Classic migraine, common migraine

Prevalence in USA: Approximately 30 million cases, 15% of the general population under 40 years of age.

Age Group: Under 18 years—0.8% of population; 18 to 44 years—4.7% of population; 45 to 64 years—5% of population; over 65 years—1.9% of population.

Male to Female Ratio

With onset at puberty, boys and girls are affected equally.
By age 40 there is a 3 to 2 predominance in women.

Principal Features

Migraine headaches may first appear in childhood but usually begin in
the late teens or early twenties; they often cease after menopause.
The migraine attack occurs in one of two patterns:

(1) Classic migraine (15% of the total) begins with an "aura" of symptoms that may precede the onset of headache by 15 to 20 minutes;
these usually consist of visual manifestations described as blind spots,
zig-zag effects or flashing lights. The attack may begin at any time
of the day or night; the headache is usually (70% of attacks) located
on one side of the head, but may spread to both sides before terminating. The pain is usually pulsating or throbbing in nature and varies in intensity from mild to severe. The migraine attack commonly
(90% of attacks) includes nausea, vomiting and increased sensitivity
to light and noise. Other associated features are scalp tenderness,
dizziness, dry mouth, tremors, sweating and chilliness.

(2) Common migraine (85% of the total) begins as a headache without
a warning "aura." Otherwise the pattern is essentially the same. Attacks may occur rarely (1 or 2 a year) or every few days; the average
frequency is 2 to 4 per month. Individual episodes usually last from
12 to 48 hours.

Causes: The exact complex of mechanisms responsible for the migraine
attack is not known. It is basically a disturbance in the autonomic
nervous system that causes instability in the control of cerebral arteries. There is a positive family history in 70% of those who experience migraine attacks. The majority of women who experience
migraine find frequent association of the episode with menstruation.
Other factors that are reported to trigger migraine attacks include
emotional stress, excessive fatigue, erratic patterns of eating and
sleeping, bright sunlight, loud noises, and the use of alcohol. The following foods are thought to be responsible for migraine attacks in
sensitive individuals: aged cheese, bananas, chicken livers, chocolate,
citrus fruits, monosodium glutamate, onions, pickled herring, pork,
red wine, excessive salt, shell fish, sodium nitrite, vinegar, yogurt.

Drugs That Can Cause This Disorder: The following drugs may induce
migrainelike headaches or aggravate existing migraine syndromes:
aminophylline
analgesics (chronic use of acetaminophen or aspirin)
antihypertensive drugs that cause vasodilation
caffeine (chronic use may cause vascular headache)
estrogens (can worsen migraine in 50% of women)
hydralazine
indomethacin
nifedipine

nitrates
oral contraceptives
prazosin
reserpine

Drugs Used to Treat This Disorder
For Prevention of Migraine Attacks
Beta-Adrenergic-Blocking Drugs (Beta Blockers)
- propranolol (Inderal).
- nadolol (Corgard).
- atenolol (Tenormin).
- timolol (Blocadren).
- metoprolol (Lopressor).

Calcium Channel-Blocking Drugs (Calcium Blockers)
- nifedipine (Procardia).
- verapamil (Calan, Isoptin).

Anti-inflammatory Drugs (Aspirin Substitutes)
- naproxen (Naprosyn).
- ibuprofen (Motrin, Rufen, Advil, etc.).
- fenoprofen (Nalfon).

Antidepressants
- amitriptyline (Elavil, Endep).
- doxepin (Sinequan, Adapin).

methysergide (Sansert)
lithium (Lithane, Lithobid, etc.)

For Abortion and Relief of Migraine Attacks
Vasoconstrictor Drugs
- ergotamine: oral (Cafergot, Wigraine); rectal (Cafergot, Wigraine suppositories); sublingual (Ergostat, Ergomar, Wigrettes); inhalant (Medihaler ergotamine).
- isometheptene (Midrin).

Anti-inflammatory Drugs
- aspirin.
- meclofenamate (Meclomen).
- ibuprofen (Motrin, Rufen, Advil, etc.).
- naproxen (Naprosyn).
- diflunisal (Dolobid).

Opioid Analgesics
- codeine.
- meperidine (Demerol).

Goals of Drug Treatment
Prompt abortion and relief of the acute migraine attack.
Reduction in the frequency and severity of recurrent migraine attacks.
A permanent cure is not available.

Drug Management
Important note: Not every drug is effective with every patient. Trial and experimentation may be necessary to determine the most effective treatment for each individual.

For fewer than 3 attacks per month of mild to moderate migraine, use abortive medications at the onset of symptoms. Ergotamine and anti-inflammatory drugs are the medications of choice.

For 3 or more attacks per month and for severe, prolonged migraine, use preventive medications on a continual basis. Beta blockers are the drugs of choice to reduce the frequency and severity of recurrent migraine attacks.

Always try to take your medication as soon as possible after the first indications of a developing migraine attack.

Isometheptene (Midrin) is a mild, well-tolerated and safer drug than ergotamine; use it first to determine its effectiveness. Go to stronger drugs only as needed.

Metoclopramide (Reglan) is an effective addition to the treatment of migraine attacks; it often controls nausea and vomiting, and it enhances the effectiveness of other oral migraine drugs.

Antidepressants may be used concurrently with other preventive drugs. They may be very effective *even in the absence of depression.*

For best results, start the preventive treatment of menstrual migraine 3 days before the onset of menstruation and continue it until all spotting has ceased.

Use of Beta Blockers

1. These are the drugs of choice for long-term prevention of migraine attacks. Propranolol (Inderal) is the most widely used; nadolol (Corgard) is a good second choice.
2. The preventive dose varies greatly and must be determined by individual trial. Effective dosage ranges from 80 mg to 320 mg daily.
3. After a period of 6 to 12 months of good headache control, the dose may be reduced gradually and the drug eventually discontinued.

Use of Calcium Blockers

1. The preventive use of this class of drugs is still experimental in this country; they have been highly effective in Europe.
2. Verapamil (Calan, Isoptin) is the most effective of this class currently available in the USA. Nifedipine (Procardia) has been found to intensify migraine attacks in some individuals. Its use is not recommended.
3. A trial of 6 to 8 weeks is usually required to determine the preventive effectiveness of these drugs.
4. Observe for the development of fluid retention and constipation.

Use of Anti-inflammatory Drugs

1. These drugs are useful in both preventing and relieving migraine attacks. They are usually well tolerated and are not habit-forming.
2. Meclofenamate (Meclomen) is the fastest acting of the class and is very effective in aborting acute migraine.
3. Naproxen (Naprosyn) and fenoprofen (Nalfon) are also effective and widely used for intermittent prevention (as in menstrual migraine).
4. The prolonged-action forms of these drugs should be used cautiously, especially in the elderly, because of their potential for reducing kidney blood flow.

Use of Antidepressants

1. The long-term use of amitriptyline (Elavil, Endep, etc.) is effective in preventing all types of chronic headaches: tension headaches, migraine attacks and mixed forms.
2. Effectiveness is not dependent upon the drug's antidepressant action; the dose required for headache control is less than the antidepressant dose.
3. For migraine patients with sleep problems, the antidepressants of choice are amitriptyline, doxepin and trazodone because of their sedative effects. The total daily requirement is best given as a single dose at bedtime.
4. Desipramine (Norpramin, Pertofrane) is usually considered to have the fewest side-effects.

Use of Methysergide

1. While very effective as a migraine preventive, this drug is inherently dangerous. It can cause serious and life-threatening adverse effects with long-term use: formation of scar tissue (fibrosis) involving the heart, lungs, blood vessels and kidneys.
2. It is usually reserved to treat severe migraine that has not responded to safer drugs.
3. Its use should be limited to courses of no more than 4 to 6 months followed by drug-free intervals of 4 to 6 weeks.
4. This drug should not be used in the presence of valvular heart disease or serious blood vessel disorders.
5. The smallest effective dose should be determined; the total daily dosage should not exceed 8 mg.

Use of Ergotamine

1. This is the most effective abortive drug if taken early in the migraine attack; it can relieve the headache in 1 to 2 hours. It tends to be less effective if taken later.
2. It may be taken orally or sublingually in tablet form, rectally in the form of suppositories, by inhalation or by injection.
3. Dosage should be limited to no more than 6 mg/24 hours or 10 mg/week to prevent serious adverse effects. (See Drug Profile.)
4. Avoid concurrent use with dopamine, erythromycins, troleandomycin and beta blockers.
5. Avoid frequent and regular use; this drug can cause dependence (see Glossary). Long-term use on a daily basis can *cause* chronic migrainelike headaches.
6. Ergotamine "rebound" (return and intensification of headache) can be prevented by allowing 48 hours between courses.

Ancillary Drug Treatment (as required)

Condition	*Drug Treatment*
For nausea and vomiting:	metoclopramide (Reglan)

For preheadache visual
disturbances: nitroglycerin, sublingual
                             isoproterenol (Isuprel), inhalation

Note: Drug selection, dosage and administration schedule must be determined
by the physician for each patient individually.

Resource for Additional Information and Services

National Headache Foundation
5252 North Western Avenue
Chicago, IL 60625
Phone: 1-800-843-2256 (outside IL); 1-800-523-8858 (inside IL); (312)
878-5558

Publications available.

MYASTHENIA GRAVIS

Other Names: MG, autoimmune myasthenia gravis, myasthenia gravis
pseudoparalytica

Prevalence in USA: Estimated to be 1 in 25,000. Approximately 24,000
documented cases. (Because many mild forms of this disorder are not
recognized or reported, it is estimated that the prevalence may approach 100,000.)

Age Group: The autoimmune form of myasthenia gravis (over 90% of all
forms of MG) can have its onset at any age from birth to 90 years.
Thirty percent of all cases begin in women between puberty and 40
years of age, with the highest incidence in the twenties. Thirty percent of all cases begin in men after the age of 40, with the highest
incidence in the fifties.

Male to Female Ratio

Age of onset under 40 years—1 to 3
Age of onset 30–50 years—1 to 1
Age of onset over 40 years—3 to 1

Principal Features: Myasthenia gravis is a chronic disorder of neuromuscular function attributed to the presence of antibodies in the blood
that impair the transmission of nerve impulses across the junction of
nerve and muscle tissue. The characteristic symptoms are periods of
fluctuating fatigue and early exhaustion of affected muscles. Involvement may be restricted to a single muscle group or may gradually
expand to affect major muscle groups throughout the body. The first
muscles to show abnormal fatigability in 50% of all cases are those
of the eye, resulting in drooping eyelids and blurred or double vision;
25% of cases first become aware of weakness while speaking, chewing
or swallowing; 20% first notice unusual weakness and fatigue in the

arms or legs. The course of the disorder varies greatly from one person to another, but the point of maximal involvement is usually reached within 3 years. Stage 1, the "active" stage, is characterized by increasing disability and fluctuation of symptoms; it may last from 5 to 10 years. Stage 2, the "inactive" stage, is marked by less variation and greater stability. Stage 3, the "burned out" stage, is usually reached 14 to 20 years after the initial onset of symptoms; it generally represents the residual pattern of the disorder that must be managed for the remaining life of the individual. Spontaneous remissions occur in fewer than 10% of cases, and these may last only 2 to 3 years.

Causes: The current belief is that myasthenia gravis is an autoimmune disorder characterized by the formation of antibodies that impair acetylcholine receptors of the nerve-muscle junctions in affected voluntary muscles. Such antibodies are present in 80% to 90% of all MG patients. Their presence implies damage or destruction of receptors by autoimmune complexes. The resulting reduction of available receptors for nerve impulse transmission is responsible for the muscle weakness and easy fatigability that characterize this disorder. The mechanisms responsible for the formation of destructive antibodies are not understood. There is no clear pattern of heredity to account for the development of MG.

Drugs That Can Cause This Disorder

The drug penicillamine (Cuprimine, Depen), used to treat rheumatoid arthritis and Wilson's disease, can cause true myasthenia gravis in about 1% of users.

The following drugs may impair neuromuscular impulse transmission and should be avoided or used with great caution in patients with myasthenia gravis:

antihistamines	morphine
barbiturates	neomycin
beta blocker drugs	opioid analgesics
calcium channel blocker drugs	phenytoin
clindamycin	polymyxin A and B
colistimethate	procainamide
colistin	quinidine
gentamycin	quinine
kanamycin	streptomycin
lidocaine	tranquilizers
lithium	trimethadione
magnesium sulfate	tubocurarine

Drugs Used to Treat This Disorder

Cholinesterase Inhibitors

- ambenonium (Mytelase).
- neostigmine (Prostigmin).
- pyridostigmine (Mestinon).

Cortisonelike Drug (Corticosteroid)
- prednisone

azathioprine (Imuran)

Goals of Drug Treatment

The primary aim is to minimize disability; cure is not possible.

Prompt determination of the optimal drug regimen for each patient individually.

Smooth control of fluctuating muscle weakness and fatigability; restoration of sustained strength and endurance.

Prevention of both myasthenic crisis and cholinergic crisis.

Achievement of remission of the disease process.

Drug Management

Dosage requirements may vary from day to day, according to the course of the disorder, the physical demands of daily routines, the emotional state of the patient, etc. Doses should be adjusted according to need, larger doses being taken at times of greatest fatigue—as just before meals, to facilitate eating.

Restoration of muscle strength and endurance beyond 80% of normal status (before MG) is usually not possible. Learn by experience the limit of your response to the drugs that work best for you and do not exceed the optimal dose.

Cholinesterase inhibitors provide only transient symptomatic relief and are of limited usefulness in most cases of moderate to severe MG. They are most useful for nonprogressive eye muscle weakness and mild limb muscle weakness.

Use caution when taking drugs concurrently that can cause low blood potassium levels (hypokalemia). Many diuretics in wide use can cause potassium loss and thereby increase muscle weakness and fatigue.

Use of Cholinesterase Inhibitors

1. These drugs are generally used first to treat the newly diagnosed case of MG. A trial of 1 to 3 months is usually sufficient to determine their effectiveness.

2. The drug of choice must be determined for each patient individually by trial and error, as must the optimal dose and administration schedule.

3. Pyridostigmine (Mestinon) is usually preferred by most patients with ocular or mild nonprogressive MG.

4. These drugs are prone to irregular absorption and consequent variation in therapeutic effect. They are best taken with food to reduce stomach upset.

5. Careful dosage adjustment is mandatory. Underdosage can result in myasthenic crisis. Overdosage can result in cholinergic crisis. Both reactions can cause sudden muscle weakness and be life-threatening if respiration is seriously impaired. Sudden weakness occurring 1 hour after taking medication usually indicates overdosage (cholinergic crisis).

6. After prolonged use, these drugs may lose their effectiveness. Your ability to respond to them can be restored by reducing the dose or withdrawing them for several days. ***However, this must be done under the supervision of your physician.***

7. Long-term treatment with high doses of these drugs may itself cause permanent changes in the motor end-plates and adversely affect neuromuscular transmission.

Use of Cortisonelike Drugs (Corticosteroids)

1. These drugs have become more widely used within the past 5 years for treating MG. Some physicians initiate treatment with prednisone if there are no contraindications. The usual course of treatment is 2 years, to minimize the possibility of relapse.

2. Prednisone is given initially in high doses daily until improvement begins, then changed to an alternate-day schedule. With sustained improvement and stabilization of function, the dose is gradually reduced to the smallest effective maintenance level.

3. A trial period of 60 days is usually necessary to determine the effectiveness of prednisone therapy for MG. For those who respond favorably, marked improvement occurs within 3 months and maximal improvement is usually attained within 9 months. Favorable results are reported in 80% of patients, with remissions in 25% to 35%.

4. Significant worsening of symptoms can occur in 48% of patients during the early phase of high-dose prednisone treatment. For this reason a trial of prednisone is best initiated in the hospital.

5. Approximately 90% of patients remain dependent upon long-term prednisone treatment for sustained improvement. Only 10% can withdraw successfully and remain in remission.

6. Observe carefully for the possible development of adverse effects that often accompany long-term use of cortisonelike drugs. See the Drug Profile of Prednisone in Section Three.

7. Some experts now recommend that thymectomy be done in serious cases *before* corticosteroids are used. A consensus is emerging that long-term corticosteroid therapy should be avoided if possible.

Use of Azathioprine (Imuran)

1. It is now felt that azathioprine is significantly less toxic than long-term steroid therapy. It is useful in reducing steroid requirement, and can produce improvement or remission when used alone.

2. It may be used alone or in conjunction with cortisonelike drugs to treat advanced stages of MG with severe disability.

3. For those who respond favorably, improvement usually begins within 3 to 12 months; maximal improvement may require continual treatment for 12 to 36 months. Approximately 53% of patients show some improvement using azathioprine alone, with 40% achieving temporary remission. However, continued improvement usually requires high doses.

4. Only 10% of patients show sustained improvement following discontinuation of this drug.

5. Observe carefully for the development of serious adverse effects. See the Drug Profile of Azathioprine in Section Three.

Ancillary Drug Treatment (as required)

Condition	*Drug Treatment*
For apathy, lethargy:	ephedrine
For hypokalemia:	potassium supplements (see Drug Profile)
For diarrhea:	diphenoxylate (Imodium)

Note: Drug selection, dosage and administration schedule must be determined by the physician for each patient individually.

Resource for Additional Information and Services

Myasthenia Gravis Foundation
53 West Jackson Boulevard, Suite 909
Chicago, IL 60604
Phone: (312) 427-6252

Sponsors 52 state groups and low-cost pharmacy service.
Publications: physicians' and nurses' manuals, patient handbooks, brochures, pamphlets.

OSTEOARTHRITIS

Other Names: Osteoarthrosis, degenerative arthritis, degenerative joint disease, hypertrophic arthritis

Prevalence in USA: 16 million—8.7% of the adult population; 10% of the elderly population.

Age Group: 55 years and over.

Male to Female Ratio: Same incidence in men and women.

Principal Features: Osteoarthritis is the most common joint disease and the major cause of disability of our older population. It is an insidious, slowly progressive deterioration of the surface cartilage on the ends of bones where they come together to form joints. During the early phases of change, there are no symptoms. With progressive destruction of protective cartilage, bone surface becomes exposed and irritated; this results in pain, stiffness and muscle spasm. As the central area of cartilage is destroyed, new bone and cartilage begin to form on the edges of the joint (spur formation). These degenerative changes can start as early as the fourth decade of life; they usually begin to cause symptoms in sixth and seventh decades; by age 75, all individuals have some degree of osteoarthritis in one or more joints.

The most commonly involved joints are: fingers, thumb, shoulders, hips, knees, base of the first toe, neck and lower (lumbar) spine. Progressive changes in the weight-bearing joints, principally the lower spine, hips and knees, eventually give rise to pain, deep ache and muscle spasm. Discomfort grows worse after prolonged activity that involves diseased joints.

Causes: There is no apparent initiating cause for primary osteoarthritis. The disorder does have a familial pattern, and it is thought that genetic biochemical defects in cartilage structure predispose some individuals to excessive "wear and tear" deterioration of vulnerable joints. Secondary osteoarthritis is due to congenital joint malformations, joint injuries and infections and other infrequent causes of bone and cartilage deterioration.

Drugs That Can Cause This Disorder: Although some drugs are capable of causing joint aches and pains (e.g., barbiturates, "sulfa" drugs, oral contraceptives, isoniazid, pyrazinamide), no drugs cause the bone and cartilage destruction characteristic of osteoarthritis. Rarely the systemic (internal) use of cortisonelike steroid drugs can cause aseptic necrosis of bone (destruction without infection); this can initiate a secondary form of osteoarthritis.

Drugs Used to Treat This Disorder

There are no drugs that can prevent, halt the progression of or reverse the degenerative changes of osteoarthritis. The following drugs are used to relieve pain, stiffness and muscle spasm.

Nonsteroidal Anti-inflammatory Drugs (NSAIDs)
Salicylates
- aspirin (Bufferin, Ascriptin, Cama, etc.).
- aspirin, enteric-coated (Easprin, Ecotrin, etc.).
- aspirin, zero-order-release (Zorpin).
- magnesium salicylate (Magan, Mobidin).
- choline magnesium salicylate (Trisilate).
- salsalate (Disalcid).
- diflunisal (Dolobid).
- sodium salicylate.

Indole Derivatives
- indomethacin (Indocin).
- sulindac (Clinoril).
- tolmetin (Tolectin).

Propionic Acid Derivatives
- fenoprofen (Nalfon).
- flurbiprofen (Ansaid).
- ibuprofen (Motrin, Rufen, Advil, etc.).
- ketoprofen (Orudis).
- naproxen (Naprosyn).
- suprofen (Suprol).

Fenamic Acid Derivatives
- meclofenamate (Meclomen).

- mefenamic acid (Ponstel).

Oxicam Derivative
- piroxicam (Feldene).

Phenylacetic Acid Derivative
- diclofenac (Voltaren).

Simple Analgesics
- acetaminophen (Tylenol, Panadol, etc.).
- propoxyphene (Darvon, etc.).
- codeine (Tylenol with codeine, etc.).
- hydrocodone (Vicodin, etc.).
- oxycodone (Percodan, Percocet, Tylox).

Muscle Relaxants
- carisoprodol (Soma).
- cyclobenzaprine (Flexeril).
- diazepam (Valium).
- methocarbamol (Robaxin).
- orphenadrine (Norflex).

Goals of Drug Treatment

Relief of pain and stiffness sufficient to permit continued activity, therapeutic exercise and physiotherapy.

Relief of associated anxiety and/or depression.

Drug Management

General Principles

Osteoarthritis is a chronic but slowly progressive disorder; although there is no curative treatment available, the symptoms are generally mild for long periods of time and can usually be relieved satisfactorily with available drugs.

Nonsteroidal anti-inflammatory drugs (NSAIDs) are the primary drugs of choice for managing osteoarthritis. Their principal actions are within the tissues of the diseased joint.

Simple analgesics, such as propoxyphene, codeine, oxycodone, etc., suppress pain perception in the brain; they are used to supplement the analgesic effects of NSAIDs.

Cortisonelike steroids by mouth should not be used in the management of osteoarthritis. They may be helpful when injected directly into osteoarthritis joints, sometimes providing prompt and lasting relief of pain and swelling. If effective, steroid injections may be repeated at intervals of 4 to 6 months for a limited number of times.

Symptomatic drug treatment will be more effective if it is supplemented by appropriate physiotherapy and the use of physical aids, such as canes, crutches, walkers, railings, etc.

Avoid prolonged and repeated overuse of diseased joints to (1) slow the progression of joint destruction and (2) minimize requirements for analgesic drugs.

Excessive body weight (obesity) can accelerate deterioration of weight-bearing joints. Prudent weight reduction programs are a most important part of treatment for osteoarthritis of the lower spine, hips and knees.

Use of Nonsteroidal Anti-inflammatory Drugs (NSAIDs)

1. These drugs are not thought to be able to favorably influence the natural course of osteoarthritis, but they can relieve pain and inflammation and thereby improve joint function and mobility.
2. Treatment is usually initiated with aspirin (lowest cost). Unfortunately, large doses (2 to 4 tablets of 325 mg each, 3 to 4 times daily) are often necessary to achieve satisfactory relief. The high blood levels required can cause ringing in the ears (tinnitus) and loss of hearing, especially in the elderly. Measurements of salicylate blood levels can be most helpful in establishing correct dosage. (See Therapeutic Drug Monitoring in Section One.)
3. Soluble aspirin preparations (regular aspirin, Bufferin, Ascriptin, etc.) often cause stomach ulceration and bleeding; they should be taken with food to minimize this effect.
4. The preferred forms of aspirin for continual use in large doses include (1) enteric-coated preparations and (2) zero-order-release tablets. (See list above.)
5. Salicylates other than aspirin can also be used. (See list above.) These cause significantly less stomach irritation; some are effective with twice daily dosage.
6. All NSAID aspirin substitutes are better tolerated than aspirin. However, they may share a cross-sensitivity in individuals who are allergic to aspirin and may induce asthmatic reactions.
7. An NSAID should be used on a regular schedule for a trial period of 3 to 4 weeks; if it is not effective, another one should be tried in sequence (selecting one from a different chemical group). An attempt is made to find the NSAID that provides the best relief with the fewest side-effects.
8. Authorities do not recommend the use of NSAIDs in combination with each other. A small dose of aspirin taken along with an NSAID may provide additional relief of pain.
9. NSAIDs have a potential for injuring the kidney and impairing kidney function. They should be used with caution in individuals over 50 years old, in those with hypertension, diabetes, congestive heart failure and especially in those taking diuretics.
10. NSAIDs can increase the effects of oral antidiabetic drugs (sulfonylureas) and anticoagulants. Dosage adjustments may be necessary.

Use of Narcoticlike Analgesics

1. In advanced cases of osteoarthritis, mild analgesics such as acetaminophen or propoxyphene may not provide adequate pain relief. Codeine, hydrocodone and oxycodone may be tried cautiously on an intermittent schedule to avoid tolerance and dependence.
2. The use of stronger narcotic (opioid) analgesics (morphine, meperidine, etc.) should be avoided completely. Their potential for causing dependence (addiction) precludes repetitious, long-term use in chronically painful disorders like osteoarthritis.

Use of Muscle Relaxants
1. Muscle spasm prevents exercise and use of affected joints. The cautious use of muscle relaxants in conjunction with physiotherapy may be beneficial in preserving joint mobility and muscle strength.
2. Muscle relaxants are most useful in managing osteoarthritis of the lower spine with associated lumbo-sacral muscle spasm.

Ancillary Drug Treatment (as required)

Condition	Drug Treatment
For anxiety and/or mild depression:	alprazolam (Xanax), for intermittent, short-term use
For moderate or severe depression:	trazodone (Desyrel) (see Profile of Depression in this section)
For drug-induced constipation:	docusate with casanthranol (Peri-Colace)

Note: Drug selection, dosage and administration schedule must be determined by the physician for each patient individually.

Resources for Additional Information and Services

Arthritis Foundation
1314 Spring Street, N.W.
Atlanta, GA 30309
Phone: (404) 872-7100

Publications available.

Association for People With Arthritis
P.O. Box 954
6 Commercial Street
Hicksville, NY 11802
Phone: 1-800-323-2243

Publications available.

OSTEOPOROSIS

Other Names: Osteopenia, type I postmenopausal or spinal osteoporosis (95% of all cases), type II senile osteoporosis

Prevalence in USA: 24 million—approximately 25% of white women over 60 years of age have osteoporosis; 1.3 million fractures due to osteoporosis occur annually.

Age Group: Type I osteoporosis—50 to 65 years. Type II osteoporosis—65 years and over.

Male to Female Ratio: Much higher incidence in women: 8 to 1.

Principal Features: Osteoporosis is a major disorder of bone in the elderly, occurring most often in postmenopausal women. As ovarian function declines and estrogen is withdrawn, the natural loss of bone mass is accelerated. This eventually weakens bone structure and predisposes to fractures that can result from minimal trauma. Osteoporosis can be localized in a single bone (a leg immobilized in a cast), but it is usually more widely distributed, with most fractures occurring in the spine, wrist and hip. The basic defect is a relative increase in the rate of bone destruction without a compensating increase in the reformation of new bone. There are usually no symptoms prior to the occurrence of a spontaneous or traumatic fracture. A sudden compression fracture of a vertebra in the middle or lower section of the spine can result from such minor strains as bending, lifting or sneezing; it causes immediate pain and disability lasting several weeks. Gradual compression of the vertebrae (usually painless) causes loss of height and the development of a stooped, rounded back ("dowager's hump"). A spontaneous fracture of a hip (femur) can occur on arising from a chair or while walking. Untreated osteoporosis can cause a loss of 30% to 60% of bone mass.

Causes: Primary osteoporosis is a normal consequence of aging. A woman loses approximately 50% of bone mass, and a man approximately 25%, during a normal life span. Type I primary osteoporosis refers to the estrogen withdrawal syndrome following menopause. Type II primary osteoporosis occurs later as a feature of senility. Secondary osteoporosis refers to the bone loss that is associated with other diseases and disorders: hyperthyroidism, hyperparathyroidism, adrenal cortical hormone excess (Cushing's syndrome or drug-induced), multiple myeloma, diabetes, and alcoholism.

Drugs That Can Cause This Disorder
- Cortisonelike steroids, especially in immobilized women over 50 years of age receiving large doses.
- Heparin, when used in long-term therapy.
- Methotrexate, when used in prepubertal children for long-term therapy.

Drugs Used to Treat This Disorder
Estrogens ("Natural-type" Estrogens Are Preferred)
- conjugated estrogens (Genisis, Premarin).
- esterified estrogens (Evex, Menest).
- estradiol cypionate (Depo-Estradiol, injection).
- estradiol valerate (Delestrogen, injection).
- estriol (Hormonin, a mixture of estriol, estradiol and estrone).
- piperazine estrone sulfate (Ogen).

- micronized 17-B estadiol (Estrace).
- transdermal estradiol skin patch (Estraderm-50 and 100).

Calcium Preparations
- calcium carbonate (40% calcium) (generic tablets, Alka-2, Biocal, Caltrate, OsCal-500, Tums).
- calcium gluconate (9% calcium) (generic tablets).
- calcium lactate (13% calcium) (generic tablets).
- dibasic calcium phosphate (31% calcium) (generic tablets).

Vitamin D Analogs
- calcifediol (Calderol).
- calcitriol (Rocaltrol).

Other Drugs
- calcitonin (Calcimar).
- fluorides (investigational).

Goals of Drug Treatment

Primary prevention: early initiation of estrogen therapy—during or immediately after menopause—to prevent acceleration of natural bone loss.

Secondary prevention: initiation of estrogen therapy 3 or more years following menopause (after some degree of osteoporosis is present) to arrest or retard progressive bone loss.

Prevention of osteoporosis-related fractures.

Relief of pain and muscle spasm associated with fracture of osteoporotic bone.

Drug Management

General Principles

It is now firmly established that excessive bone loss (osteoporosis) following menopause can be prevented or significantly reduced by the timely administration of low-dose estrogen.

Accurate assessment of bone mass for the detection of osteoporosis can be made by quantitative CAT scan of vertebrae and by photon absorptiometry of wrist bones. However, these procedures are expensive and not generally available.

Currently it is not feasible to screen all postmenopausal women for osteoporosis. To identify those who may benefit from estrogen used preventively, the following "risk factors" characterize the candidates for postmenopausal osteoporosis:

1. slender build, light-boned, white or Oriental race
2. a sedentary life style or restricted physical activity
3. a family history of osteoporosis (grandmother, mother, aunt or sister)
4. a high-protein diet
5. a low-sodium diet (also likely to be a low-calcium diet)
6. lifelong avoidance of dairy products
7. heavy smoking
8. excessive use of antacids that contain aluminum
9. long-term use of cortisonelike steroid drugs

10. habitual use of carbonated beverages
11. excessive consumption of alcohol
12. increased urinary excretion of calcium

Thyroid replacement therapy (in appropriate dosage) may increase bone loss and predispose to the development of osteoporosis in the vertebrae of the lower spine. If you are taking a thyroid preparation to correct hypothyroidism, consult your physician regarding a possible need for calcium and vitamin D supplements to prevent potential bone loss.

Use of Estrogens

1. Estrogen increases the absorption of dietary calcium and reduces the rate of calcium loss from bone. Recent studies have shown that estrogen can reduce the risk of hip fractures by as much as 66%.
2. Estrogen does not substantially increase bone mass; it does not enhance restoration of bone following loss.
3. To be effective in preventing significant osteoporosis, estrogen therapy must begin within 3 years after menopause. Available evidence seems to indicate that continued protection against the development of osteoporosis requires ongoing use of estrogen—probably for life by those at risk.
4. Fifty percent of women are protected by 0.3 mg of conjugated estrogens daily; close to 100% are protected by 0.625 mg daily. Your physician can advise the dose most appropriate for you.
5. For detailed information regarding the use of estrogen, see the Profile of Menopause in this section and the Drug Profile of Estrogen in Section Three.

Use of Calcium Preparations

1. Calcium supplementation of the diet is appropriate for preventing or treating osteoporosis because the calcium content of the diet is usually less than the ongoing requirement for the maintenance of normal bone density. The average dietary intake of calcium by women is 500 to 600 mg daily. The daily requirement for the postmenopausal woman is 1500 to 2000 mg (all sources).
2. There is some evidence that calcium supplements (taken alone) may reduce the rate of bone loss and the incidence of fracture, but further proof is needed. Calcium is most effective when taken in conjunction with vitamin D and estrogen.
3. Supplemental calcium must not be taken in excessive doses. The recommended daily intake of calcium is approximately 1000 mg if taking estrogen and 1500 mg if not taking estrogen.
4. Excessive intake of supplemental calcium (more than 2000 mg daily) can cause abnormal increases in the blood and urine levels of calcium and predispose to kidney stone formation.
5. The most appropriate calcium preparations to use for supplementation are listed above.
6. Calcium supplements made from bone meal or mineral clay (dolomite, montmorillomite) may contain lead or other toxic metals and should be avoided.

7. Calcium supplements may be more effective if taken as a single late-evening dose to suppress the normal nocturnal rise in parathyroid hormone that increases bone loss.
8. Calcium may decrease the effects of aspirin (and other salicylates), calcium channel-blocking drugs, iron and tetracyclines. Do not take calcium preparations within 2 hours of taking other drugs.

Use of Vitamin D Analogs

1. Elderly individuals with osteoporosis who have a normal life style are not likely to a have a vitamin D deficiency; they usually have an adequate supply from their diet and exposure to sunlight.
2. Shut-ins (those confined to home, nursing home or hospital) probably need a supplement of vitamin D. Currently recommended sources include Calderol and Rocaltrol.
3. When vitamin D is used, limit calcium intake to 600 to 700 mg daily to prevent excessive absorption and abnormally high calcium levels in blood and urine.

Use of Calcitonin (a Thyroid Hormone That Reduces Bone Loss)

1. Studies to date show that calcitonin in doses of 100 units daily can produce an increase in total body calcium (99% in bone) after 2 years of treatment. A favorable response was achieved in 70% of users.
2. Calcitonin is given by injection and is used in conjunction with calcium and vitamin D.
3. Studies using other dosage forms of calcitonin—oral, buccal (cheek), intranasal—are under way.

Use of Fluoride

1. The use of fluoride in the prevention and treatment of osteoporosis is still investigational. Directions for its optimal use have not been established.
2. A dose of 40 to 65 mg/day is required to stimulate bone formation. Adverse effects occur in over 30% of users; these include nausea, stomach pain, gastrointestinal bleeding, bone and joint pain and severe foot discomfort, often intense enought to preclude compliance with treatment.
3. Calcium must always be used concurrently with fluoride to avoid the development of osteomalacia (abnormal mineral composition of bone).

Ancillary Drug Treatment (as required)

Condition	*Drug Treatment*
For calcium-induced constipation:	docusate (Colace, etc.) docusate with casanthranol (Peri-Colace, etc.)

For fracture pain: acetaminaphen with codeine (Tylenol with codeine)
acetaminophen with propoxyphene (Darvocet-N 100)
Avoid opiate analgesics stronger than codeine.

For muscle spasm: diazepam (Valium)

For mild depression: alprazolam (Xanax), for intermittent, short-term use

For marked depression: trazodone (Desyrel)

Note: Drug selection, dosage and administration schedule must be determined by the physician for each patient individually.

Resources for Additional Information and Services

National Institute of Arthritis and Musculoskeletal and Skin Diseases Information Office: Building 31, Room 4C32B
9000 Rockville Pike
Bethesda, MD 20892
Phone: Information Specialist, (301) 496-8188

Handles inquiries on arthritis, bone diseases (including osteoporosis), and skin diseases.

National Osteoporosis Foundation
1625 Eye Street, N.W., Suite 822
Washington, DC 20006
Phone: (202) 223-2226

Publications available.

WARM (Women's Association for Research in Menopause)
128 East 56th Street
New York, NY 10022
Phone: (212) 418-0610

Gathers and disseminates information on menopause-related subjects.

PARKINSON'S DISEASE

Other Names: Paralysis agitans, parkinsonism, parkinsonian syndrome

Prevalence in USA: Approximately 1.5 million—50,000 new cases annually; 1% of the population over 50 years old.

Age Group: 10% of cases under 40 years old; 20% of cases 40 to 50 years old; 70% of cases 50 years old and over. The mean age at onset is 58 to 62 years.

Male to Female Ratio: More common in men, 3 to 2.

Principal Features: Parkinson's disease is a slowly progressive, debilitating disorder of certain brain centers that contribute to the control and regulation of body movement. The earliest symptoms begin very insidiously; one arm or one leg (or the arm and leg on one side) will gradually develop a sense of weakness, retarded movement and stiffness. A fine tremor in a hand or foot will appear in 70% of cases; this occurs at rest and disappears with intentional use of the affected limb and while asleep. Symptoms may remain mild for years or they may progress steadily. Eventually the principal features of the disorder become generalized; the tremor spreads, most of the body musculature becomes rigid, the posture is stooped, movement is slow and jerky, the gait is shuffling and unsteady. Facial expression is lost; the voice grows weak and speech indistinct. Withdrawal and depression may occur as disability advances. Loss of mental acuity occurs in 30% of cases within 7 to 10 years. Currently available drug therapy can slow the progress of the disorder significantly for many, and life expectancy has been extended to equal the norms.

Causes: Primary Parkinson's disease is due to degeneration of the nerve cells in the brain that produce dopamine, one of the major nerve impulse transmitters. In most instances, the initiating cause of the cellular degeneration is unknown. Infrequently a virus infection of the brain (encephalitis) can initiate the degenerative process. Secondary parkinsonism can be caused by hardening of brain arteries, strokes, brain tumors, trauma, carbon monoxide or manganese poisoning and a few rare degenerative disorders of brain tissue.

Drugs That Can Cause This Disorder: The following drugs can block the action of dopamine and cause a form of secondary parkinsonism with features that are indistinguishable from primary Parkinson's disease: phenothiazines, droperidol, haloperidol, reserpine, chlorprothixene, thiothixene, methyldopa, metoclopramide, lithium. (See respective Drug Profiles in Section Three or Drug Classes in Section Four.)

Drugs Used to Treat This Disorder
- levodopa (Dopar, Larodopa).
- levodopa + carbidopa (Sinemet).
- levodopa + bensarazide (Prolopa in Canada).
- amantadine (Symmetrel).
- anticholinergics (atropinelike drugs): benztropine (Cogentin), diphenhydramine (Benadryl), trihexyphenidyl (Artane).
- bromocriptine (Parlodel).
- pergolide (Permax).
- selegiline (Eldepryl).

New Drugs in Development for Treating This Disorder: Sinemet CR-4, a new slow-release formulation of Sinemet, is now being tested in clinical trials. It is designed to reduce or eliminate the wearing-off phenomenon or end-of-dose failure that some individuals experience with standard Sinemet. Dosing frequency can be reduced by 25% to 50% and fluctuations in drug response minimized or eliminated throughout the day.

Goals of Drug Treatment

Improvement of overall function and mobility.
Reduction of muscular rigidity and tremor.
Reversal of slowed movement.
Improvement of posture, balance, gait, speech and writing.

Drug Management

General Principles

The symptoms of Parkinson's disease are due to a relative increase in the effects of acetylcholine in the brain centers that regulate body movement. The exaggerated acetylcholine effects are the result of a reduced supply of dopamine (primary Parkinson's disease) or to a blocking of dopamine action (drug-induced parkinsonism).

Drugs used to manage parkinsonism utilize three distinct mechanisms of action: (1) anticholinergic drugs reduce the excessive effects of acetylcholine; (2) levodopa is converted to dopamine in the brain, increasing its supply to restore a balance closer to normal; (3) bromocriptine serves as a substitute for dopamine by stimulating its receptor cells directly. Amantadine is thought to have both anticholinergic and direct-stimulating effects.

Appropriate drugs, properly used, can improve function and mobility for significant periods of time; up to 50% of those treated have no major disabilities after 10 years of disease.

The optimal drug program—either one drug used alone or two or more used in combination—is that which provides satisfactory relief of symptoms or the most acceptable compromise between symptom relief and drug side-effects. (Complete relief of symptoms may not be possible.)

Drug selection and dosage schedules *must be carefully individualized;* adjustments will be necessary throughout the course of this disorder. Daily fluctuations in symptoms and drug responses occur in almost every individual and vary greatly from person to person. A "trial-and-error" process is unavoidable in determining the best drug(s) and the best dosage schedule. For the best treatment results, keep your physician informed regarding all aspects of your response to the drugs prescribed.

Combinations of several drugs taken in small doses are often more beneficial than a single drug taken in large doses.

Use of Levodopa

1. Only 25% of levodopa taken alone by mouth enters the brain. The large doses required to be effective often cause unacceptable side-effects. To prevent this, levodopa is combined with carbidopa; the combination (marketed as Sinemet) permits a 75% dosage reduction of levodopa.

2. Levodopa is the most effective drug available in the USA and has been the drug of choice for managing primary parkinsonism for the past 15 years. Approximately 80% of users achieve 80% improvement in muscular rigidity and retarded movement.

3. Levodopa may be tried at any time during the course of this disorder. It is most effective during the first 2 to 5 years of use. However, authorities differ in their opinions as to the best time to use levodopa. Some advise early use—within the first year of symptoms—to obtain the fullest benefit possible. Others advise later use to delay the onset of side-effects and adverse effects that develop with long-term use of levodopa.

4. Levodopa is more completely absorbed when taken on an empty stomach. However, it may be necessary to take it following food to prevent nausea. If so, avoid meat when possible; proteins can interfere with absorption of levodopa.

5. After a year or more of continual use of levodopa, 80% of users will develop abnormal involuntary movements (dyskinesias) of various muscle groups—jerks and twitches of the head and face or semi-purposeful movement of the extremities. In 30% of the users these may be severe enough to interfere with normal functioning. They last for a few minutes to several hours and seem to coincide with the times of both high and low blood levels of levodopa.

6. Another 20% of users will experience "on-off" episodes—changes from relatively good function and mobility (drug effects "on") to marked loss of function and mobility (drug effects "off"). To minimize these periods of fluctuating effectiveness, levodopa may be taken in small doses every 1 to 3 hours throughout the day to maintain a more constant blood level.

7. Levodopa can cause a variety of mental disturbances: euphoria, hypomania, depression, confusion, nightmares, vivid hallucinations.

8. Levodopa should not be used concurrently with those antipsychotic drugs that block the action of dopamine; or with monoamine oxidase (MAO) inhibitors that increase the risk of a hypertensive crisis.

9. Some authorities advocate the use of "drug holidays" to reduce the toxic manifestations of levodopa. The very gradual withdrawal and reintroduction of the drug are essential to success.

Use of Amantadine

1. This drug probably releases dopamine from nerve cells and increases its availability. It may also seve as a dopamine substitute and stimulate receptor cells directly. It has anticholinergic effects that contribute to its effectiveness.

2. Amantadine may be tried first in all patients. It can produce a 15% to 25% improvement in 60% of users. A trial period of 1 week is usually adequate; if not beneficial or if mentality is adversely affected, discontinue use.

3. Amantadine may also be used in conjunction with anticholinergics and levodopa. It is usually well tolerated by the elderly.

4. This drug has a low incidence of side-effects. Ankle swelling and a reddish-blue mottling of the arms or legs may occur after 1 month to 1 year of use. These are not serious and are reversible.

5. Doses over 200 mg can cause excitement, increased tremor, jerkiness, insomnia and nightmares in sensitive individuals.

6. Amantadine may lose some of its effectiveness after 6 to 12 weeks of continual use.

7. In very rare cases the long-term use of this drug is associated with the unexpected development of congestive heart failure. If shortness of breath appears during exertion or while lying down or rouses you from sleep, report this promptly.

8. Recent reports indicate that this drug should not be stopped abruptly in the elderly patient (over 70 years of age). Sudden withdrawal can result in the prompt return of parkinsonian features and rapid deterioration.

Use of Anticholinergic Drugs

1. These atropinelike drugs are often used to initiate treatment when symptoms are mild. They can produce a 20% to 30% improvement by suppressing effects due to overactivity of acetylcholine: tremor, excessive salivation, rigidity and slow movement.

2. They may be used alone as long as symptoms remain mild. They may be combined with any of the other drugs used and at any stage of the disorder.

3. These drugs are not well tolerated by individuals over 70 years old. They can provoke latent glaucoma and can aggravate urinary retention in men with prostatism (see Glossary).

4. Unavoidable side-effects include blurring of near vision, dry mouth, constipation and urinary hesitancy. High doses may cause drowsiness, confusion, impaired memory, hallucinations and nightmares.

5. Following long-term use, these drugs must be discontinued very gradually to avoid a dangerous withdrawal syndrome.

Use of Bromocriptine

1. This drug may be used alone but is usually added to the treatment program at a later stage. It is the drug of choice for alleviating the abnormal involuntary movements associated with long-term levodopa use. It can also have a stabilizing effect when the "on-off" effects of levodopa therapy become apparent.

2. Bromocriptine is initiated with very small doses, and the dose is increased very slowly. Some individuals develop extreme hypotension (low blood pressure) with the first doses. It is advisable to try a test dose at bedtime for several days to determine individual blood pressure response.

3. This drug may not be effective in severe Parkinson's disease or in those with a poor response to levodopa.

4. High doses can cause acute personality changes, mood swings and other intolerable adverse effects; 40% of users discontinue this drug because of undesirable reactions.

5. This drug is an ergot derivative; it should be used with caution in the presence of angina, hypertension or any form of peripheral vascular disease.

Current Controversies in Drug Management

The difference of opinion among authorities regarding the best time to begin treatment with levodopa (Sinemet) has not been resolved to date. Those advocating early use—when symptoms are causing only mild disability—argue that the individual's quality of life is significantly improved and that his or her period of productive functioning is prolonged. Those advocating late introduction of levodopa—when symptoms are causing moderate to severe disability—argue that the early use of levodopa hastens the onset of adverse levodopa effects (abnormal involuntary movements, "wearing-off" effects, "on-off" effects). They propose the use of amantadine and/or anticholinergic drugs to manage the early period of mild disability and the later use of levodopa only if and when progression of symptoms requires greater relief. Studies to date have not been sufficiently conclusive to resolve the controversy.

One recently published study, however, does show that levodopa treatment started early (1 to 3 years after the onset of symptoms) significantly reduces mortality rates, especially those related to the disease itself.

Comment: The decision as to when levodopa therapy is to be started must be made jointly by the patient and the physician on an individual, case-by-case basis. The patient should be informed of the issues involved in making the decision and should share the resposibility for making the best decision for all concerned.

Ancillary Drug Treatment (as required)

Condition	*Drug Treatment*
For levodopa-induced drowsiness:	methylphenidate (Ritalin)
For levodopa-induced nausea:	diphenidol (Vontrol)
For action tremor:	propranolol (Inderal)
For muscle spasm and rigidity:	diazepam (Valium)
For nocturnal leg cramps:	quinine (Quinamm) at bedtime
For constipation:	docusate (Colace)
	docusate with casanthranol (Peri-Colace)
For insomnia:	chloral hydrate (Noctec, Somnos)
For ankle swelling:	hydrochlorothiazide (generic)
For depression:	amitriptyline (Elavil)
	desipramine (Norpramin)
	imipramine (Tofranil)

| | trazodone (Desyrel) |
| | fluoxetine (Prozac) |

For action tremor (that
accompanies resting
tremor):   propranolol (Inderal)

Note: Drug selection, dosage and administration schedule must be determined
by the physician for each patient individually.

Resources for Additional Information and Services

American Parkinson Disease Association
116 John Street, Suite 417
New York, NY 10038
Phone: 1-800-223-2732; (212) 732-9550

Available 8:30 a.m.–5:00 p.m. EST, M–F.
Provides publications, referrals, references and answers to inquiries regarding research and treatment.

Parkinson's Disease Foundation
Columbia Presbyterian Medical Center
640 West 168th Street
New York, NY 10032
Phone: (212) 923-4700

Serves as a source of information to patients and physicians on all aspects of Parkinson's disease.

United Parkinson Foundation
220 South State Street
Chicago, IL 60604
Phone: (312) 922-9734

Serves 28,000 members (patients, family members, medical personnel);
publishes reliable information on all aspects of Parkinson's disease.

PEPTIC ULCER

Other Names: Peptic ulcer disease, duodenal ulcer, gastric ulcer

Prevalence in USA: Approximately 20 million; 10% of the general population will have a symptomatic peptic ulcer sometime during life;
25% of men and 16% of women have scars of peptic ulcer disease on
autopsy examination.

Age Group: Duodenal ulcer occurs most commonly between 25 and 40
years. Gastric ulcer occurs most commonly between 40 and 55 years.
Of all ulcers, 1.9% occur under 18 years; 43% occur between 18 and

44 years; 36% occur between 45 and 64 years; 12.8% occur between 65 and 74 years; 6.3% occur at 75 years and over.

Male to Female Ratio: Duodenal ulcer: higher incidence in men—2 to 1. Gastric ulcer: same incidence in men and women.

Principal Features: Peptic ulcer disease refers to an intermittent disorder of the stomach and first portion of the small intestine (duodenum) that is characterized by the formation of ulcers in the lining of these organs. The tissues subject to ulceration are constantly bathed in digestive juices produced in the stomach; the principal components of these juices include hydrochloric acid and the digestive enzyme pepsin (hence "peptic" ulcer). Most individuals with peptic ulcer disease produce excessive amounts of acid and pepsin, which overwhelm the normal protection of the lining tissues and cause erosion (ulceration). The singular feature of an active duodenal ulcer is a gnawing or burning pain in the upper mid-abdomen that usually occurs between meals and in the early morning hours—when acid secretion is high. The pain is characteristically relieved by food or antacids. The pattern of pain-food-relief typifies active duodenal ulcer. Episodes of ulcer activation occur unpredictably, but are often more frequent and troublesome in the spring and fall of the year. By nature, peptic ulcer disease is a chronically recurrent disorder. The recurrence rate of duodenal ulcer is approximately 70% within 1 year and 90% within 2 years. Frequent recurrence predisposes to serious complications in 30% of ulcer patients, 10% to 15% will experience bleeding, 5% to 10% will suffer perforation of the duodenal wall and 5% will develop obstruction at the stomach outlet (pylorus) due to the extensive scarring that follows ulcer healing.

Causes: A predisposition to develop peptic ulcer disease appears to be hereditary. The primary initiating cause of ulceration is not known. Those individuals who produce excessive amounts of stomach acid and pepsin are often prone to the development of duodenal ulcer. Others with normal amounts of acid and pepsin develop ulceration because the protective mechanisms in the lining tissues are defective and inadequate. Certain states of physical stress (burns, trauma, surgery) can increase the incidence of peptic ulcer.

Drugs That Can Cause This Disorder: The following drugs can initiate ulceration of the stomach or duodenum in susceptible individuals or aggravate existing ulcers:

alcohol	cortisonelike steroids
aminophylline	phenylbutazone
aspirin and other nonsteroidal anti-inflammatory drugs	reserpine (?)

Drugs Used to Treat This Disorder
- antacids (Delcid, Maalox TC, Mylanta II, etc.).
- cimetidine (Tagamet).

- famotidine (Pepcid).
- misoprostol (Cytotec). Used for prevention and treatment.
- nizatidine (Axid).
- ranitidine (Zantac).
- sucralfate (Carafate).
- anticholinergic drugs (Darbid, Pro-Banthine, Robinul) for adjunctive use.

New Drugs in Development for Treating This Disorder: Current studies in 13 countries are showing that a new antiulcer drug, omeprazole (Losec), relieves symptoms and promotes ulcer healing more rapidly than other treatments in general use. Approval for marketing is expected within the next year.

Goals of Drug Treatment

Short-term control of stomach acidity sufficient to relieve pain and promote ulcer healing.

Long-term control of stomach acidity to prevent ulcer recurrence.

Prevention of complications.

Drug Management

General Principles

Most cases of peptic ulcer disease can be managed successfully by appropriate drug therapy. A treatment program of 4 to 6 weeks will heal up to 90% of duodenal ulcers. Surgery is needed only for the management of ulcer complications: uncontrolled bleeding, perforation, obstruction, persistent pain.

The four principal drugs used to promote healing of duodenal ulcer are all equally effective when taken in adequate dosage for 4 to 6 weeks. However, some individuals may respond more favorably to 2 (or more) drugs used concurrently. In the treatment of gastric ulcer, antacids are less effective than cimetidine, ranitidine, or sucralfate.

Anticholinergic (atropinelike) drugs are used only when ulcer symptoms are not adequately controlled by antacids and/or cimetidine or ranitidine.

Tranquilizers and sedatives should not be used routinely but only as necessary to relieve significant anxiety and nervous tension that could possibly contribute to hyperacidity.

If possible, it is advisable to avoid cortisonelike steroid therapy in the presence of active peptic ulcer or in those individuals who are subject to recurrently active peptic ulcer disease. If steroid treatment is necessary, antacids and/or cimetidine (or ranitidine) should be used protectively.

The chronic use of aspirin (and substitute nonsteroidal anti-inflammatory drugs) increases the chance of developing active peptic ulcer.

Cigarette smoking doubles the chance of developing peptic ulcer disease; it also delays healing significantly.

Caffeine-containing beverages (coffee, tea, cola) can stimulate stomach acid production and aggravate an existing ulcer.

Alcohol (in excess) can aggravate gastric ulcer and increase the risk of bleeding.

Use of Antacids

1. These drugs are used to neutralize stomach acids and thereby (1) relieve pain, heartburn and acid indigestion; and (2) correct hyperacidity and promote ulcer healing.

2. The antacids of choice are composed of magnesium aluminum hydroxide (Delcid, Maalox TC, Mylanta II). The optimal treatment schedule is 1 ounce taken 1 hour and 3 hours after meals and at bedtime until free of pain for 2 weeks; then 1 hour after meals and at bedtime for an additional 4 weeks.

3. Avoid long-term use of aluminum hydroxide and magnesium trisilicate preparations; they may cause depletion of phosphate and increase the risk of osteomalacia (softening of bones).

4. Avoid calcium-containing antacids (Alka-2, Titralac, Tums); these stimulate secretion of gastrin, a stomach hormone that in turn stimulates production of hydrochloric acid and pepsin, referred to as rebound hyperacidity.

5. When practical, antacid liquids (suspensions) are more effective than tablets.

6. Antacids can interfere with the absorption of cimetidine (but not ranitidine), digoxin, iron, isoniazid and tetracyclines.

Use of Histamine (H-2)-Blocking Drugs

1. These drugs reduce the production of hydrochloric acid by blocking the stomach's response to stimulation by histamine. They promote healing of peptic ulcer in 70% to 80% of cases when taken for 4 to 6 weeks.

2. Treatment with one of these drugs alone is a reasonable alternative to high-dose antacid therapy.

3. Cimetidine may cause confusion and unsteadiness in the elderly, especially those with impaired kidney function; infrequently it can cause breast enlargement and impotence in men; it increases the effects of warfarin when taken concurrently.

4. Ranitidine taken in a single dose at bedtime is as effective as other multidose drug regimens for healing peptic ulcer.

5. Ranitidine is less likely to cause confusion, unsteadiness, breast changes or altered sexual functions; in addition, it does not appear to be involved in any significant drug-drug interactions.

6. In the presence of liver disease or impaired liver function, avoid the concurrent use of ranitidine and acetaminophen to reduce the risk of liver toxicity.

7. Drugs of this class taken once daily at bedtime, can reduce the recurrence rate (in 1 year) for duodenal ulcer from 70% to 10%, and for gastric ulcer from 56% to 20%.

Use of Sucralfate

1. This drug is used for short-term (8 weeks') treatment of active duodenal ulcer. It promotes ulcer healing by forming a dense coating over the ulcer that protects it from the erosive action of hydro-

chloric acid. Its effectiveness is comparable to antacids and histamine blockers (cimetidine and ranitidine) when used alone.
2. Sucralfate should not be used in conjunction with antacids or histamine blockers.
3. Food may impair the effectiveness of sucralfate. The recommended schedule is as follows:
    (1) If other drugs are being used concurrently, take these 1 hour before sucralfate.
    (2) Take sucralfate on an empty stomach, 1 hour before meals and at bedtime.
    (3) Food may be taken 1 hour after sucralfate.
4. This drug is very safe; it has no contraindications and minimal side-effects—constipation (2%).
5. It can interfere with the absorption of tetracyclines and phenytoin.

Current Controversies in Drug Management

Should histamine (H-2)-blocking drugs (see above) be used intermittently or continuously in treating peptic ulcer disease?

Recently completed studies (219 patients followed for 5 years) have shown that continuous treatment with cimetidine (Tagamet) is significantly more effective than intermittent treatment in preventing recurrence of ulcer activity. Current recommendations call for continuous treatment (daily bedtime maintenance dosing) of anyone who has two or more relapses within two years.

Comments: Such long-term treatment must be individualized; consult your physician regarding its advisability for you. The optimal duration of such treatment and the long-term effects of chronic histamine (H-2)-blocking drug use have not been determined.

Ancillary Drug Treatment (as required)

Condition	*Drug Treatment*
For persistant nocturnal ulcer pain:	isopropamide (Combid, Darbid) taken at bedtime
For constipation:	docusate (Colace, etc.)
	docusate with casanthranol (Peri-Colace, etc.)
For anxiety or nervous tension:	buspirone (Buspar)
	diazepam (Valium)
For headache, minor aches and pains:	acetaminophen (Tylenol, etc.)
	propoxyphene (Darvon)
	Avoid aspirin.

Note: Drug selection, dosage and administration schedule must be determined by the physician for each patient individually.

Resources for Additional Information and Services

American Digestive Disease Society
7720 Wisconsin Avenue
Bethesda, MD 20814
Phone: (301) 652-9293

Telecommunications services: Gutline, available to the public every Tuesday evening from 7:30 to 9:00 p.m., EST.
Publications available.

National Ulcer Foundation
675 Main Street
Melrose, MA 02176
Phone: (617) 665-6210

Publication: newsletter concerning peptic ulcer disease.

PSORIASIS

Other Name: Psoriasis vulgaris

Prevalence in USA: 2% to 4% of the white population; less than 1% of the black population. 6% to 7% of individuals with psoriasis have associated arthritis (psoriatic arthritis).

Age Group: The usual onset is between 10 and 40 years of age. However, psoriasis may begin at any age.

Male to Female Ratio: Slightly more common in men in all age groups.

Principal Features

Psoriasis is the most common type of chronic, recurrent scaling dermatitis. It begins gradually, often with one or two small patches, and follows a course of irregular and unpredictable remissions and recurrences throughout life. The characteristic skin change consists of a well-demarcated pink to reddish patch (plaque), one to three inches in size, which is covered almost completely by dry, silvery scales. Removal of the scales exposes numerous small, red bleeding points. Itching, if present at all, is usually mild. The size, number and distribution of the patches varies greatly. They may remain localized to a few small areas or they may spread to involve the entire body surface. The areas most commonly involved include the scalp, back of the neck and the outer surfaces of the arms and legs, especially the elbows, knees and shins. Less commonly psoriasis may involve the eyebrows, armpits, palms of the hands, soles of the feet, finger nails, umbilicus and the anal and genital areas. A rare form may involve the back, hips and thighs. Very rarely patches may occur in the mouth or on the tongue. During remission the patches fade and clear, the skin heals without scarring and there is no alteration of hair in involved areas. Permanent remission is rare. Currently there is no curative treatment, but most cases can be controlled satisfactorily.

Usually the general health is not affected. Infrequently a more serious and extensive form of psoriasis may develop. An acute, generalized, pustular form with fever, weakness and systemic debility can occur. Another unusual type causes extensive inflammation and peeling of the skin. Approximately 7% of cases will develop a form of arthritis that resembles rheumatoid arthritis; this varies in severity from relatively mild to permanently disabling.

Causes: The primary, fundamental cause is unknown. Psoriasis is a genetically determined, hereditary defect of the factors that regulate skin growth. The characteristic scaly patch is caused by a ten-fold increase in the turnover rate of the surface cells of the skin. Precipitating factors that can "trigger" the development of psoriasis plaques include excessive sunburn, acute respiratory infections (such as "strep" throat), local injury to the skin, surgical incisions and vaccination.

Drugs That Can Cause This Disorder: Drugs cannot cause or initiate psoriasis in an individual with normal skin (hereditary defect absent). However, a few drugs can exacerbate existing psoriasis. These include beta blockers, chloroquine, hydroxychloroquine, lithium, quinidine and the withdrawal of cortisonelike drugs.

Drugs Used to Treat This Disorder

Lubricants: lotions, creams, ointments; used to reduce water loss from psoriasis plaques. Examples: Lac-Hydrin, Moisturel lotion, Eucerin Creme, Aquaphor Creme, Vaseline Petroleum Jelly.

Keratolytic agents: used to remove scale. Examples: 6% salicylic acid (Keralyt Gel), 10% to 20% urea in petrolatum.

Coal tar preparations: used with and without ultraviolet light. Examples: Aquatar, Estar, Fototar, psoriGel, P&S Plus.

Anthralin preparations: used with and without ultraviolet light. Examples: Dithroceme, Lasan.

Cortisonelike preparations: topical creams, gels and ointments for local use. Examples: Aristocort, Cyclocort, Diprolene, Kenalog, Lidex, Topicort, Valisone, others.

Psoralen preparations: used with ultraviolet light. Example: methoxsalen, topical and oral forms.

Methotrexate: see Drug Profile, Section Three.

Etretinate: see Drug Profile, Section Three.

Fish oil containing eicosapentanoic acid (EPA): for relief of itching and inflammation.

New Drugs in Development for Treating This Disorder

Vitamin A derivatives similar to etretinate and isotretinoin are currently under investigation.

Cyclosporine, a drug in current use to prevent rejection in organ transplant surgery, appears to be effective for psoriasis when used in small doses; this use is currently under investigation. It can cause dramatic clearing of generalized psoriasis, but its long-term adverse effects preclude its use except in very severe and resistant cases.

Goals of Drug Treatment

Acceleration of clearing of active plaques; this can usually be achieved in close to 90% of cases.

Prevention of recurrence of plaques; while remissions of several months can be achieved, permanent remission is not possible with currently available drugs.

Drug Management

Topical Use of Drugs

1. Coal tar preparations: method of action is not fully known. Available in solutions, bath oils, shampoos, lotions and ointments.

    When used in conjunction with ultraviolet light (UVL), they can produce remissions lasting 6 to 12 months.

    Can cause burning, stinging reactions ("tar smarts") in skin on exposure to sun or large doses of UVL.

2. Anthralin preparations: interfere with DNA synthesis and skin cell reproduction.

    Available in creams, ointments and paste.

    Apply only to psoriasis plaques; can irritate normal skin and stain it brown.

    More effective when used in conjunction with UVL.

3. Cortisonelike preparations for local use: reduce inflammation, swelling and itching of psoriasis plaques.

    These are the drugs most commonly used in the current management of mild to moderate psoriasis.

    Available in lotions, creams and ointments. Lotions are preferred for treating the scalp; creams are preferred for treating the armpits and groin; ointments are preferred for remaining skin areas. The ointment is more effective when used under occlusive dressings.

    These drugs are used primarily when (1) the skin is "sore" and vulnerable to the irritant effects of other drugs; (2) other drugs are unacceptable for cosmetic reasons; (3) results with coal tar or anthralin preparations alone are unsatisfactory.

    Prolonged use without interruption can cause skin atrophy and loss of drug effectiveness.

    Possible side-effects: rosacealike skin changes, excessive hair growth (at point of application), lowered resistance to infection, systemic absorption, glaucoma (when applied around eyes).

Systemic Use of Drugs

1. Psoralens: inhibit DNA synthesis and suppress skin cell reproduction.

Available as methoxsalen and trioxsalen for both local and systemic use.

These are photosensitizing drugs and are used in conjunction with ultraviolet light in the A range; the combined treatment program is referred to as PUVA. The drug is taken orally 2 hours before UVL exposure; food impairs absorption and should be avoided. Treatments are given 2 to 4 times per week until the skin is clear. Maintenance treatment is given every 1 to 3 weeks to prevent recurrence. Protective glasses should be worn during treatment and for 8 hours following treatment to prevent cataracts.

Side-effects include itching, nausea and accelerated aging of the skin.

When properly used, this form of treatment produces improvement in 2 to 3 weeks and clearance of plaques within 1 to 3 months in 75% to 80% of cases.

2. Methotrexate: reduces the turnover rate of superficial skin cells.

This drug is reserved for use in treating severe, resistant cases of psoriasis, especially the generalized pustular forms and those with chronic extensive plaque formation that have not responded to safer treatment measures. It may also be beneficial in cases of psoriatic arthritis.

This drug can be highly effective. However, it has very serious potential toxicity. It can depress bone marrow function, damage liver tissue and impair kidney function.

Avoid alcohol, aspirin and aspirin substitutes while taking this drug.

See the Drug Profile in Section Three for a complete discussion.

3. Etretinate:

This vitamin A derivative may be used alone or in conjunction with other appropriate treatments, especially PUVA. It provides excellent relief in severe pustular psoriasis and when there is involvement of the palms and soles.

This drug should be used only to treat severe, resistant forms of psoriasis that have failed to respond to standard treatments. It can cause major birth defects, significant elevations of blood triglycerides and toxic effects on bone marrow, liver and kidney tissue.

See the Drug Profile in Section Three for a complete discussion.

Current Controversies in Drug Management

Should doses of psoralen and ultraviolet light (PUVA) and the duration of treatment be reduced to lessen the long-term risk of developing skin cancer?

Comments: PUVA treatment is an established, highly effective therapy for severe psoriasis. The best results are obtained when relatively high doses and extended treatment periods are used. Two recently published research reports demonstrate a significantly increased risk of developing two types of skin cancer five years after initial treatment with PUVA. The risk for squamous cell skin cancer was 12 times greater for those who received over 260 PUVA treatments than for those who received 160 or fewer treatments. The risk for basal cell skin cancer was moderately increased and also dose-related. It is recommended that PUVA treatment dosage be reduced by alternating it with other treatment methods, even if this means less than complete clearing of the skin.

Ancillary Drug Treatment (as required)

Condition	Drug Treatment
For itching:	hydroxyzine (Atarax, Vistaril)

Note: Drug selection, dosage and administration schedule must be determined by the physician for each patient individually.

Resources for Additional Information and Services

National Institute of Arthritis and Musculoskeletal and Skin Diseases
Information Office: Building 31, Room 4C32B
9000 Rockville Pike
Bethesda, MD 20892
Phone: Information Specialist, (301) 496-8188

Handles inquiries on arthritis, bone diseases, and skin diseases (including psoriasis).

Psoriasis Research Association
107 Vista del Grande
San Carlos, CA 94070
Phone: (415) 593-1394

Publications available.

RHEUMATOID ARTHRITIS

Other Names: Atrophic arthritis, chronic inflammatory arthritis, proliferative arthritis

Prevalence in USA: Approximately 7 million—2% to 3% of the general population.

Age Group: Affects all ages—infancy to senescence. Usual onset is between 20 and 50 years. Mean age at onset is 30 to 40 years.

Male to Female Ratio: In 20-to-50-year age group—more common in women, 3 to 1. Over 50 years—same incidence in men and women.

Principal Features: Rheumatoid arthritis is a highly complex inflammatory disorder that can affect several systems of the body simultaneously. It is quite variable in its manifestations: it may last a few days or up to 50 years; it may affect a single joint or up to 60 joints; it may involve the skin, the eyes, the nervous system, the lungs, the heart and blood vessels and the spleen; it can be mild, moderately severe or life-threatening in its most virulent forms. It usually begins with fatigue, poor appetite, loss of weight, morning stiffness and joint pains. Initially the small joints of the hands, wrists and feet are affected; larger joints may be affected later. The painful and destructive disease of the joints is the major feature of this disorder. The disease process begins with a severe inflammation of the joint lining (synovial membrane). This is followed by the formation of thick granulation tissue that ultimately destroys joint cartilage, bone and adjacent ligaments. The affected joints are swollen, warm, tender, stiff and painful to use; after a sustained period of active disease, joint destruction results in irreversible deformity. All of the joints that are affected will show evidence of disease within the first 2 years. Ten percent of cases will have a spontaneous complete remission (recovery) within 6 to 24 months after the onset of symptoms.

Causes: A specific definitive cause for rheumatoid arthritis has not been established. However, there is evidence to support the theory that the disease process is initiated by a virus that infects the joints of individuals who are genetically susceptible because of a defective immune system.

Drugs That Can Cause This Disorder: There are no drugs that induce true rheumatoid arthritis. The following drugs may aggravate an active or latent arthritis: iron dextran, isoniazid and pyrazinamide (in combination), oral contraceptives (?).

Drugs Used to Treat This Disorder: There are no drugs that can cure rheumatoid arthritis. The drugs currently available for use in managing this form of arthritis fall into 2 groups: (1) those that relieve symptoms but do not alter the basic disease process—do not produce remission; (2) those that may retard or arrest the disease and initiate remission.

Drugs Used to Relieve Symptoms
Salicylates
- aspirin (Bufferin, Ascriptin, Cama, etc.).
- aspirin, enteric-coated (Easprin, Ecotrin, etc.).
- aspirin, zero-order-release (Zorprin).
- magnesium salicylate (Magan, Mobidin).
- choline magnesium salicylate (Trisilate).
- salsalate (Disalcid).
- diflunisal (Dolobid).
- sodium salicylate (Pabalate).

Other Nonsteroidal Anti-inflammatory Drugs (NSAIDs)
Indole derivatives:
- indomethacin (Indocin).
- sulindac (Clinoril).
- tolmetin (Tolectin).

Propionic acid derivatives:
- fenoprofen (Nalfon).
- flurbiprofen (Ansaid).
- ibuprofen (Motrin, Rufen, etc.).
- ketoprofen (Orudis).
- naproxen (Naprosyn).
- suprofen (Suprol).

Fenamic acid derivative: meclofenamate (Meclomen).
Oxicam derivative: piroxicam (Feldene).
Phenylacetic acid derivative: diclofenac (Voltaren).
Cortisonelike Steroid Drugs
- prednisone.
- triamcinolone (Aristocort).
- dexamethasone (Decadron).
- methylprednisolone (Medrol).

Immunosuppressive Drugs
- azathioprine (Imuran).
- chlorambucil (Leukeran).
- cyclophosphamide (Cytoxan).
- methotrexate (Mexate).

Drugs Used to Produce Remission
Gold Preparations
- auranofin (Ridaura).
- aurothioglucose (Solganal).
- gold sodium thiomalate (Myochrysine).

hydroxychloroquine (Plaquenil)
penicillamine (Cuprimine, Depen)

Goals of Drug Treatment
Relief of pain, tenderness and stiffness.
Control of inflammation in joint tissues.
Production of remission; arrest of active disease.
Prevention of joint destruction; preservation of joint function.

Drug Management
General Principles
Rheumatoid arthritis can be the most difficult of all arthritic disorders
to control; in its more severe forms, it is the most damaging to joint
tissues. Its course is usually intermittent to chronic. No cure is
known. If adequate treatment is started early, severe crippling can
often be prevented or minimized.

Every case of rheumatoid arthritis is a unique, individual problem; successful management depends upon a treatment program that is carefully individualized.

Many drugs are available to treat rheumatoid arthritis. None is curative, and none is effective in all cases. Drugs that control inflammation can provide symptomatic relief but do not modify the underlying disease process; they cannot induce a remission. Disease-altering drugs are used in an attempt to modify the actual disease process and thereby initiate a remission. If successful, maintenance drug treatment may be continued for months or years.

Treatment is usually started with the safest and best tolerated drugs. There is marked individual variation in response to most drugs; this is very apparent with the use of the nonsteroidal anti-inflammatory drugs (aspirin substitutes). Trial-and-error experimentation is necessary to find the most effective and acceptable anti-inflammatory drug for each person.

Drug treatment of rheumatoid arthritis often requires a combination of drugs. The more severe forms of this arthritis respond more favorably when a disease-modifying drug is added to an established program of salicylates or NSAIDs. (See drugs listed above.)

Use of Salicylates

1. Aspirin is often the first drug used to provide adequate anti-inflammatory effects; it must be taken in large doses. A trial of salicylates is indicated in all cases of rheumatoid arthritis. (Avoid if there is a history of aspirin allergy, peptic ulcer disease, gastritis or gastrointestinal bleeding.)
2. Aspirin preparations that are designed for absorption in the small intestine (instead of in the stomach) are preferred: Disalcid, Easprin, Ecotrin, Zorprin.
3. The measurement of salicylate blood levels is advisable to determine the optimal dose of the salicylate used and to avoid serious toxicity.
4. Warning symptoms of early salicylate toxicity are ringing in the ears (tinnitus) and loss of hearing. However, these may not occur in the very young or in the elderly.
5. Approximately 50% of patients cannot tolerate the large doses of aspirin required to achieve adequate anti-inflammatory effects. Other salicylates may be tried or a nonsteroidal anti-inflammatory drug may be substituted.

Use of Other Nonsteroidal Anti-inflammatory Drugs (NSAIDs)

1. These may be used as substitutes for aspirin by those who cannot tolerate (or should not take) salicylates; or they may be used to initiate treatment at the outset.
2. As a group, the NSAIDs are not superior to salicylates in anti-inflammatory effect, but they are generally better tolerated.
3. These drugs produce significant decrease in morning stiffness, improve comfort and function and may be more effective than aspirin for some.
4. Fenoprofen and naproxen are among the more active NSAIDs; a trial of 2 weeks will identify those who can respond favorably.

5. Response to NSAIDs is highly variable from person to person. If an NSAID from one chemical class proves to be ineffective or unacceptable, a drug from another class within the NSAID group should be tried. A trial of 2 weeks is usually adequate to determine effectiveness and tolerance. (See drugs listed above.)

Use of Cortisonelike Steroid Drugs

1. Steroids are used infrequently and for short periods of time in both acute and chronic stages of rheumatoid arthritis. They are always added to existing drug programs as needed. Their use is justified, in small doses, to control acute "flares" of inflammation that prevent any degree of mobility in severely diseased joints.

2. Steroids provide a powerful anti-inflammatory effect, but they do not alter the underlying disease process or induce remission. They should be used to provide short-term comfort as necessary but not to abolish all symptoms.

3. Long-term maintenance use of steroids—even in small doses—must be avoided. Risks of excessive use include cataracts, osteoporosis, muscle wasting, atherosclerosis.

Use of Immunosuppressive Drugs

1. These highly toxic and hazardous drugs are used only when arthritis activity persists in spite of combined treatment with NSAIDs and disease-modifying agents. They are used in an attempt to prevent further joint destruction, deformity and disability.

2. Cyclophosphamide is the most effective drug of this group. Its use is reserved for patients with disabling systemic complications of rheumatoid arthritis.

3. Methotrexate is often the first choice of this group to try in the treatment of severe rheumatoid arthritis that has not responded to conventional therapy. In low dosage it can be very effective in approximately 50% of patients. Potential risks include severe depression of the bone marrow, liver damage, ulceration of the mouth and intestine and birth defects. Avoid alcohol and salicylates during methotrexate therapy.

Use of Gold Preparations

1. Based upon long experience with its use, gold is the standard disease-modifying drug for treating rheumatoid arthritis. It is often the first choice to add to an established program of NSAID therapy.

2. Gold is used only when arthritis cannot be controlled with safer drugs. A trial of 6 months or longer is necessary to determine its ability to induce remission. Approximately 50% of patients respond favorably.

3. Risks of gold therapy include dermatitis, kidney damage and blood cell and bone marrow toxicity. Treatment should be stopped immediately if any of the following develop: skin rash, mouth ulcers, fever, sore throat, abnormal bleeding or bruising.

Use of Hydroxychloroquine
1. This drug is used to treat mild or moderately severe rheumatoid arthritis. It can be very effective in some cases, relieving symptoms and retarding disease activity.
2. A trial of 6 months is necessary to determine this drug's ability to induce remission.
3. After 1 year of continual use, this drug can (rarely) damage eye structures and impair vision. Corneal deposits, retinal pigmentation and optic neuritis have been reported. The estimated incidence is 1 in 1000 to 1 in 2000 patients.
4. Other possible adverse drug effects include skin rash, abnormally low white blood cell count and peripheral neuritis (see Glossary).
5. This drug can aggravate existing psoriasis.

Use of Penicillamine
1. This drug is an effective substitute for gold therapy when a disease-modifying drug is needed.
2. A trial of 6 to 12 months is necessary to determine its ability to induce remission.
3. For maximal effectiveness, this drug should be taken on an empty stomach.
4. This is a potent drug; it can cause the following adverse effects: dermatitis, kidney damage, blood cell and bone marrow toxicity, bronchiolitis (dry cough and shortness of breath) and a pattern of muscular weakness similar to myasthenia gravis.

Ancillary Drug Treatment (as required)

Condition	*Drug Treatment*
For additional analgesia:	propoxyphene (Darvon)
	hydrocodone (Vicodin) (for short-term, intermittent use only)
For night pain:	indomethacin (Indocin) (taken with food at bedtime)
For anemia:	iron preparations
	folic acid (if appropriate for type of anemia)
For anxiety and tension:	diazepam (Valium)
For depression:	tricyclic antidepressants (see Profile of Depression in this section)
For drug-induced peptic ulcer:	cimetidine (Tagamet)
	famotidine (Pepcid)
	nizatidine (Axid)
	ranitidine (Zantac) (see Profile of Peptic Ulcer in this section)

Note: Drug selection, dosage and administration schedule must be determined by the physician for each patient individually.

Resources for Additional Information and Services

American Juvenile Arthritis Organization
1314 Spring Street
Atlanta, GA 30309
Phone: (404) 872-7100

Publications available.

Arthritis Foundation (parent organization)
1314 Spring Street
Atlanta, GA 30309
Phone: (404) 872-7100

Publications available.

Association for People With Arthritis
P.O. Box 954
6 Commercial Street
Hicksville, NY 11802
Phone: 1-800-323-2243

Publications available.

SCHIZOPHRENIA

Other Name: Dementia praecox

Prevalence in USA: Approximately 2.4 million—1% of the general population; 100,000 new cases annually.

Age Group: Onset most common between 16 and 25 years of age. Onset uncommon after 30 and rare after 40 years of age.

Male to Female Ratio: Equal incidence in men and women.

Principal Features: Schizophrenia refers to a group of disorders of the brain manifested by severe disturbances of the mind and personality. Cardinal features are abnormal thinking, behavior and mood; the schizophrenic pattern is characterized by misinterpretation of reality, withdrawal, delusions, hallucinations (usually auditory), bizarre or regressive behavior. It usually begins early in life, may be mild and transient in nature or may develop into a psychosis of major dimension that is intermittent or chronic for life. The first group—referred to as schizophreniform—experiences one episode of varying severity (often in response to stress), responds well to treatment and has no relapse after treatment is stopped. The second group—classical chronic schizophrenia—experiences recurrent episodes of disabling symptoms that require long-term antipsychotic drug therapy for control. Most of this group will relapse if maintenance treatment is stopped. A variety of subtypes are identified according to their dominant features: delusions of persecution and grandeur (paranoid type); primitive mentality, markedly disorganized thought and behavior (hebephrenic type); withdrawn, negativistic, uncommunicative, apathetic behavior pattern (catatonic); disorganized thinking, delusions, hallucinations accompanied by either mania or depression (schizo-affective); insidious loss of motivation and ambition, avoidance of interpersonal relationships (simple type); mixed or indefinite symptom complex (undifferentiated type). Though the presentations may vary according to type, the same group of antipsychotic drugs is used to treat all types without distinction.

Causes: The fundamental cause of schizophrenia is unknown. No anatomical or biochemical abnormality of the brain has been identified. Studies suggest that a genetic predisposition is necessary for the development of schizophrenia, rendering the subject vulnerable to disturbances of neurochemical transmission of nerve impulses or to alterations of brain circuitry. Effective antipsychotic drugs block dopamine receptors in certain brain cells; this suggests that increased dopamine activity is somehow responsible for the schizophrenic syndrome.

Drugs That Can Cause This Disorder: The following drugs may aggravate existing schizophrenia or produce schizophrenialike symptoms in normal individuals:

albuterol	cortisonelike steroids
alcohol (intoxication)	digitalis
amantadine	disopyramide
amphetamines (abuse)	disulfiram (toxicity)
anticonvulsants	indomethacin
apomorphine	isoniazid
atropinelike drugs	levodopa
bromides	methyldopa
bromocriptine	propranolol
cimetidine	tocainide
cocaine	triazolam

Drugs Used to Treat This Disorder
Phenothiazines
Aliphatic type:
  • chlorpromazine (Thorazine)
Piperidine type:
  • thioridazine (Mellaril)
  • mesoridazine (Serentil)
Piperazine type:
  • perphenazine (Trilafon)
  • trifluoperazine (Stelazine)
  • fluphenazine (Prolixin, Permitil)

Thioxanthenes
- thiothixene (Navane).

Butyrophenones
- haloperidol (Haldol).

Dibenzoxazepines
- loxapine (Loxitane).

Dihydroindolones
- molindone (Moban).

Goals of Drug Treatment

Good control of symptoms with the lowest possible dose of anti-psychotic drug.

Determination of the most effective drug and dosage schedule for each individual: intermittent dosage (as needed) versus continual long-term dosage.

Prevention of relapse (recurrent psychotic episode).

Improvement of capacity to function in society as normally as possible.

Drug Management

General Principles

The primary management of schizophrenia is based upon the rational use of antipsychotic drugs. Psychotherapy and drug therapy are considered to be complementary; psychotherapy can improve the patient's social adjustment; drug therapy can control disabling symptoms and make the situation somewhat manageable. Drug therapy is not curative.

If appropriate drug treatment is started early, 30% to 50% of patients will have a satisfactory remission; another 30% will improve sufficiently to live outside of a hospital. Drug therapy can abolish delusions, hallucinations, hyperactivity and combative behavior. Approximately 10% to 20% of patients do not respond to any drugs currently available.

The initial treatment of an acute psychotic episode consists of a course of carefully selected antipsychotic drugs taken for 6 to 12 months. Many individuals will respond favorably to one drug and not at all to another. History of previous drug use and response can be very helpful in selecting a drug for the management of recurrent episodes.

Current practice is to attempt withdrawal of antipsychotic drugs from all patients who have had a good response to drug treatment during their first episode of schizophrenia. This allows identification of those who will have a self-limited type of schizophrenia (schizophreniform disorder) and will do well without maintenance drug therapy. From 15% to 30% of patients will recover spontaneously following the initial episode and drug withdrawal. Antipsychotic drugs should be discontinued gradually over a period of 1 to 2 weeks.

The majority of schizophrenic patients will require continual drug therapy for long periods of time—possibly for life. Many will relapse rapidly and severely after drugs are discontinued. The nature of the drug maintenance program is determined by the type and frequency of continuing psychotic symptoms and the pattern of relapses experienced by each individual. When the patient complies well, maintenance drug therapy is successful in 85% of cases.

The principal action of antipsychotic drugs is to block dopamine receptors in the brain. By blocking dopamine action in the mesolimbic system, the drugs control the abnormal manifestations of schizophrenia; by blocking dopamine action in the nigrostriatal system, the drugs cause parkinsonism (and related adverse effects). Thus parkinsonism is now recognized as an *unavoidable* side-effect of most antipsychotic drugs. It is usually very responsive to the anticholinergic drugs used to treat Parkinson's disease, but not to levodopa. (See Profile of Parkinson's Disease in this section.)

It is generally recommended that antiparkinsonism drugs *not* be used routinely while taking antipsychotic drugs. Reasons given are:
(1) antiparkinsonism drugs can produce toxic brain syndromes
(2) they can interfere with the effectiveness of antipsychotic drugs
(3) they may increase the risk of developing tardive dyskinesia

Tardive dyskinesia (see Glossary) is one of the most serious adverse effects of long-term antipsychotic drug use. The reported incidence ranges from 3% after 1 year of medication to 21% after 7 years of medication. It appears to occur more frequently in elderly women.

"Drug holidays" of 4 to 6 weeks without medication are being used by some physicians treating chronic schizophrenia to reduce the risk of developing tardive dyskinesia. Among those who have been on maintenance therapy for 1 year without relapsing, 66% will not relapse within 6 months after stopping medication. For this group of patients, a "drug holiday" is feasible and possibly beneficial.

Antipsychotic drugs usually improve behavior. However, excessively high doses can cause a toxic state that worsens behavior. Drug response and tolerance vary greatly from person to person and must be monitored carefully in each individual.

Patients with schizo-affective disorders will probably require an antipsychotic drug and an additional drug for the affective component; this could be either lithium or an antidepressant.

Lithium may aggravate the neurological complications of antipsychotic drug therapy. The concurrent use of these two drugs requires caution and careful monitoring.

Use of Phenothiazines
1. Because of its numerous side-effects, chlorpromazine (the first phenothiazine) is used less frequently.
2. Because of its relatively greater sedative effects, thioridazine is favored for treatment of acute psychotic episodes. It causes parkinsonism (and possibly tardive dyskinesia) less frequently.
3. Fluphenazine is less sedating but is thought to have a higher risk for causing parkinsonism and tardive dyskinesia.
4. Trifluoperazine is thought to be preferable for the elderly schizophrenic because it has less sedative and atropinelike side-effects.

Use of Thiothixene
1. This antipsychotic drug is thought to be more effective for the retarded and regressed schizophrenic.
2. Because of its mild antidepressant effect, this drug is preferred for the schizo-affective patient who has features of depression.
3. This drug has less sedative and atropinelike side-effects, but a higher risk for causing parkinsonism.

Use of Haloperidol
1. This drug is reported to be effective in patients who are not responsive to chlorpromazine.
2. It can control aggressive behavior without causing significant sedation.
3. Although it has a relatively high potential for causing parkinsonism (and related effects), it is useful in the elderly because it is less sedating and has fewer atropinelike side-effects.

Use of Loxapine
1. This drug is especially useful in treating the paranoid schizophrenic.
2. It is less sedating than chlorpromazine and equal to haloperidol in effectiveness.

Use of Molindone
1. This is the only antipsychotic drug that appears to contribute to weight loss; many antipsychotic drugs tend to promote weight gain.
2. This drug is as effective as other major antipsychotics and is less sedating than many.

Current Controversies in Drug Management

Is "low-dose" antipsychotic drug therapy feasible for maintenance following release from the hospital?

The vast majority of schizophrenic individuals will experience a return of symptoms shortly after discontinuing a stabilizing maintenance dose of effective medication. Conventional practice has not favored reduction of dosage that proved effective for long-term maintenance. Recent studies have shown that many responsive and stabilized schizophrenic patients can be maintained satisfactorily at home (following hospital discharge) with one-fifth of the usually prescribed dose of injectable, long-acting fluphenazine: 5 mg every 2 weeks instead of the standard 25 mg dose. Patients on low-dose maintenane therapy adjusted better to family and work situations, were less apathetic and experienced fewer adverse drug effects. The lower dosage may also reduce the potential for the development of tardive dyskinesia (see Glossary).

Ancillary Drug Treatment (as required)

Condition	*Drug Treatment*
For anxiety:	buspirone (Buspar)
For depression:	see Profile of Depression in this section

For insomnia: chloral hydrate (Noctec, etc.)
                              temazepam (Restoril)
                              triazolam (Halcion)
For constipation: docusate (Colace, etc.)
                              docusate with casanthranol (Peri-Colace)
For parkinsonism: benztropine (Cogentin)
                              trihexyphenidyl (Artane)
For akathisia (marked
  restlessness):   propranolol (Inderal)
                              diphenhydramine (Benadryl)

Note: Drug selection, dosage and administration schedule must be determined
  by the physician for each patient individually.

Resources for Additional Information and Services

American Schizophrenia Association
900 North Federal Highway
Boca Raton, FL 33432
Phone: 1-800-847-3802

National Mental Health Association
1021 Prince Street
Alexandria, VA 22314
Phone: (703) 684-7722

Publications: *FOCUS*; also provides pamphlets and films.

National Mental Health Consumers' Association
311 South Juniper Street, Room 902
Philadelphia, PA 19107
Phone: (215) 735-2465

Publications available.

Schizophrenics Anonymous
1209 California Road
Eastchester, NY 10709
Phone: (914) 337-2252

Twenty-five local groups. A self-help organization sponsored by the
American Schizophrenia Association. Conduct meetings for discussion of all aspects of managing and coping with schizophrenia.

ULCERATIVE COLITIS

Other Names: Idiopathic proctocolitis, inflammatory bowel disease

Prevalence in USA: 1 million (includes 100,000 children); 15,000 new cases
  annually.

Age Group: Peak incidence occurs between 19 and 49 years of age; 75% of cases develop before the age of 40.

Male to Female Ratio: Same incidence in men and women.

Principal Features: Ulcerative colitis is a chronically recurrent disorder of the colon (large intestine) and rectum characterized by inflammation and ulceration. Its course follows a pattern of frequent spontaneous remissions and recurrences without apparent cause. It may be associated with disease in other organs of the body, notably the skin, joints, eye, liver and blood vessels, making it a multiple system disorder. The principle symptoms of the diseased colon are abdominal cramping and bloody diarrhea; associated symptoms include fatigue, weakness, occasional low-grade fever, weight loss, anemia and dehydration. The more severe forms of ulcerative colitis can be very difficult to control.

Causes: The basic cause of ulcerative colitis is not known. Theories of possible causes include infection, environmental toxins, psychological stress, sensitivities to foods and "autoimmunity"—a disorder of the immune system that results in the selective destruction of body tissues. There is some evidence that indicates a familial pattern, suggesting a hereditary susceptibility to a causative agent.

Drugs That Can Cause This Disorder: No drugs initiate true ulcerative colitis. However, the following anti-infective drugs can cause pseudomembranous colitis, a disorder that closely resembles an acute attack of ulcerative colitis:

amoxicillin
ampicillin
cephalosporins
chloramphenicol
clindamycin
lincomycin
penicillin
tetracycline
trimethoprim and
   sulfamethoxsazole in
   combination

Drugs Used to Treat This Disorder

Anti-inflammatory Drugs
- 5-aminosalicylic acid (5-ASA)
- mesalamine (Rowasa) rectal suspension
- sulfasalazine (Azulfidine)

Cortisonelike Steroids
- prednisone, prednisolone (generic).
- hydrocortisone enemas (Cortenema).
- methylprednisolone enema (Medrol Enpak).

Antidiarrheals
- diphenoxylate (Lomotil).
- loperamide (Imodium).

Antispasmodics
- dicyclomine (Bentyl).
- propantheline (Pro-Banthine).

Immunosuppressive Drugs
- azathioprine (Imuran).
- 6-mercatopurine (Purinethol).

Goals of Drug Treatment

Control of pain and diarrhea.

Prompt control of acute attacks; surppression of inflammation and ulceration.

Induction of a remission.

Prevention of recurrence of acute attacks.

Drug Management

General Principles

The majority (up to 90%) of cases of active ulcerative colitis respond well to medical treatment or have a spontaneous remission. Approximately 20% have a prolonged remission after the first acute attack.

Studies indicate that 55% of individuals who experience ulcerative colitis remain in remission at any given time during the course of the disorder. To minimize the risks of long-term drug use, the smallest dose of maintenance drugs (azulfidine and steroids) that prevents recurrence should be determined.

It is essential that every recurrence of acute colitis (relapse) be treated promptly and vigorously. Chronically active ulcerative colitis predisposes to a higher than normal incidence of cancer of the colon and rectum. Estimates are 3% after the first 10 years of disease, increasing to 20% per decade thereafter. Everyone subject to ulcerative colitis should have a thorough examination of the colon and rectum annually regardless of the status of the disorder.

Antidiarrheal drugs should be used with extreme caution. Excessive use can induce a paralysis of colon activity and increase the risk of developing toxic megacolon—a massive distention of the colon with air; perforation constitutes a surgical emergency.

Iron preparations for anemia should not be taken during a period of acute inflammation or active ulceration. Withhold iron therapy until a remission is established.

Use of Sulfasalazine

1. This effective and reliable drug is used to treat acute attacks of active colitis and to prevent relapse during periods of remission.

2. It is used concurrently with cortisonelike steroids during acute attacks to control inflammation and ulceration and to induce remission.

3. During the quiescent phase of colitis, it is used in small doses (up to 2 grams/day) for the long-term maintenance of remission. It may be taken indefinitely.

4. This drug is best taken with or following food to reduce stomach irritation.

5. The long-term use of this drug can impair folic acid absorption and may cause a folic acid deficiency. Consult your physician regarding the need for a supplement.

6. During long-term use, it is advisable to monitor blood cell counts to detect the development of anemia or abnormally low white blood cells.
7. Mesalamine, the active derivative of sulfasalazine, is used in the form of a rectal suspension (retention enema), taken at bedtime for night-long action. The initial course of treatment is from 3 to 6 weeks. Carefully read and follow the printed instructions that are provided with this drug.

Use of Cortisonelike Steroids

1. These drugs are the mainstay of treatment for acute, active ulcerative colitis. They can induce remission in 70% to 80% of cases.
2. Steroids should be used when there are obvious symptoms of disease activity: diarrhea, bloody stools, nocturnal bowel movements, anemia, weight loss, etc. They are also of value in treating the systemic manifestations of this disorder: dermatitis, arthritis, iritis, etc.
3. To ensure prompt and adequate control of acute inflammation, initial dosage should be high. Response usually occurs within 10 to 14 days.
4. After a remission has been induced, steroid dosage is reduced to a minimum that will stabilize the colon and prevent relapse. The long-term maintenance use of steroids is controversial. If individual circumstances warrant the continual use of low-dose steroids, it is preferable to use alternate-day dosage—a single morning dose every 48 hours. This is effective in preventing recurrence for some patients and it carries a lower risk of causing adverse effects.
5. When the inflammation and ulceration are limited to the rectum, steroids can be administered in the form of enemas, foams and suppositories for local application. This minimizes systemic effects.
6. The long-term use of steroids (even in small doses) can cause significant adverse effects:
   • susceptibility to infection.
   • mineral and water imbalance.
   • reduced tolerance for sugar, potential for diabetes.
   • cataracts.
   • hypertension.
   • acne, excessive hair growth.
   • muscle wasting.
   • mental disturbances.
   • osteoporosis.
   • peptic ulcer activation.
   • retarded growth in children.

Ancillary Drug Treatment (as required)

Condition	Drug Treatment
For abdominal cramps:	dicyclomine (Bentyl) propantheline (Pro-Banthine) Use these sparingly.
For diarrhea:	diphenoxylate (Lomotil) loperamide (Imodium) Use these sparingly.
For anxiety:	buspirone (Buspar), nonsedating diazepam (Valium), sedating
For depression:	see Profile of Depression in this section
For anemia:	iron preparations (not during acute stage of colitis) folic acid (if appropriate for type of anemia)

Note: Drug selection, dosage and administration schedule must be determined by the physician for each patient individually.

Resource for Additional Information and Services

American Digestive Disease Society
7720 Wisconsin Avenue
Bethesda, MD 20814
Phone: (301) 652-9293

Telecommunications services: Gutline, available to the public every Tuesday evening from 7:30 to 9:00 p.m.
Publications available.

DRUG PROFILES

NOTE

The designation [CD] following the brand name of any drug in these Profiles indicates a combination drug (a drug product with more than one active ingredient).

ACEBUTOLOL
(a se BYU toh lohl)

Introduced: 1973

Class: Antihypertensive, heart rhythm regulator, beta-adrenergic blocker

Prescription: USA: Yes

Controlled Drug: USA: No

Available as Generic: No

Brand Name: Sectral

BENEFITS versus RISKS

Possible Benefits	*Possible Risks*
EFFECTIVE ANTIHYPERTEN-SIVE in mild to moderate high blood pressure	CONGESTIVE HEART FAILURE in advanced heart disease Worsening of angina in coronary heart disease (abrupt withdrawal) Masking of low blood sugar (hypoglycemia) in drug-treated diabetes

---

▷ **Principal Uses**

As a Single Drug Product: The treatment of mild to moderately severe high blood pressure. May be used alone or concurrently with other antihypertensive drugs, such as diuretics. Also used to prevent premature ventricular heartbeats.

How This Drug Works: By blocking certain actions of the sympathetic nervous system, this drug

- reduces the rate and contraction force of the heart, thus lowering the ejection pressure of the blood leaving the heart.
- reduces the degree of contraction of blood vessel walls, resulting in their relaxation and expansion and consequent lowering of the blood pressure.
- prolongs the conduction time of nerve impulses through the heart, of benefit in the management of certain heart rhythm disorders.

Available Dosage Forms and Strengths
Capsules — 200 mg, 400 mg

▷ **Usual Adult Dosage Range:** Initially 400 mg daily, either as a single dose in the morning or as 200 mg taken morning and evening (12 hours apart). The usual maintenance dose is 400 to 800 mg/24 hours. The total dose should not exceed 1200 mg/24 hours, given as 600 mg twice daily. **Note: Actual dosage and administration schedule must be determined by the physician for each patient individually.**

▷ **Dosing Instructions:**   May be taken without regard to eating. Capsule may be opened for administration. Do not discontinue this drug abruptly.

Usual Duration of Use: Continual use on a regular schedule for 10 to 14 days is usually necessary to determine this drug's effectiveness in lowering the blood pressure or abolishing premature heartbeats. The long-term use of this drug will be determined by the course of your blood pressure over time and your response to the overall treatment program (weight reduction, salt restriction, smoking cessation, etc.). Consult your physician on a regular basis.

Possible Advantages of This Drug
Causes less slowing of the heart rate than most other beta blocker drugs. Less likely to cause asthma (in susceptible individuals) when used in low doses.

Currently a "Drug of Choice" for initiating treatment of hypertension with a single drug, especially for those subject to bronchial asthma or diabetes.

▷ **This Drug Should Not Be Taken If**
- you have had an allergic reaction to it previously.
- you have congestive heart failure.
- you have an abnormally slow heart rate or a serious form of heart block.
- you are taking, or have taken within the past 14 days, any monoamine oxidase (MAO) type A inhibitor drug (see Drug Class, Section Four).

▷ **Inform Your Physician Before Taking This Drug If**
- you have had an adverse reaction to any beta blocker drug in the past (see Drug Class, Section Four).
- you have a history of serious heart disease, with or without episodes of heart failure.
- you have a history of hay fever (allergic rhinitis), asthma, chronic bronchitis or emphysema.
- you have a history of overactive thyroid function (hyperthyroidism).
- you have a history of low blood sugar (hypoglycemia).
- you have impaired liver or kidney function.
- you have diabetes or myasthenia gravis.
- you are currently taking any form of digitalis, quinidine or reserpine, or any calcium blocker drug (see Drug Class, Section Four).
- you plan to have surgery under general anesthesia in the near future.

Possible Side-Effects (natural, expected and unavoidable drug actions)
Lethargy and fatigability (11%), cold extremities (0.2%), slow heart rate, light-headedness in upright position (see Orthostatic Hypotension in Glossary).

▷ **Possible Adverse Effects** (unusual, unexpected and infrequent reactions)
If any of the following develop, consult your physician promptly for guidance.

Mild Adverse Effects
   Allergic Reactions: Skin rash, itching.
   Headache, dizziness, insomnia, abnormal dreams.
   Indigestion, nausea, constipation, diarrhea.
   Joint and muscle discomfort, fluid retention (edema).
Serious Adverse Effects
   Mental depression (2%), anxiety.
   Chest pain, shortness of breath, precipitation of congestive heart failure.
   Induction of bronchial asthma (in asthmatic individuals).

▷ **Possible Effects on Sexual Function:**   Impotence (2%), decreased libido, Peyronie's disease (see Glossary).

CAUTION
   1. ***Do not discontinue this drug suddenly*** without the knowledge and guidance of your physician. Carry a notation on your person that you are taking this drug.
   2. Consult your physician or pharmacist before using nasal decongestants usually present in over-the-counter cold preparations and nose drops. These can cause sudden increases in blood pressure when taken concurrently with beta blocker drugs.
   3. Report the development of any tendency to emotional depression.

Precautions for Use
   By Infants and Children: Safety and effectiveness for use by those under 12 years of age have not been established. However, if this drug is used, observe for the development of low blood sugar (hypoglycemia) during periods of reduced food intake.
   By Those over 60 Years of Age: Proceed ***cautiously*** with all antihypertensive drugs. Unacceptably high blood pressure should be reduced without creating the risks associated with excessively low blood pressure. Start treatment with small doses, and monitor the blood pressure response frequently. Sudden, rapid and excessive reduction of blood pressure can predispose to stroke or heart attack. Total daily dosage should not exceed 800 mg. Observe for dizziness, unsteadiness, tendency to fall, confusion, hallucinations, depression or urinary frequency.

▷ **Advisability of Use During Pregnancy**
   Pregnancy Category: B (tentative). See Pregnancy Code inside back cover.
      Animal studies: No significant increase in birth defects found in rats or rabbits.
      Human studies: Information from adequate studies of pregnant women is not available.
   Use this drug only if clearly needed. Ask physician for guidance.

Advisability of Use if Breast-Feeding
   Presence of this drug in breast milk: Yes.
   Avoid drug or refrain from nursing.

Habit-Forming Potential: None.

Effects of Overdosage: Weakness, slow pulse, low blood pressure, fainting, cold and sweaty skin, congestive heart failure, possible coma and convulsions.

Possible Effects of Long-Term Use: Reduced heart reserve and eventual heart failure in susceptible individuals with advanced heart disease.

Suggested Periodic Examinations While Taking This Drug (at physician's discretion)
Measurements of blood pressure, evaluation of heart function.

▷ **While Taking This Drug, Observe the Following**
Foods: No restrictions. Avoid excessive salt intake.
Beverages: No restrictions. May be taken with milk.
▷ *Alcohol:* Use with caution until the combined effect has been determined. Alcohol may exaggerate this drug's ability to lower the blood pressure and may increase its mild sedative effect.
Tobacco Smoking: Nicotine may reduce this drug's effectiveness in treating high blood pressure. In addition, high doses of this drug may potentiate the constriction of the bronchial tubes caused by regular smoking.
▷ *Other Drugs*
Acebutolol may ***increase*** the effects of
- other antihypertensive drugs and cause excessive lowering of the blood pressure. Dosage adjustments may be necessary.
- reserpine (Ser-Ap-Es, etc.) and cause sedation, depression, slowing of the heart rate and lowering of the blood pressure.
Acebutolol ***taken concurrently*** with
- clonidine (Catapres) requires close monitoring for rebound high blood pressure if clonidine is withdrawn while acebutolol is still being taken.
- insulin requires close monitoring to avoid undetected hypoglycemia (see Glossary).
The following drugs may ***decrease*** the effects of acebutolol
- indomethacin (Indocin), and possibly other "aspirin substitutes," may impair acebutolol's antihypertensive effect.
▷ *Driving, Hazardous Activities:* Use caution until the full extent of drowsiness, lethargy and blood pressure change has been determined.
Aviation Note: The use of this drug ***is a disqualification*** for piloting. Consult a designated Aviation Medical Examiner.
Exposure to Sun: No restrictions.
Exposure to Heat: Caution advised. Hot environments can lower the blood pressure and exaggerate the effects of this drug.
Exposure to Cold: Caution advised. Cold environments can enhance the circulatory deficiency in the extremities that may occur with this drug. The elderly should take precautions to prevent hypothermia (see Glossary).

Heavy Exercise or Exertion: It is advisable to avoid exertion that produces light-headedness, excessive fatigue or muscle cramping. The use of this drug may intensify the hypertensive response to isometric exercise.

Occurrence of Unrelated Illness: The fever that accompanies systemic infections can lower the blood pressure and require adjustment of dosage. Illnesses that cause nausea or vomiting may interrupt the regular dosage schedule. Ask your physician for guidance.

Discontinuation: It is advisable to avoid sudden discontinuation of this drug in all situations. If possible, gradual reduction of dose over a period of 2 to 3 weeks is recommended. Ask your physician for specific guidance.

ACETAMINOPHEN
(a set a MEE noh fen)

Other Names: APAP, paracetamol

Introduced: 1893

Class: Mild analgesic and antipyretic

Prescription: No

Controlled Drug: No

Available as Generic: Yes

Brand Names: Actifed-A [CD], Anacin-3, Anexsia [CD], Anexsia 7.5 [CD], ♣Apo-Acetaminophen, ♣Atasol, ♣Atasol Forte, Bromo-Seltzer [CD], Children's Fevernol, Contac Severe Cold Formula Caplets [CD], CoTylenol Children's Liquid Cold Formula [CD], CoTylenol Tablets [CD], Darvocet-N 50/100 [CD], Datril Extra Strength, Demerol-APAP [CD], Dimetapp-A Preparations [CD], Dolene AP-65 [CD], Drixoral Plus [CD], ♣Empracet-30, -60 [CD], Empracet w/Codeine No. 3, 4 [CD], ♣Emtec-30 [CD], Excedrin [CD], Excedrin P.M. [CD], ♣Exdol, ♣Exdol Strong, ♣Exdol-8, -15, -30 [CD], Fioricet [CD], Hycomine Compound [CD], ♣Lenoltec w/Codeine No. 1, 2, 3, 4 [CD], Lorcet Plus [CD], Lortab [CD], Ornex [CD], ♣Oxycocet [CD], Panadol, Parafon Forte [CD], Percocet [CD], ♣Percocet-Demi [CD], Percogesic [CD], Phenaphen, Phenaphen w/Codeine No. 2, 3, 4 [CD], ♣Robaxacet [CD], ♣Robigesic, ♣Rounox, ♣Rounox w/Codeine [CD], Sine-Aid [CD], Sine-Off Extra Strength Capsules [CD], Singlet [CD], Sinubid [CD], Sinutab Maximum Strength [CD], Sinutab No Drowsiness Tablets [CD], Sinutab Tablets [CD], St. Joseph Aspirin-Free, Sudafed Sinus Maximum Strength [CD], Talacen [CD], Tapar, Tempra, Triaminicin [CD], Trigesic [CD], Tycolet [CD], Tylenol, Tylenol w/Codeine No. 1, 2, 3, 4 [CD], ♣Tylenol Sinus Medication [CD], Tylox [CD], Valadol, Vanquish [CD], Vicodin [CD], Vicodin ES [CD], Wygesic [CD], Zydone [CD]

BENEFITS versus RISKS	
Possible Benefits	*Possible Risks*
EFFECTIVE RELIEF OF MILD TO MODERATE PAIN REDUCTION OF FEVER	Rare anemia, liver or kidney damage (with prolonged or excessive use)

▷ **Principal Uses**

As a Single Drug Product: To relieve mild to moderate pain from any cause, and to reduce high fever. It is often used instead of aspirin for these purposes.

As a Combination Drug Product [CD]: Often combined with other analgesics to enhance pain relief. Also combined with antihistamines and decongestants to relieve the discomfort of respiratory tract infections; and with muscle relaxants to augment the relief of discomfort associated with muscle spasm.

How This Drug Works: The mechanism of its analgesic action is not completely known. It may reduce the tissue concentrations of prostaglandins (chemicals involved in the production of pain) more effectively in the brain than in peripheral tissues. This could explain its reasonably good analgesic effect and its weak anti-inflammatory effect.

Available Dosage Forms and Strengths

Capsules — 325 mg, 500 mg
Effervescent granules — 325 mg (buffered)
Elixir — 120 mg, 160 mg, 325 mg per 5-ml teaspoonful
Liquid — 160 mg per 5-ml teaspoonful, 500 mg per 15-ml tablespoonful
Solution — 100 mg per ml, 120 mg per 2.5 ml
Suppositories — 120 mg, 125 mg, 325 mg, 600 mg, 650 mg
Tablets — 160 mg, 325 mg, 500 mg, 650 mg
Tablets, chewable — 80 mg, 160 mg
Wafers — 120 mg

▷ **Usual Adult Dosage Range:** 325 to 650 mg/4 hours as needed, or 1000 mg (1 gram)/4 to 6 hours (not to exceed 4 times/24 hours). **Note: For long-term use, actual dosage and administration schedule must be determined by the physician for each patient individually.**

▷ **Dosing Instructions:** May be taken on empty stomach or with food or milk. Capsule may be opened for administration.

Usual Duration of Use: Continual use (at above dosage) should not exceed 10 days at a time. For long-term use under physician supervision, the daily dosage should not exceed 2600 mg/24 hours. Recently published studies reveal that uninterrupted long-term use can cause significant kidney damage. Ask your physician for guidance.

▷ **This Drug Should Not Be Taken If**
  • you have had an allergic reaction to any dosage form of it previously.

▷ **Inform Your Physician Before Taking This Drug If**
  • you have impaired liver or kidney function.
  • you are currently taking any anticoagulant drug ("blood thinner").

Possible Side-Effects (natural, expected and unavoidable drug actions)
  Drowsiness (in sensitive individuals).

▷ **Possible Adverse Effects** (unusual, unexpected and infrequent reactions)
  If any of the following develop, consult your physician promptly for guidance.
  Mild Adverse Effects
  Allergic Reactions: Skin rash, hives (rare).
  Impaired thinking and concentration.
  Serious Adverse Effects
  Allergic Reactions: Swelling of the vocal cords, difficult breathing, anaphylactic reaction (see Glossary). Hemolytic anemia (see Glossary).
  Fever, sore throat (abnormally low white blood cell count).
  Abnormal bleeding or bruising (reduced blood platelet count, see Glossary).
  Decreased urine volume, bloody urine (kidney damage).
  Jaundice (liver damage).

▷ **Possible Effects on Sexual Function:**   None reported.

  CAUTION
  1. If you have bronchial asthma and you are also allergic to aspirin, use this drug with caution until your sensitivity to it has been determined.
  2. If you are taking an oral anticoagulant drug ("blood thinner"), high-dose acetaminophen may alter your response to it and increase the risk of abnormal bleeding. Ask physician for guidance.
  3. Avoid the long-term use of this drug concurrently with aspirin or aspirin substitutes. This combination, especially in high doses, can increase the risk of kidney damage.

  Precautions for Use
  By Infants and Children: Dosage is based upon age; ask physician for guidance if in doubt. Do not exceed 5 doses/24 hours. Continual use should not exceed 5 days at a time without physician guidance.
  By Those over 60 Years of Age: Do not exceed a total dose of 2600 mg/24 hours. Prolonged use in excessive doses can cause anemia, liver damage with jaundice and kidney damage.

▷ **Advisability of Use During Pregnancy**
  Pregnancy Category: B (tentative). See Pregnancy Code inside back cover.
  Animal studies: No birth defects due to this drug have been demonstrated.

Human studies: Is used in all stages of pregnancy. No evidence of adverse effects on mother or fetus has been documented when used in recommended doses for short periods of time.

Advisability of Use if Breast-Feeding
Presence of this drug in breast milk: Yes.
No adverse effects on nursing infants reported.

Habit-Forming Potential: None.

Effects of Overdosage: Nausea, vomiting, stomach pain, drowsiness, stupor, convulsions, coma, jaundice (in 2 to 5 days after large overdose).

Possible Effects of Long-Term Use: Formation of abnormal hemoglobin (methemoglobin). Development of anemia.

Suggested Periodic Examinations While Taking This Drug (at physician's discretion)
None required for short-term use.
During long-term use, examination for abnormal hemoglobin, anemia, reduced white blood cell or platelet counts, liver and kidney function.

▷ **While Taking This Drug, Observe the Following**
Foods: No restrictions.
Beverages: No restrictions. May be taken with milk or juices.
▷   *Alcohol:* No interactions expected.
Tobacco Smoking: No interactions expected.
▷   *Other Drugs*
Acetaminophen may ***increase*** the effects of
• oral anticoagulants if the acetaminophen is taken continually in daily doses of 2000 mg or more.
The following drug may ***increase*** the effects of acetaminophen
• diflunisal (Dolobid) may increase the risk of acetaminophen toxicity.
▷   *Driving, Hazardous Activities:* Usually no restrictions. Be alert to the rare occurrence of drowsiness and/or impaired thinking, and restrict activities accordingly.
Aviation Note: Usually no restrictions. However, it is advisable to observe for the possible occurrence of drowsiness or impaired thinking and to restrict activities accordingly.
Exposure to Sun: No restrictions.

ACETAZOLAMIDE
(a set a ZOHL a mide)

Introduced: 1953

Prescription: USA: Yes
Canada: Yes

Class: Anticonvulsant, antiglaucoma, diuretic, sulfonamides

Controlled Drug: USA: No
Canada: No

Available as Generic: USA: Yes
   Canada: No

Brand Names: ✦Acetazolam, Ak-Zol, ✦Apo-Acetazolamide, Dazamide, Diamox, Diamox Sequles

---

BENEFITS versus RISKS

Possible Benefits	*Possible Risks*
REDUCTION OF INTERNAL EYE PRESSURE in selected cases of glaucoma	Acidosis with long-term use
	Increased risk of kidney stone
	Rare bone marrow, liver or
CONTROL OF ABSENCE (PETIT MAL) SEIZURES	kidney injury
TREATMENT OF PERIODIC PARALYSIS	

▷ **Principal Uses**
   As a Single Drug Product: Primarily to treat certain types of glaucoma. Also used with other anticonvulsant drugs to manage petit mal epilepsy. Used less frequently to treat familial periodic paralysis and to prevent altitude sickness.

How This Drug Works: By inhibiting the action of the enzyme carbonic anhydrase, it decreases the formation of fluid (the aqueous humor) in the eye and increases the volume of urine.

Available Dosage Forms and Strengths
   Capsules, prolonged-action — 500 mg
                Injections — 500 mg per vial
                Tablets — 125 mg, 250 mg

▷ **Usual Adult Dosage Range:**   For glaucoma: 250 to 1000 mg/24 hours, in 2 or 3 doses. For epilepsy: 250 to 1000 mg/24 hours. As a diuretic: 250 to 375 mg/24 hours, in one morning dose. **Note: Actual dosage and administration schedule must be determined by the physician for each patient individually.**

▷ **Dosing Instructions:**   Best taken with food or milk to prevent stomach irritation. Tablet may be crushed. Diamox Sequels may be opened, but do not chew or crush contents for administration.

Usual Duration of Use: Treatment of glaucoma and epilepsy require long-term use. If taken to control seizures, do not stop this drug abruptly. Consult your physician on a regular basis.

▷ **This Drug Should Not Be Taken If**
   • you have had an allergic reaction to any dosage form of it previously.
   • you have serious liver or kidney disease.
   • you have Addison's disease.

▷ **Inform Your Physician Before Taking This Drug If**
- you have had an allergic reaction to any "sulfa" drug in the past.
- you have gout or lupus erythematosus.

Possible Side-Effects (natural, expected and unavoidable drug actions)
Drowsiness, temporary nearsightedness.

▷ **Possible Adverse Effects** (unusual, unexpected and infrequent reactions)
If any of the following develop, consult your physician promptly for guidance.
Mild Adverse Effects
Allergic Reactions: Skin rash, hives, drug fever.
Reduced appetite, indigestion, nausea.
Fatigue; weakness; dizziness; tingling of face, arms or legs.
Serious Adverse Effects
Allergic Reactions: Hemolytic anemia (see Glossary), spontaneous bruising (reduced blood platelet count, see Glossary).
Bone marrow depression (see Glossary)—fatigue, weakness, fever, sore throat, abnormal bleeding or bruising.
Hepatitis with jaundice (see Glossary)—yellow eyes and skin, dark-colored urine, light-colored stools.

▷ **Possible Effects on Sexual Function:** Decreased libido (male and female), impotence (both infrequent). Effects may begin after 2 weeks of use and subside when drug is discontinued.

▷ **Adverse Effects That May Mimic Natural Diseases or Disorders**
Toxic liver reaction may suggest viral hepatitis.
Lupus erythematosus–like syndrome.

Natural Diseases or Disorders That May Be Activated by This Drug
Gout, acidosis secondary to chronic obstructive lung disease—asthma, bronchitis, emphysema.

CAUTION
1. Observe for possible loss of drug effectiveness when used as a diuretic or to control seizures.
2. Emotional depression may occur and not be recognized as an adverse effect of this drug.
3. This drug may cause an excessive loss of potassium from the body. Consult your physician regarding the need for a high-potassium diet or potassium supplements.

Precautions for Use
By Infants and Children: Excessive dosage may cause drowsiness and numbness of the face and extremities. Not recommended for use as a diuretic in children.
By Those over 60 Years of Age: Do not exceed recommended doses. Increased dosage may cause excessive loss of sodium and potassium, with resultant weakness, confusion, numbness in the extremities and

nausea. If taking a digitalis preparation (digitoxin, digoxin), consult your physician regarding the need for a high-potassium diet or potassium supplements.

▷ **Advisability of Use During Pregnancy**
Pregnancy Category: C (tentative). See Pregnancy Code inside back cover.
Animal studies: Limb and skeletal defects reported in mice and rats.
Human studies: Information from adequate studies of pregnant women is not available.
Avoid completely during the first 3 months and during labor and delivery.

Advisability of Use if Breast-Feeding
Presence of this drug in breast milk: Yes.
Diuretic effect of drug may temporarily impair milk production.
Monitor nursing infant closely and discontinue drug or nursing if adverse effects develop.

Habit-Forming Potential: None.

Effects of Overdosage: Drowsiness, numbness and tingling, thirst, nausea, vomiting, confusion, excitement, convulsions, coma.

Possible Effects of Long-Term Use: The development of low blood potassium and/or acidosis.

Suggested Periodic Examinations While Taking This Drug (at physician's discretion)
Complete blood cell counts, measurements of blood sodium, potassium and uric acid levels, liver and kidney function tests.

▷ **While Taking This Drug, Observe the Following**
Foods: Consult your physician regarding the advisability of eating a high-potassium diet. See Section Six for the Table of High Potassium Foods.
Beverages: No restrictions. May be taken with milk.
▷ *Alcohol:* Use with caution until the combined effect has been determined. Alcohol may impair the anticonvulsant effect of this drug and reduce its control of seizures.
Tobacco Smoking: No interactions expected.
▷ *Other Drugs*
Acetazolamide may ***increase*** the effects of
• quinidine.
Acetazolamide may ***decrease*** the effects of
• lithium.
▷ *Driving, Hazardous Activities:* Usually no restrictions. Be alert to the possible occurrence of drowsiness or dizziness.
Aviation Note: The use of this drug ***may be a disqualification*** for piloting. Consult a designated Aviation Medical Examiner.
Exposure to Sun: No restrictions.

ACYCLOVIR
(ay SI kloh ver)

Introduced: 1979

Class: Antiviral

Prescription: USA: Yes
Canada: Yes

Controlled Drug: USA: No
Canada: No

Available as Generic: No

Brand Name: Zovirax

BENEFITS versus RISKS

Possible Benefits	*Possible Risks*
HASTENED RECOVERY FROM INITIAL EPISODE OF GENITAL HERPES	Nausea, vomiting, diarrhea (8% in long-term use)
PREVENTION OF RECURRENCE OF GENITAL HERPES	Nervousness, depression (less than 3%)
	Joint and muscle pain (3%)

▷ **Principal Uses**

As a Single Drug Product: Treatment of initial episodes and prevention of recurrent episodes of genital herpes in selected individuals.

How This Drug Works: By inhibiting DNA replication of the herpes simplex virus, this drug arrests the multiplication and spread of the infecting virus and thus reduces the severity and duration of the herpes infection.

Available Dosage Forms and Strengths
Capsules — 200 mg
Ointment — 5%

▷ **Usual Adult Dosage Range:** For initial episode of genital herpes—200 mg/4 hours for a total of 5 capsules daily for 10 consecutive days (total dose of 50 capsules). For intermittent recurrence—200 mg/4 hours for a total of 5 capsules daily for 5 consecutive days (total dose of 25 capsules). Begin treatment at the earliest indication of recurrence. For prevention of frequent recurrence—200 mg taken 3 to 5 times daily for up to 6 months. For the ointment form—cover all infected areas every 3 hours for a total of 6 times daily for 7 consecutive days. Begin treatment at the earliest indication of infection. **Note: Actual dosage and administration schedule must be determined by the physician for each patient individually.**

▷ **Dosing Instructions:** May be taken without regard to eating. Capsule may be opened for administration. Take the full course of the exact dose prescribed. Use a finger cot or rubber glove to apply the ointment.

Usual Duration of Use: Continual use on a regular schedule for 10 days is usually necessary to determine this drug's effectiveness in reducing the severity and duration of the initial infection. Continual use for 4 to 6 months may be necessary to prevent frequent recurrence of herpes eruptions.

▷ **This Drug Should Not Be Taken If**
  • you have had an allergic reaction to any dosage form of it previously.

▷ **Inform Your Physician Before Taking This Drug If**
  • you have impaired liver or kidney function.
  • you are taking any other drugs at this time.

Possible Side-Effects (natural, expected and unavoidable drug actions)
  With use of capsules—none.
  With use of ointment—mild pain, burning or stinging at site of application (28%).

▷ **Possible Adverse Effects** (unusual, unexpected and infrequent reactions)
  If any of the following develop, consult your physician promptly for guidance.
  Mild Adverse Effects
  Allergic Reaction: Skin rash.
  Headache, dizziness, nervousness, insomnia, depression, fatigue.
  Nausea, vomiting, diarrhea.
  Joint pains, muscle cramps.
  Acne, hair loss.
  Serious Adverse Effects
  Superficial thrombophlebitis, enlarged lymph glands.

▷ **Possible Effects on Sexual Function:**   Altered timing and pattern of menstruation.

  CAUTION
  1. This drug does not eliminate all herpes virus and is not a permanent cure. Observe for possible recurrence and resume treatment at the earliest indication of active infection.
  2. Avoid sexual intercourse while herpes blisters and inflammation are visible.
  3. Do not exceed the prescribed dosage.
  4. Inform physician if the frequency and severity of recurrent infections do not improve.

Precautions for Use
  By Infants and Children: Safety and effectiveness for use by those under 12 years of age have not been established.
  By Those over 60 Years of Age: Avoid dehydration. Drink 2 to 3 quarts of liquids daily.

▷ **Advisability of Use During Pregnancy**
  Pregnancy Category: C (tentative). See Pregnancy Code inside back cover.
  Animal studies: No birth defects found in mouse, rat or rabbit studies.

Human studies: Information from adequate studies of pregnant women is not available.

Avoid use if possible. Use only if clearly needed.

Advisability of Use if Breast-Feeding
Presence of this drug in breast milk: Unknown.
Avoid drug or refrain from nursing.

Habit-Forming Potential: None.

Effects of Overdosage: Possible impairment of kidney function.

Possible Effects of Long-Term Use: Development of strains of herpes virus that are resistant to this drug.

Suggested Periodic Examinations While Taking This Drug (at physician's discretion)
Kidney function tests.

▷ **While Taking This Drug, Observe the Following**
Foods: No restrictions.
Beverages: No restrictions. May be taken with milk. Drink 2 to 3 quarts of liquids daily.
▷ *Alcohol:* Use caution until the combined effects have been determined. Dizziness or fatigue may be accentuated.
Tobacco Smoking: No interactions expected.
▷ *Other Drugs*
The following drugs may *increase* the effects of acyclovir
• probenecid (Benemid) may delay its elimination.
▷ *Driving, Hazardous Activities:* Use caution if dizziness or fatigue occurs.
Aviation Note: The use of this drug *may be a disqualification* for piloting. Consult a designated Aviation Medical Examiner.
Exposure to Sun: No restrictions.

ALBUTEROL
(al BYU ter ohl)

Other Name: Salbutamol

Introduced: 1968

Class: Antiasthmatic, bronchodilator

Prescription: USA: Yes
Canada: Yes

Controlled Drug: USA: No
Canada: No

Available as Generic: No

Brand Names: ✦Novosalmol, Proventil Inhaler, Proventil Repetabs, Proventil Tablets, Ventolin Inhaler, Ventolin Rotacaps, Ventolin Tablets

---

BENEFITS versus RISKS

Possible Benefits
VERY EFFECTIVE RELIEF OF
BRONCHOSPASM

Possible Risks
Increased blood pressure
Fine hand tremor
Irregular heart rhythm (with
    excessive use)

▷ **Principal Uses**

As a Single Drug Product: To relieve acute bronchial asthma and to reduce
the frequency and severity of chronic, recurrent asthmatic attacks.

How This Drug Works: It is thought that by increasing the production of
cyclic AMP, this drug relaxes constricted bronchial muscles to relieve
asthmatic wheezing.

Available Dosage Forms and Strengths

Aerosol — 90 mcg per actuation
Capsules for inhalation — 200 mcg
Solution for inhalation — 0.83 mg per ml, 5 mg per ml
Syrup — 2 mg per 5-ml teaspoonful
Tablets — 2 mg, 4 mg
Tablets, prolonged-action — 4 mg

▷ **Usual Adult Dosage Range:** Inhaler—1 to 2 inhalations (90 to 180 mcg)
up to 4 times daily, every 4 to 6 hours. Tablets—2 to 4 mg 3 to 4
times daily, every 4 to 6 hours. **Do not exceed** 8 inhalations (720 mcg)/
24 hours, or 32 mg (tablet form)/24 hours. **Note: Actual dosage and
administration schedule must be determined by the physician for
each patient individually.**

▷ **Dosing Instructions:** May be taken on empty stomach or with food or milk.
Tablet may be crushed. For inhaler, follow the written instructions
carefully. Do not overuse.

Usual Duration of Use: According to individual requirements. Do not use
beyond the time necessary to terminate episodes of asthma.

▷ **This Drug Should Not Be Taken If**

• you have had an allergic reaction to any dosage form of it previously.
• you currently have an irregular heart rhythm.
• you are taking, or have taken within the past 2 weeks, any monoamine oxidase (MAO) type A inhibitor drug (see Drug Class, Section
Four).

▷ **Inform Your Physician Before Taking This Drug If**

• you have any type of heart or circulatory disorder, especially high
blood pressure or coronary heart disease.
• you have diabetes.
• you are taking any form of digitalis or any stimulant drug.

Possible Side-Effects (natural, expected and unavoidable drug actions)
Aerosol—dryness or irritation of mouth or throat, altered taste.
Tablet—nervousness, palpitation.

▷ **Possible Adverse Effects** (unusual, unexpected and infrequent reactions)
If any of the following develop, consult your physician promptly for guidance.
Mild Adverse Effects
Headache (7%), dizziness (2%), restlessness, insomnia, fine tremor of hands (20%).
Nausea (2%), heartburn, vomiting.
Leg cramps (3%), flushing of skin.
Serious Adverse Effects
Rapid or irregular heart rhythm, increased blood pressure, difficult urination.

▷ **Possible Effects on Sexual Function:**   None reported.

Natural Diseases or Disorders That May Be Activated By This Drug
Latent coronary artery disease, diabetes or high blood pressure.

CAUTION
1. Concurrent use of this drug by inhalation with beclomethasone aerosol (Beclovent, Vanceril) may increase the risk of toxicity due to fluorocarbon propellants. It is advisable to use albuterol aerosol 20 to 30 minutes *before* beclomethasone aerosol. This will reduce the risk of toxicity and will enhance the penetration of beclomethasone.
2. The excessive or prolonged use of this drug by inhalation can reduce its effectiveness and cause serious heart rhythm disturbances, including cardiac arrest.

Precautions for Use
By Infants and Children: Safety and effectiveness of use in children under 12 years of age have not been established.
By Those over 60 Years of Age: Avoid excessive and continual use. If acute asthma is not relieved promptly, other drugs will have to be tried. Observe for the development of nervousness, palpitations, irregular heart rhythm and muscle tremors.

▷ **Advisability of Use During Pregnancy**
Pregnancy Category: C (tentative). See Pregnancy Code inside back cover.
Animal studies: Cleft palate reported in mice.
Human studies: Information from adequate studies of pregnant women is not available.
Avoid use during first 3 months if possible.

Advisability of Use if Breast-Feeding
Presence of this drug in breast milk: Unknown.
Avoid drug or refrain from nursing.

Habit-Forming Potential: None.

Effects of Overdosage: Nervousness, palpitation, rapid heart rate, sweating, headache, tremor, vomiting, chest pain.

Possible Effects of Long-Term Use: Loss of effectiveness.

Suggested Periodic Examinations While Taking This Drug (at physician's discretion)
Blood pressure measurements, evaluation of heart status.

▷ **While Taking This Drug, Observe the Following**
Foods: No restrictions.
Beverages: Avoid excessive use of caffeine-containing beverages—coffee, tea, cola, chocolate.
▷ *Alcohol:* No interactions expected.
Tobacco Smoking: No interactions expected.
▷ *Other Drugs*
Albuterol ***taken concurrently*** with
• monoamine oxidase (MAO) type A inhibitor drugs may cause excessive increase in blood pressure and undesirable heart stimulation.
▷ *Driving, Hazardous Activities:* Use caution if excessive nervousness or dizziness occurs.
Aviation Note: The use of this drug ***is a disqualification*** for piloting. Consult a designated Aviation Medical Examiner.
Exposure to Sun: No restrictions.
Heavy Exercise or Exertion: Use caution. Excessive exercise can induce asthma in sensitive individuals.

ALLOPURINOL
(al oh PURE i nohl)

Introduced: 1963

Class: Antigout

Prescription: USA: Yes
Canada: Yes

Controlled Drug: USA: No
Canada: No

Available as Generic: USA: Yes
Canada: No

Brand Names: ♣Alloprin, ♣Apo-Allopurinol, Lopurin, ♣Novopurol, ♣Purinol, Zurinol, Zyloprim

BENEFITS versus RISKS	
Possible Benefits	*Possible Risks*
EFFECTIVE CONTROL OF GOUT	Increased frequency of acute gout
CONTROL OF HIGH BLOOD	initially
URIC ACID due to poly-	Peripheral neuritis
cythemia, leukemia, cancer and	Allergic reactions in skin, blood
chemotherapy	vessels and liver
	Bone marrow depression
	(questionable)

▷ **Principal Uses**

As a Single Drug Product: Used primarily in the long-term management of gout to *prevent* episodes of acute gout. (It does not relieve the symptoms of acute gout attacks.) Also used to prevent abnormally high blood levels of uric acid in individuals who have recurrent uric acid kidney stones, and in those receiving chemotherapy or radiation therapy for cancer.

How This Drug Works: By inhibiting the action of the tissue enzyme xanthine oxidase, this drug decreases the conversion of purines (protein nutrients) to uric acid.

Available Dosage Forms and Strengths

Tablets — 100 mg, 300 mg (and 200 mg in Canada)

▷ **Usual Adult Dosage Range:**   Initially 100 mg/24 hours. Increase by 100 mg/24 hours at intervals of 1 week until uric acid blood level is 6 mg/dl or less. Usual dose is 200 to 300 mg/24 hours for mild gout, and 400 to 600 mg/24 hours for moderate to severe gout. Daily doses of 300 mg or less may be taken as a single dose. Doses exceeding 300 mg daily should be divided into 2 or 3 equal portions; for the high uric acid levels associated with cancer, 600 to 800 mg/24 hours, divided into 3 equal portions. **Note: Actual dosage and administration schedule must be determined by the physician for each patient individually.**

▷ **Dosing Instructions:**   Best taken with food or milk to reduce stomach irritation. Tablet may be crushed. Drink 2 to 3 quarts of liquids daily.

Usual Duration of Use: According to individual requirements. Blood uric acid levels usually begin to decrease in 48 to 72 hours and may reach a normal range in 1 to 3 weeks. Regular use for several months may be required to prevent attacks of acute gout. Continual use for many years may be necessary for adequate control. Consult your physician on a regular basis.

▷ **This Drug Should Not Be Taken If**

• you have had an allergic reaction to any dosage form of it previously.
• you are experiencing an acute attack of gout at the present time.

▷ **Inform Your Physician Before Taking This Drug If**

• you have a personal or family history of hemochromatosis.
• you have a history of liver or kidney disease.
• you have had a blood cell or bone marrow disorder.
• you have any type of convulsive disorder (epilepsy).

Possible Side-Effects (natural, expected and unavoidable drug actions)

An increase in the frequency and severity of episodes of acute gout may occur during the first several weeks of drug use. Consult your physician regarding the need for other drugs during this period.

▷ **Possible Adverse Effects** (unusual, unexpected and infrequent reactions)
  If any of the following develop, consult your physician promptly for guidance.
  Mild Adverse Effects
    Allergic Reactions: Skin rash, hives, itching, drug fever.
    Headache, dizziness, drowsiness.
    Nausea, vomiting, diarrhea, stomach cramps.
    Loss of scalp hair.
  Serious Adverse Effects
    Allergic Reactions: Severe skin reactions, high fever, chills, joint pains, swollen glands, kidney damage.
    Hepatitis with or without jaundice (see Glossary)—yellow eyes and skin, dark-colored urine, light-colored stools.
    Bone marrow depression (see Glossary)—questionable.
    Seizures, peripheral neuritis.
    Macular eye damage, cataract formation—questionable.

▷ **Possible Effects on Sexual Function:**   Less than 1% and causal relationship not established: male infertility, male breast enlargement, impotence.

▷ **Adverse Effects That May Mimic Natural Diseases or Disorders**
    Toxic liver reaction may suggest viral hepatitis.
    Severe skin reactions may resemble the Stevens-Johnson syndrome (erythema multiforme).

  CAUTION
    1. During the early weeks of treatment, the frequency of acute attacks of gout may increase. These subside with continuation of treatment.
    2. This drug will not relieve the symptoms of acute gout. It should not be started during the presence of acute gout symptoms.
    3. Vitamin C in doses of 2 grams or more daily may acidify the urine and increase the risk of kidney stone formation during the use of allopurinol.
    4. The concurrent use of thiazide diuretics (see Drug Class, Section Four) is reported to cause a possible allergic-type kidney damage. Avoid this drug combination.

  Precautions for Use
    By Infants and Children: Monitor closely for allergic skin reactions and blood cell disorders. This drug may increase the toxicity of azathioprine (Imuran) or mercaptopurine (Purinethol) in children receiving chemotherapy for cancer.
    By Those over 60 Years of Age: The natural decline in kidney function makes it advisable to use smaller initial and maintenance doses of this drug.

▷ **Advisability of Use During Pregnancy**
    Pregnancy Category: C (tentative). See Pregnancy Code inside back cover.
    Animal studies: Results are conflicting and inconclusive.

Human studies: Information from adequate studies of pregnant women is not available.

Avoid use of drug during the first 3 months. Use during the last 6 months only if clearly needed.

Advisability of Use if Breast-Feeding
Presence of this drug in breast milk: Yes.

Avoid drug or refrain from nursing.

Habit-Forming Potential: None.

Effects of Overdosage: Nausea, vomiting or diarrhea may occur as a result of individual sensitivity. No serious toxic effects expected.

Possible Effects of Long-Term Use: None identified.

Suggested Periodic Examinations While Taking This Drug (at physician's discretion)
Blood uric acid levels, complete blood cell counts, liver and kidney function tests. If appropriate, eye examinations for possible cataract formation or macular damage. A cause-and-effect relationship (see Glossary) between this drug and eye changes has not been established.

▷ **While Taking This Drug, Observe the Following**
Foods: Follow physician's advice regarding the need for a low-purine diet.
Beverages: No restrictions. May be taken with milk.
▷   *Alcohol:* No interactions expected.
Tobacco Smoking: No interactions expected.
▷   *Other Drugs*
Allopurinol may ***increase*** the effects of
- azathioprine (Imuran) and mercaptopurine (Purinethol), making it necessary to reduce their dosages.
- oral anticoagulants (see Drug Class, Section Four) in *some* individuals.
- theophylline (aminophylline, Elixophyllin, Theo-Dur, etc.)
Allopurinol ***taken concurrently*** with
- ampicillin may increase the incidence of skin rash.
▷   *Driving, Hazardous Activities:* Drowsiness may occur in some individuals. Determine sensitivity before engaging in hazardous activities.
Aviation Note: The use of this drug ***may be a disqualification*** for piloting. Consult a designated Aviation Medical Examiner.
Exposure to Sun: No restrictions.

ALPRAZOLAM
(al PRAY zoh lam)

Introduced: 1973

Class: Mild tranquilizer, benzodiazepines

Prescription: USA: Yes
Canada: Yes

Controlled Drug: USA: C-IV*
Canada: No

Available as Generic: No

Brand Name: Xanax

BENEFITS versus RISKS	
Possible Benefits	*Possible Risks*
RELIEF OF ANXIETY AND NERVOUS TENSION in 75% of users	Habit-forming potential with prolonged use
Wide margin of safety with therapeutic doses	Minor impairment of mental functions with therapeutic doses

▷ **Principal Uses**

As a Single Drug Product: Used primarily as a mild tranquilizer for the short-term relief of mild to moderate anxiety and nervous tension. It is also used to relieve anxiety associated with depression and to prevent or relieve panic attacks.

How This Drug Works: It is thought that this drug produces a calming effect by enhancing the action of the nerve transmitter gamma-aminobutyric acid (GABA), which in turn blocks the arousal of higher brain centers.

Available Dosage Forms and Strengths
Tablets — 0.25 mg, 0.5 mg, 1 mg

▷ **Usual Adult Dosage Range:** 0.25 mg to 0.5 mg 3 times daily. The maximal dose is 4 mg/24 hours, taken in divided doses. **Note: Actual dosage and administration schedule must be determined by the physician for each patient individually.**

▷ **Dosing Instructions:** May be taken on empty stomach or with food or milk. Tablet may be crushed for administration. Do not discontinue this drug abruptly if taken for more than 4 weeks.

Usual Duration of Use: Several days to several weeks. Avoid prolonged and uninterrupted use. Continual use should not exceed 8 weeks without evaluation by your physician.

*See Schedules of Controlled Drugs inside back cover.

▷ **This Drug Should Not Be Taken If**
- you have had an allergic reaction to it previously.
- you are pregnant (first 3 months).
- you have acute narrow-angle glaucoma.
- you have myasthenia gravis.

▷ **Inform Your Physician Before Taking This Drug If**
- you are allergic to other benzodiazepine drugs (see Drug Class, Section Four).
- you are pregnant (last 6 months) or planning pregnancy.
- you are breast-feeding.
- you have a history of depression or serious mental illness (psychosis).
- you have a history of alcoholism or drug abuse.
- you have impaired liver or kidney function.
- you have open-angle glaucoma.
- you have a seizure disorder (epilepsy).
- you have severe chronic lung disease.

Possible Side-Effects (natural, expected and unavoidable drug actions)
Drowsiness, light-headedness.

▷ **Possible Adverse Effects** (unusual, unexpected and infrequent reactions)
If any of the following develop, consult your physician promptly for guidance.
Mild Adverse Effects
Allergic Reactions: Skin rash, hives.
Headache, dizziness, fatigue, blurred vision, dry mouth.
Nausea, vomiting, constipation.
Serious Adverse Effects
Confusion, hallucinations, depression, unexpected excitement, agitation (paradoxical reaction).

▷ **Possible Effects on Sexual Function:** Rare but documented: inhibited female orgasm (5 mg/day); impaired ejaculation (3.5 mg/day); decreased libido, impaired erection (4.5 mg/day); altered timing and pattern of menstruation (0.75 to 4 mg/day).

CAUTION
1. This drug should not be discontinued abruptly if it has been taken continually for more than 4 weeks.
2. The concurrent use of some over-the-counter drug products that contain antihistamines (allergy and cold preparations, sleep aids) can cause excessive sedation in sensitive individuals.

Precautions for Use
By Infants and Children: Safety and effectiveness for use by those under 18 years of age have not been established.
By Those over 60 Years of Age: The starting dose should be 0.25 mg 2 or 3 times daily. Monitor for excessive drowsiness, dizziness, unsteadiness and incoordination (possible low blood pressure).

▷ **Advisability of Use During Pregnancy**

Pregnancy Category: D (tentative). See Pregnancy Code inside back cover.

Animal studies: Diazepam (a closely related benzodiazepine) can cause cleft palate in mice and skeletal defects in rats. No information available for alprazolam.

Human studies: Some studies suggest a possible association between the use of diazepam and defects such as cleft lip and heart deformities. Information from adequate studies on the use of alprazolam by pregnant women is not available.

Avoid use during entire pregnancy if possible.

Advisability of Use if Breast-Feeding

Presence of this drug in breast milk: Probably yes.

Avoid drug or refrain from nursing.

Habit-Forming Potential: This drug can produce psychological and/or physical dependence (see Glossary) if used in large doses for an extended period of time.

Effects of Overdosage: Marked drowsiness, weakness, feeling of drunkenness, staggering gait, tremor, stupor progressing to deep sleep or coma.

Possible Effects of Long-Term Use: Psychological and/or physical dependence.

Suggested Periodic Examinations While Taking This Drug (at physician's discretion)

None required for short-term use.

▷ **While Taking This Drug, Observe the Following**

Foods: No restrictions.

Beverages: Avoid excessive intake of caffeine-containing beverages: coffee, tea, cola. This drug may be taken with milk.

▷ *Alcohol:* Use with extreme caution and in very small amounts until the combined effect is determined. Alcohol may increase the sedative effects of alprazolam. Alprazolam may increase the intoxicating effects of alcohol. Avoid alcohol completely—throughout the day and night— if you find it necessary to drive or to engage in *any* hazardous activity.

Tobacco Smoking: Heavy smoking may reduce the calming action of alprazolam.

Marijuana Smoking

Occasional (once or twice weekly): Mild increase in the sedative effect of this drug.

Daily: Marked increase in the sedative effect of this drug.

▷ *Other Drugs*

Alprazolam may ***increase*** the effects of

• digoxin (Lanoxin), and cause digoxin toxicity.

Alprazolam may **decrease** the effects of
- levodopa (Sinemet, etc.), and reduce its effectiveness in treating Parkinson's disease.

The following drugs may **increase** the effects of alprazolam
- cimetidine (Tagamet).
- disulfiram (Antabuse).
- isoniazid (INH, Rifamate, etc.).
- oral contraceptives.
- valproic acid (Depakene).

The following drugs may **decrease** the effects of alprazolam
- rifampin (Rimactane, etc.).
- theophylline (aminophylline, Theo-Dur, etc.).

▷ *Driving, Hazardous Activities:* This drug can impair mental alertness, judgment, physical coordination and reaction time. Avoid hazardous activities accordingly.

Aviation Note: The use of this drug *is a disqualification* for piloting. Consult a designated Aviation Medical Examiner.

Exposure to Sun: No restrictions.

Discontinuation: If it has been necessary to use this drug for an extended period of time, do not discontinue it abruptly. Reduce dose gradually at the rate of 1 mg every 3 days.

AMANTADINE
(a MAN ta deen)

Introduced: 1966

Prescription: USA: Yes
Canada: Yes

Available as Generic: USA: Yes
Canada: No

Brand Names: Symadine, Symmetrel

Class: Antiparkinsonism, antiviral

Controlled Drug: USA: No
Canada: No

BENEFITS versus RISKS

Possible Benefits	*Possible Risks*
PARTIAL RELIEF OF RIGIDITY, TREMOR AND IMPAIRED MOTION in all forms of parkinsonism (in 60% of users) PREVENTION AND TREATMENT OF REPIRATORY TRACT INFECTIONS CAUSED BY INFLUENZA TYPE A VIRUSES*	Skin rashes, mild to severe Confusion, hallucinations Congestive heart failure Increased prostatism (see Glossary) Abnormally low white blood cell counts

---

*This drug is not effective for the prevention or treatment of viral infections other than those caused by influenza type A viruses.

▷ **Principal Uses**

As a Single Drug Product: This drug has two primary uses: (1) to treat all forms of parkinsonism, and (2) to prevent and treat respiratory tract infections caused by strains of influenza type A virus.

How This Drug Works: Not completely known. It is thought that by increasing the availability of the nerve impulse transmitter known as dopamine in certain nerve centers, this drug reduces the muscular rigidity, tremor and impaired movement associated with all forms of parkinsonism. By blocking the penetration of infectious material from virus particles into tissue cells, this drug prevents the development of influenza type A.

Available Dosage Forms and Strengths
Capsules — 100 mg
Syrup — 50 mg per 5-ml teaspoonful

▷ **Usual Adult Dosage Range:**   Antiparkinsonism: 100 mg once or twice daily. The total daily dose should not exceed 400 mg. Antiviral: 200 mg once daily; or 100 mg/12 hours. **Note: Actual dosage and administration schedule must be determined by the physician for each patient individually.**

▷ **Dosing Instructions:**   May be taken with or following meals. The capsule may be opened for administration.

Usual Duration of Use: Continual use on a regular schedule for up to 2 weeks is usually necessary to determine this drug's effectiveness in relieving the symptoms of parkinsonism. Long-term use (months to years) requires periodic evaluation of response and dosage adjustment. Consult your physician on a regular basis. Following exposure to influenza type A, maximal protection requires continual daily dosage for at least 10 days. During influenza epidemics, this drug may be given for 6 to 8 weeks.

Currently a "Drug of Choice" for prevention of influenza Type A infection (70% to 90% effective), and for treatment of such infections (50% reduction of severity and length of illness).

▷ **This Drug Should Not Be Taken If**
  • you have had an allergic reaction to it previously.

▷ **Inform Your Physician Before Taking This Drug If**
  • you have any type of seizure disorder.
  • you have a history of serious emotional or mental disorder.
  • you have a history of heart disease, especially previous heart failure.
  • you have impaired liver or kidney function.
  • you have a history of peptic ulcer disease.
  • you have eczema or recurring eczemalike skin rashes.
  • you are taking any drugs for emotional or mental disorders.

Possible Side-Effects (natural, expected and unavoidable drug actions)
Light-headedness, dizziness, weakness, feeling of impending faint in up-right position (see Orthostatic Hypotension in Glossary). Dry mouth, constipation. Reddish-blue network pattern or patchy discoloration of the skin of the legs and feet (livedo reticularis); this is transient and unimportant.

▷ **Possible Adverse Effects** (unusual, unexpected and infrequent reactions)
If any of the following develop, consult your physician promptly for guidance.
Mild Adverse Effects
Allergic Reaction: Skin rash.
Headache, nervousness, irritability, inability to concentrate, insomnia, nightmares.
Unsteadiness, visual disturbances, slurred speech.
Loss of appetite, nausea, vomiting.
Serious Adverse Effects
Allergic Reaction: Severe eczemalike skin rashes.
Idiosyncratic Reactions: Confusion, depression, hallucinations.
Swelling (fluid retention) of the arms, feet or ankles.
Development of congestive heart failure (rare).
Aggravation of prostatism (see Glossary).
Abnormally low white blood cell counts: fever, sore throat, infections.

▷ **Possible Effects on Sexual Function:**   None reported.

▷ **Adverse Effects That May Mimic Natural Diseases or Disorders**
Mood or mental changes, confusion or hallucinations may suggest a psychotic disorder.
Swelling of the legs and feet may suggest (but not necessarily be indicative of) heart, liver or kidney disorder.

Natural Diseases or Disorders That May Be Activated by This Drug
Latent epilepsy, incipient congestive heart failure.

CAUTION
  1. This drug has a narrow margin of safety. Do not exceed a total dose of 400 mg/24 hours. Observe closely for indications of adverse effects with doses over 200 mg/24 hours.
  2. After an initial period of benefit lasting 3 to 6 months, this drug may lose its effectiveness in the treatment of parkinsonism. If this occurs, consult your physician regarding dosage adjustment or drug replacement.
  3. This drug is reported to increase susceptibility to German measles. Avoid exposure to anyone with active German measles infection.
  4. Observe for early indications of congestive heart failure: shortness of breath on exertion or during the night while sleeping, mild cough, swelling of the feet and ankles. Report these developments promptly to your physician.

Precautions for Use

By Infants and Children: Safety and effectiveness for use by those under 1 year of age have not been established.

By Those over 60 Years of Age: Observe for the possible development of confusion, delirium, hallucinations and disorderly conduct. Prostatism may be aggravated by this drug.

▷ **Advisability of Use During Pregnancy**

Pregnancy Category: C (tentative). See Pregnancy Code inside back cover.

Animal studies: Birth defects reported in rat studies; no defects reported in rabbit studies.

Human studies: Information from adequate studies of pregnant women is not available. Avoid this drug during the first 3 months if possible. Ask your physician for guidance.

Advisability of Use if Breast-Feeding

Presence of this drug in breast milk: Yes.

The nursing infant may develop skin rash, vomiting or retention of urine. Avoid drug or refrain from nursing.

Habit-Forming Potential: While not habituating, this drug does have a potential for abuse because of its ability to cause euphoria, hallucinations and feelings of detachment.

Effects of Overdosage: Hyperactivity, disorientation, confusion, visual hallucinations, aggressive behavior, severe toxic psychosis, seizures, heart rhythm disturbances, drop in blood pressure.

Possible Effects of Long-Term Use: Livedo reticularis (see Possible Side-Effects above). Congestive heart failure in predisposed individuals.

Suggested Periodic Examinations While Taking This Drug (at physician's discretion)

White blood cell counts, liver and kidney function tests.

Evaluation of heart function.

▷ **While Taking This Drug, Observe the Following**

Foods: No restrictions.

Beverages: No restrictions. May be taken with milk.

▷   *Alcohol:* Use caution until combined effects have been determined. This combination may impair mental function and lower blood pressure excessively.

Tobacco Smoking: No interactions expected.

Marijuana Smoking: No interactions expected.

▷   *Other Drugs*

Amantadine may *increase* the effects of

- those atropinelike drugs that are used to treat parkinsonism, especially benztropine (Cogentin), orphenadrine (Disipal) and trihexyphenidyl (Artane). Amantadine can increase their therapeutic effectiveness. However, if doses are too large, these drugs taken concurrently with amantadine may cause mental confusion, delirium, hallucinations and nightmares.

- levodopa (Dopar, Larodopa, Sinemet, etc.), and enhance its therapeutic effectiveness. However, this combination may cause acute mental disturbances.

The following drugs may **increase** the effects of amantadine

- amphetamine and amphetaminelike stimulant drugs may cause excessive stimulation and adverse behavioral effects.

▷ *Driving, Hazardous Activities:* This drug may cause drowsiness, dizziness, blurred vision or confusion. If these drug effects occur, avoid all hazardous activities.

Aviation Note: The use of this drug **may be a disqualification** for piloting. Consult a designated Aviation Medical Examiner.

Exposure to Sun: No restrictions.

Exposure to Heat: No restrictions.

Exposure to Cold: Use caution. Excessive chilling may enhance the development of livedo reticularis (see Possible Side-Effects above).

Discontinuation: When used to treat parkinsonism, this drug should not be stopped abruptly. Sudden discontinuation may cause an acute parkinsonian crisis. When used to treat influenza A infections, this drug should be continued for 48 hours after the disappearance of all symptoms.

AMBENONIUM
(am bee NOH ni um)

Introduced: 1956

Class: Antimyasthenic

Prescription: USA: Yes
Canada: No

Controlled Drug: USA: No
Canada: No

Available as Generic: USA: No
Canada: No

Brand Name: Mytelase Caplets

BENEFITS versus RISKS

Possible Benefits	*Possible Risks*
MODERATELY EFFECTIVE TREATMENT OF OCULAR AND MILD FORMS OF MYASTHENIA GRAVIS (symptomatic relief of muscle weakness)	Cholinergic crisis (overdose): excessive salivation, nausea, vomiting, stomach cramps, diarrhea, shortness of breath (asthmalike wheezing), excessive weakness

---

▷ **Principal Uses**

As a Single Drug Product: Used primarily to treat the ocular and milder forms of myasthenia gravis by providing temporary relief of muscle weakness and fatigability. Because of its potential for serious adverse effects, its use is generally reserved for treating those individuals who cannot use neostigmine (Prostigmin) or pyridostigmine (Mestinon).

How This Drug Works: This drug inhibits cholinesterase, the enzyme that destroys acetylcholine. This results in higher levels of acetylcholine, the nerve transmitter that facilitates the stimulation of muscular activity. The net effects are increased muscle strength and endurance.

Available Dosage Forms and Strengths
Tablets — 10 mg

▷ **Usual Adult Dosage Range:** Initially: 2.5 to 5 mg 3 or 4 times daily; adjust dosage as needed and tolerated at intervals of 48 hours. Maintenance: up to 300 mg/24 hours; the average dose is 15 to 100 mg/24 hours. It is advisable to try to determine the smallest dose that will provide the greatest strength. **Note: Actual dosage and administration schedule must be determined by the physician for each patient individually.**

▷ **Dosing Instructions:** Take with food or milk to reduce the intensity of side-effects. Larger portions of the daily maintenance dosage should be timed according to the pattern of fatigue and weakness. The tablet may be crushed for administration.

Usual Duration of Use: Continual use on a regular schedule (with dosage adjustment) for 10 to 14 days is usually necessary to determine this drug's effectiveness in relieving the symptoms of myasthenia gravis. Long-term use (months to years) requires periodic evaluation of response and dosage adjustment. Consult your physician on a regular basis.

▷ **This Drug Should Not Be Taken If**
• you have had an allergic reaction to it previously.

▷ **Inform Your Physician Before Taking This Drug If**
• you have any type of seizure disorder.
• you are subject to heart rhythm disorders or bronchial asthma.
• you have recurrent urinary tract infections.
• you have prostatism (see Glossary).
• you plan to have surgery under general anesthesia in the near future.

Possible Side-Effects (natural, expected and unavoidable drug actions)
Small pupils, watering of eyes, slow pulse, low blood pressure, excessive salivation, nausea, vomiting, stomach cramps, diarrhea, urge to urinate, increased sweating.

▷ **Possible Adverse Effects** (unusual, unexpected and infrequent reactions)
If any of the following develop, consult your physician promptly for guidance.
Mild Adverse Effects
Allergic Reaction: Skin rash.
Nervousness, anxiety, unsteadiness, muscle cramps or twitching.
Serious Adverse Effects
Confusion, slurred speech, seizures, difficult breathing (asthmatic wheezing).
Increased muscle weakness or paralysis.
Excessive vomiting or diarrhea may induce abnormally low blood potassium levels (hypokalemia). This will accentuate muscle weakness.

▷ **Possible Effects on Sexual Function:**   None reported.

▷ **Adverse Effects That May Mimic Natural Diseases or Disorders**
Seizures may suggest the possibility of epilepsy.

Natural Diseases or Disorders That May Be Activated by This Drug
Latent bronchial asthma.

CAUTION
1. Certain drugs can block the action of this drug and reduce its effectiveness in treating myasthenia gravis. (See *Other Drugs* below.) Consult your physician before starting any new drug, prescription or over-the-counter.
2. The dosage schedule of this drug must be carefully individualized for each patient. Variations in response may occur from time to time. Because generalized muscle weakness is a major symptom of both myasthenia crisis (underdosage) and cholinergic crisis (overdosage), it may be difficult to recognize the correct cause. As a rule, weakness that begins within 1 hour after taking this drug probably represents overdosage; weakness that begins 3 or more hours after taking this drug is probably due to underdosage. Observe these time relationships and inform your physician.
3. During long-term use of this drug, observe for the possible development of resistance to the drug's therapeutic action (loss of effectiveness). Consult your physician regarding the advisability of discontinuing this drug for a few days to see if responsiveness can be restored.

Precautions for Use
By Infants and Children: Dosage and administration schedule should be determined by a qualified pediatric neurologist.
By Those over 60 Years of Age: Avoid high doses that are more likely to cause serious adverse effects.

▷ **Advisability of Use During Pregnancy**
Pregnancy Category: C (tentative). See Pregnancy Code inside back cover.
Animal studies: No information available.

Human studies: Information from adequate studies of pregnant women is not available.

There are no reports of birth defects due to the use of this drug during pregnancy. However, there are reports of significant muscular weakness in 10% to 20% of newborn infants whose mothers had taken this class of drugs during pregnancy. Ask your physician for guidance.

Advisability of Use if Breast-Feeding

Presence of this drug in breast milk: Probably not.

Monitor nursing infant closely and discontinue drug or nursing if adverse effects develop.

Habit-Forming Potential: None.

Effects of Overdosage: Generalized muscular weakness, blurred vision, very small pupils, slow heart rate, difficult breathing (wheezing), excessive salivation, nausea, vomiting, stomach cramps, diarrhea, muscle cramps or twitching. This syndrome constitutes the cholinergic crisis.

Possible Effects of Long-Term Use: Development of tolerance (see Glossary) with loss of therapeutic effectiveness.

Suggested Periodic Examinations While Taking This Drug (at physician's discretion)

Assessment of drug effectiveness and dosage schedule for optimal therapeutic results.

▷ **While Taking This Drug, Observe the Following**

Foods: No restrictions.

Beverages: No restrictions. May be taken with milk.

▷   *Alcohol:* Use caution until the combined effects are determined. Weakness and unsteadiness may be accentuated.

Tobacco Smoking: No interactions expected.

▷   *Other Drugs*

The following drugs may ***decrease*** the effects of ambenonium

- atropine (belladonna).
- clindamycin (Cleocin).
- guanadrel (Hylorel).
- guanethidine (Esimil, Ismelin).
- procainamide (Procan SR, Pronestyl).
- quinidine (Cardioquin, Duraquin, etc.).
- quinine (Quinamm).

▷   *Driving, Hazardous Activities:* This drug may cause blurred vision, confusion or generalized weakness. Restrict activities as necessary.

Aviation Note: The use of this drug ***is a disqualification*** for piloting. Consult a designated Aviation Medical Examiner.

Exposure to Sun: No restrictions.

Exposure to Heat: Use caution. This may cause excessive sweating and increased weakness.

Exposure to Environmental Chemicals: Avoid excessive exposure (inhalation, skin contamination) to the insecticides Baygon, Diazinon and Sevin. These can accentuate the potential toxicity of this drug.

Discontinuation: Do not discontinue this drug abruptly without your physician's knowledge and guidance.

AMILORIDE
(a MIL oh ride)

Introduced: 1967

Class: Diuretic

Prescription: USA: Yes
Canada: Yes

Controlled Drug: USA: No
Canada: No

Available as Generic: Yes

Brand Names: Midamor, ✦Moduret [CD], Moduretic [CD]

BENEFITS versus RISKS	
Possible Benefits	*Possible Risks*
EFFECTIVE DIURETIC WITHOUT LOSS OF POTASSIUM	ABNORMALLY HIGH BLOOD POTASSIUM with excessive use
	Rare bone marrow depression

▷ **Principal Uses**

As a Single Drug Product: To eliminate excessive fluid retention (edema).

As a Combination Drug Product [CD]: It is combined with other diuretics of the thiazide class primarily to prevent the loss of potassium from the body.

How This Drug Works: It is thought that this drug promotes the loss of sodium and water from the body and the retention of potassium by altering the enzyme systems of the kidney that control the formation of urine.

Available Dosage Forms and Strengths

Tablets — 5 mg

▷ **Usual Adult Dosage Range:** Initially 5 mg once daily, preferably in the morning. May increase up to 15 mg daily as needed and tolerated. Should not exceed 20 mg/24 hours. **Note: Actual dosage and administration schedule must be determined by the physician for each patient individually.**

▷ **Dosing Instructions:** Preferably taken on arising, with the stomach empty. For best results, withhold food for 4 hours. May be taken with food if necessary to reduce stomach irritation. Tablet may be crushed for administration.

Usual Duration of Use: As needed for elimination of edema or maintenance of normal blood pressure. Intermittent or alternate-day use is recommended to minimize imbalance of sodium and potassium. Consult your physician on a regular basis.

▷ **This Drug Should Not Be Taken If**
- you have had an allergic reaction to any dosage form of it previously.
- your blood potassium level is above the normal range.
- your kidneys are not producing urine.

▷ **Inform Your Physician Before Taking This Drug If**
- you have diabetes or glaucoma.
- you have a history of kidney disease or impaired kidney function.
- you are taking any other diuretic, blood pressure drug, any form of digitalis or lithium.

Possible Side-Effects (natural, expected and unavoidable drug actions)
Abnormally high blood potassium level (10% of users), abnormally low blood sodium level, dehydration, constipation.

▷ **Possible Adverse Effects** (unusual, unexpected and infrequent reactions)
If any of the following develop, consult your physician promptly for guidance.
Mild Adverse Effects
Allergic Reactions: Skin rash, itching.
Headache, dizziness, weakness, fatigue, numbness and tingling.
Dry mouth, nausea, vomiting, stomach pains, diarrhea.
Loss of scalp hair.
Serious Adverse Effects
Idiosyncratic Reactions: Joint and muscle pains.
Excessively high blood potassium level—marked fatigue and weakness, confusion, numbness and tingling of lips and extremities, slow and irregular heartbeats.
Increased internal eye pressure (of concern in glaucoma).
Mental depression, visual disturbances, ringing in ears, tremors.
Aplastic anemia (see Glossary)—unusual fatigue or weakness, fever, sore throat, abnormal bleeding or bruising.

▷ **Possible Effects on Sexual Function:**   More than 1%: decreased libido and impotence (5 to 10 mg/day).

▷ **Adverse Effects That May Mimic Natural Diseases or Disorders**
Nervousness, confusion and/or depression may resemble spontaneous mental disorder.

Natural Diseases or Disorders That May Be Activated by This Drug
Preexisting peptic ulcer, latent glaucoma.

CAUTION
1. Do not take potassium supplements, and do not increase your intake of high-potassium foods.
2. If taking any form of digitalis, report as directed for periodic measurements of your blood potassium level.
3. Do not discontinue this drug abruptly unless directed to do so by your physician.

Precautions for Use
By Infants and Children: Safety and effectiveness for use by those under 12 years of age have not been established.

By Those over 60 Years of Age: The natural decline in kidney function may predispose to excessive retention of potassium in the body. It is advisable to limit use of this drug to periods of 2 to 3 weeks if possible. Overdosage and extended use can cause excessive loss of body water, increased viscosity of the blood and an increased tendency to abnormal blood clotting (thrombosis, heart attack, stroke).

▷ **Advisability of Use During Pregnancy**
Pregnancy Category: B (tentative). See Pregnancy Code inside back cover.
Animal studies: No birth defects reported.
Human studies: Information from adequate studies of pregnant women is not available.
Use only if clearly needed.

Advisability of Use if Breast-Feeding
Presence of this drug in breast milk: Unknown, but probably present.
This drug may suppress milk production.
Avoid drug if possible. If use is necessary, monitor nursing infant closely and discontinue drug or nursing if adverse effects develop.

Habit-Forming Potential: None.

Effects of Overdosage: Thirst, drowsiness, fatigue, weakness, nausea, vomiting, confusion, numbness and tingling of face and extremities, irregular heart rhythm, shortness of breath.

Suggested Periodic Examinations While Taking This Drug (at physician's discretion)
Complete blood cell counts; measurements of blood levels of sodium, potassium and chloride; kidney function tests; and assessment of water balance (state of hydration).

▷ **While Taking This Drug, Observe the Following**
Foods: No restrictions. Avoid excessive restriction of salt. Avoid excessive amounts of high-potassium foods.
Beverages: No restrictions. May be taken with milk.
▷   *Alcohol:* Use with caution until the combined effect has been determined. Alcohol can exaggerate the blood-pressure-lowering effect of this drug and cause orthostatic hypotension (see Glossary).

Tobacco Smoking: No interactions expected.
▷ *Other Drugs*
    Amiloride may *increase* the effects of
    • other blood-pressure-lowering drugs. Dosage adjustments may be necessary.
    Amiloride may *decrease* the effects of
    • digoxin (Lanoxin, etc.), and reduce its effectiveness in treating heart failure.
    Amiloride *taken concurrently* with
    • spironolactone (Aldactone, Aldactazide) or triamterene (Dyrenium, Dyazide) may cause excessive (dangerous) increase in blood potassium levels. Avoid the concurrent use of these drugs.
    • lithium may cause lithium accumulation to toxic levels.
▷ *Driving, Hazardous Activities:* This drug may cause drowsiness, dizziness and orthostatic hypotension in sensitive individuals. If these drug effects occur, avoid hazardous activities.
Aviation Note: The use of this drug *may be a disqualification* for piloting. Consult a designated Aviation Medical Examiner.
Exposure to Sun: No restrictions.
Exposure to Heat: Caution advised. Excessive perspiration can cause water, sodium and potassium imbalance. Hot environments can cause lowering of blood pressure.
Occurrence of Unrelated Illness: Consult your physician if you contract an illness that causes vomiting or diarrhea.
Discontinuation: With high dosage or prolonged use, withdraw this drug gradually. Sudden withdrawal can cause excessive loss of potassium from the body.

AMITRIPTYLINE
(a mee TRIP ti leen)

Introduced: 1961   **Class:** Antidepressant

Prescription: USA: Yes   **Controlled Drug:** USA: No
    Canada: Yes   Canada: No

Available as Generic: Yes

Brand Names: Amitril, ✦Apo-Amitriptyline, Elavil, ✦Elavil Plus [CD], Emitrip, Endep, Etrafon [CD], Etrafon-A [CD], Etrafon-Forte [CD], ✦Levate, Limbitrol [CD], ✦Novotriptyn, Triavil [CD]

BENEFITS versus RISKS	
Possible Benefits	*Possible Risks*
EFFECTIVE RELIEF OF ENDOGENOUS DEPRESSION in 60% to 75% of users	ADVERSE BEHAVIORAL EFFECTS: Confusion, disorientation, hallucinations CONVERSION OF DEPRESSION TO MANIA in manic-depressive disorders Irregular heart rhythms Rare blood cell abnormalities

▷ **Principal Uses**

As a Single Drug Product: To relieve the symptoms associated with spontaneous (endogenous) depression, and to initiate the restoration of normal mood. This drug should be used only when a diagnosis of a true, primary depression of significant degree has been established. It should not be used to treat the symptoms of mild and transient (reactive) depression that may be associated with many life situations in the absence of a bona fide affective illness.

As a Combination Drug Product [CD]: This drug is available in combination with chlordiazepoxide, a mild tranquilizer of the benzodiazepine class. This combination is used to relieve anxiety that may accompany depression. This drug is also available in combination with perphenazine, a strong tranquilizer of the phenothiazine class. This combination is used to relieve severe agitation that may accompany depression.

How This Drug Works: It is thought that this drug relieves depression by slowly restoring to normal levels certain constituents of brain tissue (norepinephrine and serotonin) that transmit nerve impulses.

Available Dosage Forms and Strengths
Tablets — 10 mg, 25 mg, 50 mg, 75 mg, 100 mg, 150 mg

▷ **Usual Adult Dosage Range:**   Initially 25 mg 2 to 4 times daily. Dose may be increased cautiously as needed and tolerated by 10 to 25 mg daily at intervals of 1 week. Usual maintenance dose is 50 to 100 mg/24 hours. Total dose should not exceed 150 mg/24 hours. When the optimal requirement is determined, it may be taken at bedtime as one dose. **Note: Actual dosage and administration schedule must be determined by the physician for each patient individually.**

▷ **Dosing Instructions:**   May be taken without regard to meals. Tablet may be crushed for administration.

Usual Duration of Use: Some benefit may be apparent within 1 to 2 weeks, but adequate response may require continual use for 4 to 6 weeks or longer. Long-term use should not exceed 6 months without evaluation regarding the need for continuation of the drug. Consult your physician on a regular basis.

▷ **This Drug Should Not Be Taken If**
- you are allergic to any of the drugs bearing the brand names listed above.
- you are taking or have taken within the past 14 days any monoamine oxidase (MAO) type A inhibitor drug (see Drug Class, Section Four).
- you are recovering from a recent heart attack.
- you have narrow-angle glaucoma.

▷ **Inform Your Physician Before Taking This Drug If**
- you are allergic or sensitive to any other tricyclic antidepressant (see Drug Class, Section Four).
- you have a history of any of the following: diabetes, epilepsy, glaucoma, heart disease, prostate gland enlargement or overactive thyroid function.
- you plan to have surgery under general anesthesia in the near future.

Possible Side-Effects (natural, expected and unavoidable drug actions)
Drowsiness, blurred vision, dry mouth, constipation, impaired urination.

▷ **Possible Adverse Effects** (unusual, unexpected and infrequent reactions)
If any of the following develop, consult your physician promptly for guidance.
Mild Adverse Effects
Allergic Reactions: Skin rash, hives, swelling of face or tongue, drug fever (see Glossary).
Headache, dizziness, weakness, fainting, unsteady gait, tremors.
Peculiar taste, irritation of tongue or mouth, nausea, indigestion.
Fluctuation of blood sugar levels.
Serious Adverse Effects
Allergic Reactions: Hepatitis, with or without jaundice (see Glossary).
Confusion, hallucinations, agitation, restlessness, nightmares.
Heart palpitation and irregular rhythm.
Bone marrow depression (see Glossary)—fatigue, weakness, fever, sore throat, abnormal bleeding or bruising.
Peripheral neuritis (see Glossary)—numbness, tingling, pain, loss of strength in arms and legs.
Parkinson-like disorders (see Glossary)—usually mild and infrequent; more likely to occur in the elderly.

▷ **Possible Effects on Sexual Function:** Decreased libido (8%), increased libido (antidepressant effect), impotence (19%), inhibited female orgasm, inhibited ejaculation, male and female breast enlargement, milk production, swelling of testicles. These effects usually disappear within 2 to 10 days after discontinuation of the drug.

▷ **Adverse Effects That May Mimic Natural Diseases or Disorders**
Liver toxicity may suggest viral hepatitis.

Natural Diseases or Disorders That May Be Activated by This Drug
Latent diabetes, epilepsy, glaucoma, impaired urination due to prostate gland enlargement.

CAUTION
1. Dosage must be adjusted for each person individually. Report for follow-up evaluation and laboratory tests as directed by your physician.
2. It is advisable to withhold this drug if electroconvulsive therapy (ECT, "shock" treatment) is to be used to treat your depression.

Precautions for Use
By Infants and Children: Safety and effectiveness for use by those under 12 years of age have not been established.
By Those over 60 Years of Age: During the first 2 weeks of treatment, observe for the development of confusion, agitation, forgetfulness, disorientation, delusions and hallucinations. Reduction of dosage or discontinuation may be necessary. Unsteadiness may predispose to falling and injury. This drug can increase the degree of impaired urination associated with prostate gland enlargement (prostatism).

▷ **Advisability of Use During Pregnancy**
Pregnancy Category: C (tentative). See Pregnancy Code inside back cover.
Animal studies: Skull deformities reported in rabbits.
Human studies: No defects reported in 21 exposures. Information from adequate studies of pregnant women is not available.
Avoid use of drug during first 3 months. Use during last 6 months only if clearly needed.

Advisability of Use if Breast-Feeding
Presence of this drug in breast milk: Yes, in small amounts.
Monitor nursing infant closely and discontinue drug or nursing if adverse effects develop.

Habit-Forming Potential: Psychological or physical dependence is rare and unexpected.

Effects of Overdosage: Confusion, hallucinations, marked drowsiness, heart palpitations, dilated pupils, tremors, stupor, deep sleep, coma, convulsions.

Suggested Periodic Examinations While Taking This Drug (at physician's discretion)
Complete blood cell counts, liver function tests, serial blood pressure readings and electrocardiograms.

▷ **While Taking This Drug, Observe the Following**
Foods: No restrictions. This drug may increase the appetite and cause excessive weight gain.
Beverages: No restrictions. May be taken with milk.

▷ *Alcohol:* Avoid completely. This drug can markedly increase the intoxicating effects of alcohol and accentuate its depressant action on brain function.

Tobacco Smoking: May hasten the elimination of this drug. Higher doses may be necessary.

▷ *Other Drugs*

Amitriptyline may *increase* the effects of
- atropinelike drugs (see Drug Class, Section Four).

Amitriptyline may *decrease* the effects of
- clonidine (Catapres).
- guanethidine (Ismelin).

Amitriptyline *taken concurrently* with
- monoamine oxidase (MAO) type A inhibitor drugs may cause high fever, delirium and convulsions (see Drug Class, Section Four).
- thyroid preparations may impair heart rhythm and function. Ask physician for guidance regarding adjustment of thyroid dose.

▷ *Driving, Hazardous Activities:* This drug may impair mental alertness, judgment, physical coordination and reaction time. Avoid hazardous activities.

Aviation Note: The use of this drug *is a disqualification* for piloting. Consult a designated Aviation Medical Examiner.

Exposure to Sun: Use caution until sensitivity to sun has been determined. This drug may cause photosensitivity (see Glossary).

Exposure to Heat: This drug can inhibit sweating and impair the body's adaptation to hot environments, increasing the risk of heat stroke. Avoid saunas.

Exposure to Cold: The elderly should use caution and avoid conditions conducive to hypothermia (see Glossary).

Discontinuation: It is advisable to discontinue this drug gradually. Abrupt withdrawal after long-term use can cause headache, malaise and nausea.

AMOXAPINE
(a MOX a peen)

Introduced: 1970

Class: Antidepressant

Prescription: USA: Yes
Canada: Yes

Controlled Drug: USA: No
Canada: No

Available as Generic: No

Brand Name: Asendin

BENEFITS versus RISKS

Possible Benefits	*Possible Risks*
EFFECTIVE RELIEF OF PRIMARY DEPRESSIONS: Endogenous, neurotic, reactive	ADVERSE BEHAVIORAL EFFECTS: Confusion, delusions, disorientation, hallucinations
Well tolerated by most persons	CONVERSION OF DEPRESSION TO MANIA in manic-depressive disorders
	Rare blood cell abnormalities

▷ **Principal Uses**

As a Single Drug Product: To provide symptomatic relief in all types of depression, and to initiate the restoration of normal mood.

How This Drug Works: It is thought that by increasing the availability of certain nerve impulse transmitters (norepinephrine and serotonin) in brain tissue, this drug relieves the symptoms associated with depression.

Available Dosage Forms and Strengths

Tablets — 25 mg, 50 mg, 100 mg, 150 mg

▷ **Usual Adult Dosage Range:**   Initially 50 mg 3 times daily. Dose may be increased cautiously on the third day as needed and tolerated to 100 mg 3 times daily. Usual maintenance dose is 200 to 300 mg/24 hours. Total dosage should not exceed 400 mg/24 hours. When determined, the optimal requirement may be taken at bedtime as one dose, not to exceed 300 mg. **Note: Actual dosage and administration schedule must be determined by the physician for each patient individually.**

▷ **Dosing Instructions:**   May be taken without regard to meals. Tablet may be crushed for administration.

Usual Duration of Use: Benefit may be apparent within 4 to 7 days in some individuals, but continual use on a regular schedule for 2 to 3 weeks is usually necessary to determine this drug's effectiveness. Long-term use should not exceed 6 months without evaluation regarding the need for continuation. Consult your physician on a regular basis.

▷ **This Drug Should Not Be Taken If**
- you have had an allergic reaction to it previously.
- you are taking or have taken within the past 14 days any monoamine oxidase (MAO) type A inhibitor drug (see Drug Class, Section Four).
- you are recovering from a recent heart attack.

▷ **Inform Your Physician Before Taking This Drug If**
- you are allergic or overly sensitive to other antidepressant drugs.
- you have a history of any of the following: diabetes, epilepsy, glaucoma, heart disease, paranoia, prostate gland enlargement, schizophrenia or overactive thyroid function.
- you plan to have surgery under general anesthesia in the near future.

Possible Side-Effects (natural, expected and unavoidable drug actions)
Drowsiness, blurred vision, dry mouth, constipation, impaired urination.

▷ **Possible Adverse Effects** (unusual, unexpected and infrequent reactions)
If any of the following develop, consult your physician promptly for guidance.

Mild Adverse Effects
Allergic Reactions: Skin rash, hives, swellings, drug fever (see Glossary).
Insomnia, nervousness, palpitations, dizziness, unsteadiness, tremors, fainting.
Peculiar taste, indigestion, nausea, vomiting.

Serious Adverse Effects
Behavioral effects: anxiety, confusion, excitement, disorientation, hallucinations, delusions.
Aggravation of paranoid psychosis and schizophrenia.
Aggravation of epilepsy (seizures).
Parkinson-like disorders (see Glossary).
Peripheral neuritis (see Glossary)—numbness, tingling, pain, loss of strength in arms and legs.
Reduced white blood cell count—fever, sore throat.

▷ **Possible Effects on Sexual Function:** Decreased libido (150 mg/day), increased libido (antidepressant effect), inhibited ejaculation (75 to 150 mg/day), painful ejaculation (75 mg/day), inhibited female orgasm (100 mg/day), female breast enlargement/milk production (300 mg/day), altered menstrual timing and pattern (300 mg/day), swelling of testicles. These effects usually disappear within 2 to 10 days after discontinuation of the drug.

Natural Diseases or Disorders That May Be Activated by This Drug
Latent epilepsy, glaucoma, prostatism.

CAUTION
1. The dosage of this drug must be adjusted carefully for each person individually. This requires observation of symptom improvement and, in some instances, the measurement of drug levels in the blood.
2. Observe for early indications of toxicity: confusion, agitation, rapid heartbeat.
3. It is advisable to withhold this drug if electroconvulsive therapy (ECT, "shock" treatment) is to be used.

Precautions for Use
By Infants and Children: Safety and effectiveness for use by those under 16 years of age have not been established.
By Those over 60 Years of Age: During the first 2 weeks of treatment, observe for the development of confusion, restlessness, agitation, forgetfulness, disorientation, delusions and hallucinations. Reduction of dosage or discontinuation may be necessary. Observe for unsteadiness that may predispose to falling and injury. This drug can increase the

degree of impaired urination associated with prostate gland enlargement (prostatism). It is advisable to take the total dose at bedtime to reduce the risk of postural hypotension (see Glossary).

▷ **Advisability of Use During Pregnancy**
Pregnancy Category: C (tentative). See Pregnancy Code inside back cover.
Animal studies: Reveal toxic effects on the embryo in rats and rabbits but no birth defects in the newborn.
Human studies: Information from adequate studies of pregnant women is not available.
Avoid drug during first 3 months. Use during the last 6 months only if clearly needed.

Advisability of Use if Breast-Feeding
Presence of this drug in breast milk: Yes, in small amounts.
Monitor nursing infant closely and discontinue drug or nursing if adverse effects develop.

Habit-Forming Potential: None.

Effects of Overdosage: Confusion, hallucinations, marked drowsiness, tremors, dilated pupils, cold skin, stupor, coma, convulsions, rapid heartbeat, low blood pressure.

Suggested Periodic Examinations While Taking This Drug (at physician's discretion)
Complete blood cell counts, serial blood pressure readings and electrocardiograms.

▷ **While Taking This Drug, Observe the Following**
Foods: No restrictions. Drug may increase appetite and cause excessive weight gain.
Beverages: No restrictions. May be taken with milk.
▷   *Alcohol:* Avoid completely. This drug can markedly increase the intoxicating effects of alcohol and accentuate its depressant action on brain function.
Tobacco Smoking: May hasten the elimination of this drug. Higher doses may be necessary.
▷   *Other Drugs*
Amoxapine may **increase** the effects of
• atropinelike drugs (see Drug Class, Section Four).
Amoxapine may **decrease** the effects of
• clonidine (Catapres).
• guanethidine (Ismelin).
Amoxapine **taken concurrently** with
• monoamine oxidase (MAO) type A inhibitor drugs may cause high fever, delirium and convulsions (see Drug Class, Section Four).
• thyroid preparations may impair heart rhythm and function. Ask physician for guidance regarding adjustment of thyroid dose.

▷ *Driving, Hazardous Activities:* This drug may impair mental alertness, judgment, physical coordination and reaction time. Avoid hazardous activities.

Aviation Note: The use of this drug **is a disqualification** for piloting. Consult a designated Aviation Medical Examiner.

Exposure to Sun: Use caution until sensitivity to sun has been determined. This drug may cause photosensitivity (see Glossary).

Exposure to Heat: This drug can inhibit sweating and impair the body's adaptation to hot environments, increasing the risk of heat stroke. Avoid saunas.

Exposure to Cold: The elderly should use caution and avoid conditions conducive to hypothermia (see Glossary).

Discontinuation: It is advisable to discontinue this drug gradually. Abrupt withdrawal after long-term use can cause headache, malaise and nausea.

AMOXICILLIN
(a mox i SIL in)

Introduced: 1969

Prescription: USA: Yes
Canada: Yes

Available as Generic: USA: Yes
Canada: No

Class: Antibiotic, penicillins

Controlled Drug: USA: No
Canada: No

Brand Names: Amoxil, ✦Apo-Amoxi, Augmentin [CD], ✦Clavulin [CD], Larotid, ✦Novamoxin, Polymox, Trimox, Utimox, Wymox

BENEFITS versus RISKS	
Possible Benefits	*Possible Risks*
EFFECTIVE TREATMENT OF INFECTIONS due to susceptible microorganisms	ALLERGIC REACTIONS, mild to severe, in 3% of the general population and 15% of allergic individuals
	Superinfections (yeast)
	Drug-induced colitis

▷ **Principal Uses**

As a Single Drug Product: To treat certain infections of the skin and soft tissues; of the ear, nose and throat; and of the genitourinary tract, including gonorrhea.

How This Drug Works: This drug destroys susceptible infecting bacteria by interfering with their ability to produce new protective cell walls as they multiply and grow.

Available Dosage Forms and Strengths
     Capsules — 150 mg, 500 mg
   Chewable tablets — 125 mg, 250 mg
   Oral suspension — 125 mg, 250 mg per 5-ml teaspoonful
   Pediatric drops — 50 mg per ml

▷ **Usual Adult Dosage Range:** 250 to 500 mg/8 hours. The usual maximal dose is 4500 mg/24 hours. **Note: Actual dosage and administration schedule must be determined by the physician for each patient individually.**

▷ **Dosing Instructions:** May be taken on an empty stomach or with food, milk, fruit juice, ginger ale or other cold drinks. Capsule may be opened for administration.

Usual Duration of Use: For all streptococcal infections—not less than 10 consecutive days (without interruption) to reduce the possibility of developing rheumatic fever or glomerulonephritis. For all other infections—as long as necessary to eradicate the infection.

▷ **This Drug Should Not Be Taken If**
- you have had an allergic reaction to any dosage form of it previously.
- you are certain you are allergic to **any** form of penicillin.

▷ **Inform Your Physician Before Taking This Drug If**
- you suspect you may be allergic to penicillin or you have a history of a previous "reaction" to penicillin.
- you are allergic to cephalosporin antibiotics (Ancef, Ceporan, Ceporex, Kafocin, Keflex, Keflin, Kefzol, Loridine).
- you are allergic by nature (hay fever, asthma, hives, eczema).

Possible Side-Effects (natural, expected and unavoidable drug actions)
Superinfections (see Glossary), often due to yeast organisms.

▷ **Possible Adverse Effects** (unusual, unexpected and infrequent reactions)
 If any of the following develop, consult your physician promptly for guidance.
Mild Adverse Effects
Allergic Reactions: Skin rashes, hives, itching.
Irritations of mouth and tongue, "black tongue," nausea, vomiting, mild diarrhea, dizziness (rare).
Serious Adverse Effects
Allergic Reactions: Anaphylactic reaction (see Glossary), severe skin reactions, drug fever, swollen painful joints, sore throat, abnormal bleeding or bruising.

▷ **Possible Effects on Sexual Function:** None reported.

CAUTION
1. Take the exact dose and the full course prescribed.
2. This drug should not be used concurrently with antibiotics like erythromycin or tetracycline.

Precautions for Use

By Infants and Children: A generalized rash occurs in approximately 90% of individuals who take this drug during an episode of infectious mononucleosis. This drug may cause diarrhea, which sometimes necessitates discontinuation.

By Those over 60 Years of Age: Natural changes in the skin may predispose to prolonged itching reactions in the genital and anal regions. Report such reactions promptly.

▷ **Advisability of Use During Pregnancy**

Pregnancy Category: B (tentative). See Pregnancy Code inside back cover.
Animal studies: No information available.
Human studies: Information from adequate studies of pregnant women indicates no increased risk of birth defects in 3546 pregnancies exposed to penicillin derivatives.
Ask physician for guidance.

Advisability of Use if Breast-Feeding

Presence of this drug in breast milk: Yes.
The nursing infant may be sensitized to penicillin and may be at risk for developing diarrhea or yeast infections.
Avoid drug if possible or refrain from nursing.

Habit-Forming Potential: None.

Effects of Overdosage: Possible nausea, vomiting and/or diarrhea.

Possible Effects of Long-Term Use: Superinfections, often due to yeast organisms.

Suggested Periodic Examinations While Taking This Drug (at physician's discretion)
Complete blood cell counts.

▷ **While Taking This Drug, Observe the Following**

Foods: No restrictions.
Beverages: No restrictions. May be taken with milk, fruit juices or carbonated drinks.

▷ *Alcohol:* No interactions expected.
Tobacco Smoking: No interactions expected.

▷ *Other Drugs*
Amoxicillin may *decrease* the effects of
• oral contraceptives in some women, and impair their effectiveness in preventing pregnancy.

The following drugs may *decrease* the effects of amoxicillin
- antacids reduce the absorption of amoxicillin.
- chloramphenicol (Chloromycetin).
- erythromycin (Erythrocin, E-Mycin, etc.).
- tetracyclines (Achromycin, Declomycin, Minocin, etc.). (See Drug Class, Section Four.)

▷ *Driving, Hazardous Activities:* Usually no restrictions. Be alert to the rare occurrence of dizziness and/or nausea, and restrict activities accordingly.

Aviation Note: The use of this drug *may be a disqualification* for piloting. Consult a designated Aviation Medical Examiner.

Exposure to Sun: No restrictions.

Special Storage Instructions: Oral suspension and pediatric drops should be refrigerated.

Observe the Following Expiration Times: Do not take the oral suspension or drops of this drug if older than 7 days when kept at room temperature or 14 days when kept refrigerated.

AMPICILLIN
(am pi SIL in)

Introduced: 1961

Class: Antibiotic, penicillins

Prescription: USA: Yes
Canada: Yes

Controlled Drug: USA: No
Canada: No

Available as Generic: Yes

Brand Names: Amcill, ✦Ampicin, ✦Ampicin PRB [CD], ✦Ampilean, ✦Apo-Ampi, 500 Kit [CD], ✦Novo-Ampicillin, Omnipen, Omnipen Pediatric Drops, ✦Penbritin, Polycillin, Polycillin Pediatric Drops, Polycillin-PRB [CD], Principen, Probampacin [CD], ✦Pro-Biosan, Totacillin

---

BENEFITS versus RISKS

Possible Benefits	*Possible Risks*
EFFECTIVE TREATMENT OF INFECTIONS due to susceptible microorganisms	ALLERGIC REACTIONS, mild to severe, in 3% of the general population and 15% of allergic individuals
	Superinfections (yeast)
	Drug-induced colitis

▷ **Principal Uses**

As a Single Drug Product: To treat certain infections of the skin and soft tissues, of the respiratory tract, of the gastrointestinal tract, and of the genitourinary tract (including gonorrhea in females). Also used to treat certain types of septicemia and meningitis.

As a Combination Drug Product [CD]: May be combined with probenecid (Benemid) to delay the elimination of ampicillin by the kidney and thereby increase its level in the blood. This combination drug is designed primarily for the treatment of gonorrhea in males and females.

How This Drug Works: This drug destroys susceptible infecting bacteria by interfering with their ability to produce new protective cell walls as they multiply and grow.

Available Dosage Forms and Strengths

Capsules — 250 mg, 500 mg

Oral suspension — 100 mg per ml, 125 mg, 250 mg, 500 mg per 5-ml teaspoonful

Pediatric drops — 100 mg per ml

▷ **Usual Adult Dosage Range:**   250 to 500 mg/6 hours. The usual maximal dose is 6000 mg/24 hours. **Note: Actual dosage and administration schedule must be determined by the physician for each patient individually.**

▷ **Dosing Instructions:**   Best taken on an empty stomach, 1 hour before or 2 hours after eating. Capsule may be opened for administration.

Usual Duration of Use: For all streptococcal infections—not less than 10 consecutive days (without interruption) to reduce the possibility of developing rheumatic fever or glomerulonephritis. For all other infections—as long as necessary to eradicate the infection.

▷ **This Drug Should Not Be Taken If**
- you have had an allergic reaction to any dosage form of it previously.
- you are certain you are allergic to *any* form of penicillin.

▷ **Inform Your Physician Before Taking This Drug If**
- you suspect you may be allergic to penicillin or you have a history of a previous "reaction" to penicillin.
- you are allergic to cephalosporin antibiotics (Ancef, Ceporan, Ceporex, Kafocin, Keflex, Keflin, Kefzol, Loridine).
- you are allergic by nature (hay fever, asthma, hives, eczema).

Possible Side-Effects (natural, expected and unavoidable drug actions)
Superinfections (see Glossary), often due to yeast organisms.

▷ **Possible Adverse Effects** (unusual, unexpected and infrequent reactions)
If any of the following develop, consult your physician promptly for guidance.
Mild Adverse Effects
Allergic Reactions: Skin rashes, hives, itching.
Irritations of mouth and tongue, "black tongue," nausea, vomiting, mild diarrhea, dizziness (rare).

Serious Adverse Effects

Allergic Reactions: Anaphylactic reaction (see Glossary), severe skin reactions, drug fever, swollen painful joints, sore throat, abnormal bleeding or bruising.

▷ **Possible Effects on Sexual Function:**   None reported.

CAUTION

1. Take the exact dose and the full course prescribed.
2. This drug should not be used concurrently with antibiotics like erythromycin or tetracycline.

Precautions for Use

By Infants and Children: A generalized rash occurs in approximately 90% of individuals who take this drug during an episode of infectious mononucleosis. This drug may cause diarrhea, which sometimes necessitates discontinuation.

By Those over 60 Years of Age: Natural changes in the skin may predispose to prolonged itching reactions in the genital and anal regions. Report such reactions promptly.

▷ **Advisability of Use During Pregnancy**

Pregnancy Category: B (tentative). See Pregnancy Code inside back cover.
Animal studies: No birth defects due to this drug found in mice or rats.
Human studies: Information from adequate studies of pregnant women indicates no increased risk of birth defects in 3546 pregnancies exposed to penicillin derivatives.
Ask physician for guidance.

Advisability of Use if Breast-Feeding

Presence of this drug in breast milk: Yes, in small amounts.
The nursing infant may be sensitized to penicillin and may be at risk for developing diarrhea or yeast infections.
Avoid drug if possible or refrain from nursing.

Habit-Forming Potential: None.

Effects of Overdosage: Possible nausea, vomiting and/or diarrhea.

Possible Effects of Long-Term Use: Superinfections, often due to yeast organisms.

Suggested Periodic Examinations While Taking This Drug (at physician's discretion)
Complete blood cell counts.

▷ **While Taking This Drug, Observe the Following**

Foods: No restrictions.
Beverages: No restrictions. May be taken with milk.
▷ *Alcohol:* No interactions expected.
Tobacco Smoking: No interactions expected.

▷   *Other Drugs*
>   Ampicillin may ***decrease*** the effects of
>   • oral contraceptives in some women, and impair their effectiveness in preventing pregnancy.
>   The following drugs may ***decrease*** the effects of ampicillin
>   • antacids reduce the absorption of amoxicillin.
>   • chloramphenicol (Chloromycetin).
>   • erythromycin (Erythrocin, E-Mycin, etc.).
>   • tetracyclines (Achromycin, Declomycin, Minocin, etc.). (See Drug Class, Section Four.)

▷   *Driving, Hazardous Activities:* Usually no restrictions. Be alert to the rare occurrence of dizziness and/or nausea, and restrict activities accordingly.
>   *Aviation Note:* The use of this drug ***may be a disqualification*** for piloting. Consult a designated Aviation Medical Examiner.
>   *Exposure to Sun:* No restrictions.
>   *Special Storage Instructions:* Oral suspension and pediatric drops should be refrigerated.
>   *Observe the Following Expiration Times:* Do not take the oral suspension or drops of this drug if older than 7 days when kept at room temperature or 14 days when kept refrigerated.

ASPIRIN*
(AS pir in)

Other Names: ASA, acetylsalicylic acid

Introduced: 1899

Class: Mild analgesic, antiinflammatory, antipyretic, salicylates

Prescription: USA: No
Canada: No

Controlled Drug: USA: No
Canada: No

Available as Generic: Yes

*In the United States *aspirin* is an official generic designation. In Canada *Aspirin* is the Registered Trade Mark of the Bayer Company Division of Sterling Drug Limited.

Brand Names: Alka-Seltzer Effervescent Pain Reliever & Antacid [CD], Alka-Seltzer Plus [CD], Anacin [CD], Anacin Maximum Strength [CD], ✦Anacin w/Codeine [CD], ✦Ancasal, A.S.A. Enseals, ✦Asasantine [CD], Ascriptin [CD], Ascriptin A/D [CD], Aspergum, ✦Aspirin*, ✦Astrin, Axotal [CD], Azdone [CD], Bayer Aspirin, Bayer Children's Chewable Aspirin, Bufferin [CD], Bufferin Arthritis Strength [CD], Bufferin Extra Strength [CD], Bufferin w/Codeine [CD], Cama Arthritis Pain Reliever [CD], Cope [CD], ✦Coryphen, ✦Coryphen-Codeine [CD], Darvon Compound [CD], Darvon Compound-65 [CD], Darvon w/ASA [CD], ✦Darvon-N Compound [CD], Darvon-N w/ASA [CD], Dolene Compound-65 [CD], Easprin, Ecotrin Preparations, 8-Hour Bayer, Empirin, Empirin w/Codeine No. 2, 4 [CD], ✦Entrophen, Excedrin [CD], Fiorinal [CD], Fiorinal w/Codeine [CD], ✦Fiorinal-C 1/4, -C 1/2 [CD], 4-Way Cold Tablets [CD], Lortab ASA [CD], Maximum Bayer Aspirin, Measurin, Midol Caplets [CD], Norgesic [CD], Norgesic Forte [CD], ✦Novasen, ✦Novopropoxyn Compound [CD], ✦Oxycodan [CD], Percodan [CD], Percodan-Demi [CD], ✦Phenaphen [CD], ✦Phenaphen No. 2, 3, 4 [CD], ✦Riphen-10, Robaxisal [CD], ✦Robaxisal-C [CD], ✦Sal-Adult, ✦Sal-Infant, Sine-Off Tablets [CD], St. Joseph Children's Aspirin, ✦Supasa, Synalgos [CD], Synalgos-DC [CD], Talwin Compound [CD], Talwin Compound-50 [CD], ✦Triaphen-10, Trigesic [CD]

BENEFITS versus RISKS

Possible Benefits	*Possible Risks*
EFFECTIVE RELIEF OF MILD TO MODERATE PAIN and INFLAMMATION	Stomach irritation, bleeding, and/or ulceration
REDUCTION OF FEVER	Hearing loss
PREVENTION OF BLOOD CLOTS (as in heart attack, phlebitis and stroke)	Decreased numbers of white blood cells and platelets
	Hemolytic anemia

▷ **Principal Uses**

As a Single Drug Product: To relieve mild to moderate pain from any cause, to provide symptomatic relief in conditions characterized by inflammation and to reduce high fever. A major use is to treat musculoskeletal disorders, especially acute and chronic arthritis. It is also used selectively in low dosage to prevent platelet embolism to the brain (in men) and to reduce the risk of thromboembolism in patients recovering from a recent heart attack, in those with artificial heart valves and in those undergoing hip surgery. (See Blood Platelets in the Glossary.)

---

*In the United States *aspirin* is an official generic designation. In Canada *Aspirin* is the Registered Trade Mark of the Bayer Company Division of Sterling Drug Limited.

As a Combination Drug Product [CD]: Frequently combined with other mild or strong analgesic drugs to enhance pain relief. Also combined with antihistamines and decongestants in many cold preparations to relieve the headache and general discomfort that often accompany respiratory infections.

How This Drug Works: Aspirin reduces the tissue concentrations of prostaglandins, chemicals involved in the production of inflammation and pain. By modifying the temperature-regulating center in the brain, dilating blood vessels in the skin, and increasing sweating, aspirin hastens the loss of body heat and reduces fever. By preventing the production of thromboxane in blood platelets, aspirin inhibits the aggregation of platelets and the initiation of blood clots.

Available Dosage Forms and Strengths

Capsules, enteric-coated — 500 mg
Capsules, enteric-coated granules — 325 mg
Gum tablets — 227.5 mg
Suppositories — 60 mg, 120 mg, 125 mg, 130 mg, 195 mg, 200 mg, 300 mg, 325 mg, 600 mg, 650 mg, 1.2 grams
Tablets — 65 mg, 81 mg, 325 mg, 500 mg
Tablets, chewable — 81 mg
Tablets, enteric-coated — 325 mg, 500 mg, 650 mg, 975 mg
Tablets, prolonged-action — 650 mg, 800 mg

▷ **Usual Adult Dosage Range:** For pain or fever—325 to 650 mg/4 hours as needed. For arthritis (and related conditions)—3600 to 5400 mg daily in divided doses. For the prevention of blood clots—80 to 150 mg/24 to 48 hours. **Note: For long-term use, actual dosage and administration schedule must be determined by the physician for each patient individually.**

▷ **Dosing Instructions:** Take with food, milk, or a full glass of water to reduce stomach irritation. Regular tablets may be crushed and capsules opened for administration. Enteric-coated tablets, prolonged-action tablets, A.S.A. Enseals, Cama tablets and Ecotrin tablets should not be crushed.

Usual Duration of Use: Short-term use is recommended—3 to 5 days. Daily use should not exceed 10 days without physician supervision. Continual use on a regular schedule for 1 week is usually necessary to determine this drug's effectiveness in relieving the symptoms of chronic arthritis. Long-term use requires periodic evaluation of response and dosage adjustment. Consult your physician on a regular basis.

▷ **This Drug Should Not Be Taken If**
  • you have had an allergic reaction or unfavorable response to any form of aspirin previously.

- you have any type of bleeding disorder (such as hemophilia).
- you have active peptic ulcer disease.
- it has an odor resembling vinegar. This is due to the presence of acetic acid and indicates the decomposition of aspirin.

▷ **Inform Your Physician Before Taking This Drug If**
  - you are taking any anticoagulant drug.
  - you are taking oral antidiabetic drugs.
  - you have a history of peptic ulcer disease or gout.
  - you have lupus erythematosus.
  - you are pregnant or planning pregnancy.
  - you plan to have surgery of any kind in the near future.

Possible Side-Effects (natural, expected and unavoidable drug actions)
Mild drowsiness in sensitive individuals.

▷ **Possible Adverse Effects** (unusual, unexpected and infrequent reactions)
  If any of the following develop, consult your physician promptly for guidance.
  Mild Adverse Effects
  Allergic Reactions: Skin rash, hives, nasal discharge (resembling hay fever), nasal polyps.
  Stomach irritation, heartburn, nausea, vomiting, constipation.
  Serious Adverse Effects
  Allergic Reactions: Acute anaphylactic reaction (see Glossary), asthma, unusual bruising due to allergic destruction of blood platelets (see Glossary).
  Idiosyncratic Reactions: Hemolytic anemia (see Glossary).
  Erosion of stomach lining, with silent bleeding.
  Activation of peptic ulcer, with or without hemorrhage.
  Bone marrow depression (see Glossary)—fatigue, weakness, fever, sore throat, abnormal bleeding or bruising.
  Hepatitis with jaundice (see Glossary)—yellow skin and eyes, dark-colored urine, light-colored stool (very rare).
  Kidney damage, if used in large doses or for a prolonged period of time.

▷ **Possible Effects on Sexual Function:**   None reported.

▷ **Adverse Effects That May Mimic Natural Diseases or Disorders**
  Liver damage may suggest viral hepatitis.

CAUTION
  1. It is most important to understand that aspirin is a drug. While it is one of our most useful drugs, we have an unrealistic sense of safety and unconcern regarding its action within the body and its potential for adverse effects.
  2. In order to know if you are taking aspirin, make it a point to learn the contents of all drugs you take—those prescribed by your physician and those you purchase over-the-counter (OTC) without prescription.

3. Limit the dose of aspirin to no more than 3 tablets (975 mg) at one time, allow at least 4 hours between doses and take no more than 10 tablets (3250 mg) in 24 hours without physician supervision.
4. Remember that aspirin can
   - cause new illnesses.
   - complicate existing illnesses.
   - complicate pregnancy.
   - complicate surgery.
   - interact unfavorably with other drugs.
5. When your physician asks "Are you taking any drugs?" the answer is yes if you are taking aspirin. This also applies to *any* nonprescription drug you may be taking. (See OTC Drugs in the Glossary.)

Precautions for Use

By Infants and Children: Reye syndrome (brain and liver damage in children, often fatal) can follow flu or chicken pox in children and teenagers. While the exact cause and nature of the syndrome are not known, some reports suggest that the use of aspirin by children with flu or chicken pox can increase the risk of developing this complication. Consult your physician before giving aspirin to a child or teenager with chicken pox, flu or similar infection.

Usual dosage schedule for children:

Up to 2 years of age—consult physician.
2 to 4 years of age—160 mg/4 hours, up to 5 doses/24 hours.
4 to 6 years of age—240 mg/4 hours, up to 5 doses/24 hours.
6 to 9 years of age—320 mg/4 hours, up to 5 doses/24 hours.
9 to 11 years of age—400 mg/4 hours, up to 5 doses/24 hours.
11 to 12 years of age—480 mg/4 hours, up to 5 doses/24 hours.

Do not exceed 5 days of continual use without consulting your physician.

Give all doses with food, milk or a full glass of water.

By Those over 60 Years of Age: The natural decline in kidney function can reduce your tolerance for aspirin. Observe for indications of excessive dosage: nervous irritabilty, confusion, ringing in the ears, deafness, loss of appetite, nausea and stomach irritation. Aspirin can cause excessive bleeding from the stomach in sensitive individuals. This can occur as "silent" bleeding of small amounts over an extended period of time, resulting in anemia. In addition, sudden hemorrhage can occur, even without a history of stomach ulcer. Observe stools for gray to black discoloration—an indication of stomach bleeding.

▷ Advisability of Use During Pregnancy

Pregnancy Category: D (tentative). See Pregnancy Code inside back cover.

Animal studies: Significant birth defects due to this drug have been reported.

Human studies: Information from studies of pregnant women indicates no increased risk of birth defects in 32,164 pregnancies exposed to aspirin. However, studies show that the regular use of salicylates during pregnancy is often detrimental to the health of the mother and to the welfare of the fetus. Excessive use of salicylate drugs can cause anemia, hemorrhage before and after delivery and an increased incidence of stillbirths and newborn deaths. It is advisable to limit the use of aspirin during pregnancy to small doses and for brief periods of time, and to avoid aspirin altogether during the last 3 months.

Advisability of Use if Breast-Feeding
Presence of this drug in breast milk: Yes.
Avoid drug or refrain from nursing.

Habit-Forming Potential: Use of this drug in large doses for a prolonged period of time may cause a form of psychological dependence (see Glossary).

Effects of Overdosage: Stomach distress, nausea, vomiting, ringing in the ears, dizziness, impaired hearing, sweating, stupor, fever, deep and rapid breathing, muscular twitching, delirium, hallucinations, convulsions.

Possible Effects of Long-Term Use
A form of psychological dependence (see Glossary).
Anemia due to chronic blood loss from erosion of stomach lining.
The development of stomach ulcer.
The development of "aspirin allergy"—nasal discharge, nasal polyps, asthma.
Kidney damage.
Excessive prolongation of bleeding time, of major importance in the event of injury or surgery.

Suggested Periodic Examinations While Taking This Drug (at physician's discretion)
Complete blood cell counts.
Kidney function tests and urine analyses.
Liver function tests.

▷ While Taking This Drug, Observe the Following
Foods: No restrictions.
Nutritional Support: If supplementing the diet with vitamin C, take no more than the recommended daily allowance. Do not take large doses of vitamin C while taking aspirin on a regular basis.
Beverages: No restrictions. May be taken with milk.
▷   *Alcohol:* No interactions expected. However, the concurrent use of alcohol and aspirin may significantly increase the possibility of erosion and ulceration of the stomach lining and may result in bleeding.
Tobacco Smoking: No interactions expected.
▷   *Other Drugs*
Aspirin may *increase* the effects of
• oral anticoagulants, and cause abnormal bleeding. Dosage adjustment is often necessary.

- oral antidiabetic drugs and insulin, and cause hypoglycemia (see Glossary). Dosage adjustment is often necessary.
- heparin, and cause abnormal bleeding.
- methotrexate, and increase its toxic effects.
- valproic acid (Depakene).

Aspirin may *decrease* the effects of

- beta-adrenergic-blocking drugs (see Drug Class, Section Four).
- captopril (Capoten).
- probenecid (Benemid), and reduce its effectiveness in the treatment of gout—with aspirin doses of less than 2 grams/24 hours.
- spironolactone (Aldactone), and reduce its diuretic effect.
- sulfinpyrazone (Anturane), and reduce its effectiveness in the treatment of gout—with aspirin doses of less than 2 grams/24 hours.

The following drugs may *increase* the effects of aspirin

- acetazolamide (Diamox).
- para-aminobenzoic acid (Pabalate).
- vitamin C, taken as ascorbic acid and in large doses, may acidify the urine in some individuals and cause aspirin accumulation and toxicity.

The following drugs may *decrease* the effects of aspirin

- antacids, in regular continual use.
- cortisonelike drugs (see Drug Class, Section Four).
- urinary alkalizers (sodium bicarbonate, sodium citrate).

▷ *Driving, Hazardous Activities:* No restrictions or precautions.

Aviation Note: Usually no restrictions. However, it is advisable to observe for the possible occurrence of mild drowsiness and to restrict activities accordingly.

Exposure to Sun: No restrictions.

Discontinuation: The use of aspirin should be discontinued completely at least 1 week before surgery of any kind.

ATENOLOL
(a TEN oh lohl)

Introduced: 1973

Class: Antianginal, antihypertensive, beta-adrenergic blocker

Prescription: USA: Yes
　　Canada: Yes

Controlled Drug: USA: No
　　Canada: No

Available as Generic: No

Brand Names: Tenoretic [CD], Tenormin

```
┌─────────────────────────────────────────────────────────────┐
│                    BENEFITS versus RISKS                      │
│                                                               │
│        Possible Benefits              Possible Risks          │
│  EFFECTIVE ANTIANGINAL          CONGESTIVE HEART FAILURE       │
│    DRUG in the management of       in advanced heart disease  │
│    effort-induced angina        Worsening of angina in coronary│
│  EFFECTIVE, WELL-TOLERATED        heart disease (abrupt        │
│  ANTIHYPERTENSIVE in mild         withdrawal)                 │
│    to moderate high blood       Masking of low blood sugar    │
│    pressure                       (hypoglycemia) in drug-treated│
│                                   diabetes                    │
│                                 Provocation of bronchial asthma│
│                                   (with high doses)           │
└─────────────────────────────────────────────────────────────┘
```

▷ **Principal Uses**

As a Single Drug Product: Used primarily to treat (1) classical, effort-induced angina pectoris; (2) mild to moderately severe high blood pressure. May be used alone or concurrently with other antihypertensive drugs, such as diuretics.

How This Drug Works: By blocking certain actions of the sympathetic nervous system, this drug

- reduces the rate and contraction force of the heart, thus lowering the ejection pressure of the blood leaving the heart and reducing the oxygen requirement for heart function.
- reduces the degree of contraction of blood vessel walls, resulting in their relaxation and expansion and consequent lowering of blood pressure.

Available Dosage Forms and Strengths

Tablets — 50 mg, 100 mg

▷ **Usual Adult Dosage Range:** Initially 50 mg once daily. Dose may be increased gradually at intervals of 7 to 10 days as needed and tolerated up to 100 mg/24 hours. The usual maintenance dose is 50 to 100 mg/24 hours. The total dose should not exceed 100 mg/24 hours. **Note: Actual dosage and administration schedule must be determined by the physician for each patient individually.**

▷ **Dosing Instructions:** May be taken without regard to eating. Tablet may be crushed for administration. Do not discontinue this drug abruptly.

Usual Duration of Use: Continual use on a regular schedule for 10 to 14 days is usually necessary to determine this drug's effectiveness in lowering blood pressure. The long-term use of this drug will be determined by the course of your blood pressure over time and your response to the overall treatment program (weight reduction, salt restriction, smoking cessation, etc.). Consult your physician on a regular basis.

Possible Advantages of This Drug: The least likely of all beta blocker drugs to cause central nervous system adverse effects: confusion, hallucinations, nervousness, nightmares.

Currently a "Drug of Choice" for initiating treatment of hypertension with a single drug, especially for those subject to bronchial asthma or diabetes.

▷ **This Drug Should Not Be Taken If**
- you have had an allergic reaction to it previously.
- you have congestive heart failure.
- you have an abnormally slow heart rate or a serious form of heart block.
- you are taking, or have taken within the past 14 days, any monoamine oxidase (MAO) type A inhibitor drug (see Drug Class, Section Four).

▷ **Inform Your Physician Before Taking This Drug If**
- you have had an adverse reaction to any beta blocker drug in the past (see Drug Class, Section Four).
- you have a history of serious heart disease, with or without episodes of heart failure.
- you have a history of hay fever (allergic rhinitis), asthma, chronic bronchitis or emphysema.
- you have a history of overactive thyroid function (hyperthyroidism).
- you have a history of low blood sugar (hypoglycemia).
- you have impaired liver or kidney function.
- you have diabetes or myasthenia gravis.
- you are currently taking any form of digitalis, quinidine or reserpine, or any calcium blocker drug (see Drug Class, Section Four).
- you plan to have surgery under general anesthesia in the near future.

Possible Side-Effects (natural, expected and unavoidable drug actions)
Lethargy, fatigability, cold extremities, slow heart rate, light-headedness in upright position (see Orthostatic Hypotension in Glossary).

▷ **Possible Adverse Effects** (unusual, unexpected and infrequent reactions)
If any of the following develop, consult your physician promptly for guidance.
Mild Adverse Effects
Allergic Reactions: Skin rash, itching.
Headache, dizziness, drowsiness, abnormal dreams.
Indigestion, nausea, diarrhea.
Joint and muscle discomfort, fluid retention (edema).
Serious Adverse Effects
Mental depression, anxiety.
Chest pain, shortness of breath, precipitation of congestive heart failure.
Induction of bronchial asthma (in asthmatic individuals).

▷ **Possible Effects on Sexual Function:**   Decreased libido and impaired potency (50 to 100 mg/day). This beta blocker is less likely to cause reduced erectile capacity than most other drugs of this class.

CAUTION

1. **Do not discontinue this drug suddenly** without the knowledge and guidance of your physician. Carry a notation on your person that you are taking this drug.
2. Consult your physician or pharmacist before using nasal decongestants usually present in over-the-counter cold preparations and nose drops. These can cause sudden increases in blood pressure when taken concurrently with beta blocker drugs.
3. Report the development of any tendency to emotional depression.

Precautions for Use

By Infants and Children: Safety and effectiveness for use by those under 12 years of age have not been established. However, if this drug is used, observe for the development of low blood sugar (hypoglycemia) during periods of reduced food intake.

By Those over 60 Years of Age: Proceed **cautiously** with all antihypertensive drugs. Unacceptably high blood pressure should be reduced without creating the risks associated with excessively low blood pressure. Start treatment with small doses, and monitor the blood pressure response frequently. Sudden, rapid and excessive reduction of blood pressure can predispose to stroke or heart attack. Total daily dosage should not exceed 100 mg. Observe for dizziness, unsteadiness, tendency to fall, confusion, hallucinations, depression or urinary frequency.

▷ Advisability of Use During Pregnancy

Pregnancy Category: C (tentative). See Pregnancy Code inside back cover.

Animal studies: Increased resorptions of embryo and fetus reported in rats, but no birth defects.

Human studies: Information from adequate studies of pregnant women is not available.

Avoid use of drug during the first 3 months if possible. Avoid use during labor and delivery because of the possible effects on the newborn infant.

Advisability of Use if Breast-Feeding

Presence of this drug in breast milk: Yes.

Avoid drug if possible. If drug is necessary, observe nursing infant for slow heart rate and indications of low blood sugar.

Habit-Forming Potential: None.

Effects of Overdosage: Weakness, slow pulse, low blood pressure, fainting, cold and sweaty skin, congestive heart failure, possible coma and convulsions.

Possible Effects of Long-Term Use: Reduced heart reserve and eventual heart failure in susceptible individuals with advanced heart disease.

Suggested Periodic Examinations While Taking This Drug (at physician's discretion)
Measurements of blood pressure, evaluation of heart function.

▷ **While Taking This Drug, Observe the Following**
Foods: No restrictions. Avoid excessive salt intake.
Beverages: No restrictions. May be taken with milk.
▷ *Alcohol:* Use with caution until the combined effect has been determined. Alcohol may exaggerate this drug's ability to lower blood pressure and may increase its mild sedative effect.
Tobacco Smoking: Nicotine may reduce this drug's effectiveness in treating high blood pressure. In addition, high doses of this drug may potentiate the constriction of the bronchial tubes caused by regular smoking.
▷ *Other Drugs*
Atenolol may ***increase*** the effects of
• other antihypertensive drugs and cause excessive lowering of blood pressure. Dosage adjustments may be necessary.
• reserpine (Ser-Ap-Es, etc.) and cause sedation, depression, slowing of heart rate and lowering of blood pressure.
Atenolol ***taken concurrently*** with
• clonidine (Catapres) requires close monitoring for rebound high blood pressure if clonidine is withdrawn while atenolol is still being taken.
• insulin requires close monitoring to avoid undetected hypoglycemia (see Glossary).
The following drugs may ***decrease*** the effects of atenolol
• indomethacin (Indocin), and possibly other "aspirin substitutes," may impair atenolol's antihypertensive effect.
▷ *Driving, Hazardous Activities:* Use caution until the full extent of drowsiness, lethargy, and blood pressure change has been determined.
Aviation Note: The use of this drug ***is a disqualification*** for piloting. Consult a designated Aviation Medical Examiner.
Exposure to Sun: No restrictions.
Exposure to Heat: Caution advised. Hot environments can lower blood pressure and exaggerate the effects of this drug.
Exposure to Cold: Caution advised. Cold environments can enhance the circulatory deficiency in the extremities that may occur with this drug. The elderly should take precautions to prevent hypothermia (see Glossary).
Heavy Exercise or Exertion: It is advisable to avoid exertion that produces light-headedness, excessive fatigue, or muscle cramping. The use of this drug may intensify the hypertensive response to isometric exercise.
Occurrence of Unrelated Illness: The fever that accompanies systemic infections can lower blood pressure and require adjustment of dosage. Illnesses that cause nausea or vomiting may interrupt the regular dosage schedule. Ask your physician for guidance.

Discontinuation: It is advisable to avoid sudden discontinuation of this drug in all situations. If possible, gradual reduction of dose over a period of 2 to 3 weeks is recommended. Ask your physician for specific guidance.

ATROPINE*
(A troh peen)

Other Names: Belladonna alkaloids, hyoscyamine, scopolamine

Introduced: 1831

Class: Antispasmodic, atropinelike drugs, anticholinergics

Prescription: USA: Yes
          Canada: No

Controlled Drug: USA: No
          Canada: No

Available as Generic: Yes

Brand Names: Barbidonna [CD], Barbidonna Elixir [CD], Belladenal [CD], Belladenal-S [CD], ✦Belladenal Spacetabs [CD], ✦Bellergal [CD], Bellergal-S [CD], ✦Bellergal Spacetabs [CD], Butibel [CD], Cafergot P-B [CD], Chardonna-2 [CD], Donnagel [CD], ✦Donnagel w/Neomycin [CD], Kinesed [CD], Lomotil [CD], Pyridium Plus [CD], Urised [CD], ✦Wigraine [CD]

+---+
| **BENEFITS versus RISKS** |
| |
| *Possible Benefits*   *Possible Risks* |
| EFFECTIVE ANTISPASMODIC   Increased internal eye pressure |
| ACTION in spastic disorders of   (important in glaucoma) |
| the stomach and intestine   Constipation (may be quite |
| marked) |
| Urinary retention (in predisposed |
| persons) |
+---+

▷ **Principal Uses**

As a Single Drug Product: Used primarily for its antispasmodic effect in the treatment of spastic disorders of the digestive tract and lower urinary tract.

As a Combination Drug Product [CD]: Frequently combined with mild sedatives (especially barbiturates) to utilize their calming effects in the management of functional disorders associated with anxiety and nervous tension. The combination of a mild tranquilizer and an antispasmodic medication is more effective than either drug used alone.

---

*Atropine, hyoscyamine and scopolamine are the principal belladonna alkaloids. The characteristics of atropine are representative of the group.

How This Drug Works: By blocking the action of the chemical (acetylcholine) that transmits impulses at parasympathetic nerve endings, this drug prevents stimulation of muscular contraction and glandular secrection within the organs involved. This results in reduced overall activity, including the prevention or relief of muscle spasm.

Available Dosage Forms and Strengths
> Injection — 0.05 mg, 0.1 mg, 0.3 mg, 0.4 mg, 0.5 mg, 0.8 mg, 1 mg, 1.2 mg, all per ml
> Tablets — 0.4 mg
> Tablets, soluble — 0.3 mg, 0.4 mg, 0.6 mg

▷ **Usual Adult Dosage Range:**   0.3 to 1.2 mg/4 to 6 hours. **Note: Actual dosage and administration schedule must be determined by the physician for each patient individually.**

▷ **Dosing Instructions:**   For maximal absorption and effect, this drug should be taken 30 to 60 minutes before eating. Regular tablets may be crushed and regular capsules may be opened for administration. Prolonged-action and sustained-release dosage forms should be taken whole (neither crushed nor opened).

Usual Duration of Use: Continual use on a regular schedule for 2 to 5 days is usually necessary to determine this drug's effectiveness in relieving the symptoms of spastic disorders of the digestive system. Limit use to the relief of symptoms as necessary. Ask physician for guidance regarding long-term use.

▷ **This Drug Should Not Be Taken If**
- you have had an allergic reaction or unfavorable response to any atropine or belladonna preparation in the past.
- your stomach cannot empty properly into the intestine (pyloric obstruction).
- you are unable to empty the urinary bladder completely.
- you have glaucoma (narrow-angle type).
- you have severe ulcerative colitis.

▷ **Inform Your Physician Before Taking This Drug If**
- you have glaucoma (open-angle type).
- you have angina or coronary heart disease.
- you have chronic bronchitis.
- you have a hiatal hernia or peptic ulcer disease.
- you have enlargement of the prostate gland.
- you have myasthenia gravis.
- you plan to have surgery under general anesthesia in the near future.

Possible Side-Effects (natural, expected and unavoidable drug actions)
> Blurring of near vision (impairment of focus), dryness of mouth and throat, constipation, hesitancy in urination.

▷ **Possible Adverse Effects** (unusual, unexpected and infrequent reactions)
   **If any of the following develop, consult your physician promptly for
   guidance.**
   Mild Adverse Effects
   Allergic Reactions: Skin rash, hives.
   Light-headedness, dizziness, unsteadiness.
   Dilation of pupils, causing sensitivity to light.
   Flushing and dryness of skin, reduced sweating.
   Serious Adverse Effects
   Allergic Reactions: Severe skin reactions—exfoliative dermatitis.
   Idiosyncratic Reactions: Paradoxical excitement, nervousness, confu-
   sion, delirium.
   Increased internal eye pressure, development of glaucoma in suscepti-
   ble individuals.

▷ **Possible Effects on Sexual Function:** Inhibited female orgasm, reduced
   male fertility (0.4 to 0.6 mg/dose).

Natural Diseases or Disorders That May Be Activated by This Drug
   Latent glaucoma (narrow-angle type), latent myasthenia gravis.

CAUTION
   1. Use cautiously in the presence of asthma and chronic bronchitis.
      This drug can thicken bronchial secretions and promote retention
      of mucous plugs.
   2. Many over-the-counter medications (see OTC Drugs in the Glossary)
      for allergies, colds and coughs contain antihistamines that can aug-
      ment this drug's drying effects. Ask your physician or pharmacist
      for guidance before using such preparations.

Precautions for Use
   By Infants and Children: Children are particularly vulnerable to atropine
      toxicity. Start with low doses and increase cautiously as needed and
      tolerated. Observe for idiosyncratic reactions consisting of flushing,
      high fever, agitation, rapid pulse and breathing. Children with Down's
      syndrome or brain damage are more susceptible to this type of re-
      action.
   By Those over 60 Years of Age: Observe for agitation, confusion, loss of
      short-term memory, disorientation, visual and auditory hallucina-
      tions, delirium. This drug can increase the degree of impaired uri-
      nation associated with prostate gland enlargement (prostatism).

▷ **Advisability of Use During Pregnancy**
   Pregnancy Category: C (tentative). See Pregnancy Code inside back cover.
      Animal studies: Birth defects reported in mouse studies.
      Human studies: No increase in birth defects reported in 1198 exposures
      to this drug. Information from adequate studies of pregnant women
      is not available.
   Avoid drug completely during first 3 months.

Advisability of Use if Breast-Feeding
Presence of this drug in breast milk: Yes, in very small amounts.
Monitor nursing infant closely and discontinue drug or nursing if adverse effects develop.

Habit-Forming Potential: None.

Effects of Overdosage: Dilated pupils, blurring of near vision, dryness of mouth and throat, heart palpitation, impaired urination, high fever, hot skin, excitement, confusion, hallucinations, delirium, convulsions, coma.

Possible Effects of Long-Term Use: Chronic constipation, severe enough to result in fecal impaction. (Constipation should be treated promptly with effective laxatives.)

Suggested Periodic Examinations While Taking This Drug (at physician's discretion)
Measurement of internal eye pressure to detect any significant increase that could indicate developing glaucoma.

▷ **While Taking This Drug, Observe the Following**
Foods: Avoid constipating foods, such as cheeses. Follow the diet prescribed by your physician.
Beverages: Avoid large amounts of tea (may be constipating).
▷ *Alcohol:* No interactions expected.
Tobacco Smoking: No interactions expected.
▷ *Other Drugs*
Atropine may ***increase*** the effects of
• all other drugs having atropinelike actions (see Drug Class, Section Four).
Atropine may ***decrease*** the effects of
• haloperidol (Haldol), and reduce its effectiveness.
• phenothiazines (Thorazine, etc.), and reduce their effectiveness.
• pilocarpine eye drops, and reduce their effectiveness in lowering internal eye pressure in the treatment of glaucoma.
▷ *Driving, Hazardous Activities:* This drug may cause drowsiness, dizziness or blurred vision. Avoid hazardous activities if these drug effects occur.
Aviation Note: The use of this drug ***is a disqualification*** for piloting. Consult a designated Aviation Medical Examiner.
Exposure to Sun: No restrictions.
Exposure to Heat: Use extreme caution. The use of this drug in hot environments may significantly increase the risk of heat stroke.
Heavy Exercise or Exertion: Use caution in warm or hot environments. This drug may impair normal perspiration (heat loss) and interfere with the regulation of body temperature.
Discontinuation: Avoid prolonged and unnecessary use of this drug. When symptoms have been controlled for an adequate period of time, and

discontinuation appears possible, reduce the dose gradually over a period of several days.

AURANOFIN
(aw RAY noh fin)

Introduced: 1976

Class: Antiarthritic, gold compounds

Prescription: USA: Yes
Canada: Yes

Controlled Drug: USA: No
Canada: No

Available as Generic: No

Brand Name: Ridaura

BENEFITS versus RISKS

Possible Benefits	*Possible Risks*
REDUCTION OF JOINT PAIN, TENDERNESS AND SWELLING in active, severe RHEUMATOID ARTHRITIS Medication effective when taken by mouth	SIGNIFICANTLY REDUCED LEVELS OF RED AND WHITE BLOOD CELLS AND BLOOD PLATELETS (1% to 3%) LIVER DAMAGE WITH JAUNDICE (less than 0.1%) Diarrhea (47%), ulcerative colitis (less than 0.1%) Skin rash (24%) Mouth sores (13%)

▷ **Principal Uses**

As a Single Drug Product: Used *only* for the treatment of adults with active, severe rheumatoid arthritis who have had an inadequate and disappointing response to aspirin, aspirin substitutes and other antiarthritic drugs and treatment programs. It is usually added to a well-established program of antiarthritic drugs of the aspirin-substitute class.

How This Drug Works: Its method of action is unknown. It suppresses but does not cure arthritis and associated synovitis.

Available Dosage Forms and Strengths
Capsules — 3 mg

▷ **Usual Adult Dosage Range:** 6 mg daily, taken either as one dose every 24 hours or as two doses of 3 mg each every 12 hours. If response is inadequate after 6 months of regular continual use, the dose may be increased to 9 mg daily, taken as 3 doses of 3 mg each. If response remains inadequate after 3 months of 9 mg daily, this drug should be discontinued. **Note: Actual dosage and administration schedule must be determined by the physician for each patient individually.**

▷ **Dosing Instructions:** Take with or following food to reduce stomach irritation. Take the capsule whole with milk or a full glass of water.

Usual Duration of Use: Continual use on a regular schedule for 3 to 4 months is usually necessary to determine this drug's effectiveness in reducing the joint pain, tenderness and swelling associated with rheumatoid arthritis. The extent of long-term use will be determined by the degree of benefit and the pattern of adverse effects experienced by the individual patient. Consult your physician on a regular basis.

▷ **This Drug Should Not Be Taken If**
- you have had an allergic reaction or serious adverse effect from previous use of gold.
- you have active ulcerative colitis.
- you have a current blood cell or bone marrow disorder.
- you have active liver or kidney disease.
- you are pregnant or breast-feeding.
- you are taking penicillamine or antimalarial drugs for your arthritis.

▷ **Inform Your Physician Before Taking This Drug If**
- you are allergic by nature, or have a history of allergic reactions to drugs.
- you have diabetes.
- you have a history of heart disease, high blood pressure, circulatory disorders, liver or kidney disease, or ulcerative colitis.
- you are taking any other drugs at this time.
- you are planning pregnancy in the near future.

Possible Side-Effects (natural, expected and unavoidable drug actions)
Metallic taste.

▷ **Possible Adverse Effects** (unusual, unexpected and infrequent reactions)
If any of the following develop, consult your physician promptly for guidance.
Mild Adverse Effects
Allergic Reactions: Itching, skin rash.
Sores in mouth and throat and on tongue, loss of appetite, nausea, vomiting, stomach cramps, diarrhea.
Headache, partial or complete hair loss.
Serious Adverse Effects
Allergic Reactions: Severe skin reactions, exfoliative dermatitis.
Fever, cough, shortness of breath, drug-induced pneumonia and lung damage.
Liver damage with jaundice, ulcerative colitis.
Kidney damage.

Blood cell and bone marrow toxicity—fatigue, weakness, sore throat, abnormal bleeding or bruising.

Peripheral neuritis—pain, numbness, weakness of arms and legs.

▷ **Possible Effects on Sexual Function:**   None reported.

Possible Delayed Adverse Effects: Adverse effects from gold may occur many months after treatment has been discontinued. This is due to accumulation of gold in body tissues and its slow elimination. Report any indications of possible toxicity to your physician promptly.

▷ **Adverse Effects That May Mimic Natural Diseases or Disorders**

Fever, cough and chest discomfort may suggest respiratory tract infections such as bronchitis or pneumonia.

Liver damage may suggest viral hepatitis.

CAUTION

1. Periodic examinations (blood and urine tests) are mandatory during the use of this drug. Keep all appointments as directed by your physician.
2. Inform your physician promptly of any indications of possible toxic reactions. If there is a delay in reaching your physician, discontinue this drug until you obtain medical guidance.

Precautions for Use

By Infants and Children: Safety and effectiveness for use by those under 12 years of age have not been established.

By Those over 60 Years of Age: Tolerance to gold usually decreases with advancing age. Use small doses initially and observe closely for indications of adverse effects.

▷ **Advisability of Use During Pregnancy**

Pregnancy Category: C (tentative). See Pregnancy Code inside back cover.

Animal studies: Rabbit studies revealed an increase in resorptions, abortions and birth defects.

Human studies: Information from adequate studies of pregnant women is not available.

The manufacturer does not recommend the use of this drug during pregnancy.

Advisability of Use if Breast-Feeding

Presence of this drug in breast milk: Yes.

Avoid drug or refrain from nursing.

Habit-Forming Potential: None.

Effects of Overdosage: Nausea, vomiting, diarrhea, confusion, delirium, peripheral neuritis.

Suggested Periodic Examinations While Taking This Drug (at physician's discretion)

Complete blood cell counts, urine analyses, liver and kidney function tests.

▷ **While Taking This Drug, Observe the Following**
  Foods: No restrictions.
  Beverages: No restrictions. May be taken with milk.
▷ *Alcohol:* Use caution until the combined effects have been determined. Alcohol may intensify the irritant effect of this drug on the gastrointestinal tract.
  Tobacco Smoking: No interactions expected.
▷ *Other Drugs*
  Auranofin may *increase* the effects of
  • phenytoin (Dilantin), by increasing its blood level. Monitor closely for indications of phenytoin toxicity.
▷ *Driving, Hazardous Activities:* Usually no restrictions.
  Aviation Note: The use of this drug **may be a disqualification** for piloting. Consult a designated Aviation Medical Examiner.
  Exposure to Sun: Use caution. This drug may cause photosensitivity (see Glossary). Avoid sun and sun lamps if a drug-induced rash occurs.

AZATADINE
(a ZA ta deen)

Introduced: 1977

Class: Antihistamines

Prescription: USA: Yes
  Canada: Yes

Controlled Drug: USA: No
  Canada: No

Available as Generic: No

Brand Names: Optimine, Trinalin Repetabs [CD]

BENEFITS versus RISKS	
Possible Benefits	*Possible Risks*
EFFECTIVE RELIEF OF ALLERGIC RHINITIS AND ALLERGIC SKIN DISORDERS	Mild sedation Atropinelike effects Rare blood cell disorders: hemolytic anemia, abnormally low white blood cell and platelet counts

▷ **Principal Uses**
  As a Single Drug Product: Used primarily to provide symptomatic relief in allergic and related disorders: seasonal and perennial allergic rhinitis (hay fever), allergic conjunctivitis, and vasomotor rhinitis; also in hives and localized swellings (angioedema) of allergic origin.

As a Combination Drug Product [CD]: This drug is combined with a decongestant drug to enhance its ability to reduce tissue swelling and secretions in allergic and infectious disorders of the upper respiratory tract—hay fever, head colds and sinusitis.

How This Drug Works: Antihistamines reduce the intensity of the allergic response by blocking the action of histamine after it has been released from sensitized tissue cells in the eyes, nose and skin.

Available Dosage Forms and Strengths
Tablets — 1 mg

▷ **Usual Adult Dosage Range:**   1 to 2 mg/12 hours as needed (twice daily). **Note: Actual dosage and administration schedule must be determined by the physician for each patient individually.**

▷ **Dosing Instructions:**   Take with food or milk to prevent stomach irritation. The prolonged-action (combination) tablet should be swallowed whole (not crushed or chewed).

Usual Duration of Use: Continual use on a regular schedule for 2 to 3 days is usually necessary to determine this drug's effectiveness in relieving the symptoms of allergic rhinitis and dermatosis. It may be necessary to take this drug throughout the entire pollen season, depending upon individual sensitivity. However, antihistamines should not be taken continually (without interruption) for long-term use. Limit their use to periods that require symptomatic relief.

▷ **This Drug Should Not Be Taken If**
- you have had an allergic reaction to any dosage form of it previously.
- you are currently undergoing allergy skin tests.
- you are taking, or have taken within the past 14 days, any monoamine oxidase (MAO) type A inhibitor drug (see Drug Class, Section Four).

▷ **Inform Your Physician Before Taking This Drug If**
- you have had any allergic reactions or unfavorable responses to the previous use of antihistamines.
- you have glaucoma (narrow-angle type) or asthma.
- you have difficulty emptying the urinary bladder, especially if due to prostate gland enlargement.
- you are taking an anticoagulant at this time.
- you plan to have surgery under general anesthesia in the near future.

Possible Side-Effects (natural, expected and unavoidable drug actions)
Drowsiness; sense of weakness; blurred vision; dryness of the nose, mouth and throat; impaired urination.

▷ **Possible Adverse Effects** (unusual, unexpected and infrequent reactions)
If any of the following develop, consult your physician promptly for guidance.

Mild Adverse Effects
  Allergic Reaction: Skin rash.
  Headache, nervous agitation, dizziness, confusion.
  Reduced tolerance for contact lenses.
  Thickening of bronchial secretions in asthma or bronchitis.
  Indigestion, nausea, vomiting.
Serious Adverse Effects
  Hemolytic anemia (see Glossary).
  Abnormally low white blood cell count—fever, sore throat, infections.
  Abnormally low blood platelet count—abnormal bleeding or bruising.

▷ **Possible Effects on Sexual Function:** Shortened menstrual cycle (early arrival of expected menstrual onset).

CAUTION
  1. Discontinue this drug 4 days before diagnostic skin testing procedures in order to prevent false negative test results.
  2. Do not use this drug if you have active bronchial asthma, bronchitis or pneumonia. It can thicken bronchial mucus and make it more difficult to remove (by absorption or coughing).

Precautions for Use
  By Infants and Children: Safety and effectiveness for use by those under 12 years of age have not been established.
  By Those over 60 Years of Age: You may be more susceptible to the development of drowsiness, dizziness, and unsteadiness, and to impairment of thinking, judgment and memory. This drug can increase the degree of impaired urination associated with prostate gland enlargement (prostatism).

▷ **Advisability of Use During Pregnancy**
  Pregnancy Category: B (tentative). See Pregnancy Code inside back cover.
    Animal studies: Reproduction studies of rats and rabbits revealed no increase in birth defects.
    Human studies: Information from adequate studies of pregnant women is not available.
    Avoid this drug during the last 3 months because of the potential risk for serious adverse effects on the newborn infant.

Advisability of Use if Breast-Feeding
  Presence of this drug in breast milk: Unknown.
  Avoid drug or refrain from nursing.

Habit-Forming Potential: None.

Effects of Overdosage: Drowsiness; unsteadiness; faintness; marked dryness of mouth, nose and throat; flushing of face; shortness of breath; hallucinations; convulsions.

Possible Effects of Long-Term Use: Tardive dyskinesia (see Glossary) has been reported in association with the long-term use of several widely used antihistamines. It is advisable to avoid the prolonged, continual use of antihistamines without interruption.

Suggested Periodic Examinations While Taking This Drug (at physician's discretion)
Complete blood cell counts.

▷ **While Taking This Drug, Observe the Following**
Foods: No restrictions.
Beverages: No restrictions. May be taken with milk.
▷   *Alcohol:* Use with extreme caution until the combined effects have been determined. The combination of antihistamine and alcohol can produce rapid and marked sedation.
Tobacco Smoking: No interactions expected.
▷   *Other Drugs*
    Azatadine may ***increase*** the effects of
    • all sedatives, sleep-inducing drugs, tranquilizers, analgesics, and narcotic drugs, and produce oversedation.
    Azatadine may ***decrease*** the effects of
    • oral anticoagulants (Warfarin, etc.), by hastening their elimination from the body. Consult physician regarding prothrombin time testing and dosage adjustment.
    The following drugs may ***increase*** the effects of azatadine
    • monoamine oxidase (MAO) type A inhibitor drugs (see Drug Class, Section Four) may prolong the action of antihistamines.
▷   *Driving, Hazardous Activities:* This drug can impair mental alertness, judgment, coordination and reaction time. Avoid hazardous activities until the full sedative effects have been determined.
Aviation Note: The use of this drug ***may be a disqualification*** for piloting. Consult a designated Aviation Medical Examiner.
Exposure to Sun: Use caution. This drug may cause photosensitivity in some individuals (see Glossary).

AZATHIOPRINE
(ay za THI oh preen)

Introduced: 1965

Class: Antiarthritic, immunosuppressive

Prescription: USA: Yes
Canada: Yes

Controlled Drug: USA: No
Canada: No

Available as Generic: No

Brand Name: Imuran

```
┌─────────────────────────────────────────────────────────────┐
│                    BENEFITS versus RISKS                     │
│                                                              │
│      Possible Benefits            Possible Risks             │
│   REDUCTION OF JOINT PAIN,     UNACCEPTABLE ADVERSE          │
│     TENDERNESS AND               EFFECTS IN 15% OF USERS     │
│     SWELLING in active, severe REDUCED LEVELS OF WHITE       │
│     RHEUMATOID ARTHRITIS         BLOOD CELLS (28% in         │
│     (66% of users)               rheumatoid arthritis, 50% in│
│   PREVENTION OF REJECTION        kidney transplants)         │
│     IN ORGAN                   REDUCED LEVELS OF RED         │
│     TRANSPLANTATION              BLOOD CELLS AND             │
│                                  PLATELETS                   │
│                                LIVER DAMAGE WITH            │
│                                  JAUNDICE (less than 1%)    │
│                                POSSIBLE INCREASED RISK OF   │
│                                  MALIGNANCY (3%)            │
└─────────────────────────────────────────────────────────────┘
```

▷ **Principal Uses**

As a Single Drug Product: Used primarily as an immunosuppressant to prevent rejection in organ transplantation (mainly kidney transplants). Also used to manage active, severe rheumatoid arthritis (in adults) that has failed to respond adequately to conventional treatment. Progression of the arthritic process may be slowed or even stopped. Lesser uses include treatment of lupus erythematosus, ulcerative colitis, chronic active hepatitis and other "autoimmune" disorders.

How This Drug Works: Not fully known. It is thought that by impairing purine metabolism, blocking production of DNA and RNA, and inhibiting cell multiplication, this drug suppresses the immune reaction that is responsible for such "autoimmune" disorders as rheumatoid arthritis, lupus erythematosus, etc.

Available Dosage Forms and Strengths
Injection — 100 mg per 20-ml vial
Tablets — 50 mg

▷ **Usual Adult Dosage Range:** As immunosuppressant—3 to 5 mg/kilogram of body weight daily, 1 to 3 days before transplantation surgery; for postoperative maintenance—1 to 2 mg/kilogram of body weight daily. As antiarthritic—1 mg/kilogram of body weight daily for 6 to 8 weeks; increase dose by 0.5 mg/kilogram of body weight every 4 weeks as needed and tolerated. Maximal daily dose is 2.5 mg/kilogram of body weight. Total dose may be taken once daily or divided into 2 equal doses taken 12 hours apart. **Note: Actual dosage and administration schedule must be determined by the physician for each patient individually.**

▷ **Dosing Instructions:** Take with or following food to reduce stomach irritation. Tablet may be crushed for administration.

Usual Duration of Use: Continual use on a regular schedule for 12 weeks is usually necessary to determine this drug's effectiveness in favorably modifying the course of rheumatoid arthritis. This drug has been used successfully for periods of up to 11 years. Consult your physician on a regular basis.

▷ **This Drug Should Not Be Taken If**
- you have had an allergic reaction to it previously.
- you are pregnant, and this drug is prescribed to treat rheumatoid arthritis.
- you have an active blood cell or bone marrow disorder.
- you are taking, or have recently taken, any form of chlorambucil (Leukeran), cyclophosphamide (Cytoxan) or melphalan (Alkeran).

▷ **Inform Your Physician Before Taking This Drug If**
- you have any kind of active infection.
- you have any form of cancer.
- you have gout or are taking allopurinol (Zyloprim).
- you have a history of blood cell or bone marrow disorders.
- you have impaired liver or kidney function.
- you are taking any form of gold, penicillamine or an antimalarial drug for arthritis.
- you plan pregnancy in the near future.

Possible Side-Effects (natural, expected and unavoidable drug actions)
Development of infection (2.4%).

▷ **Possible Adverse Effects** (unusual, unexpected and infrequent reactions)
If any of the following develop, consult your physician promptly for guidance.
Mild Adverse Effects
Allergic Reaction: Skin rash (2%).
Loss of appetite, nausea, vomiting, diarrhea (19%).
Sores on lips and in mouth.
Serious Adverse Effects
Allergic Reactions: Drug fever (see Glossary), joint and muscle pain.
Pancreatitis—severe stomach pain with nausea and vomiting (0.18%).
Bone marrow depression (see Glossary)—fatigue, weakness, fever, sore throat, abnormal bleeding or bruising.
Liver damage—yellow eyes and skin, dark-colored urine, light-colored stools (0.37%). (See Hepatitis and Jaundice in Glossary.)
Drug-induced pneumonia—cough, shortness of breath.
Development of cancer—skin cancer, reticulum-cell sarcoma, lymphoma, leukemia (3.3%).

▷ **Possible Effects on Sexual Function:** Reversal of male infertility that is due to the body's production of autoantibodies to sperm; this drug suppresses the formation of autoantibodies and permits the normal accumulation of sperm as they are produced.

Possible Delayed Adverse Effects: Bone marrow depression may become apparent many weeks after discontinuing this drug.

▷ **Adverse Effects That May Mimic Natural Diseases or Disorders**
Liver damage may suggest viral hepatitis.

CAUTION
1. Report promptly any indications of a developing infection—fever, chills, lip or mouth sores, etc.
2. Inform your physician promptly if you become pregnant.
3. Periodic blood counts are mandatory for the safe use of this drug. Report for examinations as directed.

Precautions for Use
By Infants and Children: Safety and effectiveness for use by those under 12 years of age have not been established.
By Those over 60 Years of Age: To reduce the risk of possible toxic reactions, the minimal effective dose should be determined and maintained.

▷ **Advisability of Use During Pregnancy**
Pregnancy Category: D (tentative). See Pregnancy Code inside back cover.
Animal studies: Birth defects reported in rodent studies.
Human studies: Two incidents of birth defects reported.
Information from adequate studies of pregnant women is not available.
Avoid completely during entire pregnancy if possible.

Advisability of Use if Breast-Feeding
Presence of this drug in breast milk: Unknown.
Avoid drug or refrain from nursing.

Habit-Forming Potential: None.

Effects of Overdosage: Immediate—nausea, vomiting, diarrhea. Delayed—lowered white blood cell and platelet counts.

Possible Effects of Long-Term Use: Susceptibility to infection, bone marrow depression, development of malignancies.

Suggested Periodic Examinations While Taking This Drug (at physician's discretion)
Complete blood cell counts, liver function tests.

▷ **While Taking This Drug, Observe the Following**
Foods: No restrictions.
Beverages: No restrictions. May be taken with milk.
▷ *Alcohol:* No interactions expected.
Tobacco Smoking: No interactions expected.

▷ *Other Drugs*

Azathioprine may **decrease** the effects of
- oral anticoagulants (warfarin, etc.), and make it necessary to increase their dosage.
- certain muscle relaxants (gallamine, pancuronium, tubocurarine), and make it necessary to increase their dosage.

The following drugs may **increase** the effects of azathioprine
- allopurinol (Zyloprim) may increase its activity and toxicity and make it necessary to reduce its dosage.

▷ *Driving, Hazardous Activities:* No restrictions.

Aviation Note: The use of this drug **may be a disqualification** for piloting. Consult a designated Aviation Medical Examiner.

Exposure to Sun: No restrictions.

Discontinuation: If possible, do not discontinue this drug suddenly. A gradual reduction in dosage is preferable. Consult your physician for a withdrawal schedule.

BACAMPICILLIN
(bak am pi SIL in)

Introduced: 1979

Class: Antibiotic, penicillins

Prescription: USA: Yes
Canada: Yes

Controlled Drug: USA: No
Canada: No

Available as Generic: No

Brand Names: ✦Penglobe, Spectrobid

BENEFITS versus RISKS	
Possible Benefits	*Possible Risks*
EFFECTIVE TREATMENT OF INFECTIONS due to susceptible microorganisms	ALLERGIC REACTIONS, mild to severe, in 3% of the general population and 15% of allergic individuals
	Superinfections (yeast)
	Drug-induced colitis

▷ **Principal Uses**

As a Single Drug Product: To treat certain infections of the skin and skin structures, of the upper and lower respiratory tract, and of the genitourinary tract, including gonorrhea.

How This Drug Works: During its absorption from the gastrointestinal tract, bacampicillin is converted to ampicillin. The unique chemical modification that characterizes bacampicillin permits its more rapid and complete absorption than ampicillin. When given in equivalent doses, bacampicillin provides peak blood levels that are 3 times higher than the levels provided by unmodified ampicillin. Thus bacampicillin can be effective when given every 12 hours; ampicillin requires a dosage schedule of every 6 hours. (See the Drug Profile of ampicillin.)

Available Dosage Forms and Strengths
Oral suspension — 125 mg per 5-ml teaspoonful
Tablets — 400 mg

▷ **Usual Adult Dosage Range:** 400 to 800 mg/12 hours. **Note: Actual dosage and administration schedule must be determined by the physician for each patient individually.**

▷ **Dosing Instructions:** Tablets may be taken without regard to eating. The oral suspension should be taken on an empty stomach, 1 hour before or 2 hours after eating. The tablet may be crushed for administration.

Usual Duration of Use: Continual use on a regular schedule for 5 to 7 days is usually necessary to determine this drug's effectiveness in eradicating the infection. Treatment is usually continued for 2 to 3 days after all indications of infection are gone. Treatment for all streptococcal infections should be for no less than 10 consecutive days (without interruption) to reduce the possibility of developing rheumatic fever or glomerulonephritis.

▷ **While Taking This Drug, Observe the Following**
▷ *Other Drugs*
Bacampicillin *taken concurrently* with
• allopurinol (Zyloprim) substantially increases the incidence of skin rash.
• disulfiram (Antabuse) can cause a disulfiramlike reaction (see Glossary). Avoid the concurrent use of these 2 drugs.
The following drugs may *decrease* the effects of bacampicillin
• chloramphenicol (Chloromycetin).
• erythromycins (E-Mycin, Erythrocin, etc.).
• sulfonamides ("Sulfa" drugs, see Drug Class, Section Four).
• tetracyclines (see Drug Class, Section Four).

Note: The information categories provided in this Profile are appropriate for bacampicillin. For specific information that is normally found in those categories that have been omitted from this Profile, the reader is referred to the Drug Profile of ampicillin.

BECLOMETHASONE
(be kloh METH a sohn)

Introduced: 1976

Class: Antiallergic, antiasthmatic, cortisonelike drugs

Prescription: USA: Yes
Canada: Yes

Controlled Drug: USA: No
Canada: No

Available as Generic: No

Brand Names: Beclovent, ♣Beclovent Rotacaps, ♣Beclovent Rotahaler, Beconase AQ Nasal Spray, Beconase Nasal Inhaler, ♣Propaderm, Vancenase AQ Nasal Spray, Vancenase Nasal Inhaler, Vanceril

BENEFITS versus RISKS	
Possible Benefits	*Possible Risks*
EFFECTIVE RELIEF OF ALLERGIC RHINITIS	FUNGUS INFECTIONS OF THE MOUTH AND THROAT
EFFECTIVE CONTROL OF SEVERE, CHRONIC ASTHMA	Localized areas of "allergic" pneumonia

▷ **Principal Uses**

As a Single Drug Product: Used primarily to treat bronchial asthma in those individuals who do not respond to bronchodilators and who require cortisonelike drugs for asthma control. This inhalation dosage form is significantly more advantageous than cortisone taken by mouth (swallowed) or by injection in that it works locally on the tissues of the respiratory tract and does not require absorption and systemic distribution. This prevents the more serious adverse effects that usually result from the long-term use of cortisone taken for systemic effects.

How This Drug Works: Not established. One possibility is that by increasing the amount of cyclic AMP in appropriate tissues, this drug may thereby increase the concentration of epinephrine, which is an effective bronchodilator and antiasthmatic. Additional benefit may be due to the drug's ability to reduce local inflammation in the lining tissues of the respiratory tract.

Available Dosage Forms and Strengths

Nasal inhaler — 16.8 grams (200 doses of 42 mcg each)
Nasal spray — 0.042%
Oral inhaler — 16.8 grams (200 doses of 42 mcg each)

▷ **Usual Adult Dosage Range:**   Nasal inhaler—1 inhalation (42 mcg) 2 to 4 times daily. Oral inhaler—2 inhalations (84 mcg) 3 or 4 times daily. For severe asthma—12 to 16 inhalations daily. The maximal daily dose should not exceed 20 inhalations. **Note: Actual dosage and administration schedule must be determined by the physician for each patient individually.**

▷ **Dosing Instructions:**   May be used as needed without regard to eating. Rinse the mouth and throat (gargle) with water thoroughly after each inhalation.

Usual Duration of Use: Continual use on a regular schedule for 1 to 4 weeks is usually necessary to determine this drug's effectiveness in

relieving severe, chronic allergic rhinitis and in controlling severe, chronic asthma. Long-term use requires the supervision and guidance of the physician. Consult your physician on a regular basis.

▷ **This Drug Should Not Be Taken If**
- you have had an allergic reaction to any of the drugs bearing the brand names listed above.
- you are experiencing severe acute asthma or status asthmaticus that requires more intense treatment for prompt relief.
- your asthma can be controlled by bronchodilators and other antiasthmatic drugs that are not related to cortisone.
- your asthma requires cortisonelike drugs infrequently for control.
- you have a form of nonallergic bronchitis with asthmatic features.

▷ **Inform Your Physician Before Taking This Drug If**
- you are now taking or have recently taken any cortisone-related drug (including ACTH by injection) for any reason (see Drug Class, Section Four).
- you have a history of tuberculosis of the lungs.
- you have chronic bronchitis or bronchiectasis.
- you think you may have an active infection of any kind, especially a respiratory infection.

Possible Side-Effects (natural, expected and unavoidable drug actions)
Fungus infections (thrush) of the mouth and throat.

▷ **Possible Adverse Effects** (unusual, unexpected and infrequent reactions)
If any of the following develop, consult your physician promptly for guidance.
Mild Adverse Effects
Allergic Reaction: Skin rash (rare).
Dryness of mouth, hoarseness, sore throat.
Serious Adverse Effects
Allergic Reaction: Localized areas of "allergic" pneumonitis (lung inflammation).
Bronchospasm, asthmatic wheezing (rare).

▷ **Possible Effects on Sexual Function:** None reported.

Natural Diseases or Disorders That May Be Activated by This Drug
Cortisone-related drugs that have systemic effects can impair immunity and lead to reactivation of "healed" or quiescent tuberculosis of the lungs. Individuals with a history of tuberculosis must be observed closely during use of this drug by inhalation.

CAUTION
1. This drug does not act primarily as a brochodilator and should not be relied upon for the immediate relief of acute asthma.
2. If you were using any cortisone-related drugs for treatment of your asthma **before** transferring to this inhaler drug, it may be necessary

to resume the former cortisone-related drug if you experience injury or infection of any kind, or if you require surgery. Be sure to notify your attending physician of your prior use of cortisone-related drugs taken either by mouth or by injection.

3. If you experience a return of severe asthma while using this drug, notify your physician immediately so that additional supportive treatment with cortisone-related drugs by mouth or injection can be provided as needed.

4. It is advisable to carry a card of personal identification with a notation (if applicable) that you have used cortisone-related drugs within the past year. During periods of stress it may be necessary to resume cortisone treatment in adequate dosage.

5. An interval of approximately 5 to 10 minutes should separate the inhalation of bronchodilators such as epinephrine, isoetharine, or isoproterenol (which should be used first) and the inhalation of this drug. This sequence will permit greater penetration of beclomethasone into the bronchial tubes. The delay between inhalations will also reduce the possibility of adverse effects from the propellants used in the two inhalers.

Precautions for Use

By Infants and Children: Safety and effectiveness for use of the nasal inhaler by those under 12 years of age have not been established. Safety and effectiveness for use of the oral inhaler by those under 6 years of age have not been established. The maximal daily dose in children 6 to 12 years of age should not exceed 10 inhalations.

By Those over 60 Years of Age: Individuals with bronchiectasis should be observed closely for the development of lung infections.

▷ Advisability of Use During Pregnancy

Pregnancy Category: C (tentative). See Pregnancy Code inside back cover.

Animal studies: Mouse, rat and rabbit studies reveal significant birth defects due to this drug.

Human studies: Information from adequate studies of pregnant women is not available.

Avoid drug during the first 3 months. Use infrequently and only as clearly needed during the last 6 months.

Advisability of Use if Breast-Feeding

Presence of this drug in breast milk: Probably yes.

Avoid drug or refrain from nursing.

Habit-Forming Potential: With recommended dosage, a state of functional dependence (see Glossary) is not likely to develop.

Effects of Overdosage: Indications of cortisone excess (due to systemic absorption)—fluid retention, flushing of the face, stomach irritation, nervousness.

Suggested Periodic Examinations While Taking This Drug (at physician's discretion)

Inspection of nose, mouth and throat for evidence of fungus infection.

Assessment of the status of adrenal function in individuals who have used cortisone-related drugs over an extended period of time prior to using this drug.

X-ray examination of the lungs of individuals with a prior history of tuberculosis.

▷ **While Taking This Drug, Observe the Following**

Foods: No specific restrictions beyond those advised by your physician.

Beverages: No specific restrictions.

▷ *Alcohol:* No interactions expected.

Tobacco Smoking: No interactions expected. However, smoking can affect the condition under treatment and reduce the effectiveness of this drug. Follow your physician's advice.

▷ *Other Drugs*

The following drugs may **increase** the effects of beclomethasone

- inhalant bronchodilators—epinephrine, isoetharine, isoproterenol.
- oral bronchodilators—aminophylline, ephedrine, terbutaline, theophylline, etc.

▷ *Driving, Hazardous Activities:* No restrictions.

Aviation Note: The use of this drug and the disorder for which this drug is prescribed **may be disqualifications** for piloting. Consult a designated Aviation Medical Examiner.

Exposure to Sun: No restrictions.

Occurrence of Unrelated Illness: Acute infections, serious injuries, and surgical procedures can create an urgent need for the administration of additional supportive cortisone-related drugs given by mouth and/or injection. Notify your physician immediately in the event of new illness or injury of any kind.

Discontinuation: If the regular use of this drug has made it possible to reduce or discontinue maintenance doses of cortisonelike drugs by mouth, **do not** discontinue this drug abruptly. If you find it necessary to discontinue this drug for any reason, consult your physician promptly. It may be necessary to resume cortisone preparations and to institute other measures for satisfactory management.

Special Storage Instructions : Store at room temperature. Avoid exposure to temperatures above 120 degrees F (49 degrees C). Do not store or use this inhaler near heat or open flame. Protect from light.

BENZTROPINE
(BENZ troh peen)

Introduced: 1954

Prescription: USA: Yes
Canada: No

Class: Antiparkinsonism, atropine-like drugs

Controlled Drug: USA: No
Canada: No

Available as Generic: USA: No
    Canada: Yes

Brand Names: ✦Apo-Benztropine, ✦Bensylate, Cogentin, ✦PMS Benztropine

BENEFITS versus RISKS	
Possible Benefits	*Possible Risks*
PARTIAL RELIEF OF SYMPTOMS OF PARKINSON'S DISEASE	Atropinelike side-effects: blurred vision, dry mouth, constipation, impaired urination

▷ **Principal Uses**

As a Single Drug Product: Used adjunctively in the management of all types of parkinsonism to relieve the characteristic rigidity, tremor and sluggish movement. Should it fail to provide adequate relief, it may be supplemented with more potent drugs such as levodopa and bromocriptine. This drug is also used to control the parkinsonian reactions that can result from the use of certain antipsychotic drugs, such as the phenothiazines and related compounds.

How This Drug Works: By restoring a more normal balance of the chemical activities responsible for the transmission of nerve impulses within the basal ganglia of the brain, this drug relieves the symptoms of parkinsonism.

Available Dosage Forms and Strengths
    Injection — 1 mg per ml
    Tablets — 0.5 mg, 1 mg, 2 mg

▷ **Usual Adult Dosage Range:**   For Parkinson's disease—0.5 to 2 mg daily, taken in a single dose at bedtime. For drug-induced parkinsonian reactions—1 to 4 mg daily, either in a single dose or in 2 to 3 divided doses. The total daily dose should not exceed 6 mg. **Note: Actual dosage and administration schedule must be determined by the physician for each patient individually.**

▷ **Dosing Instructions:**   May be taken with or following food to reduce stomach irritation. Tablet may be crushed for administration.

Usual Duration of Use: Continual use on a regular schedule for 2 to 4 weeks is usually necessary to determine this drug's effectiveness in relieving the symptoms of parkinsonism and to determine the optimal dosage schedule. Long-term use (months to years) requires physician supervision and guidance. Consult your physician on a regular basis.

▷ **This Drug Should Not Be Taken If**
    • you have had an allergic reaction to any dosage form of it previously.
    • it is prescribed for a child under 3 years of age.

▷ **Inform Your Physician Before Taking This Drug If**
- you have experienced an unfavorable reaction to atropine or atropinelike drugs in the past.
- you have glaucoma or myasthenia gravis.
- you have heart disease or high blood pressure.
- you have a history of liver or kidney disease.
- you have difficulty emptying the urinary bladder, especially if due to an enlarged prostate gland.
- you are taking, or have taken within the past 2 weeks, any monoamine oxidase (MAO) type A inhibitor drug (see Drug Class, Section Four).

Possible Side-Effects (natural, expected and unavoidable drug actions)
Nervousness, blurring of vision, dryness of mouth, constipation, impaired urination. (These often subside as drug use continues.)

▷ **Possible Adverse Effects** (unusual, unexpected and infrequent reactions)
If any of the following develop, consult your physician promptly for guidance.
Mild Adverse Effects
Allergic Reaction: Skin rashes.
Headache, dizziness, drowsiness, muscle cramps.
Indigestion, nausea, vomiting.
Serious Adverse Effects
Idiosyncratic Reactions: Abnormal behavior, confusion, delusions, hallucinations, agitation.

▷ **Possible Effects on Sexual Function**
Reversal of male impotence due to the use of fluphenazine (a phenothiazine antipsychotic drug).
Male infertility (0.5 to 6 mg/day).

Natural Diseases or Disorders That May Be Activated by This Drug
Latent glaucoma, latent myasthenia gravis.

CAUTION
1. Many over-the-counter (OTC) medications for allergies, colds and coughs contain drugs that can interact unfavorably with this drug. Ask your physician or pharmacist for guidance before using such preparations.
2. This drug may aggravate tardive dyskinesia (see Glossary). Ask physician for guidance.

Precautions for Use
By Infants and Children: Safety and effectiveness for use by those under 3 years of age have not been established. Children are especially susceptible to the atropinelike effects of this drug.
By Those over 60 Years of Age: Small doses are advisable until your response has been determined. You may be more susceptible to the development of impaired thinking, confusion, nightmares, hallucina-

tions, increased internal eye pressure (glaucoma) and impaired urination associated with prostate gland enlargement (prostatism).

▷ **Advisability of Use During Pregnancy**
Pregnancy Category: C (tentative). See Pregnancy Code inside back cover.
Animal studies: No data available.
Human studies: Information from adequate studies of pregnant women is not available.
Avoid use if possible, especially close to delivery. This drug can impair the proper functioning of the infant's intestinal tract following birth.

Advisability of Use if Breast-Feeding
Presence of this drug in breast milk: Unknown.
Avoid drug or refrain from nursing.

Habit-Forming Potential: None with recommended doses. At higher doses it may cause euphoria and hallucinations, creating a potential for abuse.

Effects of Overdosage: Weakness; drowsiness; stupor; impaired vision; rapid pulse; excitement; confusion; hallucinations; dry, hot skin; skin rash; dilated pupils.

Possible Effects of Long-Term Use: Increased internal eye pressure—possible glaucoma, especially in the elderly.

Suggested Periodic Examinations While Taking This Drug (at physician's discretion)
Measurement of internal eye pressure at regular intervals.

▷ **While Taking This Drug, Observe the Following**
Foods: No restrictions.
Beverages: No restrictions.
▷   *Alcohol:* Use caution until the combined effects have been determined. Alcohol may increase the sedative effects of this drug.
Tobacco Smoking: No interactions expected.
▷   *Other Drugs*
Benztropine may ***decrease*** the effects of
• haloperidol (Haldol), and reduce its effectiveness.
• phenothiazines (Thorazine, etc.), and reduce their effectiveness.
The following drugs may ***increase*** the effects of benztropine
• antihistamines may add to the dryness of mouth and throat.
• tricyclic antidepressants (Elavil, etc.) may add to the effects on the eye and further increase internal eye pressure (dangerous in glaucoma).
• monoamine oxidase (MAO) type A inhibitor drugs may intensify all effects of this drug (see Drug Class, Section Four).
▷   *Driving, Hazardous Activities:* Drowsiness and dizziness may occur in sensitive individuals. Avoid hazardous activities until full effects and tolerance have been determined.

Aviation Note: The use of this drug ***is a disqualification*** for piloting. Consult a designated Aviation Medical Examiner.

Exposure to Sun: No restrictions.

Exposure to Heat: Use caution. This drug may reduce sweating, cause an increase in body temperature, and contribute to the development of heat stroke.

Heavy Exercise or Exertion: Use caution. Avoid in hot environments.

Discontinuation: Do not discontinue this drug abruptly. Ask physician for guidance in reducing the dose gradually.

BITOLTEROL
(bi TOHL ter ohl)

Introduced: 1985

Class: Antiasthmatic, bronchodilator

Prescription: Yes

Controlled Drug: No

Available as Generic: No

Brand Name: Tornalate

BENEFITS versus RISKS	
Possible Benefits	*Possible Risks*
EFFECTIVE PREVENTION AND RELIEF OF ASTHMA for 5 to 8 hours	Fine hand tremor (14%)
	Nervousness (5%)
	Throat irritation (5%)
	Irregular heart rhythm (with excessive use)

▷ **Principal Uses**

As a Single Drug Product: To relieve acute bronchial asthma and to reduce the frequency and severity of chronic, recurrent asthmatic attacks.

How This Drug Works: It is thought that by increasing the production of cyclic AMP, this drug relaxes constricted bronchial muscles to relieve asthmatic wheezing.

Available Dosage Forms and Strengths

Aerosol inhaler — 15 ml (300 inhalations of 0.37 mg each)

▷ **Usual Adult Dosage Range:** For acute bronchospasm—2 inhalations at intervals of 1 to 3 minutes, followed by a third inhalation in 3 to 4 minutes if needed. For prevention of bronchospasm—2 inhalations/8 hours. **Note: Actual dosage and administration schedule must be determined by the physician for each patient individually.**

▷ **Dosing Instructions:** May be used without regard to eating. Follow the written directions for use carefully. Do not overuse.

Usual Duration of Use: According to individual requirements. Do not use beyond the time necessary to terminate episodes of acute asthma. Ask physician for guidance regarding duration of use for prevention of asthma attacks.

▷ **This Drug Should Not Be Taken If**
- you have had an allergic reaction to it previously.
- you currently have an irregular heart rhythm.
- you are taking, or have taken within the past 2 weeks, any mono-amine oxidase (MAO) type A inhibitor drug (see Drug Class, Section Four).

▷ **Inform Your Physician Before Taking This Drug If**
- you have any type of heart or circulatory disorder, especially high blood pressure or coronary heart disease.
- you have diabetes, epilepsy or an overactive thyroid gland.
- you are taking any form of digitalis or any stimulant drug.

Possible Side-Effects (natural, expected and unavoidable drug actions)
Dryness or irritation of mouth or throat (5%).

▷ **Possible Adverse Effects** (unusual, unexpected and infrequent reactions)
If any of the following develop, consult your physician promptly for guidance.
Mild Adverse Effects
Headache (4%), dizziness (3%), nervousness (5%), insomnia (less than 1%), fine tremor of hands (14%).
Nausea (3%), indigestion.
Serious Adverse Effects
Rapid or irregular heart rhythm or increased blood pressure can occur with excessive use.

▷ **Possible Effects on Sexual Function:** None reported.

Natural Diseases or Disorders That May Be Activated by This Drug
Latent coronary artery disease, diabetes or high blood pressure.

CAUTION
1. Concurrent use of this drug by inhalation with beclomethasone aerosol (Beclovent, Vanceril) may increase the risk of toxicity due to fluorocarbon propellants. It is advisable to use bitolterol aerosol 20 to 30 minutes *before* beclomethasone aerosol. This will reduce the risk of toxicity and will enhance the penetration of beclomethasone.
2. The excessive or prolonged use of this drug by inhalation can reduce its effectiveness and cause serious heart rhythm disturbances.

Precautions for Use
By Infants and Children: Safety and effectiveness for use by children under 12 years of age have not been established.

By Those over 60 Years of Age: Avoid excessive and continual use. If acute asthma is not relieved promptly, other drugs will have to be tried. Observe for the development of nervousness, palpitations, irregular heart rhythm and muscle tremors.

▷ **Advisability of Use During Pregnancy**
Pregnancy Category: C (tentative). See Pregnancy Code inside back cover.
Animal studies: Cleft palate reported in mice.
Human studies: Information from adequate studies of pregnant women is not available.
Avoid use during first 3 months if possible.

Advisability of Use if Breast-Feeding
Presence of this drug in breast milk: Unknown.
Avoid drug or refrain from nursing.

Habit-Forming Potential: None.

Effects of Overdosage: Nervousness, palpitation, rapid heart rate, sweating, headache, tremor, vomiting, chest pain.

Possible Effects of Long-Term Use: Loss of effectiveness.

Suggested Periodic Examinations While Taking This Drug (at physician's discretion)
Blood pressure measurements, evaluation of heart status.

▷ **While Taking This Drug, Observe the Following**
Foods: No restrictions.
Beverages: Avoid excessive use of caffeine-containing beverages—coffee, tea, cola, chocolate.
▷   *Alcohol:* No interactions expected.
Tobacco Smoking: No interactions expected.
▷   *Other Drugs*
Bitolterol *taken concurrently* with
• monoamine oxidase (MAO) type A inhibitor drugs (see Drug Class, Section Four) may cause excessive increase in blood pressure and undesirable heart stimulation.
▷   *Driving, Hazardous Activities:* Use caution if excessive nervousness or dizziness occurs.
Aviation Note: The use of this drug *is a disqualification* for piloting. Consult a designated Aviation Medical Examiner.
Exposure to Sun: No restrictions.
Heavy Exercise or Exertion: Use caution. Excessive exercise can induce asthma in sensitive individuals.

BROMOCRIPTINE
(broh moh KRIP teen)

Introduced: 1975

Class: Antiparkinsonism, dopamine agonist, ergot derivative

Prescription: USA: Yes
Canada: Yes

Controlled Drug: USA: No
Canada: No

Available as Generic: No

Brand Name: Parlodel

BENEFITS versus RISKS

Possible Benefits	*Possible Risks*
PARTIAL RELIEF OF SYMPTOMS OF PARKINSON'S DISEASE	ABNORMAL INVOLUNTARY MOVEMENTS AND ALTERED BEHAVIOR in 20% to 35% of users taking high doses
PREVENTION OF LACTATION following childbirth	Raynaud's phenomenon (see Glossary) in 30% to 60% of users taking high doses
CORRECTION OF INFERTILITY AND ABSENT MENSTRUATION in women with high prolactin levels	

▷ **Principal Uses**

As a Single Drug Product: This drug is used primarily to

1. Treat the manifestations of Parkinson's disease. It may be used as the initial drug in treating those with early-stage symptoms. More often it is used in conjunction with levodopa when it is found that levodopa is losing its effectiveness, or the patient cannot tolerate the adverse effects of levodopa and dosage adjustment or withdrawal is necessary.

2. Suppress the production of milk and thereby prevent the breast congestion and engorgement that normally follow childbirth.

3. Treat those disorders that are due to excessive production of prolactin by the pituitary gland: absence of menstruation, infertility, and inappropriate production of milk.

How This Drug Works: By directly stimulating the dopamine receptor sites in the corpus striatum of the brain, this drug helps to offset the deficiency of dopamine that is responsible for the rigidity, tremor, and sluggish movement characteristic of Parkinson's disease. By inhibiting the production of the hormone prolactin by the anterior pituitary gland, this drug

• reduces the amount of prolactin in the blood to below the level required to stimulate the breast glands to produce milk.

- reduces abnormally high levels of prolactin in the blood, restoring it to normal levels that permit menstrual regularity and fertility.

Available Dosage Forms and Strengths
Capsules — 5 mg
Tablets — 2.5 mg

▷ **Usual Adult Dosage Range:**   For Parkinson's disease—initially 1.25 to 2.5 mg once daily; for maintenance, 2.5 to 100 mg daily in divided doses. Increase dose by no more than 2.5 to 5 mg on alternate days. The usual dosage range is 10 to 40 mg daily. Do not exceed 300 mg daily. For suppression of lactation—2.5 mg 2 times a day for 14 days; may extend to 21 days if needed. For absent menstruation and infertility— initially 1.25 to 2.5 mg daily; for maintenance, 2.5 mg 2 or 3 times a day. **Note: Actual dosage and administration schedule must be determined by the physician for each patient individually.**

▷ **Dosing Instructions:**   Take with food or milk to reduce stomach irritation. Capsule may be opened and tablet may be crushed for administration.

Usual Duration of Use: Continual use on a regular schedule for 3 to 4 months is usually necessary to determine this drug's effectiveness in controlling the symptoms of Parkinson's disease. Treatment for 4 to 12 weeks restores fertility and normal menstruation in most women; however, treatment may be necessary for 6 to 12 months. Long-term use (up to 3 years or more) must be under physician supervision and guidance. Consult your physician on a regular basis.

▷ **This Drug Should Not Be Taken If**
- you have had an allergic reaction to it previously.
- you have had a serious adverse effect from any ergot preparation in the past.
- you have severe coronary artery disease or peripheral vascular disease.
- you are pregnant.

▷ **Inform Your Physician Before Taking This Drug If**
- you have constitutionally low blood pressure.
- you are taking any antihypertensive drugs or phenothiazines (see Drug Classes, Section Four).
- you have any degree of coronary artery disease, especially with a history of a "heart attack" (myocardial infarction).
- you have a history of heart rhythm abnormalities.
- you have impaired liver function.
- you have a seizure disorder (epilepsy).

Possible Side-Effects (natural, expected and unavoidable drug actions)
Fatigue, lethargy, light-headedness in upright position (see Orthostatic Hypotension in Glossary).

▷ **Possible Adverse Effects** (unusual, unexpected and infrequent reactions)
If any of the following develop, consult your physician promptly for guidance.

Mild Adverse Effects

Allergic Reaction: Skin rash.

Headache, drowsiness, dizziness, fainting, nervousness, nightmares.

Nasal congestion, dry mouth, loss of appetite, nausea, vomiting, stomach cramps, constipation, diarrhea.

Serious Adverse Effects

Abnormal involuntary movements, confusion, hallucinations, incoordination, visual disturbances, depression, seizures.

Swelling of feet and ankles (edema).

Loss of urinary bladder control, inability to empty bladder.

Indications of "ergotism": numbness and tingling of fingers, cold hands and feet, muscle cramps of legs and feet.

Vomiting blood, bloody or black stools (gastrointestinal bleeding).

▷ **Possible Effects on Sexual Function:**   Rare occurrence of impotence. However, this drug can correct impotence and reduced libido when these conditions are due to increased blood levels of prolactin (a pituitary hormone).

▷ **Adverse Effects That May Mimic Natural Diseases or Disorders**

Effects on mental function and behavior may resemble psychotic disorders.

Natural Diseases or Disorders That May Be Activated by This Drug

Coronary artery disease with anginal syndrome, Raynaud's syndrome.

CAUTION

1. During treatment of parkinsonism, avoid excessive and hurried activity as improvement occurs; this will reduce the risk of falls and injury.
2. The neurological and psychiatric disturbances due to this drug may last for 2 to 6 weeks after stopping it.
3. During treatment to reduce the blood level of prolactin and restore normal menstruation and fertility, it is mandatory that you use a barrier method of contraception to prevent pregnancy. Oral contraceptives should not be used while taking bromocriptine.
4. If pregnancy occurs, notify your physician immediately.

Precautions for Use

By Infants and Children: Safety and effectiveness for use by those under 15 years of age have not been established.

By Those over 60 Years of Age: Your initial test dose should be 1.25 mg. Observe closely for any tendency to light-headedness or faintness on attempting to stand after this first dose. You may be more susceptible to the development of impaired thinking, confusion, agitation, nightmares, hallucinations, nausea or vomiting. Close monitoring and careful dosage adjustments are mandatory.

▷ **Advisability of Use During Pregnancy**

Pregnancy Category: X (tentative). See Pregnancy Code inside back cover.
Animal studies: Rabbit studies reveal an increase in cleft lip.

Human studies: Serious birth defects have been reported in infants
whose mothers took this drug during early pregnancy. Because the
incidence of these defects (3.3%) does not exceed that reported for the
general population, a cause-and-effect relationship is uncertain. Information from adequate studies of pregnant women is not available.

Pending further studies, it is recommended that this drug not be taken
during the entire pregnancy.

Advisability of Use if Breast-Feeding

This drug prevents the production of milk and makes nursing impossible.

Habit-Forming Potential: None.

Effects of Overdosage: Weakness, low blood pressure, nausea, vomiting,
diarrhea, confusion, agitation, hallucinations, loss of consciousness.

Possible Effects of Long-Term Use: Drug-induced changes in the lung tissue, thickening of the pleura and pleural effusion (fluid formation
within the chest cage). These effects appear to be reversible after discontinuation of the drug. Fibrosis (scar tissue formation) in the back
wall of the abdominal cavity and contractures of the extremities have
also been reported.

Suggested Periodic Examinations While Taking This Drug (at physician's
discretion)

Blood pressure measurements; CAT scan of the pituitary gland for enlargement due to tumor; pregnancy test; blood tests for anemia; evaluation of heart, lung and liver functions.

▷ **While Taking This Drug, Observe the Following**

Foods: No restrictions.

Beverages: No restrictions. May be taken with milk.

▷ *Alcohol:* Use caution until the combined effects have been determined.
Alcohol can exaggerate the blood-pressure-lowering effects and sedative effects of this drug.

▷ *Other Drugs*

Bromocriptine *taken concurrently* with

• antihypertensive drugs (and other drugs that can lower blood pressure) requires careful monitoring for excessive drops in pressure. Dosage adjustments may be necessary.

The following drugs may *decrease* the effects of bromocriptine

• phenothiazines (see Drug Class, Section Four). Theoretically, bromocriptine and phenothiazines have opposite effects on the utilization
of dopamine in the brain. It is probably best to avoid the concurrent
use of these drugs until the results of further studies are available.

▷ *Driving, Hazardous Activities:* Be alert to the possible occurrence of orthostatic hypotension, dizziness, drowsiness or impaired coordination.

Aviation Note: Parkinsonism *is a disqualification* for piloting. The use of this drug otherwise *may be a disqualification* for piloting. Consult a designated Aviation Medical Examiner.

Exposure to Sun: No restrictions.

BROMPHENIRAMINE
(brohm fen IR a meen)

Introduced: 1957

Class: Antihistamines

Prescription: USA: Varies
Canada: No

Controlled Drug: USA: No
Canada: No

Available as Generic: USA: Yes
Canada: No

Brand Names: ✦Dimedrine [CD], Dimetane, Dimetane Cough Syrup-DC [CD], Dimetane-DC [CD], Dimetane Decongestant Elixir [CD], Dimetane Decongestant Tablets [CD], Dimetane-DX [CD], ✦Dimetane Expectorant [CD], ✦Dimetane Expectorant-C [CD], ✦Dimetane Expectorant-DC [CD], Dimetane Extentabs, Dimetane-Ten, Dimetapp Preparations [CD], ✦Dimetapp-A Preparations [CD], ✦Dimetapp-C [CD], ✦Dimetapp w/Codeine [CD], ✦Dimetapp-DM [CD], ✦Dimetapp Infant Drops [CD], Disophrol [CD], Drixoral Plus [CD], Drixoral Syrup [CD], Drixoral Tablets [CD], ✦Drixtab, Veltane

---

BENEFITS versus RISKS

Possible Benefits	*Possible Risks*
EFFECTIVE RELIEF OF ALLERGIC RHINITIS AND ALLERGIC SKIN DISORDERS	Mild sedation (23%) Atropinelike effects Rare blood cell disorders: abnormally low white blood cell and platelet counts

---

▷ **Principal Uses**

As a Single Drug Product: Used primarily to provide symptomatic relief in allergic and related disorders: seasonal and perennial allergic rhinitis (hay fever), allergic conjunctivitis and vasomotor rhinitis; also in hives and localized swellings (angioedema) of allergic origin.

As a Combination Drug Product [CD]: This drug is combined with a decongestant drug to enhance its ability to reduce tissue swelling and secretions in allergic and infectious disorders of the upper respiratory tract—hay fever, head colds and sinusitis. It is also combined with decongestants, expectorants and codeine to increase their effectiveness in the symptomatic treatment of allergic and infectious disorders of the lower respiratory tract, often with associated coughing.

How This Drug Works: Antihistamines reduce the intensity of the allergic response by blocking the action of histamine after it has been released from sensitized tissue cells in the eyes, nose, respiratory passages and skin.

Available Dosage Forms and Strengths

> Elixir — 2 mg per 5-ml teaspoonful
> Injection — 10 mg per ml, 100 mg per ml
> Tablets — 4 mg
> Tablets, prolonged-action — 8 mg, 12 mg

▷ **Usual Adult Dosage Range:**   4 mg/4 to 6 hours, or 8 to 12 mg (prolonged-action form)/12 hours. Total daily dosage should not exceed 24 mg. **Note: Actual dosage and administration schedule must be determined by the physician for each patient individually.**

▷ **Dosing Instructions:**   Take with food or milk to prevent stomach irritation. The prolonged-action forms should be swallowed whole (not crushed or chewed).

Usual Duration of Use: Continual use on a regular schedule for 2 to 3 days is usually necessary to determine this drug's effectiveness in relieving the symptoms of allergic rhinitis and dermatosis. It may be necessary to take this drug throughout the entire pollen season, depending upon individual sensitivity. However, antihistamines should not be taken continually (without interruption) for long-term use. Limit their use to periods that require symptomatic relief.

▷ **This Drug Should Not Be Taken If**
- you have had an allergic reaction to any dosage form of it previously.
- you are currently undergoing allergy skin tests.
- you are taking, or have taken within the past 14 days, any monoamine oxidase (MAO) type A inhibitor drug (see Drug Class, Section Four).

▷ **Inform Your Physician Before Taking This Drug If**
- you have had any allergic reactions or unfavorable responses to the previous use of antihistamines.
- you have glaucoma (narrow-angle type) or asthma.
- you have epilepsy or a seizure disorder.
- you have difficulty emptying the urinary bladder, especially if due to prostate gland enlargement.
- you plan to have surgery under general anesthesia in the near future.

Possible Side-Effects (natural, expected and unavoidable drug actions)
Drowsiness; sense of weakness; blurred vision; dryness of the nose, mouth and throat; impaired urination.

▷ **Possible Adverse Effects** (unusual, unexpected and infrequent reactions)
If any of the following develop, consult your physician promptly for guidance.
Mild Adverse Effects
Allergic Reaction: Skin rash.
Headache, nervous agitation, dizziness, confusion, tremor, blurred or double vision, ringing in ears.
Reduced tolerance for contact lenses.
Thickening of bronchial secretions in asthma or bronchitis.
Indigestion, nausea, vomiting, diarrhea.
Serious Adverse Effects
Hemolytic anemia (see Glossary).
Abnormally low white blood cell count—fever, sore throat, infections.
Abnormally low blood platelet count—abnormal bleeding or bruising.

▷ **Possible Effects on Sexual Function**
No adverse effects reported.
This drug has been used successfully to correct retrograde (backward) ejaculation, a condition that occurs occasionally in some men with diabetes.

Natural Diseases or Disorders That May Be Activated by This Drug
Latent epilepsy, glaucoma, prostatism (see Glossary).

CAUTION
1. Discontinue this drug 4 days before diagnostic skin testing procedures in order to prevent false negative test results.
2. Do not use this drug if you have active bronchial asthma, bronchitis or pneumonia. It can thicken bronchial mucus and make it more difficult to remove (by absorption or coughing).

Precautions for Use
By Infants and Children: This drug should not be used in premature or full-term newborn infants. Doses for children should be small. The young child is especially sensitive to the effects of antihistamines on the brain and nervous system.
By Those over 60 Years of Age: You may be more susceptible to the development of drowsiness, dizziness, and unsteadiness, and to impairment of thinking, judgment and memory. This drug can increase the degree of impaired urination associated with prostate gland enlargement (prostatism). The sedative effects of antihistamines in the elderly can cause a syndrome of underactivity that may be misinterpreted as senility or emotional depression.

▷ **Advisability of Use During Pregnancy**
Pregnancy Category: B (tentative). See Pregnancy Code inside back cover.
Animal studies: No information available.

Human studies: Information from adequate studies of pregnant women is not available. Birth defects have been reported in 10 infants whose mothers used this drug during the first 3 months of pregnancy.

Avoid this drug during the first 3 months, and the last 3 months because of the potential risk for serious adverse effects on the newborn infant.

Advisability of Use if Breast-Feeding

Presence of this drug in breast milk: Yes, in small amounts.

Avoid drug or refrain from nursing.

Habit-Forming Potential: None.

Effects of Overdosage: Drowsiness; unsteadiness; faintness; marked dryness of mouth, nose and throat; flushing of face; shortness of breath; hallucinations; convulsions; stupor progressing to coma.

Possible Effects of Long-Term Use: Tardive dyskinesia (see Glossary) has been reported in association with the long-term use of several widely used antihistamines. It is advisable to avoid the prolonged, continual use of antihistamines without interruption.

Suggested Periodic Examinations While Taking This Drug (at physician's discretion)

Complete blood cell counts.

▷ **While Taking This Drug, Observe the Following**

Foods: No restrictions.

Beverages: No restrictions. May be taken with milk.

▷ *Alcohol:* Use with extreme caution until the combined effects have been determined. The combination of antihistamine and alcohol can produce rapid and marked sedation.

Tobacco Smoking: No interactions expected.

▷ *Other Drugs*

Brompheniramine may *increase* the effects of

- all sedatives, sleep-inducing drugs, tranquilizers, analgesics and narcotic drugs, and produce oversedation.

The following drugs may *increase* the effects of brompheniramine

- monoamine oxidase (MAO) type A inhibitor drugs (see Drug Class, Section Four) may prolong the action of antihistamines.

▷ *Driving, Hazardous Activities:* This drug can impair mental alertness, judgment, coordination and reaction time. Avoid hazardous activities until the full sedative effects have been determined.

Aviation Note: The use of this drug *is a disqualification* for piloting. Consult a designated Aviation Medical Examiner.

Exposure to Sun: Use caution. Some drugs of this class can cause photosensitivity (see Glossary).

BUMETANIDE
(byu MET a nide)

Introduced: 1983

Prescription: USA: Yes

Available as Generic: No

Brand Name: Bumex

Class: Diuretic

Controlled Drug: USA: No

BENEFITS versus RISKS

Possible Benefits	*Possible Risks*
POTENT, EFFECTIVE DIURETIC BY MOUTH OR INJECTION	ABNORMALLY LOW BLOOD POTASSIUM with excessive use Impaired sexual function

---

▷ **Principal Uses**

As a Single Drug Product: To relieve edema (fluid retention) associated with congestive heart failure, liver disease or kidney disease.

How This Drug Works: By increasing the elimination of salt and water from the body (through increased urine production), this drug reduces the volume of fluid in the blood and body tissues and lowers the sodium content throughout the body.

Available Dosage Forms and Strengths

Injection — 0.25 mg per ml (2-ml ampules)

Tablets — 0.5 mg, 1 mg, 2 mg

▷ **Usual Adult Dosage Range:** 0.5 to 2 mg daily, usually taken in the morning as a single dose. If needed, an additional second or third dose may be taken later in the day at 4- to 5-hour intervals. The total daily dose should not exceed 10 mg. Alternate-day dosage (taken every other day) may be adequate for some individuals. **Note: Actual dosage and administration schedule must be determined by the physician for each patient individually.**

▷ **Dosing Instructions:** May be taken with or following food to reduce stomach irritation. Tablet may be crushed for administration.

Usual Duration of Use: Continual use on a regular schedule for 2 to 3 days is usually necessary to determine this drug's effectiveness in relieving edema. After maximal benefit has been achieved, intermittent use will reduce the risk of sodium, potassium and water imbalance. Long-term use requires the supervision and guidance of the physician. Consult your physician on a regular basis.

▷ **This Drug Should Not Be Taken If**

- you have had an allergic reaction to either dosage form previously.
- your kidneys are unable to produce urine.

▷ **Inform Your Physician Before Taking This Drug If**
- you are allergic to any form of "sulfa" drug.
- you are pregnant or planning pregnancy.
- you have impaired liver or kidney function.
- you have diabetes or a tendency to diabetes.
- you have a history of gout.
- you have impaired hearing.
- you are taking any form of cortisone, digitalis, oral antidiabetic drugs, insulin, probenecid (Benemid), indomethacin (Indocin), lithium or drugs for high blood pressure.
- you plan to have surgery under general anesthesia in the near future.

Possible Side-Effects (natural, expected and unavoidable drug actions)
Light-headedness on arising from sitting or lying position (see Orthostatic Hypotension in Glossary).
Increase in level of blood sugar, affecting control of diabetes.
Increase in level of blood uric acid, affecting control of gout.
Decrease in levels of blood potassium and sodium, resulting in muscle weakness and cramping.

▷ **Possible Adverse Effects** (unusual, unexpected and infrequent reactions)
If any of the following develop, consult your physician promptly for guidance.
Mild Adverse Effects
Allergic Reactions: Skin rashes, hives, itching.
Headache, dizziness, vertigo, fatigue, weakness, sweating, earache.
Nausea, vomiting, stomach pain, diarrhea.
Breast nipple tenderness, joint and muscle pains.
Serious Adverse Effects
Impaired hearing, precipitation of liver coma (in preexisting liver disease).

▷ **Possible Effects on Sexual Function:**   Difficulty maintaining an erection; premature ejaculation (0.5 to 2 mg/day).

Natural Diseases or Disorders That May Be Activated by This Drug
Latent diabetes, gout.

CAUTION
1. Do not exceed recommended doses. Increased dosage can cause excessive excretion of water, sodium and potassium, with resultant loss of appetite, nausea, weakness, confusion and profound drop in blood pressure (circulatory collapse).
2. If you are also taking a digitalis preparation (digitoxin, digoxin), ensure an adequate intake of high-potassium foods to prevent potassium deficiency—a potential cause of digitalis toxicity.
3. If you are being treated for cirrhosis of the liver, do not increase your dose without consulting your physician. Excessive dosage can alter blood chemistry significantly and induce liver coma.

Precautions for Use

By Infants and Children: Safety and effectiveness for use by those under 18 years of age have not been established.

By Those over 60 Years of Age: Small doses are advisable until your individual response has been determined. You may be more susceptible to the development of impaired thinking, orthostatic hypotension, potassium loss and elevation of blood sugar. Overdosage and prolonged use of this drug can cause excessive loss of body water, thickening of the blood, and an increased tendency of the blood to clot, predisposing to stroke, heart attack or thrombophlebitis.

▷ **Advisability of Use During Pregnancy**

Pregnancy Category: C (tentative). See Pregnancy Code inside back cover.

Animal studies: High-dose studies of rats and rabbits reveal defects in bone development.

Human studies: Information from adequate studies of pregnant women is not available.

This drug should not be used during pregnancy unless a very serious complication of pregnancy occurs for which this drug is significantly beneficial.

Advisability of Use if Breast-Feeding

Presence of this drug in breast milk: Unknown.

Avoid drug or refrain from nursing.

Habit-Forming Potential: None.

Effects of Overdosage: Weakness, lethargy, dizziness, confusion, nausea, vomiting, muscle cramps, thirst, drowsiness progressing to deep sleep or coma, weak and rapid pulse.

Possible Effects of Long-Term Use: Impaired balance of water, salt, and potassium in blood and body tissues. Dehydration with resultant increase in blood viscosity and potential for abnormal clotting. Development of diabetes in predisposed individuals.

Suggested Periodic Examinations While Taking This Drug (at physician's discretion)

Complete blood cell counts; measurements of blood levels of sodium, potassium, chloride, sugar, uric acid; liver and kidney function tests.

▷ **While Taking This Drug, Observe the Following**

Foods: Consult your physician regarding the advisability of eating a high-potassium diet. See Section Six for the Table of High Potassium Foods. Follow your physician's instructions regarding the use of salt.

Beverages: No restrictions unless directed by your physician. May be taken with milk.

▷   *Alcohol:* Use with caution until the combined effect has been determined. Alcohol can exaggerate the blood-pressure-lowering effect of this drug and cause orthostatic hypotension (see Glossary).

Tobacco Smoking: No interactions expected. Follow your physician's advice regarding smoking.

▷ *Other Drugs*

Bumetanide may *increase* the effects of

- antihypertensive drugs. Careful adjustment of dosages is necessary to prevent excessive lowering of the blood pressure.

Bumetanide *taken concurrently* with

- aminoglycoside antibiotics (amikacin, gentamicin, kanamycin, neomycin, streptomycin, tobramycin, viomycin) may increase the risk of hearing loss.
- cortisone-related drugs may cause excessive loss of potassium from the body.
- digitalis-related drugs requires very careful monitoring and dosage adjustments to prevent serious disturbances of heart rhythm.
- lithium may increase the risk of lithium toxicity.

The following drugs may *decrease* the effects of bumetanide

- indomethacin (Indocin) may reduce its diuretic effect.

▷ *Driving, Hazardous Activities:* Use caution until the possible occurrence of dizziness, weakness or orthostatic hypotension (see Glossary) has been determined.

Aviation Note: The use of this drug *may be a disqualification* for piloting. Consult a designated Aviation Medical Examiner.

Exposure to Sun: No restrictions.

Occurrence of Unrelated Illness: Illnesses that cause vomiting or diarrhea can produce a serious imbalance of important body chemistry. Report such illnesses promptly.

Discontinuation: It may be advisable to discontinue this drug 5 to 7 days before major surgery. Consult your physician, surgeon, or anesthesiologist for guidance regarding dosage reduction or withdrawal.

BUSPIRONE

(byu SPI rohn)

Introduced: 1979   **Class:** Mild tranquilizer

Prescription: USA: Yes   **Controlled Drug:** USA: No

Available as Generic: No

Brand Name: Buspar

BENEFITS versus RISKS	
Possible Benefits	*Possible Risks*
EFFECTIVE RELIEF OF MILD TO MODERATE ANXIETY without significant sedation or risk of dependence	Mild dizziness, faintness or headache (uncommon) Rare restlessness, tremor and rigidity (with high doses)

▷ **Principal Uses**

As a Single Drug Product: Used to relieve anxiety and nervous tension states of mild to moderate severity. Because of its lack of significant sedative effects and of abuse potential, it is particularly useful in the elderly, the alcoholic and the addiction-prone individual.

How This Drug Works: Not completely established. This drug is thought to be a "mid-brain modulator" with effects on dopamine, norepinephrine and serotonin transmission activities. Its exact method of action is not understood.

Available Dosage Forms and Strengths

Tablets — 5 mg, 10 mg

▷ **Usual Adult Dosage Range:**   20 to 30 mg/day, in divided doses. Initially, 5 mg 3 times/day; if needed, increase dose by 5 to 10 mg/day every 3 to 4 days, with individual doses every 6 to 8 hours. The total daily dose should not exceed 60 mg. **Note: Actual dosage and administration schedule must be determined by the physician for each patient individually.**

▷ **Dosing Instructions:**   May be taken without regard to food. The tablet may be crushed for administration.

Usual Duration of Use: Continual use on a regular schedule for 7 to 10 days is usually necessary to determine this drug's effectiveness in relieving anxiety and nervous tension. Use intermittently and only as necessary; avoid prolonged and uninterrupted use.

Possible Advantages of This Drug

Relieves anxiety and nervous tension without causing significant sedation.

Does not cause withdrawal symptoms upon discontinuation.

▷ **This Drug Should Not Be Taken If**
- you have had an allergic reaction to it previously.

▷ **Inform Your Physician Before Taking This Drug If**
- you are taking other drugs that affect the function of the brain and nervous system: tranquilizers, sedatives, hypnotics, analgesics, narcotics, antidepressants, antipsychotic drugs, anticonvulsants or drugs for parkinsonism.
- you have impaired liver or kidney function.

Possible Side-Effects (natural, expected and unavoidable drug actions)

Infrequent and mild drowsiness (less than with benzodiazepines), lethargy, fatigue.

▷ **Possible Adverse Effects** (unusual, unexpected and infrequent reactions)

If any of the following develop, consult your physician promptly for guidance.

Mild Adverse Effects
Headache, dizziness, faintness, excitement, nausea.
Serious Adverse Effects
Depression (3%).
With high doses: restlessness, rigidity, tremors.

▷ **Possible Effects on Sexual Function:** Increased or decreased libido, inhibited ejaculation, impotence, breast milk production, altered timing and pattern of menstruation (10 to 40 mg/day).

CAUTION
Although this drug is reported to have no significant (or very mild) sedative effects and no potential for causing dependence, it should be used with caution and only when clearly needed. It has not been used by large numbers of people for long periods of time; some unexpected side-effects or adverse effects may become apparent after general use for several years.

Precautions for Use
By Infants and Children: Safety and effectiveness for use by those under 18 years of age have not been established.
By Those over 60 Years of Age: This drug should be tolerated much better than benzodiazepines and barbiturates when used by this age group. Observe for some possible increase in dizziness and/or weakness; use caution to avoid falls.

▷ **Advisability of Use During Pregnancy**
Pregnancy Category: B (tentative). See Pregnancy Code inside back cover.
Animal studies: No birth defects found in rat and rabbit studies.
Human studies: Information from adequate studies of pregnant women is not available.
Use this drug during pregnancy only when clearly needed. Until more experience has been gained from wider use, it is advisable to avoid this drug during the first 3 months of pregnancy.

Advisability of Use if Breast-Feeding
Presence of this drug in breast milk: Unknown; probably yes.
Avoid drug or refrain from nursing.

Habit-Forming Potential: None demonstrated in premarketing trials.

Effects of Overdosage: No experience reported. Probable effects would be increased dizziness, weakness and lethargy.

Possible Effects of Long-Term Use: None reported.

Suggested Periodic Examinations While Taking This Drug (at physician's discretion)
None required or recommended at the time of this writing.

▷ **While Taking This Drug, Observe the Following**
   Foods: No restrictions.
   Beverages: No restrictions.
▷ *Alcohol:* No interactions expected.
   Tobacco Smoking: No interactions expected.
▷ *Other Drugs:* No significant drug interactions have been reported at the
     time of this writing.
▷ *Driving, Hazardous Activities:* This drug may cause dizziness, faintness or
     fatigue. Restrict activities as necessary.
   Aviation Note: The use of this drug **may be a disqualification** for piloting.
     Consult a designated Aviation Medical Examiner.
   Exposure to Sun: No restrictions.

BUTALBITAL
(byu TAL bi tal)

Introduced: 1954

Class: Mild sedative, hypnotic,
barbiturates

Prescription: USA: Yes
Canada: Yes

Controlled Drug: USA: C-III*
Canada: C

Available as Generic: No

Brand Names: Axotal [CD], Fioricet [CD], Fiorinal [CD], ✦Fiorinal-C1/4,
C1/2 [CD], Fiorinal w/Codeine No. 1, 2, 3 [CD]

BENEFITS versus RISKS	
Possible Benefits	*Possible Risks*
RELIEF OF ANXIETY AND NERVOUS TENSION	HABIT-FORMING POTENTIAL WITH EXCESSIVE USE
	Minor impairment of mental functions with usual doses
	Allergic skin rashes and hepatitis
	Rare blood cell changes: abnormally low white blood cell and blood platelet counts

▷ **Principal Uses**
   As a Single Drug Product: This barbiturate, with short to intermediate
     duration of action, is a mild sedative that is infrequently used alone
     to relieve anxiety and nervous tension.

*See Schedules of Controlled Drugs inside back cover.

As a Combination Drug Product [CD]: This drug is used primarily in combination with aspirin, caffeine and codeine to treat headaches associated with nervous tension. Because of the significant emotional component in the perception of pain, the addition of a mild sedative to a mixture of analgesics renders the combination more effective in relieving pain.

How This Drug Works: Not completely established. It is thought that this drug relieves nervous tension by reducing the amount of available norepinephrine, one of the chemicals responsible for nerve impulse transmission in the brain.

Available Dosage Forms and Strengths
Capsules — 50 mg (in combination)
Tablets — 50 mg (in combination)

▷ **Usual Adult Dosage Range:**   50 mg (in combination capsule or tablet)/4 hours as needed. Total daily dose should not exceed 6 capsules or tablets. **Note: Actual dosage and administration schedule must be determined by the physician for each patient individually.**

▷ **Dosing Instructions:**   Take with food or milk to prevent stomach irritation. The tablet may be crushed or the capsule opened for administration.

Usual Duration of Use: For short-term use only. Take only as needed to abort or relieve tension headaches. Avoid prolonged and uninterrupted use.

▷ **This Drug Should Not Be Taken If**
- you have had an allergic reaction to any dosage form of it previously.
- you have a history of porphyria.

▷ **Inform Your Physician Before Taking This Drug If**
- you are allergic or overly sensitive to any barbiturate drug.
- you are taking any other sedative drugs, tranquilizers, antihistamines or pain relievers.
- you have epilepsy.
- you have a history of liver or kidney disease.
- you plan to have surgery under general anesthesia in the near future.

Possible Side-Effects (natural, expected and unavoidable drug actions)
Drowsiness, lethargy and sense of mental and physical sluggishness as "hangover" effect.

▷ **Possible Adverse Effects** (unusual, unexpected and infrequent reactions)
If any of the following develop, consult your physician promptly for guidance.
Mild Adverse Effects
Allergic Reactions: Skin rash; hives; localized swellings of eyelids, face or lips; drug fever (see Glossary).

Headache, dizziness.

Nausea, vomiting, diarrhea.

Serious Adverse Effects

Allergic Reactions: Drug-induced hepatitis, with or without jaundice (see Glossary).

Idiosyncratic Reactions: Paradoxical excitement and delirium (rather than sedation). This is more likely to occur in the presence of pain and in the elderly.

Abnormally low white blood cell count—infection, fever, sore throat.

Abnormally low blood platelet count—abnormal bleeding or bruising.

▷ **Possible Effects on Sexual Function:**   None reported.

▷ **Adverse Effects That May Mimic Natural Diseases or Disorders**

Drug-induced jaundice may suggest viral hepatitis.

Natural Diseases or Disorders That May Be Activated by This Drug

Acute intermittent porphyria.

CAUTION

This drug is most commonly used in combination with caffeine and/or aspirin. For complete information, be sure to read the Profiles of these two drugs.

Precautions for Use

By Infants and Children: Observe for possible paradoxical excitement and hyperactivity. Barbiturates should not be given to the hyperkinetic child.

By Those over 60 Years of Age: Small doses are advisable until tolerance has been determined. The elderly or debilitated may experience agitation, excitement, confusion and delirium with standard doses. This drug may also cause excessive lowering of body temperature (hypothermia). Keep dosage to a minimum during cold weather; dress warmly.

▷ **Advisability of Use During Pregnancy**

Pregnancy Category: D (tentative). See Pregnancy Code inside back cover.

Animal studies: No information available.

Human studies: Information from adequate studies of pregnant women is not available. However, some studies suggest that barbiturates taken during pregnancy are associated with a higher incidence of fetal abnormalities. This drug should be avoided during entire pregnancy.

Advisability of Use if Breast-Feeding

Presence of this drug in breast milk: Probably yes.

Avoid drug or refrain from nursing.

Habit-Forming Potential: If used for an extended period of time, this drug can cause both psychological and physical dependence (see Glossary).

Effects of Overdosage: Behavior similar to alcoholic intoxication: confusion, slurred speech, incoordination, staggering gait, drowsiness, deepening sleep, coma.

Possible Effects of Long-Term Use: Psychological and/or physical dependence. If dose is excessive, a form of chronic intoxication can occur: headache, impaired vision, slurred speech and depression.

Suggested Periodic Examinations While Taking This Drug (at physician's discretion)
   With frequent or continual use, complete blood cell counts and liver function tests are desirable.

▷ **While Taking This Drug, Observe the Following**
   Foods: No restrictions.
   Beverages: No restrictions.
▷ *Alcohol:* Avoid completely. Alcohol can increase greatly the sedative and depressant actions of this drug on brain function.
   Tobacco Smoking: No interactions expected.
▷ *Other Drugs*
   Butalbital may **increase** the effects of
   • other sedatives, hypnotics, tranquilizers, antihistamines and pain relievers, and cause oversedation. Ask your physician for guidance regarding dosage adjustments.
   Butalbital may **decrease** the effects of
   • oral anticoagulants of the coumarin drug class. Ask physician for guidance regarding prothrombin time testing and adjustment of the anticoagulant dose.
   • beta blocker drugs (see Drug Class, Section Four).
   • oral contraceptives (see Drug Profile, Section Three).
   • cortisonelike drugs (see Drug Class, Section Four).
   • doxycycline (Vibramycin, etc.).
   • griseofulvin (Fulvicin, Grisactin, etc.).
   • phenmetrazine (Preludin).
   • quinidine (Quinaglute, Quinidex, etc.).
   • theophylline (Bronkotabs, Quibron, Theo-Dur, etc.).
   Butalbital **taken concurrently** with
   • anticonvulsants may cause a change in the pattern of epileptic seizures. Dosage adjustments may be necessary to achieve a balance of drug actions that will give the best protection from seizures.
▷ *Driving, Hazardous Activities:* This drug can cause drowsiness and can impair mental alertness, judgment, physical coordination and reaction time. Avoid hazardous activities until its full sedative effects have been determined.
   Aviation Note: The use of this drug **is a disqualification** for piloting. Consult a designated Aviation Medical Examiner.
   Exposure to Sun: Use caution until sensitivity has been determined. Some barbiturates can cause photosensitivity (see Glossary).

Discontinuation: If it has been necessary to use this drug for an extended
period of time, do not discontinue it abruptly. Ask physician for guidance during gradual withdrawal. It may also be necessary to adjust
the doses of other drugs taken concurrently with it.

CAFFEINE
(KAF een)

Introduced: 4700 B.C. (tea)

Class: Stimulant, xanthines

Prescription: USA: No
Canada: No

Controlled Drug: USA: No
Canada: No

Available as Generic: USA: Yes
Canada: No

Brand Names: Anacin [CD], Anacin Maximum Strength [CD], ♦Anacin w/
Codeine [CD], Cafergot [CD], Cafergot-PB [CD], Cope [CD], Darvon
Compound [CD], Darvon Compound-65 [CD], Darvon-N Compound
[CD], Dolene Compound-65 [CD], Ercaf [CD], ♦Ergodryl [CD], Exced-
rin [CD], ♦Exdol-8, -15, -30 [CD], Fioricet [CD], Fiorinal [CD],
♦Fiorinal-C 1/4, -C 1/2 [CD], Fiorinal w/Codeine No. 1, 2, 3 [CD], Hy-
comine Compound [CD], ♦Lenoltec No. 1, 2, 3 [CD], Midol Caplets
[CD], NoDoz, Norgesic [CD], Norgesic Forte [CD], ♦Novopropoxyn
Compound [CD], Synalgos [CD], Synalgos-DC [CD], ♦Talwin Com-
pound-50 [CD], Trigesic [CD], ♦Tylenol No. 1 [CD], ♦Tylenol No. 1
Forte [CD], ♦Tylenol w/Codeine No. 2, 3 [CD], Vivarin, Wigraine [CD],
♦Wigraine [CD]

BENEFITS versus RISKS	
Possible Benefits	*Possible Risks*
RELIEF OF DROWSINESS AND FATIGUE	Nervousness, insomnia
	Irritability
RELIEF OF MIGRAINE AND RELATED HEADACHES (in combination drugs)	Impaired thinking
	Stomach irritation, heartburn, ulcer

▷ **Principal Uses**

As a Single Drug Product: This stimulant of brain activity is used primarily
to prolong wakefulness and delay the onset of sleep.

As a Combination Drug Product [CD]: This drug is used most commonly
in combination with ergotamine to treat vascular headaches, such as
migraine and cluster headaches. Caffeine increases the absorption of
ergotamine and renders it more effective.

How This Drug Works: By increasing the energy level of the chemical systems responsible for nerve tissue activity, this drug induces wakefulness and improves alertness and mental acuity. By constricting the walls of blood vessels, this drug corrects the excessive expansion (dilation) responsible for the pain of vascular headache.

Available Dosage Forms and Strengths
> Capsules, prolonged-action — 200 mg, 250 mg
> Tablets — 65 mg, 100 mg, 150 mg, 200 mg

▷ **Usual Adult Dosage Range:**   100 to 200 mg/4 hours, as needed. Prolonged-action forms: 200 to 250 mg/6 hours, as needed. **Note: For frequent or long-term use, actual dosage and administration schedule must be determined by the physician for each patient individually.**

▷ **Dosing Instructions:**   If necessary, take with food or milk to prevent stomach irritation. The prolonged-action forms should be taken whole (not crushed or chewed). Do not take within 6 hours of retiring.

Usual Duration of Use: Short-term use advised. Avoid frequent or prolonged use without physician supervision.

▷ **This Drug Should Not Be Taken If**
- you have had an allergic reaction to any dosage form of it previously.
- you have severe heart disease.
- you have an active peptic ulcer.

▷ **Inform Your Physician Before Taking This Drug If**
- you have serious disturbances of heart rhythm.
- you have a history of peptic ulcer disease.
- you are subject to hypoglycemia.
- you have epilepsy.

Possible Side-Effects (natural, expected and unavoidable drug actions)
> Nervousness, insomnia, increased urine output. (Nature and degree of side-effects depend upon the size of the dose and the susceptibility of the individual.)

▷ **Possible Adverse Effects** (unusual, unexpected and infrequent reactions)
> **If any of the following develop, consult your physician promptly for guidance.**
> *Mild Adverse Effects*
> Headache, irritability, light-headedness, feeling of drunkenness, impaired thinking and concentration.
> Rapid, forceful heart action; palpitation.
> Indigestion, stomach irritation, heartburn, nausea.
> *Serious Adverse Effects*
> Development of peptic ulcer (in susceptible individuals).

▷ **Possible Effects on Sexual Function:**   None reported.

CAUTION
1. Do not exceed 250 mg/dose or 500 mg/24 hours.
2. Caffeine in excessive amounts can provoke migraine headache in susceptible individuals.

Precautions for Use

By Infants and Children: Use not recommended.

By Those over 60 Years of Age: Tolerance for caffeine often decreases after 60. You may be more susceptible to caffeine-induced nervousness, irritability, impaired thinking, tremor, insomnia, disturbed heart rhythm and acid indigestion.

▷ **Advisability of Use During Pregnancy**

Pregnancy Category: C (tentative). See Pregnancy Code inside back cover.

Animal studies: Significant birth defects are attributed to this drug.

Human studies: Information from studies of pregnant women indicates no increased birth defects in 12,696 exposures to this drug.

Avoid completely during first 3 months. Because caffeine reaches the same level in fetal tissues as in maternal tissues and is associated with fetal loss, premature deliveries and low birth weights, it is advisable to avoid caffeine throughout pregnancy.

Advisability of Use if Breast-Feeding

Presence of this drug in breast milk: Yes, in small amounts.

Monitor nursing infant closely and discontinue drug or nursing if adverse effects develop.

Habit-Forming Potential: Varying degrees of tolerance and psychological dependence (see Glossary) may occur with prolonged use.

Effects of Overdosage: Nervousness, restlessness, insomnia (followed by depression in some individuals), tremor, sweating, ringing in ears, spots before eyes, heart palpitation, diarrhea, excitement, delirium, hallucinations, seizures.

Possible Effects of Long-Term Use: Development of tolerance and psychological dependence; stomach irritation (gastritis), peptic ulcer.

Suggested Periodic Examinations While Taking This Drug (at physician's discretion)

None.

▷ **While Taking This Drug, Observe the Following**

Foods: No restrictions. Note: Chocolate contains 5 to 10 mg of caffeine per ounce.

Beverages: Keep in mind that caffeine beverages (coffee, tea, cola) will add to the total intake of caffeine taken in medicinal form. Avoid possible overdosage. The approximate caffeine content of popular beverages is as follows:

Regular coffee (average cup) 100–150 mg

Instant coffee (average cup) 80–100 mg
Coffee-grain blends (average cup) 14–37 mg
Decaffeinated coffee (average cup) 3–5 mg
Tea (average cup) 60–75 mg
Regular cola (6 ounces) 36 mg
Diet cola (6 ounces) 18 mg
Cocoa (6 ounces) 10 mg

▷ *Alcohol:* No interactions expected.

Tobacco Smoking: Consult physician regarding possible adverse effects of combined nicotine and caffeine. Smoking can hasten the elimination of caffeine and shorten its period of effectiveness.

▷ *Other Drugs*

Caffeine may ***decrease*** the effects of
- sedatives, tranquilizers, hypnotics and pain relievers.

The following drugs may ***increase*** the effects of caffeine
- cimetidine (tagamet).
- oral contraceptives.

▷ *Driving, Hazardous Activities:* No restrictions.

Aviation Note: No restrictions.

Exposure to Sun: No restrictions.

Discontinuation: Sudden discontinuation of this drug after extended use can produce a "caffeine-withdrawal" headache. This is readily relieved by coffee or caffeine in medicinal form.

CALCIUM CARBONATE
(KAL see um KAR boh nayt)

Other Name: Antacid

Introduced: 1825

Class: Antacid, calcium supplements

Prescription: USA: No
Canada: No

Controlled Drug: USA: No
Canada: No

Available as Generic: Yes

Brand Names: Alka-Mints, Alkets [CD], ✦Apo-Cal, BioCal, Bisodol Tablets [CD], ✦Calcite 500, ✦Calcium-Sandoz [CD], ✦Calsan, Cal.Sup, Caltrate 600, Camalox [CD], ✦DiCal-D [CD], Dicarbosil, Di-Gel Advanced Formula [CD], ✦Gramcal [CD], Marblen [CD], ✦Os-Cal, ✦Os-Cal D [CD], Os-Cal + D [CD], Os-Cal 500 + D [CD], Os-Cal 250 [CD], Os-Cal 500, Titralac, Tums, Tums Extra Strength, Tums with Simethicone [CD]

BENEFITS versus RISKS	
Possible Benefits	*Possible Risks*
EFFECTIVE RELIEF OF ACID INDIGESTION	Constipation
CORRECTION OF CALCIUM DEFICIENCY	Predisposition to calcified kidney stones and kidney damage (excessive use)

▷ **Principal Uses**

As a Single Drug Product: Used primarily to (1) relieve acid indigestion, heartburn and sour stomach, and (2) supplement the diet to meet the body's requirements for calcium in the formation and maintenance of normal bone. Used primarily in children to prevent or treat rickets, and in adults to prevent or treat osteoporosis or osteomalacia.

As a Combination Drug Product [CD]: Often combined with other antacids to enhance the product's ability to neutralize stomach acids. Also combined with vitamin D, which increases the intestinal absorption of calcium. Also available in combination with the entire spectrum of essential vitamins and minerals.

How This Drug Works: By neutralizing some of the hydrochloric acid in the stomach and by reducing the action of the digestive enzyme pepsin, antacids lessen the irritant effect of digestive juices on inflamed tissues and create a more favorable environment for the healing of peptic ulcers.

Available Dosage Forms and Strengths

Capsules — 364 mg

Capsules, soft gel — 1512 mg

Chewing gum — 500 mg

Oral suspension — 1000 mg, 1250 mg per 5-ml teaspoonful

Tablets — 250 mg, 280 mg, 650 mg, 667 mg, 750 mg, 1250 mg, 1500 mg

Tablets, chewable — 350 mg, 420 mg, 500 mg, 625 mg, 650 mg, 750 mg, 850 mg, 1250 mg, 1500 mg

▷ **Usual Adult Dosage Range:**   (1) As antacid: 500 mg to 2 grams after meals and at bedtime, or as needed. Total daily dosage should not exceed 8 grams. (2) As supplement, the recommended daily dietary allowances are as follows:

Infants up to 6 months of age: 360 mg.

Infants 6 months to 1 year of age: 540 mg.

Children 1 to 10 years of age: 800 mg.

Males 11 to 18 years of age: 1200 mg.

Males 19 years of age and older: 800 mg.

Females 11 to 18 years of age: 1200 mg.

Females 19 to 50 years of age: 800 mg.

Females after 50 years of age (postmenopausal): 1500 mg.

During pregnancy: 1200 mg.

While breast-feeding: 1200 mg.
Note: For long-term use, actual dosage and administration schedule must be determined by the physician for each patient individually.

▷ **Dosing Instructions:**   As antacid for treatment of peptic ulcer disease, take 1 to 3 hours after meals and at bedtime. As supplement, take 1 to 2 hours after meals. Chewable tablets should be chewed thoroughly before swallowing. Shake suspension well before measuring dose. Do not take within 2 hours of other oral medications.

Usual Duration of Use: If used for the treatment of peptic ulcer disease, continual use on a regular schedule is recommended for 4 to 6 weeks after all symptoms of ulcer activity have disappeared. Long-term use, as antacid or supplement, should be under physician supervision. Consult your physician on a regular basis.

▷ **This Drug Should Not Be Taken If**
- your calcium blood level is abnormally high.
- you have severe kidney disease.
- you have calcified kidney stones.
- you are immobilized for an extended period of time.

▷ **Inform Your Physician Before Taking This Drug If**
- you have a history of kidney stones or impaired kidney function.
- you have any form of heart disease.
- you have sarcoidosis.
- you have deficient or absent stomach acid.
- you are prone to constipation.
- you are taking any other oral medications at this time, especially thiazide diuretics, quinidine or tetracycline.

Possible Side-Effects (natural, expected and unavoidable drug actions)
Constipation (may be severe with large doses).

▷ **Possible Adverse Effects** (unusual, unexpected and infrequent reactions)
If any of the following develop, consult your physician promptly for guidance.
Mild Adverse Effects
Chalky taste in mouth, belching, intestinal gas.
Serious Adverse Effects
With normal dosage—none.
With excessive dosage—abnormally high level of blood calcium: headache, fatigue, weakness, loss of appetite, nausea, vomiting.

▷ **Possible Effects on Sexual Function:**   None reported.

CAUTION
1. Calcium can interfere with the absorption of many drugs. Do not take any other oral medication within 2 hours of a dose of calcium carbonate.

2. Avoid large doses of vitamin D while taking any form of calcium. Ask physician for guidance regarding vitamin D dosage.

Precautions for Use
By Infants and Children: May cause constipation with frequent or chronic use. Limit use to short-term schedules.

By Those over 60 Years of Age: This drug should be avoided because of its potential for raising the blood calcium level and predisposing to kidney stones and impairment of kidney function.

▷ **Advisability of Use During Pregnancy**
Pregnancy Category: C (tentative). See Pregnancy Code inside back cover.
Animal studies: No information available.

Human studies: Information from adequate studies of pregnant women is not available.

This drug is considered safe for use during the last 6 months of pregnancy in doses not to exceed 1200 mg daily. The calcium content of the diet must be considered.

Advisability of Use if Breast-Feeding
Presence of this drug in breast milk: Calcium is a normal constituent of breast milk. This drug does not increase the calcium content of milk to any significant degree, but does prevent deficiency.

Habit-Forming Potential: None.

Effects of Overdosage: Headache, fatigue, weakness, nervousness, muscle twitching, stomach pain, nausea, vomiting, constipation, mental disturbance, delirium, coma.

Possible Effects of Long-Term Use: Development of calcium-containing kidney stones.

Suggested Periodic Examinations While Taking This Drug (at physician's discretion)
Measurement of blood calcium levels (chronic use).

▷ **While Taking This Drug, Observe the Following**
Foods: Avoid frequent and excessive intake of spinach, rhubarb, bran and whole grain cereals; these can interfere with the absorption of calcium.

Beverages: Avoid large quantities of milk while taking calcium.
▷   *Alcohol:* No interactions.

Tobacco Smoking: No interactions.
▷   *Other Drugs*
Calcium may ***increase*** the effects of
• quinidine by delaying its elimination.
Calcium may ***decrease*** the effects of
• iron preparations.
• salicylates (aspirin, etc.).

- tetracyclines.

Calcium *taken concurrently* with

- thiazide diuretics (see Drug Class, Section Four) may cause abnormally high blood levels of calcium.

▷ *Driving, Hazardous Activities:* No restrictions.

CAPTOPRIL
(KAP toh pril)

Introduced: 1979

Class: Antihypertensive, ACE inhibitor

Prescription: USA: Yes
Canada: Yes

Controlled Drug: USA: No
Canada: No

Available as Generic: No

Brand Names: Capoten, Capozide [CD]

BENEFITS versus RISKS	
Possible Benefits	*Possible Risks*
EFFECTIVE CONTROL OF MILD TO SEVERE HIGH BLOOD PRESSURE	Rash, itching, fever (10%)
	Lost or altered taste (7%)
USEFUL ADJUNCTIVE TREATMENT FOR CONGESTIVE HEART FAILURE	Impaired white blood cell production (0.3%)
	Bone marrow depression (rare)
	Kidney damage (rare)
	Liver damage (rare)

▷ **Principal Uses**

As a Single Drug Product: Used primarily to treat all degrees of high blood pressure. Mild to moderate high blood pressure usually responds to low doses; severe high blood pressure requires higher doses, with greater risk of serious adverse effects. Also used to treat selected cases of advanced heart failure that have not responded to conventional treatment with digitalis and diuretics.

How This Drug Works: Not completely known. It is thought that by blocking certain enzyme systems that influence arterial function, this drug contributes to the relaxation of arterial walls throughout the body and thus lowers the resistance to blood flow that causes high blood pressure. This, in turn, reduces the workload of the heart and improves its performance.

Available Dosage Forms and Strengths
Tablets — 12.5 mg, 25 mg, 50 mg, 100 mg

▷ **Usual Adult Dosage Range:** Initially 12.5 to 25 mg 2 or 3 times daily for 2 weeks. If necessary, dose may be increased to 50 mg 3 times daily. Usual maintenance dose is 50 to 100 mg 3 times daily. Total daily dose should not exceed 450 mg. **Note: Actual dosage and administration schedule must be determined by the physician for each patient individually.**

▷ **Dosing Instructions:** Take on empty stomach, 1 hour before meals, at same time each day. Tablet may be crushed for administration.

Usual Duration of Use: Continual use on a regular schedule for several weeks is usually necessary to determine this drug's effectiveness in controlling high blood pressure. The proper treatment of high blood pressure usually requires the long-term use of effective medications. Consult your physician on a regular basis.

▷ **This Drug Should Not Be Taken If**
- you have had an allergic reaction to it previously.
- you currently have a blood cell or bone marrow disorder.
- you have active liver disease.
- you have an abnormally high level of blood potassium.

▷ **Inform Your Physician Before Taking This Drug If**
- you have a history of kidney disease or impaired kidney function.
- you have scleroderma or systemic lupus erythematosus.
- you have any form of heart disease.
- you have diabetes.
- you are taking any of the following drugs: other antihypertensives, diuretics, nitrates, allopurinol (Zyloprim), Indocin or potassium supplements.
- you plan to have surgery under general anesthesia in the near future.

Possible Side-Effects (natural, expected and unavoidable drug actions)
Dizziness, light-headedness, fainting (excessive drop in blood pressure).

▷ **Possible Adverse Effects** (unusual, unexpected and infrequent reactions)
If any of the following develop, consult your physician promptly for guidance.
Mild Adverse Effects
Allergic Reactions: Skin rash; swelling of face, hands or feet; fever.
Lost or altered taste, mouth or tongue sores.
Rapid heart rate, palpitation.
Serious Adverse Effects
Bone marrow depression—fatigue, weakness, fever, sore throat, abnormal bleeding or bruising.
Kidney damage—water retention (edema).
Liver damage—with or without jaundice.

▷ **Possible Effects on Sexual Function:**   Decreased male libido (20% to 30%) with recommended dosage.

CAUTION
1. If possible, it is advisable to discontinue all other antihypertensive drugs (especially diuretics) for 1 week before starting captopril.
2. **Report promptly** any indications of infection (fever, sore throat), and any indications of water retention (weight gain, puffiness, swollen feet or ankles).
3. Do not use a salt substitute without your physician's knowledge and approval. (Many salt substitutes contain potassium.)
4. It is advisable to obtain blood cell counts and urine analyses **before** starting this drug.

Precautions for Use
By Infants and Children: Safety and effectiveness for use by those in this age group have not been established.

By Those over 60 Years of Age: Small doses are advisable until tolerance has been determined. Sudden and excessive lowering of blood pressure can predispose to stroke or heart attack in those with impaired brain circulation or coronary artery heart disease.

▷ **Advisability of Use During Pregnancy**
Pregnancy Category: C (tentative). See Pregnancy Code inside back cover.
Animal studies: No birth defects found in rat, rabbit or hamster studies. However, this drug was shown to be toxic to the embryo and newborn.
Human studies: Information from adequate studies of pregnant women is not available.
Avoid during first 3 months if possible. Use only if clearly needed during last 6 months.

Advisability of Use if Breast-Feeding
Presence of this drug in breast milk: Yes, in small amounts.
Monitor nursing infant closely and discontinue drug or nursing if adverse effects develop.

Habit-Forming Potential: None.

Effects of Overdosage: Excessive drop in blood pressure—light-headedness, dizziness, fainting.

Possible Effects of Long-Term Use: Gradual increase in blood potassium level.

Suggested Periodic Examinations While Taking This Drug (at physician's discretion)
Before starting drug: Complete blood cell counts; urine analysis with measurement of protein content, blood potassium level. During use of drug: Blood cell counts every 2 weeks during the first 3 months of treatment, then periodically for duration of use. Urine protein meas-

urements every month during the first 9 months of treatment, then periodically for duration of use. Periodic measurements of blood potassium.

▷ **While Taking This Drug, Observe the Following**
Foods: Consult physician regarding salt intake.
Nutritional Support: **Do not take** potassium supplements unless directed by your physician.
Beverages: No restrictions. May be taken with milk.
▷ *Alcohol:* Use caution until combined effect has been determined. Alcohol may enhance the blood-pressure-lowering effect of this drug.
Tobacco Smoking: No interactions expected.
▷ *Other Drugs*
Captopril *taken concurrently* with
- potassium preparations (K-Lyte, Slow-K, etc.) may cause increased blood levels of potassium with risk of serious heart rhythm disturbances.
- potassium-sparing diuretics: amiloride (Moduretic), spironolactone (Aldactazide), triamterene (Dyazide) may cause increased blood levels of potassium with risk of serious heart rhythm disturbances.
The following drugs may *decrease* the effects of captopril
- indomethacin (Indocin).
- salicylates (aspirin, etc.).
▷ *Driving, Hazardous Activities:* Usually no restrictions. Be aware of possible drops in blood pressure with resultant dizziness or faintness.
Aviation Note: The use of this drug **may be a disqualification** for piloting. Consult a designated Aviation Medical Examiner.
Exposure to Sun: Caution advised. This drug can cause photosensitivity.
Exposure to Heat: Caution advised. Avoid excessive perspiring with resultant loss of body water and drop in blood pressure.
Occurrence of Unrelated Illness: Report promptly any disorder that causes nausea, vomiting or diarrhea. Fluid and chemical imbalances must be corrected as soon as possible.

CARBAMAZEPINE
(kar ba MAZ e peen)

Introduced: 1962

Class: Anticonvulsant, antineuralgic

Prescription: USA: Yes
Canada: Yes

Controlled Drug: USA: No
Canada: No

Available as Generic: Yes

Brand Names: ✦Apo-Carbamazepine, Epitol, ✦Mazepine, ✦PMS-Carbamazepine, Tegretol

```
┌─────────────────────────────────────────────────────────────┐
│                   BENEFITS versus RISKS                       │
│                                                               │
│       Possible Benefits              Possible Risks           │
│   RELIEF OF PAIN IN              RARE BONE MARROW             │
│     TRIGEMINAL NEURALGIA           DEPRESSION (reduced        │
│   EFFECTIVE CONTROL OF             formation of all blood cells)│
│     CERTAIN TYPES OF             Liver damage with jaundice   │
│     EPILEPTIC SEIZURES                                        │
│   Relief of pain in some rare forms                           │
│     of neuralgia                                              │
└─────────────────────────────────────────────────────────────┘
```

▷ **Principal Uses**

    As a Single Drug Product: This drug is used primarily in the management of two uncommon but serious disorders: (1) for relief of pain in true trigeminal neuralgia (tic douloureux) and glossopharyngeal neuralgia; (2) for control of several types of epilepsy, namely grand mal, psychomotor or temporal lobe, and mixed seizure patterns. Because of its potential for serious toxic effects, precise diagnosis and careful management are mandatory for its proper use.

How This Drug Works: Not completely known. It is thought that by reducing the transmission of impulses at certain nerve terminals, this drug relieves or reduces pain (of trigeminal neuralgia) and also reduces the excitability of certain nerve fibers in the brain and thereby inhibits the repetitious spread of electrical impulses along nerve pathways. This action may prevent seizures altogether or reduce their frequency and severity.

Available Dosage Forms and Strengths
    Oral suspension — 100 mg per 5-ml teaspoonful
            Tablets — 200 mg
    Tablets, chewable — 100 mg

▷ **Usual Adult Dosage Range:** Initially 200 mg/12 hours. Dose may be increased by 200 mg/24 hours as needed and tolerated. Total daily dosage should not exceed 1200 mg. **Note: Actual dosage and administration schedule must be determined by the physician for each patient individually.**

▷ **Dosing Instructions:** Take at same time each day, with or following food to reduce stomach irritation. Tablet may be crushed for administration.

Usual Duration of Use: Continual use on a regular schedule for 3 months is usually necessary to determine this drug's effectiveness in relieving the pain of trigeminal neuralgia. Longer periods, with dosage adjustment, may be required to determine its ability to control epileptic seizures. Careful evaluation of each individual's tolerance and response should be made every 3 months during long-term treatment. Consult your physician on a regular basis.

▷ **This Drug Should Not Be Taken If**
  - you have had an allergic reaction to it previously.
  - you have active liver disease.
  - you currently have a blood cell or bone marrow disorder.
  - you are currently taking, or have taken within the past 14 days, any monoamine oxidase (MAO) type A inhibitor drug (see Drug Class, Section Four).

▷ **Inform Your Physician Before Taking This Drug If**
  - you have had an allergic reaction to any tricyclic antidepressant drug (see Drug Class, Section Four).
  - you have taken this drug in the past.
  - you have a history of any kind of blood cell or bone marrow disorder, especially one due to a drug.
  - you have a history of liver or kidney disease.
  - you have had serious mental depression or other mental disorder.
  - you have had thrombophlebitis.
  - you have high blood pressure, heart disease or glaucoma.
  - you take more than 2 alcoholic drinks a day.

Possible Side-Effects (natural, expected and unavoidable drug actions)
  Dry mouth and throat, constipation, impaired urination.

▷ **Possible Adverse Effects** (unusual, unexpected and infrequent reactions)
  If any of the following develop, consult your physician promptly for guidance.
  Mild Adverse Effects
  Allergic Reactions: Skin rash, hives, itching, drug fever.
  Headache, dizziness, drowsiness, unsteadiness, fatigue, blurred vision, confusion.
  Exaggerated hearing, ringing in ears.
  Loss of appetite, nausea, vomiting, indigestion, diarrhea.
  Water retention (edema), frequent urination.
  Changes in skin pigmentation, hair loss.
  Aching of muscles and joints, leg cramps.
  Serious Adverse Effects
  Allergic Reactions: Severe dermatitis with peeling of skin, irritation of mouth and tongue, swelling of lymph glands.
  Idiosyncratic Reactions: Lung inflammation (pneumonitis): cough, shortness of breath.
  Bone marrow depression (see Glossary)—fatigue, weakness, fever, sore throat, abnormal bleeding or bruising.
  Liver damage with jaundice (see Glossary)—yellow eyes and skin, dark-colored urine, light-colored stools.
  Kidney damage—reduced urine volume, uremic poisoning.
  Mental depression and agitation.
  Double vision, visual hallucinations, speech disturbances, peripheral neuritis (see Glossary).
  Thrombophlebitis.

▷ **Possible Effects on Sexual Function**

Decreased libido and/or impotence (13%), male infertility.

This drug is used to control hypersexuality (exaggerated sexual behavior) that can result from injury to the temporal lobe of the brain.

▷ **Adverse Effects That May Mimic Natural Diseases or Disorders**

Liver reactions may suggest viral hepatitis.

Rare lung reactions may suggest interstitial pneumonitis.

Natural Diseases or Disorders That May Be Activated by This Drug

Latent psychosis, systemic lupus erythematosus.

CAUTION

1. Because this drug can cause serious adverse effects, it should be used only after a trial of less hazardous drugs has been ineffective.
2. *Before* the first dose is taken, pretreatment blood cell counts, liver function tests and kidney function tests should be performed.
3. Careful periodic testing for early indications of blood cell or bone marrow toxicity is *mandatory.*
4. During periods of spontaneous remission from trigeminal neuralgia, this drug *should not be used* to prevent recurrence.
5. If used to control epileptic seizures, *do not discontinue this drug suddenly.*

Precautions for Use

By Infants and Children: Because of the high frequency of adverse effects (up to 25%), careful testing of blood cell production, liver function and kidney function must be performed regularly. This drug can reduce the effectiveness of other anticonvulsant drugs. Blood levels of all anticonvulsant drugs should be monitored when this drug is added to the treatment program.

By Those over 60 Years of Age: This drug can cause confusion and agitation. Observe for the possible aggravation of glaucoma, coronary artery disease (angina) or prostatism (see Glossary).

▷ **Advisability of Use During Pregnancy**

Pregnancy Category: C (tentative). See Pregnancy Code inside back cover.

Animal studies: Rat studies reveal significant birth defects.

Human studies: Information from adequate studies of pregnant women is not available.

Avoid completely during the first 3 months. Use during the last 6 months only if clearly needed.

Advisability of Use if Breast-Feeding

Presence of this drug in breast milk: Yes.

Avoid drug or refrain from nursing.

Habit-Forming Potential: None.

Effects of Overdosage: Dizziness, unsteadiness, drowsiness, disorientation, tremor, involuntary movements, nausea, vomiting, flushed skin, dilated pupils, stupor progressing to coma.

Possible Effects of Long-Term Use: Water retention (edema), impaired kidney function, possible liver damage with jaundice.

Suggested Periodic Examinations While Taking This Drug (at physician's discretion)
Complete blood cell counts weekly during the first 3 months of treatment, and monthly thereafter until the drug is discontinued. Liver and kidney function tests. Complete eye examinations.

▷ **While Taking This Drug, Observe the Following**
Foods: No restrictions.
Beverages: No restrictions. May be taken with milk.
▷   *Alcohol:* Use caution until the combined effect has been determined. This drug may increase the sedative effect of alcohol.
Tobacco Smoking: No interactions expected.
▷   *Other Drugs*
Carbamazepine may *increase* the effects of
  • sedatives, tranquilizers, hypnotics, narcotics, and enhance their sedative effects.
Carbamazepine may *decrease* the effects of
  • doxycycline (Doxy-II, Vibramycin, etc.).
  • warfarin (Coumadin, Panwarfin, etc.).
Carbamazepine *taken concurrently* with
  • lithium may cause serious neurological disturbances: confusion, drowsiness, weakness, unsteadiness, tremors, muscle twitching.
  • monoamine oxidase (MAO) type A inhibitor drugs (see Drug Class, Section Four) may cause severe toxic reactions.
The following drugs may *increase* the effects of carbamazepine
  • erythromycin (E.E.S., E-Mycin, etc.).
  • isoniazid (INH).
  • propoxyphene (Darvon, Darvocet, etc.).
  • troleandomycin (Tao).
▷   *Driving, Hazardous Activities:* This drug can cause dizziness and drowsiness. Adjust activities accordingly.
Aviation Note: The use of this drug *is a disqualification* for piloting. Consult a designated Aviation Medical Examiner.
Exposure to Sun: This drug can cause photosensitivity (see Glossary). Use caution until sensitivity to sun has been determined.
Heavy Exercise or Exertion: Use caution if you have coronary artery disease. This drug can intensify angina and reduce tolerance for physical activity.
Occurrence of Unrelated Illness: Because of this drug's potential for serious adverse effects, it is mandatory that you inform each physician and dentist you consult that you are taking carbamazepine.
Discontinuation: If used to treat trigeminal neuralgia, attempt should be made every 3 months to reduce the maintenance dose or to discontinue this drug altogether. If used to control epilepsy, this drug *must not be discontinued abruptly.*

CARBENICILLIN
(kar ben i SIL in)

Introduced: 1964

Class: Antibiotic, penicillins

Prescription: USA: Yes
Canada: Yes

Controlled Drug: USA: No
Canada: No

Available as Generic: No

Brand Names: Geocillin, Geopen, ✦Geopen Oral, Pyopen

BENEFITS versus RISKS	
Possible Benefits	*Possible Risks*
EFFECTIVE TREATMENT OF INFECTIONS due to susceptible microorganisms	ALLERGIC REACTIONS, mild to severe Superinfections (yeast) Drug-induced colitis Rare blood cell disorders

▷ **Principal Uses**

As a Single Drug Product: Oral tablets are used to treat certain infections of the urinary tract and prostate gland. Injections are used to treat a wider variety of more serious infections.

How This Drug Works: This drug destroys susceptible infecting bacteria by interfering with their ability to produce new protective cell walls as they multiply and grow.

Available Dosage Forms and Strengths

Injections — Vials of 1 gram, 2 grams, 5 grams
Tablets, film-coated — 382 mg

▷ **Usual Adult Dosage Range:** 382 to 764 mg/6 hours (4 doses/24 hours). **Note: Actual dosage and administration schedule must be determined by the physician for each patient individually.**

▷ **Dosing Instructions:** Take on an empty stomach, 1 hour before or 2 hours after eating, at same times each day. Tablet be crushed for administration, but drug has a bitter taste.

Usual Duration of Use: For urinary tract infections—10 days. For prostate gland infections—2 to 4 weeks. Recurrent and chronic infections require longer periods of treatment.

▷ **This Drug Should Not Be Taken If**
- you have had an allergic reaction to any dosage form of it previously.
- you are certain you are allergic to **any** form of penicillin.

▷ **Inform Your Physician Before Taking This Drug If**
- you suspect you may be allergic to penicillin or you have a history of a previous "reaction" to penicillin.
- you are allergic to cephalosporin antibiotics (Ancef, Ceporan, Ceporex, Kafocin, Keflex, Keflin, Kefzol, Loridine).
- you are allergic by nature—hay fever, asthma, hives, eczema.
- you have a history of a bleeding disorder, kidney disease, regional enteritis or ulcerative colitis.

Possible Side-Effects (natural, expected and unavoidable drug actions)
Superinfections (see Glossary), often due to yeast organisms.

▷ **Possible Adverse Effects** (unusual, unexpected and infrequent reactions)
If any of the following develop, consult your physician promptly for guidance.
Mild Adverse Effects
Allergic Reactions: Skin rashes, hives, itching.
Irritations of mouth and tongue, unpleasant taste, nausea, vomiting, mild diarrhea.
Serious Adverse Effects
Allergic Reactions: Anaphylactic reaction (see Glossary), severe skin reactions, drug fever, swollen painful joints, sore throat, abnormal bleeding or bruising.
Hemolytic anemia (see Glossary).
Pseudomembranous colitis—severe diarrhea.

▷ **Possible Effects on Sexual Function:**   None reported.

CAUTION
1. Take the exact dose and the full course prescribed.
2. This drug should not be used concurrently with antibiotics like erythromycin or tetracycline.

Precautions for Use
By Infants and Children: Safety and effectiveness for use by those under 12 years of age have not been established.
By Those over 60 Years of Age: It is advisable to evaluate kidney function before and during use of this drug to determine the need for dosage adjustment. Natural changes in the skin may predispose to prolonged itching reactions in the genital and anal regions. Report such reactions promptly.

▷ **Advisability of Use During Pregnancy**
Pregnancy Category: B (tentative). See Pregnancy Code inside back cover.
Animal studies: No information available.
Human studies: Information from adequate studies of pregnant women indicates no increased risk of birth defects in 3546 pregnancies exposed to penicillin derivatives.
Ask physician for guidance.

Advisability of Use if Breast-Feeding
Presence of this drug in breast milk: Probably yes.
The nursing infant may be sensitized to penicillin and be at risk for developing diarrhea or yeast infections.
Avoid drug if possible or refrain from nursing.

Habit-Forming Potential: None.

Effects of Overdosage: Possible nausea, vomiting and/or diarrhea.

Possible Effects of Long-Term Use: Superinfections, often due to yeast organisms.

Suggested Periodic Examinations While Taking This Drug (at physician's discretion)
Complete blood cell counts. Liver and kidney function tests with long-term use.

▷ **While Taking This Drug, Observe the Following**
Foods: No restrictions.
Beverages: No restrictions.
▷ *Alcohol:* No interactions expected.
Tobacco Smoking: No interactions expected.
▷ *Other Drugs*
Carbenicillin may *decrease* the effects of
- oral contraceptives in some women, and impair their effectiveness in preventing pregnancy.
The following drugs may *decrease* the effects of carbenicillin
- antacids may reduce the absorption of carbenicillin.
- chloramphenicol (Chloromycetin).
- erythromycin (Erythrocin, E-Mycin, etc.).
- tetracyclines (Achromycin, Declomycin, Minocin, etc.). (See Drug Class, Section Four.)
▷ *Driving, Hazardous Activities:* Usually no restrictions.
Aviation Note: The use of this drug *may be a disqualification* for piloting. Consult a designated Aviation Medical Examiner.
Exposure to Sun: No restrictions.

CEFACLOR
(SEF a klor)

Introduced: 1979

Class: Antibiotic, cephalosporins

Prescription: USA: Yes
Canada: Yes

Controlled Drug: USA: No
Canada: No

Available as Generic: No

Brand Name: Ceclor

BENEFITS versus RISKS

Possible Benefits	*Possible Risks*
EFFECTIVE TREATMENT OF INFECTIONS due to susceptible microorganisms	ALLERGIC REACTIONS mild to severe (up to 5% of general population, up to 16% of those allergic to penicillin) Drug-induced colitis (rare) Superinfections (see Glossary)

▷ **Principal Uses**

As a Single Drug Product: To treat certain infections of the skin and skin structures, the upper and lower respiratory tract (including middle ear infections and "strep" throat) and certain infections of the urinary tract.

How This Drug Works: This drug destroys susceptible infecting bacteria by interfering with their ability to produce new protective cell walls as they multiply and grow.

Available Dosage Forms and Strengths
Capsules — 250 mg, 500 mg
Oral suspension — 125 mg, 250 mg per 5-ml teaspoonful

▷ **Usual Adult Dosage Range:** 250 to 500 mg/8 hours. Total daily dose should not exceed 4 grams. **Note: Actual dosage and administration schedule must be determined by the physician for each patient individually.**

▷ **Dosing Instructions:** May be taken on an empty stomach or with food if stomach irritation occurs. Capsule may be opened for administration. Shake suspension well before measuring dose. Take the full course prescribed.

Usual Duration of Use: Continual use on a regular schedule for 3 to 5 days is usually necessary to determine this drug's effectiveness in controlling the infection under treatment. Response varies with the nature of the infection. Total treatment time will vary from 1 to 4 weeks. Certain infections require that this drug be taken for 10 consecutive days to prevent the development of rheumatic fever. Follow your physician's instructions regarding duration of use.

▷ **This Drug Should Not Be Taken If**
- you are allergic to any cephalosporin antibiotic (see Drug Class, Section Four).

▷ **Inform Your Physician Before Taking This Drug If**
- you have a history of allergy to any form of penicillin (see Drug Class, Section Four).

- you have a history of regional enteritis or ulcerative colitis.
- you have impaired kidney function.

Possible Side-Effects (natural, expected and unavoidable drug actions)
Superinfections (see Glossary).

▷ **Possible Adverse Effects** (unusual, unexpected and infrequent reactions)
If any of the following develop, consult your physician promptly for guidance.
Mild Adverse Effects
Allergic Reactions: Skin rash, itching, hives.
Nausea and vomiting (1 in 90), mild diarrhea (1 in 70), sore mouth or tongue.
Serious Adverse Effects
Allergic Reactions: Drug fever (see Glossary), joint aches and pains, anaphylactic reaction (see Glossary).
Idiosyncratic Reactions: Minor and temporary changes in white blood cell counts and liver function tests (infrequent).
Genital itching (may represent a fungus superinfection).
Severe diarrhea, possibly indicating a drug-induced form of colitis (rare).

▷ **Possible Effects on Sexual Function:** None reported.

▷ **Adverse Effects That May Mimic Natural Diseases or Disorders**
Skin rash and fever may resemble measles.

CAUTION
In the management of diabetes it should be noted that this drug can cause a false positive test result for urine sugar when using Clinitest tablets, Benedict's solution or Fehling's solution, but not with Tes-Tape.

Precautions for Use
By Infants and Children: Not recommended for use in infants less than 1 month old. The maximal dose in children should not exceed 1 gram/24 hours.
By Those over 60 Years of Age: Dosage must be carefully individualized and based upon evaluation of kidney function. Natural changes in the skin may predispose to severe and prolonged itching reactions in the genital and anal regions. Such reactions should be reported promptly.

▷ **Advisability of Use During Pregnancy**
Pregnancy Category: B (tentative). See Pregnancy Code inside back cover.
Animal studies: No birth defects reported.
Human studies: Information from adequate studies of pregnant women is not available.
Generally considered to be safe. Ask physician for guidance.

Advisability of Use if Breast-Feeding
Presence of this drug in breast milk: Yes, in small amounts.
Avoid drug or refrain from nursing.

Habit-Forming Potential: None.

Effects of Overdosage: Nausea, vomiting, stomach cramps and/or diarrhea.

Possible Effects of Long-Term Use: Superinfections (see Glossary).

Suggested Periodic Examinations While Taking This Drug (at physician's discretion)
Complete blood cell counts.

▷ **While Taking This Drug, Observe the Following**
Foods: No restrictions.
Beverages: No restrictions. May be taken with milk.
▷ *Alcohol:* No interactions expected.
Tobacco Smoking: No interactions expected.
▷ *Other Drugs*
Cefaclor *taken concurrently* with
• probenecid (Benemid) will slow the elimination of cefaclor, resulting in higher blood levels and prolonged effect.
▷ *Driving, Hazardous Activities:* Usually no restrictions.
Aviation Note: The use of this drug *may be a disqualification* for piloting. Consult a designated Aviation Medical Examiner.
Exposure to Sun: No restrictions.
Special Storage Instructions: Oral suspension should be refrigerated.
Observe the Following Expiration Times: Do not take the oral suspension of this drug if it is older than 14 days.

CEFADROXIL
(sef a DROX il)

Introduced: 1977

Class: Antibiotic, cephalosporins

Prescription: USA: Yes
Canada: Yes

Controlled Drug: USA: No
Canada: No

Available as Generic: No

Brand Names: Duricef, Ultracef

BENEFITS versus RISKS	
Possible Benefits	*Possible Risks*
EFFECTIVE TREATMENT OF INFECTIONS due to susceptible microorganisms	ALLERGIC REACTIONS mild to severe (up to 5% of general population, up to 16% of those allergic to penicillin) Drug-induced colitis (rare) Superinfections (see Glossary)

▷ **Principal Uses**

As a Single Drug Product: To treat certain infections of the skin and skin structures, the upper respiratory tract (including tonsillitis and "strep" throat) and certain infections of the urinary tract.

How This Drug Works: This drug destroys susceptible infecting bacteria by interfering with their ability to produce new protective cell walls as they multiply and grow.

Available Dosage Forms and Strengths
Capsules — 500 mg
Oral suspension — 125 mg, 250 mg, 500 mg per 5-ml teaspoonful
Tablets — 1000 mg (1 gram)

▷ **Usual Adult Dosage Range:** Skin infections—500 mg/12 hours, or 1 gram daily. "Strep" throat—500 mg/12 hours for 10 days. Urinary tract infections—500 mg to 1 gram/12 hours, or 1 to 2 grams daily. Total daily dosage should not exceed 6 grams. **Note: Actual dosage and administration schedule must be determined by the physician for each patient individually.**

▷ **Dosing Instructions:** May be taken on an empty stomach or with food if stomach irritation occurs. Capsule may be opened for administration. Shake suspension well before measuring dose. Take the full course prescribed.

Usual Duration of Use: Continual use on a regular schedule for 3 to 5 days is usually necessary to determine this drug's effectiveness in controlling the infection under treatment. Response varies with the nature of the infection. Total treatment time will vary from 1 to 4 weeks. Certain infections require that this drug be taken for 10 consecutive days to prevent the development of rheumatic fever. Follow your physician's instructions regarding duration of use.

▷ **This Drug Should Not Be Taken If**
• you are allergic to any cephalosporin antibiotic (see Drug Class, Section Four).

▷ **Inform Your Physician Before Taking This Drug If**
• you have a history of allergy to any form of penicillin (see Drug Class, Section Four).
• you have a history of regional enteritis or ulcerative colitis.
• you have impaired kidney function.

Possible Side-Effects (natural, expected and unavoidable drug actions)
Superinfections (see Glossary).

▷ **Possible Adverse Effects** (unusual, unexpected and infrequent reactions)
If any of the following develop, consult your physician promptly for guidance.

Mild Adverse Effects
 Allergic Reactions: Skin rash, itching, hives, localized swellings.
 Headache, drowsiness, dizziness.
 Indigestion, stomach cramping, nausea, vomiting, mild diarrhea, sore
  mouth or tongue.
Serious Adverse Effects
 Allergic Reactions: Drug fever (see Glossary), joint aches and pains,
  anaphylactic reaction (see Glossary).
 Idiosyncratic Reactions: Minor and temporary changes in white blood
  cell counts and liver function tests (infrequent).
 Genital itching (may represent a fungus superinfection).
 Severe diarrhea, possibly indicating a drug-induced form of colitis
  (rare).

▷ **Possible Effects on Sexual Function:**   None reported.

▷ **Adverse Effects That May Mimic Natural Diseases or Disorders**
 Skin rash and fever may resemble measles.

CAUTION
 In the management of diabetes it should be noted that this drug can
 cause a false positive test result for urine sugar when using Clinitest
 tablets, Benedict's solution or Fehling's solution, but not with Tes-
 Tape.

Precautions for Use
 By Infants and Children: Dosage is based upon weight, and must be determined by the physician for each individual. Follow your physician's instructions exactly.
 By Those over 60 Years of Age: Dosage must be carefully individualized
  and based upon evaluation of kidney function. Natural changes in the
  skin may predispose to severe and prolonged itching reactions in the
  genital and anal regions. Such reactions should be reported promptly.

▷ **Advisability of Use During Pregnancy**
 Pregnancy Category: B (tentative). See Pregnancy Code inside back cover.
  Animal studies: No birth defects reported.
  Human studies: Information from adequate studies of pregnant women
  is not available.
  Generally considered to be safe. Ask physician for guidance.

Advisability of Use if Breast-Feeding
 Presence of this drug in breast milk: Yes, in small amounts.
 Avoid drug or refrain from nursing.

Habit-Forming Potential: None.

Effects of Overdosage: Nausea, vomiting, stomach cramps and/or diarrhea.

Possible Effects of Long-Term Use: Superinfections (see Glossary).

Suggested Periodic Examinations While Taking This Drug (at physician's
   discretion)
   Complete blood cell counts. Liver and kidney function tests.

▷ **While Taking This Drug, Observe the Following**
   Foods: No restrictions.
   Beverages: No restrictions. May be taken with milk.
▷   *Alcohol:* No interactions expected.
   Tobacco Smoking: No interactions expected.
▷   *Other Drugs*
      Cefadroxil *taken concurrently* with
      • probenecid (Benemid) will slow the elimination of cefadroxil, result-
         ing in higher blood levels and prolonged effect.
▷   *Driving, Hazardous Activities:* Usually no restrictions. If drowsiness or diz-
         ziness occurs, restrict activities accordingly.
      Aviation Note: The use of this drug *may be a disqualification* for piloting.
         Consult a designated Aviation Medical Examiner.
      Exposure to Sun: No restrictions.
      Special Storage Instructions: Oral suspension should be refrigerated.
      Observe the Following Expiration Times: Do not take the oral suspension
         of this drug if it is older than 14 days.

CEFUROXIME
(sef yur OX eem)

Introduced: 1976

Class: Antibiotic, cephalosporins

Prescription: USA: Yes

Controlled Drug: USA: No

Available as Generic: No

Brand Name: Ceftin

BENEFITS versus RISKS	
Possible Benefits	*Possible Risks*
EFFECTIVE TREATMENT OF INFECTIONS due to susceptible microorganisms	ALLERGIC REACTIONS mild to severe (up to 1% of general population, up to 2.9% of those allergic to penicillin) Drug-induced colitis (rare) Superinfections (see Glossary)

▷ **Principal Uses**
   As a Single Drug Product: Used primarily to treat certain infections of the
      middle ear, tonsils, throat, bronchial tubes, urinary tract and skin.

How This Drug Works: This drug destroys susceptible infecting bacteria by interfering with their ability to produce new protective cell walls as they multiply and grow.

Available Dosage Forms and Strengths
Tablets — 125 mg, 250 mg, 500 mg

▷ **Usual Adult Dosage Range:** 250 to 500 mg/12 hrs. Total daily dosage should not exceed 4 grams. **Note: Actual dosage and administration schedule must be determined by the physician for each patient individually.**

▷ **Dosing Instructions:** May be taken on an empty stomach or with food if stomach irritation occurs. The tablet may be crushed and mixed with food (such as applesauce or ice cream) if necessary to facilitate swallowing. (Note: The crushed tablet has a persistent, bitter taste.) Take the full course prescribed.

Usual Duration of Use: Continual use on a regular schedule for 3 to 5 days is usually necessary to determine this drug's effectiveness in controlling the infection under treatment. Response varies with the nature of the infection. Total treatment time will vary from 1 to 4 weeks. Certain infections require that this drug be taken for 10 consecutive days to prevent the development of rheumatic fever. Follow your physician's instructions regarding duration of use.

▷ **This Drug Should Not Be Taken If**
- you are allergic to any cephalosporin antibiotic (see Drug Class, Section Four).

▷ **Inform Your Physician Before Taking This Drug If**
- you have a history of allergy to any form of penicillin (see Drug Class, Section Four).
- you have a history of regional enteritis or ulcerative colitis.
- you have impaired kidney function.

Possible Side-Effects (natural, expected and unavoidable drug actions)
Superinfections (see Glossary): vaginitis (1.9%).

▷ **Possible Adverse Effects** (unusual, unexpected and infrequent reactions)
If any of the following develop, consult your physician promptly for guidance.
Mild Adverse Effects
Allergic Reactions: Skin rash (0.6%), hives (0.2%), itching (0.3%).
Nausea (2.4%), vomiting (2.0%), loose stools (1.3%), mild diarrhea (3.5%).
Headache (0.7%), dizziness (0.2%).
Serious Adverse Effects
Severe diarrhea, possibly indicating a drug-induced form of colitis (rare).

▷ **Possible Effects on Sexual Function:** None reported.

▷ **Adverse Effects That May Mimic Natural Diseases or Disorders**
Skin rash may resemble measles.

CAUTION
In the management of diabetes it should be noted that this drug can cause a false positive test result for urine sugar when using Clinitest tablets, Benedict's solution or Fehling's solution, but not with Clinistix or Tes-Tape.

Precautions for Use
By Infants and Children: The usual dose is 125 mg/12 hours. For middle ear infection, the recommended dose for those under 2 years of age is 125 mg/12 hours, and 250 mg/12 hours for those over 2 years of age.
By Those over 60 Years of Age: Dosage must be carefully individualized and based upon evaluation of kidney function. Natural changes in the skin may predispose to severe and prolonged itching reactions in the genital and anal regions. Such reactions should be reported promptly.

▷ **Advisability of Use During Pregnancy**
Pregnancy Category: B (tentative). See Pregnancy Code inside back cover.
Animal studies: No birth defects due to this drug reported in mouse and rat studies.
Human studies: Information from adequate studies of pregnant women is not available.
Generally considered to be safe. Ask physician for guidance.

Advisability of Use if Breast-Feeding
Presence of this drug in breast milk: Yes, in small amounts.
Avoid drug or refrain from nursing.

Habit-Forming Potential: None.

Effects of Overdosage: Nausea, vomiting, stomach cramps and/or diarrhea.

Possible Effects of Long-Term Use: Superinfections (see Glossary).

Suggested Periodic Examinations While Taking This Drug (at physician's discretion)
None.

▷ **While Taking This Drug, Observe the Following**
Foods: No restrictions. Food enhances the absorption of this drug.
Beverages: No restrictions. May be taken with milk.
▷   *Alcohol:* No interactions expected.
Tobacco Smoking: No interactions expected.
▷   *Other Drugs*
Cefuroxime **taken concurrently** with
• probenecid (Benemid) will slow the elimination of cefuroxime, resulting in higher blood levels and prolonged effect.

▷ *Driving, Hazardous Activities:* Usually no restrictions. Observe for the rare occurrence of dizziness.
   Aviation Note: The use of this drug **may be a disqualification** for piloting. Consult a designated Aviation Medical Examiner.
   Exposure to Sun: No restrictions.

CEPHALEXIN
(sef a LEX in)

Introduced: 1969

Class: Antibiotic, cephalosporins

Prescription: USA: Yes
   Canada: Yes

Controlled Drug: USA: No
   Canada: No

Available as Generic: Yes

Brand Names: ✦Ceporex, Keflet, Keflex, Keftab, ✦Novolexin

BENEFITS versus RISKS	
Possible Benefits	*Possible Risks*
EFFECTIVE TREATMENT OF INFECTIONS due to susceptible microorganisms	ALLERGIC REACTIONS mild to severe (up to 5% of general population, up to 16% of those allergic to penicillin) Drug-induced colitis (rare) Superinfections (see Glossary)

▷ **Principal Uses**
   As a Single Drug Product: To treat certain infections of the skin and skin structures, the upper respiratory tract (including middle ear infections and "strep" throat), the genitourinary tract and certain infections involving bones and joints.

   How This Drug Works: This drug destroys susceptible infecting bacteria by interfering with their ability to produce new protective cell walls as they multiply and grow.

   Available Dosage Forms and Strengths
   Capsules — 250 mg, 500 mg
   Oral suspension — 125 mg, 250 mg per 5-ml teaspoonful
   Pediatric oral suspension — 100 mg per ml
   Tablets — 250 mg, 500 mg, 1000 mg (1 gram)

▷ **Usual Adult Dosage Range:** 250 to 500 mg/6 hours. Total daily dose should not exceed 4 grams. **Note: Actual dosage and administration schedule must be determined by the physician for each patient individually.**

▷ **Dosing Instructions:** May be taken on an empty stomach or with food if stomach irritation occurs. Capsule may be opened and tablet may be crushed for administration. Shake suspension well before measuring dose. Take the full course prescribed.

Usual Duration of Use: Continual use on a regular schedule for 3 to 5 days is usually necessary to determine this drug's effectiveness in controlling the infection under treatment. Response varies with the nature of the infection. Total treatment time will vary from 1 to 4 weeks. Certain infections require that this drug be taken for 10 consecutive days to prevent the development of rheumatic fever. Follow your physician's instructions regarding duration of use.

▷ **This Drug Should Not Be Taken If**
- you are allergic to any cephalosporin antibiotic (see Drug Class, Section Four).

▷ **Inform Your Physician Before Taking This Drug If**
- you have a history of allergy to any form of penicillin (see Drug Class, Section Four).
- you have a history of regional enteritis or ulcerative colitis.
- you have impaired kidney function.

Possible Side-Effects (natural, expected and unavoidable drug actions)
Superinfections (see Glossary).

▷ **Possible Adverse Effects** (unusual, unexpected and infrequent reactions)
If any of the following develop, consult your physician promptly for guidance.
Mild Adverse Effects
Allergic Reactions: Skin rash (0.8%), itching, hives (0.3%).
Headache, drowsiness, dizziness.
Irritation of mouth or tongue, indigestion, stomach cramping, nausea, vomiting (1.8%), diarrhea (1.1%).
Serious Adverse Effects
Allergic Reactions: Drug fever (see Glossary), joint aches and pains, anaphylactic reaction (see Glossary).
Idiosyncratic Reactions: Minor and temporary changes in white blood cell counts and liver function tests (infrequent).
Genital itching (may represent a fungus superinfection).
Severe diarrhea, possibly indicating a drug-induced form of colitis (rare).

▷ **Possible Effects on Sexual Function:** None reported.

▷ **Adverse Effects That May Mimic Natural Diseases or Disorders**
Skin rash and fever may resemble measles.

CAUTION
1. In the management of diabetes it should be noted that this drug can cause a false positive test result for urine sugar when using

Clinitest tablets, Benedict's solution or Fehling's solution, but not with Tes-Tape.

2. Do not use this drug concurrently with other antibiotics such as erythromycin or tetracyclines.

Precautions for Use
By Infants and Children: Not recommended for use in infants less than 1 year old. Monitor allergic children closely for evidence of developing allergy to this drug.

By Those over 60 Years of Age: Dosage must be carefully individualized and based upon evaluation of kidney function. Natural changes in the skin may predispose to severe and prolonged itching reactions in the genital and anal regions. Such reactions should be reported promptly.

▷ Advisability of Use During Pregnancy
Pregnancy Category: B (tentative). See Pregnancy Code inside back cover.
Animal studies: No birth defects reported.
Human studies: Information from adequate studies of pregnant women is not available.
Generally considered to be safe. Ask physician for guidance.

Advisability of Use if Breast-Feeding
Presence of this drug in breast milk: Yes, in small amounts.
Avoid drug or refrain from nursing.

Habit-Forming Potential: None.

Effects of Overdosage: Nausea, vomiting, stomach cramps and/or diarrhea.

Possible Effects of Long-Term Use: Superinfections (see Glossary).

Suggested Periodic Examinations While Taking This Drug (at physician's discretion)
Complete blood cell counts. Liver and kidney function tests.

▷ While Taking This Drug, Observe the Following
Foods: No restrictions.
Beverages: No restrictions. May be taken with milk.
▷   *Alcohol:* No interactions expected.
Tobacco Smoking: No interactions expected.
▷   *Other Drugs*
Cephalexin *taken concurrently* with
• probenecid (Benemid) will slow the elimination of cephalexin, resulting in higher blood levels and prolonged effect.
▷   *Driving, Hazardous Activities:* Usually no restrictions. Use caution if drowsiness or dizziness occurs.
Aviation Note: The use of this drug *may be a disqualification* for piloting. Consult a designated Aviation Medical Examiner.
Exposure to Sun: No restrictions.

Special Storage Instructions: Oral suspension should be refrigerated.
Observe the Following Expiration Times: Do not take the oral suspension
of this drug if it is older than 14 days.

CHLORAL HYDRATE
(klor al HI drayt)

Introduced: 1832

Prescription: USA: Yes
Canada: Yes

Available as Generic: Yes

Class: Sedative, hypnotic

Controlled Drug: USA: C-IV*
Canada: No

Brand Names: Aquachloral Supprettes, Noctec, ◆Novochlorhydrate

---

BENEFITS versus RISKS

Possible Benefits	*Possible Risks*
EFFECTIVE HYPNOTIC for short-term use (2 weeks)	DRUG DEPENDENCE with prolonged use
Effective daytime sedative for intermittent use	Severe allergic skin reactions
	Paradoxical excitement, delirium, psychotic behavior (infrequent)

▷ **Principal Uses**

As a Single Drug Product: Used primarily as a bedtime sedative in sufficient dosage to induce sleep. It is the drug of choice for use in the
elderly because it produces less "hangover" effect and is less likely to
cause the confusion so commonly seen with use of barbiturates.

How This Drug Works: Not completely known. It is converted into an
alcohol, which is thought to have a sedative effect on the wake-sleep
centers of the brain.

Available Dosage Forms and Strengths
Capsules — 250 mg, 500 mg
Suppositories — 324 mg, 500 mg, 648 mg
Syrup — 250 mg, 500 mg per 5-ml teaspoonful

▷ **Usual Adult Dosage Range:** As sedative—250 mg 3 times daily. As hypnotic—500 to 1000 mg, 15 to 30 minutes before bedtime. Total daily
dosage should not exceed 2000 mg (2 grams). **Note: Actual dosage
and administration schedule must be determined by the physician
for each patient individually.**

---

*See Schedules of Controlled Drugs inside back cover.

▷ **Dosing Instructions:**   Take capsules whole (unopened) with a full glass of water, fruit juice or ginger ale to prevent stomach irritation. Mix the elixir or syrup in half a glass of water, fruit juice or ginger ale. Daytime doses are best taken after meals.

Usual Duration of Use: As sedative, use intermittently and not on a regular basis. As hypnotic, limit use to periods of 7 to 10 days. Avoid continual and prolonged use. Duration of use should not exceed 14 days without drug-free periods of several days, and reappraisal of continued need.

▷ **This Drug Should Not Be Taken If**
  • you have had an allergic or unfavorable reaction to it previously.
  • you have severely impaired liver or kidney function.
  • you have severe heart disease.
  • you have active gastritis or peptic ulcer disease.
  • you have a history of intermittent porphyria.

▷ **Inform Your Physician Before Taking This Drug If**
  • you have a history of heart disease or peptic ulcer disease.
  • you are taking other sedatives, hypnotics, tranquilizers or narcotic drugs of any kind.
  • you plan to have surgery under general anesthesia in the near future.

Possible Side-Effects (natural, expected and unavoidable drug actions)
Light-headedness in upright position, unsteadiness, weakness.
"Hangover" effect following nighttime use as hypnotic.

▷ **Possible Adverse Effects** (unusual, unexpected and infrequent reactions)
If any of the following develop, consult your physician promptly for guidance.
Mild Adverse Effects
Allergic Reactions: Skin rashes, hives, conjunctivitis.
Dizziness, confusion, hallucinations, nightmares.
Unpleasant taste, stomach irritation, nausea, vomiting, diarrhea.
Serious Adverse Effects
Allergic Reactions: Severe forms of dermatitis.
Idiosyncratic Reactions: Sleepwalking, delirium, disorientation, paranoid behavior.
Double vision, temporary blindness.
Reduced formation of white blood cells.

▷ **Possible Effects on Sexual Function:**   None reported.

Possible Delayed Adverse Effects: Allergic skin reactions may occur up to 10 days following the last dose.

▷ **Adverse Effects That May Mimic Natural Diseases or Disorders**
Paradoxical excitement or delirium may suggest latent psychosis.

Natural Diseases or Disorders That May Be Activated by This Drug
Intermittent porphyria.

CAUTION
1. Use with caution in the presence of bronchial asthma. Avoid high and frequent doses.
2. Take all doses well diluted with water, milk, fruit juice or ginger ale to prevent stomach irritation.

Precautions for Use
By Infants and Children: Avoid concurrent use with other drugs that have a sedative effect. Use very cautiously in asthmatic children.

By Those over 60 Years of Age: Small doses are advisable until your individual response has been determined. You may be more susceptible to the development of "hangover" effect, dizziness, confused thinking, impaired memory, unsteadiness, loss of bladder control or constipation.

▷ ### Advisability of Use During Pregnancy
Pregnancy Category: C (tentative). See Pregnancy Code inside back cover.
Animal studies: No information available.
Human studies: Information from adequate studies of pregnant women is not available.
Use this drug only if clearly needed. Continual use during pregnancy can cause withdrawal symptoms in the newborn infant.

Advisability of Use if Breast-Feeding
Presence of this drug in breast milk: Yes.
Monitor nursing infant closely and discontinue drug or nursing if adverse effects develop.

Habit-Forming Potential: This drug can cause psychological and/or physical dependence (see Glossary). Avoid large doses and continual use.

Effects of Overdosage: Marked drowsiness, confusion, incoordination, slurred speech, staggering gait, weakness, vomiting, stupor, deep sleep.

Possible Effects of Long-Term Use: Psychological and/or physical dependence, toxic psychosis, liver and kidney damage.

Suggested Periodic Examinations While Taking This Drug (at physician's discretion)
Complete blood cell counts. Liver and kidney function tests.

▷ ### While Taking This Drug, Observe the Following
Foods: No restrictions.
Beverages: No restrictions. May be taken with milk.
▷ *Alcohol:* Avoid completely for at least 6 hours before taking this drug. Alcohol can greatly increase the sedative and depressant actions of this drug on brain function.
Tobacco Smoking: No interactions expected.
Marijuana Smoking: Increased drowsiness, impaired mental and physical performance.

▷ *Other Drugs*

Chloral hydrate may ***increase*** the effects of

- oral anticoagulants (Coumadin, etc.), and cause abnormal bleeding or hemorrhage. Consult physician regarding prothrombin time testing and dosage adjustment.

▷ *Driving, Hazardous Activities:* This drug can impair mental alertness, judgment, physical coordination and reaction time. Avoid hazardous activities until all sensation of drowsiness has disappeared.

Aviation Note: The use of this drug ***is a disqualification*** for piloting. Consult a designated Aviation Medical Examiner.

Exposure to Sun: No restrictions.

Discontinuation: If this drug has been used continually over an extended period of time, it should be discontinued gradually under physician supervision.

CHLORAMPHENICOL
(klor am FEN i kohl)

Introduced: 1947

Class: Antibiotic

Prescription: USA: Yes
Canada: Yes

Controlled Drug: USA: No
Canada: No

Available as Generic: USA: Yes
Canada: No

Brand Names: Ak-Chlor, Chloromycetin, Chloroptic, ✦Fenicol, ✦Isopto Fenicol, ✦Minims, ✦Nova-Phenicol, ✦Novochlorocap, Ophthochlor, ✦Pentamycetin

BENEFITS versus RISKS	
Possible Benefits	*Possible Risks*
VERY EFFECTIVE TREATMENT OF INFECTIONS due to susceptible microorganisms	BONE MARROW DEPRESSION APLASTIC ANEMIA (see Glossary) Peripheral neuritis (see Glossary) Liver damage, jaundice

▷ **Principal Uses**

As a Single Drug Product: This drug is quite effective in a broad spectrum of serious infections. However, because of its potential for serious toxicity (fatal aplastic anemia), its use is now reserved for life-threatening infections caused by organisms that are resistant to safer antibiotics, and for infections in individuals who, for one reason or another, cannot take other appropriate anti-infective drugs.

How This Drug Works: This drug prevents the growth and multiplication of susceptible microorganisms by interfering with their formation of essential proteins.

Available Dosage Forms and Strengths
               Capsules — 250 mg, 500 mg
                  Cream — 1%
        Eye/ear solutions — 0.5%
          Eye ointment — 1%
               Injection — 100 mg per ml
        Oral suspension — 150 mg per 5-ml teaspoonful

▷ **Usual Adult Dosage Range:**   Total daily dose is 250 mg for each 10 pounds of body weight, given in 4 equally divided doses, 6 hours apart. Total daily dose should not exceed 500 mg for each 10 pounds of body weight. **Note: Actual dosage and administration schedule must be determined by the physician for each patient individually.**

▷ **Dosing Instructions:**   Take with a full glass of water on an empty stomach, 1 hour before or 2 hours after eating. Capsule may be opened for administration. Shake oral suspension well before measuring dose.

Usual Duration of Use: Continual use on a regular schedule for 3 to 5 days is usually necessary to determine this drug's effectiveness in controlling the infection. Limit use to the time required to eradicate the infection. Avoid repeated courses of treatment if possible.

▷ **This Drug Should Not Be Taken If**
   • you have had an allergic reaction to it previously.
   • you have an active blood cell or bone marrow disorder.
   • it is prescribed for a mild or trivial infection such as a cold, sore throat or "flulike" illness.
   • it is prescribed for a premature or newborn infant (under 2 weeks of age).

▷ **Inform Your Physician Before Taking This Drug If**
   • you have a history of a blood cell or bone marrow disorder.
   • you have impaired liver or kidney function.
   • you are taking anticoagulants.

Possible Side-Effects (natural, expected and unavoidable drug actions)
   Superinfections (see Glossary).

▷ **Possible Adverse Effects** (unusual, unexpected and infrequent reactions)
   If any of the following develop, consult your physician promptly for guidance.
   Mild Adverse Effects
   Allergic Reactions: Skin rashes, hives, swelling of face or extremities, fever.

Headache, confusion, peripheral neuritis (see Glossary)—numbness, pain, weakness in hands and/or feet.

Sore mouth or tongue, "black tongue," nausea, vomiting, diarrhea.

Serious Adverse Effects

Allergic Reactions: Anaphylactic reaction (see Glossary), liver damage with jaundice (rare).

Bone marrow depression (see Glossary)—fatigue, weakness, fever, sore throat, abnormal bleeding or bruising.

▷ **Possible Effects on Sexual Function:**   None reported.

▷ **Adverse Effects That May Mimic Natural Diseases or Disorders**
Liver reaction with jaundice may suggest viral hepatitis.

CAUTION

1. This drug can cause serious bone marrow depression and aplastic anemia (see Glossary). It must not be used to treat trivial infections or as a preventive medication under any circumstances. Its use must be restricted to the treatment of serious or life-threatening infections that fail to respond to other anti-infective drugs.
2. Troublesome and persistent diarrhea can develop in sensitive individuals. If diarrhea persists for more than 24 hours, discontinue this drug and consult your physician.

Precautions for Use

By Infants and Children: Follow prescribed dosage exactly. Blood cell counts should be monitored twice a week. Long-term use of this drug can cause optic neuritis. This may be prevented by taking supplemental vitamin B complex during treatment. Idiosyncratic aplastic anemia is rare (1 in 40,000 users), but may occur weeks or months after discontinuation of this drug.

By Those over 60 Years of Age: The natural decline in liver and kidney function after 60 may require reduction in dosage and adjustment of dosage interval. Natural changes in the skin after 60 may predispose to severe and prolonged itching reactions in the genital and anal regions. Report such reactions promptly.

▷ **Advisability of Use During Pregnancy**
Pregnancy Category: C (tentative). See Pregnancy Code inside back cover.
Animal studies: Results are inconclusive.
Human studies: Information from adequate studies of pregnant women is not available. Limited studies (348 exposures) indicate that this drug does not cause birth defects. However, it has been shown to be potentially toxic for the fetus and newborn. Ask physician for guidance.

Advisability of Use if Breast-Feeding

Presence of this drug in breast milk: Yes.
Avoid drug or refrain from nursing.

Habit-Forming Potential: None.

Effects of Overdosage: Possible nausea, vomiting, diarrhea.

Possible Effects of Long-Term Use: Superinfections, impaired vision, bone marrow depression.

Suggested Periodic Examinations While Taking This Drug (at physician's discretion)
Complete blood cell counts—before treatment is started and every 2 to 3 days during administration of drug.
Liver and kidney function tests.

▷ **While Taking This Drug, Observe the Following**
Foods: No restrictions.
Nutritional Support: Supplemental vitamins B-2, B-6 and B-12 are recommended.
Beverages: No restrictions. May be taken with milk.
▷ *Alcohol:* Avoid completely if you have liver disease. Use cautiously until the combined effect has been determined. Some sensitive individuals may develop a disulfiramlike reaction (see Glossary).
Tobacco Smoking: No interactions expected.
▷ *Other Drugs*
Chloramphenicol may ***increase*** the effects of
- oral anticoagulants (Coumadin, dicumarol, etc.), and increase the risk of bleeding.
- barbiturates (phenobarbital, etc.), and cause excessive sedation.
- phenytoin (Dilantin), and cause phenytoin toxicity.
- sulfonylureas (Diabinese, Dymelor, Orinase, Tolinase), and cause hypoglycemia (see Glossary).
Chloramphenicol may ***decrease*** the effects of
- iron preparations, used to treat anemia.
- penicillins.
- vitamin B-12.
The following drugs may ***decrease*** the effects of chloramphenicol
- barbiturates (phenobarbital, etc.).
- rifampin (Rifadin, Rimactane, etc.).
▷ *Driving, Hazardous Activities:* Usually no restrictions. Be alert to the rare occurrence of confusion, and restrict activities accordingly.
Aviation Note: The use of this drug ***may be a disqualification*** for piloting. Consult a designated Aviation Medical Examiner.
Exposure to Sun: No restrictions.

CHLORDIAZEPOXIDE
(klor di az e POX ide)

Introduced: 1960

Class: Mild tranquilizer, benzodi-azepines

Prescription: USA: Yes
Canada: Yes

Controlled Drug: USA: C-IV*
Canada: No

Available as Generic: Yes

Brand Names: ✦Apo-Chlorax [CD], ✦Apo-Chlordiazepoxide, ✦Corium [CD], Librax [CD], Libritabs, Librium, Lidox [CD], Limbitrol [CD], Lipox-ide, Menrium [CD], ✦Novopoxide, ✦Pentrium [CD], ✦Solium

---

BENEFITS versus RISKS

Possible Benefits	*Possible Risks*
RELIEF OF ANXIETY AND NERVOUS TENSION in 70% to 80% of users	Habit-forming potential with prolonged use
Wide margin of safety with therapeutic doses	Minor impairment of mental functions
Very few drug interactions	Very rare jaundice
	Very rare blood cell disorders

▷ **Principal Uses**

As a Single Drug Product: Used primarily to (1) provide short-term relief of mild to moderate anxiety, and (2) relieve the symptoms of acute alcohol withdrawal: agitation, tremors, hallucinations, incipient delirium tremens.

As a Combination Drug Product [CD]: Used in combination with amitriptyline (an antidepressant) to allay the anxiety that is often a troublesome feature in the agitated and depressed individual. Also used in combination with clidinium (a synthetic atropinelike antispasmodic) to treat peptic ulcer disease and irritable bowel syndrome.

How This Drug Works: It is thought that this drug produces a calming effect by enhancing the action of the nerve transmitter gamma-aminobutyric acid (GABA), which in turn blocks the arousal of higher brain centers.

Available Dosage Forms and Strengths
Capsules — 5 mg, 10 mg, 25 mg
Injection — 100 mg/ampul
Tablets — 5 mg, 10 mg, 25 mg

*See Schedules of Controlled Drugs inside back cover.

▷ **Usual Adult Dosage Range:** 5 to 25 mg, 3 or 4 times daily. Dose may be increased cautiously as needed and tolerated. After 1 week of continual use, the total daily dose may be taken at bedtime. Total daily dose should not exceed 150 mg for anxiety and tension, or 300 mg for alcohol withdrawal. **Note: Actual dosage and administration schedule must be determined by the physician for each patient individually.**

▷ **Dosing Instructions:** May be taken on empty stomach or with food or milk. Capsule may be opened and tablet may be crushed for administration. Do not discontinue this drug abruptly if taken for more than 4 weeks.

Usual Duration of Use: Continual use on a regular schedule for 3 to 5 days is usually necessary to determine this drug's effectiveness in relieving moderate anxiety. Limit continual use to 1 to 3 weeks. Avoid uninterrupted and prolonged use.

▷ **This Drug Should Not Be Taken If**
- you have had an allergic reaction to any dosage form of it previously.
- you have acute narrow-angle glaucoma.
- it is prescribed for a child under 6 years of age.

▷ **Inform Your Physician Before Taking This Drug If**
- you are allergic to any benzodiazepine drug (see Drug Class, Section Four).
- you have a history of alcoholism or drug abuse.
- you are pregnant or planning pregnancy.
- you have impaired liver or kidney function.
- you have a history of serious depression or mental disorder.
- you have any of the following: asthma, emphysema, epilepsy, myasthenia gravis, porphyria.

Possible Side-Effects (natural, expected and unavoidable drug actions)
Drowsiness (3.9%), lethargy, unsteadiness; "hangover" effects on the day following bedtime use.

▷ **Possible Adverse Effects** (unusual, unexpected and infrequent reactions)
If any of the following develop, consult your physician promptly for guidance.
Mild Adverse Effects
Allergic Reactions: Rashes, fixed skin eruptions, bruising.
Dizziness, fainting, blurred vision, double vision, slurred speech, sweating, nausea.
Serious Adverse Effects
Allergic Reactions: Liver damage with jaundice (see Glossary), abnormally low blood platelet count.
Idiosyncratic Reaction: Acute hepatic porphyria.
Bone marrow depression—impaired production of red and white blood cells.
Paradoxical responses of excitement, agitation, anger, rage.

▷ **Possible Effects on Sexual Function**

Decreased libido with high doses, increased libido with low doses (antianxiety effect); rare report of inhibited ejaculation.

Altered timing and pattern of menstruation; female breast enlargement and milk production.

▷ **Adverse Effects That May Mimic Natural Diseases or Disorders**

Liver reaction with jaundice may suggest viral hepatitis.

Natural Diseases or Disorders That May Be Activated by This Drug

Acute intermittent hepatic porphyria, systemic lupus erythematosus–like syndrome.

CAUTION

1. This drug should not be discontinued abruptly if it has been taken continually for more than 4 weeks.
2. The concurrent use of some over-the-counter drug products that contain antihistamines (allergy and cold preparations, sleep aids) can cause excessive sedation in sensitive individuals.

Precautions for Use

By Infants and Children: Safety and effectiveness for use by those under 6 years of age have not been established. This drug should not be used in the hyperactive or psychotic child of any age.

By Those over 60 Years of Age: It is advisable to use smaller doses at longer intervals to avoid overdosage. Observe for the possible development of lethargy, indifference, fatigue, weakness, unsteadiness, disturbing dreams, nightmares and paradoxical reactions of excitement, agitation, anger, hostility and rage.

▷ **Advisability of Use During Pregnancy**

Pregnancy Category: D (tentative). See Pregnancy Code inside back cover.

Animal studies: Cleft palate reported in mice.

Human studies: Available information is conflicting and inconclusive. Some studies found a fourfold increase in serious birth defects associated with the use of this drug. Other studies have found no significant increase in birth defects.

Frequent use in late pregnancy can cause the "floppy infant" syndrome in the newborn: weakness, lethargy, unresponsiveness, depressed breathing, low body temperature.

Avoid use during entire pregnancy if possible.

Advisability of Use if Breast-Feeding

Presence of this drug in breast milk: Yes, in small amounts.

Monitor nursing infant closely and discontinue drug or nursing if adverse effects develop.

Habit-Forming Potential: This drug can produce psychological and/or physical dependence (see Glossary) if used in large doses for an extended period of time.

Effects of Overdosage: Marked drowsiness, weakness, feeling of drunkenness, staggering gait, tremor, stupor progressing to deep sleep or coma.

Possible Effects of Long-Term Use: Psychological and/or physical dependence, rare blood cell disorders.

Suggested Periodic Examinations While Taking This Drug (at physician's discretion)
Complete blood cell counts during long-term use.

▷ **While Taking This Drug, Observe the Following**
Foods: No restrictions.
Beverages: Avoid excessive intake of caffeine-containing beverages: coffee, tea, cola. May be taken with milk.

▷ *Alcohol:* Use with extreme caution until the combined effect is determined. Alcohol may increase the absorption of this drug and add to its depressant effects on the brain. It is advisable to avoid alcohol completely—throughout the day and night—if it is necessary to drive or to engage in any hazardous activity.
Tobacco Smoking: Heavy smoking may reduce the calming action of this drug.
Marijuana Smoking: Increased sedation and significant impairment of intellectual and physical performance.

▷ *Other Drugs*
Chlordiazepoxide may *increase* the effects of
• digoxin (Lanoxin), and cause digoxin toxicity.
Chlordiazepoxide may *decrease* the effects of
• levodopa (Sinemet, etc.), and reduce its effectiveness in treating Parkinson's disease.
The following drugs may *increase* the effects of chlordiazepoxide
• cimetidine (Tagamet).
• disulfiram (Antabuse).
• isoniazid (INH, Rifamate, etc.).
• oral contraceptives.
• valproic acid (Depakene).
The following drugs may *decrease* the effects of chlordiazepoxide
• rifampin (Rimactane, etc.).
• theophylline (aminophylline, Theo-Dur, etc.).

▷ *Driving, Hazardous Activities:* This drug can impair mental alertness, judgment, physical coordination and reaction time. Avoid hazardous activities accordingly.
Aviation Note: The use of this drug *is a disqualification* for piloting. Consult a designated Aviation Medical Examiner.
Exposure to Sun: Use caution until sensitivity is determined. A photoallergic skin reaction may occur rarely.
Discontinuation: Avoid sudden discontinuation if this drug has been taken for over 4 weeks. Dosage should be tapered gradually to prevent a withdrawal syndrome that could include depression, confusion, hal-

lucinations, tremor, seizures, muscle cramping, sweating and vomiting.

CHLOROTHIAZIDE
(klor oh THI a zide)

Introduced: 1957

Class: Antihypertensive, diuretic, thiazides

Prescription: USA: Yes

Controlled Drug: USA: No

Available as Generic: USA: Yes

Brand Names: Aldoclor [CD], Diachlor, Diupres [CD], Diurigen, Diuril

---

BENEFITS versus RISKS

Possible Benefits	*Possible Risks*
EFFECTIVE, WELL-TOLERATED DIURETIC	Loss of body potassium
POSSIBLY EFFECTIVE IN MILD HYPERTENSION	Increased blood sugar
ENHANCES EFFECTIVENESS OF OTHER ANTIHYPERTENSIVES	Increased blood uric acid
Beneficial in treatment of diabetes insipidus	Increased blood calcium
	Rare blood cell disorders

▷ **Principal Uses**

As a Single Drug Product: Thiazide diuretics are used primarily to (1) increase the volume of urine (diuresis) to correct the excessive fluid retention associated with congestive heart failure and certain types of liver and kidney disease; and (2) initiate treatment for high blood pressure (hypertension). They are often the first drugs tried in treating mild to moderate hypertension. Less frequent uses include the treatment of diabetes insipidus and the prevention of kidney stones that contain calcium.

As a Combination Drug Product [CD]: When this drug is used alone to treat hypertension, it is referred to as a "step 1" antihypertensive. Should it fail to reduce the blood pressure adequately, a "step 2" antihypertensive drug is added to be taken concurrently with the "step 1" drug. These drugs may be combined into one drug product. Thiazides are available in combination with beta blockers, hydralazine, methyldopa, reserpine and other diuretics to increase their effectiveness in treating hypertension.

How This Drug Works: By increasing the elimination of salt and water from the body (through increased urine production), this drug reduces the volume of fluid in the blood and body tissues and lowers the sodium content throughout the body. By relaxing the walls of smaller arteries and allowing them to expand, this drug increases the total capacity of the arterial system. The combined effect of these two actions (reduced blood volume in expanded space) results in lowering of the blood pressure.

Available Dosage Forms and Strengths
Injection — 500 mg per 20 ml
Oral suspension — 250 mg per 5-ml teaspoonful
Tablets — 250 mg, 500 mg

▷ **Usual Adult Dosage Range:** As antihypertensive: 500 to 1000 mg/day initially; 500 to 2000 mg/day for maintenance. As diuretic: 500 to 2000 mg/day initially; the smallest effective dose should be determined. The total daily dose should not exceed 2000 mg. **Note: Actual dosage and administration schedule must be determined by the physician for each patient individually.**

▷ **Dosing Instructions:** May be taken with or following meals to reduce stomach irritation. Best taken in the morning to avoid nighttime urination. The tablet may be crushed for administration.

Usual Duration of Use: Continual use on a regular schedule for 2 to 3 weeks is usually necessary to determine this drug's effectiveness in lowering high blood pressure. Long-term use (months to years) requires periodic evaluation of response and possible dosage adjustment. Use as a diuretic should be intermittent with "drug holidays" (no drug taken) to reduce the risk of sodium and potassium imbalance. Consult your physician on a regular basis.

▷ **This Drug Should Not Be Taken If**
• you have had an allergic reaction to any dosage form of it previously.

▷ **Inform Your Physician Before Taking This Drug If**
• you are allergic to any form of "sulfa" drug.
• you are pregnant or planning pregnancy.
• you have a history of kidney or liver disease.
• you have diabetes, gout or lupus erythematosus.
• you are taking any form of cortisone, digitalis, oral antidiabetic drug or insulin.
• you plan to have surgery under general anesthesia in the near future.

Possible Side-Effects (natural, expected and unavoidable drug actions)
Light-headedness on arising from sitting or lying position (see Orthostatic Hypotension in Glossary).
Increase in blood sugar level, affecting control of diabetes.
Increase in blood uric acid level, affecting control of gout.

Decrease in blood potassium level, causing muscle weakness and cramping.

▷ **Possible Adverse Effects** (unusual, unexpected and infrequent reactions)
If any of the following develop, consult your physician promptly for guidance.

Mild Adverse Effects
Allergic Reactions: Skin rashes, hives, drug fever.
Headache, dizziness, blurred or yellow vision.
Reduced appetite, indigestion, nausea, vomiting, diarrhea.

Serious Adverse Effects
Allergic Reactions: Hepatitis with jaundice (see Glossary), anaphylactic reaction (see Glossary), severe skin reactions.
Inflammation of the pancreas—severe abdominal pain.
Bone marrow depression (see Glossary)—fatigue, weakness, fever, sore throat, abnormal bleeding or bruising.

▷ **Possible Effects on Sexual Function:**   Impotence (500 to 2000 mg/day).

▷ **Adverse Effects That May Mimic Natural Diseases or Disorders**
Liver reaction may suggest viral hepatitis.

Natural Diseases or Disorders That May Be Activated by This Drug
Diabetes, gout, systemic lupus erythematosus.

CAUTION
1. Do not exceed recommended doses. Increased dosage can cause excessive loss of sodium and potassium, with resultant loss of appetite, nausea, fatigue, weakness, confusion and tingling in the extremities.
2. If you are also taking a digitalis preparation (digitoxin, digoxin), ensure an adequate intake of high-potassium foods to prevent potassium deficiency—a potential cause of digitalis toxicity. (See Table of High Potassium Foods in Section Six.)

Precautions for Use
By Infants and Children: Avoid overdosage that could cause serious dehydration. Significant potassium loss can occur within the first 2 weeks of drug use.
By Those over 60 Years of Age: Small doses are advisable until your individual response has been determined. You may be more susceptible to the development of impaired thinking, orthostatic hypotension, potassium loss and blood sugar increase. Overdosage and extended use of this drug can cause excessive loss of body water, thickening (increased viscosity) of the blood and an increased tendency for the blood to clot—predisposing to stroke, heart attack or thrombophlebitis (vein inflammation with blood clot).

▷ **Advisability of Use During Pregnancy**
Pregnancy Category: D (tentative). See Pregnancy Code inside back cover.
Animal studies: No birth defects found in rat studies.

Human studies: Reports are conflicting and inconclusive. This drug does not seem to carry the risk of birth defects that has been found with other related diuretics. However, other types of fetal injury are possible with this drug. It should not be used during pregnancy unless a very serious complication occurs for which this drug is significantly beneficial. Ask physician for guidance.

Advisability of Use if Breast-Feeding
Presence of this drug in breast milk: Yes, in small amounts.
Avoid drug or refrain from nursing.

Habit-Forming Potential: None.

Effects of Overdosage: Dry mouth, thirst, lethargy, weakness, muscle cramping, nausea, vomiting, drowsiness progressing to stupor or coma.

Possible Effects of Long-Term Use: Impaired balance of water, salt and potassium in blood and body tissues. Development of diabetes in predisposed individuals. Pathological changes in parathyroid glands with increased blood calcium levels and decreased blood phosphate levels.

Suggested Periodic Examinations While Taking This Drug (at physician's discretion)
Complete blood cell counts, measurements of blood levels of sodium, potassium, chloride, sugar and uric acid.
Kidney and liver function tests.

▷ **While Taking This Drug, Observe the Following**
Foods: Consult your physician regarding the advisability of eating foods rich in potassium. If so advised, see the Table of High Potassium Foods in Section Six. Follow physician's advice regarding the use of salt.
Beverages: No restrictions. This drug may be taken with milk.
▷   *Alcohol:* Use with caution until the combined effects have been determined. Alcohol may exaggerate the blood-pressure-lowering effects of this drug and cause orthostatic hypotension.
Tobacco Smoking: No interactions expected. Follow physician's advice.
▷   *Other Drugs*
Chlorothiazide may ***increase*** the effects of
- other antihypertensive drugs; dosage adjustments may be necessary to prevent excessive lowering of blood pressure.
- lithium, and cause lithium toxicity.
Chlorothiazide may ***decrease*** the effects of
- oral antidiabetic drugs (sulfonylureas); dosage adjustments may be necessary for proper control of blood sugar.
Chlorothiazide ***taken concurrently*** with
- digitalis preparations (digitoxin, digoxin) requires very careful monitoring and dosage adjustments to prevent fluctuations of blood potassium levels and serious disturbances of heart rhythm.

The following drugs may *decrease* the effects of chlorothiazide
- cholestyramine (Cuemid, Questran) may interfere with its absorption.
- colestipol (Colestid) may interfere with its absorption.

Take cholestyramine and colestipol 1 hour before any oral diuretic.

▷ *Driving, Hazardous Activities:* Use caution until the possible occurrence of orthostatic hypotension, dizziness or impaired vision has been determined.

Aviation Note: The use of this drug *may be a disqualification* for piloting. Consult a designated Aviation Medical Examiner.

Exposure to Sun: Use caution until sensitivity has been determined. This drug can cause photosensitivity (see Glossary).

Exposure to Heat: Avoid excessive perspiring, which could cause additional loss of salt and water from the body.

Heavy Exercise or Exertion: Avoid exertion that produces light-headedness, excessive fatigue or muscle cramping. Isometric exercises—the "overload" technique for strengthening individual muscles—can raise blood pressure significantly. Ask physician for guidance regarding participation in this form of exercise.

Occurrence of Unrelated Illness: Illnesses that cause vomiting or diarrhea can produce a serious imbalance of important body chemistry. Consult your physician for guidance.

Discontinuation: This drug should not be stopped abruptly following long-term use; serious thiazide-withdrawal fluid retention (edema) can develop after sudden withdrawal. The dose should be reduced gradually. It may be advisable to discontinue this drug 5 to 7 days before major surgery. Ask your physician, surgeon and/or anesthesiologist for guidance regarding dosage adjustment or drug withdrawal.

CHLORPHENIRAMINE
(klor fen IR a meen)

Introduced: 1949

Prescription: USA: Varies
Canada: No

Available as Generic: USA: Yes
Canada: Yes

Class: Antihistamines

Controlled Drug: USA: No
Canada: No

Brand Names: Alka-Seltzer Plus [CD], Allerest Tablets [CD], Chlor-Trimeton, ✦Chlor-Tripolon, ✦Chlor-Tripolon Decongestant [CD], Contac Severe Cold Formula Caplets [CD], Contac 12-Hour Capsules [CD], ✦Corsym [CD], CoTylenol Children's Liquid Cold Formula [CD], CoTylenol Cold Caplets & Tablets [CD], CoTylenol Liquid [CD], CoTylenol Tablets [CD], Deconamine [CD], Demazin [CD], Fedahist [CD], Fedahist Expectorant [CD], 4-Way Cold Tablets [CD], ✦Histapan-P [CD], Hycomine Compound [CD], Isoclor [CD], Naldecon [CD], ✦Neo-Nasol [CD], Novafed A [CD], ✦Novahistex Cold Capsules [CD], ✦Novopheniram, Ornade [CD], ✦Ornade-A.F. [CD], ✦Ornade-DM [CD], ✦Ornade Expectorant [CD], Penntuss [CD], Polaramine*, Rynatan [CD], Sine-Off Extra Strength Capsules [CD], Sine-Off Tablets [CD], Singlet [CD], Sinutab Maximum Strength Capsules & Tablets [CD], Sinutab Tablets [CD], Sudafed Plus [CD], Teldrin, Triaminic Allergy Tablets [CD], Triaminic Chewable Tablets [CD], Triaminic Cold Syrup & Tablets [CD], Tiaminicin [CD]

BENEFITS versus RISKS

Possible Benefits	*Possible Risks*
EFFECTIVE RELIEF OF ALLERGIC RHINITIS AND ALLERGIC SKIN DISORDERS	Mild sedation
	Atropinelike effects
	Very rare blood cell disorders

▷ **Principal Uses**

As a Single Drug Product: Used primarily to provide symptomatic relief in allergic and related disorders: seasonal and perennial allergic rhinitis (hay fever), allergic conjunctivitis and vasomotor rhinitis; also in hives and localized swellings (angioedema) of allergic origin.

As a Combination Drug Product [CD]: This drug is combined with a decongestant drug to enhance its ability to reduce tissue swelling and secretions in allergic and infectious disorders of the upper respiratory tract—hay fever, head colds and sinusitis. It is also combined with decongestants, expectorants and codeine to increase their effectiveness in the symptomatic treatment of allergic and infectious disorders of the lower respiratory tract, often with associated coughing.

How This Drug Works: Antihistamines reduce the intensity of the allergic response by blocking the action of histamine after it has been released from sensitized tissue cells in the eyes, nose, respiratory passages and skin.

Available Dosage Forms and Strengths

Capsules, prolonged-action — 8 mg, 12 mg

Injection — 10 mg, 100 mg per ml

Syrup — 2 mg per 5-ml teaspoonful (7% alcohol)

---

*A brand of the closely related generic drug dexchlorpheniramine.

> Tablets — 4 mg
> Tablets, chewable — 2 mg
> Tablets, prolonged-action — 8 mg, 12 mg

▷ **Usual Adult Dosage Range:**   4 mg/4 to 6 hours, or 8 to 12 mg (prolonged-action form)/12 hours. Total daily dosage should not exceed 24 mg. **Note: Actual dosage and administration schedule must be determined by the physician for each patient individually.**

▷ **Dosing Instructions:**   Take with food or milk to prevent stomach irritation. The prolonged-action forms should be swallowed whole (not crushed or chewed).

Usual Duration of Use: Continual use on a regular schedule for 2 to 3 days is usually necessary to determine this drug's effectiveness in relieving the symptoms of allergic rhinitis and dermatosis. It may be necessary to take this drug throughout the entire pollen season, depending upon individual sensitivity. However, antihistamines should not be taken continually (without interruption) for long-term use. Limit their use to periods that require symptomatic relief.

▷ **This Drug Should Not Be Taken If**
  • you have had an allergic reaction to any dosage form of it previously.
  • you are currently undergoing allergy skin tests.
  • you are taking, or have taken within the past 14 days, any monoamine oxidase (MAO) type A inhibitor drug (see Drug Class, Section Four).

▷ **Inform Your Physician Before Taking This Drug If**
  • you have had any allergic reactions or unfavorable responses to the previous use of antihistamines.
  • you have glaucoma (narrow-angle type) or asthma.
  • you have epilepsy or a seizure disorder.
  • you have difficulty emptying the urinary bladder, especially if due to prostate gland enlargement.
  • you plan to have surgery under general anesthesia in the near future.

Possible Side-Effects (natural, expected and unavoidable drug actions)
  Drowsiness; sense of weakness; blurred vision; dryness of the nose, mouth and throat; impaired urination.

▷ **Possible Adverse Effects** (unusual, unexpected and infrequent reactions)
  If any of the following develop, consult your physician promptly for guidance.
  Mild Adverse Effects
  Allergic Reactions: Skin rash, hives.
  Headache, nervous agitation, dizziness, confusion, tremor, blurred or double vision, ringing in ears.
  Reduced tolerance for contact lenses.
  Thickening of bronchial secretions in asthma or bronchitis.
  Indigestion, nausea, vomiting, diarrhea.

Serious Adverse Effects
Allergic Reaction: Anaphylactic reaction (see Glossary).
Idiosyncratic Reactions: Euphoria, hysteria, depression, nightmares.
Hemolytic anemia (see Glossary).
Abnormally low white blood cell count—fever, sore throat, infections.
Abnormally low blood platelet count—abnormal bleeding or bruising.

▷ **Possible Effects on Sexual Function:** Shortened menstrual cycle (early arrival of expected menstrual onset).

Natural Diseases or Disorders That May Be Activated by This Drug
Latent epilepsy, glaucoma, prostatism (see Glossary).

CAUTION
1. Discontinue this drug 4 days before diagnostic skin testing procedures in order to prevent false negative test results.
2. Do not use this drug if you have active bronchial asthma, bronchitis or pneumonia. It can thicken bronchial mucus and make it more difficult to remove (by absorption or coughing).

Precautions for Use
By Infants and Children: This drug should not be used in premature or full-term newborn infants. Doses for children should be small. The young child is especially sensitive to the effects of antihistamines on the brain and nervous system.
By Those over 60 Years of Age: You may be more susceptible to the development of drowsiness, dizziness and unsteadiness, and to impairment of thinking, judgment and memory. This drug can increase the degree of impaired urination associated with prostate gland enlargement (prostatism). The sedative effects of antihistamines in the elderly can cause a syndrome of underactivity that may be misinterpreted as senility or emotional depression.

▷ **Advisability of Use During Pregnancy**
Pregnancy Category: B (tentative). See Pregnancy Code inside back cover.
Animal studies: No birth defects reported in mice.
Human studies: Information from studies of pregnant women indicates no significant increase in defects in 3931 exposures to this drug. However, this drug may cause seizures and other adverse effects in newborn infants if used during pregnancy.
Use this drug only if clearly needed. Avoid during the last 3 months. Ask physician for guidance.

Advisability of Use if Breast-Feeding
Presence of this drug in breast milk: Yes, in small amounts.
Avoid drug or refrain from nursing.

Habit-Forming Potential: None.

Effects of Overdosage: Drowsiness; unsteadiness; faintness; marked dryness of mouth, nose and throat; flushing of face; shortness of breath; hallucinations; convulsions; stupor progressing to coma.

Possible Effects of Long-Term Use: Tardive dyskinesia (see Glossary) has been reported in association with the long-term use of several widely used antihistamines. It is advisable to avoid the prolonged, continual use of antihistamines without interruption.

Suggested Periodic Examinations While Taking This Drug (at physician's discretion)
Complete blood cell counts.

▷ **While Taking This Drug, Observe the Following**
Foods: No restrictions.
Beverages: No restrictions. May be taken with milk.
▷ *Alcohol:* Use with extreme caution until the combined effects have been determined. The combination of antihistamine and alcohol can produce rapid and marked sedation.
Tobacco Smoking: No interactions expected.
▷ *Other Drugs*
Chlorpheniramine may ***increase*** the effects of
• all sedatives, sleep-inducing drugs, tranquilizers, analgesics and narcotic drugs, and produce oversedation.
Chlorpheniramine ***taken concurrently*** with
• phenytoin (Dantoin, Dilantin) may cause phenytoin toxicity, and may alter the pattern of seizures. Dosage adjustments may be necessary.
The following drugs may ***increase*** the effects of chlorpheniramine
• monoamine oxidase (MAO) type A inhibitor drugs (see Drug Class, Section Four) may prolong the action of antihistamines.
▷ *Driving, Hazardous Activities:* This drug can impair mental alertness, judgment, coordination and reaction time. Avoid hazardous activities until the full sedative effects have been determined.
Aviation Note: The use of this drug ***is a disqualification*** for piloting. Consult a designated Aviation Medical Examiner.
Exposure to Sun: Use caution. Some drugs of this class can cause photosensitivity (see Glossary).

CHLORPROMAZINE
(klor PROH ma zeen)

Introduced: 1952

Class: Strong tranquilizer, phenothiazines

Prescription: USA: Yes
Canada: Yes

Controlled Drug: USA: No
Canada: No

Available as Generic: Yes

Brand Names: ✤Chlorpromanyl, ✤Largactil, ✤Novochlorpromazine, Promapar, Sonazine, Thorazine

BENEFITS versus RISKS

Possible Benefits	*Possible Risks*
EFFECTIVE CONTROL OF ACUTE MENTAL DISORDERS in the majority of patients	SERIOUS TOXIC EFFECTS ON BRAIN with long-term use
Beneficial effects on thinking, mood and behavior	Liver damage with jaundice (less than 0.5%)
Moderately effective control of nausea and vomiting	Rare blood cell disorders: hemolytic anemia, abnormally low white blood cell count

▷ **Principal Uses**

As a Single Drug Product: This antipsychotic drug is used primarily to treat acute and chronic psychotic disorders such as agitated depression, schizophrenia and similar states of mental dysfunction. It may be used as a tranquilizer in the management of agitated and disruptive behavior in the absence of true psychosis. Less frequently it may be used to relieve severe nausea or vomiting.

How This Drug Works: Not completely established. Present theory is that by inhibiting the action of dopamine, this drug acts to correct an imbalance of nerve impulse transmissions that is thought to be responsible for certain mental disorders.

Available Dosage Forms and Strengths

Capsules, prolonged-action — 30 mg, 75 mg, 150 mg, 200 mg, 300 mg
Concentrate — 30 mg per ml, 100 mg per ml
Injection — 25 mg per ml
Suppositories — 25 mg, 100 mg
Syrup — 10 mg per 5-ml teaspoonful
Tablets — 10 mg, 25 mg, 50 mg, 100 mg, 200 mg

▷ **Usual Adult Dosage Range:** Initially 10 to 25 mg 3 or 4 times daily. Dose may be increased by 20 to 50 mg at 3- to 4-day intervals as needed and tolerated. Usual dosage range is 300 to 800 mg daily. Extreme range is 25 to 2000 mg daily. Total daily dosage should not exceed 2000 mg. **Note: Actual dosage and administration schedule must be determined by the physician for each patient individually.**

▷ **Dosing Instructions:** May be taken with or following meals to reduce stomach irritation. Tablets may be crushed for administration. Prolonged-action capsules may be opened, but do not crush or chew contents.

Usual Duration of Use: Continual use on a regular schedule for several weeks is usually necessary to determine this drug's effectiveness in controlling psychotic disorders. If not significantly beneficial within 6 weeks, it should be discontinued. Long-term use (months to years) requires periodic evaluation of response, appropriate dosage adjustment and consideration of continued need. Consult your physician on a regular basis.

▷ **This Drug Should Not Be Taken If**
- you are allergic to any of the drugs bearing the brand names listed above.
- you have active liver disease.
- you have cancer of the breast.
- you have a current blood cell or bone marrow disorder.

▷ **Inform Your Physician Before Taking This Drug If**
- you are allergic or abnormally sensitive to any phenothiazine drug (see Drug Class, Section Four).
- you have impaired liver or kidney function.
- you have any type of seizure disorder.
- you have diabetes, glaucoma or heart disease.
- you have a history of lupus erythematosus.
- you are taking any drug with sedative effects.
- you plan to have surgery under general or spinal anesthesia in the near future.

Possible Side-Effects (natural, expected and unavoidable drug actions)
Drowsiness (usually during the first 2 weeks), orthostatic hypotension (see Glossary), blurred vision, dry mouth, nasal congestion, constipation, impaired urination.
Pink or purple coloration of urine, of no significance.

▷ **Possible Adverse Effects** (unusual, unexpected and infrequent reactions)
If any of the following develop, consult your physician promptly for guidance.
Mild Adverse Effects
Allergic Reactions: Skin rash, hives, low-grade fever.
Lowering of body temperature, especially in the elderly.
Increased appetite and weight gain.
Weakness, agitation, insomnia, impaired day and night vision.
Chronic constipation, fecal impaction.
Serious Adverse Effects
Allergic Reactions: Hepatitis with jaundice (see Glossary), usually between second and fourth week; high fever; asthma; anaphylactic reaction (see Glossary).
Depression, disorientation, seizures.
Disturbances of heart rhythm, rapid heart rate.
Hemolytic anemia (see Glossary), impaired production of white blood cells—fever, sore throat, infections.
Parkinson-like disorders (see Glossary); muscle spasms of face, jaw, neck, back, extremities.
Prolonged drop in blood pressure with weakness, perspiration and fainting.

▷ **Possible Effects on Sexual Function**
Decreased libido and impotence (1200 mg/day); inhibited ejaculation (400 mg/day); priapism (see Glossary) (250 mg/day); male infertility

(30 to 800 mg/day); enlargement of male breasts, enlargement of female breasts with milk production, cessation of menstruation (30 to 800 mg/day).

This drug may also cause a false positive pregnancy test.

▷ **Adverse Effects That May Mimic Natural Diseases or Disorders**
Nervous system reactions may suggest Parkinson's disease.
Liver reactions may suggest viral hepatitis.
Reactions resembling systemic lupus erythematosus can occur.

Natural Diseases or Disorders That May Be Activated by This Drug
Latent epilepsy, glaucoma, diabetes mellitus (25%), prostatism (see Glossary).

CAUTION
1. Many over-the-counter medications (see OTC Drugs in Glossary) for allergies, colds and coughs contain drugs that can interact unfavorably with this drug. Ask your physician or pharmacist for guidance before using any such medications.
2. Antacids that contain aluminum and/or magnesium can prevent the absorption of this drug and reduce its effectiveness.
3. Obtain prompt evaluation of any change or disturbance of vision.
4. This drug can cause false positive pregnancy tests.

Precautions for Use
By Infants and Children: Do not use this drug in infants under 6 months of age, or in children of any age with symptoms suggestive of Reye syndrome (see Glossary). Monitor carefully for blood cell changes.
By Those over 60 Years of Age: Small doses are advisable until individual response has been determined. You may be more susceptible to the development of drowsiness, lethargy, constipation, lowering of body temperature (hypothermia) and orthostatic hypotension (see Glossary). This drug can enhance existing prostatism (see Glossary). You may also be more susceptible to the development of Parkinson-like reactions and/or tardive dyskinesia (see discussion of these terms in Glossary). These reactions must be recognized early since they may become unresponsive to treatment and irreversible.

▷ **Advisability of Use During Pregnancy**
Pregnancy Category: C (tentative). See Pregnancy Code inside back cover.
Animal studies: No birth defects reported in rodent studies. However, rodent studies suggest possible permanent neurological damage to the fetus.
Human studies: No increase in birth defects reported in 284 exposures. Information from adequate studies of pregnant women is not available.
Limit use to small and infrequent doses only when clearly needed. Avoid drug during the last month because of possible adverse effects on the newborn infant.

Advisability of Use if Breast-Feeding
Presence of this drug in breast milk: Yes, in small amounts.
Avoid drug or refrain from nursing.

Habit-Forming Potential: None.

Effects of Overdosage: Marked drowsiness, weakness, tremor, agitation, unsteadiness, deep sleep, coma, convulsions.

Possible Effects of Long-Term Use: Tardive dyskinesia in 10% to 20% (see Glossary); eye changes—cataracts and pigmentation of retina; gray to violet pigmentation of skin in exposed areas, more common in women; severe ulcerative colitis.

Suggested Periodic Examinations While Taking This Drug (at physician's discretion)
Complete blood cell counts, especially between the fourth and tenth weeks of treatment.
Liver function tests, electrocardiograms.
Complete eye examinations—eye structures and vision.
Careful inspection of the tongue for early evidence of fine, involuntary, wavelike movements that could indicate the beginning of tardive dyskinesia.

▷ **While Taking This Drug, Observe the Following**
Foods: No restrictions.
Nutritional Support: A riboflavin (vitamin B-2) supplement should be taken with long-term use.
Beverages: No restrictions. May be taken with milk.
▷ *Alcohol:* Avoid completely. Alcohol can increase the sedative action of phenothiazines and accentuate their depressant effects on brain function and blood pressure. Phenothiazines can increase the intoxicating effects of alcohol.
Tobacco Smoking: Possible reduction of drowsiness from drug.
Marijuana Smoking: Moderate increase in drowsiness; accentuation of orthostatic hypotension; increased risk of precipitating latent psychoses, confusing the interpretation of mental status and drug responses.
▷ *Other Drugs*
Chlorpromazine may *increase* the effects of
• all sedative drugs, especially meperidine (Demerol), and cause excessive sedation.
• all atropinelike drugs, and cause nervous system toxicity.
Chlorpromazine may *decrease* the effects of
• guanethidine (Ismelin, Esimil), and reduce its effectiveness in lowering blood pressure.
Chlorpromazine *taken concurrently* with
• propranolol (Inderal) may cause increased effects of both drugs; monitor drug effects closely and adjust dosages as necessary.
The following drugs may *decrease* the effects of chlorpromazine

- antacids containing aluminum and/or magnesium.
- benztropine (Cogentin).
- trihexyphenidyl (Artane).

▷ *Driving, Hazardous Activities:* This drug can impair mental alertness, judgment and physical coordination. Avoid hazardous activities.

Aviation Note: The use of this drug **is a disqualification** for piloting. Consult a designated Aviation Medical Examiner.

Exposure to Sun: Use caution until sensitivity has been determined. Some phenothiazines can cause photosensitivity (see Glossary).

Exposure to Heat: Use caution and avoid excessive heat as much as possible. This drug may impair the regulation of body temperature and increase the risk of heat stroke.

Exposure to Cold: Use caution and dress warmly. This drug can increase the risk of hypothermia in the elderly.

Discontinuation: After a period of long-term use, do not discontinue this drug suddenly. Gradual withdrawal over 2 to 3 weeks under physician supervision is recommended. Do not discontinue this drug without your physician's knowledge and approval. The relapse rate of schizophrenia after discontinuation is 50% to 60%.

CHLORPROPAMIDE
(klor PROH pa mide)

Introduced: 1958

Class: Antidiabetic, sulfonylureas

Prescription: USA: Yes
Canada: Yes

Controlled Drug: USA: No
Canada: No

Available as Generic: Yes

Brand Names: ✦Apo-Chlorpropamide, ✦Chloronase, Diabinese, ✦Novopropamide

---

BENEFITS versus RISKS

Possible Benefits	*Possible Risks*
Assistance in regulating blood sugar in noninsulin-dependent diabetes (adjunctive to appropriate diet and weight control)	HYPOGLYCEMIA, severe and prolonged Allergic skin reactions (some severe) Water retention Liver damage Rare blood cell and bone marrow disorders

---

▷ **Principal Uses**

As a Single Drug Product: To assist in the control of mild to moderately severe type II diabetes mellitus (adult, maturity-onset) that does not require insulin, but that cannot be adequately controlled by diet alone.

How This Drug Works: It is thought that this drug (1) stimulates the secretion of insulin (by a pancreas that is capable of responding to stimulation), and (2) enhances the utilization of insulin by appropriate tissues.

Available Dosage Forms and Strengths
Tablets — 100 mg, 250 mg

▷ **Usual Adult Dosage Range:** Initially 250 mg daily with breakfast. After 5 to 7 days, dose may be increased to 500 mg daily if needed and tolerated. Total daily dosage should not exceed 750 mg. A "loading" or priming dose is not necessary and should not be given. **Note: Actual dosage and administration schedule must be determined by the physician for each patient individually.**

▷ **Dosing Instructions:** May be taken with food to reduce stomach irritation. Tablet may be crushed for administration.

Usual Duration of Use: Continual use on a regular schedule for 1 to 2 weeks is usually necessary to determine this drug's effectiveness in controlling diabetes. Failure to respond to maximal doses within 1 month constitutes a primary failure. Up to 15% of those who respond initially may develop secondary failure of the drug within the first year of use. The duration of effective use can only be determined by periodic measurement of the blood sugar. Consult your physician on a regular basis.

▷ **This Drug Should Not Be Taken If**
- you have had an allergic reaction to it previously.
- you have severe impairment of liver or kidney function.
- you are pregnant.

▷ **Inform Your Physician Before Taking This Drug If**
- you are allergic to other sulfonylurea drugs or to "sulfa" drugs.
- your diabetes has been unstable or "brittle" in the past.
- you do not know how to recognize or treat hypoglycemia (see Glossary).
- you have a history of congestive heart failure, peptic ulcer disease, cirrhosis of the liver, hypothyroidism or porphyria.

Possible Side-Effects (natural, expected and unavoidable drug actions)
If drug dosage is excessive or food intake is delayed or inadequate, abnormally low blood sugar (hypoglycemia) will occur as a predictable drug effect.

▷ **Possible Adverse Effects** (unusual, unexpected and infrequent reactions)
If any of the following develop, consult your physician promptly for guidance.
Mild Adverse Effects
Allergic Reactions: Skin rash, hives, itching, drug fever.
Headache, ringing in ears, weakness, numbness and tingling.
Indigestion, nausea, vomiting, diarrhea (may be severe).
Serious Adverse Effects
Allergic Reactions: Hepatitis with jaundice (see Glossary), severe skin reactions.
Idiosyncratic Reaction: Hemolytic anemia (see Glossary).
Disulfiramlike reaction with concurrent use of alcohol (see Glossary).
Water retention (edema), weight gain.
Bone marrow depression (see Glossary)—fatigue, weakness, fever, sore throat, abnormal bleeding or bruising.

▷ **Possible Effects on Sexual Function:** None reported.

▷ **Adverse Effects That May Mimic Natural Diseases or Disorders**
Liver reactions may suggest viral hepatitis.

Natural Diseases or Disorders That May Be Activated by This Drug
Acute intermittent porphyria, congestive heart failure (in predisposed individuals), peptic ulcer disease.

CAUTION
1. This drug must be regarded as only one part of the total program for the management of your diabetes. It is not a substitute for a properly prescribed diet and regular exercise.
2. Over a period of time (usually several months), this drug may lose its effectiveness in controlling blood sugar levels. Periodic follow-up examinations are necessary to monitor all aspects of response to drug treatment.
3. This drug has a long duration of action (up to 60 hours) and therefore can be cumulative in its effects. It can produce severe and prolonged hypoglycemia in some individuals, especially the elderly.

Precautions for Use
By Infants and Children: This drug is not effective in type I (juvenile, growth-onset) insulin-dependent diabetes.
By Those over 60 Years of Age: This drug is best avoided in this age group. Due to its long duration of action it can accumulate and cause marked and prolonged hypoglycemia. Repeated episodes of hypoglycemia in the elderly can cause brain damage.

▷ **Advisability of Use During Pregnancy**
Pregnancy Category: X (tentative). See Pregnancy Code inside back cover.
Animal studies: This class of drugs has been shown to cause birth defects in animals.

Human studies: Information from adequate studies of pregnant women is not available.

The manufacturer states that this drug is contraindicated during entire pregnancy.

Advisability of Use if Breast-Feeding

Presence of this drug in breast milk: Yes.

Avoid drug or refrain from nursing.

Habit-Forming Potential: None.

Effects of Overdosage: Symptoms of mild to severe hypoglycemia: headache, light-headedness, faintness, nervousness, confusion, tremor, sweating, heart palpitation, weakness, hunger, nausea, vomiting, stupor progressing to coma.

Possible Effects of Long-Term Use: Reduced function of the thyroid gland (hypothyroidism). Reports of increased frequency and severity of heart and blood vessel diseases associated with long-term use of this class of drugs are highly controversial and inconclusive. A direct cause-and-effect relationship (see Glossary) is tenuous. Ask your physician for guidance.

Suggested Periodic Examinations While Taking This Drug (at physician's discretion)

Complete blood cell counts, liver function tests, thyroid function tests, periodic evaluation of heart and circulatory system.

▷ **While Taking This Drug, Observe the Following**

Foods: Follow the diabetic diet prescribed by your physician.

Beverages: As directed in the diabetic diet. May be taken with milk.

▷   *Alcohol:* Use with extreme caution until the combined effect has been determined. Alcohol can exaggerate this drug's hypoglycemic effect. This drug can cause a marked intolerance of alcohol resulting in a disulfiramlike reaction (see Glossary): facial flushing, sweating, palpitation.

Tobacco Smoking: No interactions expected.

▷   *Other Drugs*

The following drugs may ***increase*** the effects of chlorpropamide

- ammonium chloride.
- aspirin, and other salicylates.
- chloramphenicol (Chloromycetin).
- clofibrate (Atromid S).
- dicumarol.
- fenfluramine (Pondimin).
- monoamine oxidase (MAO) type A inhibitor drugs (see Drug Class, Section Four).
- phenylbutazone (Butazolidin).
- some "sulfa" drugs: sulfamethoxazole (Gantanol), sulfisoxazole (Gantrisin).

The following drugs may *decrease* the effects of chlorpropamide
- diazoxide (Proglycem).
- propranolol (Inderal).
- rifampin (Rifidin, Rimactane).
- sodium bicarbonate.
- thiazide diuretics (see Drug Class, Section Four).

▷ *Driving, Hazardous Activities:* Regulate your dosage schedule, eating schedule and physical activities very carefully to prevent hypoglycemia. Be able to recognize the early symptoms of hypoglycemia so you can avoid hazardous activities and take corrective measures.

Aviation Note: Diabetes *is a disqualification* for piloting. Consult a designated Aviation Medical Examiner.

Exposure to Sun: Use caution until sensitivity has been determined. Some drugs of this class can cause photosensitivity (see Glossary).

Occurrence of Unrelated Illness: Acute infections, illnesses causing vomiting or diarrhea, serious injuries and surgical procedures can interfere with diabetic control and may require the use of insulin. If any of these conditions occur, consult your physician promptly.

Discontinuation: It is estimated that no more than 12% of patients remain well controlled by this drug for more than 6 to 7 years. Because of the high incidence of secondary failures, it is advisable to evaluate the continued benefit of this drug every 6 months.

CHLORTHALIDONE
(klor THAL i dohn)

Introduced: 1960

Class: Antihypertensive, diuretic

Prescription: USA: Yes
Canada: Yes

Controlled Drug: USA: No
Canada: No

Available as Generic: USA: Yes
Canada: Yes

Brand Names: ✦Apo-Chlorthalidone, Combipres [CD], Demi-Regroton [CD], Hygroton, ✦Hygroton-Reserpine [CD], Hylidone, ✦Novothalidone, Regroton [CD], Tenoretic [CD], Thalitone, ✦Uridon

---

BENEFITS versus RISKS

Possible Benefits	*Possible Risks*
EFFECTIVE, WELL-TOLERATED DIURETIC	Loss of body potassium
POSSIBLY EFFECTIVE IN MILD HYPERTENSION	Increased blood sugar
	Increased blood uric acid
ENHANCES EFFECTIVENESS OF OTHER ANTIHYPERTENSIVES	Increased blood calcium
	Rare blood cell disorders
Beneficial in treatment of diabetes insipidus	

▷ **Principal Uses**

As a Single Drug Product: Thiazidelike diuretics are used primarily to (1) increase the volume of urine (diuresis) to correct the excessive fluid retention associated with congestive heart failure and certain types of liver and kidney disease; and (2) initiate treatment for high blood pressure (hypertension). They are often the first drugs tried in treating mild to moderate hypertension. Less frequent uses include the treatment of diabetes insipidus and the prevention of kidney stones that contain calcium.

As a Combination Drug Product [CD]: When this drug is used alone to treat hypertension, it is referred to as a "step 1" antihypertensive. Should it fail to reduce the blood pressure adequately, a "step 2" antihypertensive drug is added to be taken concurrently with the "step 1" drug. These drugs may be combined into one drug product. This drug is available in combination with atenolol, clonidine and reserpine to increase their effectiveness in treating hypertension.

How This Drug Works: By increasing the elimination of salt and water from the body (through increased urine production), this drug reduces the volume of fluid in the blood and body tissues and lowers the sodium content throughout the body. By relaxing the walls of smaller arteries and allowing them to expand, this drug increases the total capacity of the arterial system. The combined effect of these two actions (reduced blood volume in expanded space) results in lowering of blood pressure.

Available Dosage Forms and Strengths
Tablets — 25 mg, 50 mg, 100 mg

▷ **Usual Adult Dosage Range:** As antihypertensive: 25 to 50 mg/day initially; 50 to 100 mg/day for maintenance. As diuretic: 50 to 100 mg/day initially; the smallest effective dose should be determined. The total daily dose should not exceed 200 mg. **Note: Actual dosage and administration schedule must be determined by the physician for each patient individually.**

▷ **Dosing Instructions:** May be taken with or following meals to reduce stomach irritation. Best taken in the morning to avoid nighttime urination. The tablet may be crushed for administration.

Usual Duration of Use: Continual use on a regular schedule for 2 to 3 weeks is usually necessary to determine this drug's effectiveness in lowering high blood pressure. Long-term use (months to years) requires periodic evaluation of response and possible dosage adjustment. Use as a diuretic should be intermittent with "drug holidays" (no drug taken) to reduce the risk of sodium and potassium imbalance. Consult your physician on a regular basis.

▷ **This Drug Should Not Be Taken If**
• you have had an allergic reaction to it previously.

▷ **Inform Your Physician Before Taking This Drug If**
- you are allergic to any form of "sulfa" drug.
- you are pregnant or planning pregnancy.
- you have a history of kidney or liver disease.
- you have diabetes, gout or lupus erythematosus.
- you are taking any form of cortisone, digitalis, oral antidiabetic drug or insulin.
- you plan to have surgery under general anesthesia in the near future.

Possible Side-Effects (natural, expected and unavoidable drug actions)
Light-headedness on arising from sitting or lying position (see Orthostatic Hypotension in Glossary).
Increase in blood sugar level, affecting control of diabetes.
Increase in blood uric acid level, affecting control of gout.
Decrease in blood potassium level, causing muscle weakness and cramping.

▷ **Possible Adverse Effects** (unusual, unexpected and infrequent reactions)
If any of the following develop, consult your physician promptly for guidance.
Mild Adverse Effects
Allergic Reactions: Skin rashes, hives, drug fever.
Headache, dizziness, blurred or yellow vision.
Reduced appetite, indigestion, nausea, vomiting, diarrhea.
Serious Adverse Effects
Allergic Reactions: Hepatitis with jaundice (see Glossary), anaphylactic reaction (see Glossary), severe skin reactions.
Inflammation of the pancreas—severe abdominal pain.
Bone marrow depression (see Glossary)—fatigue, weakness, fever, sore throat, abnormal bleeding or bruising.

▷ **Possible Effects on Sexual Function:**   Decreased libido and impotence, beginning from 2 weeks to several months after starting drug (100 mg/day).

▷ **Adverse Effects That May Mimic Natural Diseases or Disorders**
Liver reaction may suggest viral hepatitis.

Natural Diseases or Disorders That May Be Activated by This Drug
Diabetes, gout, systemic lupus erythematosus (questionable).

CAUTION
1. Do not exceed recommended doses. Increased dosage can cause excessive loss of sodium and potassium, with resultant loss of appetite, nausea, fatigue, weakness, confusion and tingling in the extremities.
2. If you are also taking a digitalis preparation (digitoxin, digoxin), ensure an adequate intake of high-potassium foods to prevent potassium deficiency, a potential cause of digitalis toxicity. (See Table of High Potassium Foods in Section Six.)

Precautions for Use

By Infants and Children: Avoid overdosage that could cause serious dehydration. Significant potassium loss can occur within the first 2 weeks of drug use.

By Those over 60 Years of Age: Small doses are advisable until your individual response has been determined. You may be more susceptible to the development of fatigue (40%), low blood potassium (10%), elevated blood uric acid (30%), impaired thinking, orthostatic hypotension and blood sugar increase. Overdosage and extended use of this drug can cause excessive loss of body water, thickening (increased viscosity) of the blood, and an increased tendency for the blood to clot—predisposing to stroke, heart attack, or thrombophlebitis (vein inflammation with blood clot). Report promptly any type of skin reaction.

▷ **Advisability of Use During Pregnancy**

Pregnancy Category: D (tentative). See Pregnancy Code inside back cover.
Animal studies: No birth defects reported.
Human studies: Information from adequate studies of pregnant women is not available.
It should not be used during pregnancy unless a very serious complication occurs for which this drug is significantly beneficial. This drug can cause serious adverse effects in the newborn infant. Ask physician for guidance.

Advisability of Use if Breast-Feeding

Presence of this drug in breast milk: Yes.
Avoid drug or refrain from nursing.

Habit-Forming Potential: None.

Effects of Overdosage: Dry mouth, thirst, lethargy, weakness, muscle cramping, nausea, vomiting, drowsiness progressing to stupor or coma.

Possible Effects of Long-Term Use: Impaired balance of water, salt and potassium in blood and body tissues. Development of diabetes in predisposed individuals. Pathological changes in parathyroid glands with increased blood calcium levels and decreased blood phosphate levels.

Suggested Periodic Examinations While Taking This Drug (at physician's discretion)

Complete blood cell counts; measurements of blood levels of sodium, potassium, chloride, sugar and uric acid.
Kidney and liver function tests.

▷ **While Taking This Drug, Observe the Following**

Foods: Consult your physician regarding the advisability of eating foods rich in potassium. If so advised, see the Table of High Potassium

Foods in Section Six. Follow physician's advice regarding the use of salt.

Beverages: No restrictions. This drug may be taken with milk.

▷ *Alcohol:* Use with caution until the combined effects have been determined. Alcohol may exaggerate the blood-pressure-lowering effects of this drug and cause orthostatic hypotension (see Glossary).

Tobacco Smoking: No interactions expected. Follow physician's advice.

▷ *Other Drugs*

Chlorthalidone may ***increase*** the effects of
- other antihypertensive drugs; dosage adjustments may be necessary to prevent excessive lowering of blood pressure.
- lithium, and cause lithium toxicity.

Chlorthalidone may ***decrease*** the effects of
- oral antidiabetic drugs (sulfonylureas); dosage adjustments may be necessary for proper control of blood sugar.

Chlorthalidone ***taken concurrently*** with
- digitalis preparations (digitoxin, digoxin) requires very careful monitoring and dosage adjustments to prevent fluctuations of blood potassium levels and serious disturbances of heart rhythm.

The following drugs may ***decrease*** the effects of chlorthalidone
- cholestyramine (Cuemid, Questran) may interfere with its absorption.
- colestipol (Colestid) may interfere with its absorption.

Take cholestyramine and colestipol 1 hour before any oral diuretic.

▷ *Driving, Hazardous Activities:* Use caution until the possible occurrence of orthostatic hypotension, dizziness or impaired vision has been determined.

Aviation Note: The use of this drug ***may be a disqualification*** for piloting. Consult a designated Aviation Medical Examiner.

Exposure to Sun: Use caution until sensitivity has been determined. This drug can cause photosensitivity (see Glossary).

Exposure to Heat: Avoid excessive perspiring which could cause additional loss of salt and water from the body.

Heavy Exercise or Exertion: Avoid exertion that produces light-headedness, excessive fatigue or muscle cramping. Isometric exercises—the "overload" technique for strengthening individual muscles—can raise the blood pressure significantly. Ask physician for guidance regarding participation in this form of exercise.

Occurrence of Unrelated Illness: Illnesses that cause vomiting or diarrhea can produce a serious imbalance of important body chemistry. Consult your physician for guidance.

Discontinuation: It may be advisable to discontinue this drug 5 to 7 days before major surgery. Ask your physician, surgeon and/or anesthesiologist for guidance regarding dosage adjustment or drug withdrawal. Following long-term use, this drug should be withdrawn gradually to prevent the occurrence of rebound edema.

CHLORZOXAZONE
(klor ZOX a zohn)

Introduced: 1958

Class: Muscle relaxant

Prescription: USA: Yes
    Canada: No

Controlled Drug: USA: No
    Canada: No

Available as Generic: USA: Yes
    Canada: No

Brand Names: Paraflex, Parafon Forte [CD]

BENEFITS versus RISKS	
Possible Benefits	***Possible Risks***
Mild to moderate relief of discomfort due to spasm of voluntary muscles	Red and white blood cell disorders
	Gastrointestinal bleeding
	Liver damage, jaundice (questionable)
	(All rare)

▷ **Principal Uses**

As a Single Drug Product: Used primarily to relieve the pain and stiffness associated with spasm of voluntary muscles, such as that resulting from accidental injury of musculoskeletal structures. It is often necessary to supplement the use of this drug with other treatment measures, such as rest, support and physiotherapy.

As a Combination Drug Product [CD]: It is combined with acetaminophen to enhance its effectiveness in relieving discomfort. Acetaminophen is an effective analgesic and may be necessary to control the pain that is not relieved by chlorzoxazone alone.

How This Drug Works: Not completely established. It is thought that this drug may relieve muscle spasm and pain by blocking the transmission of nerve impulses over reflex pathways and/or by producing a sedative effect that decreases the perception of pain.

Available Dosage Forms and Strengths
    Caplets — 500 mg
    Tablets — 250 mg

▷ **Usual Adult Dosage Range:** 250 to 750 mg, 3 or 4 times daily; adjust dosage as needed and tolerated. **Note: Actual dosage and administration schedule must be determined by the physician for each patient individually.**

▷ **Dosing Instructions:** Take either on empty stomach or with food to prevent stomach irritation. Tablet may be crushed for administration.

Usual Duration of Use: Continual use on a regular schedule for 2 to 3 days is usually necessary to determine this drug's effectiveness in relieving the discomfort of muscle spasm. Evaluate need for continued use after periods of 7 to 10 days.

▷ **This Drug Should Not Be Taken If**
  • you have had an allergic reaction to it previously.
  • you have active liver disease.

▷ **Inform Your Physician Before Taking This Drug If**
  • you have experienced any unfavorable reactions to muscle relaxants in the past.
  • you have a history of liver or kidney disease.

Possible Side-Effects (natural, expected and unavoidable drug actions)
  Drowsiness, orange or reddish purple discoloration of the urine (of no significance).

▷ **Possible Adverse Effects** (unusual, unexpected and infrequent reactions)
  If any of the following develop, consult your physician promptly for guidance.
  Mild Adverse Effects
  Allergic Reactions: Skin rash, hives, itching, spontaneous bruising.
  Light-headedness, dizziness, lethargy.
  Indigestion, heartburn, nausea.
  Serious Adverse Effects
  Idiosyncratic Reactions: Nervousness, excitement, irritability.
  Anemia, abnormally low white blood cell count—weakness, fever, sore throat.
  Gastrointestinal bleeding—black- or dark-colored stools.
  Liver reaction with or without jaundice (see Glossary)—yellow eyes and skin, dark-colored urine, light-colored stools.

▷ **Possible Effects on Sexual Function:**   None reported.

▷ **Adverse Effects That May Mimic Natural Diseases or Disorders**
  Liver reaction may suggest viral hepatitis.

Precautions for Use
  By Infants and Children: Dosage is based on the child's age and weight. Consult your physician for exact dosage schedule.
  By Those over 60 Years of Age: Small doses are advisable initially. You may be more susceptible to the development of drowsiness, dizziness, weakness, unsteadiness and falling.

▷ **Advisability of Use During Pregnancy**
  Pregnancy Category: C (tentative). See Pregnancy Code inside back cover.
  Animal studies: No data available.
  Human studies: Information from adequate studies of pregnant women is not available.
  Avoid drug if possible; use only if clearly needed.

Advisability of Use if Breast-Feeding
Presence of this drug in breast milk: Yes.
Avoid drug or refrain from nursing.

Habit-Forming Potential: None.

Effects of Overdosage: Nausea, vomiting, diarrhea, headache, drowsiness, dizziness, marked weakness, sense of paralysis of arms and legs, rapid and irregular breathing.

Possible Effects of Long-Term Use: None reported.

Suggested Periodic Examinations While Taking This Drug (at physician's discretion)
Complete blood cell counts. Liver function tests.

▷ **While Taking This Drug, Observe the Following**
Foods: No restrictions.
Beverages: No restrictions. May be taken with milk.
▷ *Alcohol:* Use with caution until the combined effect has been determined. This drug may add to the depressant action of alcohol on the brain.
Tobacco Smoking: No interactions expected.
Marijuana Smoking: Moderate to marked drowsiness, muscle weakness, incoordination, accentuation of orthostatic hypotension (see Glossary).
▷ *Other Drugs*
The following drug may *decrease* the effects of chlorzoxazone
• testosterone is reported to reduce its ability to relax muscles in spasm.
▷ *Driving, Hazardous Activities:* This drug can cause drowsiness, light-headedness or dizziness in susceptible individuals. Avoid hazardous activities if these drug effects occur.
Aviation Note: The use of this drug *is a disqualification* for piloting. Consult a designated Aviation Medical Examiner.
Exposure to Sun: No restrictions.

CHOLESTYRAMINE
(koh LES tir a meen)

Introduced: 1959

Class: Anticholesterol

Prescription: USA: Yes
Canada: No

Controlled Drug: USA: No
Canada: No

Available as Generic: USA: No
Canada: No

Brand Names: Cholybar, Questran

+--+
| **BENEFITS versus RISKS** |
| |
| *Possible Benefits*   *Possible Risks* |
| EFFECTIVE REDUCTION OF   Constipation (may be severe) |
| TOTAL CHOLESTEROL AND   Reduced absorption of fat, fat- |
| LOW DENSITY   soluble vitamins (A, D, E and |
| CHOLESTEROL IN TYPE IIa   K) and folic acid |
| CHOLESTEROL DISORDERS   Reduced formation of |
| (15% to 25% reduction of total prothrombin with resultant |
| cholesterol, 25% to 35%   bleeding |
| reduction of LDL cholesterol) |
| EFFECTIVE RELIEF OF |
| ITCHING associated with |
| biliary obstruction |
+--+

▷ **Principal Uses**

As a Single Drug Product: Used primarily to (1) reduce abnormally high blood levels of total cholesterol and low density (LDL) cholesterol in Type IIa cholesterol disorders; (2) relieve the itching due to the deposit of bile acids in the skin associated with partial biliary obstruction.

How This Drug Works: By combining with bile acids and bile salts in the intestinal tract, this drug forms insoluble complexes that are excreted in the feces. This removal of bile acids (which are necessary for food digestion) stimulates the conversion of cholesterol to bile acids to replace the loss; this in turn reduces the blood levels of cholesterol. By reducing the blood levels of bile acids, this drug hastens the absorption and clearance of bile acids deposited in the skin and thus relieves itching.

Available Dosage Forms and Strengths
     Bars — 4 grams
     Cans — 378 grams
     Packets — 9 grams

▷ **Usual Adult Dosage Range:**   9 grams of powder (equivalent to 4 grams of cholestyramine) 3 times daily. Dose may be increased slowly as needed and tolerated. The total daily dosage should not exceed 72 grams of powder (32 grams of cholestyramine). **Note: Actual dosage and administration schedule must be determined by the physician for each patient individually.**

▷ **Dosing Instructions:**   Always take just before or with a meal; this drug is ineffective when taken without food. Mix the powder thoroughly in 4 to 6 ounces of water, fruit juice, milk, thin soup or a soft food like applesauce; do not use carbonated beverages. **Do not take it in its dry form.**

Usual Duration of Use: Continual use on a regular schedule for 4 to 6 weeks is usually necessary to determine this drug's effectiveness in

lowering excessively high blood levels of cholesterol. Duration of use should not exceed 3 months if an adequate response does not occur. Long-term use (months to years) requires periodic evaluation of response and dosage adjustment. Consult your physician on a regular basis.

Currently a "Drug of Choice" for initiating treatment of elevated LDL cholesterol. See Cholesterol Disorders in Section Two.

▷ **This Drug Should Not Be Taken If**
- you have had an allergic reaction to it previously.
- you have complete biliary obstruction.

▷ **Inform Your Physician Before Taking This Drug If**
- you are prone to constipation.
- you have peptic ulcer disease.
- you have a bleeding disorder of any kind.
- you have impaired kidney function.

Possible Side-Effects (natural, expected and unavoidable drug actions)
Constipation (25%); interference with normal fat digestion and absorption; reduced absorption of vitamins A, D, E and K and folic acid.

▷ **Possible Adverse Effects** (unusual, unexpected and infrequent reactions)
If any of the following develop, consult your physician promptly for guidance.
Mild Adverse Effects
Allergic Reactions: Skin rash, hives, tongue irritation, anal itching.
Loss of appetite, indigestion, heartburn, abdominal discomfort, excessive gas, nausea, vomiting, diarrhea.
Serious Adverse Effects
Allergic Reaction: Asthmalike wheezing.
Vitamin K deficiency with resultant deficiency of prothrombin and increased bleeding tendency.
Impaired absorption of calcium; predisposition to osteoporosis.
Gallbladder colic.

▷ **Possible Effects on Sexual Function:** Increased libido (questionable).

Natural Diseases or Disorders That May Be Activated by This Drug
Peptic ulcer disease; steatorrhea (excessive fat in stools) with large doses.

CAUTION
1. The powder should never be taken in its dry form; always mix it thoroughly with a suitable liquid before swallowing.
2. Observe carefully for the development of constipation; use stool softeners and laxatives as needed.
3. This drug may bind other drugs taken concurrently and impair their absorption. It is advisable to take *all other drugs* 1 to 2 hours before or 4 to 6 hours after taking this drug.

Precautions for Use

By Infants and Children: Safety and effectiveness for use by those under 6 years of age have not been established. Observe carefully for the possible development of acidosis and vitamin A or folic acid deficiency. (Ask your physician for guidance.)

By Those over 60 Years of Age: There may be increased risk of developing severe constipation. Impaired kidney function may predispose to·the development of acidosis.

▷ **Advisability of Use During Pregnancy**

Pregnancy Category: C (tentative). See Pregnancy Code inside back cover.
Animal studies: No information available.
Human studies: Information from adequate studies of pregnant women is not available.
Use this drug only if clearly needed. Ensure adequate intake of vitamins and minerals since this drug can reduce their availability to both mother and fetus. Ask physician for guidance.

Advisability of Use if Breast-Feeding

Presence of this drug in breast milk: No.
Breast-feeding is permitted.

Habit-Forming Potential: None.

Effects of Overdosage: Progressive constipation.

Possible Effects of Long-Term Use

Deficiencies of vitamins A, D, E and K and folic acid.
Calcium deficiency, osteoporosis.
Acidosis due to excessive retention of chloride.

Suggested Periodic Examinations While Taking This Drug (at physician's discretion)

Measurements of blood levels of total cholesterol, low density (LDL) cholesterol and high density (HDL) cholesterol.
Hemoglobin and red blood cell studies for possible anemia.

▷ **While Taking This Drug, Observe the Following**

Foods: Avoid foods that tend to constipate (cheeses, etc.).
Nutritional Support: Consult your physician regarding the need for supplements of vitamins A, D, E and K, folic acid and calcium.
Beverages: Avoid carbonated beverages. Ensure adequate liquid intake (up to 2 quarts daily). This drug may be taken with milk.
▷ *Alcohol:* No interactions expected.
Tobacco Smoking: No interactions expected.
▷ *Other Drugs*

Cholestyramine may ***decrease*** the effects of
• acetaminophen; give 2 hours before cholestyramine.
• digitoxin and digoxin; give 2 hours before.
• iron preparations; give 2 to 3 hours before.

- phenobarbital; give 2 hours before.
- thiazide diuretics (see Drug Class, Section Four); give 2 hours before.
- thyroxin; give 5 hours before.
- warfarin; give 6 hours after.

▷ *Driving, Hazardous Activities:* No restrictions.

Aviation Note: The use of this drug **is usually not a disqualification** for piloting. Consult a designated Aviation Medical Examiner.

Exposure to Sun: No restrictions.

Discontinuation: The dose of any potentially toxic drug taken concurrently must be reduced appropriately when this drug is discontinued.

CIMETIDINE
(si MET i deen)

Introduced: 1976

Class: Antiulcer, H-2 receptor blocker

Prescription: USA: Yes
Canada: Yes

Controlled Drug: USA: No
Canada: No

Available as Generic: No

Brand Names: ✦Apo-Cimetidine, ✦Novocimetine, ✦Peptol, Tagamet

BENEFITS versus RISKS	
Possible Benefits	*Possible Risks*
EFFECTIVE TREATMENT OF PEPTIC ULCER DISEASE: relief of symptoms, acceleration of healing, prevention of recurrence	CONFUSIONAL STATES in the elderly and debilitated
	Rare blood cell and bone marrow disorders
CONTROL OF HYPERSECRETORY STOMACH DISORDERS	Rare pancreatitis
	Rare liver damage
Beneficial in treatment of reflux esophagitis	Rare kidney damage

▷ **Principal Uses**

As a Single Drug Product: Used primarily in the treatment of peptic ulcer disease, specifically to hasten the healing of duodenal ulcer and to prevent its recurrence. Also used to control the excessive production of stomach acid in Zollinger-Ellison syndrome. Though its effectiveness has not been fully established, this drug is also widely used in the management of stomach (gastric) ulcer, esophagitis (as with hiatal hernia) and upper gastrointestinal bleeding.

How This Drug Works: By blocking the action of histamine, this drug effectively inhibits the secretion of stomach acid and thus creates a more favorable environment for the healing of peptic ulcers.

Available Dosage Forms and Strengths
Injection — 300 mg per 2 ml
Liquid — 300 mg per 5-ml teaspoonful (2.8% alcohol)
Tablets — 200 mg, 300 mg, 400 mg, 800 mg

▷ **Usual Adult Dosage Range:** For active peptic ulcer and hypersecretory states—300 mg, 4 times daily, taken with meals and at bedtime. For prevention of recurrent ulcer—400 mg at bedtime. Total daily dosage should not exceed 1200 mg. **Note: Actual dosage and administration schedule must be determined by the physician for each patient individually.**

▷ **Dosing Instructions:** To obtain the longest period of stomach acid reduction, this drug should be taken with or immediately following meals. The tablet may be crushed for administration.

Usual Duration of Use: Continual use on a regular schedule for 4 to 6 weeks is usually necessary to determine this drug's effectiveness in healing active peptic ulcer. Continual use for up to 1 year is recommended for prevention of ulcer recurrence. Consult your physician on a regular basis.

▷ **This Drug Should Not Be Taken If**
- you have had an allergic reaction to any dosage form of it previously.

▷ **Inform Your Physician Before Taking This Drug If**
- you have impaired liver or kidney function.
- you have a low sperm count.
- you are taking any oral anticoagulant, propranolol or quinidine.

Possible Side-Effects (natural, expected and unavoidable drug actions)
None reported.

▷ **Possible Adverse Effects** (unusual, unexpected and infrequent reactions)
If any of the following develop, consult your physician promptly for guidance.
Mild Adverse Effects
Allergic Reactions: Skin rash, hives, drug fever (see Glossary).
Headache, dizziness, double vision, fatigue, muscular pains, diarrhea.
Serious Adverse Effects
Allergic Reactions: Pancreatitis, kidney damage.
Idiosyncratic Reactions: Nervous agitation, confusion, delirium, hallucinations, coma.
Slowed heart rate, liver damage.
Bone marrow depression (see Glossary)—weakness, fever, sore throat, abnormal bleeding or bruising.

▷ **Possible Effects on Sexual Function:** Decreased libido (600 mg/day); impaired erection and impotence (1000 mg/day); decreased male fertility (1200 mg/day); male breast enlargement (1000 mg/day); female breast enlargement with milk production (1600 mg/day).

▷ **Adverse Effects That May Mimic Natural Diseases or Disorders**
Liver reactions may suggest viral hepatitis.

Natural Diseases or Disorders That May Be Activated by This Drug
Psoriasis (questionable).

CAUTION
1. Do not discontinue this drug abruptly. Ulcer activation and perforation have occurred following abrupt cessation.
2. Hemodialysis can remove from 8% to 14% of this drug. Schedule the dosage to follow completion of each dialysis treatment.

Precautions for Use
By Infants and Children: Safety and effectiveness for use by those under 16 years of age have not been established. If use of this drug is deemed necessary, observe for sedation, confusion, breast enlargement, milk secretion and possible kidney damage.
By Those over 60 Years of Age: Initiate treatment with one-half the usual dose. Observe for the development of nervous agitation, depression, confusion, slurred speech or excessive drowsiness. This drug can contribute to the formation of stomach phytobezoars (masses of undigested vegetable fibers). Individuals with poor chewing ability (missing teeth) and those who have had partial gastrectomy or vagotomy (stomach surgery) are most susceptible. Observe for loss of appetite, stomach fullness, nausea and vomiting.

▷ **Advisability of Use During Pregnancy**
Pregnancy Category: B (tentative). See Pregnancy Code inside back cover.
Animal studies: No birth defects reported.
Human studies: Information from adequate studies of pregnant women is not available.
Use this drug only if clearly needed. Ask physician for guidance.

Advisability of Use if Breast-Feeding
Presence of this drug in breast milk: Yes, in large amounts.
Avoid drug or refrain from nursing.

Habit-Forming Potential: None.

Effects of Overdosage: Confusion, delirium, slurred speech, flushing, sweating, drowsiness, muscle twitching, seizures, coma.

Possible Effects of Long-Term Use: Liver damage (reversible), swelling and tenderness of breast tissue in men.

Suggested Periodic Examinations While Taking This Drug (at physician's discretion)

Complete blood cell counts, liver and kidney function tests, sperm counts, prothrombin times if an anticoagulant is taken concurrently.

▷ **While Taking This Drug, Observe the Following**

Foods: Protein-rich foods produce maximal stomach acid secretion. Follow the diet prescribed to derive optimal benefit from this drug.

Nutritional Support: This drug may inhibit the absorption of vitamin B-12. Consult physician regarding the need for B-12 supplement.

Beverages: No restrictions. May be taken with milk.

▷ *Alcohol:* No interactions with drug. However, alcoholic beverages increase stomach acidity and can reduce the effectiveness of this drug.

Marijuana Smoking: Possible accentuation of reduced sperm production due to this drug.

▷ *Other Drugs*

Cimetidine may ***increase*** the effects of

- oral anticoagulants, and increase the risk of bleeding.
- benzodiazepines (Librium, Valium, etc.), see Drug Class, Section Four.
- phenytoin (Dilantin).
- procainamide (Procan, Pronestyl).
- propranolol (Inderal).
- quinidine (Quinaglute, etc.).
- theophylline (Theo-Dur, Bronkodyl, Slo-bid, etc.).

Cimetidine ***taken concurrently*** with

- carmustine (BCNU) may cause severe bone marrow depression. Do not use these drugs concurrently.

▷ *Driving, Hazardous Activities:* This drug can cause erratic driving behavior. Use caution until it has been determined that dizziness, confusion or double vision does not occur.

Aviation Note: The use of this drug ***may be a disqualification*** for piloting. Consult a designated Aviation Medical Examiner.

Exposure to Sun: No restrictions.

Discontinuation: Do not discontinue this drug suddenly if taken for peptic ulcer disease. Consult physician for withdrawal instructions. This drug does not provide an extended protective effect. Be alert to the possibility of ulcer recurrence anytime after discontinuation.

CIPROFLOXACIN
(sip roh FLOX a sin)

Introduced: 1984

Class: Anti-infective

Prescription: USA: Yes

Controlled Drug: USA: No

Available as Generic: USA: No

Brand Name: Cipro

```
┌─────────────────────────────────────────────────────────────────────┐
│                    BENEFITS versus RISKS                            │
│                                                                     │
│        Possible Benefits                    Possible Risks          │
│   HIGHLY EFFECTIVE              Nausea (1.6%), diarrhea (1.5%),      │
│     TREATMENT FOR                 very rare drug-induced colitis     │
│     INFECTIONS OF THE LOWER     Mild allergic reactions (1.4%)       │
│     RESPIRATORY TRACT,          Very rare hallucination or seizure   │
│     URINARY TRACT, BONES,                                           │
│     JOINTS AND SKIN TISSUES                                         │
│   due to susceptible organisms                                      │
│   Effective treatment for some                                      │
│     forms of bacterial                                              │
│     gastroenteritis (diarrhea)                                      │
└─────────────────────────────────────────────────────────────────────┘
```

▷ **Principal Uses**

As a Single Drug Product: Used primarily to treat responsive infections (in adults) of: (1) the lower respiratory tract (lungs and bronchial tubes); (2) the urinary tract (kidneys, bladder, urethra and prostate gland); (3) the digestive tract (small intestine and colon); (4) bones and joints; (5) skin and related tissues.

How This Drug Works: By interfering with the bacterial enzyme DNA gyrase (which is required for DNA synthesis and cell reproduction), this drug arrests bacterial growth (in low concentrations) and destroys bacteria (in high concentrations).

Available Dosage Forms and Strengths

Tablets — 250 mg, 500 mg, 750 mg

▷ **Usual Adult Dosage Range:** 250 mg to 750 mg/12 hours, depending upon the nature and severity of the infection. The total daily dosage should not exceed 1500 mg. **Note: Actual dosage and administration schedule must be determined by the physician for each patient individually.**

▷ **Dosing Instructions:** May be taken with or without food. Preferably it should be taken 2 hours after eating. Drink fluids liberally during the entire course of treatment. Avoid antacids containing aluminum or magnesium for 2 hours before and after dosing. The tablet may be crushed for administration.

Usual Duration of Use: Continual use on a regular schedule for 7 to 14 days is usually necessary to determine this drug's effectiveness in eradicating the infection. The drug should be continued for at least 2 days after all indications of infection have disappeared. Bone and joint infections may require treatment for 6 weeks or longer. Long-term use requires periodic evaluation of response and dosage adjustment. Consult your physician on a regular basis.

Possible Advantages of This Drug

The most potent anti-infective action of the drugs in this class (quinolones).

Highly effective in treating numerous types of infection caused by a wide spectrum of bacteria (overall clinical response rate of 96%).

Capable of establishing effective drug levels throughout the prostate gland (clinical response rate of 83% in treating prostatitis).

Effective one-dose treatment for uncomplicated gonorrheal infection of the urethra.

No significant effect on kidney function.

Currently a **"Drug of Choice"** for (1) starting treatment of urinary tract infections prior to obtaining the results of urine bacterial culture and sensitivity tests; (2) treating infections due to *Pseudomonas aeruginosa*, a bacterial strain often resistant to other anti-infective drugs.

▷ **This Drug Should Not Be Taken If**

- you have had an allergic reaction to it previously.
- you are pregnant or breast-feeding.
- you have a seizure disorder that is not adequately controlled.
- it is prescribed for a person under 18 years of age.

▷ **Inform Your Physician Before Taking This Drug If**

- you are allergic to cinoxacin (Cinobac), nalidixic acid (NegGram) or norfloxacin (Noroxin).
- you have a history of a seizure disorder or a circulatory disorder of the brain.
- you have impaired liver or kidney function.
- you are taking any form of probenecid or theophylline.

Possible Side-Effects (natural, expected and unavoidable drug actions)

Superinfections (5%). (See Superinfection in the Glossary.)

▷ **Possible Adverse Effects** (unusual, unexpected and infrequent reactions)

If any of the following develop, consult your physician promptly for guidance.

Mild Adverse Effects

Allergic Reactions: Rash (0.83%), itching (0.47%), localized swelling (0.12%).

Dizziness (0.53%), headache (0.30%), weakness (0.36%), migraine (0.06%), anxiety (0.06%), abnormal vision (0.06%).

Nausea (1.6%), diarrhea (1.5%), vomiting (0.7%), indigestion (0.36%).

Serious Adverse Effects

Allergic Reactions: None reported.

Idiosyncratic Reactions: None reported.

Central nervous system stimulation: restlessness, tremor, confusion, hallucinations, seizures (all very rare).

▷ **Possible Effects on Sexual Function:**   None reported.

▷ **Natural Diseases or Disorders That May Be Activated by This Drug**
Latent epilepsy, latent gout.

CAUTION
1. With high doses or prolonged use, crystal formation in the kidney may occur. This can be prevented by drinking copious amounts of water, up to 2 quarts/24 hours.
2. Drugs of this class may decrease the formation of saliva and predispose to the development of dental cavities or gum disease. Consult your dentist if dry mouth persists.

Precautions for Use
By Infants and Children: Avoid the use of this drug completely. It can impair normal bone growth and development.
By Those over 60 Years of Age: Impaired kidney function may require dosage reduction.
If you are taking theophylline concurrently with this drug, observe closely for possible theophylline accumulation and toxicity.

▷ **Advisability of Use During Pregnancy**
Pregnancy Category: C (tentative). See Pregnancy Code inside back cover.
Animal studies: No birth defects due to this drug found in mouse, rat or rabbit studies. However, this drug can impair normal bone development in immature dogs.
Human studies: Information from adequate studies of pregnant women is not available. However, the potential for adverse effects on fetal bone development contraindicates the use of this drug during entire pregnancy.

Advisability of Use if Breast-Feeding
Presence of this drug in breast milk: Probably yes.
Avoid drug or refrain from nursing.

Habit-Forming Potential: None.

Effects of Overdosage: No information available.

Possible Effects of Long-Term Use: Superinfections (see Glossary); crystal formation in kidneys.

Suggested Periodic Examinations While Taking This Drug (at physician's discretion)
Liver function tests, urine analysis.

▷ **While Taking This Drug, Observe the Following**
Foods: No restrictions.
Beverages: No restrictions. May be taken with milk.
▷   *Alcohol:* No interactions expected.
Tobacco Smoking: No interactions expected.
▷   *Other Drugs*
Ciprofloxacin may ***increase*** the effects of

- theophylline, and cause theophylline toxicity.

The following drug may **increase** the effects of ciprofloxacin

- probenecid (Benemid).

The following drugs may **decrease** the effects of ciprofloxacin

- antacids containing aluminum or magnesium can reduce the absorption of ciprofloxacin and lessen its effectiveness.

▷ *Driving, Hazardous Activities:* This drug may cause dizziness and impair vision. Restrict activities as necessary.

Aviation Note: The use of this drug **may be a disqualification** for piloting. Consult a designated Aviation Medical Examiner.

Exposure to Sun: This drug may rarely cause photosensitivity (see Glossary). Sunglasses are advised if eyes are overly sensitive to bright light.

Discontinuation: If you experience no adverse effects from this drug, take the full course prescribed for maximal results. Consult your physician regarding termination of treatment.

CLEMASTINE
(KLEM as teen)

Introduced: 1968

Class: Antihistamines

Prescription: USA: Yes
    Canada: No

Controlled Drug: USA: No
    Canada: No

Available as Generic: USA: No
    Canada: No

Brand Names: Tavist, Tavist-D [CD], Tavist-1

BENEFITS versus RISKS	
Possible Benefits	*Possible Risks*
EFFECTIVE RELIEF OF ALLERGIC RHINITIS AND ALLERGIC SKIN DISORDERS	Mild sedation Atropinelike effects Very rare blood cell disorders

▷ **Principal Uses**

As a Single Drug Product: Used primarily to provide symptomatic relief in allergic and related disorders: seasonal and perennial allergic rhinitis (hay fever), allergic conjunctivitis and vasomotor rhinitis; also in hives and localized swellings (angioedema) of allergic origin.

As a Combination Drug Product [CD]: This drug is combined with a decongestant drug (phenylpropanolamine) to enhance its ability to reduce tissue swelling and secretions in allergic and infectious disorders of the upper respiratory tract—hay fever, head colds and sinusitis.

How This Drug Works: Antihistamines reduce the intensity of the allergic response by blocking the action of histamine after it has been released from sensitized tissue cells in the eyes, nose, respiratory passages and skin.

Available Dosage Forms and Strengths
Syrup — 0.67 mg per 5-ml teaspoonful (5.5% alcohol)
Tablets — 1.34 mg, 2.68 mg

▷ **Usual Adult Dosage Range:**   1.34 mg twice daily, or 2.68 mg 3 times daily. The total daily dosage should not exceed 8.04 mg. **Note: Actual dosage and administration schedule must be determined by the physician for each patient individually.**

▷ **Dosing Instructions:**   Take with food or milk to prevent stomach irritation. The tablet may be crushed for administration.

Usual Duration of Use: Continual use on a regular schedule for 2 to 3 days is usually necessary to determine this drug's effectiveness in relieving the symptoms of allergic rhinitis and dermatosis. It may be necessary to take this drug throughout the entire pollen season, depending upon individual sensitivity. However, antihistamines should not be taken continually (without interruption) for long-term use. Limit their use to periods that require symptomatic relief.

▷ **This Drug Should Not Be Taken If**
- you have had an allergic reaction to any dosage form of it previously.
- you are currently undergoing allergy skin tests.
- you are taking, or have taken within the past 14 days, any monoamine oxidase (MAO) type A inhibitor drug (see Drug Class, Section Four).

▷ **Inform Your Physician Before Taking This Drug If**
- you have had any allergic reactions or unfavorable responses to the previous use of antihistamines.
- you have glaucoma (narrow-angle type) or asthma.
- you have epilepsy or a seizure disorder.
- you have difficulty emptying the urinary bladder, especially if due to prostate gland enlargement (see Prostatism in Glossary).
- you plan to have surgery under general anesthesia in the near future.

Possible Side-Effects (natural, expected and unavoidable drug actions)
Drowsiness; sense of weakness; blurred vision; dryness of the nose, mouth and throat; impaired urination.

▷ **Possible Adverse Effects** (unusual, unexpected and infrequent reactions)
If any of the following develop, consult your physician promptly for guidance.
Mild Adverse Effects
Allergic Reactions: Skin rash, hives.
Headache, nervous agitation, dizziness, confusion, tremor, blurred or double vision, altered color vision, ringing in ears.

Reduced tolerance for contact lenses.

Thickening of bronchial secretions in asthma or bronchitis.

Indigestion, nausea, vomiting, diarrhea.

Serious Adverse Effects

Allergic Reaction: Anaphylactic reaction (see Glossary).

Idiosyncratic Reactions: Euphoria, hysteria, depression, nightmares.

Hemolytic anemia (see Glossary).

Abnormally low white blood cell count—fever, sore throat, infections.

Abnormally low blood platelet count—abnormal bleeding or bruising.

▷ **Possible Effects on Sexual Function:** Shortened menstrual cycle (early arrival of expected menstrual onset).

Natural Diseases or Disorders That May Be Activated by This Drug

Latent epilepsy, glaucoma, prostatism (see Glossary).

CAUTION

1. Discontinue this drug 4 days before diagnostic skin testing procedures in order to prevent false negative test results.
2. Do not use this drug if you have active bronchial asthma, bronchitis or pneumonia. It can thicken bronchial mucus and make it more difficult to remove (by absorption or coughing).

Precautions for Use

By Infants and Children: This drug should not be used in premature or full-term newborn infants. Doses for children should be small. The young child is especially sensitive to the effects of antihistamines on the brain and nervous system.

By Those over 60 Years of Age: You may be more susceptible to the development of drowsiness, dizziness and unsteadiness, and to impairment of thinking, judgment and memory. This drug can increase the degree of impaired urination associated with prostate gland enlargement (prostatism). The sedative effects of antihistamines in the elderly can cause a syndrome of underactivity that may be misinterpreted as senility or emotional depression.

▷ **Advisability of Use During Pregnancy**

Pregnancy Category: B (tentative). See Pregnancy Code inside back cover.

Animal studies: No birth defects due to this drug reported in rat and rabbit studies.

Human studies: Information from adequate studies of pregnant women is not available. However, drugs of this class can cause seizures and other adverse effects on the newborn infant.

Use this drug only if clearly needed. Avoid during the last 3 months. Ask physician for guidance.

Advisability of Use if Breast-Feeding

Presence of this drug in breast milk: Probably yes.

Avoid drug or refrain from nursing.

Habit-Forming Potential: None.

Effects of Overdosage: Drowsiness; unsteadiness; faintness; marked dryness of mouth, nose and throat; flushing of face; shortness of breath; hallucinations; convulsions; stupor progressing to coma.

Possible Effects of Long-Term Use: Tardive dyskinesia (see Glossary) has been reported in association with the long-term use of several widely used antihistamines. It is advisable to avoid the prolonged, continual use of antihistamines without interruption.

Suggested Periodic Examinations While Taking This Drug (at physician's discretion)
Complete blood cell counts.

▷ **While Taking This Drug, Observe the Following**
Foods: No restrictions.
Beverages: No restrictions. May be taken with milk.
▷ *Alcohol:* Use with extreme caution until the combined effects have been determined. The combination of antihistamine and alcohol can produce rapid and marked sedation.
Tobacco Smoking: No interactions expected.
▷ *Other Drugs*
Clemastine may ***increase*** the effects of
• all sedatives, sleep-inducing drugs, tranquilizers, analgesics and narcotic drugs, and produce oversedation.
Clemastine ***taken concurrently*** with
• phenytoin (Dantoin, Dilantin) may alter the pattern of seizures. Dosage adjustments of the anticonvulsant may be necessary.
The following drugs may ***increase*** the effects of clemastine
• monoamine oxidase (MAO) type A inhibitor drugs (see Drug Class, Section Four) may prolong the action of antihistamines.
▷ *Driving, Hazardous Activities:* This drug can impair mental alertness, judgment, coordination and reaction time. Avoid hazardous activities until the full sedative effects have been determined.
Aviation Note: The use of this drug ***is a disqualification*** for piloting. Consult a designated Aviation Medical Examiner.
Exposure to Sun: Use caution. Some drugs of this class can cause photosensitivity (see Glossary).

CLIDINIUM
(kli DIN ee um)

Introduced: 1961

Class: Antispasmodic, atropinelike

Prescription: USA: Yes
Canada: Yes

Controlled Drug: USA: No
Canada: No

Available as Generic: No

Brand Names: ✦Apo-Chlorax [CD], ✦Corium [CD], Librax [CD], Lidox [CD], Quarzan

BENEFITS versus RISKS	
Possible Benefits	*Possible Risks*
RELIEF OF SYMPTOMS DUE TO GASTROINTESTINAL SPASM AND OVERACTIVITY as in peptic ulcer disease and irritable bowel syndrome	Skin rash, hives Dizziness, unsteadiness Confusion, delirium

▷ **Principal Uses**

As a Single Drug Product: This atropinelike antispasmodic drug is used primarily in the management of peptic ulcer disease and the irritable bowel syndrome. Because it has been replaced by more effective drugs, it is seldom used alone.

As a Combination Drug Product [CD]: The major use of this drug is in combination with chlordiazepoxide. When combined, the tranquilizing effect of chlordiazepoxide and the atropinelike effects of clidinium are more effective than either drug used alone. Their actions complement each other in the treatment of peptic ulcer and functional disorders of the gastrointestinal tract.

How This Drug Works: By blocking the action of the chemical (acetylcholine) that transmits impulses at parasympathetic nerve endings, this drug prevents stimulation of muscular contraction and glandular secretion within the organs involved. This results in reduced overall activity, including the prevention or relief of muscle spasms.

Available Dosage Forms and Strengths

Capsules — 2.5 mg, 5 mg

Capsules [CD] — 2.5 mg and 5 mg of chlordiazepoxide

Note: In Canada this drug is available only in combination with chlordiazepoxide. To be fully informed on the use of Librax, read the Drug Profiles of both components.

▷ **Usual Adult Dosage Range:** For Librax—1 or 2 capsules from 1 to 4 times daily, as needed and tolerated. Total daily dosage should not exceed 8 capsules. **Note: Actual dosage and administration schedule must be determined by the physician for each patient individually.**

▷ **Dosing Instructions:** Take 30 to 60 minutes before meals and also at bedtime if necessary. The capsule may be opened for administration.

Usual Duration of Use: Continual use on a regular schedule for 3 to 5 days is usually necessary to determine this drug's effectiveness in relieving the symptoms of gastrointestinal spasm and overactivity. Long-term use (weeks to months) requires physician supervision and guidance. Consult your physician on a regular basis.

▷ **This Drug Should Not Be Taken If**
- you have had an allergic reaction to it previously.
- your stomach cannot empty properly into the intestine (pyloric obstruction).
- you are unable to empty the urinary bladder completely.
- you have narrow-angle-type glaucoma.
- you have severe ulcerative colitis.

▷ **Inform Your Physician Before Taking This Drug If**
- you have open-angle type glaucoma.
- you have angina or coronary heart disease.
- you have a history of peptic ulcer disease.
- you have chronic bronchitis, a hiatal hernia, myasthenia gravis or prostatism (see Glossary).
- you plan to have surgery under general anesthesia in the near future.

Possible Side-Effects (natural, expected and unavoidable drug actions)
Blurred vision (impaired focus), dry mouth and throat, constipation, impaired urination. (Nature and degree of side-effects depend upon individual sensitivity and drug dosage.)

▷ **Possible Adverse Effects** (unusual, unexpected and infrequent reactions)
If any of the following develop, consult your physician promptly for guidance.
Mild Adverse Effects
Allergic Reactions: Skin rash, hives.
Light-headedness, dizziness, unsteadiness.
Dilation of pupils, causing sensitivity to light.
Flushing and dryness of skin, reduced sweating.
Rapid heart action.
Serious Adverse Effects
Idiosyncratic Reactions: Confusion, delirium, abnormal behavior.
Development of acute glaucoma (in susceptible individuals).

▷ **Possible Effects on Sexual Function:**   Impotence; suppressed milk production (7.5 to 20 mg/day).

CAUTION
1. Many over-the-counter medications (see OTC Drugs in Glossary) for allergies, colds and coughs contain drugs that can interact unfavorably with this drug. Ask your physician or pharmacist for guidance before taking these drugs together.
2. Constipation should be treated promptly with stool softeners and effective laxatives.

Precautions for Use
By Infants and Children: Safety, effectiveness and dosage for use by those under 12 years of age have not been established. Ask physician for guidance.

By Those over 60 Years of Age: Initial dosage should be 1 capsule twice a day until tolerance has been determined. This drug can accentuate the symptoms of prostatism (see Glossary).

▷ **Advisability of Use During Pregnancy**
   Pregnancy Category: B (tentative). See Pregnancy Code inside back cover.
      Animal studies: No birth defects reported.
      Human studies: Information from adequate studies of pregnant women is not available.
      Note: If this drug is taken in its combination form (Librax [CD]), see the pregnancy category in the Drug Profile of Chlordiazepoxide. Ask physician for guidance.

Advisability of Use if Breast-Feeding
   Presence of this drug in breast milk: Yes.
   Avoid drug or refrain from nursing.

Habit-Forming Potential: For clidinium—none. For Librax—see Drug Profile of Chlordiazepoxide.

Effects of Overdosage: Dilated pupils, dry mouth, headache, excitement, confusion, hallucinations, delirium, hot skin, high fever, convulsions, coma.

Possible Effects of Long-Term Use: Chronic constipation, severe enough to cause fecal impaction.

Suggested Periodic Examinations While Taking This Drug (at physician's discretion)
   Measurement of internal eye pressure to detect significant increase that could indicate developing glaucoma.

▷ **While Taking This Drug, Observe the Following**
   Foods: No interactions with drug. Follow prescribed diet.
   Beverages: As allowed by prescribed diet. Drug may be taken with milk.
▷ *Alcohol:* Use caution and observe for increased sedation or dizziness.
   Tobacco Smoking: No interactions with clidinium. For Librax—see Drug Profile of Chlordiazepoxide.
▷ *Other Drugs*
      Clidinium may *increase* the effects of
      • atenolol (Tenormin), and require reduction of its dosage.
      • other drugs with atropinelike actions (see Drug Class, Section Four).
▷ *Driving, Hazardous Activities:* This drug may cause drowsiness, dizziness or blurred vision. Avoid hazardous activities if these drug effects occur.
   Aviation Note: The use of this drug *may be a disqualification* for piloting. Consult a designated Aviation Medical Examiner.
   Exposure to Sun: No restrictions.

Exposure to Heat: Use extreme caution. The use of this drug in hot environments may impair the regulation of body temperature and increase the risk of heat stroke.

CLINDAMYCIN
(klin da MI sin)

Introduced: 1973

Class: Antibiotic

Prescription: USA: Yes
Canada: Yes

Controlled Drug: USA: No
Canada: No

Available as Generic: USA: Yes
Canada: No

Brand Names: Cleocin, Cleocin T, ✦Dalacin C

BENEFITS versus RISKS

Possible Benefits	*Possible Risks*
EFFECTIVE TREATMENT FOR SERIOUS INFECTIONS OF THE LOWER RESPIRATORY TRACT, ABDOMINAL CAVITY, GENITAL TRACT IN WOMEN, BLOOD STREAM (SEPTICEMIA), SKIN AND RELATED TISSUES caused by susceptible organisms	SEVERE DRUG-INDUCED COLITIS (fatalities reported)
SPECIFIC PREVENTION AND TREATMENT FOR PNEUMOCYSTIS CARINII PNEUMONIA (PCP) ASSOCIATED WITH AIDS	Rare liver injury with jaundice
Possibly effective for the local treatment of acne	Rare reduction in white blood cell and platelet counts

---

▷ **Principal Uses**

As a Single Drug Product

Used primarily to treat serious and unusual infections of the lungs and bronchial tubes, organs and tissues within the abdominal cavity, the genital tract and pelvic organs in women, the skin and soft tissue structures and generalized infections involving the bloodstream.

A more recent use has been the prevention and treatment of pneumocystis carinii pneumonia, a frequent infection associated with AIDS.

How This Drug Works: By interfering with the formation of proteins necessary for cell growth and reproduction, this drug (in low concentrations) arrests the multiplication of bacteria and (in high concentrations) destroys bacteria.

Available Dosage Forms and Strengths
>   Capsules — 75 mg, 150 mg, 300 mg
>   Injection — 150 mg per ml
>   Oral solution — 75 mg per 5-ml teaspoonful
>   Topical solution — 10 mg per ml

▷ **Usual Adult Dosage Range:** For infections of average severity: 150 to 300 mg/6 hours; for more severe infections: 300 to 450 mg/6 hours. The total daily dosage should not exceed 1800 mg. **Note: Actual dosage and administration schedule must be determined by the physician for each patient individually.**

▷ **Dosing Instructions:** Take the capsule with a full glass of water or with food to prevent irritation of the esophagus. The capsule may be opened and the contents mixed with food for administration. Shake the oral solution well before measuring the dose. Do not refrigerate the oral solution; chilling can cause it to thicken, making administration difficult.

Usual Duration of Use: Continual use on a regular schedule for 3 to 5 days is usually necessary to determine this drug's effectiveness in controlling responsive infections. The duration of use should not exceed the time required to eliminate the infection.

Possible Advantages of This Drug: Bacterial sensitivity testing may show this drug to be more effective than commonly used antibiotics in treating some severe and unusual infections.

Currently a "Drug of Choice" for preventing and treating pneumonia due to pneumocystis carinii, a frequent complication of AIDS.

▷ **This Drug Should Not Be Taken If**
- you are allergic to either clindamycin or lincomycin.
- it is prescribed for a mild or trivial infection such as a cold, sore throat or "flulike" illness.
- you have a history of Crohn's disease or ulcerative colitis.

▷ **Inform Your Physician Before Taking This Drug If**
- you have a history of allergy to any drug.
- you have a history of drug-induced colitis.
- you are allergic by nature: hay fever, asthma, hives, eczema.
- you have a history of previous yeast infections.
- you have myasthenia gravis.
- you have impaired liver or kidney function.
- you plan to have surgery under general anesthesia in the near future.

Possible Side-Effects (natural, expected and unavoidable drug actions)
Superinfections (see Glossary).

▷ **Possible Adverse Effects** (unusual, unexpected and infrequent reactions)
If any of the following develop, consult your physician promptly for guidance.
Mild Adverse Effects
Allergic Reactions: Skin rashes (3% to 5%), hives.
Nausea, vomiting, mild diarrhea (3% to 30%), stomach pain.
Multiple joint pains (rare).
Serious Adverse Effects
Allergic Reactions: Severe skin reactions: erythema multiforme (Stevens-Johnson syndrome).
Toxic liver reaction with jaundice (see Glossary).
Severe colitis with persistent diarrhea (0.01% to 10%); stools may contain blood and/or mucus.
Rare reduction of white blood cell and platelet counts.

▷ **Possible Effects on Sexual Function:** None reported.

Possible Delayed Adverse Effects: Severe colitis with diarrhea (pseudomembranous colitis) may begin several weeks after discontinuing this drug.

▷ **Adverse Effects That May Mimic Natural Diseases or Disorders**
Liver reactions may suggest viral hepatitis.
Multiple joint pains may suggest the onset of arthritis.

▷ **Natural Diseases or Disorders That May Be Activated by This Drug**
Crohn's disease, ulcerative colitis, myasthenia gravis.

CAUTION
1. Troublesome and persistent diarrhea can develop in sensitive individuals. If diarrhea persists longer than 24 hours, discontinue this drug and consult your physician for guidance.
2. If surgery under general anesthesia is planned while taking this drug, the choice of anesthetic must be considered carefully to prevent excessive muscle relaxation and associated impairment of breathing.

Precautions for Use
By Infants and Children: Safety and effectiveness for use by those under 1 month of age have not been established. Use with caution.
By Those over 60 Years of Age: Observe closely for the possible development of diarrhea (more common in this age group). Also observe for the possible development of yeast infection of the skin in the genital and anal regions, a form of superinfection (see Glossary). Report such developments promptly to your physician.

▷ **Advisability of Use During Pregnancy**
Pregnancy Category: B (tentative). See Pregnancy Code inside back cover.
Animal studies: No birth defects due to this drug found in mouse or rat studies.
Human studies: Information from adequate studies of pregnant women is not available. Use this drug only if clearly needed. Ask your physician for guidance.

Advisability of Use if Breast-Feeding
Presence of this drug in breast milk: Yes.
Avoid drug or refrain from nursing.

Habit-Forming Potential: None.

Effects of Overdosage: Nausea, vomiting, cramping, diarrhea.

Possible Effects of Long-Term Use
Superinfections, especially from yeast organisms.
Severe colitis with persistent diarrhea.

Suggested Periodic Examinations While Taking This Drug (at physician's discretion)
Complete blood cell counts, liver function tests.

▷ **While Taking This Drug, Observe the Following**
Foods: No restrictions.
Beverages: No restrictions. May be taken with milk.
▷ *Alcohol:* No interactions expected.
Tobacco Smoking: No interactions expected.
▷ *Other Drugs*
Clindamycin *taken concurrently* with
- antidiarrheal drugs (diphenoxylate, loperamide, paregoric) may result in worsening of the underlying colitis because of impaired elimination of causative toxins.
- antimyasthenic drugs (ambenonium, neostigmine, pyridostigmine) may reduce their effectiveness in relieving the muscle weakness of myasthenia gravis.
The following drugs may *decrease* the effects of clindamycin
- chloramphenicol (Chloromycetin).
- erythromycin (E.E.S., E-Mycin, etc.).
▷ *Driving, Hazardous Activities:* This drug may cause nausea and diarrhea. Restrict activities as necessary.
Aviation Note: The use of this drug *may be a disqualification* for piloting. Consult a designated Aviation Medical Examiner.
Exposure to Sun: Use caution until sensitivity is determined.
Discontinuation: If tolerated satisfactorily, take the full course prescribed. When used to treat infections that may predispose to rheumatic fever or nephritis, take continually in full dosage for no less than 10 days.
Special Storage Instructions: Oral solution should be kept at room temperature; do not refrigerate.

Observe the Following Expiration Time: Do not take the oral solution if it is older than 14 days.

CLONIDINE
(KLOH ni deen)

Introduced: 1969

Prescription: USA: Yes
Canada: Yes

Available as Generic: USA: Yes
Canada: No

Class: Antihypertensive

Controlled Drug: USA: No
Canada: No

Brand Names: Catapres, Catapres-TTS, Combipres [CD], ✦Dixarit

---

BENEFITS versus RISKS

Possible Benefits	*Possible Risks*
EFFECTIVE ANTIHYPERTEN-SIVE in mild to moderate high blood pressure	ACUTE WITHDRAWAL SYNDROME and hypertensive "overshoot" with abrupt discontinuation
Effective control of menopausal hot flashes (in selected cases)	Raynaud's phenomenon (cold fingers or toes)

▷ **Principal Uses**

As a Single Drug Product: This antihypertensive drug is often used as a "step 2" drug in the treatment of mild to moderate high blood pressure. It is generally not used to initiate treatment, but is added when a "step 1" drug proves to be inadequate. It may also be used as a "step 3 or 4" drug in place of drugs that cause marked orthostatic hypotension (see Glossary). It is sometimes used to prevent migraine headache, to prevent hot flashes of the menopause and to treat menstrual cramps.

As a Combination Drug Product [CD]: This "step 2" antihypertensive is available in combination with the "step 1" antihypertensive drug chlorthalidone, a diuretic. The differing methods of action complement each other to make the combination a more effective antihypertensive.

How This Drug Works: By decreasing the activity of the vasomotor center in the brain, this drug reduces the ability of the sympathetic nervous system to maintain the degree of blood vessel constriction responsible for the elevation of blood pressure. This change results in relaxation of blood vessel walls and lowering of blood pressure.

Available Dosage Forms and Strengths
Patches — 0.1 mg, 0.2 mg, 0.3 mg
Tablets — 0.1 mg, 0.2 mg, 0.3 mg

▷ **Usual Adult Dosage Range:** Tablets—initially 0.1 mg twice daily. Increase by 0.1 to 0.2 mg daily as needed and tolerated. Usual range is 0.2 to 0.8 mg daily, taken in 2 doses. Total daily dosage should not exceed 2.4 mg. Medicated patches are applied once a week. **Note: Actual dosage and administration schedule must be determined by the physician for each patient individually.**

▷ **Dosing Instructions:** Tablets may be taken without regard to eating. The tablet may be crushed for administration.

Usual Duration of Use: Continual use on a regular schedule for 2 to 3 weeks is usually necessary to determine this drug's effectiveness in controlling high blood pressure. Long-term use (months to years) requires supervision and guidance by the physician. Consult your physician on a regular basis.

▷ **This Drug Should Not Be Taken If**
- you have had an allergic reaction to it previously.

▷ **Inform Your Physician Before Taking This Drug If**
- you have a circulatory disorder of the brain.
- you have angina or coronary artery disease.
- you have or have had serious emotional depression.
- you have Buerger's disease or Raynaud's phenomenon.
- you are taking any sedative or hypnotic drugs or an antidepressant.
- you plan to have surgery under general anesthesia in the near future.

Possible Side-Effects (natural, expected and unavoidable drug actions)
Drowsiness (35%), dry nose and mouth (40%), constipation (common), decreased heart rate, mild orthostatic hypotension (see Glossary).

▷ **Possible Adverse Effects** (unusual, unexpected and infrequent reactions)
If any of the following develop, consult your physician promptly for guidance.
Mild Adverse Effects
Allergic Reactions: Skin rash, hives, localized swellings, itching.
Headache, dizziness, fatigue, anxiety, nervousness, dryness and burning of eyes.
Painful parotid (salivary) gland, nausea, vomiting.
Weight gain, urinary retention.
Serious Adverse Effects
Idiosyncratic Reaction: Raynaud's phenomenon (see Glossary).
Aggravation of congestive heart failure, heart rhythm disorders, vivid dreaming, nightmares, depression, hallucinations.
Corneal ulcers (rare). Acute pancreatitis (rare).

▷ **Possible Effects on Sexual Function:** Decreased libido in 10% (0.2 to 0.8 mg/day); impotence in 8% to 24% (0.5 to 3.6 mg/day); impaired ejaculation (rare); enlargement of male breasts (0.2 to 0.8 mg/day).

CAUTION

1. ***Do not discontinue this drug suddenly.*** Sudden withdrawal can produce a severe and possibly fatal reaction.
2. Hot weather and the fever associated with infection can reduce blood pressure significantly. Dosage adjustments may be necessary.
3. Report the development of any tendency to emotional depression.

Precautions for Use

By Infants and Children: Safety and effectiveness for use by those under 12 years of age have not been established.

By Those over 60 Years of Age: ***Proceed cautiously*** with the use of any antihypertensive drug. Unacceptably high blood pressure should be reduced without creating the risks associated with excessively low blood pressure. Start treatment with small doses and monitor the blood pressure response frequently. Observe for the development of light-headedness, dizziness, unsteadiness, fainting and falling. Sedation and dry mouth occur in 50% of elderly users. Report promptly any changes in mood or behavior: depression, delusions, hallucinations.

▷ **Advisability of Use During Pregnancy**

Pregnancy Category: C (tentative). See Pregnancy Code inside back cover.

Animal studies: No birth defects reported. However, this drug is toxic to the embryo in low dosage.

Human studies: Information from adequate studies of pregnant women is not available.

The manufacturer recommends that this drug be avoided by women who are or who may become pregnant. Ask physician for guidance.

Advisability of Use if Breast-Feeding

Presence of this drug in breast milk: Yes.

This drug may impair milk production. Monitor nursing infant closely and discontinue drug or nursing if adverse effects develop.

Habit-Forming Potential: None.

Effects of Overdosage: Marked drowsiness, weakness, dry mouth, slow pulse, low blood pressure, vomiting, stupor progressing to coma.

Possible Effects of Long-Term Use: Development of tolerance (see Glossary) with loss of drug effectiveness; weight gain due to salt and water retention; temporary sexual impotence.

Suggested Periodic Examinations While Taking This Drug (at physician's discretion)

Blood pressure measurements, monitoring of body weight.

▷ **While Taking This Drug, Observe the Following**

Foods: Avoid excessive salt. Ask physician for guidance regarding degree of salt restriction.

Beverages: No restrictions. May be taken with milk.

▷ *Alcohol:* Use with extreme caution. The combined effects can cause marked drowsiness and exaggerated reduction of blood pressure.

Tobacco Smoking: No interactions expected. Follow your physician's advice regarding use of tobacco.

▷ *Other Drugs*

Clonidine may *decrease* the effects of

- levodopa (Larodopa, Sinemet, etc.), causing an increase in parkinsonism symptoms.

Clonidine *taken concurrently* with

- beta-adrenergic-blocking drugs (Inderal, Lopressor, etc.) may increase the risk of serious rebound hypertension if clonidine is discontinued first. It is advisable to discontinue the beta blocker first and then withdraw clonidine gradually.

The following drugs may *decrease* the effects of clonidine

- tricyclic antidepressants (Elavil, Sinequan, etc.) may reduce its effectiveness in lowering blood pressure.

▷ *Driving, Hazardous Activities:* Use caution. This drug can cause drowsiness and can impair mental alertness, judgment and coordination.

Aviation Note: Hypertension (high blood pressure) *is a disqualification* for piloting. Consult a designated Aviation Medical Examiner.

Exposure to Sun: No restrictions.

Exposure to Heat: Use caution. Hot environments may reduce the blood pressure significantly; be alert to the possibility of orthostatic hypotension (see Glossary).

Exposure to Cold: Use caution. This drug may cause painful blanching and numbness of the hands and feet on exposure to cold air or water (Raynaud's phenomenon).

Heavy Exercise or Exertion: Use caution. Isometric exercises—the "overload" technique for strengthening individual muscles—can raise blood pressure significantly. The use of this drug may intensify the hypertensive response to isometric exercise. Ask physician for guidance.

Occurrence of Unrelated Illness: Fever associated with infections may lower the blood pressure significantly. Repeated vomiting may prevent the regular use of this drug and result in an acute withdrawal reaction. Consult your physician.

Discontinuation: **Do not discontinue this drug suddenly.** A severe withdrawal reaction can occur within 12 to 48 hours after the last dose. The dose should be reduced gradually over 3 to 4 days, with periodic monitoring of the blood pressure.

CLORAZEPATE
(klor AZ e payt)

Introduced: 1968

Class: Mild tranquilizer, benzodiazepines

Prescription: USA: Yes
Canada: Yes

Controlled Drug: USA: C-IV*
Canada: No

Available as Generic: Yes

Brand Names: Gen-Xene, ♦Novoclopate, Tranxene, Tranxene-SD, Tranxene-SD Half Strength

---

BENEFITS versus RISKS	
Possible Benefits	*Possible Risks*
RELIEF OF ANXIETY AND NERVOUS TENSION in 70% to 80% of users	Habit-forming potential with prolonged use
Wide margin of safety with therapeutic doses	Minor impairment of mental functions
Very few drug interactions	

▷ **Principal Uses**

As a Single Drug Product: Used primarily to (1) provide short-term relief of mild to moderate anxiety, and (2) provide adjunctive treatment in controlling "partial" seizures, a type of epilepsy.

How This Drug Works: It is thought that this drug produces a calming effect by enhancing the action of the nerve transmitter gamma-aminobutyric acid (GABA), which in turn blocks the arousal of higher brain centers.

Available Dosage Forms and Strengths
Capsules — 3.75 mg, 7.5 mg, 15 mg
Tablets — 3.75 mg, 7.5 mg, 15 mg
Tablets, single dose — 11.25 mg, 22.5 mg

▷ **Usual Adult Dosage Range:** 15 to 60 mg/24 hours, in 2 to 4 divided doses or as a single dose at bedtime. The usual dose is 30 mg/24 hours. Total daily dose should not exceed 90 mg. **Note: Actual dosage and administration schedule must be determined by the physician for each patient individually.**

▷ **Dosing Instructions:** May be taken on empty stomach or with food or milk. Capsule may be opened and regular tablet may be crushed for admin-

*See Schedules of Controlled Drugs inside back cover.

istration; the single-dose tablet should not be crushed. Do not discontinue this drug abruptly if taken for more than 4 weeks.

Usual Duration of Use: Continual use on a regular schedule for 5 to 7 days is usually necessary to determine this drug's effectiveness in relieving moderate anxiety. Limit continual use to 1 to 3 weeks. Avoid uninterrupted and prolonged use.

▷ **This Drug Should Not Be Taken If**
- you have had an allergic reaction to any dosage form of it previously.
- you have acute narrow-angle glaucoma.

▷ **Inform Your Physician Before Taking This Drug If**
- you are allergic to any benzodiazepine drug (see Drug Class, Section Four).
- you have a history of alcoholism or drug abuse.
- you are pregnant or planning pregnancy.
- you have impaired liver or kidney function.
- you have a history of serious depression or mental disorder.
- you have any of the following: asthma, emphysema, epilepsy, myasthenia gravis.

Possible Side-Effects (natural, expected and unavoidable drug actions)
Drowsiness, lethargy, unsteadiness; "hangover" effects on the day following bedtime use.

▷ **Possible Adverse Effects** (unusual, unexpected and infrequent reactions)
If any of the following develop, consult your physician promptly for guidance.
Mild Adverse Effects
Allergic Reactions: Skin rash, hives.
Dizziness, fainting, blurred vision, double vision, slurred speech, sweating, nausea.
Serious Adverse Effects
Idiosyncratic Reactions: Paradoxical responses of excitement, agitation, anger, rage.

▷ **Possible Effects on Sexual Function:** Altered timing and pattern of menstruation.

CAUTION
1. This drug should not be discontinued abruptly if it has been taken continually for more than 4 weeks.
2. The concurrent use of some over-the-counter drug products that contain antihistamines (allergy and cold preparations, sleep aids) can cause excessive sedation in sensitive individuals.
3. If this drug is taken at bedtime as a hypnotic (see Glossary), significant impairment of intellectual and physical skills may persist into the following day; avoid alcohol and hazardous activities (driving, etc.).

Precautions for Use

By Infants and Children: Safety and effectiveness for use by those under 9 years of age have not been established. This drug should not be used in the hyperactive or psychotic child of any age.

By Those over 60 Years of Age: It is advisable to use smaller doses at longer intervals to avoid overdosage. Observe for the possible development of lethargy, indifference, fatigue, weakness, unsteadiness, disturbing dreams, nightmares and paradoxical reactions of excitement, agitation, anger, hostility and rage.

▷ Advisability of Use During Pregnancy

Pregnancy Category: D (tentative). See Pregnancy Code inside back cover.
Animal studies: No birth defects reported in mouse, rat and rabbit studies.

Human studies: Information from adequate studies of pregnant women is not available.

There has been one report of multiple birth defects in a fetus exposed to this drug during the first 3 months. Frequent use in late pregnancy can cause the "floppy infant" syndrome in the newborn: weakness, lethargy, unresponsiveness, depressed breathing, low body temperature. Avoid use during entire pregnancy.

Advisability of Use if Breast-Feeding

Presence of this drug in breast milk: Yes, in small amounts.
Avoid drug or refrain from nursing.

Habit-Forming Potential: This drug can produce psychological and/or physical dependence (see Glossary) if used in large doses for an extended period of time.

Effects of Overdosage: Marked drowsiness, weakness, feeling of drunkenness, staggering gait, tremor, stupor progressing to deep sleep or coma.

Possible Effects of Long-Term Use: Psychological and/or physical dependence.

Suggested Periodic Examinations While Taking This Drug (at physician's discretion)
During long-term use: Complete blood cell counts.

▷ While Taking This Drug, Observe the Following

Foods: No restrictions.
Beverages: Avoid excessive intake of caffeine-containing beverages: coffee, tea, cola. May be taken with milk.

▷   *Alcohol:* Use with extreme caution until the combined effect is determined. Alcohol may increase the absorption of this drug and add to its depressant effects on the brain. It is advisable to avoid alcohol completely—throughout the day and night—if it is necessary to drive or to engage in any hazardous activity.

Tobacco Smoking: Heavy smoking may reduce the calming action of this drug.

Marijuana Smoking: Increased sedation and significant impairment of intellectual and physical performance.

▷ *Other Drugs*

Clorazepate may ***increase*** the effects of
- digoxin (Lanoxin), and cause digoxin toxicity.

Clorazepate may ***decrease*** the effects of
- levodopa (Sinemet, etc.), and reduce its effectiveness in treating Parkinson's disease.

The following drugs may ***increase*** the effects of clorazepate
- cimetidine (Tagamet).
- disulfiram (Antabuse).
- isoniazid (INH, Rifamate, etc.).
- oral contraceptives.
- valproic acid (Depakene).

The following drugs may ***decrease*** the effects of clorazepate
- rifampin (Rimactane, etc.).
- theophylline (aminophylline, Theo-Dur, etc.).

▷ *Driving, Hazardous Activities:* This drug can impair mental alertness, judgment, physical coordination and reaction time. Avoid hazardous activities accordingly.

Aviation Note: The use of this drug ***is a disqualification*** for piloting. Consult a designated Aviation Medical Examiner.

Exposure to Sun: No restrictions.

Discontinuation: Avoid sudden discontinuation if this drug has been taken for more than 4 weeks. Dosage should be tapered gradually to prevent a withdrawal syndrome that could include depression, confusion, hallucinations, tremor, seizures, muscle cramping, sweating and vomiting.

CLOXACILLIN
(klox a SIL in)

Introduced: 1962

Class: Antibiotic, penicillins

Prescription: USA: Yes
Canada: Yes

Controlled Drug: USA: No
Canada: No

Available as Generic: USA: Yes
Canada: No

Brand Names: ✦Apo-Cloxi, ✦Bactopen, Cloxapen, ✦Novocloxin, ✦Orbenin, Tegopen

BENEFITS versus RISKS	
Possible Benefits	*Possible Risks*
EFFECTIVE TREATMENT OF INFECTIONS due to susceptible microorganisms	ALLERGIC REACTIONS, mild to severe
	Superinfections (yeast)
	Drug-induced colitis
	Rare blood cell disorders

▷ **Principal Uses**

    As a Single Drug Product: Used primarily to treat infections that are caused by bacteria (principally staphylococcus) that have developed resistance to the original types of penicillin. It is of value in treating infections of the skin and skin structures, the upper and lower respiratory tract (including "strep" throat) and infections that are widely scattered throughout the body.

How This Drug Works: This drug destroys susceptible infecting bacteria by interfering with their ability to produce new protective cell walls as they multiply and grow.

Available Dosage Forms and Strengths
    Capsules — 250 mg, 500 mg
    Oral solution — 125 mg per 5-ml teaspoonful

▷ **Usual Adult Dosage Range:** 250 to 500 mg/6 hours (4 doses/24 hours). The maximal dose is 6000 mg/24 hours. **Note: Actual dosage and administration schedule must be determined by the physician for each patient individually.**

▷ **Dosing Instructions:** Take on empty stomach, 1 hour before or 2 hours after eating, at same times each day. Capsule may be opened for administration.

Usual Duration of Use: As long as necessary to eradicate the infection. For all streptococcal infections: not less than 10 consecutive days (without interruption) to reduce the possibility of developing rheumatic fever or glomerulonephritis.

▷ **This Drug Should Not Be Taken If**
- you have had an allergic reaction to any dosage form of it previously.
- you are certain you are allergic to *any* form of penicillin.

▷ **Inform Your Physician Before Taking This Drug If**
- you suspect you may be allergic to penicillin or you have a history of a previous "reaction" to penicillin.
- you are allergic to cephalosporin antibiotics (Ancef, Ceporan, Ceporex, Duricef, Kafocin, Keflex, Keflin, Kefzol, Loridine).
- you are allergic by nature—hay fever, asthma, hives, eczema.

- you have a history of kidney disease, regional enteritis or ulcerative colitis.

Possible Side-Effects (natural, expected and unavoidable drug actions)
Superinfections (see Glossary), often due to yeast organisms.

▷ **Possible Adverse Effects** (unusual, unexpected and infrequent reactions)
If any of the following develop, consult your physician promptly for guidance.
Mild Adverse Effects
Allergic Reactions: Skin rashes, hives, itching.
Irritations of mouth and tongue, unpleasant taste, nausea, vomiting, mild diarrhea.
Serious Adverse Effects
Allergic Reactions: Anaphylactic reaction (see Glossary), severe skin reactions, drug fever, swollen painful joints, sore throat.
Pseudomembranous colitis—severe diarrhea.

▷ **Possible Effects on Sexual Function:**   None reported.

CAUTION
1. Take the exact dose and the full course prescribed.
2. This drug should not be used concurrently with antibiotics like erythromycin or tetracycline.

Precautions for Use
By Infants and Children: Dosage is based on age and weight. Consult your physician for precise dosage schedule.
By Those over 60 Years of Age: It is advisable to evaluate kidney function before and during use of this drug to determine the need for dosage adjustment. Natural changes in the skin may predispose to prolonged itching reactions in the genital and anal regions. Report such reactions promptly.

▷ **Advisability of Use During Pregnancy**
Pregnancy Category: B (tentative). See Pregnancy Code inside back cover.
Animal studies: No birth defects reported in rabbit studies.
Human studies: Information from adequate studies of pregnant women indicates no increased risk of birth defects in 3546 pregnancies exposed to penicillin derivatives.
Use only if clearly needed. Ask physician for guidance.

Advisability of Use if Breast-Feeding
Presence of this drug in breast milk: Probably yes.
The nursing infant may be sensitized to penicillin and may be at risk for diarrhea or yeast infections. Avoid drug if possible or refrain from nursing.

Habit-Forming Potential: None.

Effects of Overdosage: Possible nausea, vomiting and/or diarrhea.

Possible Effects of Long-Term Use: Superinfections, often due to yeast organisms.

Suggested Periodic Examinations While Taking This Drug (at physician's discretion)
Complete blood cell counts. Liver and kidney function tests with long-term use.

▷ **While Taking This Drug, Observe the Following**
Foods: No restrictions.
Beverages: No restrictions.
▷ *Alcohol:* No interactions expected.
Tobacco Smoking: No interactions expected.
▷ *Other Drugs*
Cloxacillin may **decrease** the effects of
• oral contraceptives in some women, and impair their effectiveness in preventing pregnancy.
The following drugs may **decrease** the effects of cloxacillin
• antacids may reduce the absorption of cloxacillin.
• chloramphenicol (Chloromycetin).
• erythromycin (Erythrocin, E-Mycin, etc.).
• tetracyclines (Achromycin, Declomycin, Minocin, etc.). (See Drug Class, Section Four.)
▷ *Driving, Hazardous Activities:* Usually no restrictions.
Aviation Note: The use of this drug **may be a disqualification** for piloting. Consult a designated Aviation Medical Examiner.
Exposure to Sun: No restrictions.
Special Storage Instructions: Keep capsules in a tightly closed container at room temperature. Keep oral solution in the refrigerator.
Observe the Following Expiration Times: Oral solution kept refrigerated is good for 14 days; when kept at room temperature, it is good for only 3 days.

CODEINE
(KOH deen)

Introduced: 1886

Class: Analgesic, narcotic

Prescription: USA: Yes
Canada: Yes

Controlled Drug: USA: C-II*
Canada: <N>

Available as Generic: Yes

*See Schedules of Controlled Drugs inside back cover.

Brand Names: Actifed w/Codeine [CD], Ambenyl Expectorant [CD], Ambenyl Syrup [CD], Atasol-8, -15, -30 [CD], Benylin Syrup w/Codeine [CD], Bufferin w/Codeine [CD], ♦Coryphen-Codeine [CD], Dimetane Cough Syrup-DC [CD], Dimetane Expectorant-C [CD], Dimetapp-C [CD], Dimetapp w/Codeine [CD], Empirin w/Codeine No. 2, 4 [CD], Empracet w/Codeine No. 3, 4 [CD], ♦Empracet-30, -60 [CD], ♦Emtec-30 [CD], ♦Exdol [CD], ♦Exdol-8, -15, -30 [CD], ♦Fiorinal-C 1/4, -C 1/2 [CD], Fiorinal w/Codeine No. 1, 2, 3 [CD], Isoclor Expectorant [CD], ♦Lenoltec w/Codeine No. 1, 2, 3, 4 [CD], Naldecon-CX [CD], ♦Novahistex C [CD], ♦Paveral, Penntuss [CD], ♦Phenaphen No. 2, 3, 4 [CD], Phenaphen w/Codeine No. 2, 3, 4 [CD], Phenergan w/Codeine [CD], Robaxisal-C [CD], ♦Rounox w/Codeine [CD], Triaminic Expectorant w/Codeine [CD], ♦Tylenol w/Codeine [CD], Tylenol w/Codeine No. 1, 2, 3, 4 [CD], ♦Tylenol w/Codeine Elixir [CD]

BENEFITS versus RISKS

Possible Benefits	*Possible Risks*
EFFECTIVE RELIEF OF MODERATE TO SEVERE PAIN	Low potential for habit formation (dependence)
EFFECTIVE CONTROL OF COUGH	Mild allergic reactions (infrequent)
	Nausea, constipation

▷ **Principal Uses**

As a Single Drug Product: Used primarily to (1) relieve moderate to severe pain; (2) control cough; (3) control diarrhea. Its widest use is as an ingredient in analgesic preparations and cough remedies. Its constipating effect is sometimes used to treat diarrhea, though better drugs are now available for this purpose.

As a Combination Drug Product [CD]: Codeine is commonly combined with other milder analgesics to enhance their effectiveness, notably aspirin and acetaminophen. It is frequently added to cough mixtures containing antihistamines, decongestants and expectorants to make these "shotgun" preparations more effective in reducing the frequency and severity of cough.

How This Drug Works: Acting primarily as a depressant of certain brain functions, this drug suppresses the perception of pain, calms the emotional response to pain, reduces the sensitivity of the cough reflex and inhibits the activity of brain centers that regulate the intestinal tract.

Available Dosage Forms and Strengths

Injection — 30 mg per ml, 60 mg per ml
Tablets — 15 mg, 30 mg, 60 mg
Tablets, soluble — 15 mg, 30 mg, 60 mg

▷ **Usual Adult Dosage Range:** As analgesic—15 to 60 mg/3 to 6 hours as needed. For cough—10 to 20 mg/4 to 6 hours as needed. For diarrhea—30 mg/6 hours as needed. Total daily dosage should not exceed 200 mg for pain or 120 mg for cough or diarrhea. **Note: Actual dosage and administration schedule must be determined by the physician for each patient individually.**

▷ **Dosing Instructions:**   May be taken with or following food to reduce stomach irritation or nausea. Tablet may be crushed for administration.

Usual Duration of Use: As required to control pain, cough or diarrhea. Continual use should not exceed 5 to 7 days without interruption and reassessment of need.

▷ **This Drug Should Not Be Taken If**
- you have had an allergic reaction to any dosage form of it previously.
- you are having an acute attack of asthma.

▷ **Inform Your Physician Before Taking This Drug If**
- you have a history of drug abuse or alcoholism.
- you have impaired liver or kidney function.
- you have gall-bladder disease, a seizure disorder or an underactive thyroid gland.
- you are taking any other drugs that have a sedative effect.
- you plan to have surgery under general anesthesia in the near future.

Possible Side-Effects (natural, expected and unavoidable drug actions)
Drowsiness, light-headedness, dry mouth, urinary retention, constipation.

▷ **Possible Adverse Effects** (unusual, unexpected and infrequent reactions)
If any of the following develop, consult your physician promptly for guidance.
Mild Adverse Effects
Allergic Reactions: Skin rash, hives, itching.
Dizziness, impaired concentration, sensation of drunkenness, confusion, depression, blurred or double vision.
Nausea, vomiting.
Serious Adverse Effects
Allergic Reactions: Anaphylaxis (rare), severe skin reactions.
Idiosyncratic Reactions: Delirium, hallucinations, excitement, increased sensitivity to pain after the analgesic effect has worn off.
Seizures (rare), impaired breathing.

▷ **Possible Effects on Sexual Function:**   None reported.

▷ **Adverse Effects That May Mimic Natural Diseases or Disorders**
Paradoxical behavioral disturbances may suggest psychotic disorder.

CAUTION
1. If you have asthma, chronic bronchitis or emphysema, excessive use of this drug may cause significant respiratory difficulty, thickening of bronchial secretions and suppression of coughing.

2. The concurrent use of this drug with atropinelike drugs can increase the risk of urinary retention and reduced intestinal function.
3. Do not take this drug following acute head injury.

Precautions for Use
By Infants and Children: Do not use this drug in children under 2 years of age because of their vulnerability to life-threatening respiratory depression.
By Those over 60 Years of Age: Use small doses initially and increase dosage as needed and tolerated. Limit use to short-term treatment only. There may be increased susceptibility to the development of drowsiness, dizziness, unsteadiness, falling, urinary retention and constipation (often leading to fecal impaction).

▷ **Advisability of Use During Pregnancy**
Pregnancy Category: C (tentative). See Pregnancy Code inside back cover.
Animal studies: Skull defects reported in hamster studies.
Human studies: Information from adequate studies of pregnant women is not available. Some studies suggest a possible increase in significant birth defects when this drug is taken during the first 6 months of pregnancy. Codeine taken during the last few weeks before delivery can cause withdrawal symptoms in the newborn infant.
Use this drug only if clearly needed and in small, infrequent doses.

Advisability of Use if Breast-Feeding
Presence of this drug in breast milk: Yes, in small amounts.
Avoid drug or refrain from nursing.

Habit-Forming Potential: Psychological and/or physical dependence can develop with use of large doses for an extended period of time. However, true dependence is infrequent and unlikely with prudent use.

Effects of Overdosage: Drowsiness, restlessness, agitation, nausea, vomiting, dry mouth, vertigo, weakness, lethargy, stupor, coma, seizures.

Possible Effects of Long-Term Use: Psychological and physical dependence, chronic constipation.

Suggested Periodic Examinations While Taking This Drug (at physician's discretion)
None.

▷ **While Taking This Drug, Observe the Following**
Foods: No restrictions.
Beverages: No restrictions. May be taken with milk.
▷ *Alcohol:* Use extreme caution until the combined effects have been determined. Codeine can intensify the intoxicating effects of alcohol, and alcohol can intensify the depressant effects of codeine on brain function, breathing and circulation.
Tobacco Smoking: No interactions expected.

Marijuana Smoking: Increase in drowsiness and pain relief; impairment of mental and physical performance.

▷ *Other Drugs*

Codeine may ***increase*** the effects of
- other drugs with sedative effects.
- atropinelike drugs, and increase the risk of constipation and urinary retention.

▷ *Driving, Hazardous Activities:* This drug can impair mental alertness, judgment, reaction time and physical coordination. Avoid hazardous activities accordingly.

Aviation Note: The use of this drug ***is a disqualification*** for piloting. Consult a designated Aviation Medical Examiner.

Exposure to Sun: No restrictions.

Discontinuation: It is advisable to limit this drug to short-term use. If it is necessary to use it for extended periods of time, discontinuation should be gradual to minimize possible effects of withdrawal (usually mild with codeine).

COLCHICINE
(KOL chi seen)

Introduced: 1763

Class: Antigout

Prescription: USA: Yes
Canada: No

Controlled Drug: USA: No
Canada: No

Available as Generic: Yes

Brand Names: Colabid [CD], ColBENEMID [CD], Proben-C [CD], ✦Verban [CD]

BENEFITS versus RISKS	
Possible Benefits	*Possible Risks*
EFFECTIVE RELIEF OF ACUTE GOUT SYMPTOMS	Loss of hair
Prevention of recurrent gout attacks	Rare bone marrow depression (see Glossary)
Prevention of attacks of Mediterranean fever	Rare peripheral neuritis (see Glossary)
	Rare liver damage

▷ **Principal Uses**

As a Single Drug Product: Used primarily to reduce the pain, swelling and inflammation associated with acute attacks of gout. It is also used in smaller doses to prevent recurrent gout attacks. An infrequent use is the prevention and control of attacks of familial Mediterranean fever.

As a Combination Drug Product [CD]: Colchicine is combined with probenecid to enhance its ability to prevent recurrent attacks of gout. While colchicine is most effective in relieving the symptoms of acute gout, it has some effect in preventing recurrent and chronic discomfort. Probenecid increases the elimination of uric acid by the kidneys and thereby reduces the blood level of uric acid to a point at which acute episodes of gout will not occur. This dual action is more effective than either drug used alone in the long-term management of gout.

How This Drug Works: It is thought that by decreasing the acidity of joint tissues, this drug reduces the deposit of uric acid crystals that cause acute inflammation and pain. (Colchicine does not lower the level of uric acid in the blood or increase the level of uric acid in the urine.)

Available Dosage Forms and Strengths
Injection — 1 mg per 2 ml
Tablets — 0.5 mg, 0.6 mg

▷ **Usual Adult Dosage Range:** For acute attack—0.5 to 1.3 mg initially, followed by 0.5 to 0.65 mg/1 to 2 hours until pain is relieved or nausea, vomiting or diarrhea occurs. The total dose should not exceed 10 mg. For prevention of recurrent attacks—0.5 to 0.65 mg, 1 to 3 times/day. **Note: Actual dosage and administration schedule must be determined by the physician for each patient individually.**

▷ **Dosing Instructions:** May be taken either on an empty stomach or with food to reduce nausea or stomach irritation. Start treatment at the earliest indication of an acute attack. Take the exact dose prescribed. The tablet may be crushed for administration.

Usual Duration of Use: For acute attack—discontinue when pain is relieved or when nausea, vomiting or diarrhea occurs; do not resume this drug for 3 days without consulting your physician. For prevention—use the smallest effective dose for long-term management; consult your physician regarding dosage schedule and duration.

▷ **This Drug Should Not Be Taken If**
  • you have had an allergic reaction to it previously.
  • you have an active stomach or duodenal ulcer.
  • you have active ulcerative colitis.

▷ **Inform Your Physician Before Taking This Drug If**
  • you have a history of peptic ulcer disease or ulcerative colitis.
  • you have any type of heart disease.
  • you have impaired liver or kidney function.
  • you plan to have surgery in the near future.

Possible Side-Effects (natural, expected and unavoidable drug actions)
Nausea, vomiting, abdominal cramping, diarrhea.

▷ **Possible Adverse Effects** (unusual, unexpected and infrequent reactions)
 If any of the following develop, consult your physician promptly for guidance.
 Mild Adverse Effects
 Allergic Reactions: Skin rash, hives, fever.
 Serious Adverse Effects
 Allergic Reaction: Anaphylactic reaction (see Glossary).
 Loss of hair.
 Bone marrow depression (see Glossary)—fatigue, weakness, fever, sore throat, abnormal bleeding or bruising.
 Peripheral neuritis (see Glossary)—numbness, tingling, pain, weakness in hands and/or feet.
 Inflammation of colon with bloody diarrhea.
 Liver damage.

▷ **Possible Effects on Sexual Function:**   None reported.

Possible Delayed Adverse Effects: Impaired production of sperm, possibly resulting in birth defects of child that was conceived while father was taking this drug.

Natural Diseases or Disorders That May Be Activated by This Drug
 Peptic ulcer disease, ulcerative colitis.

CAUTION
 1. If this drug causes vomiting and/or diarrhea before relief of joint pain, discontinue it and inform your physician.
 2. Try to limit each course of treatment for acute gout to 4 to 8 mg. Do not exceed 3 mg/24 hours or a total of 10 mg/course.
 3. Omit drug for 3 days between courses to avoid toxicity.
 4. Carry this drug with you while traveling if you are subject to attacks of acute gout.
 5. It is advisable to take colchicine preventively prior to and following surgery if you have recurrent gout. (Surgery often precipitates acute attacks of gout.) Ask your physician for proper dosage schedule.

Precautions for Use
 By Infants and Children: Dosage has not been established. Ask physician for guidance.
 By Those over 60 Years of Age: This drug has a very narrow margin of safety. Because the total dosage required to relieve the pain of acute gout often causes vomiting and/or diarrhea, extreme caution is advised when this drug is used by anyone with heart or circulatory disorders, reduced liver or kidney function or general debility.

▷ **Advisability of Use During Pregnancy**
 Pregnancy Category: D (tentative). See Pregnancy Code inside back cover.
 Animal studies: This drug causes significant birth defects in hamsters and rabbits.

Human studies: Information from adequate studies of pregnant women is not available. However, it is reported that colchicine can cause harm to the fetus.

Avoid during entire pregnancy if possible. Ask physician for guidance.

Advisability of Use if Breast-Feeding
Presence of this drug in breast milk: Unknown.
Avoid drug or refrain from nursing.

Habit-Forming Potential: None.

Effects of Overdosage: Nausea, vomiting, abdominal cramping, diarrhea (may be bloody), burning sensation in throat and skin, weak and rapid pulse, progressive paralysis, inability to breathe.

Possible Effects of Long-Term Use: Hair loss, aplastic anemia (see Glossary), peripheral neuritis (see Glossary).

Suggested Periodic Examinations While Taking This Drug (at physician's discretion)
Complete blood cell counts, uric acid blood levels to monitor status of gout, sperm analysis for quantity and condition, liver function tests.

▷ **While Taking This Drug, Observe the Following**
Foods: Follow physician's advice regarding the need for a low-purine diet.
Beverages: It is advisable to drink no less than 3 quarts of liquids/24 hours. This drug may be taken with milk. Some "herbal teas" (promoted as being beneficial for arthritis) contain phenylbutazone and other potentially toxic ingredients. Avoid herbal teas if you are not certain of their source, content and medicinal effects.
▷ *Alcohol:* No interactions expected. However, alcohol may increase the risk of gastrointestinal irritation or bleeding. It also raises uric acid blood levels and could interfere with gout management.
Tobacco Smoking: No interactions expected.
▷ *Other Drugs*
Colchicine *taken concurrently* with
  • allopurinol (Zyloprim), probenecid (Benemid) or sulfinpyrazone (Anturane) can prevent attacks of acute gout that often occur when treatment with these drugs is first started.
▷ *Driving, Hazardous Activities:* Usually no restrictions when taken continually in small (preventive) doses. Be alert to the possible occurrence of nausea, vomiting and/or diarrhea when taken in larger (treatment) doses.
Aviation Note: The use of this drug *may be a disqualification* for piloting. Consult a designated Aviation Medical Examiner.
Exposure to Sun: No restrictions.
Exposure to Cold: This drug can lower body temperature. Use caution to prevent excessive lowering (hypothermia), especially if you are over 60 years of age.

Occurrence of Unrelated Illness: Inform your physician if you are injured or if you develop any new illness or disorder. During periods of such stress you may be subject to acute attacks of gout, and it may be necessary to adjust your medication schedule.

COLESTIPOL
(koh LES ti pohl)

Introduced: 1974

Prescription: USA: Yes
   Canada: Yes

Available as Generic: USA: No
   Canada: No

Brand Name: Colestid

Class: Anticholesterol

Controlled Drug: USA: No
   Canada: No

BENEFITS versus RISKS

Possible Benefits	*Possible Risks*
EFFECTIVE REDUCTION OF TOTAL CHOLESTEROL AND LOW DENSITY CHOLESTEROL IN TYPE IIa CHOLESTEROL DISORDERS (15% to 25% reduction of total cholesterol, 25% to 35% reduction of LDL cholesterol) EFFECTIVE RELIEF OF ITCHING associated with biliary obstruction	Constipation (may be severe) Reduced absorption of fat, fat-soluble vitamins (A, D, E and K) and folic acid Reduced formation of prothrombin with resultant bleeding

---

▷ **Principal Uses**

As a Single Drug Product: Used primarily to (1) reduce abnormally high blood levels of total cholesterol and low density (LDL) cholesterol in Type IIa cholesterol disorders; (2) relieve the itching due to the deposit of bile acids in the skin associated with partial biliary obstruction.

How This Drug Works: By combining with bile acids and bile salts in the intestinal tract, this drug forms insoluble complexes that are excreted in the feces. This removal of bile acids (which are necessary for food digestion) stimulates the conversion of cholesterol to bile acids to replace the loss; this in turn reduces the blood levels of cholesterol. By reducing the blood levels of bile acids, this drug hastens the absorption and clearance of bile acids deposited in the skin and thus relieves itching.

Available Dosage Forms and Strengths
Bottles — 250 grams, 500 grams
Packets — 5 grams

▷ **Usual Adult Dosage Range:**   Initially 5 grams of powder 3 times daily. Dose may be increased slowly as needed and tolerated to 30 grams daily in 2 to 4 divided doses. **Note: Actual dosage and administration schedule must be determined by the physician for each patient individually.**

▷ **Dosing Instructions:**   Always take just before or with a meal; this drug is ineffective when taken without food. Mix the powder thoroughly in 4 to 6 ounces of water, fruit juice, tomato juice, milk, thin soup or a soft food like applesauce. **Do not take it in its dry form.**

Usual Duration of Use: Continual use on a regular schedule for 4 to 6 weeks is usually necessary to determine this drug's effectiveness in lowering excessively high blood levels of cholesterol. Duration of use should not exceed 3 months if an adequate response does not occur. Long-term use (months to years) requires periodic evaluation of response and dosage adjustment. Consult your physician on a regular basis.

Currently a "Drug of Choice" for initiating treatment of elevated LDL cholesterol. See Cholesterol Disorders in Section Two.

▷ **This Drug Should Not Be Taken If**
  • you have had an allergic reaction to it previously.
  • you have complete biliary obstruction.

▷ **Inform Your Physician Before Taking This Drug If**
  • you are prone to constipation.
  • you have peptic ulcer disease.
  • you have a bleeding disorder of any kind.
  • you have impaired kidney function.

Possible Side-Effects (natural, expected and unavoidable drug actions)
Constipation (10%); interference with normal fat digestion and absorption; reduced absorption of vitamins A, D, E and K and folic acid.

▷ **Possible Adverse Effects** (unusual, unexpected and infrequent reactions)
If any of the following develop, consult your physician promptly for guidance.
Mild Adverse Effects
Allergic Reactions: Skin rash (0.1%), hives, tongue irritation, anal itching.
Headache, dizziness, weakness, muscle and joint pains.

Loss of appetite, indigestion, heartburn, abdominal discomfort, excessive gas, nausea, vomiting, diarrhea.

Serious Adverse Effects

Vitamin K deficiency with resultant deficiency of prothrombin and increased bleeding tendency.

Impaired absorption of calcium; predisposition to osteoporosis.

Gallbladder colic (questionable).

▷ **Possible Effects on Sexual Function:**   None reported.

Natural Diseases or Disorders That May Be Activated by This Drug

Peptic ulcer disease; steatorrhea (excessive fat in stools) with large doses.

CAUTION

1. The powder should never be taken in its dry form; always mix it thoroughly with a suitable liquid before swallowing.
2. Observe carefully for the development of constipation; use stool softeners and laxatives as needed.
3. This drug may bind other drugs taken concurrently and impair their absorption. It is advisable to take *all other drugs* 1 to 2 hours before or 4 to 6 hours after taking this drug.

Precautions for Use

By Infants and Children: Safety and effectiveness for use by those under 12 years of age have not been established. Observe carefully for the possible development of acidosis and vitamin A or folic acid deficiency. (Ask your physician for guidance.)

By Those over 60 Years of Age: There may be increased risk of developing severe constipation. Impaired kidney function may predispose to the development of acidosis.

▷ **Advisability of Use During Pregnancy**

Pregnancy Category: C (tentative). See Pregnancy Code inside back cover.

Animal studies: No information available.

Human studies: Information from adequate studies of pregnant women is not available.

Use this drug only if clearly needed. Ensure adequate intake of vitamins and minerals to satisfy needs of mother and fetus.

Advisability of Use if Breast-Feeding

Presence of this drug in breast milk: No.

Breast-feeding is permitted.

Habit-Forming Potential: None.

Effects of Overdosage: Progressive constipation.

Possible Effects of Long-Term Use: Deficiencies of vitamins A, D, E and K and folic acid. Calcium deficiency, osteoporosis. Acidosis due to excessive retention of chloride.

Suggested Periodic Examinations While Taking This Drug (at physician's discretion)

Measurements of blood levels of total cholesterol, low density (LDL) cholesterol and high density (HDL) cholesterol.

Hemoglobin and red blood cell studies for possible anemia.

▷ **While Taking This Drug, Observe the Following**

Foods: Avoid foods that tend to constipate (cheeses, etc.).

Nutritional Support: Consult your physician regarding the need for supplements of vitamins A, D, E and K, folic acid and calcium.

Beverages: Ensure adequate liquid intake (up to 2 quarts daily). This drug may be taken with milk.

▷ *Alcohol:* No interactions expected.

Tobacco Smoking: No interactions expected.

▷ *Other Drugs*

Colestipol may ***decrease*** the effects of

- acetaminophen; give 2 hours before colestipol.
- aspirin; give 2 hours before.
- digitoxin and digoxin; give 2 hours before.
- iron preparations; give 2 to 3 hours before.
- penicillin G; give 2 hours before.
- phenobarbital; give 2 hours before.
- tetracycline; give 2 hours before.
- thiazide diuretics (see Drug Class, Section Four); give 2 hours before.
- thyroxin; give 5 hours before.
- warfarin; give 6 hours after.

▷ *Driving, Hazardous Activities:* No restrictions.

Aviation Note: The use of this drug **is usually not a disqualification** for piloting. Consult a designated Aviation Medical Examiner.

Exposure to Sun: No restrictions.

Discontinuation: The dose of any potentially toxic drug taken concurrently must be reduced appropriately when this drug is discontinued. Following discontinuation of this drug, cholesterol blood levels usually return to pretreatment levels in approximately 1 month.

CROMOLYN
(KROH moh lin)

Other Names: Cromolyn sodium, sodium cromoglycate

Introduced: 1968

Class: Asthma preventive, rhinitis preventive

Prescription: USA: Yes
Canada: Yes

Controlled Drug: USA: No
Canada: No

Available as Generic: USA: No
Canada: No

Brand Names: ◆Fivent, Intal, ◆Nalcrom, Nasalcrom, Opticrom, ◆Rynacrom, ◆Vistacrom

---

BENEFITS versus RISKS

Possible Benefits	*Possible Risks*
LONG-TERM PREVENTION OF RECURRENT ASTHMA ATTACKS (70% to 75% effective)	Rare anaphylactic reaction (see Glossary)
Prevention of acute asthma due to allergens or exercise	Rare spasm of bronchial tubes, increased wheezing
Prevention and treatment of allergic rhinitis	Rare allergic pneumonitis (allergic reaction in lung tissue)
Relief of allergic conjunctivitis	

▷ **Principal Uses**

As a Single Drug Product: Used primarily to *prevent* allergic reactions in the nose (allergic rhinitis, hay fever) and allergic reactions in the bronchial tubes (bronchial asthma). (It is of no value in relieving asthma after the attack has begun.) It is also used to treat the symptoms of allergic rhinitis (70% effective) and conjunctivitis.

How This Drug Works: By blocking the release of histamine (and other substances) that normally occurs in allergic reactions, this drug acts to prevent the sequence of tissue changes that leads to swelling and itching of nasal membranes (allergic rhinitis) and to constriction of bronchial tubes (asthma).

Available Dosage Forms and Strengths

Eye drops — 2%, 4%
Inhalation aerosol — 0.8 mg per metered spray
Inhalation capsules (powder) — 20 mg
Inhalation solution — 20 mg per ampul
Nasal insufflation (powder) — 10 mg per cartridge
Nasal solution — 20 mg per ml, 40 mg per ml

▷ **Usual Adult Dosage Range**

Eye drops: 1 drop 4 to 6 times daily at regular intervals.

Inhalation aerosol: 1.6 mg (2 inhalations) 4 times daily at regular intervals for long-term prevention of asthma, or as a single dose 10 to 15 minutes before exposure to prevent acute allergen-induced or exercise-induced asthma.

Inhalation powder: 20 mg (1 capsule) 4 times daily at regular intervals for long-term prevention of asthma; 20 mg (1 capsule) as a single dose 10 to 15 minutes before exposure to prevent acute allergen-induced or exercise-induced asthma. Total daily dosage should not exceed 160 mg (8 capsules).

Inhalation solution: Same as inhalation powder.

Nasal insufflation: Initially 10 mg in each nostril every 4 to 6 hours as needed; reduce to every 8 to 12 hours for maintenance.

Nasal solution: 2.6 mg to 5.2 mg in each nostril 3 to 6 times daily as needed.

Note: Actual dosage and administration schedule must be determined by the physician for each patient individually.

▷ **Dosing Instructions:** Follow carefully the dosing instructions provided with each of the above dosage forms, especially the inhalers. Do not swallow the capsules; the powder is intended for inhalation into the air passages of the lungs. (If the capsule is swallowed inadvertently, the drug will cause no beneficial or adverse effects.)

Usual Duration of Use: Continual use on a regular schedule for 4 to 6 weeks is usually necessary to determine this drug's effectiveness in preventing recurrent attacks of asthma or allergic rhinitis. Long-term use (months to years) requires periodic evaluation of response and dosage adjustment. Consult your physician on a regular basis.

Possible Advantages of This Drug
May be quite effective in the young asthmatic.
Usually well tolerated.
Serious adverse effects are very rare.

▷ **This Drug Should Not Be Taken If**
- you have had an allergic reaction to any dosage form of it previously.

▷ **Inform Your Physician Before Taking This Drug If**
- you are allergic to milk, milk products or lactose. (The inhalation powder contains lactose.)
- you have impaired liver or kidney function.
- you have angina or a heart rhythm disorder. (The inhalation aerosol contains propellants that could be hazardous.)

Possible Side-Effects (natural, expected and unavoidable drug actions)
Unpleasant taste with use of inhalation aerosol.
Mild throat irritation, hoarseness, cough. (These can be minimized by a few swallows of water after each inhalation of powder.)

▷ **Possible Adverse Effects** (unusual, unexpected and infrequent reactions)
If any of the following develop, consult your physician promptly for guidance.
Mild Adverse Effects
Allergic Reactions: Skin rash, hives, itching.
Headache, dizziness.
Nausea, vomiting, urinary urgency and pain, joint and muscle pain.

Serious Adverse Effects

Allergic Reactions: Anaphylactic reaction (see Glossary). Allergic pneumonitis (allergic reaction in lung tissue).

▷ **Possible Effects on Sexual Function:**   None reported.

CAUTION

1. Remember that this drug acts solely as a *preventive* in the management of bronchial asthma; its effectiveness is limited to the pretreatment phase of asthma—*before* the onset of acute bronchial constriction (asthmatic wheezing).
2. **Do not** use this drug during an acute attack of asthma; it could worsen and prolong asthmatic wheezing.
3. This drug does **not** interfere with the actions of those drugs used to relieve the acute asthma attack after it has begun. Cromolyn is used **before and between** acute attacks to prevent their development; bronchodilators are used **during** acute attacks to relieve them.
4. If you are also using a bronchodilator drug by inhalation, it is advisable to take it about 5 minutes before inhaling cromolyn.

Precautions for Use

By Infants and Children: Safety and effectiveness for use by those under 5 years of age have not been established. Young children may find it easier to use the nebulized solution than the powder.

By Those over 60 Years of Age: This drug is not effective in the management of chronic bronchitis or emphysema.

▷ **Advisability of Use During Pregnancy**

Pregnancy Category: B (tentative). See Pregnancy Code inside back cover.

Animal studies: Mouse, rat and rabbit studies revealed no birth defects due to this drug.

Human studies: Information from adequate studies of pregnant women is not available.

Use this drug only if clearly needed.

Advisability of Use if Breast-Feeding

Presence of this drug in breast milk: Unknown.

Avoid drug or refrain from nursing.

Habit-Forming Potential: None.

Effects of Overdosage: No significant effects reported.

Possible Effects of Long-Term Use: Allergic reaction of lung tissue (allergic pneumonitis, very rare).

Suggested Periodic Examinations While Taking This Drug (at physician's discretion)

Examination of lungs by sputum analysis and X-ray if symptoms suggest allergic pneumonitis.

▷ **While Taking This Drug, Observe the Following**

Foods: Follow diet prescribed by your physician. Avoid all foods to which you may be allergic.

Beverages: Avoid all beverages to which you may be allergic.

▷ *Alcohol:* No interactions expected.

Tobacco Smoking: Follow your physician's advice regarding smoking.

▷ *Other Drugs:* Cromolyn may make it possible to reduce the dosage of cortisonelike drugs in the management of chronic asthma. Consult your physician regarding dosage adjustment.

▷ *Driving, Hazardous Activities:* This drug may cause dizziness. Restrict activities as necessary.

Aviation Note: The use of this drug **may be a disqualification** for piloting. Consult a designated Aviation Medical Examiner.

Exposure to Sun: No restrictions.

Heavy Exercise or Exertion: This drug may be effective in preventing exercise-induced asthma if taken 10 to 15 minutes before exertion. It is most effective in young individuals.

Discontinuation: If the regular use of cromolyn has made it possible to reduce or discontinue maintenance doses of cortisonelike drugs, and you find it necessary to discontinue cromolyn for any reason, observe closely for a sudden return of asthma. It may be necessary to resume a cortisonelike drug and to institute other measures for satisfactory control of asthma.

Special Storage Instructions: Keep the powder cartridges in a dry, tightly closed container. Store in a cool place but not in the refrigerator. Do not handle the cartridges or the inhaler when hands are wet.

CYCLOBENZAPRINE
(si kloh BENZ a preen)

Introduced: 1977

Class: Muscle relaxant

Prescription: USA: Yes
Canada: Yes

Controlled Drug: USA: No
Canada: No

Available as Generic: USA: No
Canada: No

Brand Name: Flexeril

BENEFITS versus RISKS	
Possible Benefits	*Possible Risks*
Mild to moderate relief of discomfort due to spasm of voluntary muscles	Confusion, depression Impaired urination Allergic reactions: skin rash, hives, swelling of face or tongue

▷ **Principal Uses**

As a Single Drug Product: Used primarily to relieve the pain and stiffness associated with spasm of voluntary muscles, such as that resulting from accidental injury of musculoskeletal structures. It is often necessary to supplement the use of this drug with other treatment measures, such as rest, support and physiotherapy.

How This Drug Works: Not completely established. It is thought that this drug may relieve muscle spasm and pain by blocking the transmission of nerve impulses over reflex pathways and/or by producing a sedative effect that decreases the perception of pain.

Available Dosage Forms and Strengths
Tablets — 10 mg

▷ **Usual Adult Dosage Range:**   10 mg, 2 to 4 times daily; adjust dosage as needed and tolerated. Total daily dosage should not exceed 60 mg. **Note: Actual dosage and administration schedule must be determined by the physician for each patient individually.**

▷ **Dosing Instructions:**   Take either on empty stomach or with food to prevent stomach irritation. Tablet may be crushed for administration.

Usual Duration of Use: Continual use on a regular schedule for 7 to 10 days is usually necessary to determine this drug's effectiveness in relieving the discomfort of muscle spasm. Evaluate need for continued use after periods of 2 to 3 weeks.

▷ **This Drug Should Not Be Taken If**
- you have had an allergic reaction to it previously.
- you have taken any monoamine oxidase (MAO) type A inhibitor drug within the past 14 days (see Drug Class, Section Four).
- you are recovering from a recent heart attack.
- you have congestive heart failure or a serious heart rhythm disorder.
- you have uncorrected hyperthyroidism (overactive thyroid function).

▷ **Inform Your Physician Before Taking This Drug If**
- you have experienced any unfavorable reactions to other muscle relaxants or to tricyclic antidepressants (see Drug Class, Section Four) in the past.
- you have a history of heart disease or heart rhythm disorder.
- you have glaucoma or prostatism (see Glossary).
- you are currently taking any drugs with atropinelike effects or sedative effects.

Possible Side-Effects (natural, expected and unavoidable drug actions)
Drowsiness (40%), dizziness (11%), dry mouth (28%), constipation (3%).

▷ **Possible Adverse Effects** (unusual, unexpected and infrequent reactions)
If any of the following develop, consult your physician promptly for guidance.

Mild Adverse Effects
Allergic Reactions: Skin rash, hives, swelling of face and tongue.
Headache, fatigue, weakness, numbness, blurred vision, slurred speech, unsteadiness.
Unpleasant taste, indigestion, nausea.
Serious Adverse Effects
Idiosyncratic Reactions: Euphoria, confusion, disorientation, hallucinations, depression.
Impaired urination (urine retention).

▷ **Possible Effects on Sexual Function:** Increased or decreased libido, impotence, swelling of testicles, enlargement of male breasts, enlargement of female breasts with milk production. (Any effect may occur with dosage of 30 to 60 mg/day.)

▷ **Adverse Effects That May Mimic Natural Diseases or Disorders**
Mental and behavioral reactions may suggest acute psychosis.

Precautions for Use
By Infants and Children: Safety and effectiveness for use by those under 15 years of age have not been established.
By Those over 60 Years of Age: Small doses are advisable initially. You may be more susceptible to the development of drowsiness, dizziness, weakness, unsteadiness and falling. This drug can aggravate existing prostatism (see Glossary).

▷ **Advisability of Use During Pregnancy**
Pregnancy Category: B (tentative). See Pregnancy Code inside back cover.
Animal studies: No birth defects reported in mice, rats or rabbits.
Human studies: Information from adequate studies of pregnant women is not available.
Avoid drug if possible; use only if clearly needed.

Advisability of Use if Breast-Feeding
Presence of this drug in breast milk: Probably yes.
Avoid drug or refrain from nursing.

Habit-Forming Potential: None.

Effects of Overdosage: Excessive drowsiness, confusion, impaired concentration, visual disturbances, vomiting, stupor progressing to coma, seizures, weak and rapid pulse.

Possible Effects of Long-Term Use: None reported.

Suggested Periodic Examinations While Taking This Drug (at physician's discretion)
Measurements of internal eye pressure (if any predisposition to glaucoma).

▷ **While Taking This Drug, Observe the Following**

Foods: No restrictions.

Beverages: No restrictions. May be taken with milk.

▷   *Alcohol:* Use with caution until the combined effect has been determined. This drug may add to the depressant action of alcohol on the brain.

Tobacco Smoking: No interactions expected.

Marijuana Smoking: Moderate to marked drowsiness, muscle weakness, incoordination, impairment of intellectual and physical performance. All hazardous activities should be avoided.

▷   *Other Drugs*

Cyclobenzaprine may *increase* the effects of

• atropinelike drugs (see Drug Class, Section Four).

• all drugs with sedative effects, and cause excessive sedation.

Cyclobenzaprine *taken concurrently* with

• monoamine oxidase (MAO) type A inhibitor drugs may cause high fever, seizures and life-threatening reactions (theoretical).

▷   *Driving, Hazardous Activities:* This drug may cause drowsiness, dizziness and incoordination in susceptible individuals. Avoid hazardous activities if these drug effects occur.

Aviation Note: The use of this drug *is a disqualification* for piloting. Consult a designated Aviation Medical Examiner.

Exposure to Sun: Use caution until sensitivity to sun has been determined. Other drugs closely related to this drug can cause photosensitivity (see Glossary).

Exposure to Heat: Use caution in hot environments. This drug may increase the risk of heat stroke.

CYCLOPHOSPHAMIDE
(si kloh FOSS fa mide)

Introduced: 1959

Class: Anticancer, immunosuppressive

Prescription: USA: Yes
Canada: Yes

Controlled Drug: USA: No
Canada: No

Available as Generic: No

Brand Names: Cytoxan, Neosar, ✦Procytox

BENEFITS versus RISKS

Possible Benefits	*Possible Risks*
CURE OR CONTROL OF CERTAIN TYPES OF CANCER	REDUCED WHITE BLOOD CELL COUNT
PREVENTION OF REJECTION IN ORGAN TRANSPLANTATION	SECONDARY INFECTION
	URINARY BLADDER BLEEDING
	HEART, LUNG, LIVER OR KIDNEY DAMAGE
Possibly beneficial in the treatment of rheumatoid arthritis and lupus erythematosus	Loss of hair
Possibly beneficial in selected cases of nephrotic syndrome in children	

▷ **Principal Uses**

As a Single Drug Product: Used primarily in the treatment of various forms of cancer, notably malignant lymphomas, multiple myeloma, leukemias and cancers of the breast and ovary. Because this drug exerts a suppressant effect on the immune system, it is also used to prevent rejection in organ transplantation and to treat certain autoimmune disorders. It is also approved for treating certain resistant forms of nephrotic syndrome in children.

How This Drug Works: Not completely known. Because of its ability to kill cancer cells during all phases of their development and reproduction, this drug suppresses the primary growth and secondary spread (metastasis) of certain types of cancer.

Available Dosage Forms and Strengths

Injection — vials of 100 mg, 200 mg, 500 mg, 1 gram, 2 grams

Tablets — 25 mg, 50 mg

▷ **Usual Adult Dosage Range:**   1 to 5 mg per kg of body weight daily. **Note: Actual dosage and administration schedule must be determined by the physician for each patient individually.**

▷ **Dosing Instructions:**   It is preferable to take the tablet on an empty stomach. However, if nausea or indigestion occurs, this drug may be taken with or following food. The total liquid intake should be no less than 3 quarts/24 hours to reduce the risk of bladder irritation. Tablets may be crushed for administration.

Usual Duration of Use: Continual use on a regular schedule is required to achieve and maintain a significant remission of the cancer under treatment. Actual duration of use depends upon the response of the cancer and the tolerance of the patient to the effects of the drug. Consult your physician on a regular basis.

▷ **This Drug Should Not Be Taken If**
- you have had an allergic reaction to any dosage form of it previously.
- you have an active infection of any kind.
- you have bloody urine for any reason.

▷ **Inform Your Physician Before Taking This Drug If**
- you have impaired liver or kidney function.
- you have a blood cell or bone marrow disorder.
- you have had previous chemotherapy or X-ray therapy for any type of cancer.
- you are now taking, or have taken within the past year, any cortisonelike drug (adrenal corticosteroids).
- you have diabetes.
- you plan to have surgery under general anesthesia in the near future.

Possible Side-Effects (natural, expected and unavoidable drug actions)
Bone marrow depression (see Glossary)—impaired production of primarily white blood cells and, to a lesser degree, red blood cells and blood platelets (see Glossary). Possible effects include fever, chills, sore throat, fatigue, weakness, abnormal bleeding or bruising.
Impairment of natural resistance (immunity) to infection.

▷ **Possible Adverse Effects** (unusual, unexpected and infrequent reactions)
If any of the following develop, consult your physician promptly for guidance.
Mild Adverse Effects
Allergic Reaction: Skin rash (rare).
Headache, dizziness.
Loss of scalp hair (50% of users), darkening of skin and fingernails, transverse ridging of nails.
Loss of appetite, nausea (30%), vomiting (25%), ulceration of mouth, diarrhea (may be bloody).
Serious Adverse Effects
Idiosyncratic Reaction: Hemolytic anemia (see Glossary).
Liver damage with jaundice—yellow eyes and skin, dark-colored urine, light-colored stools.
Kidney damage—impaired kidney function, reduced urine volume, bloody urine.
Severe inflammation of bladder (10%)—painful urination, bloody urine.
Drug-induced damage of heart and lung tissue.

▷ **Possible Effects on Sexual Function**
Suppression of ovarian function—irregular menstrual pattern or cessation of menstruation (18% to 57% of users depending upon dosage and duration of use).
Suppression of testicular function—reduction or cessation of sperm production (100% of users).

Possible Delayed Adverse Effects

Development of other types of cancer (secondary malignancies).
Development of severe cystitis with bleeding from the bladder wall. (This may occur many months after the last dose.)

CAUTION

1. This drug may interfere with the normal healing of wounds.
2. This drug can cause significant changes (mutations) in the chromosome structure of both sperm and eggs (ova). Any man or woman taking this drug should understand its potential for causing serious defects in children that are conceived during or following the course of medication.
3. This drug can suppress natural resistance (immunity) to infection, resulting in life-threatening illness.
4. Avoid live-virus vaccines while taking this drug.

Precautions for Use

By Infants and Children: This drug should not be given if the child is dehydrated. Provide adequate fluid intake to ensure a copious urine volume for 4 hours following each dose. Prevent exposure of child to anyone with active chicken pox or shingles. This drug may cause ovarian or testicular sterility.

By Those over 60 Years of Age: To reduce the risk of developing serious chemical cystitis, it is necessary to maintain a copious volume of urine. This may increase the risk of urinary retention in the man with prostatism (see Glossary).

▷ **Advisability of Use During Pregnancy**

Pregnancy Category: D (tentative). See Pregnancy Code inside back cover.
Animal studies: Significant birth defects reported in mice, rat and rabbit studies.
Human studies: Information from studies of pregnant women indicates that this drug can cause serious birth defects or fetal death.
Avoid completely during the first 3 months. Use of this drug during the last 6 months must be carefully individualized.

Advisability of Use if Breast-Feeding

Presence of this drug in breast milk: Yes.
Avoid drug or refrain from nursing.

Habit-Forming Potential: None.

Effects of Overdosage: Nausea, vomiting, diarrhea, bloody urine, water retention, weight gain, severe bone marrow depression, severe infections.

Possible Effects of Long-Term Use: Development of fibrous tissue in lungs; secondary malignancies.

Suggested Periodic Examinations While Taking This Drug (at physician's discretion)

Complete blood cell counts, every 2 to 4 days during initial treatment; then every 3 to 4 weeks during maintenance treatment.

Liver and kidney function tests.

Thyroid function tests (if symptoms warrant).

▷ **While Taking This Drug, Observe the Following**

Foods: No restrictions.

Beverages: No restrictions. May be taken with milk.

▷ *Alcohol:* No interactions expected.

Tobacco Smoking: No interactions expected.

▷ *Other Drugs*

Cyclophosphamide **taken concurrently** with

• allopurinol (Zyloprim) may increase the degree of bone marrow depression.

▷ *Driving, Hazardous Activities:* Use caution if dizziness occurs.

Aviation Note: The use of this drug **may be a disqualification** for piloting. Consult a designated Aviation Medical Examiner.

Exposure to Sun: No restrictions.

Occurrence of Unrelated Illness: Report promptly the development of any indications of infection—fever, chills, sore throat, cough, flulike symptoms. It may be necessary to discontinue this drug until the infection is controlled. Consult your physician.

DEMECLOCYCLINE
(dem e kloh SI kleen)

Introduced: 1959

Class: Antibiotic, tetracyclines

Prescription: USA: Yes
    Canada: Yes

Controlled Drug: USA: No
    Canada: No

Available as Generic: No

Brand Name: Declomycin

BENEFITS versus RISKS	
Possible Benefits	*Possible Risks*
EFFECTIVE TREATMENT OF INFECTIONS due to susceptible microorganisms	Allergic reactions
	Drug-induced colitis
	Drug-induced diabetes insipidus (water diabetes)
	Fungal superinfections

▷ **Principal Uses**

As a Single Drug Product: This member of the tetracycline drug class is used primarily to (1) treat a broad range of infections caused by susceptible bacteria and protozoa and (2) treat the syndrome of inappropriate secretion of antidiuretic hormone, a condition that reduces the normal production of urine.

How This Drug Works: This drug prevents the growth and multiplication of susceptible bacteria by interfering with their formation of essential proteins.

Available Dosage Forms and Strengths
Capsules — 150 mg
Tablets, film-coated — 150 mg, 300 mg

▷ **Usual Adult Dosage Range:**   150 mg/6 hours or 300 mg/12 hours. Total daily dosage should not exceed 2400 mg. **Note: Actual dosage and administration schedule must be determined by the physician for each patient individually.**

▷ **Dosing Instructions:**   Preferably taken on an empty stomach, 1 hour before or 2 hours after eating. However, if stomach irritation occurs, it may be taken with crackers or light food (not milk or milk products). Take at same time each day, with a full glass of water. Take the full course prescribed. The tablet may be crushed and the capsule may be opened for administration.

Usual Duration of Use: The time required to control the infection and be free of fever and symptoms for 48 hours. This varies with the nature of the infection.

▷ **This Drug Should Not Be Taken If**
- you are allergic to any tetracycline drug (see Drug Class, Section Four).
- you are pregnant or breast-feeding.

▷ **Inform Your Physician Before Taking This Drug If**
- it is prescribed for a child under 8 years of age.
- you have a history of liver or kidney disease.
- you have systemic lupus erythematosus.
- you are taking any penicillin drug.
- you are taking any anticoagulant drug.
- you plan to have surgery under general anesthesia in the near future.

Possible Side-Effects (natural, expected and unavoidable drug actions)
Superinfections (see Glossary), often due to yeast organisms. These can occur in the mouth, intestinal tract, rectum and/or vagina, resulting in rectal and vaginal itching.

▷ **Possible Adverse Effects** (unusual, unexpected and infrequent reactions)
If any of the following develop, consult your physician promptly for guidance.

Mild Adverse Effects
Allergic Reactions: Skin rash, hives, itching of hands and feet, swelling of face or extremities.
Loss of appetite, nausea, vomiting, diarrhea.
Irritation of mouth or tongue, "black tongue," sore throat, abdominal cramping or pain.

Serious Adverse Effects
Allergic Reactions: Anaphylactic reaction (see Glossary), asthma, fever, swollen joints, abnormal bleeding or bruising, jaundice (see Glossary).
Permanent discoloration and/or malformation of teeth when taken under 8 years of age, including unborn child and infant.
Drug-induced diabetes insipidus (water diabetes).

▷ **Possible Effects on Sexual Function:** Questionable decrease of libido (1 report only).

Natural Diseases or Disorders That May Be Activated by This Drug
Systemic lupus erythematosus.

CAUTION
1. Antacids, dairy products and preparations containing aluminum, bismuth, calcium, iron, magnesium or zinc can prevent adequate absorption of this drug and reduce its effectiveness significantly.
2. Troublesome and persistent diarrhea can develop in sensitive individuals. If diarrhea persists for more than 24 hours, discontinue this drug and consult your physician.
3. If surgery under general anesthesia is required while taking this drug, the choice of anesthetic agent must be considered carefully to prevent serious kidney damage.

Precautions for Use
By Infants and Children: If possible, tetracyclines should not be given to children under 8 years of age because of the risk of permanent discoloration and deformity of the teeth. Rarely, young infants may develop increased intracranial pressure within the first 4 days of receiving this drug. Tetracyclines may inhibit normal bone growth and development.
By Those over 60 Years of Age: Dosage must be carefully individualized and based upon determinations of kidney function. Natural skin changes may predispose to severe and prolonged itching reactions in the genital and anal regions.

▷ **Advisability of Use During Pregnancy**
Pregnancy Category: D (tentative). See Pregnancy Code inside back cover.
Animal studies: Tetracycline causes limb defects in rats, rabbits and chickens.
Human studies: Information from studies of pregnant women indicates that this drug can cause impaired development and discoloration of teeth and other developmental defects.
It is advisable to avoid this drug completely during entire pregnancy.

Advisability of Use if Breast-Feeding
Presence of this drug in breast milk: Yes.
Avoid drug or refrain from nursing.

Habit-Forming Potential: None.

Effects of Overdosage: Nausea, vomiting, diarrhea, acute liver damage (rare).

Possible Effects of Long-Term Use: Superinfections; rarely, impairment of bone marrow, liver or kidney function.

Suggested Periodic Examinations While Taking This Drug (at physician's discretion)
Complete blood cell counts, liver and kidney function tests.
During extended use, sputum and stool examinations may detect early superinfection due to yeast organisms.

▷ **While Taking This Drug, Observe the Following**
Foods: Avoid cheeses, yogurt, ice cream, iron-fortified cereals and supplements and meats for 2 hours before and after taking this drug.
Beverages: Avoid all forms of milk for 2 hours before and after taking this drug.
▷   *Alcohol:* No interactions expected. However, it is best avoided if you have active liver disease.
Tobacco Smoking: No interactions expected.
▷   *Other Drugs*
Tetracyclines may ***increase*** the effects of
- oral anticoagulants, and make it necessary to reduce their dosage.
- digoxin (Lanoxin), and cause digitalis toxicity.
- lithium (Eskalith, Lithane, etc.), and increase the risk of lithium toxicity.
Tetracyclines may ***decrease*** the effects of
- oral contraceptives, and impair their effectiveness in preventing pregnancy.
- penicillins, and impair their effectiveness in treating infections.
Tetracyclines ***taken concurrently*** with
- methoxyflurane anesthesia may impair kidney function.
The following drugs may ***decrease*** the effects of tetracyclines
- antacids (aluminum and magnesium preparations, sodium bicarbonate, etc.) may reduce drug absorption.
- iron and mineral preparations may reduce drug absorption.
▷   *Driving, Hazardous Activities:* Usually no restrictions. Be alert to the possible occurrence of nausea or diarrhea.
Aviation Note: The use of this drug ***may be a disqualification*** for piloting. Consult a designated Aviation Medical Examiner.
Exposure to Sun: Use caution until sensitivity has been determined. Tetracyclines can cause photosensitivity (see Glossary).

DESIPRAMINE
(des IP ra meen)

Introduced: 1964

Prescription: USA: Yes
  Canada: Yes

Available as Generic: USA: No
  Canada: No

Brand Names: Norpramin, Pertofrane

Class: Antidepressant

Controlled Drug: USA: No
  Canada: No

BENEFITS versus RISKS

Possible Benefits	*Possible Risks*
EFFECTIVE RELIEF OF ENDOGENOUS DEPRESSION	ADVERSE BEHAVIORAL EFFECTS: confusion, disorientation, delusions, hallucinations
Possibly beneficial in other depressive disorders	CONVERSION OF DEPRESSION TO MANIA in bipolar affective disorders
	Aggravation of paranoia and schizophrenia
	Drug-induced heart rhythm disorders
	Abnormally low white blood cell and platelet counts

▷ **Principal Uses**

As a Single Drug Product: Used primarily to relieve severe emotional depression and to initiate gradual restoration of normal mood. This drug is more likely to be effective in primary (endogenous) depression than in secondary, reactive (exogenous) depression. It is also being used to treat attention deficit disorder in children over 6 years of age and in adolescents.

How This Drug Works: Not completely established. It is thought that by increasing brain tissue concentrations of certain nerve impulse transmitters (norepinephrine and serotonin), this drug relieves the symptoms associated with depression.

Available Dosage Forms and Strengths
  Capsules — 25 mg, 50 mg
  Tablets — 10 mg, 25 mg, 50 mg, 75 mg, 100 mg, 150 mg

▷ **Usual Adult Dosage Range:** Initially 25 mg 2 to 4 times daily. Dose may be increased cautiously as needed and tolerated by 25 mg daily at intervals of 1 week. The usual maintenance dose is 100 mg to 200 mg/24 hours. The total daily dosage should not exceed 300 mg. (When determined, the optimal daily requirement may be given at bedtime as a single dose.) **Note: Actual dosage and administration schedule must be determined by the physician for each patient individually.**

▷ **Dosing Instructions:** May be taken without regard to meals. The capsule may be opened and the tablet may be crushed for administration.

Usual Duration of Use: Continual use on a regular schedule for 3 to 4 weeks is usually necessary to determine this drug's effectiveness in relieving depression; optimal response may require 3 months of use. Long-term use (months to years) requires periodic evaluation of response and dosage adjustment. Consult your physician on a regular basis.

▷ **This Drug Should Not Be Taken If**
- you have had an allergic reaction to it previously.
- you are taking, or have taken within the past 14 days, any monoamine oxidase (MAO) type A inhibitor drug (see Drug Class, Section Four).
- you have had a recent heart attack (myocardial infarction).
- you have narrow-angle glaucoma.

▷ **Inform Your Physician Before Taking This Drug If**
- you have had an adverse reaction to any other antidepressant drug.
- you have any type of seizure disorder.
- you have increased internal eye pressure.
- you have any type of heart disease, especially a heart rhythm disorder.
- you have any type of thyroid disorder or are taking thyroid medication.
- you have diabetes or sugar intolerance.
- you have prostatism (see Glossary).
- you plan to have surgery under general anesthesia in the near future.

Possible Side-Effects (natural, expected and unavoidable drug actions)
Mild drowsiness, light-headedness (low blood pressure), blurred vision, dry mouth, constipation, impaired urination.

▷ **Possible Adverse Effects** (unusual, unexpected and infrequent reactions)
If any of the following develop, consult your physician promptly for guidance.
Mild Adverse Effects
Allergic Reactions: Skin rash, hives, swelling of face or tongue, drug fever (see Glossary).
Headache, dizziness, weakness, unsteadiness, tremors, fainting.
Irritation of tongue or mouth, altered taste, indigestion, nausea.
Fluctuations of blood sugar.
Serious Adverse Effects
Allergic Reactions: Drug-induced hepatitis, with or without jaundice; anaphylactoid reaction (see terms in Glossary).

Adverse behavioral effects: confusion, disorientation, delusions, hallucinations.

Seizures; reduced control of epilepsy.

Aggravation of paranoid psychoses and schizophrenia.

Heart rhythm disturbances.

Parkinsonlike disorders, peripheral neuritis (see both terms in Glossary).

Abnormally low white blood cell and platelet counts: fever, sore throat, infections, abnormal bleeding or bruising.

▷ **Possible Effects on Sexual Function:** Decreased libido, increased libido (antidepressant effect), impotence, painful male orgasm, male breast enlargement, female breast enlargement with milk production, swelling of testicles.

▷ **Adverse Effects That May Mimic Natural Diseases or Disorders**
Liver toxicity may suggest viral hepatitis.

Natural Diseases or Disorders That May Be Activated by This Drug
Latent diabetes, epilepsy, glaucoma, prostatism.

CAUTION
1. This drug should be used only when a true, primary, endogenous depression has been diagnosed. It should *not* be used to treat the symptoms of reactive depression that may be associated with many life situations in the absence of a true bona fide affective illness.
2. Observe for early indications of toxicity or overdosage: confusion, agitation, rapid heart rate, heart irregularity. Measurement of the blood level of the drug will clarify the situation.
3. It is advisable to withhold this drug if electroconvulsive therapy (ECT) is to be used to treat the depression.

Precautions for Use
By Infants and Children: Safety and effectiveness for use by those under 6 years of age have not been established. This drug is being used experimentally to treat children who have attention deficit syndrome, with or without hyperactivity. Dosage and management must be supervised by a properly trained pediatrician.

By Those over 60 Years of Age: Initiate treatment with 25 mg 1 or 2 times daily to evaluate tolerance. During the first 2 weeks of treatment, observe for confusional reactions—restlessness, agitation, forgetfulness, disorientation, delusions or hallucinations. Also observe for unsteadiness and instability that may predispose to falling. This drug may aggravate prostatism.

▷ **Advisability of Use During Pregnancy**
Pregnancy Category: C (tentative). See Pregnancy Code inside back cover.
Animal studies: Birth defects reported in rat and rabbit studies.
Human studies: Information from adequate studies of pregnant women is not available.

Use only if clearly needed. Avoid during the first 3 months if possible.

Advisability of Use if Breast-Feeding
Presence of this drug in breast milk: Yes, in small amounts.
Monitor nursing infant closely and discontinue drug or nursing if adverse effects develop.

Habit-Forming Potential: Psychological or physical dependence is rare and unexpected. This drug is not liable to abuse.

Effects of Overdosage: Confusion, hallucinations, drowsiness, tremors, heart irregularity, seizures, stupor, hypothermia (see Glossary).

Possible Effects of Long-Term Use: None reported.

Suggested Periodic Examinations While Taking This Drug (at physician's discretion)
Complete blood cell counts, liver function tests.
Serial blood pressure readings and electrocardiograms.

▷ **While Taking This Drug, Observe the Following**
Foods: No specific restrictions. May need to limit food intake to avoid excessive weight gain.
Beverages: No restrictions. May be taken with milk.
▷ *Alcohol:* Avoid completely. This drug can markedly increase the intoxicating effects of alcohol; the combination can depress brain function significantly.
Tobacco Smoking: May accelerate the elimination of this drug and require increased dosage.
Marijuana Smoking
Occasional (once or twice weekly): Transient increase in drowsiness and mouth dryness.
Daily: Persistent drowsiness and mouth dryness; possible reduced effectiveness of this drug.
▷ *Other Drugs*
Desipramine may *increase* the effects of
• all drugs with sedative effects; observe for excessive sedation.
• all drugs with atropinelike effects (see Drug Class, Section Four).
Desipramine may *decrease* the effects of
• clonidine (Catapres).
• guanethidine (Ismelin, Esimil).
Desipramine *taken concurrently* with
• anticonvulsants requires careful monitoring for changes in seizure patterns and need to adjust anticonvulsant dosage.
• ethchlorvynol (Placidyl) may cause delirium; avoid concurrent use.
• monoamine oxidase (MAO) type A inhibitor drugs (see Drug Class, Section Four) may cause high fever, seizures and excessive rise in blood pressure; avoid concurrent use of these drugs and provide periods of 14 days between administration of either.
• stimulant drugs (amphetamine, cocaine, epinephrine, phenylpropanolamine, etc.) may cause severe high blood pressure and/or high fever.
• thyroid preparations may increase the risk of heart rhythm disorders.

The following drugs may *increase* the effects of desipramine
- methylphenidate (Ritalin).
- phenothiazines (see Drug Class, Section Four).

The following drugs may *decrease* the effects of desipramine
- barbiturates (see Drug Class, Section Four).
- chloral hydrate (Noctec, Somnos, etc.).
- estrogen (see Drug Profile for brand names).
- lithium (Lithobid, Lithotab, etc.).
- oral contraceptives (see Drug Profile for brand names).
- reserpine (Serpasil, Ser-Ap-Es, etc.).

▷ *Driving, Hazardous Activities:* This drug may impair mental alertness, judgment, physical coordination and reaction time. Restrict activities as necessary.

Aviation Note: The use of this drug *is a disqualification* for piloting. Consult a designated Aviation Medical Examiner.

Exposure to Sun: Use caution until sensitivity has been determined. This drug may cause photosensitivity (see Glossary).

Exposure to Heat: Use caution. This drug can inhibit sweating and impair the body's adaptation to hot environments, increasing the risk of heat stroke. Avoid saunas.

Exposure to Cold: The elderly should use caution and avoid conditions conducive to hypothermia (see Glossary).

Exposure to Environmental Chemicals: This drug may mask the symptoms of poisoning due to handling certain insecticides (organophosphorus types). Read their labels carefully.

Discontinuation: It is advisable to discontinue this drug gradually. Abrupt withdrawal after prolonged use may cause headache, malaise and nausea. When this drug is stopped, it may be necessary to adjust the dosages of other drugs taken concurrently.

DEXAMETHASONE
(dex a METH a sohn)

Introduced: 1958

Class: Cortisonelike drugs

Prescription: USA: Yes
Canada: Yes

Controlled Drug: USA: No
Canada: No

Available as Generic: USA: Yes
Canada: Yes

Brand Names: ✦Ak-Dex, Decaderm, Decadron, Decadron-LA, Decadron Phosphate Ophthalmic, Decadron Phosphate Respihaler, Decadron Phosphate Turbinaire, Decadron w/Xylocaine [CD], Decaspray, ✦Deronil, Dexasone, Dexone, Hexadrol, Maxidex

```
┌─────────────────────────────────────────────────────────────┐
│                   BENEFITS versus RISKS                       │
│                                                               │
│      Possible Benefits              Possible Risks            │
│  EFFECTIVE RELIEF OF            Short-term use (up to 10 days) is│
│    SYMPTOMS IN A WIDE             usually well tolerated       │
│    VARIETY OF INFLAMMATORY     Long-term use (exceeding 2     │
│    AND ALLERGIC DISORDERS        weeks) is associated with many│
│  EFFECTIVE                       possible adverse effects:    │
│    IMMUNOSUPPRESSION in         ALTERED MOOD AND              │
│  selected benign and malignant    PERSONALITY                 │
│  disorders                      CATARACTS, GLAUCOMA           │
│                                 HYPERTENSION                   │
│                                 OSTEOPOROSIS                   │
│                                 ASEPTIC BONE NECROSIS         │
│                                 INCREASED SUSCEPTIBIL-        │
│                                   ITY TO INFECTIONS           │
│                                 (See Possible Adverse Effects │
│                                   and Possible Effects of Long-│
│                                   Term Use below)             │
└─────────────────────────────────────────────────────────────┘
```

▷ **Principal Uses**

As a Single Drug Product: This potent drug of the cortisone class is used in the treatment of a wide variety of allergic and inflammatory conditions. It is used most commonly in the management of serious skin disorders, asthma, regional enteritis, ulcerative colitis and all types of major rheumatic disorders including bursitis, tendonitis and most forms of arthritis.

How This Drug Works: Not fully established. It is thought that this drug's anti-inflammatory effect is due to its ability to inhibit the normal defensive functions of certain white blood cells. Its immunosuppressant effect is attributed to a reduced production of lymphocytes and antibodies.

Available Dosage Forms and Strengths

Aerosol — 0.01%, 0.04%

Aerosol inhaler — 84 mcg per spray

Cream — 0.1%

Elixir — 0.5 mg per 5-ml teaspoonful

Eye ointment — 0.05%

Gel — 0.1%

Injection — 4 mg per ml, 8 mg per ml, 10 mg per ml, 16 mg per ml, 20 mg per ml, 24 mg per ml

Oral solution — 0.5 mg per 0.5 ml, 0.5 mg per 5 ml

Solution — 0.1%

Suspension — 0.1%

Tablets — 0.25 mg, 0.5 mg, 0.75 mg, 1 mg, 1.5 mg, 2 mg, 4 mg, 6 mg

▷ **Usual Adult Dosage Range:**   0.5 to 9 mg daily as a single dose or in divided doses. **Note: Actual dosage and administration schedule must be determined by the physician for each patient individually.**

▷ **Dosing Instructions:**   Take with or following food to prevent stomach irritation, preferably in the morning. The tablet may be crushed for administration.

Usual Duration of Use: For acute disorders: 4 to 10 days. For chronic disorders: according to individual requirements. The duration of use should not exceed the time necessary to obtain adequate symptomatic relief in acute self-limiting conditions; or the time required to stabilize a chronic condition and permit gradual withdrawal. Because of its long duration of action, this drug is not appropriate for alternate day administration. Consult your physician on a regular basis.

▷ **This Drug Should Not Be Taken If**
- you have had an allergic reaction to any dosage form of it previously.
- you have active peptic ulcer disease.
- you have an active infection of the eye caused by the herpes simplex virus.
- you have active tuberculosis.

▷ **Inform Your Physician Before Taking This Drug If**
- you have had an unfavorable reaction to any cortisonelike drug in the past.
- you have a history of peptic ulcer disease, thrombophlebitis or tuberculosis.
- you have any of the following: diabetes, glaucoma, high blood pressure, deficient thyroid function or myasthenia gravis.
- you plan to have surgery of any kind in the near future.

Possible Side-Effects (natural, expected and unavoidable drug actions)
Increased appetite, weight gain, retention of salt and water, excretion of potassium, increased susceptibility to infection.

▷ **Possible Adverse Effects** (unusual, unexpected and infrequent reactions)
If any of the following develop, consult your physician promptly for guidance.
Mild Adverse Effects
Allergic Reaction: Skin rash.
Headache, dizziness, insomnia.
Acid indigestion, abdominal distention.
Muscle cramping and weakness.
Acne, excessive growth of facial hair.
Serious Adverse Effects
Mental and emotional disturbances of serious magnitude.
Reactivation of latent tuberculosis.
Development of peptic ulcer.
Increased blood pressure.

Development of inflammation of the pancreas.

Thrombophlebitis (inflammation of a vein with the formation of blood clot)—pain or tenderness in thigh or leg, with or without swelling of the foot, ankle or leg.

Pulmonary embolism (movement of a blood clot to the lung)—sudden shortness of breath, pain in the chest, coughing, bloody sputum.

▷ **Possible Effects on Sexual Function:**   Altered timing and pattern of menstruation.

▷ **Adverse Effects That May Mimic Natural Diseases or Disorders**

Pattern of symptoms and signs resembling Cushing's syndrome.

Natural Diseases or Disorders That May Be Activated by This Drug

Latent diabetes, glaucoma, peptic ulcer disease, tuberculosis.

CAUTION

1. It is advisable to carry a card of personal identification with a notation that you are taking this drug, if your course of treatment is to exceed 1 week.
2. Do not discontinue this drug abruptly if you are using it for long-term treatment.
3. If vaccination against measles, rabies, smallpox or yellow fever is required, discontinue this drug 72 hours before vaccination and do not resume it for at least 14 days after vaccination.

Precautions for Use

By Infants and Children: Avoid prolonged use if possible. During long-term use, observe for suppression of normal growth and the possibility of increased intracranial pressure. Following long-term use, the child may be at risk for adrenal gland deficiency during stress for as long as 18 months after cessation of this drug.

By Those over 60 Years of Age: Cortisonelike drugs should be used very sparingly after 60 and only when the disorder under treatment is unresponsive to adequate trials of unrelated drugs. Avoid prolonged use of this drug. Continual use (even in small doses) can increase the severity of diabetes, enhance fluid retention, raise blood pressure, weaken resistance to infection, induce stomach ulcer and accelerate the development of cataract and osteoporosis.

▷ **Advisability of Use During Pregnancy**

Pregnancy Category: C (tentative). See Pregnancy Code inside back cover.

Animal studies: Birth defects reported in mice, rats and rabbits.

Human studies: Information from adequate studies of pregnant women is not available.

Avoid completely during the first 3 months. Limit use during the last 6 months as much as possible. If used, examine infant for possible deficiency of adrenal gland function.

Advisability of Use if Breast-Feeding

Presence of this drug in breast milk: Yes.

Avoid drug or refrain from nursing.

Habit-Forming Potential: Use of this drug to suppress symptoms over an extended period of time may produce a state of functional dependence (see Glossary). In the treatment of conditions like asthma and rheumatoid arthritis, it is advisable to keep the dose as small as possible and to attempt drug withdrawal after periods of reasonable improvement. Such procedures may reduce the degree of "steroid rebound"— the return of symptoms as the drug is withdrawn.

Effects of Overdosage: Fatigue, muscle weakness, stomach irritation, acid indigestion, excessive sweating, facial flushing, fluid retention, swelling of extremities, increased blood pressure.

Possible Effects of Long-Term Use: Increased blood sugar (possible diabetes), increased fat deposits on the trunk of the body ("buffalo hump"), rounding of the face ("moon face"), thinning and fragility of skin, loss of texture and strength of bones (osteoporosis, aseptic necrosis), cataracts, glaucoma, retarded growth and development in children.

Suggested Periodic Examinations While Taking This Drug (at physician's discretion)

Measurements of blood pressure, blood sugar and potassium levels.

Complete eye examinations at regular intervals.

Chest X-ray if history of tuberculosis.

Determination of the rate of development of the growing child to detect retardation of normal growth.

▷ **While Taking This Drug, Observe the Following**

Foods: No interactions expected. Ask physician regarding need to restrict salt intake or to eat potassium-rich foods. During long-term use of this drug, it is advisable to eat a high-protein diet.

Nutritional Support: During long-term use, take a vitamin D supplement. During wound repair, take a zinc supplement.

Beverages: No restrictions. Drink all forms of milk liberally.

▷   *Alcohol:* No interactions expected. Use caution if you are prone to peptic ulcer disease.

Tobacco Smoking: Nicotine increases the blood levels of naturally produced cortisone and related hormones. Heavy smoking may add to the expected actions of this drug and requires close observation for excessive effects.

Marijuana Smoking: May cause additional impairment of immunity.

▷   *Other Drugs*

Dexamethasone may ***decrease*** the effects of

- isoniazid (INH, Niconyl, etc.)
- salicylates (aspirin, sodium salicylate, etc.)

Dexamethasone *taken concurrently* with
- oral anticoagulants may either increase or decrease their effectiveness; consult physician regarding the need for prothrombin time testing and dosage adjustment.

The following drugs may *decrease* the effects of dexamethasone
- antacids may reduce its absorption.
- barbiturates (Amytal, Butisol, phenobarbital, etc.).
- phenytoin (Dilantin, etc.).
- rifampin (Rifadin, Rimactane, etc.).

▷ *Driving, Hazardous Activities:* Usually no restrictions. Be alert to the rare occurrence of dizziness.

Aviation Note: The use of this drug *may be a disqualification* for piloting. Consult a designated Aviation Medical Examiner.

Exposure to Sun: No restrictions.

Occurrence of Unrelated Illness: This drug may decrease natural resistance to infection. Inform your physician if you develop an infection of any kind. It may also reduce your body's ability to respond to the stress of acute illness, injury or surgery. Keep your physician fully informed of any significant changes in your state of health.

Discontinuation: If you have been taking this drug for an extended period of time, do not discontinue it abruptly. Ask physician for guidance regarding gradual withdrawal. For a period of 2 years after discontinuing this drug, it is essential in the event of illness, injury or surgery that you inform attending medical personnel that you have used this drug in the past. The period of impaired response to stress following the use of cortisonelike drugs may last for 1 to 2 years.

DIAZEPAM
(di AZ e pam)

Introduced: 1963

Class: Mild tranquilizer, benzodiazepines

Prescription: USA: Yes
Canada: Yes

Controlled Drug: USA: C-IV*
Canada: No

Available as Generic: Yes

Brand Names: ✦Apo-Diazepam, ✦Diazemuls, Diazepam Intensol, ✦E-Pam, ✦Meval, ✦Novodipam, ✦Rival, Valium, Valrelease, Vazepam, ✦Vivol

*See Schedules of Controlled Drugs inside back cover.

```
┌─────────────────────────────────────────────────────────────┐
│                   BENEFITS versus RISKS                        │
│                                                                │
│      Possible Benefits              Possible Risks             │
│  RELIEF OF ANXIETY AND          Habit-forming potential with   │
│    NERVOUS TENSION in 70% to      prolonged use                │
│    80% of users                 Minor impairment of mental     │
│  Wide margin of safety with       functions                    │
│    therapeutic doses            Very rare jaundice             │
│  Very few drug interactions     Very rare blood cell disorders │
└─────────────────────────────────────────────────────────────┘
```

▷ **Principal Uses**

As a Single Drug Product: Used primarily to (1) provide short-term relief of mild to moderate anxiety; (2) relieve the symptoms of acute alcohol withdrawal: agitation, tremors, hallucinations, incipient delirium tremens; (3) relieve skeletal muscle spasm; (4) provide short-term control of certain types of seizures (epilepsy).

How This Drug Works: It is thought that this drug produces a calming effect by enhancing the action of the nerve transmitter gamma-aminobutyric acid (GABA), which in turn blocks the arousal of higher brain centers.

Available Dosage Forms and Strengths

Capsules, prolonged-action — 15 mg
Concentrate — 5 mg per ml
Injection — 5 mg per ml
Oral solution — 5 mg per ml, 5 mg per 5-ml teaspoonful
Tablets — 2 mg, 5 mg, 10 mg

▷ **Usual Adult Dosage Range:** 2 to 10 mg, 2 to 4 times daily. Dose may be increased cautiously as needed and tolerated. After 1 week of continual use, the total daily dose may be taken at bedtime. Total daily dose should not exceed 60 mg. **Note: Actual dosage and administration schedule must be determined by the physician for each patient individually.**

▷ **Dosing Instructions:** May be taken on empty stomach or with food or milk. The prolonged-action capsule should not be opened, but the tablet may be crushed for administration. Do not discontinue this drug abruptly if taken for more than 4 weeks.

Usual Duration of Use: Continual use on a regular schedule for 3 to 5 days is usually necessary to determine this drug's effectiveness in relieving moderate anxiety. Limit continual use to 1 to 3 weeks. Avoid uninterrupted and prolonged use.

▷ **This Drug Should Not Be Taken If**
- you have had an allergic reaction to any dosage form of it previously.
- you have acute narrow-angle glaucoma.
- it is prescribed for a child under 6 months of age.

▷ **Inform Your Physician Before Taking This Drug If**
- you are allergic to any benzodiazepine drug (see Drug Class, Section Four).
- you have a history of alcoholism or drug abuse.
- you are pregnant or planning pregnancy.
- you have impaired liver or kidney function.
- you have a history of serious depression or mental disorder.
- you have any of the following: asthma, emphysema, epilepsy, myasthenia gravis.

Possible Side-Effects (natural, expected and unavoidable drug actions)
Drowsiness (5%), lethargy, unsteadiness (0.2%), "hangover" effects on the day following bedtime use.

▷ **Possible Adverse Effects** (unusual, unexpected and infrequent reactions)
If any of the following develop, consult your physician promptly for guidance.
Mild Adverse Effects
Allergic Reactions: Rashes (0.4%), hives.
Dizziness, fainting, blurred vision, double vision, slurred speech, sweating, nausea.
Serious Adverse Effects
Allergic Reactions: Liver damage with jaundice (see Glossary), abnormally low blood platelet count.
Bone marrow depression—impaired production of white blood cells, fever, sore throat.
Paradoxical responses of excitement, agitation, anger, rage.

▷ **Possible Effects on Sexual Function**
Altered timing and pattern of menstruation.
Small doses (2 to 5 mg/day) are used to allay the anxiety that accounts for many cases of impotence in the male and inhibited sexual responsiveness in the female.
Larger doses (10 mg/day or more) can decrease libido, impair potency in the male and inhibit orgasm in the female.

▷ **Adverse Effects That May Mimic Natural Diseases or Disorders**
Liver reaction with jaundice may suggest viral hepatitis.

CAUTION
1. This drug should not be discontinued abruptly if it has been taken continually for more than 4 weeks.
2. The concurrent use of some over-the-counter drug products that contain antihistamines (allergy and cold preparations, sleep aids) can cause excessive sedation in sensitive individuals.

Precautions for Use
By Infants and Children: Safety and effectiveness for use by those under 6 months of age have not been established. This drug should not be

used in the hyperactive or psychotic child of any age. Observe for excessive sedation and incoordination.

By Those over 60 Years of Age: It is advisable to use smaller doses at longer intervals to avoid overdosage. Observe for the possible development of lethargy, indifference, fatigue, weakness, unsteadiness, disturbing dreams, nightmares and paradoxical reactions of excitement, agitation, anger, hostility and rage.

▷ **Advisability of Use During Pregnancy**

Pregnancy Category: D (tentative). See Pregnancy Code inside back cover.

Animal studies: Cleft palate reported in mice; skeletal defects reported in rats.

Human studies: Available information is conflicting and inconclusive. Some studies found an increase in serious birth defects associated with the use of this drug. Other studies have found no significant increase in birth defects.

Frequent use in late pregnancy can cause the "floppy infant" syndrome in the newborn: weakness, lethargy, unresponsiveness, depressed breathing, low body temperature.

Avoid use during entire pregnancy.

Advisability of Use if Breast-Feeding

Presence of this drug in breast milk: Yes.

Avoid drug or refrain from nursing.

Habit-Forming Potential: This drug can produce psychological and/or physical dependence (see Glossary) if used in large doses for an extended period of time.

Effects of Overdosage: Marked drowsiness, weakness, feeling of drunkenness, staggering gait, tremor, stupor progressing to deep sleep or coma.

Possible Effects of Long-Term Use: Psychological and/or physical dependence, rare blood cell disorders.

Suggested Periodic Examinations While Taking This Drug (at physician's discretion)

Complete blood cell counts during long-term use.

▷ **While Taking This Drug, Observe the Following**

Foods: No restrictions.

Beverages: Avoid excessive intake of caffeine-containing beverages: coffee, tea, cola. May be taken with milk.

▷   *Alcohol:* Use with extreme caution until the combined effect is determined. Alcohol may increase the absorption of this drug and add to its depressant effects on the brain. It is advisable to avoid alcohol completely—throughout the day and night—if it is necessary to drive or to engage in any hazardous activity.

Tobacco Smoking: Heavy smoking may reduce the calming action of this drug.

Marijuana Smoking: Increased sedation and significant impairment of intellectual and physical performance.

▷ *Other Drugs*

Diazepam may *increase* the effects of
- digoxin (Lanoxin), and cause digoxin toxicity.
- phenytoin (Dilantin), and cause phenytoin toxicity.

Diazepam may *decrease* the effects of
- levodopa (Sinemet, etc.), and reduce its effectiveness in treating Parkinson's disease.

The following drugs may *increase* the effects of diazepam
- cimetidine (Tagamet).
- disulfiram (Antabuse).
- isoniazid (INH, Rifamate, etc.).
- oral contraceptives.
- valproic acid (Depakene).

The following drugs may *decrease* the effects of diazepam
- rifampin (Rimactane, etc.).
- theophylline (aminophylline, Theo-Dur, etc.).

▷ *Driving, Hazardous Activities:* This drug can impair mental alertness, judgment, physical coordination and reaction time. Avoid hazardous activities accordingly.

Aviation Note: The use of this drug *is a disqualification* for piloting. Consult a designated Aviation Medical Examiner.

Exposure to Sun: No restrictions.

Exposure to Heat: Use caution until the effect of excessive perspiration is determined. Because of reduced urine volume, this drug may accumulate in the body and produce effects of overdosage.

Discontinuation: Avoid sudden discontinuation if this drug has been taken for over 4 weeks without interruption. Dosage should be tapered gradually to prevent a withdrawal syndrome that could include depression, confusion, hallucinations, tremor, seizures, muscle cramping, sweating and vomiting.

DICLOFENAC
(di KLOH fen ak)

Introduced: 1976

Class: Mild analgesic, anti-inflammatory

Prescription: USA: Yes
Canada: Yes

Controlled Drug: USA: No
Canada: No

Available as Generic: USA: No
Canada: No

Brand Name: Voltaren

BENEFITS versus RISKS

Possible Benefits	*Possible Risks*
EFFECTIVE RELIEF OF SYMPTOMS ASSOCIATED WITH MAJOR TYPES OF ARTHRITIS	PEPTIC ULCER DISEASE (less than 2%); associated bleeding and perforation
Effective relief of symptoms associated with bursitis, tendinitis and related conditions	Liver toxicity with jaundice (less than 1%)
	Rare aplastic anemia (see Glossary)
Effective relief of menstrual cramps	Water retention
	Rare kidney toxicity

▷ **Principal Uses**

As a Single Drug Product: Used primarily to relieve the symptoms associated with (1) rheumatoid arthritis, osteoarthritis and ankylosing spondylitis; (2) bursitis, tendinitis, capsulitis and tenosynovitis; (3) painful menstruation.

How This Drug Works: Not completely established. It is thought that this drug reduces the tissue concentrations of prostaglandins (and related compounds), chemicals involved in the production of inflammation and pain.

Available Dosage Forms and Strengths

Suppositories (Canada) — 50 mg, 100 mg
Tablets, enteric-coated — 25 mg, 50 mg, 75 mg
Tablets, prolonged-action (Canada) — 100 mg

▷ **Usual Adult Dosage Range:**   Initially 100 to 200 mg/24 hours, in 2 to 5 divided doses. After a satisfactory response has been achieved, dosage should be reduced to the minimum that will sustain adequate relief. The usual maintenance dose is 50 to 100 mg/24 hours. **Note: Actual dosage and administration schedule must be determined by the physician for each patient individually.**

▷ **Dosing Instructions:**   Take either on an empty stomach or with food or milk if necessary to prevent stomach irritation. Take with a full glass of water and remain upright (do not lie down) for 15 to 30 minutes to prevent lodging of the tablet in the esophagus (food tube). Take the tablet whole; do not crush for administration.

Usual Duration of Use: Continual use on a regular schedule for 1 to 2 weeks is usually necessary to determine this drug's effectiveness in relieving the symptoms of arthritis, bursitis, etc. Severe arthritis may require continual use for 3 to 4 weeks to obtain maximal relief. Long-term use (months to years) requires periodic evaluation of response and dosage adjustment. Consult your physician on a regular basis.

▷ **This Drug Should Not Be Taken If**
  • you have had an allergic reaction to it previously.
  • you are subject to asthma or nasal polyps caused by aspirin.
  • you have active peptic ulcer disease or any form of gastrointestinal bleeding.
  • you have active liver disease.
  • you have a bleeding disorder or a blood cell disorder.
  • you have severe impairment of kidney function.
  • you have porphyria (see Glossary).

▷ **Inform Your Physician Before Taking This Drug If**
  • you are allergic to aspirin or to other aspirin substitutes.
  • you have a history of peptic ulcer disease or any type of bleeding disorder.
  • you have impaired liver or kidney function.
  • you have high blood pressure or a history of heart failure.
  • you have systemic lupus erythematosus (SLE).
  • you are taking any of the following drugs: acetaminophen, aspirin or other aspirin substitutes, anticoagulants, cyclosporine, digoxin, diuretics, insulin, lithium, methotrexate, oral antidiabetic drugs.

  Possible Side-Effects (natural, expected and unavoidable drug actions)
  Fluid retention (weight gain).

▷ **Possible Adverse Effects** (unusual, unexpected and infrequent reactions)
  If any of the following develop, consult your physician promptly for guidance.
  Mild Adverse Effects
  Allergic Reactions: Skin rash, hives, itching.
  Headache, dizziness, drowsiness, depression, anxiety, insomnia, blurred vision, double vision, reversible hearing loss, ear ringing, altered taste.
  Mouth soreness, stomach discomfort, nausea, vomiting, indigestion, constipation, diarrhea.
  Serious Adverse Effects
  Allergic Reactions: Severe skin reactions, eczema, bruising, erythema multiforme, Stevens-Johnson syndrome, hair loss; swelling of lips, tongue, vocal cords; anaphylactoid reaction (see Glossary).
  Drug-induced peptic ulcers, with bleeding and perforation; colitis with bloody diarrhea.
  Abnormally low red blood cell, white blood cell and blood platelet counts; rare aplastic anemia (see Glossary).
  Liver injury with jaundice.
  Kidney injury with significantly impaired function.

▷ **Possible Effects on Sexual Function:** Impotence reported (less than 1%), but causal relationship not established.

  Possible Delayed Adverse Effects: Mild anemia due to "silent" blood loss from the stomach (less than that caused by aspirin).

▷ **Adverse Effects That May Mimic Natural Diseases or Disorders**
Liver reactions may suggest viral hepatitis.

▷ **Natural Diseases or Disorders That May Be Activated by This Drug**
Peptic ulcer disease, Crohn's disease, ulcerative colitis, porphyria, kidney failure associated with systemic lupus erythematosus.

CAUTION
1. Dosage should always be limited to the smallest amount that produces reasonable improvement.
2. This drug may mask early indications of infection. Inform your physician if you think you are developing an infection of any kind.
3. Observe for a pattern of symptoms that may indicate the development of liver toxicity: fatigue, lethargy, "flulike" symptoms, nausea, itching, tenderness under the right rib cage, jaundice (see Glossary). Report such symptoms promptly.
4. Observe for possible drug-induced bleeding in the gastrointestinal tract: bloody (reddish) or tarry (black) stools.

Precautions for Use
By Infants and Children: Safety and effectiveness for use by those under 12 years of age have not been established.
By Those over 60 Years of Age: Small doses are advisable initially until tolerance is determined. Observe for any indications of liver or kidney toxicity, fluid retention, dizziness, confusion, impaired memory, stomach bleeding or constipation.

▷ **Advisability of Use During Pregnancy**
Pregnancy Category: B (tentative). See Pregnancy Code inside back cover.
Animal studies: Mouse, rat and rabbit studies reveal toxic effects on the embryo but no birth defects due to this drug.
Human studies: Information from adequate studies of pregnant women is not available.
Avoid this drug completely during the last 3 months. Use it during the first 6 months only if clearly needed. Ask your physician for guidance.

Advisability of Use if Breast-Feeding
Presence of this drug in breast milk: Yes.
Avoid drug or refrain from nursing.

Habit-Forming Potential: None.

Effects of Overdosage: Probable drowsiness, dizziness, ear ringing, nausea, vomiting, diarrhea, confusion, unsteadiness, stupor.

Possible Effects of Long-Term Use: Secondary anemia (chronic blood loss from stomach), fluid retention, elevated blood pressure.

Suggested Periodic Examinations While Taking This Drug (at physician's discretion)

Complete blood cell counts; liver function tests within the first 8 weeks of use and periodically thereafter; kidney function tests.

Complete eye examinations if vision is altered in any way.

▷ **While Taking This Drug, Observe the Following**

Foods: No restrictions.

Nutritional Support: Supplemental iron if anemia develops.

Beverages: No restrictions. May be taken with milk.

▷ *Alcohol:* Use sparingly and with caution. The irritant action of alcohol on the stomach lining, added to the irritant action of this drug in sensitive individuals, can increase the risk of stomach ulceration and/or bleeding.

Tobacco Smoking: No interactions expected.

▷ *Other Drugs*

Diclofenac may ***increase*** the effects of

- acetaminophen (Tylenol, etc.), and increase the risk of liver or kidney damage; avoid prolonged use of this combination.
- anticoagulants (Coumadin, etc.), and increase the risk of bleeding; monitor prothrombin time, adjust dose accordingly.
- aspirin, and increase the risk of stomach ulceration and/or bleeding; avoid this combination.

Diclofenac may ***decrease*** the effects of

- amiloride (Midamor, Moduretic), and raise blood potassium levels.
- oral antidiabetic drugs (see Drug Class, Section Four), and alter control of blood sugar unpredictably.
- bumetanide (Bumex).
- chlorthalidone (Hygroton, etc.).
- ethacrynic acid (Edecrin).
- furosemide (Lasix).
- indapamide (Lozol).
- metolazone (Diulo, Zaroxolyn).
- spironolactone (Aldactone, Aldactazide), and raise blood potassium levels.
- thiazide diuretics (see Drug Class, Section Four).
- triamterene (Dyazide, Maxzide), and raise blood potassium levels.

Diclofenac ***taken concurrently*** with the following drugs may increase the risk of bleeding (antiplatelet effect); monitor these combinations closely:

- aspirin.
- colchicine (ColBenemid, etc.).
- dipyridamole (Persantine).
- indomethacin (Indocin).
- sulfinpyrazone (Anturane).
- valproic acid (Depakene).

Diclofenac ***taken concurrently*** with the following drugs may increase their toxicity; monitor these combinations closely:

- cyclosporine (Sandimmune).
- digoxin (Lanoxin).
- lithium (Lithane, etc.).
- methotrexate (Folex, Mexate).

The following drug may **increase** the effects of diclofenac

- probenecid (Benemid), by slowing its elimination.

▷ *Driving, Hazardous Activities:* This drug may cause dizziness, drowsiness or blurred vision. Restrict activities as necessary.

Aviation Note: The use of this drug **may be a disqualification** for piloting. Consult a designated Aviation Medical Examiner.

Exposure to Sun: Use caution until sensitivity is determined. Photosensitivity (see Glossary) has been reported.

DICYCLOMINE
(di SI kloh meen)

Introduced: 1952

Class: Antispasmodic, atropinelike drugs

Prescription: USA: Yes
Canada: No

Controlled Drug: USA: No
Canada: No

Available as Generic: Yes

Brand Names: Bentyl, ✦Bentylol, Byclomine, ✦Formulex, ✦Lomine, ✦Protylol, ✦Spasmoban, ✦Viscerol

BENEFITS versus RISKS	
Possible Benefits	*Possible Risks*
EFFECTIVE RELIEF OF GASTROINTESTINAL SPASM	Increased internal eye pressure (important in glaucoma) Constipation Urinary retention (in predisposed persons)

▷ **Principal Uses**

As a Single Drug Product: Used primarily for its atropinelike antispasmodic effect in the management of functional disorders of the gastrointestinal tract, notably the irritable bowel syndrome (spastic colon). It is also used to relieve cramping and pain in infant colic.

How This Drug Works: Not completely established. It has been suggested that this drug may relax gastrointestinal muscle by means of a local anesthetic action that blocks reflex activity responsible for contraction and motility.

Available Dosage Forms and Strengths
Capsules — 10 mg, 20 mg
Injection — 10 mg per ml
Syrup — 10 mg per 5-ml teaspoonful
Tablets — 20 mg

▷ **Usual Adult Dosage Range:** 10 to 20 mg, 3 or 4 times daily. Total daily dosage should not exceed 160 mg. **Note: Actual dosage and administration schedule must be determined by the physician for each patient individually.**

▷ **Dosing Instructions:** May be taken with or following food to prevent stomach irritation. The syrup may be diluted with an equal amount of water. The capsule may be opened and the tablet may be crushed for administration.

Usual Duration of Use: Continual use on a regular schedule for 2 to 5 days is usually necessary to determine this drug's effectiveness in relieving the symptoms of spastic disorders of the digestive system. Limit use to the relief of symptoms as necessary. Ask physician for guidance regarding long-term use.

▷ **This Drug Should Not Be Taken If**
- you have had an allergic reaction to any dosage form of it previously.
- your stomach cannot empty properly into the intestine (pyloric obstruction).
- you are unable to empty the urinary bladder completely.
- you have ulcerative colitis.

▷ **Inform Your Physician Before Taking This Drug If**
- you have a history of peptic ulcer disease.
- you have impaired liver or kidney function.
- you have glaucoma, myasthenia gravis or prostatism (see Glossary).

Possible Side-Effects (natural, expected and unavoidable drug actions)
Dryness of the mouth, blurred vision, constipation.

▷ **Possible Adverse Effects** (unusual, unexpected and infrequent reactions)
If any of the following develop, consult your physician promptly for guidance.
Mild Adverse Effects
Allergic Reactions: Skin rash, hives.
Headache, dizziness, drowsiness, weakness.
Reduced appetite, nausea, vomiting.
Difficult urination.
Serious Adverse Effects
Allergic Reaction: Anaphylactic reaction (see Glossary).
Idiosyncratic Reactions: Excitement, confusion, disturbed behavior.
Increased internal eye pressure (significant in glaucoma).

▷ **Possible Effects on Sexual Function**
>
> Impotence (6-hour effect following dosage).
> Suppression of milk production.

Natural Diseases or Disorders That May Be Activated by This Drug

> Glaucoma, prostatism (see Glossary).

CAUTION

> Many over-the-counter medications (see OTC drugs in Glossary) for allergies, colds and coughs contain drugs that can interact unfavorably with this drug. Ask your physician or pharmacist for guidance before using any such medications.

Precautions for Use

> *By Infants and Children:* Use extreme care in giving syrup to infants so as to prevent aspiration (inhalation) of the drug. Serious reactions have occurred as a result of this accident during administration.
>
> *By Those over 60 Years of Age:* Begin treatment with small doses until tolerance is determined. You may be more susceptible to the development of confusion, excitement, constipation and prostatism.

▷ **Advisability of Use During Pregnancy**

> *Pregnancy Category:* B (tentative). See Pregnancy Code inside back cover.
> Animal studies: No birth defects reported.
> Human studies: Information from adequate studies of pregnant women is not available.
> Use only if clearly needed. Ask physician for guidance.

Advisability of Use if Breast-Feeding

> Presence of this drug in breast milk: Unknown.
> Avoid drug or refrain from nursing.

Habit-Forming Potential: None.

Effects of Overdosage: Headache, dizziness, nausea, dry mouth, difficulty in swallowing, excitement, restlessness, dilated pupils, hot and dry skin.

Possible Effects of Long-Term Use: None reported.

Suggested Periodic Examinations While Taking This Drug (at physician's discretion)

> Measurements of internal eye pressure (in presence of glaucoma or suspected glaucoma).

▷ **While Taking This Drug, Observe the Following**

> *Foods:* No interactions. Follow prescribed diet.
> *Beverages:* No interactions. May be taken with milk.
▷   *Alcohol:* Use caution until combined effects have been determined. Observe for increased drowsiness.
> *Tobacco Smoking:* No interactions expected. Follow physician's advice regarding smoking.

Marijuana Smoking: Possible increase in drowsiness and dryness of mouth.
▷ *Other Drugs*
Dicyclomine may **increase** the effects of
- other drugs that have atropinelike actions (see Drug Class, Section Four).

Dicyclomine may **decrease** the effects of
- levodopa (Larodopa, Sinemet, etc.).
▷ *Driving, Hazardous Activities:* This drug may cause drowsiness, dizziness or blurred vision. Restrict activities accordingly.
Aviation Note: The use of this drug **may be a disqualification** for piloting. Consult a designated Aviation Medical Examiner.
Exposure to Sun: No restrictions.
Exposure to Heat: Use caution. The use of this drug in hot environments may impair normal perspiration and interfere with the regulation of body temperature, thus increasing the risk of heat stroke.

DIFLUNISAL
(di FLOO ni sal)

Introduced: 1977

Class: Mild analgesic, anti-inflammatory

Prescription: USA: Yes
Canada: Yes

Controlled Drug: USA: No
Canada: No

Available as Generic: No

Brand Name: Dolobid

BENEFITS versus RISKS	
Possible Benefits	*Possible Risks*
EFFECTIVE RELIEF OF MILD TO MODERATE PAIN AND INFLAMMATION	Gastrointestinal pain, ulceration, bleeding (rare) Rare liver or kidney damage Rare fluid retention

▷ **Principal Uses**
As a Single Drug Product: Used primarily to relieve mild to moderately severe pain associated with (1) musculoskeletal injuries; (2) acute and chronic rheumatoid arthritis and osteoarthritis; and (3) dental, obstetrical and orthopedic surgery.

How This Drug Works: Not completely established. It is thought that this drug reduces the tissue concentrations of prostaglandins (and related compounds), chemicals involved in the production of inflammation and pain.

Available Dosage Forms and Strengths
Tablets — 250 mg, 500 mg

▷ **Usual Adult Dosage Range:**   Initially 500 to 1000 mg (loading dose), then 250 to 500 mg/8 to 12 hours. Total daily dosage should not exceed 1500 mg. **Note: Actual dosage and administration schedule must be determined by the physician for each patient individually.**

▷ **Dosing Instructions:**   Take either on an empty stomach or with food or milk to prevent stomach irritation. Swallow tablets whole; do not crush or chew. Take with a full glass of water and remain upright (do not lie down) for 30 minutes.

Usual Duration of Use: Continual use on a regular schedule for 1 to 2 weeks is usually necessary to determine this drug's effectiveness in relieving the discomfort of arthritis. Long-term use requires supervision and periodic evaluation by the physician. Consult your physician on a regular basis.

▷ **This Drug Should Not Be Taken If**
- you have had an allergic reaction to it previously.
- you are subject to asthma or nasal polyps caused by aspirin.
- you have active peptic ulcer disease or any form of gastrointestinal bleeding.

▷ **Inform Your Physician Before Taking This Drug If**
- you are allergic to aspirin or to other aspirin substitutes.
- you have a history of peptic ulcer disease or any type of bleeding disorder.
- you have impaired liver or kidney function.
- you have high blood pressure or a history of heart failure.
- you are pregnant.
- you are taking any of the following: acetaminophen, aspirin or other aspirin substitutes, anticoagulants, oral antidiabetic drugs.

Possible Side-Effects (natural, expected and unavoidable drug actions)
Drowsiness, ringing in ears, fluid retention.

▷ **Possible Adverse Effects** (unusual, unexpected and infrequent reactions)
If any of the following develop, consult your physician promptly for guidance.
Mild Adverse Effects
Allergic Reactions: Skin rash, hives, itching.
Headache, dizziness, altered or blurred vision, depression.
Mouth sores, indigestion, nausea, vomiting, constipation, diarrhea.
Serious Adverse Effects
Allergic Reactions: Severe skin reactions, swollen lymph glands, drug fever (see Glossary), asthma, anaphylaxis (see Glossary).

Active peptic ulcer, with or without bleeding.
Liver damage with jaundice (see Glossary).
Kidney damage with painful urination, bloody urine, reduced urine formation.
Reduced blood platelet (see Glossary) count with abnormal bleeding or bruising.

▷ **Possible Effects on Sexual Function:** None reported.

▷ **Adverse Effects That May Mimic Natural Diseases or Disorders**
Liver reaction may suggest viral hepatitis.

Natural Diseases or Disorders That May Be Activated by This Drug
Peptic ulcer disease, ulcerative colitis.

CAUTION
1. Inform your physician promptly if flulike symptoms develop in association with a skin rash; this could represent a serious allergic reaction.
2. This drug may mask early indications of infection. Inform your physician if you think you are developing an infection of any kind.

Precautions for Use
By Infants and Children: Safety and effectiveness for use by those under 12 years of age have not been established.
By Those over 60 Years of Age: Small doses are advisable until tolerance is determined. Observe for any indications of liver or kidney toxicity.

▷ **Advisability of Use During Pregnancy**
Pregnancy Category: C (tentative). See Pregnancy Code inside back cover.
Animal studies: Skeletal birth defects reported in rabbits.
Human studies: Information from adequate studies of pregnant women is not available.
Avoid this drug during the first and last 3 months. Use it during the middle 3 months only if clearly needed. Ask physician for guidance.

Advisability of Use if Breast-Feeding
Presence of this drug in breast milk: Yes.
Avoid drug or refrain from nursing.

Habit-Forming Potential: None.

Effects of Overdosage: Drowsiness, confusion, disorientation, nausea, vomiting, stupor.

Possible Effects of Long-Term Use: None reported.

Suggested Periodic Examinations While Taking This Drug (at physician's discretion)
Complete blood cell counts, liver and kidney function tests.
Complete eye examinations if vision is altered in any way.

▷ **While Taking This Drug, Observe the Following**
  Foods: No restrictions.
  Beverages: No restrictions. May be taken with milk.
▷   *Alcohol:* Use with caution. The irritant action of alcohol on the stomach lining, added to the irritant action of this drug in sensitive individuals, can increase the risk of stomach ulceration and/or bleeding.
  Tobacco Smoking: No interactions expected.
▷   *Other Drugs*
  Diflunisal may *increase* the effects of
  • acetaminophen (Tylenol, etc.), and increase the risk of liver damage; avoid this combination.
  • anticoagulants (Coumadin, etc.), and increase the risk of bleeding; monitor prothrombin time, adjust dose accordingly.
  • hydrochlorothiazide (Esidrix, HydroDiuril, etc.).
  Diflunisal *taken concurrently* with the following drugs may increase the risk of bleeding; avoid these combinations:
  • aspirin.
  • dipyridamole (Persantine).
  • indomethacin (Indocin).
  • sulfinpyrazone (Anturane).
  • valproic acid (Depakene).
  The following drugs may *decrease* the effects of diflunisal
  • aluminum antacids may decrease its absorption.
▷   *Driving, Hazardous Activities:* This drug may cause drowsiness, dizziness or altered vision. Restrict activities as necessary.
  Aviation Note: The use of this drug *may be a disqualification* for piloting. Consult a designated Aviation Medical Examiner.
  Exposure to Sun: Use caution until sensitivity is determined. This drug may cause photosensitivity (see Glossary).

DIGOXIN
(di JOX in)

Introduced: 1934   **Class:** Digitalis preparations

Prescription: USA: Yes   **Controlled Drug:** USA: No
  Canada: No   Canada: No

Available as Generic: Yes

Brand Names: Lanoxicaps, Lanoxin, ✦Novodigoxin

BENEFITS versus RISKS

Possible Benefits	*Possible Risks*
EFFECTIVE HEART STIMULANT IN CONGESTIVE HEART FAILURE	NARROW TREATMENT RANGE (treatment dose is 60% of toxic dose)
EFFECTIVE PREVENTION AND TREATMENT OF CERTAIN HEART RHYTHM DISORDERS	Frequent and sometimes serious disturbances of heart rhythm

---

▷ **Principal Uses**

As a Single Drug Product: This drug has two primary uses: (1) the treatment of congestive heart failure; (2) the restoration and maintenance of normal heart rate and rhythm in such disorders as atrial fibrillation, atrial flutter and atrial/supraventricular tachycardia.

How This Drug Works: By increasing the availability of calcium within the heart muscle, this drug improves the efficiency of the conversion of chemical energy to mechanical energy, thus increasing the force of heart muscle contraction. By slowing the activity of the pacemaker and delaying the transmission of electrical impulses through the conduction system of the heart, this drug assists in restoring normal heart rate and rhythm.

Available Dosage Forms and Strengths

    Elixir, pediatric — 0.05 mg per ml
          Capsules — 0.05 mg, 0.1 mg, 0.2 mg
          Injection — 0.1 mg per ml, 0.25 mg per ml
          Tablets — 0.125 mg, 0.25 mg, 0.5 mg

▷ **Usual Adult Dosage Range:** Rapid digitalization—1 to 1.5 mg divided into 2 or 3 doses given every 6 to 8 hours in 1 day. Slow digitalization—0.125 to 0.5 mg/day for 7 days. Maintenance—0.125 to 0.5 mg/day. Total daily dosage should not exceed 2 mg. **Note: Actual dosage and administration schedule must be determined by the physician for each patient individually.**

▷ **Dosing Instructions:** Take at the same time each day, or preferably on an empty stomach to ensure uniform absorption. May be taken with or following food if desired (not milk or dairy products). The tablet may be crushed for administration; the capsule should be swallowed whole.

Usual Duration of Use: Continual use on a regular schedule for 7 to 10 days is usually necessary to determine this drug's effectiveness in relieving heart failure or controlling heart rhythm disorders. Long-term use requires physician supervision and periodic assessment of continued need. The use of this drug is not necessarily "for life." Consult your physician on a regular basis.

▷ **This Drug Should Not Be Taken If**
- you have had an allergic reaction to any dosage form of it previously.

▷ **Inform Your Physician Before Taking This Drug If**
- you have experienced any unfavorable reaction to a digitalis preparation in the past.
- you have taken any digitalis preparation within the past 2 weeks.
- you are now taking (or have recently taken) any diuretic (urine-producing) drug.
- you have impaired liver or kidney function.
- you have a history of thyroid function disorder.

Possible Side-Effects (natural, expected and unavoidable drug actions)
Slow heart rate, rare enlargement and/or sensitivity of the male breast tissue.

▷ **Possible Adverse Effects** (unusual, unexpected and infrequent reactions)
If any of the following develop, consult your physician promptly for guidance.
Mild Adverse Effects
Allergic Reactions: Skin rash, hives.
Headache, drowsiness, lethargy, confusion, changes in vision: "halo" effect, blurring, spots, double vision, yellow-green vision.
Loss of appetite, nausea, vomiting, diarrhea—early indications of toxicity in adults.
Serious Adverse Effects
Idiosyncratic Reactions: Hallucinations, facial neuralgias, peripheral neuralgias, blindness (very rare).
Disorientation, most common in the elderly.
Heart rhythm disturbances.

▷ **Possible Effects on Sexual Function**
Decreased libido and impotence in 35% of male users.
Enlargement and tenderness of male breasts.
Both effects are attributed to digoxin's estrogenlike action.

▷ **Adverse Effects That May Mimic Natural Diseases or Disorders**
Drug-induced mental disturbances in the elderly may be mistaken for senile dementia or psychosis.

Natural Diseases or Disorders That May Be Activated by This Drug
Digitalis may induce a systemic lupus erythematosus–like syndrome.

CAUTION
1. This drug has a narrow margin of safe use. Adhere strictly to prescribed dosage schedules. Do not raise or lower the dose without first consulting your physician.
2. If you are taking calcium supplements, ask your physician for guidance. Avoid large doses.
3. It is advisable to carry a card of personal identification with a notation that you are taking this drug.

4. Avoid taking over-the-counter antacids and cold, cough and allergy remedies without consulting your physician.

Precautions for Use

By Infants and Children: Observe carefully for indications of toxicity: slow heart rate (below 60 beats/minute), irregular heart rhythms.

By Those over 60 Years of Age: You may have a reduced tolerance for this drug; smaller doses are advisable. Observe for indications of early toxicity: headache, dizziness, fatigue, weakness, lethargy, depression, confusion, nervousness, agitation, delusions, difficulty with reading. Report the development of any of these effects promptly to your physician.

▷ **Advisability of Use During Pregnancy**

Pregnancy Category: C (tentative). See Pregnancy Code inside back cover.
Animal studies: No birth defects reported.
Human studies: Information from adequate studies of pregnant women is not available. However, no birth defects attributable to the therapeutic use of this drug have been reported.
Use this drug only if clearly needed. Overdosage can be harmful to the fetus.

Advisability of Use if Breast-Feeding

Presence of this drug in breast milk: Yes.
Monitor nursing infant closely and discontinue drug or nursing if adverse effects develop.

Habit-Forming Potential: None.

Effects of Overdosage: Loss of appetite, excessive saliva, nausea, vomiting, diarrhea, serious disturbances of heart rate and rhythm, intestinal bleeding, drowsiness, headache, confusion, delirium, hallucinations, convulsions.

Possible Effects of Long-Term Use: None reported.

Suggested Periodic Examinations While Taking This Drug (at physician's discretion)
Measurements of blood levels of digoxin, calcium, magnesium and potassium; electrocardiograms.

▷ **While Taking This Drug, Observe the Following**

Foods: Avoid all cheeses, yogurt and ice cream for 2 hours before and after taking this drug. Consult physician regarding the advisability of eating high-potassium foods.

Beverages: Avoid all forms of milk for 2 hours before and after taking this drug. Avoid excessive amounts of caffeine-containing beverages: coffee, tea, cola.

▷ *Alcohol:* No interactions expected.

Tobacco Smoking: Nicotine can cause irritability of the heart muscle and can predispose to serious rhythm disturbances. It is advisable to abstain from all forms of tobacco.

Marijuana Smoking: Possible accentuation of heart failure; reduced digoxin effect; possible changes in electrocardiogram, confusing interpretation.

▷   *Other Drugs*

Digoxin ***taken concurrently*** with

- diuretics (other than spironolactone and triamterene) may result in serious heart rhythm disturbances due to excessive loss of potassium.
- quinidine may result in decreased digoxin effectiveness and increased digoxin toxicity; careful dosage adjustments are necessary.

The following drugs may ***increase*** the effects of digoxin

- amiodarone (Cordarone).
- benzodiazepines (Librium, Valium, etc.; see Drug Class, Section Four).
- captopril (Capoten, Capazide).
- diltiazem (Cardizem).
- erythromycin (EES, Erythrocin, etc.).
- flecainide (Tambocor).
- hydroxychloroquine.
- ibuprofen (Advil, Medipren, Motrin, Nuprin, etc.).
- indomethacin (Indocin).
- methimazole (Tapazole).
- nifedipine (Adalat, Procardia).
- propylthiouracil (Propacil).
- quinine.
- tetracyclines (see Drug Class, Section Four).
- tolbutamide (Orinase).
- verapamil (Isoptin).

The following drugs may ***decrease*** the effects of digoxin

- aluminum-containing antacids (Amphojel, Maalox, etc.).
- bleomycin (Blenoxane).
- carmustine (Bicnu).
- cholestyramine (Questran).
- colestipol (Colestid).
- cyclophosphamide (Cytoxan).
- cytarabine (Cytosar).
- doxorubicin (Adriamycin).
- methotrexate (Mexate).
- penicillamine (Cuprimine, Depen).
- procarbazine (Matulane).
- thyroid hormones.
- vincristine (Oncovin).

▷   *Driving, Hazardous Activities:* Usually no restrictions. However, this drug may cause drowsiness, vision changes and nausea. Restrict activities as necessary.

Aviation Note: Heart function disorders **are a disqualification** for piloting. Consult a designated Aviation Medical Examiner.

Exposure to Sun: No restrictions.

Occurrence of Unrelated Illness: Any illness that causes vomiting or diarrhea can seriously alter this drug's effectiveness. Notify your physician promptly.

Discontinuation: This drug must be continued indefinitely. Do not discontinue it without consulting your physician.

DILTIAZEM
(dil TI a zem)

Introduced: 1977

Class: Antianginal, antihypertensive, calcium channel blocker

Prescription: USA: Yes
Canada: Yes

Controlled Drug: USA: No
Canada: No

Available as Generic: No

Brand Names: Cardizem, Cardizem SR

BENEFITS versus RISKS	
Possible Benefits	*Possible Risks*
EFFECTIVE PREVENTION OF BOTH MAJOR TYPES OF ANGINA	Depression, confusion
	Low blood pressure
	Heart rhythm disturbance (2%)
EFFECTIVE CONTROL OF MILD TO MODERATE HYPERTENSION	Fluid retention (2.4%)
	Liver damage (very rare)

▷ **Principal Uses**

As a Single Drug Product: Used primarily to treat (1) angina pectoris due to coronary artery spasm (Prinzmetal's variant angina) that occurs spontaneously and is not associated with exertion; (2) classical angina-of-effort (due to atherosclerotic disease of the coronary arteries) in individuals who have not responded to or cannot tolerate the nitrates and beta blocker drugs customarily used to treat this disorder; (3) mild to moderately severe hypertension.

How This Drug Works: Not completely established. It is thought that by blocking the normal passage of calcium through certain cell walls (which is necessary for the function of nerve and muscle tissue), this drug slows the spread of electrical activity through the conduction system of the heart and inhibits the contraction of coronary arteries and peripheral arterioles. As a result of these combined effects, this drug

- prevents spontaneous spasm of the coronary arteries (Prinzmetal's type of angina).
- reduces the rate and contraction force of the heart during exertion, thus lowering the oxygen requirement of the heart muscle; this reduces the occurrence of effort-induced angina (classical angina pectoris).
- reduces the degree of contraction of peripheral arterial walls, resulting in their relaxation and consequent lowering of blood pressure. This further reduces the work load of the heart during exertion and contributes to the prevention of angina.

Available Dosage Forms and Strengths
Tablets — 30 mg, 60 mg, 90 mg, 120 mg
Capsules, prolonged-action — 60 mg, 90 mg, 120 mg

▷ **Usual Adult Dosage Range:**   Initially 30 mg, 3 or 4 times daily. Dose may be increased gradually at 1- to 2-day intervals as needed and tolerated. Total daily dosage should not exceed 360 mg. **Note: Actual dosage and administration schedule must be determined by the physician for each patient individually.**

▷ **Dosing Instructions:**   Preferably taken before meals and at bedtime. Tablet may be crushed for administration.

Usual Duration of Use: Continual use on a regular schedule for 2 to 4 weeks is usually necessary to determine this drug's effectiveness in reducing the frequency and severity of angina and in lowering elevated blood pressure. For long-term use (months to years), determine the smallest effective dose. Consult your physician on a regular basis.

Possible Advantages of This Drug
Often effective as single drug therapy.
Does not reduce blood supply to kidneys.
Does not raise blood cholesterol levels.
Does not induce asthma in susceptible individuals.

▷ **This Drug Should Not Be Taken If**
- you have had an allergic reaction to it previously.
- you have a "sick sinus" syndrome (and are not wearing an artificial pacemaker).
- you have been told that you have a second-degree or third-degree heart block.
- you have low blood pressure—systolic pressure below 90.

▷ **Inform Your Physician Before Taking This Drug If**
- you have had an unfavorable response to any calcium blocker drug in the past.
- you are currently taking any form of digitalis or a beta blocker drug (see Drug Class, Section Four).

- you have a history of congestive heart failure.
- you have impaired liver or kidney function.
- you have a history of drug-induced liver damage.

Possible Side-Effects (natural, expected and unavoidable drug actions)
Fatigue (1.2%), light-headedness, heart rate and rhythm changes in pre-disposed individuals (1.1%).

▷ **Possible Adverse Effects** (unusual, unexpected and infrequent reactions)
If any of the following develop, consult your physician promptly for guidance.
Mild Adverse Effects
Allergic Reactions: Skin rash (1.3%), hives, itching.
Headache (2.1%), drowsiness, dizziness (1.5%), nervousness, insomnia, depression, confusion, hallucinations.
Flushing, palpitations, fainting, slow heart rate, low blood pressure.
Nausea (1.9%), indigestion, heartburn, vomiting, diarrhea, constipation.
Serious Adverse Effects
Serious disturbances of heart rate and/or rhythm, fluid retention (edema) (2.4%), congestive heart failure.
Drug-induced liver damage (very rare).

▷ **Possible Effects on Sexual Function:** Impotence is reported in less than 1% of users.

CAUTION
1. Be sure to inform all physicians and dentists you consult that you are taking this drug. Note the use of this drug on your card of personal identification.
2. You may use nitroglycerin and other nitrate drugs as needed to relieve acute episodes of angina pain. However, if you detect that your angina attacks are becoming more frequent or intense, notify your physician promptly.

Precautions for Use
By Infants and Children: Safety and effectiveness for use by those under 12 years of age have not been established.
By Those over 60 Years of Age: You may be more susceptible to the development of weakness, dizziness, fainting and falling. Take necessary precautions to prevent injury. Report promptly any changes in your pattern of thirst and urination.

▷ **Advisability of Use During Pregnancy**
Pregnancy Category: C (tentative). See Pregnancy Code inside back cover.
Animal studies: Embryo and fetal deaths and skeletal birth defects reported in mice, rats and rabbits.
Human studies: Information from adequate studies of pregnant women is not available.
Avoid this drug during the first 3 months.

Use during the last 6 months only if clearly needed. Ask physician for guidance.

Advisability of Use if Breast-Feeding
Presence of this drug in breast milk: Yes.
Avoid drug or refrain from nursing.

Habit-Forming Potential: None.

Effects of Overdosage: Weakness, light-headedness, fainting, slow pulse, low blood pressure, shortness of breath, congestive heart failure.

Possible Effects of Long-Term Use: None reported.

Suggested Periodic Examinations While Taking This Drug (at physician's discretion)
Evaluations of heart function, including electrocardiograms; liver and kidney function tests, with long-term use.

▷ **While Taking This Drug, Observe the Following**
Foods: No restrictions. Avoid excessive salt intake.
Beverages: No restrictions. May be taken with milk.
▷ *Alcohol:* Use with caution until combined effects have been determined. Alcohol may exaggerate the drop in blood pressure experienced by some individuals.
Tobacco Smoking: Nicotine may reduce the effectiveness of this drug. Follow your physician's advice regarding smoking.
Marijuana Smoking: Possible reduced effectiveness of this drug; mild to moderate increase in angina; possible changes in electrocardiogram, confusing interpretation.
▷ *Other Drugs*
Diltiazem *taken concurrently* with
• beta blocker drugs or digitalis preparations (see Drug Classes, Section Four) may affect heart rate and rhythm adversely. Careful monitoring by your physician is necessary if these drugs are taken concurrently.
The following drugs may *increase* the effects of diltiazem
• cimetidine (Tagamet).
▷ *Driving, Hazardous Activities:* Usually no restrictions. This drug may cause drowsiness or dizziness. Restrict activities as necessary.
Aviation Note: Coronary artery disease *is a disqualification* for piloting. Consult a designated Aviation Medical Examiner.
Exposure to Sun: Use caution until sensitivity has been determined. This drug may cause photosensitivity (see Glossary).
Exposure to Heat: Caution advised. Hot environments can exaggerate the blood-pressure-lowering effects of this drug. Observe for light-headedness or weakness.
Heavy Exercise or Exertion: This drug may improve your ability to be more active without resulting angina pain. Use caution and avoid excessive exercise that could impair heart function in the absence of warning pain.

Discontinuation: Do not discontinue this drug abruptly. Consult your physician regarding gradual withdrawal.

DIPHENHYDRAMINE
(di fen HI dra meen)

Introduced: 1946

Class: Hypnotic, antihistamines

Prescription: USA: Varies
Canada: No

Controlled Drug: USA: No*
Canada: No

Available as Generic: Yes

Brand Names: ✦Allerdryl, ✦Ambenyl Expectorant [CD], Ambenyl Syrup [CD], Benadryl, Benadryl 25, Benylin, ✦Benylin Decongestant [CD], ✦Benylin Pediatric Syrup, ✦Benylin Syrup w/Codeine [CD], ✦Caladryl [CD], Compoz, ✦Ergodryl [CD], Excedrin P.M. [CD], Genahist, ✦Insomnal, ✦Mandrax [CD], Nytol, Sleep-Eze 3, Sominex 2, Twilite, Valdrene

---

BENEFITS versus RISKS

Possible Benefits	*Possible Risks*
EFFECTIVE RELIEF OF ALLERGIC RHINITIS AND ALLERGIC SKIN DISORDERS	Marked sedation (50%)
	Atropinelike effects
EFFECTIVE, NONADDICTIVE SEDATIVE AND HYPNOTIC	Accentuation of prostatism (see Glossary)
Prevention and relief of motion sickness	Rare blood cell disorders: abnormally low white blood cell and platelet counts
Partial relief of symptoms of Parkinson's disease	

▷ **Principal Uses**

As a Single Drug Product: This versatile antihistamine is used primarily for (1) the safe and effective induction of sleep (mild to moderate sedation); (2) the prevention and treatment of motion sickness (control of dizziness, nausea and vomiting); (3) the relief of symptoms associated with Parkinson's disease; (4) the treatment of drug-induced parkinsonian reactions, especially in children and the elderly.

As a Combination Drug Product [CD]: This drug may have a mild suppressant effect on coughing, but its actual effectiveness is questionable. It is combined with expectorants and either codeine or dextromethorphan in some cough preparations.

*Ambenyl Syrup is C-V. See Schedules of Controlled Drugs inside back cover.

How This Drug Works: This drug reduces the intensity of allergic response by blocking the action of histamine after it has been released from sensitized tissue cells. Its natural side-effects are used to advantage: its sedative action is used to induce drowsiness and sleep; its atropinelike action is used in the management of motion sickness and Parkinson-related disorders.

Available Dosage Forms and Strengths
Capsules — 25 mg, 50 mg
  Cream — 1%
   Elixir — 12.5 mg per 5-ml teaspoonful (14% alcohol)
   Syrup — 12.5 mg, 13.3 mg per 5-ml teaspoonful
  Tablets — 25 mg, 50 mg

▷ **Usual Adult Dosage Range:**   25 to 50 mg/4 to 6 hours. Total daily dosage should not exceed 300 mg. **Note: Actual dosage and administration schedule must be determined by the physician for each patient individually.**

▷ **Dosing Instructions:**   Preferably taken with or following food to reduce stomach irritation. Tablet may be crushed and capsule may be opened for administration.

Usual Duration of Use: Continual use on a regular schedule for 2 to 3 days is usually necessary to determine this drug's effectiveness in relieving the symptoms of allergic rhinitis and dermatosis. If not effective after 5 days, this drug should be discontinued. As a bedtime sedative (hypnotic), use only as needed. Avoid long-term use without interruption.

▷ **This Drug Should Not Be Taken If**
  • you have had an allergic reaction to any dosage form of it previously.
  • you are taking, or have taken during the past 2 weeks, any monoamine oxidase (MAO) type A inhibitor drug (see Drug Class, Section Four).

▷ **Inform Your Physician Before Taking This Drug If**
  • you have had an unfavorable response to any antihistamine drug in the past.
  • you have narrow-angle glaucoma.
  • you have peptic ulcer disease, with any degree of pyloric obstruction.
  • you have prostatism (see Glossary).
  • you are subject to bronchial asthma or seizures (epilepsy).

Possible Side-Effects (natural, expected and unavoidable drug actions)
Drowsiness; sense of weakness; dryness of nose, mouth and throat; constipation.

▷ **Possible Adverse Effects** (unusual, unexpected and infrequent reactions)
If any of the following develop, consult your physician promptly for guidance.

Mild Adverse Effects
Allergic Reactions: Skin rash, hives.
Headache, dizziness, inability to concentrate, nervousness, blurred or double vision, difficult urination.
Reduced tolerance for contact lenses.
Nausea, vomiting, diarrhea.
Serious Adverse Effects
Allergic Reaction: Anaphylactic reaction (see Glossary).
Idiosyncratic Reactions: Insomnia, excitement, confusion.
Hemolytic anemia (see Glossary).
Reduced white blood cell count—fever, sore throat, infections.
Blood platelet destruction (see Glossary)—abnormal bleeding or bruising.

▷ **Possible Effects on Sexual Function:**   Shortened menstrual cycle (early arrival of expected menstrual onset).

Natural Diseases or Disorders That May Be Activated by This Drug
Latent epilepsy, glaucoma, prostatism.

CAUTION
1. Discontinue this drug 5 days before diagnostic skin testing procedures in order to prevent false negative test results.
2. Do not use this drug if you have active bronchial asthma, bronchitis or pneumonia. It can thicken bronchial mucous and make it more difficult to remove (by absorption or coughing).

Precautions for Use
By Infants and Children: This drug should not be used in premature or full-term newborn infants. Doses for children should be small. The young child is especially sensitive to the effects of antihistamines on the brain and nervous system. Avoid the use of this drug in the child with chicken pox or a flulike infection; although unproven, this drug may adversely affect the course of Reye syndrome should the child develop it during the course of illness.
By Those over 60 Years of Age: You may be more susceptible to the development of drowsiness, dizziness and unsteadiness, and to impairment of thinking, judgment and memory. This drug can increase the degree of impaired urination associated with prostate gland enlargement (prostatism). The sedative effects of antihistamines in the elderly can cause a syndrome of underactivity that may be misinterpreted as senility or emotional depression.

▷ **Advisability of Use During Pregnancy**
Pregnancy Category: B (tentative). See Pregnancy Code inside back cover.
Animal studies: No birth defects reported in rats or rabbits.
Human studies: Information from studies of pregnant women indicates no significant increase in birth defects in 2948 exposures to this drug. A withdrawal syndrome of tremor and diarrhea has been reported in

a 5-day-old infant whose mother used this drug (150 mg daily) during pregnancy.

Avoid drug during the last 3 months. Use sparingly during the first 6 months only if clearly needed.

Advisability of Use if Breast-Feeding
Presence of this drug in breast milk: Yes.
Avoid drug or refrain from nursing.

Habit-Forming Potential: None.

Effects of Overdosage: Marked drowsiness, confusion, incoordination, unsteadiness, muscle tremors, stupor, coma, seizures, fever, flushed face, dilated pupils, weak pulse, shallow breathing.

Possible Effects of Long-Term Use: The development of tolerance (see Glossary) and reduced effectiveness of drug.

Suggested Periodic Examinations While Taking This Drug (at physician's discretion)
Complete blood cell counts.

▷ **While Taking This Drug, Observe the Following**
Foods: No restrictions.
Beverages: No restrictions. May be taken with milk.
▷ *Alcohol:* Use with extreme caution until the combined effect has been determined. The combination of alcohol and antihistamines can cause rapid and marked sedation.
Tobacco Smoking: No interactions expected.
Marijuana Smoking: Increased drowsiness and mouth dryness; possible accentuation of impaired thinking.
▷ *Other Drugs*
Diphenhydramine may **increase** the effects of
• all drugs with a sedative effect, and cause oversedation.
• atropine and atropinelike drugs (see Drug Class, Section Four).
The following drugs may **increase** the effects of diphenhydramine
• monoamine oxidase (MAO) type A inhibitor drugs (see Drug Class, Section Four) may delay its elimination, thus exaggerating and prolonging its action.
▷ *Driving, Hazardous Activities:* This drug may impair mental alertness, judgment, physical coordination and reaction time. Restrict activities as necessary.
Aviation Note: The use of this drug **is a disqualification** for piloting. Consult a designated Aviation Medical Examiner.
Exposure to Sun: Use caution until sensitivity has been determined. This drug may cause photosensitivity (see Glossary).
Exposure to Environmental Chemicals: The insecticides Aldrin, Dieldrin and Chlordane may decrease the effectiveness of this drug. The insecticide Sevin may increase the sedative effects of this drug.

DIPHENOXYLATE
(di fen OX i layt)

Introduced: 1960

Class: Antidiarrheal

Prescription: USA: Yes
Canada: Yes

Controlled Drug: USA: C-V*
Canada: <N>

Available as Generic: USA: Yes
Canada: No

Brand Names: Lomotil [CD], ✦Lomotil

BENEFITS versus RISKS	
Possible Benefits	*Possible Risks*
EFFECTIVE RELIEF OF INTESTINAL CRAMPING AND DIARRHEA	Drowsiness Constipation Low habit-forming potential

▷ **Principal Uses**

As a Single Drug Product: Used primarily for the control of overactivity of the intestinal tract, cramping and diarrhea. Because of its potential for abuse, this drug is not marketed as a single-entity product in the USA.

As a Combination Drug Product [CD]: This drug, in therapeutically effective dosage, is combined with a small amount of atropine to discourage abusive overdosage. The accumulative effects of atropine overdosage would make the combination intolerable.

How This Drug Works: Not completely established. It is thought that this drug acts directly on the nerve supply of the gastrointestinal tract to reduce its motility and propulsive contractions, thus relieving cramping and diarrhea.

Available Dosage Forms and Strengths
Liquid — 2.5 mg (+ 0.025 mg atropine) per 5-ml teaspoonful
Tablets — 2.5 mg (+ 0.025 mg atropine)

▷ **Usual Adult Dosage Range:** Initially 2.5 to 5 mg/4 hours as needed for acute diarrhea; then 2.5 mg/6 to 8 hours as needed for chronic diarrhea. **Note: Actual dosage and administration schedule must be determined by the physician for each patient individually.**

▷ **Dosing Instructions:** May be taken on an empty stomach or with food if stomach irritation occurs. Tablet may be crushed for administration.

Usual Duration of Use: Continual use on a regular schedule for 24 to 36 hours is usually necessary to determine this drug's effectiveness in

*See Schedules of Controlled Drugs inside back cover.

controlling acute diarrhea. If diarrhea persists, consult your physician. Avoid prolonged and uninterrupted use.

▷ **This Drug Should Not Be Taken If**
- you are allergic to either component of this combination drug (single component in Canada).
- you have active liver disease.
- it is prescribed for a child under 2 years of age.

▷ **Inform Your Physician Before Taking This Drug If**
- you have a history of liver disease or impaired liver function.
- you have regional enteritis or ulcerative colitis.
- you have chronic lung disease of any kind.

Possible Side-Effects (natural, expected and unavoidable drug actions)
Drowsiness, constipation.

▷ **Possible Adverse Effects** (unusual, unexpected and infrequent reactions)
If any of the following develop, consult your physician promptly for guidance.
Mild Adverse Effects
Allergic Reactions: Skin rash, hives, localized swellings, itching.
Headache, dizziness, weakness, euphoria.
Reduced appetite, nausea, vomiting, bloating.
Serious Adverse Effects
"Toxic megacolon" (distended, immobile colon with fluid retention) may develop in acute ulcerative colitis.

▷ **Possible Effects on Sexual Function:**   None reported.

CAUTION
1. Do not exceed recommended doses.
2. Use with caution in the presence of chronic lung disease (asthma, bronchitis, emphysema). This drug may impair respiration.
3. If used to treat chronic diarrhea, report promptly any development of bloating, abdominal distension, nausea, vomiting, constipation or abdominal pain.

Precautions for Use
By Infants and Children: Do not use in those under 2 years of age. Use with caution (especially in children with Down's syndrome); observe closely for any indications of atropine overdosage: excitement, overactivity, hallucinations, fever, flushed face, dilated pupils.
By Those over 60 Years of Age: Start treatment with small doses. You may be more sensitive to the sedative and constipating effects of this drug.

▷ **Advisability of Use During Pregnancy**
Pregnancy Category: C (tentative). See Pregnancy Code inside back cover.
Animal studies: No information available.

Human studies: Information from adequate studies of pregnant women is not available.

Use sparingly and only if clearly needed. Ask physician for guidance.

Advisability of Use if Breast-Feeding
Presence of this drug in breast milk: Yes.
Avoid drug or refrain from nursing.

Habit-Forming Potential: Because of its similarity to meperidine, this drug may cause physical dependence (see Glossary) if used in large doses over an extended period of time.

Effects of Overdosage: Marked drowsiness, lethargy, depression, numbness in arms and legs, dry skin and mouth, flushing, fever, rapid pulse, slow and shallow breathing, stupor progressing to coma.

Possible Effects of Long-Term Use: The development of tolerance with loss of drug effectiveness. Physical dependence is a remote possibility.

Suggested Periodic Examinations While Taking This Drug (at physician's discretion)
None required.

▷ **While Taking This Drug, Observe the Following**
Foods: No restrictions. Follow prescribed diet.
Beverages: No restrictions. May be taken with milk.
▷ *Alcohol:* Use with extreme caution until combined effects have been determined. This drug may increase the depressant action of alcohol on the brain.
Tobacco Smoking: No interactions expected.
▷ *Other Drugs*
Diphenoxylate may *increase* the effects of
• all drugs with a sedative effect, and cause oversedation.
Diphenoxylate *taken concurrently* with
• monoamine oxidase (MAO) type A inhibitor drugs (see Drug Class, Section Four) will require close observation for excessive rise in blood pressure.
▷ *Driving, Hazardous Activities:* This drug may cause drowsiness or dizziness. Restrict activities as necessary.
Aviation Note: The use of this drug *is a disqualification* for piloting. Consult a designated Aviation Medical Examiner.
Exposure to Sun: No restrictions.

DIPYRIDAMOLE
(di peer ID a mohl)

Introduced: 1959

Prescription: USA: Yes
Canada: No

Class: Platelet inhibitor

Controlled Drug: USA: No
Canada: No

Available as Generic: USA: Yes
 Canada: No

Brand Names: ✦Apo-Dipyridamole, ✦Asasantine [CD], Persantine, Pyridamole

```
┌─────────────────────────────────────────────────────────────────┐
│                    BENEFITS versus RISKS                          │
│                                                                   │
│        Possible Benefits              Possible Risks              │
│    EFFECTIVE PREVENTION OF      Mild low blood pressure with      │
│      THROMBOEMBOLISM              dizziness and fainting           │
│    (BLOOD CLOTS) FOLLOWING        (infrequent)                    │
│    HEART VALVE SURGERY          Mild indigestion                  │
└─────────────────────────────────────────────────────────────────┘
```

▷ **Principal Uses**
  As a Single Drug Product: This drug is used primarily for (1) the prevention of thromboembolism (blood clot formation and migration) following heart valve surgery; (2) the prevention of thromboembolism thought to be responsible for transient ischemic attacks in brain circulation (ministrokes). It may be used together with aspirin or with anticoagulants such as warfarin (Coumadin).

  How This Drug Works: Not completely established. It is thought that by inhibiting the actions of certain enzymes, this drug prevents the aggregation of blood platelets (see Glossary) and thereby reduces the tendency to blood clot formation.

  Available Dosage Forms and Strengths
  Tablets — 25 mg, 50 mg, 75 mg

▷ **Usual Adult Dosage Range:**   50 to 100 mg, 3 or 4 times daily. Total daily dosage should not exceed 400 mg. **Note: Actual dosage and administration schedule must be determined by the physician for each patient individually.**

▷ **Dosing Instructions:**   Preferably taken with a full glass of water on an empty stomach, 1 hour before or 2 hours after eating. However, it may be taken with or following food to reduce stomach irritation. The tablet may be crushed for administration.

  Usual Duration of Use: Significant reduction in platelet aggregation is thought to occur in 1 week. Long-term use (months to years) requires supervision and periodic evaluation by your physician.

▷ **This Drug Should Not Be Taken If**
  • you have had an allergic reaction to it previously.
  • you have just experienced an acute heart attack (myocardial infarction).
  • you have uncontrolled high blood pressure.

▷ **Inform Your Physician Before Taking This Drug If**
- you have low blood pressure.
- you have impaired liver function.
- you have any type of bleeding disorder.

Possible Side-Effects (natural, expected and unavoidable drug actions)
Flushing, light-headedness, weakness.

▷ **Possible Adverse Effects** (unusual, unexpected and infrequent reactions)
If any of the following develop, consult your physician promptly for guidance.
Mild Adverse Effects
Allergic Reaction: Skin rash.
Headache, dizziness, fainting.
Stomach irritation, nausea, diarrhea.
Serious Adverse Effects
Significant low blood pressure with large doses.
Paradoxical increase in angina on starting treatment (infrequent).
Aggravation of migraine headaches.

▷ **Possible Effects on Sexual Function:**   None reported.

CAUTION
1. Occasionally this drug may cause an ***increase*** in the frequency and/or severity of preexisting angina. If this response occurs, inform your physician promptly.
2. Anyone with low blood pressure should avoid large doses of this drug.

Precautions for Use
By Infants and Children: Observe closely for indications of excessively low blood pressure.
By Those over 60 Years of Age: Begin treatment with small doses (25 mg twice daily) to evaluate effect on blood pressure. Avoid doses that cause excessively low blood pressure. Observe for any tendency to develop hypothermia (see Glossary) in cold environments.

▷ **Advisability of Use During Pregnancy**
Pregnancy Category: B (tentative). See Pregnancy Code inside back cover.
Animal studies: Mouse, rat and rabbit studies show no birth defects due to this drug.
Human studies: Information from adequate studies of pregnant women is not available.
Use this drug only if clearly needed. If possible, avoid use during the last month of pregnancy and during labor and delivery because of possible prolongation of bleeding following delivery.

Advisability of Use if Breast-Feeding
Presence of this drug in breast milk: Yes, in small amounts.
Monitor nursing infant closely and discontinue drug or nursing if adverse effects develop.

Habit-Forming Potential: None.

Effects of Overdosage: Flushing, stomach irritation, nausea, vomiting, stomach cramps, diarrhea, rapid heart rate, low blood pressure, weakness, fainting.

Possible Effects of Long-Term Use: None reported.

Suggested Periodic Examinations While Taking This Drug (at physician's discretion)
Measurements of blood pressure in lying, sitting and standing positions.

▷ **While Taking This Drug, Observe the Following**
Foods: No restrictions.
Beverages: No restrictions. May be taken with milk.
▷   *Alcohol:* Use with caution until the combined effect has been determined. Alcohol may enhance the ability of this drug to lower blood pressure.
Tobacco Smoking: Nicotine can reduce the effectiveness of this drug. Follow physician's advice regarding smoking.
Marijuana Smoking: Possible reduced effectiveness of this drug; mild to moderate increase in angina; possible changes in electrocardiogram, confusing interpretation.
▷   *Other Drugs*
Dipyridamole may ***increase*** the effects of
- oral anticoagulants (warfarin, etc.), when doses of dipyridamole approach or exceed 400 mg/day; observe for abnormal bleeding or bruising.
- other drugs that inhibit platelet activity; observe for abnormal bleeding or bruising.
Dipyridamole ***taken concurrently*** with
- aspirin makes it possible to reduce the dose of dipyridamole and thus lessen any side-effects that may occur.
▷   *Driving, Hazardous Activities:* This drug may cause light-headedness or dizziness. Restrict activities as necessary.
Aviation Note: The use of this drug ***may be a disqualification*** for piloting. Consult a designated Aviation Medical Examiner.
Exposure to Sun: No restrictions.
Exposure to Heat: Use caution. Hot environments can cause significant drop in blood pressure.
Exposure to Cold: Use caution. This drug may increase the risk of hypothermia (see Glossary) in the elderly.
Discontinuation: Following long-term use, this drug should not be discontinued abruptly. It should be withdrawn gradually over a period of 2 to 3 weeks. Ask your physician for guidance.

DISOPYRAMIDE
(di so PEER a mide)

Introduced: 1969

Class: Antiarrhythmic

Prescription: USA: Yes
  Canada: Yes

Controlled Drug: USA: No
  Canada: No

Available as Generic: USA: Yes
  Canada: No

Brand Names: Napamide, Norpace, Norpace CR, ✦Rythmodan, ✦Rythmodan-LA

BENEFITS versus RISKS

Possible Benefits	*Possible Risks*
EFFECTIVE TREATMENT OF SELECTED HEART RHYTHM DISORDERS	NARROW TREATMENT RANGE FREQUENT ADVERSE EFFECTS (10–40%) LOW BLOOD PRESSURE CONGESTIVE HEART FAILURE Heart conduction and rhythm abnormalities Frequent atropinelike side-effects

---

▷ **Principal Uses**

  As a Single Drug Product: This drug is classified as a Type 1 antiarrhythmic agent, similar to procainamide and quinidine in its actions. It is used primarily to abolish and prevent the recurrence of premature beats arising in the atria (upper chambers) and the ventricles (lower chambers) of the heart. It is also useful in the treatment and prevention of abnormally rapid heart rates (tachycardia) that originate in the atria or the ventricles.

How This Drug Works: By slowing the activity of the pacemaker and delaying the transmission of electrical impulses through the conduction system and muscle of the heart, this drug assists in restoring normal heart rate and rhythm.

Available Dosage Forms and Strengths
Capsules — 100 mg, 150 mg
Capsules, prolonged-action — 100 mg, 150 mg

▷ **Usual Adult Dosage Range:** 100 to 200 mg/6 hours. Dosage should not exceed 200 mg/6 hours or 800 mg/24 hours (1600 mg/24 hours have been used occasionally). **Note: Actual dosage and administration schedule must be determined by the physician for each patient individually.**

▷ **Dosing Instructions:**   Preferably taken on an empty stomach, 1 hour before or 2 hours after eating. However, it may be taken with or following food to reduce stomach irritation. The regular capsules may be opened for administration; however, the prolonged-action capsules should not be opened, chewed or crushed.

Usual Duration of Use: Continual use on a regular schedule for 2 to 4 days is usually necessary to determine this drug's effectiveness in correcting or preventing responsive rhythm disorders. Long-term use requires supervision and periodic evaluation by your physician.

▷ **This Drug Should Not Be Taken If**
- you have had an allergic reaction to it previously.
- you have second-degree or third-degree heart block (determined by electrocardiogram).

▷ **Inform Your Physician Before Taking This Drug If**
- you have had any unfavorable reactions to other antiarrhythmic drugs in the past.
- you have a history of heart disease of any kind, especially "heart block."
- you have a history of low blood pressure.
- you have impaired liver or kidney function.
- you have glaucoma, or a family history of glaucoma.
- you have an enlarged prostate gland.
- you have myasthenia gravis.
- you are taking any form of digitalis or any diuretic drug that can cause excessive loss of body potassium (ask physician).

Possible Side-Effects (natural, expected and unavoidable drug actions)
Drop in blood pressure in susceptible individuals.
Dry mouth (32%), constipation (11%), blurred vision (3–9%), impaired urination (14%).

▷ **Possible Adverse Effects** (unusual, unexpected and infrequent reactions)
If any of the following develop, consult your physician promptly for guidance.
Mild Adverse Effects
Allergic Reactions: Skin rash (1–3%), itching.
Headache, nervousness, fatigue, muscular weakness, mild aches.
Loss of appetite, indigestion, nausea, vomiting, diarrhea.
Lowered blood sugar level (hypoglycemia).
Serious Adverse Effects
Idiosyncratic Reaction: Acute psychotic behavior (rare).
Severe drop in blood pressure, fainting.
Progressive heart weakness, predisposing to congestive heart failure.
Inability to empty urinary bladder, prostatism (see Glossary).
Jaundice (see Glossary).
Abnormally low white blood cell count (rare).

▷ **Possible Effects on Sexual Function:** Rare reports of impotence (300 mg/day); enlargement and tenderness of male breasts.

▷ **Adverse Effects That May Mimic Natural Diseases or Disorders**
Reversible jaundice may suggest viral hepatitis.

Natural Diseases or Disorders That May Be Activated by This Drug
Glaucoma, myasthenia gravis.

CAUTION
1. Thorough evaluation of your heart function (including electrocardiograms) is necessary prior to using this drug.
2. Periodic evaluation of your heart function is necessary to determine your response to this drug. Some individuals may experience worsening of their heart rhythm disorder and/or deterioration of heart function. Close monitoring of heart rate, rhythm and overall performance is essential.
3. Dosage must be adjusted carefully for each individual. Do not change your dosage without the knowledge and supervision of your physician.
4. Do not take any other antiarrhythmic drug while taking this drug unless directed to do so by your physician.

Precautions for Use
By Infants and Children: Safety and effectiveness for use by those under 12 years of age have not been established. Initial use of this drug requires hospitalization and supervision by a qualified pediatrician.
By Those over 60 Years of Age: Reduced kidney function may require reduction in dosage. This drug can aggravate existing prostatism (see Glossary) and promote constipation. Observe carefully for light-headedness, dizziness, unsteadiness and tendency to fall.

▷ **Advisability of Use During Pregnancy**
Pregnancy Category: B (tentative). See Pregnancy Code inside back cover.
Animal studies: No birth defects reported in rats and rabbits.
Human studies: Information from adequate studies of pregnant women is not available. It has been reported that this drug can cause contractions of the pregnant uterus.
Use this drug only if clearly needed. Ask your physician for guidance.

Advisability of Use if Breast-Feeding
Presence of this drug in breast milk: Yes.
Avoid drug or refrain from nursing.

Habit-Forming Potential: None.

Effects of Overdosage: Dryness of eyes, nose, mouth and throat; impaired urination; constipation; marked drop in blood pressure; abnormal heart rhythms; congestive heart failure.

Possible Effects of Long-Term Use: None reported.

Suggested Periodic Examinations While Taking This Drug (at physician's discretion)

Electrocardiograms, complete blood cell counts, measurements of potassium blood levels.

▷ **While Taking This Drug, Observe the Following**

Foods: No restrictions. Ask physician regarding need for salt restriction and advisability of eating potassium-rich foods.

Beverages: No restrictions. May be taken with milk.

▷ *Alcohol:* Use caution until the combined effects have been determined. Alcohol can increase the blood-pressure-lowering effects and the blood-sugar-lowering effects of this drug.

Tobacco Smoking: Nicotine can cause irritability of the heart and reduce the effectiveness of this drug. Follow physician's advice regarding smoking.

▷ *Other Drugs*

Disopyramide may ***increase*** the effects of

- antihypertensive drugs, and cause excessive lowering of blood pressure.
- atropinelike drugs (see Drug Class, Section Four).
- warfarin (Coumadin, etc.); monitor prothrombin times, adjust dosage accordingly.

Disopyramide may ***decrease*** the effects of

- ambenonium (Mytelase).
- neostigmine (Prostigmin).
- pyridostigmine (Mestinon).

The beneficial effects of these three drugs in the treatment of myasthenia gravis may be reduced.

The following drugs may ***decrease*** the effects of disopyramide

- all diuretics that promote potassium loss.
- rifampin (Rimactane, Rifadin).

▷ *Driving, Hazardous Activities:* This drug may cause dizziness or blurred vision. Restrict activities as necessary.

Aviation Note: The use of this drug ***may be a disqualification*** for piloting. Consult a designated Aviation Medical Examiner.

Exposure to Sun: Use caution. This drug is reported to cause photosensitization (see Glossary) in susceptible individuals.

Exposure to Heat: Use caution. The use of this drug in hot environments may increase the risk of heat stroke.

Occurrence of Unrelated Illness: Disorders that cause vomiting, diarrhea or dehydration can affect this drug's action adversely. Report such developments promptly.

Discontinuation: This drug should not be discontinued abruptly following long-term use. Ask your physician for guidance regarding gradual dose reduction.

DISULFIRAM
(di SULF i ram)

Introduced: 1948

Class: Antialcoholism

Prescription: USA: Yes
Canada: Yes

Controlled Drug: USA: No
Canada: No

Available as Generic: USA: Yes
Canada: No

Brand Name: Antabuse

BENEFITS versus RISKS

Possible Benefits	*Possible Risks*
EFFECTIVE ADJUNCT IN THE TREATMENT OF CHRONIC ALCOHOLISM	DANGEROUS REACTIONS WITH ALCOHOL INGESTION Acute psychotic reactions (uncommon) Drug-induced liver damage (rare) Drug-induced optic and/or peripheral neuritis (rare)

▷ **Principal Uses**

As a Single Drug Product: This drug is used for one purpose only—to deter the abusive drinking of alcoholic beverages. It does not abolish the craving or impulse to drink. It is of value in the treatment of alcoholism because of the psychological reinforcement it provides by reminding the patient of the dire consequences of ingesting alcohol.

How This Drug Works: Following the ingestion of alcohol, this drug interrupts normal liver enzyme activity after the conversion of alcohol to acetaldehyde. This causes excessive accumulation of acetaldehyde, a highly toxic substance that produces the disulfiram (Antabuse) reaction (see Glossary).

Available Dosage Forms and Strengths
Tablets — 250 mg, 500 mg

▷ **Usual Adult Dosage Range:** In the absence of all signs of alcoholic intoxication and no less than 12 hours after the last ingestion of alcohol, treatment is started with a single dose of 500 mg/day for 1 to 2 weeks. This is followed by a maintenance dose of 250 mg/day. The range of the maintenance dose is 125 mg to 500 mg/day and is determined by experience with each patient individually. The total daily dosage should not exceed 1000 mg. **Note: Actual dosage and administration schedule must be determined by the physician for each patient individually.**

▷ **Dosing Instructions:**   May be taken with or following food to reduce stomach irritation. Tablet may be crushed for administration.

Usual Duration of Use: Continual use on a regular schedule for several months is usually necessary to determine this drug's effectiveness in deterring the drinking of alcohol. If tolerated well, use should continue until a basis for permanent self-control and sobriety is established. Consult your physician on a regular basis.

▷ **This Drug Should Not Be Taken If**
- you have experienced a severe allergic reaction to disulfiram in the past. (Note: The interaction of disulfiram and alcohol is **not an allergic** reaction.)
- you have ingested any form of alcohol in any amount within the past 12 hours.
- you are pregnant.
- you are taking (or have taken recently) metronidazole (Flagyl).
- you have coronary heart disease or a serious heart rhythm disorder.

▷ **Inform Your Physician Before Taking This Drug If**
- you have used disulfiram in the past.
- you do not intend to avoid alcohol completely while taking this drug.
- you have not been given a full explanation of the reaction you will experience if you drink alcohol while taking this drug.
- you are planning pregnancy in the near future.
- you have a history of diabetes, epilepsy, kidney or liver disease.
- you are currently taking oral anticoagulants, digitalis, isoniazid, paraldehyde or phenytoin (Dilantin).
- you plan to have surgery under general anesthesia while taking this drug.

Possible Side-Effects (natural, expected and unavoidable drug actions)
Drowsiness, lethargy during early use.
Offensive breath and body odor.

▷ **Possible Adverse Effects** (unusual, unexpected and infrequent reactions)
If any of the following develop, consult your physician promptly for guidance.
Mild Adverse Effects
Allergic Reactions: Skin rash, hives.
Headache, dizziness, restlessness, tremor.
Metallic or garliclike taste, indigestion. (These usually subside after 2 weeks of use.)
Serious Adverse Effects
Allergic Reactions: Severe skin rashes, drug-induced hepatitis (rare).
Idiosyncratic Reaction: Acute toxic effect on brain; psychotic behavior.
Optic or peripheral neuritis (see Glossary).

▷ **Possible Effects on Sexual Function:**   Decreased libido and/or impaired erection in 30% of users taking recommended doses of 125 to 500 mg/day.

▷ **Adverse Effects That May Mimic Natural Diseases or Disorders**
> Liver reaction may suggest viral hepatitis.
> Brain toxicity may suggest spontaneous psychosis.

CAUTION
1. This drug should never be taken by anyone who is in a state of alcoholic intoxication.
2. The patient should be fully informed regarding the purpose and actions of this drug *before* treatment is started.
3. During long-term use of this drug, examine for any indication of reduced thyroid function.
4. Carry a card of personal identification with the notation that you are taking this drug.

Precautions for Use
> *By Infants and Children:* Safety and effectiveness for use by those under 12 years of age have not been established.
> *By Those over 60 Years of Age:* Observe for excessive sedation during the early use of this drug. *Do not* perform an "alcohol trial" to determine the effects of this drug.

▷ **Advisability of Use During Pregnancy**
> *Pregnancy Category:* X (tentative). See Pregnancy Code inside back cover.
> Animal studies: No defects reported in rats and hamsters.
> Human studies: Two reports indicate that 4 of 8 fetuses exposed to this drug had serious birth defects. Information from adequate studies of pregnant women is not available.
> Avoid this drug completely if possible.

Advisability of Use if Breast-Feeding
> Presence of this drug in breast milk: Unknown.
> Avoid drug or refrain from nursing.

Habit-Forming Potential: None.

Effects of Overdosage: Marked lethargy, impaired memory, altered behavior, confusion, unsteadiness, weakness, stomach pain, nausea, vomiting, diarrhea.

Possible Effects of Long-Term Use: Decreased function of thyroid gland.

Suggested Periodic Examinations While Taking This Drug (at physician's discretion)
> Visual acuity, liver function tests.

▷ **While Taking This Drug, Observe the Following**
> *Foods:* Avoid all foods prepared with alcohol, including sauces, marinades, vinegars, desserts, etc. Inquire when dining out regarding the use of alcohol in food preparation.
> *Beverages:* Avoid all punches, fruit drinks, etc., that may contain alcohol. This drug may be taken with milk.

▷   *Alcohol:* **Avoid completely in all forms** while taking this drug and for 14
days following the last dose. The combination of disulfiram and alcohol—even in small amounts—produces the disulfiram (Antabuse)
reaction. This begins within 5 to 10 minutes after ingesting alcohol
and consists of intense flushing and warming of the face, a severe
throbbing headache, shortness of breath, chest pains, nausea, repeated vomiting, sweating and weakness. If the amount of alcohol
ingested is large enough, the reaction may progress to blurred vision,
vertigo, confusion, marked drop in blood pressure and loss of consciousness. Severe reactions may lead to convulsions and death. The
reaction may last from 30 minutes to several hours, depending upon
the amount of alcohol and disulfiram in the body. As the symptoms
subside, the individual is exhausted and usually sleeps for several
hours.

Tobacco Smoking: No interactions expected.

Marijuana Smoking: Possible increase in drowsiness and lethargy.

▷   *Other Drugs*

Disulfiram may ***increase*** the effects of

- oral anticoagulants (warfarin, etc.), and increase the risk of bleeding;
dosage adjustments may be necessary.
- barbiturates, and cause oversedation (see Drug Class, Section Four).
- chlordiazepoxide (Librium) and diazepam (Valium), and cause
oversedation.
- paraldehyde, and cause excessive depression of brain function.
- phenytoin (Dilantin), and cause toxic effects on the brain; dosage adjustments may be necessary.

Disulfiram may ***decrease*** the effects of

- perphenazine (Tilafon, etc.).

Disulfiram ***taken concurrently*** with

- isoniazid (INH, etc.) may cause acute mental disturbance and incoordination, making it necessary to discontinue treatment.
- metronidazole (Flagyl) may cause acute mental and behavioral disturbances, making it necessary to discontinue treatment.
- OTC cough syrups, tonics, etc., containing alcohol may cause a disulfiram (Antabuse) reaction; avoid concurrent use. (See OTC Drugs
in Glossary.)

The following drugs may ***increase*** the effects of disulfiram

- amitriptyline (Elavil) may enhance the disulfiram + alcohol interaction; avoid concurrent use of these drugs.

▷   *Driving, Hazardous Activities:* This drug may cause drowsiness or dizziness. Restrict activities as necessary.

Aviation Note: Alcoholism **is a disqualification** for piloting. Consult a designated Aviation Medical Examiner.

Exposure to Sun: No restrictions.

Exposure to Environmental Chemicals: Thiram, a pesticide, and carbon
disulfide, a pesticide and industrial solvent, can have additive toxic
effects during use of this drug. Observe for toxic effects on the brain
and nervous system.

Discontinuation: Treatment with this drug is only part of your total treatment program. Do not discontinue it without the knowledge and guidance of your physician. Abrupt withdrawal does not cause any symptoms. However, no alcohol should be ingested for 14 days following discontinuation.

DOXEPIN
(DOX e pin)

Introduced: 1969

Class: Antidepressant

Prescription: USA: Yes
    Canada: Yes

Controlled Drug: USA: No
    Canada: No

Available as Generic: USA: Yes
    Canada: No

Brand Names: Adapin, Sinequan, ✦Triadapin

BENEFITS versus RISKS

Possible Benefits	*Possible Risks*
EFFECTIVE RELIEF OF ENDOGENOUS DEPRESSION	ADVERSE BEHAVIORAL EFFECTS: confusion, disorientation, hallucinations, delusions
EFFECTIVE RELIEF OF ANXIETY AND NERVOUS TENSION	CONVERSION OF DEPRESSION TO MANIA in manic-depressive disorder
Possibly beneficial in other depressive disorders	Aggravation of schizophrenia and paranoia
	Rare blood cell disorders

▷ **Principal Uses**

As a Single Drug Product: To relieve the symptoms associated with spontaneous (endogenous) depression, and to initiate the restoration of normal mood. This drug should be used only when a diagnosis of a true, primary depression of significant degree has been established. It should not be used to treat the symptoms of mild and transient (reactive) depression that may be associated with many life situations in the absence of a bona fide affective illness.

How This Drug Works: Not completely established. It is thought that this drug relieves depression by slowly restoring to normal levels certain constituents of brain tissue (norepinephrine and serotonin) that transmit nerve impulses.

Available Dosage Forms and Strengths
Capsules — 10 mg, 25 mg, 50 mg, 75 mg, 100 mg, 150 mg
Oral concentrate — 10 mg per ml

▷ **Usual Adult Dosage Range:**   Initially 25 mg 2 to 4 times daily. Dose may be increased cautiously as needed and tolerated by 10 to 25 mg daily at intervals of 1 week. Usual maintenance dose is 75 to 150 mg/24 hours. Total dose should not exceed 300 mg/24 hours. When the optimal requirement is determined, it may be taken at bedtime as one dose. **Note: Actual dosage and administration schedule must be determined by the physician for each patient individually.**

▷ **Dosing Instructions:**   May be taken without regard to meals. Capsule may be opened for administration.

Usual Duration of Use: Some benefit may be apparent within 1 to 2 weeks, but adequate response may require continual use for 10 to 12 weeks or longer. Long-term use should not exceed 6 months without evaluation regarding the need for continuation of the drug. Consult your physician on a regular basis.

▷ **This Drug Should Not Be Taken If**
- you have had an allergic reaction to it previously.
- you are taking or have taken within the past 14 days any monoamine oxidase (MAO) type A inhibitor drug (see Drug Class, Section Four).
- you are recovering from a recent heart attack.
- you have narrow-angle glaucoma.

▷ **Inform Your Physician Before Taking This Drug If**
- you are allergic or sensitive to any other tricyclic antidepressant (see Drug Class, Section Four).
- you have a history of any of the following: diabetes, epilepsy, glaucoma, heart disease, prostate gland enlargement or overactive thyroid function.
- you plan to have surgery under general anesthesia in the near future.

Possible Side-Effects (natural, expected and unavoidable drug actions)
Drowsiness, blurred vision, dry mouth, constipation, impaired urination.

▷ **Possible Adverse Effects** (unusual, unexpected and infrequent reactions)
If any of the following develop, consult your physician promptly for guidance.
Mild Adverse Effects
Allergic Reactions: Skin rash, hives, swelling of face or tongue, drug fever (see Glossary).
Headache, dizziness, weakness, fainting, unsteady gait, tremors.
Peculiar taste, irritation of tongue or mouth, nausea, indigestion.
Fluctuation of blood sugar levels.

Serious Adverse Effects
Allergic Reactions: Hepatitis, with or without jaundice (see Glossary).
Confusion, hallucinations, agitation, restlessness, delusions.
Bone marrow depression (see Glossary)—fatigue, weakness, fever, sore throat, abnormal bleeding or bruising (reported for other drugs of this class).
Peripheral neuritis (see Glossary)—numbness, tingling, pain, loss of strength in arms and legs.
Parkinson-like disorders (see Glossary)—usually mild and infrequent; more likely to occur in the elderly.

▷ **Possible Effects on Sexual Function:**   Female breast enlargement with milk production; swelling of testicles.

▷ **Adverse Effects That May Mimic Natural Diseases or Disorders**
Liver toxicity may suggest viral hepatitis.

Natural Diseases or Disorders That May Be Activated by This Drug
Latent diabetes, epilepsy, glaucoma, impaired urination due to prostate gland enlargement (prostatism, see Glossary).

CAUTION
1. Dosage must be adjusted for each person individually. Report for follow-up evaluation and laboratory tests as directed by your physician.
2. It is advisable to withhold this drug if electroconvulsive therapy (ECT, "shock" treatment) is to be used to treat your depression.

Precautions for Use
By Infants and Children: Safety and effectiveness for use by those under 12 years of age have not been established.
By Those over 60 Years of Age: During the first 2 weeks of treatment, observe for the development of confusion, agitation, forgetfulness, disorientation, delusions and hallucinations. Reduction of dosage or discontinuation may be necessary. Unsteadiness may predispose to falling and injury. This drug can increase the degree of impaired urination associated with prostate gland enlargement (prostatism).

▷ **Advisability of Use During Pregnancy**
Pregnancy Category: B (tentative). See Pregnancy Code inside back cover.
Animal studies: No birth defects reported in rats, rabbits, dogs or monkeys.
Human studies: Information from adequate studies of pregnant women is not available.
Use this drug only if clearly needed. If possible, avoid use during the first 3 months and the last month. Ask physician for guidance.

Advisability of Use if Breast-Feeding
Presence of this drug in breast milk: Yes, in small amounts.
Monitor nursing infant closely and discontinue drug or nursing if adverse effects develop.

Habit-Forming Potential: None.

Effects of Overdosage: Confusion, hallucinations, marked drowsiness, heart palpitations, dilated pupils, tremors, stupor, deep sleep, coma, convulsions.

Suggested Periodic Examinations While Taking This Drug (at physician's discretion)
Complete blood cell counts, liver function tests, serial blood pressure readings and electrocardiograms.

▷ **While Taking This Drug, Observe the Following**
Foods: No restrictions. This drug may increase the appetite and cause excessive weight gain.
Beverages: No restrictions. May be taken with milk.
▷ *Alcohol:* Avoid completely. This drug can markedly increase the intoxicating effects of alcohol and accentuate its depressant action on brain function.
Tobacco Smoking: May hasten the elimination of this drug. Higher doses may be necessary.
▷ *Other Drugs*
Doxepin may *increase* the effects of
• atropinelike drugs (see Drug Class, Section Four).
• dicumarol, and increase the risk of bleeding; dosage adjustments may be necessary.
• thyroid hormones.
Doxepin may *decrease* the effects of
• clonidine (Catapres).
• guanethidine (Ismelin).
Doxepin *taken concurrently* with
• monoamine oxidase (MAO) type A inhibitor drugs may cause high fever, delirium and convulsions (see Drug Class, Section Four).
▷ *Driving, Hazardous Activities:* This drug may impair mental alertness, judgment, physical coordination and reaction time. Avoid hazardous activities.
Aviation Note: The use of this drug *is a disqualification* for piloting. Consult a designated Aviation Medical Examiner.
Exposure to Sun: Use caution until sensitivity to sun has been determined. This drug may cause photosensitivity (see Glossary).
Exposure to Heat: This drug can inhibit sweating and impair the body's adaptation to hot environments, increasing the risk of heat stroke. Avoid saunas.
Exposure to Cold: The elderly should use caution and avoid conditions conducive to hypothermia (see Glossary).
Discontinuation: It is advisable to discontinue this drug gradually. Abrupt withdrawal after long-term use can cause headache, malaise and nausea.

DOXYCYCLINE
(dox ee SI kleen)

Introduced: 1967

Class: Antibiotic, tetracyclines

Prescription: USA: Yes
  Canada: Yes

Controlled Drug: USA: No
  Canada: No

Available as Generic: USA: Yes
  Canada: No

Brand Names: Doryx, Doxychel, Vibramycin, Vibra-Tabs, Vivox

BENEFITS versus RISKS

Possible Benefits	*Possible Risks*
EFFECTIVE TREATMENT OF INFECTIONS due to susceptible microorganisms	ALLERGIC REACTIONS, mild to severe Liver reaction with jaundice (rare) Fungal superinfections Drug-induced colitis Blood cell disorders

---

▷ **Principal Uses**

As a Single Drug Product: This member of the tetracycline drug class is used primarily to (1) treat a broad range of infections caused by susceptible bacteria and protozoa; (2) treat and prevent "traveler's diarrhea." It is often used to treat acute and chronic sinusitis and bronchitis.

How This Drug Works: This drug prevents the growth and multiplication of susceptible bacteria by interfering with their formation of essential proteins.

Available Dosage Forms and Strengths

Capsules — 50 mg, 100 mg
Capsules, coated pellets — 100 mg
Injection — 100 mg per vial, 200 mg per vial
Oral suspension — 25 mg per 5-ml teaspoonful
Syrup — 50 mg per 5-ml teaspoonful
Tablets — 50 mg, 100 mg

▷ **Usual Adult Dosage Range:** 100 mg/12 hours the first day; then 100 to 200 mg once daily or 50 to 100 mg/12 hours. Total daily dosage should not exceed 300 mg. **Note: Actual dosage and administration schedule must be determined by the physician for each patient individually.**

▷ **Dosing Instructions:** Preferably taken on an empty stomach, 1 hour before or 2 hours after eating. However, if stomach irritation occurs, it may be taken with food or milk. Take at same time each day, with a full glass of water. Take the full course prescribed. The tablet may be crushed and the capsule may be opened for administration.

Usual Duration of Use: The time required to control the infection and be free of fever and symptoms for 48 hours. This varies with the nature of the infection.

▷ **This Drug Should Not Be Taken If**
- you are allergic to any tetracycline drug (see Drug Class, Section Four).
- you are pregnant or breast-feeding.

▷ **Inform Your Physician Before Taking This Drug If**
- it is prescribed for a child under 8 years of age.
- you have a history of liver or kidney disease.
- you have systemic lupus erythematosus.
- you are taking any penicillin drug.
- you are taking any anticoagulant drug.
- you plan to have surgery under general anesthesia in the near future.

Possible Side-Effects (natural, expected and unavoidable drug actions)
Superinfections (see Glossary), often due to yeast organisms. These can occur in the mouth, intestinal tract, rectum and/or vagina, resulting in rectal and vaginal itching.

▷ **Possible Adverse Effects** (unusual, unexpected and infrequent reactions)
If any of the following develop, consult your physician promptly for guidance.
Mild Adverse Effects
Allergic Reactions: Skin rash, hives, itching of hands and feet, swelling of face or extremities.
Loss of appetite, nausea, vomiting, diarrhea.
Irritation of mouth or tongue, "black tongue," sore throat, abdominal cramping or pain.
Serious Adverse Effects
Allergic Reactions: Anaphylactic reaction (see Glossary), asthma, fever, swollen joints, abnormal bleeding or bruising, jaundice (see Glossary).
Permanent discoloration and/or malformation of teeth when taken by children under 8 years of age, including unborn child and infant.

▷ **Possible Effects on Sexual Function:**   None reported.

Natural Diseases or Disorders That May Be Activated by This Drug
Systemic lupus erythematosus.

CAUTION
1. Antacids and preparations containing aluminum, bismuth, iron, magnesium or zinc can prevent adequate absorption of this drug and reduce its effectiveness significantly.

2. Troublesome and persistent diarrhea can develop in sensitive individuals. If diarrhea persists for more than 24 hours, discontinue this drug and consult your physician.

Precautions for Use

By Infants and Children: If possible, tetracyclines should not be given to children under 8 years of age because of the risk of permanent discoloration and deformity of the teeth. Rarely, young infants may develop increased intracranial pressure within the first 4 days of receiving this drug. Tetracyclines may inhibit normal bone growth and development.

By Those over 60 Years of Age: Natural skin changes may predispose to severe and prolonged itching reactions in the genital and anal regions.

▷ Advisability of Use During Pregnancy

Pregnancy Category: D (tentative). See Pregnancy Code inside back cover.
Animal studies: Tetracycline causes limb defects in rats, rabbits and chickens.
Human studies: Information from studies of pregnant women indicates that drugs of this class can cause impaired development and discoloration of teeth and other developmental defects.
It is advisable to avoid this drug completely during entire pregnancy.

Advisability of Use if Breast-Feeding

Presence of this drug in breast milk: Yes.
Avoid drug or refrain from nursing.

Habit-Forming Potential: None.

Effects of Overdosage: Nausea, vomiting, diarrhea, acute liver damage (rare).

Possible Effects of Long-Term Use: Superinfections (see Glossary), prolongation of prothrombin time.

Suggested Periodic Examinations While Taking This Drug (at physician's discretion)

Complete blood cell counts, liver and kidney function tests.
During extended use, sputum and stool examinations may detect early superinfection due to yeast organisms.

▷ While Taking This Drug, Observe the Following

Foods: Avoid meats and iron-fortified cereals and supplements for 2 hours before and after taking this drug.
Beverages: No restrictions. May be taken with milk.
▷ *Alcohol:* No interactions expected. However, it is best avoided if you have active liver disease.
Tobacco Smoking: No interactions expected.

▷ *Other Drugs*
    Doxycycline may *increase* the effects of
- oral anticoagulants, and make it necessary to reduce their dosage.
- digoxin (Lanoxin), and cause digitalis toxicity.
- lithium (Eskalith, Lithane, etc.), and increase the risk of lithium toxicity.

Doxycycline may *decrease* the effects of
- oral contraceptives, and impair their effectiveness in preventing pregnancy.
- penicillins, and impair their effectiveness in treating infections.

The following drugs may *decrease* the effects of doxycycline
- antacids (aluminum and magnesium preparations, sodium bicarbonate, etc.) may reduce drug absorption.
- barbiturates (see Drug Class, Section Four).
- bismuth preparations (Pepto-Bismol, etc.).
- carbamazepine (Tegretol).
- cimetidine (Tagamet).
- phenytoin (Dilantin).
- iron and mineral preparations may reduce drug absorption.

▷ *Driving, Hazardous Activities:* Usually no restrictions. Be alert to the possible occurrence of nausea or diarrhea.
    Aviation Note: The use of this drug *may be a disqualification* for piloting. Consult a designated Aviation Medical Examiner.
    Exposure to Sun: Use caution until sensitivity has been determined. Tetracyclines can cause photosensitivity (see Glossary).

ENALAPRIL
(e NAL a pril)

Introduced: 1981   **Class:** Antihypertensive, ACE
                                                inhibitor

Prescription: USA: Yes   **Controlled Drug:** USA: No

Available as Generic: No

Brand Names: Vaseretic [CD], Vasotec

BENEFITS versus RISKS	
Possible Benefits	*Possible Risks*
EFFECTIVE CONTROL OF MILD TO SEVERE HIGH BLOOD PRESSURE	Headache (4.8%), dizziness (4.6%), fatigue (2.8%)
Possibly beneficial as adjunctive treatment in selected cases of congestive heart failure	Low blood pressure (2.3%)
	Bone marrow depression (rare)
	Allergic swelling of face, tongue or vocal cords (0.2%)

▷ **Principal Uses**

As a Single Drug Product

Used primarily to treat all degrees of high blood pressure. Mild to moderate high blood pressure usually responds to low doses; severe high blood pressure may require higher doses, with greater risk of serious adverse effects.

This drug is also used adjunctively to treat heart failure that is not responding adequately to digitalis and diuretics.

How This Drug Works: Not completely known. It is thought that by blocking certain enzyme systems that influence arterial function, this drug contributes to the relaxation of arterial walls throughout the body and thus lowers the resistance to blood flow that causes high blood pressure. This, in turn, reduces the workload of the heart and improves its performance.

Available Dosage Forms and Strengths

Tablets — 5 mg, 10 mg, 20 mg

▷ **Usual Adult Dosage Range:**   Initially 5 mg once daily for 2 weeks. Usual maintenance dose is 10 to 40 mg/day in a single dose or in 2 divided doses. Total daily dose should not exceed 40 mg if kidney function is impaired. **Note: Actual dosage and administration schedule must be determined by the physician for each patient individually.**

▷ **Dosing Instructions:**   Take on an empty stomach or with food, at same time each day. Tablet may be crushed for administration.

Usual Duration of Use: Continual use on a regular schedule for several weeks is usually necessary to determine this drug's effectiveness in controlling high blood pressure. The proper treatment of high blood pressure usually requires the long-term use of effective medications. Consult your physician on a regular basis.

▷ **This Drug Should Not Be Taken If**
- you have had an allergic reaction to it previously.
- you currently have a blood cell or bone marrow disorder.
- you have active liver disease.
- you have an abnormally high level of blood potassium.

▷ **Inform Your Physician Before Taking This Drug If**
- you have a history of kidney disease or impaired kidney function.
- you have scleroderma or systemic lupus erythematosus.
- you have any form of heart disease.
- you have diabetes.
- you are taking any of the following drugs: other antihypertensives, diuretics, nitrates or potassium supplements.
- you plan to have surgery under general anesthesia in the near future.

Possible Side-Effects (natural, expected and unavoidable drug actions)

Dizziness, light-headedness, fainting (excessive drop in blood pressure).

▷ **Possible Adverse Effects** (unusual, unexpected and infrequent reactions)
If any of the following develop, consult your physician promptly for guidance.
Mild Adverse Effects
Allergic Reactions: Skin rash, itching.
Headache, fatigue, drowsiness, nervousness, numbness and tingling, insomnia.
Rapid heart rate, palpitation.
Indigestion, stomach pain, nausea, vomiting, diarrhea.
Excessive sweating, muscle cramps.
Serious Adverse Effects
Allergic Reactions: Swelling (angioedema) of face, tongue and/or vocal cords: can be life threatening.
Bone marrow depression—fatigue, weakness, fever, sore throat, abnormal bleeding or bruising.

▷ **Possible Effects on Sexual Function:**   Rare report of impotence.

CAUTION
1. Consult your physician regarding the advisability of discontinuing other antihypertensive drugs (especially diuretics) for 1 week before starting this drug.
2. **Report promptly** any indications of infection (fever, sore throat), and any indications of water retention (weight gain, puffiness, swollen feet or ankles).
3. Do not use a salt substitute without your physician's knowledge and approval. (Many salt substitutes contain potassium.)
4. It is advisable to obtain blood cell counts and urine analyses **before** starting this drug.

Precautions for Use
By Infants and Children: Safety and effectiveness for use by those in this age group have not been established.
By Those over 60 Years of Age: Small doses are advisable until tolerance has been determined. Sudden and excessive lowering of blood pressure can predispose to stroke or heart attack in those with impaired brain circulation or coronary artery heart disease.

▷ **Advisability of Use During Pregnancy**
Pregnancy Category: C (tentative). See Pregnancy Code inside back cover.
Animal studies: No birth defects found in rat or rabbit studies.
Human studies: Information from adequate studies of pregnant women is not available.
Avoid during first 3 months if possible.

Advisability of Use if Breast-Feeding
Presence of this drug in breast milk: Not known.
Monitor nursing infant closely and discontinue drug or nursing if adverse effects develop.

Habit-Forming Potential: None.

Effects of Overdosage: Excessive drop in blood pressure—light-headedness, dizziness, fainting.

Possible Effects of Long-Term Use: Gradual increase in blood potassium level.

Suggested Periodic Examinations While Taking This Drug (at physician's discretion)
>Before starting drug: Complete blood cell counts; urine analysis with measurement of protein content; blood potassium level.
>During use of drug: Blood cell counts; measurements of blood potassium.

▷ **While Taking This Drug, Observe the Following**
Foods: Consult physician regarding salt intake.
*Nutritional Support: **Do not take*** potassium supplements unless directed by your physician.
Beverages: No restrictions. May be taken with milk.
▷   *Alcohol:* Use caution until combined effect has been determined. Alcohol may enhance the blood-pressure-lowering effect of this drug.
Tobacco Smoking: No interactions expected.
▷   *Other Drugs*
>Enalapril *taken concurrently* with
>- potassium preparations (K-Lyte, Slow-K, etc.) may cause increased blood levels of potassium with risk of serious heart rhythm disturbances.
>- potassium-sparing diuretics: amiloride (Moduretic), spironolactone (Aldactazide), triamterene (Dyazide) may cause increased blood levels of potassium with risk of serious heart rhythm disturbances.

▷   *Driving, Hazardous Activities:* Usually no restrictions. Be aware of possible drops in blood pressure with resultant dizziness or faintness.
Aviation Note: The use of this drug *may be a disqualification* for piloting. Consult a designated Aviation Medical Examiner.
Exposure to Sun: Caution advised. A similar drug of this class can cause photosensitivity.
Exposure to Heat: Caution advised. Avoid excessive perspiring with resultant loss of body water and drop in blood pressure.
Occurrence of Unrelated Illness: Report promptly any disorder that causes nausea, vomiting or diarrhea. Fluid and chemical imbalances must be corrected as soon as possible.

EPINEPHRINE
(ep i NEF rin)

Other Name: Adrenaline

Introduced: 1900

Class: Antiasthmatic, antiglau-coma, decongestant

Prescription: USA: Varies
Canada: No

Controlled Drug: USA: No
Canada: No

Available as Generic: USA: Yes
Canada: No

Brand Names: Adrenalin, Bronkaid Mist, ✦Bronkaid Mistometer, ✦Dysne-Inhal, Epifrin, E-Pilo Preparations [CD], Epitrate, Glaucon, Medi-haler-Epi Preparations, Primatene Mist, Sus-Phrine, Vaponefrin

---

BENEFITS versus RISKS

Possible Benefits	*Possible Risks*
EFFECTIVE RELIEF OF SEVERE ALLERGIC (ANAPHYLACTIC) REACTIONS	Significant increase in blood pressure (in sensitive individuals)
TEMPORARY RELIEF OF ACUTE BRONCHIAL ASTHMA	Idiosyncratic reaction: pulmonary edema (fluid formation in lungs)
Reduction of internal eye pressure (treatment of glaucoma)	Heart rhythm disorders (in sensitive individuals)
Relief of allergic congestion of the nose and sinuses	

▷ **Principal Uses**

As a Single Drug Product: This drug is used most commonly by inhalation to relieve acute attacks of bronchial asthma. It is used less frequently as a decongestant for symptomatic relief of allergic nasal congestion and as eye drops in the management of glaucoma.

How This Drug Works: By stimulating certain sympathetic nerve termi-nals, this drug acts to

- contract blood vessel walls and raise the blood pressure.
- inhibit the release of harmful amounts of histamine into the skin and internal organs.
- dilate those bronchial tubes that are in sustained constriction, thereby increasing the size of the airways and improving the ability to breathe.
- decrease the formation of fluid within the eye, increase its outflow from the eye and thereby reduce internal eye pressure.
- decrease the volume of blood in nasal tissue, thereby shrinking the tissue mass (decongestion) and expanding the nasal airway.

Available Dosage Forms and Strengths

Aerosol — 0.2 mg, 0.27 mg, 0.3 mg per spray
Eye drops — 0.1%, 0.25%, 0.5%, 1%, 2%

Injection — 0.01 mg, 0.1 mg, 1 mg, 5 mg per ml
Nose drops — 0.1%
Solution for nebulizer — 1%, 1.25%, 2.25%

▷ **Usual Adult Dosage Range:** Aerosols: 1 inhalation, repeated in 1 to 2 minutes if needed; wait 4 hours before next inhalation. Eye drops: 1 drop/12 hours. Dosage may vary with product; follow printed instructions and label directions. **Note: Actual dosage and administration schedule must be determined by the physician for each patient individually.**

▷ **Dosing Instructions:** Aerosols and inhalation solutions: After first inhalation, wait 1 to 2 minutes to determine if a second inhalation is necessary. If relief does not occur within 20 minutes of use, and difficult breathing persists, discontinue this drug and seek medical attention promptly. Avoid prolonged and excessive use. Eye drops: During instillation of drops and for 2 minutes following, press finger against the tear sac (inner corner of eye) to prevent rapid absorption of drug into body circulation.

   Usual Duration of Use: According to individual needs. Long-term use requires supervision and periodic evaluation by your physician.

▷ **This Drug Should Not Be Taken If**
   • you have had an allergic reaction to any dosage form of it previously.
   • you have narrow-angle glaucoma.
   • you have experienced a recent stroke or heart attack.

▷ **Inform Your Physician Before Taking This Drug If**
   • you have any degree of high blood pressure.
   • you have any form of heart disease, especially coronary heart disease (with or without angina), or a heart rhythm disorder.
   • you have diabetes or overactive thyroid function (hyperthyroidism).
   • you have a history of stroke.
   • you are taking any of the following drugs: monoamine oxidase (MAO) type A inhibitors, phenothiazines (see Drug Classes, Section Four), digitalis preparations or quinidine.

   Possible Side-Effects (natural, expected and unavoidable drug actions)
      In sensitive individuals—restlessness, anxiety, headache, tremor, palpitation, coldness of hands and feet, dryness of mouth and throat (with use of aerosol).

▷ **Possible Adverse Effects** (unusual, unexpected and infrequent reactions)
      If any of the following develop, consult your physician promptly for guidance.
   Mild Adverse Effects
      Allergic Reactions: Skin rash; eye drops may cause redness, swelling and itching of the eyelids.
      Weakness, dizziness, pallor.

Serious Adverse Effects
   Idiosyncratic Reaction: Sudden development of excessive fluid in the lungs (pulmonary edema).
   In predisposed individuals—excessive rise in blood pressure with risk of stroke (cerebral hemorrhage).

▷ **Possible Effects on Sexual Function:**   None reported.

CAUTION
   1. The frequently repeated use of this drug at short intervals can produce a condition of unresponsiveness and result in medication failure. If this develops, avoid use completely for 12 hours, at which time a normal response should return.
   2. Excessive use of aerosol preparations in the treatment of asthma has been associated with sudden death.
   3. This drug can cause significant irritability of the nerve pathways (conduction system) and muscles of the heart, predisposing to serious heart rhythm disorders. If you have any form of heart disorder, consult your physician.
   4. This drug can increase the blood sugar level. If you have diabetes, test for urine sugar frequently to detect significant changes.
   5. If you become unresponsive to this drug and you intend to substitute isoproterenol (Isuprel), allow an interval of 4 hours between using these two drugs.
   6. Promptly discard all preparations of this drug at the first appearance of discoloration (pink to red to brown) or cloudiness (precipitation). Such changes indicate drug deterioration.

Precautions for Use
   By Infants and Children: Use cautiously in small doses until tolerance is determined. Observe for any indications of weakness, light-headedness or inclination to faint.
   By Those over 60 Years of Age: Use cautiously in small doses until tolerance is determined. Observe for excessive stimulation: nervousness, headache, tremor, rapid heart rate. If you have hardening of the arteries (arteriosclerosis), heart disease, high blood pressure, Parkinson's disease or prostatism (see Glossary), this drug may aggravate your disorder. Ask your physician for guidance.

▷ **Advisability of Use During Pregnancy**
   Pregnancy Category: C (tentative). See Pregnancy Code inside back cover.
   Animal studies: Birth defects reported in rats.
   Human studies: Information from adequate studies of pregnant women is not available.
   This drug can cause significant reduction of oxygen supply to the fetus. Use it only if clearly needed and in small, infrequent doses. Avoid during the first 3 months and during labor and delivery.

Advisability of Use if Breast-Feeding
   Presence of this drug in breast milk: Yes.
   Avoid drug or refrain from nursing.

Habit-Forming Potential: Tolerance to this drug can develop with frequent use (see Glossary), but dependence does not occur.

Effects of Overdosage: Nervousness, throbbing headache, dizziness, tremor, palpitation, disturbance of heart rhythm, difficult breathing, abdominal pain, vomiting of blood.

Possible Effects of Long-Term Use: "Epinephrine-fastness": loss of ability to respond to this drug's bronchodilator effect. With long-term treatment of glaucoma: pigment deposits on eyeball and eyelids, possible damage to retina, impaired vision, blockage of tear ducts.

Suggested Periodic Examinations While Taking This Drug (at physician's discretion)
Blood pressure measurements; blood or urine sugar measurements in presence of diabetes; vision testing and measurement of internal eye pressure in presence of glaucoma.

▷ **While Taking This Drug, Observe the Following**
Foods: No restrictions, except those that have been shown to cause you to have asthma.
Beverages: No restrictions.
▷ *Alcohol:* Alcoholic beverages can increase the urinary excretion of this drug.
Tobacco Smoking: No interactions expected. Follow physician's advice regarding smoking as it affects the condition under treatment.
▷ *Other Drugs*
Epinephrine **taken concurrently** with
- certain beta blocker drugs (nadolol, propranolol) may cause increased blood pressure and decreased heart rate.
- chlorpromazine (Thorazine) may cause decreased blood pressure and increased heart rate.
- furazolidone (Furoxone) may cause increased blood pressure and high fever.
- guanethidine (Esimil, Ismelin) may cause increased blood pressure.
- tricyclic antidepressants (amitriptyline, etc.) may cause increased blood pressure and heart rhythm disturbances.
▷ *Driving, Hazardous Activities:* This drug may cause dizziness or excessive nervousness. Restrict activities as necessary.
Aviation Note: The use of this drug **may be a disqualification** for piloting. Consult a designated Aviation Medical Examiner.
Exposure to Sun: No restrictions.
Heavy Exercise or Exertion: No interactions expected. However, exercise can induce asthma in sensitive individuals.
Occurrence of Unrelated Illness: Use caution in presence of severe burns. This drug can increase drainage from burned tissue and cause significant loss of tissue fluids and blood proteins.
Discontinuation: If this drug fails to provide relief after an adequate trial, discontinue it and consult your physician. It is dangerous to increase the dosage or frequency of use.

Special Storage Instructions: Protect drug from exposure to air, light and heat. Keep in a cool place, preferably in the refrigerator.

ERGOLOID MESYLATES
(ER goh loyd MESS i lates)

Other Name: Dihydrogenated ergot alkaloids

Introduced: 1949

Class: Ergot preparations

Prescription: USA: Yes
Canada: Yes

Controlled Drug: USA: No
Canada: No

Available as Generic: USA: Yes
Canada: No

Brand Names: Deapril-ST, Hydergine, Hydergine LC

BENEFITS versus RISKS	
Possible Benefits	*Possible Risks*
Limited relief of symptoms associated with deteriorating brain function (in some individuals)	Low blood pressure, fainting Slow heart rate Worsening of symptoms (instead of relief)

▷ **Principal Uses**

As a Single Drug Product: The use of this drug is limited to the treatment of the aging individual with symptoms indicative of deteriorating brain function. Its benefit is unpredictable, and its use must be monitored carefully and adjusted appropriately for each individual.

How This Drug Works: Not completely established. Present theory is that by stimulating brain cell metabolism, this drug increases the brain's ability to utilize oxygen and nutrients. The resulting improvement in brain function is thought to contribute to the benefit seen in responsive individuals.

Available Dosage Forms and Strengths
Capsules, liquid — 1 mg
Liquid — 1 mg per ml
Tablets — 1 mg
Tablets, sublingual — 0.5 mg, 1 mg

▷ **Usual Adult Dosage Range:** 1 to 2 mg, 3 times/day. **Note: Actual dosage and administration schedule must be determined by the physician for each patient individually.**

▷ **Dosing Instructions:**   May be taken on an empty stomach or with food to reduce stomach irritation. The regular tablet may be crushed for administration. The sublingual tablet should be dissolved under the tongue and not swallowed. The liquid capsule should be taken whole (unopened).

Usual Duration of Use: Continual use on a regular schedule for 3 to 4 weeks is usually necessary to determine this drug's effectiveness in relieving the symptoms of mental deterioration. Long-term use requires supervision and periodic evaluation by your physician. Consult your physician on a regular basis.

▷ **This Drug Should Not Be Taken If**
- you have had an allergic reaction to any dosage form of it previously.
- your pulse rate is below 60 beats/minute or your systolic blood pressure is consistently below 100.
- you have an active psychosis.

▷ **Inform Your Physician Before Taking This Drug If**
- you have a history of low blood pressure.
- you are taking any of the following: antihypertensive drugs, a beta blocker drug or any form of digitalis.

Possible Side-Effects (natural, expected and unavoidable drug actions)
Orthostatic hypotension (see Glossary).

▷ **Possible Adverse Effects** (unusual, unexpected and infrequent reactions)
If any of the following develop, consult your physician promptly for guidance.
Mild Adverse Effects
Allergic Reactions: Skin rash, drug fever (see Glossary).
Headache, dizziness, flushing, blurred vision.
Nasal stuffiness, reduced appetite, nausea, vomiting, stomach cramping.
Serious Adverse Effects
Marked drop in blood pressure, falling, fainting.
Marked slowing of the heart rate (40 to 50 beats/minute).
Reduced activity, sluggishness, drowsiness, emotional withdrawal, apathy.

▷ **Possible Effects on Sexual Function:**   None reported.

Natural Diseases or Disorders That May Be Activated by This Drug
Ergot alkaloids can precipitate attacks of acute intermittent porphyria in susceptible individuals.

CAUTION
While numerous studies have demonstrated that this drug can be beneficial in relieving many complaints of the elderly related to memory, intellectual performance and social adjustment, others have not con-

firmed this. It is important to remember that the causes of such symptoms are poorly understood, that they can occur whether or not drugs are being taken and that behavioral changes in the elderly are often frequent and unpredictable. It is therefore advisable to monitor the response to this drug very closely and to notify the physician if any significant adverse personality changes occur. In some instances, the development of nervousness, hostility, confusion and depression may be related to the use of this drug.

Precautions for Use

By Those over 60 Years of Age: It is not possible to predict in advance the nature of your response to this drug. It may relieve your symptoms, have no significant effect or make your symptoms worse. Dosage must be carefully individualized.

Habit-Forming Potential: None.

Effects of Overdosage: Headache, flushing, nasal stuffiness, weakness, nausea, vomiting, collapse, coma.

Possible Effects of Long-Term Use: None reported.

Suggested Periodic Examinations While Taking This Drug (at physician's discretion)

Pulse counts and blood pressure measurements on a regular basis.

▷ **While Taking This Drug, Observe the Following**

Foods: No restrictions.

Beverages: No restrictions.

▷ *Alcohol:* Use with caution until the combined effects have been determined. Sensitive individuals may experience an excessive drop in blood pressure.

Tobacco Smoking: No interactions expected.

▷ *Other Drugs*

Ergoloid mesylates may ***increase*** the effects of

- antihypertensive drugs, and cause excessive lowering of blood pressure.

Ergoloid mesylates ***taken concurrently*** with

- beta blocker drugs (see Drug Class, Section Four) may cause excessive slowing of heart rate and/or excessive lowering of blood pressure.
- digitalis preparations (Lanoxin, etc.) may cause excessive slowing of heart rate.

▷ *Driving, Hazardous Activities:* This drug may cause dizziness or blurred vision. Restrict activities as necessary.

Aviation Note: Brain function disorder ***is a disqualification*** for piloting. Consult a designated Aviation Medical Examiner.

Exposure to Sun: No restrictions.

Exposure to Cold: Use caution. Avoid exposure that could lower body temperature, impair metabolism and induce hypothermia (see Glossary).

ERGOTAMINE
(er GOT a meen)

Introduced: 1926

Class: Antimigraine, ergot preparations

Prescription: USA: Yes
  Canada: Yes

Controlled Drug: USA: No
  Canada: No

Available as Generic: No

Brand Names: ✦Bellergal [CD], Bellergal-S [CD], ✦Bellergal Spacetabs [CD], Cafergot [CD], Cafergot P-B [CD], Ercaf [CD], ✦Ergodryl [CD], Ergomar, Ergostat, ✦Gynergen, Medihaler Ergotamine, Wigraine [CD], Wigrettes

---

BENEFITS versus RISKS	
Possible Benefits	**Possible Risks**
PREVENTION AND RELIEF OF VASCULAR HEADACHES: MIGRAINE, MIGRAINELIKE AND HISTAMINE HEADACHES	GANGRENE OF THE FINGERS, TOES OR INTESTINE AGGRAVATION OF CORONARY ARTERY DISEASE (ANGINA) ABORTION

▷ **Principal Uses**

As a Single Drug Product: This drug is used primarily in the treatment of vascular headaches, especially migraine and "cluster" headaches. It should not be used on a continual basis to prevent migraine attacks, but it is often effective in terminating the headache if taken within the first hour following the onset of pain. It may be used on a short-term basis in an attempt to prevent or abort "cluster" headaches during the period of their occurrence. The inhalation form provides rapid onset of action.

As a Combination Drug Product [CD]: This drug is combined with caffeine to take advantage of caffeine's ability to enhance its absorption. This permits a smaller dose of ergotamine to be effective and reduces the risk of adverse effects with repeated use. This drug is also combined with belladonna (atropine) and one of the barbiturates to provide preparations that are useful in relieving the symptoms of premenstrual tension and the menopausal syndrome: nervousness, nausea, hot flushes and sweating.

How This Drug Works: Not completely established. It is thought that by constricting the walls of blood vessels in the head, this drug prevents or relieves the excessive expansion (dilation) that is responsible for the pain of migrainelike headaches.

Available Dosage Forms and Strengths
>   Aerosol — 9 mg per ml (0.36 mg/inhalation)
>   Suppositories — 2 mg (in combination with caffeine)
> Tablets, sublingual — 2 mg

▷ **Usual Adult Dosage Range:**   Inhalation: 1 spray (0.36 mg) at the onset of headache; repeat 1 spray every 5 to 10 minutes as needed for relief, up to a maximum of 6 sprays/24 hours. Do not exceed 15 sprays/week. Sublingual tablets: Dissolve 1 mg under tongue at the onset of headache; repeat 1 mg every 30 to 60 minutes as needed, up to a maximum of 5 mg/attack. Do not exceed 5 mg/24 hours or 10 mg/week. Try to determine the optimal dose required (up to 5 mg) that will abort the headache when taken as a single dose at the onset of pain. **Note: Actual dosage and administration schedule must be determined by the physician for each patient individually.**

▷ **Dosing Instructions:**   Follow written instructions carefully. Do not exceed prescribed doses. The regular tablets (combination drug) may be crushed for administration; the sustained-release tablets should be taken whole (not crushed). Sublingual tablets should be dissolved under the tongue, not swallowed.

Usual Duration of Use: Continual use on a regular schedule for several episodes of headache is usually necessary to determine this drug's effectiveness in aborting or relieving the pain of vascular headache. Do not exceed recommended dosage schedules. If headaches are not controlled after several trials of maximal doses, consult your physician for alternative treatment.

▷ **This Drug Should Not Be Taken If**
- you have had an allergic reaction to any dosage form of it previously.
- you are pregnant.
- you have a severe infection.
- you have any of the following conditions:
  angina pectoris (coronary artery disease)
  Buerger's disease
  hardening of the arteries (arteriosclerosis)
  high blood pressure (severe hypertension)
  kidney disease or impaired kidney function
  liver disease or impaired liver function
  Raynaud's phenomenon
  thrombophlebitis
  severe itching

▷ **Inform Your Physician Before Taking This Drug If**
- you are allergic or overly sensitive to *any* ergot preparation.

Possible Side-Effects (natural, expected and unavoidable drug actions)
Usually infrequent and mild with recommended doses.
Susceptible individuals may notice a sensation of cold hands and feet, with mild numbness and tingling.

▷ **Possible Adverse Effects** (unusual, unexpected and infrequent reactions)
If any of the following develop, consult your physician promptly for guidance.
Mild Adverse Effects
Allergic Reactions: Localized swellings (angioedema), itching.
Headache, drowsiness, dizziness, confusion.
Chest pain, numbness and tingling of fingers and toes, muscle pains in arms or legs.
Nausea, vomiting, diarrhea.
Serious Adverse Effects
Gangrene of the extremities—coldness; numbness; pain; dark discoloration; eventual loss of fingers, toes or feet.
Gangrene of the intestine—severe abdominal pain and swelling; emergency surgery required.

▷ **Possible Effects on Sexual Function:** None reported.

Natural Diseases or Disorders That May Be Activated by This Drug
Angina pectoris (coronary artery insufficiency), Buerger's disease, Raynaud's syndrome.

CAUTION
1. The excessive use of this drug can actually provoke migraine headache and increase the frequency of its occurrence.
2. Do not exceed a total dose of 5 mg/24 hours or 10 mg/week.
3. Individual sensitivity to the effects of this drug vary greatly. Some may experience early toxic effects even while taking recommended doses. Report promptly any indications of impaired circulation: numbness in fingers or toes, muscle cramping, chest pain.

Precautions for Use
By Infants and Children: Safety and effectiveness for use by those under 12 years of age have not been established.
By Those over 60 Years of Age: Natural changes in blood vessels and circulation may make you more susceptible to the serious adverse effects of this drug. See the preceding list of disorders that are contraindications for the use of this drug.

▷ **Advisability of Use During Pregnancy**
Pregnancy Category: X. See Pregnancy Code inside back cover.
Animal studies: Fetal deaths reported due to this drug.
Human studies: Information from studies of pregnant women indicates that this drug can cause abortion.
This drug should be avoided during the entire pregnancy.

Advisability of Use if Breast-Feeding
Presence of this drug in breast milk: Yes.
Avoid drug or refrain from nursing.

Habit-Forming Potential: None.

Effects of Overdosage: Manifestations of "ergotism": coldness of skin, severe muscle pains, tingling and burning pain in hands and feet, loss of blood supply to extremities resulting in tissue death (gangrene) in fingers and toes. Acute ergot poisoning: nausea, vomiting, diarrhea, cold skin, numbness extremities, confusion, seizures, coma.

Possible Effects of Long-Term Use: A form of functional dependence (see Glossary) may develop, resulting in withdrawal headaches when the drug is discontinued.

Suggested Periodic Examinations While Taking This Drug (at physician's discretion)
Evaluation of circulation (blood flow) to the extremities.

▷ **While Taking This Drug, Observe the Following**
Foods: No interactions expected. Avoid all foods to which you are allergic; some migraine headaches are due to food allergies.
Beverages: No restrictions.
▷ *Alcohol:* Best avoided; alcohol can intensify vascular headache.
Tobacco Smoking: Best avoided; nicotine can further reduce the restricted blood flow produced by this drug.
Marijuana Smoking: Best avoided; additive effects can increase the coldness of hands and feet.
▷ *Other Drugs*
Ergotamine may ***decrease*** the effects of
• nitroglycerin, and reduce its effectiveness in preventing or relieving angina pain.
The following drugs may ***increase*** the effects of ergotamine
• erythromycin (E-Mycin, Eryc, etc.).
• troleandomycin (TAO).
▷ *Driving, Hazardous Activities:* This drug may cause drowsiness or dizziness. Restrict activities as necessary.
Aviation Note: Vascular headache **is a disqualification** for piloting. Consult a designated Aviation Medical Examiner.
Exposure to Sun: No restrictions.
Exposure to Cold: Avoid as much as possible. Cold environments and handling cold objects will further reduce the restricted blood flow to the extremities.
Discontinuation: Following long-term use, it may be necessary to withdraw this drug gradually to prevent withdrawal headache. Ask physician for guidance.

ERYTHROMYCIN
(er ith roh MY sin)

Introduced: 1952	**Class:** Antibiotic, erythromycins
Prescription: USA: Yes	**Controlled Drug:** USA: No
Canada: Yes	Canada: No

Available as Generic: Yes

Brand Names: ✦Apo-Erythro Base, ✦Apo-Erythro-ES, ✦Apo-Erythro-S, E.E.S., E-Mycin, E-Mycin E, E-Mycin 333, Eryc, Eryderm, Erypar, EryPed, Ery-Tab, Erythrocin, ✦Erythromid, Ilosone, Ilotycin, ✦Novorythro, PCE Dispertab, Pediamycin, Pediazole [CD], Robimycin, Wyamycin E, Wyamycin S

BENEFITS versus RISKS

Possible Benefits	*Possible Risks*
EFFECTIVE TREATMENT OF INFECTIONS DUE TO SUSCEPTIBLE MICROORGANISMS	Allergic reactions, mild and infrequent
	Liver reaction (most common with erythromycin estolate)
	Drug-induced colitis (rare)
	Superinfections (rare)

▷ **Principal Uses**

As a Single Drug Product: This well-tolerated and versatile antibiotic is used to treat a broad variety of common infections. The more important among these are (1) skin and skin structure infections; (2) upper and lower respiratory tract infections, including "strep" throat, diphtheria and several types of pneumonia; (3) gonorrhea and syphilis; and (4) amebic dysentery. It is also used for the long-term prevention of recurrences of rheumatic fever. Effective use requires the precise identification of the causative organism and determination of its sensitivity to erythromycin.

How This Drug Works: This drug prevents the growth and multiplication of susceptible organisms by interfering with their formation of essential proteins.

Available Dosage Forms and Strengths

Capsules — 125 mg, 250 mg
Capsules, enteric-coated — 125 mg, 250 mg
Drops — 100 mg per ml
Eye ointment — 5 mg per gram
Oral suspension — 125 mg, 250 mg per 5-ml teaspoonful
Skin ointment — 2%
Tablets — 500 mg
Tablets, chewable — 125 mg, 250 mg
Tablets, enteric-coated — 250 mg, 333 mg, 500 mg
Tablets, film-coated — 250 mg, 500 mg
Topical solution — 1.5%, 2%

▷ **Usual Adult Dosage Range:** 250 to 1000 mg/6 hours, according to nature and severity of infection. Total daily dosage should not exceed 8 grams. For endocarditis prophylaxis: 1 gram 2 hours before procedure and 500 mg 6 hours later. **Note: Actual dosage and administration schedule must be determined by the physician for each patient individually.**

▷ **Dosing Instructions:** Nonenteric-coated preparations should be taken 1 hour before or 2 hours after eating. Enteric-coated preparations may be taken without regard to food. Regular uncoated capsules may be opened and tablets may be crushed for administration; coated and prolonged-action preparations should be swallowed whole. Ask pharmacist for guidance.

Usual Duration of Use: Continual use on a regular schedule for 3 to 5 days is usually necessary to determine this drug's effectiveness in controlling responsive infections. For streptococcal infections: not less than 10 consecutive days (without interruption) to reduce the possibility of developing rheumatic fever or glomerulonephritis. The duration of use should not exceed the time required to eliminate the infection.

▷ **This Drug Should Not Be Taken If**
  • you have had an allergic reaction to any form of erythromycin previously.
  • you have active liver disease.

▷ **Inform Your Physician Before Taking This Drug If**
  • you have a history of a previous "reaction" to erythromycin.
  • you are allergic by nature: hay fever, asthma, hives, eczema.
  • you have taken the estolate form of erythromycin previously.

Possible Side-Effects (natural, expected and unavoidable drug actions)
  Superinfections (see Glossary).

▷ **Possible Adverse Effects** (unusual, unexpected and infrequent reactions)
  If any of the following develop, consult your physician promptly for guidance.
  Mild Adverse Effects
  Allergic Reactions: Skin rash, hives, itching.
  Nausea, vomiting, diarrhea, abdominal cramping.
  Serious Adverse Effects
  Allergic Reaction: Rare anaphylactic reaction (see Glossary).
  Idiosyncratic Reactions: Liver reaction—nausea, vomiting, fever, jaundice (usually but not exclusively associated with erythromycin estolate).
  Drug-induced colitis, transient loss of hearing.

▷ **Possible Effects on Sexual Function:** None reported.

▷ **Adverse Effects That May Mimic Natural Diseases or Disorders**
  Liver toxicity may resemble acute gallbladder disease or viral hepatitis.

CAUTION
1. Take the full dosage prescribed to prevent the possible emergence of resistant bacterial strains.
2. If you have a history of liver disease or impaired liver function, avoid any form of erythromycin estolate.
3. If diarrhea develops and continues for more than 24 hours, consult your physician promptly.

Precautions for Use
By Infants and Children: Observe allergic children closely for indications of developing allergy to this drug. Observe also for evidence of gastrointestinal irritation.

By Those over 60 Years of Age: Observe for indications of itching reactions in the genital and anal regions, often due to yeast superinfections. Observe also for evidence of hearing loss. Report such developments promptly.

▷ **Advisability of Use During Pregnancy**
Pregnancy Category: B (tentative). See Pregnancy Code inside back cover.
  Animal studies: Studies of rats are inconclusive.
  Human studies: No increase in birth defects reported in 230 exposures. Information from adequate studies of pregnant women is not available.
  Generally thought to be safe during entire pregnancy, *except for erythromycin estolate*; this form of erythromycin can cause toxic liver reactions during pregnancy and should be avoided.

Advisability of Use if Breast-Feeding
Presence of this drug in breast milk: Yes.
Monitor nursing infant closely and discontinue drug or nursing if adverse effects develop.

Habit-Forming Potential: None.

Effects of Overdosage: Possible nausea, vomiting, diarrhea and abdominal discomfort.

Possible Effects of Long-Term Use: Superinfections (see Glossary).

Suggested Periodic Examinations While Taking This Drug (at physician's discretion)
Liver function tests if the estolate form is used.

▷ **While Taking This Drug, Observe the Following**
Foods: No restrictions.
Beverages: Avoid fruit juices and carbonated beverages for 1 hour after taking any nonenteric-coated preparation. May be taken with milk.
▷ *Alcohol:* Avoid if you have impaired liver function or are taking the estolate form of this drug.
Tobacco Smoking: No interactions expected.

▷ *Other Drugs*

Erythromycin may *increase* the effects of

- carbamazepine (Tegretol), and cause toxicity.
- digoxin (Lanoxin), and cause toxicity.
- ergotamine (Cafergot, Ergostat, etc.), and cause impaired circulation to extremities.
- methylprednisolone (Medrol), and cause excess steroid effects.
- theophylline (aminophylline, Theo-Dur, etc.), and cause toxicity.
- warfarin (Coumadin), and increase the risk of bleeding.

Erythromycin may *decrease* the effects of

- clindamycin.
- lincomycin.
- penicillins.

▷ *Driving, Hazardous Activities:* This drug may cause nausea and/or diarrhea. Restrict activities as necessary.

Aviation Note: The use of this drug *may be a disqualification* for piloting. Consult a designated Aviation Medical Examiner.

Exposure to Sun: No restrictions.

Special Storage Instructions: Keep liquid forms refrigerated.

Observe the Following Expiration Times: Freshly mixed oral suspension—14 days. Premixed oral suspension—18 months. Ask pharmacist for guidance.

ESTROGENS
(ES troh jenz)

Other Names: Chlorotrianisene, conjugated estrogens, esterified estrogens, estradiol, estriol, estrone, estropipate, quinestrol

Introduced: 1933

Class: Female sex hormones

Prescription: USA: Yes
    Canada: Yes

Controlled Drug: USA: No
    Canada: No

Available as Generic: USA: Yes
    Canada: No

Brand Names: ✚C.E.S., ✚Climestrone, ✚Delestrogen, DV, Estinyl, Estrace, Estraderm, Estraguard, Estratab, Estrovis, Feminone, ✚Femogen, ✚Femogex, Menest, Menrium [CD], Milprem [CD], ✚Oestrilin, Ogen, PMB [CD], Premarin, TACE

BENEFITS versus RISKS

Possible Benefits

EFFECTIVE RELIEF OF
MENOPAUSAL HOT FLUSHES
AND NIGHT SWEATS
PREVENTION OR RELIEF OF
ATROPHIC VAGINITIS,
ATROPHY OF THE VULVA
AND URETHRA
PREVENTION OF
OSTEOPOROSIS
Prevention of thinning of the skin
Mental tonic effect

Possible Risks

INCREASED RISK OF CANCER
OF THE UTERUS with 3+
years of continual use
Increased frequency of gallstones
Accelerated growth of preexisting
fibroid tumors of the uterus
Fluid retention
Postmenopausal bleeding
Deep vein thrombophlebitis and
thromboembolism (less likely
with conjugated estrogens,
more likely with synthetic
unconjugated hormones)
Increased blood pressure (rare)
Decreased sugar tolerance (rare)

▷ **Principal Uses**

As a Single Drug Product: This widely used hormone is very effective when administered in proper dosage and carefully supervised. Its primary use is supplemental ("replacement" therapy) when used to treat the following conditions: (1) ovarian failure or removal in the young woman; (2) the menopausal syndrome; (3) postmenopausal atrophy of genital tissues; and (4) postmenopausal osteoporosis. It is also used in selected cases of breast cancer and prostate cancer.

As a Combination Drug Product [CD]: Estrogen is available in combination with chlordiazepoxide (Librium) and with meprobamate (Equanil, Miltown). These mild tranquilizers are added to provide a calming effect that makes the combination more effective in treating selected cases of the menopausal syndrome. See the Drug Profile of the Oral Contraceptives for a discussion of the combination of estrogens and progestins.

How This Drug Works: When used to correct hormonal deficiency states, estrogens restore normal cellular activity by increasing the synthesis of chromatin, RNA and cellular proteins. The frequency and intensity of menopausal symptoms are significantly reduced when normal tissue levels of estrogen are restored.

Available Dosage Forms and Strengths

Capsules — 12 mg, 25 mg, 72 mg (TACE)
Tablets — 0.02 mg, 0.05 mg, 0.1 mg, 0.3 mg, 0.5 mg, 0.625 mg, 0.9 mg, 1.25 mg, 2.5 mg, 5 mg
Transdermal patch — 0.05 mg, 0.1 mg
Vaginal cream — 0.1 mg, 0.625 mg, 1.5 mg per gram

▷ **Usual Adult Dosage Range:**   For conjugated and esterified estrogens: 0.3 to 1.25 mg daily for 21 days. Omit for 7 days. Repeat cyclically as needed. For other forms of estrogen: consult your physician. **Note: Actual dosage and administration schedule must be determined by the physician for each patient individually.**

▷ **Dosing Instructions:**   May be taken without regard to food. The tablets may be crushed for administration. The capsules should be taken whole.

Usual Duration of Use: Continual use on a regular schedule for 10 to 20 days is usually necessary to determine this drug's effectiveness in relieving menopausal symptoms. Long-term use requires supervision and periodic evaluation by your physician every 6 months. Consult your physician on a regular basis.

▷ **This Drug Should Not Be Taken If**
- you have had a significant allergic reaction to any dosage form of it previously.
- you have a history of thrombophlebitis, embolism, heart attack or stroke.
- you have seriously impaired liver function.
- you have abnormal and unexplained vaginal bleeding.
- you have sickle cell disease.
- you are pregnant.

▷ **Inform Your Physician Before Taking This Drug If**
- you have had an unfavorable reaction to estrogen therapy previously.
- you have a history of cancer of the breast or reproductive organs.
- you have any of the following conditions: fibrocystic breast changes, fibroid tumors of the uterus, endometriosis, migrainelike headaches, epilepsy, asthma, heart disease, high blood pressure, gallbladder disease, diabetes or porphyria.
- you smoke tobacco on a regular basis.
- you plan to have surgery in the near future.

Possible Side-Effects (natural, expected and unavoidable drug actions)
Fluid retention, weight gain, "breakthrough" bleeding (spotting in middle of menstrual cycle), altered menstrual pattern, resumption of menstrual flow (bleeding from the uterus) after a period of natural cessation (postmenopausal bleeding), increased susceptibility to yeast infection of the genital tissues.

▷ **Possible Adverse Effects** (unusual, unexpected and infrequent reactions)
If any of the following develop, consult your physician promptly for guidance.
Mild Adverse Effects
Allergic Reactions: Skin rash, hives, itching.
Headache, nervous tension, irritability, accentuation of migraine headaches.

Nausea, vomiting, bloating, diarrhea.

Tannish pigmentation of the face.

Serious Adverse Effects

Idiosyncratic Reaction: Cutaneous porphyria—fragility and scarring of the skin.

Emotional depression, rise in blood pressure (in susceptible individuals).

Gallbladder disease, benign liver tumors, jaundice, rise in blood sugar.

Erosion of uterine cervix, enlargement of uterine fibroid tumors.

Thrombophlebitis (inflammation of a vein with formation of blood clot)—pain or tenderness in thigh or leg, with or without swelling of foot or leg.

Pulmonary embolism (movement of blood clot to lung)—sudden shortness of breath, pain in chest, coughing, bloody sputum.

Stroke (blood clot in brain)—headaches, blackout, sudden weakness or paralysis of any part of the body, severe dizziness, altered vision, slurred speech, inability to speak.

Retinal thrombosis (blood clot in eye vessels)—sudden impairment or loss of vision.

Heart attack (blood clot in coronary artery)—sudden pain in chest, neck, jaw or arm; weakness; sweating; nausea.

▷ **Possible Effects on Sexual Function**

Swelling and tenderness of breasts, milk production.

Increased vaginal secretions.

Possible Delayed Adverse Effects: Estrogens taken during pregnancy can predispose the female child to the later development of cancer of the vagina or cervix following puberty.

▷ **Adverse Effects That May Mimic Natural Diseases or Disorders**

Liver reactions may suggest viral hepatitis.

Natural Diseases or Disorders That May Be Activated by This Drug

Latent hypertension, diabetes mellitus, acute intermittent porphyria.

CAUTION

1. To avoid prolonged (uninterrupted) stimulation of breast and uterine tissues, estrogen should be taken in cycles of 3 weeks on and 1 week off of medication.
2. The estrogen in estrogen vaginal creams is absorbed systemically by the woman. It may also be absorbed through the penis during sexual intercourse and can cause enlargement and tenderness of male breast tissue.

Precautions for Use

By Those over 60 Years of Age: This drug has very limited usefulness after 60. Its use should be restricted to those women who are at increased risk for developing osteoporosis. In this age group, it is advisable to attempt relief of hot flushes with nonestrogenic medications. During use, report promptly any indications of impaired circulation: speech disturbances, altered vision, sudden hearing loss, vertigo, sudden weakness or paralysis, angina, leg pains.

▷ **Advisability of Use During Pregnancy**
Pregnancy Category: X. See Pregnancy Code inside back cover.
Animal studies: Genital defects reported in mice and guinea pigs; cleft palate reported in rodents.
Human studies: Information from studies of pregnant women indicates that estrogens can masculinize the female fetus. In addition, limb defects and heart malformations have been reported.
It is now known that estrogens taken during pregnancy can predispose the female child to the development of cancer of the vagina or cervix following puberty. *Avoid estrogens completely during entire pregnancy.*

Advisability of Use if Breast-Feeding
Presence of this drug in breast milk: Yes, in minute amounts.
Estrogens in large doses can suppress milk formation.
Breast-feeding is considered to be safe during the use of estrogens.

Habit-Forming Potential: None.

Effects of Overdosage: Headache, drowsiness, nausea, vomiting, fluid retention, abnormal vaginal bleeding, breast enlargement and discomfort.

Possible Effects of Long-Term Use: High blood pressure, gallbladder disease with gallstone formation, increased growth of benign fibroid tumors of the uterus. Several reports suggest possible association between the long-term use (3 + years) of estrogens and the development of cancer of the lining of the uterus. Further studies are needed to establish a definite cause-and-effect relationship (see Glossary). Prudence dictates that women with uterus intact should use estrogens only when symptoms justify it and with proper supervision. See the profile of menopause in Section Two.

Suggested Periodic Examinations While Taking This Drug (at physician's discretion)
Regular (every 6 months) evaluation of the breasts and pelvic organs, including Pap smears. Liver function tests as indicated.

▷ **While Taking This Drug, Observe the Following**
Foods: Avoid excessive use of salt if fluid retention occurs.
Beverages: No restrictions. May be taken with milk.
▷ *Alcohol:* No interactions expected.
Tobacco Smoking: Recent studies indicate that heavy smoking (15 or more cigarettes daily) in association with the use of estrogen-containing oral contraceptives significantly increases the risk of heart attack (coronary thrombosis). Avoid heavy smoking during long-term estrogen therapy.

▷   *Other Drugs*

Estrogens *taken concurrently* with

- antidiabetic drugs may cause unpredictable fluctuations of blood sugar.
- tricyclic antidepressants (Elavil, Sinequan, etc.) may enhance their adverse effects and reduce their antidepressant effectiveness.
- warfarin (Coumadin) may cause unpredictable alterations of prothrombin activity.

The following drugs may *decrease* the effects of estrogens

- carbamazepine (Tegretol).
- phenobarbital.
- phenytoin (Dilantin).
- primidone (Mysoline).
- rifampin (Rifadin, Rimactane).

▷ *Driving, Hazardous Activities:* Usually no restrictions. Consult your physician for assessment of individual risk and for guidance regarding specific restrictions.

Aviation Note: Usually no restrictions. However, it is advisable to observe for the rare occurrence of disturbed vision and to restrict activities accordingly. Consult a designated Aviation Medical Examiner.

Exposure to Sun: Use caution until full effect is known. These drugs can cause photosensitivity (see Glossary).

Discontinuation: It is advisable to discontinue estrogens periodically to determine if a need for them still exists. Reduce the dose gradually to prevent acute withdrawal hot flushes. Avoid continual, uninterrupted use of large doses. Discontinue altogether when a definite indication for replacement therapy no longer exists. Ask your physician for guidance.

ETHOSUXIMIDE
(eth oh SUX i mide)

Introduced: 1960

Class: Anticonvulsant, succinimides

Prescription: USA: Yes
    Canada: Yes

Controlled Drug: USA: No
    Canada: No

Available as Generic: No

Brand Name: Zarontin

BENEFITS versus RISKS

Possible Benefits	*Possible Risks*
EFFECTIVE CONTROL OF ABSENCE SEIZURES (PETIT MAL EPILEPSY) in 70% of cases	RARE APLASTIC ANEMIA (See Aplastic Anemia and Bone Marrow Depression in Glossary)
EFFECTIVE CONTROL OF MYOCLONIC AND AKINETIC EPILEPSY in some individuals	Rare decrease in white blood cells and blood platelets

---

▷ **Principal Uses**

As a Single Drug Product: This is the drug of first choice by many physicians for the management of absence seizures. It causes serious adverse effects less frequently than other drugs used for this disorder, and it is quite effective in the presence of structural abnormalities of the brain.

How This Drug Works: Not completely established. It is thought that by altering the transmission of certain nerve impulses, this drug suppresses the abnormal showers of electrical activity responsible for the absence seizures of petit mal epilepsy.

Available Dosage Forms and Strengths

Capsules — 250 mg

Syrup — 250 mg per 5-ml teaspoonful

▷ **Usual Adult Dosage Range:**   20 to 40 mg per kilogram of body weight/24 hours. Initially 500 mg/24 hours. Dosage may be increased cautiously by 250 mg every 4 to 7 days until satisfactory control is achieved. The total daily dosage should not exceed 1500 mg. **Note: Actual dosage and administration schedule must be determined by the physician for each patient individually.**

▷ **Dosing Instructions:**   May be taken with food to reduce stomach irritation. Capsule may be opened for administration.

Usual Duration of Use: Continual use on a regular schedule for 1 to 2 weeks is usually necessary to determine this drug's effectiveness in reducing the frequency of absence seizures. Long-term use requires supervision and periodic evaluation by your physician. Consult your physician on a regular basis.

▷ **This Drug Should Not Be Taken If**

- you are allergic to this or any other succinimide: methsuximide (Celontin), phenfuximide (Milontin).
- you have active liver disease.
- you currently have a blood cell or bone marrow disorder.

▷ **Inform Your Physician Before Taking This Drug If**
  • you have a history of liver or kidney disease.
  • you have a history of any type of blood cell disorder, especially one induced by drugs.
  • you have a history of serious depression or other mental illness.

Possible Side-Effects (natural, expected and unavoidable drug actions)
  Drowsiness, lethargy, fatigue.

▷ **Possible Adverse Effects** (unusual, unexpected and infrequent reactions)
  If any of the following develop, consult your physician promptly for guidance.
  Mild Adverse Effects
  Allergic Reactions: Skin rash, hives.
  Headache, dizziness, unsteadiness, euphoria, impaired vision, numbness and tingling in extremities.
  Loss of appetite, nausea, vomiting, hiccups, stomach pain, diarrhea.
  Excessive growth of hair.
  Serious Adverse Effects
  Allergic Reaction: Swelling of tongue.
  Thickening and overgrowth of gums.
  Nervousness, hyperactivity, disturbed sleep, night terrors.
  Aggravation of emotional depression and paranoid mental disorders.
  Severe bone marrow depression—fatigue, weakness, fever, sore throat, abnormal bleeding or bruising.

▷ **Possible Effects on Sexual Function:**   Increased libido (questionable); nonmenstrual vaginal bleeding.

Natural Diseases or Disorders That May Be Activated by This Drug
  Latent psychosis, systemic lupus erythematosus.

CAUTION
  1. This drug may increase the frequency of grand mal seizures in individuals with mixed seizure disorders.
  2. It is mandatory that you comply with your physician's request for periodic blood counts and other tests that are deemed necessary.

Precautions for Use
  By Infants and Children: If a single daily dose causes nausea or vomiting, give in 2 or 3 divided doses 8 to 12 hours apart. Marked individual variation in response occurs; the use of blood levels for monitoring is advised. Observe for a possible lupuslike reaction: fever, rash, arthritis.
  By Those over 60 Years of Age: Rarely used in this age group.

▷ **Advisability of Use During Pregnancy**
  Pregnancy Category: C (tentative). See Pregnancy Code inside back cover.
  Animal studies: Bone defects reported in rodents.

Human studies: Three instances of birth defects have been reported. Information from adequate studies of pregnant women is not available.

Avoid during first 3 months. Use only if clearly needed during the last 6 months.

Advisability of Use if Breast-Feeding

Presence of this drug in breast milk: Yes.

Monitor nursing infant closely and discontinue drug or nursing if adverse effects develop. If mother requires high doses, refrain from nursing. Ask physician for guidance.

Habit-Forming Potential: None.

Effects of Overdosage: Increased drowsiness, lethargy, weakness, dizziness, unsteadiness, nausea, vomiting, stupor progressing to coma.

Possible Effects of Long-Term Use: Systemic lupus erythematosus.

Suggested Periodic Examinations While Taking This Drug (at physician's discretion)

Complete blood cell counts every 2 weeks during the first 3 months of use, then monthly thereafter; liver and kidney function tests.

▷ **While Taking This Drug, Observe the Following**

Foods: No restrictions.

Beverages: No restrictions. May be taken with milk.

▷ *Alcohol:* Use caution until the combined effects have been determined. This drug may increase the sedative effects of alcohol. Excessive alcohol may precipitate seizures.

Tobacco Smoking: No interactions expected.

▷ *Other Drugs*

Ethosuximide may ***increase*** the effects of

- phenytoin (Dilantin), by slowing its elimination.

Ethosuximide ***taken concurrently*** with

- valproic acid (Depakene) may alter the effects of ethosuximide unpredictably.

The following drugs may ***increase*** the effects of ethosuximide

- isoniazid (INH, Niconyl, etc.).

▷ *Driving, Hazardous Activities:* This drug may cause drowsiness, dizziness, unsteadiness and impaired vision. Restrict activities as necessary.

Aviation Note: Seizure disorders and the use of this drug ***are disqualifications*** for piloting. Consult a designated Aviation Medical Examiner.

Exposure to Sun: No restrictions.

Discontinuation: Do not stop taking this drug abruptly. Ask your physician for guidance regarding gradual reduction of dosage.

ETRETINATE
(e TRET i nayt)

Introduced: 1976

Class: Antipsoriasis

Prescription: USA: Yes
    Canada: Yes

Controlled Drug: USA: No
    Canada: No

Available as Generic: USA: No
    Canada: No

Brand Name: Tegison

BENEFITS versus RISKS

Possible Benefits	*Possible Risks*
EFFECTIVE TREATMENT FOR SEVERE, RESISTANT PSORIASIS in the majority of all cases treated	MAJOR DRUG-INDUCED BIRTH DEFECTS RARE DRUG-INDUCED HEPATITIS Adverse effects on eyes and vision Adverse effects on musculoskeletal structures Adverse effects on blood cholesterol and triglycerides Increased intracranial pressure (very rare)

▷ **Principal Uses**

As a Single Drug Product: Used primarily to treat severe, generalized forms of psoriasis (and related skin disorders) that have failed to respond to conventional, less hazardous treatments.

How This Drug Works: Not completely established. Its principal action is the regulation of cell differentiation in the skin; this results in a more normal pattern of cell growth, with reduction of inflammation and scale formation.

Available Dosage Forms and Strengths
Capsules — 10 mg, 25 mg

▷ **Usual Adult Dosage Range:** Initially 0.75 to 1 mg/kg/day, in divided doses, until satisfactory response is obtained (usually 8 to 16 weeks). Maintenance: 0.5 to 0.75 mg/kg/day, beginning after initial response. Total daily dosage should not exceed 75 mg. **Note: Actual dosage and administration schedule must be determined by the physician for each patient individually.**

▷ **Dosing Instructions:** Take with or immediately following meals, preferably with whole milk. Do not suck or chew the capsule; swallow it whole.

Usual Duration of Use: Continual use on a regular schedule for 2 to 4 weeks is usually necessary to determine this drug's effectiveness in reversing the skin changes of psoriasis. The full effect of treatment may not be apparent until after 2 to 3 months of continual use. Long-term use (months to years) requires periodic evaluation of response and dosage adjustment. Due to the potential for drug accumulation and toxicity with long-term use, this drug should be temporarily discontinued after 18 months of treatment; it may be resumed as needed. Consult your physician on a regular basis.

Possible Advantages of This Drug: When used in conjunction with other antipsoriasis drugs and procedures, this drug can enhance the therapeutic response and reduce the total dosage and length of treatment required for satisfactory management.

▷ **This Drug Should Not Be Taken If**
- you have had an allergic reaction to any dosage form of it previously.
- you are pregnant or breast-feeding.
- you plan to donate blood in the near future.

▷ **Inform Your Physician Before Taking This Drug If**
- you are allergic to vitamin A or other vitamin A derivatives: isotretinoin (Accutane), tretinoin (Retin-A).
- you are allergic to parabens (preservatives).
- you have cerebral or coronary artery disease.
- you have high blood cholesterol or triglyceride levels.
- you have diabetes.
- you have impaired liver or kidney function.
- you have alcoholism.
- you have a history of Crohn's disease or ulcerative colitis.

Possible Side-Effects (natural, expected and unavoidable drug actions)
Dry nose, nosebleed, dry lips, sore mouth and tongue, bleeding gums.
Loss of hair, skin peeling of hands and feet, dry skin, itching, bruising, nail deformities.
Thickening of bone (hyperostosis), calcification of tendons and ligaments, bone and joint pain.

▷ **Possible Adverse Effects** (unusual, unexpected and infrequent reactions)
If any of the following develop, consult your physician promptly for guidance.
Mild Adverse Effects
Allergic Reactions: Skin rash, hives, itching.
Headache, dizziness, fatigue, fever, emotional irritability.
Eye irritation, blurred or double vision, sensitivity to bright light, decreased tolerance for contact lenses, earache, impaired hearing.
Altered taste, loss of appetite, nausea, stomach pain, constipation, diarrhea.
Painful urination.

Serious Adverse Effects

Increased intracranial pressure (less than 1%): headache, nausea, vomiting, visual disturbances.

Hepatitis (1.5%); 4 reported deaths worldwide.

Eye reactions: corneal erosion, abrasion, staining; cataract; retinal hemorrhage; visual field defects; reduced night vision.

Inflammatory bowel disease (Crohn's disease), rare.

Altered blood fat levels: increased triglycerides (45%), increased total cholesterol (16%), decreased HDL cholesterol (37%); any of these changes may increase the risk for the development of atherosclerotic heart disease.

▷ **Possible Effects on Sexual Function:**   Altered timing and pattern of menstruation.

Possible Delayed Adverse Effects: This drug has been found in the blood 2.9 years following termination of its use and has the potential for inducing birth defects during this time. It has not been determined how long pregnancy should be avoided after discontinuation of treatment.

▷ **Adverse Effects That May Mimic Natural Diseases or Disorders**

Increased intracranial pressure may suggest brain tumor.

Liver reactions may suggest viral hepatitis.

Joint pains due to calcification of ligaments and tendons may suggest the onset of arthritis.

Natural Diseases or Disorders That May Be Activated by This Drug

Angina may develop in the presence of coronary artery heart disease. Heart attack (myocardial infarction) has been associated with the use of this drug.

CAUTION

1. ***This drug should not be taken during pregnancy.*** A pregnancy test should be performed within 2 weeks prior to taking this drug. In the absence of pregnancy, the drug should be started on the second or third day of the next normal menstrual period. An effective form of contraception should be used for 1 month before the drug is started, during the entire period of treatment, and for an indefinite period (minimum of 3 years) after the drug is discontinued. If pregnancy does occur, discontinue this drug immediately and consult your physician.

2. ***Do not donate blood to a blood bank if you are taking this drug.*** Blood containing this drug could pose a serious risk to the developing fetus of a pregnant patient who received it. Avoid blood donation for a minimum of 3 years if use of the blood is beyond your control.

3. *Comply fully with your physician's recommendations for periodic examinations before, during and following treatment with this drug.* These are mandatory for safe and effective use.
4. Avoid the concurrent use of vitamin A supplements while taking this drug.
5. If you experience significant eye reactions or altered vision, consult your physician promptly.
6. Your psoriasis may appear to worsen during the early period of treatment with this drug. This is a common response. Consult your physician if symptoms become severe or prolonged.
7. If dry mouth or sore and bleeding gums persist, consult your dentist.

Precautions for Use

By Infants and Children: This drug should be used only after all less hazardous treatments have failed. It is advisable to obtain pretreatment X-rays to determine bone age and to monitor bone growth and development by yearly X-ray studies. This drug can impair normal bone maturation.

By Those over 60 Years of Age: Monitor for the possible development of anemia, impaired kidney function and fluctuation of blood potassium levels.

▷ Advisability of Use During Pregnancy

Pregnancy Category: X. See Pregnancy Code inside back cover.

Animal studies: No information available.

Human studies: Major birth defects occur in association with the use of this drug: malformations of the skull, vertebrae, face, extremities, brain and spinal cord.

Avoid this drug completely during entire pregnancy. See *CAUTION.*

Advisability of Use if Breast-Feeding

Presence of this drug in breast milk: Unknown.

Avoid drug or refrain from nursing.

Habit-Forming Potential: None.

Effects of Overdosage: Severe headache, irritability, drowsiness, itching, nausea, vomiting.

Possible Effects of Long-Term Use: Hyperostosis (84%): abnormal thickening of bone (pelvis), calcification of ligaments and tendons (knees and ankles).

Suggested Periodic Examinations While Taking This Drug (at physician's discretion)

Complete blood cell counts; measurements of blood sugar, potassium, sodium and chloride.

Blood cholesterol profiles, before and during treatment.
Liver and kidney function tests.
Complete eye examinations.
Bone X-rays, especially children.

▷ **While Taking This Drug, Observe the Following**
    Foods: No restrictions. High-fat foods increase absorption of this drug.
    Beverages: No restrictions. Whole milk increases absorption of this drug.
▷   *Alcohol:* No interactions expected. Use moderately; excessive intake can
        increase blood triglyceride levels.
    Tobacco Smoking: No interactions expected.
▷   *Other Drugs*
        Etretinate may *increase* the effects of
        • vitamin A and its derivatives (isotretinoin and tretinoin) and increase
          the risk of vitamin A toxicity.
        Etretinate *taken concurrently* with
        • methotrexate may increase the risk of liver toxicity.
        • tetracyclines may increase the risk of elevated intracranial pressure.
▷   *Driving, Hazardous Activities:* This drug may cause dizziness and blurred
        vision. Restrict activities as necessary.
    Aviation Note: The use of this drug *may be a disqualification* for piloting.
    Consult a designated Aviation Medical Examiner.
    Exposure to Sun: Use caution. This drug can cause photosensitivity (see
    Glossary).
    Discontinuation: If this drug is not significantly beneficial after 4 months
    of continual use, it should be discontinued. If response is adequate
    to justify its long-term use, it should be discontinued temporarily
    ("drug holiday") after 18 months of continual treatment. Once the skin
    has cleared satisfactorily, this drug should be discontinued. The ma-
    jority of individuals will experience some degree of recurrence by the
    end of 2 months. Subsequent treatment courses of 4 to 9 months can
    be instituted as required.

FAMOTIDINE
(fa MOH te deen)

Introduced: 1986

Class: Antiulcer, H-2 receptor
blocker

Prescription: USA: Yes

Controlled Drug: USA: No

Available as Generic: USA: No

Brand Name: Pepcid

```
┌─────────────────────────────────────────────────────────────┐
│                    BENEFITS versus RISKS                    │
│                                                             │
│      Possible Benefits                   Possible Risks     │
│   EFFECTIVE TREATMENT OF          Headache, dizziness       │
│     PEPTIC ULCER DISEASE:                                   │
│     relief of symptoms, acceleration                        │
│     of healing, prevention of                               │
│     recurrence                                              │
│   CONTROL OF                                                │
│     HYPERSECRETORY                                          │
│     STOMACH DISORDERS                                       │
│   Beneficial in treatment of reflux                         │
│     esophagitis                                             │
└─────────────────────────────────────────────────────────────┘
```

▷ **Principal Uses**

As a Single Drug Product: Used primarily in the treatment of peptic ulcer disease, both benign stomach (gastric) ulcer and duodenal ulcer. It is used specifically to hasten the healing of ulcer and to prevent recurrence. Also used to control the excessive production of stomach acid in the Zollinger-Ellison syndrome. Though its effectiveness has not been fully established, this drug is also used in the management of esophagitis (as with hiatal hernia) and upper gastrointestinal bleeding.

How This Drug Works: By blocking the action of histamine, this drug effectively inhibits the secretion of stomach acid and thus creates a more favorable environment for the healing of peptic ulcers.

Available Dosage Forms and Strengths

Injection — 10 mg per ml
Oral suspension — 40 mg per 5-ml teaspoonful
Tablets — 20 mg, 40 mg

▷ **Usual Adult Dosage Range:**   For active peptic ulcer: 20 mg twice daily, or 40 mg at bedtime. For prevention of recurrent ulcer: 20 mg at bedtime. For hypersecretory states: 20 mg/6 hours. **Note: Actual dosage and administration schedule must be determined by the physician for each patient individually.**

▷ **Dosing Instructions:**   To obtain the longest period of stomach acid reduction, this drug should be taken with or immediately following food. The tablet may be crushed for administration. If needed, antacids may be taken concurrently with this drug to relieve ulcer pain.

Usual Duration of Use: Continual use on a regular schedule for 4 to 6 weeks is usually necessary to determine this drug's effectiveness in healing active peptic ulcer. Long-term use (months to years) for prevention of ulcer recurrence requires individual consideration by your physician.

▷ **This Drug Should Not Be Taken If**
- you have had an allergic reaction to any dosage form of it previously.

▷ **Inform Your Physician Before Taking This Drug If**
- you are allergic to cimetidine (Tagamet) or ranitidine (Zantac).
- you have impaired liver or kidney function.

Possible Side-Effects (natural, expected and unavoidable drug actions)
None reported.

▷ **Possible Adverse Effects** (unusual, unexpected and infrequent reactions)
If any of the following develop, consult your physician promptly for guidance.
Mild Adverse Effects
Allergic Reactions: Skin rash, swelling of eyelids.
Headache (4.7%), dizziness (1.3%), fatigue.
Nausea, constipation (1.2%), diarrhea (1.7%).
Serious Adverse Effects
Rare decrease in blood platelet counts: abnormal bleeding or bruising (questionable).

▷ **Possible Effects on Sexual Function:** Decreased libido.

CAUTION
1. Do not discontinue this drug abruptly. (Ulcer activation and perforation have occurred following abrupt cessation of cimetidine, a closely related drug.)
2. After discontinuation of this drug, inform your physician promptly if you experience a return of symptoms indicative of ulcer reactivation.
3. Inform your allergist that you are taking this drug if allergy skin tests are to be done; this drug may interfere with skin testing and cause false negative results.

Precautions for Use
By Infants and Children: Safety and effectiveness for use by those under 12 years of age have not been established.
By Those over 60 Years of Age: This drug may contribute to the formation of stomach phytobezoars (masses of undigested vegetable fibers). Individuals with poor chewing ability (missing teeth) and those who have had partial gastrectomy or vagotomy (stomach surgery) are most susceptible. Observe for loss of appetite, stomach fullness, nausea and vomiting.

▷ **Advisability of Use During Pregnancy**
Pregnancy Category: B (tentative). See Pregnancy Code inside back cover.
Animal studies: No birth defects reported.
Human studies: Information from adequate studies of pregnant women is not available.
Use this drug only if clearly needed. Ask physician for guidance.

Advisability of Use if Breast-Feeding
Presence of this drug in breast milk: Probably yes.
Avoid drug or refrain from nursing.

Habit-Forming Potential: None.

Effects of Overdosage: Related drugs (cimetidine, ranitidine) may cause confusion, delirium, slurred speech, flushing, sweating, drowsiness, muscle twitching, seizures, coma.

Possible Effects of Long-Term Use: Impaired absorption of vitamin B-12.

Suggested Periodic Examinations While Taking This Drug (at physician's discretion)
Complete blood cell counts.

▷ **While Taking This Drug, Observe the Following**
Foods: Protein-rich foods produce maximal stomach acid secretion. Follow the diet prescribed to derive optimal benefit from this drug.
Beverages: No restrictions. May be taken with milk.
▷ *Alcohol:* No interactions with drug. However, alcoholic beverages increase stomach acidity and can reduce the effectiveness of this drug.
Tobacco Smoking: Decreased effectiveness of this drug, especially in its ability to reduce nocturnal stomach acid secretion. Avoid smoking during periods of active peptic ulcer disease.
▷ *Other Drugs:* No significant drug interactions reported to date.
▷ *Driving, Hazardous Activities:* This drug may cause dizziness. Restrict activities as necessary.
Aviation Note: The use of this drug **may be a disqualification** for piloting. Consult a designated Aviation Medical Examiner.
Exposure to Sun: No restrictions.
Discontinuation: Do not discontinue this drug suddenly if taken for peptic ulcer disease. Consult physician for withdrawal instructions. This drug does not provide an extended protective effect. Be alert to the possibility of ulcer recurrence anytime after discontinuation.

FENOPROFEN
(fen oh PROH fen)

Introduced: 1976

Class: Mild analgesic, anti-inflammatory

Prescription: USA: Yes
Canada: Yes

Controlled Drug: USA: No
Canada: No

Available as Generic: Yes

Brand Name: Nalfon

BENEFITS versus RISKS

Possible Benefits	*Possible Risks*
EFFECTIVE RELIEF OF MILD TO MODERATE PAIN AND INFLAMMATION	Gastrointestinal pain, ulceration, bleeding (rare) Rare liver or kidney damage Rare fluid retention Rare bone marrow depression

---

▷ **Principal Uses**

As a Single Drug Product: Used primarily to relieve mild to moderately severe pain associated with (1) musculoskeletal injuries; (2) acute and chronic gout, rheumatoid arthritis and osteoarthritis; (3) dental, obstetrical and orthopedic surgery; (4) menstrual cramps; and (5) vascular (migrainelike) headaches.

How This Drug Works: Not completely established. It is thought that this drug reduces the tissue concentrations of prostaglandins (and related compounds), chemicals involved in the production of inflammation and pain.

Available Dosage Forms and Strengths
Capsules — 200 mg, 300 mg
Tablets — 600 mg

▷ **Usual Adult Dosage Range:** 300 to 600 mg 3 or 4 times/day. Total daily dosage should not exceed 3200 mg. **Note: Actual dosage and administration schedule must be determined by the physician for each patient individually.**

▷ **Dosing Instructions:** Take either on an empty stomach or with food or milk to prevent stomach irritation. Take with a full glass of water and remain upright (do not lie down) for 30 minutes. The tablet may be crushed and the capsule may be opened for administration.

Usual Duration of Use: Continual use on a regular schedule for 2 to 3 weeks is usually necessary to determine this drug's effectiveness in relieving the discomfort of arthritis. Long-term use requires supervision and periodic evaluation by the physician. Consult your physician on a regular basis.

▷ **This Drug Should Not Be Taken If**
- you have had an allergic reaction to it previously.
- you are subject to asthma or nasal polyps caused by aspirin.
- you have active peptic ulcer disease or any form of gastrointestinal bleeding.
- you have a bleeding disorder or a blood cell disorder.
- you have severe impairment of kidney function.

▷ **Inform Your Physician Before Taking This Drug If**
- you are allergic to aspirin or to other aspirin substitutes.
- you have a history of peptic ulcer disease or any type of bleeding disorder.
- you have impaired liver or kidney function.
- you have high blood pressure or a history of heart failure.
- you are taking any of the following: acetaminophen, aspirin or other aspirin substitutes, anticoagulants, oral antidiabetic drugs.

Possible Side-Effects (natural, expected and unavoidable drug actions)
Drowsiness (15%), ringing in ears, fluid retention.

▷ **Possible Adverse Effects** (unusual, unexpected and infrequent reactions)
If any of the following develop, consult your physician promptly for guidance.
Mild Adverse Effects
Allergic Reactions: Skin rash, hives, itching (9%).
Headache (15%), dizziness, altered or blurred vision, depression.
Mouth sores, indigestion, nausea, vomiting, constipation, diarrhea.
Serious Adverse Effects
Allergic Reaction: Anaphylaxis (see Glossary).
Blurred vision, impaired hearing.
Active peptic ulcer, with or without bleeding.
Liver damage with jaundice (see Glossary).
Kidney damage with painful urination, bloody urine, reduced urine formation.
Rare bone marrow depression (see Glossary)—fatigue, weakness, fever, sore throat, abnormal bleeding or bruising.

▷ **Possible Effects on Sexual Function:**   None reported.

Possible Delayed Adverse Effects: Mild anemia due to "silent" blood loss from the stomach (less than that caused by aspirin).

▷ **Adverse Effects That May Mimic Natural Diseases or Disorders**
Liver reaction may suggest viral hepatitis.

Natural Diseases or Disorders That May Be Activated by This Drug
Peptic ulcer disease, ulcerative colitis.

CAUTION
1. Dosage should always be limited to the smallest amount that produces reasonable improvement.
2. This drug may mask early indications of infection. Inform your physician if you think you are developing an infection of any kind.

Precautions for Use
By Infants and Children: Safety and effectiveness for use by those under 12 years of age have not been established.
By Those over 60 Years of Age: Small doses are advisable until tolerance is determined. Observe for any indications of liver or kidney toxicity,

fluid retention, dizziness, confusion, impaired memory, stomach bleeding or constipation.

▷ **Advisability of Use During Pregnancy**
Pregnancy Category: B (tentative). See Pregnancy Code inside back cover.
Animal studies: No birth defects reported.
Human studies: Information from adequate studies of pregnant women is not available.
Avoid this drug during the last 3 months. Use it during the first 6 months only if clearly needed. Ask physician for guidance.
The manufacturer does not recommend the use of this drug during pregnancy.

Advisability of Use if Breast-Feeding
Presence of this drug in breast milk: Yes, in minute amounts.
Avoid drug or refrain from nursing.

Habit-Forming Potential: None.

Effects of Overdosage: Drowsiness, nausea, vomiting, diarrhea.

Possible Effects of Long-Term Use: Cataracts have been reported, but a definite cause-and-effect relationship (see Glossary) has not been established.

Suggested Periodic Examinations While Taking This Drug (at physician's discretion)
Complete blood cell counts, liver and kidney function tests, complete eye examinations if vision is altered in any way.

▷ **While Taking This Drug, Observe the Following**
Foods: No restrictions.
Beverages: No restrictions. May be taken with milk.
▷ *Alcohol:* Use with caution. The irritant action of alcohol on the stomach lining, added to the irritant action of this drug in sensitive individuals, can increase the risk of stomach ulceration and/or bleeding.
Tobacco Smoking: No interactions expected.
▷ *Other Drugs*
Fenoprofen may ***increase*** the effects of
- acetaminophen (Tylenol, etc.), and increase the risk of kidney damage; avoid prolonged use of this combination.
- anticoagulants (Coumadin, etc.), and increase the risk of bleeding; monitor prothrombin time, adjust dose accordingly.

Fenoprofen ***taken concurrently*** with the following drugs may increase the risk of bleeding; avoid these combinations:
- aspirin.
- dipyridamole (Persantine).
- indomethacin (Indocin).
- sulfinpyrazone (Anturane).
- valproic acid (Depakene).

▷   *Driving, Hazardous Activities:* This drug may cause drowsiness or dizziness. Restrict activities as necessary.
 Aviation Note: The use of this drug **may be a disqualification** for piloting. Consult a designated Aviation Medical Examiner.
 Exposure to Sun: No restrictions.

FLECAINIDE
(FLEK a nide)

Introduced: 1982

Class: Antiarrhythmic

Prescription: USA: Yes

Controlled Drug: USA: No

Available as Generic: USA: No

Brand Name: Tambocor

BENEFITS versus RISKS	
Possible Benefits	*Possible Risks*
EFFECTIVE TREATMENT (72%) OF SELECTED HEART RHYTHM DISORDERS	DRUG-INDUCED HEART RHYTHM DISORDERS (7%) CONGESTIVE HEART FAILURE (5%) Rare blood cell disorders Rare liver damage with jaundice

▷ **Principal Uses**
 As a Single Drug Product: This drug is classified as a Type 1 antiarrhythmic agent, similar to procainamide and quinidine in its actions. It is used primarily to correct and prevent the recurrence of life-threatening rapid heart rates (tachycardia) that arise in the ventricles (lower heart chambers).

 How This Drug Works: By slowing the transmission of electrical impulses throughout the conduction system of the heart, this drug assists in restoring normal heart rate and rhythm.

 Available Dosage Forms and Strengths
 Tablets — 50 mg, 100 mg, 150 mg

▷ **Usual Adult Dosage Range:** Do not take a loading dose. Initiate treatment with 100 mg/12 hours. At intervals of 4 days, increase dose by 50-mg increments to 150 mg/12 hours, then to 200 mg/12 hours if necessary. Total daily dosage should not exceed 400 mg. Measurement of drug blood levels is advised to determine the optimal dose and schedule.

Note: Actual dosage and administration schedule must be determined by the physician for each patient individually.

▷ **Dosing Instructions:** May be taken without regard to meals. Take at same time each day to obtain uniform results. Tablet may be crushed for administration.

Usual Duration of Use: Continual use on a regular schedule for 1 to 2 weeks is usually necessary to determine this drug's effectiveness in correcting or preventing responsive rhythm disorders. Long-term use requires supervision and periodic evaluation by your physician. Consult your physician on a regular basis.

▷ **This Drug Should Not Be Taken If**
- you have had an allergic reaction to it previously.
- you have second-degree or third-degree heart block (determined by electrocardiogram).

▷ **Inform Your Physician Before Taking This Drug If**
- you have had any unfavorable reactions to other antiarrhythmic drugs in the past.
- you have a history of heart disease of any kind, especially "heart block."
- you have impaired liver or kidney function.
- you are taking any form of digitalis, a potassium supplement or any diuretic drug that can cause excessive loss of body potassium (ask physician).

Possible Side-Effects (natural, expected and unavoidable drug actions)
Flushing, increased sweating, light-headedness.

▷ **Possible Adverse Effects** (unusual, unexpected and infrequent reactions)
If any of the following develop, consult your physician promptly for guidance.
Mild Adverse Effects
Allergic Reactions: Skin rash (1% to 3%), hives, itching.
Headache (9%), dizziness (18%), visual disturbance (15%), fatigue (7%), weakness (4%), tremor (4%).
Loss of appetite, indigestion, nausea (8%), vomiting, constipation (4%), abdominal pain (3%).
Serious Adverse Effects
Idiosyncratic Reactions: Depression, confusion, amnesia, euphoria (less than 1%).
Drug-induced heart rhythm disorders (7%), congestive heart failure (5%), shortness of breath (10%), palpitations (6%), chest pain (5%), swelling of feet (3%).
Urinary retention.
Jaundice (see Glossary).
Abnormally low white blood cell and blood platelet counts (rare): fever, sore throat, abnormal bleeding or bruising.

▷ **Possible Effects on Sexual Function:** Decreased libido; impaired erection with doses of 200 mg/day; complete impotence with doses of 400 mg/day.

▷ **Adverse Effects That May Mimic Natural Diseases or Disorders**
Reversible jaundice may suggest viral hepatitis.

CAUTION
1. Thorough evaluation of your heart function (including electrocardiograms) is necessary prior to using this drug.
2. Periodic evaluation of your heart function is necessary to determine your response to this drug. Some individuals may experience worsening of their heart rhythm disorder and/or deterioration of heart function. Close monitoring of heart rate, rhythm and overall performance is essential.
3. Dosage must be adjusted carefully for each individual. Do not change your dosage without the knowledge and supervision of your physician.
4. Do not take any other antiarrhythmic drug while taking this drug unless directed to do so by your physician.

Precautions for Use
By Infants and Children: Safety and effectiveness for use by those under 18 years of age have not been established. Initial use of this drug requires hospitalization and supervision by a qualified cardiologist.
By Those over 60 Years of Age: Reduced kidney function may require reduction in dosage. Observe carefully for light-headedness, dizziness, unsteadiness and tendency to fall.

▷ **Advisability of Use During Pregnancy**
Pregnancy Category: C (tentative). See Pregnancy Code inside back cover.
Animal studies: Birth defects reported in one species of rabbit.
Human studies: Information from adequate studies of pregnant women is not available.
Avoid during first 3 months. Use this drug only if clearly needed. Ask physician for guidance.

Advisability of Use if Breast-Feeding
Presence of this drug in breast milk: Unknown.
Avoid drug or refrain from nursing.

Habit-Forming Potential: None.

Effects of Overdosage: Impaired urination, constipation, marked drop in blood pressure, abnormal heart rhythms, slow heart rate, congestive heart failure.

Possible Effects of Long-Term Use: None reported.

Suggested Periodic Examinations While Taking This Drug (at physician's discretion)

Electrocardiograms, complete blood cell counts, measurements of potassium blood levels.

▷ **While Taking This Drug, Observe the Following**

Foods: No restrictions. Ask physician regarding need for salt restriction and advisability of eating potassium-rich foods.

Beverages: No restrictions. May be taken with milk.

▷ *Alcohol:* Use caution until the combined effects have been determined. Alcohol can increase the blood-pressure-lowering effects of this drug.

Tobacco Smoking: Nicotine can cause irritability of the heart and reduce the effectiveness of this drug. Follow physician's advice regarding smoking.

▷ *Other Drugs*

Flecainide may ***increase*** the effects of

- antihypertensive drugs, and cause excessive lowering of blood pressure.
- beta blocker drugs (see Drug Class, Section Four).

The following drugs may ***decrease*** the effects of flecainide

- diuretics that promote potassium loss.

▷ *Driving, Hazardous Activities:* This drug may cause drowsiness, dizziness or blurred vision. Restrict activities as necessary.

Aviation Note: The use of this drug **may be a disqualification** for piloting. Consult a designated Aviation Medical Examiner.

Exposure to Sun: No restrictions.

Occurrence of Unrelated Illness: Disorders that cause vomiting, diarrhea or dehydration can affect this drug's action adversely. Report such developments promptly.

Discontinuation: This drug should not be discontinued abruptly following long-term use. Ask your physician for guidance regarding gradual dose reduction.

FLUOXETINE

(flu OX e teen)

Introduced: 1978

Class: Antidepressant

Prescription: USA: Yes

Controlled Drug: USA: No

Available as Generic: USA: No

Brand Name: Prozac

BENEFITS versus RISKS	
Possible Benefits	*Possible Risks*
EFFECTIVE TREATMENT OF MAJOR DEPRESSIVE DISORDERS in 60% to 75% of cases	Serious allergic reactions (4%)
	Conversion of depression to mania in manic-depressive disorders (1%)
Possibly effective in relieving the symptoms of obsessive-compulsive disorder	Seizures (0.2%)

▷ **Principal Uses**

As a Single Drug Product: Used primarily to treat major forms of depression that have not responded well to other therapies. This drug should be used only when a diagnosis of a true, primary depression of significant degree has been established. It should not be used to treat the symptoms of mild and transient (reactive) depression that may be associated with many life situations in the absence of a bona fide affective illness.

How This Drug Works: It is thought that this drug relieves depression by slowly restoring to normal levels a specific constituent of brain tissue (serotonin) that transmits nerve impulses.

Available Dosage Forms and Strengths

Capsules — 20 mg

▷ **Usual Adult Dosage Range:** Initially 20 mg daily as a single morning dose; if no improvement after 3 weeks of treatment, the dose may be increased by 20 mg/day as needed and tolerated. Doses over 20 mg/day should be taken in 2 divided doses, early morning and noon. Total daily dosage should not exceed 80 mg. **Note: Actual dosage and administration schedule must be determined by the physician for each patient individually.**

▷ **Dosing Instructions:** May be taken without regard to food. The capsule may be opened for administration and the contents mixed with any convenient food.

Usual Duration of Use: Continual use on a regular schedule for up to 3 weeks is usually necessary to determine this drug's effectiveness in relieving depression. Long-term use (months to years) requires periodic evaluation of response and dosage adjustment. Consult your physician on a regular basis.

Possible Advantages of This Drug

Does not cause weight gain, a common side-effect of tricyclic antidepressants.

Less likely to cause dry mouth, constipation, urinary retention, ortho-static hypotension (see Glossary) and heart rhythm disturbances than tricyclic antidepressants.
Does not cause Parkinson-like reactions.

▷ **This Drug Should Not Be Taken If**
- you have had an allergic reaction to any dosage form of it previously.
- you are currently taking or have taken within the past 14 days any monoamine oxidase (MAO) type A inhibitor drug (see Drug Class, Section Four).

▷ **Inform Your Physician Before Taking This Drug If**
- you have experienced any adverse effects from antidepressant drugs used in the past.
- you have impaired liver or kidney function.
- you have a seizure disorder.

Possible Side-Effects (natural, expected and unavoidable drug actions)
Decreased appetite (8.7%), weight loss (13%).

▷ **Possible Adverse Effects** (unusual, unexpected and infrequent reactions)
If any of the following develop, consult your physician promptly for guidance.
Mild Adverse Effects
Allergic Reactions: Skin rash (2.7%), hives (2%), itching (2.4%).
Headache (20%), nervousness (14%), insomnia (13%), drowsiness (11%), tremor (7%), dizziness (5%), fatigue (4%), impaired concentration (1.5%).
Altered taste (1.8%), nausea (21%), vomiting (2.4%), diarrhea (12%).
Serious Adverse Effects
Allergic Reactions: Serum sickness–like syndrome (2% to 3%): fever, weakness, joint pain and swelling, swollen lymph glands, fluid reten-tion, skin rash and/or hives.
Drug-induced seizures (0.2%).

▷ **Possible Effects on Sexual Function:**   Impaired erection (1.9%).

Natural Diseases or Disorders That May Be Activated by This Drug
Latent epilepsy.

CAUTION
1. If any type of skin reaction develops (rash, hives, etc.), discontinue this drug and inform your physician promptly.
2. If dryness of the mouth develops and persists for more than 2 weeks, consult your dentist for guidance.
3. Consult your physician before taking any other prescription or over-the-counter drug while taking this drug.
4. If you are advised to take any monoamine oxidase (MAO) type A inhibitor drug (see Drug Class, Section Four), allow an interval of 5 weeks after discontinuing this drug before starting the MAO in-hibitor.

5. It is advisable to withhold this drug if electroconvulsive therapy (ECT, "shock" treatment) is to be used to treat your depression.

Precautions for Use
By Infants and Children: Safety and effectiveness for use by those under 12 years of age have not been established.

By Those over 60 Years of Age: Total daily dosage should not exceed 60 mg.

▷ Advisability of Use During Pregnancy
Pregnancy Category: B (tentative). See Pregnancy Code inside back cover.
  Animal studies: No birth defects due to this drug found in rat or rabbit studies.
  Human studies: Information from adequate studies of pregnant women is not available.
  Use this drug only if clearly needed.

Advisability of Use if Breast-Feeding
Presence of this drug in breast milk: Unknown.
Avoid drug or refrain from nursing.

Habit-Forming Potential:　None.

Effects of Overdosage:　Agitation, restlessness, excitement, nausea, vomiting, seizures.

Possible Effects of Long-Term Use:　None reported.

Suggested Periodic Examinations While Taking This Drug (at physician's discretion)
None.

▷ While Taking This Drug, Observe the Following
Foods: No restrictions.

Beverages: No restrictions. May be taken with milk.

▷ *Alcohol:* Avoid completely.

Tobacco Smoking: No interactions expected.

▷ *Other Drugs*
  Fluoxetine may ***increase*** the effects of
  • diazepam (Valium).
  • digitalis preparations (digitoxin, digoxin).
  • warfarin (Coumadin) and related oral anticoagulants.
  Fluoxetine ***taken concurrently*** with
  • monoamine oxidase (MAO) type A inhibitor drugs may cause confusion, agitation, high fever, seizures and dangerous elevations of blood pressure. Avoid the concurrent use of these drugs.

▷ *Driving, Hazardous Activities:* This drug may cause drowsiness, dizziness, impaired judgment and delayed reaction time. Restrict activities as necessary.

Aviation Note: The use of this drug ***is a disqualification*** for piloting. Consult a designated Aviation Medical Examiner.

Exposure to Sun: No restrictions.

Discontinuation: The slow elimination of this drug from the body makes it unlikely that any withdrawal effects will result from abrupt discontinuation. However, consult your physician if you plan to discontinue this drug for any reason.

FLUPHENAZINE
(flu FEN a zeen)

Introduced: 1959

Class: Strong tranquilizer, phenothiazines

Prescription: USA: Yes
　　　Canada: Yes

Controlled Drug: USA: No
　　　Canada: No

Available as Generic: USA: No
　　　Canada: Yes

Brand Names: ♦Apo-Fluphenazine, ♦Modecate, ♦Moditen, Permitil, Prolixin

BENEFITS versus RISKS	
Possible Benefits	*Possible Risks*
EFFECTIVE CONTROL OF ACUTE MENTAL DISORDERS in the majority of patients	SERIOUS TOXIC EFFECTS ON BRAIN with long-term use
Beneficial effects on thinking, mood and behavior	Liver damage with jaundice (less than 0.5%)
	Rare blood cell disorders: abnormally low white blood cell counts

▷ **Principal Uses**

As a Single Drug Product: This antipsychotic drug is used primarily to treat acute and chronic psychotic disorders such as schizophrenia, mania and similar states of mental dysfunction.

How This Drug Works: Not completely established. Present theory is that by inhibiting the action of dopamine, this drug acts to correct an imbalance of nerve impulse transmissions that is thought to be responsible for certain mental disorders.

Available Dosage Forms and Strengths

　　Concentrate — 5 mg per ml (1% alcohol)
　　　　Elixir — 2.5 mg per 5-ml teaspoonful (14% alcohol)
　　Injection — 2.5 mg per ml
　　　Tablets — 1 mg, 2.5 mg, 5 mg, 10 mg

▷ **Usual Adult Dosage Range:**   0.5 to 2.5 mg 1 to 4 times/day; adjust dosage as needed and tolerated. Total daily dosage should not exceed 20 mg. **Note: Actual dosage and administration schedule must be determined by the physician for each patient individually.**

▷ **Dosing Instructions:**   May be taken with or following meals to reduce stomach irritation. Regular tablets may be crushed for administration. Prolonged-action tablets should be swallowed whole (not crushed). The concentrate must be diluted in 4 to 6 ounces of water, milk, fruit juice or carbonated beverage.

   Usual Duration of Use: Continual use on a regular schedule for several weeks is usually necessary to determine this drug's effectiveness in controlling psychotic disorders. If not significantly beneficial within 6 weeks, it should be discontinued. Long-term use (months to years) requires periodic evaluation of response, appropriate dosage adjustment and consideration of continued need. Consult your physician on a regular basis.

▷ **This Drug Should Not Be Taken If**
   • you are allergic to any of the drugs bearing the brand names listed above.
   • you have a history of brain damage.
   • you have active liver disease.
   • you have cancer of the breast.
   • you have a current blood cell or bone marrow disorder.

▷ **Inform Your Physician Before Taking This Drug If**
   • you are allergic or abnormally sensitive to any phenothiazine drug (see Drug Class, Section Four).
   • you have impaired liver or kidney function.
   • you have any type of seizure disorder.
   • you have diabetes, glaucoma, heart disease or chronic lung disease.
   • you have a history of lupus erythematosus.
   • you are taking any drug with sedative effects.
   • you plan to have surgery under general or spinal anesthesia in the near future.

   Possible Side-Effects (natural, expected and unavoidable drug actions)
      Drowsiness (usually during the first 2 weeks), orthostatic hypotension (see Glossary), blurred vision, dry mouth, nasal congestion, constipation, impaired urination (all mild).

▷ **Possible Adverse Effects** (unusual, unexpected and infrequent reactions)
      If any of the following develop, consult your physician promptly for guidance.
      Mild Adverse Effects
      Allergic Reactions: Skin rash, hives, itching.
      Lowering of body temperature, especially in the elderly.

Headache, dizziness, weakness, excitement, restlessness, unusual dreaming.

Increased appetite and weight gain.

Serious Adverse Effects

Allergic Reactions: Hepatitis with jaundice (see Glossary), usually between second and fourth week; anaphylactic reaction (see Glossary).

Idiosyncratic Reaction: High fever.

Impaired production of white blood cells—fever, sore throat, infections.

Parkinson-like disorders (see Glossary); muscle spasms of face, jaw, neck, back, extremities.

Prolonged drop in blood pressure with weakness, perspiration and fainting.

▷ **Possible Effects on Sexual Function**

Decreased male libido; increased female libido.

Impaired erection (38% to 42%); complete impotence.

Inhibited male orgasm (58%); inhibited female orgasm (22% to 33%).

Inhibited ejaculation (46%).

Altered timing and pattern of menstruation (91%).

Female breast enlargement and milk production.

Male breast enlargement and tenderness.

▷ **Adverse Effects That May Mimic Natural Diseases or Disorders**

Nervous system reactions may suggest Parkinson's disease.

Liver reactions may suggest viral hepatitis.

Reactions resembling systemic lupus erythematosus may occur.

Natural Diseases or Disorders That May Be Activated by This Drug

Latent epilepsy, glaucoma, prostatism (see Glossary).

CAUTION

1. Many over-the-counter medications (see OTC Drugs in Glossary) for allergies, colds and coughs contain drugs that can interact unfavorably with this drug. Ask your physician or pharmacist for guidance before using any such medications.
2. Antacids that contain aluminum and/or magnesium can prevent the absorption of this drug and reduce its effectiveness.
3. Obtain prompt evaluation of any change or disturbance of vision.

Precautions for Use

By Infants and Children: Do not use this drug in infants under 6 months of age, or in children of any age with symptoms suggestive of Reye syndrome (see Glossary). Monitor carefully for blood cell changes.

By Those over 60 Years of Age: Small doses are advisable until individual response has been determined. You may be more susceptible to the development of drowsiness, lethargy, constipation, lowering of body temperature (hypothermia) and orthostatic hypotension (see Glossary). This drug can enhance existing prostatism (see Glossary). You may also be more susceptible to the development of Parkinson-like reactions and/or tardive dyskinesia (see discussion of these terms in

Glossary). These reactions must be recognized early since they may become unresponsive to treatment and irreversible.

▷ **Advisability of Use During Pregnancy**
Pregnancy Category: C (tentative). See Pregnancy Code inside back cover.
Animal studies: Significant birth defects reported in mice.
Human studies: Information from adequate studies of pregnant women is not available.
Avoid drug during the first 3 months and during the last month because of possible effects on the newborn infant.

Advisability of Use if Breast-Feeding
Presence of this drug in breast milk: Unknown.
Avoid drug or refrain from nursing.

Habit-Forming Potential: None.

Effects of Overdosage: Marked drowsiness, weakness, tremor, agitation, unsteadiness, deep sleep, coma, convulsions.

Possible Effects of Long-Term Use: Tardive dyskinesia (see Glossary); eye changes—cataracts and pigmentation of retina; gray to violet pigmentation of skin in exposed areas, more common in women.

Suggested Periodic Examinations While Taking This Drug (at physician's discretion)
Complete blood cell counts, especially between the fourth and tenth weeks of treatment.
Liver function tests, electrocardiograms.
Complete eye examinations—eye structures and vision.
Careful inspection of the tongue for early evidence of fine, involuntary, wavelike movements that could indicate the beginning of tardive dyskinesia.

▷ **While Taking This Drug, Observe the Following**
Foods: No restrictions.
Beverages: No restrictions. May be taken with milk.
▷ *Alcohol:* Avoid completely. Alcohol can increase the sedative action of phenothiazines and accentuate their depressant effects on brain function and blood pressure. Phenothiazines can increase the intoxicating effects of alcohol.
Tobacco Smoking: Possible reduction of drowsiness from drug.
Marijuana Smoking: Moderate increase in drowsiness; accentuation of orthostatic hypotension; increased risk of precipitating latent psychoses, confusing the interpretation of mental status and drug responses.
▷ *Other Drugs*
Fluphenazine may ***increase*** the effects of
• all sedative drugs, and cause excessive sedation.
• all atropinelike drugs, and cause nervous system toxicity.

Fluphenazine may *decrease* the effects of
- guanethidine (Ismelin, Esimil), and reduce its effectiveness in lowering blood pressure.

Fluphenazine *taken concurrently* with
- beta blocker drugs (see Drug Class, Section Four) may cause increased effects of both drugs; monitor drug effects closely and adjust dosages as necessary.

The following drugs may *decrease* the effects of fluphenazine
- antacids containing aluminum and/or magnesium.
- benztropine (Cogentin).
- trihexyphenidyl (Artane).

▷ *Driving, Hazardous Activities:* This drug can impair mental alertness, judgment and physical coordination. Avoid hazardous activities.

Aviation Note: The use of this drug *is a disqualification* for piloting. Consult a designated Aviation Medical Examiner.

Exposure to Sun: Use caution until sensitivity has been determined. Some phenothiazines can cause photosensitivity (see Glossary).

Exposure to Heat: Use caution and avoid excessive heat as much as possible. This drug may impair the regulation of body temperature and increase the risk of heat stroke.

Exposure to Cold: Use caution and dress warmly. This drug can increase the risk of hypothermia in the elderly.

Discontinuation: After a period of long-term use, do not discontinue this drug suddenly. Gradual withdrawal over 2 to 3 weeks under physician supervision is recommended. Do not discontinue this drug without your physician's knowledge and approval. The relapse rate of schizophrenia after discontinuation is 50% to 60%.

FLURAZEPAM
(floor AZ e pam)

Introduced: 1970

Class: Hypnotic, benzodiazepines

Prescription: USA: Yes
 Canada: Yes

Controlled Drug: USA: C-IV*
 Canada: No

Available as Generic: USA: Yes
 Canada: No

Brand Names: ✦Apo-Flurazepam, Dalmane, Durapam, ✦Novoflupam, ✦Somnol, ✦Som-Pam

*See Schedules of Controlled Drugs inside back cover.

```
┌─────────────────────────────────────────────────────────────┐
│                    BENEFITS versus RISKS                    │
│                                                             │
│       Possible Benefits              Possible Risks         │
│  EFFECTIVE HYPNOTIC after 2      Habit-forming potential with│
│    weeks of continual use          long-term use           │
│  NO SUPPRESSION OF REM           Minor impairment of mental │
│    (RAPID EYE MOVEMENT)            functions ("hangover" effect)│
│    SLEEP                          Very rare jaundice        │
│  NO REM SLEEP REBOUND after      Very rare blood cell disorder│
│    discontinuation               Suppression of stage-4 sleep with│
│  Wide margin of safety with        reduced "quality" of sleep│
│    therapeutic doses                                        │
└─────────────────────────────────────────────────────────────┘
```

▷ **Principal Uses**

> *As a Single Drug Product:* This member of the benzodiazepine class of "minor tranquilizers" is used exclusively as a bedtime sedative to induce sleep.

How This Drug Works: It is thought that this drug produces calming effect by enhancing the action of the nerve transmitter gamma-aminobutyric acid (GABA), which in turn blocks the arousal of higher brain centers and helps to induce sleep.

Available Dosage Forms and Strengths
> Capsules — 15 mg, 30 mg

▷ **Usual Adult Dosage Range:**   15 to 30 mg at bedtime. Total daily dosage should not exceed 90 mg. **Note: Actual dosage and administration schedule must be determined by the physician for each patient individually.**

▷ **Dosing Instructions:**   May be taken on an empty stomach or with food or milk. The capsule may be opened for administration. Do not discontinue this drug abruptly if taken for more than 4 weeks.

Usual Duration of Use: Periods of 3 to 5 nights intermittently, repeated as needed with appropriate dosage adjustment. Avoid uninterrupted and prolonged use. The duration of use should not exceed 2 weeks without reappraisal of continued need.

▷ **This Drug Should Not Be Taken If**
- you have had an allergic reaction to it previously.
- you have acute narrow-angle glaucoma.

▷ **Inform Your Physician Before Taking This Drug If**
- you are allergic to any benzodiazepine drug (see Drug Class, Section Four).
- you have a history of alcoholism or drug abuse.
- you are pregnant or planning pregnancy.
- you have impaired liver or kidney function.

- you have a history of serious depression or mental disorder.
- you are taking other drugs with sedative effects.
- you have any of the following: asthma, emphysema, epilepsy, myasthenia gravis.

Possible Side-Effects (natural, expected and unavoidable drug actions)
   "Hangover" effects on arising: drowsiness, lethargy and unsteadiness.

▷ **Possible Adverse Effects** (unusual, unexpected and infrequent reactions)
   If any of the following develop, consult your physician promptly for guidance.
   Mild Adverse Effects
   Allergic Reactions: Skin rash, hives, burning eyes, swelling of tongue.
   Dizziness, fainting, blurred vision, double vision, slurred speech, nausea, indigestion.
   Serious Adverse Effects
   Allergic Reactions: Liver damage with jaundice (see Glossary).
   Idiosyncratic Reactions: Nervousness, talkativeness, irritability, apprehension, euphoria, excitement, hallucinations.
   Bone marrow depression—impaired production of white blood cells, fever, sore throat.

▷ **Possible Effects on Sexual Function:**   None reported.

▷ **Adverse Effects That May Mimic Natural Diseases or Disorders**
   Liver reaction with jaundice may suggest viral hepatitis.

CAUTION
   1. This drug should not be discontinued abruptly if it has been taken continually for more than 4 weeks.
   2. The concurrent use of some over-the-counter drug products that contain antihistamines (allergy and cold preparations, sleep aids) can cause excessive sedation in sensitive individuals.
   3. Regular nightly use of any hypnotic drug should be avoided.
   4. This drug is transformed by the liver into long-acting forms that can persist in the body for 24 hours or more. With continual use of this drug daily, these active drug forms accumulate and produce increasing sedation. If you experience a "hangover" effect, avoid hazardous activities (driving, etc.) and the use of alcohol.

Precautions for Use
   By Infants and Children: Safety and effectiveness for use by those under 15 years of age have not been established.
   By Those over 60 Years of Age: It is advisable to use smaller doses at longer intervals to avoid overdosage. Observe for the possible development of lethargy, indifference, fatigue, weakness, unsteadiness, disturbing dreams, nightmares and paradoxical reactions of excitement, agitation, anger, hostility and rage.

▷ **Advisability of Use During Pregnancy**
   Pregnancy Category: C (tentative). See Pregnancy Code inside back cover.
      Animal studies: No birth defects reported in rat and rabbit studies.
      Human studies: Information from adequate studies of pregnant women
         is not available.
      Frequent use in late pregnancy can cause the "floppy infant" syndrome
         in the newborn: weakness, lethargy, unresponsiveness, depressed
         breathing, low body temperature.
      Avoid use during entire pregnancy if possible. Ask physician for guid-
         ance.

Advisability of Use if Breast-Feeding
   Presence of this drug in breast milk: Probably yes.
   Avoid drug or refrain from nursing.

Habit-Forming Potential: This drug can produce psychological and/or
   physical dependence (see Glossary) if used in large doses for an extended period of time. Avoid continual use.

Effects of Overdosage: Marked drowsiness, weakness, feeling of drunkenness, staggering gait, tremor, stupor progressing to deep sleep or
   coma.

Possible Effects of Long-Term Use: Psychological and/or physical dependence, impaired liver function.

Suggested Periodic Examinations While Taking This Drug (at physician's
   discretion)
   Complete blood cell counts and liver function tests during long-term
   use.

▷ **While Taking This Drug, Observe the Following**
   Foods: No restrictions.
   Beverages: Avoid excessive intake of caffeine-containing beverages (coffee,
      tea, cola) within 4 hours of taking this drug. May be taken with milk.
▷ *Alcohol:* Use with extreme caution until the combined effect is deter-
      mined. Alcohol may increase the absorption of this drug and add to
      its depressant effects on the brain. It is advisable to avoid alcohol
      completely—throughout the day and night—if it is necessary to drive
      or to engage in any hazardous activity.
   Tobacco Smoking: Heavy smoking may reduce the hypnotic action of this
      drug.
   Marijuana Smoking: Increased sedation and significant impairment of in-
      tellectual and physical performance.
▷ *Other Drugs*
      Flurazepam may ***increase*** the effects of
      • digoxin (Lanoxin), and cause digoxin toxicity.
      • phenytoin (Dilantin), and cause phenytoin toxicity.
      Flurazepam may ***decrease*** the effects of

- levodopa (Sinemet, etc.), and reduce its effectiveness in treating Parkinson's disease.

The following drugs may **increase** the effects of flurazepam

- cimetidine (Tagamet).
- disulfiram (Antabuse).
- isoniazid (INH, Rifamate, etc.).
- oral contraceptives.
- valproic acid (Depakene).

The following drugs may **decrease** the effects of flurazepam

- rifampin (Rimactane, etc.).
- theophylline (aminophylline, Theo-Dur, etc.).

▷ *Driving, Hazardous Activities:* This drug can impair mental alertness, judgment, physical coordination and reaction time. Avoid hazardous activities accordingly.

Aviation Note: The use of this drug **is a disqualification** for piloting. Consult a designated Aviation Medical Examiner.

Exposure to Sun: No restrictions.

Exposure to Heat: Use caution until the effect of excessive perspiration is determined. Because of reduced urine volume, this drug may accumulate in the body and produce effects of overdosage.

Discontinuation: Avoid sudden discontinuation if this drug has been taken for over 4 weeks without interruption. Dosage should be tapered gradually to prevent a withdrawal syndrome that could include depression, confusion, hallucinations, tremor, seizures, muscle cramping, sweating and vomiting.

FLURBIPROFEN
(floor BI pro fen)

Introduced: 1977

Class: Mild analgesic, anti-inflammatory

Prescription: USA: Yes
Canada: Yes

Controlled Drug: USA: No
Canada: No

Available as Generic: USA: No
Canada: No

Brand Names: Ansaid, ✦Froben

BENEFITS versus RISKS	
Possible Benefits	***Possible Risks***
EFFECTIVE RELIEF OF SYMPTOMS ASSOCIATED WITH MAJOR TYPES OF ARTHRITIS	PEPTIC ULCER DISEASE (1% to 4%) with associated bleeding and perforation
Effective relief of symptoms associated with bursitis, tendinitis and related conditions	Liver toxicity with jaundice (less than 1%)
	Water retention
	Rare kidney toxicity
Effective relief of menstrual cramps	Rare aplastic anemia (see Glossary)

▷ **Principal Uses**

As a Single Drug Product: Used primarily to relieve the symptoms associated with (1) rheumatoid arthritis, osteoarthritis and ankylosing spondylitis; (2) bursitis, tendinitis, capsulitis and tenosynovitis; (3) painful menstruation.

How This Drug Works: Not completely established. It is thought that this drug reduces the tissue concentrations of prostaglandins (and related compounds), chemicals involved in the production of inflammation and pain.

Available Dosage Forms and Strengths

Tablets — 50 mg (Canada), 100 mg

▷ **Usual Adult Dosage Range:** Initially 100 to 200 mg/24 hours, in 2 to 4 divided doses. After a satisfactory response has been achieved, dosage should be reduced to the minimum that will sustain adequate relief. Total daily dosage should not exceed 300 mg. **Note: Actual dosage and administration schedule must be determined by the physician for each patient individually.**

▷ **Dosing Instructions:** Take either on an empty stomach or with food or milk if necessary to prevent stomach irritation. Take with a full glass of water and remain upright (do not lie down) for 15 to 30 minutes to prevent lodging of the tablet in the esophagus (food tube). The tablet may be crushed for administration.

Usual Duration of Use: Continual use on a regular schedule for 1 to 2 weeks is usually necessary to determine this drug's effectiveness in relieving the symptoms of arthritis, bursitis, etc. Severe arthritis may require continual use for 3 to 4 weeks to obtain maximal relief. Long-term use (months to years) requires periodic evaluation of response and dosage adjustment. Consult your physician on a regular basis.

▷ **This Drug Should Not Be Taken If**
- you have had an allergic reaction to it previously.
- you are subject to asthma or nasal polyps caused by aspirin.

- you have active peptic ulcer disease or any form of gastrointestinal bleeding.
- you have active liver disease.
- you have a bleeding disorder or a blood cell disorder.
- you have severe impairment of kidney function.

▷ **Inform Your Physician Before Taking This Drug If**
- you are allergic to aspirin or to other aspirin substitutes.
- you have a history of peptic ulcer disease or any type of bleeding disorder.
- you have a history of gout.
- you have impaired liver or kidney function.
- you have high blood pressure or a history of heart failure.
- you have systemic lupus erythematosus (SLE).
- you are taking any of the following drugs: acetaminophen, aspirin or other aspirin substitutes, anticoagulants, diuretics, insulin, lithium, methotrexate, oral antidiabetic drugs.

Possible Side-Effects (natural, expected and unavoidable drug actions)
Fluid retention (1%), increased blood uric acid levels.

▷ **Possible Adverse Effects** (unusual, unexpected and infrequent reactions)
If any of the following develop, consult your physician promptly for guidance.
Mild Adverse Effects
Allergic Reactions: Skin rash (1.4%), hives (0.1%), itching (0.6%).
Headache (1%), dizziness (1%), drowsiness, depression (0.1%), anxiety (0.1%), insomnia (0.3%), blurred vision (1.6%), double vision, reversible hearing loss, ear ringing (1.7%), altered taste (0.2%).
Mouth soreness (0.4%), stomach discomfort (4%), nausea (3.5%), vomiting (0.5%), indigestion (6.9%), constipation (2%), diarrhea (3.8%).
Serious Adverse Effects
Allergic Reactions: Severe skin reactions, eczema, bruising (0.1%), erythema multiforme, Stevens-Johnson syndrome, hair loss; swelling of lips, tongue, vocal cords; anaphylactoid reaction (see Glossary).
Drug-induced gastrointestinal ulceration, with bleeding and perforation (1% after 3 to 6 months of use, up to 4% after 1 year); colitis with bloody diarrhea.
Abnormally low red blood cell (0.3%), white blood cell and blood platelet counts; rare aplastic anemia (see Glossary).
Liver injury with jaundice (0.2%).
Kidney injury with significantly impaired function.

▷ **Possible Effects on Sexual Function:** None reported to date.

Possible Delayed Adverse Effects: Mild anemia due to "silent" blood loss from the stomach (less than that caused by aspirin).

▷ **Adverse Effects That May Mimic Natural Diseases or Disorders**
Liver reactions may suggest viral hepatitis.

▷ **Natural Diseases or Disorders That May Be Activated by This Drug**
Peptic ulcer disease, Crohn's disease, ulcerative colitis, gout, kidney failure associated with systemic lupus erythematosus.

CAUTION
1. Dosage should always be limited to the smallest amount that produces reasonable improvement.
2. This drug may mask early indications of infection. Inform your physician if you think you are developing an infection of any kind.
3. Observe for a pattern of symptoms that may indicate the development of liver toxicity: fatigue, lethargy, "flulike" symptoms, nausea, itching, tenderness under the right rib cage, jaundice (see Glossary). Report such symptoms promptly.
4. Observe for possible drug-induced bleeding in the gastrointestinal tract: bloody (reddish) or tarry (black) stools.

Precautions for Use
By Infants and Children: Safety and effectiveness for use by those under 12 years of age have not been established.
By Those over 60 Years of Age: Small doses are advisable initially until tolerance is determined. Observe for any indications of liver or kidney toxicity, fluid retention, dizziness, confusion, impaired memory, stomach bleeding or constipation.

▷ **Advisability of Use During Pregnancy**
Pregnancy Category: B (tentative). See Pregnancy Code inside back cover.
Animal studies: Mouse, rat and rabbit studies reveal no birth defects due to this drug.
Human studies: Information from adequate studies of pregnant women is not available.
The manufacturer does not recommend the use of this drug during pregnancy.

Advisability of Use if Breast-Feeding
Presence of this drug in breast milk: Unknown.
Avoid drug or refrain from nursing.

Habit-Forming Potential: None.

Effects of Overdosage: Probable drowsiness, dizziness, ear ringing, nausea, vomiting, diarrhea, confusion, unsteadiness, stupor.

Possible Effects of Long-Term Use: Secondary anemia (chronic blood loss from stomach), fluid retention, elevated blood pressure.

Suggested Periodic Examinations While Taking This Drug (at physician's discretion)
Complete blood cell counts; liver function tests within the first 8 weeks of use and periodically thereafter; kidney function tests.
Complete eye examinations if vision is altered in any way.

▷ **While Taking This Drug, Observe the Following**

Foods: No restrictions.

Nutritional Support: Supplemental iron if anemia develops.

Beverages: No restrictions. May be taken with milk.

▷ *Alcohol:* Use sparingly and with caution. The irritant action of alcohol on the stomach lining, added to the irritant action of this drug in sensitive individuals, can increase the risk of stomach ulceration and/or bleeding.

Tobacco Smoking: No interactions expected.

▷ *Other Drugs*

Flurbiprofen may ***increase*** the effects of

- acetaminophen (Tylenol, etc.), and increase the risk of liver or kidney damage; avoid prolonged use of this combination.
- anticoagulants (Coumadin, etc.), and increase the risk of bleeding; monitor prothrombin and bleeding times, adjust dose accordingly.
- oral antidiabetic drugs, and alter control of blood sugar levels unpredictably.
- aspirin, and increase the risk of stomach ulceration and/or bleeding; avoid this combination.

Flurbiprofen may ***decrease*** the effects of

- amiloride (Midamor, Moduretic).
- bumetanide (Bumex).
- chlorthalidone (Hygroton, etc.).
- ethacrynic acid (Edecrin).
- furosemide (Lasix).
- indapamide (Lozol).
- metolazone (Diulo, Zaroxolyn).
- spironolactone (Aldactone, Aldactazide).
- thiazide diuretics (see Drug Class, Section Four).
- triamterene (Dyazide, Maxzide).

Flurbiprofen ***taken concurrently*** with the following drugs may increase the risk of bleeding (antiplatelet effect); monitor these combinations closely:

- aspirin.
- colchicine (ColBenemid, etc.).
- dipyridamole (Persantine).
- indomethacin (Indocin).
- sulfinpyrazone (Anturane).
- valproic acid (Depakene).

Flurbiprofen ***taken concurrently*** with the following drugs may increase their toxicity; monitor these combinations closely:

- lithium (Lithane, etc.).
- methotrexate (Folex, Mexate).

The following drug may ***increase*** the effects of flurbiprofen

- probenecid (Benemid), by slowing its elimination.

▷ *Driving, Hazardous Activities:* This drug may cause dizziness, drowsiness or blurred vision. Restrict activities as necessary.

Aviation Note: The use of this drug **may be a disqualification** for piloting. Consult a designated Aviation Medical Examiner.

Exposure to Sun: Use caution until sensitivity is determined. Photosensitivity (see Glossary) has been reported.

FUROSEMIDE
(fur OH se mide)

Introduced: 1964

Class: Antihypertensive, diuretic

Prescription: USA: Yes
 Canada: Yes

Controlled Drug: USA: No
 Canada: No

Available as Generic: USA: Yes
 Canada: Yes

Brand Names: ✦Apo-Furosemide, ✦Furoside, Lasix, ✦Novosemide, ✦Uritol

BENEFITS versus RISKS	
Possible Benefits	*Possible Risks*
PROMPT, EFFECTIVE, RELIABLE DIURETIC	WATER AND ELECTROLYTE DEPLETION with excessive use
MODEST ANTIHYPERTENSIVE IN MILD TO MODERATE HYPERTENSION	Excessive potassium loss
	Increased blood sugar level
	Increased blood uric acid level
ENHANCES EFFECTIVENESS OF OTHER ANTIHYPERTENSIVES	Decreased blood calcium level
	Rare liver damage
	Rare blood cell disorder

▷ **Principal Uses**

As a Single Drug Product: This powerful diuretic is used primarily to increase the volume of urine and thereby relieve the body of excessive water retention (edema) that is commonly associated with congestive heart failure and some forms of liver disease and kidney disease. It is also used in the treatment of high blood pressure, but usually in conjunction with other antihypertensive drugs. A less frequent use is to increase the amount of calcium excreted the urine when the blood level of calcium is abnormally high.

How This Drug Works: By increasing the elimination of salt and water from the body (through increased urine production), this drug reduces the volume of fluid in the blood and body tissues and lowers the sodium content throughout the body. These changes contribute to lowering blood pressure.

Available Dosage Forms and Strengths
    Injection — 10 mg per ml
    Solution — 10 mg per ml, 40 mg per 5-ml teaspoonful
    Tablets — 20 mg, 40 mg, 80 mg

▷ **Usual Adult Dosage Range:** As antihypertensive: 40 mg/12 hours initially; increase dose as needed and tolerated. As diuretic: 20 to 80 mg in a single dose initially; if necessary, increase the dose by 20 to 40 mg/ 6 to 8 hours. The smallest effective dose should be determined. The total daily dose should not exceed 600 mg. **Note: Actual dosage and administration schedule must be determined by the physician for each patient individually.**

▷ **Dosing Instructions:** May be taken with or following meals to reduce stomach irritation. Best taken in the morning to avoid nighttime urination. The tablet may be crushed for administration.

Usual Duration of Use: Continual use on a regular schedule for 2 to 3 weeks is usually necessary to determine this drug's effectiveness in lowering high blood pressure. Long-term use (months to years) requires periodic evaluation of response and possible dosage adjustment. Use as a diuretic should be intermittent with "drug holidays" (no drug taken) to reduce the risk of sodium and potassium imbalance. Consult your physician on a regular basis.

▷ **This Drug Should Not Be Taken If**
    • you have had an allergic reaction to any dosage form of it previously.

▷ **Inform Your Physician Before Taking This Drug If**
    • you are allergic to any form of "sulfa" drug.
    • you are pregnant or planning pregnancy.
    • you have a history of kidney or liver disease.
    • you have diabetes, gout or lupus erythematosus.
    • you are taking any form of cortisone, digitalis, oral antidiabetic drug or insulin.
    • you plan to have surgery under general anesthesia in the near future.

Possible Side-Effects (natural, expected and unavoidable drug actions)
    Light-headedness on arising from sitting or lying position (see Orthostatic Hypotension in Glossary).
    Increase in blood sugar level, affecting control of diabetes.
    Increase in blood uric acid level, affecting control of gout.
    Decrease in blood potassium level, causing muscle weakness and cramping.

▷ **Possible Adverse Effects** (unusual, unexpected and infrequent reactions)
    If any of the following develop, consult your physician promptly for guidance.

Mild Adverse Effects

Allergic Reactions: Skin rashes, hives, drug fever.

Headache, dizziness, blurred or yellow vision, ringing in ears, numbness and tingling.

Reduced appetite, indigestion, nausea, vomiting, diarrhea.

Serious Adverse Effects

Allergic Reactions: Hepatitis with jaundice (see Glossary), anaphylactic reaction (see Glossary), severe skin reactions.

Idiosyncratic Reaction: Fluid accumulation in lungs.

Temporary hearing loss.

Inflammation of the pancreas—severe abdominal pain.

Bone marrow depression (see Glossary)—fatigue, weakness, fever, sore throat, abnormal bleeding or bruising.

▷ **Possible Effects on Sexual Function:** Impotence (5%) using recommended dosage of 20 to 80 mg/day.

▷ **Adverse Effects That May Mimic Natural Diseases or Disorders**

Liver reaction may suggest viral hepatitis.

Natural Diseases or Disorders That May Be Activated by This Drug

Diabetes, gout, systemic lupus erythematosus.

CAUTION

1. Do not exceed recommended doses. Increased dosage can cause excessive loss of sodium and potassium, with resultant loss of appetite, nausea, fatigue, weakness, confusion and tingling in the extremities.

2. If you are also taking a digitalis preparation (digitoxin, digoxin), ensure an adequate intake of high-potassium foods to prevent potassium deficiency—a potential cause of digitalis toxicity. (See Table of High Potassium Foods in Section Six.)

Precautions for Use

By Infants and Children: Avoid overdosage that could cause serious dehydration. Significant potassium loss can occur within the first 2 weeks of drug use.

By Those over 60 Years of Age: Small doses are advisable until your individual response has been determined. You may be more susceptible to the development of impaired thinking, orthostatic hypotension, potassium loss and blood sugar increase. Overdosage and extended use of this drug can cause excessive loss of body water, thickening (increased viscosity) of the blood and an increased tendency for the blood to clot—predisposing to stroke, heart attack or thrombophlebitis (vein inflammation with blood clot).

▷ **Advisability of Use During Pregnancy**

Pregnancy Category: C (tentative). See Pregnancy Code inside back cover.

Animal studies: Significant birth defects have been reported.

Human studies: Information from adequate studies of pregnant women is not available.

It should not be used during pregnancy unless a very serious complication occurs for which this drug is significantly beneficial. Avoid completely during the first 3 months. Ask physician for guidance.

Advisability of Use if Breast-Feeding
Presence of this drug in breast milk: Yes.
Avoid drug or refrain from nursing.

Habit-Forming Potential: None.

Effects of Overdosage: Dry mouth, thirst, lethargy, weakness, muscle cramping, nausea, vomiting, drowsiness progressing to stupor or coma.

Possible Effects of Long-Term Use: Impaired balance of water, salt and potassium in blood and body tissues; dehydration and increased blood coagulability, with predisposition to thromboembolic disorders. Development of diabetes in predisposed individuals.

Suggested Periodic Examinations While Taking This Drug (at physician's discretion)
Complete blood cell counts, measurements of blood levels of sodium, potassium, chloride, sugar and uric acid.
Kidney and liver function tests.

▷ **While Taking This Drug, Observe the Following**
Foods: Consult your physician regarding the advisability of eating foods rich in potassium. If so advised, see the Table of High Potassium Foods in Section Six. Follow physician's advice regarding the use of salt.
Beverages: No restrictions. This drug may be taken with milk.
▷ *Alcohol:* Use with caution until the combined effects have been determined. Alcohol may exaggerate the blood-pressure-lowering effects of this drug and cause orthostatic hypotension.
Tobacco Smoking: No interactions expected. Follow physician's advice.
▷ *Other Drugs*
Furosemide may ***increase*** the effects of
- other antihypertensive drugs; dosage adjustments may be necessary to prevent excessive lowering of blood pressure.
- lithium, and cause lithium toxicity.

Furosemide may ***decrease*** the effects of
- oral antidiabetic drugs (sulfonylureas); dosage adjustments may be necessary for proper control of blood sugar.

Furosemide ***taken concurrently*** with
- digitalis preparations (digitoxin, digoxin) requires very careful monitoring and dosage adjustments to prevent fluctuations of blood potassium levels and serious disturbances of heart rhythm.

The following drug may **decrease** the effects of furosemide
- indomethacin (Indocin).

▷ *Driving, Hazardous Activities:* Use caution until the possible occurrence of orthostatic hypotension, dizziness or impaired vision has been determined.

Aviation Note: The use of this drug **may be a disqualification** for piloting. Consult a designated Aviation Medical Examiner.

Exposure to Sun: Use caution until sensitivity has been determined. This drug may cause photosensitivity (see Glossary).

Exposure to Heat: Avoid excessive perspiring, which could cause additional loss of salt and water from the body.

Heavy Exercise or Exertion: Avoid exertion that produces light-headedness, excessive fatigue or muscle cramping. Isometric exercises—the "overload" technique for strengthening individual muscles—can raise blood pressure significantly. Ask physician for guidance regarding participation in this form of exercise.

Occurrence of Unrelated Illness: Illnesses that cause vomiting or diarrhea can produce a serious imbalance of important body chemistry. Consult your physician for guidance.

Discontinuation: It may be advisable to discontinue this drug 5 to 7 days before major surgery. Ask your physician, surgeon and/or anesthesiologist for guidance regarding dosage adjustment or drug withdrawal.

GEMFIBROZIL
(jem FI broh zil)

Introduced: 1976

Prescription: USA: Yes
Canada: Yes

Available as Generic: USA: No
Canada: No

Brand Name: Lopid

Class: Anticholesterol

Controlled Drug: USA: No
Canada: No

BENEFITS versus RISKS	
Possible Benefits	*Possible Risks*
EFFECTIVE REDUCTION OF TRIGLYCERIDE BLOOD LEVELS AND ELEVATION OF HIGH DENSITY (HDL) CHOLESTEROL BLOOD LEVELS (40% to 50% reduction of triglycerides; 25% to 30% elevation of HDL cholesterol)	May elevate total cholesterol levels in one third of users Gallstone formation with long-term use Increased susceptibility to viral and bacterial infections

▷ **Principal Uses**

As a Single Drug Product: Used primarily to reduce abnormally high blood levels of triglycerides in Types IV and V blood lipid (fat) disorders. Its use is recommended as an adjunct to appropriate dietary adjustment in those individuals who are considered to be at high risk for developing coronary artery heart disease.

How This Drug Works: Not completely known. It is thought that this drug reduces blood levels of triglycerides by inhibiting their production in the liver. It addition, it may hasten removal of cholesterol from the liver and increase its excretion in the stool.

Available Dosage Forms and Strengths

Capsules — 300 mg
Tablets — 600 mg

▷ **Usual Adult Dosage Range:**   900 mg to 1500 mg daily in 2 divided doses. The average dose is 1200 mg/24 hours. Dose increases should be made gradually over a period of 2 to 3 months. **Note: Actual dosage and administration schedule must be determined by the physician for each patient individually.**

▷ **Dosing Instructions:**   Take 30 minutes before the morning and evening meals. The capsule may be opened for administration.

Usual Duration of Use: Continual use on a regular schedule for 4 to 8 weeks is usually necessary to determine this drug's effectiveness in reducing blood levels of triglycerides. Long-term use (months to years) requires periodic evaluation of response and dosage adjustment. Consult your physician on a regular basis.

Currently a "Drug of Choice" for initiating treatment of elevated LDL cholesterol and VLDL triglycerides. See Cholesterol Disorders in Section Two.

▷ **This Drug Should Not Be Taken If**
- you have had an allergic reaction to it previously.
- you have biliary cirrhosis of the liver.

▷ **Inform Your Physician Before Taking This Drug If**
- you have impaired liver or kidney function.
- you have gallbladder disease or gallstones.

Possible Side-Effects (natural, expected and unavoidable drug actions)
Moderate increase in blood sugar levels.

▷ **Possible Adverse Effects** (unusual, unexpected and infrequent reactions)
If any of the following develop, consult your physician promptly for guidance.
Mild Adverse Effects
Allergic Reactions: Skin rash, hives, itching.
Headache, dizziness, blurred vision, fatigue, muscle aches and cramps.

Indigestion, excessive gas, stomach discomfort (6%), nausea (4%), vomiting (1.6%), diarrhea (5%).

Serious Adverse Effects

Abnormally low white blood cell count: fever, chills, sore throat.

Formation of gallstones with long-term use.

▷ **Possible Effects on Sexual Function:**   Decreased libido.

Natural Diseases or Disorders That May Be Activated by This Drug

Latent diabetes, latent urinary tract infections.

CAUTION

1. This drug should be used only after nondrug methods (primarily diet) have been ineffective in lowering triglyceride levels.
2. If you used the drug clofibrate (Atromid-S) in the past, inform your physician fully regarding your experience.
3. Comply fully with all recommendations for periodic measurements of blood triglyceride and cholesterol levels. These are essential to the proper management of drug therapy for your disorder.

Precautions for Use

By Infants and Children: Safety and effectiveness for use by those under 12 years of age have not been established.

By Those over 60 Years of Age: Observe for any increased tendency to infection; treat all infections promptly.

▷ **Advisability of Use During Pregnancy**

Pregnancy Category: B (tentative). See Pregnancy Code inside back cover.

Animal studies: No significant birth defects found due to this drug.

Human studies: Information from adequate studies of pregnant women is not available.

Use only if clearly needed. Ask your physician for guidance.

Advisability of Use if Breast-Feeding

Presence of this drug in breast milk: Unknown.

Avoid drug or refrain from nursing.

Habit-Forming Potential: None.

Effects of Overdosage: Abdominal pain, nausea, vomiting, diarrhea.

Possible Effects of Long-Term Use: Formation of gallstones.

Suggested Periodic Examinations While Taking This Drug (at physician's discretion)

Complete blood cell counts.

Measurements of blood levels of total cholesterol, HDL and LDL cholesterol fractions, triglycerides and sugar.

Liver function tests.

▷ **While Taking This Drug, Observe the Following**

Foods: Follow the diet prescribed by your physician.

Beverages: No restrictions. May be taken with milk.

▷ *Alcohol:* No interactions expected.
  Tobacco Smoking: No interactions expected.
▷ *Other Drugs*
  Gemfibrozil may **increase** the effects of
  • warfarin (Coumadin), and increase the risk of bleeding; frequent pro-
    thrombin time measurements and dosage adjustments are necessary.
  Gemfibrozil may **decrease** the effects of
  • chenodiol (Chenix), and reduce its effectiveness in the treatment of
    gallstones.
▷ *Driving, Hazardous Activities:* This drug may cause dizziness and blurred
    vision. Restrict activities as necessary.
  Aviation Note: The use of this drug **is usually not a disqualification** for
    piloting. Consult a designated Aviation Medical Examiner.
  Exposure to Sun: No restrictions.
  Discontinuation: If adequate reduction of triglycerides does not occur
    after 3 months of treatment, this drug should be discontinued. Fol-
    lowing withdrawal, blood cholesterol and triglyceride will return to
    pretreatment levels.

GLIPIZIDE
(GLIP i zide)

Introduced: 1972

Prescription: USA: Yes

Available as Generic: No

Brand Name: Glucotrol

Class: Antidiabetic, sulfonylureas

Controlled Drug: USA: No

BENEFITS versus RISKS

Possible Benefits	*Possible Risks*
Assistance in regulating blood sugar in noninsulin-dependent diabetes (adjunctive to appropriate diet and weight control)	HYPOGLYCEMIA, severe and prolonged Allergic skin reactions (some severe) Water retention Rare liver damage Rare blood cell and bone marrow disorders

---

▷ **Principal Uses**
  As a Single Drug Product: To assist in the control of mild to moderately
    severe type II diabetes mellitus (adult, maturity-onset) that does not

require insulin, but that cannot be adequately controlled by diet alone.

How This Drug Works: It is thought that this drug (1) stimulates the secretion of insulin (by a pancreas that is capable of responding to stimulation), and (2) enhances the utilization of insulin by appropriate tissues.

Available Dosage Forms and Strengths
Tablets — 5 mg, 10 mg

▷ **Usual Adult Dosage Range:** Initially 5 mg daily with breakfast. At 7 day intervals, the dose may be increased by increments of 2.5 to 5 mg daily as needed and tolerated. Total daily dosage should not exceed 40 mg. A "loading" or priming dose is not necessary and should not be given. **Note: Actual dosage and administration schedule must be determined by the physician for each patient individually.**

▷ **Dosing Instructions:** If the daily maintenance dose is found to be 15 mg or more, the total dose should be divided into 2 equal doses: the first taken with the morning meal, the second with the evening meal. The tablet may be crushed for administration.

Usual Duration of Use: Continual use on a regular schedule for 1 to 2 weeks is usually necessary to determine this drug's effectiveness in controlling diabetes. Failure to respond to maximal doses within 1 month constitutes a primary failure. Up to 10% of those who respond initially may develop secondary failure of the drug later. The duration of effective use can only be determined by periodic measurement of the blood sugar. Consult your physician on a regular basis.

Possible Advantages of This Drug
Effective with once-daily dosing.
Onset of action within 30 minutes.
Near-normal insulin response to eating.
Well tolerated by the elderly diabetic.

Currently a "Drug of Choice" for initiating treatment in noninsulin-dependent diabetes when diet and weight control fail.

▷ **This Drug Should Not Be Taken If**
- you have had an allergic reaction to it previously.
- you have severe impairment of liver or kidney function.
- you are pregnant.

▷ **Inform Your Physician Before Taking This Drug If**
- you are allergic to other sulfonylurea drugs or to "sulfa" drugs.
- your diabetes has been unstable or "brittle" in the past.
- you do not know how to recognize or treat hypoglycemia (see Glossary).

- you have a history of congestive heart failure, peptic ulcer disease, cirrhosis of the liver, hypothyroidism or porphyria.

Possible Side-Effects (natural, expected and unavoidable drug actions)
> If drug dosage is excessive or food intake is delayed or inadequate, abnormally low blood sugar (hypoglycemia) will occur as a predictable drug effect.

▷ **Possible Adverse Effects** (unusual, unexpected and infrequent reactions)
> **If any of the following develop, consult your physician promptly for guidance.**

Mild Adverse Effects
Allergic Reactions: Skin rash, hives, itching.
Headache (1.25%), drowsiness (1.75%), dizziness (2.25%), fatigue (2.13%), sweating (1.25%).
Indigestion, nausea (1.38%), vomiting, diarrhea (1.25%).

Serious Adverse Effects
Allergic Reactions: Hepatitis with jaundice (see Glossary), severe skin reactions.
Idiosyncratic Reaction: Hemolytic anemia (see Glossary).
Disulfiramlike reaction with concurrent use of alcohol (see Glossary), infrequent with this drug.
Water retention (edema), weight gain.
Bone marrow depression (see Glossary)—fatigue, weakness, fever, sore throat, abnormal bleeding or bruising.

▷ **Possible Effects on Sexual Function:**   None reported.

▷ **Adverse Effects That May Mimic Natural Diseases or Disorders**
Liver reactions may suggest viral hepatitis.

CAUTION
1. This drug must be regarded as only one part of the total program for the management of your diabetes. It is not a substitute for a properly prescribed diet and regular exercise.
2. Over a period of time (usually several months), this drug may lose its effectiveness in controlling blood sugar levels. Periodic follow-up examinations are necessary to monitor all aspects of response to drug treatment.

Precautions for Use
By Infants and Children: This drug is not effective in type I (juvenile, growth-onset) insulin-dependent diabetes.
By Those over 60 Years of Age: This drug should be used with caution in this age group. Start treatment with 2.5 mg/day; increase dosage cautiously and monitor closely to prevent hypoglycemic reactions. Repeated episodes of hypoglycemia in the elderly can cause brain damage.

▷ **Advisability of Use During Pregnancy**
> *Pregnancy Category:* C (tentative). See Pregnancy Code inside back cover.
> Animal studies: No birth defects reported in rats and rabbits.
> Human studies: Information from adequate studies of pregnant women is not available.
> Because uncontrolled blood sugar levels during pregnancy are associated with a higher incidence of birth defects, many experts recommend that insulin (instead of an oral agent) be used as necessary to control diabetes during the entire pregnancy.

Advisability of Use if Breast-Feeding
> Presence of this drug in breast milk: Unknown.
> Avoid drug or refrain from nursing.

Habit-Forming Potential: None.

Effects of Overdosage: Symptoms of mild to severe hypoglycemia: headache, light-headedness, faintness, nervousness, confusion, tremor, sweating, heart palpitation, weakness, hunger, nausea, vomiting, stupor progressing to coma.

Possible Effects of Long-Term Use: Reduced function of the thyroid gland (hypothyroidism). Reports of increased frequency and severity of heart and blood vessel diseases associated with long-term use of this class of drugs are highly controversial and inconclusive. A direct cause-and-effect relationship (see Glossary) is tenuous. Ask your physician for guidance.

Suggested Periodic Examinations While Taking This Drug (at physician's discretion)
> Complete blood cell counts, liver function tests, thyroid function tests, periodic evaluation of heart and circulatory system.

▷ **While Taking This Drug, Observe the Following**
> *Foods:* Follow the diabetic diet prescribed by your physician.
> *Beverages:* As directed in the diabetic diet. May be taken with milk.
▷ *Alcohol:* Use with extreme caution until the combined effect has been determined. Alcohol can exaggerate this drug's hypoglycemic effect. This drug infrequently causes a marked intolerance of alcohol, resulting in a disulfiramlike reaction (see Glossary): facial flushing, sweating, palpitation.
> *Tobacco Smoking:* No interactions expected.
▷ *Other Drugs*
> The following drugs may ***increase*** the effects of glipizide
> - aspirin, and other salicylates.
> - cimetidine (Tagamet).
> - clofibrate (Atromid S).
> - fenfluramine (Pondimin).
> - monoamine oxidase (MAO) type A inhibitor drugs (see Drug Class, Section Four).

- phenylbutazone (Butazolidin).
- ranitidine (Zantac).

The following drugs may **decrease** the effects of glipizide

- beta blocker drugs (see Drug Class, Section Four).
- bumetanide (Bumex).
- diazoxide (Proglycem).
- ethacrynic acid (Edecrin).
- furosemide (Lasix).
- phenytoin (Dilantin).
- thiazide diuretics (see Drug Class, Section Four).

▷ *Driving, Hazardous Activities:* Regulate your dosage schedule, eating schedule and physical activities very carefully to prevent hypoglycemia. Be able to recognize the early symptoms of hypoglycemia so you can avoid hazardous activities and take corrective measures.

Aviation Note: Diabetes **is a disqualification** for piloting. Consult a designated Aviation Medical Examiner.

Exposure to Sun: Use caution until sensitivity has been determined. Some drugs of this class can cause photosensitivity (see Glossary).

Occurrence of Unrelated Illness: Acute infections, illnesses causing vomiting or diarrhea, serious injuries and surgical procedures can interfere with diabetic control and may require the use of insulin. If any of these conditions occur, consult your physician promptly.

Discontinuation: Because of the possibility of secondary failure, it is advisable to evaluate the continued benefit of this drug every 6 months.

GLYBURIDE
(GLI byoor ide)

Other Name: Glibenclamide

Introduced: 1970

Class: Antidiabetic, sulfonylureas

Prescription: USA: Yes
Canada: Yes

Controlled Drug: USA: No
Canada: No

Available as Generic: No

Brand Names: DiaBeta, ✦Euglucon, Micronase

BENEFITS versus RISKS	
Possible Benefits	*Possible Risks*
Assistance in regulating blood sugar in noninsulin-dependent diabetes (adjunctive to appropriate diet and weight control)	HYPOGLYCEMIA, severe and prolonged Allergic skin reactions (some severe) Rare liver damage Rare blood cell and bone marrow disorders

▷ **Principal Uses**
> *As a Single Drug Product:* To assist in the control of mild to moderately severe type II diabetes mellitus (adult, maturity-onset) that does not require insulin, but that cannot be adequately controlled by diet alone.

How This Drug Works: It is thought that this drug (1) stimulates the secretion of insulin (by a pancreas that is capable of responding to stimulation), and (2) enhances the utilization of insulin by appropriate tissues.

Available Dosage Forms and Strengths
> Tablets — 1.25 mg, 2.5 mg, 5 mg

▷ **Usual Adult Dosage Range:**   Initially 2.5 to 5 mg daily with breakfast. At 7-day intervals the dose may be increased by increments of 2.5 mg daily as needed and tolerated. Total daily dosage should not exceed 20 mg. A "loading" or priming dose is not necessary and should not be given. **Note: Actual dosage and administration schedule must be determined by the physician for each patient individually.**

▷ **Dosing Instructions:**   If the daily maintenance dose is found to be 10 mg or more, the total dose should be divided into 2 equal doses: the first taken with the morning meal, the second with the evening meal. The tablet may be crushed for administration.

Usual Duration of Use: Continual use on a regular schedule for 1 to 2 weeks is usually necessary to determine this drug's effectiveness in controlling diabetes. Failure to respond to maximal doses within 1 month constitutes a primary failure. Up to 10% of those who respond initially may develop secondary failure of the drug later. The duration of effective use can only be determined by periodic measurement of the blood sugar. Consult your physician on a regular basis.

▷ **This Drug Should Not Be Taken If**
- you have had an allergic reaction to it previously.
- you have severe impairment of liver and kidney function.
- you are pregnant.

▷ **Inform Your Physician Before Taking This Drug If**
- you are allergic to other sulfonylurea drugs or to "sulfa" drugs.
- your diabetes has been unstable or "brittle" in the past.
- you do not know how to recognize or treat hypoglycemia (see Glossary).
- you have a history of congestive heart failure, peptic ulcer disease, cirrhosis of the liver, hypothyroidism or porphyria.

Possible Side-Effects (natural, expected and unavoidable drug actions)
> If drug dosage is excessive or food intake is delayed or inadequate, abnormally low blood sugar (hypoglycemia) will occur as a predictable drug effect.

▷ **Possible Adverse Effects** (unusual, unexpected and infrequent reactions)
  If any of the following develop, consult your physician promptly for guidance.
  Mild Adverse Effects
  Allergic Reactions: Skin rash, hives, itching.
  Headache, drowsiness, dizziness, fatigue.
  Indigestion, heartburn, nausea.
  Serious Adverse Effects
  Allergic Reactions: Hepatitis with jaundice (see Glossary), severe skin reactions.
  Idiosyncratic Reaction: Hemolytic anemia (see Glossary).
  Disulfiramlike reaction with concurrent use of alcohol (see Glossary), infrequent with this drug.
  Bone marrow depression (see Glossary)—fatigue, weakness, fever, sore throat, abnormal bleeding or bruising.

▷ **Possible Effects on Sexual Function:**   None reported.

▷ **Adverse Effects That May Mimic Natural Diseases or Disorders**
  Liver reactions may suggest viral hepatitis.

CAUTION
  1. This drug must be regarded as only one part of the total program for the management of your diabetes. It is not a substitute for a properly prescribed diet and regular exercise.
  2. Over a period of time (usually several months), this drug may lose its effectiveness in controlling blood sugar levels. Periodic follow-up examinations are necessary to monitor all aspects of response to drug treatment.

Precautions for Use
  By Infants and Children: This drug is not effective in type I (juvenile, growth-onset) insulin-dependent diabetes.
  By Those over 60 Years of Age: This drug should be used with caution in this age group. Start treatment with 1.25 mg/day; increase dosage cautiously and monitor closely to prevent hypoglycemic reactions. Repeated episodes of hypoglycemia in the elderly can cause brain damage.

▷ **Advisability of Use During Pregnancy**
  Pregnancy Category: B (tentative). See Pregnancy Code inside back cover.
  Animal studies: No birth defects reported in rats and rabbits.
  Human studies: Information from adequate studies of pregnant women is not available.
  Because uncontrolled blood sugar levels during pregnancy are associated with a higher incidence of birth defects, many experts recommend that insulin (instead of an oral agent) be used as necessary to control diabetes during the entire pregnancy.

Advisability of Use if Breast-Feeding
Presence of this drug in breast milk: Unknown.
Avoid drug or refrain from nursing.

Habit-Forming Potential: None.

Effects of Overdosage: Symptoms of mild to severe hypoglycemia: headache, light-headedness, faintness, nervousness, confusion, tremor, sweating, heart palpitation, weakness, hunger, nausea, vomiting, stupor progressing to coma.

Possible Effects of Long-Term Use: Reduced function of the thyroid gland (hypothyroidism). Reports of increased frequency and severity of heart and blood vessel diseases associated with long-term use of this class of drugs are highly controversial and inconclusive. A direct cause-and-effect relationship (see Glossary) is tenuous. Ask your physician for guidance.

Suggested Periodic Examinations While Taking This Drug (at physician's discretion)
Complete blood cell counts, liver function tests, thyroid function tests, periodic evaluation of heart and circulatory system.

▷ **While Taking This Drug, Observe the Following**
Foods: Follow the diabetic diet prescribed by your physician.
Beverages: As directed in the diabetic diet. May be taken with milk.
▷   *Alcohol:* Use with extreme caution until the combined effect has been determined. Alcohol can exaggerate this drug's hypoglycemic effect. This drug infrequently causes a marked intolerance of alcohol, resulting in a disulfiramlike reaction (see Glossary): facial flushing, sweating, palpitation.
Tobacco Smoking: No interactions expected.
▷   *Other Drugs*
The following drugs may ***increase*** the effects of glyburide
• aspirin, and other salicylates.
• cimetidine (Tagamet).
• clofibrate (Atromid S).
• fenfluramine (Pondimin).
• monoamine oxidase (MAO) type A inhibitor drugs (see Drug Class, Section Four).
• phenylbutazone (Butazolidin).
• ranitidine (Zantac).
The following drugs may ***decrease*** the effects of glyburide
• beta blocker drugs (see Drug Class, Section Four).
• bumetanide (Bumex).
• diazoxide (Proglycem).
• ethacrynic acid (Edecrin).
• furosemide (Lasix).
• phenytoin (Dilantin).
• thiazide diuretics (see Drug Class, Section Four).

▷ *Driving, Hazardous Activities:* Regulate your dosage schedule, eating schedule and physical activities very carefully to prevent hypoglycemia. Be able to recognize the early symptoms of hypoglycemia so you can avoid hazardous activities and take corrective measures.

Aviation Note: Diabetes **is a disqualification** for piloting. Consult a designated Aviation Medical Examiner.

Exposure to Sun: Use caution until sensitivity has been determined. Some drugs of this class can cause photosensitivity (see Glossary).

Occurrence of Unrelated Illness: Acute infections, illnesses causing vomiting or diarrhea, serious injuries and surgical procedures can interfere with diabetic control and may require the use of insulin. If any of these conditions occur, consult your physician promptly.

Discontinuation: Because of the possibility of secondary failure, it is advisable to evaluate the continued benefit of this drug every 6 months.

GUANFACINE
(GWAHN fa seen)

Introduced: 1980

Class: Antihypertensive

Prescription: USA: Yes

Controlled Drug: USA: No

Available as Generic: USA: No

Brand Name: Tenex

BENEFITS versus RISKS	
Possible Benefits	*Possible Risks*
EFFECTIVE ANTIHYPERTENSIVE in mild to moderate high blood pressure	Amnesia, confusion, mental depression (3% or less)

▷ **Principal Uses**

As a Single Drug Product: This antihypertensive drug is often used as a "step 2" drug in the treatment of mild to moderate high blood pressure. It is generally not used to initiate treatment, but is added when a "step 1" drug proves to be inadequate. It may also be used as a "step 3 or 4" drug in place of drugs that cause marked orthostatic hypotension (see Glossary).

How This Drug Works: By decreasing the activity of the vasomotor center in the brain, this drug reduces the ability of the sympathetic nervous system to maintain the degree of blood vessel constriction responsible for the elevation of blood pressure. This change results in relaxation of blood vessel walls and lowering of blood pressure.

Available Dosage Forms and Strengths
Tablets — 1 mg

▷ **Usual Adult Dosage Range:** Initially 1 mg once daily taken at bedtime. The dose may be increased after 3 to 4 weeks to 2 mg daily, as needed and tolerated. If needed, the dose may be increased again after 3 to 4 weeks to 3 mg daily. The total daily requirement may be taken in 2 divided doses if necessary for stable blood pressure control. **Note: Actual dosage and administration schedule must be determined by the physician for each patient individually.**

▷ **Dosing Instructions:** Tablets may be taken without regard to eating. It is recommended that the daily dose be taken at bedtime to reduce the side-effect of daytime drowsiness. The tablet may be crushed for administration.

Usual Duration of Use: Continual use on a regular schedule for 4 to 6 weeks is usually necessary to determine this drug's effectiveness in controlling high blood pressure. Long-term use (months to years) requires supervision and guidance by the physician. Consult your physician on a regular basis.

▷ **This Drug Should Not Be Taken If**
- you have had an allergic reaction to it previously.

▷ **Inform Your Physician Before Taking This Drug If**
- you have a circulatory disorder of the brain.
- you have angina or coronary artery disease.
- you have or have had serious emotional depression.
- you have impaired liver or kidney function.
- you are taking any sedative or hypnotic drugs or an antidepressant.
- you plan to have surgery under general anesthesia in the near future.

Possible Side-Effects (natural, expected and unavoidable drug actions)
Drowsiness (21%), dry nose and mouth (30%), constipation (10%), decreased heart rate, mild orthostatic hypotension (see Glossary).

▷ **Possible Adverse Effects** (unusual, unexpected and infrequent reactions)
If any of the following develop, consult your physician promptly for guidance.
Mild Adverse Effects
Allergic Reactions: Skin rash, itching.
Headache (4%), dizziness (11%), fatigue (9%), insomnia (4%).
Indigestion, nausea, diarrhea.

Serious Adverse Effects
Amnesia, confusion, depression.

▷ **Possible Effects on Sexual Function:**   Decreased libido, impotence.

CAUTION
1. ***Do not discontinue this drug suddenly.*** Sudden withdrawal can produce anxiety, nervousness, tremors, fast or irregular heart action, nausea, stomach cramps, vomiting and rebound hypertension.
2. Hot weather and the fever associated with infection can reduce blood pressure significantly. Dosage adjustments may be necessary.
3. Report the development of any tendency to emotional depression.

Precautions for Use
By Infants and Children: Safety and effectiveness for use by those under 12 years of age have not been established.
By Those over 60 Years of Age: ***Proceed cautiously*** with the use of any antihypertensive drug. Unacceptably high blood pressure should be reduced without creating the risks associated with excessively low blood pressure. Start treatment with small doses and monitor the blood pressure response frequently. Observe for the development of light-headedness, dizziness, unsteadiness, fainting and falling. Sedation and dry mouth occur commonly in elderly users. Report promptly any changes in mood or behavior: depression, delusions, hallucinations.

▷ **Advisability of Use During Pregnancy**
Pregnancy Category: B (tentative). See Pregnancy Code inside back cover.
Animal studies: No birth defects due to this drug reported in rat and rabbit studies.
Human studies: Information from adequate studies of pregnant women is not available.
Use this drug only if clearly needed. Ask your physician for guidance.

Advisability of Use if Breast-Feeding
Presence of this drug in breast milk: Probably yes.
Avoid drug or refrain from nursing.

Habit-Forming Potential: None.

Effects of Overdosage: Marked drowsiness, weakness, dry mouth, slow pulse, low blood pressure, vomiting, stupor progressing to coma.

Possible Effects of Long-Term Use: Development of tolerance (see Glossary) with loss of drug effectiveness.

Suggested Periodic Examinations While Taking This Drug (at physician's discretion)
Blood pressure measurements.

▷ **While Taking This Drug, Observe the Following**

    Foods: Avoid excessive salt. Ask physician for guidance regarding degree of salt restriction.

    Beverages: No restrictions. May be taken with milk.

▷   *Alcohol:* Use with extreme caution. The combined effects can cause marked drowsiness and exaggerated reduction of blood pressure.

    Tobacco Smoking: No interactions expected. Follow your physician's advice regarding use of tobacco.

▷   *Other Drugs:* No significant drug interactions reported to date.

▷   *Driving, Hazardous Activities:* Use caution. This drug can cause drowsiness and can impair mental alertness, judgment and coordination.

    Aviation Note: Hypertension (high blood pressure) **is a disqualification** for piloting. Consult a designated Aviation Medical Examiner.

    Exposure to Sun: No restrictions.

    Exposure to Heat: Use caution. Hot environments may reduce the blood pressure significantly; be alert to the possibility of orthostatic hypotension (see Glossary).

    Heavy Exercise or Exertion: Use caution. Isometric exercises—the "overload" technique for strengthening individual muscles—can raise blood pressure significantly. The use of this drug may intensify the hypertensive response to isometric exercise. Ask physician for guidance.

    Occurrence of Unrelated Illness: Fever associated with infections may lower the blood pressure significantly. Repeated vomiting may prevent the regular use of this drug and result in an acute withdrawal reaction. Consult your physician.

    Discontinuation: **Do not discontinue this drug suddenly.** A significant withdrawal reaction can occur within 2 to 7 days after the last dose. The dose should be reduced gradually over 3 to 4 days, with periodic monitoring of the blood pressure.

HALOPERIDOL
(hal oh PER i dohl)

Introduced: 1958

Class: Strong tranquilizer, butyrophenones

Prescription: USA: Yes
Canada: Yes

Controlled Drug: USA: No
Canada: No

Available as Generic: USA: Yes
Canada: No

Brand Names: ✦Apo-Haloperidol, Haldol, ✦Haldol LA, Halperon, ✦Novoperidol, ✦Peridol

> **BENEFITS versus RISKS**
>
> | *Possible Benefits* | *Possible Risks* |
> |---|---|
> | EFFECTIVE CONTROL OF ACUTE FREQUENT PSYCHOSES in majority of patients: beneficial effects on thinking, mood and behavior | FREQUENT PARKINSON-LIKE SIDE-EFFECTS |
> | | SERIOUS TOXIC EFFECTS ON BRAIN with long-term use |
> | EFFECTIVE CONTROL OF SOME CASES OF TOURETTE'S DISORDER | Rare blood cell disorders |
> | | Abnormally low white blood cell count |
> | Beneficial in the management of the hyperactive child | |

▷ **Principal Uses**

As a Single Drug Product: Used primarily to control the psychotic thinking and abnormal behavior associated with acute psychosis of unknown nature, acute schizophrenia, paranoid states and the manic phase of manic-depressive disorders. It is also used to treat the hyperactivity syndrome in children. A less frequent use is to control the tics and offensive language characteristic of Gilles de la Tourette's syndrome.

How This Drug Works: Not completely established. It is thought that by interfering with the action of dopamine as nerve impulse transmitter in certain areas of the brain, this drug reduces anxiety and agitation, improves coherence and organization of thinking and abolishes delusions and hallucinations.

Available Dosage Forms and Strengths

Concentrate — 2 mg per ml
Injection — 5 mg per ml, 50 mg per ml
Tablets — 0.5 mg, 1 mg, 2 mg, 5 mg, 10 mg, 20 mg

▷ **Usual Adult Dosage Range:**   Initially 0.5 to 2 mg 2 or 3 times daily. Dose may be increased by 0.5 mg/day at 3- to 4-day intervals as needed and tolerated. The usual dosage range is 0.5 to 30 mg/24 hours. The total daily dosage should not exceed 100 mg. **Note: Actual dosage and administration schedule must be determined by the physician for each patient individually.**

▷ **Dosing Instructions:**   May be taken with or following food to reduce stomach irritation. The concentrate may be diluted in 2 ounces of water or fruit juice; do not add it to coffee or tea. The tablet may be crushed for administration.

Usual Duration of Use: Continual use on a regular schedule for several weeks is usually necessary to determine this drug's effectiveness in controlling the symptoms of psychotic or psychoneurotic behavior. If not significantly beneficial within 6 weeks, it should be discontinued.

Long-term use requires supervision and periodic evaluation by your physician. Consult your physician on a regular basis.

▷ **This Drug Should Not Be Taken If**
- you have had an allergic reaction to any dosage form of it previously.
- you are experiencing mental depression.
- you have any form of Parkinson's disease.
- you have cancer of the breast.
- you have active liver disease.
- you currently have a bone marrow or blood cell disorder.

▷ **Inform Your Physician Before Taking This Drug If**
- you are allergic or abnormally sensitive to phenothiazine drugs.
- you have a history of mental depression.
- you have any type of heart disease.
- you have impaired liver or kidney function.
- you have low blood pressure, epilepsy or glaucoma.
- you are taking any drugs with a sedative effect.
- you plan to have surgery under general or spinal anesthesia in the near future.

Possible Side-Effects (natural, expected and unavoidable drug actions)
Mild drowsiness, low blood pressure, blurred vision, dry mouth, constipation, marked and frequent Parkinson-like reactions (see Glossary).

▷ **Possible Adverse Effects** (unusual, unexpected and infrequent reactions)
If any of the following develop, consult your physician promptly for guidance.
Mild Adverse Effects
Allergic Reactions: Skin rash, hives.
Dizziness, weakness, agitation, insomnia.
Loss of appetite, indigestion, nausea, vomiting, diarrhea.
Urinary retention.
Serious Adverse Effects
Allergic Reactions: Rare liver reaction with jaundice, asthma, spasm of vocal cords.
Idiosyncratic Reactions: High fever, weakness, fast heart rate, muscle stiffness, seizures (rare neuroleptic malignant syndrome).
Depression, disorientation, eye damage (deposits in cornea, lens and retina).
Blood cell disorders: anemia, fluctuation in number of white blood cells.
Nervous system reactions: rigidity of extremities, tremors, restlessness, constant movement, facial grimacing, eye-rolling, spasm of neck muscles, tardive dyskinesia (see Glossary).

▷ **Possible Effects on Sexual Function**
Decreased libido; impotence (10% to 20%); painful ejaculation; priapism (see Glossary).

Male breast enlargement and tenderness; female breast enlargement with milk production.

Altered timing and pattern of menstruation.

▷ **Adverse Effects That May Mimic Natural Diseases or Disorders**

Liver reaction may suggest viral hepatitis.

Nervous system reactions may suggest Parkinson's disease or Reye syndrome.

Natural Diseases or Disorders That May Be Activated by This Drug

Latent epilepsy, glaucoma, diabetes.

CAUTION

1. It is advisable to use the smallest dose that is effective for long-term treatment.
2. Use with extreme caution in epilepsy; this drug can alter the pattern of seizures.
3. Individuals with lupus erythematosus and those taking prednisone are more susceptible to nervous system reactions.
4. Do not use levodopa to treat Parkinson-like reactions; it can cause agitation and worsening of the psychotic disorder.
5. Obtain prompt evaluation of any change or disturbance in vision.

Precautions for Use

By Infants and Children: This drug should not be used in children under 3 years of age or 15 kilograms in weight. Avoid this drug in the presence of symptoms suggestive of Reye syndrome. Children are quite susceptible to nervous system reactions induced by this drug.

By Those over 60 Years of Age: Initiate treatment with small doses. This drug can cause significant changes in mood and behavior; observe for confusion, disorientation, agitation, restlessness, aggression and paranoia. You may be more susceptible to the development of drowsiness, lethargy, orthostatic hypotension (see Glossary), hypothermia (see Glossary), Parkinson-like reactions and prostatism (see Glossary).

▷ **Advisability of Use During Pregnancy**

Pregnancy Category: C (tentative). See Pregnancy Code inside back cover.

Animal studies: Cleft palate reported in mouse studies.

Human studies: No increase in birth defects reported in 100 exposures. Information from adequate studies of pregnant women is not available.

Avoid during the first trimester. Use only if clearly needed. Ask physician for guidance.

Advisability of Use if Breast-Feeding

Presence of this drug in breast milk: Yes.

Monitor nursing infant closely and discontinue drug or nursing if adverse effects develop.

Habit-Forming Potential: None.

Effects of Overdosage: Marked drowsiness, weakness, tremor, unsteadiness, agitation, stupor, coma, convulsions.

Possible Effects of Long-Term Use: Eye damage: deposits in cornea, lens or retina; tardive dyskinesia (see Glossary).

Suggested Periodic Examinations While Taking This Drug (at physician's discretion)
Complete blood cell counts, liver function tests, eye examinations, electrocardiograms.
Careful inspection of the tongue for early evidence of fine, involuntary, wavelike movements that could indicate the beginning of tardive dyskinesia.

▷ **While Taking This Drug, Observe the Following**
Foods: No restrictions.
Beverages: No restrictions. May be taken with milk.
▷   *Alcohol:* Avoid completely. Alcohol can increase the sedative action of haloperidol and accentuate its depressant effects on brain function. Haloperidol can increase the intoxicating effects of alcohol.
Tobacco Smoking: No interactions expected.
Marijuana Smoking: Moderate increase in drowsiness; accentuation of orthostatic hypotension; increased risk of precipitating latent psychosis, confusing interpretation of mental status and of drug response.
▷   *Other Drugs*
Haloperidol may **increase** the effects of
• all drugs with sedative actions, and cause excessive sedation.
• some antihypertensive drugs, and cause excessive lowering of blood pressure; monitor the combined effects carefully.
Haloperidol may **decrease** the effects of
• guanethidine (Esimil, Ismelin), and reduce its antihypertensive effect.
Haloperidol **taken concurrently** with
• beta blocker drugs may cause excessive lowering of blood pressure.
• lithium may cause toxic effects on the brain and nervous system.
• methyldopa (Aldomet) may cause serious dementia.
The following drugs may **decrease** the effects of haloperidol
• antacids containing aluminum and/or magnesium may reduce its absorption.
• barbiturates.
• benztropine (Cogentin).
• phenytoin (Dilantin).
• trihexyphenidyl (Artane).
▷   *Driving, Hazardous Activities:* This drug may impair mental alertness, judgment and physical coordination. Restrict activities as necessary.
Aviation Note: The use of this drug **is a disqualification** for piloting. Consult a designated Aviation Medical Examiner.
Exposure to Sun: Use caution until sensitivity has been determined. This drug can cause photosensitivity.

Exposure to Heat: Use caution in hot environments. This drug may impair the regulation of body temperature and increase the risk of heat stroke.

Exposure to Cold: The elderly are advised to use caution; this drug can increase the risk of hypothermia (see Glossary).

Discontinuation: This drug should not be discontinued abruptly following long-term use. Gradual withdrawal over a period of 2 to 3 weeks is advised. Ask physician for guidance.

HYDRALAZINE
(hi DRAL a zeen)

Introduced: 1950

Prescription: USA: Yes
Canada: Yes

Available as Generic: USA: Yes
Canada: No

Class: Antihypertensive

Controlled Drug: USA: No
Canada: No

Brand Names: Alazine, Apresazide [CD], Apresoline, Apresoline-Esidrix [CD], Ser-Ap-Es [CD], Serpasil-Apresoline [CD], Unipres [CD]

BENEFITS versus RISKS

Possible Benefits	*Possible Risks*
EFFECTIVE STEP 2 OR 3 ANTIHYPERTENSIVE FOR MODERATE TO SEVERE HYPERTENSION when used adjunctively with other antihypertensive drugs Possibly beneficial in the management of severe congestive heart failure	DRUG-INDUCED LUPUS ERYTHEMATOSUS–LIKE SYNDROME (up to 13%) Intensification of angina pectoris Rare blood cell disorders Rare liver damage

---

▷ **Principal Uses**

As a Single Drug Product: Used primarily as a step 2 or antihypertensive drug in conjunction with other antihypertensives in the treatment of moderate to severe high blood pressure.

As a Combination Drug Product [CD]: This drug is available in combination with hydrochlorothiazide (a diuretic) and with reserpine (another type of antihypertensive). When used in combination, several different types of drug action occur concurrently to reduce blood pressure: hydralazine relaxes and expands blood vessel walls; the diuretic reduces the amount of water and sodium in the body; reserpine reduces the rate and contraction force of the heart and enhances the expansion of blood vessels.

How This Drug Works: By causing direct relaxation of arterial walls (mechanism unknown), this drug dilates peripheral blood vessels, with resultant lowering of blood pressure. The dilation of blood vessels can also be beneficial in some cases of heart failure by reducing the workload of the heart and increasing its output.

Available Dosage Forms and Strengths
Tablets — 10 mg, 25 mg, 50 mg, 100 mg

▷ **Usual Adult Dosage Range:** Initially 10 mg 4 times daily for 2 to 4 days; then increase to 25 mg 4 times daily for the balance of the first week. During the second week the dose may be increased to 50 mg 4 times daily if needed and tolerated. The total daily dosage should not exceed 300 mg for fast acetylators or 200 mg for slow acetylators. Ask your physician for guidance. **Note: Actual dosage and administration schedule must be determined by the physician for each patient individually.**

▷ **Dosing Instructions:** Preferably taken with or following meals to enhance absorption and reduce stomach irritation. The tablet may be crushed and the capsule [CD] may be opened for administration.

Usual Duration of Use: Continual use on a regular schedule for several weeks is usually necessary to determine this drug's effectiveness in lowering blood pressure. Long-term use requires supervision and periodic evaluation by your physician. Consult your physician on a regular basis.

▷ **This Drug Should Not Be Taken If**
- you have had an allergic reaction to it previously.
- you have active angina pectoris.
- you have mitral valvular heart disease.

▷ **Inform Your Physician Before Taking This Drug If**
- you have a history of any type of heart disease.
- you have lupus erythematosus.
- you have impaired brain circulation.
- you are subject to migraine headaches.
- you have impaired kidney function.
- you have a history of liver sensitivity to other drugs.
- you plan to have surgery under general anesthesia in the near future.

Possible Side-Effects (natural, expected and unavoidable drug actions)
Orthostatic hypotension (see Glossary), nasal congestion, constipation, delayed or impaired urination, increased heart rate of 10 to 25 beats/minute.

▷ **Possible Adverse Effects** (unusual, unexpected and infrequent reactions)
If any of the following develop, consult your physician promptly for guidance.

Mild Adverse Effects
Allergic Reactions: Skin rash, hives, itching, drug fever.
Headache, dizziness, flushing of face, palpitation.
Loss of appetite, nausea, vomiting, diarrhea.
Tremors, muscle cramps.

Serious Adverse Effects
Allergic Reactions: Liver reaction, with or without jaundice.
Idiosyncratic Reactions: Behavioral changes: nervousness, confusion, emotional depression. Bleeding into lung tissue: densities found on X-ray examination. A syndrome resembling rheumatoid arthritis or lupus erythematosus (see Glossary).
Intensification of coronary artery disease.
Peripheral neuropathy (see Glossary): weakness, numbness and/or pain in extremities.
Rare bone marrow depression (see Glossary): fatigue, weakness, fever, sore throat, abnormal bleeding or bruising.

▷ **Possible Effects on Sexual Function:**   Rare reports of impotence and priapism (see Glossary).

▷ **Adverse Effects That May Mimic Natural Diseases or Disorders**
Drug fever may suggest systemic infection. Liver reaction may suggest viral hepatitis. Skin and joint symptoms may suggest lupus erythematosus.

Natural Diseases or Disorders That May Be Activated by This Drug
Latent coronary artery disease.

CAUTION
1. Toxic reactions are more likely to occur with large doses. Adhere strictly to prescribed dosage schedules. Keep appointments for periodic follow-up examinations.
2. Report the development of any tendency to emotional depression.
3. This drug can cause salt and water retention if a diuretic is not taken concurrently.
4. This drug can provoke migraine headache.

Precautions for Use
By Infants and Children: Dosage is based upon age, weight and kidney function status. Observe for the possible development of a lupus erythematosus–like reaction.
By Those over 60 Years of Age: Initiate treatment with low doses and proceed cautiously. Unacceptably high blood pressure should be reduced without creating the risks associated with excessively low blood pressure. Sudden, rapid and excessive reduction of blood pressure can predispose to stroke or heart attack. Observe for possible dizziness, unsteadiness, fainting or falling. Headache, palpitation and rapid

heart rates are more common in the elderly and can mimic acute anxiety states.

▷ **Advisability of Use During Pregnancy**
Pregnancy Category: C (tentative). See Pregnancy Code inside back cover.
Animal studies: Birth defects of head and facial bones reported in mice.
Human studies: Information from adequate studies of pregnant women is not available.
Avoid use during the first and last 3 months; if taken late in pregnancy, this drug can cause a deficiency of blood platelets (see Glossary) in the newborn infant.

Advisability of Use if Breast-Feeding
Presence of this drug in breast milk: Yes.
Avoid drug or refrain from nursing.

Habit-Forming Potential: None.

Effects of Overdosage: Marked light-headedness, dizziness, headache, flushing of skin, nausea, vomiting, collapse of circulation: loss of consciousness, cold and sweaty skin, weak and rapid pulse, irregular heart rhythm.

Possible Effects of Long-Term Use: An acute or subacute syndrome resembling rheumatoid arthritis or lupus erythematosus, usually seen in slow acetylators taking daily doses of over 200 mg.

Suggested Periodic Examinations While Taking This Drug (at physician's discretion)
Complete blood cell counts, liver function tests, blood tests for evidence of lupus erythematosus.

▷ **While Taking This Drug, Observe the Following**
Foods: No restrictions.
Nutritional Support: Monitor for peripheral neuropathy and take a supplement of pyridoxine (vitamin B-6) as needed. Ask physician for guidance.
Beverages: No restrictions. May be taken with milk.
▷   *Alcohol:* Use with extreme caution until the combined effect has been determined. Alcohol can exaggerate the blood-pressure-lowering effect of this drug and cause excessive reduction.
Tobacco Smoking: Avoid completely. Nicotine can contribute significantly to this drug's ability to intensify angina in susceptible individuals.
▷   *Other Drugs*
Hydralazine may *increase* the effects of
• metoprolol (Lopressor).
• oxprenolol (Trasicor).
• propranolol (Inderal).
▷   *Driving, Hazardous Activities:* This drug may cause light-headedness or dizziness. Restrict activities as necessary.

Aviation Note: Hypertension and the use of this drug **are *disqualifications*** for piloting. Consult a designated Aviation Medical Examiner.

Exposure to Sun: No restrictions.

Exposure to Heat: Caution advised. Hot environments may reduce blood pressure significantly.

Exposure to Cold: Caution advised. Cold environments may increase this drug's ability to cause angina in susceptible individuals.

Heavy Exercise or Exertion: Caution advised. Excessive exertion can increase this drug's ability to cause angina in susceptible individuals. Also, isometric exercises can raise blood pressure significantly.

HYDROCHLOROTHIAZIDE
(hi droh klor oh THI a zide)

Introduced: 1959

Class: Antihypertensive, diuretic, thiazides

Prescription: USA: Yes
Canada: Yes

Controlled Drug: USA: No
Canada: No

Available as Generic: USA: Yes
Canada: Yes

Brand Names: Aldactazide [CD], Aldoril-15/25 [CD], Aldoril D30/D50 [CD], ✦Apo-Hydro, ✦Apo-Methazide [CD], ✦Apo-Triazide [CD], Apresazide [CD], Apresoline-Esidrix [CD], Capozide [CD], ✦Co-Betaloc [CD], ✦Diuchlor H, Dyazide [CD], Esidrix, Hydral [CD], HydroDIURIL, Hydropres [CD], Hydro-Z-50, Inderide [CD], Inderide LA [CD], ✦Ismelin-Esidrix [CD], Lopressor HCT [CD], Maxzide [CD], Maxzide-25 [CD], ✦Moduret [CD], Moduretic [CD], ✦Natrimax, ✦Neo-Codema, Normozide [CD], ✦Novodoparil [CD], ✦Novohydrazide, ✦Novospirozine [CD], ✦Novotriamzide [CD], Oretic, Oreticyl [CD], ✦PMS Dopazide [CD], Prinzide [CD], Ser-Ap-Es [CD], Serpasil-Esidrix [CD], Thiuretic, Timolide [CD], Trandate HCT [CD], Unipres [CD], ✦Urozide, Vaseretic [CD], ✦Viskazide [CD], Zestoretic [CD], Zide

BENEFITS versus RISKS	
Possible Benefits	*Possible Risks*
EFFECTIVE, WELL-TOLERATED DIURETIC	Loss of body potassium
POSSIBLY EFFECTIVE IN MILD HYPERTENSION	Increased blood sugar
ENHANCES EFFECTIVENESS OF OTHER ANTIHYPERTENSIVES	Increased blood uric acid
Beneficial in treatment of diabetes insipidus	Increased blood calcium
	Rare blood cell disorders

▷ **Principal Uses**

As a Single Drug Product: Thiazide diuretics are used primarily to (1) increase the volume of urine (diuresis) to correct the excessive fluid retention associated with congestive heart failure and certain types of liver and kidney disease; and (2) initiate treatment for high blood pressure (hypertension). They are often the first drugs tried in treating mild to moderate hypertension. Less frequent uses include the treatment of diabetes insipidus and the prevention of kidney stones that contain calcium.

As a Combination Drug Product [CD]: When this drug is used alone to treat hypertension, it is referred to as a "step 1" antihypertensive. Should it fail to reduce the blood pressure adequately, a "step 2" antihypertensive drug is added to be taken concurrently with the "step 1" drug. These drugs may be combined into one drug product. Thiazides are available in combination with beta blockers, hydralazine, methyldopa, reserpine and other diuretics to increase their effectiveness in treating hypertension.

How This Drug Works: By increasing the elimination of salt and water from the body (through increased urine production), this drug reduces the volume of fluid in the blood and body tissues and lowers the sodium content throughout the body. By relaxing the walls of smaller arteries and allowing them to expand, this drug increases the total capacity of the arterial system. The combined effect of these two actions (reduced blood volume in expanded space) results in lowering of the blood pressure.

Available Dosage Forms and Strengths

Solution — 50 mg per 5-ml teaspoonful
Solution, intensol — 100 mg per ml
Tablets — 25 mg, 50 mg, 100 mg

▷ **Usual Adult Dosage Range:**   As antihypertensive: 50 to 100 mg/day initially; 50 to 200 mg/day for maintenance. As diuretic: 50 to 200 mg/day initially; the smallest effective dose should be determined. The total daily dose should not exceed 200 mg. **Note: Actual dosage and administration schedule must be determined by the physician for each patient individually.**

▷ **Dosing Instructions:**   May be taken with or following meals to reduce stomach irritation. Best taken in the morning to avoid nighttime urination. The tablet may be crushed for administration.

Usual Duration of Use: Continual use on a regular schedule for 2 to 3 weeks is usually necessary to determine this drug's effectiveness in lowering high blood pressure. Long-term use (months to years) requires periodic evaluation of response and possible dosage adjustment. Use as a diuretic should be intermittent with "drug holidays" (no drug taken) to reduce the risk of sodium and potassium imbalance. Consult your physician on a regular basis.

▷ **This Drug Should Not Be Taken If**
- you have had an allergic reaction to any dosage form of it previously.

▷ **Inform Your Physician Before Taking This Drug If**
- you are allergic to any form of "sulfa" drug.
- you are pregnant or planning pregnancy.
- you have a history of kidney or liver disease.
- you have a history of pancreatitis.
- you have diabetes, gout or lupus erythematosus.
- you are taking any form of cortisone, digitalis, oral antidiabetic drug or insulin.
- you plan to have surgery under general anesthesia in the near future.

Possible Side-Effects (natural, expected and unavoidable drug actions)
Light-headedness on arising from sitting or lying position (see Orthostatic Hypotension in Glossary).
Increase in blood sugar level, affecting control of diabetes.
Increase in blood uric acid level, affecting control of gout.
Decrease in blood potassium level, causing muscle weakness and cramping.

▷ **Possible Adverse Effects** (unusual, unexpected and infrequent reactions)
If any of the following develop, consult your physician promptly for guidance.
Mild Adverse Effects
Allergic Reactions: Skin rashes, hives, drug fever.
Headache, dizziness, blurred or yellow vision.
Reduced appetite, indigestion, nausea, vomiting, diarrhea.
Serious Adverse Effects
Allergic Reactions: Hepatitis with jaundice (see Glossary), anaphylactic reaction (see Glossary), severe skin reactions.
Inflammation of the pancreas—severe abdominal pain.
Bone marrow depression (see Glossary)—fatigue, weakness, fever, sore throat, abnormal bleeding or bruising.

▷ **Possible Effects on Sexual Function:**   Decreased libido (12%); impotence (3%).

▷ **Adverse Effects That May Mimic Natural Diseases or Disorders**
Liver reaction may suggest viral hepatitis.

Natural Diseases or Disorders That May Be Activated by This Drug
Diabetes, gout, systemic lupus erythematosus.

CAUTION
1. Do not exceed recommended doses. Increased dosage can cause excessive loss of sodium and potassium, with resultant loss of appetite, nausea, fatigue, weakness, confusion and tingling in the extremities.
2. If you are also taking a digitalis preparation (digitoxin, digoxin), ensure an adequate intake of high-potassium foods to prevent po-

tassium deficiency—a potential cause of digitalis toxicity. (See Table of High Potassium Foods in Section Six.)

Precautions for Use

By Infants and Children: Avoid overdosage that could cause serious dehydration. Significant potassium loss can occur within the first 2 weeks of drug use.

By Those over 60 Years of Age: Small doses are advisable until your individual response has been determined. You may be more susceptible to the development of impaired thinking, orthostatic hypotension, potassium loss and blood sugar increase. Overdosage and extended use of this drug can cause excessive loss of body water, thickening (increased viscosity) of the blood and an increased tendency for the blood to clot—predisposing to stroke, heart attack or thrombophlebitis (vein inflammation with blood clot).

▷ **Advisability of Use During Pregnancy**

Pregnancy Category: D (tentative). See Pregnancy Code inside back cover. Animal studies: No birth defects found in rat studies.

Human studies: Reports are conflicting and inconclusive. This drug does not seem to carry the risk of birth defects that has been found with other related diuretics. However, other types of fetal injury are possible with this drug. It should not be used during pregnancy unless a very serious complication occurs for which this drug is significantly beneficial. Ask physician for guidance.

Advisability of Use if Breast-Feeding

Presence of this drug in breast milk: Yes.
Avoid drug or refrain from nursing.

Habit-Forming Potential: None.

Effects of Overdosage: Dry mouth, thirst, lethargy, weakness, muscle cramping, nausea, vomiting, drowsiness progressing to stupor or coma.

Possible Effects of Long-Term Use: Impaired balance of water, salt and potassium in blood and body tissues. Development of diabetes in predisposed individuals. Pathological changes in parathyroid glands with increased blood calcium levels and decreased blood phosphate levels.

Suggested Periodic Examinations While Taking This Drug (at physician's discretion)

Complete blood cell counts, measurements of blood levels of sodium, potassium, chloride, sugar and uric acid.
Kidney and liver function tests.

▷ **While Taking This Drug, Observe the Following**

Foods: Consult your physician regarding the advisability of eating foods rich in potassium. If so advised, see the Table of High Potassium

Foods in Section Six. Follow physician's advice regarding the use of salt.

Beverages: No restrictions. This drug may be taken with milk.

▷ *Alcohol:* Use with caution until the combined effects have been determined. Alcohol may exaggerate the blood-pressure-lowering effects of this drug and cause orthostatic hypotension.

Tobacco Smoking: No interactions expected. Follow physician's advice.

▷ *Other Drugs*

Hydrochlorothiazide may *increase* the effects of

- other antihypertensive drugs; dosage adjustments may be necessary to prevent excessive lowering of blood pressure.
- lithium, and cause lithium toxicity.

Hydrochlorothiazide may *decrease* the effects of

- oral antidiabetic drugs (sulfonylureas); dosage adjustments may be necessary for proper control of blood sugar.

Hydrochlorothiazide *taken concurrently* with

- digitalis preparations (digitoxin, digoxin) requires very careful monitoring and dosage adjustments to prevent fluctuations of blood potassium levels and serious disturbances of heart rhythm.

The following drugs may *decrease* the effects of hydrochlorothiazide

- cholestyramine (Cuemid, Questran) may interfere with its absorption.
- colestipol (Colestid) may interfere with its absorption.

Take cholestyramine and colestipol 1 hour before any oral diuretic.

▷ *Driving, Hazardous Activities:* Use caution until the possible occurrence of orthostatic hypotension, dizziness or impaired vision has been determined.

Aviation Note: The use of this drug *may be a disqualification* for piloting. Consult a designated Aviation Medical Examiner.

Exposure to Sun: Use caution until sensitivity has been determined. This drug can cause photosensitivity (see Glossary).

Exposure to Heat: Avoid excessive perspiring, which could cause additional loss of salt and water from the body.

Heavy Exercise or Exertion: Avoid exertion that produces light-headedness, excessive fatigue or muscle cramping. Isometric exercises—the "overload" technique for strengthening individual muscles—can raise blood pressure significantly. Ask physician for guidance regarding participation in this form of exercise.

Occurrence of Unrelated Illness: Illnesses that cause vomiting or diarrhea can produce a serious imbalance of important body chemistry. Consult your physician for guidance.

Discontinuation: This drug should not be stopped abruptly following longterm use; sudden discontinuation can cause serious thiazide-withdrawal fluid retention (edema). The dose should be reduced gradually. It may be advisable to discontinue this drug 5 to 7 days before major surgery. Ask your physician, surgeon and/or anesthesiologist for guidance regarding dosage adjustment or drug withdrawal.

HYDROCODONE
(hi droh KOH dohn)

Other Name: Dihydrocodeinone

Introduced: 1951

Class: Analgesic, narcotic; cough suppressant

Prescription: USA: Yes
Canada: Yes

Controlled Drug: USA: C-III*
Canada: <N>

Available as Generic: USA: Yes
Canada: No

Brand Names: Anexsia [CD], Anexsia 7.5 [CD], Azdone, ♦Biohisdex DHC [CD], ♦Biohisdine DHC [CD], Dimetane Expectorant-DC [CD], ♦Hycodan, Hycodan [CD], ♦Hycomine [CD], Hycomine Compound [CD], Hycomine Pediatric Syrup [CD], ♦Hycomine-S [CD], Hycomine Syrup [CD], Hycotuss Expectorant [CD], Lorcet Plus [CD], Lortab [CD], Lortab ASA [CD], ♦Novahistex DH [CD], ♦Novahistine DH [CD], ♦Robidone, Triaminic Expectorant DH [CD], Tussend [CD], Tussend Expectorant [CD], Tussionex [CD], Tycolet [CD], Vicodin [CD], Vicodin ES [CD], Zydone [CD]

BENEFITS versus RISKS

Possible Benefits	Possible Risks
EFFECTIVE RELIEF OF MILD TO MODERATE PAIN	Low potential for habit formation (dependence)
EFFECTIVE CONTROL OF COUGH	Mild allergic reactions (infrequent)
	Nausea, constipation

▷ **Principal Uses**

As a Single Drug Product: Used primarily to (1) control cough; (2) relieve mild to moderate pain. Its widest use is as an ingredient in cough remedies.

As a Combination Drug Product [CD]: Hydrocodone is frequently added to cough mixtures containing antihistamines, decongestants and expectorants to make these "shotgun" preparations more effective in reducing the frequency and severity of cough. It is also combined with milder analgesics, such as acetaminophen and aspirin, to enhance pain relief.

How This Drug Works: Acting primarily as a depressant of certain brain functions, this drug suppresses the perception of pain, calms the emotional response to pain and reduces the sensitivity of the cough reflex.

*See Schedules of Controlled Drugs inside back cover.

Available Dosage Forms and Strengths
Syrup — 5 mg per 5-ml teaspoonful
Tablets — 5 mg

▷ **Usual Adult Dosage Range:** As analgesic—5 to 10 mg/4 to 6 hours as needed. For cough—5 mg/4 to 6 hours as needed. Total daily dosage should not exceed 60 mg. **Note: Actual dosage and administration schedule must be determined by the physician for each patient individually.**

▷ **Dosing Instructions:** May be taken with or following food to reduce stomach irritation or nausea. Tablet may be crushed for administration.

Usual Duration of Use: As required, to control pain or cough. Continual use should not exceed 5 to 7 days without interruption and reassessment of need.

▷ **This Drug Should Not Be Taken If**
- you have had an allergic reaction to any dosage form of it previously.
- you are having an acute attack of asthma.

▷ **Inform Your Physician Before Taking This Drug If**
- you have had an unfavorable reaction to any narcotic drug in the past.
- you have a history of drug abuse or alcoholism.
- you have chronic lung disease with impaired breathing.
- you have impaired liver or kidney function.
- you have gallbladder disease, a seizure disorder or an underactive thyroid gland.
- you have difficulty emptying the urinary bladder.
- you are taking any other drugs that have a sedative effect.
- you plan to have surgery under general anesthesia in the near future.

Possible Side-Effects (natural, expected and unavoidable drug actions)
Drowsiness, light-headedness, dry mouth, urinary retention, constipation.

▷ **Possible Adverse Effects** (unusual, unexpected and infrequent reactions)
If any of the following develop, consult your physician promptly for guidance.
Mild Adverse Effects
Allergic Reactions: Skin rash, hives, itching.
Dizziness, impaired concentration, sensation of drunkenness, confusion, depression, blurred or double vision, facial flushing, sweating.
Nausea, vomiting.
Serious Adverse Effects
Allergic Reactions: Anaphylaxis (rare), severe skin reactions.
Idiosyncratic Reactions: Delirium, hallucinations, excitement, increased sensitivity to pain after the analgesic effect has worn off.
Seizures (rare), impaired breathing.

▷ **Possible Effects on Sexual Function:**   None reported.

▷ **Adverse Effects That May Mimic Natural Diseases or Disorders**
Paradoxical behavioral disturbances may suggest psychotic disorder.

CAUTION
1. If you have asthma, chronic bronchitis or emphysema, the excessive use of this drug may cause significant respiratory difficulty, thickening of bronchial secretions and suppression of coughing.
2. The concurrent use of this drug with atropinelike drugs can increase the risk of urinary retention and reduced intestinal function.
3. Do not take this drug following acute head injury.

Precautions for Use
By Infants and Children: Do not use this drug in children under 2 years of age because of their vulnerability to life-threatening respiratory depression.
By Those over 60 Years of Age: Use small doses initially and increase dosage as needed and tolerated. Limit use to short-term treatment only. There may be increased susceptibility to the development of drowsiness, dizziness, unsteadiness, falling, urinary retention and constipation (often leading to fecal impaction).

▷ **Advisability of Use During Pregnancy**
Pregnancy Category: C (tentative). See Pregnancy Code inside back cover.
Animal studies: Birth defects reported in hamster studies.
Human studies: Information from adequate studies of pregnant women is not available. Hydrocodone taken repeatedly during the last few weeks before delivery may cause withdrawal symptoms in the newborn infant.
Use this drug only if clearly needed and in small, infrequent doses.

Advisability of Use if Breast-Feeding
Presence of this drug in breast milk: Unknown.
Monitor nursing infant closely and discontinue drug or nursing if adverse effects develop. Ask physician for guidance.

Habit-Forming Potential: Psychological and/or physical dependence can develop with use of large doses for an extended period of time. However, true dependence is infrequent and unlikely with prudent use.

Effects of Overdosage: Drowsiness, restlessness, agitation, nausea, vomiting, dry mouth, vertigo, weakness, lethargy, stupor, coma, seizures.

Possible Effects of Long-Term Use: Psychological and physical dependence, chronic constipation.

Suggested Periodic Examinations While Taking This Drug (at physician's discretion)
None.

▷ **While Taking This Drug, Observe the Following**

Foods: No restrictions.

Beverages: No restrictions. May be taken with milk.

▷ *Alcohol:* Use extreme caution until the combined effects have been determined. Hydrocodone can intensify the intoxicating effects of alcohol, and alcohol can intensify the depressant effects of hydrocodone on brain function, breathing and circulation.

Tobacco Smoking: No interactions expected.

Marijuana Smoking: Increase in drowsiness and pain relief; impairment of mental and physical performance.

▷ *Other Drugs*

Hydrocodone may ***increase*** the effects of

• other drugs with sedative effects.

• atropinelike drugs, and increase the risk of constipation and urinary retention.

▷ *Driving, Hazardous Activities:* This drug can impair mental alertness, judgment, reaction time and physical coordination. Avoid hazardous activities accordingly.

Aviation Note: The use of this drug ***is a disqualification*** for piloting. Consult a designated Aviation Medical Examiner.

Exposure to Sun: No restrictions.

Discontinuation: It is advisable to limit this drug to short-term use. If it is necessary to use it for extended periods of time, discontinuation should be gradual to minimize possible effects of withdrawal (usually mild with this drug).

HYDROXYZINE
(hi DROX i zeen)

Introduced: 1953

Class: Mild tranquilizer, antihistamines

Prescription: USA: Yes
Canada: Yes

Controlled Drug: USA: No
Canada: No

Available as Generic: USA: Yes
Canada: No

Brand Names: ✦Apo-Hydroxyzine, Atarax, Marax [CD], Marax DF [CD], ✦Multipax, Vistaril, Vistrax [CD],

```
┌─────────────────────────────────────────────────────────────┐
│                  BENEFITS versus RISKS                        │
│                                                               │
│      Possible Benefits              Possible Risks            │
│  EFFECTIVE RELIEF OF          Mild atropinelike effects       │
│    ITCHING DUE TO HIVES       Potentiation of other sedative  │
│  Moderately effective relief of   drugs                       │
│    itching due to allergic skin   Impaired control of seizure │
│    disorders                        disorders (epilepsy)      │
│  Moderately effective relief of mild                          │
│    to moderate anxiety and                                    │
│    nervous tension                                            │
└─────────────────────────────────────────────────────────────┘
```

▷ **Principal Uses**

> *As a Single Drug Product:* Used primarily as a mild tranquilizer to relieve anxiety and nervous tension, whether occurring independently or in association with a physical disorder. Also used frequently to relieve itching due to allergic skin conditions.

> *As a Combination Drug Product* [CD]: Combined with antispasmodic drugs, this drug helps to allay the anxiety that is conducive to functional disorders of the gastrointestinal tract. Combined with ephedrine and theophylline (bronchodilator drugs), this drug controls the anxiety that is often associated with bronchial spasm in asthma, bronchitis and emphysema.

How This Drug Works: Not completely established. It is thought that this drug may reduce excessive activity in those brain systems that determine the emotional state.

Available Dosage Forms and Strengths

> Capsules — 25 mg, 50 mg, 100 mg
> Injection — 25 mg per ml, 50 mg per ml
> Oral suspension — 25 mg per 5-ml teaspoonful
> Syrup — 10 mg per 5-ml teaspoonful
> Tablets — 10 mg, 25 mg, 50 mg, 100 mg

▷ **Usual Adult Dosage Range:**   25 to 100 mg 3 or 4 times daily. The total daily dosage should not exceed 600 mg. **Note: Actual dosage and administration schedule must be determined by the physician for each patient individually.**

▷ **Dosing Instructions:**   May be taken without regard to eating. The tablet may be crushed and the capsule may be opened for administration.

Usual Duration of Use: Continual use on a regular schedule for 1 to 3 weeks is usually necessary to determine this drug's effectiveness in relieving anxiety and tension. Relief of itching is usually apparent in 2 to 3 days. Duration of use as a tranquilizer should not exceed 4 months without reappraisal of continued need. Consult your physician on a regular basis.

▷ **This Drug Should Not Be Taken If**
- you have had an allergic reaction to any dosage form of it previously.

▷ **Inform Your Physician Before Taking This Drug If**
- you have a seizure disorder (epilepsy).
- you have prostatism (see Glossary).
- you are taking any drugs with sedative effects.
- you plan to have surgery under general anesthesia in the near future.

Possible Side-Effects (natural, expected and unavoidable drug actions)
Drowsiness (may subside with continued use); "hangover" effect if taken at bedtime for sleep; dry mouth.

▷ **Possible Adverse Effects** (unusual, unexpected and infrequent reactions)
If any of the following develop, consult your physician promptly for guidance.
Mild Adverse Effects
Allergic Reaction: Itching.
Headache.
Serious Adverse Effects
Idiosyncratic Reactions: Involuntary movements, tremors, seizures (with excessive dosage).

▷ **Possible Effects on Sexual Function:**   None reported.

Natural Diseases or Disorders That May Be Activated by This Drug
Latent epilepsy.

CAUTION
1. This drug can cause excessive sedation if taken concurrently with other sedative drugs.
2. Use very cautiously if you have a seizure disorder. This drug may increase the frequency of seizures.
3. If pregnancy occurs, discontinue this drug immediately and inform your physician.

Precautions for Use
By Infants and Children: Observe for evidence of excessive sedation.
By Those over 60 Years of Age: There may be increased susceptibility to the development of drowsiness, dizziness and lethargy, and to impairment of thinking, judgment and memory. A pattern of underactivity may be misinterpreted as senility or emotional depression. Observe also for orthostatic hypotension and prostatism (see Glossary).

▷ **Advisability of Use During Pregnancy**
Pregnancy Category: C (tentative). See Pregnancy Code inside back cover.
Animal studies: Facial bone defects reported in mice, rats and dogs.
Human studies: Information from adequate studies of pregnant women is not available.
Avoid completely during the first 3 months. During the last 6 months, use only if clearly needed. Ask physician for guidance.

Advisability of Use if Breast-Feeding
Presence of this drug in breast milk: Yes.
Monitor nursing infant closely and discontinue drug or nursing if adverse effects (sedation, poor feeding) develop.

Habit-Forming Potential: None.

Effects of Overdosage: Drowsiness, unsteadiness, dry mouth, delirium, stupor, tremors, seizures.

Possible Effects of Long-Term Use: Loss of drug effectiveness due to development of tolerance (see Glossary).

Suggested Periodic Examinations While Taking This Drug (at physician's discretion)
None required.

▷ **While Taking This Drug, Observe the Following**
Foods: No restrictions.
Beverages: Avoid large amounts of caffeine-containing beverages: coffee, tea, cola, chocolate. May be taken with milk.
▷ *Alcohol:* Use with extreme caution until the combined effects have been determined. Alcohol can increase the sedative action of hydroxyzine. Hydroxyzine can increase the intoxicating effect of alcohol.
Tobacco Smoking: No interactions expected.
Marijuana Smoking: Increased sedative effects.
▷ *Other Drugs*
Hydroxyzine may ***increase*** the effects of
• ketamine (intravenous anesthetic), and prolong the recovery time.
• other drugs with sedative effects, and cause excessive sedation.
Hydroxyzine may ***decrease*** the effects of
• phenothiazines (see Drug Class, Section Four), and reduce their antipsychotic effectiveness.
▷ *Driving, Hazardous Activities:* This drug may impair mental alertness, judgment, coordination and reaction time. Restrict activities as necessary.
Aviation Note: The use of this drug ***is a disqualification*** for piloting. Consult a designated Aviation Medical Examiner.
Exposure to Sun: No restrictions.

IBUPROFEN
(i BYU proh fen)

Introduced: 1969	**Class:** Mild analgesic, anti-inflammatory
Prescription: USA: Varies Canada: Yes	**Controlled Drug:** USA: No Canada: No

Available as Generic: Yes

Brand Names: Advil, ♣Amersol, ♣Apo-Ibuprofen, Haltran, Ibu-Tab, Medipren, Motrin, ♣Novoprofen, Nuprin, Rufen

---

BENEFITS versus RISKS

Possible Benefits	*Possible Risks*
EFFECTIVE RELIEF OF MILD TO MODERATE PAIN AND INFLAMMATION	Gastrointestinal pain, ulceration, bleeding (rare) Rare kidney damage Rare fluid retention Rare bone marrow depression (less than 1%)

▷ **Principal Uses**

As a Single Drug Product: Used primarily to relieve mild to moderately severe pain associated with (1) musculoskeletal injuries; (2) acute and chronic gout, rheumatoid arthritis and osteoarthritis; (3) dental, obstetrical and orthopedic surgery; (4) menstrual cramps; (5) vascular (migrainelike) headaches; and (6) to reduce fever.

How This Drug Works: Not completely established. It is thought that this drug reduces the tissue concentrations of prostaglandins (and related compounds), chemicals involved in the production of inflammation and pain.

Available Dosage Forms and Strengths

Tablets — 200 mg, 300 mg, 400 mg, 600 mg, 800 mg

▷ **Usual Adult Dosage Range:**   200 to 800 mg 3 or 4 times/day. Total daily dosage should not exceed 3200 mg (3600 mg in selected individuals). **Note: Actual dosage and administration schedule must be determined by the physician for each patient individually.**

▷ **Dosing Instructions:**   Take either on an empty stomach or with food or milk to prevent stomach irritation. Take with a full glass of water and remain upright (do not lie down) for 30 minutes. The tablet may be crushed for administration.

Usual Duration of Use: Continual use on a regular schedule for 1 to 2 weeks is usually necessary to determine this drug's effectiveness in relieving the discomfort of arthritis. Long-term use requires supervision and periodic evaluation by the physician. Consult your physician on a regular basis.

▷ **This Drug Should Not Be Taken If**
- you have had an allergic reaction to it previously.
- you are subject to asthma or nasal polyps caused by aspirin.
- you have active peptic ulcer disease or any form of gastrointestinal bleeding.

- you have a bleeding disorder or a blood cell disorder.
- you have severe impairment of kidney function.

▷ **Inform Your Physician Before Taking This Drug If**
- you are allergic to aspirin or to other aspirin substitutes.
- you have a history of peptic ulcer disease or any type of bleeding disorder.
- you have impaired liver or kidney function.
- you have high blood pressure or a history of heart failure.
- you are taking any of the following: acetaminophen, aspirin or other aspirin substitutes, anticoagulants, oral antidiabetic drugs.

Possible Side-Effects (natural, expected and unavoidable drug actions)
Fluid retention (weight gain); pink, red, purple or rust coloration of urine (of no significance).

▷ **Possible Adverse Effects** (unusual, unexpected and infrequent reactions)
If any of the following develop, consult your physician promptly for guidance.

Mild Adverse Effects
Allergic Reactions: Skin rash, hives, itching.
Headache, dizziness, altered or blurred vision, ringing in the ears, depression.
Mouth sores, indigestion, nausea, vomiting, constipation, diarrhea.

Serious Adverse Effects
Allergic Reactions: Anaphylaxis (see Glossary), severe skin reactions.
Idiosyncratic Reactions: Drug-induced meningitis with fever and coma.
Active peptic ulcer, with or without bleeding.
Liver damage with jaundice (see Glossary).
Kidney damage with painful urination, bloody urine, reduced urine formation.
Rare bone marrow depression (see Glossary)—fatigue, weakness, fever, sore throat, abnormal bleeding or bruising.

▷ **Possible Effects on Sexual Function**
Altered timing and pattern of menstruation (30%); excessive menstrual bleeding.
Male breast enlargement and tenderness.

Possible Delayed Adverse Effects: Mild anemia due to "silent" blood loss from the stomach (less than that caused by aspirin).

▷ **Adverse Effects That May Mimic Natural Diseases or Disorders**
Liver reaction may suggest viral hepatitis.

Natural Diseases or Disorders That May Be Activated by This Drug
Peptic ulcer disease, ulcerative colitis.

CAUTION
1. Dosage should always be limited to the smallest amount that produces reasonable improvement.

2. This drug may mask early indications of infection. Inform your physician if you think you are developing an infection of any kind.

Precautions for Use
By Infants and Children: Safety and effectiveness for use by those under 12 years of age have not been established.

By Those over 60 Years of Age: Small doses are advisable until tolerance is determined. Observe for any indications of liver or kidney toxicity, fluid retention, dizziness, confusion, impaired memory, stomach bleeding or constipation.

▷ Advisability of Use During Pregnancy
Pregnancy Category: B (tentative). See Pregnancy Code inside back cover.
Animal studies: No birth defects reported in rats or rabbits.
Human studies: Information from adequate studies of pregnant women is not available.
Avoid this drug during the last 3 months. Use it during the first 6 months only if clearly needed. Ask physician for guidance.
The manufacturer does not recommend the use of this drug during pregnancy.

Advisability of Use if Breast-Feeding
Presence of this drug in breast milk: Yes, in minute amounts.
Avoid drug or refrain from nursing.

Habit-Forming Potential: None.

Effects of Overdosage: Drowsiness, dizziness, ringing in the ears, nausea, vomiting, diarrhea, confusion, unsteadiness, stupor progressing to coma.

Possible Effects of Long-Term Use: Fluid retention.

Suggested Periodic Examinations While Taking This Drug (at physician's discretion)
Complete blood cell counts, liver and kidney function tests, complete eye examinations if vision is altered in any way.

▷ While Taking This Drug, Observe the Following
Foods: No restrictions.
Beverages: No restrictions. May be taken with milk.
▷ *Alcohol:* Use with caution. The irritant action of alcohol on the stomach lining, added to the irritant action of this drug in sensitive individuals, can increase the risk of stomach ulceration and/or bleeding.
Tobacco Smoking: No interactions expected.
▷ *Other Drugs*
Ibuprofen may ***increase*** the effects of
- acetaminophen (Tylenol, etc.), and increase the risk of kidney damage; avoid prolonged use of this combination.
- anticoagulants (Coumadin, etc.), and increase the risk of bleeding; monitor prothrombin time, adjust dose accordingly.

Ibuprofen **taken concurrently** with the following drugs may increase the risk of bleeding; avoid these combinations:
- aspirin.
- dipyridamole (Persantine).
- indomethacin (Indocin).
- sulfinpyrazone (Anturane).
- valproic acid (Depakene).

▷ *Driving, Hazardous Activities:* This drug may cause drowsiness or dizziness. Restrict activities as necessary.

Aviation Note: The use of this drug **may be a disqualification** for piloting. Consult a designated Aviation Medical Examiner.

Exposure to Sun: Use caution until sensitivity is determined. Questionable photosensitivity (see Glossary) has been reported.

INDAPAMIDE
(in DAP a mide)

Introduced: 1974

Prescription: USA: Yes
Canada: Yes

Available as Generic: No

Brand Names: ✦Lozide, Lozol

Class: Antihypertensive, diuretic

Controlled Drug: USA: No
Canada: No

BENEFITS versus RISKS	
Possible Benefits	*Possible Risks*
EFFECTIVE ONCE-A-DAY TREATMENT OF MILD TO MODERATE HYPERTENSION	Excessive loss of blood potassium (14%)
EFFECTIVE, MILD DIURETIC	Increased blood sugar level
	Increased blood uric acid level

▷ **Principal Uses**

As a Single Drug Product: Used primarily to (1) increase the volume of urine (diuresis) to correct the excessive fluid retention associated with congestive heart failure; and (2) initiate treatment for high blood pressure (hypertension). It may be the first drug tried in treating mild to moderate hypertension.

How This Drug Works: By increasing the elimination of salt and water from the body (through increased urine production), this drug reduces the volume of fluid in the blood and body tissues and lowers the sodium content throughout the body. By relaxing the walls of smaller arteries and allowing them to expand, this drug increases the total capacity of the arterial system. The combined effect of these two actions (reduced blood volume in expanded space) results in lowering of blood pressure.

Available Dosage Forms and Strengths
Tablets — 2.5 mg

▷ **Usual Adult Dosage Range:**   Initially 2.5 mg/day, taken as a single dose in the morning. If necessary, the dose may be increased to 5 mg/day after 1 week (for diuresis) or after 4 weeks (for hypertension). The total daily dosage should not exceed 5 mg. (In Canada, the total daily dosage limit is given as 2.5 mg.) **Note: Actual dosage and administration schedule must be determined by the physician for each patient individually.**

▷ **Dosing Instructions:**   May be taken with or following food to reduce stomach irritation. Best taken in the morning to avoid nighttime urination. The tablet may be crushed for administration.

Usual Duration of Use: Continual use on a regular schedule for 2 to 4 weeks is usually necessary to determine this drug's effectiveness in lowering high blood pressure. Long-term use (months to years) requires periodic evaluation of response and possible dosage adjustment. Use as a diuretic should be intermittent with "drug holidays" (no drug taken) to reduce the risk of sodium and potassium imbalance. Consult your physician on a regular basis.

Possible Advantages of This Drug
Causes no significant increase in blood cholesterol levels.
Less likely to cause significant loss of potassium.

▷ **This Drug Should Not Be Taken If**
- you have had an allergic reaction to it previously.

▷ **Inform Your Physician Before Taking This Drug If**
- you are allergic to any form of "sulfa" drug.
- you are pregnant or planning pregnancy.
- you have a history of kidney or liver disease.
- you have diabetes, gout or lupus erythematosus.
- you are taking any form of cortisone, digitalis, oral antidiabetic drug or insulin.
- you plan to have surgery under general anesthesia in the near future.

Possible Side-Effects (natural, expected and unavoidable drug actions)
Light-headedness on arising from sitting or lying position (see Orthostatic Hypotension in Glossary).
Increase in blood sugar level, affecting control of diabetes.
Increase in blood uric acid level, affecting control of gout.
Decrease in blood potassium level, causing muscle weakness and cramping.

▷ **Possible Adverse Effects** (unusual, unexpected and infrequent reactions)
If any of the following develop, consult your physician promptly for guidance.
Mild Adverse Effects
Allergic Reactions: Skin rashes, hives, itching.
Headache, dizziness, drowsiness, weakness, lethargy, visual disturbance.
Reduced appetite, indigestion, nausea, vomiting, diarrhea.
Serious Adverse Effects
None reported.

▷ **Possible Effects on Sexual Function:**   Decreased libido (4%); impotence (less than 1%).

Natural Diseases or Disorders That May Be Activated by This Drug
Diabetes, gout, systemic lupus erythematosus.

CAUTION
1. Do not exceed recommended doses. Increased dosage can cause excessive loss of sodium and potassium, with resultant loss of appetite, nausea, fatigue, weakness, confusion and tingling in the extremities.
2. If you are also taking a digitalis preparation (digitoxin, digoxin), ensure an adequate intake of high-potassium foods to prevent potassium deficiency—a potential cause of digitalis toxicity. (See Table of High Potassium Foods in Section Six.)

Precautions for Use
By Infants and Children: Safety and effectiveness for use by those under 12 years of age have not been established.
By Those over 60 Years of Age: Small doses are advisable until your individual response has been determined. You may be more susceptible to the development of impaired thinking, orthostatic hypotension, potassium loss and blood sugar increase. Overdosage and extended use of this drug can cause excessive loss of body water, thickening (increased viscosity) of the blood and an increased tendency for the blood to clot—predisposing to stroke, heart attack or thrombophlebitis (vein inflammation with blood clot).

▷ **Advisability of Use During Pregnancy**
Pregnancy Category: B (tentative). See Pregnancy Code inside back cover.
Animal studies: No birth defects reported.
Human studies: Information from adequate studies of pregnant women is not available.
This drug should not be used during pregnancy unless a very serious complication occurs for which this drug is significantly beneficial. Ask physician for guidance.

Advisability of Use if Breast-Feeding
Presence of this drug in breast milk: Unknown.
Avoid drug or refrain from nursing.

Habit-Forming Potential: None.

Effects of Overdosage: Dry mouth, thirst, lethargy, weakness, muscle cramping, nausea, vomiting, drowsiness progressing to stupor or coma.

Possible Effects of Long-Term Use: Impaired balance of water, salt and potassium in blood and body tissues. Development of diabetes in predisposed individuals.

Suggested Periodic Examinations While Taking This Drug (at physician's discretion)
Measurements of blood levels of sodium, potassium, chloride, sugar and uric acid.

▷ **While Taking This Drug, Observe the Following**
Foods: Consult your physician regarding the advisability of eating foods rich in potassium. If so advised, see the Table of High Potassium Foods in Section Six. Follow physician's advice regarding the use of salt.
Beverages: No restrictions. This drug may be taken with milk.
▷ *Alcohol:* Use with caution until the combined effects have been determined. Alcohol may exaggerate the blood-pressure-lowering effects of this drug and cause orthostatic hypotension.
Tobacco Smoking: No interactions expected. Follow physician's advice.
▷ *Other Drugs*
Indapamide may ***increase*** the effects of
- other antihypertensive drugs; dosage adjustments may be necessary to prevent excessive lowering of blood pressure.
- lithium, and cause lithium toxicity.
Indapamide may ***decrease*** the effects of
- oral antidiabetic drugs (sulfonylureas); dosage adjustments may be necessary for proper control of blood sugar.
Indapamide ***taken concurrently*** with
- digitalis preparations (digitoxin, digoxin) requires very careful monitoring and dosage adjustments to prevent fluctuations of blood potassium levels and serious disturbances of heart rhythm.
The following drugs may ***decrease*** the effects of indapamide
- cholestyramine (Cuemid, Questran) may interfere with its absorption.
- colestipol (Colestid) may interfere with its absorption.
Take cholestyramine and colestipol 1 hour before any oral diuretic.
▷ *Driving, Hazardous Activities:* Use caution until the possible occurrence of orthostatic hypotension, drowsiness, dizziness or impaired vision has been determined.
Aviation Note: The use of this drug ***may be a disqualification*** for piloting. Consult a designated Aviation Medical Examiner.
Exposure to Sun: No restrictions.
Exposure to Heat: Avoid excessive perspiring, which could cause additional loss of salt and water from the body.

Heavy Exercise or Exertion: Avoid exertion that produces light-headedness, excessive fatigue or muscle cramping. Isometric exercises—the "overload" technique for strengthening individual muscles—can raise blood pressure significantly. Ask physician for guidance regarding participation in this form of exercise.

Occurrence of Unrelated Illness: Illnesses that cause vomiting or diarrhea can produce a serious imbalance of important body chemistry. Consult your physician for guidance.

Discontinuation: It may be advisable to discontinue this drug 5 to 7 days before major surgery. Ask your physician, surgeon and/or anesthesiologist for guidance regarding dosage adjustment or drug withdrawal.

INDOMETHACIN
(in doh METH a sin)

Introduced: 1963

Class: Mild analgesic, anti-inflammatory

Prescription: USA: Yes
Canada: Yes

Controlled Drug: USA: No
Canada: No

Available as Generic: USA: Yes
Canada: No

Brand Names: ✦Apo-Indomethacin, Indameth, ✦Indocid, ✦Indocid PDA, Indocin, Indocin-SR, ✦Novomethacin

---

BENEFITS versus RISKS

Possible Benefits	*Possible Risks*
EFFECTIVE RELIEF OF MILD TO MODERATE PAIN AND INFLAMMATION	Gastrointestinal pain, ulceration, bleeding (rare)
	Rare liver or kidney damage
	Rare fluid retention
	Rare bone marrow depression
	Mental depression, confusion

▷ **Principal Uses**

As a Single Drug Product: Used primarily to relieve mild to moderately severe pain associated with (1) musculoskeletal injuries; (2) acute and chronic gout, rheumatoid arthritis and osteoarthritis; (3) dental, obstetrical and orthopedic surgery; (4) menstrual cramps; and (5) vascular (migrainelike) headaches.

How This Drug Works: Not completely established. It is thought that this drug reduces the tissue concentrations of prostaglandins (and related compounds), chemicals involved in the production of inflammation and pain.

Available Dosage Forms and Strengths
Capsules — 25 mg, 50 mg, 75 mg
Capsules, prolonged-action — 75 mg
Oral suspension — 25 mg per 5-ml teaspoonful
Suppositories — 50 mg

▷ **Usual Adult Dosage Range:**   For arthritis and related conditions: 25 to 50 mg 2 to 4 times daily. If needed and tolerated, dose may be increased by 25 or 50 mg/day at intervals of 1 week. For acute gout: 100 mg initially; then 50 mg 3 times/day until pain is relieved. Total daily dosage should not exceed 200 mg. **Note: Actual dosage and administration schedule must be determined by the physician for each patient individually.**

▷ **Dosing Instructions:**   Take with or following food to prevent stomach irritation. Take with a full glass of water and remain upright (do not lie down) for 30 minutes. The regular capsule may be opened for administration, but not the prolonged-action capsule.

Usual Duration of Use: Continual use on a regular schedule for 1 to 2 weeks is usually necessary to determine this drug's effectiveness in relieving the discomfort of arthritis. The usual length of treatment for bursitis or tendinitis is 7 to 14 days. Long-term use requires supervision and periodic evaluation by the physician. Consult your physician on a regular basis.

▷ **This Drug Should Not Be Taken If**
  • you have had an allergic reaction to it previously.
  • you are subject to asthma or nasal polyps caused by aspirin.
  • you are pregnant or breast-feeding.
  • you have active peptic ulcer disease or any form of gastrointestinal ulceration or bleeding.
  • you have a bleeding disorder or a blood cell disorder.
  • you have severe impairment of kidney function.

▷ **Inform Your Physician Before Taking This Drug If**
  • you are allergic to aspirin or to other aspirin substitutes.
  • you have a history of peptic ulcer disease, Crohn's disease, ulcerative colitis or any type of bleeding disorder.
  • you have a history of epilepsy, Parkinson's disease or mental illness (psychosis).
  • you have impaired liver or kidney function.
  • you have high blood pressure or a history of heart failure.
  • you are taking any of the following: acetaminophen, aspirin or other aspirin substitutes, anticoagulants, oral antidiabetic drugs.

Possible Side-Effects (natural, expected and unavoidable drug actions)
Drowsiness, ringing in ears, fluid retention.

▷ **Possible Adverse Effects** (unusual, unexpected and infrequent reactions)
   If any of the following develop, consult your physician promptly for guidance.

Mild Adverse Effects
   Allergic Reactions: Skin rash, hives, itching, localized swellings of face and/or extremities.
   Headache, dizziness, feelings of detachment.
   Mouth sores, indigestion, nausea, vomiting, diarrhea.
   Temporary loss of hair.

Serious Adverse Effects
   Allergic Reactions: Asthma, difficult breathing, mouth irritation.
   Blurred vision, confusion, depression.
   Active peptic ulcer, with or without bleeding.
   Liver damage with jaundice (see Glossary).
   Kidney damage with painful urination, bloody urine, reduced urine formation.
   Rare bone marrow depression (see Glossary)—fatigue, weakness, fever, sore throat, abnormal bleeding or bruising.
   Peripheral neuritis (see Glossary)—numbness, pain or weakness in extremities.

▷ **Possible Effects on Sexual Function**
   Enlargement and tenderness of both male and female breasts.
   Nonmenstrual vaginal bleeding.

Possible Delayed Adverse Effects: Mild anemia due to "silent" blood loss from the stomach (less than that caused by aspirin).

▷ **Adverse Effects That May Mimic Natural Diseases or Disorders**
   Liver reaction may suggest viral hepatitis.

Natural Diseases or Disorders That May Be Activated by This Drug
   Peptic ulcer disease, ulcerative colitis.

CAUTION
   1. Dosage should always be limited to the smallest amount that produces reasonable improvement.
   2. This drug may mask early indications of infection. Inform your physician if you think you are developing an infection of any kind.

Precautions for Use
   By Infants and Children: This drug frequently causes impairment of kidney function in infants. Fatal liver reactions have occurred in children between 6 and 12 years of age; avoid the use of this drug in this age group.
   By Those over 60 Years of Age: Adverse effects are very common in this age group. Small doses are advisable until tolerance is determined. Observe for any indications of liver or kidney toxicity, fluid retention, dizziness, confusion, impaired memory, depression, peptic ulcer or diarrhea, often with rectal bleeding.

▷ **Advisability of Use During Pregnancy**

Pregnancy Category: D (tentative). See Pregnancy Code inside back cover.

Animal studies: Significant toxicity and birth defects reported in mice and rats.

Human studies: Information from adequate studies of pregnant women is not available. However, birth defects have been attributed to the use of this drug during pregnancy.

The manufacturer recommends that this drug not be taken during pregnancy.

Advisability of Use if Breast-Feeding

Presence of this drug in breast milk: Yes.

Avoid drug or refrain from nursing.

The manufacturer recommends that this drug not be taken while breast-feeding.

Habit-Forming Potential: None.

Effects of Overdosage: Drowsiness, agitation, confusion, nausea, vomiting, diarrhea, disorientation, seizures, coma.

Possible Effects of Long-Term Use: Eye changes: deposits in the cornea, alterations in the retina.

Suggested Periodic Examinations While Taking This Drug (at physician's discretion)

Complete blood cell counts, liver and kidney function tests, complete eye examinations if vision is altered in any way.

▷ **While Taking This Drug, Observe the Following**

Foods: No restrictions.

Nutritional Support: Take 50 mg of vitamin C (ascorbic acid) daily.

Beverages: No restrictions. May be taken with milk.

▷   *Alcohol:* Use with caution. The irritant action of alcohol on the stomach lining, added to the irritant action of this drug in sensitive individuals, can increase the risk of stomach ulceration and/or bleeding.

Tobacco Smoking: No interactions expected.

▷   *Other Drugs*

Indomethacin may ***increase*** the effects of

• acetaminophen (Tylenol, etc.), and increase the risk of kidney damage; avoid prolonged use of this combination.

• anticoagulants (Coumadin, etc.), and increase the risk of bleeding; monitor prothrombin time, adjust dose accordingly.

• lithium, and cause lithium toxicity.

Indomethacin may ***decrease*** the effects of

• beta blocker drugs (see Drug Class, Section Four), and reduce their antihypertensive effectiveness.

• bumetanide (Bumex).

• captopril (Capoten).

• ethacrynic acid (Edecrin).

- furosemide (Lasix).

Indomethacin **taken concurrently** with the following drugs may increase the risk of bleeding; avoid these combinations:

- aspirin.
- diflunisal (Dolobid).
- dipyridamole (Persantine).
- sulfinpyrazone (Anturane).
- valproic acid (Depakene).

▷ *Driving, Hazardous Activities:* This drug may cause drowsiness, dizziness or impaired vision. Restrict activities as necessary.

Aviation Note: The use of this drug **may be a disqualification** for piloting. Consult a designated Aviation Medical Examiner.

Exposure to Sun: No restrictions.

INSULIN
(IN suh lin)

Introduced: 1922

Class: Antidiabetic

Prescription: USA: No
Canada: No

Controlled Drug: USA: No
Canada: No

Available as Generic: Yes

Brand Names: Humulin BR, Humulin L, Humulin N, Humulin R, Humulin U, Humulin U Ultralente, Iletin I NPH, ✦Initard, Insulatard NPH, ✦Insulin-Toronto, Lente Iletin I, Lente Iletin II Beef, Lente Iletin II Pork, Lente Insulin, Mixtard, Novolin L, Novolin N, NovolinPen, Novolin R, ✦Novolin-Lente, ✦Novolin-NPH, ✦Novolin-30/70, ✦Novolin-Toronto, ✦Novolin-Ultralente, NPH Iletin I, NPH Iletin II Beef, NPH Iletin II Pork, NPH Insulin, NPH Purified Pork, Protamine, Zinc & Iletin I, Protamine, Zinc & Iletin II Beef, Protamine, Zinc & Iletin II Pork, Regular Iletin I, Regular Iletin II Beef, Regular Iletin II Pork, Regular Iletin II U-500, Regular Insulin, Regular Purified Pork Insulin, Semilente Iletin I, Semilente Insulin, Semilente Purified Pork, Ultralente Iletin I, Ultralente Insulin, Ultralente Purified Beef, Velosulin

BENEFITS versus RISKS	
Possible Benefits	*Possible Risks*
EFFECTIVE CONTROL OF TYPE I (INSULIN-DEPENDENT) DIABETES MELLITUS	HYPOGLYCEMIA WITH EXCESSIVE DOSAGE Infrequent allergic reactions

▷ **Principal Uses**

As a Single Drug Product: Insulin is used to control diabetes mellitus in those individuals whose diabetes has been shown to be insulin-dependent. Proper use involves selection of the most appropriate type of insulin for the individual and determination of the optimal dosage schedule for the continuous regulation of blood sugar levels.

How This Drug Works: Not completely established. By direct action on certain cell membranes, insulin facilitates the transport of sugar through the cell wall to the interior of the cell where it is utilized. This occurs primarily in the brain, the voluntary muscles, the heart muscle and the liver.

Available Dosage Forms and Strengths

Injections — 40 units, 100 units, 500 units per ml
PenFil cartridges — 150 units

▷ **Usual Adult Dosage Range:** According to individual requirements for the optimal regulation of blood sugar on a 24-hour basis. **Note: Actual dosage and administration schedule must be determined by the physician for each patient individually.**

▷ **Dosing Instructions:** Inject insulin subcutaneously according to the schedule prescribed by your physician. The timing and frequency of injections will vary with the type of insulin precribed. The following table of insulin actions (according to type) will help you understand the treatment schedule prescribed for you.

Insulin Type	Action Onset	Peak	Duration
Regular	0.5–1 hr	2–4 hrs	5–7 hrs
Isophane (NPH)	3–4 hrs	6–12 hrs	18–28 hrs
Regular 30%/NPH 70%	0.5 hr	4–8 hrs	24 hrs
Semilente	1–3 hrs	2–8 hrs	12–16 hrs
Lente	1–3 hrs	8–12 hrs	18–28 hrs
Ultralente	4–6 hrs	18–24 hrs	36 hrs
Protamine Zinc	4–6 hrs	14–24 hrs	36 hrs

Usual Duration of Use: Type I insulin-dependent (juvenile-onset) diabetes mellitus usually requires insulin treatment for life. Type II noninsulin-dependent (maturity-onset) diabetes is usually controlled by oral antidiabetic drugs and/or diet but may, on occasion, require insulin for adequate control. Such occasions include serious infections, injuries, burns, surgical procedures and other forms of physical stress. Insulin is used as needed on a temporary basis to regulate and normalize the body's use of sugar until recovery is complete and basic health is restored. Consult your physician on a regular basis.

▷ **This Drug Should Not Be Taken If**

• the need for it and its correct dosage schedule have not been established by a properly qualified physician.

▷ **Inform Your Physician Before Taking This Drug If**
- you have a history of allergic reaction to any form of insulin on previous use.
- you do not know how to recognize and treat abnormally low blood sugar (see Hypoglycemia in Glossary).
- you are taking any of the following drugs: aspirin, beta blockers, fenfluramine (Pondimin), monoamine oxidase (MAO) type A inhibitors (see respective Drug Classes, Section Four).

Possible Side-Effects (natural, expected and unavoidable drug actions)
In the management of stable diabetes, no side-effects occur when insulin dose, diet and physical activity are correctly balanced and maintained.
In the management of unstable ("brittle") diabetes, unexpected drops in blood sugar levels can occur, resulting in periods of hypoglycemia (see Glossary).

▷ **Possible Adverse Effects** (unusual, unexpected and infrequent reactions)
If any of the following develop, consult your physician promptly for guidance.
Mild Adverse Effects
Allergic Reactions: Local redness, swelling and itching at site of injection. Occasional hives.
Thinning of subcutaneous tissue at sites of injection.
Serious Adverse Effects
Allergic Reaction: Anaphylactic reactions (see Glossary).
Severe, prolonged hypoglycemia.

▷ **Possible Effects on Sexual Function:** None reported.

▷ **Adverse Effects That May Mimic Natural Diseases or Disorders**
The early manifestations of hypoglycemia may be mistaken for alcoholic intoxication.

CAUTION
1. It is most important that you carry with you a card of personal identification with a notation that you have diabetes and are taking insulin.
2. Be sure that you know how to recognize the onset of hypoglycemia and how to treat it. Always carry with you a readily available form of sugar, such as hard candy or sugar cubes. Report all episodes of hypoglycemia to your physician; it may be necessary to adjust your insulin dosage or schedule.
3. Improvement in vision may occur during the first several weeks of insulin treatment. It is advisable to defer examination for glasses for 6 weeks after starting insulin.
4. The rates of insulin absorption vary significantly from one anatomic site to another. Absorption is 80% greater from the abdominal wall than from the leg, and 30% greater than from the arm. Individuals with unstable diabetes may achieve better control of

blood sugar levels by rotating the injection site within the same anatomic region rather than by rotating from one anatomic region to another.

Precautions for Use

By Infants and Children: Insulin dosages and schedules are modified according to patient size. Adhere strictly to the physician's prescribed routine.

By Those over 60 Years of Age: Insulin requirements may change with aging. Periodic evaluation of individual status is necessary to determine correct insulin dosage and scheduling. The aging brain adapts well to higher blood sugar levels. Attempts to maintain strictly "normal" blood sugar levels may result in episodes of unrecognized hypoglycemia that is manifested by confusion and abnormal behavior. Repeated episodes of hypoglycemia (especially if severe) in the elderly may cause brain damage.

▷ **Advisability of Use During Pregnancy**

Pregnancy Category: B (tentative). See Pregnancy Code inside back cover. Animal studies: Inconclusive.

Human studies: Information from adequate studies of pregnant women is not available. It is known that birth defects occur 2 to 4 times more frequently in infants of diabetic mothers than in infants of mothers who do not have diabetes. The exact causes of this are not known.

Insulin is the drug of choice for managing diabetes during pregnancy. To preserve the health of the mother and the welfare of the fetus, every effort must be made to establish the optimal dosage of insulin necessary for "good control" and to prevent episodes of hypoglycemia.

Advisability of Use if Breast-Feeding

Presence of this drug in breast milk: No.

Insulin treatment of the mother has no adverse effect on the nursing infant.

Breast-feeding may decrease insulin requirements; dosage adjustment may be necessary.

Habit-Forming Potential: None.

Effects of Overdosage: Hypoglycemia: fatigue, weakness, headache, nervousness, irritability, sweating, tremors, hunger, confusion, delirium, abnormal behavior (resembling alcoholic intoxication), loss of consciousness, seizures.

Possible Effects of Long-Term Use: Thinning of subcutaneous fat tissue at sites of insulin injection.

Suggested Periodic Examinations While Taking This Drug (at physician's discretion)

Monitoring of urine sugar content as a guide to adjustment of diet and insulin dosage. Measurement of blood sugar levels at intervals recommended by physician.

▷ **While Taking This Drug, Observe the Following**

Foods: Follow your prescribed diabetic diet conscientiously. Do not omit snack foods in midafternoon or at bedtime if they are prescribed to prevent hypoglycemia.

Beverages: According to prescribed diabetic diet.

▷ *Alcohol:* Use with caution until the combined effect has been determined. Used excessively, alcohol can induce severe hypoglycemia, resulting in brain damage.

Tobacco Smoking: Regular smoking can decrease insulin absorption and increase insulin requirements by 30%. It is advisable to refrain from smoking altogether.

Marijuana Smoking: Possible increase in blood sugar levels.

▷ *Other Drugs*

The following drugs may ***increase*** the effects of insulin

- aspirin, and other salicylates.
- some beta blocker drugs (especially the nonselective ones) may prolong insulin-induced hypoglycemia. (See Drug Class, Section Four.)
- fenfluramine (Pondimin).
- monoamine oxidase (MAO) type A inhibitor drugs (see Drug Class, Section Four).

The following drugs may ***decrease*** the effects of insulin (by raising blood sugar levels)

- chlorthalidone (Hygroton).
- cortisonelike drugs (see Drug Class, Section Four).
- furosemide (Lasix).
- oral contraceptives.
- phenytoin (Dilantin, etc.).
- thiazide diuretics (see Drug Class, Section Four).
- thyroid preparations.

▷ *Driving, Hazardous Activities:* Usually no restrictions. However, be prepared to stop and take corrective action if indications of impending hypoglycemia develop.

Aviation Note: Diabetes and the use of this drug ***are disqualifications*** for piloting. Consult a designated Aviation Medical Examiner.

Exposure to Sun: No restrictions.

Exposure to Heat: Use caution. Sauna baths can signficantly increase the rate of insulin absorption and cause hypoglycemia.

Heavy Exercise or Exertion: Use caution. Periods of unusual or unplanned heavy physical activity will hasten the utilization of blood sugar and predispose to hypoglycemia.

Occurrence of Unrelated Illness: Report all illnesses that prevent regular eating. The omission of meals as a result of nausea, vomiting or injury may lead to hypoglycemia. Untreated infections can increase insulin requirements. Consult physician for guidance.

Discontinuation: Do not discontinue this drug without consulting your physician. Diabetes that is insulin-dependent requires continual treatment on a regular basis. Omission of insulin may result in life-threatening coma.

Special Storage Instructions: Keep in a cool place, preferably in the refrigerator. Protect from freezing. Protect from strong light and high temperatures when not refrigerated.

Observe the Following Expiration Times: Do not use this drug if it is older than the expiration date on the vial. Always use fresh, "within date" insulin.

ISONIAZID
(i soh NI a zid)

Other Names: Isonicotinic acid hydrazide, INH

Introduced: 1956

Class: Antitubercular

Prescription: USA: Yes
Canada: Yes

Controlled Drug: USA: No
Canada: No

Available as Generic: USA: Yes
Canada: No

Brand Names: ✦Isotamine, Laniazid, Nydrazid, P-I-N Forte [CD], ✦PMS Isoniazid, Rifamate [CD], Rimactane/INH Dual Pack [CD], Teebaconin, Teebaconin and Vitamin B-6 [CD]

BENEFITS versus RISKS

Possible Benefits	*Possible Risks*
EFFECTIVE PREVENTION AND TREATMENT OF ACTIVE TUBERCULOSIS	ALLERGIC LIVER REACTION (1% to 2%) Peripheral neuropathy (see Glossary) Bone marrow depression (see Glossary) Mental and behavioral disturbances

---

▷ **Principal Uses**

As a Single Drug Product: Used alone to prevent the development of active tuberculous infection in individuals who are considered to be at high risk because of known exposure to infection or recent conversion of a negative tuberculin skin test to positive.

As a Combination Drug Product [CD]: This drug is available in combination with rifampin, another antitubercular drug that has a different mechanism of action. This combination is more effective than either drug used alone. Isoniazid can cause a deficiency of pyridoxine (vitamin B-6); for this reason, a combination of the two drugs is available in tablet form.

How This Drug Works: Not completely established. It is thought that this drug destroys susceptible tuberculosis organisms by interfering with several of their essential metabolic activities and by disrupting their cell wall.

Available Dosage Forms and Strengths
Injection — 100 mg per ml
Syrup — 50 mg per 5-ml teaspoonful
Tablets — 50 mg, 100 mg, 300 mg

▷ **Usual Adult Dosage Range:**   For prevention: 300 mg once daily. For treatment: 5 mg per kilogram of body weight daily. The total daily dosage should not exceed 600 mg. **Note: Actual dosage and administration schedule must be determined by the physician for each patient individually.**

▷ **Dosing Instructions:**   May be taken with food to prevent stomach irritation. The tablet may be crushed for administration.

Usual Duration of Use: Continual use on a regular schedule for 1 or more years is often necessary, depending upon the nature of the infection. Shorter courses of intermittent high dosage may be adequate in some cases. Consult your physician on a regular basis.

▷ **This Drug Should Not Be Taken If**
- you have had an allergic reaction (especially a liver reaction) to any dosage form of it previously.
- you have active liver disease.

▷ **Inform Your Physician Before Taking This Drug If**
- you have serious impairment of liver or kidney function.
- you drink an alcoholic beverage daily.
- you have a seizure disorder.
- you are taking any other drugs on a long-term basis, especially phenytoin (Dilantin).
- you plan to have surgery under general anesthesia in the near future.

Possible Side-Effects (natural, expected and unavoidable drug actions)
None.

▷ **Possible Adverse Effects** (unusual, unexpected and infrequent reactions)
If any of the following develop, consult your physician promptly for guidance.
Mild Adverse Effects
Allergic Reactions: Skin rash, fever, swollen glands, painful muscles and joints.
Dizziness, indigestion, nausea, vomiting.
Serious Adverse Effects
Allergic Reactions: Drug-induced hepatitis (see Glossary): loss of appetite, nausea, fatigue, fever, itching, dark-colored urine, yellow discoloration of eyes and skin.

Peripheral neuritis (see Glossary): numbness, tingling, pain, weakness in hands and/or feet.

Acute mental and behavioral disturbances, impaired vision, increase in epileptic seizures.

Bone marrow depression (see Glossary): fatigue, weakness, fever, sore throat, abnormal bleeding or bruising.

▷ **Possible Effects on Sexual Function:** Male breast enlargement and tenderness.

Possible Delayed Adverse Effects: An increase in the frequency of cirrhosis of the liver has been reported.

▷ **Adverse Effects That May Mimic Natural Diseases or Disorders**
Drug-induced hepatitis may suggest viral hepatitis.

Natural Diseases or Disorders That May Be Activated by This Drug
Latent epilepsy, systemic lupus erythematosus (questionable).

CAUTION
1. Consult your physician regarding the advisability of determining if you are a "slow" or "rapid" inactivator (acetylator) of isoniazid. This has a bearing on your predisposition to developing adverse effects from this drug.
2. Copper sulfate tests for urine sugar may give a false positive test result. (Diabetics please note.)

Precautions for Use
By Infants and Children: Use with caution in children with seizure disorders. "Slow acetylators" are more prone to adverse drug effects. It is advisable to give supplemental pyridoxine (vitamin B-6).
By Those over 60 Years of Age: There is a greater incidence of liver damage in this age group; the liver status should be monitored carefully. Observe for any indications of an "acute brain syndrome" consisting of confusion, delirium and seizures.

▷ **Advisability of Use During Pregnancy**
Pregnancy Category: C (tentative). See Pregnancy Code inside back cover.
Animal studies: No birth defects reported in mice, rats or rabbits.
Human studies: Information from adequate studies of pregnant women is not available.
Earlier reports of human birth defects due to this drug have not been substantiated by later studies. If clearly needed, this drug is now used at any time during pregnancy. Ask your physician for guidance.

Advisability of Use if Breast-Feeding
Presence of this drug in breast milk: Yes.
Avoid drug or refrain from nursing.

Habit-Forming Potential: None.

Effects of Overdosage: Nausea, vomiting, dizziness, blurred vision, hallucinations, slurred speech, stupor, coma, seizures.

Possible Effects of Long-Term Use: Peripheral neuritis due to a deficiency of pyridoxine (vitamin B-6).

Suggested Periodic Examinations While Taking This Drug (at physician's discretion)
Complete blood cell counts, liver function tests, complete eye examinations.

▷ **While Taking This Drug, Observe the Following**
Foods: Eat the following foods cautiously until your tolerance is determined: Swiss and Cheshire cheeses, tuna fish, skipjack fish and Sardinella species. These may interact with the drug to produce skin rash, itching, sweating, chills, headache, light-headedness or rapid heart rate.
Nutritional Support: It is advisable to take a supplement of pyridoxine (vitamin B-6) to prevent peripheral neuritis. Ask your physician for dosage.
Beverages: No restrictions. May be taken with milk.
▷ *Alcohol:* Avoid completely or use very sparingly. Alcohol may reduce the effectiveness of this drug and increase the risk of liver toxicity.
Tobacco Smoking: No interactions expected.
▷ *Other Drugs*
Isoniazid may *increase* the effects of
• carbamazepine (Tegretol), and cause toxicity.
• phenytoin (Dilantin), and cause toxicity.
The following drugs may *decrease* the effects of isoniazid
• cortisonelike drugs (see Drug Class, Section Four).
▷ *Driving, Hazardous Activities:* Usually no restrictions. This drug may cause dizziness. Restrict activities as necessary.
Aviation Note: The use of this drug *may be a disqualification* for piloting. Consult a designated Aviation Medical Examiner.
Exposure to Sun: No restrictions.
Discontinuation: Long-term treatment is required. Do not discontinue this drug without consulting your physician.

ISOSORBIDE DINITRATE
(i soh SOHR bide di NI trayt)

Other Name: Sorbide nitrate

Introduced: 1959   **Class:** Antianginal, nitrates

Prescription: USA: Yes   **Controlled Drug:** USA: No
  Canada: No   Canada: No

Available as Generic: USA: Yes
Canada: No

Brand Names: ✦Apo-ISDN, ✦Coronex, Dilatrate-SR, Isonate, Isordil, Isordil Tembids, Isordil Titradose, ✦Novosorbide, Sorbitrate

---

BENEFITS versus RISKS

Possible Benefits	*Possible Risks*
EFFECTIVE RELIEF AND PREVENTION OF ANGINA EFFECTIVE ADJUNCTIVE TREATMENT IN SELECTED CASES OF CONGESTIVE HEART FAILURE	Orthostatic hypotension (see Glossary) Rare skin reactions (severe peeling)

▷ **Principal Uses**

As a Single Drug Product: The sublingual (under-the-tongue) tablets and the chewable tablets are used to prevent and to relieve acute attacks of anginal pain. The longer-acting tablets and capsules are used to prevent the development of angina, but are not effective in relieving acute episodes of anginal pain. This drug is also used to improve heart function in selected cases of congestive heart failure.

How This Drug Works: By direct action on the muscle in blood vessel walls, this drug relaxes and dilates both arteries and veins. It is thought that its beneficial effects in treating angina and heart failure are due to (1) dilation of coronary arteries, and (2) dilation of systemic veins with consequent reduction of volume and pressure of blood in the heart. The net effects are improved blood flow to the heart muscle and reduced workload of the heart.

Available Dosage Forms and Strengths

Capsules — 40 mg
Capsules, prolonged-action — 40 mg
Tablets — 5 mg, 10 mg, 20 mg, 30 mg, 40 mg
Tablets, chewable — 5 mg, 10 mg
Tablets, prolonged-action — 40 mg
Tablets, sublingual — 2.5 mg, 5 mg, 10 mg

▷ **Usual Adult Dosage Range**

Sublingual tablets: 5 to 10 mg dissolved under tongue every 2 to 3 hours; use for relief of acute attack and for prevention of anticipated attack.

Chewable tablets: Initially, 5 mg chewed to evaluate tolerance; increase dose to 5 or 10 mg every 2 to 3 hours as needed and tolerated; use for relief of acute attack and for prevention of anticipated attack.

Tablets: 5 to 30 mg 4 times daily to prevent acute attack; usual dose is 10 to 20 mg 4 times/day.

Prolonged-action capsules and tablets: 40 mg/6 to 12 hours as needed to prevent acute attacks.

The total daily dosage should not exceed 120 mg.

Note: Actual dosage and administration schedule must be determined by the physician for each patient individually.

▷ **Dosing Instructions:**   Capsules and tablets to be swallowed are best taken on an empty stomach to achieve maximal blood levels. Regular tablets may be crushed for administration; prolonged-action capsules and tablets should be taken whole and not altered.

Usual Duration of Use: Continual use on a regular schedule for 3 to 7 days is usually necessary to (1) determine this drug's effectiveness in preventing or relieving acute anginal pain, and (2) establish the optimal dosage shedule. Long-term use (months to years) requires supervision and periodic evaluation by your physician. Consult your physician on a regular basis.

▷ **This Drug Should Not Be Taken If**
- you have had an allergic reaction to any dosage form of it previously.
- you have had a very recent heart attack (myocardial infarction).

▷ **Inform Your Physician Before Taking This Drug If**
- you have had an unfavorable response to other nitrate drugs or vasodilators in the past.
- you have a history of low blood pressure.
- you have any form of glaucoma.

Possible Side-Effects (natural, expected and unavoidable drug actions)
Flushing of face, throbbing in head, palpitation, rapid heart rate, orthostatic hypotension (see Glossary).

▷ **Possible Adverse Effects** (unusual, unexpected and infrequent reactions)
If any of the following develop, consult your physician promptly for guidance.
Mild Adverse Effects
Allergic Reaction: Skin rash.
Headache (may be severe and persistent), dizziness, fainting.
Nausea, vomiting.
Serious Adverse Effects
Allergic Reaction: Severe dermatitis with peeling of skin.
Transient ischemic attacks (TIAs) in presence of impaired circulation within the brain: dizziness, fainting, impaired vision or speech, localized numbness or weakness.

▷ **Possible Effects on Sexual Function:**   None reported.

▷ **Adverse Effects That May Mimic Natural Diseases or Disorders**
Spells of low blood pressure (due to this drug) may be mistaken for late-onset epilepsy.

CAUTION

1. The development of tolerance (see Glossary) to long-acting forms of nitrates may render the sublingual tablets of nitroglycerin less effective for the relief of acute anginal attacks. Antianginal effectiveness is restored after 1 week of abstinence from long-acting nitrates.
2. Many over-the-counter (OTC) medications for allergies, colds and coughs contain drugs that may counteract the desired effects of this drug. Ask your physician or pharmacist for guidance before using such medications.

Precautions for Use

By Those over 60 Years of Age: Small doses are advisable until your tolerance has been determined. You may be more susceptible to the development of low blood pressure and associated "blackout" spells, fainting and falling. Throbbing headaches and flushing may be more apparent.

▷ Advisability of Use During Pregnancy

Pregnancy Category: C (tentative). See Pregnancy Code inside back cover.
Animal studies: No information available.
Human studies: Information from adequate studies of pregnant women is not available.
Use this drug only if clearly needed.

Advisability of Use if Breast-Feeding

Presence of this drug in breast milk: Unknown.
If drug is thought to be necessary, monitor the nursing infant for low blood pressure and poor feeding.

Habit-Forming Potential: None.

Effects of Overdosage: Headache, dizziness, marked flushing of face and skin, vomiting, weakness, fainting, difficult breathing, coma.

Possible Effects of Long-Term Use: Development of tolerance with temporary loss of effectiveness at recommended doses. Development of abnormal hemoglobin (red blood cell pigment).

Suggested Periodic Examinations While Taking This Drug (at physician's discretion)
Measurement of internal eye pressure. Red blood cell counts and hemoglobin evaluation.

▷ While Taking This Drug, Observe the Following

Foods: No restrictions.
Beverages: No restrictions. May be taken with milk.
▷   *Alcohol:* Use extreme caution until the combined effects have been determined. Avoid alcohol completely in the presence of any side-effects or adverse effects of this drug. Alcohol may exaggerate the blood-pressure-lowering effect of this drug.

Tobacco Smoking: Nicotine can reduce the effectiveness of this drug. Avoid all forms of tobacco.

Marijuana Smoking: Possible reduced effectiveness of this drug; mild to moderate increase in angina; possible changes in electrocardiogram, confusing interpretation.

▷ *Other Drugs*

Isosorbide dinitrate **taken concurrently** with

• antihypertensive drugs may cause excessive lowering of blood pressure; dosage adjustments may be necessary.

▷ *Driving, Hazardous Activities:* Usually no restrictions. This drug may cause dizziness or spells of low blood pressure. Restrict activities as necessary.

Aviation Note: Coronary artery disease **is a disqualification** for piloting. Consult a designated Aviation Medical Examiner.

Exposure to Sun: No restrictions.

Exposure to Heat: Use caution. Hot environments can cause a significant drop in blood pressure.

Exposure to Cold: Cold environments can increase the need for this drug and limit its effectiveness.

Heavy Exercise or Exertion: This drug may improve your ability to be more active without anginal pain. Use caution and avoid excessive exertion.

Discontinuation: It is advisable to withdraw this drug gradually after long-term use. The dosage and frequency of prolonged-action dosage forms should be reduced gradually over a period of 4 to 6 weeks.

ISOTRETINOIN
(i soh TRET i noin)

Introduced: 1979

Class: Antiacne

Prescription: USA: Yes
Canada: Yes

Controlled Drug: USA: No
Canada: No

Available as Generic: No

Brand Name: Accutane

BENEFITS versus RISKS

Possible Benefits	*Possible Risks*
EFFECTIVE TREATMENT OF SEVERE CYSTIC ACNE	MAJOR BIRTH DEFECTS
	Initial worsening of acne (transient)
	Inflammation of lips (90%)
	Dry skin, nose and mouth
	Musculoskeletal discomfort
	Corneal opacities (rare)

▷ **Principal Uses**

As a Single Drug Product: This drug is reserved to treat severe nodular and cystic acne that has failed to respond to all other forms of standard therapy. *It should not be used to treat mild forms of acne.* It is also used to treat some less common conditions of the skin that are due to disorders of keratin production.

How This Drug Works: Not completely established. By an unknown action, this drug reduces the size of sebaceous glands and inhibits their production of sebum (skin oil). This helps to correct the major feature of acne and its complications.

Available Dosage Forms and Strengths

Capsules — 10 mg, 20 mg, 40 mg

▷ **Usual Adult Dosage Range:**   Initial dosage is individualized according to the patient's weight and the severity of the acne; the usual dose is 1 to 2 mg per kilogram of body weight daily, taken in 2 divided doses for 15 to 20 weeks. After 2 weeks of treatment, the dose should be adjusted according to the response of the acne and the development of adverse effects. **Note: Actual dosage and administration schedule must be determined by the physician for each patient individually.**

▷ **Dosing Instructions:**   Take with meals (morning and evening) to achieve optimal blood levels. The capsule should not be opened for administration.

Usual Duration of Use: Continual use on a regular schedule for 15 to 20 weeks is usually necessary to determine this drug's effectiveness in clearing or improving severe cystic acne. The drug may be discontinued earlier if the total cyst count is reduced by more than 70%. If a repeat course of treatment is necessary, it should not be started until after a period of 2 months without this drug. Long-term use (months to years) requires supervision and periodic evaluation by your physician. Consult your physician on a regular basis.

▷ **This Drug Should Not Be Taken If**

- you are allergic to parabens, additives that are used to preserve the drug product.
- you are pregnant, or planning pregnancy.

▷ **Inform Your Physician Before Taking This Drug If**

- you have had an allergic reaction to any form of vitamin A in the past.
- you have diabetes mellitus.
- you have a cholesterol or triglyceride disorder.
- you have a history of liver or kidney disease.

Possible Side-Effects (natural, expected and unavoidable drug actions)

Dryness of the nose and mouth (80%), inflammation of the lips (90%), dryness of the skin with itching (80%), peeling of the palms and soles (5%).

▷ **Possible Adverse Effects** (unusual, unexpected and infrequent reactions)
   If any of the following develop, consult your physician promptly for guidance.
   Mild Adverse Effects
   Allergic Reaction: Skin rash (less than 10%).
   Thinning of hair, conjunctivitis, intolerance of contact lenses, muscular and joint aches, headache, fatigue, indigestion.
   Serious Adverse Effects
   Skin infections, worsening of arthritis, inflammatory bowel disorders.
   Abnormal acceleration of bone development in children.
   Development of opacities in the cornea of the eye.
   Reduced red blood cell and white blood cell counts; increased blood platelet count.
   Increased pressure within the head, with associated headache, visual disturbances, nausea and vomiting.

▷ **Possible Effects on Sexual Function**
   Decreased male libido (7%), decreased female libido (13%) beginning after 1 month of drug use.
   Impotence (3%) beginning after 3 months of drug use.
   Decreased vaginal secretions (43%).
   Altered timing and pattern of menstruation (22%).
   Female breast discharge (rare).

CAUTION
   1. This drug should not be used to treat mild forms of acne.
   2. A transient worsening of your acne may occur during the first few weeks of treatment; this will subside with continued use of the drug.
   3. Do not take any other form of vitamin A while taking this drug. (Observe contents of multiple vitamin preparations.)
   4. Women with potential for pregnancy should have a pregnancy test before taking this drug and should use an effective form of contraception during its use. It is recommended that contraception be continued until normal menstruation resumes after discontinuing this drug.
   5. This drug may cause increased blood levels of cholesterol and triglycerides.
   6. If repeated courses of this drug are prescribed, wait a minimum of 2 months between courses before resuming medication.

Precautions for Use
   By Infants and Children: Long-term use (6 to 12 months) may cause abnormal acceleration of bone growth and development. Your physician can monitor this possibility by periodic X-ray examination of long bones.

▷ **Advisability of Use During Pregnancy**
Pregnancy Category: X. See Pregnancy Code inside back cover.
Animal studies: Birth defects of skull, brain and vertebral column found in rats; skeletal birth defects found in rabbits.
Human studies: Information from adequate studies of pregnant women is not available. However, serious birth defects of fetal brain development (thought to be due to this drug) have been reported.
Avoid this drug completely during entire pregnancy.

Advisability of Use if Breast-Feeding
Presence of this drug in breast milk: Unknown.
Avoid drug or refrain from nursing.

Habit-Forming Potential: None.

Effects of Overdosage: No experience with overdosage in humans to date.

Suggested Periodic Examinations While Taking This Drug (at physician's discretion)
Complete blood cell counts, including platelet counts.
Measurements of blood cholesterol and triglyceride levels.
Complete eye examinations.
Liver and kidney function tests.

▷ **While Taking This Drug, Observe the Following**
Foods: No restrictions.
Beverages: No restrictions.
▷   *Alcohol:* No interactions expected.
Tobacco Smoking: No interactions expected.
▷   *Other Drugs:* No interactions reported to date.
▷   *Driving, Hazardous Activities:* No restrictions.
Exposure to Sun: This drug can cause photosensitivity (see Glossary).
Avoid excessive exposure to sun until your sensitivity is determined.

KETOPROFEN
(kee toh PROH fen)

Introduced: 1973

Class: Mild analgesic, anti-inflammatory

Prescription: USA: Yes
Canada: Yes

Controlled Drug: USA: No
Canada: No

Available as Generic: No

Brand Names: Orudis, ✦Orudis E-50

BENEFITS versus RISKS	
Possible Benefits	*Possible Risks*
EFFECTIVE RELIEF OF MILD TO MODERATE PAIN AND INFLAMMATION	Gastrointestinal pain, ulceration, bleeding (rare) Rare liver or kidney damage Rare fluid retention Rare bone marrow depression

▷ **Principal Uses**

As a Single Drug Product: Used primarily to relieve mild to moderately severe pain associated with (1) rheumatoid arthritis and osteoarthritis; (2) acute gouty arthritis; (3) acute bursitis, tendinitis and related conditions; and (4) menstrual cramps.

How This Drug Works: Not completely established. It is thought that this drug reduces the tissue concentrations of prostaglandins (and related compounds), chemicals involved in the production of inflammation and pain.

Available Dosage Forms and Strengths

Capsules — 50 mg, 75 mg

Suppositories — 100 mg (in Canada)

Tablets, enteric-coated — 50 mg (in Canada)

▷ **Usual Adult Dosage Range:** Initially, 75 mg 3 times/day or 50 mg 4 times/day. Usual daily dose is 150 to 300 mg divided into 3 or 4 doses. Total daily dosage should not exceed 300 mg. **Note: Actual dosage and administration schedule must be determined by the physician for each patient individually.**

▷ **Dosing Instructions:** Take either on an empty stomach or with food or milk to prevent stomach irritation. Take with a full glass of water and remain upright (do not lie down) for 30 minutes. The capsule may be opened for administration; the tablet should not be crushed or altered.

Usual Duration of Use: Continual use on a regular schedule for 1 to 3 weeks is usually necessary to determine this drug's effectiveness in relieving the discomfort of arthritis. Long-term use (months to years) requires supervision and periodic evaluation by the physician. Consult your physician on a regular basis.

▷ **This Drug Should Not Be Taken If**

- you have had an allergic reaction to it previously.
- you are subject to asthma or nasal polyps caused by aspirin.
- you have active peptic ulcer disease or any form of gastrointestinal ulceration or bleeding.
- you have a bleeding disorder or a blood cell disorder.
- you have severe impairment of kidney function.
- you have active liver disease.

▷ **Inform Your Physician Before Taking This Drug If**
  • you are allergic to aspirin or to other aspirin substitutes.
  • you have a history of peptic ulcer disease or any type of bleeding disorder.
  • you have impaired liver or kidney function.
  • you have high blood pressure or a history of heart failure.
  • you are taking any of the following: acetaminophen, aspirin or other aspirin substitutes, anticoagulants, oral antidiabetic drugs, or probenecid.

Possible Side-Effects (natural, expected and unavoidable drug actions)
  Drowsiness (1% to 3%), ringing in ears (1% to 3%), fluid retention (3%).

▷ **Possible Adverse Effects** (unusual, unexpected and infrequent reactions)
  If any of the following develop, consult your physician promptly for guidance.
  Mild Adverse Effects
  Allergic Reactions: Skin rash (1% to 3%), hives, itching.
  Headache (less than 1%), dizziness, altered or blurred vision, depression, confusion, impaired memory.
  Mouth sores, indigestion (11%), nausea, vomiting, constipation, diarrhea.
  Serious Adverse Effects
  Allergic Reaction: Anaphylaxis (see Glossary).
  Impaired hearing.
  Active peptic ulcer, with or without bleeding (2%).
  Rare liver damage with jaundice (see Glossary).
  Kidney damage with painful urination, bloody urine, reduced urine formation.
  Rare bone marrow depression (see Glossary)—fatigue, weakness, fever, sore throat, abnormal bleeding or bruising.

▷ **Possible Effects on Sexual Function**
  Decreased libido, impotence, male breast enlargement.
  Altered timing and pattern of menstruation, excessive menstrual bleeding.

Possible Delayed Adverse Effects: Mild anemia due to "silent" blood loss from the stomach (less than that caused by aspirin).

▷ **Adverse Effects That May Mimic Natural Diseases or Disorders**
  Liver reaction may suggest viral hepatitis.

Natural Diseases or Disorders That May Be Activated by This Drug
  Peptic ulcer disease, ulcerative colitis.

CAUTION
  1. Dosage should always be limited to the smallest amount that produces reasonable improvement.
  2. This drug may mask early indications of infection. Inform your physician if you think you are developing an infection of any kind.

Precautions for Use

By Infants and Children: Safety and effectiveness for use by those under 12 years of age have not been established.

By Those over 60 Years of Age: Small doses are advisable until tolerance is determined. Observe for any indications of liver or kidney toxicity, fluid retention, dizziness, confusion, impaired memory, stomach bleeding or constipation.

▷ **Advisability of Use During Pregnancy**

Pregnancy Category: B (tentative). See Pregnancy Code inside back cover.

Animal studies: No birth defects reported in mouse, rat or rabbit studies.

Human studies: Information from adequate studies of pregnant women is not available.

Avoid this drug during the last 3 months. Use it during the first 6 months only if clearly needed. Ask physician for guidance.

Advisability of Use if Breast-Feeding

Presence of this drug in breast milk: Unknown.

Avoid drug or refrain from nursing.

Habit-Forming Potential: None.

Effects of Overdosage: Drowsiness, nausea, vomiting, diarrhea.

Possible Effects of Long-Term Use: None reported.

Suggested Periodic Examinations While Taking This Drug (at physician's discretion)

Complete blood cell counts, liver and kidney function tests, complete eye examinations if vision is altered in any way.

▷ **While Taking This Drug, Observe the Following**

Foods: No restrictions.

Beverages: No restrictions. May be taken with milk.

▷ *Alcohol:* Use with caution. The irritant action of alcohol on the stomach lining, added to the irritant action of this drug in sensitive individuals, can increase the risk of stomach ulceration and/or bleeding.

Tobacco Smoking: No interactions expected.

▷ *Other Drugs*

Ketoprofen may *increase* the effects of
- acetaminophen (Tylenol, etc.), and increase the risk of kidney damage; avoid prolonged use of this combination.
- anticoagulants (Coumadin, etc.), and increase the risk of bleeding; monitor prothrombin time, adjust dose accordingly.

Ketoprofen *taken concurrently* with the following drugs may increase the risk of bleeding; avoid these combinations:
- aspirin.
- dipyridamole (Persantine).
- indomethacin (Indocin).

- sulfinpyrazone (Anturane).
- valproic acid (Depakene).

▷ *Driving, Hazardous Activities:* This drug may cause drowsiness or dizziness. Restrict activities as necessary.

Aviation Note: The use of this drug **may be a disqualification** for piloting. Consult a designated Aviation Medical Examiner.

Exposure to Sun: This drug can cause photosensitivity (see Glossary). Avoid excessive exposure to sun until tolerance has been determined.

LABETALOL
(la BET a lohl)

Introduced: 1978

Class: Antihypertensive, alpha- and beta-adrenergic blocker

Prescription: USA: Yes
Canada: Yes

Controlled Drug: USA: No
Canada: No

Available as Generic: No

Brand Names: Normodyne, Normozide [CD], Trandate, Trandate HCT [CD]

BENEFITS versus RISKS

Possible Benefits	*Possible Risks*
EFFECTIVE, WELL-TOLERATED ANTIHYPERTENSIVE in mild to moderate high blood pressure	CONGESTIVE HEART FAILURE in advanced heart disease Worsening of angina in coronary heart disease (if drug is abruptly withdrawn) Masking of low blood sugar (hypoglycemia) in drug-treated diabetes

---

▷ **Principal Uses**

As a Single Drug Product: The treatment of mild to moderately severe high blood pressure. May be used alone or concurrently with other antihypertensive drugs, such as diuretics.

How This Drug Works: By blocking certain actions of the sympathetic nervous system, this drug

- reduces the rate and contraction force of the heart, thus lowering the ejection pressure of blood leaving the heart.
- reduces the degree of contraction of blood vessel walls, resulting in their relaxation and expansion and consequent lowering of blood pressure.

Available Dosage Forms and Strengths
Injection — 5 mg per ml
Tablets — 100 mg, 200 mg, 300 mg

▷ **Usual Adult Dosage Range:**   Initially, 100 mg twice daily, 12 hours apart; the dose may be increased by 100 mg twice daily every 2 to 3 days as required to reduce blood pressure. The usual maintenance dose is 200 to 400 mg twice daily. The total dose should not exceed 2400 mg/ 24 hours, given as 800 mg 3 times daily. **Note: Actual dosage and administration schedule must be determined by the physician for each patient individually.**

▷ **Dosing Instructions:**   Take at the same times each day, preferably following the morning and evening meals. The tablet may be crushed for administration. Do not discontinue this drug abruptly.

Usual Duration of Use: Continual use on a regular schedule for 10 to 14 days is usually necessary to determine this drug's effectiveness in lowering blood pressure. The long-term use (months to years) of this drug will be determined by the course of your blood pressure over time and your response to the overall treatment program (weight reduction, salt restriction, smoking cessation, etc.). Consult your physician on a regular basis.

Possible Advantages of This Drug
Decreases blood pressure more promptly than other beta blocker drugs. Can be used to treat hypertensive emergencies.

Currently a "Drug of Choice" for initiating treatment of hypertension with a single drug.

▷ **This Drug Should Not Be Taken If**
  • you have had an allergic reaction to it previously.
  • you have active bronchial asthma.
  • you have congestive heart failure.
  • you have an abnormally slow heart rate or a serious form of heart block.

▷ **Inform Your Physician Before Taking This Drug If**
  • you have had an adverse reaction to any beta blocker drug in the past (see Drug Class, Section Four).
  • you have a history of serious heart disease, with or without episodes of heart failure.
  • you have a history of hay fever (allergic rhinitis), asthma, chronic bronchitis or emphysema.
  • you have a history of overactive thyroid function (hyperthyroidism).
  • you have a history of low blood sugar (hypoglycemia).
  • you have impaired liver or kidney function.
  • you have diabetes or myasthenia gravis.

- you are currently taking any form of digitalis, quinidine or reserpine, or any calcium blocker drug (see Drug Class, Section Four).
- you plan to have surgery under general anesthesia in the near future.

Possible Side-Effects (natural, expected and unavoidable drug actions)
Lethargy and fatigability (11%), light-headedness in upright position (see Orthostatic Hypotension in Glossary).

▷ **Possible Adverse Effects** (unusual, unexpected and infrequent reactions)
If any of the following develop, consult your physician promptly for guidance.
Mild Adverse Effects
Allergic Reactions: Skin rash, itching.
Headache, drowsiness, dizziness (20%), scalp tingling (during early treatment).
Indigestion, nausea, diarrhea.
Joint and muscle discomfort, fluid retention (edema).
Serious Adverse Effects
Chest pain, shortness of breath, precipitation of congestive heart failure.
Induction of bronchial asthma (in asthmatic individuals).
Liver damage with jaundice (rare).
Difficult urination (urinary bladder retention).

▷ **Possible Effects on Sexual Function**
Impotence (10%), inhibited ejaculation (10%), prolonged erection following orgasm (related to higher doses), Peyronie's disease (see Glossary).
Decreased vaginal secretions (with low doses), inhibited female orgasm (related to higher doses).

CAUTION
1. ***Do not discontinue this drug suddenly*** without the knowledge and guidance of your physician. Carry a notation on your person that you are taking this drug.
2. Consult your physician or pharmacist before using nasal decongestants usually present in over-the-counter cold preparations and nose drops. These can cause sudden increases in blood pressure when taken concurrently with beta blocker drugs.
3. Report the development of any tendency to emotional depression.

Precautions for Use
By Infants and Children: Safety and effectiveness for use by those under 12 years of age have not been established. However, if this drug is used, observe for the development of low blood sugar (hypoglycemia) during periods of reduced food intake.
By Those over 60 Years of Age: Proceed **cautiously** with all antihypertensive drugs. Unacceptably high blood pressure should be reduced without creating the risks associated with excessively low blood pressure. Start treatment with small doses, and monitor the blood pressure response frequently. Sudden, rapid and excessive reduction of blood

pressure can predispose to stroke or heart attack. Observe for dizziness, unsteadiness, tendency to fall, confusion, hallucinations, depression or urinary frequency.

▷ **Advisability of Use During Pregnancy**
Pregnancy Category: C (tentative). See Pregnancy Code inside back cover.
Animal studies: No significant increase in birth defects found in rats or rabbits; some increase in fetal deaths reported.
Human studies: Information from adequate studies of pregnant women is not available.
Use this drug only if clearly needed. Ask physician for guidance.

Advisability of Use if Breast-Feeding
Presence of this drug in breast milk: Yes, in very small amounts.
Avoid drug or refrain from nursing.

Habit-Forming Potential: None.

Effects of Overdosage: Weakness, slow pulse, low blood pressure, fainting, cold and sweaty skin, congestive heart failure, possible coma and convulsions.

Possible Effects of Long-Term Use: Reduced heart reserve and eventual heart failure in susceptible individuals with advanced heart disease.

Suggested Periodic Examinations While Taking This Drug (at physician's discretion)
Measurements of blood pressure, evaluation of heart function.

▷ **While Taking This Drug, Observe the Following**
Foods: No restrictions. Avoid excessive salt intake.
Beverages: No restrictions. May be taken with milk.
▷ *Alcohol:* Use with caution until the combined effect has been determined. Alcohol may exaggerate this drug's ability to lower blood pressure and may increase its mild sedative effect.
Tobacco Smoking: Nicotine may reduce this drug's effectiveness in treating high blood pressure. In addition, high doses of this drug may potentiate the constriction of the bronchial tubes caused by regular smoking.
▷ *Other Drugs*
Labetalol may ***increase*** the effects of
• other antihypertensive drugs and cause excessive lowering of blood pressure. Dosage adjustments may be necessary.
Labetalol ***taken concurrently*** with
• clonidine (Catapres) requires close monitoring for rebound high blood pressure if clonidine is withdrawn while labetalol is still being taken.
• insulin requires close monitoring to avoid undetected hypoglycemia (see Glossary).
▷ *Driving, Hazardous Activities:* Use caution until the full extent of fatigue, dizziness and blood pressure change has been determined.

Aviation Note: The use of this drug *is a disqualification* for piloting. Consult a designated Aviation Medical Examiner.

Exposure to Sun: No restrictions.

Exposure to Heat: Caution advised. Hot environments can lower the blood pressure and exaggerate the effects of this drug.

Exposure to Cold: Caution advised. Cold environments can enhance the circulatory deficiency in the extremities that may occur with some beta blocker drugs. The elderly should take precautions to prevent hypothermia (see Glossary).

Heavy Exercise or Exertion: It is advisable to avoid exertion that produces light-headedness, excessive fatigue or muscle cramping. The use of this drug may intensify the hypertensive response to isometric exercise.

Occurrence of Unrelated Illness: The fever that accompanies systemic infections can lower the blood pressure and require adjustment of dosage. Illnesses that cause nausea or vomiting may interrupt the regular dosage schedule. Ask your physician for guidance.

Discontinuation: It is advisable to avoid sudden discontinuation of this drug in all situations. If possible, gradual reduction of dose over a period of 2 to 3 weeks is recommended. Ask your physician for specific guidance.

LEVODOPA
(lee voh DOH pa)

Introduced: 1967

Class: Antiparkinsonism

Prescription: USA: Yes
Canada: Yes

Controlled Drug: USA: No
Canada: No

Available as Generic: USA: Yes
Canada: No

Brand Names: Dopar, Larodopa, ✦Prolopa [CD], Sinemet [CD]

BENEFITS versus RISKS

Possible Benefits	*Possible Risks*
EFFECTIVE RELIEF OF SYMPTOMS IN 80% OF CASES OF IDIOPATHIC PARKINSON'S DISEASE	Emotional depression, confusion, abnormal thinking and behavior
	Abnormal involuntary movements
	Heart rhythm disturbance
	Urinary bladder retention
	Induction of peptic ulcer (rare)
	Blood cell abnormalities: hemolytic anemia, reduced white blood cell count (both rare)

▷ **Principal Uses**

As a Single Drug Product: Used exclusively to treat the major types of Parkinson's disease: paralysis agitans ("shaking palsy" of unknown cause), the type that follows encephalitis, the parkinsonism that develops with aging (associated with hardening of the brain arteries), and the forms of parkinsonism that follow poisoning by carbon monoxide or manganese.

As a Combination Drug Product [CD]: This drug is available in combination with carbidopa, a chemical that prevents the decomposition of levodopa before it reaches its site of action in the brain. The addition of carbidopa reduces the amount of levodopa required by 75%. This combination is more effective in smaller doses and reduces the frequency and severity of adverse effects.

How This Drug Works: Not completely established. Present thinking is that levodopa enters the brain tissue and is converted to dopamine. After sufficient dosage, this corrects the deficiency of dopamine (that is thought to be the cause of parkinsonism) and restores a more normal balance of the chemicals responsible for transmission of nerve impulses in appropriate control centers of the brain.

Available Dosage Forms and Strengths
Capsules — 100 mg, 250 mg, 500 mg
Tablets — 100 mg, 250 mg, 500 mg

▷ **Usual Adult Dosage Range:** Initially, 250 mg 2 to 4 times/day. The dose may be increased cautiously by increments of 100 to 750 mg at 3- to 7-day intervals as needed and tolerated. The total dosage should not exceed 8000 mg/24 hours. If the combination drug Sinemet is used, the total levodopa requirement will be considerably less. **Note: Actual dosage and administration schedule must be determined by the physician for each patient individually.**

▷ **Dosing Instructions:** Preferably taken with or following carbohydrate foods to reduce stomach irritation; when possible, do not take this drug concurrently with high-protein foods. The tablet may be crushed for administration.

Usual Duration of Use: Continual use on a regular schedule for 3 to 6 weeks is usually necessary to determine this drug's effectiveness in relieving the major symptoms of parkinsonism. The determination of maximal effectiveness may require continual use for 6 months. Long-term use (months to years) requires supervision and periodic evaluation by your physician; dosage adjustments will be necessary and unavoidable during the course of the disorder. Consult your physician on a regular basis.

▷ **This Drug Should Not Be Taken If**
- you are allergic to any of the drugs bearing the brand names listed.
- you have narrow-angle glaucoma (inadequately controlled).

- you are taking, or have taken within the past 14 days, any monoamine oxidase (MAO) type A inhibitor drug (see Drug Class, Section Four).

▷ **Inform Your Physician Before Taking This Drug If**
- you have diabetes, epilepsy, heart disease, high blood pressure or chronic lung disease.
- you have impaired liver or kidney function.
- you have a history of peptic ulcer disease or malignant melanoma.
- you plan to have surgery under general anesthesia in the near future.

Possible Side-Effects (natural, expected and unavoidable drug actions)
Fatigue, lethargy, altered taste, offensive body odor, orthostatic hypotension (see Glossary).
Pink to red coloration of urine, turning black on exposure to air (of no significance).

▷ **Possible Adverse Effects** (unusual, unexpected and infrequent reactions)
If any of the following develop, consult your physician promptly for guidance.
Mild Adverse Effects
Allergic Reactions: Skin rash, itching.
Headache, dizziness, numbness, unsteadiness, insomnia, nightmares, blurred vision, double vision.
Loss of appetite, nausea, vomiting, dry mouth, difficult swallowing, excessive gas, diarrhea, constipation.
Loss of hair (rare).
Serious Adverse Effects
Idiosyncratic Reaction: Hemolytic anemia (see Glossary).
Confusion, delusions, hallucinations, agitation, paranoia, depression, psychotic episodes, seizures.
Abnormal involuntary movements of the head, face and extremities.
Disturbances of heart rhythm, high blood pressure (rare).
Development of peptic ulcer, gastrointestinal bleeding.
Urinary bladder retention.
Abnormally low white blood cell count—lowered resistance to infection, fever, sore throat.

▷ **Possible Effects on Sexual Function:** Increased libido reported by both males and females (24% to 36%); inhibited ejaculation (rare); priapism (see Glossary).

▷ **Adverse Effects That May Mimic Natural Diseases or Disorders**
Mental reactions may resemble idiopathic psychosis.

Natural Diseases or Disorders That May Be Activated by This Drug
Latent peptic ulcer.

CAUTION
1. To reduce the high frequency of serious adverse effects, it is advisable to begin treatment with small doses, and to increase dosage gradually until the desired response is achieved.

2. As improvement occurs, avoid excessive and hurried activity (which often causes falls and injury).

Precautions for Use

By Infants and Children: This drug can cause precocious puberty when taken by the prepubertal boy. Observe closely for hypersexual behavior and for premature growth of the genital organs.

By Those over 60 Years of Age: Treatment should begin with half of the usual adult dose; dosage increases should be made cautiously in small increments as needed and tolerated. Observe for the possible development of significant behavioral changes: depression or inappropriate elation, acute confusion, agitation, paranoia, dementia, nightmares and hallucinations. Abnormal involuntary movements may also occur.

▷ Advisability of Use During Pregnancy

Pregnancy Category: C (tentative). See Pregnancy Code inside back cover.
Animal studies: Significant birth defects reported in rodent studies.
Human studies: Information from adequate studies of pregnant women is not available.
Avoid use of drug during the first 3 months. Use only if clearly needed during the last 6 months.

Advisability of Use if Breast-Feeding

Presence of this drug in breast milk: Yes.
Avoid drug or refrain from nursing.

Habit-Forming Potential: None.

Effects of Overdosage: Muscle twitching, spastic closure of eyelids, nausea, vomiting, diarrhea, weakness, fainting, confusion, agitation, hallucinations.

Possible Effects of Long-Term Use: Development of abnormal involuntary movements involving the head, face, mouth and extremities. These may be reversible and may gradually subside as the drug is withdrawn.

Suggested Periodic Examinations While Taking This Drug (at physician's discretion)

Complete blood cell counts; measurements of internal eye pressure; blood pressure measurements in lying, sitting and standing positions.

▷ While Taking This Drug, Observe the Following

Foods: No restrictions. Insofar as possible, do not take concurrently with protein foods; proteins compete for absorption.

Nutritional Support: If taken alone (without carbidopa), monitor for the development of peripheral neuritis and take small supplements of pyridoxine (vitamin B-6) if needed: 10 mg or less; larger doses can decrease the effectiveness of levodopa. If taken in combination with carbidopa (Sinemet), supplemental pyridoxine is not required.

Beverages: No restrictions. May be taken with milk.

▷ *Alcohol:* No interactions expected.

Tobacco Smoking: No interactions expected.

Marijuana Smoking: Increased fatigue and lethargy; possible accentuation of orthostatic hypotension (see Glossary).

▷ *Other Drugs*

Levodopa *taken concurrently* with

- monoamine oxidase (MAO) type A inhibitor drugs (see Drug Class, Section Four) may cause a dangerous rise in blood pressure and body temperature. Do not use these drugs concurrently.

The following drugs may *decrease* the effects of levodopa

- papaverine (Cerespan, Pavabid, Vasospan, etc.).
- phenytoin (Dilantin, etc.).
- pyridoxine (vitamin B-6).

▷ *Driving, Hazardous Activities:* This drug may cause dizziness, impaired vision and orthostatic hypotension. Restrict activities as necessary.

Aviation Note: Parkinson's disease *is a disqualification* for piloting. Consult a designated Aviation Medical Examiner.

Exposure to Sun: No restrictions.

Exposure to Heat: Use caution. This drug can cause flushing and excessive sweating and predispose to heat exhaustion.

Occurrence of Unrelated Illness: Suspicious dark-colored skin lesions should be evaluated carefully to exclude the possibility of malignant melanoma. During the course of any intercurrent infection, monitor the white blood cell count carefully for normal response.

LISINOPRIL
(li SIN oh pril)

Introduced: 1988

Class: Antihypertensive, ACE inhibitor

Prescription: USA: Yes

Controlled Drug: USA: No

Available as Generic: No

Brand Names: Prinivil, Prinzide [CD], Zestoretic [CD], Zestril

BENEFITS versus RISKS	
Possible Benefits	*Possible Risks*
EFFECTIVE CONTROL OF MILD TO SEVERE HIGH BLOOD PRESSURE	Headache (5.3%), dizziness (6.3%), fatigue (3.3%)
	Low blood pressure (1.8%)
	Allergic swelling of face, tongue, throat, vocal cords (0.1%)

▷ **Principal Uses**

As a Single Drug Product: Used primarily to treat all degrees of high blood pressure. Mild to moderate high blood pressure usually responds to low doses; severe high blood pressure may require higher doses and the concurrent use of a thiazide or other class of antihypertensive drug.

How This Drug Works: Not completely known. It is thought that by blocking certain enzyme systems that influence arterial function, this drug contributes to the relaxation of arterial walls throughout the body and thus lowers the resistance to blood flow that causes high blood pressure. This, in turn, reduces the workload of the heart and improves its performance.

Available Dosage Forms and Strengths

Tablets — 5 mg, 10 mg, 20 mg, 40 mg

▷ **Usual Adult Dosage Range:**   Initially 10 mg once daily for those not taking a diuretic; 5 mg once daily for those taking a diuretic. Usual maintenance dose is 20 to 40 mg/day taken in a single dose. Total daily dosage should not exceed 80 mg. **Note: Actual dosage and administration schedule must be determined by the physician for each patient individually.**

▷ **Dosing Instructions:**   Take on an empty stomach or with food, at same time each day. The tablet may be crushed for administration.

Usual Duration of Use: Continual use on a regular schedule for several weeks is usually necessary to determine this drug's effectiveness in controlling high blood pressure. The proper treatment of high blood pressure usually requires the long-term use of effective medications. Consult your physician on a regular basis.

Possible Advantages of This Drug

Controls blood pressure effectively with one daily dose.
Relatively low incidence of adverse effects.
No adverse influence on asthma, cholesterol blood levels or diabetes.
Sudden withdrawal does not result in a rapid increase in blood pressure.

▷ **This Drug Should Not Be Taken If**

- you have had an allergic reaction to it previously.
- you currently have a blood cell or bone marrow disorder.
- you have an abnormally high level of blood potassium.

▷ **Inform Your Physician Before Taking This Drug If**

- you have a history of kidney disease or impaired kidney function.
- you have scleroderma or systemic lupus erythematosus.
- you have cerebral artery disease.
- you have any form of heart disease.

- you are taking any of the following drugs: other antihypertensives, diuretics, nitrates or potassium supplements.
- you plan to have surgery under general anesthesia in the near future.

Possible Side-Effects (natural, expected and unavoidable drug actions)
Dizziness (6.3%), orthostatic hypotension (1.4%) (see Glossary), increased blood potassium level (2.2%).

▷ **Possible Adverse Effects** (unusual, unexpected and infrequent reactions)
If any of the following develop, consult your physician promptly for guidance.
Mild Adverse Effects
Allergic Reactions: Skin rash (1.5%), itching (0.3% to 1.0%).
Headache (5.3%), fatigue (3.3%), numbness and tingling (0.8%), weakness (1.3%).
Chest pain (1.3%), palpitation (0.3% to 1.0%), cough (2.9%).
Indigestion (1.0%), nausea (2.3%), vomiting (1.3%), diarrhea (3.2%).
Serious Adverse Effects
Allergic Reactions: Swelling (angioedema) of face, tongue and/or vocal cords (less than 0.1%); can be life-threatening.
Impairment of kidney function (0.3% to 1.0%).

▷ **Possible Effects on Sexual Function:** Decreased libido (0.2%), impotence (0.7%).

CAUTION
1. Consult your physician regarding the advisability of discontinuing other antihypertensive drugs (especially diuretics) for 1 week before starting this drug.
2. **Report promptly** any indications of infection (fever, sore throat), and any indications of water retention (weight gain, puffiness, swollen feet or ankles).
3. Do not use a salt substitute without your physician's knowledge and approval. (Many salt substitutes contain potassium.)
4. It is advisable to obtain blood cell counts and urine analyses **before** starting this drug.

Precautions for Use
By Infants and Children: Safety and effectiveness for use by those in this age group have not been established.
By Those over 60 Years of Age: Small doses are advisable until tolerance has been determined. Sudden and excessive lowering of blood pressure can predispose to stroke or heart attack in those with impaired brain circulation or coronary artery heart disease.

▷ **Advisability of Use During Pregnancy**
Pregnancy Category: C (tentative). See Pregnancy Code inside back cover.
Animal studies: No birth defects found in mouse or rat studies. Impaired bone formation found in rabbit studies.

Human studies: Information from adequate studies of pregnant women is not available.

Avoid during first 3 months if possible.

Advisability of Use if Breast-Feeding
Presence of this drug in breast milk: Unknown.
Avoid drug or refrain from nursing.

Habit-Forming Potential: None.

Effects of Overdosage: Excessive drop in blood pressure, light-headedness, dizziness, fainting.

Possible Effects of Long-Term Use: Gradual increase in blood potassium level.

Suggested Periodic Examinations While Taking This Drug (at physician's discretion)
Before starting drug: Complete blood cell counts; urine analysis with measurement of protein content; blood potassium level.
During use of drug: Blood cell counts; measurements of blood potassium.

▷ **While Taking This Drug, Observe the Following**
Foods: Consult physician regarding salt intake.
Nutritional Support: **Do not take** potassium supplements unless directed by your physician.
Beverages: No restrictions. May be taken with milk.
▷   *Alcohol:* Use caution until combined effect has been determined. Alcohol may enhance the blood-pressure-lowering effect of this drug.
Tobacco Smoking: No interactions expected.
▷   *Other Drugs*
Lisinopril *taken concurrently* with
   • potassium preparations (K-Lyte, Slow-K, etc.) may cause increased blood levels of potassium with risk of serious heart rhythm disturbances.
   • potassium-sparing diuretics: amiloride (Moduretic), spironolactone (Aldactazide), triamterene (Dyazide) may cause increased blood levels of potassium with risk of serious heart rhythm disturbances.
▷   *Driving, Hazardous Activities:* Usually no restrictions. Be aware of possible drops in blood pressure with resultant dizziness or faintness.
Aviation Note: The use of this drug **may be a disqualification** for piloting. Consult a designated Aviation Medical Examiner.
Exposure to Sun: Caution advised. A similar drug of this class can cause photosensitivity.
Exposure to Heat: Caution advised. Avoid excessive perspiring with resultant loss of body water and drop in blood pressure.
Occurrence of Unrelated Illness: Report promptly any disorder that causes nausea, vomiting or diarrhea. Fluid and chemical imbalances must be corrected as soon as possible.

Discontinuation: This drug may be stopped abruptly without causing a sudden increase in blood pressure. However, you should consult your physician regarding withdrawal of this drug for any reason.

LITHIUM
(LITH i um)

Introduced: 1949

Class: Antidepressant, antimanic

Prescription: USA: Yes
  Canada: Yes

Controlled Drug: USA: No
  Canada: No

Available as Generic: USA: Yes
  Canada: No

Brand Names: ✦Carbolith, Cibalith-S, ✦Duralith, Eskalith, Lithane, ✦Lithizine, Lithobid, Lithonate, Lithotabs

---

BENEFITS versus RISKS

Possible Benefits	*Possible Risks*
RAPID REVERSAL OF ACUTE MANIA in 80% of users	VERY NARROW MARGIN BETWEEN TREATMENT AND TOXIC BLOOD LEVELS
STABILIZATION OF MOOD in 60% to 70% of users with manic-depressive disorder	POTENTIALLY FATAL TOXICITY with inadequate monitoring
Prevention of recurrent depression in "responders"	Infrequent induction of diabetes mellitus, hypothyroidism
	Diabetes insipidus–like syndrome (excessive dilute urine without sugar)

▷ **Principal Uses**

As a Single Drug Product: Used primarily in the management of manic-depressive disorders. While its principal use is the prompt correction of acute mania, it is also used to stabilize these disorders by reducing the frequency and severity of recurrent manic-depressive mood swings. It is also beneficial in treating the depression phase of these disorders in individuals who do not experience the manic phase. Additional uses (experimental) include the prevention of cluster headaches and the stimulation of production of white blood cells.

How This Drug Works: Not completely established. It is thought that lithium may act to correct chemical imbalances in certain nerve impulse transmitters (dopamine and norepinephrine) that influence emotional status and behavior.

Available Dosage Forms and Strengths
Capsules — 150 mg, 300 mg, 600 mg
Syrup — 8 mEq per 5-ml teaspoonful
Tablets — 300 mg
Tablets, prolonged-action — 300 mg, 450 mg

▷ **Usual Adult Dosage Range:**   First day: 300 mg taken 3 times, 6 hours apart; second day and thereafter: increase dose to 1200 mg/24 hours and later to 1800 mg/24 hours if needed and tolerated. The usual maintenance dose is 600 to 1200 mg/24 hours taken in 3 divided doses. The total daily dosage should not exceed 3600 mg. **Note: Actual dosage and administration schedule must be determined by the physician for each patient individually.**

▷ **Dosing Instructions:**   May be taken after meals to reduce stomach irritation. The capsules may be opened and the regular tablets may be crushed for administration; the prolonged-action tablets should be swallowed whole and not altered.

Usual Duration of Use: Continual use on a regular schedule for 1 to 3 weeks is usually necessary to determine this drug's effectiveness in correcting acute mania; several months of continual treatment may be required to correct depression. Long-term use (months to years) requires supervision and periodic evaluation by your physician. Consult your physician on a regular basis.

Currently a "Drug of Choice" for the treatment of acute mania in bipolar manic-depressive disorders.

▷ **This Drug Should Not Be Taken If**
- you have had an allergic reaction to any dosage form of it previously.
- you have uncontrolled diabetes or uncorrected hypothyroidism.
- you are breast-feeding.
- you will be unable to comply with the need for regular monitoring of lithium blood levels.

▷ **Inform Your Physician Before Taking This Drug If**
- you have a history of a schizophreniclike thought disorder.
- you have any type of organic brain disease, or a history of grand mal epilepsy.
- you have diabetes, heart disease, hypothyroidism or impaired kidney function.
- you are on a salt-restricted diet.
- you are pregnant or planning pregnancy.
- you are taking any diuretic drug or a cortisonelike steroid preparation.

Possible Side-Effects (natural, expected and unavoidable drug actions)
Increased thirst and urine volume may occur in 60% of initial users and in 20% of long-term maintenance users. Weight gain may occur in

first few months of use. Drowsiness and lethargy may occur in sensitive individuals.

▷ **Possible Adverse Effects** (unusual, unexpected and infrequent reactions)
If any of the following develop, consult your physician promptly for guidance.
Mild Adverse Effects
Allergic Reactions: Skin rashes, generalized itching.
Skin dryness, loss of hair.
Headache, dullness, dizziness, weakness, blurred vision, ringing in ears, fine hand tremor, unsteadiness.
Metallic taste, loss of appetite, stomach irritation, nausea, vomiting, diarrhea.
Serious Adverse Effects
"Blackout" spells, confusion, stupor, slurred speech, spasmodic movements of extremities, epilepticlike seizures.
Loss of bladder or rectal control.
Diabetes insipidus–like syndrome: loss of kidney concentrating power, excessive dilute urine.

▷ **Possible Effects on Sexual Function:** Decreased libido (blood level of 0.7 to 0.9 meq/L); inhibited erection: 30% of users (0.6 to 0.8 meq/L); male infertility; female breast swelling with milk production.

▷ **Adverse Effects That May Mimic Natural Diseases or Disorders**
Painful discoloration and coldness of the hands and feet may resemble Raynaud's syndrome.

Natural Diseases or Disorders That May Be Activated by This Drug
Diabetes mellitus may be worsened. Psoriasis may be intensified. Myasthenia gravis may be induced (1 case).

CAUTION
1. This drug has a very narrow margin of safe use. The blood level of drug required to be effective is quite close to the level that can cause toxic effects. Periodic measurements of blood lithium levels are mandatory for appropriate adjustments of dosage. Follow instructions exactly regarding drug dosage and periodic blood examinations.
2. Lithium should be discontinued at the first signs of toxicity: drowsiness, sluggishness, muscle twitching, vomiting or diarrhea.
3. The major causes of lithium toxicity are
   • accidental overdose (sometimes due to inadequate monitoring of blood levels).
   • impaired kidney function.
   • salt restriction.
   • inadequate fluid intake, dehydration.
   • concurrent use of diuretics.
   • intercurrent illness.
   • childbirth (rapid decrease in kidney clearance of lithium).

- initiation of treatment with a new drug.
4. Over-the-counter preparations that contain iodides (some cough products and vitamin-mineral supplements) should be avoided because of the added antithyroid effect when taken with lithium.

Precautions for Use

By Infants and Children: Safety and effectiveness for use by those under 12 years of age have not been established. Follow physician's instructions exactly.

By Those over 60 Years of Age: Initial and maintenance doses should be smaller than standard doses for younger adults; treatment should start with a "test" dose of 75 to 150 mg daily. Observe closely for early indications of toxic effects, especially if on a low-salt diet and using diuretics. Parkinsonian reactions (abnormal gait and movements) occur with greater frequency; coma can develop without warning symptoms.

▷ Advisability of Use During Pregnancy

Pregnancy Category: D (tentative). See Pregnancy Code inside back cover.

Animal studies: Cleft palate reported in mice; eye, ear and palate defects reported in rats.

Human studies: Information from adequate studies of pregnant women is not available. However, cardiovascular defects and goiter in newborn infants (of mothers using lithium) have been reported. If the infant's blood level of lithium approaches the toxic range before delivery, the newborn may suffer the "floppy infant" syndrome: weakness, lethargy, unresponsiveness, low body temperature, weak cry and poor feeding ability.

Avoid use of drug during the first 3 months. Use only if clearly necessary during the last 6 months. Monitor mother's blood lithium levels carefully to avoid possible toxicity.

Advisability of Use if Breast-Feeding

Presence of this drug in breast milk: Yes, in significant amounts.

Avoid drug or refrain from nursing.

Habit-Forming Potential: None.

Effects of Overdosage: Drowsiness, weakness, lack of coordination, nausea, vomiting, diarrhea, muscle spasms, blurred vision, dizziness, staggering gait, slurred speech, confusion, stupor, coma, seizures.

Possible Effects of Long-Term Use: Hypothyroidism (5%), goiter, reduced sugar tolerance, diabetes insipidus–like syndrome, serious kidney damage.

Suggested Periodic Examinations While Taking This Drug (at physician's discretion)

Regular determinations of blood lithium levels are absolutely essential to the safe and effective use of this drug.

Periodic evaluation of thyroid gland size and function.
Complete blood cell counts; kidney function tests.

▷ **While Taking This Drug, Observe the Following**

Foods: Maintain a normal diet; **do not** restrict your use of salt.

Beverages: No restrictions. Drink at least 2.5 to 3 quarts of liquids/24 hours. This drug may be taken with milk.

▷ *Alcohol:* Use with caution until the combined effects have been determined. Avoid alcohol completely if any symptoms of lithium toxicity develop.

Tobacco Smoking: No interactions expected.

Marijuana Smoking: Possible increase in apathy, lethargy, drowsiness or sluggishness; accentuation of lithium-induced tremor; possible increased risk of precipitating psychotic behavior.

▷ *Other Drugs* Lithium **taken concurrently** with
- carbamazepine (Tegretol) or with
- chlorpromazine (Thorazine, etc.) or with
- haloperidol (Haldol) is usually well tolerated; however, it may cause a severe neurotoxic reaction in susceptible individuals. These combinations should be used very cautiously.
- diazepam (Valium) may cause hypothermia.

The following drugs may **increase** the effects of lithium
- indomethacin (Indocin).
- piroxicam (Feldene).
- thiazide diuretics (see Drug Class, Section Four).

The following drugs may **decrease** the effects of lithium
- sodium bicarbonate.
- theophylline (Theo-Dur, etc.) and related drugs.

▷ *Driving, Hazardous Activities:* This drug may impair mental alertness, judgment, physical coordination and reaction time. Restrict activities as necessary.

Aviation Note: The use of this drug **is a disqualification** for piloting. Consult a designated Aviation Medical Examiner.

Exposure to Sun: No restrictions.

Exposure to Heat: Excessive sweating can cause significant depletion of salt and water and resultant lithium toxicity. Avoid sauna baths.

Occurrence of Unrelated Illness: Any illness that causes fever, sweating, vomiting or diarrhea can result in significant alterations of blood and tissue lithium concentrations. Close monitoring of your physical condition and blood lithium levels is necessary to prevent serious toxicity.

Discontinuation: Sudden discontinuation does not cause withdrawal symptoms. Avoid premature discontinuation; some individuals may require continual treatment for up to a year to achieve maximal response. Discontinuation by "responders" may result in recurrence of either mania or depression. Lithium should be discontinued if symptoms of brain toxicity appear or if an uncorrectable diabetes insipidus–like syndrome develops.

LOPERAMIDE
(loh PER a mide)

Introduced: 1977

Class: Antidiarrheal

Prescription: USA: Yes
  Canada: No

Controlled Drug: USA: No
  Canada: No

Available as Generic: No

Brand Names: Imodium, Imodium A-D

BENEFITS versus RISKS	
Possible Benefits	*Possible Risks*
EFFECTIVE RELIEF OF INTESTINAL CRAMPING AND DIARRHEA	Drowsiness Constipation Induction of toxic megacolon

▷ **Principal Uses**

As a Single Drug Product: Used primarily for the control of cramping and diarrhea associated with acute gastroenteritis and chronic enteritis and colitis. Also used to reduce the volume of discharge from ileostomies.

How This Drug Works: Not completely established. It is thought that this drug acts directly on the nerve supply of the gastrointestinal tract to reduce its motility and propulsive contractions, thus relieving cramping and diarrhea.

Available Dosage Forms and Strengths

Capsules — 2 mg
Liquid — 1 mg per 5-ml teaspoonful (alcohol 5.25%)

▷ **Usual Adult Dosage Range:** For acute diarrhea: 4 mg initially, then 2 mg after each unformed stool until diarrhea is controlled. For chronic diarrhea: 4 to 8 mg/day in divided doses, taken 8 to 12 hours apart. The total daily dosage should not exceed 16 mg. **Note: Actual dosage and administration schedule must be determined by the physician for each patient individually.**

▷ **Dosing Instructions:** May be taken on an empty stomach or with food if stomach irritation occurs. The capsule may be opened for administration.

Usual Duration of Use: Continual use on a regular schedule for 48 hours is usually necessary to determine this drug's effectiveness in controlling acute diarrhea; continual use for 10 days may be needed to evaluate its effectiveness in controlling chronic diarrhea. If diarrhea persists, consult your physician.

▷ **This Drug Should Not Be Taken If**
- you have had an allergic reaction to it previously.
- it is prescribed for a child under 2 years of age.

▷ **Inform Your Physician Before Taking This Drug If**
- you have a history of liver disease or impaired liver function.
- you have regional enteritis or ulcerative colitis.

Possible Side-Effects (natural, expected and unavoidable drug actions)
Drowsiness, constipation.

▷ **Possible Adverse Effects** (unusual, unexpected and infrequent reactions)
If any of the following develop, consult your physician promptly for guidance.
Mild Adverse Effects
Allergic Reaction: Skin rash.
Fatigue, dizziness.
Reduced appetite, dry mouth, nausea, vomiting, stomach pain, bloating.
Serious Adverse Effects
"Toxic megacolon" (distended, immobile colon with fluid retention) may develop while treating acute ulcerative colitis.

▷ **Possible Effects on Sexual Function:** None reported.

CAUTION
1. Do not exceed recommended doses.
2. If used to treat chronic diarrhea, report promptly any development of bloating, abdominal distension, nausea, vomiting, constipation or abdominal pain.

Precautions for Use
By Infants and Children: Do not use in those under 2 years of age. Follow physician's instructions exactly regarding dosage. Observe for drowsiness, irritability, personality changes and altered behavior.
By Those over 60 Years of Age: Start treatment with small doses. You may be more sensitive to the sedative and constipating effects of this drug.

▷ **Advisability of Use During Pregnancy**
Pregnancy Category: B (tentative). See Pregnancy Code inside back cover.
Animal studies: No birth defects found in rat and rabbit studies.
Human studies: Information from adequate studies of pregnant women is not available.
Use sparingly and only if clearly needed. Ask physician for guidance.

Advisability of Use if Breast-Feeding
Presence of this drug in breast milk: Unknown.
Avoid drug or refrain from nursing.

Habit-Forming Potential: None.

Effects of Overdosage: Drowsiness, lethargy, depression, dry mouth.

Possible Effects of Long-Term Use: None identified.

Suggested Periodic Examinations While Taking This Drug (at physician's discretion)
None required.

▷ **While Taking This Drug, Observe the Following**
Foods: No restrictions. Follow prescribed diet.
Beverages: No restrictions. May be taken with milk.
▷ *Alcohol:* Use with caution until combined effects have been determined. This drug may increase the depressant action of alcohol on the brain.
Tobacco Smoking: No interactions expected.
▷ *Other Drugs:* No significant drug interactions reported.
▷ *Driving, Hazardous Activities:* This drug may cause drowsiness or dizziness. Restrict activities as necessary.
Aviation Note: The use of this drug *is a disqualification* for piloting. Consult a designated Aviation Medical Examiner.
Exposure to Sun: No restrictions.

LORAZEPAM
(lor AZ e pam)

Introduced: 1971

Class: Mild tranquilizer, benzodiazepines

Prescription: USA: Yes
Canada: Yes

Controlled Drug: USA: C-IV*
Canada: No

Available as Generic: USA: Yes
Canada: No

Brand Names: Alzapam, ✦Apo-Lorazepam, Ativan, Loraz, ✦Novolorazepam

---

BENEFITS versus RISKS

Possible Benefits	*Possible Risks*
RELIEF OF ANXIETY AND NERVOUS TENSION in 70% to 80% of users	Habit-forming potential with prolonged use
Wide margin of safety with therapeutic doses	Minor impairment of mental functions
Very few drug interactions	

---

*See Schedules of Controlled Drugs inside back cover.

▷ **Principal Uses**

As a Single Drug Product: Used primarily to provide short-term relief of mild to moderate anxiety. While it is less sedative than the barbiturates, it is also used at bedtime to produce a calming effect that permits natural sleep.

How This Drug Works: It is thought that this drug produces a calming effect by enhancing the action of the nerve transmitter gamma-aminobutyric acid (GABA), which in turn blocks the arousal of higher brain centers.

Available Dosage Forms and Strengths

Injection — 2 mg per ml, 4 mg per ml

Tablets — 0.5 mg, 1 mg, 2 mg

▷ **Usual Adult Dosage Range:**   1 to 10 mg/24 hours. For anxiety: 2 to 3 mg, 2 or 3 times/day. For insomnia: 2 to 4 mg at bedtime. The total daily dose should not exceed 10 mg. **Note: Actual dosage and administration schedule must be determined by the physician for each patient individually.**

▷ **Dosing Instructions:**   May be taken on empty stomach or with food or milk. The tablet may be crushed for administration. Do not discontinue this drug abruptly if taken for more than 4 weeks.

Usual Duration of Use: Continual use on a regular schedule for 3 to 5 days is usually necessary to determine this drug's effectiveness in relieving moderate anxiety. Limit continual use to 1 to 3 weeks. Avoid uninterrupted and prolonged use.

▷ **This Drug Should Not Be Taken If**

- you have had an allergic reaction to any dosage form of it previously.
- you have acute narrow-angle glaucoma.
- it is prescribed for a child under 12 years of age.

▷ **Inform Your Physician Before Taking This Drug If**

- you are allergic to any benzodiazepine drug (see Drug Class, Section Four).
- you have a history of alcoholism or drug abuse.
- you are pregnant or planning pregnancy.
- you have impaired liver or kidney function.
- you have a history of serious depression or mental disorder.
- you have any of the following: asthma, emphysema, epilepsy, myasthenia gravis.

Possible Side-Effects (natural, expected and unavoidable drug actions)

Drowsiness, lethargy, unsteadiness, "hangover" effects on the day following bedtime use.

▷ **Possible Adverse Effects** (unusual, unexpected and infrequent reactions)

If any of the following develop, consult your physician promptly for guidance.

Mild Adverse Effects
Allergic Reaction: Skin rash.
Dizziness (6%), fainting, blurred vision, double vision, slurred speech, headache, sweating, nausea, indigestion.
Serious Adverse Effects
Disorientation, emotional depression, agitation, disturbed sleep, periodic amnesia.

▷ **Possible Effects on Sexual Function:** Antianxiety effect can relieve nervous tension that is often responsible for male impotence and female vaginismus (painful spasm of vagina), thus improving sexual performance. (Impaired sexual functioning relieved in 40%.)

CAUTION
1. This drug should not be discontinued abruptly if it has been taken continually for more than 4 weeks.
2. The concurrent use of some over-the-counter drug products that contain antihistamines (allergy and cold preparations, sleep aids) can cause excessive sedation in sensitive individuals.
3. If this drug is taken at bedtime as a hypnotic, significant impairment of intellectual and motor functions may persist into the following day; avoid hazardous activities and the use of alcohol.

Precautions for Use
By Infants and Children: Safety and effectiveness for use by those under 12 years of age have not been established. This drug should not be used in the hyperactive or psychotic child of any age. Observe for excessive sedation and incoordination.
By Those over 60 Years of Age: It is advisable to use smaller doses at longer intervals to avoid overdosage. Observe for the possible development of lethargy, indifference, fatigue, weakness, unsteadiness, disturbing dreams, nightmares and paradoxical reactions of excitement, agitation, anger, hostility and rage.

▷ **Advisability of Use During Pregnancy**
Pregnancy Category: C (tentative). See Pregnancy Code inside back cover.
Animal studies: Skeletal and eye defects reported in rabbits.
Human studies: Information from adequate studies of pregnant women is not available. No birth defects have been reported with the use of this drug.
Avoid drug completely during the first 3 months; avoid during the last 6 months if possible. Frequent use in late pregnancy may cause the "floppy infant" syndrome in the newborn: weakness, lethargy, unresponsiveness, depressed breathing, low body temperature.

Advisability of Use if Breast-Feeding
Presence of this drug in breast milk: Yes, in small amounts.
Monitor nursing infant closely and discontinue drug or nursing if adverse effects develop.

Habit-Forming Potential: This drug can produce psychological and/or physical dependence (see Glossary) if used in large doses for an extended period of time.

Effects of Overdosage: Marked drowsiness, weakness, feeling of drunkenness, staggering gait, tremor, stupor progressing to deep sleep or coma.

Possible Effects of Long-Term Use: Psychological and/or physical dependence.

Suggested Periodic Examinations While Taking This Drug (at physician's discretion)

Complete blood cell counts and liver function tests during long-term use. (Other drugs of this class are known to cause blood cell and liver function disorders rarely.)

▷ **While Taking This Drug, Observe the Following**

Foods: No restrictions.

Beverages: Avoid excessive intake of caffeine-containing beverages: coffee, tea, cola. May be taken with milk.

▷ *Alcohol:* Use with extreme caution until the combined effect is determined. Alcohol may increase the absorption of this drug and add to its depressant effects on the brain. It is advisable to avoid alcohol completely—throughout the day and night—if it is necessary to drive or to engage in any hazardous activity.

Tobacco Smoking: Heavy smoking may reduce the calming action of this drug.

Marijuana Smoking: Increased sedation and significant impairment of intellectual and physical performance.

▷ *Other Drugs*

Lorazepam may ***increase*** the effects of

• other sedatives, hypnotics, tranquilizers, anticonvulsants and narcotic drugs; excessive sedation may result.

▷ *Driving, Hazardous Activities:* This drug can impair mental alertness, judgment, physical coordination and reaction time. Avoid hazardous activities accordingly.

Aviation Note: The use of this drug ***is a disqualification*** for piloting. Consult a designated Aviation Medical Examiner.

Exposure to Sun: No restrictions.

Exposure to Heat: Use caution until the effect of excessive perspiration is determined. Because of reduced urine volume, this drug may accumulate in the body and produce effects of overdosage.

Discontinuation: Avoid sudden discontinuation if this drug has been taken for over 4 weeks without interruption. Dosage should be tapered gradually to prevent a withdrawal syndrome that could include depression, confusion, hallucinations, tremor, seizures, muscle cramping, sweating and vomiting.

LOVASTATIN
(loh vah STA tin)

Introduced: 1987

Prescription: USA: Yes

Available as Generic: USA: No

Brand Name: Mevacor

Class: Anticholesterol

Controlled Drug: USA: No

BENEFITS versus RISKS

Possible Benefits	*Possible Risks*
EFFECTIVE REDUCTION OF TOTAL BLOOD CHOLESTEROL in selected individuals	Drug-induced hepatitis (without jaundice) 1.9% Drug-induced myositis (muscle inflammation) 0.5% Drug-induced stomach ulceration (rare)

▷ **Principal Uses**

As a Single Drug Product: Used primarily to reduce abnormally high total blood cholesterol levels in individuals with Types IIa and IIb hypercholesterolemia. It is used in conjunction with a cholesterol-lowering diet. It should not be used until a trial of nondrug methods for lowering cholesterol has proved to be inadequate.

How This Drug Works: This drug is converted in the body to mevolinic acid, which inhibits the liver enzyme that initiates the production of cholesterol. Its principal action is the reduction of low-density lipoproteins (LDL), the fraction of total blood cholesterol that is thought to increase the risk of coronary heart disease. This drug may or may not increase the level of high-density lipoproteins (HDL), the cholesterol fraction that is thought to reduce the risk of heart disease.

Available Dosage Forms and Strengths

Tablets — 20 mg, 40 mg

▷ **Usual Adult Dosage Range:** Initially 20 mg once a day; dose may be increased up to 40 mg twice a day as needed and tolerated. Dosage adjustments should be made at 4-week intervals. The total daily dosage should not exceed 80 mg. **Note: Actual dosage and administration schedule must be determined by the physician for each patient individually.**

▷ **Dosing Instructions:** Take with food, preferably with the evening meal for maximal effectiveness. (The highest rates of cholesterol production occur between midnight and 5 a.m.) The tablet may be crushed for administration.

Usual Duration of Use: Continual use on a regular schedule for 4 to 6 weeks is usually necessary to determine this drug's effectiveness in reducing blood levels of total and LDL cholesterol. Long-term use (months to years) requires periodic evaluation of response and dosage adjustment. Consult your physician on a regular basis.

Possible Advantages of This Drug: Recent studies indicate that this drug is more effective and better tolerated than other drugs currently available for reducing total and LDL cholesterol. Its long-term effects are yet to be determined. See Cholesterol Disorders in Section Two.

▷ **This Drug Should Not Be Taken If**
 • you have had an allergic reaction to it previously.
 • you have active liver disease.
 • you have active peptic ulcer disease.
 • you are pregnant or breast-feeding.

▷ **Inform Your Physician Before Taking This Drug If**
 • you have a history of liver disease or impaired liver function.
 • you have a history of peptic ulcer disease or upper gastrointestinal bleeding.
 • you are not using any method of birth control, or you are planning pregnancy.
 • you regularly consume substantial amounts of alcohol.
 • you have cataracts or impaired vision.
 • you have any type of chronic muscular disorder.

Possible Side-Effects (natural, expected and unavoidable drug actions)
 Development of abnormal liver function tests without associated symptoms.

▷ **Possible Adverse Effects** (unusual, unexpected and infrequent reactions)
 If any of the following develop, consult your physician promptly for guidance.
 Mild Adverse Effects
 Allergic Reactions: Skin rash, itching (5.2%).
 Headache (9.3%), dizziness (2.0%), blurred vision (1.5%), altered taste (0.8%).
 Indigestion (3.9%), stomach pain (5.7%), nausea (4.7%), excessive gas (6.4%), constipation (4.9%), diarrhea (5.5%).
 Muscle cramps and/or pain (2.4%).
 Serious Adverse Effects
 Marked and persistent abnormal liver function tests with focal hepatitis (without jaundice) occurred in 1.9% after 1 year of use.
 Acute myositis (muscle pain and tenderness) occurred in 0.5% during long-term use.
 Cataracts occurred in 8% after 5 to 15 months of continual use; a cause-and-effect relationship (see Glossary) has not been established.
 Stomach and duodenal ulceration with bleeding have been reported in a few cases.

▷ **Possible Effects on Sexual Function:**   None reported.

Possible Delayed Adverse Effects: None reported to date.

Natural Diseases or Disorders That May Be Activated by This Drug
Latent liver disease; latent peptic ulcer disease; latent cataracts (possibly).

CAUTION
1. If pregnancy occurs while taking this drug, discontinue it immediately and consult your physician.
2. Report promptly any development of muscle pain or tenderness, especially if accompanied by fever or malaise.
3. Report promptly the development of altered or impaired vision so that appropriate evaluation can be made.

Precautions for Use
By Infants and Children: Safety and effectiveness for use by those under 20 years of age have not been established.
By Those over 60 Years of Age: Inform your physician regarding any personal or family history of cataracts. Comply with all recommendations regarding periodic eye examinations. Report promptly any alterations in vision.

▷ **Advisability of Use During Pregnancy**
Pregnancy Category: X. See Pregnancy Code inside back cover.
Animal studies: Mouse and rat studies reveal skeletal birth defects due to this drug.
Human studies: Information from adequate studies of pregnant women is not available.
This drug should be avoided during entire pregnancy.

Advisability of Use if Breast-Feeding
Presence of this drug in breast milk: Probably yes.
Avoid drug or refrain from nursing.

Habit-Forming Potential: None.

Effects of Overdosage: Increased indigestion, stomach distress, nausea, diarrhea.

Possible Effects of Long-Term Use: Abnormal liver function with focal hepatitis.

Suggested Periodic Examinations While Taking This Drug (at physician's discretion)
Blood cholesterol studies: total cholesterol, HDL and LDL fractions.
Liver function tests every 4 to 6 weeks during the first 15 months of use and periodically thereafter.
Complete eye examination at beginning of treatment and periodically thereafter. Ask your physician for guidance.

▷ **While Taking This Drug, Observe the Following**

Foods: Follow a standard low-cholesterol diet.

Beverages: No restrictions. May be taken with milk.

▷ *Alcohol:* No interactions expected. Use sparingly.

Tobacco Smoking: No interactions expected.

▷ *Driving, Hazardous Activities:* This drug may cause dizziness or impaired vision. Restrict activities as necessary.

Aviation Note: The use of this drug **may be a disqualification** for piloting. Consult a designated Aviation Medical Examiner.

Exposure to Sun: No restrictions.

Discontinuation: Do not discontinue this drug without your physician's knowledge and guidance.

MAPROTILINE
(ma PROH ti leen)

Introduced: 1974

Prescription: USA: Yes
Canada: Yes

Available as Generic: No

Brand Name: Ludiomil

Class: Antidepressant

Controlled Drug: USA: No
Canada: No

BENEFITS versus RISKS

Possible Benefits	*Possible Risks*
EFFECTIVE RELIEF OF ALL TYPES OF DEPRESSION	ADVERSE BEHAVIORAL EFFECTS: confusion, disorientation, hallucinations
	CONVERSION OF DEPRESSION TO MANIA in manic-depressive disorders
	Irregular heart rhythms
	Rare liver toxicity with jaundice

▷ **Principal Uses**

As a Single Drug Product: To relieve the symptoms associated with spontaneous (endogenous) depression and with reactive depressions, and to initiate the restoration of normal mood. This drug should be used only when a diagnosis of true depression of significant degree has been established. It should not be used to treat mild and transient despondency that may be associated with many life situations in the absence of a bona fide affective illness.

How This Drug Works: It is thought that this drug relieves depression by slowly restoring the nerve impulse transmitter norepinephrine to normal levels within brain tissue.

Available Dosage Forms and Strengths
Tablets — 10 mg (in Canada), 25 mg, 50 mg, 75 mg

▷ **Usual Adult Dosage Range:**   Initially 25 mg 3 times daily. Dose may be increased cautiously as needed and tolerated by 10 to 25 mg daily at intervals of 1 week. Usual maintenance dose is 50 to 100 mg/24 hours. The total daily dose should not exceed 150 mg. When the optimal requirement is determined, it may be taken at bedtime as one dose. **Note: Actual dosage and administration schedule must be determined by the physician for each patient individually.**

▷ **Dosing Instructions:**   May be taken without regard to meals. Tablet may be crushed for administration.

Usual Duration of Use: Some benefit may be apparent within 1 to 2 weeks, but adequate response may require continual use for 4 to 6 weeks or longer. Long-term use should not exceed 6 months without evaluation regarding the need for continuation of the drug. Consult your physician on a regular basis.

▷ **This Drug Should Not Be Taken If**
 • you have had an allergic reaction to it previously.
 • you are taking or have taken within the past 14 days any monoamine oxidase (MAO) type A inhibitor drug (see Drug Class, Section Four).
 • you are recovering from a recent heart attack.

▷ **Inform Your Physician Before Taking This Drug If**
 • you are allergic or overly sensitive to any tricyclic antidepressant (see Drug Class, Section Four).
 • you have a history of any of the following: alcoholism, asthma, epilepsy, glaucoma, heart disease, paranoia, prostate gland enlargement, schizophrenia or overactive thyroid function.
 • you have impaired liver function.
 • you plan to have surgery under general anesthesia in the near future.

Possible Side-Effects (natural, expected and unavoidable drug actions)
Drowsiness, blurred vision, dry mouth, constipation, impaired urination.

▷ **Possible Adverse Effects** (unusual, unexpected and infrequent reactions)
If any of the following develop, consult your physician promptly for guidance.
Mild Adverse Effects
Allergic Reactions: Skin rash, itching.
Insomnia, nervousness, palpitations, dizziness, unsteadiness, tremors, fainting, weakness.

Nausea, vomiting, acid indigestion, diarrhea.
Increased sweating.
Serious Adverse Effects
Behavioral effects: anxiety, confusion, hallucinations.
Aggravation of paranoid psychosis and schizophrenia.
Aggravation of seizure disorders (epilepsy).
Liver toxicity with jaundice (see Glossary).

▷ **Possible Effects on Sexual Function:** Decreased libido, increased libido (antidepressant effect), impotence, male breast enlargement and tenderness, female breast enlargement with milk production, swelling of testicles.

▷ **Adverse Effects That May Mimic Natural Diseases or Disorders**
The development of jaundice may suggest viral hepatitis.

Natural Diseases or Disorders That May Be Activated by This Drug
Latent epilepsy, glaucoma, prostatism (see Glossary).

CAUTION
1. Dosage must be adjusted for each person individually. Report for follow-up evaluation and laboratory tests as directed by your physician.
2. Observe for early indications of toxicity: confusion, agitation, rapid heartbeat.
3. It is advisable to withhold this drug if electroconvulsive therapy (ECT, "shock" treatment) is to be used to treat your depression.

Precautions for Use
By Infants and Children: Safety and effectiveness for use by those under 18 years of age have not been established.
By Those over 60 Years of Age: During the first 2 weeks of treatment, observe for the development of confusion, agitation, forgetfulness, disorientation, delusions and hallucinations. Reduction of dosage or discontinuation may be necessary. Unsteadiness may predispose to falling and injury. This drug can increase the degree of impaired urination associated with prostate gland enlargement (prostatism).

▷ **Advisability of Use During Pregnancy**
Pregnancy Category: B (tentative). See Pregnancy Code inside back cover.
Animal studies: No birth defects found in mouse, rat or rabbit studies.
Human studies: Information from adequate studies of pregnant women is not available.
Avoid use of drug during first 3 months. Use during the last 6 months only if clearly needed.

Advisability of Use if Breast-Feeding
Presence of this drug in breast milk: Yes.
Monitor nursing infant closely for drowsiness or failure to feed properly; discontinue drug or nursing if adverse effects develop.

Habit-Forming Potential: None.

Effects of Overdosage: Confusion, hallucinations, marked drowsiness, heart palpitations, dilated pupils, tremors, stupor, deep sleep, coma, convulsions.

Suggested Periodic Examinations While Taking This Drug (at physician's discretion)

Complete blood cell counts, liver function tests, serial blood pressure readings and electrocardiograms.

▷ **While Taking This Drug, Observe the Following**

Foods: No restrictions.

Beverages: No restrictions. May be taken with milk.

▷   *Alcohol:* Avoid completely. This drug can markedly increase the intoxicating effects of alcohol and accentuate its depressant action on brain function.

Tobacco Smoking: No interactions expected.

Marijuana Smoking: Increased drowsiness and dryness of mouth; possible reduced effectiveness of this drug.

▷   *Other Drugs*

Maprotiline may ***increase*** the effects of

• atropinelike drugs (see Drug Class, Section Four).

• all drugs with sedative effects, and cause excessive sedation.

Maprotiline may ***decrease*** the effects of

• clonidine (Catapres).

• guanethidine (Ismelin).

• methyldopa (Aldomet).

• reserpine (Serpasil, Ser-Ap-Es, etc.).

Maprotiline ***taken concurrently*** with

• amphetaminelike drugs may cause severe high blood pressure and/or high fever (see Drug Class, Section Four).

• antiseizure drugs requires careful monitoring for change in seizure patterns; dosage adjustments may be necessary.

• ethchlorvynol (Placidyl) may cause delirium; avoid concurrent use.

• monoamine oxidase (MAO) type A inhibitor drugs may cause high fever, delirium and convulsions (see Drug Class, Section Four).

• thyroid preparations may impair heart rhythm and function.

Ask physician for guidance regarding adjustment of thyroid dose.

The following drugs may ***decrease*** the effects of maprotiline

• estrogens.

• oral contraceptives.

▷   *Driving, Hazardous Activities:* This drug may impair mental alertness, judgment, physical coordination and reaction time. Avoid hazardous activities.

Aviation Note: The use of this drug ***is a disqualification*** for piloting. Consult a designated Aviation Medical Examiner.

Exposure to Sun: Use caution until sensitivity to sun has been determined. This drug may cause photosensitivity (see Glossary).

Exposure to Heat: This drug can inhibit sweating and impair the body's adaptation to hot environments, increasing the risk of heat stroke. Avoid saunas.

Exposure to Cold: The elderly should use caution and avoid conditions conducive to hypothermia (see Glossary).

Discontinuation: It is advisable to discontinue this drug gradually. Abrupt withdrawal after long-term use may cause headache, malaise and nausea.

MECLIZINE
(MEK li zeen)

Other Name: Meclozine

Introduced: 1951

Class: Antinausea, antivertigo, antihistamines

Prescription: USA: Varies
    Canada: Yes

Controlled Drug: USA: No
    Canada: No

Available as Generic: USA: Yes
    Canada: No

Brand Names: Antivert, ✦Bonamine, Bonine, Ru-Vert-M

BENEFITS versus RISKS

Possible Benefits	*Possible Risks*
EFFECTIVE PREVENTION OF MOTION SICKNESS	Mild sedation
Moderately effective relief of nausea and vertigo	Mild atropinelike effects

---

▷ **Principal Uses**

As a Single Drug Product: Used primarily to control dizziness and vertigo associated with disorders of the inner ear. Also used to prevent or relieve the nausea, vomiting and dizziness characteristic of motion sickness.

As a Combination Drug Product [CD]: This drug is available in Canada in combination with niacin (nicotinic acid), which is added because of its ability to dilate blood vessels and (theoretically) improve circulation.

How This Drug Works: Not completely established. It is thought that this drug reduces the sensitivity of the nerve pathways connecting the organ of equilibrium in the inner ear with the vomiting center in the brain; this prevents or reduces the occurrence of nausea, vomiting and vertigo.

Available Dosage Forms and Strengths
>   Tablets — 12.5 mg, 25 mg, 50 mg
>   Tablets, chewable — 25 mg

▷ **Usual Adult Dosage Range:**   12.5 to 25 mg, once or twice daily as needed for vertigo. For motion sickness: 25 to 50 mg taken 1 hour before travel; repeat once daily if needed. Total daily dosage should not exceed 100 mg. **Note: Actual dosage and administration schedule must be determined by the physician for each patient individually.**

▷ **Dosing Instructions:**   May be taken without regard to food. The regular tablet may be crushed for administration.

Usual Duration of Use: Continual use on a regular schedule for 2 to 4 days is usually necessary to determine this drug's effectiveness in relieving vertigo or preventing motion sickness. Duration of use should not exceed 5 days if this drug is not effective.

▷ **This Drug Should Not Be Taken If**
- you have had an allergic reaction to it previously.
- you are taking, or have taken within the past 14 days, any monoamine oxidase (MAO) type A inhibitor drug (see Drug Class, Section Four).
- you are, or think you may be, pregnant.

▷ **Inform Your Physician Before Taking This Drug If**
- you have had an unfavorable response to any antihistamine drug in the past.
- you have any of the following: asthma, epilepsy, glaucoma, peptic ulcer disease, prostate gland enlargement.

Possible Side-Effects (natural, expected and unavoidable drug actions)
Mild drowsiness, lethargy, impaired concentration, dry mouth, constipation.

▷ **Possible Adverse Effects** (unusual, unexpected and infrequent reactions)
If any of the following develop, consult your physician promptly for guidance.
Mild Adverse Effects
Allergic Reactions: No significant reactions identified.
Blurred vision.
Serious Adverse Effects
Possible increase in prostatism (see Glossary).

▷ **Possible Effects on Sexual Function:**   None reported.

Natural Diseases or Disorders That May Be Activated by This Drug
Latent epilepsy, glaucoma, prostatism.

CAUTION
1. Discontinue this drug 5 days before diagnostic skin testing for allergies.
2. Avoid this drug completely in children with flulike infections or chicken pox. Although a cause-and-effect relationship has not been established, this drug may contribute to the development of Reye syndrome (see Glossary) in susceptible children.

Precautions for Use
By Infants and Children: Safety and effectiveness for use by those under 12 years of age have not been established. See *CAUTION.*

By Those over 60 Years of Age: Observe for increased susceptibility to drowsiness, dizziness and impaired thinking, judgment and memory; the antihistamine-sedative effect can cause a hypoactive syndrome that may be mistaken for emotional depression or senility.

▷ Advisability of Use During Pregnancy
Pregnancy Category: C (tentative). See Pregnancy Code inside back cover.
Animal studies: Significant birth defects reported in mouse, rat and ferret studies.
Human studies: Information from studies of pregnant women is inconclusive. No increase in birth defects was reported in 2076 exposures in 2 studies; 12 cleft lips or palates were reported in 3333 exposures in another study.
Avoid this drug completely during the first 3 months. Use it during the last 6 months only if clearly needed. **Note:** This drug is *contraindicated* during pregnancy by one manufacturer.

Advisability of Use if Breast-Feeding
Presence of this drug in breast milk: Unknown.
Avoid drug or refrain from nursing.

Habit-Forming Potential: None.

Effects of Overdosage: Marked drowsiness, confusion, unsteadiness, tremors, stupor progressing to coma; in children: excitement, hallucinations, overactivity, seizures.

Possible Effects of Long-Term Use: Development of tolerance and loss of effectiveness.

Suggested Periodic Examinations While Taking This Drug (at physician's discretion)
None required.

▷ While Taking This Drug, Observe the Following
Foods: No restrictions.
Beverages: No restrictions. May be taken with milk.
▷ *Alcohol:* Use with extreme caution until the combined effects have been determined. The combination of alcohol and antihistamines can cause rapid and marked sedation.

Tobacco Smoking: No interactions expected.

▷ *Other Drugs*

Meclizine may ***increase*** the effects of
- all other drugs with atropinelike effects.
- all other drugs with sedative effects.

The following drugs may ***increase*** the effects of meclizine:
- monoamine oxidase (MAO) type A inhibitor drugs may prolong its atropinelike effects (see Drug Class, Section Four).

▷ *Driving, Hazardous Activities:* This drug may impair mental alertness, judgment, physical coordination and reaction time. Restrict activities as necessary.

Aviation Note: The use of this drug ***is a disqualification*** for piloting. Consult a designated Aviation Medical Examiner.

Exposure to Sun: No restrictions.

MECLOFENAMATE
(me kloh fen AM ayt)

Introduced: 1977

Class: Mild analgesic, anti-inflammatory

Prescription: USA: Yes

Controlled Drug: USA: No

Available as Generic: Yes

Brand Names: Meclodium, Meclomen

BENEFITS versus RISKS

Possible Benefits	*Possible Risks*
EFFECTIVE RELIEF OF MILD TO MODERATE PAIN AND INFLAMMATION	Gastrointestinal pain, ulceration, bleeding (rare)
	Rare liver or kidney damage
	Rare fluid retention
	Rare bone marrow depression

▷ **Principal Uses**

As a Single Drug Product: Used primarily to relieve mild to moderately severe pain and inflammation associated with acute and chronic rheumatoid arthritis and osteoarthritis. Also used to relieve mild to moderate pain of any cause.

How This Drug Works: Not completely established. It is thought that this drug reduces the tissue concentrations of prostaglandins (and related compounds), chemicals involved in the production of inflammation and pain.

Available Dosage Forms and Strengths
Capsules — 50 mg, 100 mg

▷ **Usual Adult Dosage Range:** 200 to 400 mg daily, in 3 or 4 divided doses. Total daily dosage should not exceed 400 mg. **Note: Actual dosage and administration schedule must be determined by the physician for each patient individually.**

▷ **Dosing Instructions:** Take with food or milk to prevent stomach irritation. Take with a full glass of water and remain upright (do not lie down) for 30 minutes. The capsule may be opened for administration.

Usual Duration of Use: Continual use on a regular schedule for 2 to 3 weeks is usually necessary to determine this drug's effectiveness in relieving the discomfort of arthritis. Long-term use (months to years) requires supervision and periodic evaluation by your physician. Consult your physician on a regular basis.

▷ **This Drug Should Not Be Taken If**
- you have had an allergic reaction to it previously.
- you are subject to asthma or nasal polyps caused by aspirin.
- you have active peptic ulcer disease, regional enteritis, ulcerative colitis or any form of gastrointestinal bleeding.
- you have a bleeding disorder or a blood cell disorder.
- you have severe impairment of kidney function.

▷ **Inform Your Physician Before Taking This Drug If**
- you are allergic to aspirin or to other aspirin substitutes.
- you have a history of peptic ulcer disease, regional enteritis or ulcerative colitis.
- you have a history of any type of bleeding disorder.
- you have impaired liver or kidney function.
- you have high blood pressure or a history of heart failure.
- you are taking any of the following: acetaminophen, aspirin or other aspirin substitutes, anticoagulants, oral antidiabetic drugs or cortisonelike drugs.

Possible Side-Effects (natural, expected and unavoidable drug actions)
Ringing in ears, fluid retention.

▷ **Possible Adverse Effects** (unusual, unexpected and infrequent reactions)
If any of the following develop, consult your physician promptly for guidance.
Mild Adverse Effects
Allergic Reactions: Skin rash, hives, itching.
Headache, dizziness, altered or blurred vision, depression.
Mouth sores, indigestion, nausea, vomiting (11%), diarrhea (10% to 33%).
Serious Adverse Effects
Allergic Reactions: Severe skin reactions, drug fever (see Glossary).
Active peptic ulcer, with or without bleeding.

Liver damage with jaundice (see Glossary).

Kidney damage with painful urination, bloody urine, reduced urine formation.

Rare bone marrow depression (see Glossary)—fatigue, weakness, fever, sore throat, abnormal bleeding or bruising.

▷ **Possible Effects on Sexual Function**   None reported.

Possible Delayed Adverse Effects: Mild anemia due to "silent" blood loss from the stomach (less than that caused by aspirin).

▷ **Adverse Effects That May Mimic Natural Diseases or Disorders**

Liver reaction may suggest viral hepatitis.

Natural Diseases or Disorders That May Be Activated by This Drug

Peptic ulcer disease, ulcerative colitis.

CAUTION

1. Dosage should always be limited to the smallest amount that produces reasonable improvement.
2. This drug may mask early indications of infection. Inform your physician if you think you are developing an infection of any kind.

Precautions for Use

By Infants and Children: Safety and effectiveness for use by those under 14 years of age have not been established.

By Those over 60 Years of Age: Small doses are advisable until tolerance is determined. Observe for any indications of liver or kidney toxicity, fluid retention, dizziness, confusion, impaired memory, stomach bleeding or diarrhea.

▷ **Advisability of Use During Pregnancy**

Pregnancy Category: B (tentative). See Pregnancy Code inside back cover.

Animal studies: Some minor birth defects reported in rodents.

Human studies: Information from adequate studies of pregnant women is not available.

Avoid this drug during the first and last 3 months. Use it during the second 3 months only if clearly needed. Ask physician for guidance.

The manufacturer does not recommend the use of this drug during pregnancy.

Advisability of Use if Breast-Feeding

Presence of this drug in breast milk: Unknown.

Avoid drug or refrain from nursing.

Habit-Forming Potential: None.

Effects of Overdosage: Drowsiness, nausea, vomiting, diarrhea, marked agitation, irrational behavior, seizures.

Possible Effects of Long-Term Use: None identified.

Suggested Periodic Examinations While Taking This Drug (at physician's discretion)
Complete blood cell counts, liver and kidney function tests, complete eye examinations if vision is altered in any way.

▷ **While Taking This Drug, Observe the Following**
Foods: No restrictions.
Beverages: No restrictions. May be taken with milk.
▷ *Alcohol:* Use with caution. The irritant action of alcohol on the stomach lining, added to the irritant action of this drug in sensitive individuals, can increase the risk of stomach ulceration and/or bleeding.
Tobacco Smoking: No interactions expected.
▷ *Other Drugs*
Meclofenamate may *increase* the effects of
- acetaminophen (Tylenol, etc.), and increase the risk of kidney damage; avoid prolonged use of this combination.
- anticoagulants (Coumadin, etc.), and increase the risk of bleeding; monitor prothrombin time, adjust dose accordingly.

Meclofenamate *taken concurrently* with the following drugs may increase the risk of bleeding; avoid these combinations:
- aspirin.
- dipyridamole (Persantine).
- sulfinpyrazone (Anturane).
- valproic acid (Depakene).

▷ *Driving, Hazardous Activities:* This drug may cause dizziness or altered vision. Restrict activities as necessary.
Aviation Note: The use of this drug *may be a disqualification* for piloting. Consult a designated Aviation Medical Examiner.
Exposure to Sun: No restrictions.

MEDROXYPROGESTERONE
(me DROX ee proh JESS te rohn)

Introduced: 1959

Class: Female sex hormones, progestins

Prescription: USA: Yes
Canada: Yes

Controlled Drug: USA: No
Canada: No

Available as Generic: Yes

Brand Names: Amen, Curretab, Provera

```
┌─────────────────────────────────────────────────────────────────┐
│                      BENEFITS versus RISKS                        │
│                                                                   │
│      Possible Benefits                    Possible Risks          │
│   EFFECTIVE TREATMENT OF          Thrombophlebitis (rare)         │
│     ABSENT OR ABNORMAL           Pulmonary embolism (rare)        │
│     MENSTRUATION due to          Liver reaction with jaundice     │
│     hormone imbalance              (rare)                         │
│   EFFECTIVE CONTRACEPTION        Drug-induced birth defects       │
│     when given by injection                                       │
│   Useful adjunctive therapy in                                    │
│     selected cases of uterine and                                 │
│     kidney cancer                                                 │
└─────────────────────────────────────────────────────────────────┘
```

▷ **Principal Uses**

As a Single Drug Product: Used primarily to initiate and regulate menstruation and to correct abnormal patterns of menstrual bleeding caused by hormonal imbalance (and not by organic disease). The injectable form of this drug is a very effective contraceptive (but is not approved for this use in the USA).

How This Drug Works: By inducing and maintaining a lining in the uterus that resembles pregnancy, this drug can prevent uterine bleeding until it is withdrawn. By suppressing the release of the pituitary gland hormone that induces ovulation, and by stimulating the secretion of mucus by the uterine cervix (to resist the passage of sperm), this drug can prevent pregnancy.

Available Dosage Forms and Strengths

Tablets — 2.5 mg, 5 mg, 10 mg

▷ **Usual Adult Dosage Range:** To initiate menstruation: 5 to 10 mg/day for 5 to 10 days, started at any time; to correct abnormal bleeding: 5 to 10 mg/day for 5 to 10 days, started on the sixteenth or twenty-first day of the menstrual cycle. Withdrawal bleeding usually begins within 3 to 7 days after stopping the drug. **Note: Actual dosage and administration schedule must be determined by the physician for each patient individually.**

▷ **Dosing Instructions:** Take on an empty stomach or with food to prevent nausea. The tablet may be crushed for administration.

Usual Duration of Use: Continual use on a regular schedule for 2 or 3 menstrual cycles is usually necessary to determine this drug's effectiveness in correcting abnormal patterns of menstrual bleeding. Consult your physician on a regular basis.

▷ **This Drug Should Not Be Taken If**

- you have had an allergic reaction to it previously.
- you are pregnant.
- you have seriously impaired liver function.

- you have a history of cancer of the breast or reproductive organs.
- you have a history of thrombophlebitis, embolism or stroke.
- you have abnormal and unexplained vaginal bleeding.

▷ **Inform Your Physician Before Taking This Drug If**
- you have impaired kidney function.
- you have any of the following disorders: asthma, diabetes, emotional depression, epilepsy, heart disease, migraine headaches.

Possible Side-Effects (natural, expected and unavoidable drug actions)
Fluid retention, weight gain, changes in menstrual timing and flow, spotting between periods.

▷ **Possible Adverse Effects** (unusual, unexpected and infrequent reactions)
If any of the following develop, consult your physician promptly for guidance.
Mild Adverse Effects
Allergic Reactions: Skin rash, hives, itching.
Fatigue, weakness, nausea.
Acne, excessive hair growth.
Serious Adverse Effects
Liver toxicity with jaundice (see Glossary): yellow eyes and skin, dark-colored urine, light-colored stools.
Thrombophlebitis (inflammation of a vein with blood clot formation): pain or tenderness in thigh or leg, with or without swelling of the foot, ankle or leg.
Pulmonary embolism (movement of blood clot to lung): sudden shortness of breath, chest pain, cough, bloody sputum.
Stroke (blood clot in the brain): sudden headache, blackouts, sudden weakness or paralysis of any part of the body, severe dizziness, double vision, slurred speech, inability to speak.
Retinal thrombosis (blood clot in principal blood vessel to the eye): sudden impairment or loss of vision.

▷ **Possible Effects on Sexual Function**
Altered timing and pattern of menstruation.
Female breast tenderness and secretion.
Decreased vaginal secretions.

▷ **Adverse Effects That May Mimic Natural Diseases or Disorders**
Liver toxicity may suggest viral hepatitis.

CAUTION
1. There is an increased risk of birth defects in children whose mothers take this drug during the first 4 months of pregnancy.
2. Inform your physician promptly if you think you may be pregnant.
3. This drug should not be used as a test for pregnancy.

Precautions for Use

By Infants and Children: Not used in this age group.

By Those over 60 Years of Age: Used selectively as adjunctive therapy in treating cancer of the breast, uterus and kidney. Observe for excessive fluid retention.

▷ **Advisability of Use During Pregnancy**

Pregnancy Category: X. See Pregnancy Code inside back cover.

Animal studies: Genital defects reported in rat and rabbit studies; masculinization of the female rodent fetus; various defects in chick embryo and rabbit.

Human studies: Masculinization of the female genitals: enlargement of the clitoris, fusion of the labia. Increased risk of heart, nervous system and limb defects also reported.

Avoid this drug completely during entire pregnancy.

Advisability of Use if Breast-Feeding

Presence of this drug in breast milk: Yes.

Avoid drug or refrain from nursing.

Habit-Forming Potential: None.

Effects of Overdosage: Nausea, vomiting, fluid retention, breast enlargement and discomfort, abnormal vaginal bleeding.

Possible Effects of Long-Term Use: None reported in humans.

Suggested Periodic Examinations While Taking This Drug (at physician's discretion)

Regular examinations (every 6 to 12 months) of the breasts and reproductive organs (pelvic examination of the uterus and ovaries, including Pap smear).

▷ **While Taking This Drug, Observe the Following**

Foods: No restrictions.

Beverages: No restrictions.

▷ *Alcohol:* No interactions expected.

Tobacco Smoking: It is advisable to smoke lightly or not at all.

▷ *Other Drugs*

The following drugs may **decrease** the effects of medroxyprogesterone
  • rifampin (Rifadin, Rimactane, etc.) may hasten its elimination.

▷ *Driving, Hazardous Activities:* Usually no restrictions. Consult your physician for assessment of individual risk and for guidance regarding specific restrictions.

Aviation Note: The use of this drug **may be a disqualification** for piloting. Consult a designated Aviation Medical Examiner.

Exposure to Sun: No restrictions.

MEPERIDINE
(me PER i deen)

Other Name: Pethidine

Introduced: 1939

Class: Strong analgesic, opioids

Prescription: USA: Yes
    Canada: Yes

Controlled Drug: USA: C-II*
    Canada: <N>

Available as Generic: Yes

Brand Names: Demerol, Demerol APAP [CD], Pethadol

BENEFITS versus RISKS	
Possible Benefits	*Possible Risks*
EFFECTIVE RELIEF OF MODERATE TO SEVERE PAIN	POTENTIAL FOR HABIT FORMATION (DEPENDENCE) Weakness, fainting Disorientation, hallucinations Interference with urination

▷ **Principal Uses**

As a Single Drug Product: This potent analgesic is used by mouth or injection to relieve moderate to severe pain of any cause.

As a Combination Drug Product [CD]: This drug is available in combination with acetaminophen (APAP) to create a dosage form that utilizes two pain relievers, one of which also reduces fever.

How This Drug Works: Acting primarily as a depressant of certain brain functions, this drug suppresses the perception of pain and calms the emotional response to pain.

Available Dosage Forms and Strengths

Injection — 10 mg per ml, 25 mg per ml, 50 mg per ml, 75 mg per ml, 100 mg per ml

Syrup — 50 mg per 5-ml teaspoonful

Tablets — 50 mg, 100 mg

▷ **Usual Adult Dosage Range:** Taken by mouth: 50 to 150 mg/3 to 4 hours as needed to relieve pain; the usual dose is 100 mg. The total daily dosage should not exceed 900 mg. **Note: Actual dosage and administration schedule must be determined by the physician for each patient individually.**

▷ **Dosing Instructions:** May be taken with or following food to reduce stomach irritation or nausea. The tablet may be crushed for administration. The syrup may be diluted in 4 ounces of water to reduce the numbing effect on the tongue and mouth tissues.

*See Schedules of Controlled Drugs inside back cover.

Usual Duration of Use: As required to control pain. Continual use should not exceed 5 to 7 days without interruption and reassessment of need.

▷ **This Drug Should Not Be Taken If**
- you have had an allergic reaction to any dosage form of it previously.
- you are having an acute attack of asthma.
- you are taking, or have taken within the past 14 days, any monoamine oxidase (MAO) type A inhibitor drug (see Drug Class, Section Four).

▷ **Inform Your Physician Before Taking This Drug If**
- you have a history of drug abuse or alcoholism.
- you have impaired liver or kidney function.
- you have a history of asthma, epilepsy or glaucoma.
- you are taking any other drugs that have a sedative effect.
- you plan to have surgery under general anesthesia in the near future.

Possible Side-Effects (natural, expected and unavoidable drug actions)
Drowsiness, light-headedness, weakness, euphoria, dry mouth, urinary retention, constipation.

▷ **Possible Adverse Effects** (unusual, unexpected and infrequent reactions)
If any of the following develop, consult your physician promptly for guidance.
Mild Adverse Effects
Allergic Reactions: Skin rash, hives, itching.
Headache, dizziness, impaired concentration, sensation of drunkenness, confusion, depression, blurred or double vision.
Facial flushing, sweating, heart palpitation.
Nausea, vomiting.
Serious Adverse Effects
Drop in blood pressure, causing severe weakness and fainting.
Disorientation, hallucinations, unstable gait, tremor, muscle twitching.

▷ **Possible Effects on Sexual Function:**   None reported.

▷ **Adverse Effects That May Mimic Natural Diseases or Disorders**
Paradoxical behavioral disturbances may suggest psychotic disorder.

CAUTION
1. If you have asthma, chronic bronchitis or emphysema, the excessive use of this drug may cause significant respiratory difficulty, thickening of bronchial secretions and suppression of coughing.
2. The concurrent use of this drug with atropinelike drugs can increase the risk of urinary retention and reduced intestinal function.
3. Do not take this drug following acute head injury.

Precautions for Use
By Infants and Children: Do not use this drug in infants under 1 year of age because of their vulnerability to life-threatening respiratory depression.

By Those over 60 Years of Age: Use small doses initially and increase dosage as needed and tolerated. Limit use to short-term treatment only if possible. There may be increased susceptibility to the development of drowsiness, dizziness, unsteadiness, falling, urinary retention and constipation (often leading to fecal impaction).

▷ **Advisability of Use During Pregnancy**
Pregnancy Category: C (tentative). See Pregnancy Code inside back cover.
Animal studies: Significant birth defects reported in hamster studies.
Human studies: Information from adequate studies of pregnant women is not available. However, no significant increase in birth defects was found in 1100 exposures to this drug.
Avoid during the first 3 months. Use sparingly and in small doses during the last 6 months only if clearly needed.

Advisability of Use if Breast-Feeding
Presence of this drug in breast milk: Yes.
Avoid drug or refrain from nursing.

Habit-Forming Potential: This drug can cause psychological and physical dependence (see Glossary).

Effects of Overdosage: Marked drowsiness, confusion, tremors, convulsions, stupor progressing to coma.

Possible Effects of Long-Term Use: Psychological and physical dependence, chronic constipation.

Suggested Periodic Examinations While Taking This Drug (at physician's discretion)
None.

▷ **While Taking This Drug, Observe the Following**
Foods: No restrictions.
Beverages: No restrictions. May be taken with milk.
▷ *Alcohol:* Use extreme caution until the combined effects have been determined. Opioid analgesics can intensify the intoxicating effects of alcohol, and alcohol can intensify the depressant effects of opioids on brain function, breathing and circulation. Alcohol is best avoided.
Tobacco Smoking: No interactions expected.
Marijuana Smoking: Increase in drowsiness and pain relief; impairment of mental and physical performance.
▷ *Other Drugs*
Meperidine may ***increase*** the effects of
• other drugs with sedative effects.
• atropinelike drugs, and increase the risk of constipation and urinary retention.
Meperidine ***taken concurrently*** with
• monoamine oxidase (MAO) type A inhibitor drugs (see Drug Class, Section Four) can cause the equivalent of an acute narcotic overdose:

unconsciousness; severe depression of breathing, heart action and circulation. A variation of this reaction can be excitability, convulsions,
high fever and rapid heart action.

- phenothiazines (see Drug Class, Section Four) can cause excessive and
prolonged depression of brain functions, breathing and circulation.

▷ *Driving, Hazardous Activities:* This drug can impair mental alertness, judgment, reaction time and physical coordination. Avoid hazardous activities.

Aviation Note: The use of this drug *is a disqualification* for piloting. Consult a designated Aviation Medical Examiner.

Exposure to Sun: No restrictions.

Discontinuation: It is advisable to limit this drug to short-term use. If it
is necessary to use it for extended periods of time, discontinuation
should be gradual to minimize possible effects of withdrawal.

METAPROTERENOL
(met a proh TER e nohl)

Other Name: Orciprenaline

Introduced: 1964

Class: Antiasthmatic,
bronchodilator

Prescription: USA: Yes
Canada: Yes

Controlled Drug: USA: No
Canada: No

Available as Generic: Yes

Brand Names: Alupent, Metaprel

BENEFITS versus RISKS	
Possible Benefits	*Possible Risks*
VERY EFFECTIVE RELIEF OF BRONCHOSPASM	Increased blood pressure
	Fine hand tremor
	Irregular heart rhythm (with excessive use)

▷ **Principal Uses**

As a Single Drug Product: To relieve acute bronchial asthma and to reduce
the frequency and severity of chronic, recurrent asthmatic attacks;
also used to relieve reversible bronchospasm associated with chronic
bronchitis and emphysema.

How This Drug Works: By stimulating certain sympathetic nerve terminals, this drug acts to dilate those bronchial tubes that are in sus-

tained constriction, thereby increasing the size of the airway and improving the ability to breathe.

Available Dosage Forms and Strengths
Powder for inhalation — 0.65 mg/inhalation
Solution for nebulizer — 0.6%, 5%
Syrup — 10 mg per 5-ml teaspoonful
Tablets — 10 mg, 20 mg

▷ **Usual Adult Dosage Range:** Inhaler: 2 or 3 inhalations/3 to 4 hours; do not exceed 12 inhalations/day. Hand nebulizer: 5 to 15 inhalations/4 hours; do not exceed 40 inhalations/day. Syrup and tablets: 20 mg/6 to 8 hours. **Note: Actual dosage and administration schedule must be determined by the physician for each patient individually.**

▷ **Dosing Instructions:** May be taken on empty stomach or with food or milk. Tablets should not be crushed for administration. For aerosol and nebulizer, follow the written instructions carefully. Do not overuse.

Usual Duration of Use: According to individual requirements. Do not use beyond the time necessary to terminate episodes of asthma.

▷ **This Drug Should Not Be Taken If**
- you have had an allergic reaction to any dosage form of it previously.
- you currently have an irregular heart rhythm.
- you are taking, or have taken within the past 2 weeks, any monoamine oxidase (MAO) type A inhibitor drug (see Drug Class, Section Four).

▷ **Inform Your Physician Before Taking This Drug If**
- you are overly sensitive to other drugs that stimulate the sympathetic nervous system.
- you are currently using epinephrine (Adrenalin, Primatene Mist, etc.) to relieve asthmatic breathing.
- you have any type of heart or circulatory disorder, especially high blood pressure or coronary heart disease.
- you have diabetes or an overactive thyroid gland (hyperthyroidism).
- you are taking any form of digitalis or any stimulant drug.

Possible Side-Effects (natural, expected and unavoidable drug actions)
Aerosol—dryness or irritation of mouth or throat, altered taste.
Tablet—nervousness, palpitation.

▷ **Possible Adverse Effects** (unusual, unexpected and infrequent reactions)
If any of the following develop, consult your physician promptly for guidance.
Mild Adverse Effects
Headache, dizziness, restlessness, insomnia, fine tremor of hands.
Rapid, pounding heartbeat; increased sweating; muscle cramps in arms and legs.
Nausea, heartburn, vomiting.

Serious Adverse Effects

Rapid or irregular heart rhythm, intensification of angina, increased blood pressure.

▷ **Possible Effects on Sexual Function:**   None reported.

Natural Diseases or Disorders That May Be Activated By This Drug

Latent coronary artery disease, diabetes or high blood pressure.

CAUTION

1. Concurrent use of this drug by aerosol inhalation with beclomethasone aerosol (Beclovent, Vanceril) may increase the risk of toxicity due to fluorocarbon propellants. It is advisable to use this aerosol 20 to 30 minutes *before* beclomethasone aerosol. This will reduce the risk of toxicity and will enhance the penetration of beclomethasone.

2. ***Avoid excessive use of aerosol inhalation.*** The excessive or prolonged use of this drug by inhalation can reduce its effectiveness and cause serious heart rhythm disturbances, including cardiac arrest.

3. Do not use this drug concurrently with epinephrine. These two drugs may be used alternately if an interval of 4 hours is allowed between doses.

4. If you do not respond to your usually effective dose, ask your physician for guidance. Do not increase the size or frequency of the dose without your physician's approval.

Precautions for Use

By Infants and Children: Safety and effectiveness of use of the aerosol and nebulized solution have not been established for children under 12 years of age. Safety and effectiveness of use of the syrup and tablet have not been established for children under 6 years of age.

By Those over 60 Years of Age: Avoid excessive and continual use. If acute asthma is not relieved promptly, other drugs will have to be tried. Observe for the development of nervousness, palpitations, irregular heart rhythm and muscle tremors. Use with extreme caution if you have hardening of the arteries, heart disease or high blood pressure.

▷ **Advisability of Use During Pregnancy**

Pregnancy Category: C (tentative). See Pregnancy Code inside back cover.

Animal studies: Significant birth defects reported in rabbit studies.

Human studies: Information from adequate studies of pregnant women is not available.

Avoid use during first 3 months. Use during the last 6 months only if clearly needed.

Advisability of Use if Breast-Feeding

Presence of this drug in breast milk: Unknown.

Avoid drug or refrain from nursing.

Habit-Forming Potential: None.

Effects of Overdosage: Nervousness, palpitation, rapid heart rate, sweating, headache, tremor, vomiting, chest pain.

Possible Effects of Long-Term Use: Loss of effectiveness. See *CAUTION* category.

Suggested Periodic Examinations While Taking This Drug (at physician's discretion)
Blood pressure measurements, evaluation of heart status.

▷ **While Taking This Drug, Observe the Following**
Foods: No restrictions.
Beverages: Avoid excessive use of caffeine-containing beverages: coffee, tea, cola, chocolate.
▷ *Alcohol:* No interactions expected.
Tobacco Smoking: No interactions expected.
▷ *Other Drugs*
Metaproterenol **taken concurrently** with
• monoamine oxidase (MAO) type A inhibitor drugs may cause excessive increase in blood pressure and undesirable heart stimulation.
▷ *Driving, Hazardous Activities:* Usually no restrictions. Use caution if excessive nervousness or dizziness occurs.
Aviation Note: The use of this drug **is a disqualification** for piloting. Consult a designated Aviation Medical Examiner.
Exposure to Sun: No restrictions.
Heavy Exercise or Exertion: Use caution. Excessive exercise can induce asthma in sensitive individuals.

METHADONE
(METH a dohn)

Introduced: 1948

Prescription: USA: Yes

Available as Generic: Yes

Brand Name: Dolophine

Class: Strong analgesic, opioids

Controlled Drug: USA: C-II*

BENEFITS versus RISKS	
Possible Benefits	*Possible Risks*
EFFECTIVE RELIEF OF MODERATE TO SEVERE PAIN	POTENTIAL FOR HABIT FORMATION (DEPENDENCE) Weakness, fainting Disorientation, hallucinations Interference with urination

*See Schedules of Controlled Drugs inside back cover.

▷ **Principal Uses**

As a Single Drug Product: This potent analgesic is used by mouth or injection to relieve moderate to severe pain of any cause. Its primary use today is to provide an appropriate substitute for heroin in treatment programs for drug addiction.

How This Drug Works: Acting primarily as a depressant of certain brain functions, this drug suppresses the perception of pain and calms the emotional response to pain.

Available Dosage Forms and Strengths

Concentrate — 10 mg per ml
Injection — 10 mg per ml
Oral solution — 5 mg, 10 mg per 5-ml teaspoonful (8% alcohol)
Tablets — 5 mg, 10 mg
Tablets, dispersible — 40 mg

▷ **Usual Adult Dosage Range:** Taken by mouth: 2.5 to 10 mg/3 to 4 hours as needed to relieve pain. The total daily dosage should not exceed 80 mg. (Dosage schedules for maintenance treatment during heroin withdrawal must be individualized.) **Note: Actual dosage and administration schedule must be determined by the physician for each patient individually.**

▷ **Dosing Instructions:** May be taken with or following food to reduce stomach irritation or nausea. The tablet may be crushed for administration. The concentrate must be diluted in 3 ounces (or more) of water before swallowing.

Usual Duration of Use: As required to control pain. Continual use should not exceed 5 to 7 days without interruption and reassessment of need.

▷ **This Drug Should Not Be Taken If**
- you have had an allergic reaction to any dosage form of it previously.
- you are having an acute attack of asthma.

▷ **Inform Your Physician Before Taking This Drug If**
- you have a history of drug abuse or alcoholism.
- you have impaired liver or kidney function.
- you have a history of asthma or other chronic lung disease.
- you are taking any other drugs that have a sedative effect.
- you are taking, or have taken within the past 14 days, any monoamine oxidase (MAO) type A inhibitor drug (see Drug Class, Section Four).
- you plan to have surgery under general anesthesia in the near future.

Possible Side-Effects (natural, expected and unavoidable drug actions)
Drowsiness, light-headedness, weakness, euphoria, dry mouth, urinary retention, constipation.

▷ **Possible Adverse Effects** (unusual, unexpected and infrequent reactions)
If any of the following develop, consult your physician promptly for guidance.

Mild Adverse Effects
Allergic Reactions: Skin rash, hives, itching.
Headache, dizziness, impaired concentration, sensation of drunkenness, confusion, depression, blurred or double vision.
Facial flushing, sweating, heart palpitation.
Nausea, vomiting.
Serious Adverse Effects
Drop in blood pressure, causing severe weakness and fainting.
Disorientation, hallucinations, unstable gait, tremor, muscle twitching.

▷ **Possible Effects on Sexual Function:**   Decreased libido, impotence, delayed ejaculation, inhibited female orgasm, male infertility, loss of menstruation. (These effects do not occur with short-term use for pain relief; however, they are very common with long-term use and addiction.)

▷ **Adverse Effects That May Mimic Natural Diseases or Disorders**
Paradoxical behavioral disturbances may suggest psychotic disorder.

CAUTION
1. If you have asthma, chronic bronchitis or emphysema, the excessive use of this drug may cause significant respiratory difficulty, thickening of bronchial secretions and suppression of coughing.
2. The concurrent use of this drug with atropinelike drugs can increase the risk of urinary retention and reduced intestinal function.
3. Do not take this drug following acute head injury.

Precautions for Use
By Infants and Children: Do not use this drug in infants under 1 year of age because of their vulnerability to life-threatening respiratory depression.
By Those over 60 Years of Age: Use small doses initially and increase dosage as needed and tolerated. Limit use to short-term treatment only if possible. There may be increased susceptibility to the development of drowsiness, dizziness, unsteadiness, falling, urinary retention and constipation (often leading to fecal impaction).

▷ **Advisability of Use During Pregnancy**
Pregnancy Category: C (tentative). See Pregnancy Code inside back cover.
Animal studies: Significant birth defects reported in mice and hamster studies.
Human studies: Information from adequate studies of pregnant women is not available.
Avoid during the first 3 months. Use sparingly and in small doses during the last 6 months only if clearly needed.

Advisability of Use if Breast-Feeding
Presence of this drug in breast milk: Yes.
Avoid drug or refrain from nursing.

Habit-Forming Potential: This drug can cause psychological and physical dependence (see Glossary).

Effects of Overdosage: Marked drowsiness, confusion, tremors, convulsions, stupor progressing to coma.

Possible Effects of Long-Term Use: Psychological and physical dependence, chronic constipation.

Suggested Periodic Examinations While Taking This Drug (at physician's discretion)
   None.

▷ **While Taking This Drug, Observe the Following**
Foods: No restrictions.
Beverages: No restrictions. May be taken with milk.
▷ *Alcohol:* Use extreme caution until the combined effects have been determined. Opioid analgesics can intensify the intoxicating effects of alcohol, and alcohol can intensify the depressant effects of opioids on brain function, breathing and circulation. Alcohol is best avoided.
Tobacco Smoking: No interactions expected.
Marijuana Smoking: Increase in drowsiness and pain relief; impairment of mental and physical performance.
▷ *Other Drugs*
   Methadone may ***increase*** the effects of
   • other drugs with sedative effects, and cause excessive sedation.
   Methadone ***taken concurrently*** with
   • monoamine oxidase (MAO) type A inhibitor drugs (see Drug Class, Section Four) requires cautious observation for indications of nervous system toxicity.
   The following drugs may ***decrease*** the effects of methadone
   • phenytoin (Dilantin, etc.).
   • rifampin (Rifadin, Rimactane, etc.).
▷ *Driving, Hazardous Activities:* This drug can impair mental alertness, judgment, reaction time and physical coordination. Avoid hazardous activities.
Aviation Note: The use of this drug ***is a disqualification*** for piloting. Consult a designated Aviation Medical Examiner.
Exposure to Sun: No restrictions.
Discontinuation: It is advisable to limit this drug to short-term use. If it is necessary to use it for extended periods of time, discontinuation should be gradual to minimize possible effects of withdrawal (stomach cramps, tearing eyes, nasal discharge, chills and tremors.

METHOCARBAMOL
(meth oh KAR ba mohl)

Introduced: 1957

Prescription: USA: Yes
   Canada: No

Class: Muscle relaxant

Controlled Drug: USA: No
   Canada: No

Available as Generic: USA: Yes
Canada: No

Brand Names: ✦Robaxacet [CD], Robaxin, Robaxin-750, Robaxisal [CD], ✦Robaxisal-C [CD]

BENEFITS versus RISKS

Possible Benefits	*Possible Risks*
Mild to moderate relief of discomfort due to spasm of voluntary muscles	White blood cell reduction (rare) Drowsiness, weakness Blurred or double vision

---

▷ **Principal Uses**

As a Single Drug Product: Used primarily to relieve the pain and stiffness associated with spasm of voluntary muscles, such as that resulting from accidental injury of musculoskeletal structures. It is often necessary to supplement the use of this drug with other treatment measures, such as rest, support and physiotherapy.

As a Combination Drug Product [CD]: It is combined with aspirin (and with codeine in Canada) to enhance its effectiveness in relieving discomfort. Aspirin and codeine are effective analgesics and may be necessary to control the pain that is not relieved by methocarbamol alone.

How This Drug Works: Not completely established. It is thought that this drug may relieve muscle spasm and pain by blocking the transmission of nerve impulses over reflex pathways and/or by producing a sedative effect that decreases the perception of pain.

Available Dosage Forms and Strengths

Injection — 100 mg per ml
Tablets — 500 mg, 750 mg

▷ **Usual Adult Dosage Range:**   Initially, 1500 mg 4 times/day for the first 2 to 3 days; for maintenance, 750 to 1000 mg 4 times/day, or 1500 mg 3 times/day. The total daily dose should not exceed 8000 mg. **Actual dosage and administration schedule must be determined by the physician for each patient individually.**

▷ **Dosing Instructions:**   Take either on empty stomach or with food to prevent stomach irritation. The tablet may be crushed for administration.

Usual Duration of Use: Continual use on a regular schedule for 2 to 3 days is usually necessary to determine this drug's effectiveness in relieving the discomfort of muscle spasm. Evaluate need for continued use after periods of 7 to 10 days.

▷ **This Drug Should Not Be Taken If**

• you have had an allergic reaction to it previously.
• you have active liver disease.

▷ **Inform Your Physician Before Taking This Drug If**
- you have experienced any unfavorable reactions to muscle relaxants in the past.
- you have epilepsy or myasthenia gravis.
- you have a history of liver or kidney disease.

Possible Side-Effects (natural, expected and unavoidable drug actions)
Drowsiness, light-headedness, weakness.
Brown, black, green or blue discoloration of the urine (of no significance).

▷ **Possible Adverse Effects** (unusual, unexpected and infrequent reactions)
If any of the following develop, consult your physician promptly for guidance.
Mild Adverse Effects
Allergic Reactions: Skin rash, hives, itching, fever.
Headache, dizziness, faintness, unsteadiness, blurred or double vision, red eyes, congested nose.
Indigestion, heartburn, nausea, vomiting.
Serious Adverse Effects
Abnormally low white blood cell count: fever, sore throat, infections.

▷ **Possible Effects on Sexual Function:**   None reported.

CAUTION
All muscle relaxants cause some degree of sedation. Use caution if other sedatives, tranquilizers or pain relievers are taken concurrently with this drug.

Precautions for Use
By Infants and Children: Dosage is based on the child's age and weight. Consult your physician for exact dosage schedule.
By Those over 60 Years of Age: Small doses are advisable initially. You may be more susceptible to the development of drowsiness, dizziness, weakness, unsteadiness and falling.

▷ **Advisability of Use During Pregnancy**
Pregnancy Category: C (tentative). See Pregnancy Code inside back cover.
Animal studies: No data available.
Human studies: Information from adequate studies of pregnant women is not available.
Avoid drug if possible; use only if clearly needed.

Advisability of Use if Breast-Feeding
Presence of this drug in breast milk: Yes, in small amounts.
Avoid drug or refrain from nursing.

Habit-Forming Potential: None.

Effects of Overdosage: Nausea, vomiting, diarrhea, headache, drowsiness, dizziness, marked weakness, impaired coordination, sense of paral-

ysis of arms and legs, rapid and weak pulse, shallow breathing, cold
and sweaty skin.

Possible Effects of Long-Term Use: None reported.

Suggested Periodic Examinations While Taking This Drug (at physician's
 discretion)
 Complete blood cell counts.

▷ **While Taking This Drug, Observe the Following**
 Foods: No restrictions.
 Beverages: No restrictions. May be taken with milk.
▷   *Alcohol:* Use with caution until the combined effect has been determined.
 This drug may add to the depressant action of alcohol on the brain.
 Tobacco Smoking: No interactions expected.
 Marijuana Smoking: Moderate to marked drowsiness, muscle weakness,
 incoordination, accentuation of orthostatic hypotension (see Glos-
 sary).
▷   *Other Drugs*
 Methocarbamol may ***increase*** the effects of
 • all other drugs with sedative effects and cause excessive sedation.
▷   *Driving, Hazardous Activities:* This drug may cause drowsiness, light-head-
 edness or dizziness in susceptible individuals. Avoid hazardous activ-
 ities if these drug effects occur.
 Aviation Note: The use of this drug ***is a disqualification*** for piloting. Consult a designated Aviation Medical Examiner.
 Exposure to Sun: No restrictions.

METHOTREXATE
(meth oh TREX ayt)

Other Names: Amethopterin, MTX

Introduced: 1948   **Class:**   Anticancer drugs,
 antipsoriasis

Prescription: USA: Yes   **Controlled Drug:**   USA: No
 Canada: Yes   Canada: No

Available as Generic: Yes

Brand Names: Folex, Mexate, Rheumatrex Dose Pack

BENEFITS versus RISKS

Possible Benefits	*Possible Risks*
EFFECTIVE TREATMENT OF SOME CASES OF SEVERE DISABLING PSORIASIS	GASTROINTESTINAL ULCERATION AND BLEEDING
EFFECTIVE TREATMENT OF CERTAIN ADULT AND CHILDHOOD CANCERS	MOUTH AND THROAT ULCERATION
PREVENTION OF REJECTION OF BONE MARROW TRANSPLANTS	SEVERE BONE MARROW DEPRESSION
Helpful adjunctive therapy in severe, refractory rheumatoid arthritis and related disorders	DAMAGE TO LUNGS, LIVER AND KIDNEYS
	Loss of hair

▷ **Principal Uses**

As a Single Drug Product: This very potent drug is used to treat (1) severe and widespread forms of disabling psoriasis that have failed to respond to all standard treatment procedures; (2) various types of both adult and childhood cancer. In addition, it is used to prevent rejection of transplanted bone marrow. More recently, it is being used in the treatment of connective tissue disorders such as rheumatoid arthritis, scleroderma and related conditions. Its use in rheumatoid arthritis is restricted to the treatment of selected adults with severe active disease that has failed to respond to conventional therapy.

How This Drug Works: By interfering with the normal utilization of folic acid in tissue cell reproduction, this drug retards abnormally rapid tissue growth (as in psoriasis and cancer).

Available Dosage Forms and Strengths

Injections — 2.5 mg per ml, 25 mg per ml
Injections (preservative-free) — 25 mg per ml
Tablets — 2.5 mg

▷ **Usual Adult Dosage Range**

For psoriasis (alternate schedules): (1) 10 to 50 mg once/week; (2) 2.5 to 5 mg/12 hours for 3 doses, or every 8 hours for 4 doses, once a week up to a maximum of 30 mg/week; (3) 2.5 mg/day for 5 days, followed by 2 days without drug, with gradual increase in dosage to a maximum of 6.25 mg/day.

For rheumatoid arthritis (alternate schedules): (1) single oral dose of 7.5 mg once weekly; (2) divided doses of 2.5 mg every 12 hours for 3 doses per week. Dosage may be increased gradually as needed and tolerated. Do not exceed a weekly dose of 20 mg.

Note: Actual dosage and administration schedule must be determined by the physician for each patient individually.

▷ **Dosing Instructions:** May be taken with food to reduce stomach irritation. Drink at least 2 to 3 quarts of liquids daily. The tablet may be crushed for administration.

Usual Duration of Use: Continual use on a regular schedule for several weeks is usually necessary to determine this drug's effectiveness in reducing the severity and extent of psoriasis. Response in rheumatoid arthritis usually begins after 3 to 6 weeks of treatment. When a favorable response has been achieved, the dosage should be reduced to the smallest amount that will maintain acceptable improvement. Long-term use (months to years) requires supervision and periodic evaluation by your physician. Consult your physician on a regular basis.

▷ **This Drug Should Not Be Taken If**
- you have had an allergic reaction to it previously.
- you currently have, or have had a recent exposure to, either chicken pox or shingles (herpes zoster).
- you are pregnant or planning pregnancy in the near future, and you are taking this drug to treat psoriasis or rheumatoid arthritis.
- you have active liver disease, peptic ulcer, regional enteritis or ulcerative colitis.
- you currently have a blood cell or bone marrow disorder.

▷ **Inform Your Physician Before Taking This Drug If**
- you have a chronic infection of any kind.
- you have impaired liver or kidney function.
- you have a history of bone marrow impairment of any kind, especially drug-induced bone marrow depression.
- you have a history of gout, peptic ulcer disease, regional enteritis or ulcerative colitis.

Possible Side-Effects (natural, expected and unavoidable drug actions)
The following are due to the pharmacological actions of this drug. **Report such developments to your physician promptly.**
Sores on the lips, in the mouth or throat; vomiting; intestinal cramping; diarrhea (may be bloody); painful urination; bloody urine.
Reduced resistance to infection, fatigue, weakness, fever, abnormal bleeding or bruising (bone marrow depression).

▷ **Possible Adverse Effects** (unusual, unexpected and infrequent reactions)
If any of the following develop, consult your physician promptly for guidance.
Mild Adverse Effects
Allergic Reactions: Skin rash, hives, itching.
Headache, drowsiness, blurred vision.
Loss of appetite, nausea, vomiting.
Loss of hair, loss of skin pigmentation, acne.

Serious Adverse Effects

Allergic Reactions: Drug-induced pneumonia: cough, chest pain, shortness of breath.

Nervous system toxicity: speech disturbances, paralysis, seizures.

Liver toxicity with jaundice (see Glossary).

Kidney toxicity: reduced urine volume, kidney failure.

▷ **Possible Effects on Sexual Function:** Altered timing and pattern of menstruation.

Possible Delayed Adverse Effects: Some reports suggest that methotrexate therapy may contribute to the later development of secondary cancers. Other studies have not confirmed this.

CAUTION

1. This drug has a high potential for serious toxicity. Its use must be monitored carefully and continually by a physician who is skilled in its proper administration. Request the Patient Package Insert that is available with this drug (Rheumatrex Dose Pack) and read it thoroughly.
2. Appropriate laboratory examinations, performed before and during the use of this drug, are mandatory. Comply fully with your physician's instructions regarding periodic studies.
3. Women with potential for pregnancy should have a pregnancy test before taking this drug and should use an effective form of contraception during its use and for 8 weeks following its discontinuation.
4. Administration of live virus vaccines should be avoided during use of this drug. Because immune functions are suppressed by this drug, live virus vaccines could actually produce infection rather than stimulate an immune response.

Precautions for Use

By Those over 60 Years of Age: Careful evaluation of kidney function should be made before starting treatment and during the entire course of therapy.

▷ **Advisability of Use During Pregnancy**

Pregnancy Category: D (tentative). See Pregnancy Code inside back cover.

Animal studies: Skull and facial defects reported in mice.

Human studies: This drug is known to cause fetal deaths and birth defects.

Its use during pregnancy to treat psoriasis or rheumatoid arthritis cannot be justified. If its use during pregnancy is deemed necessary to treat a responsive type of cancer, it should be avoided during the first 3 months if possible.

Advisability of Use if Breast-Feeding

Presence of this drug in breast milk: Yes.

Avoid drug or refrain from nursing.

Habit-Forming Potential: None.

Effects of Overdosage: The side-effects and adverse effects listed previously develop earlier and with greater severity.

Possible Effects of Long-Term Use: Liver fibrosis and cirrhosis occur in 3% to 5% of long-term users (35 to 49 months).

Suggested Periodic Examinations While Taking This Drug (at physician's discretion)
Complete blood cell counts, liver and kidney function tests, blood uric acid levels, chest X-ray examinations.

▷ **While Taking This Drug, Observe the Following**
   Foods: Avoid highly seasoned foods that could be irritating. Between courses of treatment, eat liberally of the following foods: beef, chicken, lamb and pork liver, asparagus, navy beans, kale and spinach.
   Beverages: No restrictions. This drug may be taken with milk.
▷ *Alcohol:* Avoid completely.
   Tobacco Smoking: No interactions expected.
▷ *Other Drugs Methotrexate may **decrease** the effects of*
   • digoxin (Lanoxin).
   • phenytoin (Dilantin).
   The following drugs may **increase** the effects of methotrexate and enhance its toxicity
   • aspirin and other salicylates.
   • probenecid (Benemid).
▷ *Driving, Hazardous Activities:* This drug may cause drowsiness, dizziness or blurred vision. Restrict activities as necessary.
   Aviation Note: The use of this drug **is a disqualification** for piloting. Consult a designated Aviation Medical Examiner.
   Exposure to Sun: Use caution until skin sensitivity has been determined. This drug can cause photosensitivity. Avoid ultraviolet lamps.

METHYCLOTHIAZIDE
(METH ee kloh THI a zide)

Introduced: 1960

Class: Antihypertensive, diuretic, thiazides

Prescription: USA: Yes
Canada: Yes

Controlled Drug: USA: No
Canada: No

Available as Generic: USA: Yes
Canada: No

Brand Names: Aquatensen, Diutensen [CD], Diutensen-R [CD], ✦Duretic, ✦Dureticyl [CD], Enduron, Enduronyl [CD], Enduronyl Forte [CD]

BENEFITS versus RISKS

Possible Benefits	*Possible Risks*
EFFECTIVE, WELL-TOLERATED DIURETIC	Loss of body potassium
POSSIBLY EFFECTIVE IN MILD HYPERTENSION	Increased blood sugar
ENHANCES EFFECTIVENESS OF OTHER ANTIHYPERTENSIVES	Increased blood uric acid
Beneficial in treatment of diabetes insipidus	Increased blood calcium
	Rare blood cell disorders

▷ **Principal Uses**

As a Single Drug Product: Thiazide diuretics are used primarily to (1) increase the volume of urine (diuresis) to correct the excessive fluid retention associated with congestive heart failure and certain types of liver and kidney disease; and (2) initiate treatment for high blood pressure (hypertension). They are often the first drugs tried in treating mild to moderate hypertension. Less frequent uses include the treatment of diabetes insipidus and the prevention of kidney stones that contain calcium.

As a Combination Drug Product [CD]: When this drug is used alone to treat hypertension, it is referred to as a "step 1" antihypertensive. Should it fail to reduce the blood pressure adequately, a "step 2" antihypertensive drug is added to be taken concurrently with the step 1 drug. These drugs may be combined into one drug product. Thiazides are available in combination with beta blockers, hydralazine, methyldopa, reserpine and other diuretics to increase their effectiveness in treating hypertension.

How This Drug Works: By increasing the elimination of salt and water from the body (through increased urine production), this drug reduces the volume of fluid in the blood and body tissues and lowers the sodium content throughout the body. By relaxing the walls of smaller arteries and allowing them to expand, this drug increases the total capacity of the arterial system. The combined effect of these two actions (reduced blood volume in expanded space) results in lowering of blood pressure.

Available Dosage Forms and Strengths

Tablets — 2.5 mg, 5 mg

▷ **Usual Adult Dosage Range:** As antihypertensive: 2.5 to 5 mg/day initially; 2.5 to 10 mg/day for maintenance. As diuretic: 2.5 to 10 mg/day initially; the smallest effective dose should be determined. The total daily dose should not exceed 10 mg. **Note: Actual dosage and administration schedule must be determined by the physician for each patient individually.**

▷ **Dosing Instructions:**   May be taken with or following meals to reduce stomach irritation. Best taken in the morning to avoid nighttime urination. The tablet may be crushed for administration.

Usual Duration of Use: Continual use on a regular schedule for 2 to 3 weeks is usually necessary to determine this drug's effectiveness in lowering high blood pressure. Long-term use (months to years) requires periodic evaluation of response and possible dosage adjustment. Use as a diuretic should be intermittent with "drug holidays" (no drug taken) to reduce the risk of sodium and potassium imbalance. Consult your physician on a regular basis.

▷ **This Drug Should Not Be Taken If**
  • you have had an allergic reaction to any dosage form of it previously.

▷ **Inform Your Physician Before Taking This Drug If**
  • you are allergic to any form of "sulfa" drug.
  • you are pregnant or planning pregnancy.
  • you have a history of kidney or liver disease.
  • you have diabetes, gout or lupus erythematosus.
  • you are taking any form of cortisone, digitalis, oral antidiabetic drug or insulin.
  • you plan to have surgery under general anesthesia in the near future.

Possible Side-Effects (natural, expected and unavoidable drug actions)
  Light-headedness on arising from sitting or lying position (see Orthostatic Hypotension in Glossary).
  Increase in blood sugar level, affecting control of diabetes.
  Increase in blood uric acid level, affecting control of gout.
  Decrease in blood potassium level, causing muscle weakness and cramping.

▷ **Possible Adverse Effects** (unusual, unexpected and infrequent reactions)
  If any of the following develop, consult your physician promptly for guidance.
  Mild Adverse Effects
  Allergic Reactions: Skin rashes, hives, drug fever.
  Headache, dizziness, blurred or yellow vision.
  Reduced appetite, indigestion, nausea, vomiting, diarrhea.
  Serious Adverse Effects
  Allergic Reactions: Hepatitis with jaundice (see Glossary), anaphylactic reaction (see Glossary), severe skin reactions.
  Inflammation of the pancreas—severe abdominal pain.
  Bone marrow depression (see Glossary)—fatigue, weakness, fever, sore throat, abnormal bleeding or bruising.

▷ **Possible Effects on Sexual Function:**   Impotence (rare) with recommended dosage.

▷ **Adverse Effects That May Mimic Natural Diseases or Disorders**
  Liver reaction may suggest viral hepatitis.

Natural Diseases or Disorders That May Be Activated by This Drug
Diabetes, gout, systemic lupus erythematosus.

CAUTION

1. Do not exceed recommended doses. Increased dosage can cause excessive loss of sodium and potassium, with resultant loss of appetite, nausea, fatigue, weakness, confusion and tingling in the extremities.
2. If you are also taking a digitalis preparation (digitoxin, digoxin), ensure an adequate intake of high-potassium foods to prevent potassium deficiency—a potential cause of digitalis toxicity. (See Table of High Potassium Foods in Section Six.)

Precautions for Use

By Infants and Children: Avoid overdosage that could cause serious dehydration. Significant potassium loss can occur within the first 2 weeks of drug use.

By Those over 60 Years of Age: Small doses are advisable until your individual response has been determined. You may be more susceptible to the development of impaired thinking, orthostatic hypotension, potassium loss and blood sugar increase. Overdosage and extended use of this drug can cause excessive loss of body water, thickening (increased viscosity) of the blood and an increased tendency for the blood to clot—predisposing to stroke, heart attack or thrombophlebitis (vein inflammation with blood clot).

▷ **Advisability of Use During Pregnancy**
Pregnancy Category: D (tentative). See Pregnancy Code inside back cover.
Animal studies: No information available.
Human studies: Information from adequate studies of pregnant women is not available.
This drug should not be used during pregnancy unless a very serious complication occurs for which this drug is significantly beneficial. Ask physician for guidance.

Advisability of Use if Breast-Feeding

Presence of this drug in breast milk: Yes, in small amounts.
Avoid drug or refrain from nursing.

Habit-Forming Potential: None.

Effects of Overdosage: Dry mouth, thirst, lethargy, weakness, muscle cramping, nausea, vomiting, drowsiness progressing to stupor or coma.

Possible Effects of Long-Term Use: Impaired balance of water, salt and potassium in blood and body tissues. Development of diabetes in predisposed individuals. Pathological changes in parathyroid glands with increased blood calcium levels and decreased blood phosphate levels.

Suggested Periodic Examinations While Taking This Drug (at physician's discretion)

Complete blood cell counts, measurements of blood levels of sodium, potassium, chloride, sugar and uric acid.

Kidney and liver function tests.

▷ **While Taking This Drug, Observe the Following**

Foods: Consult your physician regarding the advisability of eating foods rich in potassium. If so advised, see the Table of High Potassium Foods in Section Six. Follow physician's advice regarding the use of salt.

Beverages: No restrictions. This drug may be taken with milk.

▷　*Alcohol:* Use with caution until the combined effects have been determined. Alcohol may exaggerate the blood-pressure-lowering effects of this drug and cause orthostatic hypotension.

Tobacco Smoking: No interactions expected. Follow physician's advice.

▷　*Other Drugs*

Methyclothiazide may *increase* the effects of

- other antihypertensive drugs; dosage adjustments may be necessary to prevent excessive lowering of blood pressure.
- lithium, and cause lithium toxicity.

Methyclothiazide may *decrease* the effects of

- oral antidiabetic drugs (sulfonylureas); dosage adjustments may be necessary for proper control of blood sugar.

Methyclothiazide *taken concurrently* with

- digitalis preparations (digitoxin, digoxin) requires very careful monitoring and dosage adjustments to prevent fluctuations of blood potassium levels and serious disturbances of heart rhythm.

The following drugs may *decrease* the effects of methyclothiazide

- cholestyramine (Cuemid, Questran) may interfere with its absorption.
- colestipol (Colestid) may interfere with its absorption.

Take cholestyramine and colestipol 1 hour before any oral diuretic.

▷　*Driving, Hazardous Activities:* Use caution until the possible occurrence of orthostatic hypotension, dizziness or impaired vision has been determined.

Aviation Note: The use of this drug *may be a disqualification* for piloting. Consult a designated Aviation Medical Examiner.

Exposure to Sun: Use caution until sensitivity has been determined. This drug can cause photosensitivity (see Glossary).

Exposure to Heat: Avoid excessive perspiring, which could cause additional loss of salt and water from the body.

Heavy Exercise or Exertion: Avoid exertion that produces light-headedness, excessive fatigue or muscle cramping. Isometric exercises—the "overload" technique for strengthening individual muscles—can raise blood pressure significantly. Ask physician for guidance regarding participation in this form of exercise.

Occurrence of Unrelated Illness: Illnesses that cause vomiting or diarrhea can produce a serious imbalance of important body chemistry. Consult your physician for guidance.

Discontinuation: This drug should not be stopped abruptly following long-term use; serious thiazide-withdrawal fluid retention (edema) can develop after sudden withdrawal. The dose should be reduced gradually. It may be advisable to discontinue this drug 5 to 7 days before major surgery. Ask your physician, surgeon and/or anesthesiologist for guidance regarding dosage adjustment or drug withdrawal.

METHYLDOPA
(meth il DOH pa)

Other Name: Alpha-methyldopa

Introduced: 1963

Class: Antihypertensive

Prescription: USA: Yes
Canada: Yes

Controlled Drug: USA: No
Canada: No

Available as Generic: Yes

Brand Names: Aldochlor-150/250 [CD], Aldomet, Aldoril-15/25 [CD], Aldoril D30/D50 [CD], ♣Apo-Methazide [CD], ♣Apo-Methyldopa, ♣Dopamet, ♣Medimet-250, ♣Novodoparil [CD], ♣Novomedopa, ♣PMS Dopazide [CD]

BENEFITS versus RISKS

Possible Benefits	*Possible Risks*
EFFECTIVE STEP-2 OR -3 ANTIHYPERTENSIVE IN 66% OF CASES OF MILD TO SEVERE HYPERTENSION when used adjunctively with other drugs	LIVER TOXICITY (may be severe)
	Mental depression
	Water retention
	Hemolytic anemia (less than 1%)
	Drug fever
Symptomatic relief in cases of Raynaud's disease	Blood cell disorders (rare)

▷ **Principal Uses**

As a Single Drug Product: Used as a "step 2" or "step 3" medication in conjunction with other antihypertensive drugs in the treatment of moderate to severe high blood pressure.

As a Combination Drug Product [CD]: This drug is available in combination with chlorothiazide and with hydrochlorothiazide, mild diuretics that represent "step 1" antihypertensive drugs. Combinations of "step 1" and "step 2" drugs are more effective and more convenient for long-term use.

How This Drug Works: By decreasing the activity of the vasomotor center in the brain, this drug reduces the ability of the sympathetic nervous system to maintain the degree of blood vessel constriction that is responsible for blood pressure elevation. This change results in relaxation of blood vessel walls and lowering of blood pressure.

Available Dosage Forms and Strengths

Injection — 250 mg per 5 ml
Oral suspension — 250 mg per 5-ml teaspoonful (1% alcohol)
Tablets — 125 mg, 250 mg, 500 mg

▷ **Usual Adult Dosage Range:**   Initially, 250 mg 2 or 3 times/day for 2 days; increase dose as needed and tolerated. For maintenance, 500 to 2000 mg/day in 2 to 4 divided doses. The total daily dose should not exceed 3000 mg. **Note: Actual dosage and administration schedule must be determined by the physician for each patient individually.**

▷ **Dosing Instructions:**   May be taken without regard to meals. The tablet may be crushed for administration.

Usual Duration of Use: Continual use on a regular schedule for 2 to 4 weeks is usually necessary to determine this drug's effectiveness in controlling high blood pressure. Long-term use (months to years) requires supervision and periodic evaluation by your physician. Consult your physician on a regular basis.

▷ **This Drug Should Not Be Taken If**
- you have had an allergic reaction to it previously.
- you have active liver disease.
- you have a mild and uncomplicated case of hypertension.

▷ **Inform Your Physician Before Taking This Drug If**
- you have a history of liver disease or impaired liver function.
- you have a history of mental depression or porphyria.
- you are taking any monoamine oxidase (MAO) type A inhibitor drugs, phenothiazines or tricyclic antidepressant drugs (see Drug Classes, Section Four).
- you plan to have surgery under general anesthesia in the near future.

Possible Side-Effects (natural, expected and unavoidable drug actions)
Drowsiness, lethargy and weakness; these may occur during the first few weeks and then subside.
Light-headedness in upright position (see Orthostatic Hypotension in Glossary).
Nasal stuffiness, dry mouth.

▷ **Possible Adverse Effects** (unusual, unexpected and infrequent reactions)
If any of the following develop, consult your physician promptly for guidance.

Mild Adverse Effects
   Allergic Reactions: Skin rash, joint and muscle discomfort, fever.
   Headache, dizziness.
   Irritation of tongue, nausea, vomiting, diarrhea.
   Water retention, weight gain.
Serious Adverse Effects
   Allergic Reactions: Hepatitis with jaundice (see Glossary).
   Idiosyncratic Reaction: Episodes of high fever (not due to infection), 1%
      of users.
   Bone marrow depression (see Glossary): fatigue, weakness, fever, sore
      throat, abnormal bleeding or bruising.
   Inflammation of the pancreas: abdominal pain, fever, nausea, vomiting.
   Parkinson-like disorders (see Glossary).
   Behavioral changes: depression, confusion, nightmares.

▷ **Possible Effects on Sexual Function:** Decreased male and female libido
      (14%), impotence (24% to 80%), inhibited ejaculation (rare), inhibited
      female orgasm (related to higher doses), male breast enlargement and
      tenderness, female breast enlargement with milk production (26%),
      loss of menstruation.

▷ **Adverse Effects That May Mimic Natural Diseases or Disorders**
   Liver toxicity may suggest viral hepatitis.
   Idiosyncratic fever may suggest a viral flulike infection.
   Abnormal involuntary movements of extremities may suggest Hunting-
      ton's disease.

Natural Diseases or Disorders That May Be Activated by This Drug
   Porphyria, latent coronary artery insufficiency, lupus erythematosus–
      like syndrome.

CAUTION
   1. If this drug is used as the sole agent, the blood pressure may be
      very erratic. Observe for the development of tolerance and loss of
      effectiveness.
   2. This drug is most effective when combined with a diuretic.
   3. Avoid concurrent use with other drugs known to depress bone mar-
      row function.
   4. Report the development of any tendency to emotional depression.

Precautions for Use
   By Infants and Children: Observe for the development of hemolytic ane-
      mia, abnormal liver function, excessive sedation and nightmares.
   By Those over 60 Years of Age: The basic rule in treating hypertension
      after 60 is to proceed cautiously. Unacceptably high blood pressure
      should be reduced without creating risks associated with excessively
      low blood pressure. Sudden, rapid and excessive reduction of blood
      pressure can predispose to stroke or heart attack. Adverse effects are
      common: drowsiness (50%), depression (10%), forgetfulness, reduced

mental acuity, nasal congestion, dry mouth, hallucinations. This drug can cause parkinsonism or intensify existing parkinsonism.

▷ **Advisability of Use During Pregnancy**
Pregnancy Category: B (tentative). See Pregnancy Code inside back cover.
Animal studies: No birth defects reported in mice, rats or rabbits.
Human studies: Information from adequate studies of pregnant women is not available.
Use this drug only if clearly needed. Use the minimal effective dose.

Advisability of Use if Breast-Feeding
Presence of this drug in breast milk: Yes.
If drug is necessary, monitor infant for drowsiness and inadequate feeding.

Habit-Forming Potential: None.

Effects of Overdosage: Marked drowsiness, weakness, confusion, nausea, vomiting, stupor progressing to coma.

Possible Effects of Long-Term Use: Water retention (if not taken with a diuretic). Development of hemolytic anemia (see Glossary).

Suggested Periodic Examinations While Taking This Drug (at physician's discretion)
Complete blood cell counts, liver function tests.

▷ **While Taking This Drug, Observe the Following**
Foods: Avoid excessive salt. When possible, avoid high-protein foods at the time this drug is taken; this drug competes with proteins for absorption.
Beverages: No restrictions. May be taken with milk.
▷ *Alcohol:* Use with extreme caution until the combined effects have been determined. This combination can cause marked sedation and exaggerated drop in blood pressure.
Tobacco Smoking: No interactions expected.
▷ *Other Drugs*
Methyldopa may *increase* the effects of
• tolbutamide (Orinase), and cause excessive hypoglycemia.
• other drugs with sedative effects, and cause excessive sedation.
Methyldopa *taken concurrently* with
• beta blocker drugs may rarely cause hypertensive reactions (see Drug Class, Section Four).
• haloperidol (Haldol) may cause dementia, disorientation and abnormal behavior.
• monoamine oxidase (MAO) type A inhibitor drugs may cause hallucinations and hypertension (see Drug Class, Section Four).
• phenothiazines may cause hypertension (see Drug Class, Section Four).
The following drugs may *decrease* the effects of methyldopa
• tricyclic antidepressants (see Drug Class, Section Four).

▷   *Driving, Hazardous Activities:* This drug may cause drowsiness and fatigue. Restrict activities as necessary.

Aviation Note: The use of this drug **may be a disqualification** for piloting. Consult a designated Aviation Medical Examiner.

Exposure to Sun: No restrictions.

Heavy Exercise or Exertion: Use caution. Excessive physical activity may increase the possibility of orthostatic hypotension. Isometric exercises—the "overload" technique for strengthening individual muscles—can raise blood pressure significantly. Ask your physician for guidance.

Discontinuation: It may be advisable to discontinue this drug 5 to 7 days before surgery under general anesthesia. Consult your surgeon and/ or anesthesiologist regarding dosage adjustment or withdrawal of this drug prior to surgery.

METHYLPHENIDATE
(meth il FEN i dayt)

Introduced: 1956

Class: Stimulant, amphetaminelike drugs

Prescription: USA: Yes
Canada: Yes

Controlled Drug: USA: C-II*
Canada: \<C\>

Available as Generic: USA: Yes
Canada: No

Brand Names: Ritalin, Ritalin-SR

BENEFITS versus RISKS	
Possible Benefits	*Possible Risks*
EFFECTIVE CONTROL OF NARCOLEPSY	POTENTIAL FOR SERIOUS PSYCHOLOGICAL DEPENDENCE
USEFUL AS ADJUNCTIVE TREATMENT IN THE ATTENTION DEFICIT DISORDERS OF CHILDHOOD	SUPPRESSION OF GROWTH IN CHILDHOOD
Useful in treatment of mild to moderate depression	Abnormal behavior
Useful in some cases of emotional withdrawal in the elderly	Rare blood cell disorders

*See Schedules of Controlled Drugs inside back cover.

▷ **Principal Uses**

As a Single Drug Product: Used primarily to treat (1) narcolepsy, recurrent spells of uncontrollable drowsiness and sleep; and (2) attention-deficit disorders of childhood, formerly known as the hyperactive child syndrome, minimal brain damage and minimal brain dysfunction. Additional uses include the treatment of mild to moderate depression, and the management of apathetic and withdrawal states in the elderly.

How This Drug Works: Not completely established. It is thought that this drug may increase the release of the nerve impulse transmitter norepinephrine. The resulting stimulation of brain function improves alertness and concentration, and increases learning ability and attention span. The primary action that calms the overactive child is not known.

Available Dosage Forms and Strengths
Tablets — 5 mg, 10 mg, 20 mg
Tablets, prolonged-action — 20 mg

▷ **Usual Adult Dosage Range:** 5 to 20 mg 2 or 3 times/day. **Note: Actual dosage and administration schedule must be determined by the physician for each patient individually.**

▷ **Dosing Instructions:** Take tablet 30 to 45 minutes before meals. The regular tablet may be crushed for administration; the prolonged-action tablet should be taken whole, not crushed.

Usual Duration of Use: Continual use on a regular schedule for 3 to 4 weeks is usually necessary to determine this drug's effectiveness in controlling the symptoms of narcolepsy or improving the behavior of attention-deficit children. Long-term use (months to years) requires supervision and periodic evaluation by your physician. Consult your physician on a regular basis.

▷ **This Drug Should Not Be Taken If**
- you have had an allergic reaction to it previously.
- you have glaucoma (inadequately treated).
- you are experiencing a period of severe anxiety, nervous tension or emotional depression.

▷ **Inform Your Physician Before Taking This Drug If**
- you have high blood pressure, angina or epilepsy.
- you are taking, or have taken within the past 14 days, any monoamine oxidase (MAO) type A inhibitor drug (see Drug Class, Section Four).

Possible Side-Effects (natural, expected and unavoidable drug actions)
Nervousness, insomnia.

▷ **Possible Adverse Effects** (unusual, unexpected and infrequent reactions)
If any of the following develop, consult your physician promptly for guidance.

Mild Adverse Effects
  Allergic Reactions: Skin rash, hives, drug fever, joint pains.
  Headache, dizziness, rapid and forceful heart palpitation.
  Reduced appetite, nausea, abdominal discomfort.
Serious Adverse Effects
  Allergic Reactions: Severe skin reactions, extensive bruising due to allergic destruction of blood platelets (see Glossary).
  Idiosyncratic Reaction: Abnormal patterns of behavior.
  Abnormally low red blood cell and white blood cell counts.

▷ **Possible Effects on Sexual Function:**   None reported.

Natural Diseases or Disorders That May Be Activated by This Drug
  Latent epilepsy.

CAUTION
  1. Careful dosage adjustments on an individual basis are mandatory.
  2. Paradoxical reactions (see Glossary) can occur, causing aggravation of initial symptoms for which this drug was prescribed.

Precautions for Use
  By Infants and Children: Safety and effectiveness for use by those under 6 years of age have not been established. If this drug is not benefical in managing an attention deficit disorder after a trial of one month, it should be discontinued. During long-term use, monitor the child for normal growth and development.
  By Those over 60 Years of Age: Start with small doses to determine your tolerance for this drug. You may be more susceptible to the development of nervousness, agitation, insomnia, high blood pressure, angina or disturbance of heart rhythm.

▷ **Advisability of Use During Pregnancy**
  Pregnancy Category: B (tentative). See Pregnancy Code inside back cover.
  Animal studies: No birth defects found in mouse studies.
  Human studies: Information from adequate studies of pregnant women is not available.
  Use this drug only if clearly needed. Ask physician for guidance.

Advisability of Use if Breast-Feeding
  Presence of this drug in breast milk: Unknown.
  Avoid drug or refrain from nursing.

Habit-Forming Potential: This drug can produce tolerance and cause serious psychological dependence (see Glossary), a potentially dangerous characteristic of amphetaminelike drugs (see Drug Class, Section Four).

Effects of Overdosage: Headache, vomiting, agitation, tremors, muscle twitching, dry mouth, sweating, fever, confusion, hallucinations, seizures, coma.

Possible Effects of Long-Term Use: Suppression of growth (in weight and/or height) has been reported in children during long-term use of this drug.

Suggested Periodic Examinations While Taking This Drug (at physician's discretion)
Complete blood cell counts, blood pressure measurements.

▷ **While Taking This Drug, Observe the Following**
Foods: Avoid foods rich in tyramine (see Glossary); this drug in combination with tyramine may cause an excessive rise in blood pressure.
Beverages: Avoid beverages prepared from meat or meat extracts. This drug may be taken with milk.
▷ *Alcohol:* Avoid beer, Chianti wines and vermouth.
Tobacco Smoking: No interactions expected.
▷ *Other Drugs*
Methylphenidate may *increase* the effects of
• tricyclic antidepressants, and enhance their toxic effects (see Drug Class, Section Four).
Methylphenidate may *decrease* the effects of
• guanethidine (Ismelin), and impair its ability to lower blood pressure.
Methylphenidate *taken concurrently* with
• anticonvulsants may cause a significant change in the pattern of epileptic seizures; dosage adjustments may be necessary for proper control.
• monoamine oxidase (MAO) type A inhibitor drugs (see Drug Class, Section Four) may cause a significant rise in blood pressure. Avoid the concurrent use of these drugs.
▷ *Driving, Hazardous Activities:* This drug may cause dizziness or drowsiness. Restrict activities as necessary.
Aviation Note: The use of this drug *is a disqualification* for piloting. Consult a designated Aviation Medical Examiner.
Exposure to Sun: No restrictions.
Discontinuation: If it has been necessary to use this drug for an extended period of time, do not discontinue it abruptly. Careful supervision is necessary during withdrawal to prevent severe depression and erratic behavior.

METHYLPREDNISOLONE
(meth il pred NIS oh lohn)

Introduced: 1957   **Class:** Cortisonelike drugs

Prescription: USA: Yes   **Controlled Drug:** USA: No
       Canada: Yes   Canada: No

Available as Generic: USA: Yes
          Canada: No

Brand Names: Medrol, Medrol Enpak

BENEFITS versus RISKS

Possible Benefits	*Possible Risks*
EFFECTIVE RELIEF OF SYMPTOMS IN A WIDE VARIETY OF INFLAMMATORY AND ALLERGIC DISORDERS	Short-term use (up to 10 days) is usually well tolerated
EFFECTIVE IMMUNO-SUPPRESSION in selected benign and malignant disorders	Long-term use (exceeding 2 weeks) is associated with many possible adverse effects:

Short-term use (up to 10 days) is usually well tolerated
Long-term use (exceeding 2 weeks) is associated with many possible adverse effects:
ALTERED MOOD AND PERSONALITY
CATARACTS, GLAUCOMA
HYPERTENSION
OSTEOPOROSIS
ASEPTIC BONE NECROSIS
INCREASED SUSCEPTIBILITY TO INFECTIONS
(See Possible Adverse Effects and Possible Effects of Long-Term Use)

▷ **Principal Uses**

As a Single Drug Product: This potent drug of the cortisone class is used in the treatment of a wide variety of allergic and inflammatory conditions. It is used most commonly in the management of serious skin disorders, asthma, regional enteritis, ulcerative colitis and all types of major rheumatic disorders including bursitis, tendinitis and most forms of arthritis.

How This Drug Works: Not fully established. It is thought that this drug's anti-inflammatory effect is due to its ability to inhibit the normal defensive functions of certain white blood cells. Its immunosuppressant effect is attributed to a reduced production of lymphocytes and antibodies.

Available Dosage Forms and Strengths
          Ointment — 0.25%, 1%
    Retention enema — 40 mg/bottle
          Tablets — 2 mg, 4 mg, 8 mg, 16 mg, 24 mg, 32 mg

▷ **Usual Adult Dosage Range:**   4 to 48 mg daily as a single dose or in divided doses. **Note: Actual dosage and administration schedule must be determined by the physician for each patient individually.**

▷ **Dosing Instructions:**   Take with or following food to prevent stomach irritation, preferably in the morning. The tablet may be crushed for administration.

Usual Duration of Use: For acute disorders: 4 to 10 days. For chronic disorders: according to individual requirements. The duration of use should not exceed the time necessary to obtain adequate symptomatic relief in acute self-limiting conditions, or the time required to stabilize a chronic condition and permit gradual withdrawal. Because of its intermediate duration of action, this drug is appropriate for alternate-day administration. Consult your physician on a regular basis.

▷ **This Drug Should Not Be Taken If**
- you have had an allergic reaction to any dosage form of it previously.
- you have active peptic ulcer disease.
- you have an active infection of the eye caused by the herpes simplex virus.
- you have active tuberculosis.

▷ **Inform Your Physician Before Taking This Drug If**
- you have had an unfavorable reaction to any cortisonelike drug in the past.
- you have a history of peptic ulcer disease, thrombophlebitis or tuberculosis.
- you have any of the following: diabetes, glaucoma, high blood pressure, deficient thyroid function or myasthenia gravis.
- you plan to have surgery of any kind in the near future.

Possible Side-Effects (natural, expected and unavoidable drug actions)
Increased appetite, weight gain, retention of salt and water, excretion of potassium, increased susceptibility to infection.

▷ **Possible Adverse Effects** (unusual, unexpected and infrequent reactions)
If any of the following develop, consult your physician promptly for guidance.
Mild Adverse Effects
Allergic Reaction: Skin rash.
Headache, dizziness, insomnia.
Acid indigestion, abdominal distension.
Muscle cramping and weakness.
Acne, excessive growth of facial hair.
Serious Adverse Effects
Mental and emotional disturbances of serious magnitude.
Reactivation of latent tuberculosis.
Development of peptic ulcer.
Increased blood pressure.
Development of inflammation of the pancreas.

Thrombophlebitis (inflammation of a vein with the formation of blood clot)—pain or tenderness in thigh or leg, with or without swelling of the foot, ankle or leg.

Pulmonary embolism (movement of a blood clot to the lung)—sudden shortness of breath, pain in the chest, coughing, bloody sputum.

▷ **Possible Effects on Sexual Function:** Altered timing and pattern of menstruation.

▷ **Adverse Effects That May Mimic Natural Diseases or Disorders**

Pattern of symptoms and signs resembling Cushing's syndrome.

Natural Diseases or Disorders That May Be Activated by This Drug

Latent diabetes, glaucoma, peptic ulcer disease, tuberculosis.

CAUTION

1. It is advisable to carry a card of personal identification with a notation that you are taking this drug, if your course of treatment is to exceed 1 week.
2. Do not discontinue this drug abruptly if you are using it for long-term treatment.
3. If vaccination against measles, rabies, smallpox or yellow fever is required, discontinue this drug 72 hours before vaccination and do not resume it for at least 14 days after vaccination.

Precautions for Use

By Infants and Children: Avoid prolonged use if possible. During long-term use, observe for suppression of normal growth and the possibility of increased intracranial pressure. Following long-term use, the child may be at risk for adrenal gland deficiency during stress for as long as 18 months after cessation of this drug.

By Those over 60 Years of Age: Cortisonelike drugs should be used very sparingly after 60 and only when the disorder under treatment is unresponsive to adequate trials of unrelated drugs. Avoid prolonged use of this drug. Continual use (even in small doses) can increase the severity of diabetes, enhance fluid retention, raise blood pressure, weaken resistance to infection, induce stomach ulcer and accelerate the development of cataract and osteoporosis.

▷ **Advisability of Use During Pregnancy**

Pregnancy Category: C (tentative). See Pregnancy Code inside back cover.

Animal studies: Birth defects reported in mice, rats and rabbits.

Human studies: Information from adequate studies of pregnant women is not available.

Avoid completely during the first 3 months. Limit use during the last 6 months as much as possible. If used, examine infant for possible deficiency of adrenal gland function.

Advisability of Use if Breast-Feeding

Presence of this drug in breast milk: Yes.

Avoid drug or refrain from nursing.

Habit-Forming Potential: Use of this drug to suppress symptoms over an extended period of time may produce a state of functional dependence (see Glossary). In the treatment of conditions like asthma and rheumatoid arthritis, it is advisable to keep the dose as small as possible and to attempt drug withdrawal after periods of reasonable improvement. Such procedures may reduce the degree of "steroid rebound"—the return of symptoms as the drug is withdrawn.

Effects of Overdosage: Fatigue, muscle weakness, stomach irritation, acid indigestion, excessive sweating, facial flushing, fluid retention, swelling of extremities, increased blood pressure.

Possible Effects of Long-Term Use: Increased blood sugar (possible diabetes), increased fat deposits on the trunk of the body ("buffalo hump"), rounding of the face ("moon face"), thinning and fragility of skin, loss of texture and strength of bones (osteoporosis, aseptic necrosis), cataracts, glaucoma, retarded growth and development in children.

Suggested Periodic Examinations While Taking This Drug (at physician's discretion)
Measurements of blood pressure, blood sugar and potassium levels.
Complete eye examinations at regular intervals.
Chest X-ray if history of tuberculosis.
Determination of the rate of development of the growing child to detect retardation of normal growth.

▷ **While Taking This Drug, Observe the Following**
Foods: No interactions expected. Ask physician regarding need to restrict salt intake or to eat potassium-rich foods. During long-term use of this drug, it is advisable to eat a high-protein diet.
Nutritional Support: During long-term use, take a vitamin D supplement. During wound repair, take a zinc supplement.
Beverages: No restrictions. Drink all forms of milk liberally.
▷   *Alcohol:* No interactions expected. Use caution if you are prone to peptic ulcer disease.
Tobacco Smoking: Nicotine increases the blood levels of naturally produced cortisone and related hormones. Heavy smoking may add to the expected actions of this drug and requires close observation for excessive effects.
Marijuana Smoking: May cause additional impairment of immunity.
▷   *Other Drugs*
Methylprednisolone may **decrease** the effects of
• isoniazid (INH, Niconyl, etc.).
• salicylates (aspirin, sodium salicylate, etc.).
Methylprednisolone **taken concurrently** with
• oral anticoagulants may either increase or decrease their effectiveness; consult physician regarding the need for prothrombin time testing and dosage adjustment.

The following drugs may **decrease** the effects of methylprednisolone
- antacids may reduce its absorption.
- barbiturates (Amytal, Butisol, phenobarbital, etc.).
- phenytoin (Dilantin, etc.).
- rifampin (Rifadin, Rimactane, etc.).

▷ *Driving, Hazardous Activities:* Usually no restrictions. Be alert to the rare occurrence of dizziness.

Aviation Note: The use of this drug **may be a disqualification** for piloting. Consult a designated Aviation Medical Examiner.

Exposure to Sun: No restrictions.

Occurrence of Unrelated Illness: This drug may decrease natural resistance to infection. Inform your physician if you develop an infection of any kind. It may also reduce your body's ability to respond to the stress of acute illness, injury or surgery. Keep your physician fully informed of any significant changes in your state of health.

Discontinuation: If you have been taking this drug for an extended period of time, do not discontinue it abruptly. Ask physician for guidance regarding gradual withdrawal. For a period of 2 years after discontinuing this drug, it is essential in the event of illness, injury or surgery that you inform attending medical personnel that you have used this drug in the past. The period of impaired response to stress following the use of cortisonelike drugs may last for 1 to 2 years.

METOCLOPRAMIDE
(met oh kloh PRA mide)

Introduced: 1973

Class: Gastrointestinal stimulant, antivomiting agent

Prescription: USA: Yes
Canada: Yes

Controlled Drug: USA: No
Canada: No

Available as Generic: No

Brand Names: ✦Emex, ✦Maxeran, Maxolon, Reglan

BENEFITS versus RISKS	
Possible Benefits	*Possible Risks*
EFFECTIVE STOMACH STIMULANT FOR CORRECTING DELAYED EMPTYING	Sedation and fatigue (10%)
	Parkinson-like reactions (see Glossary), 1 in 500
Symptomatic relief in reflux esophagitis	Tardive dyskinesia (see Glossary), rare
Relief of nausea and vomiting associated with migraine headache	

▷ **Principal Uses**

As a Single Drug Product: Used primarily to stimulate contractions of the stomach and thereby facilitate timely emptying of the stomach in disorders such as (1) the stomach retention (gastroparesis) associated with diabetes; (2) acid reflux from the stomach into the esophagus (esophagitis); (3) the nausea and vomiting associated with migraine headaches; and (4) the nausea and vomiting induced by anticancer drugs.

How This Drug Works: Not completely established. It is thought that this drug inhibits relaxation of the stomach muscles and enhances the stimulation of the parasympathetic nervous system that is responsible for stomach muscle contractions. This action accelerates emptying of the stomach into the intestine.

Available Dosage Forms and Strengths
Injection — 5 mg per ml, 10 mg per ml
Syrup — 5 mg per 5-ml teaspoonful
Tablets — 5 mg, 10 mg

▷ **Usual Adult Dosage Range:**   10 to 15 mg 4 times/day. The total daily dose should not exceed 0.5 mg per kilogram of body weight. **Note: Actual dosage and administration schedule must be determined by the physician for each patient individually.**

▷ **Dosing Instructions:**   Take tablet or syrup 30 minutes before each meal and at bedtime. The tablet may be crushed for administration.

Usual Duration of Use: Continual use on a regular schedule for 5 to 7 days is usually necessary to determine this drug's effectiveness in accelerating stomach emptying and relieving symptoms of heartburn, fullness and belching. Long-term use (months to years) requires supervision and periodic evaluation by your physician. Consult your physician on a regular basis.

▷ **This Drug Should Not Be Taken If**
- you have had an allergic reaction to it previously.
- you have a seizure disorder of any kind.
- you have active gastrointestinal bleeding.
- you have a pheochromocytoma (adrenaline-producing tumor).

▷ **Inform Your Physician Before Taking This Drug If**
- you are allergic or overly sensitive to procaine or procainamide.
- you have impaired liver or kidney function.
- you have Parkinson's disease.
- you are taking any atropinelike drugs, antipsychotic drugs or opioid analgesics (see Drug Classes, Section Four).

Possible Side-Effects (natural, expected and unavoidable drug actions)
Drowsiness and lethargy (10%), breast tenderness and swelling, milk production.

▷ **Possible Adverse Effects** (unusual, unexpected and infrequent reactions)
If any of the following develop, consult your physician promptly for guidance.
Mild Adverse Effects
Allergic Reaction: Skin rash.
Headache, dizziness, restlessness, depression, insomnia.
Dry mouth, nausea, diarrhea, constipation.
Serious Adverse Effects
Parkinson-like reactions (see Glossary).
Tardive dyskinesia (see Glossary).

▷ **Possible Effects on Sexual Function**
Decreased libido (80%), impaired erection (60%), decreased sperm count.
Altered timing and pattern of menstruation.

Precautions for Use
By Infants and Children: Observe for the early development of Parkinson-like reactions soon after starting treatment. Use the smallest effective dose to minimize such reactions.
By Those over 60 Years of Age: Parkinson-like reactions and tardive dyskinesias are more likely to occur with the use of high doses over an extended period of time. Determine the smallest effective dose and use this only when clearly needed.

▷ **Advisability of Use During Pregnancy**
Pregnancy Category: B (tentative). See Pregnancy Code inside back cover.
Animal studies: No birth defects found due to this drug.
Human studies: Information from adequate studies of pregnant women is not available.
Use this drug only if clearly needed.

Advisability of Use if Breast-Feeding
Presence of this drug in breast milk: Yes.
Avoid drug or refrain from nursing.

Habit-Forming Potential: None.

Effects of Overdosage: Marked drowsiness, confusion, muscle spasms, jerking movements of head and face, tremors, shuffling gait.

Possible Effects of Long-Term Use: Parkinson-like reactions may appear within several months of use. Tardive dyskinesias usually occur after a year of continual use; they may persist after this drug is discontinued.

Suggested Periodic Examinations While Taking This Drug (at physician's discretion)
During long-term use, observe for the development of fine, wormlike movements on the surface of the tongue; these may be the first indications of an emerging tardive dyskinesia.

▷ **While Taking This Drug, Observe the Following**

Foods: No restrictions.

Beverages: No restrictions. May be taken with milk.

▷   *Alcohol:* Use with extreme caution. Combined effects can result in excessive sedation and marked intoxication. Alcohol is best avoided.

Tobacco Smoking: No interactions expected.

▷   *Other Drugs*

Metoclopramide may *decrease* the effects of

- cimetidine (Tagamet).
- digoxin (slow-dissolving dosage forms), and reduce its effectiveness.

Metoclopramide *taken concurrently* with

- major antipsychotic drugs (phenothiazines, thiothixenes, haloperidol, etc.) may increase the risk of developing Parkinson-like reactions.

The following drugs may *decrease* the effects of metoclopramide

- atropinelike drugs.
- opioid analgesics (see Drug Class, Section Four).

▷   *Driving, Hazardous Activities:* This drug may cause drowsiness and dizziness. Restrict activities as necessary.

Aviation Note: The use of this drug *may be a disqualification* for piloting. Consult a designated Aviation Medical Examiner.

Exposure to Sun: No restrictions.

METOLAZONE
(me TOHL a zohn)

Introduced: 1974

Class: Antihypertensive, diuretic, sulfonamides

Prescription: USA: Yes
Canada: Yes

Controlled Drug: USA: No
Canada: No

Available as Generic: USA: No
Canada: No

Brand Names: Diulo, Microx, Zaroxolyn

BENEFITS versus RISKS	
Possible Benefits	*Possible Risks*
EFFECTIVE, WELL-TOLERATED DIURETIC	Loss of body potassium
POSSIBLY EFFECTIVE IN MILD HYPERTENSION	Increased blood sugar
ENHANCES EFFECTIVENESS OF OTHER ANTIHYPERTENSIVES	Increased blood uric acid
	Rare liver damage, jaundice
	Rare blood cell disorder: abnormally low white blood cell count

▷ **Principal Uses**

> *As a Single Drug Product:* Diuretics of this class are used to primarily to (1) increase the volume of urine (diuresis) to correct the excessive fluid retention associated with congestive heart failure and certain types of liver and kidney disease; and (2) initiate treatment for high blood pressure (hypertension). They are often the first drugs tried ("step 1") in treating mild to moderate hypertension.

> **How This Drug Works:** By increasing the elimination of salt and water from the body (through increased urine production), this drug reduces the volume of fluid in the blood and body tissues and lowers the sodium content throughout the body. By relaxing the walls of smaller arteries and allowing them to expand, this drug increases the total capacity of the arterial system. The combined effect of these two actions (reduced blood volume in expanded space) results in lowering of blood pressure.

Available Dosage Forms and Strengths
> Tablets — 0.5 mg, 2.5 mg, 5 mg, 10 mg

▷ **Usual Adult Dosage Range:** As antihypertensive: 2.5 to 5 mg/day initially; 2.5 to 10 mg/day for maintenance. As diuretic: 2.5 to 10 mg/day initially; the smallest effective dose should be determined. The total daily dose should not exceed 20 mg. **Note: Actual dosage and administration schedule must be determined by the physician for each patient individually.**

▷ **Dosing Instructions:** May be taken with or following food to reduce stomach irritation. Best taken as one dose in the morning to avoid nighttime urination. The tablet may be crushed for administration.

> **Usual Duration of Use:** Continual use on a regular schedule for 2 to 3 weeks is usually necessary to determine this drug's effectiveness in lowering high blood pressure. Long-term use (months to years) requires periodic evaluation of response and possible dosage adjustment. Use as a diuretic should be intermittent with "drug holidays" (no drug taken) to reduce the risk of sodium and potassium imbalance. Consult your physician on a regular basis.

▷ **This Drug Should Not Be Taken If**
> • you have had an allergic reaction to it previously.

▷ **Inform Your Physician Before Taking This Drug If**
> • you are allergic to any form of "sulfa" drug.
> • you are pregnant or planning pregnancy.
> • you have a history of kidney or liver disease.
> • you have diabetes, gout or lupus erythematosus.
> • you are taking any form of cortisone, digitalis, oral antidiabetic drug or insulin.
> • you plan to have surgery under general anesthesia in the near future.

Possible Side-Effects (natural, expected and unavoidable drug actions)
Light-headedness on arising from sitting or lying position (see Orthostatic Hypotension in Glossary).
Increase in blood sugar level, affecting control of diabetes.
Increase in blood uric acid level, affecting control of gout.
Decrease in blood potassium level, causing muscle weakness and cramping.

▷ **Possible Adverse Effects** (unusual, unexpected and infrequent reactions)
If any of the following develop, consult your physician promptly for guidance.
Mild Adverse Effects
Allergic Reactions: Skin rashes, hives.
Headache, dizziness, blurred vision.
Reduced appetite, indigestion, nausea, vomiting, diarrhea.
Serious Adverse Effects
Allergic Reactions: Hepatitis with jaundice (see Glossary).
Idiosyncratic Reactions: Muscle pains and cramping, seizures, collapse.
Acute gout attacks (in susceptible individuals).
Acute to chronic muscle disorders (due to potassium loss).
Abnormally low white blood cell count: fever, sore throat, infections.

▷ **Possible Effects on Sexual Function:**   None reported.

▷ **Adverse Effects That May Mimic Natural Diseases or Disorders**
Liver reaction may suggest viral hepatitis.

Natural Diseases or Disorders That May Be Activated by This Drug
Diabetes, gout, systemic lupus erythematosus (questionable).

CAUTION
1. Do not exceed recommended doses. Increased dosage can cause excessive loss of sodium and potassium, with resultant loss of appetite, nausea, fatigue, weakness, confusion and tingling in the extremities.
2. If you are also taking a digitalis preparation (digitoxin, digoxin), ensure an adequate intake of high-potassium foods to prevent potassium deficiency—a potential cause of digitalis toxicity. (See Table of High Potassium Foods in Section Six).

Precautions for Use
By Infants and Children: Safety and effectiveness for use by those under 12 years of age have not been established. Avoid overdosage that could cause serious dehydration. Significant potassium loss can occur within the first 2 weeks of drug use.
By Those over 60 Years of Age: Small doses are advisable until your individual response has been determined. You may be more susceptible to the development of impaired thinking, orthostatic hypotension, potassium loss and blood sugar increase. Overdosage and extended use of this drug can cause excessive loss of body water, thickening (in-

creased viscosity) of the blood and an increased tendency for the blood to clot—predisposing to stroke, heart attack or thrombophlebitis (vein inflammation with blood clot).

▷ **Advisability of Use During Pregnancy**
Pregnancy Category: B (tentative). See Pregnancy Code inside back cover.
Animal studies: No birth defects reported in mouse, rat or rabbit studies.
Human studies: Information from adequate studies of pregnant women is not available.
This drug should not be used during pregnancy unless a very serious complication occurs for which this drug is significantly beneficial. Ask physician for guidance.

Advisability of Use if Breast-Feeding
Presence of this drug in breast milk: Yes.
Avoid drug if possible. If use is necessary, monitor nursing infant closely and discontinue drug or nursing if adverse effects develop.

Habit-Forming Potential: None.

Effects of Overdosage: Dry mouth, thirst, lethargy, weakness, muscle cramping, nausea, vomiting, drowsiness progressing to stupor or coma.

Possible Effects of Long-Term Use: Impaired balance of water, salt and potassium in blood and body tissues. Development of diabetes in predisposed individuals. Pathological changes in the parathyroid glands (with increased blood calcium levels and decreased blood phosphate levels) have been reported with long-term use of thiazide diuretics, a class chemically related to this diuretic.

Suggested Periodic Examinations While Taking This Drug (at physician's discretion)
Complete blood cell counts, measurements of blood levels of sodium, potassium, chloride, sugar and uric acid.
Kidney and liver function tests.

▷ **While Taking This Drug, Observe the Following**
Foods: Consult your physician regarding the advisability of eating foods rich in potassium. If so advised, see the Table of High Potassium Foods in Section Six. Follow physician's advice regarding the use of salt.
Beverages: No restrictions. This drug may be taken with milk.
▷   *Alcohol:* Use with caution until the combined effects have been determined. Alcohol may exaggerate the blood-pressure-lowering effects of this drug and cause orthostatic hypotension.
Tobacco Smoking: No interactions expected. Follow physician's advice.
▷   *Other Drugs*
Metolazone may ***increase*** the effects of
• other antihypertensive drugs; dosage adjustments may be necessary

to prevent excessive lowering of blood pressure.

- lithium, and cause lithium toxicity.

Metolazone may *decrease* the effects of

- oral antidiabetic drugs (sulfonylureas); dosage adjustments may be necessary for proper control of blood sugar.

Metolazone *taken concurrently* with

- digitalis preparations (digitoxin, digoxin) requires very careful monitoring and dosage adjustments to prevent fluctuations of blood potassium levels and serious disturbances of heart rhythm.

The following drugs may *decrease* the effects of metolazone

- cholestyramine (Cuemid, Questran) may interfere with its absorption.
- colestipol (Colestid) may interfere with its absorption.

Take cholestyramine and colestipol 1 hour before any oral diuretic.

▷ *Driving, Hazardous Activities:* Use caution until the possible occurrence of orthostatic hypotension, dizziness or impaired vision has been determined.

Aviation Note: The use of this drug *may be a disqualification* for piloting. Consult a designated Aviation Medical Examiner.

Exposure to Sun: Use caution until sensitivity has been determined. This drug may cause photosensitivity (see Glossary).

Exposure to Heat: Avoid excessive perspiring, which could cause additional loss of salt and water from the body.

Heavy Exercise or Exertion: Avoid exertion that produces light-headedness, excessive fatigue or muscle cramping. Isometric exercises—the "overload" technique for strengthening individual muscles—can raise blood pressure significantly. Ask physician for guidance regarding participation in this form of exercise.

Occurrence of Unrelated Illness: Illnesses that cause vomiting or diarrhea can produce a serious imbalance of important body chemistry. Consult your physician for guidance.

Discontinuation: This drug should not be stopped abruptly following long-term use; serious diuretic-withdrawal fluid retention (edema) can develop after sudden discontinuation. The dose should be reduced gradually. It may be advisable to discontinue this drug 5 to 7 days before major surgery. Ask your physician, surgeon and/or anesthesiologist for guidance regarding dosage adjustment or drug withdrawal.

METOPROLOL
(me TOH proh lohl)

Introduced: 1974

Class: Antihypertensive, beta-adrenergic blocker

Prescription: USA: Yes
Canada: Yes

Controlled Drug: USA: No
Canada: No

Available as Generic: No

Brand Names: ✦Apo-Metoprolol, ✦Betaloc, ✦Co-Betaloc [CD], Lopressor, Lopressor HCT [CD], ✦Novometoprol

BENEFITS versus RISKS	
Possible Benefits	*Possible Risks*
EFFECTIVE, WELL-TOLERATED ANTIHYPERTENSIVE in mild to moderate high blood pressure	CONGESTIVE HEART FAILURE in advanced heart disease
	Worsening of angina in coronary heart disease (abrupt withdrawal)
	Masking of low blood sugar (hypoglycemia) in drug-treated diabetes
	Provocation of asthma (with high doses)

▷ **Principal Uses**

As a Single Drug Product: The treatment of mild to moderately severe high blood pressure. May be used alone or concurrently with other antihypertensive drugs, such as diuretics. Also used to reduce the risk of recurrent heart attack.

How This Drug Works: By blocking certain actions of the sympathetic nervous system, this drug
- reduces the rate the contraction force of the heart, thus lowering the ejection pressure of the blood leaving the heart.
- reduces the degree of contraction of blood vessel walls, resulting in their relaxation and expansion and consequent lowering of blood pressure.
- prolongs the conduction time of nerve impulses through the heart, of benefit in the management of certain heart rhythm disorders.

Available Dosage Forms and Strengths
Injection — 1 mg per ml
Tablets — 50 mg, 100 mg

▷ **Usual Adult Dosage Range:**   Initially, 50 mg twice daily (12 hours apart). The dose may be increased gradually at intervals of 7 to 10 days as needed and tolerated, up to 300 mg/day. For maintenance, 100 mg twice/day. The total daily dose should not exceed 450 mg. **Note: Actual dosage and administration schedule must be determined by the physician for each patient individually.**

▷ **Dosing Instructions:**   May be taken without regard to eating. The tablet may be crushed for administration. Do not discontinue this drug abruptly.

Usual Duration of Use: Continual use on a regular schedule for 10 to 14 days is usually necessary to determine this drug's effectiveness in lowering blood pressure. The long-term use of this drug (months to years) will be determined by the course of your blood pressure over time and your response to the overall treatment program (weight reduction, salt restriction, smoking cessation, etc.). Consult your physician on a regular basis.

Currently a "Drug of Choice" for initiating treatment of hypertension with a single drug, especially for those subject to bronchial asthma or diabetes.

▷ **This Drug Should Not Be Taken If**
- you have had an allergic reaction to it previously.
- you have congestive heart failure.
- you have an abnormally slow heart rate or a serious form of heart block.
- you are taking, or have taken within the past 14 days, any monoamine oxidase (MAO) type A inhibitor drug (see Drug Class, Section Four).

▷ **Inform Your Physician Before Taking This Drug If**
- you have had an adverse reaction to any beta blocker drug in the past (see Drug Class, Section Four).
- you have a history of serious heart disease, with or without episodes of heart failure.
- you have a history of hay fever (allergic rhinitis), asthma, chronic bronchitis or emphysema.
- you have a history of overactive thyroid function (hyperthyroidism).
- you have a history of low blood sugar (hypoglycemia).
- you have impaired liver or kidney function.
- you have diabetes or myasthenia gravis.
- you are currently taking any form of digitalis, quinidine or reserpine, or any calcium blocker drug (see Drug Class, Section Four).
- you plan to have surgery under general anesthesia in the near future.

Possible Side-Effects (natural, expected and unavoidable drug actions)
Lethargy and fatigability (10%), cold extremities, slow heart rate (15%), light-headedness in upright position (see Orthostatic Hypotension in Glossary).

▷ **Possible Adverse Effects** (unusual, unexpected and infrequent reactions)
If any of the following develop, consult your physician promptly for guidance.
Mild Adverse Effects
Allergic Reactions: Skin rash, itching.
Headache, dizziness (10%), insomnia, abnormal dreams.
Indigestion, nausea, vomiting, constipation, diarrhea.
Joint and muscle discomfort, fluid retention (edema).

Serious Adverse Effects
Mental depression (5%), anxiety.
Chest pain, shortness of breath, precipitation of congestive heart failure.
Induction of bronchial asthma (in asthmatic individuals).

▷ **Possible Effects on Sexual Function:** Decreased libido (4 times more common in men); impaired erection (less common with this drug than with most other beta blockers); Peyronie's disease (see Glossary).

CAUTION
1. ***Do not discontinue this drug suddenly*** without the knowledge and guidance of your physician. Carry a notation on your person that you are taking this drug.
2. Consult your physician or pharmacist before using nasal decongestants usually present in over-the-counter cold preparations and nose drops. These can cause sudden increases in blood pressure when taken concurrently with beta blocker drugs.
3. Report the development of any tendency to emotional depression.

Precautions for Use
By Infants and Children: Safety and effectiveness for use by those under 12 years of age have not been established. However, if this drug is used, observe for the development of low blood sugar (hypoglycemia) during periods of reduced food intake.
By Those over 60 Years of Age: Proceed ***cautiously*** with all antihypertensive drugs. Unacceptably high blood pressure should be reduced without creating the risks associated with excessively low blood pressure. Start treatment with small doses, and monitor the blood pressure response frequently. Sudden, rapid and excessive reduction of blood pressure can predispose to stroke or heart attack. Observe for dizziness, unsteadiness, tendency to fall, confusion, hallucinations, depression or urinary frequency.

▷ **Advisability of Use During Pregnancy**
Pregnancy Category: B (tentative). See Pregnancy Code inside back cover.
Animal studies: No significant increase in birth defects due to this drug.
Human studies: Information from adequate studies of pregnant women is not available.
Use this drug only if clearly needed. Ask physician for guidance.

Advisability of Use if Breast-Feeding
Presence of this drug in breast milk: Yes, in large amounts.
Avoid drug or refrain from nursing.

Habit-Forming Potential: None.

Effects of Overdosage: Weakness, slow pulse, low blood pressure, fainting, cold and sweaty skin, congestive heart failure, possible coma and convulsions.

Possible Effects of Long-Term Use: Reduced heart reserve and eventual heart failure in susceptible individuals with advanced heart disease.

Suggested Periodic Examinations While Taking This Drug (at physician's discretion)
Measurements of blood pressure, evaluation of heart function.

▷ **While Taking This Drug, Observe the Following**
Foods: No restrictions. Avoid excessive salt intake.
Beverages: No restrictions. May be taken with milk.
▷   *Alcohol:* Use with caution until the combined effect has been determined. Alcohol may exaggerate this drug's ability to lower the blood pressure and may increase its mild sedative effect.
Tobacco Smoking: Nicotine may reduce this drug's effectiveness in treating high blood pressure. In addition, high doses of this drug may potentiate the constriction of the bronchial tubes caused by regular smoking.
▷   *Other Drugs*
Metoprolol may ***increase*** the effects of
• other antihypertensive drugs, and cause excessive lowering of the blood pressure. Dosage adjustments may be necessary.
• reserpine (Ser-Ap-Es, etc.), and cause sedation, depression, slowing of the heart rate and lowering of the blood pressure.
• verapamil (Calan, Isoptin), and cause excessive depression of heart function; monitor this combination closely.
Metoprolol ***taken concurrently*** with
• clonidine (Catapres) requires close monitoring for rebound high blood pressure if clonidine is withdrawn while metoprolol is still being taken.
• insulin requires close monitoring to avoid undetected hypoglycemia (see Glossary).
The following drugs may ***increase*** the effects of metoprolol
• cimetidine (Tagamet).
• methimazole (Tapazole).
• oral contraceptives.
• propylthiouracil (Propacil).
The following drugs may ***decrease*** the effects of metoprolol
• barbiturates (phenobarbital, etc.).
• indomethacin (Indocin), and possibly other "aspirin substitutes," may impair metoprolol's antihypertensive effect.
• rifampin (Rifadin, Rimactane).
▷   *Driving, Hazardous Activities:* Use caution until the full extent of drowsiness, lethargy and blood pressure change has been determined.
Aviation Note: The use of this drug ***is a disqualification*** for piloting. Consult a designated Aviation Medical Examiner.
Exposure to Sun: No restrictions.
Exposure to Heat: Caution advised. Hot environments can lower the blood pressure and exaggerate the effects of this drug.

Exposure to Cold: Caution advised. Cold environments can enhance the circulatory deficiency in the extremities that may occur with this drug. The elderly should take precautions to prevent hypothermia (see Glossary).

Heavy Exercise or Exertion: It is advisable to avoid exertion that produces light-headedness, excessive fatigue or muscle cramping. The use of this drug may intensify the hypertensive response to isometric exercise.

Occurrence of Unrelated Illness: The fever that accompanies systemic infections can lower the blood pressure and require adjustment of dosage. Illnesses that cause nausea or vomiting may interrupt the regular dosage schedule. Ask your physician for guidance.

Discontinuation: It is advisable to avoid sudden discontinuation of this drug in all situations. If possible, gradual reduction of dose over a period of 2 to 3 weeks is recommended. Ask your physician for specific guidance.

METRONIDAZOLE
(me troh NI da zohl)

Introduced: 1960

Class: Anti-infective

Prescription: USA: Yes
  Canada: Yes

Controlled Drug: USA: No
  Canada: No

Available as Generic: Yes

Brand Names: ✦Apo-Metronidazole, Flagyl, Metizol, MetroGel, Metryl, ✦Neo-Tric, ✦Novonidazole, ✦PMS-Metronidazole, Protostat

---

BENEFITS versus RISKS	
Possible Benefits	*Possible Risks*
EFFECTIVE TREATMENT FOR TRICHOMONAS INFECTIONS, AMEBIC DYSENTERY AND GIARDIASIS	Superinfection with yeast organisms
	Peripheral neuropathy (see Glossary)
Effective treatment for some anaerobic bacterial infections	Abnormally low white blood cell count (transient)
Effective local treatment for rosacea	Aggravation of epilepsy

---

▷ **Principal Uses**

As a Single Drug Product: Used primarily to treat trichomonas infections of the vaginal canal and cervix and of the male urethra. It is also used to treat amebic dysentery, giardia infections of the intestine and serious infections caused by certain strains of anaerobic bacteria. A more recent use is the treatment of rosacea with local application of a gel dosage form.

How This Drug Works: By interacting with DNA, this drug destroys essential components of the nucleus that are necessary for the cell life and growth of infecting organisms.

Available Dosage Forms and Strengths
        Gel — 0.75%
    Injection — 500 mg per 100 ml
    Tablets — 250 mg, 500 mg

▷ **Usual Adult Dosage Range:**   Varies with infection to be treated.
    For trichomoniasis: One-day course—2 grams as a single dose; or 1 gram for 2 doses 12 hours apart. Seven-day course—250 mg 3 times/day for 7 consecutive days. (The 7-day course is preferred.)
    For amebiasis: 500 to 750 mg 3 times/day for 5 to 10 consecutive days.
    For giardiasis: 2 grams once/day for 3 days; or 250 to 500 mg 3 times/day for 5 to 7 days.
    The total daily dosage should not exceed 4 grams (4000 mg).
    Note: Actual dosage and administration schedule must be determined by the physician for each patient individually.

▷ **Dosing Instructions:**   May be taken with or following food to reduce stomach irritation. The tablet may be crushed for administration.

    Usual Duration of Use: Continual use on a regular schedule as outlined is necessary to ensure this drug's effectiveness. Do not repeat the course of treatment without your physician's approval.

▷ **This Drug Should Not Be Taken If**
    • you have had an allergic reaction to it previously.
    • you currently have a bone marrow or blood cell disorder.
    • you have any type of central nervous system disorder, including epilepsy.

▷ **Inform Your Physician Before Taking This Drug If**
    • you have a history of any type of blood cell disorder, especially one induced by drugs.
    • you have impaired liver or kidney function.
    • you are pregnant or breast-feeding.

    Possible Side-Effects (natural, expected and unavoidable drug actions)
    A sharp, metallic, unpleasant taste.
    Dark discoloration of the urine (of no significance).
    Superinfection (see Glossary) by yeast organisms in the mouth or vagina.

▷ **Possible Adverse Effects** (unusual, unexpected and infrequent reactions)
    If any of the following develop, consult your physician promptly for guidance.

Mild Adverse Effects
 Allergic Reactions: Skin rash, hives, flushing, itching.
 Headache, dizziness, incoordination, unsteadiness.
 Loss of appetite, nausea, vomiting, abdominal cramps, diarrhea.
 Irritation of mouth and tongue, possibly due to yeast infection.
Serious Adverse Effects
 Idiosyncratic Reactions: Abnormal behavior, confusion, depression.
 Peripheral neuropathy (see Glossary).
 Abnormally low white blood cell count (transient): fever, sore throat,
   infections.

▷ **Possible Effects on Sexual Function:**   Decreased libido; decreased vaginal
   secretions (difficult or painful intercourse).

Possible Delayed Adverse Effects: Studies have shown that this drug can
   cause cancer in mice and possibly in rats. There is no evidence to
   date that this drug causes cancer in man when used in the dosages
   specified earlier. Follow your physician's instructions exactly. Avoid
   unnecessary or prolonged use.

▷ **Adverse Effects That May Mimic Natural Diseases or Disorders**
   Behavioral changes may suggest spontaneous psychosis.

Natural Diseases or Disorders That May Be Activated by This Drug
   Latent yeast infections.

CAUTION
 1. Troublesome and persistent diarrhea can develop in sensitive in-
    dividuals. If diarrhea persists for more than 24 hours, discontinue
    this drug and consult with your physician.
 2. Discontinue this drug immediately if you develop any indications
    of toxic effects on the brain or nervous system: confusion, irrita-
    bility, dizziness, incoordination, unsteady stance or gait, muscle
    jerking or twitching, numbness or weakness in the extremities.

Precautions for Use
 By Infants and Children: Avoid use in those with a history of bone marrow
   or blood cell disorders.
 By Those over 60 Years of Age: Natural changes in the skin may predispose
   to yeast infections in the genital and anal regions. Report the development of rashes and itching promptly.

▷ **Advisability of Use During Pregnancy**
 Pregnancy Category: X (tentative). See Pregnancy Code inside back cover.
   Animal studies: No birth defects reported in rat studies. However, this
     drug is known to cause cancer in mice and possibly in rats.
   Human studies: No increase in birth defects reported in 206 exposures
     to this drug during the first 3 months. However, information from
     adequate studies of pregnant women is not available.

The manufacturer advises against the use of this drug during the first 3 months. Use during the last 6 months is not advised unless it is absolutely essential to the mother's health.

Advisability of Use if Breast-Feeding
Presence of this drug in breast milk: Yes.
Avoid drug or refrain from nursing.

Habit-Forming Potential: None.

Effects of Overdosage: Weakness, stomach irritation, nausea, vomiting, confusion, disorientation.

Possible Effects of Long-Term Use: None reported. Avoid long-term use.

Suggested Periodic Examinations While Taking This Drug (at physician's discretion)
Complete blood cell counts.

▷ **While Taking This Drug, Observe the Following**
Foods: No restrictions.
Beverages: No restrictions. May be taken with milk.
▷ *Alcohol:* Use caution until combined effects have been determined. A disulfiramlike reaction has been reported (see Glossary).
Tobacco Smoking: No interactions expected.
▷ *Other Drugs*
Metronidazole may *increase* the effects of
• warfarin (Coumadin, etc.), and cause abnormal bleeding. The prothrombin time should be monitored closely, especially during the first 10 days of concurrent use.
Metronidazole *taken concurrently* with
• disulfiram (Antabuse) may cause severe emotional and behavioral disturbances.
▷ *Driving, Hazardous Activities:* This drug may cause dizziness or incoordination. Restrict activities as necessary.
Aviation Note: The use of this drug *may be a disqualification* for piloting. Consult a designated Aviation Medical Examiner.
Exposure to Sun: No restrictions.

MEXILETINE
(mex IL e teen)

Introduced: 1973

Class: Antiarrhythmic

Prescription: USA: Yes
Canada: Yes

Controlled Drug: USA: No
Canada: No

Available as Generic: No

Brand Name: Mexitil

```
┌──────────────────────────────────────────────────────────────────┐
│                      BENEFITS versus RISKS                         │
│                                                                    │
│       Possible Benefits                  Possible Risks            │
│    EFFECTIVE TREATMENT IN          NARROW TREATMENT RANGE          │
│      30% OF SELECTED HEART         FREQUENT ADVERSE EFFECTS        │
│      RHYTHM DISORDERS                (up to 40% of users)          │
│                                    WORSENING OF SOME               │
│                                      ARRHYTHMIAS                   │
│                                    Rare seizures, liver injury and │
│                                      reduced white blood cell count│
└──────────────────────────────────────────────────────────────────┘
```

▷ **Principal Uses**

As a Single Drug Product: This drug is classified as a Class 1B agent, similar to lidocaine in its actions. It is used primarily to correct and prevent the recurrence of (1) abnormally rapid heart rates (tachycardia) that arise in the ventricles (lower heart chambers); and (2) premature beats arising in the ventricles.

How This Drug Works: By slowing the transmission of electrical impulses throughout the conduction system of the heart, this drug assists in restoring normal heart rate and rhythm in selected types of arrhythmia.

Available Dosage Forms and Strengths

Capsules — 150 mg, 200 mg, 250 mg

▷ **Usual Adult Dosage Range:**   Initiate treatment with 200 mg/8 hours. At intervals of 2 to 3 days, increase dose by 50 to 100 mg as needed and tolerated. The total daily dosage should not exceed 1200 mg. Measurement of drug blood levels is advised (when available) to determine the optimal dose and schedule. **Note: Actual dosage and administration schedule must be determined by the physician for each patient individually.**

▷ **Dosing Instructions:**   Take with food or antacid to reduce stomach irritation. Take at same times each day to obtain uniform results. The capsule may be opened for administration.

Usual Duration of Use: Continual use on a regular schedule for 1 to 2 weeks is usually necessary to determine this drug's effectiveness in correcting or preventing responsive rhythm disorders. Long-term use requires supervision and periodic evaluation by your physician. Consult your physician on a regular basis.

▷ **This Drug Should Not Be Taken If**
  • you have had an allergic reaction to it previously.
  • you have second-degree or third-degree heart block (determined by electrocardiogram), uncorrected by a pacemaker.

▷ **Inform Your Physician Before Taking This Drug If**
- you have had any unfavorable reactions to other antiarrhythmic drugs in the past.
- you have a history of heart disease of any kind, especially "heart block" or heart failure.
- you have impaired liver function.
- you have a seizure disorder of any kind.
- you are taking any form of digitalis, a potassium supplement or any diuretic drug that can cause excessive loss of body potassium (ask physician).

Possible Side-Effects (natural, expected and unavoidable drug actions)
Nervousness (11%), light-headedness (10%).

▷ **Possible Adverse Effects** (unusual, unexpected and infrequent reactions)
If any of the following develop, consult your physician promptly for guidance.
Mild Adverse Effects
Allergic Reaction: Skin rash (4%).
Headache (7%), dizziness (26%), visual disturbance (7%), fatigue (3%), weakness (5%), tremor (13%).
Loss of appetite, indigestion, nausea (39%), vomiting, constipation (4%), diarrhea (5%), abdominal pain (1%).
Serious Adverse Effects
Idiosyncratic Reactions: Depression, confusion, amnesia, hallucinations, seizures (all rare).
Drug-induced heart rhythm disorders (1%), shortness of breath (5%), palpitations (7%), chest pain (7%), swelling of feet.
Urinary retention.
Liver damage with jaundice (see Glossary).
Abnormally low white blood cell and blood platelet counts (rare): fever, sore throat, abnormal bleeding or bruising.

▷ **Possible Effects on Sexual Function:** Decreased libido, impotence (rare).

▷ **Adverse Effects That May Mimic Natural Diseases or Disorders**
Liver toxicity may suggest viral hepatitis.

Natural Diseases or Disorders That May Be Activated by This Drug
Latent epilepsy.

CAUTION
1. Thorough evaluation of your heart function (including electrocardiograms) is necessary prior to using this drug.
2. Periodic evaluation of your heart function is necessary to determine your response to this drug. Some individuals may experience worsening of their heart rhythm disorder and/or deterioration of heart function. Close monitoring of heart rate, rhythm and overall performance is essential.

3. Dosage must be adjusted carefully for each individual. Do not change your dosage without the knowledge and supervision of your physician.
4. Do not take any other antiarrhythmic drug while taking this drug unless you are directed to do so by your physician.
5. Carry a card of personal identification with the notation that you are taking this drug. Inform all attending medical personnel that you are taking this drug, especially if you require surgery of any kind.

Precautions for Use
By Infants and Children: Safety and effectiveness for use by those under 12 years of age have not been established. Initial use of this drug requires hospitalization and supervision by a qualified cardiologist.
By Those over 60 Years of Age: Reduced liver function may require reduction in dosage. Observe carefully for light-headedness, dizziness, unsteadiness and tendency to fall.

▷ Advisability of Use During Pregnancy
Pregnancy Category: C (tentative). See Pregnancy Code inside back cover.
Animal studies: No birth defects reported in mice, rats or rabbits. However, an increased rate of fetal resorption was found.
Human studies: Information from adequate studies of pregnant women is not available.
Avoid during first 3 months. Use this drug only if clearly needed. Ask physician for guidance.

Advisability of Use if Breast-Feeding
Presence of this drug in breast milk: Yes.
Avoid drug or refrain from nursing.

Habit-Forming Potential: None.

Effects of Overdosage: Impaired urination, constipation, marked drop in blood pressure, abnormal heart rhythms, congestive heart failure, dizziness, incoordination, seizures.

Possible Effects of Long-Term Use: None reported.

Suggested Periodic Examinations While Taking This Drug (at physician's discretion)
Electrocardiograms, complete blood cell counts, liver function tests.

▷ While Taking This Drug, Observe the Following
Foods: No restrictions. Ask physician regarding need for salt restriction.
Beverages: No restrictions. May be taken with milk.
▷   *Alcohol:* Use caution until the combined effects have been determined. Alcohol can increase the blood-pressure-lowering effects of this drug.
Tobacco Smoking: Nicotine can cause irritability of the heart and reduce the effectiveness of this drug. Follow physician's advice regarding smoking.

▷ *Other Drugs*

Mexiletine may ***increase*** the effects of
* antihypertensive drugs, and cause excessive lowering of blood pressure.
* beta blocker drugs (see Drug Class, Section Four).

The following drugs may ***decrease*** the effects of mexiletine
* phenytoin (Dilantin, etc.).
* rifampin (Rifadin, Rimactane).

▷ *Driving, Hazardous Activities:* This drug may cause weakness, dizziness or blurred vision. Restrict activities as necessary.

Aviation Note: The use of this drug ***may be a disqualification*** for piloting. Consult a designated Aviation Medical Examiner.

Exposure to Sun: No restrictions.

Occurrence of Unrelated Illness: Disorders that cause vomiting, diarrhea or dehydration can affect this drug's action adversely. Report such developments promptly.

Discontinuation: This drug should not be discontinued abruptly following long-term use. Ask your physician for guidance regarding gradual dose reduction.

MINOCYCLINE
(min oh SI kleen)

Introduced: 1970

Class: Antibiotic, tetracyclines

Prescription: USA: Yes
Canada: Yes

Controlled Drug: USA: No
Canada: No

Available as Generic: No

Brand Name: Minocin

BENEFITS versus RISKS	
Possible Benefits	*Possible Risks*
EFFECTIVE TREATMENT OF INFECTIONS due to susceptible microorganisms	Allergic reactions
	Drug-induced colitis
	Drug-induced dizziness and unsteadiness
	Fungal superinfections

▷ **Principal Uses**

As a Single Drug Product: This member of the tetracycline drug class is used primarily to treat (1) a broad range of infections caused by susceptible bacteria and protozoa, and (2) severe, resistant pustular acne.

How This Drug Works: This drug prevents the growth and multiplication of susceptible bacteria by interfering with their formation of essential proteins.

Available Dosage Forms and Strengths
Capsules — 50 mg, 100 mg
Oral suspension — 50 mg per 5-ml teaspoonful (5% alcohol)
Tablets, film-coated — 50 mg, 100 mg

▷ **Usual Adult Dosage Range:**   Initially, 200 mg; then 100 mg/12 hours or 50 mg/6 hours. The total daily dosage should not exceed 350 mg the first day or 200 mg thereafter. **Note: Actual dosage and administration schedule must be determined by the physician for each patient individually.**

▷ **Dosing Instructions:**   May be taken without regard to food. Take at same time each day, with a full glass of water or milk. Take the full course prescribed. The tablet may be crushed and the capsule may be opened for administration.

Usual Duration of Use: The time required to control the infection and be free of fever and symptoms for 48 hours. This varies with the nature of the infection.

▷ **This Drug Should Not Be Taken If**
- you are allergic to any tetracycline drug (see Drug Class, Section Four).
- you are pregnant or breast-feeding.

▷ **Inform Your Physician Before Taking This Drug If**
- it is prescribed for a child under 8 years of age.
- you have a history of liver or kidney disease.
- you have systemic lupus erythematosus.
- you are taking any penicillin drug.
- you are taking any anticoagulant drug.
- you plan to have surgery under general anesthesia in the near future.

Possible Side-Effects (natural, expected and unavoidable drug actions)
Superinfections (see Glossary), often due to yeast organisms. These can occur in the mouth, intestinal tract, rectum and/or vagina, resulting in rectal and vaginal itching.

▷ **Possible Adverse Effects** (unusual, unexpected and infrequent reactions)
If any of the following develop, consult your physician promptly for guidance.
Mild Adverse Effects
Allergic Reactions: Skin rash, hives, itching of hands and feet, swelling of face or extremities.
Marked dizziness, unsteadiness, incoordination (usually occurs during the first 3 days).

Pigmentation of skin.

Loss of appetite, stomach irritation, nausea, vomiting, diarrhea.

Irritation of mouth or tongue, "black tongue," sore throat, abdominal cramping or pain.

Serious Adverse Effects

Allergic Reactions: Anaphylactic reaction (see Glossary), asthma, fever, swollen joints, abnormal bleeding or bruising.

Permanent discoloration and/or malformation of teeth when taken under 8 years of age, including unborn child and infant.

▷ **Possible Effects on Sexual Function:** None reported.

Natural Diseases or Disorders That May Be Activated by This Drug
Systemic lupus erythematosus.

CAUTION

1. Antacids, dairy products and preparations containing aluminum, bismuth, calcium, iron, magnesium or zinc can prevent adequate absorption of this drug and reduce its effectiveness significantly.
2. Troublesome and persistent diarrhea can develop in sensitive individuals. If diarrhea persists for more than 24 hours, discontinue this drug and consult your physician.
3. If surgery under general anesthesia is required while taking this drug, the choice of anesthetic agent must be considered carefully to prevent serious kidney damage.

Precautions for Use
By Infants and Children: If possible, tetracyclines should not be given to children under 8 years of age because of the risk of permanent discoloration and deformity of the teeth. Rarely, young infants may develop increased intracranial pressure within the first 4 days of receiving this drug. Tetracyclines may inhibit normal bone growth and development.

By Those over 60 Years of Age: Dosage must be carefully individualized and based upon determinations of kidney function. Natural skin changes may predispose to severe and prolonged itching reactions in the genital and anal regions.

▷ **Advisability of Use During Pregnancy**
Pregnancy Category: D (tentative). See Pregnancy Code inside back cover.
Animal studies: Tetracycline causes limb defects in rats, rabbits and chickens.
Human studies: Information from studies of pregnant women indicates that this drug can cause impaired development and discoloration of teeth and other developmental defects.
It is advisable to avoid this drug completely during entire pregnancy.

Advisability of Use if Breast-Feeding
Presence of this drug in breast milk: Yes.
Avoid drug or refrain from nursing.

Habit-Forming Potential: None.

Effects of Overdosage: Dizziness, nausea, vomiting, diarrhea.

Possible Effects of Long-Term Use: Superinfections; rarely, impairment of bone marrow, liver or kidney function.

Suggested Periodic Examinations While Taking This Drug (at physician's discretion)
Complete blood cell counts, liver and kidney function tests.
During extended use, sputum and stool examinations may detect early superinfection due to yeast organisms.

▷ **While Taking This Drug, Observe the Following**
Foods: No restrictions.
Beverages: No restrictions.
▷ *Alcohol:* No interactions expected. However, it is best avoided if you have active liver disease.
Tobacco Smoking: No interactions expected.
▷ *Other Drugs*
Tetracyclines may ***increase*** the effects of
- oral anticoagulants, and make it necessary to reduce their dosage.
- digoxin (Lanoxin), and cause digitalis toxicity.
- lithium (Eskalith, Lithane, etc.), and increase the risk of lithium toxicity.

Tetracyclines may ***decrease*** the effects of
- oral contraceptives, and impair their effectiveness in preventing pregnancy.
- penicillins, and impair their effectiveness in treating infections.

Tetracyclines ***taken concurrently*** with
- methoxyflurane anesthesia may impair kidney function.

The following drugs may ***decrease*** the effects of tetracyclines
- antacids (aluminum and magnesium preparations, sodium bicarbonate, etc.) may reduce drug absorption.
- iron and mineral preparations may reduce drug absorption.

▷ *Driving, Hazardous Activities:* This drug may cause marked dizziness or incoordination. Restrict activities as necessary.
Aviation Note: The use of this drug ***may be a disqualification*** for piloting. Consult a designated Aviation Medical Examiner.
Exposure to Sun: Use caution until sensitivity has been determined. Some tetracyclines can cause photosensitivity (see Glossary).

MINOXIDIL
(min OX i dil)

Introduced: 1972

Class: Antihypertensive, hair growth stimulant

Prescription: USA: Yes
Canada: Yes

Controlled Drug: USA: No
Canada: No

Available as Generic: Yes

Brand Names: Loniten, Minodyl, Rogaine

BENEFITS versus RISKS

Possible Benefits	*Possible Risks*
A POTENT, LONG-ACTING ANTIHYPERTENSIVE	EXCESSIVE BODY HAIR GROWTH (in 80% of users)
EFFECTIVE IN 75% OF CASES OF SEVERE HYPERTENSION	SALT AND WATER RETENTION
EFFECTIVE IN ACCELERATED AND MALIGNANT HYPERTENSION	Excessively rapid heart rate
	Aggravation of angina
	Local scalp irritation (topical use)
Moderately effective in treating male-pattern baldness in 39% of users	

▷ **Principal Uses**

As a Single Drug Product: Principal uses include (1) the treatment of severe high blood pressure that cannot be controlled by conventional therapy; (2) the treatment of male-pattern baldness, using a topical solution applied to the scalp.

How This Drug Works: (1) By causing direct relaxation of the constricted muscles within the walls of small arteries throughout the body, this drug permits expansion of the arteries with resultant lowering of blood pressure. (2) The exact mechanism by which this drug stimulates hair growth is not completely known. It is thought that it may increase the size of previously closed small blood vessels in the scalp (improve blood flow) and restore small hair follicles to normal size and activity.

Available Dosage Forms and Strengths
Tablets — 2.5 mg, 10 mg
Topical solution — 2%

▷ **Usual Adult Dosage Range:** For hypertension: Initially, 5 mg/24 hours in one dose. Gradually increase dose to 10 mg, 20 mg, then 40 mg/24 hours, taken in 1 or 2 divided doses daily, as needed and tolerated. The usual maintenance dose is 10 to 40 mg/24 hours. The total daily dosage should not exceed 50 mg. For male-pattern baldness: Apply thinly 1 ml of topical solution to the balding area of the scalp twice daily. The total daily dosage should not exceed 2 ml. **Note: Actual dosage and administration schedule must be determined by the physician for each patient individually.**

▷ **Dosing Instructions:** For hypertension: Tablets may be taken with or following food to prevent nausea. Take at the same time each day. The tablet may be crushed for administration. For baldness: ***The topical solution is for external, local use only; it is not to be swallowed.*** Begin application at the center of the bald area; apply thinly to cover the entire area. The scalp and hair must be dry at the time of application. Follow carefully the instructions that accompany the applicator you have purchased.

Usual Duration of Use: Continual use on a regular schedule for 3 to 7 days is usually necessary to determine this drug's effectiveness in controlling severe hypertension. Continual use of the topical solution for at least 4 months is necessary to determine its ability to promote hair growth. Long-term use (months to years) of both dosage forms requires supervision and periodic evaluation by your physician. Consult your physician on a regular basis.

▷ **This Drug Should Not Be Taken If**
- you have had an allergic reaction to it previously.
- you are known to have a pheochromocytoma (an adrenaline-producing tumor).
- you have pulmonary hypertension due to mitral valve stenosis.

▷ **Inform Your Physician Before Taking This Drug If**
- you are pregnant or planning pregnancy.
- you have a history of coronary artery disease or impaired heart function.
- you have a history of stroke or impaired brain circulation.
- you have impaired liver or kidney function.

Possible Side-Effects (natural, expected and unavoidable drug actions)
Increased heart rate, fluid retention with weight gain (7%), excessive hair growth on face, arms, legs and back (80%).

▷ **Possible Adverse Effects** (unusual, unexpected and infrequent reactions)
If any of the following develop, consult your physician promptly for guidance.
Mild Adverse Effects
Allergic Reactions: Skin rash (less than 1%). Localized dermatitis at site of application of topical solution.
Headache, dizziness, fainting (1% to 2%).
Nausea, increased thirst.
Serious Adverse Effects
Idiosyncratic Reaction: Fluid formation around the heart (pericardial effusion) (3%).
Development of angina pectoris; development of high blood pressure in the lung circulation (pulmonary hypertension).

▷ **Possible Effects on Sexual Function:**   Breast tenderness (less than 1%).

Natural Diseases or Disorders That May Be Activated by This Drug
Latent coronary artery disease with symptomatic angina.

CAUTION
1. The long-term use of this drug for hypertension usually requires the concurrent use of an effective diuretic to counteract salt and water retention.
2. The long-term use of this drug for hypertension often requires the concurrent use of a beta blocker drug to control excessive acceleration of the heart rate.
3. It is best to avoid the concurrent use of this drug and guanethidine; the combination can cause severe orthostatic hypotension (see Glossary).
4. Consult your physician regarding the advisability of using a "no salt added" diet.
5. Only very small amounts of this drug are absorbed into the general circulation when the topical solution is applied to the scalp. However, some systemic effects have been reported. Inform your physician promptly if you experience any unusual symptoms while using the topical solution.

Precautions for Use
By Infants and Children: Dosage schedules should be determined by a qualified pediatrician. Monitor closely for salt and water retention.
By Those over 60 Years of Age: This drug must be used very cautiously by this age group. Start treatment with small doses and limit the total daily dose to 75 mg. Headache, palpitation and rapid heart rate due to this drug are more common in this age group and can mimic acute anxiety states. Observe for dizziness, unsteadiness, fainting and falling.

▷ **Advisability of Use During Pregnancy**
Pregnancy Category: C (tentative). See Pregnancy Code inside back cover.
Animal studies: No birth defects reported in rats or rabbits. However, studies did reveal decreased fertility and increased fetal deaths.
Human studies: Information from adequate studies of pregnant women is not available.
Avoid during the first 3 months. Use only if clearly needed during the last 6 months.

Advisability of Use if Breast-Feeding
Presence of this drug in breast milk: Yes.
Avoid drug or refrain from nursing.

Habit-Forming Potential: None.

Effects of Overdosage: Headache, dizziness, weakness, nausea, marked low blood pressure, weak and rapid pulse, loss of consciousness.

Possible Effects of Long-Term Use: Excessive growth of body hair occurs in 80% of users after 1 to 2 months of continual treatment for hypertension. Close to 100% of users will experience this effect after 1 year of continual treatment. This may be accompanied by darkening of the skin and coarsening of facial features.

Suggested Periodic Examinations While Taking This Drug (at physician's discretion)

Body weight measurement for insidious gain due to water retention.
Electrocardiographic and echocardiographic heart examinations.

▷ **While Taking This Drug, Observe the Following**

Foods: Avoid excessive salt and heavily salted foods.

Beverages: No restrictions. May be taken with milk.

▷ *Alcohol:* Use with extreme caution until combined effects have been determined. Alcohol can exaggerate the blood-pressure-lowering effects of this drug.

Tobacco Smoking: Best avoided. Nicotine can contribute significantly to the development of angina in susceptible individuals.

▷ *Other Drugs*

Minoxidil may *increase* the effects of

- all other antihypertensive drugs; careful dosage adjustments are mandatory.

Minoxidil *taken concurrently* with

- guanethidine (Ismelin, Esimil) may cause severe orthostatic hypotension; avoid this combination.

▷ *Driving, Hazardous Activities:* This drug may cause dizziness and fatigue. Restrict activities as necessary.

Aviation Note: The use of this drug *is a disqualification* for piloting. Consult a designated Aviation Medical Examiner.

Exposure to Sun: No restrictions.

Discontinuation: This drug should not be stopped abruptly. If it is to be discontinued, consult your physician regarding gradual reduction in dosage and appropriate replacement with other drugs for the management of hypertension. Following discontinuation of the topical solution, the pretreatment pattern of baldness may return within 3 to 4 months.

MISOPROSTOL
(mi soh PROH stohl)

Introduced: 1987

Class: Stomach ulcer preventive, antiulcer

Prescription: USA: Yes
Canada: Yes

Controlled Drug: USA: No
Canada: No

Available as Generic: USA: No
Canada: No

Brand Name: Cytotec

```
┌─────────────────────────────────────────────────────────────────────┐
│                        BENEFITS versus RISKS                        │
│                                                                     │
│      Possible Benefits                    Possible Risks            │
│  EFFECTIVE PREVENTION OF          ABORTION (11%)                    │
│     STOMACH ULCERATION            Diarrhea (14% to 40%), transient  │
│     WHILE TAKING ANTI-                                              │
│     INFLAMMATORY DRUGS (93%                                         │
│     reduction of ulcer development)                                │
│  Effective treatment of duodenal                                   │
│     ulcer                                                           │
└─────────────────────────────────────────────────────────────────────┘
```

▷ **Principal Uses**

As a Single Drug Product: Used primarily to prevent development of stomach ulcers during long-term use of anti-inflammatory drugs as therapy for arthritis and related conditions. Also used (in Canada and other countries) for treatment of active duodenal ulcer unrelated to use of anti-inflammatory drugs.

How This Drug Works: This drug protects the lining tissues of the stomach and duodenum and prevents ulceration due to anti-inflammatory drugs by using several mechanisms: (1) replacing tissue prostaglandins that are depleted by anti-inflammatory drugs; (2) inhibiting the secretion of stomach acid; (3) increasing the local production of bicarbonate (to neutralize acids) and of mucus (to protect stomach and duodenal tissues). The combined effects prevent new ulcer formation and promote healing of existing ulcer(s).

Available Dosage Forms and Strengths

Tablets — 200 mcg

▷ **Usual Adult Dosage Range**

For prevention of stomach ulcer—100 to 200 mcg 4 times daily, taken concurrently during the use of any anti-inflammatory drug (see Antiarthritic/Anti-inflammatory Drug Class, Section Four).

For treatment of duodenal ulcer—200 mcg 4 times daily for 4 to 8 weeks.

Note: Actual dosage and administration schedule must be determined by the physician for each patient individually.

▷ **Dosing Instructions:** Take the prescribed dose with each of 3 daily meals; take the last (fourth) dose of the day with food at bedtime. The tablet may be crushed for administration.

Usual Duration of Use: For prevention of stomach ulcer, continual use on a regular schedule is recommended for the entire period of anti-inflammatory drug use. For treatment of duodenal ulcer, continual use on a regular schedule for 4 weeks is recommended; if ulcer healing is not complete, a second course of 4 weeks is advised. Long-term use (months to years) requires periodic evaluation of response and dosage adjustment. Consult your physician on a regular basis.

Possible Advantages of This Drug: Significantly more effective than histamine (H-2)-blocking drugs (cimetidine, famotidine, nizatidine, ranitidine) or sucralfate in preventing the development of stomach ulcers.

Currently a "Drug of Choice" for the routine prevention of stomach ulcers induced by long-term use of antiarthritic/anti-inflammatory drugs.

▷ **This Drug Should Not Be Taken If**
- you have had an allergic reaction to it previously.
- you are allergic to any type of prostaglandin.
- you are pregnant or breast-feeding.
- you are not able or willing to use effective contraception (oral contraceptives or intrauterine device) while taking this drug.

▷ **Inform Your Physician Before Taking This Drug If**
- you have a history of peptic ulcer disease or Crohn's disease.
- you have impaired kidney function.
- you have a seizure disorder.

Possible Side-Effects (natural, expected and unavoidable drug actions)
Diarrhea (14% to 40% of users), usually beginning after 13 days of use and subsiding spontaneously after 8 days.
Abortion (miscarriage) of pregnancy (11% of users); this is often incomplete and accompanied by serious uterine bleeding that may require hospitalization and urgent treatment.

▷ **Possible Adverse Effects** (unusual, unexpected and infrequent reactions)
If any of the following develop, consult your physician promptly for guidance.
Mild Adverse Effects
Allergic Reaction: Skin rash.
Headache (2.4%), dizziness.
Abdominal pain (12.8%), indigestion (2%), nausea (3.2%), vomiting (1.3%), flatulence (2.9%), constipation (1.1%).
Menstrual irregularity (0.3%), menstrual cramps (0.6%), heavy menstrual flow (0.5%), spotting between periods (0.7%).
Serious Adverse Effects
Allergic Reactions: None reported.
Post-menopausal vaginal bleeding; this may require further evaluation.

▷ **Possible Effects on Sexual Function:**   Reduced libido and impotence reported rarely, but causal relationship not established.

▷ **Natural Diseases or Disorders That May Be Activated by This Drug**
Latent epilepsy.

CAUTION

1. Do not take this drug if you are pregnant. It can cause abortion.
2. Do not make this drug available to others who may be pregnant or who may become pregnant.
3. If your physician prescribes this drug for you, it is advisable that you have a negative serum pregnancy test within 2 weeks before starting treatment.
4. Start taking this drug only on the second or third day of your next normal menstrual period.
5. Also initiate effective contraceptive measures when you begin to take this drug. Discuss the use of oral contraceptives or intrauterine devices with your physician.
6. Should pregnancy occur while you are taking this drug, discontinue it immediately and inform your physician.

Precautions for Use

By Infants and Children: Safety and effectiveness for use by those under 18 years of age have not been established.

By Those over 60 Years of Age: This drug is usually well tolerated by this age group. However, some forms of prostaglandins can cause drops in blood pressure; observe for periods of light-headedness or faintness that may indicate low blood pressure. Report any such development to your physician.

▷ ### Advisability of Use During Pregnancy

Pregnancy Category: X. See Pregnancy Code inside back cover.

Animal studies: No birth defects due to this drug found in rat or rabbit studies.

Human studies: Information from studies of pregnant women confirms that this drug can cause abortion, sometimes incomplete; unpassed products of conception can cause life-threatening complications.

Avoid this drug completely.

Advisability of Use if Breast-Feeding

Presence of this drug in breast milk: Unknown.

Avoid drug or refrain from nursing.

Habit-Forming Potential: None.

Effects of Overdosage: Abdominal pain, diarrhea, fever, drowsiness, weakness, tremor, convulsions, difficult breathing.

Possible Effects of Long-Term Use: Unknown at this time.

Suggested Periodic Examinations While Taking This Drug (at physician's discretion)

Monitoring for accidental pregnancy.

▷ ### While Taking This Drug, Observe the Following

Foods: No restrictions.

Beverages: No restrictions. May be taken with milk.

▷   *Alcohol:* No interactions expected. However, use sparingly if at all; alcohol can promote the development of stomach ulcer and reduce the effectiveness of this drug.

    Tobacco Smoking: No interactions expected. However, nicotine is conducive to the development of stomach ulcer. Smoking should be avoided.

▷   *Other Drugs*

    Misoprostol **taken concurrently** with

     • antacids that contain magnesium may increase the risk of diarrhea; avoid this combination.

▷   *Driving, Hazardous Activities:* This drug may cause dizziness, light-headedness, stomach pain or diarrhea. Restrict activities as necessary.

    Aviation Note: The use of this drug **may be a disqualification** for piloting. Consult a designated Aviation Medical Examiner.

    Exposure to Sun: No restrictions.

    Discontinuation: This drug should be taken concurrently while you are taking antiarthritic/anti-inflammatory drugs that can induce stomach ulceration. Consult your physician if you have reason to discontinue it prematurely.

MOLINDONE
(moh LIN dohn)

Introduced: 1971

Class: Strong tranquilizer, antipsychotic

Prescription: USA: Yes

Controlled Drug: USA: No

Available as Generic: No

Brand Name: Moban

BENEFITS versus RISKS	
Possible Benefits	*Possible Risks*
EFFECTIVE TREATMENT OF SOME CASES OF ACUTE AND CHRONIC SCHIZOPHRENIA	NARROW TREATMENT MARGIN SERIOUS TOXIC EFFECTS ON BRAIN:
May be effective in schizophrenia that has not responded to other drugs	PARKINSON-LIKE REACTIONS SEVERE RESTLESSNESS ABNORMAL INVOLUNTARY MOVEMENTS TARDIVE DYSKINESIAS (see Glossary)
	Liver toxicity, jaundice
	Atropinelike side-effects

▷ **Principal Uses**

As a Single Drug Product: Used primarily in the management of acute and chronic schizophrenia to control thought disorder, disorientation, hallucinations, perceptual distortions and hostility. It is sometimes effective in chronic schizophrenic individuals who have not responded to other antipsychotic drugs.

How This Drug Works: Not completely established. It is thought that by decreasing dopamine activity in the reticular activating system of the brain, this drug improves distorted patterns of thinking and behavior.

Available Dosage Forms and Strengths

Concentrate — 20 mg per ml
Tablets — 5 mg, 10 mg, 25 mg, 50 mg, 100 mg

▷ **Usual Adult Dosage Range:** Initially, 50 to 75 mg/day in 3 or 4 divided doses; dose may be increased gradually in 3 to 4 days to 100 mg/day as needed and tolerated. For maintenance: mild psychosis—5 to 15 mg, 3 or 4 times/day; moderate psychosis—10 to 25 mg, 3 or 4 times/day; severe psychosis—up to 225 mg/day, in 3 or 4 divided doses. The total daily dosage should not exceed 225 mg. **Note: Actual dosage and administration schedule must be determined by the physician for each patient individually.**

▷ **Dosing Instructions:** Take with food or milk to reduce stomach irritation. The liquid concentrate may be diluted with water, milk, fruit juice or carbonated beverages. The tablet may be crushed for administration.

Usual Duration of Use: Continual use on a regular schedule for 3 to 6 weeks is usually necessary to determine this drug's effectiveness in controlling the features of schizophrenia. Long-term use (months to years) requires supervision and periodic evaluation by your physician. Consult your physician on a regular basis.

▷ **This Drug Should Not Be Taken If**
- you have had an allergic reaction to it previously.
- you have acute alcoholic intoxication.

▷ **Inform Your Physician Before Taking This Drug If**
- you are taking any drugs that have sedative effects.
- you use alcohol excessively.
- you have any type of seizure disorder.
- you have any type of glaucoma.
- you have Parkinson's disease or an enlarged prostate gland.
- you have impaired liver or kidney function.
- you have a history of breast cancer.

Possible Side-Effects (natural, expected and unavoidable drug actions)

Drowsiness, dry mouth, nasal congestion, constipation, impaired urination.
Parkinson-like reactions (see Glossary).

▷ **Possible Adverse Effects** (unusual, unexpected and infrequent reactions)
If any of the following develop, consult your physician promptly for guidance.

Mild Adverse Effects

Allergic Reaction: Skin rash.

Headache, dizziness, blurred vision, lethargy, unsteadiness, insomnia, depression, euphoria, ringing in ears.

Rapid heartbeat, low blood pressure, fainting.

Loss of appetite, indigestion, nausea.

Serious Adverse Effects

Allergic Reactions: Liver reaction with jaundice.

Spasms of face and neck muscles, abnormal involuntary movements of extremities, severe restlessness.

Development of tardive dyskinesias (see Glossary).

Neuroleptic malignant syndrome: high fever, fast heart rate, difficult breathing, severe muscle rigidity, loss of bladder control, seizures.

▷ **Possible Effects on Sexual Function**

Increased libido; male breast enlargement and tenderness; female breast enlargement with milk formation.

Altered timing and pattern of menstruation.

▷ **Adverse Effects That May Mimic Natural Diseases or Disorders**

Parkinson-like reactions may be mistaken for naturally occurring Parkinson's disease.

Liver reactions may suggest viral hepatitis.

CAUTION

1. This drug may alter the pattern of epileptic seizures and require dosage adjustments of anticonvulsant drugs.
2. Obtain prompt evaluation of any change or disturbance of vision.
3. There is a very narrow margin between the effective therapeutic dose and the dose that can cause Parkinson-like reactions. Inform your physician promptly if suggestive symptoms develop.

Precautions for Use

By Infants and Children: Safety and effectiveness for use by those under 12 years of age have not been established.

By Those over 60 Years of Age: Start treatment with small doses. This drug can aggravate an existing prostatism (see Glossary). You may be more susceptible to the development of Parkinson-like reactions or tardive dyskinesia. Report any suggestive symptoms promptly.

▷ **Advisability of Use During Pregnancy**

Pregnancy Category: B (tentative). See Pregnancy Code inside back cover.

Animal studies: No birth defects reported in mice, rats or rabbits.

Human studies: Information from adequate studies of pregnant women is not available.

Because of its inherent toxicity for brain tissue, avoid use during pregnancy if possible.

Advisability of Use if Breast-Feeding
Presence of this drug in breast milk: Unknown.
Avoid drug or refrain from nursing.

Habit-Forming Potential: None.

Effects of Overdosage: Marked drowsiness, weakness, tremor, agitation, impaired stance and gait, stupor progressing to coma, possible seizures.

Possible Effects of Long-Term Use: Development of tardive dyskinesias.

Suggested Periodic Examinations While Taking This Drug (at physician's discretion)
Complete blood cell counts, liver function tests.

▷ **While Taking This Drug, Observe the Following**
Foods: No restrictions.
Beverages: No restrictions. May be taken with milk.
▷   *Alcohol:* Avoid completely. Alcohol can increase the sedative action of this drug and enhance its depressant effects on brain function. Also, this drug can increase the intoxicating effects of alcohol.
Tobacco Smoking: No interactions expected.
▷   *Other Drugs*
Molindone may ***increase*** the effects of
- all drugs containing atropine or having atropinelike effects (see Drug Class, Section Four).
- all drugs with sedative effects, and cause excessive sedation.

Molindone ***taken concurrently*** with
- antiepileptic drugs (anticonvulsants) may require close monitoring for changes in seizure patterns and need for dosage adjustments.
▷   *Driving, Hazardous Activities:* This drug may cause dizziness and drowsiness. Restrict activities as necessary.
Aviation Note: The use of this drug ***is a disqualification*** for piloting. Consult a designated Aviation Medical Examiner.
Exposure to Sun: No restrictions.
Exposure to Heat: Use caution and avoid excessive heat as much as possible. This drug may impair the regulation of body temperature and increase the risk of heat stroke.
Discontinuation: Do not stop taking this drug suddenly after long-term use. Ask your physician for guidance regarding gradual dosage reduction and withdrawal.

NADOLOL
(nay DOH lohl)

Introduced: 1976

Class: Antianginal, antihypertensive, beta-adrenergic blocker

Prescription: USA: Yes
Canada: Yes

Controlled Drug: USA: No
Canada: No

Available as Generic: No

Brand Names: Corgard, Corzide [CD]

BENEFITS versus RISKS

Possible Benefits	*Possible Risks*
EFFECTIVE, WELL-TOLERATED ANTIHYPERTENSIVE in mild to moderate high blood pressure	CONGESTIVE HEART FAILURE in advanced heart disease
EFFECTIVE ANTIANGINAL DRUG IN CLASSICAL CORONARY ARTERY DISEASE with moderate to severe angina	Provocation of asthma (in predisposed individuals) Masking of hypoglycemia in drug-dependent diabetes Worsening of angina following abrupt withdrawal

---

▷ **Principal Uses**

As a Single Drug Product: This beta blocker drug is used primarily to (1) treat moderately high blood pressure, and (2) contribute to the management of coronary artery disease by preventing attacks of effort-induced angina. (This drug is contraindicated in Prinzmetal's vasospastic angina.)

As a Combination Drug Product [CD]: This drug is available in combination with bendroflumethiazide, a mild diuretic "step 1" antihypertensive drug. This combination product is more effective and more convenient for long-term use.

How This Drug Works: By blocking certain actions of the sympathetic nervous system, this drug

- reduces the rate and contraction force of the heart, thus lowering the oxygen requirement of the heart muscle and reducing the ejection pressure of the blood leaving the heart; these actions reduce the frequency of angina and lower blood pressure.
- reduces the degree of contraction of blood vessel walls, resulting in their relaxation and expansion and consequent lowering of blood pressure.
- prolongs the conduction time of nerve impulses through the heart, of benefit in the management of certain heart rhythm disorders.

Available Dosage Forms and Strengths
Tablets — 40 mg, 80 mg, 120 mg, 160 mg

▷ **Usual Adult Dosage Range:** For hypertension: Initially, 40 mg daily in one dose; this may be increased gradually as needed and tolerated, up to 640 mg/24 hours. The usual maintenance dose is 80 to 320 mg/24 hours. The total daily dosage should not exceed 640 mg. For angina: Initially, 40 mg daily in one dose; increase gradually at intervals of 3 to 7 days up to 240 mg/24 hours. The usual maintenance dose is 80 to 240 mg/24 hours. The total daily dose should not exceed 240 mg. **Note: Actual dosage and administration schedule must be determined by the physician for each patient individually.**

▷ **Dosing Instructions:** May be taken without regard to eating. The tablet may be crushed for administration. Do not discontinue this drug abruptly.

Usual Duration of Use: Continual use on a regular schedule for 10 to 14 days is usually necessary to determine this drug's effectiveness in lowering blood pressure and preventing effort-induced angina. The long-term use of this drug (months to years) will be determined by the course of your blood pressure and angina over time and your response to the overall treatment program (weight reduction, salt restriction, smoking cessation, etc.). Consult your physician on a regular basis.

Possible Advantages of This Drug
Does not reduce blood flow to the kidney.
Can be used concurrently with other drugs that may reduce blood flow to the kidney (such as most anti-inflammatory aspirin substitutes).

Currently a "Drug of Choice" for initiating treatment of hypertension with a single drug.

▷ **This Drug Should Not Be Taken If**
- you have had an allergic reaction to it previously.
- you have congestive heart failure.
- you have an abnormally slow heart rate or a serious form of heart block.
- you are subject to bronchial asthma.
- you are presently experiencing seasonal hay fever.
- you are taking, or have taken within the past 14 days, any monoamine oxidase (MAO) type A inhibitor drug (see Drug Class, Section Four).

▷ **Inform Your Physician Before Taking This Drug If**
- you have had an adverse reaction to any beta blocker drug in the past (see Drug Class, Section Four).
- you have a history of serious heart disease, with or without episodes of heart failure.
- you have a history of hay fever (allergic rhinitis), asthma, chronic bronchitis or emphysema.

- you have a history of overactive thyroid function (hyperthyroidism).
- you have a history of low blood sugar (hypoglycemia).
- you have impaired liver or kidney function.
- you have diabetes or myasthenia gravis.
- you are currently taking any form of digitalis, quinidine or reserpine, or any calcium blocker drug (see Drug Class, Section Four).
- you plan to have surgery under general anesthesia in the near future.

Possible Side-Effects (natural, expected and unavoidable drug actions)
>   Lethargy and fatigability, cold extremities, slow heart rate, light-headedness in upright position (see Orthostatic Hypotension in Glossary).

▷ **Possible Adverse Effects** (unusual, unexpected and infrequent reactions)
>   **If any of the following develop, consult your physician promptly for guidance.**
>
>   *Mild Adverse Effects*
>   Allergic Reactions: Skin rash, itching, drug fever.
>   Headache, dizziness, insomnia, vivid dreaming, visual disturbances, ringing in ears, slurred speech.
>   Indigestion, nausea, vomiting, diarrhea, abdominal pain.
>   Numbness and tingling of extremities.
>   *Serious Adverse Effects*
>   Allergic Reaction: Facial swelling.
>   Chest pain, shortness of breath, precipitation of congestive heart failure.
>   Intensification of heart block.
>   Induction of bronchial asthma (in asthmatic individuals).
>   Masking of warning indications of acute hypoglycemia in drug-treated diabetes.

▷ **Possible Effects on Sexual Function:**   Decreased libido, impotence (4%), impaired erection (36%).

▷ **Adverse Effects That May Mimic Natural Diseases or Disorders**
>   Impaired circulation to the extremities may resemble Raynaud's phenomenon.

Natural Diseases or Disorders That May Be Activated by This Drug
>   Bronchial asthma, Prinzmetal's variant (vasospastic) angina, latent Raynaud's disease, myasthenia gravis (questionable).

CAUTION
1. ***Do not discontinue this drug suddenly*** without the knowledge and guidance of your physician. Carry a notation on your person that you are taking this drug.
2. Consult your physician or pharmacist before using nasal decongestants usually present in over-the-counter cold preparations and nose drops. These can cause sudden increases in blood pressure when taken concurrently with beta blocker drugs.
3. Report the development of any tendency to emotional depression.

Precautions for Use

By Infants and Children: Safety and effectiveness for use by those under 12 years of age have not been established. However, if this drug is used, observe for the development of low blood sugar (hypoglycemia) during periods of reduced food intake.

By Those over 60 Years of Age: Proceed **cautiously** with all antihypertensive drugs. Unacceptably high blood pressure should be reduced without creating the risks associated with excessively low blood pressure. Start treatment with small doses, and monitor the blood pressure response frequently. Sudden, rapid and excessive reduction of blood pressure can predispose to stroke or heart attack. Observe for dizziness, unsteadiness, tendency to fall, confusion, hallucinations, depression or urinary frequency.

▷ **Advisability of Use During Pregnancy**

Pregnancy Category: C (tentative). See Pregnancy Code inside back cover.

Animal studies: No significant increase in birth defects due to this drug, but embryotoxicity reported in rabbits.

Human studies: Information from adequate studies of pregnant women is not available.

Avoid use during the first 3 months if possible. Use this drug only if clearly needed. Ask physician for guidance.

Advisability of Use if Breast-Feeding

Presence of this drug in breast milk: Yes, in large amounts.

Avoid drug or refrain from nursing.

Habit-Forming Potential: None.

Effects of Overdosage: Weakness, slow pulse, low blood pressure, fainting, cold and sweaty skin, congestive heart failure, possible coma and convulsions.

Possible Effects of Long-Term Use: Reduced heart reserve and eventual heart failure in susceptible individuals with advanced heart disease.

Suggested Periodic Examinations While Taking This Drug (at physician's discretion)

Measurements of blood pressure, evaluation of heart function.

▷ **While Taking This Drug, Observe the Following**

Foods: No restrictions. Avoid excessive salt intake.

Beverages: No restrictions. May be taken with milk.

▷   *Alcohol:* Use with caution until the combined effect has been determined. Alcohol may exaggerate this drug's ability to lower blood pressure and may increase its mild sedative effect.

Tobacco Smoking: Nicotine may reduce this drug's effectiveness in treating high blood pressure and angina. In addition, high doses of this drug may potentiate the constriction of the bronchial tubes caused by regular smoking.

▷ *Other Drugs*

Nadolol may ***increase*** the effects of

- other antihypertensive drugs, and cause excessive lowering of blood pressure. Dosage adjustments may be necessary.
- reserpine (Ser-Ap-Es, etc.), and cause sedation, depression, slowing of the heart rate and lowering of blood pressure.
- verapamil (Calan, Isoptin), and cause excessive depression of heart function; monitor this combination closely.

Nadolol may ***decrease*** the effects of

- theophyllines (Aminophyllin, Theo-Dur, etc.), and reduce their effectiveness in treating asthma.

Nadolol ***taken concurrently*** with

- clonidine (Catapres) requires close monitoring for rebound high blood pressure if clonidine is withdrawn while nadolol is still being taken.
- insulin requires close monitoring to avoid undetected hypoglycemia (see Glossary).

The following drugs may ***decrease*** the effects of nadolol

- indomethacin (Indocin), and possibly other "aspirin substitutes," may impair nadolol's antihypertensive effect.

▷ *Driving, Hazardous Activities:* Use caution until the full extent of drowsiness, lethargy and blood pressure change has been determined.

Aviation Note: The use of this drug ***is a disqualification*** for piloting. Consult a designated Aviation Medical Examiner.

Exposure to Sun: No restrictions.

Exposure to Heat: Caution advised. Hot environments can lower the blood pressure and exaggerate the effects of this drug.

Exposure to Cold: Caution advised. Cold environments can enhance the circulatory deficiency in the extremities that may occur with this drug. The elderly should take precautions to prevent hypothermia (see Glossary).

Heavy Exercise or Exertion: It is advisable to avoid exertion that produces light-headedness, excessive fatigue or muscle cramping. The use of this drug may intensify the hypertensive response to isometric exercise.

Occurrence of Unrelated Illness: The fever that accompanies systemic infections can lower the blood pressure and require adjustment of dosage. Illnesses that cause nausea or vomiting may interrupt the regular dosage schedule. Ask your physician for guidance.

Discontinuation: It is advisable to avoid sudden discontinuation of this drug in all situations. If possible, gradual reduction of dose over a period of 2 to 3 weeks is recommended. Ask your physician for specific guidance.

NAPROXEN
(na PROX en)

Introduced: 1974

Class: Mild analgesic, anti-inflammatory

Prescription: USA: Yes
Canada: Yes

Controlled Drug: USA: No
Canada: No

Available as Generic: No

Brand Names: Anaprox, Anaprox DS, ♣Apo-Naproxen, Naprosyn, ♣Naxen, ♣Novoanaprox

---

BENEFITS versus RISKS

Possible Benefits	*Possible Risks*
EFFECTIVE RELIEF OF MILD TO MODERATE PAIN AND INFLAMMATION	Gastrointestinal pain, ulceration, bleeding (rare)
	Drug-induced hepatitis with jaundice (rare)
	Rare kidney damage
	Mild fluid retention
	Reduced white blood cell and platelet counts

▷ **Principal Uses**

As a Single Drug Product: Used primarily to relieve mild to moderately severe pain associated with (1) musculoskeletal injuries; (2) acute and chronic gout, rheumatoid arthritis and osteoarthritis; (3) dental, obstetrical and orthopedic surgery; and (4) menstrual cramps. It is also used to prevent and relieve migrainelike headaches.

How This Drug Works: Not completely established. It is thought that this drug reduces the tissue concentrations of prostaglandins (and related compounds), chemicals involved in the production of inflammation and pain.

Available Dosage Forms and Strengths

Oral suspension — 125 mg per 5-ml teaspoonful
Tablets — 250 mg, 275 mg, 375 mg, 500 mg, 550 mg

▷ **Usual Adult Dosage Range**

As analgesic: initially, 500 mg; then 250 mg every 6 to 8 hours as needed.
As antiarthritic: 250, 375 or 500 mg twice/day, 12 hours apart.
As antigout: initially, 750 mg; then 250 mg/8 hours until acute attack is relieved.
For menstrual pain: initially, 500 mg; then 250 mg every 6 to 8 hours as needed.

The total daily dosage should not exceed 1650 mg.

Note: Actual dosage and administration schedule must be determined by the physician for each patient individually.

▷ **Dosing Instructions:**   Take either on an empty stomach or with food or milk to prevent stomach irritation. Take with a full glass of water and remain upright (do not lie down) for 30 minutes. The tablet may be crushed for administration.

Usual Duration of Use: Continual use on a regular schedule for 1 to 2 weeks is usually necessary to determine this drug's effectiveness in relieving the discomfort of arthritis. Long-term use requires supervision and periodic evaluation by the physician. Consult your physician on a regular basis.

▷ **This Drug Should Not Be Taken If**
- you have had an allergic reaction to it previously.
- you are subject to asthma or nasal polyps caused by aspirin.
- you have active peptic ulcer disease or any form of gastrointestinal bleeding.
- you have a bleeding disorder or a blood cell disorder.
- you have active liver disease.
- you have severe impairment of kidney function.

▷ **Inform Your Physician Before Taking This Drug If**
- you are allergic to aspirin or to other aspirin substitutes.
- you have a history of peptic ulcer disease or any type of bleeding disorder.
- you have impaired liver or kidney function.
- you have high blood pressure or a history of heart failure.
- you are taking any of the following: acetaminophen, aspirin or other aspirin substitutes, anticoagulants, oral antidiabetic drugs.

Possible Side-Effects (natural, expected and unavoidable drug actions)
Fluid retention (weight gain), prolongation of bleeding time.

▷ **Possible Adverse Effects** (unusual, unexpected and infrequent reactions)
If any of the following develop, consult your physician promptly for guidance.
Mild Adverse Effects
Allergic Reactions: Skin rash, hives, itching, localized swellings, spontaneous bruising.
Headache, dizziness, altered or blurred vision, ringing in the ears, drowsiness, fatigue, inability to concentrate.
Mouth sores, indigestion, nausea, vomiting, abdominal pain, diarrhea.
Serious Adverse Effects
Active peptic ulcer, stomach or intestinal bleeding, diverticulitis.
Liver damage with jaundice (see Glossary).
Kidney damage with painful urination, bloody urine, reduced urine formation.

Visual disturbances due to corneal changes, lens opacities, retinal changes.
Impaired hearing.
Reduction of white blood cell and/or platelet counts.

▷ **Possible Effects on Sexual Function**
Inhibited ejaculation (1 report).
Altered timing and pattern of menstruation.

Possible Delayed Adverse Effects: Mild anemia due to "silent" blood loss from the stomach (less than that caused by aspirin).

▷ **Adverse Effects That May Mimic Natural Diseases or Disorders**
Liver reaction may suggest viral hepatitis.

Natural Diseases or Disorders That May Be Activated by This Drug
Peptic ulcer disease, ulcerative colitis.

CAUTION
1. Dosage should always be limited to the smallest amount that produces reasonable improvement.
2. This drug may mask early indications of infection. Inform your physician if you think you are developing an infection of any kind.

Precautions for Use
By Infants and Children: Indications and dosage recommendations for use by those under 12 years of age have not been established.
By Those over 60 Years of Age: Small doses are advisable until tolerance is determined. Observe for any indications of liver or kidney toxicity, fluid retention, dizziness, confusion, impaired memory, stomach bleeding or constipation.

▷ **Advisability of Use During Pregnancy**
Pregnancy Category: B (tentative). See Pregnancy Code inside back cover.
Animal studies: No birth defects reported in mice, rats or rabbits.
Human studies: Information from adequate studies of pregnant women is not available.
Avoid this drug during the last 3 months. Use it during the first 6 months only if clearly needed. Ask physician for guidance.

Advisability of Use if Breast-Feeding
Presence of this drug in breast milk: Yes, in minute amounts.
Avoid drug or refrain from nursing.

Habit-Forming Potential: None.

Effects of Overdosage: Possible drowsiness, dizziness, ringing in the ears, nausea, vomiting, indigestion.

Possible Effects of Long-Term Use: Eye changes such as opacities in the cornea or lens, retinal changes in the macular area. Kidney damage.

Suggested Periodic Examinations While Taking This Drug (at physician's discretion)

Complete blood cell counts, liver and kidney function tests.

Complete eye examinations if vision is altered in any way.

Hearing examinations if ringing in the ears or hearing loss develops.

▷ **While Taking This Drug, Observe the Following**

Foods: No restrictions.

Beverages: No restrictions. May be taken with milk.

▷ *Alcohol:* Use with caution. The irritant action of alcohol on the stomach lining, added to the irritant action of this drug in sensitive individuals, can increase the risk of stomach ulceration and/or bleeding.

Tobacco Smoking: No interactions expected.

▷ *Other Drugs*

Naproxen may *increase* the effects of

- acetaminophen (Tylenol, etc.), and increase the risk of kidney damage; avoid prolonged use of this combination.
- anticoagulants (Coumadin, etc.), and increase the risk of bleeding; monitor prothrombin time and adjust dose accordingly.

Naproxen *taken concurrently* with the following drugs may increase the risk of bleeding; avoid these combinations:

- aspirin.
- dipyridamole (Persantine).
- indomethacin (Indocin).
- sulfinpyrazone (Anturane).
- valproic acid (Depakene).

▷ *Driving, Hazardous Activities:* This drug may cause drowsiness or dizziness. Restrict activities as necessary.

Aviation Note: The use of this drug *may be a disqualification* for piloting. Consult a designated Aviation Medical Examiner.

Exposure to Sun: No restrictions.

NEOSTIGMINE
(nee oh STIG meen)

Introduced: 1931

Class: Antimyasthenic

Prescription: USA: Yes
Canada: No

Controlled Drug: USA: No
Canada: No

Available as Generic: USA: Yes
Canada: No

Brand Name: Prostigmin

BENEFITS versus RISKS	
Possible Benefits	***Possible Risks***
MODERATELY EFFECTIVE TREATMENT OF OCULAR AND MILD FORMS OF MYASTHENIA GRAVIS (symptomatic relief of muscle weakness)	Cholinergic crisis (overdose): excessive salivation, nausea, vomiting, stomach cramps, diarrhea, shortness of breath (asthmalike wheezing), excessive weakness

▷ **Principal Uses**

As a Single Drug Product: Used primarily to treat the ocular and milder forms of myasthenia gravis by providing temporary relief of muscle weakness and fatigability. It is most useful in long-term treatment when there is little or no difficulty in swallowing.

How This Drug Works: This drug inhibits cholinesterase, the enzyme that destroys acetylcholine. This results in higher levels of acetylcholine, the nerve transmitter that facilitates the stimulation of muscular activity. The net effects are increased muscle strength and endurance.

Available Dosage Forms and Strengths
Injection — 0.25, 0.5, 1.0 mg per ml
Tablets — 15 mg

▷ **Usual Adult Dosage Range:** Initially: 15 mg/3 to 4 hours; adjust dosage as needed and tolerated. Maintenance: up to 300 mg/24 hours; the average dose is 75 to 150 mg/24 hours. **Note: Actual dosage and administration schedule must be determined by the physician for each patient individually.**

▷ **Dosing Instructions:** Take with food or milk to reduce the intensity of side-effects. Larger portions of the daily maintenance dosage should be timed according to the pattern of fatigue and weakness. The tablet may be crushed for administration.

Usual Duration of Use: Continual use on a regular schedule (with dosage adjustment) for 10 to 14 days is usually necessary to determine this drug's effectiveness in relieving the symptoms of myasthenia gravis. Long-term use (months to years) requires periodic evaluation of response and dosage adjustment. Consult your physician on a regular basis.

▷ **This Drug Should Not Be Taken If**
- you have had an allergic reaction to it previously.
- you are known to be allergic to bromide compounds.

▷ **Inform Your Physician Before Taking This Drug If**
- you have any type of seizure disorder.
- you are subject to heart rhythm disorders or bronchial asthma.

- you have recurrent urinary tract infections.
- you have prostatism (see Glossary).
- you plan to have surgery under general anesthesia in the near future.

Possible Side-Effects (natural, expected and unavoidable drug actions)
Small pupils, watering of eyes, slow pulse, excessive salivation, nausea, vomiting, stomach cramps, diarrhea, urge to urinate, increased sweating.

▷ **Possible Adverse Effects** (unusual, unexpected and infrequent reactions)
If any of the following develop, consult your physician promptly for guidance.
Mild Adverse Effects
Allergic Reaction: Skin rash.
Nervousness, anxiety, unsteadiness, muscle cramps or twitching.
Serious Adverse Effects
Confusion, slurred speech, seizures, difficult breathing (asthmatic wheezing).
Increased muscle weakness or paralysis.
Excessive vomiting or diarrhea may induce abnormally low blood potassium levels (hypokalemia). This will accentuate muscle weakness.

▷ **Possible Effects on Sexual Function:**   None reported.

▷ **Adverse Effects That May Mimic Natural Diseases or Disorders**
Seizures may suggest the possibility of epilepsy.

Natural Diseases or Disorders That May Be Activated by This Drug
Latent bronchial asthma.

CAUTION
1. Certain drugs can block the action of this drug and reduce its effectiveness in treating myasthenia gravis. (See *Other Drugs* below.) Consult your physician before starting any new drug, prescription or over-the-counter.
2. The dosage schedule of this drug must be carefully individualized for each patient. Variations in response may occur from time to time. Because generalized muscle weakness is a major symptom of both myasthenia crisis (underdosage) and cholinergic crisis (overdosage), it may be difficult to recognize the correct cause. As a rule, weakness that begins within 1 hour after taking this drug probably represents overdosage; weakness that begins 3 or more hours after taking this drug is probably due to underdosage. Observe these time relationships and inform your physician.
3. During long-term use of this drug, observe for the possible development of resistance to the drug's therapeutic action (loss of effectiveness). Consult your physician regarding the advisability of discontinuing this drug for a few days to see if responsiveness can be restored.

Precautions for Use

By Infants and Children: Dosage and administration schedule must be modified if kidney function is severely impaired.

By Those over 60 Years of Age: The natural decline of kidney function with aging may require smaller doses to prevent accumulation of this drug to toxic levels.

▷ **Advisability of Use During Pregnancy**

Pregnancy Category: C (tentative). See Pregnancy Code inside back cover.

Animal studies: No information available.

Human studies: Information from adequate studies of pregnant women is not available.

There are no reports of birth defects due to the use of this drug during pregnancy. However, there are reports of significant muscular weakness in 20% of newborn infants whose mothers had taken this drug during pregnancy. Ask your physician for guidance.

Advisability of Use if Breast-Feeding

Presence of this drug in breast milk: Probably not.

Monitor nursing infant closely and discontinue drug or nursing if adverse effects develop.

Habit-Forming Potential: None.

Effects of Overdosage: Generalized muscular weakness, blurred vision, very small pupils, slow heart rate, difficult breathing (wheezing), excessive salivation, nausea, vomiting, stomach cramps, diarrhea, muscle cramps or twitching. This syndrome constitutes the cholinergic crisis.

Possible Effects of Long-Term Use: Development of tolerance (see Glossary) with loss of therapeutic effectiveness.

Suggested Periodic Examinations While Taking This Drug (at physician's discretion)

Assessment of drug effectiveness and dosage schedule for optimal therapeutic results.

▷ **While Taking This Drug, Observe the Following**

Foods: No restrictions.

Beverages: No restrictions. May be taken with milk.

▷ *Alcohol:* Use caution until the combined effects are determined. Weakness and unsteadiness may be accentuated.

Tobacco Smoking: No interactions expected.

▷ *Other Drugs*

The following drugs may *decrease* the effects of neostigmine

- atropine (belladonna).
- clindamycin (Cleocin).
- guanadrel (Hylorel).
- guanethidine (Esimil, Ismelin).

- procainamide (Procan SR, Pronestyl).
- quinidine (Cardioquin, Duraquin, etc.).
- quinine (Quinamm).

▷ *Driving, Hazardous Activities:* This drug may cause blurred vision, confusion or generalized weakness. Restrict activities as necessary.

Aviation Note: The use of this drug *is a disqualification* for piloting. Consult a designated Aviation Medical Examiner.

Exposure to Sun: No restrictions.

Exposure to Heat: Use caution. This may cause excessive sweating and increased weakness.

Exposure to Environmental Chemicals: Avoid excessive exposure (inhalation, skin contamination) to the insecticides Baygon, Diazinon and Sevin. These can accentuate the potential toxicity of this drug.

Discontinuation: Do not discontinue this drug abruptly without your physician's knowledge and guidance.

NIACIN
(NI a sin)

Other Names: Nicotinic acid, vitamin B-3

Introduced: 1937

Class: Anticholesterol, vasodilator, vitamins

Prescription: USA: Tablets and liquid—no; capsules—yes
Canada: No

Controlled Drug: USA: No
Canada: No

Available as Generic: USA: Yes
Canada: Yes

Brand Names: ✦Antivert [CD], Niac, Nicobid, Nico-400, Nicolar, Nicotinex, ✦Novoniacin, Slo-Niacin, Span-Niacin-150

BENEFITS versus RISKS

Possible Benefits	*Possible Risks*
EFFECTIVE REDUCTION OF TOTAL CHOLESTEROL, LOW DENSITY CHOLESTEROL AND TRIGLYCERIDES IN TYPES II, III, IV AND V CHOLESTEROL DISORDERS (25% reduction of total cholesterol, 35% reduction of LDL cholesterol, and 20% elevation of HDL cholesterol, a beneficial effect)	Activation of peptic ulcer Drug-induced hepatitis Aggravation of diabetes or gout
Specific prevention and treatment of pellagra (niacin-deficiency disease)	

▷ **Principal Uses**

As a Single Drug Product: This drug is used to treat three unrelated disorders: (1) certain patterns of abnormally high blood levels of cholesterol and triglycerides in individuals considered to be at high risk for the development of coronary artery heart disease; (2) pellagra, a niacin (vitamin B-3) deficiency disorder characterized by dementia, dermatitis and diarrhea; and (3) certain types of vertigo and tinnitus (ringing in the ears).

As a Combination Drug Product [CD]: In Canada this drug is combined with meclizine to enhance its effectiveness in the treatment of motion sickness and vertigo.

How This Drug Works

The mechanism by which this drug reduces cholesterol and triglyceride blood levels is not completely known. It is thought that it may inhibit the initial production of triglycerides and impair the conversion of fatty tissue to cholesterol and triglycerides.

This drug corrects the specific deficiency of vitamin B-3 that is responsible for the symptoms of pellagra.

This drug causes direct dilation of peripheral blood vessels in the skin of the face and neck; for this reason it has been used to increase the blood flow to the inner ear in an attempt to relieve some types of vertigo and ringing in the ears. The effectiveness of this application is questionable.

Available Dosage Forms and Strengths

Capsules, prolonged-action — 125 mg, 250 mg, 300 mg, 400 mg, 500 mg

Oral solution — 50 mg per 5-ml teaspoonful

Tablets — 20 mg, 25 mg, 50 mg, 100 mg, 500 mg
Tablets, prolonged-action — 150 mg, 250 mg, 500 mg, 750 mg

▷ **Usual Adult Dosage Range**

For cholesterol disorders: Initially 100 mg 3 times daily. Dose may be increased in increments of 300 mg daily at intervals of 4 to 7 days as needed and tolerated. The usual maintenance dose is 1 to 2 grams 3 times daily. The total daily dosage should not exceed 6 grams.

For prevention of pellagra: 10 to 20 mg daily.

For treatment of pellagra: 50 mg 3 to 10 times daily.

Note: Actual dosage and administration schedule must be determined by the physician for each patient individually.

▷ **Dosing Instructions:**   Take with or immediately following meals to prevent stomach irritation. Also take one-half of an adult's aspirin tablet or 1 children's aspirin tablet with each dose of niacin to prevent facial flushing and itching. Dosage should be increased very slowly over 2 to 3 months as needed. The prolonged-action form of niacin is preferable to improve tolerance. The regular tablet may be crushed for administration, but the prolonged-action capsules and tablets should not be altered.

Usual Duration of Use: Continual use on a regular schedule for 3 to 5 weeks is usually necessary to determine this drug's effectiveness in reducing elevated levels of cholesterol and triglycerides. Long-term use (months to years) requires periodic evaluation of response and dosage adjustment. Consult your physician on a regular basis.

Currently a "Drug of Choice" for initiating treatment of elevated LDL cholesterol and VLDL triglycerides. See Cholesterol Disorders in Section Two.

▷ **This Drug Should Not Be Taken If**

- you have had an allergic reaction to it previously.
- you have active peptic ulcer disease or inflammatory bowel disease.
- you have active liver disease.

▷ **Inform Your Physician Before Taking This Drug If**

- you are prone to low blood pressure.
- you have a heart rhythm disorder of any kind.
- you have a history of peptic ulcer disease, inflammatory bowel disease, liver disease, jaundice or gallbladder disease (with or without gallstones).
- you have diabetes or gout.

Possible Side-Effects (natural, expected and unavoidable drug actions)

Flushing, itching, tingling and feeling of warmth usually in the face and neck. Sensitive individuals may experience orthostatic hypotension (see Glossary).

▷ **Possible Adverse Effects** (unusual, unexpected and infrequent reactions)
   If any of the following develop, consult your physician promptly for guidance.
   Mild Adverse Effects
   Allergic Reactions: Skin rash, itching, hives.
   Headache, dizziness, faintness, impaired vision.
   Indigestion, nausea, vomiting, diarrhea.
   Dryness of skin, grayish-black pigmentation of skin folds.
   Serious Adverse Effects
   Drug-induced hepatitis with jaundice (see Glossary): yellow eyes and skin, dark-colored urine, light-colored stools.
   Worsening of diabetes and gout.
   Development of heart rhythm disorders.

▷ **Possible Effects on Sexual Function:**   None reported.

▷ **Adverse Effects That May Mimic Natural Diseases or Disorders**
   Liver reactions may suggest viral hepatitis.

Natural Diseases or Disorders That May Be Activated by This Drug
   Latent diabetes, gout, inflammatory bowel disease or peptic ulcer.

CAUTION
   1. Large doses may cause significant increases in blood levels of sugar and uric acid. Those who have diabetes or gout should monitor their status regularly.
   2. Comply fully with all recommendations for periodic measurements of blood cholesterol and triglyceride levels. These are essential to monitoring your response to treatment and determining the need for changes in dosage or medication.

Precautions for Use
   By Infants and Children: Safety and effectiveness for use of large doses by those under 12 years of age have not been established.
   By Those over 60 Years of Age: Observe for the possible development of low blood pressure (light-headedness, dizziness, faintness) and heart rhythm disorders.

▷ **Advisability of Use During Pregnancy**
   Pregnancy Category: C (tentative). See Pregnancy Code inside back cover.
   Animal studies: Significant birth defects due to this drug were found in chicks.
   Human studies: Information from adequate studies of pregnant women is not available.
   Use this drug only if clearly needed. Avoid completely during the first 3 months.

Advisability of Use if Breast-Feeding
   Presence of this drug in breast milk: Unknown.
   Avoid drug or refrain from nursing.

Habit-Forming Potential: None.

Effects of Overdosage: Generalized flushing, nausea, vomiting, stomach cramps, diarrhea, weakness, fainting.

Possible Effects of Long-Term Use: Increased blood levels of sugar and uric acid; liver damage.

Suggested Periodic Examinations While Taking This Drug (at physician's discretion)
Measurements of blood levels of total cholesterol, HDL and LDL cholesterol fractions, triglycerides, sugar and uric acid.
Liver function tests.

▷ **While Taking This Drug, Observe the Following**
Foods: Follow the low-cholesterol diet prescribed by your physician.
Beverages: No restrictions. May be taken with milk.
▷ *Alcohol:* Use with caution until the combined effects have been determined. Alcohol used with large doses of this drug may cause excessive lowering of blood pressure.
Tobacco Smoking: No interactions expected.
▷ *Other Drugs*
Niacin may ***increase*** the effects of
• some antihypertensive drugs, and cause excessive lowering of blood pressure.
Niacin may ***decrease*** the effects of
• antidiabetic drugs (insulin and sulfonylureas), by raising the level of blood sugar.
• probenecid (Benemid) and sulfinpyrazone (Anturane), by raising the level of blood uric acid.
▷ *Driving, Hazardous Activities:* This drug may cause dizziness and faintness. Restrict activities as necessary.
Aviation Note: The use of this drug ***may be a disqualification*** for piloting. Consult a designated Aviation Medical Examiner.
Exposure to Sun: No restrictions.
Discontinuation: Do not discontinue this drug without your physician's knowledge and guidance. Abrupt withdrawal may be followed by excessive increase in blood cholesterol and triglyceride levels.

NICARDIPINE
(ni KAR de peen)

Introduced: 1984

Prescription: USA: Yes

Class: Antianginal, antihypertensive, calcium channel blocker

Controlled Drug: USA: No

Available as Generic: USA: No

Brand Name: Cardene

BENEFITS versus RISKS	
Possible Benefits	***Possible Risks***
EFFECTIVE PREVENTION OF CLASSICAL ANGINA-OF-EFFORT EFFECTIVE TREATMENT OF HYPERTENSION	Increase in angina upon starting treatment (7%) Water retention, ankle swelling (8%)

▷ **Principal Uses**

As a Single Drug Product: Used primarily to treat (1) classical angina-of-effort (due to atherosclerotic disease of the coronary arteries) in individuals who have not responded to or cannot tolerate the nitrates and beta blocker drugs customarily used to treat this disorder; (2) mild to moderately severe hypertension.

How This Drug Works: Not completely established. It is thought that by blocking the normal passage of calcium through certain cell walls (which is necessary for the function of nerve and muscle tissue), this drug inhibits the contraction of coronary arteries and peripheral arterioles. As a result of these effects, this drug

- promotes dilation of the coronary arteries (antianginal effect).
- reduces the degree of contraction of peripheral arterial walls, resulting in their relaxation and consequent lowering of blood pressure. This further reduces the workload of the heart during exertion and contributes to the prevention of angina.

Available Dosage Forms and Strengths

Capsules — 20 mg, 30 mg

▷ **Usual Adult Dosage Range:**   Initially 20 mg 3 times daily, 6 to 8 hours apart. Dose may be increased gradually at 3-day intervals (as needed and tolerated) up to 40 mg 3 times daily. The total daily dosage should not exceed 120 mg. **Note: Actual dosage and administration schedule must be determined by the physician for each patient individually.**

▷ **Dosing Instructions:**   May be taken with or following food to reduce stomach irritation. However, if taken after a high-fat meal, total absorption of this drug may be reduced by 20% to 30%. The capsule should be swallowed whole (not altered).

Usual Duration of Use: Continual use on a regular schedule for 2 to 4 weeks is usually necessary to determine this drug's effectiveness in reducing the frequency and severity of angina or controlling hypertension. For long-term use (months to years), determine the smallest effective dose. Supervision and periodic evaluation are essential. Consult your physician on a regular basis.

▷ **This Drug Should Not Be Taken If**
- you have had an allergic reaction to it previously.
- you have advanced aortic stenosis.

▷ **Inform Your Physician Before Taking This Drug If**
- you have had an unfavorable response to any calcium blocker drug in the past (see Drug Class, Section Four).
- you are currently taking any form of digitalis or a beta blocker drug (see Drug Class, Section Four).
- you are taking any drugs that lower blood pressure.
- you are taking cimetidine (Tagamet) or cyclosporine (Sandimmune).
- you have a history of congestive heart failure, heart attack or stroke.
- you are subject to disturbances of heart rhythm.
- you have impaired liver or kidney function.

Possible Side-Effects (natural, expected and unavoidable drug actions)
Rapid heart rate (3.4%), swelling of the feet and ankles (8%), flushing and sensation of warmth (9.7%).

▷ **Possible Adverse Effects** (unusual, unexpected and infrequent reactions)
If any of the following develop, consult your physician promptly for guidance.
Mild Adverse Effects
Allergic Reaction: Skin rash (0.4% to 1.2%).
Headache (6.4% to 8.2%), dizziness (4% to 6.9%), weakness (4.2% to 5.8%), nervousness (0.6%), blurred vision, confusion.
Palpitation (3.3% to 4.1%), shortness of breath (0.6%).
Indigestion (0.8% to 1.5%), nausea (1.9% to 2.2%), vomiting (0.4%), constipation (0.6%).
Serious Adverse Effects
Allergic Reactions: None reported.
Increased frequency or severity of angina on initiation of treatment or following an increase in dose (7%).
Marked drop in blood pressure with fainting (0.8%).

▷ **Possible Effects on Sexual Function:**   Rare impotence (less than 1%).

▷ **Adverse Effects That May Mimic Natural Diseases or Disorders**
Flushing and warmth may resemble menopausal "hot flushes."

CAUTION
1. If you are monitoring your own blood pressure, make your measurements just before each dose and 1–2 hours after each dose to obtain an accurate picture of this drug's effect. This will detect excessive fluctuations between high and low readings.
2. Be sure to inform all physicians and dentists you consult that you are taking this drug. Note the use of this drug on your card of personal identification.

3. You may use nitroglycerin and other nitrate drugs as needed to relieve acute episodes of angina pain. However, if you detect that your angina attacks are becoming more frequent or intense, notify your physician promptly.

Precautions for Use
By Infants and Children: Safety and effectiveness for use by those under 18 years of age have not been established.

By Those over 60 Years of Age: Usually well tolerated by this age group. However, observe for the development of weakness, dizziness, fainting and falling. Take necessary precautions to prevent injury. Report promptly any changes in your pattern of thirst and urination.

▷ Advisability of Use During Pregnancy
Pregnancy Category: C (tentative). See Pregnancy Code inside back cover.
Animal studies: Embryo and fetal toxicity reported in small animals, but no birth defects due to this drug.
Human studies: Information from adequate studies of pregnant women is not available.
Avoid this drug during the first 3 months. Use during the last 6 months only if clearly needed. Ask physician for guidance.

Advisability of Use if Breast-Feeding
Presence of this drug in breast milk: Probably yes.
Avoid drug or refrain from nursing.

Habit-Forming Potential: None.

Effects of Overdosage: Weakness, light-headedness, fainting, fast pulse, low blood pressure, shortness of breath, flushed and warm skin, tremors.

Possible Effects of Long-Term Use: None reported.

Suggested Periodic Examinations While Taking This Drug (at physician's discretion)
Evaluations of heart function, including electrocardiograms; measurements of blood pressure in supine, sitting and standing positions.

▷ While Taking This Drug, Observe the Following
Foods: No restrictions. Avoid excessive salt intake.
Beverages: No restrictions. May be taken with milk.
▷ *Alcohol:* Use with caution until combined effects have been determined. Alcohol may exaggerate the drop in blood pressure experienced by some individuals.
Tobacco Smoking: Nicotine may reduce the effectiveness of this drug. Follow your physician's advice regarding smoking.
Marijuana Smoking: Possible reduced effectiveness of this drug; mild to moderate increase in angina; possible changes in electrocardiogram, confusing interpretation.

▷   *Other Drugs*
    Nicardipine may ***increase*** the effects of
    • cyclosporine (Sandimmune), and cause kidney toxicity.
    Nicardipine ***taken concurrently*** with
    • beta blocker drugs or digitalis preparations (see Drug Classes, Section
        Four) may affect heart rate and rhythm adversely. Careful monitoring
        by your physician is necessary if these drugs are taken concurrently.
    The following drugs may ***increase*** the effects of nicardipine
    • cimetidine (Tagamet).
▷   *Driving, Hazardous Activities:* Usually no restrictions. This drug may cause
    drowsiness or dizziness. Restrict activities as necessary.
    Aviation Note: Coronary artery disease and hypertension ***are disqualifi-***
        cations for piloting. Consult a designated Aviation Medical Examiner.
    Exposure to Sun: No restrictions.
    Exposure to Heat: Caution advised. Hot environments can exaggerate the
        blood-pressure-lowering effects of this drug. Observe for light-head-
        edness or weakness.
    Heavy Exercise or Exertion: This drug may improve your ability to be more
        active without resulting angina pain. Use caution and avoid excessive
        exercise that could impair heart function in the absence of warning
        pain.
    Discontinuation: Do not discontinue this drug abruptly. Consult your phy-
        sician regarding gradual withdrawal. Observe for the possible devel-
        opment of rebound angina.

NIFEDIPINE
(ni FED i peen)

Introduced: 1972

Class: Antianginal, calcium
        channel blocker

Prescription: USA: Yes
        Canada: Yes

Controlled Drug: USA: No
        Canada: No

Available as Generic: No

Brand Names: Adalat, Procardia

BENEFITS versus RISKS	
Possible Benefits	*Possible Risks*
EFFECTIVE PREVENTION OF BOTH MAJOR TYPES OF ANGINA	Rare increase in angina upon starting treatment
	Rare precipitation of congestive heart failure
	Very rare drug-induced hepatitis

▷ **Principal Uses**

As a Single Drug Product: Used primarily to treat (1) angina pectoris due to coronary artery spasm (Prinzmetal's variant angina) that occurs spontaneously and is not associated with exertion; and (2) classical angina-of-effort (due to atherosclerotic disease of the coronary arteries) in individuals who have not responded to or cannot tolerate the nitrates and beta blocker drugs customarily used to treat this disorder.

How This Drug Works: Not completely established. It is thought that by blocking the normal passage of calcium through certain cell walls (which is necessary for the function of nerve and muscle tissue), this drug slows the spread of electrical activity through the conduction system of the heart and inhibits the contraction of coronary arteries and peripheral arterioles. As a result of these combined effects, this drug

- prevents spontaneous spasm of the coronary arteries (Prinzmetal's type of angina).
- reduces the rate and contraction force of the heart during exertion, thus lowering the oxygen requirement of the heart muscle; this reduces the occurrence of effort-induced angina (classical angina pectoris).
- reduces the degree of contraction of peripheral arterial walls, resulting in their relaxation and consequent lowering of blood pressure. This further reduces the workload of the heart during exertion and contributes to the prevention of angina.

Available Dosage Forms and Strengths
Capsules — 10 mg, 20 mg

▷ **Usual Adult Dosage Range:**   Initially, 10 mg 3 times daily. Dose may be increased gradually at 7- to 14-day intervals (as needed and tolerated) up to 30 mg 3 or 4 times/day. The usual maintenance dose is 10 to 20 mg 3 times/day. The total daily dosage should not exceed 180 mg. **Note: Actual dosage and administration schedule must be determined by the physician for each patient individually.**

▷ **Dosing Instructions:**   May be taken with or following food to reduce stomach irritation. The capsule should be swallowed whole (not altered).

Usual Duration of Use: Continual use on a regular schedule for 2 to 4 weeks is usually necessary to determine this drug's effectiveness in reducing the frequency and severity of angina. For long-term use (months to years), determine the smallest effective dose. Supervision and periodic evaluation by your physician are essential. Consult your physician on a regular basis.

▷ **This Drug Should Not Be Taken If**
- you have had an allergic reaction to it previously.
- you have active liver disease.
- you have low blood pressure—systolic pressure below 90.

▷ **Inform Your Physician Before Taking This Drug If**
- you have had an unfavorable response to any calcium blocker drug in the past.
- you are currently taking any form of digitalis or a beta blocker drug (see Drug Class, Section Four).
- you are taking any drugs that lower blood pressure.
- you have a history of congestive heart failure, heart attack or stroke.
- you are subject to disturbances of heart rhythm.
- you have impaired liver or kidney function.
- you have diabetes.
- you have a history of drug-induced liver damage.

Possible Side-Effects (natural, expected and unavoidable drug actions)
Low blood pressure, rapid heart rate, swelling of the feet and ankles (7%), flushing and sensation of warmth (25%), sweating.

▷ **Possible Adverse Effects** (unusual, unexpected and infrequent reactions)
If any of the following develop, consult your physician promptly for guidance.
Mild Adverse Effects
Allergic Reactions: Skin rash, hives, itching, fever.
Headache (23%), dizziness (27%), weakness (12%), nervousness (7%), blurred vision.
Palpitation (7%), shortness of breath, wheezing (6%), cough.
Heartburn (11%), nausea, cramps, diarrhea (2%).
Tremors, muscle cramps (8%).
Serious Adverse Effects
Allergic Reaction: Drug-induced hepatitis (very rare).
Idiosyncratic Reactions: Joint stiffness and inflammation.
Increased frequency or severity of angina on initiation of treatment or following an increase in dose.
Marked drop in blood pressure with fainting.

▷ **Possible Effects on Sexual Function:** Altered timing and pattern of menstruation; excessive menstrual bleeding.

▷ **Adverse Effects That May Mimic Natural Diseases or Disorders**
An allergic rash and swelling of the legs may resemble erysipelas.
Drug-induced hepatitis may suggest viral hepatitis.

CAUTION
1. Be sure to inform all physicians and dentists you consult that you are taking this drug. Note the use of this drug on your card of personal identification.
2. You may use nitroglycerin and other nitrate drugs as needed to relieve acute episodes of angina pain. However, if you detect that your angina attacks are becoming more frequent or intense, notify your physician promptly.

Precautions for Use

By Infants and Children: Safety and effectiveness for use by those under 12 years of age have not been established.

By Those over 60 Years of Age: You may be more susceptible to the development of weakness, dizziness, fainting and falling. Take necessary precautions to prevent injury. Report promptly any changes in your pattern of thirst and urination.

▷ **Advisability of Use During Pregnancy**

Pregnancy Category: C (tentative). See Pregnancy Code inside back cover.

Animal studies: Embryo and fetal deaths reported in mice, rats and rabbits; birth defects reported in rats.

Human studies: Information from adequate studies of pregnant women is not available.

Avoid this drug during the first 3 months. Use during the last 6 months only if clearly needed. Ask physician for guidance.

Advisability of Use if Breast-Feeding

Presence of this drug in breast milk: Unknown.

Avoid drug or refrain from nursing.

Habit-Forming Potential: None.

Effects of Overdosage: Weakness, light-headedness, fainting, fast pulse, low blood pressure, shortness of breath, flushed and warm skin, tremors.

Possible Effects of Long-Term Use: None reported.

Suggested Periodic Examinations While Taking This Drug (at physician's discretion)

Evaluations of heart function, including electrocardiograms; measurements of blood pressure in supine, sitting and standing positions.

▷ **While Taking This Drug, Observe the Following**

Foods: No restrictions. Avoid excessive salt intake.

Beverages: No restrictions. May be taken with milk.

▷ *Alcohol:* Use with caution until combined effects have been determined. Alcohol may exaggerate the drop in blood pressure experienced by some individuals.

Tobacco Smoking: Nicotine may reduce the effectiveness of this drug. Follow your physician's advice regarding smoking.

Marijuana Smoking: Possible reduced effectiveness of this drug; mild to moderate increase in angina; possible changes in electrocardiogram, confusing interpretation.

▷ *Other Drugs*

Nifedipine *taken concurrently* with

• beta blocker drugs or digitalis preparations (see Drug Classes, Section Four) may affect heart rate and rhythm adversely. Careful monitoring by your physician is necessary if these drugs are taken concurrently.

The following drugs may *increase* the effects of nifedipine
- cimetidine (Tagamet).

▷ *Driving, Hazardous Activities:* Usually no restrictions. This drug may cause drowsiness or dizziness. Restrict activities as necessary.

Aviation Note: Coronary artery disease *is a disqualification* for piloting. Consult a designated Aviation Medical Examiner.

Exposure to Sun: No restrictions.

Exposure to Heat: Caution advised. Hot environments can exaggerate the blood-pressure-lowering effects of this drug. Observe for light-headedness or weakness.

Heavy Exercise or Exertion: This drug may improve your ability to be more active without resulting angina pain. Use caution and avoid excessive exercise that could impair heart function in the absence of warning pain.

Discontinuation: Do not discontinue this drug abruptly. Consult your physician regarding gradual withdrawal. Observe for the possible development of rebound angina.

NITROFURANTOIN
(ni troh fyur AN toin)

Introduced: 1953

Class: Urinary anti-infective

Prescription: USA: Yes
Canada: Yes

Controlled Drug: USA: No
Canada: No

Available as Generic: Yes

Brand Names: ✦Apo-Nitrofurantoin, Furadantin, Furalan, Macrodantin, Macrodantin MACPAC, ✦Nephronex, ✦Novofuran

BENEFITS versus RISKS	
Possible Benefits	*Possible Risks*
EFFECTIVE TREATMENT OF SOME URINARY TRACT INFECTIONS	ALLERGIC REACTIONS: Anaphylaxis Rashes, hives Repetitive asthma Lung inflammation Drug-induced hepatitis Peripheral neuropathy (see Glossary) Blood cell disorders: hemolytic anemia (see Glossary) Reduced white blood cell count Superinfections

▷ **Principal Uses**

As a Single Drug Product: Because this drug is concentrated in the urine and attains only low levels in the blood, its use is limited to the prevention or treatment of infections in the urinary tract.

How This Drug Works: Not completely established. It is thought that by interfering with some bacterial enzyme systems, this drug is bacteriostatic (growth retarding) in low to moderate concentrations and bactericidal (killing) in high concentrations.

Available Dosage Forms and Strengths

Capsules — 25 mg, 50 mg, 100 mg
Oral suspension — 25 mg per 5-ml teaspoonful
Tablets — 50 mg, 100 mg

▷ **Usual Adult Dosage Range:** For treatment of active infections: 50 to 100 mg/6 hours. For prevention: 50 to 100 mg once/day at bedtime. The total daily dosage should not exceed 600 mg. **Note: Actual dosage and administration schedule must be determined by the physician for each patient individually.**

▷ **Dosing Instructions:** Preferably taken with or following food to facilitate absorption and reduce stomach irritation. The tablet may be crushed and the capsule opened for administration, but this drug can stain the teeth yellow on contact.

Usual Duration of Use: Continual use on a regular schedule for 7 to 10 days is usually necessary to determine this drug's effectiveness in curing urinary tract infections. Long-term use for prevention (months to years) requires supervision and periodic evaluation by your physician. Consult your physician on a regular basis.

▷ **This Drug Should Not Be Taken If**
- you have had an allergic reaction to it previously.
- you have severely impaired kidney function.
- you have active liver disease.
- you are in the last month of pregnancy.

▷ **Inform Your Physician Before Taking This Drug If**
- you are allergic to any nitrofuran drug.
- you have impaired liver or kidney function.
- you have a deficiency of glucose-6-phosphate dehydrogenase in your red blood cells.
- you have chronic anemia or diabetes.

Possible Side-Effects (natural, expected and unavoidable drug actions)
Superinfections (see Glossary) in the urinary tract.
Brown discoloration of the urine, of no significance.

▷ **Possible Adverse Effects** (unusual, unexpected and infrequent reactions)
If any of the following develop, consult your physician promptly for guidance.

Mild Adverse Effects

Allergic Reactions: Skin rashes, hives, localized swellings, itching, fever.

Headache, dizziness, drowsiness, burning and tearing of eyes, impaired color vision, muscle aching, loss of hair.

Loss of appetite, nausea, vomiting, diarrhea, abdominal cramping.

Serious Adverse Effects

Allergic Reactions: Anaphylaxis (see Glossary), interstitial pneumonitis (lung inflammation), asthma, hepatitis.

Idiosyncratic Reaction: Hemolytic anemia (see Glossary).

Peripheral neuropathy (see Glossary).

Blood cell disorders: reduced red and white blood cell counts.

▷ **Possible Effects on Sexual Function:**   None reported.

▷ **Adverse Effects That May Mimic Natural Diseases or Disorders**

Allergic pneumonitis may suggest an infectious pneumonia.

Allergic hepatitis may suggest viral hepatitis.

Natural Diseases or Disorders That May Be Activated by This Drug

Latent asthma.

CAUTION

Troublesome and persistent diarrhea can develop in sensitive individuals. If diarrhea persists for more than 24 hours, discontinue this drug and consult your physician.

Precautions for Use

By Infants and Children: This drug should not be used in infants under 1 month of age. Observe closely for the possible development of increased intracranial pressure.

By Those over 60 Years of Age: Dosage must be carefully individualized on the basis of kidney function. This age group is more susceptible to skin rashes, nausea, vomiting and constipation.

▷ **Advisability of Use During Pregnancy**

Pregnancy Category: C (tentative). See Pregnancy Code inside back cover.

Animal studies: No information available.

Human studies: No significant increase in birth defects reported in 590 exposures. Information from adequate studies of pregnant women is not available.

Avoid use of drug during the last few weeks of pregnancy. Use otherwise only if clearly needed. Ask your physician for guidance.

Advisability of Use if Breast-Feeding

Presence of this drug in breast milk: Yes, in small amounts.

Avoid drug or refrain from nursing.

Habit-Forming Potential: None.

Effects of Overdosage: Nausea, vomiting, diarrhea.

Possible Effects of Long-Term Use: Allergic reactions in lungs or liver, peripheral neuropathy, superinfections within the urinary tract.

Suggested Periodic Examinations While Taking This Drug (at physician's discretion)
Complete blood cell counts, liver function tests, X-ray examinations of lungs during long-term use.

▷ **While Taking This Drug, Observe the Following**
Foods: No restrictions. Eat liberally of the following foods: beef, chicken, lamb and pork liver, asparagus, navy beans (good sources of folic acid).
Beverages: No restrictions. May be taken with milk.
▷ *Alcohol:* Use with extreme caution until the combined effects have been determined. This drug, in combination with alcohol, may cause a disulfiramlike reaction (see Glossary) in sensitive individuals.
Tobacco Smoking: No interactions expected.
▷ *Other Drugs*
The following drugs may **decrease** the effects of nitrofurantoin
• antacids that contain magnesium can prevent the absorption of nitrofurantoin and reduce its effectiveness.
▷ *Driving, Hazardous Activities:* This drug may cause dizziness. Restrict activities as necessary.
Aviation Note: The use of this drug **may be a disqualification** for piloting. Consult a designated Aviation Medical Examiner.
Exposure to Sun: No restrictions.

NITROGLYCERIN
(ni troh GLIS er in)

Introduced: 1847

Class: Antianginal, nitrates

Prescription: USA: Yes
Canada: No

Controlled Drug: USA: No
Canada: No

Available as Generic: Yes

Brand Names: Deponit, Minitran Transdermal Delivery System, Nitro-Bid, Nitrodisc, Nitro-Dur, Nitro-Dur II, Nitrogard, ✦Nitrogard-SR, Nitroglyn, Nitrol, Nitrolingual Spray, Nitrong, ✦Nitrong SR, Nitrospan, ✦Nitrostabilin, Nitrostat, Transderm-Nitro, ✦Tridil

BENEFITS versus RISKS	
Possible Benefits	*Possible Risks*
EFFECTIVE RELIEF AND PREVENTION OF ANGINA EFFECTIVE ADJUNCTIVE TREATMENT IN SELECTED CASES OF CONGESTIVE HEART FAILURE	Orthostatic hypotension (see Glossary) with and without fainting Skin rash (rare) Altered hemoglobin with large doses (very rare)

▷ **Principal Uses**

 As a Single Drug Product: Used primarily in the treatment of symptomatic coronary artery disease. The rapid-action forms are used to relieve acute attacks of anginal pain at their onset. The sustained-action forms are used to prevent the development of angina.

How This Drug Works: By direct action on the muscles in blood vessel walls, this drug relaxes and dilates both arteries and veins. Its beneficial effects in the management of angina are due to two mechanisms of action: (1) dilation of narrowed coronary arteries; (2) dilation of veins in the general circulation, with consequent reduction of the volume and pressure of blood entering the heart. The net effects are improved blood supply to the heart muscle and reduced workload for the heart. Both actions reduce the frequency and severity of angina.

Available Dosage Forms and Strengths

 Canisters, translingual spray — 13.8 grams (200 doses), 0.4 mg per metered dose

 Capsules, prolonged-action — 2.5 mg, 2.6 mg, 6.5 mg, 9 mg

 Ointment — 2%

 Tablets, buccal — 1 mg, 2 mg, 3 mg

 Tablets, prolonged-action — 2.6 mg, 6.5 mg, 9 mg

 Tablets, sublingual — 0.15 mg, 0.3 mg, 0.4 mg, 0.6 mg

 Transdermal systems — 2.5 mg, 5 mg, 7.5 mg, 10 mg, 15 mg

▷ **Usual Adult Dosage Range:** According to dosage form:

 Sublingual spray—1 metered spray (0.4 mg) under tongue/3 to 5 minutes, up to 3 doses within 15 minutes, to relieve acute angina. To prevent angina, 1 spray taken 5 to 10 minutes before exertion.

 Sublingual tablets—0.15 to 0.6 mg dissolved under tongue at 5-minute intervals to relieve acute angina.

 Prolonged-action tablets—1.3 to 6.5 mg at 8- to 12-hour intervals to prevent angina.

 Prolonged-action capsules—2.5 to 9 mg at 8- to 12-hour intervals to prevent angina.

 Ointment—2.5 to 5 cm (1 to 2 inches, 15 to 30 mg) applied in a thin, even layer of uniform size to hairless skin at 3- to 4-hour intervals to prevent angina.

Buccal tablets—1 to 2 mg/4 to 5 hours placed between cheek and gum.
Transdermal patches—5-sq.-cm to 30-sq.-cm patch applied to hairless skin once/24 hours to prevent angina.
Note: Actual dosage and administration schedule must be determined by the physician for each patient individually.

▷ **Dosing Instructions:** Dosage forms to be swallowed are best taken when stomach is empty (1 hour before or 2 hours after eating) to obtain maximal blood levels. Tablets should not be crushed for administration. Capsules may be opened, but the contents should not be crushed or chewed before swallowing.

Usual Duration of Use: Continual use on a regular schedule for 3 to 5 days is usually necessary to determine this drug's effectiveness in preventing and relieving acute anginal attacks. Individual dosage adjustments will be necessary for optimal results. Long-term use (months to years) requires supervision and periodic evaluation by your physician. Consult your physician on a regular basis.

▷ **This Drug Should Not Be Taken If**
  • you have had an allergic reaction to it previously.
  • you are severely anemic.
  • you have closed-angle glaucoma (inadequately treated).

▷ **Inform Your Physician Before Taking This Drug If**
  • you have had an unfavorable response to other nitrate drugs in the past.
  • you have low blood pressure.
  • you have any form of glaucoma.

Possible Side-Effects (natural, expected and unavoidable drug actions)
  Flushing of face, headaches (50%), orthostatic hypotension (see Glossary), rapid heart rate, palpitation.

▷ **Possible Adverse Effects** (unusual, unexpected and infrequent reactions)
  If any of the following develop, consult your physician promptly for guidance.
  Mild Adverse Effects
  Allergic Reaction: Skin rash.
  Throbbing headaches (may be severe and persistent), dizziness, fainting. Nausea, vomiting.
  Serious Adverse Effects
  Allergic Reactions: Severe skin reactions with peeling.
  Idiosyncratic Reaction: Methemoglobinemia (very rare).

▷ **Possible Effects on Sexual Function**
  Correction of impotence (1 report following sublingual use).
  The preventive use of nitroglycerin prior to sexual activity has been recommended to eliminate or reduce the risk of angina. Consult your physician for guidance.

▷ **Adverse Effects That May Mimic Natural Diseases or Disorders**
> Hypotensive spells (sudden drops in blood pressure) due to this drug may be mistaken for late-onset epilepsy.

CAUTION
1. This drug can provoke migraine headaches in susceptible individuals.
2. In the presence of impaired brain circulation (cerebral arteriosclerosis), this drug can cause transient ischemic attacks—periods of temporary speech impairment, paralysis, numbness, etc.
3. The development of tolerance to long-acting forms of nitrates will render the sublingual tablets ineffective for the relief of acute angina. Sensitivity to the drug's antianginal effect is restored after one week of abstinence from the long-acting forms.
4. Many over-the-counter (OTC) drug products for allergies, colds and coughs contain drugs that may counteract the desired effects of this drug. Ask your physician or pharmacist for guidance before using any such medications.

Precautions for Use
> *By Infants and Children:* Limited usefulness and experience in this age group. Dosage schedules not established.
> *By Those over 60 Years of Age:* Begin treatment with small doses and increase dose cautiously as needed and tolerated. You may be more susceptible to the development of flushing, throbbing headache, dizziness, "blackout" spells, fainting and falling.

▷ **Advisability of Use During Pregnancy**
> *Pregnancy Category:* C (tentative). See Pregnancy Code inside back cover.
> Animal studies: No information available.
> Human studies: Information from adequate studies of pregnant women is not available.
> Use this drug only if clearly needed. Ask physician for guidance.

Advisability of Use if Breast-Feeding
> Presence of this drug in breast milk: Unknown.
> Monitor nursing infant closely and discontinue drug or nursing if adverse effects develop.

Habit-Forming Potential: None.

Effects of Overdosage: Throbbing headache, dizziness, marked flushing, nausea, vomiting, abdominal cramps, confusion, delirium, paralysis, seizures, circulatory collapse.

Possible Effects of Long-Term Use: The development of tolerance (see Glossary) and the temporary loss of effectiveness.

Suggested Periodic Examinations While Taking This Drug (at physician's discretion)
> Measurements of blood pressure and internal eye pressures.
> Evaluation of hemoglobin.

▷ **While Taking This Drug, Observe the Following**

Foods: No restrictions.

Beverages: No restrictions. May be taken with milk.

▷ *Alcohol:* Use extreme caution until the combined effects have been determined. Avoid alcohol completely in the presence of any side-effects or adverse effects from nitroglycerin. Never use alcohol in the presence of a nitroglycerin headache.

Tobacco Smoking: Nicotine can reduce the effectiveness of this drug. Follow your physician's advice regarding smoking.

Marijuana Smoking: Possible reduced effectiveness of this drug; mild to moderate increase in angina; possible changes in the electrocardiogram, confusing interpretation.

▷ *Other Drugs*

Nitroglycerin *taken concurrently* with

- antihypertensive drugs may cause excessive lowering of blood pressure. Careful dosage adjustments may be necessary.

The following drugs may *increase* the effects of nitroglycerin

- aspirin, in analgesic doses (500 mg or more).

▷ *Driving, Hazardous Activities:* Usually no restrictions. This drug may cause dizziness or faintness. Restrict activities as necessary.

Aviation Note: Coronary artery disease *is a disqualification* for piloting. Consult a designated Aviation Medical Examiner.

Exposure to Sun: No restrictions.

Exposure to Heat: Use caution. Hot environments can cause significant lowering of blood pressure.

Exposure to Cold: Cold environments can increase the need for this drug and limit its effectiveness.

Heavy Exercise or Exertion: This drug can increase your tolerance for exercise. Use good judgment regarding excessive exertion in the absence of anginal pain.

Discontinuation: Do not stop this drug abruptly after long-term use. It is advisable to reduce the dose (of the prolonged-action dosage forms) gradually over a period of 4 to 6 weeks. Observe for rebound angina.

Special Storage Instructions: For sublingual tablets, to prevent loss of strength

- keep tablets in the original glass container.
- do not transfer tablets to a plastic or metallic container (such as a pillbox).
- do not place absorbent cotton, paper (such as the prescription label), or other material inside the container.
- do not store other drugs in the same container.
- close the container tightly immediately after each use.
- store at room temperature.

NIZATIDINE
(ni ZA te deen)

Introduced: 1986

Class: Antiulcer, H-2 receptor blocker

Prescription: USA: Yes

Controlled Drug: USA: No

Available as Generic: No

Brand Name: Axid

BENEFITS versus RISKS

Possible Benefits	*Possible Risks*
EFFECTIVE TREATMENT OF PEPTIC ULCER DISEASE: relief of symptoms, acceleration of healing (in 80% to 90% of cases), prevention of recurrence (in 65% to 80% of cases)	Drug-induced liver damage (rare) Abnormally low blood platelet count (rare)
CONTROL OF HYPERSECRETORY STOMACH DISORDERS	
Beneficial in treatment of reflux esophagitis	

▷ **Principal Uses**

As a Single Drug Product: Used primarily in the treatment of peptic ulcer disease, both benign stomach (gastric) ulcer and duodenal ulcer. It is used specifically to hasten the healing of ulcer and to prevent recurrence. Also used to control the excessive production of stomach acid in the Zollinger-Ellison syndrome. Though its effectiveness has not been fully established, this drug is also used in the management of esophagitis (as with hiatal hernia) and upper gastrointestinal bleeding.

How This Drug Works: By blocking the action of histamine, this drug effectively inhibits the secretion of stomach acid and thus creates a more favorable environment for the healing of peptic ulcers.

Available Dosage Forms and Strengths
Capsules — 150 mg, 300 mg

▷ **Usual Adult Dosage Range:** For active peptic ulcer: 150 mg 2 times daily, 12 hours apart; or 300 mg once daily at bedtime. For prevention of recurrent ulcer: 150 mg at bedtime. **Note: Actual dosage and administration schedule must be determined by the physician for each patient individually.**

▷ **Dosing Instructions:**   To obtain the longest period of stomach acid reduction, this drug should be taken with or immediately following food. The capsule may be opened for administration.

Usual Duration of Use: Continual use on a regular schedule for 4 to 6 weeks is usually necessary to determine this drug's effectiveness in healing active peptic ulcer. Long-term use (months to years) for prevention of ulcer recurrence requires individual consideration by your physician.

Possible Advantages of This Drug
Effective ulcer treatment with once-a-day dosage.
Minimal adverse effects.
Does not cause confusion; does not reduce sperm count or sexual potency.
No significant drug interactions.

▷ **This Drug Should Not Be Taken If**
- you have had an allergic reaction to any dosage form of it previously.

▷ **Inform Your Physician Before Taking This Drug If**
- you are allergic to other H-2 receptor blockers: cimetidine (Tagamet), famotidine (Pepcid), ranitidine (Zantac).
- you have impaired liver or kidney function.
- you are taking large doses of aspirin.

Possible Side-Effects (natural, expected and unavoidable drug actions)
None reported.

▷ **Possible Adverse Effects** (unusual, unexpected and infrequent reactions)
If any of the following develop, consult your physician promptly for guidance.
Mild Adverse Effects
Allergic Reaction: Skin rash, hives (0.5%).
Drowsiness (2.4%), sweating (1.0%).
Serious Adverse Effects
Allergic Reaction: Exfoliative dermatitis.
Drug-induced liver injury (without jaundice), reversible.
Reduced blood platelet count: abnormal bleeding or bruising (rare).

▷ **Possible Effects on Sexual Function:**   Male breast enlargement (rare).

CAUTION
1. Do not discontinue this drug abruptly. (Ulcer activation and perforation have occurred following abrupt cessation of cimetidine, a closely related drug.)
2. After discontinuation of this drug, inform your physician promptly if you experience a return of symptoms indicative of ulcer reactivation.

Precautions for Use

By Infants and Children: Safety and effectiveness for use by those under 12 years of age have not been established.

By Those over 60 Years of Age: This drug may contribute to the formation of stomach phytobezoars (masses of undigested vegetable fibers). Individuals with poor chewing ability (missing teeth) and those who have had partial gastrectomy or vagotomy (stomach surgery) are most susceptible. Observe for loss of appetite, stomach fullness, nausea and vomiting.

▷ **Advisability of Use During Pregnancy**

Pregnancy Category: C (tentative). See Pregnancy Code inside back cover.
   Animal studies: Rabbit studies revealed significant birth defects of the heart, brain and spinal cord.
   Human studies: Information from adequate studies of pregnant women is not available.
   Avoid drug during the first 3 months if possible. Use this drug only if clearly needed. Ask physician for guidance.

Advisability of Use if Breast-Feeding

Presence of this drug in breast milk: Probably yes.
Avoid drug or refrain from nursing.

Habit-Forming Potential: None.

Effects of Overdosage: Based on animal studies: excessive tearing, salivation, vomiting, diarrhea.

Possible Effects of Long-Term Use: None reported.

Suggested Periodic Examinations While Taking This Drug (at physician's discretion)
Complete blood cell counts, liver function tests.

▷ **While Taking This Drug, Observe the Following**

Foods: Protein-rich foods produce maximal stomach acid secretion. Follow the diet prescribed to derive optimal benefit from this drug.

Beverages: No restrictions. May be taken with milk.

▷   *Alcohol:* No interactions with drug. However, alcoholic beverages increase stomach acidity and can reduce the effectiveness of this drug.

▷   *Other Drugs*
   Nizatidine may ***increase*** the effects of
   • aspirin (when aspirin is taken in large doses—3900 mg/day).
   The following drugs may ***decrease*** the effects of nizatidine
   • antacids containing aluminum and magnesium hydroxide can reduce absorption of nizatidine by 10%. Avoid antacids for 2 hours before and after taking nizatidine.

▷   *Driving, Hazardous Activities:* This drug may cause drowsiness. Restrict activities as necessary.

Aviation Note: The use of this drug ***may be a disqualification*** for piloting. Consult a designated Aviation Medical Examiner.

Exposure to Sun: No restrictions.

Discontinuation: Do not discontinue this drug suddenly if taken for peptic ulcer disease. Consult physician for withdrawal instructions. This drug does not provide an extended protective effect. Be alert to the possibility of ulcer recurrence anytime after discontinuation.

NORFLOXACIN
(nor FLOX a sin)

Introduced: 1986

Class: Anti-infectives

Prescription: USA: Yes
   Canada: Yes

Controlled Drug: USA: No
   Canada: No

Available as Generic: USA: No
   Canada: No

Brand Name: Noroxin

BENEFITS versus RISKS	
Possible Benefits	*Possible Risks*
HIGH CURE RATE (95%) IN TREATMENT OF URINARY TRACT INFECTIONS	Infrequent nausea, indigestion
	Rare impairment of vision
Effective treatment of bacterial gastroenteritis and gonorrhea	Rare seizure

▷ **Principal Uses**

As a Single Drug Product: Used primarily to treat urinary tract infections (in adults) caused by a wide variety of bacteria sensitive to the action of this drug. It is also used to treat acute gastroenteritis caused by certain bacteria, to prevent traveler's diarrhea and to treat gonorrhea.

How This Drug Works: By inhibiting essential enzyme systems of bacterial nucleic acids (DNA), this drug prevents bacterial reproduction (with low doses) and destroys bacteria (with higher doses).

Available Dosage Forms and Strengths
Tablets — 400 mg

▷ **Usual Adult Dosage Range:** Uncomplicated urinary tract infections—400 mg/12 hours for 3 days. Complicated urinary tract infections—400 mg/12 hours for 10 to 21 days. Total daily dosage should not exceed 800 mg. **Note: Actual dosage and administration schedule must be determined by the physician for each patient individually.**

▷ **Dosing Instructions:** Preferably taken with a full glass of water 1 hour before or 2 hours after eating. Avoid antacids for 2 hours after taking this drug. The tablet may be crushed for administration. Take the full course prescribed.

Usual Duration of Use: Continual use on a regular schedule for 3 to 21 days (depending upon the nature of the infection) is usually necessary to determine this drug's effectiveness in eradicating the infection.

Possible Advantages of This Drug: Highly effective in treating adults with urinary tract infections due to virtually all varieties of causative bacteria. This drug kills bacteria rapidly, preventing the development of bacterial resistance to the action of the drug.

Currently a "Drug of Choice" for starting anti-infective treatment prior to obtaining the results of urine bacterial culture and sensitivity tests.

▷ **This Drug Should Not Be Taken If**
- you have had an allergic reaction to any dosage form of it previously.
- you are pregnant or breast-feeding.
- it is prescribed for a child under 18 years of age.

▷ **Inform Your Physician Before Taking This Drug If**
- you are allergic to cinoxacin (Cinobac) or nalidixic acid (NegGram).
- you have a seizure disorder.
- you have impaired liver or kidney function.

Possible Side-Effects (natural, expected and unavoidable drug actions)
None reported.

▷ **Possible Adverse Effects** (unusual, unexpected and infrequent reactions)
If any of the following develop, consult your physician promptly for guidance.
Mild Adverse Effects
Allergic Reactions: Skin rash (0.4%), hives (0.1%), localized swelling, itching (0.1%).
Headache (1.6%), dizziness (1.2%), mental depression (4 reports), seizures (3 reports).
Drowsiness, mood alterations, nervousness, insomnia, hallucinations (all less than 1%).
Visual disturbances: blurred or double vision, altered color vision, increased sensitivity to light (all less than 0.1%).
Dry mouth, decreased appetite (0.1%), nausea (2%), indigestion (0.3%), vomiting, (0.2%), diarrhea (0.2%).
Swollen or painful tendons and joints (0.1%).
Serious Adverse Effects
Allergic Reactions: Exfoliative dermatitis (1 report), anaphylactic reaction (see Glossary; 1 report).

▷ **Possible Effects on Sexual Function:** None reported.

Natural Diseases or Disorders That May Be Activated by This Drug
Latent epilepsy.

CAUTION
1. With high doses or prolonged use, crystal formation in the kidney can occur. This can be prevented by drinking copious amounts of water, up to 2 quarts/24 hours.
2. This drug may decrease the formation of saliva and predispose to the formation of dental cavities or gum disease. Consult your dentist if mouth dryness persists.

Precautions for Use
By Infants and Children: Safety for use by those who have not attained complete bone growth has not been established. This drug can impair normal bone growth and development in test animals. Avoid its use in children until complete bone development is assured.
By Those over 60 Years of Age: Impaired kidney function may require dosage reduction. Consult your physician.

▷ **Advisability of Use During Pregnancy**
Pregnancy Category: C (tentative). See Pregnancy Code inside back cover.
Animal studies: Mouse, rat, rabbit and monkey studies reveal no birth defects due to this drug. However, this drug can cause impaired bone development in immature dogs.
Human studies: Information from adequate studies of pregnant women is not available.
This drug should be avoided during entire pregnancy.

Advisability of Use if Breast-Feeding
Presence of this drug in breast milk: Unknown.
Avoid drug or refrain from nursing.

Habit-Forming Potential: None.

Effects of Overdosage: No information available.

Possible Effects of Long-Term Use: Crystal formation in kidneys with high doses and inadequate fluid intake.

Suggested Periodic Examinations While Taking This Drug (at physician's discretion)
Liver function tests, urine analysis.

▷ **While Taking This Drug, Observe the Following**
Foods: No restrictions.
Beverages: No restrictions.
▷ *Alcohol:* No interactions expected.
Tobacco Smoking: No interactions expected.
▷ *Other Drugs*
Nitrofurantoin (Macrodantin, etc.) **taken concurrently** with norfloxacin may antagonize the antibacterial action of norfloxacin in the urinary tract. Avoid this combination.

The following drug may *increase* the effects of norfloxacin
- probenecid (Benemid).

The following drugs may *decrease* the effects of norfloxacin
- antacids may reduce its absorption.

▷ *Driving, Hazardous Activities:* This drug may cause dizziness or impaired vision. Restrict activities as necessary.

Aviation Note: The use of this drug *may be a disqualification* for piloting. Consult a designated Aviation Medical Examiner.

Exposure to Sun: Sunglasses advised if eyes are overly sensitive to bright light.

Discontinuation: If you experience no adverse effects from this drug, take the full course prescribed for maximal results. Consult your physician regarding termination of treatment.

NORTRIPTYLINE
(nor TRIP ti leen)

Introduced: 1963

Class: Antidepressant

Prescription: USA: Yes
  Canada: Yes

Controlled Drug: USA: No
  Canada: No

Available as Generic: USA: No
  Canada: No

Brand Names: Aventyl, Pamelor

BENEFITS versus RISKS

Possible Benefits	*Possible Risks*
EFFECTIVE RELIEF OF ENDOGENOUS DEPRESSION	ADVERSE BEHAVIORAL EFFECTS: confusion, disorientation, hallucinations, delusions
Possibly beneficial in other depressive disorders	CONVERSION OF DEPRESSION TO MANIA in manic-depressive disorders
Possibly beneficial in the management of some types of chronic, severe pain	Aggravation of schizophrenia
	Irregular heart rhythms
	Rare blood cell abnormalities

▷ **Principal Uses**

As a Single Drug Product

Used primarily to relieve the symptoms associated with spontaneous (endogenous) depression, and to initiate the restoration of normal mood. This drug should be used only when a diagnosis of a true, primary depression of significant degree has been established. It should not be used to treat the symptoms of mild and transient (reactive) depression that may be associated with many life situations in the absence of a bona fide affective illness.

It is also used in conjunction with other drugs to manage chronic, severe pain associated with such conditions as cancer, migraine headache, severe arthritis, peripheral neuropathy, AIDS, etc.

How This Drug Works: It is thought that this drug relieves depression by slowly restoring to normal levels certain constituents of brain tissue (norepinephrine and serotonin) that transmit nerve impulses.

Available Dosage Forms and Strengths
     Capsules — 10 mg, 25 mg, 50 mg, 75 mg
Oral solution — 10 mg per 5-ml teaspoonful (alcohol 4%)

▷ **Usual Adult Dosage Range:**   Initially 25 mg 3 or 4 times daily. Dose may be increased cautiously as needed and tolerated by 10 to 25 mg daily at intervals of 1 week. Usual maintenance dose is 50 to 100 mg/24 hours. Total dose should not exceed 150 mg/24 hours. When the optimal requirement is determined, it may be taken at bedtime as one dose. **Note: Actual dosage and administration schedule must be determined by the physician for each patient individually.**

▷ **Dosing Instructions:**   May be taken without regard to meals. The capsule may be opened for administration.

Usual Duration of Use: Some benefit may be apparent within 1 to 2 weeks, but adequate response may require continual use for 3 months or longer. Long-term use should not exceed 6 months without evaluation regarding the need for continuation of the drug. Consult your physician on a regular basis.

▷ **This Drug Should Not Be Taken If**
- you have had an allergic reaction to it previously.
- you are taking or have taken within the past 14 days any monoamine oxidase (MAO) type A inhibitor drug (see Drug Class, Section Four).
- you are recovering from a recent heart attack.
- you have narrow-angle glaucoma.

▷ **Inform Your Physician Before Taking This Drug If**
- you are allergic or sensitive to any other tricyclic antidepressant (see Drug Class, Section Four).
- you have a history of any of the following: diabetes, epilepsy, glaucoma, heart disease, prostate gland enlargement or overactive thyroid function.
- you plan to have surgery under general anesthesia in the near future.

Possible Side-Effects (natural, expected and unavoidable drug actions)
Light-headedness, drowsiness, blurred vision, dry mouth, constipation, impaired urination (see Prostatism in Glossary).

▷ **Possible Adverse Effects** (unusual, unexpected and infrequent reactions)
If any of the following develop, consult your physician promptly for guidance.
Mild Adverse Effects
Allergic Reactions: Skin rash, hives, swelling of face or tongue, drug fever (see Glossary).
Headache, dizziness, weakness, fainting, unsteady gait, tremors.
Peculiar taste, irritation of tongue or mouth, nausea, indigestion.
Fluctuation of blood sugar levels.
Serious Adverse Effects
Allergic Reactions: Hepatitis, with or without jaundice (see Glossary).
Confusion, disorientation, hallucinations, delusions.
Aggravation of paranoid psychoses and schizophrenia; seizures.
Heart palpitation and irregular rhythm.
Bone marrow depression (see Glossary)—fatigue, weakness, fever, sore throat, abnormal bleeding or bruising.
Peripheral neuritis (see Glossary)—numbness, tingling, pain, loss of strength in arms and legs.
Parkinson-like disorders (see Glossary)—usually mild and infrequent; more likely to occur in the elderly.

▷ **Possible Effects on Sexual Function:** Decreased libido, increased libido (antidepressant effect), male impotence, inhibited female orgasm, male and female breast enlargement, milk production, swelling of testicles.

▷ **Adverse Effects That May Mimic Natural Diseases or Disorders**
Liver toxicity may suggest viral hepatitis.

Natural Diseases or Disorders That May Be Activated by This Drug
Latent diabetes, epilepsy, glaucoma, prostatism.

CAUTION
1. Dosage must be adjusted for each person individually. Report for follow-up evaluation and laboratory tests as directed by your physician.
2. It is advisable to withhold this drug if electroconvulsive therapy (ECT, "shock" treatment) is to be used to treat your depression.

Precautions for Use
By Infants and Children: Safety and effectiveness for use by those under 6 years of age have not been established.
By Those over 60 Years of Age: Usual dosage is 30 to 50 mg daily in divided doses. During the first 2 weeks of treatment, observe for the development of confusion, agitation, forgetfulness, disorientation, delusions and hallucinations. Reduction of dosage or discontinuation may be necessary. Unsteadiness may predispose to falling and injury. This drug can increase the degree of impaired urination associated with prostate gland enlargement (prostatism).

▷ **Advisability of Use During Pregnancy**
    Pregnancy Category: C (tentative). See Pregnancy Code inside back cover.
    Animal studies: Results are inconclusive.
    Human studies: No defects reported in 21 exposures to amitriptyline,
    a closely related drug. Information from adequate studies of pregnant
    women is not available for this drug.
    Avoid use of drug during first 3 months. Use during last 6 months only
    if clearly needed. Ask your physician for guidance.

Advisability of Use if Breast-Feeding
    Presence of this drug in breast milk: Yes, in small amounts.
    Monitor nursing infant closely and discontinue drug or nursing if ad-
    verse effects develop: excessive drowsiness and failure to feed.

Habit-Forming Potential: Psychological or physical dependence is rare
    and unexpected.

Effects of Overdosage: Confusion, hallucinations, marked drowsiness,
    heart palpitations, dilated pupils, tremors, stupor, deep sleep, coma,
    convulsions.

Suggested Periodic Examinations While Taking This Drug (at physician's
    discretion)
    Complete blood cell counts, liver function tests, serial blood pressure
    readings and electrocardiograms.

▷ **While Taking This Drug, Observe the Following**
    Foods: No restrictions. This drug may increase the appetite and cause
    excessive weight gain.
    Beverages: No restrictions. May be taken with milk.
▷   *Alcohol:* Avoid completely. This drug can markedly increase the intoxi-
    cating effects of alcohol and accentuate its depressant action on brain
    function.
    Tobacco Smoking: May hasten the elimination of this drug. Higher doses
    may be necessary.
▷   *Other Drugs*
    Nortriptyline may ***increase*** the effects of
    • atropinelike drugs (see Drug Class, Section Four).
    • dicoumarol, and increase the risk of bleeding.
    • epinephrine (Adrenalin).
    Nortriptyline may ***decrease*** the effects of
    • clonidine (Catapres).
    • ephedrine (Primatene tablets).
    • guanethidine (Ismelin).
    Nortriptyline ***taken concurrently*** with
    • disulfiram (Antabuse) may cause acute dementia: confusion, diso-
    rientation, hallucinations.
    • monoamine oxidase (MAO) type A inhibitor drugs may cause high
    fever, delirium and convulsions (see Drug Class, Section Four).

- thyroid preparations may impair heart rhythm and function. Ask physician for guidance regarding adjustment of thyroid dose.

The following drugs may *increase* the effects of nortriptyline
- cimetidine (Tagamet), and cause nortriptyline toxicity.
- quinidine (Quinaglute, etc,), and cause nortriptyline toxicity.

The following drugs may *decrease* the effects of nortriptyline
- barbiturates (see Drug Class, Section Four), and reduce its effectiveness.

▷ *Driving, Hazardous Activities:* This drug may impair mental alertness, judgment, physical coordination and reaction time. Avoid hazardous activities.

Aviation Note: The use of this drug *is a disqualification* for piloting. Consult a designated Aviation Medical Examiner.

Exposure to Sun: Use caution until sensitivity to sun has been determined. This drug may cause photosensitivity (see Glossary).

Exposure to Heat: This drug can inhibit sweating and impair the body's adaptation to hot environments, increasing the risk of heat stroke. Avoid saunas.

Exposure to Cold: The elderly should use caution and avoid conditions conducive to hypothermia (see Glossary).

Discontinuation: It is advisable to discontinue this drug gradually. Abrupt withdrawal after long-term use can cause headache, malaise and nausea.

ORAL CONTRACEPTIVES
(or al kon tra SEP tivs)

Other Names: Estrogens/progestins

Introduced: 1956   **Class:** Female sex hormones

Prescription: USA: Yes   **Controlled Drug:** USA: No
    Canada: Yes   Canada: No

Available as Generic: USA: No
    Canada: No

Brand Names: Brevicon, Demulen, Enovid, Levlen, Loestrin, Lo/Ovral, Micronor*, ♣Minestrin 1/20, Modicon, Nelova, Nelova 10/11, Nordette, Norethin 1/35E, Norethin 1/50M, Norinyl, Norlestrin, Nor-Q.D.*, Ortho-Novum, Ovcon, Ovral, Ovrette*, ♣Synphasic, Tri-Levlen, Tri-Norinyl, Triphasil

*"Mini-Pill" type, contains progestin only.

```
┌─────────────────────────────────────────────────────────────┐
│                   BENEFITS versus RISKS                       │
│                                                               │
│     Possible Benefits                  Possible Risks         │
│  HIGHLY EFFECTIVE FOR          SERIOUS, LIFE-THREATENING       │
│     CONTRACEPTIVE                 THROMBOEMBOLIC              │
│     PROTECTION                     DISORDERS in susceptible    │
│  Moderately effective as adjunctive   individuals             │
│     treatment in management of    Hypertension                │
│     excessive menses and          Fluid retention             │
│     endometriosis                 Intensification of migrainelike │
│                                      headaches                │
│                                   Intensification of fibrocystic │
│                                      breast changes           │
│                                   Accelerated growth of uterine │
│                                      fibroid tumors           │
│                                   Drug-induced hepatitis with │
│                                      jaundice                 │
│                                   Benign liver tumors (rare)  │
└─────────────────────────────────────────────────────────────┘
```

▷ **Principal Uses**

As a Single Drug Product: The "Mini-Pill" contains only one component— a progestin. This has been shown to be slightly less effective than the combination of estrogen and progestin in preventing pregnancy.

As a Combination Drug Product [CD]: Most oral contraceptives consist of a combination of a type of estrogen and a type of progestin. These products are the most effective form of contraception available. While used primarily to prevent pregnancy, they are sometimes used to treat menstrual irregularity, excessively heavy menstrual flow and endometriosis.

How This Drug Works: When the combination of an estrogen and a progestin is taken in sufficient dosage and on a regular basis, the blood and tissue levels of these hormones increase to resemble those that occur during pregnancy. This results in suppression of the two pituitary gland hormones that normally produce ovulation (the formation and release of an egg by the ovary). In addition, these drugs may (1) alter the cervical mucus so that it resists the passage of sperm, and (2) alter the lining of the uterus so that it resists implantation of the egg (if ovulation occurs).

Available Dosage Forms and Strengths

Tablets — several combinations of synthetic estrogens and progestins in varying strengths; see the package label of the brand prescribed.

▷ **Usual Adult Dosage Range:** Initiate treatment with the first tablet on the fifth day after the onset of menstruation. Follow with 1 tablet daily (taken at the same time each day) for 21 consecutive days. Resume treatment on the eighth day following the last tablet taken during the preceding cycle. The schedule is to take the drug daily for 3 weeks and to omit it for 1 week. For the Mini-Pill (progestin only), initiate treatment on the first day of menstruation and take 1 tablet daily, every day, throughout the year (no interruption). **Note: Actual dosage and administration schedule must be determined by the physician for each patient individually.**

▷ **Dosing Instructions:**   May be taken with or after food to reduce stomach irritation. To ensure regular (every day) use and uniform blood levels, it is advisable to take the tablet at the same time daily. The tablets may be crushed for administration.

Usual Duration of Use: According to individual needs and circumstances. Long-term use (months to years) requires supervision and periodic evaluation by your physician every 6 months.

▷ **This Drug Should Not Be Taken If**
  • you have had a significant allergic reaction to any dosage form of it previously.
  • you have a history of thrombophlebitis, embolism, heart attack or stroke.
  • you have breast cancer.
  • you have active liver disease, seriously impaired liver function or a history of liver tumor.
  • you have abnormal and unexplained vaginal bleeding.
  • you have sickle cell disease.
  • you are pregnant.

▷ **Inform Your Physician Before Taking This Drug If**
  • you have had an unfavorable reaction to any oral contraceptive previously.
  • you have a history of cancer of the breast or reproductive organs.
  • you have any of the following conditions: fibrocystic breast changes, fibroid tumors of the uterus, endometriosis, migrainelike headaches, epilepsy, asthma, heart disease, high blood pressure, gallbladder disease, diabetes or porphyria.
  • you smoke tobacco on a regular basis.
  • you plan to have surgery in the near future.

Possible Side-Effects (natural, expected and unavoidable drug actions)
  Fluid retention, weight gain, "breakthrough" bleeding (spotting in middle of menstrual cycle), altered menstrual pattern, lack of menstruation (during and following cessation of drug), increased susceptibility to yeast infection of the genital tissues.

▷ **Possible Adverse Effects** (unusual, unexpected and infrequent reactions)
  If any of the following develop, consult your physician promptly for guidance.

Mild Adverse Effects
Allergic Reactions: Skin rash, hives, itching.
Headache, nervous tension, irritability, accentuation of migraine headaches.
Nausea, vomiting, bloating, diarrhea.
Tannish pigmentation of the face.
Reduced tolerance to contact lenses.
Impaired color vision: blue tinge to objects, blue halo around lights.
Serious Adverse Effects
Allergic Reactions: Erythema multiforme and nodosum (skin reactions), loss of scalp hair.
Idiosyncratic Reactions: Joint and muscle pains.
Emotional depression, rise in blood pressure (in susceptible individuals).
Eye changes: optic neuritis, retinal thrombosis, altered curvature of the cornea, cataracts.
Gallbladder disease, benign liver tumors, jaundice, rise in blood sugar.
Erosion of uterine cervix, enlargement of uterine fibroid tumors, cystitislike syndrome.
Thrombophlebitis (inflammation of a vein with formation of blood clot)—pain or tenderness in thigh or leg, with or without swelling of foot or leg.
Pulmonary embolism (movement of blood clot to lung)—sudden shortness of breath, pain in chest, coughing, bloody sputum.
Stroke (blood clot in brain)—headaches, blackout, sudden weakness or paralysis of any part of the body, severe dizziness, altered vision, slurred speech, inability to speak.
Heart attack (blood clot in coronary artery)—sudden pain in chest, neck, jaw or arm; weakness; sweating; nausea.
Mesenteric thrombosis—blood clot in abdominal artery.

▷ **Possible Effects on Sexual Function**
Decreased libido (14% to 50%).
Altered character of menstruation; midcycle spotting.
Breast enlargement and tenderness with milk production.
Absent menstruation and infertility (temporary) after discontinuation of drug.

Possible Delayed Adverse Effects: Estrogens taken during pregnancy can predispose the female child to the later development of cancer of the vagina or cervix following puberty.

▷ **Adverse Effects That May Mimic Natural Diseases or Disorders**
Liver reactions may suggest viral hepatitis.

Natural Diseases or Disorders That May Be Activated by This Drug
Latent hypertension, diabetes mellitus, acute intermittent porphyria, lupus erythematosus–like syndrome.

CAUTION

1. The incidence of serious adverse effects due to the use of these drugs is very low. However, any unusual development should be reported and evaluated promptly.
2. Studies indicate that women over 30 years of age who smoke and use oral contraceptives are at significantly greater risk of having a serious cardiovascular event than are nonusers.
3. The risk of thromboembolism increases with the amount of estrogen in the product and with the age of the user. Low-estrogen combinations are advised.
4. It is advisable to discontinue these drugs 1 month prior to elective surgery to reduce the risk of postsurgical thromboembolism.
5. Investigate promptly any alteration or disturbance of vision that occurs during the use of these drugs.
6. Investigate promptly the nature of recurrent, persistent or severe headaches that develop while taking these drugs.
7. Observe for significant change of mood. Discontinue this drug if depression develops.
8. Certain commonly used drugs may reduce the effectiveness of oral contraceptives. Some of these are listed in the category of *Other Drugs.*
9. Diarrhea lasting more than a few hours (and occurring during the days the drug is taken) can prevent adequate absorption of these drugs and impair their effectiveness as contraceptives.
10. If 2 consecutive menstrual periods are missed, consult your physician regarding the advisability of performing a pregnancy test. Do not continue to use these drugs until your pregnancy status is determined.

▷ **Advisability of Use During Pregnancy**

Pregnancy Category: X. See Pregnancy Code inside back cover.

Animal studies: Genital defects reported in mice and guinea pigs; cleft palate reported in rodents.

Human studies: Information from studies of pregnant women indicates that estrogens can masculinize the female fetus. In addition, limb defects and heart malformations have been reported.

It is now known that estrogens taken during pregnancy can predispose the female child to the development of cancer of the vagina or cervix following puberty. **Avoid these drugs completely during entire pregnancy.**

Advisability of Use if Breast-Feeding

Presence of these drugs in breast milk: Yes, in minute amounts.

These drugs may suppress milk formation if started early following delivery.

Breast-feeding is considered to be safe during the use of oral contraceptives.

Habit-Forming Potential: None.

Effects of Overdosage: Headache, drowsiness, nausea, vomiting, fluid retention, abnormal vaginal bleeding, breast enlargement and discomfort.

Possible Effects of Long-Term Use: High blood pressure, gallbladder disease with stones, accelerated growth of uterine fibroid tumors, absent menstruation and impaired fertility after discontinuation of drug.

Suggested Periodic Examinations While Taking This Drug (at physician's discretion)
Regular (every 6 months) evaluation of the breasts and pelvic organs, including Pap smears. Liver function tests as indicated.

▷ **While Taking This Drug, Observe the Following**
Foods: Avoid excessive use of salt if fluid retention occurs.
Beverages: No restrictions. May be taken with milk.
▷   *Alcohol:* No interactions expected.
Tobacco Smoking: Recent studies indicate that heavy smoking (15 or more cigarettes daily) in association with the use of oral contraceptives significantly increases the risk of heart attack (coronary thrombosis). Heavy smoking should be considered a contraindication to the use of oral contraceptives.
▷   *Other Drugs*
Oral contraceptives may ***increase*** the effects of
• some benzodiazepines, and cause excessive sedation.
• metoprolol (Lopressor), and cause excessive beta blocker effects.
• prednisolone and prednisone, and cause excessive cortisonelike effects.
• theophyllines, and increase the risk of toxic effects.
Oral contraceptives ***taken concurrently*** with
• antidiabetic drugs may cause unpredictable fluctuations of blood sugar.
• tricyclic antidepressants (Elavil, Sinequan, etc.) may enhance their adverse effects and reduce their antidepressant effectiveness.
• troleandomycin (TAO) may increase the incidence of liver toxicity and jaundice.
• warfarin (Coumadin) may cause unpredictable alterations of prothrombin activity.
The following drugs may ***decrease*** the effects of oral contraceptives (and impair their effectiveness)
• barbiturates (phenobarbital, etc.; see Drug Class, Section Four).
• carbamazepine (Tegretol).
• griseofulvin (Fulvicin, etc.).
• penicillins (ampicillin, penicillin V).
• phenytoin (Dilantin).
• primidone (Mysoline).
• rifampin (Rifadin, Rimactane).
• tetracyclines (see Drug Class, Section Four).

▷ *Driving, Hazardous Activities:* Usually no restrictions. Consult your physician for assessment of individual risk and for guidance regarding specific restrictions.

Aviation Note: Usually no restrictions. However, it is advisable to observe for the rare occurrence of disturbed vision and to restrict activities accordingly. Consult a designated Aviation Medical Examiner.

Exposure to Sun: Use caution until full effect is known. These drugs can cause photosensitivity (see Glossary).

Discontinuation: Do not discontinue this drug if "breakthrough" bleeding occurs. If spotting or bleeding continues, consult your physician. A preparation with a higher estrogen content may be required. Remember: Omitting this drug for only 1 day may allow pregnancy to occur. It is advisable to avoid pregnancy for 3 to 6 months after discontinuing these drugs; aborted fetuses from women who became pregnant within 6 months after discontinuation reveal significantly increased chromosome abnormalities.

OXAZEPAM
(ox AZ e pam)

Introduced: 1965

Class: Mild tranquilizer, benzodiazepines

Prescription: USA: Yes
Canada: Yes

Controlled Drug: USA: C-IV*
Canada: No

Available as Generic: USA: Yes
Canada: Yes

Brand Names: ✚Apo-Oxazepam, ✚Novoxapam, ✚Oxpam, Serax, ✚Zapex, Zaxopam

BENEFITS versus RISKS	
Possible Benefits	*Possible Risks*
RELIEF OF ANXIETY AND NERVOUS TENSION in 70% to 80% of users	Habit-forming potential with prolonged use
Wide margin of safety with therapeutic doses	Minor impairment of mental functions
Very few drug interactions	Very rare jaundice
	Very rare blood cell disorders

▷ **Principal Uses**

As a Single Drug Product: Used primarily to (1) provide short-term relief of mild to moderate anxiety; (2) relieve the symptoms of acute alcohol

*See Schedules of Controlled Drugs inside back cover.

withdrawal: agitation, tremors, hallucinations, incipient delirium tremens.

How This Drug Works: It is thought that this drug produces a calming effect by enhancing the action of the nerve transmitter gamma-aminobutyric acid (GABA), which in turn blocks the arousal of higher brain centers.

Available Dosage Forms and Strengths
Capsules — 10 mg, 15 mg, 30 mg
Tablets — 15 mg

▷ **Usual Adult Dosage Range:**   30 to 120 mg/24 hours, in 3 or 4 divided doses. The total daily dosage should not exceed 180 mg. **Note: Actual dosage and administration schedule must be determined by the physician for each patient individually.**

▷ **Dosing Instructions:**   May be taken on empty stomach or with food or milk as needed to prevent stomach irritation. The tablet may be crushed and the capsule may be opened for administration. Do not discontinue this drug abruptly if taken for more than 4 weeks.

Usual Duration of Use: Continual use on a regular schedule for 3 to 5 days is usually necessary to determine this drug's effectiveness in relieving moderate anxiety. Limit continual use to 1 to 3 weeks. Avoid uninterrupted and prolonged use.

▷ **This Drug Should Not Be Taken If**
- you have had an allergic reaction to any dosage form of it previously.
- you have acute narrow-angle glaucoma.
- it is prescribed for a child under 6 years of age.

▷ **Inform Your Physician Before Taking This Drug If**
- you are allergic to any benzodiazepine drug (see Drug Class, Section Four).
- you have a history of alcoholism or drug abuse.
- you are pregnant or planning pregnancy.
- you have impaired liver or kidney function.
- you have a history of serious depression or mental disorder.
- you have any of the following: asthma, emphysema, epilepsy, myasthenia gravis.
- you are taking any drugs with sedative effects.

Possible Side-Effects (natural, expected and unavoidable drug actions)
Drowsiness, lethargy, unsteadiness, "hangover" effects on the day following bedtime use.

▷ **Possible Adverse Effects** (unusual, unexpected and infrequent reactions)
If any of the following develop, consult your physician promptly for guidance.

Mild Adverse Effects
Allergic Reactions: Skin rashes, hives.
Dizziness, fainting, blurred vision, double vision, slurred speech, sweating, nausea.
Serious Adverse Effects
Allergic Reactions: Liver reaction with jaundice (see Glossary).
Abnormally low white blood cell count: fever, sore throat, infections.
Paradoxical responses of excitement, agitation, anger, rage.

▷ **Possible Effects on Sexual Function:** Altered timing and pattern of menstruation.

▷ **Adverse Effects That May Mimic Natural Diseases or Disorders**
Liver reaction with jaundice may suggest viral hepatitis.

CAUTION
1. This drug should not be discontinued abruptly if it has been taken continually for more than 4 weeks.
2. The concurrent use of some over-the-counter drug products that contain antihistamines (allergy and cold preparations, sleep aids) can cause excessive sedation in sensitive individuals.

Precautions for Use
By Infants and Children: Safety and effectiveness for use by those under 6 years of age have not been established. This drug should not be used in the hyperactive or psychotic child of any age. Observe for excessive sedation and incoordination.
By Those over 60 Years of Age: It is advisable to use smaller doses at longer intervals to avoid overdosage. Observe for the possible development of lethargy, indifference, fatigue, weakness, unsteadiness, disturbing dreams, nightmares and paradoxical reactions of excitement, agitation, anger, hostility and rage.

▷ **Advisability of Use During Pregnancy**
Pregnancy Category: C (tentative). See Pregnancy Code inside back cover.
Animal studies: No birth defects found in mice, rats or rabbits.
Human studies: Information from adequate studies of pregnant women is not available. No birth defects have been reported with the use of this drug. However, available information regarding the use of other drugs of this class (benzodiazepines) is conflicting and inconclusive. Some studies found an increase in serious birth defects associated with the use of 2 benzodiazepines. Other studies have found no significant increase in birth defects.
Frequent use in late pregnancy can cause the "floppy infant" syndrome in the newborn: weakness, lethargy, unresponsiveness, depressed breathing, low body temperature. Avoid use during entire pregnancy if possible.

Advisability of Use if Breast-Feeding
Presence of this drug in breast milk: Yes.
Avoid drug or refrain from nursing.

Habit-Forming Potential: This drug can produce psychological and/or physical dependence (see Glossary) if used in large doses for an extended period of time.

Effects of Overdosage: Marked drowsiness, weakness, feeling of drunkenness, staggering gait, tremor, stupor progressing to deep sleep or coma.

Possible Effects of Long-Term Use: Psychological and/or physical dependence, rare blood cell disorders.

Suggested Periodic Examinations While Taking This Drug (at physician's discretion)
Complete blood cell counts during long-term use.
Liver function tests.

▷ **While Taking This Drug, Observe the Following**
Foods: No restrictions.
Beverages: Avoid excessive intake of caffeine-containing beverages: coffee, tea, cola. May be taken with milk.
▷ *Alcohol:* Use with extreme caution until the combined effect is determined. Alcohol may increase the depressant effects of this drug on the brain. It is advisable to avoid alcohol completely—throughout the day and night—if it is necessary to drive or to engage in any hazardous activity.
Tobacco Smoking: Heavy smoking may reduce the calming action of this drug.
Marijuana Smoking: Increased sedation and significant impairment of intellectual and physical performance.
▷ *Other Drugs*
Oxazepam may *increase* the effects of
• digoxin (Lanoxin), and cause digoxin toxicity.
• phenytoin (Dilantin), and cause phenytoin toxicity.
Oxazepam may *decrease* the effects of
• levodopa (Sinemet, etc.), and reduce its effectiveness in treating Parkinson's disease.
The following drugs may *decrease* the effects of oxazepam
• oral contraceptives.
• theophylline (Aminophylline, Theo-Dur, etc.).
▷ *Driving, Hazardous Activities:* This drug can impair mental alertness, judgment, physical coordination and reaction time. Avoid hazardous activities accordingly.
Aviation Note: The use of this drug *is a disqualification* for piloting. Consult a designated Aviation Medical Examiner.
Exposure to Sun: No restrictions.
Exposure to Heat: Use caution until the effect of excessive perspiration is determined. Because of reduced urine volume, this drug may accumulate in the body and produce effects of overdosage.
Discontinuation: Avoid sudden discontinuation if this drug has been taken for over 4 weeks without interruption. Dosage should be tapered grad-

ually to prevent a withdrawal syndrome that could include depression, confusion, hallucinations, tremor, seizures, muscle cramping, sweating and vomiting.

OXYCODONE
(ox ee KOH dohn)

Introduced: 1950

Class: Analgesic, narcotic

Prescription: USA: Yes
Canada: Yes

Controlled Drug: USA: C-II*
Canada: <N>

Available as Generic: USA: Yes
Canada: No

Brand Names: ✦Oxycocet [CD], ✦Oxycodan [CD], Percocet [CD], ✦Percocet-Demi [CD], Percodan [CD], Percodan-Demi [CD], Roxicodone, ✦Supeudol, Tylox [CD]

BENEFITS versus RISKS

Possible Benefits	*Possible Risks*
EFFECTIVE RELIEF OF MODERATE TO SEVERE PAIN	POTENTIAL FOR HABIT FORMATION (DEPENDENCE) Sedative effects Mild allergic reactions (infrequent) Nausea, constipation

---

▷ **Principal Uses**

As a Single Drug Product: Used primarily in tablet and suppository form (Canada) to relieve moderate to severe pain.

As a Combination Drug Product [CD]: Oxycodone is available in combinations with acetaminophen and with aspirin. These milder pain relievers are added to enhance the analgesic effect and to reduce fever when present.

How This Drug Works: Acting primarily as a depressant of certain brain functions, this drug suppresses the perception of pain and calms the emotional response to pain.

Available Dosage Forms and Strengths
Solution — 5 mg per 5-ml teaspoonful
Suppositories — 10 mg, 20 mg (Canada)
Tablets — 5 mg, 10 mg (Canada)

*See Schedules of Controlled Drugs inside back cover.

Tablets — 2.44 mg, 4.88 mg (in combination drugs)

▷ **Usual Adult Dosage Range:** 5 mg/3 to 6 hours as needed. May be increased to 10 mg/4 hours if needed for severe pain. The total daily dosage should not exceed 60 mg. **Note: Actual dosage and administration schedule must be determined by the physician for each patient individually.**

▷ **Dosing Instructions:** May be taken with or following food to reduce stomach irritation or nausea. The tablet may be crushed for administration.

 Usual Duration of Use: As required to control pain. Continual use should not exceed 5 to 7 days without interruption and reassessment of need.

▷ **This Drug Should Not Be Taken If**
  • you have had an allergic reaction to any dosage form of it previously.
  • you are having an acute attack of asthma.

▷ **Inform Your Physician Before Taking This Drug If**
  • you have had an unfavorable reaction to any narcotic drug in the past.
  • you have a history of drug abuse or alcoholism.
  • you have chronic lung disease with impaired breathing.
  • you have impaired liver or kidney function.
  • you have gallbladder disease, a seizure disorder or an underactive thyroid gland.
  • you have difficulty emptying the urinary bladder.
  • you are taking any other drugs that have a sedative effect.
  • you plan to have surgery under general anesthesia in the near future.

 Possible Side-Effects (natural, expected and unavoidable drug actions)
 Drowsiness, light-headedness, dry mouth, urinary retention, constipation.

▷ **Possible Adverse Effects** (unusual, unexpected and infrequent reactions)
 If any of the following develop, consult your physician promptly for guidance.
 Mild Adverse Effects
 Allergic Reactions: Skin rash, hives, itching.
 Idiosyncratic Reactions: Skin rash and itching when combined with dairy products (milk or cheese).
 Dizziness, impaired concentration, sensation of drunkenness, confusion, depression, blurred or double vision.
 Nausea, vomiting.
 Serious Adverse Effects
 Impaired breathing: use with caution in chronic lung disease.

▷ **Possible Effects on Sexual Function:** None reported.

CAUTION

1. If you have asthma, chronic bronchitis or emphysema, the excessive use of this drug may cause significant respiratory difficulty, thickening of bronchial secretions and suppression of coughing.
2. The concurrent use of this drug with atropinelike drugs can increase the risk of urinary retention and reduced intestinal function.
3. Do not take this drug following acute head injury.

Precautions for Use

By Infants and Children: Do not use this drug in children under 2 years of age because of their vulnerability to life-threatening respiratory depression.

By Those over 60 Years of Age: Use small doses initially and increase dosage as needed and tolerated. Limit use to short-term treatment only. There may be increased susceptibility to the development of drowsiness, dizziness, unsteadiness, falling, urinary retention and constipation (often leading to fecal impaction).

▷ **Advisability of Use During Pregnancy**

Pregnancy Category: C (tentative). See Pregnancy Code inside back cover.
Animal studies: No information available.
Human studies: Information from adequate studies of pregnant women is not available. Oxycodone taken repeatedly during the last few weeks before delivery may cause withdrawal symptoms in the newborn infant.
Use this drug only if clearly needed and in small, infrequent doses.

Advisability of Use if Breast-Feeding

Presence of this drug in breast milk: Unknown.
Avoid drug or refrain from nursing.

Habit-Forming Potential: Psychological and/or physical dependence can develop with use of large doses for an extended period of time.

Effects of Overdosage: Drowsiness, restlessness, agitation, nausea, vomiting, dry mouth, vertigo, weakness, lethargy, stupor, coma, seizures.

Possible Effects of Long-Term Use: Psychological and physical dependence, chronic constipation.

Suggested Periodic Examinations While Taking This Drug (at physician's discretion)
None.

▷ **While Taking This Drug, Observe the Following**

Foods: No restrictions.
Beverages: No restrictions. May be taken with milk.
▷ *Alcohol:* Use extreme caution until the combined effects have been determined. Oxycodone can intensify the intoxicating effects of alcohol, and alcohol can intensify the depressant effects of oxycodone on brain function, breathing and circulation.

Tobacco Smoking: No interactions expected.

Marijuana Smoking: Increase in drowsiness and pain relief; impairment of mental and physical performance.

▷ *Other Drugs*

Oxycodone may ***increase*** the effects of

- other drugs with sedative effects.
- atropinelike drugs, and increase the risk of constipation and urinary retention.

▷ *Driving, Hazardous Activities:* This drug can impair mental alertness, judgment, reaction time and physical coordination. Avoid hazardous activities accordingly.

Aviation Note: The use of this drug ***is a disqualification*** for piloting. Consult a designated Aviation Medical Examiner.

Exposure to Sun: No restrictions.

Discontinuation: It is advisable to limit this drug to short-term use. If it is necessary to use it for extended periods of time, discontinuation should be gradual to minimize possible effects of withdrawal.

OXYMETAZOLINE
(ox ee met AZ oh leen)

Introduced: 1964

Class: Decongestant

Prescription: USA: No
Canada: No

Controlled Drug: USA: No
Canada: No

Available as Generic: USA: Yes
Canada: No

Brand Names: Afrin, Allerest 12 Hour Nasal, Coricidin Nasal Mist, Dristan Long Lasting, Duramist Plus, Duration, 4-Way Long Acting Nasal Spray, ✦Nafrine, Neo-Synephrine 12 Hour, Nostrilla, NTZ Long Acting Nasal, Ocuclear, Sinarest 12-Hour Nasal Spray, Sinex Long Acting

---

BENEFITS versus RISKS

Possible Benefits	*Possible Risks*
EFFECTIVE, LONG-LASTING DECONGESTION OF NASAL AND SINUS TISSUES EFFECTIVE DECONGESTION OF INFLAMED EYES	"REBOUND" CONGESTION WITH EXCESSIVE USE Mild irritation of ocular or nasal tissues Systemic effects (via absorption with excessive use): nervousness, insomnia, hypertension

---

▷ **Principal Uses**

As a Single Drug Product: Used primarily as a decongestant nose drop or spray to relieve swelling and congestion of the nasal membranes due to colds or allergy. It is also used as an eye drop to relieve inflammation and swelling of the conjunctival membranes ("red eyes") due to allergy or chemical irritation.

How This Drug Works: By contracting the walls of arterioles and thus reducing their size, this drug decreases the volume of blood in the tissues, resulting in shrinkage of tissue mass (decongestion). This expands the nasal airway and enlarges the openings into the sinuses and eustachian tubes. The same action on the conjunctival vessels in the eye results in clearing of the capillary congestion (redness) and swelling.

Available Dosage Forms and Strengths

Eye drops — 0.025%

Nasal spray — 0.05%

Nose drops — 0.05%

Pediatric nose drops — 0.025%

▷ **Usual Adult Dosage Range:** Eye drops: 1 or 2 drops in affected eye/6 to 8 hours. Nose drops and spray: 2 or 3 drops or sprays into each nostril twice/day, morning and evening, 12 hours apart. For long-term use, consult your physician.

▷ **Dosing Instructions:** Do not exceed the recommended doses. The nasal spray is more effective than the drops and is less likely to cause systemic absorption.

Usual Duration of Use: Continual use on a regular schedule for 3 to 5 days is usually necessary to determine this drug's effectiveness in relieving eye and nasal congestion. If there is no significant improvement after 1 week of use, consult your physician for further evaluation.

▷ **This Drug Should Not Be Taken If**
- you have had an allergic reaction to it previously.
- for the eye drops: you have untreated narrow-angle glaucoma or an active eye infection.

▷ **Inform Your Physician Before Taking This Drug If**
- you have high blood pressure or heart disease.
- you have diabetes or an overactive thyroid gland (hyperthyroidism).
- you are taking any beta blocker drug (see Drug Class, Section Four).
- you are taking, or have taken within the past 14 days, any monoamine oxidase (MAO) type A inhibitor drug (see Drug Class, Section Four).

Possible Side-Effects (natural, expected and unavoidable drug actions)
Dryness or irritation of the nose, nervousness, insomnia.

▷ **Possible Adverse Effects** (unusual, unexpected and infrequent reactions)
If any of the following develop, consult your physician promptly for guidance.
Mild Adverse Effects
Headache, light-headedness, burning or stinging of the nose, heart palpitation, tremors.
Serious Adverse Effects
None reported.

▷ **Possible Effects on Sexual Function:**   None reported.

CAUTION
1. Too frequent use, or extended use, of nose drops or sprays containing this drug may cause a secondary rebound congestion resulting in a form of functional dependence (see Glossary).
2. Many over-the-counter drug products for allergies, colds and coughs contain drugs that may interact unfavorably with this drug. Ask your physician or pharmacist for guidance before using such medications.

Precautions for Use
By Infants and Children: Children may be especially susceptible to systemic absorption of this drug. Avoid excessive use.
By Those over 60 Years of Age: Use small doses until your tolerance has been determined. Observe for possible nervousness, insomnia or palpitation.

▷ **Advisability of Use During Pregnancy**
Pregnancy Category: C (tentative). See Pregnancy Code inside back cover.
Animal studies: No information available.
Human studies: Information from adequate studies of pregnant women is not available.
Limit use to small, infrequent doses.

Advisability of Use if Breast-Feeding
Presence of this drug in breast milk: Unknown.
Monitor nursing infant closely and discontinue drug or nursing if adverse effects develop.

Habit-Forming Potential: Frequent or excessive use may cause functional dependence (see Glossary).

Effects of Overdosage: Headache, restlessness, anxiety, agitation, palpitation, sweating.

Possible Effects of Long-Term Use: Secondary rebound congestion and chemical irritation of nasal tissues.

Suggested Periodic Examinations While Taking This Drug (at physician's discretion)
None required.

▷ **While Taking This Drug, Observe the Following**

Foods: No restrictions.

Beverages: Heavy use of coffee or tea may add to the nervousness or insomnia experienced by sensitive individuals.

▷   *Alcohol:* No interactions expected.

Tobacco Smoking: No interactions expected.

▷   *Other Drugs*

Oxymetazoline **taken concurrently** with

- beta blocker drugs or monoamine oxidase (MAO) type A inhibitor drugs may cause dangerous elevations of blood pressure. Observe for headache or palpitation.

▷   *Driving, Hazardous Activities:* No restrictions.

Aviation Note: The use of this drug **may be a disqualification** for piloting. Consult a designated Aviation Medical Examiner.

Exposure to Sun: No restrictions.

PENBUTOLOL
(pen BYU toh lohl)

Introduced: 1976

Class: Antihypertensive, beta-adrenergic blocker

Prescription: USA: Yes

Controlled Drug: USA: No

Available as Generic: No

Brand Name: Levatol

BENEFITS versus RISKS

Possible Benefits	*Possible Risks*
EFFECTIVE, WELL-TOLERATED ANTIHYPERTENSIVE in mild to moderate high blood pressure	CONGESTIVE HEART FAILURE in advanced heart disease Worsening of angina in coronary heart disease (abrupt withdrawal) Masking of low blood sugar (hypoglycemia) in drug-treated diabetes Provocation of asthma

---

▷ **Principal Uses**

As a Single Drug Product: The treatment of mild to moderately severe high blood pressure. May be used alone or concurrently with other antihypertensive drugs, such as diuretics.

How This Drug Works: By blocking certain actions of the sympathetic nervous system, this drug
- reduces the rate and contraction force of the heart, thus lowering the ejection pressure of the blood leaving the heart.
- reduces the degree of contraction of blood vessel walls, resulting in their relaxation and expansion and consequent lowering of blood pressure.

Available Dosage Forms and Strengths
Tablets — 20 mg

▷ **Usual Adult Dosage Range:** Initially 20 mg once daily. The dose may be increased gradually by 10 mg/day at intervals of 2 weeks as needed and tolerated up to 80 mg/day. For maintenance, 20 to 40 mg once daily is usually adequate. The total daily dose should not exceed 80 mg. **Note: Actual dosage and administration schedule must be determined by the physician for each patient individually.**

▷ **Dosing Instructions:** May be taken without regard to eating. The tablet may be crushed for administration. Do not discontinue this drug abruptly.

Usual Duration of Use: Continual use on a regular schedule for 2 to 3 weeks is usually necessary to determine this drug's effectiveness in lowering blood pressure. The long-term use of this drug (months to years) will be determined by the course of your blood pressure over time and your response to the overall treatment program (weight reduction, salt restriction, smoking cessation, etc.). Consult your physician on a regular basis.

Possible Advantages of This Drug
Adequate control of blood pressure with a single daily dose.
Causes less slowing of the heart rate than most other beta blocker drugs.

Currently a "Drug of Choice" for initiating treatment of hypertension with a single drug.

▷ **This Drug Should Not Be Taken If**
- you have had an allergic reaction to it previously.
- you have congestive heart failure.
- you have an abnormally slow heart rate or a serious form of heart block.
- you are subject to bronchial asthma.

▷ **Inform Your Physician Before Taking This Drug If**
- you have had an adverse reaction to any beta blocker drug in the past (see Drug Class, Section Four).
- you have a history of serious heart disease, with or without episodes of heart failure.
- you have a history of hay fever (allergic rhinitis), asthma, chronic bronchitis or emphysema.

- you have a history of overactive thyroid function (hyperthyroidism).
- you have a history of low blood sugar (hypoglycemia).
- you have impaired liver or kidney function.
- you have diabetes or myasthenia gravis.
- you have impaired circulation in the extremities (Raynaud's disorder, claudication pains in legs).
- you are currently taking any form of digitalis, quinidine or reserpine, or any calcium blocker drug (see Drug Class, Section Four).
- you plan to have surgery under general anesthesia in the near future.

Possible Side-Effects (natural, expected and unavoidable drug actions)
Lethargy and fatigability, cold extremities, slow heart rate, light-headedness in upright position (see Orthostatic Hypotension in Glossary).

▷ **Possible Adverse Effects** (unusual, unexpected and infrequent reactions)
If any of the following develop, consult your physician promptly for guidance.
Mild Adverse Effects
Allergic Reactions: Skin rash, itching, reversible hair loss.
Headache, dizziness, blurred vision, insomnia, abnormal dreams.
Indigestion, nausea, vomiting, constipation, diarrhea.
Joint and muscle discomfort.
Serious Adverse Effects
Allergic Reactions: Anaphylactoid reaction (see Glossary).
Mental depression, anxiety, disorientation, short-term memory loss, hallucinations.
Chest pain, shortness of breath, precipitation of congestive heart failure.
Induction of bronchial asthma (in asthmatic individuals).
Aggravation of myasthenia gravis.
Abnormally low white blood cell and platelet counts: fever, sore throat, abnormal bleeding or bruising.

▷ **Possible Effects on Sexual Function:** Decreased libido and impotence, rare but more common with higher doses; Peyronie's disease (see Glossary).

▷ **Adverse Effects That May Mimic Natural Diseases or Disorders**
Reduced blood flow to extremities may resemble Raynaud's phenomenon (see Glossary).

Natural Diseases or Disorders That May Be Activated by This Drug
Raynaud's disease, intermittent claudication, myasthenia gravis.

CAUTION
1. ***Do not discontinue this drug suddenly*** without the knowledge and guidance of your physician. Carry a notation on your person that you are taking this drug.
2. Consult your physician or pharmacist before using nasal decongestants usually present in over-the-counter cold preparations and

nose drops. These can cause sudden increases in blood pressure when taken concurrently with beta blocker drugs.

3. Report the development of any tendency to emotional depression.

Precautions for Use

By Infants and Children: Safety and effectiveness for use by those under 12 years of age have not been established. However, if this drug is used, observe for the development of low blood sugar (hypoglycemia) during periods of reduced food intake.

By Those over 60 Years of Age: Proceed **cautiously** with all antihypertensive drugs. Unacceptably high blood pressure should be reduced without creating the risks associated with excessively low blood pressure. Start treatment with small doses, and monitor the blood pressure response frequently. Sudden, rapid and excessive reduction of blood pressure can predispose to stroke or heart attack. Observe for dizziness, unsteadiness, tendency to fall, confusion, hallucinations, depression or urinary frequency.

▷ **Advisability of Use During Pregnancy**

Pregnancy Category: C (tentative). See Pregnancy Code inside back cover.

Animal studies: No birth defects due to this drug found in rat or rabbit studies.

Human studies: Information from adequate studies of pregnant women is not available.

Use this drug only if clearly needed. Ask physician for guidance.

Advisability of Use if Breast-Feeding

Presence of this drug in breast milk: Unknown.

Avoid drug or refrain from nursing.

Habit-Forming Potential: None.

Effects of Overdosage: Weakness, slow pulse, low blood pressure, fainting, cold and sweaty skin, congestive heart failure, possible coma and convulsions.

Possible Effects of Long-Term Use: Reduced heart reserve and eventual heart failure in susceptible individuals with advanced heart disease.

Suggested Periodic Examinations While Taking This Drug (at physician's discretion)

Measurements of blood pressure, evaluation of heart function.

Complete blood cell counts.

▷ **While Taking This Drug, Observe the Following**

Foods: No restrictions. Avoid excessive salt intake.

Beverages: No restrictions. May be taken with milk.

▷   *Alcohol:* Use with caution until the combined effect has been determined. Alcohol may exaggerate this drug's ability to lower the blood pressure and may increase its mild sedative effect.

Tobacco Smoking: Nicotine may reduce this drug's effectiveness in treating high blood pressure. In addition, high doses of this drug may potentiate the constriction of the bronchial tubes caused by regular smoking.

▷ *Other Drugs*

Penbutolol may ***increase*** the effects of

- other antihypertensive drugs, and cause excessive lowering of the blood pressure. Dosage adjustments may be necessary.
- reserpine (Ser-Ap-Es, etc.), and cause sedation, depression, slowing of the heart rate and lowering of the blood pressure. This combination is best avoided.
- verapamil (Calan, Isoptin), and cause excessive depression of heart function; monitor this combination closely.

Penbutolol ***taken concurrently*** with

- clonidine (Catapres) requires close monitoring for rebound high blood pressure if clonidine is withdrawn while penbutolol is still being taken.
- insulin requires close monitoring to avoid undetected hypoglycemia (see Glossary).

The following drugs may ***increase*** the effects of penbutolol

- methimazole (Tapazole).
- oral contraceptives.
- propylthiouracil (Propacil).

The following drugs may ***decrease*** the effects of penbutolol

- barbiturates (phenobarbital, etc.).
- indomethacin (Indocin), and possibly other "aspirin substitutes," may impair pindolol's antihypertensive effect.
- rifampin (Rifadin, Rimactane).

▷ *Driving, Hazardous Activities:* Use caution until the full extent of fatigue, dizziness and blood pressure change have been determined.

Aviation Note: The use of this drug ***is a disqualification*** for piloting. Consult a designated Aviation Medical Examiner.

Exposure to Sun: No restrictions.

Exposure to Heat: Caution advised. Hot environments can lower the blood pressure and exaggerate the effects of this drug.

Exposure to Cold: Caution advised. Cold environments can enhance the circulatory deficiency in the extremities that may occur with this drug. The elderly should take precautions to prevent hypothermia (see Glossary).

Heavy Exercise or Exertion: It is advisable to avoid exertion that produces light-headedness, excessive fatigue or muscle cramping. The use of this drug may intensify the hypertensive response to isometric exercise.

Occurrence of Unrelated Illness: The fever that accompanies systemic infections can lower the blood pressure and require adjustment of dosage. Illnesses that cause nausea or vomiting may interrupt the regular dosage schedule. Ask your physician for guidance.

Discontinuation: It is advisable to avoid sudden discontinuation of this drug in all situations. If possible, gradual reduction of dose over a period of 2 to 3 weeks is recommended. Ask your physician for specific guidance.

PENICILLIN V
(pen i SIL in VEE)

Introduced: 1953

Class: Antibiotic, penicillins

Prescription: USA: Yes
Canada: Yes

Controlled Drug: USA: No
Canada: No

Available as Generic: USA: Yes
Canada: Yes

Brand Names: ✦Apo-Penicillin VK, Beepen VK, Betapen-VK, Ledercillin VK, ✦Nadopen-V, ✦Novopen-VK, Penapar VK, ✦Pen-Vee, Pen-Vee K, ✦PVF, ✦PVF K, Robicillin VK, Uticillin VK, V-Cillin K, ✦VC-K 500, Veetids

BENEFITS versus RISKS	
Possible Benefits	***Possible Risks***
EFFECTIVE TREATMENT OF INFECTIONS due to susceptible microorganisms	ALLERGIC REACTIONS, mild to severe, in 3% of the general population and 15% of allergic individuals
	Superinfections (yeast)
	Drug-induced colitis

▷ **Principal Uses**

As a Single Drug Product: This type of penicillin is used primarily to treat responsive infections of the upper and lower respiratory tract, the middle ear and the skin. Equally important uses are the prevention of rheumatic fever and the prevention of bacterial endocarditis in individuals with valvular heart disease.

How This Drug Works: This drug destroys susceptible infecting bacteria by interfering with their ability to produce new protective cell walls as they multiply and grow.

Available Dosage Forms and Strengths

Oral solution — 125 mg, 250 mg per 5-ml teaspoonful
Tablets — 125 mg, 250 mg, 500 mg

▷ **Usual Adult Dosage Range:** Dosage is based upon the results of sensitivity testing of the causative organism, the severity of the infection and the response of the patient. Depending upon the specific infection, the dosage range is 125 to 500 mg/6 to 8 hours. For the prevention of bacterial endocarditis: 2 grams (2000 mg) taken 1 hour before the procedure, followed by 1 gram 6 hours later. The total daily dosage should not exceed 7 grams (7000 mg). **Note: Actual dosage and administration schedule must be determined by the physician for each patient individually.**

▷ **Dosing Instructions:** May be taken on an empty stomach or with food or milk. Absorption may be slightly faster if taken when stomach is empty. The tablet may be crushed for administration.

Usual Duration of Use: For all streptococcal infections—not less than 10 consecutive days (without interruption) to reduce the possibility of developing rheumatic fever or glomerulonephritis. For all other infections—as long as necessary to eradicate the infection.

▷ **This Drug Should Not Be Taken If**
- you have had an allergic reaction to any dosage form of it previously.
- you are certain you are allergic to **any** form of penicillin.

▷ **Inform Your Physician Before Taking This Drug If**
- you suspect you may be allergic to penicillin or you have a history of a previous "reaction" of any type to penicillin.
- you are allergic to any cephalosporin antibiotic (Ancef, Anspor, Ceclor, Ceporan, Ceporex, Kafocin, Keflex, Keflin, Kefzol, Loridine, Ultracef, Velosef; see Drug Class, Section Four).
- you are allergic by nature (hay fever, asthma, hives, eczema).

Possible Side-Effects (natural, expected and unavoidable drug actions)
Superinfections (see Glossary), often due to yeast organisms.

▷ **Possible Adverse Effects** (unusual, unexpected and infrequent reactions)
If any of the following develop, consult your physician promptly for guidance.
Mild Adverse Effects
Allergic Reactions: Skin rashes, hives, itching.
Irritations of mouth and tongue, "black tongue," nausea, vomiting, mild diarrhea, dizziness (rare).
Serious Adverse Effects
Allergic Reactions: Anaphylactic reaction (see Glossary), severe skin reactions, drug fever, swollen painful joints, sore throat, abnormal bleeding or bruising.
Drug-induced colitis.

▷ **Possible Effects on Sexual Function:** None reported.

CAUTION
1. Take the exact dose and the full course prescribed.
2. This drug should not be used concurrently with antibiotics like erythromycin or tetracycline.

Precautions for Use
By Infants and Children: Observe the allergic child closely for evidence of a developing allergy to penicillin. This drug may cause diarrhea, which sometimes necessitates discontinuation.
By Those over 60 Years of Age: Natural changes in the skin may predispose to prolonged itching reactions in the genital and anal regions. Report such reactions promptly.

▷ **Advisability of Use During Pregnancy**
Pregnancy Category: B (tentative). See Pregnancy Code inside back cover.
Animal studies: Birth defects of the limbs reported in mice. (Not confirmed in other studies.)
Human studies: Information from adequate studies of pregnant women indicates no increased risk of birth defects in 3546 pregnancies exposed to penicillin derivatives.
This drug is considered safe for use during any period of pregnancy.

Advisability of Use if Breast-Feeding
Presence of this drug in breast milk: Yes.
The nursing infant may be sensitized to penicillin and be at risk for developing diarrhea or yeast infections.
Avoid drug if possible or refrain from nursing.

Habit-Forming Potential: None.

Effects of Overdosage: Possible nausea, vomiting and/or diarrhea.

Possible Effects of Long-Term Use: Superinfections, often due to yeast organisms.

Suggested Periodic Examinations While Taking This Drug (at physician's discretion)
Complete blood cell counts, kidney function tests.

▷ **While Taking This Drug, Observe the Following**
Foods: No restrictions.
Beverages: No restrictions. May be taken with milk.
▷   *Alcohol:* No interactions expected.
Tobacco Smoking: No interactions expected.
▷   *Other Drugs*
Penicillin V may ***decrease*** the effects of
• oral contraceptives in some women, and impair their effectiveness in preventing pregnancy.
The following drugs may ***decrease*** the effects of penicillin V
• antacids may reduce the absorption of penicillin V.

- chloramphenicol (Chloromycetin).
- erythromycin (Erythrocin, E-Mycin, etc.).
- tetracyclines (Achromycin, Declomycin, Minocin, etc.). (See Drug Class, Section Four.)

▷ *Driving, Hazardous Activities:* Usually no restrictions. Be alert to the rare occurrence of dizziness and/or nausea, and restrict activities accordingly.

Aviation Note: The use of this drug *may be a disqualification* for piloting. Consult a designated Aviation Medical Examiner.

Exposure to Sun: No restrictions.

Special Storage Instructions: Oral solutions should be refrigerated.

Observe the Following Expiration Times: Do not take the oral solution of this drug if older than 7 days when kept at room temperature or 14 days when kept refrigerated.

PENTAZOCINE
(pen TAZ oh seen)

Introduced: 1967

Class: Analgesic, narcotic

Prescription: USA: Yes
Canada: Yes

Controlled Drug: USA: C-IV*
Canada: <N>

Available as Generic: USA: No
Canada: No

Brand Names: Talacen [CD], Talwin, Talwin Compound [CD], ✦Talwin Compound-50 [CD], Talwin Nx [CD]

BENEFITS versus RISKS

Possible Benefits	*Possible Risks*
EFFECTIVE RELIEF OF MODERATE TO SEVERE PAIN	POTENTIAL FOR HABIT FORMATION (DEPENDENCE) Sedative effects Mental and behavioral disturbances Low blood pressure, fainting Nausea, constipation

---

▷ **Principal Uses**

As a Single Drug Product: Used exclusively to relieve acute or chronic pain of moderate to severe degree from any cause.

*See Schedules of Controlled Drugs inside back cover.

As a Combination Drug Product [CD]: Pentazocine is available in combinations with acetaminophen and with aspirin. These milder pain relievers are added to enhance the analgesic effect and to reduce fever when present. In the USA the tablet form of pentazocine also contains naloxone (Talwin Nx), a narcotic antagonist that renders the drug ineffective if abused.

How This Drug Works: Acting primarily as a depressant of certain brain functions, this drug suppresses the perception of pain and calms the emotional response to pain.

Available Dosage Forms and Strengths
  Injection — 30 mg per ml
  Tablets — 50 mg (Canada)
  Tablets — 50 mg with 0.5 mg of naloxone (USA)

▷ **Usual Adult Dosage Range:**   50 mg/3 to 4 hours as needed. May be increased to 100 mg/4 hours if needed for severe pain. The total daily dosage should not exceed 600 mg. **Note: Actual dosage and administration schedule must be determined by the physician for each patient individually.**

▷ **Dosing Instructions:**   May be taken with or following food to reduce stomach irritation or nausea. The tablet may be crushed for administration.

Usual Duration of Use: As required to control pain. Continual use should not exceed 5 to 7 days without interruption and reassessment of need.

▷ **This Drug Should Not Be Taken If**
  • you have had an allergic reaction to any dosage form of it previously.
  • you are having an acute attack of asthma.

▷ **Inform Your Physician Before Taking This Drug If**
  • you have had an unfavorable reaction to any narcotic drug in the past.
  • you have a history of drug abuse or alcoholism.
  • you have chronic lung disease with impaired breathing.
  • you have impaired liver or kidney function.
  • you have gallbladder disease, a seizure disorder or an underactive thyroid gland.
  • you have difficulty emptying the urinary bladder.
  • you are taking any other drugs that have a sedative effect.
  • you plan to have surgery under general anesthesia in the near future.

Possible Side-Effects (natural, expected and unavoidable drug actions)
  Drowsiness, light-headedness, weakness, urinary retention, constipation.

▷ **Possible Adverse Effects** (unusual, unexpected and infrequent reactions)
  If any of the following develop, consult your physician promptly for guidance.

Mild Adverse Effects
   Allergic Reactions: Skin rash, hives, itching, swelling of face.
   Headache, dizziness, impaired concentration, sensation of drunkenness,
      blurred or double vision, flushing, sweating.
   Nausea, vomiting, indigestion, diarrhea.
Serious Adverse Effects
   Marked drop in blood pressure, possible fainting.
   Impaired breathing: use with caution in chronic lung disease.
   Mental and behavioral disturbances, hallucinations, tremor.
   Bone marrow depression (see Glossary) of a mild and reversible nature
      (rare).
   Aggravation of prostatism (see Glossary).

▷ **Possible Effects on Sexual Function:**   None reported.

CAUTION
   1. The use of this drug with atropinelike drugs may increase the risk
      of urinary retention and reduced intestinal function.
   2. Do not take this drug following acute head injury.

Precautions for Use
   By Infants and Children: Safety and effectiveness for use by those under
      12 years of age have not been established.
   By Those over 60 Years of Age: Use small doses initially and increase dos-
      age as needed and tolerated. Limit use to short-term treatment only.
      There may be increased susceptibility to the development of drow-
      siness, dizziness, unsteadiness, falling, urinary retention and consti-
      pation.

▷ **Advisability of Use During Pregnancy**
   Pregnancy Category: C (tentative). See Pregnancy Code inside back cover.
      Animal studies: Significant birth defects reported in hamsters.
      Human studies: Information from adequate studies of pregnant women
      is not available. Pentazocine taken repeatedly during the last few
      weeks before delivery may cause withdrawal symptoms in the new-
      born infant.
      Avoid this drug during the first 3 months. Use only if clearly needed
      and in small, infrequent doses during the last 6 months.

Advisability of Use if Breast-Feeding
   Presence of this drug in breast milk: Unknown.
   Avoid drug or refrain from nursing.

Habit-Forming Potential: Psychological and/or physical dependence can
      develop with use of large doses for an extended period of time.

Effects of Overdosage: Anxiety, disturbed thoughts, hallucinations, pro-
      gressive drowsiness, stupor, depressed breathing.

Possible Effects of Long-Term Use: Psychological and physical depen-
      dence, chronic constipation.

Suggested Periodic Examinations While Taking This Drug (at physician's
   discretion)
   Complete blood cell counts, if used for an extended period of time.

▷ **While Taking This Drug, Observe the Following**
   Foods: No restrictions.
   Beverages: No restrictions. May be taken with milk.
▷ *Alcohol:* Use extreme caution until the combined effects have been deter-
      mined. Pentazocine can intensify the intoxicating effects of alcohol,
      and alcohol can intensify the depressant effects of pentazocine on
      brain function, breathing and circulation.
   Tobacco Smoking: Heavy smoking may reduce the effectiveness of pen-
      tazocine and make larger doses necessary.
   Marijuana Smoking: Increase in drowsiness and pain relief; impairment
      of mental and physical performance.
▷ *Other Drugs*
      Pentazocine may ***increase*** the effects of
      • other drugs with sedative effects.
      • atropinelike drugs, and increase the risk of constipation and urinary
        retention.
▷ *Driving, Hazardous Activities:* This drug can impair mental alertness, judg-
      ment, reaction time and physical coordination. Avoid hazardous ac-
      tivities accordingly.
   Aviation Note: The use of this drug ***is a disqualification*** for piloting. Con-
      sult a designated Aviation Medical Examiner.
   Exposure to Sun: No restrictions.
   Discontinuation: It is advisable to limit this drug to short-term use. If it
      is necessary to use it for extended periods of time, discontinuation
      should be gradual to minimize possible effects of withdrawal.

PENTOXIFYLLINE
(pen tox I fi leen)

Other Name: Oxpentifylline

Introduced: 1972   **Class:** Blood flow agent, xanthines

Prescription: USA: Yes   **Controlled Drug:** USA: No
      Canada: Yes   Canada: No

Available as Generic: No

Brand Name: Trental

BENEFITS versus RISKS	
Possible Benefits	*Possible Risks*
IMPROVED BLOOD FLOW IN PERIPHERAL ARTERIAL DISEASE	Reduced blood pressure, angina, abnormal heart rhythms (in susceptible individuals)
REDUCTION OF INTERMITTENT CLAUDICATION PAIN	Indigestion, nausea, vomiting Dizziness, flushing

▷ **Principal Uses**

As a Single Drug Product: Used primarily (as adjunctive treatment) in the management of peripheral obstructive arterial disease to improve arterial blood flow and reduce the frequency and severity of muscle pain due to intermittent claudication.

How This Drug Works: This drug is thought to improve blood flow through the microcirculation and to increase the oxygen supply to working muscles by way of three mechanisms: (1) reduction of blood viscosity due to decreased levels of fibrinogen in the blood; (2) increased flexibility of the red blood cells (carrying oxygen) due to an increase in cyclic AMP (enzyme) within red blood cells; this permits easier passage through the minute blood vessels of the microcirculation; and (3) prevention of red blood cell and platelet aggregation.

Available Dosage Forms and Strengths

Tablets, prolonged-action — 400 mg

▷ **Usual Adult Dosage Range:** 400 mg 3 times/day. If adverse nervous system or gastrointestinal effects occur, reduce the dose to 400 mg twice/day. **Note: Actual dosage and administration schedule must be determined by the physician for each patient individually.**

▷ **Dosing Instructions:** Take with or following food to reduce stomach irritation. Swallow the tablet whole without breaking, crushing or chewing.

Usual Duration of Use: Continual use on a regular schedule for 2 to 4 weeks is usually necessary to determine this drug's effectiveness in preventing or delaying the pains of intermittent claudication associated with walking. Treatment for 2 to 3 months is recommended to determine full effectiveness. Long-term use (months to years) requires supervision and periodic evaluation by your physician. Consult your physician on a regular basis.

Possible Advantages of This Drug

Reduces blood viscosity and thereby improves blood flow through small vessels.

Increases supply of oxygen to working muscles.

Currently a "Drug of Choice" for treating peripheral arterial disease and reducing the frequency and severity of intermittent claudication pain.

▷ **This Drug Should Not Be Taken If**
- you have had an allergic reaction to it previously.

▷ **Inform Your Physician Before Taking This Drug If**
- you are allergic to other xanthine drugs: caffeine, theophylline, theobromine.
- you have impaired kidney function.
- you have low blood pressure, impaired brain circulation or coronary artery disease.
- you smoke tobacco.
- you are taking any antihypertensive drugs.

Possible Side-Effects (natural, expected and unavoidable drug actions)
Usually none with recommended doses.

▷ **Possible Adverse Effects** (unusual, unexpected and infrequent reactions)
If any of the following develop, consult your physician promptly for guidance.
Mild Adverse Effects
Allergic Reaction: Skin rash.
Headache (1.2%), dizziness (1.9%), tremor.
Indigestion (2.8%), nausea (2.2%), vomiting (1.2%).
Serious Adverse Effects
Development of angina or heart rhythm disorders in the presence of coronary artery disease.

▷ **Possible Effects on Sexual Function:** None reported.

CAUTION
Use this drug with caution in the presence of impaired circulation within the brain (cerebral arteriosclerosis) or coronary artery disease. If any related symptoms develop, consult your physician for prompt evaluation.

Precautions for Use
By Infants and Children: Safety and effectiveness for use by those under 18 years of age have not been established. Use by this age group is not anticipated.
By Those over 60 Years of Age: You may be more susceptible to the adverse effects listed. Observe closely for any indications of dizziness or chest pain and report these promptly.

▷ **Advisability of Use During Pregnancy**
Pregnancy Category: C (tentative). See Pregnancy Code inside back cover.
Animal studies: Increased fetal resorptions reported in rats, but no birth defects found in rats or rabbits.
Human studies: Information from adequate studies of pregnant women is not available.

Avoid use during the first 3 months. Use otherwise only if clearly needed.

Advisability of Use if Breast-Feeding
Presence of this drug in breast milk: Yes.
Avoid drug or refrain from nursing.

Habit-Forming Potential: None.

Effects of Overdosage: Drowsiness, flushing, faintness, excitement, seizures.

Possible Effects of Long-Term Use: None reported.

Suggested Periodic Examinations While Taking This Drug (at physician's discretion)
Blood pressure measurements, evaluation of heart status.

▷ **While Taking This Drug, Observe the Following**
Foods: No restrictions.
Beverages: No restrictions. May be taken with milk.
▷ *Alcohol:* Use caution until the combined effects have been determined. Alcohol may increase the blood-pressure-lowering effect of this drug.
Tobacco Smoking: Nicotine constricts arteries and will impair the effectiveness of this drug significantly. Avoid all use of tobacco.
▷ *Other Drugs*
Pentoxifylline may ***increase*** the effects of
 • antihypertensive drugs, and cause excessive lowering of blood pressure.
 • warfarin (Coumadin, etc.), and increase the possibility of unwanted bleeding; monitor prothrombin times as appropriate.
▷ *Driving, Hazardous Activities:* This drug may cause drowsiness or dizziness. Restrict activities as necessary.
Aviation Note: The use of this drug ***may be a disqualification*** for piloting. Consult a designated Aviation Medical Examiner.
Exposure to Sun: No restrictions.

PERGOLIDE
(PER go lide)

Introduced: 1980

Class: Antiparkinsonism, dopamine agonist, ergot derivative

Prescription: USA: Yes (Expected to become available in 1989)

Controlled Drug: USA: No

Available as Generic: USA: No

Brand Name: Permax

```
╔══════════════════════════════════════════════════════════════╗
║                    BENEFITS versus RISKS                       ║
║                                                                ║
║      Possible Benefits                 Possible Risks          ║
║   ADDITIVE RELIEF OF             ABNORMAL INVOLUNTARY           ║
║     SYMPTOMS OF PARKINSON'S        MOVEMENTS (62%)             ║
║     DISEASE when used            HALLUCINATIONS (14%)          ║
║     concurrently with levodopa/  INITIAL FALL IN BLOOD         ║
║     carbidopa (Sinemet)            PRESSURE/ORTHOSTATIC        ║
║   PERMITS A 5% TO 30%              HYPOTENSION (10%)           ║
║     REDUCTION IN SINEMET                                       ║
║     DOSAGE                                                     ║
╚══════════════════════════════════════════════════════════════╝
```

▷ **Principal Uses**

As a Single Drug Product: Used solely as an adjunct to levodopa/carbidopa treatment of Parkinson's disease for those individuals who experience intolerable abnormal movements (dyskinesia) and/or increasing "on-off" episodes due to levodopa. The addition of pergolide (1) permits reduction of the daily dose of levodopa with consequent lessening of dyskinesia and erratic drug response, and (2) provides additional relief of parkinsonian symptoms.

How This Drug Works: By directly stimulating the dopamine receptor sites in the corpus striatum of the brain, this drug helps to compensate for the deficiency of dopamine that is responsible for the rigidity, tremor and sluggish movement characteristic of Parkinson's disease.

Available Dosage Forms and Strengths

Tablets — 0.05 mg, 0.25 mg, 1 mg

▷ **Usual Adult Dosage Range**

Initially 0.05 mg daily for the first 2 days; gradually increase the daily dose by 0.1 mg or 0.15 mg every third day over the next 12 days. If needed and tolerated, the daily dose may be increased further by 0.25 mg every third day until an optimal respose is achieved. The total daily dosage should be divided into 3 equal portions and given at 6 to 8 hour intervals. The usual maintenance dose is 3 mg/24 hours; do not exceed 5 mg/24 hours.

During the gradual introduction of pergolide, the concurrent dose of levodopa/carbidopa (Sinemet) may be cautiously decreased in accord with your physician's instructions.

Note: Actual dosage and administration schedule must be determined by the physician for each patient individually.

▷ **Dosing Instructions:**   Take with food or milk to reduce stomach irritation. The tablet may be crushed for administration.

Usual Duration of Use: Continual use on a regular schedule for 4 to 6 weeks is usually necessary to determine this drug's effectiveness in

controlling the symptoms of Parkinson's disease and permitting reduction of levodopa/carbidopa dosage. Long-term use (months to years) requires periodic evaluation of response and dosage adjustment. Consult your physician on a regular basis.

Possible Advantages of This Drug: It may provide a more effective and uniform control of parkinsonian symptoms and a significant reduction of some adverse effects of long-term levodopa therapy.

▷ **This Drug Should Not Be Taken If**
  - you have had an allergic reaction to it previously.
  - you have had a serious adverse effect from any ergot preparation in the past.
  - you have severe coronary artery disease or peripheral vascular disease.

▷ **Inform Your Physician Before Taking This Drug If**
  - you have constitutionally low blood pressure.
  - you are pregnant or breast-feeding.
  - you are taking any antihypertensive drugs or antipsychotic drugs (see Drug Classes, Section Four).
  - you have any degree of coronary artery disease, especially angina or a history of heart attack.
  - you have any type of heart rhythm disorder.
  - you have impaired liver or kidney function.
  - you have a seizure disorder.

Possible Side-Effects (natural, expected and unavoidable drug actions)
  Weakness (4.2%), chest pain—possibly anginal (3.7%), peripheral edema (7.4%), orthostatic hypotension (see Glossary) (10%).

▷ **Possible Adverse Effects** (unusual, unexpected and infrequent reactions)
  If any of the following develop, consult your physician promptly for guidance.
  Mild Adverse Effects
  Allergic Reactions: Skin rash (3.2%), facial swelling (1.1%).
  Headache (5.3%), dizziness (19%), hallucinations (14%), confusion (11%), drowsiness (10%), insomnia (8%), anxiety (6%), double vision (2%).
  Nasal congestion (12%), shortness of breath (5%), palpitation (2%), fainting (2%).
  Altered taste (1.6%), loss of appetite (4.8%), dry mouth (3.7%), indigestion (6.4%), nausea (24%), vomiting (2.7%), constipation (10%), diarrhea (6.4%).
  Serious Adverse Effects
  Allergic Reactions: None reported.
  Idiosyncratic Reactions: "Flulike" symptoms (3%).
  Abnormal involuntary movements (dyskinesia) (62%), psychotic behavior (2%).

▷ **Possible Effects on Sexual Function:**   Infrequent reports of altered libido (both increased and decreased), impotence, breast pain, priapism (see Glossary).

▷ **Adverse Effects That May Mimic Natural Diseases or Disorders**
Effects on mental function and behavior may resemble psychotic disorders.

▷ **Natural Diseases or Disorders That May Be Activated by This Drug**
Coronary artery disease with anginal syndrome, heart rhythm disorders, Raynaud's syndrome (see Glossary), seizure disorders.

CAUTION
1. This drug can initiate dyskinesias and can intensify existing dyskinesias. Observe carefully for the development of tremors, twitching or abnormal, involuntary movements of any kind. Report these promptly.
2. Begin treatment with low doses to prevent the possibility of excessive drop in blood pressure. See dosage routine outlined above.
3. Inform your physician promptly if you become pregnant or plan pregnancy. This drug has been reported (rarely) to cause abortion and birth defects.

Precautions for Use
By Infants and Children: This drug is not utilized by this age group.
By Those over 60 Years of Age: Small initial doses are mandatory. Observe closely for any tendency to light-headedness or faintness, especially on arising from a lying or sitting position. You may be more susceptible to the development of impaired thinking, confusion, agitation, nightmares or hallucinations.

▷ **Advisability of Use During Pregnancy**
Pregnancy Category: B (tentative). See Pregnancy Code inside back cover.
Animal studies: No birth defects due to this drug were found in mouse or rabbit studies.
Human studies: Information from adequate studies of pregnant women is not available. However, there are four reports of birth defects associated with the use of this drug and infrequent reports of abortion. Causal relationships have not been established, but prudence advises against the use of this drug during pregnancy. Consult your physician for guidance.

Advisability of Use if Breast-Feeding
Presence of this drug in breast milk: Unknown.
Avoid drug or refrain from nursing.

Habit-Forming Potential: None.

Effects of Overdosage: Nausea, vomiting, palpitations, low blood pressure, agitation, severe involuntary movements, hallucinations, seizures.

Possible Effects of Long-Term Use: Increased risk of developing dyskinesias.

Suggested Periodic Examinations While Taking This Drug (at physician's discretion)
Regular evaluation of drug response, heart function and blood pressure status.

▷ **While Taking This Drug, Observe the Following**
Foods: No restrictions.
Beverages: No restrictions. May be taken with milk.
▷   *Alcohol:* Use caution until the combined effects have been determined. Alcohol can exaggerate the blood-pressure-lowering and sedative effects of this drug.
Tobacco Smoking: No interactions expected.
▷   *Other Drugs*
Pergolide **taken concurrently** with
• antihypertensive drugs (and other drugs that can lower blood pressure) requires careful monitoring for excessive drops in pressure. Dosage adjustments may be necessary.
The following drugs may **decrease** the effects of pergolide and diminish its effectiveness
• chlorprothixene (Taractan).
• haloperidol (Haldol).
• metoclopramide (Reglan).
• phenothiazines (see Drug Class, Section Four).
• thiothixene (Navane).
▷   *Driving, Hazardous Activities:* This drug may cause dizziness, drowsiness, impaired coordination or fainting. Restrict activities as necessary.
Aviation Note: The use of this drug **is a disqualification** for piloting. Consult a designated Aviation Medical Examiner.
Exposure to Sun: No restrictions.
Exposure to Heat: Use caution until the combined effects have been determined. Hot environments can cause lowering of blood pressure.
Discontinuation: Do not discontinue this drug abruptly. Sudden withdrawal can cause confusion, paranoid thinking and severe hallucinations. Consult your physician regarding a schedule for gradual withdrawal.

PERPHENAZINE
(per FEN a zeen)

Introduced: 1957

Class: Strong tranquilizer, phenothiazines

Prescription: USA: Yes
Canada: Yes

Controlled Drug: USA: No
Canada: No

Available as Generic: USA: No
Canada: Yes

Brand Names: ✦Apo-Perphenazine, ✦Elavil Plus [CD], Etrafon [CD], Etrafon-A [CD], Etrafon Forte [CD], ✦Phenazine, ✦PMS Levazine, Triavil [CD], Trilafon

BENEFITS versus RISKS	
Possible Benefits	*Possible Risks*
EFFECTIVE CONTROL OF ACUTE MENTAL DISORDERS in the majority of patients	SERIOUS TOXIC EFFECTS ON BRAIN with long-term use
Beneficial effects on thinking, mood and behavior	Liver damage with jaundice (infrequent)
Relief of anxiety and tension	Rare blood cell disorders: hemolytic anemia, abnormally low white blood cell and platelet counts
Moderately effective control of nausea and vomiting	

▷ **Principal Uses**

As a Single Drug Product: This antipsychotic drug is used primarily to treat acute and chronic psychotic disorders such as agitated depression, schizophrenia and similar states of mental dysfunction. It may be used as a tranquilizer in the management of agitated and disruptive behavior in the absence of true psychosis. Less frequently, it may be used to relieve severe nausea or vomiting.

As a Combination Drug Product [CD]: This drug is available in combination with amitriptyline, an effective antidepressant. In some cases of severe agitated depression, the combination of a specific antipsychotic drug and a specific antidepressant drug will be more effective than either drug used alone.

How This Drug Works: Not completely established. Present theory is that by inhibiting the action of dopamine, this drug acts to correct an imbalance of nerve impulse transmissions that is thought to be responsible for certain mental disorders.

Available Dosage Forms and Strengths
Concentrate — 16 mg per 5-ml teaspoonful
Injection — 5 mg per ml
Tablets — 2 mg, 4 mg, 8 mg, 16 mg
Tablets, prolonged-action — 8 mg

▷ **Usual Adult Dosage Range:** Initially 2 to 16 mg 2 to 4 times daily. Dose may be increased by 4 mg at 3- to 4-day intervals as needed and tolerated. Usual dosage range is 8 to 24 mg daily. The total daily dosage should not exceed 64 mg. **Note: Actual dosage and administration schedule must be determined by the physician for each patient individually.**

▷ **Dosing Instructions:** May be taken with or following meals to reduce stomach irritation. The regular tablets may be crushed for administration; the prolonged-action tablets should be taken whole, not broken, crushed or chewed.

Usual Duration of Use: Continual use on a regular schedule for several weeks is usually necessary to determine this drug's effectiveness in controlling psychotic disorders. If it is not significantly beneficial within 6 weeks, it should be discontinued. Long-term use (months to years) requires periodic evaluation of response, appropriate dosage adjustment and consideration of continued need. Consult your physician on a regular basis.

▷ **This Drug Should Not Be Taken If**
- you are allergic to any of the drugs bearing the brand names listed.
- you have active liver disease.
- you have cancer of the breast.
- you have a current blood cell or bone marrow disorder.

▷ **Inform Your Physician Before Taking This Drug If**
- you are allergic or abnormally sensitive to any phenothiazine drug (see Drug Class, Section Four).
- you have impaired liver or kidney function.
- you have any type of seizure disorder.
- you have diabetes, glaucoma or heart disease.
- you have a history of lupus erythematosus.
- you are taking any drug with sedative effects.
- you plan to have surgery under general or spinal anesthesia in the near future.

Possible Side-Effects (natural, expected and unavoidable drug actions)
Drowsiness (usually during the first 2 weeks), orthostatic hypotension (see Glossary), blurred vision, dry mouth, nasal congestion, constipation, impaired urination.
Pink or purple coloration of urine, of no significance.

▷ **Possible Adverse Effects** (unusual, unexpected and infrequent reactions)
If any of the following develop, consult your physician promptly for guidance.
Mild Adverse Effects
Allergic Reactions: Skin rash, hives, low-grade fever.
Lowering of body temperature, especially in the elderly. (See Hypothermia in Glossary).
Increased appetite and weight gain.
Dizziness, weakness, agitation, insomnia, impaired day and night vision.
Chronic constipation, fecal impaction.
Serious Adverse Effects
Allergic Reactions: Hepatitis with jaundice (see Glossary), severe skin reactions, anaphylactic reaction (see Glossary).

Idiosyncratic Reaction: High fever.
Depression, disorientation, seizures, deposits in cornea, lens and retina.
Rapid heart rate, heart rhythm disorders.
Blood cell disorders: hemolytic anemia, reduced white blood cell and blood platelet counts.
Nervous system reactions: Parkinson-like disorders (see Glossary), severe restlessness, muscle spasms involving the face and neck, tardive dyskinesia (see Glossary).

▷ **Possible Effects on Sexual Function**
Altered timing and pattern of menstruation.
Female breast enlargement with milk production.
Male breast enlargement and tenderness.
Inhibited ejaculation.
False positive pregnancy test results.

▷ **Adverse Effects That May Mimic Natural Diseases or Disorders**
Nervous system reactions may suggest true Parkinson's disease.
Liver reactions may suggest viral hepatitis.
Reactions resembling systemic lupus erythematosus can occur.

Natural Diseases or Disorders That May Be Activated by This Drug
Latent epilepsy, glaucoma, diabetes mellitus, prostatism (see Glossary).

CAUTION
1. Many over-the-counter medications (see OTC Drugs in Glossary) for allergies, colds and coughs contain drugs that can interact unfavorably with this drug. Ask your physician or pharmacist for guidance before using any such medications.
2. Antacids that contain aluminum and/or magnesium can prevent the absorption of this drug and reduce its effectiveness.
3. Obtain prompt evaluation of any change or disturbance of vision.

Precautions for Use
By Infants and Children: Use of this drug is not recommended in children under 12 years of age. Do not use this drug in the presence of symptoms suggestive of Reye syndrome (see Glossary). Children with acute infectious diseases (flulike infections, chicken pox, measles, etc.) are more prone to develop muscular spasms of the face, back and extremities when this drug is given to control nausea or vomiting.
By Those over 60 Years of Age: Small doses are advisable until individual response has been determined. You may be more susceptible to the development of drowsiness, lethargy, constipation, lowering of body temperature (hypothermia) and orthostatic hypotension (see Glossary). This drug can enhance existing prostatism (see Glossary). You may also be more susceptible to the development of Parkinson-like reactions and/or tardive dyskinesia (see discussion of these terms in Glossary). These reactions must be recognized early since they may become unresponsive to treatment and irreversible.

▷ **Advisability of Use During Pregnancy**
  Pregnancy Category: C (tentative). See Pregnancy Code inside back cover.
  Animal studies: Cleft palate reported in mouse and rat studies.
  Human studies: No increase in birth defects reported in 166 exposures.
    Information from adequate studies of pregnant women is not available.
  Avoid drug during the first 3 months; avoid during the last month because of possible effects on the newborn infant.

Advisability of Use if Breast-Feeding
  Presence of this drug in breast milk: Yes, in minute amounts.
  Monitor nursing infant closely and discontinue drug or nursing if adverse effects develop.

Habit-Forming Potential: None.

Effects of Overdosage: Marked drowsiness, weakness, tremor, agitation, unsteadiness, deep sleep, coma, convulsions.

Possible Effects of Long-Term Use
  Opacities in the cornea or lens of the eye, pigmentation of the retina.
  Tardive dyskinesia (see Glossary).

Suggested Periodic Examinations While Taking This Drug (at physician's discretion)
  Complete blood cell counts, especially between the fourth and tenth weeks of treatment.
  Liver function tests, electrocardiograms.
  Complete eye examinations—eye structures and vision.
  Careful inspection of the tongue for early evidence of fine, involuntary, wavelike movements that could indicate the beginning of tardive dyskinesia.

▷ **While Taking This Drug, Observe the Following**
  Foods: No restrictions.
  Nutritional Support: A riboflavin (vitamin B-2) supplement should be taken with long-term use.
  Beverages: No restrictions. May be taken with milk.
▷ *Alcohol:* Avoid completely. Alcohol can increase the sedative action of phenothiazines and accentuate their depressant effects on brain function and blood pressure. Phenothiazines can increase the intoxicating effects of alcohol.
  Tobacco Smoking: Possible reduction of drowsiness from drug.
  Marijuana Smoking: Moderate increase in drowsiness; accentuation of orthostatic hypotension; increased risk of precipitating latent psychoses, confusing the interpretation of mental status and drug responses.
▷ *Other Drugs*
  Perphenazine may ***increase*** the effects of

- all sedative drugs, especially meperidine (Demerol), and cause excessive sedation.
- all atropinelike drugs, and cause nervous system toxicity.

Perphenazine may **decrease** the effects of

- guanethidine (Ismelin, Esimil), and reduce its effectiveness in lowering blood pressure.

Perphenazine **taken concurrently** with

- lithium (Lithobid, Lithotabs) may impair the effectiveness of lithium and cause nervous system toxicity.

The following drugs may **decrease** the effects of perphenazine

- antacids containing aluminum and/or magnesium.
- barbiturates (see Drug Class, Section Four).
- benztropine (Cogentin).
- disulfiram (Antabuse).
- trihexyphenidyl (Artane).

▷ *Driving, Hazardous Activities:* This drug can impair mental alertness, judgment and physical coordination. Avoid hazardous activities.

Aviation Note: The use of this drug **is a disqualification** for piloting. Consult a designated Aviation Medical Examiner.

Exposure to Sun: Use caution until sensitivity has been determined. Some phenothiazines can cause photosensitivity (see Glossary).

Exposure to Heat: Use caution and avoid excessive heat as much as possible. This drug may impair the regulation of body temperature and increase the risk of heat stroke.

Exposure to Cold: Use caution and dress warmly. This drug can increase the risk of hypothermia in the elderly.

Discontinuation: After a period of long-term use, do not discontinue this drug suddenly. Gradual withdrawal over 2 to 3 weeks under physician supervision is recommended. Do not discontinue this drug without your physician's knowledge and approval. The relapse rate of schizophrenia after discontinuation is 50% to 60%.

PHENAZOPYRIDINE
(fen az oh PEER i deen)

Introduced: 1927

Class: Urinary analgesic

Prescription: USA: Varies
Canada: No

Controlled Drug: USA: No
Canada: No

Available as Generic: USA: Yes
Canada: No

Brand Names: Azo Gantanol [CD], Azo Gantrisin [CD], Azo-Standard, Baridium, Di-Azo, ♣Phenazo, Pyridium, Pyridium Plus [CD], ♣Pyronium, Thiosulfil-A [CD], Urobiotic-250 [CD], ♣Uro Gantanol [CD]

BENEFITS versus RISKS

Possible Benefits	*Possible Risks*
EFFECTIVE RELIEF OF URINARY URGENCY AND DISCOMFORT	DRUG-INDUCED HEPATITIS (rare) Hemolytic anemia (rare)

▷ **Principal Uses**

As a Single Drug Product: Used exclusively in the treatment of lower urinary tract infections and irritations to relieve the urgency to urinate and the discomfort that accompanies the passage of urine (as in cystitis, urethritis and prostatitis).

As a Combination Drug Product [CD]: This drug is available in combinations with several anti-infective drugs that are commonly used to treat urinary tract infections. Each combination product provides a drug to eradicate the infection and a drug to relieve the discomfort during the early period of treatment.

How This Drug Works: Not completely established. By its direct local anesthetic effect on the tissues lining the lower urinary tract, this drug provides symptomatic relief of pain, burning, pressure and the sense of urgency to void.

Available Dosage Forms and Strengths
Tablets — 100 mg, 200 mg

▷ **Usual Adult Dosage Range:** 100 to 200 mg 3 or 4 times/day, as needed and tolerated. **Note: Actual dosage and administration schedule must be determined by the physician for each patient individually.**

▷ **Dosing Instructions:** Take with or after food to reduce stomach irritation. The tablet should be taken whole, not broken or crushed for administration.

Usual Duration of Use: Continual use on a regular schedule for 12 to 24 hours is usually necessary to determine this drug's effectiveness in relieving urinary urgency and discomfort. This drug is intended for short-term use; do not continue to take it after the bladder disorder has been corrected.

▷ **This Drug Should Not Be Taken If**
- you have had an allergic reaction to it previously.
- you have active liver disease.

▷ **Inform Your Physician Before Taking This Drug If**
- you have a history of liver or kidney disease.
- you have had a drug-induced blood cell disorder in the past.

Possible Side-Effects (natural, expected and unavoidable drug actions)
Reddish-orange discoloration of the urine (of no significance).

▷ **Possible Adverse Effects** (unusual, unexpected and infrequent reactions)
If any of the following develop, consult your physician promptly for guidance.

Mild Adverse Effects

Allergic Reaction: Skin rash.

Headache, dizziness, indigestion, abdominal cramping.

Serious Adverse Effects

Allergic Reactions: Drug-induced hepatitis, with or without jaundice (see Glossary).

Idiosyncratic Reaction: Hemolytic anemia (see Glossary) in sensitive individuals; this is more likely to occur in the presence of impaired kidney function.

▷ **Possible Effects on Sexual Function:**   None reported.

▷ **Adverse Effects That May Mimic Natural Diseases or Disorders**

Liver reaction may suggest viral hepatitis.

CAUTION

It is important to understand that this drug is only an analgesic, and that its action is limited to the relief of symptoms. It has no curative effect on the underlying condition that is responsible for the symptoms. Consult your physician regarding the need for specific anti-infective therapy.

Precautions for Use

By Infants and Children: Consult your physician regarding appropriate dosage. Limit use to the time required for adequate relief of symptoms.

By Those over 60 Years of Age: The natural decline in kidney function that occurs after 60 may require that you use smaller doses. Observe for the development of a yellowish coloration of the eyes or skin—an indication of excessive drug accumulation. If this occurs, consult your physician.

▷ **Advisability of Use During Pregnancy**

Pregnancy Category: B (tentative). See Pregnancy Code inside back cover.

Animal studies: No birth defects found.

Human studies: Information from studies of pregnant women indicates no increase in birth defects in 1109 exposures to this drug.

Limit use to small doses for short periods of time. Ask your physician for guidance.

Advisability of Use if Breast-Feeding

Presence of this drug in breast milk: Unknown.

Avoid drug or refrain from nursing.

Habit-Forming Potential: None.

Effects of Overdosage: Nausea, vomiting, abdominal discomfort, skin discoloration, hemolytic anemia (in susceptible individuals), altered hemoglobin resulting in weakness and shortness of breath.

Possible Effects of Long-Term Use: Orange-yellow discoloration of the skin; hemolytic anemia.

Suggested Periodic Examinations While Taking This Drug (at physician's discretion)
None for short-term use; red blood cell counts and liver-function tests during long-term use.

▷ **While Taking This Drug, Observe the Following**
Foods: No restrictions.
Beverages: No restrictions.
▷   *Alcohol:* No interactions expected.
Tobacco Smoking: No interactions expected.
▷   *Other Drugs:* No significant interactions with other drugs have been reported.
▷   *Driving, Hazardous Activities:* Usually no restrictions. This drug may cause dizziness. Restrict activities as necessary.
Aviation Note: The use of this drug **may be a disqualification** for piloting. Consult a designated Aviation Medical Examiner.
Exposure to Sun: No restrictions.

PHENELZINE
(FEN el zeen)

Introduced: 1961

Class: Antidepressant, MAO type A inhibitor

Prescription: USA: Yes
Canada: Yes

Controlled Drug: USA: No
Canada: No

Available as Generic: No

Brand Name: Nardil

BENEFITS versus RISKS	
Possible Benefits	*Possible Risks*
EFFECTIVE RELIEF OF REACTIVE, NEUROTIC, ATYPICAL DEPRESSIONS with associated anxiety or phobia Beneficial in some depressions that are not responsive to other treatments	DANGEROUS INTERACTIONS WITH MANY DRUGS AND FOODS CONDUCIVE TO HYPERTENSIVE CRISIS DISORDERED HEART RATE AND RHYTHM Drug-induced hepatitis (rare) Mental changes: agitation, confusion, impaired memory, hypomania

▷ **Principal Uses**

As a Single Drug Product: This potent MAO type A inhibitor drug is used exclusively to treat severe situational (reactive or neurotic) depression, atypical depression, and (though less effective) severe endogenous depression. Because of the supervision required during its use and its potential for serious adverse effects, this drug is usually reserved to treat depressions that have not responded satisfactorily to other antidepressant therapy.

How This Drug Works: Not completely established. It is thought that by inhibiting the action of a certain enzyme (monoamine oxidase type A) in brain tissue, this drug produces an increase of those nerve impulse transmitters that maintain normal mood and emotional stability.

Available Dosage Forms and Strengths
Tablets — 15 mg

▷ **Usual Adult Dosage Range:** Initially, 15 mg 3 times/day; increase rapidly up to 60 mg/day, as needed and tolerated, until improvement is apparent. For maintenance, reduce dose gradually over several weeks to the smallest dose that will maintain optimal improvement; this may be as low as 15 mg daily or every other day. The total daily dosage should not exceed 90 mg. **Note: Actual dosage and administration schedule must be determined by the physician for each patient individually.**

▷ **Dosing Instructions:** May be taken on an empty stomach or with food. Do not take this drug in the late evening; it can interfere with sleep. The tablet may be crushed for administration.

Usual Duration of Use: Continual use on a regular schedule for 3 to 4 weeks is usually necessary to determine this drug's effectiveness in relieving depression. Once the optimal maintenance dose has been determined, it may be continued indefinitely. Long-term use (months to years) requires supervision and periodic evaluation by your physician. Consult your physician on a regular basis.

▷ **This Drug Should Not Be Taken If**
- you have had an allergic reaction to it previously.
- you have advanced heart disease.
- you have active liver disease or impaired liver function.
- you have an adrenaline-producing tumor (pheochromocytoma).
- you are taking any of the following drugs: another MAO type A inhibitor, a tricyclic antidepressant, carbamazepine (see Drug Classes, Section Four).

▷ **Inform Your Physician Before Taking This Drug If**
- you have high blood pressure.
- you have had a stroke, or you have impaired circulation to the brain.

- you have coronary heart disease.
- you have frequent or severe headaches.
- you have diabetes, epilepsy, schizophrenia or an overactive thyroid gland (hyperthyroidism).
- you have impaired kidney function.
- you plan to have surgery under general or spinal anesthesia in the near future.

Possible Side-Effects (natural, expected and unavoidable drug actions)
Insomnia if taken in the evening.
Orthostatic hypotension (see Glossary).
Fluid retention (swelling of feet and ankles).

▷ **Possible Adverse Effects** (unusual, unexpected and infrequent reactions)
If any of the following develop, consult your physician promptly for guidance.
Mild Adverse Effects
Allergic Reaction: Skin rash.
Headache, dizziness, drowsiness, weakness, agitation, confusion, impaired memory, tremors, muscle twitching, blurred vision, impaired red-green color vision.
Dry mouth, increased appetite, indigestion, constipation.
Serious Adverse Effects
Drug-induced hepatitis with jaundice (see Glossary).
Hypertensive crisis: rapid and extreme rise in blood pressure, severe throbbing headache, palpitation, nausea, vomiting, sweating, risk of brain hemorrhage.
Unusual excitement or nervousness.
Disturbances of heart rate and rhythm.

▷ **Possible Effects on Sexual Function**
Decreased libido (30% of males, 28% of females).
Impaired erection (50%); inhibited ejaculation (60%).
Inhibited orgasm (30% of males, 35% of females).

▷ **Adverse Effects That May Mimic Natural Diseases or Disorders**
Drug-induced hepatitis may suggest viral hepatitis.

Natural Diseases or Disorders That May Be Activated by This Drug
Latent epilepsy, schizophrenia.
This drug may convert a depression into the manic phase of a manic-depressive disorder.

CAUTION
1. Careful dosage adjustment is mandatory. Determine the lowest effective dose and do not exceed it.
2. The development of a severe headache or palpitation may indicate a dangerous elevation of blood pressure. Discontinue this drug immediately and consult your physician.

3. This drug may suppress anginal pain that would normally serve as a warning of excessive demand on the heart.
4. This drug may increase the possibility of hypoglycemic reactions if used concurrently with insulin or oral antidiabetic drugs (sulfonylureas; see Drug Class, Section Four). It may also delay recovery from hypoglycemia.
5. This drug can alter the threshold for convulsions in anyone with epilepsy or a seizure disorder. Dosages of anticonvulsant drugs may require adjustment.
6. This drug should be discontinued 2 weeks before elective surgery under general or spinal anesthesia. Consult your surgeon or anesthesiologist.
7. Many over-the-counter drug products contain ingredients that can cause serious interactions if taken concurrently with this drug. Avoid use of the following: cold and sinus medications, nasal decongestants, hay fever preparations, asthma inhalants, appetite and weight control products, "pep" pills. Consult your physician or pharmacist regarding their safe use with this drug.
8. It is advisable to carry a card of personal identification with the notation that you are taking this drug. Notify all medical personnel that may attend you that you are taking this drug.

Precautions for Use
By Infants and Children: Safety and effectiveness for use by those under 16 years of age have not been established.
By Those over 60 Years of Age: This drug is not recommended for use by anyone over 60. However, if poor response to other treatment justifies consideration of a trial of this drug, it is inadvisable to use it in the presence of high blood pressure, hardening of the arteries, impaired circulation within the brain or coronary artery disease. This drug will intensify existing prostatism (see Glossary). Fluid retention is more prominent in this age group.

▷ Advisability of Use During Pregnancy
Pregnancy Category: C (tentative). See Pregnancy Code inside back cover.
Animal studies: No information available.
Human studies: Information from adequate studies of pregnant women is not available. Birth defects have been reported with the use of this drug.
Avoid this drug completely if possible. Ask your physician for guidance.

Advisability of Use if Breast-Feeding
Presence of this drug in breast milk: Probably yes.
Avoid drug or refrain from nursing.

Habit-Forming Potential: None.

Effects of Overdosage: Overstimulation, agitation, anxiety, restlessness, insomnia, confusion, delirium, hallucinations, seizures, high fever, circulatory collapse, coma.

Possible Effects of Long-Term Use: The conversion of mental depression into a state of hypomania: excessive mental and physical activity, excitement, agitation, loud and rapid talking, delusional thinking.

Suggested Periodic Examinations While Taking This Drug (at physician's discretion)
Blood pressure measurements in lying, sitting and standing positions. Complete blood cell counts, liver function tests.

▷ **While Taking This Drug, Observe the Following**
*Foods: **All tyramine-rich foods should be avoided completely.*** See Tyramine in the Glossary for a compete list of foods and beverages to avoid while taking this drug.
Beverages: Limit coffee, tea and cola beverages to one serving daily. See Tyramine in the Glossary.
▷ *Alcohol:* Use extreme caution until the combined effects have been determined. Alcohol can increase the depressant effects of this drug on brain function.
Tobacco Smoking: No interactions expected.
▷ *Other Drugs*
Phenelzine may ***increase*** the effects of
• amphetamine and related drugs.
• appetite suppressants.
• all drugs with stimulant effects on the nervous system, and cause excessive rise in blood pressure.
• all drugs with sedative effects, and cause excessive sedation.
• insulin.
• sulfonylureas (see Drug Class, Section Four).
Phenelzine ***taken concurrently*** with
• carbamazepine (Tegretol) may cause severe toxic reactions.
• levodopa (Dopar, Sinemet) may cause a dangerous rise in blood pressure.
• meperidine (Demerol) may cause high fever, seizures and coma.
• methyldopa (Aldomet) may cause a dangerous rise in blood pressure.
• methylphenidate (Ritalin) may cause severe headache, weakness and numbness in the extremities.
• tricyclic antidepressants may cause severe toxic reactions including high fever, delirium, tremor, seizures and coma.
Note: Consult your physician before taking ***any other drugs*** while taking phenelzine.
▷ *Driving, Hazardous Activities:* This drug may cause dizziness, drowsiness and blurred vision. Restrict activities as necessary.
Aviation Note: The use of this drug ***is a disqualification*** for piloting. Consult a designated Aviation Medical Examiner.
Exposure to Sun: No restrictions.
Occurrence of Unrelated Illness: Because of the very serious and life-threatening interactions that can occur between this drug and many others, it is mandatory that you inform each physician and dentist you consult that you are taking this drug.

Discontinuation: If this drug is not effective after 4 weeks of continual use, it should be discontinued. If it is effective, continue to take it in proper dosage until advised to stop. Do not discontinue it abruptly. If another antidepressant is to be tried, a drug-free waiting period of 14 days must elapse between the discontinuation of this drug and initiation of the new one. All precautions regarding the avoidance of tyramine-rich foods and other drugs must be observed during this 14-day period.

PHENOBARBITAL
(fee noh BAR bi tawl)

Other Name: Phenobarbitone

Introduced: 1912

Class: Sedative, anticonvulsant, barbiturates

Prescription: USA: Yes
Canada: Yes

Controlled Drug: USA: C-IV*
Canada: <C>

Available as Generic: Yes

Brand Names: Barbidonna [CD], Barbidonna Elixir [CD], Barbita, Belladenal [CD], Belladenal-S [CD], ✦Belladenal Spacetabs [CD], ✦Bellergal [CD], Bellergal-S [CD], ✦Bellergal Spacetabs [CD], Bronchotabs [CD], Bronkolixir [CD], Chardonna-2 [CD], ✦Diclophen [CD], Dilantin w/Phenobarbital [CD], Donnatal [CD], Donnazyme [CD], ✦Gardenal, Kinesed [CD], Luminal, Mudrane GG Elixir & Tablets [CD], Mudrane Tablets [CD], ✦Neuro-Spasex [CD], ✦Neuro-Trasentin [CD], ✦Neuro-Trasentin Forte [CD], ✦Phenaphen Capsules [CD], ✦Phenaphen No. 2, 3, 4 [CD], Quadrinal [CD], Solfoton, Tedral Preparations [CD]

BENEFITS versus RISKS

Possible Benefits	*Possible Risks*
EFFECTIVE CONTROL OF TONIC-CLONIC SEIZURES AND ALL TYPES OF PARTIAL SEIZURES	POTENTIAL FOR DEPENDENCE LIFE-THREATENING TOXICITY WITH OVERDOSAGE
EFFECTIVE CONTROL OF FEBRILE SEIZURES OF CHILDHOOD	Drug-induced hepatitis
Effective relief of anxiety and nervous tension	Rare blood cell disorders: abnormally low red cell, white cell and platelet counts

---

*See Schedules of Controlled Drugs inside back cover.

▷ **Principal Uses**

> *As a Single Drug Product:* This barbiturate drug has two primary uses: (1) as a mild sedative to relieve anxiety, nervous tension and insomnia; and (2) as an anticonvulsant to control grand mal epilepsy and all types of partial seizures. It is also used to control febrile seizures of childhood.

> *As a Combination Drug Product* [CD]: This drug is available in many combinations with derivatives of belladonna, an antispasmodic commonly used to treat functional disorders of the gastrointestinal tract. It is also available in combination with bronchodilators for the treatment of asthma, and with ergotamine for the treatment of headaches.

How This Drug Works: Not completely established. It is thought that by impeding the transfer of sodium and potassium across cell membranes, this drug selectively blocks the transmission of nerve impulses. This could serve to produce a sedative effect and to suppress the spread of nerve impulses that are responsible for epileptic seizures.

Available Dosage Forms and Strengths
> Capsules — 16 mg
> > Elixir — 15 mg, 20 mg per 5-ml teaspoonful
> > Tablets — 8 mg, 16 mg, 32 mg, 65 mg, 100 mg

▷ **Usual Adult Dosage Range:**   As sedative: 15 to 30 mg 2 to 4 times/day. As hypnotic: 100 to 200 mg at bedtime. As anticonvulsant: 100 to 200 mg given as a single dose at bedtime. The total daily dosage should not exceed 600 mg. **Note: Actual dosage and administration schedule must be determined by the physician for each patient individually.**

▷ **Dosing Instructions:**   May be taken with or after food to reduce stomach irritation. Regular tablets may be crushed and capsules opened for administration. Prolonged-action dosage forms should be swallowed whole without alteration.

Usual Duration of Use: Continual use on a regular schedule for 3 to 5 days is usually necessary to determine this drug's effectiveness in relieving anxiety and tension, and for 4 to 6 weeks to determine its ability to control seizures. If used to treat anxiety-tension states, its use should not exceed 4 weeks without reappraisal of continued need. Long-term use for seizure control (months to years) requires supervision and periodic evaluation by your physician. Consult your physician on a regular basis.

▷ **This Drug Should Not Be Taken If**
- you have had an allergic reaction to it previously.
- you are subject to acute intermittent porphyria (see Glossary).

▷ **Inform Your Physician Before Taking This Drug If**
- you are allergic or overly sensitive to any barbiturate drug (see Drug Class, Section Four).

- you are pregnant or planning pregnancy.
- you have a history of alcohol or drug abuse.
- you are taking any drugs with sedative effects.
- you have any type of seizure disorder.
- you have myasthenia gravis.
- you have impaired liver, kidney or thyroid gland function.
- you plan to have surgery under general anesthesia in the near future.

Possible Side-Effects (natural, expected and unavoidable drug actions)
Drowsiness, impaired concentration, mental and physical sluggishness.

▷ **Possible Adverse Effects** (unusual, unexpected and infrequent reactions)
If any of the following develop, consult your physician promptly for guidance.
Mild Adverse Effects
Allergic Reactions: Skin rashes, hives, localized swellings of face, drug fever (see Glossary).
Dizziness, unsteadiness, impaired vision, double vision.
Nausea, vomiting, diarrhea.
Shoulder-hand syndrome: pain and stiffness in the shoulder, pain and swelling in the hand.
Serious Adverse Effects
Allergic Reactions: Drug-induced hepatitis with jaundice (see Glossary).
Idiosyncratic Reactions: Paradoxical excitement and delirium (instead of sedation).
Mental depression, abnormal involuntary movements.
Blood cell disorders: deficiencies of all blood cell types causing fatigue, weakness, fever, sore throat, abnormal bleeding or bruising.

▷ **Possible Effects on Sexual Function**
Decreased libido and/or impotence (16%).
Decreased effectiveness of oral contraceptives taken concurrently (71%).

▷ **Adverse Effects That May Mimic Natural Diseases or Disorders**
Liver reactions may suggest viral hepatitis.

Natural Diseases or Disorders That May Be Activated by This Drug
Acute intermittent and/or cutaneous porphyria, systemic lupus erythematosus.

CAUTION
1. Anticonvulsant drug therapy must be carefully individualized. Accurate diagnosis and classification of the seizure pattern are essential to the correct selection of the most appropriate drug for seizure control.
2. Emotional stress or physical trauma (including surgery) may require increased anticonvulsant dosage to control seizures.
3. Prolonged-action dosage forms of this drug are not appropriate for the treatment of seizures and should not be used.

Precautions for Use

By Infants and Children: This drug should not be given to the hyperkinetic child. Observe for possible paradoxical stimulation and hyperactivity; this can occur in 10% to 40% of children. Changes associated with puberty characteristically slow the metabolism of this drug and permit its gradual accumulation. Blood levels of this drug in young adolescents should be monitored every 3 months to detect rising concentrations and early toxicity. Adjust dosage as necessary.

By Those over 60 Years of Age: It is advisable to avoid all barbiturates in the elderly. If use of this drug is attempted, start with small doses until tolerance has been determined. Observe for confusion, delirium, agitation and excitement. Do not use this drug concurrently with other drugs for mental disorders. This drug is conducive to the development of hypothermia (see Glossary).

▷ **Advisability of Use During Pregnancy**

Pregnancy Category: D (tentative). See Pregnancy Code inside back cover.

Animal studies: Conflicting reports of cleft palate and skeletal defects in mouse, rat and rabbit studies.

Human studies: Information from studies of pregnant women indicates no increase in birth defects in 8037 exposures to this drug. However, it is reported that barbiturates can cause fetal damage when taken during pregnancy.

Avoid use of drug during entire pregnancy if possible. If it is clearly needed to control seizures, the mother should receive vitamin K prior to delivery and the infant should receive it at birth.

Advisability of Use if Breast-Feeding

Presence of this drug in breast milk: Yes, in small amounts.

Monitor nursing infant closely and discontinue drug or nursing if adverse effects develop.

Habit-Forming Potential: Psychological and physical dependence can occur with prolonged use of excessive doses—300 to 700 mg/day for 1 to 2 months. Dependence is not likely to occur with usual sedative or anticonvulsant doses.

Effects of Overdosage: Behavior similar to alcoholic intoxication: confusion, slurred speech, physical incoordination, staggering gait, drowsiness, stupor progressing to coma.

Possible Effects of Long-Term Use: Psychological and/or physical dependence; syndrome of chronic intoxication: headache, depression, impaired vision, dizziness, slurred speech, incoordination. Megaloblastic anemia due to folic acid deficiency. Rickets or osteomalacia due to deficiencies of vitamin D and calcium.

Suggested Periodic Examinations While Taking This Drug (at physician's discretion)

Complete blood cell counts, liver function tests.

During long-term use: blood levels of folic acid, vitamin B-12, calcium and phosphorus; skeletal X-ray studies for demineralization of bone.

▷ **While Taking This Drug, Observe the Following**
    Foods: No restrictions. Eat liberally of foods rich in folic acid: fortified breakfast cereals, liver, legumes, green leafy vegetables.
    Beverages: No restrictions. May be taken with milk or fruit juices.
▷   *Alcohol:* Avoid completely. Alcohol can increase greatly the sedative and depressant actions of this drug on brain functions.
    Tobacco Smoking: May enhance the sedative effects of this drug and increase drowsiness.
    Marijuana Smoking: Increased drowsiness, unsteadiness; significantly impaired mental and physical performance.
▷   *Other Drugs*
    Phenobarbital may *increase* the effects of
    • all other drugs with sedative effects, and cause excessive sedation.
    Phenobarbital may *decrease* the effects of
    • anticoagulants (Coumadin, etc.), and require dosage adjustments.
    • certain beta blockers (Inderal, Lopressor), and reduce their effectiveness.
    • cortisonelike drugs.
    • doxycycline (Vibramycin), and reduce its effectiveness.
    • griseofulvin (Fulvicin, etc.), and reduce its effectiveness.
    • oral contraceptives, and reduce their effectiveness in preventing pregnancy.
    • quinidine (Quinaglute, etc.), and reduce its effectiveness.
    • theophyllines (Aminophyllin, Theo-Dur, etc.), and reduce their antiasthmatic effectiveness.
    Phenobarbital *taken concurrently* with
    • phenytoin (Dilantin) may alter phenytoin blood levels: a high phenobarbital level will increase the phenytoin level; a low phenobarbital level will decrease the phenytoin level. Periodic determination of blood levels of both drugs is advised.
    The following drugs may *increase* the effects of phenobarbital
    • valproic acid (Depakene).
▷   *Driving, Hazardous Activities:* This drug may cause drowsiness and may impair mental alertness, judgment, physical coordination and reaction time. Restrict activities as necessary.
    Aviation Note: The use of this drug *is a disqualification* for piloting. Consult a designated Aviation Medical Examiner.
    Exposure to Sun: Use caution until sensitivity has been determined. This drug may cause photosensitivity.
    Exposure to Cold: Observe the elderly for possible hypothermia (see Glossary) while taking this drug.
    Discontinuation: If used as an anticonvulsant, this drug must not be discontinued abruptly. Sudden withdrawal can precipitate status epilepticus (repetitive seizures). Gradual reduction in dosage should be made over a period of 3 months. Total drug withdrawal may be attempted after a period of 3 to 5 years without a seizure. However, seizures are likely to recur in 40% of adults and in 20% to 30% of children.

PHENYLBUTAZONE
(fen il BYU ta zohn)

Introduced: 1949

Class: Mild analgesic, anti-inflammatory

Prescription: USA: Yes
Canada: Yes

Controlled Drug: USA: No
Canada: No

Available as Generic: Yes

Brand Names: ✦Apo-Phenylbutazone, Azolid, Butazolidin, ✦Butone [CD], ✦Intrabutazone, ✦Neo-Zoline-M [CD], ✦Novobutazone, ✦Phenbuff

---

BENEFITS versus RISKS

Possible Benefits	*Possible Risks*
PROMPT, EFFECTIVE RELIEF OF INFLAMMATION AND PAIN IN MODERATELY SEVERE ARTHRITIS, GOUT, BURSITIS AND SUPERFICIAL PHLEBITIS (FOR SHORT-TERM USE)	BONE MARROW DEPRESSION MAY BE SEVERE DRUG-INDUCED HEPATITIS KIDNEY DAMAGE, IMPAIRED FUNCTION GASTROINTESTINAL ULCER FORMATION AND BLEEDING HYPERTENSION HEART MUSCLE DAMAGE EYE DAMAGE: OPTIC NEURITIS EAR DAMAGE: HEARING LOSS

▷ **Principal Uses**

As a Single Drug Product: This potent anti-inflammatory drug is used primarily for the short-term relief of pain and inflammation associated with moderately severe arthritis, gout, bursitis, tendinitis and superficial phlebitis. Because of its potential for severe toxicity, it is not considered to be an "aspirin substitute." Its use should be limited to those conditions that do not respond to less toxic drugs.

How This Drug Works: Not completely established. It is thought that this drug acts somewhat like aspirin, by suppressing the formation of prostaglandins and related substances that are involved in the production of inflammation.

Available Dosage Forms and Strengths
Capsules — 100 mg
Tablets — 100 mg

▷ **Usual Adult Dosage Range:** For arthritis: Initially, 100 to 200 mg 3 times/day; for maintenance, 100 mg 1 to 4 times/day. For acute gout: Initially, 400 mg as a single dose; then 100 mg/4 hours for 4 days or until the acute attack is relieved; continual use should not exceed 1 week. Alternate course for gout: 200 mg/4 hours for 4 days or until acute attack is relieved; continual use should not exceed 2 weeks. **Note: Actual dosage and administration schedule must be determined by the physician for each patient individually.**

▷ **Dosing Instructions:**   Take with or following food to reduce stomach irritation. The tablet may be crushed and the capsule may be opened for administration.

Usual Duration of Use: Continual use on a regular schedule for 2 to 5 days is usually necessary to determine this drug's effectiveness in relieving acute pain in arthritis, gout and related conditions. This drug should be limited to short-term use only. If significant improvement does not occur within 1 week, this drug should be discontinued. The maximal period of continual use should not exceed 10 to 14 days.

▷ **This Drug Should Not Be Taken If**
- you have had an allergic reaction to it previously, or to oxyphenbutazone (Tandearil), a closely related drug.
- you have a history of serious adverse effects from drugs.
- you have a history of a blood cell or bone marrow disorder.
- you have a history of stomach or intestinal ulceration or bleeding.
- you have a history of disease or impaired function of the thyroid, heart, liver or kidneys.
- you have high blood pressure.

▷ **Inform Your Physician Before Taking This Drug If**
- you are allergic to aspirin or aspirin substitutes (anti-inflammatory analgesics).
- you are taking any other drugs at this time, either prescription or over-the-counter drugs.
- you are taking anticoagulants.
- you have glaucoma.

Possible Side-Effects (natural, expected and unavoidable drug actions)
Salt and water retention, reduced urine output.

▷ **Possible Adverse Effects** (unusual, unexpected and infrequent reactions)
If any of the following develop, consult your physician promptly for guidance.
Mild Adverse Effects
Allergic Reactions: Skin rashes, hives, itching, drug fever (see Glossary).
Headache, drowsiness, lethargy, nervousness, confusion, tremors.
Indigestion, stomach pain, nausea, vomiting, diarrhea.
Progressive gain in weight and rise in blood pressure; these are indications to discontinue this drug.
Serious Adverse Effects
Allergic Reactions: Severe skin reactions, high fever, swollen and painful joints, salivary gland enlargement, anaphylactic reaction (see Glossary).

Bone marrow depression (see Glossary): fatigue, weakness, fever, sore throat, abnormal bleeding or bruising.

Drug-induced hepatitis, with or without jaundice (see Glossary).

Kidney damage, impaired kidney function, kidney failure.

Stomach and intestinal ulceration and/or bleeding.

Damage to heart muscle (myocarditis) and heart covering (pericarditis).

Eye damage: injuries to optic nerve and retina, impaired vision.

Ear damage: loss of hearing.

▷ **Possible Effects on Sexual Function:**   None reported.

Possible Delayed Adverse Effects: The development of leukemia following the use of this drug has been reported. A cause-and-effect relationship (see Glossary) has not been established.

▷ **Adverse Effects That May Mimic Natural Diseases or Disorders**
Liver reactions may suggest viral hepatitis.

Natural Diseases or Disorders That May Be Activated by This Drug
Latent hypertension, peptic ulcer disease, ulcerative colitis.

CAUTION
1. This drug should never be used for mild and trivial conditions. It has high potential for serious and life-threatening adverse effects.
2. Follow your physician's instructions fully regarding periodic examinations while taking this drug. These are essential for the early detection of possible adverse effects.

Precautions for Use
By Infants and Children: Safety and effectiveness for use by those under 15 years of age have not been established.
By Those over 60 Years of Age: Many authorities advise that this drug should not be used by this age group. More than 60% of users over 61 years of age experience adverse effects from this drug. The elderly and the debilitated are clearly more vulnerable to the toxic effects of this drug. Its use is not recommended.

▷ **Advisability of Use During Pregnancy**
Pregnancy Category: D (tentative). See Pregnancy Code inside back cover.
Animal studies: Evidence of embryo toxicity reported.
Human studies: Information from adequate studies of pregnant women is not available. Two cases of birth defects following use of this drug have been reported. A causal relationship has not been established.
One manufacturer of this drug recommends that it not be used during pregnancy.

Advisability of Use if Breast-Feeding
Presence of this drug in breast milk: Yes.
Avoid drug or refrain from nursing.

Habit-Forming Potential: None.

Effects of Overdosage: Headache, dizziness, insomnia, mental and behavioral disturbances, hallucinations, seizures, coma.

Possible Effects of Long-Term Use: Bone marrow depression. Development of thyroid gland enlargement (goiter), with or without altered function.

Suggested Periodic Examinations While Taking This Drug (at physician's discretion)
Complete blood cell counts and urine analysis should be made before the drug is taken and during the course of treatment at intervals of 1 to 2 weeks.
Liver function tests.

▷ **While Taking This Drug, Observe the Following**
Foods: No restrictions. Avoid excessive salt.
Beverages: No restrictions. May be taken with milk.
▷ *Alcohol:* Avoid completely because of its irritant effect on the stomach, increasing the risk of ulceration and bleeding.
Tobacco Smoking: No interactions expected.
▷ *Other Drugs*
Phenylbutazone may ***increase*** the effects of
  • anticoagulants (Coumadin, etc.), and cause bleeding.
  • lithium (Lithane, Lithotabs, etc.), and increase the risk of lithium toxicity.
  • phenytoin (Dilantin), and cause phenytoin toxicity.
  • sulfonylureas (see Drug Class, Section Four), and increase the risk of hypoglycemia.
▷ *Driving, Hazardous Activities:* This drug may cause dizziness, confusion and impaired vision or hearing. Restrict activities as necessary.
Aviation Note: The use of this drug ***may be a disqualification*** for piloting. Consult a designated Aviation Medical Examiner.
Exposure to Sun: Use caution until sensitivity has been determined. This drug may cause photosensitivity (see Glossary).

PHENYTOIN
(FEN i toh in)

Other Name: Diphenylhydantoin

Introduced: 1938

Class: Anticonvulsant, hydantoins

Prescription: USA: Yes
Canada: Yes

Controlled Drug: USA: No
Canada: No

Available as Generic: USA: Yes
Canada: No

Brand Names: Dilantin, Dilantin w/Phenobarbital [CD], Diphenylan, ◆Mebroin [CD]

BENEFITS versus RISKS	
Possible Benefits	*Possible Risks*
EFFECTIVE CONTROL OF TONIC-CLONIC (GRAND MAL), PSYCHOMOTOR (TEMPORAL LOBE), MYOCLONIC AND FOCAL SEIZURES IN 80% OF USERS	VERY NARROW TREATMENT MARGIN POSSIBLE BIRTH DEFECTS Overgrowth of gums Excessive hair growth Rare blood cell disorders: impaired production of all blood cells Drug-induced hepatitis Drug-induced nephritis

---

▷ **Principal Uses**

As a Single Drug Product: Used primarily as an antiepileptic drug to control grand mal, psychomotor, myoclonic and focal seizures. Though not officially approved, this drug is also used to initiate treatment of trigeminal neuralgia; it is sometimes effective in relieving the severe facial pain of this disorder.

As a Combination Drug Product [CD]: This drug is available in combination with phenobarbital, another effective anticonvulsant. Some seizure disorders require the combined actions of these two drugs for effective control.

How This Drug Works: Not completely established. It is thought that by promoting the loss of sodium from nerve fibers, this drug lowers and stabilizes their excitability and thereby inhibits the repetitious spread of electrical impulses along nerve pathways. This action may prevent seizures altogether, or it may reduce their frequency and severity.

Available Dosage Forms and Strengths

Capsules (extended) — 30 mg, 100 mg
Capsules (prompt) — 30 mg, 100 mg
Injection — 50 mg per ml
Oral suspension — 30 mg, 125 mg per 5-ml teaspoonful
Tablets, chewable — 50 mg

▷ **Usual Adult Dosage Range:** Initially, 100 mg 3 times/day. Dose may be increased cautiously by 100 mg/week as needed and tolerated. After the optimal maintenance dose has been determined, the total daily dose may be taken as a single dose every 24 hours if Dilantin capsules are used. No other formulation is approved for once-a-day use. The total daily dosage should not exceed 600 mg. **Note: Actual dosage and administration schedule must be determined by the physician for each patient individually.**

▷ **Dosing Instructions:** May be taken with or after food to reduce stomach irritation. The capsule may be opened and the tablet may be crushed for administration.

Usual Duration of Use: Continual use on a regular schedule for 2 to 3 weeks is usually necessary to determine this drug's effectiveness in reducing the frequency and severity of seizures. Optimal control will require careful dosage adjustments over a period of several months. Long-term use (months to years) requires ongoing supervision and periodic evaluation by your physician. Consult your physician on a regular basis.

▷ **This Drug Should Not Be Taken If**
- you have had an allergic reaction to this drug or to other hydantoin drugs previously.

▷ **Inform Your Physician Before Taking This Drug If**
- you are taking any other drugs at this time.
- you have a history of liver disease or impaired liver function.
- you have low blood pressure, diabetes or any type of heart disease.
- you plan to have surgery under general anesthesia in the near future.

Possible Side-Effects (natural, expected and unavoidable drug actions)
Mild fatigue, sluggishness and drowsiness (in sensitive individuals).
Pink to red to brown coloration of urine (of no significance).

▷ **Possible Adverse Effects** (unusual, unexpected and infrequent reactions)
If any of the following develop, consult your physician promptly for guidance.
Mild Adverse Effects
Allergic Reactions: Skin rashes (5% to 10%), hives, drug fever (see Glossary).
Headache, dizziness, nervousness, insomnia, muscle twitching.
Nausea, vomiting, constipation.
Overgrowth of gum tissues (most common in children).
Excessive growth of body hair (most common in young girls).
Serious Adverse Effects
Allergic Reactions: Drug-induced hepatitis, with or without jaundice (see Glossary). Drug-induced nephritis, with acute kidney failure. Severe skin reactions. Generalized enlargement of lymph glands (pseudolymphoma).
Idiosyncratic Reaction: Hemolytic anemia (see Glossary).
Acute psychotic episodes (rare).
Bone marrow depression (see Glossary): fatigue, weakness, fever, sore throat, abnormal bleeding or bruising.
Mental confusion, unsteadiness, double vision, jerky eye movements, slurred speech.
Joint pain and swelling.
Elevated blood sugar, due to inhibition of insulin release.

▷ **Possible Effects on Sexual Function**
Decreased libido and/or impotence (11%).
Peyronie's disease (see Glossary).
Decreased effectiveness of oral contraceptives taken concurrently (24%).

▷ **Adverse Effects That May Mimic Natural Diseases or Disorders**
Drug-induced hepatitis may suggest viral hepatitis.
Skin reactions may resemble lupus erythematosus.

Natural Diseases or Disorders That May Be Activated by This Drug
Latent diabetes, porphyria, systemic lupus erythematosus.

CAUTION
1. Some brand name capsules of this drug have a significantly longer duration of action than generic name capsules of the same strength. To assure a correct dosing schedule, it is necessary to distinguish between "prompt" action and "extended" action capsules. Do not substitute one for the other without your physician's knowledge and guidance.
2. When used for the treatment of epilepsy, *this drug must not be stopped abruptly.*
3. The wide variation of this drug's action from person to person requires careful individualization of dosage schedules. Periodic measurements of blood levels of this drug can be very helpful in determining appropriate dosage. (See Therapeutic Drug Monitoring in Section One.)
4. Regularity of drug use is essential for successful management of seizure disorders. Take this drug at the same time each day.
5. Shake the suspension form of this drug thoroughly before measuring the dose. Use a standard measuring device to assure that the dose is based upon a 5-ml teaspoon.
6. Side-effects and mild adverse effects are usually most apparent during the first several days of treatment, and often subside with continued use.
7. It may be necessary to take folic acid to prevent anemia while taking this drug. Consult your physician regarding this.
8. It is advisable to carry a card of personal identification with a notation that you are taking this drug.

Precautions for Use
By Infants and Children: Elimination of this drug varies widely with age. Careful monitoring by periodic measurement of blood levels is essential for all ages. Some children will require more than one dose daily for good control. Observe for early indications of drug toxicity: jerky eye movements, unsteadiness in stance and gait, slurred speech, abnormal involuntary movements of the extremities and odd behavior.
By Those over 60 Years of Age: You may be more sensitive to all of the actions of this drug and require smaller doses. Observe closely for any indications of early toxicity: drowsiness, fatigue, confusion, unsteadiness, disturbances of vision, slurred speech, muscle twitching.

▷ **Advisability of Use During Pregnancy**

Pregnancy Category: D (tentative). See Pregnancy Code inside back cover.

Animal studies: Cleft lip and palate, skeletal and visceral defects in mice; skeletal and visceral defects in rats.

Human studies: Available information is conflicting. Some studies suggest a small but significant increase in the occurrence of birth defects associated with the use of phenytoin during pregnancy. The incidence of birth defects in children of epileptics not taking anticonvulsant drugs is 3.2%; the incidence with the use of anticonvulsant drugs during pregnancy increases to 6.4%. The "fetal hydantoin syndrome" in the newborn infant exposed to phenytoin during pregnancy consists of birth defects of the skull, face and limbs, deficient growth and development, and subnormal intelligence and performance. Other effects on the infant include reduction in blood clotting factors that predispose it to severe bruising and hemorrhage.

Discuss with your physician the advantages and possible disadvantages of using this drug during pregnancy. It is advisable to use the smallest maintenance dose that will control seizures. In addition, you should be given vitamin K during the last month of pregnancy to prevent a deficiency of blood clotting factors in the fetus.

Advisability of Use if Breast-Feeding

Presence of this drug in breast milk: Yes, in trace amounts.

Monitor nursing infant closely and discontinue drug or nursing if adverse effects develop.

Habit-Forming Potential: None.

Effects of Overdosage: Drowsiness, jerky eye movements, hand tremor, unsteadiness, slurred speech, hallucinations, delusions, nausea, vomiting, stupor progressing to coma.

Possible Effects of Long-Term Use: Low blood calcium resulting in rickets or osteomalacia; megaloblastic anemia; peripheral neuropathy (see Glossary); schizophreniclike psychosis. Lymphosarcoma, malignant lymphoma and leukemia have been associated with long-term use; a cause-and-effect relationship (see Glossary) has not been established.

Suggested Periodic Examinations While Taking This Drug (at physician's discretion)

Monitoring of blood phenytoin levels to guide dosage.

Complete blood cell counts, liver function tests.

Measurements of the following blood levels: glucose, calcium, phosphorus, folic acid, vitamin B-12.

Skeletal X-ray studies for demineralization of bone.

▷ **While Taking This Drug, Observe the Following**

Foods: No restrictions.

Nutritional Support: Supplements of folic acid, calcium, vitamin D and vitamin K may be necessary.

Beverages: No restrictions. May be taken with milk.

▷ *Alcohol:* Use extreme caution until the combined effects have been determined. Alcohol (in large quantities or with continual use) may reduce this drug's effectiveness in preventing seizures.

Tobacco Smoking: No interactions expected.

▷ *Other Drugs*

Phenytoin may ***decrease*** the effects of
- cortisonelike drugs (see Drug Class, Section Four).
- cyclosporine.
- doxycycline (Vibramycin, etc.).
- levodopa (Larodopa, Sinemet).
- methadone (Dolophine).
- mexiletine (Mexitil).
- oral contraceptives.
- quinidine (Quinaglute, etc.).

Phenytoin ***taken concurrently*** with
- oral anticoagulants (Coumadin, etc.) can either increase or decrease the anticoagulant effect; monitor this combination very closely with serial prothrombin testing.
- primidone (Mysoline) may alter primidone actions and enhance its toxicity.
- theophyllines (Aminophyllin, Theo-Dur, etc.) may cause a decrease in the effectiveness of both drugs.

The following drugs may ***increase*** the effects of phenytoin
- chloramphenicol (Chloromycetin).
- cimetidine (Tagamet).
- disulfiram (Antabuse).
- isoniazid (INH, Niconyl, etc.).
- phenacemide (Phenurone).
- phenylbutazone (Butazolidin).
- sulfonamides (see Drug Class, Section Four).
- trimethoprim (Proloprim, Trimpex).
- valproic acid (Depakene).

The following drugs may ***decrease*** the effects of phenytoin
- bleomycin.
- carmustine.
- cisplatin.
- diazoxide.
- folic acid.
- methotrexate.
- rifampin.
- vinblastine.

▷ *Driving, Hazardous Activities:* This drug may impair mental alertness, vision and coordination. Restrict activities as necessary.

Aviation Note: The use of this drug ***is a disqualification*** for piloting. Consult a designated Aviation Medical Examiner.

Exposure to Sun: Use caution. This drug may cause photosensitivity (see Glossary).

Occurrence of Unrelated Illness: Intercurrent infections may slow the elimination of this drug and increase the risk of toxicity due to higher blood levels.

Discontinuation: **This drug must not be discontinued abruptly.** Sudden withdrawal can precipitate severe and repeated seizures. If this drug is to be discontinued, gradual reduction in dosage should be made over a period of 3 months. Total drug withdrawal may be attempted after a period of 3 to 4 years without a seizure. However, seizures are likely to recur in 40% of adults and in 20% to 30% of children.

PILOCARPINE
(pi loh KAR peen)

Introduced: 1875

Prescription: USA: Yes
  Canada: No

Class: Antiglaucoma

Controlled Drug: USA: No
  Canada: No

Available as Generic: Yes

Brand Names: Almocarpine, E-Pilo Preparations [CD], Isopto Carpine, ◆Minims, ◆Miocarpine, Ocusert Pilo-20,-40, PE Preparations [CD], Pilagan, Pilocar, ◆Pilopine HS

BENEFITS versus RISKS

Possible Benefits	*Possible Risks*
EFFECTIVE REDUCTION OF INTERNAL EYE PRESSURE FOR CONTROL OF ACUTE AND CHRONIC GLAUCOMA	Mild side-effects with systemic absorption Minor eye discomfort Altered vision

---

▷ **Principal Uses**

As a Single Drug Product: This drug is used exclusively for the management of all types of glaucoma. Selection of the appropriate dosage form and strength must be carefully individualized.

As a Combination Drug Product [CD]: This drug is combined with epinephrine (in eye drop solutions) to utilize the actions of both drugs in lowering internal eye pressure. The opposite effects of these two drugs on the size of the pupil (pilocarpine constricts, epinephrine dilates) provides a balance that prevents excessive constriction or dilation.

How This Drug Works: By directly stimulating constriction of the pupil, this drug enlarges the outflow canal in the anterior chamber of the eye and promotes the drainage of excess fluid (aqueous humor), thus lowering the internal eye pressure.

Available Dosage Forms and Strengths
Eye drop solutions — 0.25%, 0.5%, 1%, 2%, 3%, 4%, 5%, 6%, 8%, 10%

Gel — 4%

Ocuserts — 20 mcg, 40 mcg

▷ **Usual Adult Dosage Range:** For chronic glaucoma: Eye drop solutions—1 drop of a 0.5% to 4% solution 4 times/day. Eye gel—apply 0.5 inch strip of gel into the eye once daily at bedtime. Ocusert—insert one into affected eye and replace every 7 days with a new one. **Note: Actual dosage and administration schedule must be determined by the physician for each patient individually.**

▷ **Dosing Instructions:** To avoid excessive absorption into the body, press finger against inner corner of the eye (to close off the tear duct) during and for 2 minutes following instillation of the eye drop. Place the gel and the Ocusert in the eye at bedtime.

Usual Duration of Use: Continual use on a regular schedule for 1 to 2 weeks is usually necessary to determine this drug's effectiveness in controlling internal eye pressure. Long-term use (months to years) requires supervision and periodic evaluation by your physician. Consult your physician on a regular basis.

▷ **This Drug Should Not Be Taken If**
- you have had an allergic reaction to it previously.
- you have active bronchial asthma.

▷ **Inform Your Physician Before Taking This Drug If**
- you have a history of bronchial asthma.
- you have a history acute iritis.

Possible Side-Effects (natural, expected and unavoidable drug actions)
Temporary impairment of vision, usually lasting 2 to 3 hours following instillation of drops.

▷ **Possible Adverse Effects** (unusual, unexpected and infrequent reactions)
If any of the following develop, consult your physician promptly for guidance.
Mild Adverse Effects
Allergic Reactions: Itching of the eyes, itching and/or swelling of the eyelids.
Headache, heart palpitation, tremors.
Serious Adverse Effects
Provocation of acute asthma in susceptible individuals.

▷ **Possible Effects on Sexual Function:** None reported.

Precautions for Use
By Those over 60 Years of Age: Maintain personal cleanliness to prevent eye infections. Report promptly any indication of possible infection involving the eyes.

▷ **Advisability of Use During Pregnancy**
Pregnancy Category: C (tentative). See Pregnancy Code inside back cover.
Animal studies: Significant birth defects due to this drug reported in rats.
Human studies: Information from adequate studies of pregnant women is not available.
Limit use to the smallest effective dose. Minimize systemic absorption (see Dosing Instructions).

Advisability of Use if Breast-Feeding
Presence of this drug in breast milk: May be present in small amounts.
Monitor nursing infant closely and discontinue drug or nursing if adverse effects develop.

Habit-Forming Potential: None.

Effects of Overdosage: Flushing of face, increased flow of saliva, sweating. If solution is swallowed: nausea, vomiting, diarrhea, profuse sweating, rapid pulse, difficult breathing, loss of consciousness.

Possible Effects of Long-Term Use: Development of tolerance (see Glossary), temporary loss of effectiveness.

Suggested Periodic Examinations While Taking This Drug (at physician's discretion)
Measurement of internal eye pressure on a regular basis.
Examination of eyes for development of cataracts.

▷ **While Taking This Drug, Observe the Following**
Foods: No restrictions.
Beverages: No restrictions.
▷ *Alcohol:* Use caution until the combined effect has been determined. If this drug is absorbed, it may prolong the effect of alcohol on the brain.
Tobacco Smoking: No interactions expected.
Marijuana Smoking: Sustained additional decrease in internal eye pressure.
▷ *Other Drugs*
The following drugs may *decrease* the effects of pilocarpine
• atropine and drugs with atropinelike actions (see Drug Class, Section Four).
▷ *Driving, Hazardous Activities:* This drug may impair your ability to focus your vision properly. Restrict activities as necessary.
Aviation Note: The use of this drug *may be a disqualification* for piloting. Consult a designated Aviation Medical Examiner.
Exposure to Sun: No restrictions.
Discontinuation: Do not discontinue the regular use of this drug without consulting your physician. Periodic discontinuation and temporary substitution of another drug may be necessary to preserve its effectiveness in treating glaucoma.

PINDOLOL
(PIN doh lohl)

Introduced: 1972

Class: Antihypertensive, beta-adrenergic blocker

Prescription: USA: Yes
Canada: Yes

Controlled Drug: USA: No
Canada: No

Available as Generic: No

Brand Names: ♦Viskazide [CD], Visken

BENEFITS versus RISKS

Possible Benefits	*Possible Risks*
EFFECTIVE, WELL-TOLERATED ANTIHYPERTENSIVE in mild to moderate high blood pressure	CONGESTIVE HEART FAILURE in advanced heart disease Worsening of angina in coronary heart disease (abrupt withdrawal) Masking of low blood sugar (hypoglycemia) in drug-treated diabetes Provocation of asthma (with high doses)

▷ **Principal Uses**

As a Single Drug Product: The treatment of mild to moderately severe high blood pressure. May be used alone or concurrently with other antihypertensive drugs, such as diuretics.

As a Combination Drug Product [CD]: This drug is available in combination with hydrochlorothiazide (in Canada). The addition of a thiazide diuretic to this beta blocker drug enhances its effectiveness as an antihypertensive.

How This Drug Works: By blocking certain actions of the sympathetic nervous system, this drug

- reduces the rate and contraction force of the heart, thus lowering the ejection pressure of the blood leaving the heart.
- reduces the degree of contraction of blood vessel walls, resulting in their relaxation and expansion and consequent lowering of blood pressure.

Available Dosage Forms and Strengths
Tablets — 5 mg, 10 mg

▷ **Usual Adult Dosage Range:** Initially, 5 mg twice daily (12 hours apart). The dose may be increased gradually by 10 mg/day at intervals of 2 to 3 weeks as needed and tolerated up to 60 mg/day. For maintenance,

5 to 10 mg 2 or 3 times/day. The total daily dose should not exceed 60 mg. **Note: Actual dosage and administration schedule must be determined by the physician for each patient individually.**

▷ **Dosing Instructions:** May be taken without regard to eating. The tablet may be crushed for administration. Do not discontinue this drug abruptly.

Usual Duration of Use: Continual use on a regular schedule for 2 to 3 weeks is usually necessary to determine this drug's effectiveness in lowering blood pressure. The long-term use of this drug (months to years) will be determined by the course of your blood pressure over time and your response to the overall treatment program (weight reduction, salt restriction, smoking cessation, etc.). Consult your physician on a regular basis.

Possible Advantages of This Drug: Causes less slowing of the heart rate than most other beta blocker drugs.

Currently a "Drug of Choice" for initiating treatment of hypertension with a single drug.

▷ **This Drug Should Not Be Taken If**
- you have had an allergic reaction to it previously.
- you have congestive heart failure.
- you have an abnormally slow heart rate or a serious form of heart block.
- you are taking, or have taken within the past 14 days, any monoamine oxidase (MAO) type A inhibitor drug (see Drug Class, Section Four).

▷ **Inform Your Physician Before Taking This Drug If**
- you have had an adverse reaction to any beta blocker drug in the past (see Drug Class, Section Four).
- you have a history of serious heart disease, with or without episodes of heart failure.
- you have a history of hay fever (allergic rhinitis), asthma, chronic bronchitis or emphysema.
- you have a history of overactive thyroid function (hyperthyroidism).
- you have a history of low blood sugar (hypoglycemia).
- you have impaired liver or kidney function.
- you have diabetes or myasthenia gravis.
- you are currently taking any form of digitalis, quinidine or reserpine, or any calcium blocker drug (see Drug Class, Section Four).
- you plan to have surgery under general anesthesia in the near future.

Possible Side-Effects (natural, expected and unavoidable drug actions)
Lethargy and fatigability (15%), cold extremities, slow heart rate, lightheadedness in upright position (see Orthostatic Hypotension in Glossary).

▷ **Possible Adverse Effects** (unusual, unexpected and infrequent reactions)
If any of the following develop, consult your physician promptly for guidance.
Mild Adverse Effects
Allergic Reactions: Skin rash, itching.
Headache (5%), dizziness (17%), insomnia (19%), abnormal dreams.
Indigestion, nausea (7%), vomiting, constipation, diarrhea.
Joint and muscle discomfort (11%), fluid retention (edema) (11%).
Serious Adverse Effects
Mental depression, anxiety.
Chest pain, shortness of breath, precipitation of congestive heart failure.
Induction of bronchial asthma (in asthmatic individuals).

▷ **Possible Effects on Sexual Function:**   Decreased libido, impaired erection (rare).

CAUTION
1. ***Do not discontinue this drug suddenly*** without the knowledge and guidance of your physician. Carry a notation on your person that you are taking this drug.
2. Consult your physician or pharmacist before using nasal decongestants usually present in over-the-counter cold preparations and nose drops. These can cause sudden increases in blood pressure when taken concurrently with beta blocker drugs.
3. Report the development of any tendency to emotional depression.

Precautions for Use
By Infants and Children: Safety and effectiveness for use by those under 12 years of age have not been established. However, if this drug is used, observe for the development of low blood sugar (hypoglycemia) during periods of reduced food intake.
By Those over 60 Years of Age: Proceed **cautiously** with all antihypertensive drugs. Unacceptably high blood pressure should be reduced without creating the risks associated with excessively low blood pressure. Start treatment with small doses, and monitor the blood pressure response frequently. Sudden, rapid and excessive reduction of blood pressure can predispose to stroke or heart attack. Observe for dizziness, unsteadiness, tendency to fall, confusion, hallucinations, depression or urinary frequency.

▷ **Advisability of Use During Pregnancy**
Pregnancy Category: B (tentative). See Pregnancy Code inside back cover.
Animal studies: No significant increase in birth defects due to this drug.
Human studies: Information from adequate studies of pregnant women is not available.
Use this drug only if clearly needed. Ask physician for guidance.

Advisability of Use if Breast-Feeding
Presence of this drug in breast milk: Yes.
Avoid drug or refrain from nursing.

Habit-Forming Potential: None.

Effects of Overdosage: Weakness, slow pulse, low blood pressure, fainting, cold and sweaty skin, congestive heart failure, possible coma and convulsions.

Possible Effects of Long-Term Use: Reduced heart reserve and eventual heart failure in susceptible individuals with advanced heart disease.

Suggested Periodic Examinations While Taking This Drug (at physician's discretion)
Measurements of blood pressure, evaluation of heart function.

▷ **While Taking This Drug, Observe the Following**
Foods: No restrictions. Avoid excessive salt intake.
Beverages: No restrictions. May be taken with milk.
▷ *Alcohol:* Use with caution until the combined effect has been determined. Alcohol may exaggerate this drug's ability to lower the blood pressure and may increase its mild sedative effect.
Tobacco Smoking: Nicotine may reduce this drug's effectiveness in treating high blood pressure. In addition, high doses of this drug may potentiate the constriction of the bronchial tubes caused by regular smoking.
▷ *Other Drugs*
Pindolol may ***increase*** the effects of
- other antihypertensive drugs, and cause excessive lowering of the blood pressure. Dosage adjustments may be necessary.
- reserpine (Ser-Ap-Es, etc.), and cause sedation, depression, slowing of the heart rate and lowering of the blood pressure.
- verapamil (Calan, Isoptin), and cause excessive depression of heart function; monitor this combination closely.
Pindolol ***taken concurrently*** with
- clonidine (Catapres) requires close monitoring for rebound high blood pressure if clonidine is withdrawn while pindolol is still being taken.
- insulin requires close monitoring to avoid undetected hypoglycemia (see Glossary).
The following drugs may ***increase*** the effects of pindolol
- cimetidine (Tagamet).
- methimazole (Tapazole).
- oral contraceptives.
- propylthiouracil (Propacil).
The following drugs may ***decrease*** the effects of pindolol
- barbiturates (phenobarbital, etc.).
- indomethacin (Indocin), and possibly other "aspirin substitutes," may impair pindolol's antihypertensive effect.
- rifampin (Rifadin, Rimactane).
▷ *Driving, Hazardous Activities:* Use caution until the full extent of fatigue, dizziness and blood pressure change have been determined.

Aviation Note: The use of this drug *is a disqualification* for piloting. Consult a designated Aviation Medical Examiner.

Exposure to Sun: No restrictions.

Exposure to Heat: Caution advised. Hot environments can lower the blood pressure and exaggerate the effects of this drug.

Exposure to Cold: Caution advised. Cold environments can enhance the circulatory deficiency in the extremities that may occur with this drug. The elderly should take precautions to prevent hypothermia (see Glossary).

Heavy Exercise or Exertion: It is advisable to avoid exertion that produces light-headedness, excessive fatigue or muscle cramping. The use of this drug may intensify the hypertensive response to isometric exercise.

Occurrence of Unrelated Illness: The fever that accompanies systemic infections can lower the blood pressure and require adjustment of dosage. Illnesses that cause nausea or vomiting may interrupt the regular dosage schedule. Ask your physician for guidance.

Discontinuation: It is advisable to avoid sudden discontinuation of this drug in all situations. If possible, gradual reduction of dose over a period of 2 to 3 weeks is recommended. Ask your physician for specific guidance.

PIROXICAM
(peer OX i kam)

Introduced: 1978

Class: Mild analgesic, anti-inflammatory

Prescription: USA: Yes
Canada: Yes

Controlled Drug: USA: No
Canada: No

Available as Generic: No

Brand Names: ✦Apo-Piroxicam, Feldene, ✦Novopirocam

BENEFITS versus RISKS	
Possible Benefits	*Possible Risks*
EFFECTIVE RELIEF OF MILD TO MODERATE PAIN AND INFLAMMATION	Gastrointestinal pain, ulceration, bleeding (rare) Drug-induced hepatitis (rare) Rare kidney damage Mild fluid retention Reduced white blood cell and platelet counts

▷ **Principal Uses**

As a Single Drug Product: Used primarily to relieve mild to moderately severe pain and inflammation associated with (1) rheumatoid arthritis, (2) osteoarthritis and (3) acute and chronic gout.

How This Drug Works: Not completely established. It is thought that this drug suppresses the formation of prostaglandins (and related compounds), chemicals involved in the production of inflammation and pain.

Available Dosage Forms and Strengths

Capsules — 10 mg, 20 mg

▷ **Usual Adult Dosage Range:** As antiarthritic: 10 mg twice daily, 12 hours apart; or 20 mg once daily. The total daily dosage should not exceed 40 mg, and then for no more than 5 days. **Note: Actual dosage and administration schedule must be determined by the physician for each patient individually.**

▷ **Dosing Instructions:** Take with or following food to prevent stomach irritation. Take with a full glass of water and remain upright (do not lie down) for 30 minutes. The capsule may be opened for administration.

Usual Duration of Use: Continual use on a regular schedule for 2 weeks is usually necessary to determine this drug's effectiveness in relieving the discomfort of arthritis. Long-term use (months to years) requires supervision and periodic evaluation by your physician. Consult your physician on a regular basis.

▷ **This Drug Should Not Be Taken If**
- you have had an allergic reaction to it previously.
- you are subject to asthma or nasal polyps caused by aspirin.
- you have active peptic ulcer disease or any form of gastrointestinal bleeding.
- you have a bleeding disorder or a blood cell disorder.
- you have active liver disease.
- you have severe impairment of kidney function.

▷ **Inform Your Physician Before Taking This Drug If**
- you are allergic to aspirin or to other aspirin substitutes.
- you have a history of peptic ulcer disease, regional enteritis or ulcerative colitis.
- you have a history of any type of bleeding disorder.
- you have impaired liver or kidney function.
- you have high blood pressure or a history of heart failure.
- you are taking any of the following: acetaminophen, aspirin or other aspirin substitutes, anticoagulants, oral antidiabetic drugs.
- you plan to have surgery of any type in the near future.

Possible Side-Effects (natural, expected and unavoidable drug actions)
Fluid retention (weight gain), prolongation of bleeding time.

▷ **Possible Adverse Effects** (unusual, unexpected and infrequent reactions)
If any of the following develop, consult your physician promptly for guidance.
Mild Adverse Effects
Allergic Reactions: Skin rash, itching, spontaneous bruising.
Headache, dizziness, altered or blurred vision, ringing in the ears, drowsiness, fatigue, inability to concentrate.
Indigestion, nausea, vomiting, abdominal pain, diarrhea.
Serious Adverse Effects
Active peptic ulcer, stomach or intestinal bleeding.
Drug-induced liver damage.
Kidney damage with painful urination, bloody urine, reduced urine formation.
Rare bone marrow depression (see Glossary): fatigue, weakness, fever, sore throat, abnormal bleeding or bruising.

▷ **Possible Effects on Sexual Function:**   None reported.

Possible Delayed Adverse Effects: Mild anemia due to "silent" blood loss from the stomach (less than that caused by aspirin).

▷ **Adverse Effects That May Mimic Natural Diseases or Disorders**
Liver reaction may suggest viral hepatitis.

Natural Diseases or Disorders That May Be Activated by This Drug
Peptic ulcer disease, ulcerative colitis.

CAUTION
1. Dosage should always be limited to the smallest amount that produces reasonable improvement.
2. This drug may mask early indications of infection. Inform your physician if you think you are developing an infection of any kind.

Precautions for Use
By Infants and Children: Indications and dosage recommendations for use by those under 12 years of age have not been established.
By Those over 60 Years of Age: Small doses are advisable until tolerance is determined. Observe for any indications of liver or kidney toxicity, fluid retention, dizziness, confusion, impaired memory, stomach bleeding or constipation.

▷ **Advisability of Use During Pregnancy**
Pregnancy Category: B (tentative). See Pregnancy Code inside back cover.
Animal studies: No birth defects reported due to this drug.
Human studies: Information from adequate studies of pregnant women is not available.
The manufacturer does not recommend the use of this drug during pregnancy.

Advisability of Use if Breast-Feeding
Presence of this drug in breast milk: Unknown.
Avoid drug or refrain from nursing.

Habit-Forming Potential: None.

Effects of Overdosage: Possible drowsiness, dizziness, ringing in the ears, nausea, vomiting, indigestion.

Possible Effects of Long-Term Use: Development of anemia due to "silent" bleeding from the gastrointestinal tract.

Suggested Periodic Examinations While Taking This Drug (at physician's discretion)
Complete blood cell counts, liver and kidney function tests.
Complete eye examinations if vision is altered in any way.
Hearing examinations if ringing in the ears or hearing loss develops.

▷ **While Taking This Drug, Observe the Following**
Foods: No restrictions.
Beverages: No restrictions. May be taken with milk.
▷ *Alcohol:* Use with caution. The irritant action of alcohol on the stomach lining, added to the irritant action of this drug in sensitive individuals, can increase the risk of stomach ulceration and/or bleeding.
Tobacco Smoking: No interactions expected.
▷ *Other Drugs*
Piroxicam may ***increase*** the effects of
- acetaminophen (Tylenol, etc.), and increase the risk of kidney damage; avoid prolonged use of this combination.
- anticoagulants (Coumadin, etc.), and increase the risk of bleeding; monitor prothrombin time, adjust dose accordingly.

Piroxicam ***taken concurrently*** with the following drugs may increase the risk of bleeding; avoid these combinations:
- aspirin.
- dipyridamole (Persantine).
- indomethacin (Indocin).
- sulfinpyrazone (Anturane).
- valproic acid (Depakene).

▷ *Driving, Hazardous Activities:* This drug may cause drowsiness or dizziness. Restrict activities as necessary.
Aviation Note: The use of this drug ***may be a disqualification*** for piloting. Consult a designated Aviation Medical Examiner.
Exposure to Sun: No restrictions.

POTASSIUM
(poh TAS ee um)

Introduced: 1939

Prescription: USA: Yes
Canada: No

Class: Potassium preparations

Controlled Drug: USA: No
Canada: No

Available as Generic: Yes

Brand Names: ✦Apo-K, Kaochlor, Kaochlor-Eff, Kaon, Kaon-Cl, Kay Ciel, K-Lor, Klorvess, Klotrix, K-Lyte, K-Lyte/Cl, K-Lyte DS, K + 10, K-Tab, Micro-K, Micro-K Extencaps, Micro-K LS, ✦Neo-K, Slow-K, Ten-K, Trikates

---

BENEFITS versus RISKS

Possible Benefits	*Possible Risks*
EFFECTIVE PREVENTION AND TREATMENT OF POTASSIUM DEFICIENCY (HYPOKALEMIA)	DEVELOPMENT OF EXCESSIVE POTASSIUM (HYPERKALEMIA) Ulceration and perforation of stomach or intestine with use of slow-release or enteric-coated tablets (these forms no longer recommended)

▷ **Principal Uses**

As a Single Drug Product: This drug is used primarily in conjunction with those diuretics that cause excessive loss of potassium from the body. Potassium preparations are usually given to stabilize the blood level within the normal range. Dosage adjustments may be necessary from time to time.

How This Drug Works: By maintaining or replenishing the normal potassium content of cells, this drug preserves or restores such normal cellular functions as the transmission of nerve impulses, the contraction of muscle fibers, the regulation of kidney function and the secretion of stomach juices.

Available Dosage Forms and Strengths

Capsules, prolonged-action — 8 mEq, 10 mEq

Liquids — 10 mEq, 15 mEq, 20 mEq, 30 mEq, 40 mEq, 45 mEq per 15-ml tablespoonful

Powders — 15 mEq, 20 mEq, 25 mEq per packet

Suspension, prolonged-action — 20 mEq per packet

Tablets — 2 mEq, 2.5 mEq, 5 mEq

Tablets, chewable — 1 mEq, 2.5 mEq

Tablets, effervescent — 20 mEq, 25 mEq, 50 mEq

Tablets, enteric-coated — 4 mEq

Tablets, prolonged-action — 6.7 mEq, 8 mEq, 10 mEq

Tablets, wax matrix — 6.7 mEq, 8 mEq, 10 mEq

▷ **Usual Adult Dosage Range:**   Depends upon the dosage form prescribed. Follow your physician's prescribed dose exactly. **Note: Actual dosage and administration schedule must be determined by the physician for each patient individually.**

▷ **Dosing Instructions:**   Take each dose with food or immediately following a meal to reduce stomach irritation. Regular tablets should be swallowed whole. Soluble tablets and powders should be dissolved completely in 4 ounces of cold water or juice and sipped slowly over a period of 5 to 10 minutes. Liquid forms should be diluted in 4 ounces of water or juice. The prolonged-action capsules should be swallowed whole and not opened for administration. Wax matrix and enteric-coated tablets are not recommended because of their potential for causing localized erosion and ulceration of gastrointestinal tissues.

Usual Duration of Use: This must be determined by your physician. Periods of use will depend upon your concurrent use of diuretics, the potassium content of your diet and periodic measurement of your blood potassium level. Consult your physician on a regular basis.

▷ **This Drug Should Not Be Taken If**
- you have had an allergic reaction to it previously.
- you have severe impairment of kidney function.
- you are taking any drug that contains amiloride, spironolactone or triamterene.

▷ **Inform Your Physician Before Taking This Drug If**
- you are taking any of the following: a cortisonelike drug, a digitalis preparation, a diuretic (see Drug Classes, Section Four).
- you have Addison's disease (adrenal gland deficiency).
- you have diabetes or any form of heart disease.
- you have a history of kidney disease or impaired kidney function.
- you have a history of familial periodic paralysis.

Possible Side-Effects (natural, expected and unavoidable drug actions)
A mild laxative effect for some individuals.

▷ **Possible Adverse Effects** (unusual, unexpected and infrequent reactions)
If any of the following develop, consult your physician promptly for guidance.
Mild Adverse Effects
Nausea, vomiting, abdominal discomfort, diarrhea. (These usually occur if potassium is taken undiluted or on an empty stomach.)
Serious Adverse Effects
Potassium accumulation, resulting in abnormally high blood levels. Immediate treatment is mandatory.
Potassium in enteric-coated tablets or slow-release (wax matrix) tablets can cause ulceration of the stomach or intestine with risk of bleeding and/or perforation.

▷ **Possible Effects on Sexual Function:**   None reported.

CAUTION
1. Dosage must be carefully individualized. Periodic evaluation of overall condition and blood potassium levels is essential to safe and

effective management. Excessively high blood levels of potassium can occur without warning. Do not exceed the prescribed dose.

2. Inform your physician promptly if you are taking a tablet form of this drug and you become aware of any difficulty in swallowing.

3. If you have chronic constipation, it is advisable that you avoid potassium in tablet form.

4. Some salt substitutes contain a large amount of potassium. If you are using a salt substitute, consult your physician regarding its continued use or any necessary adjustment in the dosage of your potassium preparation.

Precautions for Use

By Those over 60 Years of Age: Your potassium balance must be maintained within strict limitations. Serious adverse effects can occur when the potassium level is either above or below the normal range. Adhere to your dosage schedule exactly.

▷ Advisability of Use During Pregnancy

Pregnancy Category: A (tentative). See Pregnancy Code inside back cover.
Animal studies: No information available.
Human studies: Information from adequate studies of pregnant women is not available.

Potassium is a normal and essential constituent of body tissues. Potassium preparations can be used safely during pregnancy. Adhere strictly to prescribed dosage schedules.

Advisability of Use if Breast-Feeding

Presence of this drug in breast milk: Yes.
Monitor nursing infant closely and discontinue drug or nursing if adverse effects develop.

Habit-Forming Potential: None.

Effects of Overdosage: Lethargy, weakness and heaviness of legs, numbness and tingling in the extremities, confusion, irregular heart rhythm, drop in blood pressure, seizures, coma, heart arrest.

Possible Effects of Long-Term Use: Reduced absorption of vitamin B-12, resulting in anemia in some individuals.

Suggested Periodic Examinations While Taking This Drug (at physician's discretion)

Measurement of blood potassium levels.

▷ While Taking This Drug, Observe the Following

Foods: No restrictions. Consult your physician regarding any special modifications of your diet.
Beverages: No restrictions.
▷   *Alcohol:* No interactions expected.
Tobacco Smoking: No interactions expected.

▷ *Other Drugs*
   Potassium *taken concurrently* with
   - amiloride, spironolactone or triamterene may cause an excessive rise in blood potassium levels. This can be extremely dangerous; avoid the concurrent use of these diuretics and any form of potassium.
   - digitalis preparations requires very careful monitoring of dosage and heart status.

▷ *Driving, Hazardous Activities:* No restrictions.
   Aviation Note: The use of this drug *may be a disqualification* for piloting. Consult a designated Aviation Medical Examiner.
   Exposure to Sun: No restrictions.
   Discontinuation: Do not discontinue this drug suddenly if you are taking digitalis. Ask your physician for guidance if you find it necessary to discontinue potassium medication for any reason.

PRAZEPAM
(PRA ze pam)

Introduced: 1969

Prescription: USA: Yes

Available as Generic: USA: No

Brand Name: Centrax

Class: Mild tranquilizer, benzodiazepines

Controlled Drug: USA: C-IV*

BENEFITS versus RISKS

Possible Benefits	*Possible Risks*
RELIEF OF ANXIETY AND NERVOUS TENSION in 70% to 80% of users	Habit-forming potential with prolonged use
Wide margin of safety with therapeutic doses	Minor impairment of mental functions
Very few drug interactions	

▷ **Principal Uses**
   As a Single Drug Product: Used primarily to (1) provide short-term relief of mild to moderate anxiety; (2) relieve the symptoms of acute alcohol withdrawal: agitation, tremors, hallucinations, incipient delirium tremens.

   How This Drug Works: It is thought that this drug produces a calming effect by enhancing the action of the nerve transmitter gamma-ami-

*See Schedules of Controlled Drugs inside back cover.

nobutyric acid (GABA), which in turn blocks the arousal of higher brain centers.

Available Dosage Forms and Strengths
Capsules — 5 mg, 10 mg, 20 mg
Tablets — 10 mg

▷ **Usual Adult Dosage Range:** 20 to 60 mg/24 hours, in 3 or 4 divided doses. The total daily dosage should not exceed 60 mg. **Note: Actual dosage and administration schedule must be determined by the physician for each patient individually.**

▷ **Dosing Instructions:** May be taken on empty stomach or with food or milk as needed to prevent stomach irritation. The tablet may be crushed and the capsule may be opened for administration. Do not discontinue this drug abruptly if taken for more than 4 weeks.

Usual Duration of Use: Continual use on a regular schedule for 3 to 5 days is usually necessary to determine this drug's effectiveness in relieving moderate anxiety. Limit continual use to 1 to 3 weeks. Avoid uninterrupted and prolonged use.

▷ **This Drug Should Not Be Taken If**
- you have had an allergic reaction to any dosage form of it previously.
- you have acute narrow-angle glaucoma.
- it is prescribed for a child under 18 years of age.

▷ **Inform Your Physician Before Taking This Drug If**
- you are allergic to any benzodiazepine drug (see Drug Class, Section Four).
- you have a history of alcoholism or drug abuse.
- you are pregnant or planning pregnancy.
- you have impaired liver or kidney function.
- you have a history of serious depression or mental disorder.
- you have any of the following: asthma, emphysema, epilepsy, myasthenia gravis.
- you are taking any drugs with sedative effects.

Possible Side-Effects (natural, expected and unavoidable drug actions)
Drowsiness (6%), lethargy (11%), unsteadiness (5%), "hangover" effects on the day following bedtime use.

▷ **Possible Adverse Effects** (unusual, unexpected and infrequent reactions)
If any of the following develop, consult your physician promptly for guidance.
Mild Adverse Effects
Allergic Reactions: Skin rashes, hives, itching.
Dizziness (8%), fainting, weakness (7%), confusion, blurred vision, double vision, slurred speech, sweating, nausea.

Serious Adverse Effects
Paradoxical responses of excitement, agitation, anger, rage.

▷ **Possible Effects on Sexual Function:** None reported.

CAUTION
1. This drug should not be discontinued abruptly if it has been taken continually for more than 4 weeks.
2. The concurrent use of some over-the-counter drug products that contain antihistamines (allergy and cold preparations, sleep aids) can cause excessive sedation in sensitive individuals.

Precautions for Use
By Infants and Children: Safety and effectiveness for use by those under 18 years of age have not been established. This drug should not be used in the hyperactive or psychotic child of any age. Observe for excessive sedation and incoordination.
By Those over 60 Years of Age: It is advisable to use smaller doses at longer intervals to avoid overdosage. Observe for the possible development of lethargy, indifference, fatigue, weakness, unsteadiness, disturbing dreams, nightmares and paradoxical reactions of excitement, agitation, anger, hostility and rage.

▷ **Advisability of Use During Pregnancy**
Pregnancy Category: C (tentative). See Pregnancy Code inside back cover.
Animal studies: No information available.
Human studies: Information from adequate studies of pregnant women is not available. No birth defects have been reported with the use of this drug. However, available information regarding the use of other drugs of this class (benzodiazepines) is conflicting and inconclusive. Some studies found an increase in serious birth defects associated with the use of 2 benzodiazepines. Other studies have found no significant increase in birth defects.
Frequent use in late pregnancy can cause the "floppy infant" syndrome in the newborn: weakness, lethargy, unresponsiveness, depressed breathing, low body temperature.
Avoid use during entire pregnancy if possible.

Advisability of Use if Breast-Feeding
Presence of this drug in breast milk: Probably yes.
Avoid drug or refrain from nursing.

Habit-Forming Potential: This drug can produce psychological and/or physical dependence (see Glossary) if used in large doses for an extended period of time.

Effects of Overdosage: Marked drowsiness, weakness, feeling of drunkenness, staggering gait, tremor, stupor progressing to deep sleep or coma.

Possible Effects of Long-Term Use: Psychological and/or physical dependence.

Suggested Periodic Examinations While Taking This Drug (at physician's discretion)
Complete blood cell counts during long-term use.

▷ **While Taking This Drug, Observe the Following**
Foods: No restrictions.
Beverages: Avoid excessive intake of caffeine-containing beverages: coffee, tea, cola. May be taken with milk.

▷ *Alcohol:* Use with extreme caution until the combined effect has been determined. Alcohol may increase the depressant effects of this drug on the brain. It is advisable to avoid alcohol completely—throughout the day and night—if it is necessary to drive or to engage in any hazardous activity.
Tobacco Smoking: Heavy smoking may reduce the calming action of this drug.
Marijuana Smoking: Increased sedation and significant impairment of intellectual and physical performance.

▷ *Other Drugs*
The following drugs may ***increase*** the effects of prazepam
• cimetidine (Tagamet).
• disulfiram (Antabuse).
• oral contraceptives.

▷ *Driving, Hazardous Activities:* This drug can impair mental alertness, judgment, physical coordination and reaction time. Avoid hazardous activities accordingly.
Aviation Note: The use of this drug *is a disqualification* for piloting. Consult a designated Aviation Medical Examiner.
Exposure to Sun: No restrictions.
Exposure to Heat: Use caution until the effect of excessive perspiration is determined. Because of reduced urine volume, this drug may accumulate in the body and produce effects of overdosage.
Exposure to Cold: The elderly should dress warmly and avoid situations and environments conducive to hypothermia (see Glossary).
Discontinuation: Avoid sudden discontinuation if this drug has been taken for over 4 weeks without interruption. Dosage should be tapered gradually to prevent a withdrawal syndrome that could include depression, confusion, hallucinations, tremor, seizures, muscle cramping, sweating and vomiting.

PRAZOSIN
(PRA zoh sin)

Introduced: 1970   **Class:** Antihypertensive
Prescription: USA: Yes   **Controlled Drug:** USA: No
   Canada: Yes   Canada: No

Available as Generic: Yes

Brand Names: Minipress, Minizide [CD]

BENEFITS versus RISKS

Possible Benefits	*Possible Risks*
EFFECTIVE INITIAL THERAPY FOR MILD TO MODERATE HYPERTENSION	"First dose" drop in blood pressure with fainting (0.15%)
EFFECTIVE "STEP 2 OR 3" ANTIHYPERTENSIVE IN 60% TO 70% OF CASES OF MODERATE TO SEVERE HYPERTENSION when used adjunctively with other antihypertensive drugs	Induction of paroxysmal tachycardia (rare)
EFFECTIVE CONTROL OF HYPERTENSION IN PHEOCHROMOCYTOMA	
Effective in presence of impaired kidney function	

▷ **Principal Uses**

As a Single Drug Product: Used primarily to initiate treatment in mild to moderate hypertension. Also used as a "step 2" or "step 3" anti-hypertensive drug, in conjunction with other drugs, to treat moderate to severe hypertension.

As a Combination Drug Product [CD]: This drug is available in combination with polythiazide, a diuretic of the thiazide class of drugs that are usually used as "step 1" medications to initiate treatment for hypertension. By utilizing two different methods of drug action, this combination product is more effective and more convenient for long-term use.

How This Drug Works: It is thought that by blocking certain actions of the sympathetic nervous system, this drug causes direct relaxation and expansion of blood vessel walls, thus lowering the pressure of the blood within the vessels.

Available Dosage Forms and Strengths

Capsules — 1 mg, 2 mg, 5 mg

▷ **Usual Adult Dosage Range:** Initiate treatment with a "test dose" of 1 mg to determine the patient's response within the first 2 hours. If tolerated satisfactorily, increase dose cautiously up to 15 mg/24 hours in 2 or 3 divided doses. The total daily dosage should not exceed 20 mg. Note: **Actual dosage and administration schedule must be determined by the physician for each patient individually.**

▷ **Dosing Instructions:** May be taken without regard to food. The capsule may be opened for administration.

Usual Duration of Use: Continual use on a regular schedule for 4 to 6 weeks is usually necessary to determine this drug's effectiveness in controlling hypertension. Long-term use (months to years) requires supervision and periodic evaluation by your physician. Consult your physician on a regular basis.

Possible Advantages of This Drug
Effective initial treatment of hypertension.
Does not alter blood cholesterol, potassium or sugar levels.

▷ **This Drug Should Not Be Taken If**
- you have had an allergic reaction to it previously.
- you are experiencing mental depression.
- you have angina (active coronary artery disease) and you are not taking a beta-blocking drug. (Consult your physician.)

▷ **Inform Your Physician Before Taking This Drug If**
- you have experienced orthostatic hypotension (see Glossary) when using other antihypertensive drugs.
- you have a history of mental depression.
- you have impaired circulation to the brain, or a history of stroke.
- you have coronary artery disease.
- you have active liver disease or impaired liver function.
- you plan to have surgery under general anesthesia in the near future.

Possible Side-Effects (natural, expected and unavoidable drug actions)
Orthostatic hypotension, drowsiness (7%), salt and water retention, dry mouth, nasal congestion, constipation.

▷ **Possible Adverse Effects** (unusual, unexpected and infrequent reactions)
If any of the following develop, consult your physician promptly for guidance.
Mild Adverse Effects
Allergic Reactions: Skin rash, itching.
Headache (7.8%), dizziness (10.3%), fatigue (6.9%), weakness (6.5%), nervousness, sweating, numbness and tingling, blurred vision, reddened eyes, ringing in the ears.
Palpitation (5.3%), rapid heart rate, shortness of breath.
Nausea (4.9%), vomiting, diarrhea, abdominal pain.
Urinary frequency and incontinence.
Serious Adverse Effects
Mental depression, sleep disturbance.
Paroxysmal tachycardia (heart rates of 120 to 160).

▷ **Possible Effects on Sexual Function**
> Decreased libido (14%); impotence (less than 1%).
> Priapism (see Glossary).

Natural Diseases or Disorders That May Be Activated by This Drug
Latent coronary artery insufficiency.

CAUTION
1. Observe for the possible "first dose" response of precipitous drop in blood pressue, with or without fainting; this usually occurs within 30 to 90 minutes. Limit initial doses to 1 mg taken at bedtime for the first 3 days; remain supine after taking these trial doses.
2. Impaired kidney function may increase your sensitivity to this drug and require smaller than usual doses.

Precautions for Use
By Infants and Children: Safety and effectiveness for use by those under 12 years of age have not been established.
By Those over 60 Years of Age: Begin treatment with no more than 1 mg/day for the first 3 days. Subsequent increases in dose must be very gradual and carefully supervised by your physician. The occurrence of orthostatic hypotension can cause unexpected falls and injury; sit or lie down promptly if you feel light-headed or dizzy. Report any indications of dizziness or chest pain promptly.

▷ **Advisability of Use During Pregnancy**
Pregnancy Category: C (tentative). See Pregnancy Code inside back cover.
Animal studies: No birth defects found.
Human studies: Information from adequate studies of pregnant women is not available.
Use this drug only if clearly needed. Ask your physician for guidance.

Advisability of Use if Breast-Feeding
Presence of this drug in breast milk: Yes, in small amounts.
Monitor nursing infant closely and discontinue drug or nursing if adverse effects develop.

Habit-Forming Potential: None.

Effects of Overdosage: Orthostatic hypotension, headache, generalized flushing, rapid heart rate, extreme weakness, irregular heart rhythm, circulatory collapse.

Possible Effects of Long-Term Use: None reported.

Suggested Periodic Examinations While Taking This Drug (at physician's discretion)
Measurements of blood pressure in lying, sitting and standing positions.
Measurements of body weight to detect fluid retention.

▷ **While Taking This Drug, Observe the Following**

Foods: No restrictions. Avoid excessive salt intake.

Beverages: No restrictions. May be taken with milk.

▷ *Alcohol:* Use with extreme caution until the combined effects have been determined. Alcohol can exaggerate the blood-pressure-lowering actions of this drug and cause excessive reduction.

Tobacco Smoking: Nicotine can contribute significantly to this drug's ability to intensify coronary insufficiency in susceptible individuals. All forms of tobacco should be avoided.

▷ *Other Drugs*

The following drugs may ***increase*** the effects of prazosin

• beta-adrenergic-blocking drugs (see Drug Class, Section Four); the severity and duration of the "first dose" hypotensive response may be increased.

▷ *Driving, Hazardous Activities:* This drug may cause dizziness or drowsiness. Restrict activities as necessary.

Aviation Note: The use of this drug ***is a disqualification*** for piloting. Consult a designated Aviation Medical Examiner.

Exposure to Sun: No restrictions.

Exposure to Cold: Use caution until combined effect has been determined. Cold environments may increase this drug's ability to cause coronary insufficiency (angina) in susceptible individuals.

Heavy Exercise or Exertion: Excessive exertion can augment this drug's ability to induce angina. See Profile of Angina in Section Two.

Discontinuation: If you are taking this drug as part of your treatment program for congestive heart failure, do not discontinue it abruptly. Ask your physician for guidance.

PREDNISOLONE
(pred NIS oh lohn)

Introduced: 1955

Class: Cortisonelike drugs

Prescription: USA: Yes
  Canada: Yes

Controlled Drug: USA: No
  Canada: No

Available as Generic: USA: Yes
  Canada: Yes

Brand Names: ✦Ak-Cide [CD], ✦Ak-Tate, Delta-Cortef, ✦Inflamase, ✦Inflamase Forte, ✦Nova-Pred, ✦Novoprednisolone, ✦Pred Forte, ✦Pred Mild, Prelone

```
┌─────────────────────────────────────────────────────────────┐
```

BENEFITS versus RISKS

Possible Benefits	*Possible Risks*
EFFECTIVE RELIEF OF SYMPTOMS IN A WIDE VARIETY OF INFLAMMATORY AND ALLERGIC DISORDERS	Short-term use (up to 10 days) is usually well tolerated
EFFECTIVE IMMUNO-SUPPRESSION in selected benign and malignant disorders	Long-term use (exceeding 2 weeks) is associated with many possible adverse effects:
Prevention of rejection in organ transplantation	ALTERED MOOD AND PERSONALITY
	CATARACTS, GLAUCOMA
	HYPERTENSION
	OSTEOPOROSIS
	ASEPTIC BONE NECROSIS
	INCREASED SUSCEPTIBILITY TO INFECTIONS
	(See Possible Adverse Effects and Possible Effects of Long-Term Use below)

▷ **Principal Uses**

As a Single Drug Product: This potent drug of the cortisone class is used in the treatment of a wide variety of allergic and inflammatory conditions. It is used most commonly in the management of serious skin disorders, asthma, regional enteritis, ulcerative colitis and all types of major rheumatic disorders including bursitis, tendinitis and most forms of arthritis.

How This Drug Works: Not fully established. It is thought that this drug's anti-inflammatory effect is due to its ability to inhibit the normal defensive functions of certain white blood cells. Its immunosuppressant effect is attributed to a reduced production of lymphocytes and antibodies.

Available Dosage Forms and Strengths

Syrup — 15 mg per 5-ml teaspoonful

Tablets — 5 mg

▷ **Usual Adult Dosage Range:** 5 to 60 mg daily as a single dose or in divided doses. The total daily dosage should not exceed 250 mg. **Note: Actual dosage and administration schedule must be determined by the physician for each patient individually.**

▷ **Dosing Instructions:** Take with or following food to prevent stomach irritation, preferably in the morning. The tablet may be crushed for administration.

Usual Duration of Use: For acute disorders: 4 to 10 days. For chronic disorders: according to individual requirements. The duration of use should not exceed the time necessary to obtain adequate symptomatic relief in acute self-limiting conditions; or the time required to stabilize a chronic condition and permit gradual withdrawal. Because of its intermediate duration of action, this drug is appropriate for alternate day administration. Consult your physician on a regular basis.

▷ **This Drug Should Not Be Taken If**
- you have had an allergic reaction to any dosage form of it previously.
- you have active peptic ulcer disease.
- you have an active infection of the eye caused by the herpes simplex virus.
- you have active tuberculosis.

▷ **Inform Your Physician Before Taking This Drug If**
- you have had an unfavorable reaction to any cortisonelike drug in the past.
- you have a history of peptic ulcer disease, thrombophlebitis or tuberculosis.
- you have any of the following: diabetes, glaucoma, high blood pressure, deficient thyroid function or myasthenia gravis.
- you plan to have surgery of any kind in the near future.

Possible Side-Effects (natural, expected and unavoidable drug actions)
Increased appetite, weight gain, retention of salt and water, excretion of potassium, increased susceptibility to infection.

▷ **Possible Adverse Effects** (unusual, unexpected and infrequent reactions)
If any of the following develop, consult your physician promptly for guidance.
Mild Adverse Effects
Allergic Reaction: Skin rash.
Headache, dizziness, insomnia.
Acid indigestion, abdominal distention.
Muscle cramping and weakness.
Acne, excessive growth of facial hair.
Serious Adverse Effects
Mental and emotional disturbances of serious magnitude.
Reactivation of latent tuberculosis.
Development of peptic ulcer.
Increased blood pressure.
Development of inflammation of the pancreas.
Thrombophlebitis (inflammation of a vein with the formation of blood clot)—pain or tenderness in thigh or leg, with or without swelling of the foot, ankle or leg.
Pulmonary embolism (movement of a blood clot to the lung)—sudden shortness of breath, pain in the chest, coughing, bloody sputum.

▷ **Adverse Effects That May Mimic Natural Diseases or Disorders**
Pattern of symptoms and signs resembling Cushing's syndrome.

▷ **Possible Effects on Sexual Function**

Altered timing and pattern of menstruation.

Correction of male infertility when due to autoantibodies that suppress sperm activity.

Natural Diseases or Disorders That May Be Activated by This Drug

Latent diabetes, glaucoma, peptic ulcer disease, tuberculosis.

CAUTION

1. It is advisable to carry a card of personal identification with a notation that you are taking this drug, if your course of treatment is to exceed 1 week.
2. Do not discontinue this drug abruptly if you are using it for long-term treatment.
3. If vaccination against measles, rabies, smallpox or yellow fever is required, discontinue this drug 72 hours before vaccination and do not resume it for at least 14 days after vaccination.

Precautions for Use

By Infants and Children: Avoid prolonged use if possible. During long-term use, observe for suppression of normal growth and the possibility of increased intracranial pressure. Following long-term use, the child may be at risk for adrenal gland deficiency during stress for as long as 18 months after cessation of this drug.

By Those over 60 Years of Age: Cortisonelike drugs should be used very sparingly after 60 and only when the disorder under treatment is unresponsive to adequate trials of unrelated drugs. Avoid prolonged use of this drug. Continual use (even in small doses) can increase the severity of diabetes, enhance fluid retention, raise blood pressure, weaken resistance to infection, induce stomach ulcer and accelerate the development of cataract and osteoporosis.

▷ **Advisability of Use During Pregnancy**

Pregnancy Category: C (tentative). See Pregnancy Code inside back cover.

Animal studies: Birth defects reported in mice, rats and rabbits.

Human studies: Information from adequate studies of pregnant women is not available.

Avoid completely during the first 3 months. Limit use during the last 6 months as much as possible. If used, examine infant for possible deficiency of adrenal gland function.

Advisability of Use if Breast-Feeding

Presence of this drug in breast milk: Yes.

Avoid drug or refrain from nursing.

Habit-Forming Potential: Use of this drug to suppress symptoms over an extended period of time may produce a state of functional dependence (see Glossary). In the treatment of conditions like asthma and rheumatoid arthritis, it is advisable to keep the dose as small as possible and to attempt drug withdrawal after periods of reasonable improvement. Such procedures may reduce the degree of "steroid rebound"—the return of symptoms as the drug is withdrawn.

Effects of Overdosage: Fatigue, muscle weakness, stomach irritation, acid indigestion, excessive sweating, facial flushing, fluid retention, swelling of extremities, increased blood pressure.

Possible Effects of Long-Term Use: Increased blood sugar (possible diabetes), increased fat deposits on the trunk of the body ("buffalo hump"), rounding of the face ("moon face"), thinning and fragility of skin, loss of texture and strength of bones (osteoporosis, aseptic necrosis), cataracts, glaucoma, retarded growth and development in children.

Suggested Periodic Examinations While Taking This Drug (at physician's discretion)

Measurements of blood pressure, blood sugar and potassium levels.
Complete eye examinations at regular intervals.
Chest X-ray if history of tuberculosis.
Determination of the rate of development of the growing child to detect retardation of normal growth.

▷ **While Taking This Drug, Observe the Following**

Foods: No interactions expected. Ask physician regarding need to restrict salt intake or to eat potassium-rich foods. During long-term use of this drug, it is advisable to eat a high-protein diet.

Nutritional Support: During long-term use, take a vitamin D supplement. During wound repair, take a zinc supplement.

Beverages: No restrictions. Drink all forms of milk liberally.

▷   *Alcohol:* No interactions expected. Use caution if you are prone to peptic ulcer disease.

Tobacco Smoking: Nicotine increases the blood levels of naturally produced cortisone and related hormones. Heavy smoking may add to the expected actions of this drug and requires close observation for excessive effects.

Marijuana Smoking: May cause additional impairment of immunity.

▷   *Other Drugs*

Prednisolone may *decrease* the effects of
- isoniazid (INH, Niconyl, etc.).
- salicylates (aspirin, sodium salicylate, etc.).

Prednisolone *taken concurrently* with
- oral anticoagulants may either increase or decrease their effectiveness; consult physician regarding the need for prothrombin time testing and dosage adjustment.

The following drugs may *decrease* the effects of prednisolone
- antacids may reduce its absorption.
- barbiturates (Amytal, Butisol, phenobarbital, etc.).
- phenytoin (Dilantin, etc.).
- rifampin (Rifadin, Rimactane, etc.).

▷ *Driving, Hazardous Activities:* Usually no restrictions. Be alert to the rare occurrence of dizziness.

Aviation Note: The use of this drug **may be a disqualification** for piloting. Consult a designated Aviation Medical Examiner.

Exposure to Sun: No restrictions.

Occurrence of Unrelated Illness: This drug may decrease natural resistance to infection. Inform your physician if you develop an infection of any kind. It may also reduce your body's ability to respond to the stress of acute illness, injury or surgery. Keep your physician fully informed of any significant changes in your state of health.

Discontinuation: If you have been taking this drug for an extended period of time, do not discontinue it abruptly. Ask physician for guidance regarding gradual withdrawal. For a period of 2 years after discontinuing this drug, it is essential in the event of illness, injury or surgery that you inform attending medical personnel that you have used this drug in the past. The period of impaired response to stress following the use of cortisonelike drugs may last for 1 to 2 years.

PREDNISONE
(PRED ni sohn)

Introduced: 1955

Prescription: USA: Yes
    Canada: Yes

Available as Generic: USA: Yes
    Canada: Yes

Class: Cortisonelike drugs

Controlled Drug: USA: No
    Canada: No

Brand Names: ✦Apo-Prednisone, Deltasone, Meticorten, ✦Novoprednisone, Orasone, ✦Winpred

```
┌─────────────────────────────────────────────────────────────────────┐
│                       BENEFITS versus RISKS                           │
│                                                                       │
│        Possible Benefits                    Possible Risks            │
│  EFFECTIVE RELIEF OF              Short-term use (up to 10 days) is    │
│    SYMPTOMS IN A WIDE               usually well tolerated             │
│    VARIETY OF INFLAMMATORY        Long-term use (exceeding 2           │
│    AND ALLERGIC DISORDERS           weeks) is associated with many     │
│  EFFECTIVE                          possible adverse effects:          │
│    IMMUNOSUPPRESSION in           ALTERED MOOD AND                     │
│    selected benign and malignant    PERSONALITY                       │
│    disorders                      CATARACTS, GLAUCOMA                  │
│  Prevention of rejection in organ HYPERTENSION                        │
│    transplantation                OSTEOPOROSIS                         │
│                                   ASEPTIC BONE NECROSIS                │
│                                   INCREASED SUSCEPTIBILITY             │
│                                     TO INFECTIONS                      │
│                                   (See Possible Adverse Effects and    │
│                                    Possible Effects of Long-Term       │
│                                    Use below)                          │
└─────────────────────────────────────────────────────────────────────┘
```

▷ **Principal Uses**

As a Single Drug Product: This potent drug of the cortisone class is used in the treatment of a wide variety of allergic and inflammatory conditions. It is used most commonly in the management of serious skin disorders, asthma, regional enteritis, ulcerative colitis and all types of major rheumatic disorders including bursitis, tendinitis and most forms of arthritis.

How This Drug Works: Not fully established. It is thought that this drug's anti-inflammatory effect is due to its ability to inhibit the normal defensive functions of certain white blood cells. Its immunosuppressant effect is attributed to a reduced production of lymphocytes and antibodies.

Available Dosage Forms and Strengths
Oral solution — 5 mg per 5-ml teaspoonful
Syrup — 5 mg per 5-ml teaspoonful (alcohol 5%)
Tablets — 1 mg, 2.5 mg, 5 mg, 10 mg, 20 mg, 25 mg, 50 mg

▷ **Usual Adult Dosage Range:**   5 to 60 mg daily as a single dose or in divided doses. The total daily dosage should not exceed 250 mg. **Note: Actual dosage and administration schedule must be determined by the physician for each patient individually.**

▷ **Dosing Instructions:**   Take with or following food to prevent stomach irritation, preferably in the morning. The tablet may be crushed for administration.

Usual Duration of Use: For acute disorders: 4 to 10 days. For chronic disorders: according to individual requirements. The duration of use should not exceed the time necessary to obtain adequate symptomatic relief in acute self-limiting conditions; or the time required to stabilize a chronic condition and permit gradual withdrawal. Because of its intermediate duration of action, this drug is appropriate for alternate day administration. Consult your physician on a regular basis.

▷ **This Drug Should Not Be Taken If**
- you have had an allergic reaction to any dosage form of it previously.
- you have active peptic ulcer disease.
- you have an active infection of the eye caused by the herpes simplex virus.
- you have active tuberculosis.

▷ **Inform Your Physician Before Taking This Drug If**
- you have had an unfavorable reaction to any cortisonelike drug in the past.
- you have a history of peptic ulcer disease, thrombophlebitis or tuberculosis.
- you have any of the following: diabetes, glaucoma, high blood pressure, deficient thyroid function or myasthenia gravis.
- you plan to have surgery of any kind in the near future.

Possible Side-Effects (natural, expected and unavoidable drug actions)
Increased appetite, weight gain, retention of salt and water, excretion of potassium, increased susceptibility to infection.

▷ **Possible Adverse Effects** (unusual, unexpected and infrequent reactions)
If any of the following develop, consult your physician promptly for guidance.
Mild Adverse Effects
Allergic Reaction: Skin rash.
Headache, dizziness, insomnia.
Acid indigestion, abdominal distention.
Muscle cramping and weakness.
Acne, excessive growth of facial hair.
Serious Adverse Effects
Mental and emotional disturbances of serious magnitude.
Reactivation of latent tuberculosis.
Development of peptic ulcer.
Increased blood pressure.
Development of inflammation of the pancreas.
Thrombophlebitis (inflammation of a vein with the formation of blood clot)—pain or tenderness in thigh or leg, with or without swelling of the foot, ankle or leg.
Pulmonary embolism (movement of a blood clot to the lung)—sudden shortness of breath, pain in the chest, coughing, bloody sputum.

▷ **Possible Effects on Sexual Function**

Altered timing and pattern of menstruation.

Correction of male infertility when due to autoantibodies that suppress sperm activity.

▷ **Adverse Effects That May Mimic Natural Diseases or Disorders**

Pattern of symptoms and signs resembling Cushing's syndrome.

Natural Diseases or Disorders That May Be Activated by This Drug

Latent diabetes, glaucoma, peptic ulcer disease, tuberculosis.

CAUTION

1. It is advisable to carry a card of personal identification with a notation that you are taking this drug, if your course of treatment is to exceed 1 week.
2. Do not discontinue this drug abruptly if you are using it for long-term treatment.
3. If vaccination against measles, rabies, smallpox or yellow fever is required, discontinue this drug 72 hours before vaccination and do not resume it for at least 14 days after vaccination.

Precautions for Use

By Infants and Children: Avoid prolonged use if possible. During long-term use, observe for suppression of normal growth and the possibility of increased intracranial pressure. Following long-term use, the child may be at risk for adrenal gland deficiency during stress for as long as 18 months after cessation of this drug.

By Those over 60 Years of Age: Cortisonelike drugs should be used very sparingly after 60 and only when the disorder under treatment is unresponsive to adequate trials of unrelated drugs. Avoid the prolonged use of this drug. Continual use (even in small doses) can increase the severity of diabetes, enhance fluid retention, raise blood pressure, weaken resistance to infection, induce stomach ulcer and accelerate development of cataract and osteoporosis.

▷ **Advisability of Use During Pregnancy**

Pregnancy Category: C (tentative). See Pregnancy Code inside back cover.

Animal studies: Birth defects reported in mice, rats and rabbits.

Human studies: Information from adequate studies of pregnant women is not available.

Avoid completely during the first 3 months. Limit use during the last 6 months as much as possible. If used, examine infant for possible deficiency of adrenal gland function.

Advisability of Use if Breast-Feeding

Presence of this drug in breast milk: Yes.

Avoid drug or refrain from nursing.

Habit-Forming Potential: Use of this drug to suppress symptoms over an extended period of time may produce a state of functional dependence (see Glossary). In the treatment of conditions like asthma and rheumatoid arthritis, it is advisable to keep the dose as small as possible and to attempt drug withdrawal after periods of reasonable improvement. Such procedures may reduce the degree of "steroid rebound"—the return of symptoms as the drug is withdrawn.

Effects of Overdosage: Fatigue, muscle weakness, stomach irritation, acid indigestion, excessive sweating, facial flushing, fluid retention, swelling of extremities, increased blood pressure.

Possible Effects of Long-Term Use: Increased blood sugar (possible diabetes), increased fat deposits on the trunk of the body ("buffalo hump"), rounding of the face ("moon face"), thinning and fragility of skin, loss of texture and strength of bones (osteoporosis, aseptic necrosis), cataracts, glaucoma, retarded growth and development in children.

Suggested Periodic Examinations While Taking This Drug (at physician's discretion)
Measurements of blood pressure, blood sugar and potassium levels.
Complete eye examinations at regular intervals.
Chest X-ray if history of tuberculosis.
Determination of the rate of development of the growing child to detect retardation of normal growth.

▷ **While Taking This Drug, Observe the Following**
Foods: No interactions expected. Ask physician regarding need to restrict salt intake or to eat potassium-rich foods. During long-term use of this drug, it is advisable to eat a high-protein diet.
Nutritional Support: During long-term use, take a vitamin D supplement. During wound repair, take a zinc supplement.
Beverages: No restrictions. Drink all forms of milk liberally.
▷ *Alcohol:* No interactions expected. Use caution if you are prone to peptic ulcer disease.
Tobacco Smoking: Nicotine increases the blood levels of naturally produced cortisone and related hormones. Heavy smoking may add to the expected actions of this drug and requires close observation for excessive effects.
Marijuana Smoking: May cause additional impairment of immunity.
▷ *Other Drugs*
Prednisone may ***decrease*** the effects of
• isoniazid (INH, Niconyl, etc.).
• salicylates (aspirin, sodium salicylate, etc.).
Prednisone ***taken concurrently*** with
• oral anticoagulants may either increase or decrease their effectiveness; consult physician regarding the need for prothrombin time testing and dosage adjustment.
The following drugs may ***decrease*** the effects of prednisone
• antacids may reduce its absorption.

- barbiturates (Amytal, Butisol, phenobarbital, etc.).
- phenytoin (Dilantin, etc.).
- rifampin (Rifadin, Rimactane, etc.).

▷ *Driving, Hazardous Activities:* Usually no restrictions. Be alert to the rare occurrence of dizziness.

Aviation Note: The use of this drug **may be a disqualification** for piloting. Consult a designated Aviation Medical Examiner.

Exposure to Sun: No restrictions.

Occurrence of Unrelated Illness: This drug may decrease natural resistance to infection. Inform your physician if you develop an infection of any kind. It may also reduce your body's ability to respond to the stress of acute illness, injury or surgery. Keep your physician fully informed of any significant changes in your state of health.

Discontinuation: If you have been taking this drug for an extended period of time, do not discontinue it abruptly. Ask physician for guidance regarding gradual withdrawal. For a period of 2 years after discontinuing this drug, it is essential in the event of illness, injury or surgery that you inform attending medical personnel that you have used this drug in the past. The period of impaired response to stress following the use of cortisonelike drugs may last for 1 to 2 years.

PRIMIDONE
(PRI mi dohn)

Introduced: 1953

Class: Anticonvulsant

Prescription: USA: Yes
Canada: Yes

Controlled Drug: USA: No
Canada: No

Available as Generic: USA: Yes
Canada: Yes

Brand Names: ✦Apo-Primidone, Myidone, Mysoline, ✦Sertan

BENEFITS versus RISKS	
Possible Benefits	*Possible Risks*
EFFECTIVE CONTROL OF TONIC-CLONIC (GRAND MAL) AND ALL TYPES OF PARTIAL SEIZURES	Allergic skin reactions Rare blood cell disorders: megaloblastic anemia, deficient white blood cells and platelets

▷ **Principal Uses**

As a Single Drug Product: This drug is used exclusively to control generalized grand mal seizures and all types of partial seizures. It can be used to supplement the anticonvulsant action of phenytoin.

How This Drug Works: Not completely established. This drug reduces and stabilizes the excitability of nerve fibers and inhibits the repetitious spread of electrical impulses along nerve pathways. This action may prevent seizures altogether, or it may reduce their frequency and severity. (Part of this drug's action is attributable to phenobarbital, one of its conversion products in the body.)

Available Dosage Forms and Strengths
> Oral suspensions — 250 mg per 5-ml teaspoonful
> Tablets — 50 mg, 250 mg

▷ **Usual Adult Dosage Range:**   Initially, 250 mg/24 hours as a single dose at bedtime for 1 week; 2nd week, 250 mg/12 hours; 3rd week, 250 mg 3 times/day, 6 to 8 hours apart; 4th week, 250 mg 4 times/day, 4 to 6 hours apart. The total daily dosage should not exceed 2000 mg. **Note: Actual dosage and administration schedule must be determined by the physician for each patient individually.**

▷ **Dosing Instructions:**   May be taken with or following food to reduce stomach irritation. The tablet may be crushed for administration. Shake the suspension well before measuring the dose.

Usual Duration of Use: Continual use on a regular schedule for 2 to 4 weeks is usually necessary to determine this drug's effectiveness in reducing the frequency and severity of seizures. Long-term use (months to years) requires supervision and periodic evaluation by your physician. Consult your physician on a regular basis.

▷ **This Drug Should Not Be Taken If**
- you have had an allergic reaction to it previously.
- you are allergic to phenobarbital.
- you have a history of porphyria.

▷ **Inform Your Physician Before Taking This Drug If**
- you have had an allergic or idiosyncratic reaction to any barbiturate drug in the past.
- you have a family history of intermittent porphyria.
- you have impaired liver, kidney or thyroid gland function.
- you have asthma, emphysema or myasthenia gravis.
- you are pregnant or planning pregnancy.
- you plan to have surgery under general anesthesia in the near future.

Possible Side-Effects (natural, expected and unavoidable drug actions)
> Drowsiness, impaired concentration, mental and physical sluggishness.

▷ **Possible Adverse Effects** (unusual, unexpected and infrequent reactions)
> **If any of the following develop, consult your physician promptly for guidance.**
> *Mild Adverse Effects*
> Allergic Reactions: Skin rashes, hives, localized swellings.
> "Hangover" effect, dizziness, unsteadiness, impaired vision, double vision, fatigue, emotional disturbances.

Low blood pressure, faintness.

Nausea, vomiting, thirst, increased urine volume.

Serious Adverse Effects

Allergic Reaction: Swelling of lymph glands.

Idiosyncratic Reactions: Paradoxical anxiety, agitation, restlessness, rage.

Visual hallucinations.

Blood cell disorders: megaloblastic anemia due to folic acid depletion; deficient production of white blood cells and blood platelets.

▷ **Possible Effects on Sexual Function**

Decreased libido and/or impotence (22%).

Decreased effectiveness of oral contraceptives taken concurrently.

▷ **Adverse Effects That May Mimic Natural Diseases or Disorders**

Allergic swelling of lymph glands may suggest a naturally occurring lymphoma.

Natural Diseases or Disorders That May Be Activated by This Drug

Acute intermittent and/or cutaneous porphyria (see Glossary).

Systemic lupus erythematosus.

CAUTION

1. This drug must not be stopped abruptly.
2. The wide variation of this drug's action from person to person requires careful individualization of dosage schedules.
3. Regularity of drug use is essential for the successful management of seizure disorders. Take your medication at the same time each day.
4. Side-effects and mild adverse effects are usually most apparent during the first several weeks of treatment and often subside with continued use.
5. It may be necessary to take folic acid to prevent anemia while taking this drug. Consult your physician.
6. It is advisable to carry a card of personal identification with a notation that you are taking this drug.

Precautions for Use

By Infants and Children: This drug should be used with caution in the hyperkinetic (overactive) child. Observe for possible paradoxical hyperactivity. Changes associated with puberty characteristically slow the metabolism of phenobarbital and permit its gradual accumulation. Measurements of blood levels in young adolescents can detect rising concentrations of this drug that could lead to toxicity. (See Therapeutic Drug Monitoring in Section One.)

By Those over 60 Years of Age: It is advisable to avoid all barbiturates in the elderly. If use of this drug is attempted, start with small doses until tolerance has been determined. Observe for confusion, delirium, agitation or paradoxical excitement. This drug may be conducive to hypothermia (see Glossary).

▷ **Advisability of Use During Pregnancy**

Pregnancy Category: D (tentative). See Pregnancy Code inside back cover. Animal studies: Birth defects due to this drug reported in mice.

Human studies: Information from adequate studies of pregnant women is not available. However, recent reports suggest a possible association between the use of this drug during the first 3 months of pregnancy and the development of birth defects in the fetus. Discuss with your physician the advantages and possible disadvantages of using this drug during pregnancy. If it is used, determine the smallest maintenance dose that will prevent seizures.

The newborn infants of mothers who take this drug during pregnancy may develop abnormal bleeding or bruising due to the deficiency of certain blood clotting factors in the blood. Consult your physician regarding the need to take vitamin K during the last month of pregnancy.

Advisability of Use if Breast-Feeding

Presence of this drug in breast milk: Yes.

Monitor nursing infant closely and discontinue drug or nursing if adverse effects develop.

Habit-Forming Potential: None.

Effects of Overdosage: Drowsiness, jerky eye movements, blurred vision, staggering gait, incoordination, slurred speech, stupor progressing to coma.

Possible Effects of Long-Term Use: Enlargement of lymph glands; enlargement of thyroid gland. Megaloblastic anemia due to folic acid deficiency. Reduced blood levels of calcium and phosphorus, leading to rickets in children and loss of bone texture (osteomalacia) in adults.

Suggested Periodic Examinations While Taking This Drug (at physician's discretion)

Complete blood cell counts. Measurements of blood levels of calcium and phosphorus. Evaluation of lymph and thyroid glands. Skeletal X-ray examinations for bone demineralization during long-term use.

▷ **While Taking This Drug, Observe the Following**

Foods: No restrictions.

Nutritional Support: Consult your physician regarding the need for supplements of calcium, vitamin D, folic acid and vitamin K.

Beverages: No restrictions. May be taken with milk or fruit juice.

▷ *Alcohol:* Avoid completely. Alcohol can increase greatly the sedative and depressant effects of this drug on brain function.

Tobacco Smoking: May enhance the sedative effects of this drug and increase drowsiness.

▷ *Other Drugs*

Note: 15% of primidone is converted to phenobarbital in the body. See the Drug Profile of Phenobarbital for possible interactions with other drugs.

▷ *Driving, Hazardous Activities:* This drug may cause drowsiness and dizziness; it can also impair mental alertness, vision and physical coordination. Restrict activities as necessary.

Aviation Note: The use of this drug **is a disqualification** for piloting. Consult a designated Aviation Medical Examiner.

Exposure to Sun: No restrictions.

Occurrence of Unrelated Illness: Notify your physician of any illness or injury that prevents the use of this drug according to your regular dosage schedule.

Discontinuation: Do not discontinue this drug without your physician's knowledge and approval. Sudden withdrawal of any anticonvulsant drug can cause severe and repeated seizures.

PROBENECID
(proh BEN e sid)

Introduced: 1951

Prescription: USA: Yes
Canada: No

Available as Generic: USA: Yes
Canada: No

Class: Antigout

Controlled Drug: USA: No
Canada: No

Brand Names: ✦Ampicin PRB [CD], Benemid, ✦Benuryl, ColBenemid [CD], Polycillin-PRB [CD], Probalan, ✦Pro-Biosan 500 Kit [CD]

BENEFITS versus RISKS	
Possible Benefits	***Possible Risks***
EFFECTIVE LONG-TERM PREVENTION OF ACUTE ATTACKS OF GOUT	Formation of uric acid kidney stones
Useful adjunct to penicillin therapy (to achieve high blood and tissue levels of penicillin)	Bone marrow depression (aplastic anemia) (rare)
	Drug-induced liver and kidney damage (both rare)

▷ **Principal Uses**

As a Single Drug Product: Used primarily in the long-term management of gout to prevent acute attacks. While effective for prevention, it has no beneficial effects in relieving the joint inflammation and pain of the acute episode. In fact, it may aggravate and prolong the symptoms of acute gout.

As a Combination Drug Product [CD]: This drug is available in combination with colchicine, a drug often used for the treatment of acute gout. Each drug has a different mechanism of action; when used in combination they provide both relief of the acute manifestations of gout and some measure of protection from recurrence of acute attacks.

How This Drug Works: By acting on the tubular systems of the kidney to increase the amount of uric acid excreted in the urine, this drug reduces the levels of uric acid in the blood and body tissues. By acting on the tubular systems of the kidney to decrease the amount of penicillin excreted in the urine, this drug prolongs the presence of penicillin in the blood and helps achieve higher concentrations in body tissues.

Available Dosage Forms and Strengths
Tablets — 500 mg

▷ **Usual Adult Dosage Range:**   Antigout: Initially, 250 mg twice/day for 1 week; then 500 mg twice/day. Adjunct to penicillin therapy: 500 mg 4 times/day. **Note: Actual dosage and administration schedule must be determined by the physician for each patient individually.**

▷ **Dosing Instructions:**   Take with or following food to reduce stomach irritation. Drink 2.5 to 3 quarts of liquids daily. The tablet may be crushed for administration.

Usual Duration of Use: Continual use on a regular schedule for several months is usually necessary to determine this drug's effectiveness in preventing acute attacks of gout. Long-term use (months to years) requires supervision and periodic evaluation by your physician. Consult your physician on a regular basis.

▷ **This Drug Should Not Be Taken If**
  • you have had an allergic reaction to it previously.
  • you have active liver disease.
  • you have an active blood cell or bone marrow disorder.
  • you are experiencing an attack of acute gout at the present time.

▷ **Inform Your Physician Before Taking This Drug If**
  • you have a history of kidney disease or kidney stones.
  • you have a history of liver disease or impaired liver function.
  • you have a history of peptic ulcer disease.
  • you have a history of a blood cell or bone marrow disorder.
  • you are taking any drug product that contains aspirin or aspirinlike drugs.

Possible Side-Effects (natural, expected and unavoidable drug actions)
Development of kidney stones (composed of uric acid); this is preventable. Consult your physician regarding the use of sodium bicarbonate (or other urine alkalizer) to prevent stone formation.

▷ **Possible Adverse Effects** (unusual, unexpected and infrequent reactions)
   If any of the following develop, consult your physician promptly for guidance.
   Mild Adverse Effects
   Allergic Reactions: Skin rash, itching, drug fever (see Glossary).
   Headache, dizziness, flushing of face.
   Reduced appetite, sore gums, nausea, vomiting.
   Serious Adverse Effects
   Allergic Reaction: Anaphylactic reaction (see Glossary).
   Idiosyncratic Reaction: Hemolytic anemia (see Glossary).
   Bone marrow depression (see Glossary): fatigue, weakness, fever, sore throat, abnormal bleeding or bruising.
   Drug-induced liver damage with jaundice (see Glossary).
   Drug-induced kidney damage: marked fluid retention, reduced urine formation.

▷ **Possible Effects on Sexual Function:**   None reported.

▷ **Adverse Effects That May Mimic Natural Diseases or Disorders**
   Liver reactions may suggest viral hepatitis.
   Kidney reactions may suggest nephrosis.

CAUTION
   1. This drug should not be started until 2 to 3 weeks after an acute attack of gout has subsided.
   2. This drug may increase the frequency of acute attacks of gout during the first few months of treatment. Concurrent use of colchicine is advised to prevent acute attacks. See the Profile of Gout in Section Two.
   3. Aspirin (and aspirin-containing drug products) can reduce the effectiveness of this drug. Use acetaminophen or a nonaspirin analgesic for pain relief as needed.

Precautions for Use
   By Infants and Children: Safety and effectiveness for use by those under 2 years of age have not been established.
   By Those over 60 Years of Age: The natural decline in kidney function that occurs after 60 may require adjustment of your dosage. You may be more susceptible to the serious adverse effects of this drug. Report any unusual symptoms promptly for evaluation.

▷ **Advisability of Use During Pregnancy**
   Pregnancy Category: C (tentative). See Pregnancy Code inside back cover.
   Animal studies: No information available.
   Human studies: Information from adequate studies of pregnant women is not available.
   This drug has been used during pregnancy with no reports of birth defects or adverse effects on the fetus. Ask your physician for guidance.

Advisability of Use if Breast-Feeding
Presence of this drug in breast milk: Unknown.
Avoid drug or refrain from nursing.

Habit-Forming Potential: None.

Effects of Overdosage: Stomach irritation, nausea, vomiting, nervous agitation, delirium, seizures, coma.

Possible Effects of Long-Term Use: Formation of kidney stones. Kidney damage in sensitive individuals.

Suggested Periodic Examinations While Taking This Drug (at physician's discretion)
Complete blood cell counts, measurements of blood uric acid, liver and kidney function tests.

▷ **While Taking This Drug, Observe the Following**
Foods: Follow physician's advice regarding the need for a low-purine diet.
Beverages: A large intake of coffee, tea or cola beverages may reduce the effectiveness of treatment.
▷   *Alcohol:* No interactions expected. However, large amounts of alcohol can raise the blood uric acid level and reduce the effectiveness of treatment.
Tobacco Smoking: No interactions expected.
▷   *Other Drugs*
Probenecid may *increase* the effects of
• clofibrate (Atromid S).
• dyphylline (Neothylline).
• methotrexate (Mexate), and increase its toxicity.
• thiopental (Pentothal), and prolong its anesthetic effect.
Probenecid *taken concurrently* with
• penicillins may cause a threefold to fivefold increase in penicillin blood levels, greatly increasing the effectiveness of each penicillin dose.
The following drugs may *decrease* the effects of probenecid
• aspirin and other salicylates may reduce its effectiveness in promoting the excretion of uric acid.
▷   *Driving, Hazardous Activities:* This drug may cause dizziness. Restrict activities as necessary.
Aviation Note: The use of this drug *may be a disqualification* for piloting. Consult a designated Aviation Medical Examiner.
Exposure to Sun: No restrictions.
Discontinuation: Do not discontinue this drug without consulting your physician.

PROBUCOL
(PROH byu kohl)

Introduced: 1971

Prescription: USA: Yes
Canada: Yes

Available as Generic: USA: No
Canada: No

Brand Name: Lorelco

Class: Anticholesterol

Controlled Drug: USA: No
Canada: No

BENEFITS versus RISKS

Possible Benefits	*Possible Risks*
EFFECTIVE REDUCTION OF TOTAL CHOLESTEROL AND LOW DENSITY CHOLESTEROL IN TYPE IIa CHOLESTEROL DISORDERS (15% to 20% reduction of total cholesterol, 10% to 15% reduction of LDL cholesterol when used in conjunction with a low-cholesterol diet)	CONCURRENT REDUCTION (22% to 25%) OF HIGH DENSITY (HDL) CHOLESTEROL (This is thought to be undesirable in the prevention and treatment of atherosclerosis.) Diarrhea, indigestion (10%)

▷ **Principal Uses**
As a Single Drug Product: Used for the reduction of abnormally high blood levels of cholesterol (type IIa) that have not responded to adequate control of diet, weight, diabetes and hypothyroidism.

How This Drug Works: Not completely known. It is thought that this drug may inhibit the absorption of dietary cholesterol, may inhibit the early stages of cholesterol production in the liver and may increase the rate of LDL cholesterol destruction and elimination.

Available Dosage Forms and Strengths
Tablets — 250 mg, 500 mg

▷ **Usual Adult Dosage Range:** 250 mg to 500 mg twice daily. **Note: Actual dosage and administration schedule must be determined by the physician for each patient individually.**

▷ **Dosing Instructions:** Take with the morning and evening meals. The tablet may be crushed for administration.

Usual Duration of Use: Continual use on a regular schedule for 3 to 6 months is usually necessary to determine this drug's effectiveness in lowering cholesterol blood levels. Long-term use (months to years) requires periodic evaluation of response and dosage adjustment. Consult your physician on a regular basis.

▷ **This Drug Should Not Be Taken If**
- you have had an allergic reaction to it previously.
- you have had a heart attack (myocardial infarction) recently.

▷ **Inform Your Physician Before Taking This Drug If**
- you are pregnant.
- you have a history of heart disease, heart rhythm disorder or abnormal electrocardiogram.
- you have impaired liver function or gallstones.

Possible Side-Effects (natural, expected and unavoidable drug actions)
None.

▷ **Possible Adverse Effects** (unusual, unexpected and infrequent reactions)
If any of the following develop, consult your physician promptly for guidance.
Mild Adverse Effects
Allergic Reactions: Rash, itching, swelling (angioedema) of face, mouth, hands or feet.
Headache, dizziness, numbness or tingling in extremities.
Indigestion, excessive gas, abdominal discomfort, nausea, vomiting, diarrhea.
Serious Adverse Effects
Idiosyncratic Reactions: Dizziness, fainting, chest pain, heart palpitations.
Altered electrocardiogram in some individuals.

▷ **Possible Effects on Sexual Function**
Altered timing and pattern of menstruation.
Impotence (rare).

CAUTION
1. Report promptly the development of chest pain, heart palpitations, dizziness or faintness.
2. Comply fully with all recommendations for periodic measurements of blood cholesterol and triglyceride levels. These are essential to monitoring your response to treatment and determining the need for changes in dosage or medication.

Precautions for Use
By Infants and Children: Safety and effectiveness for use by those under 12 years of age have not been established.
By Those over 60 Years of Age: It is advisable to have an electrocardiogram before starting this drug and at intervals of 6 months until it is determined that there is no drug-induced alteration of heart function.

▷ **Advisability of Use During Pregnancy**
Pregnancy Category: B (tentative). See Pregnancy Code inside back cover.
Animal studies: No drug-induced birth defects found in rodents.

Human studies: Information from adequate studies of pregnant women is not available.

Use this drug only if clearly needed. Because of the long persistence of this drug in body tissues, it is recommended that the drug be discontinued and that birth control be used for 6 months before attempting to establish pregnancy.

The manufacturer does not recommend the use of this drug during pregnancy.

Advisability of Use if Breast-Feeding
Presence of this drug in breast milk: Unknown.
Avoid drug or refrain from nursing.

Habit-Forming Potential: None.

Effects of Overdosage: Abdominal distress, nausea, vomiting, diarrhea.

Possible Effects of Long-Term Use: Decrease in high density (HDL) cholesterol blood levels; increase in triglyceride blood levels.

Suggested Periodic Examinations While Taking This Drug (at physician's discretion)
Measurements of blood levels of total cholesterol, HDL and LDL cholesterol fractions and triglycerides.
Electrocardiograms (selectively).

▷ **While Taking This Drug, Observe the Following**
Foods: Follow the low-cholesterol diet prescribed by your physician.
Beverages: No restrictions.
▷   *Alcohol:* No interactions expected.
Tobacco Smoking: No interactions expected.
▷   *Other Drugs*
Probucol may *decrease* the effects of
• chenodiol (Chenix), and impair its effectiveness in the treatment of gallstones.
▷   *Driving, Hazardous Activities:* This drug may cause dizziness or faintness in sensitive individuals. Restrict activities as necessary.
Aviation Note: The use of this drug *is usually not a disqualification* for piloting. Consult a designated Aviation Medical Examiner.
Exposure to Sun: No restrictions.
Discontinuation: Do not discontinue this drug without your physician's knowledge and guidance. Abrupt withdrawal may be followed by prompt and excessive increase in blood cholesterol levels.

PROCAINAMIDE
(proh kayn A mide)

Introduced: 1950

Class: Antiarrhythmic

Prescription: USA: Yes
Canada: Yes

Controlled Drug: USA: No
Canada: No

Available as Generic: USA: Yes
Canada: No

Brand Names: Procamide SR, Procan SR, Pronestyl, Pronestyl-SR

<table>
<tr><td colspan="2" align="center">BENEFITS versus RISKS</td></tr>
<tr><td align="center">Possible Benefits</td><td align="center">Possible Risks</td></tr>
<tr><td>EFFECTIVE TREATMENT OF SELECTED HEART RHYTHM DISORDERS</td><td>NARROW TREATMENT RANGE INDUCTION OF SYSTEMIC LUPUS ERYTHEMATOSUS SYNDROME in 20% of long-term users
Provocation of abnormal heart rhythms
Blood cell disorders: insufficient white blood cells and platelets</td></tr>
</table>

▷ **Principal Uses**

As a Single Drug Product: This drug is classified as a Type 1 anti-arrhythmic agent, similar to disopyramide and quinidine in its actions. It is used primarily to abolish and prevent the recurrence of premature beats arising in the atria (upper chambers) and the ventricles (lower chambers) of the heart. It is also useful in the treatment and prevention of atrial fibrillation, atrial flutter and abnormally rapid heart rates (tachycardia) that originate in the atria or the ventricles.

How This Drug Works: By slowing the activity of the pacemaker and delaying the transmission of electrical impulses through the conduction system and muscle of the heart, this drug assists in restoring normal heart rate and rhythm.

Available Dosage Forms and Strengths

Capsules — 250 mg, 375 mg, 500 mg
Injections — 100 mg per ml, 500 mg per ml
Tablets — 250 mg, 375 mg, 500 mg
Tablets, prolonged-action — 250 mg, 500 mg, 750 mg, 1000 mg

▷ **Usual Adult Dosage Range:**   Dose varies according to indication for use. Premature atrial or ventricular contractions: 250 to 500 mg/3 hours. Paroxysmal atrial tachycardia: initially, 1250 mg, followed in 1 hour by 750 mg; then 500 to 1000 mg/2 hours as needed and tolerated. Atrial fibrillation and flutter: the heart should be digitalized first; then initiate procainamide with 1250 mg, followed in 1 hour by 750 mg; follow with 500 to 1000 mg/2 hours as needed and tolerated. For maintenance: 500 to 1000 mg/4 to 6 hours. The total daily dosage should not exceed 6000 mg. **Note: Actual dosage and administration schedule must be determined by the physician for each patient individually.**

▷ **Dosing Instructions:**   Preferably taken on an empty stomach, 1 hour before or 2 hours after eating. However, it may be taken with or following food to reduce stomach irritation. The regular capsules may be opened and the regular tablets may be crushed for administration; however, the prolonged-action tablets should be swallowed whole without alteration.

Usual Duration of Use: Continual use on a regular schedule for 24 to 48 hours is usually necessary to determine this drug's effectiveness in correcting or preventing responsive rhythm disorders. Long-term use requires supervision and periodic evaluation by your physician. Consult your physician on a regular basis.

▷ **This Drug Should Not Be Taken If**
- you have had an allergic reaction to it previously.
- you have second-degree or third-degree heart block (determined by electrocardiogram).

▷ **Inform Your Physician Before Taking This Drug If**
- you are allergic to procaine (Novocain) or to other local anesthetics of the "-caine" drug class, such as those commonly used for glaucoma testing and for dental procedures.
- you have had any unfavorable reactions to other antiarrhythmic drugs in the past.
- you have a history of heart disease of any kind, especially "heart block."
- you have a history of low blood pressure.
- you have a history of lupus erythematosus.
- you have a history of abnormally low blood platelet counts from any cause.
- you have impaired liver or kidney function.
- you have myasthenia gravis.
- you have an enlarged prostate gland.
- you are taking any form of digitalis or any diuretic drug that can cause excessive loss of body potassium (ask physician).
- you plan to have surgery under general anesthesia in the near future.

Possible Side-Effects (natural, expected and unavoidable drug actions)
Drop in blood pressure in susceptible individuals.

▷ **Possible Adverse Effects** (unusual, unexpected and infrequent reactions)
If any of the following develop, consult your physician promptly for guidance.
Mild Adverse Effects
Allergic Reactions: Skin rash, hives, itching, drug fever (see Glossary).
Weakness, light-headedness.
Loss of appetite, bitter taste, indigestion, nausea, vomiting, diarrhea.
Serious Adverse Effects
Allergic Reactions: Systemic lupus erythematosuslike syndrome: fever, skin eruptions, joint and muscle pains, pleurisy. (This is reported to occur in at least 20% of users.)

Idiosyncratic Reactions: Mental depression, hallucinations, psychotic behavior, hemolytic anemia (see Glossary).

Severe drop in blood pressure, fainting.

Asthmalike breathing difficulties.

Induction of new heart rhythm disturbances.

Inability to empty urinary bladder, prostatism (see Glossary).

Blood cell disorders: abnormally low white blood cell count, causing fever, sore throat, infections; abnormally low blood platelet count, causing abnormal bleeding or bruising.

▷ **Possible Effects on Sexual Function:**   None reported.

▷ **Adverse Effects That May Mimic Natural Diseases or Disorders**
Rare liver reaction may suggest viral hepatitis.

Natural Diseases or Disorders That May Be Activated by This Drug
Systemic lupus erythematosus, myasthenia gravis.

CAUTION
1. Thorough evaluation of your heart function (including electrocardiograms) is necessary prior to using this drug.
2. Periodic evaluation of your heart function is necessary to determine your response to this drug. Some individuals may experience worsening of their heart rhythm disorder and/or deterioration of heart function. Close monitoring of heart rate, rhythm and overall performance is essential.
3. Dosage must be adjusted carefully for each individual. Do not change your dosage without the knowledge and supervision of your physician.
4. Do not take any other antiarrhythmic drug while taking this drug unless directed to do so by your physician.

Precautions for Use
By Infants and Children: Blood cell counts should be monitored for loss of white blood cells.
By Those over 60 Years of Age: Reduced kidney function may require reduction in dosage. Observe carefully for light-headedness, dizziness, unsteadiness and tendency to fall.

▷ **Advisability of Use During Pregnancy**
Pregnancy Category: C (tentative). See Pregnancy Code inside back cover.
Animal studies: No information available.
Human studies: Information from adequate studies of pregnant women is not available.
Use this drug only if clearly needed.

Advisability of Use if Breast-Feeding
Presence of this drug in breast milk: Unknown.
Avoid drug or refrain from nursing.

Habit-Forming Potential: None.

Effects of Overdosage: Loss of appetite, nausea, vomiting, weakness, faintness, irregular heart rhythm, stupor, circulatory collapse, heart arrest.

Possible Effects of Long-Term Use: Lupus erythematosus–like syndrome (see above).

Suggested Periodic Examinations While Taking This Drug (at physician's discretion)
Complete blood cell counts.
Blood tests for the development of lupus erythematosus (LE) cells and antinuclear antibodies.
Electrocardiograms to monitor the full effect of this drug on the mechanisms that influence heart rate and rhythm.

▷ **While Taking This Drug, Observe the Following**
Foods: No restrictions.
Beverages: Avoid excessive intake of coffee, tea and cola beverages. Avoid iced drinks. May be taken with milk.
▷   *Alcohol:* Use caution until the combined effects have been determined. Alcohol can increase the blood-pressure-lowering effects of this drug.
Tobacco Smoking: Nicotine can cause irritability of the heart and reduce the effectiveness of this drug. Follow physician's advice regarding smoking.
▷   *Other Drugs*
Procainamide may *increase* the effects of
• antihypertensive drugs, and cause excessive lowering of blood pressure.
The following drugs may *increase* the effects of procainamide
• amiodirone.
• cimetidine (Tagamet).
▷   *Driving, Hazardous Activities:* This drug may cause dizziness or weakness. Restrict activities as necessary.
Aviation Note: The use of this drug *may be a disqualification* for piloting. Consult a designated Aviation Medical Examiner.
Exposure to Sun: No restrictions.
Exposure to Heat: Use caution. Hot environments are conducive to lower blood pressure.
Occurrence of Unrelated Illness: Disorders that cause vomiting, diarrhea or dehydration can affect this drug's action adversely. Report such developments promptly.
Discontinuation: This drug should not be discontinued abruptly following long-term use. Ask your physician for guidance regarding gradual dose reduction.

PROCHLORPERAZINE
(proh klor PER a zeen)

Introduced: 1956

Class: Strong tranquilizer, antiemetic, phenothiazines

Prescription: USA: Yes
Canada: Yes

Controlled Drug: USA: No
Canada: No

Available as Generic: USA: Yes
Canada: No

Brand Names: ✦Combid [CD], Compazine, ✦Stemetil

BENEFITS versus RISKS

Possible Benefits	*Possible Risks*
EFFECTIVE CONTROL OF ACUTE MENTAL DISORDERS in the majority of patients: beneficial effects on thinking, mood and behavior EFFECTIVE CONTROL OF NAUSEA AND VOMITING Relief of anxiety and nervous tension	SERIOUS TOXIC EFFECTS ON BRAIN with long-term use Liver damage with jaundice (infrequent) Rare blood cell disorders: abnormally low white cell and platelet counts

---

▷ **Principal Uses**

As a Single Drug Product: This member of the phenothiazine class is used primarily to relieve severe nausea and vomiting. Although it has sedative and antipsychotic effects characteristic of this class, it is used less often as a major tranquilizer.

How This Drug Works: Not completely established. Present theory is that by inhibiting the action of dopamine, this drug acts to correct an imbalance of nerve impulse transmissions that is thought to be responsible for certain mental disorders. By blocking the action of dopamine in the chemoreceptor trigger zone of the brain, this drug prevents excessive stimulation of the vomiting center.

Available Dosage Forms and Strengths

Capsules, prolonged-action — 10 mg, 15 mg, 30 mg
Injection — 5 mg per ml
Suppositories — 2.5 mg, 5 mg, 25 mg
Syrup — 5 mg per 5-ml teaspoonful
Tablets — 5 mg, 10 mg, 25 mg

▷ **Usual Adult Dosage Range:** Initially, 5 mg/6 to 8 hours. If needed and tolerated, dose may be increased by 5 mg at intervals of 3 to 4 days. Usual range is 35 to 60 mg/24 hours. The total daily dosage should not exceed 150 mg. **Note: Actual dosage and administration schedule must be determined by the physician for each patient individually.**

▷ **Dosing Instructions:**   May be taken with or following food to reduce stomach irritation. The tablets may be crushed for administration. Prolonged-action capsules should be swallowed whole without alteration.

Duration of Use: Continual use on a regular schedule for 12 to 24 hours is usually necessary to determine this drug's effectiveness in controlling nausea and vomiting. If used for severe anxiety-tension states or acute psychotic behavior, a trial of several weeks is usually necessary to determine effectiveness. If not significantly beneficial within 6 weeks, it should be discontinued. Consult your physician on a regular basis.

▷ **This Drug Should Not Be Taken If**
   • you have had an allergic reaction to it previously.
   • you have active liver disease.
   • you have cancer of the breast.
   • you have a current blood cell or bone marrow disorder.

▷ **Inform Your Physician Before Taking This Drug If**
   • you are allergic or abnormally sensitive to any phenothiazine drug (see Drug Class, Section Four).
   • you have impaired liver or kidney function.
   • you have any type of seizure disorder.
   • you have diabetes, glaucoma or heart disease.
   • you have a history of lupus erythematosus.
   • you are taking any drug with sedative effects.
   • you plan to have surgery under general or spinal anesthesia in the near future.

Possible Side-Effects (natural, expected and unavoidable drug actions)
   Drowsiness (usually during the first 2 weeks), orthostatic hypotension (see Glossary), blurred vision, dry mouth, nasal congestion, constipation, impaired urination.
   Pink or purple coloration of urine, of no significance.

▷ **Possible Adverse Effects** (unusual, unexpected and infrequent reactions)
   If any of the following develop, consult your physician promptly for guidance.
   Mild Adverse Effects
   Allergic Reactions: Skin rash, hives, low-grade fever.
   Lowering of body temperature, especially in the elderly. (See Hypothermia in Glossary.)
   Increased appetite and weight gain.
   Dizziness, weakness, agitation, insomnia, impaired day and night vision.
   Chronic constipation, fecal impaction.

Serious Adverse Effects

Allergic Reactions: Hepatitis with jaundice (see Glossary), usually between second and fourth week; high fever; asthma; anaphylactic reaction (see Glossary).

Idiosyncratic Reaction: Toxic dermatitis.

Depression, disorientation, seizures.

Disturbances of heart rhythm, rapid heart rate.

Bone marrow depression (see Glossary): fever, sore throat, abnormal bleeding or bruising.

Parkinson-like disorders (see Glossary); muscle spasms of face, jaw, neck, back, extremities; extreme restlessness; slowed movements, muscle rigidity, tremors; tardive dyskinesias (see Glossary).

▷ **Possible Effects on Sexual Function**

Altered timing and pattern of menstruation.

Female breast enlargement with milk production.

Male breast enlargement and tenderness.

Inhibited ejaculation; priapism (see Glossary).

Causes false positive pregnancy test result.

▷ **Adverse Effects That May Mimic Natural Diseases or Disorders**

Nervous system reactions may suggest Parkinson's disease.

Liver reactions may suggest viral hepatitis.

Reactions resembling systemic lupus erythematosus can occur.

Natural Diseases or Disorders That May Be Activated by This Drug

Latent epilepsy, glaucoma, diabetes mellitus, prostatism (see Glossary).

CAUTION

1. Many over-the-counter medications (see OTC Drugs in Glossary) for allergies, colds and coughs contain drugs that can interact unfavorably with this drug. Ask your physician or pharmacist for guidance before using any such medications.
2. Antacids that contain aluminum and/or magnesium can prevent the absorption of this drug and reduce its effectiveness.
3. Obtain prompt evaluation of any change or disturbance of vision.

Precautions for Use

By Infants and Children: Do not use this drug in infants under 2 years of age, or in children of any age with symptoms suggestive of Reye syndrome (see Glossary). Children with acute illnesses ("flulike" infections, measles, chicken pox, etc.) are very susceptible to adverse effects when this drug is given to control nausea and vomiting.

By Those over 60 Years of Age: Small doses are advisable until individual response has been determined. You may be more susceptible to the development of drowsiness, lethargy, constipation, lowering of body temperature (hypothermia) and orthostatic hypotension (see Glossary). This drug can enhance existing prostatism (see Glossary). You may also be more susceptible to the development of Parkinson-like reactions and/or tardive dyskinesia (see discussion of these terms in

Glossary). These reactions must be recognized early since they may become unresponsive to treatment and irreversible.

▷ **Advisability of Use During Pregnancy**
Pregnancy Category: C (tentative). See Pregnancy Code inside back cover.
Animal studies: Cleft palate reported in mouse and rat studies.
Human studies: No increase in birth defects reported in 2023 exposures. Information from adequate studies of pregnant women is not available.
Limit use to small and infrequent doses. Avoid drug during the last month because of possible effects on the newborn infant.

Advisability of Use if Breast-Feeding
Presence of this drug in breast milk: Yes, in small amounts.
Monitor nursing infant closely and discontinue drug or nursing if adverse effects develop.

Habit-Forming Potential: None.

Effects of Overdosage: Marked drowsiness, weakness, tremor, agitation, unsteadiness, deep sleep, coma, convulsions.

Possible Effects of Long-Term Use: Tardive dyskinesias. Eye changes: opacities in cornea or lens, retinal pigmentation.

Suggested Periodic Examinations While Taking This Drug (at physician's discretion)
Complete blood cell counts, especially between the fourth and tenth weeks of treatment.
Liver function tests, electrocardiograms.
Complete eye examinations—eye structures and vision.
Careful inspection of the tongue for early evidence of fine, involuntary, wavelike movements that could indicate the beginning of tardive dyskinesia.

▷ **While Taking This Drug, Observe the Following**
Foods: No restrictions.
Nutritional Support: A riboflavin (vitamin B-2) supplement should be taken with long-term use.
Beverages: No restrictions. May be taken with milk.
▷   *Alcohol:* Avoid completely. Alcohol can increase the sedative action of phenothiazines and accentuate their depressant effects on brain function and blood pressure. Phenothiazines can increase the intoxicating effects of alcohol.
Tobacco Smoking: Possible reduction of drowsiness from drug.
Marijuana Smoking: Moderate increase in drowsiness; accentuation of orthostatic hypotension; increased risk of precipitating latent psychoses, confusing the interpretation of mental status and drug responses.

▷ *Other Drugs*
Prochlorperazine may *increase* the effects of
- all sedative drugs, especially meperidine (Demerol), and cause excessive sedation.
- all atropinelike drugs, and cause nervous system toxicity.

Prochlorperazine may *decrease* the effects of
- guanethidine (Ismelin, Esimil), and reduce its effectiveness in lowering blood pressure.

Prochlorperazine *taken concurrently* with
- propranolol (Inderal) may cause increased effects of both drugs; monitor drug effects closely and adjust dosages as necessary.

The following drugs may *decrease* the effects of prochlorperazine
- antacids containing aluminum and/or magnesium.
- benztropine (Cogentin).
- trihexyphenidyl (Artane).

▷ *Driving, Hazardous Activities:* This drug can impair mental alertness, judgment and physical coordination. Avoid hazardous activities.

Aviation Note: The use of this drug *is a disqualification* for piloting. Consult a designated Aviation Medical Examiner.

Exposure to Sun: Use caution until sensitivity has been determined. Some phenothiazines can cause photosensitivity (see Glossary).

Exposure to Heat: Use caution and avoid excessive heat as much as possible. This drug may impair the regulation of body temperature and increase the risk of heat stroke.

Exposure to Cold: Use caution and dress warmly. This drug can increase the risk of hypothermia in the elderly.

Discontinuation: After a period of long-term use, do not discontinue this drug suddenly. Gradual withdrawal over 2 to 3 weeks under physician supervision is recommended.

PROMETHAZINE
(proh METH a zeen)

Introduced: 1945

Class: Antiemetic, antihistamines, phenothiazines

Prescription: USA: Yes
Canada: No

Controlled Drug: USA: No
Canada: No

Available as Generic: USA: Yes
Canada: Yes

Brand Names: ✦Histanil, K-Phen, Pentazine, Phenergan, Phenergan-D [CD], Phenergan w/Codeine [CD], ✦PMS Promethazine, Prorex

```
┌─────────────────────────────────────────────────────────────┐
│                   BENEFITS versus RISKS                      │
│                                                              │
│      Possible Benefits              Possible Risks           │
│   EFFECTIVE SYMPTOMATIC          EXCESSIVE SEDATION in        │
│     RELIEF OF ALLERGIC             sensitive individuals     │
│     RHINITIS AND DERMATOSIS      Atropinelike effects        │
│   Moderately effective prevention  Rare blood cell disorders:│
│     and treatment of motion          abnormally low white cell and │
│     sickness, nausea and vomiting    platelet counts         │
│   Effective as mild sedative and                             │
│     hypnotic                                                 │
└─────────────────────────────────────────────────────────────┘
```

▷ **Principal Uses**

As a Single Drug Product: This versatile drug shares the characteristics of two major drug classes, the antihistamines and the phenothiazines. It is used to provide symptomatic relief in allergic disorders (hay fever, hives, etc.), to control nausea and vomiting and to produce mild sedation.

As a Combination Drug Product [CD]: This drug is often combined with analgesics such as aspirin or codeine to enhance their pain-relieving action by producing mild sedation. It is also used in cough mixtures for its drying (antihistaminic) effect.

How This Drug Works: Not completely established. This drug reduces the intensity of the allergic response by blocking the action of histamine after it has been released from sensitized tissue cells. It reduces the sensitivity of the nerve endings in the labyrinth (inner ear) and blocks the transmission of excessive nerve impulses to the vomiting center in the brain. The way this drug produces sedation and light sleep is not known.

Available Dosage Forms and Strengths

Injections — 25 mg per ml, 50 mg per ml

Suppositories — 12.5 mg, 25 mg, 50 mg

Syrups — 6.25 mg per 5-ml teaspoonful (alcohol 7%), 25 mg per 5-ml teaspoonful (alcohol 1.5%)

Tablets — 12.5 mg, 25 mg, 50 mg

▷ **Usual Adult Dosage Range:** 12.5 to 25 mg/4 to 6 hours as needed. The total daily dosage should not exceed 150 mg. **Note: Actual dosage and administration schedule must be determined by the physician for each patient individually.**

▷ **Dosing Instructions:** Preferably taken with or following food to reduce stomach irritation. The tablets may be crushed for administration.

Usual Duration of Use: Continual use on a regular schedule for 3 to 5 days is usually necessary to determine this drug's effectiveness in relieving allergic symptoms or controlling vomiting. If not effective within 5 days, it should be discontinued.

▷ **This Drug Should Not Be Taken If**
- you have had an allergic reaction to it previously.
- you have a blood cell or bone marrow disorder.
- you have narrow-angle glaucoma (not adequately treated).

▷ **Inform Your Physician Before Taking This Drug If**
- you are allergic or overly sensitive to any phenothiazine drug (see Drug Class, Section Four).
- you are taking any drugs with sedative effects.
- you have a seizure disorder or bronchial asthma.
- you have impaired liver function.
- you have a history of peptic ulcer disease.
- you have an enlarged prostate gland or prostatism (see Glossary).

Possible Side-Effects (natural, expected and unavoidable drug actions)
Drowsiness (25% of users), lethargy, impaired concentration, dry mouth, constipation, impaired urination, reduced tolerance for contact lenses.

▷ **Possible Adverse Effects** (unusual, unexpected and infrequent reactions)
If any of the following develop, consult your physician promptly for guidance.
Mild Adverse Effects
Allergic Reactions: Skin rash, hives.
Headache, dizziness, unsteadiness, confusion, nervousness, excitation, irritability, tremor, insomnia, numbness and tingling, blurred vision, double vision, ringing in ears.
Loss of appetite, stomach irritation, nausea, vomiting, diarrhea.
Rapid heart rate, palpitation, low blood pressure.
Chest tightness, asthmatic wheezing, thickening of bronchial secretions.
Serious Adverse Effects
Allergic Reactions: Drug-induced hepatitis with jaundice (see Glossary).
Idiosyncratic Reactions: Euphoria, hysteria.
Nervous system reactions: Muscle spasms of the face, neck, back and extremities: rolling of the eyes, twisting of the neck, arching of the back, spasms of the hands and feet.
Blood cell disorders: abnormally low white blood cell and blood platelet counts, causing fever, sore throat, infections, abnormal bleeding or bruising (all very rare).

▷ **Possible Effects on Sexual Function:**   None reported.

▷ **Adverse Effects That May Mimic Natural Diseases or Disorders**
Drug-induced hepatitis may suggest viral hepatitis.

Natural Diseases or Disorders That May Be Activated by This Drug
Latent epilepsy, glaucoma, prostatism (see Glossary).

CAUTION
1. This drug should not be used alone to treat symptoms of lower respiratory tract disease, including asthma.

2. Avoid this drug for at least 5 days before skin testing for possible allergens.

Precautions for Use

By Infants and Children: This drug should not be used in premature or full-term newborn infants. The young child is especially sensitive to the nervous system effects of antihistamines and phenothiazines. Children with acute illnesses ("flulike" infections, measles, chicken pox, etc.) are very susceptible to muscular spasms of the face, neck, back or extremities when this drug is used to control nausea and vomiting. Avoid this drug completely during such infections; there is evidence to suggest that it may contribute to the development of Reye syndrome (see Glossary).

By Those over 60 Years of Age: You may be more susceptible to the development of drowsiness, dizziness and lethargy and to impaired thinking, judgment and memory. The sedative effect of this drug can cause a hypoactive syndrome that may be misinterpreted as senility or emotional depression. This drug can increase the symptoms of prostatism (see Glossary).

▷ Advisability of Use During Pregnancy

Pregnancy Category: B (tentative). See Pregnancy Code inside back cover.
Animal studies: No birth defects reported in rats.
Human studies: No significant increase in birth defects reported in 746 exposures to this drug.
Avoid use of this drug during the last 3 months; it can reduce certain blood clotting factors in the fetus and cause bleeding in the newborn infant.

Advisability of Use if Breast-Feeding

Presence of this drug in breast milk: Yes.
Avoid drug or refrain from nursing.

Habit-Forming Potential: None.

Effects of Overdosage: Marked drowsiness, weakness, unsteadiness, agitation, delirium, deep sleep, coma, seizures.

Possible Effects of Long-Term Use: The development of tolerance and loss of effectiveness.

Suggested Periodic Examinations While Taking This Drug (at physician's discretion)

Complete blood cell counts.

▷ While Taking This Drug, Observe the Following

Foods: No restrictions.
Beverages: No restrictions. May be taken with milk.
▷ *Alcohol:* Use extreme caution until the combined effects have been determined. The combination of alcohol and antihistamines can cause rapid and marked sedation.

Tobacco Smoking: No interactions expected.

▷ *Other Drugs*

Promethazine may **increase** the effects of
- all sedative drugs, and cause excessive sedation.
- atropine and atropinelike drugs (see Drug Class, Section Four).

▷ *Driving, Hazardous Activities:* This drug may cause dizziness or drowsiness. Restrict activities as necessary.

Aviation Note: The use of this drug **is a disqualification** for piloting. Consult a designated Aviation Medical Examiner.

Exposure to Sun: Use caution until sensitivity has been determined. This drug may cause photosensitivity (see Glossary).

PROPOXYPHENE
(proh POX i feen)

Introduced: 1955

Class: Analgesic, narcotic

Prescription: USA: Yes
Canada: Yes

Controlled Drug: USA: C-IV*
Canada: <N>

Available as Generic: Yes

Brand Names: Darvocet-N 50/100 [CD], Darvon, Darvon-N, Darvon w/ASA [CD], Darvon Compound [CD], Darvon Compound-65 [CD], Darvon-N w/ASA [CD], ✦Darvon-N Compound [CD], Dolene, Dolene AP-65 [CD], Dolene Compound-65 [CD], ✦Novopropoxyn, ✦Novopropoxyn Compound [CD], ✦642, Wygesic [CD]

BENEFITS versus RISKS

Possible Benefits	*Possible Risks*
EFFECTIVE RELIEF OF MILD TO MODERATE PAIN	POTENTIAL FOR HABIT FORMATION (DEPENDENCE)
	Sedative effects
	Drug-induced hepatitis (very rare)

▷ **Principal Uses**

As a Single Drug Product: This drug is used exclusively as an analgesic to relieve mild to moderate pain.

As a Combination Drug Product [CD]: It is available in combinations with acetaminophen and with aspirin. These milder pain relievers are added to enhance the analgesic effect and to reduce fever when present. Some combinations also contain caffeine to counteract the sedative effects of the analgesics.

*See Schedules of Controlled Drugs inside back cover.

How This Drug Works: Acting primarily as a depressant of certain brain functions, this drug suppresses the perception of pain and calms the emotional response to pain.

Available Dosage Forms and Strengths
Capsules — 32 mg, 65 mg
Oral suspension — 50 mg per 5-ml teaspoonful
Tablets — 100 mg

▷ **Usual Adult Dosage Range:**   For propoxyphene: 65 mg/4 hours as needed. The total daily dosage should not exceed 390 mg. For propoxyphene napsylate (Darvon-N): 100 mg/4 hours as needed. The total daily dose should not exceed 600 mg. **Note: Actual dosage and administration schedule must be determined by the physician for each patient individually.**

▷ **Dosing Instructions:**   May be taken with or following food to reduce stomach irritation or nausea. The tablet may be crushed and the capsule may be opened for administration.

Usual Duration of Use: As required to control pain. Continual use should not exceed 5 to 7 days without interruption and reassessment of need.

▷ **This Drug Should Not Be Taken If**
• you have had an allergic reaction to any dosage form of it previously.
• you are having an acute attack of asthma.

▷ **Inform Your Physician Before Taking This Drug If**
• you have had an unfavorable reaction to any narcotic drug in the past.
• you have a history of drug abuse or alcoholism.
• you have chronic lung disease with impaired breathing.
• you have impaired liver or kidney function.
• you are taking any other drugs that have a sedative effect.

Possible Side-Effects (natural, expected and unavoidable drug actions)
Drowsiness, light-headedness, constipation.

▷ **Possible Adverse Effects** (unusual, unexpected and infrequent reactions)
If any of the following develop, consult your physician promptly for guidance.
Mild Adverse Effects
Allergic Reactions: Skin rash, itching.
Headache, dizziness, weakness, confusion, blurred vision.
Nausea, vomiting, abdominal discomfort.
Serious Adverse Effects
Allergic Reactions: Hepatitis with jaundice (see Glossary).
Paradoxical excitement, agitation, insomnia.

▷ **Possible Effects on Sexual Function:**   None reported.

▷ **Precautions for Use**

By Infants and Children: Safety and effectiveness for use by those under 12 years of age have not been established.

By Those over 60 Years of Age: Use small doses initially and increase dosage as needed and tolerated. Limit use to short-term treatment only. There may be increased susceptibility to the development of drowsiness, dizziness, unsteadiness, falling and constipation (possibly leading to fecal impaction).

▷ **Advisability of Use During Pregnancy**

Pregnancy Category: C (tentative). See Pregnancy Code inside back cover.

Animal studies: No birth defects due to this drug were found.

Human studies: Information from studies of pregnant women indicates no significant increase in birth defects in 2914 exposures to this drug.

Use this drug only if clearly needed and in small, infrequent doses.

Advisability of Use if Breast-Feeding

Presence of this drug in breast milk: Yes, in small amounts.

Monitor nursing infant closely and discontinue drug or nursing if adverse effects develop.

Habit-Forming Potential: Psychological and/or physical dependence can develop with use of large doses for an extended period of time.

Effects of Overdosage: Drowsiness, restlessness, agitation, nausea, vomiting, dry mouth, vertigo, weakness, lethargy, stupor, coma, seizures.

Possible Effects of Long-Term Use: Psychological and physical dependence, chronic constipation.

Suggested Periodic Examinations While Taking This Drug (at physician's discretion)

None.

▷ **While Taking This Drug, Observe the Following**

Foods: No restrictions.

Beverages: No restrictions. May be taken with milk.

▷ *Alcohol:* Use extreme caution until the combined effects have been determined. Propoxyphene can intensify the intoxicating effects of alcohol, and alcohol can intensify the depressant effects of propoxyphene on brain function.

Tobacco Smoking: Heavy smoking may reduce the effectiveness of this drug.

Marijuana Smoking: Increase in drowsiness and pain relief; impairment of mental and physical performance.

▷ *Other Drugs*

Propoxyphene may ***increase*** the effects of

• other drugs with sedative effects.

• oral anticoagulants (Coumadin, etc.), and increase the risk of bleeding.

- carbamazepine (Tegretol), and increase its toxicity.
- doxepin (Sinequan), and increase its toxicity.

▷ *Driving, Hazardous Activities:* This drug can impair mental alertness, judgment, reaction time and physical coordination. Avoid hazardous activities accordingly.

Aviation Note: The use of this drug **is a disqualification** for piloting. Consult a designated Aviation Medical Examiner.

Exposure to Sun: No restrictions.

Discontinuation: It is advisable to limit this drug to short-term use. If it is necessary to use it for extended periods of time, discontinuation should be gradual to minimize possible effects of withdrawal.

PROPRANOLOL
(proh PRAN oh lohl)

Introduced: 1966

Class: Antianginal, anti-arrhythmic, antihypertensive, migraine preventive, beta-adrenergic blocker

Prescription: USA: Yes
Canada: Yes

Controlled Drug: USA: No
Canada: No

Available as Generic: Yes

Brand Names: ✦Apo-Propranolol, ✦Detensol, Inderal, Inderal-LA, Inderide [CD], Inderide LA [CD], Ipran, ✦Novopranol, ✦PMS Propranolol

---

BENEFITS versus RISKS

Possible Benefits	*Possible Risks*
EFFECTIVE, WELL-TOLERATED AS: ANTIANGINAL DRUG in effort-induced angina; ANTIARRHYTHMIC DRUG in certain heart rhythm disorders; ANTIHYPERTENSIVE DRUG in mild to moderate hypertension	CONGESTIVE HEART FAILURE in advanced heart disease
	Worsening of angina in coronary heart disease (if drug is abruptly withdrawn)
	Masking of low blood sugar (hypoglycemia) in drug-treated diabetes
EFFECTIVE PREVENTION OF MIGRAINE HEADACHES	Provocation of asthma
Effective adjunct in the prevention of recurrent heart attack (myocardial infarction)	Rare blood cell disorders: low white cell and platelet counts
Effective adjunct in the management of pheochromocytoma	

▷ **Principal Uses**

As a Single Drug Product: This first beta blocker drug is used primarily to treat several serious cardiovascular disorders: classical effort-induced angina, certain types of heart rhythm disturbance and high blood pressure. It is also beneficial in preventing the recurrence of heart attacks (myocardial infarction). In addition, it is used to reduce the frequency and severity of migraine headaches. Other uses (not "officially approved" at this time) include the control of physical manifestations of anxiety and nervous tension (as in stage fright), the control of familial tremors and the control of symptoms associated with markedly overactive thyroid gland function (thyrotoxicosis).

As a Combination Drug Product [CD]: This drug is available in combination with hydrochlorothiazide for the treatment of hypertension. This combination product includes two "step 1" drugs with different mechanisms of action; it is intended to provide greater effectiveness and convenience for long-term use.

How This Drug Works: By blocking certain actions of the sympathetic nervous system, this drug

• reduces the rate and contraction force of the heart, thus lowering the ejection pressure of the blood leaving the heart and reducing the oxygen requirement for heart function.

• reduces the degree of contraction of blood vessel walls, resulting in their relaxation and expansion and consequent lowering of blood pressure.

• prolongs the conduction time of nerve impulses through the heart, of benefit in the management of certain heart rhythm disorders.

Available Dosage Forms and Strengths

Capsules, prolonged-action — 80 mg, 120 mg, 160 mg

Concentrate — 80 mg/ml

Injection — 1 mg per ml

Oral solution — 4 mg/ml, 8 mg/ml

Tablets — 10 mg, 20 mg, 40 mg, 60 mg, 80 mg, 90 mg

▷ **Usual Adult Dosage Range:** Varies with indication.

Antianginal: Initially, 10 to 20 mg 3 or 4 times/day; increase dose gradually every 3 to 7 days as needed and tolerated. The total daily dosage should not exceed 320 mg.

Antiarrhythmic: 10 to 30 mg 3 or 4 times/day as needed and tolerated.

Antihypertensive: Initially, 40 mg twice/day; increase dose gradually as needed and tolerated. The total daily dosage should not exceed 640 mg.

Migraine headache prevention: Initially, 20 mg 4 times/day; increase dose gradually as needed and tolerated. The total daily dosage should not exceed 240 mg.

Note: Actual dosage and administration schedule must be determined by the physician for each patient individually.

▷ **Dosing Instructions:** Preferably taken 1 hour before eating to maximize absorption. The tablet may be crushed for administration; to prevent a possible numbing effect (harmless), mix with soft food and swallow promptly. The prolonged-action capsules should be swallowed whole without alteration. Do not discontinue this drug abruptly.

Usual Duration of Use: Continual use on a regular schedule for 10 to 14 days is usually necessary to determine this drug's effectiveness in preventing angina, controlling heart rhythm disorders and lowering blood pressure. Maximal effectiveness may require continual use for 6 to 8 weeks. The long-term use of this drug (months to years) will be determined by the course of your symptoms over time and your response to the overall treatment program (weight reduction, salt restriction, smoking cessation, etc.). Consult your physician on a regular basis.

▷ **This Drug Should Not Be Taken If**
- you have had an allergic reaction to it previously.
- you have Prinzmetal's variant angina (coronary artery spasm).
- you have congestive heart failure.
- you have an abnormally slow heart rate or a serious form of heart block.
- you are taking, or have taken within the past 14 days, any monoamine oxidase (MAO) type A inhibitor drug (see Drug Class, Section Four).

▷ **Inform Your Physician Before Taking This Drug If**
- you have had an adverse reaction to any beta blocker drug in the past (see Drug Class, Section Four).
- you have a history of serious heart disease, with or without episodes of heart failure.
- you have a history of hay fever (allergic rhinitis), asthma, chronic bronchitis or emphysema.
- you have a history of overactive thyroid function (hyperthyroidism).
- you have a history of low blood sugar (hypoglycemia).
- you have impaired liver or kidney function.
- you have diabetes or myasthenia gravis.
- you are currently taking any form of digitalis, quinidine or reserpine, or any calcium blocker drug (see Drug Class, Section Four).
- you plan to have surgery under general anesthesia in the near future.

Possible Side-Effects (natural, expected and unavoidable drug actions)
Lethargy and fatigability, cold extremities, slow heart rate, light-headedness in upright position (see orthostatic hypotension in Glossary).

▷ **Possible Adverse Effects** (unusual, unexpected and infrequent reactions)
If any of the following develop, consult your physician promptly for guidance.
Mild Adverse Effects
Allergic Reactions: Skin rash, temporary loss of hair, drug fever (see Glossary).

Headache, dizziness, insomnia, vivid dreams.

Indigestion, nausea, vomiting, diarrhea.

Serious Adverse Effects

Idiosyncratic Reactions: Acute behavioral disturbances: disorientation, confusion, hallucinations, amnesia.

Mental depression, anxiety.

Chest pain, shortness of breath, precipitation of congestive heart failure.

Induction of bronchial asthma (in asthmatic individuals).

Rare blood cell disorders: abnormally low white blood cell count, causing fever and sore throat; abnormally low blood platelet count, causing abnormal bleeding or bruising.

▷ **Possible Effects on Sexual Function**

Decreased libido; impaired erection (28%); impotence (15%).

This drug has been found to have the highest incidence of libido reduction and erectile impairment of all beta blocker drugs.

Male infertility (inhibited sperm motility); Peyronie's disease (see Glossary).

▷ **Adverse Effects That May Mimic Natural Diseases or Disorders**

Reduced blood flow to extremities may resemble Raynaud's phenomenon (see Glossary).

Natural Diseases or Disorders That May Be Activated by This Drug

Prinzmetal's variant angina, Raynaud's disease, intermittent claudication, myasthenia gravis (questionable).

CAUTION

1. ***Do not discontinue this drug suddenly*** without the knowledge and guidance of your physician. Carry a notation on your person that you are taking this drug.
2. Consult your physician or pharmacist before using nasal decongestants usually present in over-the-counter cold preparations and nose drops. These can cause sudden increases in blood pressure when taken concurrently with beta blocker drugs.
3. Report the development of any tendency to emotional depression.

Precautions for Use

By Infants and Children: Safety and effectiveness for use by those under 12 years of age have not been established. However, if this drug is used, observe for the development of low blood sugar (hypoglycemia) during periods of reduced food intake.

By Those over 60 Years of Age: Proceed **cautiously** with all antihypertensive drugs. Unacceptably high blood pressure should be reduced without creating the risks associated with excessively low blood pressure. Start treatment with small doses, and monitor the blood pressure response frequently. Sudden, rapid and excessive reduction of blood pressure can predispose to stroke or heart attack. Observe for dizziness, unsteadiness, tendency to fall, confusion, hallucinations, depression or urinary frequency.

▷ **Advisability of Use During Pregnancy**

Pregnancy Category: C (tentative). See Pregnancy Code inside back cover.

Animal studies: No significant increase in birth defects due to this drug. Some toxic effects on embryo reported.

Human studies: Information from adequate studies of pregnant women is not available.

Avoid use of drug during the first 3 months if possible. Use this drug only if clearly needed. Ask your physician for guidance.

Advisability of Use if Breast-Feeding

Presence of this drug in breast milk: Yes.

Monitor nursing infant closely and discontinue drug or nursing if adverse effects develop.

Habit-Forming Potential: None.

Effects of Overdosage: Weakness, slow pulse, low blood pressure, fainting, cold and sweaty skin, congestive heart failure, possible coma and convulsions.

Possible Effects of Long-Term Use: Reduced heart reserve and eventual heart failure in susceptible individuals with advanced heart disease.

Suggested Periodic Examinations While Taking This Drug (at physician's discretion)

Complete blood cell counts.

Measurements of blood pressure, evaluation of heart function.

▷ **While Taking This Drug, Observe the Following**

Foods: No restrictions. Avoid excessive salt intake.

Beverages: No restrictions. May be taken with milk.

▷ *Alcohol:* Use with caution until the combined effect has been determined. Alcohol may exaggerate this drug's ability to lower the blood pressure and may increase its mild sedative effect.

Tobacco Smoking: Nicotine may reduce this drug's effectiveness in treating angina, heart rhythm disorders and high blood pressure. Smoking increases the rate of elimination of this drug and decreases its blood levels, especially in younger individuals. In addition, high doses of this drug may potentiate the constriction of the bronchial tubes caused by regular smoking.

▷ *Other Drugs*

Propranolol may ***increase*** the effects of

- other antihypertensive drugs, and cause excessive lowering of blood pressure. Dosage adjustments may be necessary.
- lidocaine (Xylocaine, etc.).
- reserpine (Ser-Ap-Es, etc.), and cause sedation, depression, slowing of the heart rate and lowering of the blood pressure.
- verapamil (Calan, Isoptin), and cause excessive depression of heart function; monitor this combination closely.

Propranolol may ***decrease*** the effects of

- theophyllines (Aminophyllin, Theo-Dur, etc.), and reduce their antiasthmatic effectiveness.

Propranolol *taken concurrently* with

- clonidine (Catapres) requires close monitoring for rebound high blood pressure if clonidine is withdrawn while propranolol is still being taken.
- epinephrine (Adrenalin, etc.) may cause marked rise in blood pressure and slowing of the heart rate.
- insulin requires close monitoring to avoid undetected hypoglycemia (see Glossary).

The following drugs may *increase* the effects of propranolol

- chlorpromazine (Thorazine, etc.).
- cimetidine (Tagamet).
- methimazole (Tapazole).
- propylthiouracil (Propacil).

The following drugs may *decrease* the effects of propranolol

- barbiturates (phenobarbital, etc.).
- indomethacin (Indocin), and possibly other "aspirin substitutes," may impair propranolol's antihypertensive effect.
- rifampin (Rifadin, Rimactane).

▷ *Driving, Hazardous Activities:* Use caution until the full extent of drowsiness, lethargy and blood pressure change have been determined.

Aviation Note: The use of this drug *may be a disqualification* for piloting. Consult a designated Aviation Medical Examiner.

Exposure to Sun: No restrictions.

Exposure to Heat: Caution advised. Hot environments can lower blood pressure and exaggerate the effects of this drug.

Exposure to Cold: Caution advised. Cold environments can enhance the circulatory deficiency in the extremities that may occur with this drug. The elderly should take precautions to prevent hypothermia (see Glossary).

Heavy Exercise or Exertion: It is advisable to avoid exertion that produces light-headedness, excessive fatigue or muscle cramping. The use of this drug may intensify the hypertensive response to isometric exercise.

Occurrence of Unrelated Illness: The fever that accompanies systemic infections can lower blood pressure and require adjustment of dosage. Illnesses that cause nausea or vomiting may interrupt the regular dosage schedule. Ask your physician for guidance.

Discontinuation: It is advisable to avoid sudden discontinuation of this drug in all situations; this is especially true in the presence of coronary artery disease. If possible, gradual reduction of dose over a period of 2 to 3 weeks is recommended. Ask your physician for specific guidance.

PYRIDOSTIGMINE
(peer id oh STIG meen)

Introduced: 1962

Prescription: USA: Yes
Canada: No

Available as Generic: USA: No
Canada: No

Class: Antimyasthenic

Controlled Drug: USA: No
Canada: No

Brand Names: Mestinon, Mestinon Timespan, Regonol

BENEFITS versus RISKS

Possible Benefits	*Possible Risks*
MODERATELY EFFECTIVE TREATMENT OF OCULAR AND MILD FORMS OF MYASTHENIA GRAVIS (symptomatic relief of muscle weakness)	Cholinergic crisis (overdose): excessive salivation, nausea, vomiting, stomach cramps, diarrhea, shortness of breath (asthmalike wheezing), excessive weakness

---

▷ **Principal Uses**

As a Single Drug Product: Used primarily to treat the ocular and milder forms of myasthenia gravis by providing temporary relief of muscle weakness and fatigability. It is most useful in long-term treatment when there is little or no difficulty in swallowing.

How This Drug Works: This drug inhibits cholinesterase, the enzyme that destroys acetylcholine. This results in higher levels of acetylcholine, the nerve transmitter that facilitates the stimulation of muscular activity. The net effects are increased muscle strength and endurance.

Available Dosage Forms and Strengths

Syrup — 60 mg per 5-ml teaspoonful (5% alcohol)
Tablets — 60 mg
Tablets, prolonged-action — 180 mg

▷ **Usual Adult Dosage Range:**   Initially: 60 to 120 mg/3 to 4 hours; adjust dosage as needed and tolerated. Maintenance: 60 to 1500 mg/24 hours; the average dose is 600 mg/24 hours. Prolonged-action tablets: 180 to 540 mg once or twice a day, at least 6 hours apart. **Note: Actual dosage and administration schedule must be determined by the physician for each patient individually.**

▷ **Dosing Instructions:**   Take with food or milk to reduce the intensity of side-effects. Larger portions of the daily maintenance dosage should be timed according to the pattern of fatigue and weakness. The syrup will permit a finer adjustment of dosage. The regular tablet may be crushed for administration. The prolonged-action tablet should be taken whole (not altered).

Usual Duration of Use: Continual use on a regular schedule (with dosage adjustment) for 10 to 14 days is usually necessary to determine this drug's effectiveness in relieving the symptoms of myasthenia gravis. Long-term use (months to years) requires periodic evaluation of response and dosage adjustment. Consult your physician on a regular basis.

▷ **This Drug Should Not Be Taken If**
- you are known to be allergic to bromide compounds.

▷ **Inform Your Physician Before Taking This Drug If**
- you are subject to heart rhythm disorders or bronchial asthma.
- you have recurrent urinary tract infections.
- you have prostatism (see Glossary).
- you plan to have surgery under general anesthesia in the near future.

Possible Side-Effects (natural, expected and unavoidable drug actions)
Small pupils, watering of eyes, slow pulse, excessive salivation, nausea, vomiting, stomach cramps, diarrhea, urge to urinate, increased sweating.

▷ **Possible Adverse Effects** (unusual, unexpected and infrequent reactions)
If any of the following develop, consult your physician promptly for guidance.
Mild Adverse Effects
Allergic Reaction: Skin rash.
Nervousness, anxiety, unsteadiness, muscle cramps or twitching.
Loss of scalp hair.
Serious Adverse Effects
Confusion, slurred speech, seizures, difficult breathing (asthmatic wheezing).
Increased muscle weakness or paralysis.
Excessive vomiting or diarrhea may induce abnormally low blood potassium levels (hypokalemia). This will accentuate muscle weakness.

▷ **Possible Effects on Sexual Function:** None reported.

▷ **Adverse Effects That May Mimic Natural Diseases or Disorders**
Seizures may suggest the possibility of epilepsy.

Natural Diseases or Disorders That May Be Activated by This Drug
Latent bronchial asthma.

CAUTION
1. Certain drugs can block the action of this drug and reduce its effectiveness in treating myasthenia gravis. (See *Other Drugs* below.) Consult your physician before starting any new drug, prescription or over-the-counter.

2. The dosage schedule of this drug must be carefully individualized for each patient. Variations in response may occur from time to time. Because generalized muscle weakness is a major symptom of both myasthenia crisis (underdosage) and cholinergic crisis (overdosage), it may be difficult to recognize the correct cause. As a rule, weakness that begins within 1 hour after taking this drug probably represents overdosage; weakness that begins 3 or more hours after taking this drug is probably due to underdosage. Observe these time relationships and inform your physician.

3. During long-term use of this drug, observe for the possible development of resistance to the drug's therapeutic action (loss of effectiveness). Consult your physician regarding the advisability of discontinuing this drug for a few days to see if responsiveness can be restored.

Precautions for Use

By Infants and Children: The syrup form of this drug permits greater precision of dosage adjustment and ease of administration in this age group.

By Those over 60 Years of Age: The natural decline of kidney function with aging may require smaller doses to prevent accumulation of this drug to toxic levels.

▷ Advisability of Use During Pregnancy

Pregnancy Category: C (tentative). See Pregnancy Code inside back cover.
Animal studies: No information available.
Human studies: Information from adequate studies of pregnant women is not available.
There are no reports of birth defects due to the use of this drug during pregnancy. However, there are reports of significant muscular weakness in newborn infants whose mothers had taken this drug during pregnancy. Ask your physician for guidance.

Advisability of Use if Breast-Feeding

Presence of this drug in breast milk: Probably not.
Monitor nursing infant closely and discontinue drug or nursing if adverse effects develop.

Habit-Forming Potential: None.

Effects of Overdosage: Generalized muscular weakness, blurred vision, very small pupils, slow heart rate, difficult breathing (wheezing), excessive salivation, nausea, vomiting, stomach cramps, diarrhea, muscle cramps or twitching. This syndrome constitutes the cholinergic crisis.

Possible Effects of Long-Term Use: Development of tolerance (see Glossary) with loss of therapeutic effectiveness.

Suggested Periodic Examinations While Taking This Drug (at physician's discretion)

Assessment of drug effectiveness and dosage schedule for optimal therapeutic results.

▷ **While Taking This Drug, Observe the Following**

Foods: No restrictions.

Beverages: No restrictions. May be taken with milk.

▷ *Alcohol:* Use caution until the combined effects are determined. Weakness and unsteadiness may be accentuated.

Tobacco Smoking: No interactions expected.

▷ *Other Drugs*

The following drugs may *decrease* the effects of pyridostigmine

- atropine (belladonna).
- clindamycin (Cleocin).
- guanadrel (Hylorel).
- guanethidine (Esimil, Ismelin).
- procainamide (Procan SR, Pronestyl).
- quinidine (Cardioquin, Duraquin, etc.).
- quinine (Quinamm).

▷ *Driving, Hazardous Activities:* This drug may cause blurred vision, confusion or generalized weakness. Restrict activities as necessary.

Aviation Note: The use of this drug *is a disqualification* for piloting. Consult a designated Aviation Medical Examiner.

Exposure to Sun: No restrictions.

Exposure to Heat: Use caution. This may cause excessive sweating and increased weakness.

Exposure to Environmental Chemicals: Avoid excessive exposure (inhalation, skin contamination) to the insecticides Baygon, Diazinon and Sevin. These can accentuate the potential toxicity of this drug.

Discontinuation: Do not discontinue this drug abruptly without your physician's knowledge and guidance.

QUINIDINE
(KWIN i deen)

Introduced: 1918

Class: Antiarrhythmic

Prescription: USA: Yes
Canada: No

Controlled Drug: USA: No
Canada: No

Available as Generic: Yes

Brand Names: ✦Apo-Quinidine, ✦Biquin Durules, Cardioquin, Cin-Quin, Duraquin, ✦Novoquinidine, Quinaglute Dura-Tabs, ✦Quinate, Quinidex Extentabs, ✦Quinobarb [CD]*, Quinora

*Quinobarb contains phenylethylbarbiturate, a sedative of the barbiturate class.

```
┌─────────────────────────────────────────────────────────────┐
│                    BENEFITS versus RISKS                     │
│                                                              │
│      Possible Benefits              Possible Risks           │
│  EFFECTIVE TREATMENT OF       NARROW TREATMENT RANGE         │
│   SELECTED HEART RHYTHM       FREQUENT ADVERSE EFFECTS       │
│   DISORDERS                    (30% of users)               │
│                               NUMEROUS ALLERGIC AND          │
│                                IDIOSYNCRATIC REACTIONS       │
│                               Dose-related toxicity          │
│                               Provocation of abnormal heart  │
│                                rhythms                       │
│                               Abnormally low blood platelet  │
│                                count (rare)                  │
└─────────────────────────────────────────────────────────────┘
```

▷ **Principal Uses**

   As a Single Drug Product: Used primarily to control the following types of abnormal heart rhythm: atrial fibrillation and flutter, paroxysmal atrial tachycardia, paroxysmal ventricular tachycardia, premature atrial and ventricular contractions.

   As a Combination Drug Product [CD]: This drug is available (in Canada) in combination with a barbiturate, a mild sedative that is added to allay the anxiety and nervous tension that often accompany heart rhythm disorders.

How This Drug Works: By slowing the activity of the pacemaker and delaying the transmission of electrical impulses through the conduction system and muscle of the heart, this drug assists in restoring normal heart rate and rhythm.

Available Dosage Forms and Strengths

                    Capsules — 200 mg, 300 mg
                    Injections — 80 mg, 200 mg per ml
                    Tablets — 100 mg, 200 mg, 275 mg, 300 mg
     Tablets, prolonged-action — 300 mg, 324 mg, 330 mg

▷ **Usual Adult Dosage Range:** Test dose: 200 mg, then observe for 2 hours for evidence of idiosyncrasy.

   Dose varies with indication:

   Premature atrial or ventricular contractions: 200 to 300 mg 3 or 4 times/day.

   Paroxysmal atrial tachycardia: 400 to 600 mg/2 to 3 hours until paroxysm is terminated.

   Atrial flutter: digitalize first; then individualize dosage schedule as appropriate.

   Atrial fibrillation: digitalize first; then try 200 mg/2 to 3 hours for 5 to 8 doses; increase dose daily until normal rhythm is restored or toxic effects develop.

   Maintenance schedule: 200 to 300 mg 3 or 4 times/day. The total daily dosage should not exceed 4000 mg.

Note: Actual dosage and administration schedule must be determined by the physician for each patient individually.

▷ **Dosing Instructions:**   Preferably taken on an empty stomach to achieve high blood levels rapidly. However, it may be taken with or following food to reduce stomach irritation. The regular tablets may be crushed and the capsules opened for administration. The prolonged-action forms should be swallowed whole without alteration.

   Usual Duration of Use: Continual use on a regular schedule for 2 to 4 days is usually necessary to determine this drug's effectiveness in correcting or preventing responsive abnormal rhythms. Long-term use (months to years) requires supervision and periodic evaluation by your physician. Consult your physician on a regular basis.

▷ **This Drug Should Not Be Taken If**
   • you have had an allergic or idiosyncratic reaction to any dosage form of it previously.
   • you currently have an acute infection of any kind.

▷ **Inform Your Physician Before Taking This Drug If**
   • you have coronary artery disease or myasthenia gravis.
   • you have a history of hyperthyroidism.
   • you have had a deficiency of blood platelets in the past from any cause.
   • you are now taking, or have taken recently, any digitalis preparation (digitoxin, digoxin, etc.).
   • you plan to have surgery under general anesthesia in the near future.

   Possible Side-Effects (natural, expected and unavoidable drug actions)
   Drop in blood pressure, may be marked in sensitive individuals.

▷ **Possible Adverse Effects** (unusual, unexpected and infrequent reactions)
   If any of the following develop, consult your physician promptly for guidance.
   Mild Adverse Effects
   Allergic Reactions: Skin rash, hives, itching, drug fever (rare).
   Dose-related toxicity (cinchonism): blurred vision, ringing in the ears, loss of hearing, dizziness.
   Nausea, vomiting, diarrhea (20% to 30% of users).
   Serious Adverse Effects
   Allergic Reactions: Severe skin reactions, hemolytic anemia (see Glossary), joint and muscle pains, anaphylactic reaction (see Glossary), reduced blood platelet count, drug-induced hepatitis (see Glossary).
   Idiosyncratic Reactions: Skin rash, rapid heart rate, acute delirium and combative behavior, difficult breathing.
   Heart conduction abnormalities.
   Optic neuritis, impaired vision.
   Abnormally low white blood cell count: fever, sore throat, infections.

▷ **Possible Effects on Sexual Function:**   None reported.

▷ **Adverse Effects That May Mimic Natural Diseases or Disorders**
Drug-induced hepatitis may suggest viral hepatitis.

Natural Diseases or Disorders That May Be Activated by This Drug
Systemic lupus erythematosus, myasthenia gravis, psoriasis (in sensitive individuals).

CAUTION
1. The effects of this drug are very unpredictable because of the wide variation in response from person to person. Dosage adjustments must be based upon individual reaction. Notify your physician of any events that you suspect may be drug related.
2. It is advisable to carry a card of personal identification that includes a notation that you are taking this drug.

Precautions for Use
By Infants and Children: A test for drug idiosyncrasy should be made before starting treatment with this drug. If there is no beneficial response after 3 days of adequate dosage, this drug should be discontinued.
By Those over 60 Years of Age: Small doses are mandatory until your individual response has been determined. Observe for the development of light-headedness, dizziness, weakness or sense of impending faint. Use caution to prevent falls.

▷ **Advisability of Use During Pregnancy**
Pregnancy Category: C (tentative). See Pregnancy Code inside back cover.
Animal studies: No information available.
Human studies: Information from adequate studies of pregnant women is not available. No birth defects have been reported following use of this drug during pregnancy.
Use this drug only if clearly needed.

Advisability of Use if Breast-Feeding
Presence of this drug in breast milk: Yes.
Avoid drug or refrain from nursing.

Habit-Forming Potential: None.

Effects of Overdosage: Nausea, vomiting, ringing in the ears, headache, jerky eye movements, double vision, altered color vision, confusion, delirium, hot skin, seizures, coma.

Possible Effects of Long-Term Use: None reported.

Suggested Periodic Examinations While Taking This Drug (at physician's discretion)
Complete blood cell counts, electrocardiograms.

▷ **While Taking This Drug, Observe the Following**
Foods: No restrictions.
Beverages: No restrictions. May be taken with milk.

▷ *Alcohol:* Use caution until the combined effects have been determined. Alcohol may enhance the blood-pressure-lowering effects of this drug.

Tobacco Smoking: Nicotine can increase irritability of the heart and aggravate rhythm disorders. Avoid all forms of tobacco.

▷ *Other Drugs*

Quinidine may *increase* the effects of
- anticoagulants (Coumadin, etc.), and increase the risk of bleeding.
- digitoxin and digoxin (Lanoxin), and cause digitalis toxicity.

The following drugs may *increase* the effects of quinidine
- amiodarone.
- cimetidine (Tagamet).

The following drugs may *decrease* the effects of quinidine
- barbiturates (phenobarbital, etc.).
- phenytoin (Dilantin).
- rifampin (Rifadin, Rimactane).

▷ *Driving, Hazardous Activities:* This drug may cause dizziness and alter vision. Restrict activities as necessary.

Aviation Note: The use of this drug *may be a disqualification* for piloting. Consult a designated Aviation Medical Examiner.

Exposure to Sun: No restrictions.

RANITIDINE
(ra NI te deen)

Introduced: 1981

Prescription: USA: Yes
Canada: Yes

Available as Generic: No

Brand Name: Zantac

Class: Antiulcer, H-2 receptor blocker

Controlled Drug: USA: No
Canada: No

BENEFITS versus RISKS	
Possible Benefits	*Possible Risks*
EFFECTIVE TREATMENT OF PEPTIC ULCER DISEASE: relief of symptoms, acceleration of healing, prevention of recurrence	Drug-induced hepatitis (rare)
	Confusion (in severely ill elderly patients)
	Rare blood cell disorders
CONTROL OF HYPERSECRETORY STOMACH DISORDERS	
Beneficial in treatment of reflux esophagitis	

▷ **Principal Uses**

> *As a Single Drug Product:* Used primarily in the treatment of peptic ulcer disease, both benign stomach (gastric) ulcer and duodenal ulcer. It is used specifically to hasten the healing of ulcer and to prevent recurrence. Also used to control the excessive production of stomach acid in the Zollinger-Ellison syndrome. Though its effectiveness has not been fully established, this drug is also widely used in the management of esophagitis (as with hiatal hernia) and upper gastrointestinal bleeding.

How This Drug Works: By blocking the action of histamine, this drug effectively inhibits the secretion of stomach acid and thus creates a more favorable environment for the healing of peptic ulcers.

Available Dosage Forms and Strengths
> Injection — 0.5 mg per ml, 25 mg per ml
> Syrup — 15 mg per ml (7.5% alcohol)
> Tablets — 150 mg, 300 mg

▷ **Usual Adult Dosage Range:** For active peptic ulcer and hypersecretory states: 150 mg 2 times daily, 12 hours apart. For prevention of recurrent ulcer: 150 mg at bedtime. **Note: Actual dosage and administration schedule must be determined by the physician for each patient individually.**

▷ **Dosing Instructions:** To obtain the longest period of stomach acid reduction, this drug should be taken with or immediately following meals. The tablet may be crushed for administration.

Usual Duration of Use: Continual use on a regular schedule for 4 to 6 weeks is usually necessary to determine this drug's effectiveness in healing active peptic ulcer. Long-term use (months to years) for prevention of ulcer recurrence requires individual consideration by your physician.

▷ **This Drug Should Not Be Taken If**
> • you have had an allergic reaction to any dosage form of it previously.

▷ **Inform Your Physician Before Taking This Drug If**
> • you are allergic to any other histamine (H-2)-blocking drug (see Drug Class, Section Four).
> • you have impaired liver or kidney function.
> • you are taking an oral anticoagulant.

Possible Side-Effects (natural, expected and unavoidable drug actions)
> None reported.

▷ **Possible Adverse Effects** (unusual, unexpected and infrequent reactions)
> **If any of the following develop, consult your physician promptly for guidance.**

Mild Adverse Effects
　Allergic Reaction: Skin rash.
　Headache, malaise, dizziness.
　Nausea, constipation, diarrhea.
Serious Adverse Effects
　Idiosyncratic Reaction: Confusion in the elderly and debilitated.
　Drug-induced hepatitis (see Glossary).
　Bone marrow depression (see Glossary)—weakness, fever, sore throat,
　　abnormal bleeding or bruising.

▷ **Possible Effects on Sexual Function:** Decreased libido, impotence, male
　breast enlargement and tenderness (all rare).

▷ **Adverse Effects That May Mimic Natural Diseases or Disorders**
　Liver reactions may suggest viral hepatitis.

　CAUTION
　　1. Do not discontinue this drug abruptly. (Ulcer activation and per-
　　　foration have occurred following abrupt cessation of cimetidine, a
　　　closely related drug.)
　　2. After discontinuation of this drug, inform your physician promptly
　　　if you experience a return of symptoms indicative of ulcer reacti-
　　　vation.

　Precautions for Use
　　By Infants and Children: Safety and effectiveness for use by those under
　　　12 years of age have not been established.
　　By Those over 60 Years of Age: Observe for the development of nervous
　　　agitation or confusion. This drug may contribute to the formation of
　　　stomach phytobezoars (masses of undigested vegetable fibers). Indi-
　　　viduals with poor chewing ability (missing teeth) and those who have
　　　had partial gastrectomy or vagotomy (stomach surgery) are most sus-
　　　ceptible. Observe for loss of appetite, stomach fullness, nausea and
　　　vomiting.

▷ **Advisability of Use During Pregnancy**
　Pregnancy Category: B (tentative). See Pregnancy Code inside back cover.
　　Animal studies: No birth defects reported.
　　Human studies: Information from adequate studies of pregnant women
　　　is not available.
　　Use this drug only if clearly needed. Ask physician for guidance.

　Advisability of Use if Breast-Feeding
　　Presence of this drug in breast milk: Yes.
　　Avoid drug or refrain from nursing.

　Habit-Forming Potential: None.

　Effects of Overdosage: Confusion, delirium, slurred speech, flushing,
　　sweating, drowsiness, muscle twitching, seizures, coma.

Possible Effects of Long-Term Use: None reported.

Suggested Periodic Examinations While Taking This Drug (at physician's discretion)
  Complete blood cell counts, liver function tests.

▷ **While Taking This Drug, Observe the Following**
  Foods: Protein-rich foods produce maximal stomach acid secretion. Follow the diet prescribed to derive optimal benefit from this drug.
  Beverages: No restrictions. May be taken with milk.
▷ *Alcohol:* No interactions with drug. However, alcoholic beverages increase stomach acidity and can reduce the effectiveness of this drug.
▷ *Other Drugs*
    Ranitidine may ***increase*** the effects of
    • oral anticoagulants, and increase the risk of bleeding.
▷ *Driving, Hazardous Activities:* This drug may cause dizziness. Restrict activities as necessary.
  Aviation Note: The use of this drug ***may be a disqualification*** for piloting. Consult a designated Aviation Medical Examiner.
  Exposure to Sun: No restrictions.
  Discontinuation: Do not discontinue this drug suddenly if taken for peptic ulcer disease. Consult physician for withdrawal instructions. This drug does not provide an extended protective effect. Be alert to the possibility of ulcer recurrence anytime after discontinuation.

RESERPINE
(re SER peen)

Other Names: Deserpidine, rauwolfia

Introduced: 1953   **Class:** Antihypertensive

Prescription: USA: Yes   **Controlled Drug:** USA: No
    Canada: Yes   Canada: No

Available as Generic: Yes

Brand Names: Demi-Regroton [CD], Diupres [CD], Diutensin-R [CD], Dureticyl [CD], Enduronyl [CD], Enduronyl Forte [CD], Esidrix [CD], Hydropres [CD], ✦Hygroton-Reserpine [CD], ✦Novoreserpine, Oreticyl [CD], Rauzide [CD], Regroton [CD], ✦Reserfia, Ser-Ap-Es [CD], Serpalan, Serpasil, Serpasil-Apresoline [CD], Unipres [CD]

```
┌─────────────────────────────────────────────────────────────────┐
│                    BENEFITS versus RISKS                         │
│                                                                   │
│       Possible Benefits              Possible Risks              │
│  Moderately effective "step 2"    INDUCTION OF MENTAL            │
│     antihypertensive in mild to      DEPRESSION (can be severe   │
│     moderate hypertension when       and prolonged)             │
│     used concurrently with a      ACTIVATION OF PEPTIC ULCER,   │
│     diuretic                         GASTROINTESTINAL           │
│                                      BLEEDING                    │
│                                   Frequent nasal congestion and │
│                                      diarrhea                    │
│                                   Reduced libido, sexual impotence │
│                                   Mental disturbances           │
└─────────────────────────────────────────────────────────────────┘
```

▷ **Principal Uses**

As a Single Drug Product: Used primarily as a "step 2" antihypertensive drug in the treatment of mild to moderate hypertension. Originally introduced as a tranquilizer for the treatment of schizophrenia, it is seldom used for this purpose currently.

As a Combination Drug Product [CD]: This drug is available in combination with most of the thiazide diuretics, the conventional "step 1" antihypertensive medication. One popular product combines reserpine, hydrochlorothiazide and hydralazine, a "step 2 or 3" antihypertensive. These combinations are more effective for treating moderate to severe hypertension.

How This Drug Works: By depleting the nerve impulse transmitter norepinephrine from nerve terminals, this drug reduces the ability of the sympathetic nervous system to maintain the degree of blood vessel constriction that is responsible for high blood pressure. The reduced availability of norepinephrine results in relaxation of blood vessel walls and lowering of blood pressure.

Available Dosage Forms and Strengths

Tablets — 0.1 mg, 0.25 mg, 1 mg

▷ **Usual Adult Dosage Range:** As antihypertensive: Initially, 0.1 to 0.5 mg/24 hours for 1 to 2 weeks. Adjust dose as needed and tolerated. The usual maintenance dose is 0.1 to 0.25 mg/24 hours. The total daily dosage should not exceed 1.0 mg/24 hours. **Note: Actual dosage and administration schedule must be determined by the physician for each patient individually.**

▷ **Dosing Instructions:** Take with or following food to reduce stomach irritation. The tablet may be crushed for administration. The prolonged-action capsule should be swallowed whole without alteration.

Usual Duration of Use: Continual use on a regular schedule for 3 to 6 weeks is usually necessary to determine this drug's full effectiveness in controlling hypertension. Long-term use (months to years) requires supervision and periodic evaluation by your physician. Consult your physician on a regular basis.

▷ **This Drug Should Not Be Taken If**
- you have had an allergic reaction to any form of reserpine previously.
- you are mentally depressed, or you have had a depression in the past.
- you have an active peptic ulcer, or a history of peptic ulcer disease.
- you have active regional enteritis, ulcerative colitis or a history of ulcerative bowel disease.

▷ **Inform Your Physician Before Taking This Drug If**
- you have a seizure disorder.
- you are subject to migraine headaches.
- you have any form of heart disease.
- you have gallbladder disease.
- you are taking any of the following drugs: anticoagulants, a digitalis preparation, quinidine, levodopa, antidepressants, sedatives or a monoamine oxidase (MAO) type A inhibitor (see Drug Classes, Section Four).
- you plan to have surgery under general anesthesia in the near future.

Possible Side-Effects (natural, expected and unavoidable drug actions)
Drowsiness and lethargy (especially during the first few weeks), reddening of the eyes, nasal stuffiness (frequent), dry mouth, increased hunger contractions, acid indigestion, intestinal cramping, diarrhea, water retention.

▷ **Possible Adverse Effects** (unusual, unexpected and infrequent reactions)
If any of the following develop, consult your physician promptly for guidance.
Mild Adverse Effects
Allergic Reactions: Skin rashes, itching.
Headache, dizziness, nosebleeds.
Nausea, vomiting, persistent diarrhea.
Serious Adverse Effects
Allergic Reactions: Reduction of blood platelet count, with or without spontaneous bruising.
Idiosyncratic Reactions: Paradoxical nervousness, agitation, confusion, nightmares, hallucinations.
Bronchospasm, asthmatic wheezing.
Mental depression, may be severe.
Peptic ulcer activation, with or without bleeding.

▷ **Possible Effects on Sexual Function**
Decreased libido and/or impotence (33%); inhibited ejaculation (14%).
Male breast enlargement and tenderness.
Female breast enlargement with milk production.

▷ **Adverse Effects That May Mimic Natural Diseases or Disorders**
Parkinson-like muscle rigidity and lethargic behavior may suggest true Parkinson's disease.

Natural Diseases or Disorders That May Be Activated by This Drug

Migraine headaches, mental depression, peptic ulcer disease, systemic lupus erythematosus.

CAUTION

1. Discontinue this drug at the first indication of despondency, loss of appetite, early morning awakening (insomnia), or impaired sex drive or performance.
2. Avoid concurrent use of drugs with strong sedative effects, antidepressants, levodopa and monoamine oxidase (MAO) type A inhibitors.
3. If surgery is planned, consult your surgeon and/or anesthesiologist regarding the need to discontinue this drug prior to surgery.

Precautions for Use

By Infants and Children: Continual use for a minimum of 7 to 14 days is necessary to determine this drug's effectiveness as an antihypertensive. Observe carefully for excessive drowsiness, emotional instability or gastrointestinal disturbances.

By Those over 60 Years of Age: Start treatment with small doses and proceed cautiously. Unacceptably high blood pressure should be reduced without creating the risks associated with excessively low blood pressure. Sudden, rapid and excessive reduction of blood pressure can predispose to stroke or heart attack. This age group is more susceptible to the development of impaired thinking, depression (6%), confusion, nightmares and orthostatic hypotension (see Glossary).

▷ **Advisability of Use During Pregnancy**

Pregnancy Category: D (tentative). See Pregnancy Code inside back cover.

Animal studies: Significant eye defects reported in rats.

Human studies: Information from adequate studies of pregnant women is not available. Significant birth defects have been reported with the use of this drug during the first 3 months.

Use of this drug during the last month of pregnancy can cause lethargy, nasal congestion, breathing difficulties and poor feeding in the newborn infant.

Avoid this drug during the first 3 months and the last month. Use it otherwise only if clearly needed.

Advisability of Use if Breast-Feeding

Presence of this drug in breast milk: Yes.

Avoid drug or refrain from nursing.

Habit-Forming Potential: None.

Effects of Overdosage: Marked drowsiness, flushed skin, incoordination, tremors, slow and weak pulse, slow and shallow breathing, diarrhea, stupor progressing to coma.

Possible Effects of Long-Term Use: None reported.

Suggested Periodic Examinations While Taking This Drug (at physician's discretion)

Complete blood cell counts.

Assessment of emotional status for unrecognized depression.

▷ **While Taking This Drug, Observe the Following**

Foods: No restrictions. Avoid excessive salt intake.

Beverages: No restrictions. May be taken with milk.

▷ *Alcohol:* Use with extreme caution until the combined effects have been determined. This drug can increase the intoxicating effects of alcohol. Both of these drugs depress brain function.

Tobacco Smoking: No interactions expected.

Marijuana Smoking: Significant increase in drowsiness; possible accentuation of hypotension; possible precipitation of depression.

▷ *Other Drugs*

Reserpine may **decrease** the effects of
- levodopa (Dopar, Sinemet), and reduce its effectiveness in treating Parkinson's disease.

Reserpine **taken concurrently** with
- anticonvulsants may lower the convulsive threshold in susceptible individuals and alter seizure patterns.
- digitalis preparations may cause rhythm disorders in susceptible individuals.
- monoamine oxidase (MAO) type A inhibitors may cause excessive stimulation of the nervous system (theoretical).
- quinidine may cause rhythm disorders in susceptible individuals.
- warfarin (Coumadin, etc.) may cause decreased anticoagulant effect with short-term use and increased anticoagulant effect with long-term use.

▷ *Driving, Hazardous Activities:* This drug may impair mental alertness, judgment, physical coordination and reaction time. Restrict activities as necessary.

Aviation Note: The use of this drug **is a disqualification** for piloting. Consult a designated Aviation Medical Examiner.

Exposure to Sun: No restrictions.

Exposure to Cold: Use caution. Monitor the elderly for excessive hypotension and other changes conducive to hypothermia (see Glossary).

RIFAMPIN
(RIF am pin)

Other Name: Rifampicin

Introduced: 1967   **Class:** Antibiotic, rifamycins

Prescription: USA: Yes   **Controlled Drug:** USA: No
Canada: Yes   Canada: No

Available as Generic: No

Brand Names: Rifadin, Rifamate [CD], Rimactane, Rimactane/INH Dual Pack [CD], ✦Rofact

---

BENEFITS versus RISKS

Possible Benefits	*Possible Risks*
EFFECTIVE TREATMENT OF TUBERCULOSIS in combination with other drugs	DRUG-INDUCED HEPATITIS
	DRUG-INDUCED NEPHRITIS
	Flulike syndrome
EFFECTIVE PREVENTION OF MENINGITIS by the elimination of meningococcus from the throat of carriers	Rare blood cell disorder: abnormally low blood platelet count

---

▷ **Principal Uses**

As a Single Drug Product: This antibiotic drug is used primarily to treat active tuberculosis. It is usually given concurrently with other antitubercular drugs to enhance its effectiveness. It is also used to eliminate the meningitis germ (meningococcus) from the throats of healthy carriers so it cannot be spread to others. It is not effective in the treatment of active meningitis.

As a Combination Drug Product [CD]: This drug is available in combination with isoniazid, another antitubercular drug that delays the development of drug-resistant strains of the tuberculosis germ.

How This Drug Works: This drug prevents the growth and multiplication of susceptible tuberculosis organisms by blocking specific enzyme systems that are involved in the formation of essential proteins.

Available Dosage Forms and Strengths
Capsules — 150 mg, 300 mg

▷ **Usual Adult Dosage Range:**   For tuberculosis: 600 mg once/day. For meningococcus carriers: 600 mg once/day for 4 days. The total daily dosage should not exceed 600 mg. **Note: Actual dosage and administration schedule must be determined by the physician for each patient individually.**

▷ **Dosing Instructions:**   Preferably taken with 8 ounces of water on an empty stomach (1 hour before or 2 hours after eating). However, it may be taken with food if necessary to reduce stomach irritation. The capsule may be opened and the contents mixed with applesauce or jelly for administration.

Usual Duration of Use: Continual use on a regular schedule for several months is usually necessary to determine this drug's effectiveness in promoting recovery from tuberculosis. Long-term use (possibly 1 to

2 years) requires ongoing supervision and periodic evaluation by your physician. Consult your physician on a regular basis.

▷ **This Drug Should Not Be Taken If**
- you have had an allergic reaction to it previously.
- you have active liver disease.

▷ **Inform Your Physician Before Taking This Drug If**
- you are pregnant.
- you have a history of liver disease or impaired liver function.
- you consume alcohol daily.
- you are taking an oral contraceptive. (An alternate method of contraception is advised.)
- you are taking an anticoagulant.

Possible Side-Effects (natural, expected and unavoidable drug actions)
Red, orange or brown discoloration of tears, sweat, saliva, sputum, urine or stool. Yellow discoloration of the skin (not jaundice). Note: In the absence of symptoms indicating illness, any discoloration is a harmless drug effect and does not indicate toxicity.
Possible fungal superinfections (see Glossary).

▷ **Possible Adverse Effects** (unusual, unexpected and infrequent reactions)
If any of the following develop, consult your physician promptly for guidance.
Mild Adverse Effects
Allergic Reactions: Skin rash, hives, itching, drug fever (see Glossary).
Headache, drowsiness, dizziness, blurred vision, impaired hearing, vague numbness and tingling.
Loss of appetite, heartburn, nausea, vomiting, abdominal cramps, diarrhea.
Serious Adverse Effects
Flulike syndrome: fever, chills, headache, dizziness, musculoskeletal pain, difficult breathing.
Drug-induced liver damage, with or without jaundice.
Drug-induced kidney damage: impaired urine production, bloody or cloudy urine.
Excessively low blood platelet count: abnormal bleeding or bruising.

▷ **Possible Effects on Sexual Function**
Altered timing and pattern of menstruation.
Decreased effectiveness of oral contraceptives taken concurrently.

▷ **Adverse Effects That May Mimic Natural Diseases or Disorders**
Liver reactions may suggest viral hepatitis.
Kidney reactions may suggest an infectious nephritis.

CAUTION
1. This drug may permanently discolor soft contact lenses.
2. This drug may reduce the effectiveness of oral contraceptives; unplanned pregnancy could occur; an alternate method of contraception is advised.

3. When this drug is used alone in the treatment of tuberculosis, bacterial strains that are resistant to this drug can develop rapidly. This drug should only be used in conjunction with other antitubercular drugs.

4. To ensure the best possible response to treatment, take the full course of medication prescribed; this may be for several months or years.

Precautions for Use

By Infants and Children: Monitor closely for possible liver toxicity or deficiency of blood platelets.

By Those over 60 Years of Age: Natural changes in body composition and function make you more susceptible to the adverse effects of this drug. Report promptly any indications of possible drug toxicity.

▷ **Advisability of Use During Pregnancy**

Pregnancy Category: C (tentative). See Pregnancy Code inside back cover.
Animal studies: Cleft palate and spinal defects reported in rodent studies.

Human studies: Information from adequate studies of pregnant women is not available.

If possible, avoid use of drug during the first 3 months.

Advisability of Use if Breast-Feeding

Presence of this drug in breast milk: Yes.
Avoid drug or refrain from nursing.

Habit-Forming Potential: None.

Effects of Overdosage: Nausea, vomiting, drowsiness, unconsciousness, severe liver damage, jaundice.

Possible Effects of Long-Term Use: Superinfections, fungal overgrowth of mouth or tongue.

Suggested Periodic Examinations While Taking This Drug (at physician's discretion)

Complete blood cell counts, liver and kidney function tests.
Hearing acuity tests if hearing loss is suspected.

▷ **While Taking This Drug, Observe the Following**

Foods: No restrictions.

Beverages: No restrictions.

▷ *Alcohol:* It is best to avoid alcohol completely to reduce the risk of potential liver toxicity.

Tobacco Smoking: No interactions expected.

▷ *Other Drugs*

Rifampin may *decrease* the effects of
- anticoagulants (Coumadin, etc.), and reduce their effectiveness.
- beta blockers (see Drug Class, Section Four).
- cortisonelike drugs (see Drug Class, Section Four).

- cyclosporine.
- digitoxin.
- methadone (Dolophine).
- mexiletine (Mexitil).
- oral contraceptives.
- phenytoin (Dilantin).
- progestins.
- quinidine.
- sulfonylureas (see Drug Class, Section Four).
- theophyllines (Aminophyllin, Theo-Dur, etc.).

The following drug may *decrease* the effects of rifampin
- aminosalicylic acid (PAS), and reduce its antitubercular effectiveness.

▷ *Driving, Hazardous Activities:* This drug may cause dizziness, drowsiness, impaired vision and impaired hearing. Restrict activities as necessary.

Aviation Note: The use of this drug *may be a disqualification* for piloting. Consult a designated Aviation Medical Examiner.

Exposure to Sun: No restrictions.

Discontinuation: It is advisable not to interrupt or discontinue this drug without consulting your physician. Intermittent administration can increase the possibility of developing allergic reactions.

SELEGILINE
(se LEDGE i leen)

Other Name: Deprenyl

Introduced: 1981

Class: Antiparkinsonism, monoamine oxidase (MAO) type B inhibitor

Prescription: USA: Yes (Expected to become available in 1989)

Controlled Drug: USA: No

Available as Generic: USA: No

Brand Name: Eldepryl

BENEFITS versus RISKS	
Possible Benefits	*Possible Risks*
ADDITIVE RELIEF OF SYMPTOMS OF PARKINSON'S DISEASE when used concurrently with levodopa/carbidopa (Sinemet) PERMITS UP TO 30% REDUCTION IN SINEMET DOSAGE with resultant decrease in adverse effects	ABNORMAL INVOLUNTARY MOVEMENTS (12%) HALLUCINATIONS (5.4%) INITIAL FALL IN BLOOD PRESSURE/ORTHOSTATIC HYPOTENSION (1.8%)

▷ **Principal Uses**

As a Single Drug Product: Used solely as an adjunct to levodopa/carbidopa treatment of Parkinson's disease for those individuals who experience intolerable abnormal movements (dyskinesia) and/or increasing "on-off" episodes due to loss of effectiveness of levodopa. The addition of selegiline (1) permits reduction of the daily dose of levodopa (by 25% to 30%) with consequent lessening of dyskinesia and erratic drug response, and (2) provides additional relief of parkinsonian symptoms.

How This Drug Works: By (1) inhibiting monoamine oxidase type B, the enzyme that inactivates dopamine in the brain, and by (2) slowing the restorage of released dopamine at nerve terminals, this drug helps to correct the deficiency of dopamine that is responsible for the rigidity, tremor and sluggish movement characteristic of Parkinson's disease.

Available Dosage Forms and Strengths

Tablets — 5 mg

▷ **Usual Adult Dosage Range**

5 mg once or twice daily. The usual maintenance dose is 5 mg after breakfast and 5 mg after lunch. A total daily dose of 10 mg is adequate to achieve optimal benefit from this drug. Higher doses do not result in further improvement and are not advised.

During the gradual introduction of selegiline, the concurrent dose of levodopa/carbidopa (Sinemet) may be cautiously decreased in accord with your physician's instructions. Concurrent Sinemet dosage should be reduced by 10% to 20% when selegiline is started.

Note: Actual dosage and administration schedule must be determined by the physician for each patient individually.

▷ **Dosing Instructions:** Take with food or milk to reduce stomach irritation. The tablet may be crushed for administration.

Usual Duration of Use: Continual use on a regular schedule for 4 to 6 weeks is usually necessary to determine this drug's effectiveness in controlling the symptoms of Parkinson's disease and permitting reduction of levodopa/carbidopa dosage. Long-term use (months to years) requires periodic evaluation of response and dosage adjustment. Consult your physician on a regular basis.

Possible Advantages of This Drug

It may provide a more effective and uniform control of parkinsonian symptoms and a significant reduction of some adverse effects associated with long-term levodopa therapy. Fifty to 60% of users show improvement.

It does not lose its effectiveness with long-term use.

It does not require avoidance of foods containing tyramine, as is necessary with monoamine oxidase (MAO) type A inhibitors.

It causes no life-threatening or irreversible adverse effects.

▷ **This Drug Should Not Be Taken If**
- you have had an allergic reaction to it previously.
- you have Huntington's disease, hereditary (essential) tremor or tardive dyskinesia (see Glossary).
- you are pregnant or breast-feeding.

▷ **Inform Your Physician Before Taking This Drug If**
- you have constitutionally low blood pressure.
- you have peptic ulcer disease.
- you have a history of heart rhythm disorder.
- you are taking any antihypertensive drugs or antipsychotic drugs (see Drug Classes, Section Four).

Possible Side-Effects (natural, expected and unavoidable drug actions)
Weakness (0.3%), orthostatic hypotension (see Glossary) (1.8%), dry mouth (2%), insomnia (1.5%).

▷ **Possible Adverse Effects** (unusual, unexpected and infrequent reactions)
If any of the following develop, consult your physician promptly for guidance.
Mild Adverse Effects
Headache (0.3%), dizziness (2.2%), agitation (2.5%).
Palpitations (0.2%), fainting (0.1%).
Altered taste (0.1%), nausea and vomiting (7%), stomach pain (0.1%).
Serious Adverse Effects
Dyskinesias: abnormal involuntary movements (12%).
Confusion and hallucinations (5.4%), depression (0.4%), psychosis (0.2%).
Aggravation of peptic ulcer (0.2%), gastrointestinal bleeding (0.2%).

▷ **Possible Effects on Sexual Function:**   None reported.

▷ **Adverse Effects That May Mimic Natural Diseases or Disorders**
Effects on mental function and behavior may resemble psychotic disorders.

▷ **Natural Diseases or Disorders That May Be Activated by This Drug**
Peptic ulcer disease.

CAUTION
1. This drug can initiate dyskinesias and can intensify existing dyskinesias. Observe carefully for the development of tremors, twitching or abnormal, involuntary movements of any kind. Report these promptly.
2. This drug potentiates the effects of levodopa. When this drug is added to current levodopa treatment, adverse effects of levodopa may develop or be intensified. It is necessary to reduce the dose of levodopa by 10% to 20% when treatment with selegiline begins.
3. Inform your physician promptly if you become pregnant or plan pregnancy. The manufacturer does not recommend the use of this drug during pregnancy.

Precautions for Use

By Infants and Children: This drug is not utilized by this age group.

By Those over 60 Years of Age: This drug is well tolerated by the elderly. Observe closely for any tendency to light-headedness or faintness, especially on arising from a lying or sitting position.

▷ **Advisability of Use During Pregnancy**

Pregnancy Category: B (tentative). See Pregnancy Code inside back cover.

Animal studies: No birth defects due to this drug were found in rat studies.

Human studies: Information from adequate studies of pregnant women is not available. The manufacturer advises that this drug should not be taken during pregnancy.

Advisability of Use if Breast-Feeding

Presence of this drug in breast milk: Unknown.

Avoid drug or refrain from nursing.

Habit-Forming Potential: None.

Effects of Overdosage: Nausea, vomiting, palpitations, low blood pressure, agitation, severe involuntary movements, hallucinations.

Possible Effects of Long-Term Use: None reported.

Suggested Periodic Examinations While Taking This Drug (at physician's discretion)

Regular evaluation of drug response, heart function and blood pressure status.

▷ **While Taking This Drug, Observe the Following**

Foods: No restrictions.

Beverages: No restrictions. May be taken with milk.

▷   *Alcohol:* Use caution until the combined effects have been determined. Alcohol may exaggerate the blood-pressure-lowering and sedative effects of this drug.

Tobacco Smoking: No interactions expected.

▷   *Other Drugs*

Selegiline *taken concurrently* with

- antihypertensive drugs (and other drugs that can lower blood pressure) requires careful monitoring for excessive drops in pressure. Dosage adjustments may be necessary.

The following drugs may *decrease* the effects of selegiline and diminish its effectiveness

- chlorprothixene (Taractan).
- haloperidol (Haldol).
- metoclopramide (Reglan).
- phenothiazines (see Drug Class, Section Four).
- reserpine (Ser-Ap-Es, etc.), in high doses.
- thiothixene (Navane).

▷ *Driving, Hazardous Activities:* This drug may cause dizziness, drowsiness, impaired coordination or fainting. Restrict activities as necessary.

Aviation Note: The use of this drug *is a disqualification* for piloting. Consult a designated Aviation Medical Examiner.

Exposure to Sun: No restrictions.

Exposure to Heat: Use caution until the combined effects have been determined. Hot environments can cause lowering of blood pressure.

Discontinuation: Do not discontinue this drug abruptly. Sudden withdrawal can cause prompt increase in parkinsonian symptoms and deterioration of control. Consult your physician regarding a schedule for gradual withdrawal and concurrent adjustment of Sinemet or other appropriate drugs.

SPIRONOLACTONE
(speer on oh LAK tohn)

Introduced: 1959

Class: Diuretic

Prescription: USA: Yes
Canada: Yes

Controlled Drug: USA: No
Canada: No

Available as Generic: USA: Yes
Canada: No

Brand Names: Aldactone, Aldactazide [CD], Alatone, ✦Novospiroton, ✦Novospirozine [CD], ✦Sincomen

---

BENEFITS versus RISKS

Possible Benefits	*Possible Risks*
EFFECTIVE PREVENTION OF POTASSIUM LOSS when used adjunctively with other diuretics	ABNORMALLY HIGH BLOOD POTASSIUM LEVEL with excessive use
EFFECTIVE DIURETIC IN REFRACTORY CASES OF FLUID RETENTION when used adjunctively with other diuretics	Enlargement of male breast tissue Masculinization effects in women: excessive hair growth, deepening of the voice

---

▷ **Principal Uses**

As a Single Drug Product: This mild diuretic is used as part of the treatment program for the management of congestive heart failure and disorders of the liver and kidney that are accompanied by excessive fluid retention (edema). It is also used in conjunction with other measures to treat high blood pressure. It is used primarily in situations where it is advisable to prevent loss of potassium from the body.

As a Combination Drug Product [CD]: This drug is available in combination with hydrochlorothiazide, a different kind of diuretic that promotes the loss of potassium from the body. Spironolactone is used in this combination to counteract the potassium-wasting effect of the thiazide diuretic.

How This Drug Works: Not completely established. It is thought that by inhibiting the action of aldosterone (an adrenal gland hormone), this drug prevents the reabsorption of sodium and the excretion of potassium by the kidney. Thus the drug promotes the excretion of sodium (and water with it) and the retention of potassium.

Available Dosage Forms and Strengths
Tablets — 25 mg, 50 mg, 100 mg

▷ **Usual Adult Dosage Range:** Initially, 25 to 100 mg/day for 5 days. The dose is then adjusted according to individual response. The usual maintenance dose is 50 to 200 mg/day, divided into 2 to 4 doses. The total daily dosage should not exceed 400 mg. **Note: Actual dosage and administration schedule must be determined by the physician for each patient individually.**

▷ **Dosing Instructions:** May be taken with or following meals to promote absorption of the drug and to reduce stomach irritation. The tablet may be crushed for administration. Intermittent or alternate day use is recommended to minimize the possibility of sodium and potassium imbalance.

Usual Duration of Use: Continual use on a regular schedule for 5 to 10 days is usually necessary to determine this drug's effectiveness in clearing edema, and for 2 to 3 weeks to determine its effect on hypertension. Long-term use (months to years) requires supervision and periodic evaluation by your physician. Consult your physician on a regular basis.

▷ **This Drug Should Not Be Taken If**
- you have had an allergic reaction to it previously.
- you have severely impaired liver or kidney function.

▷ **Inform Your Physician Before Taking This Drug If**
- you have a history of liver or kidney disease.
- you have diabetes.
- you are taking any of the following: an anticoagulant, antihypertensives, a digitalis preparation, another diuretic, lithium or a potassium preparation.
- you plan to have surgery under general anesthesia in the near future.

Possible Side-Effects (natural, expected and unavoidable drug actions)
Abnormally high blood potassium levels (42%), abnormally low blood sodium levels (12%), dehydration (17%).

▷ **Possible Adverse Effects** (unusual, unexpected and infrequent reactions)
If any of the following develop, consult your physician promptly for guidance.

Mild Adverse Effects

Allergic Reactions: Skin rash, hives, itching, drug fever (see Glossary).

Headache, dizziness, unsteadiness, weakness, drowsiness, lethargy, confusion.

Dry mouth, nausea, vomiting, diarrhea.

Serious Adverse Effects

Allergic Reaction: Abnormally low blood platelet count (rare).

Symptomatic potassium excess: confusion, numbness and tingling in lips and extremities, fatigue, weakness, shortness of breath, slow heart rate, low blood pressure.

Masculine pattern of hair growth and deepening of the voice in women.

Stomach ulceration with bleeding (rare).

▷ **Possible Effects on Sexual Function**

Decreased libido (close to 100%); impaired erection or impotence (30%).

Male breast enlargement and tenderness (close to 100% with high doses).

Female breast enlargement (100% with high doses); altered timing and pattern of menstruation; postmenopausal bleeding.

Decreased vaginal secretion.

CAUTION

1. Do not take potassium supplements or increase your intake of potassium-rich foods while taking this drug.
2. Do not discontinue this drug abruptly unless abnormally high blood levels of potassium develop.
3. Ordinary doses of aspirin (600 mg) may reverse the diuretic effect of this drug. Observe response to this drug combination.
4. Avoid the excessive use of salt substitutes that contain potassium; these are a potential cause of potassium excess.

Precautions for Use

By Infants and Children: Limit the continual use of this drug in children to 1 month. Observe closely for indications of potassium accumulation.

By Those over 60 Years of Age: The natural decline in kidney function may predispose to potassium retention in the body. Limit continual use of this drug to periods of 2 to 3 weeks. Observe for indications of potassium excess: slow heart rate, irregular heart rhythms, low blood pressure, confusion, drowsiness. The excessive use of diuretics can cause harmful loss of body water (dehydration), increased viscosity of the blood and an increased tendency of the blood to clot, predisposing to stroke, heart attack or thrombophlebitis.

▷ **Advisability of Use During Pregnancy**

Pregnancy Category: D (tentative). See Pregnancy Code inside back cover.

Animal studies: This drug causes feminization of male rat fetuses.

Human studies: Information from adequate studies of pregnant women is not available.

This drug should not be used during pregnancy unless a very serious complication of pregnancy occurs for which this drug is significantly beneficial.

Advisability of Use if Breast-Feeding

Presence of this drug in breast milk: A metabolic by-product (canrenone) is present.

Avoid drug or refrain from nursing.

Habit-Forming Potential: None.

Effects of Overdosage: Thirst, drowsiness, fatigue, weakness, nausea, vomiting, confusion, irregular heart rhythm, low blood pressure.

Possible Effects of Long-Term Use: Potassium accumulation to abnormally high blood levels. Male breast enlargement.

Suggested Periodic Examinations While Taking This Drug (at physician's discretion)

Measurements of blood sodium, potassium and chloride levels.

Kidney function tests.

▷ **While Taking This Drug, Observe the Following**

Foods: No restrictions. Avoid excessive restriction of salt.

Beverages: No restrictions. May be taken with milk.

▷ *Alcohol:* Use with caution until the combined effects have been determined. Alcohol may enhance the drowsiness and the blood-pressure-lowering effect of this drug.

Tobacco Smoking: No interactions expected.

▷ *Other Drugs*

Spironolactone may *increase* the effects of

• digoxin (Lanoxin).

Spironolactone may *decrease* the effects of

• anticoagulants (Coumadin, etc.).

Spironolactone *taken concurrently* with

• captopril (Capoten) may cause excessively high blood potassium levels.

• digitoxin (Crystodigin) may cause either increased or decreased digitoxin effects (unpredictable).

• lithium may cause accumulation of lithium to toxic levels.

• potassium preparations may cause excessively high blood potassium levels.

The following drugs may *decrease* the effects of spironolactone

• aspirin may reduce its diuretic effectiveness.

▷ *Driving, Hazardous Activities:* This drug may cause dizziness and drowsiness. Restrict activities as necessary.

Aviation Note: The use of this drug *may be a disqualification* for piloting. Consult a designated Aviation Medical Examiner.

Exposure to Sun: No restrictions.

Discontinuation: With high dosage or prolonged use, it is advisable to withdraw this drug gradually. Ask your physician for guidance.

SUCRALFATE
(soo KRAL fayt)

Introduced: 1978

Class: Antiulcer

Prescription: USA: Yes
    Canada: Yes

Controlled Drug: USA: No
    Canada: No

Available as Generic: No

Brand Names: Carafate, ◆Sulcrate

BENEFITS versus RISKS	
Possible Benefits	*Possible Risks*
EFFECTIVE TREATMENT IN PEPTIC ULCER DISEASE No serious adverse effects No significant drug interactions	Constipation Skin rash, hives, itching

▷ **Principal Uses**

As a Single Drug Product: Used exclusively in the management of peptic ulcer disease to promote healing of both stomach (gastric) and duodenal ulcer. It is effective when used alone, but may be used in conjunction with antacids when these are needed for pain relief.

How This Drug Works: Not completely established. It is thought that this drug promotes ulcer healing by several mechanisms: (1) the formation of a protective coating over the ulcer site to prevent further erosion by stomach acid; (2) the inhibition of the digestive action of pepsin; (3) the protection of injured tissue at the ulcer margins; (4) the stimulation of active healing (tissue repair).

Available Dosage Forms and Strengths
    Tablets — 0.5 gram, 1 gram

▷ **Usual Adult Dosage Range:** 1 gram 4 times/day. **Note: Actual dosage and administration schedule must be determined by the physician for each patient individually.**

▷ **Dosing Instructions:** Take with water on an empty stomach at least 1 hour before or 2 hours after each meal and at bedtime. Swallow the tablets whole; do not alter or chew. Take the full course prescribed.

Usual Duration of Use: Continual use on a regular schedule for 6 to 8 weeks is usually necessary to determine this drug's effectiveness in promoting the healing of peptic ulcers. Use beyond 8 weeks must be determined by your physician.

▷ **This Drug Should Not Be Taken If**
   • you have had an allergic reaction to it previously.

▷ **Inform Your Physician Before Taking This Drug If**
   • you have chronic constipation.
   • you are taking any other drugs at this time.

Possible Side-Effects (natural, expected and unavoidable drug actions)
   Constipation (2.2%).

▷ **Possible Adverse Effects** (unusual, unexpected and infrequent reactions)
   If any of the following develop, consult your physician promptly for guidance.
   Mild Adverse Effects
   Allergic Reactions: Skin rash, hives, itching.
   Dizziness, light-headedness, drowsiness.
   Dry mouth, indigestion, nausea, cramping, diarrhea.
   Serious Adverse Effects
   None reported.

▷ **Possible Effects on Sexual Function:**   None reported.

   CAUTION
   1. If antacids are needed to relieve ulcer pain, do not take them within half an hour before or 1 hour after the dose of sucralfate.
   2. This drug may impair the absorption of other drugs if they are taken close together. It is advisable to avoid taking any other drugs within 2 hours of taking sucralfate. This applies especially to cimetidine (Tagamet), phenytoin (Dilantin) and tetracyclines.

▷ **Advisability of Use During Pregnancy**
   Pregnancy Category: B (tentative). See Pregnancy Code inside back cover.
   Animal studies: No birth defects due to this drug reported in mouse, rat and rabbit studies.
   Human studies: Information from adequate studies of pregnant women is not available.
   Because only very small amounts of this drug are absorbed, it is probably safe for use at any time during pregnancy. However, it should be used only if clearly needed. Ask your physician for guidance.

Advisability of Use if Breast-Feeding
   Presence of this drug in breast milk: Unknown.
   Monitor nursing infant closely and discontinue drug or nursing if adverse effects develop.

Habit-Forming Potential: None.

Effects of Overdosage: Nausea, stomach cramping, possible diarrhea.

Possible Effects of Long-Term Use: Deficiencies of vitamins A, D, E and K due to impaired absorption from the intestine.

Suggested Periodic Examinations While Taking This Drug (at physician's discretion)
None required.

▷ **While Taking This Drug, Observe the Following**
Foods: No restrictions. Follow diet prescribed by your physician.
Beverages: No restrictions. This drug is preferably taken with water.
▷   *Alcohol:* No interactions with drug expected. However, alcohol is best avoided because of its irritant effect on the stomach.
Tobacco Smoking: No interactions expected. However, nicotine can delay ulcer healing and reduce the effectiveness of this drug. Avoid all forms of tobacco.
▷   *Other Drugs*
Sucralfate may *decrease* the effects of
   • cimetidine (Tagamet).
   • digoxin (Lanoxin).
   • phenytoin (Dilantin, etc.).
   • tetracycline (Achromycin, Tetracyn, etc.).
   • warfarin (Coumadin, etc.), and reduce its effectiveness as an anti-coagulant.
▷   *Driving, Hazardous Activities:* This drug may cause dizziness or drowsiness. Restrict activities as necessary.
Aviation Note: The use of this drug *may be a disqualification* for piloting. Consult a designated Aviation Medical Examiner.
Exposure to Sun: No restrictions.

SULFAMETHOXAZOLE
(sul fa meth OX a zohl)

Introduced: 1961   **Class:** Anti-infective, sulfonamides

Prescription: USA: Yes   **Controlled Drug:** USA: No
Canada: Yes   Canada: No

Available as Generic: Yes

Brand Names: ✦Apo-Sulfamethoxazole, ✦Apo-Sulfatrim [CD], ✦Apo-Sulfatrim DS [CD], Azo Gantanol [CD], Bactrim [CD], Bactrim DS [CD], Bethaprim [CD], Comoxol [CD], Cotrim [CD], Gantanol, ✦Novotrimel [CD], ✦Novotrimel DS [CD], ✦Protrin [CD], ✦Protrin DF [CD], ✦Roubac [CD], Septra [CD], Septra DS [CD], ✦Uro Gantanol [CD], Uroplus DS [CD], Uroplus SS [CD]

BENEFITS versus RISKS

Possible Benefits	*Possible Risks*
EFFECTIVE ANTIMICROBIAL ACTION against susceptible bacteria and protozoa	Allergic reactions: mild to severe skin reactions, anaphylaxis, myocarditis Rare blood cell disorders: aplastic anemia, hemolytic anemia, abnormally low white cell and platelet counts Drug-induced liver damage Drug-induced kidney damage

---

▷ **Principal Uses**

As a Single Drug Product: This member of the sulfonamide class is used to treat a variety of bacterial and protozoal infections. It is most commonly used to treat certain infections of the urinary tract.

As a Combination Drug Product [CD]: This drug is available in combination with phenazopyridine, an analgesic drug that relieves the discomfort associated with acute infections of the urinary bladder and urethra. This combination provides early symptomatic relief while the underlying infection is being eradicated. This drug is also available in combination with another antibacterial drug—trimethoprim. This combination is quite effective in the treatment of certain types of middle ear infection, bronchitis, pneumonia and certain infections of the intestinal tract and the urinary tract.

How This Drug Works: This drug prevents the growth and multiplication of susceptible bacteria by interfering with their formation of folic acid, an essential nutrient.

Available Dosage Forms and Strengths

Oral suspension — 500 mg per 5-ml teaspoonful

Tablets — 500 mg, 1 gram

▷ **Usual Adult Dosage Range:**   Initially, 2 grams; then 1 gram every 8 to 12 hours, depending upon the severity of the infection. The total daily dosage should not exceed 3 grams. **Note: Actual dosage and administration schedule must be determined by the physician for each patient individually.**

▷ **Dosing Instructions:**   Preferably taken on an empty stomach, 1 hour before or 2 hours after eating. However, it may be taken with or following food to reduce stomach irritation. The tablet may be crushed for administration.

Usual Duration of Use: Continual use on a regular schedule for 4 to 7 days is usually necessary to determine this drug's effectiveness in controlling responsive infections. Treatment should be continued until the patient is free of symptoms for 48 hours. Limit treatment to no more than 14 days if possible.

Currently a "Drug of Choice" (when combined with trimethoprim) for preventing pneumonia (due to pneumocystis carinii) in patients with AIDS.

▷ **This Drug Should Not Be Taken If**
- you are allergic to *any* sulfonamide drug (see Drug Class, Section Four).
- you are in the last month of pregnancy.
- you are breast-feeding.

▷ **Inform Your Physician Before Taking This Drug If**
- you are allergic to any sulfonamide derivative: acetazolamide, thiazide diuretics, sulfonylurea antidiabetic drugs (see Drug Classes, Section Four).
- you are allergic by nature: history of hay fever, asthma, hives, eczema.
- you have impaired liver or kidney function.
- you have a personal or family history of porphyria.
- you have had a drug-induced blood cell or bone marrow disorder in the past.
- you are currently taking any oral anticoagulant, antidiabetic drug or phenytoin.
- you plan to have surgery under pentothal anesthesia while taking this drug.

Possible Side-Effects (natural, expected and unavoidable drug actions)
Brownish coloration of the urine, of no significance.
Superinfections, bacterial or fungal (see Glossary).

▷ **Possible Adverse Effects** (unusual, unexpected and infrequent reactions)
If any of the following develop, consult your physician promptly for guidance.
Mild Adverse Effects
Allergic Reactions: Skin rashes, hives, itching, localized swellings, reddened eyes.
Headache, dizziness, unsteadiness, ringing in the ears.
Loss of appetite, irritation of the mouth and tongue, nausea, vomiting, abdominal pain, diarrhea.
Serious Adverse Effects
Allergic Reactions: Drug fever (see Glossary), swollen glands, painful joints, anaphylaxis (see Glossary). Allergic reaction in the heart muscle (myocarditis), allergic pneumonitis, allergic hepatitis. Severe skin reactions.
Idiosyncratic Reaction: Hemolytic anemia (see Glossary).
Bone marrow depression (see Glossary): fatigue, weakness, fever, sore throat, abnormal bleeding or bruising.

Pancreatitis; kidney damage: bloody or cloudy urine, reduced urine volume.

Psychotic reactions, hallucinations, seizures, hearing loss, peripheral neuropathy (see Glossary).

▷ **Possible Effects on Sexual Function:** None reported.

▷ **Adverse Effects That May Mimic Natural Diseases or Disorders**
Liver reactions may suggest viral hepatitis.
Lung reactions may suggest an infectious pneumonia.

Natural Diseases or Disorders That May Be Activated by This Drug
Goiter, acute intermittent porphyria, polyarteritis nodosa, systemic lupus erythematosus (questionable).

CAUTION
1. A large intake of water (up to 2 quarts daily) is necessary to ensure an adequate volume of urine.
2. Shake liquid dosage forms thoroughly before measuring each dose.

Precautions for Use
By Infants and Children: This drug should not be used in infants under 2 months of age.
By Those over 60 Years of Age: Small doses taken at longer intervals often achieve adequate blood and tissue drug levels. Observe for the development of reduced urine volume, fever, sore throat, abnormal bleeding or bruising or skin irritation with itching, particularly in the anal or genital regions.

▷ **Advisability of Use During Pregnancy**
Pregnancy Category: C (tentative). See Pregnancy Code inside back cover.
Animal studies: Cleft palate and skeletal birth defects reported in mice and rats.
Human studies: No increase in birth defects reported in 4584 exposures to various sulfonamides during pregnancy.
Avoid use of drug during the last month of pregnancy because of possible adverse effects on the newborn infant.

Advisability of Use if Breast-Feeding
Presence of this drug in breast milk: Yes.
Avoid drug or refrain from nursing.

Habit-Forming Potential: None.

Effects of Overdosage: Headache, dizziness, nausea, vomiting, abdominal cramping, toxic fever, coma, jaundice, kidney failure.

Possible Effects of Long-Term Use: Superinfections, bacterial or fungal. Development of goiter, with or without hypothyroidism. Excessive loss of vitamin C via urine.

Suggested Periodic Examinations While Taking This Drug (at physician's discretion)
Complete blood cell counts, weekly for the first 8 weeks.
Urine analysis weekly.
Liver and kidney function tests.

▷ **While Taking This Drug, Observe the Following**
Foods: No restrictions.
Beverages: No restrictions. May be taken with milk.
▷ *Alcohol:* Use caution until the combined effect has been determined. Sulfonamide drugs can increase the intoxicating effects of alcohol.
Tobacco Smoking: No interactions expected.
▷ *Other Drugs*
Sulfamethoxazole may *increase* the effects of
- anticoagulants (Coumadin, etc.), and increase the risk of bleeding.
- sulfonylureas (see Drug Class, Section Four), and increase the risk of hypoglycemia.
Sulfamethoxazole may *decrease* the effects of
- cyclosporine, and reduce its immunosuppressive effect.
- penicillins.
▷ *Driving, Hazardous Activities:* This drug may cause dizziness. Restrict activities as necessary.
Aviation Note: The use of this drug *may be a disqualification* for piloting. Consult a designated Aviation Medical Examiner.
Exposure to Sun: Use caution until sensitivity has been determined. Some sulfonamide drugs can cause photosensitivity (see Glossary).

SULFASALAZINE
(sul fa SAL a zeen)

Introduced: 1949

Class: Bowel anti-inflammatory, sulfonamides

Prescription: USA: Yes
Canada: Yes

Controlled Drug: USA: No
Canada: No

Available as Generic: USA: Yes
Canada: No

Brand Names: Azaline, Azulfidine, Azulfidine EN-tabs, ✦PMS Sulfasalazine, ✦PMS Sulfasalazine E.C., ✦Salazopyrin, ✦SAS-Enema, ✦SAS Enteric-500, SAS-500

BENEFITS versus RISKS

Possible Benefits	*Possible Risks*
EFFECTIVE SUPPRESSION OF INFLAMMATORY BOWEL DISEASE	Allergic reactions: mild to severe skin reactions
SYMPTOMATIC RELIEF IN TREATMENT OF REGIONAL ENTERITIS AND ULCERATIVE COLITIS	Rare blood cell disorders: aplastic anemia, hemolytic anemia, abnormally low white cell and platelet counts
	Drug-induced liver damage
	Drug-induced kidney damage

▷ **Principal Uses**

As a Single Drug Product: This member of the sulfonamide class is used exclusively to treat inflammatory disease of the lower intestinal tract: regional enteritis (Crohn's disease) and ulcerative colitis. It is usually taken by mouth, but may also be used in retention enemas.

How This Drug Works: Not completely established. Possible methods of this drug's action include
- an anti-inflammatory action that suppresses the formation of prostaglandins (and related compounds), tissue substances that induce inflammation, tissue destruction and diarrhea.
- an anti-infective action that may prevent the growth and multiplication of certain infective agents in the intestine and colon. (This method of action is questionable.)

Available Dosage Forms and Strengths

Oral suspension — 250 mg per 5-ml teaspoonful

Tablets — 500 mg

Tablets, enteric-coated — 500 mg

▷ **Usual Adult Dosage Range:**   Initially, 1 to 2 grams every 6 to 8 hours until symptoms are adequately controlled. For maintenance, 500 mg/6 hours. The total daily dosage should not exceed 12 grams. **Note: Actual dosage and administration schedule must be determined by the physician for each patient individually.**

▷ **Dosing Instructions:**   Preferably taken with 8 ounces of water on an empty stomach, 1 hour before or 2 hours after eating. However, it may be taken with or following food to reduce stomach irritation. Intervals between doses (day and night) should be no longer than 8 hours. The regular tablet may be crushed for administration; the enteric-coated tablet should be swallowed whole without alteration.

Usual Duration of Use: Continual use on a regular schedule for 1 to 3 weeks is usually necessary to determine this drug's effectiveness in controlling the symptoms of regional enteritis or ulcerative colitis. Long-term use (months to years) requires supervision and periodic evaluation by your physician. Consult your physician on a regular basis.

▷ **This Drug Should Not Be Taken If**
- you are allergic to *any* sulfonamide drug (see Drug Class, Section Four), or to aspirin (or other salicylates).
- you are in the last month of pregnancy.
- you are breast-feeding.

▷ **Inform Your Physician Before Taking This Drug If**
- you are allergic to any sulfonamide derivative: acetazolamide, thiazide diuretics, sulfonylurea antidiabetic drugs (see Drug Classes, Section Four).
- you are allergic by nature: history of hay fever, asthma, hives, eczema.
- you have impaired liver or kidney function.
- you have a personal or family history of porphyria.
- you have had a drug-induced blood cell or bone marrow disorder in the past.
- you are currently taking any oral anticoagulant, antidiabetic drug or phenytoin.
- you plan to have surgery under pentothal anesthesia while taking this drug.

Possible Side-Effects (natural, expected and unavoidable drug actions)
Brownish coloration of the urine, of no significance.
Superinfections, bacterial or fungal (see Glossary).

▷ **Possible Adverse Effects** (unusual, unexpected and infrequent reactions)
If any of the following develop, consult your physician promptly for guidance.
Mild Adverse Effects
Allergic Reactions: Skin rashes, hives, itching.
Headache, dizziness.
Loss of appetite, irritation of the mouth and tongue, nausea, vomiting, abdominal pain, diarrhea.
Serious Adverse Effects
Allergic Reactions: Drug fever (see Glossary), swollen glands, painful joints, anaphylaxis (see Glossary). Allergic pneumonitis, allergic hepatitis. Severe skin reactions.
Idiosyncratic Reaction: Hemolytic anemia (see Glossary).
Bone marrow depression (see Glossary): fatigue, weakness, fever, sore throat, abnormal bleeding or bruising.
Pancreatitis; kidney damage: bloody or cloudy urine, reduced urine volume.
Peripheral neuropathy (see Glossary).

▷ **Possible Effects on Sexual Function:**   Decreased production of sperm, reversible infertility.

▷ **Adverse Effects That May Mimic Natural Diseases or Disorders**
Liver reactions may suggest viral hepatitis.
Lung reactions may suggest an infectious pneumonia.

Natural Diseases or Disorders That May Be Activated by This Drug
Goiter, acute intermittent porphyria.

CAUTION
1. A large intake of water (up to 2 quarts daily) is necessary to ensure an adequate volume of urine.
2. Shake liquid dosage forms thoroughly before measuring each dose.

Precautions for Use
By Infants and Children: Safety and effectiveness for use by those under 2 years of age have not been established.
By Those over 60 Years of Age: Observe for the development of reduced urine volume, fever, sore throat, abnormal bleeding or bruising or skin irritation with itching, particularly in the anal or genital regions.

▷ **Advisability of Use During Pregnancy**
Pregnancy Category: C (tentative). See Pregnancy Code inside back cover.
Animal studies: Cleft palate and skeletal birth defects due to sulfonamides reported in mice and rats.
Human studies: No increase in birth defects reported in 4584 exposures to various sulfonamides during pregnancy.
Avoid use of drug during the last month of pregnancy because of possible adverse effects on the newborn infant.

Advisability of Use if Breast-Feeding
Presence of this drug in breast milk: Yes.
Avoid drug or refrain from nursing.

Habit-Forming Potential: None.

Effects of Overdosage: Headache, dizziness, nausea, vomiting, abdominal cramping, toxic fever, coma, jaundice, kidney failure.

Possible Effects of Long-Term Use: Development of goiter, with or without hypothyroidism. An orange-yellow discoloration of the skin has been reported. This is not jaundice.

Suggested Periodic Examinations While Taking This Drug (at physician's discretion)
Complete blood cell counts, weekly for the first 8 weeks.
Urine analysis weekly.
Liver and kidney function tests.

▷ **While Taking This Drug, Observe the Following**
Foods: No restrictions. Follow prescribed diet.
Beverages: No restrictions. May be taken with milk.
▷ *Alcohol:* Use caution until the combined effect has been determined. Sulfonamide drugs can increase the intoxicating effects of alcohol.

Tobacco Smoking: No interactions expected.
▷ *Other Drugs*
  Sulfasalazine may ***increase*** the effects of
  - anticoagulants (Coumadin, etc.), and increase the risk of bleeding.
  - sulfonylureas (see Drug Class, Section Four), and increase the risk of hypoglycemia.

  Sulfasalazine may ***decrease*** the effects of
  - digoxin (Lanoxin).

▷ *Driving, Hazardous Activities:* This drug may cause dizziness. Restrict activities as necessary.

Aviation Note: The use of this drug ***may be a disqualification*** for piloting. Consult a designated Aviation Medical Examiner.

Exposure to Sun: Use caution until sensitivity has been determined. Some sulfonamide drugs can cause photosensitivity (see Glossary).

SULFISOXAZOLE
(sul fi SOX a zohl)

Introduced: 1949   **Class:** Anti-infective, sulfonamides

Prescription: USA: Yes   **Controlled Drug:** USA: No
               Canada: Yes   Canada: No

Available as Generic: Yes

Brand Names: ✦Apo-Sulfisoxazole, Azo Gantrisin [CD], Gantrisin, Lipo Gantrisin, ✦Novosoxazole, Pediazole [CD]

BENEFITS versus RISKS	
Possible Benefits	***Possible Risks***
EFFECTIVE ANTIMICROBIAL ACTION against susceptible bacteria and protozoa	Allergic reactions: mild to severe skin reactions, anaphylaxis
	Rare blood cell disorders: aplastic anemia, hemolytic anemia, abnormally low white cell and platelet counts
	Drug-induced liver damage
	Drug-induced kidney damage

▷ **Principal Uses**
  As a Single Drug Product: This member of the sulfonamide class is used to treat a variety of bacterial and protozoal infections. It is most commonly used to treat certain infections of the urinary tract.

As a Combination Drug Product [CD]: This drug is available in combination with phenazopyridine, an analgesic drug that relieves the discomfort associated with acute infections of the urinary bladder and urethra. This combination provides early symptomatic relief while the underlying infection is being eradicated.

How This Drug Works: This drug prevents the growth and multiplication of susceptible bacteria by interfering with their formation of folic acid, an essential nutrient.

Available Dosage Forms and Strengths

Emulsion, prolonged-action — 1 gram per 5-ml teaspoonful
Eye drops — 4%
Eye ointment — 4%
Injection — 400 mg per ml
Pediatric suspension — 500 mg per 5-ml teaspoonful
Syrup — 500 mg per 5-ml teaspoonful
Tablets — 500 mg

▷ **Usual Adult Dosage Range:** Initially, 2 to 4 grams; then 750 to 1500 mg (1.5 grams) every 4 hours, or 1 to 2 grams every 6 hours, depending upon the severity of the infection. The total daily dosage should not exceed 12 grams. **Note: Actual dosage and administration schedule must be determined by the physician for each patient individually.**

▷ **Dosing Instructions:** Preferably taken with 8 ounces of water on an empty stomach, 1 hour before or 2 hours after eating. However, it may be taken with or following food to reduce stomach irritation. The tablet may be crushed for administration.

Usual Duration of Use: Continual use on a regular schedule for 7 to 10 days is usually necessary to determine this drug's effectiveness in controlling responsive infections. Treatment should be continued until the patient is free of symptoms for 48 hours. Limit treatment to no more than 14 days if possible.

▷ **This Drug Should Not Be Taken If**
- you are allergic to *any* sulfonamide drug (see Drug Class, Section Four).
- you are in the last month of pregnancy.
- you are breast-feeding.

▷ **Inform Your Physician Before Taking This Drug If**
- you are allergic to any sulfonamide derivative: acetazolamide, thiazide diuretics, sulfonylurea antidiabetic drugs (see Drug Classes, Section Four).
- you are allergic by nature: history of hay fever, asthma, hives, eczema.
- you have impaired liver or kidney function.
- you have a personal or family history of porphyria.

- you have had a drug-induced blood cell or bone marrow disorder in the past.
- you are currently taking any oral anticoagulant, antidiabetic drug or phenytoin.
- you plan to have surgery under pentothal anesthesia while taking this drug.

Possible Side-Effects (natural, expected and unavoidable drug actions)
Brownish coloration of the urine, of no significance.
Superinfections, bacterial or fungal (see Glossary).

▷ **Possible Adverse Effects** (unusual, unexpected and infrequent reactions)
If any of the following develop, consult your physician promptly for guidance.
Mild Adverse Effects
Allergic Reactions: Skin rashes, hives, itching, localized swellings, reddened eyes.
Headache, dizziness, unsteadiness, ringing in the ears.
Loss of appetite, irritation of the mouth and tongue, nausea, vomiting, abdominal pain, diarrhea.
Serious Adverse Effects
Allergic Reactions: Drug fever (see Glossary), swollen glands, painful joints, anaphylaxis (see Glossary). Allergic hepatitis. Severe skin reactions.
Idiosyncratic Reaction: Hemolytic anemia (see Glossary).
Bone marrow depression (see Glossary): fatigue, weakness, fever, sore throat, abnormal bleeding or bruising.
Kidney damage: bloody or cloudy urine, reduced urine volume.
Peripheral neuropathy (see Glossary).

▷ **Possible Effects on Sexual Function:**   None reported.

▷ **Adverse Effects That May Mimic Natural Diseases or Disorders**
Liver reactions may suggest viral hepatitis.

Natural Diseases or Disorders That May Be Activated by This Drug
Goiter, acute intermittent porphyria.

CAUTION
1. A large intake of water (up to 2 quarts daily) is necessary to ensure an adequate volume of urine.
2. Shake liquid dosage forms thoroughly before measuring each dose.

Precautions for Use
By Infants and Children: This drug should not be used in infants under 2 months of age.
By Those over 60 Years of Age: Small doses taken at longer intervals often achieve adequate blood and tissue drug levels. Observe for the development of reduced urine volume, fever, sore throat, abnormal bleeding or bruising or skin irritation with itching, particularly in the anal or genital regions.

▷ **Advisability of Use During Pregnancy**

Pregnancy Category: C (tentative). See Pregnancy Code inside back cover.

Animal studies: Cleft palate and skeletal birth defects due to sulfonamides reported in mice and rats.

Human studies: No increase in birth defects reported in 4287 exposures to this drug during pregnancy.

Avoid use of drug during the last month of pregnancy because of possible adverse effects on the newborn infant.

Advisability of Use if Breast-Feeding

Presence of this drug in breast milk: Yes.

Avoid drug or refrain from nursing.

Habit-Forming Potential: None.

Effects of Overdosage: Headache, dizziness, nausea, vomiting, abdominal cramping, toxic fever, coma, jaundice, kidney failure.

Possible Effects of Long-Term Use: Superinfections, bacterial or fungal. Development of goiter, with or without hypothyroidism. Excessive loss of vitamin C via urine.

Suggested Periodic Examinations While Taking This Drug (at physician's discretion)

Complete blood cell counts, weekly for the first 8 weeks.

Urine analysis weekly.

Liver and kidney function tests.

▷ **While Taking This Drug, Observe the Following**

Foods: No restrictions.

Beverages: No restrictions. May be taken with milk.

▷ *Alcohol:* Use caution until the combined effect has been determined. Sulfonamide drugs can increase the intoxicating effects of alcohol.

Tobacco Smoking: No interactions expected.

▷ *Other Drugs*

Sulfisoxazole may ***increase*** the effects of

- anticoagulants (Coumadin, etc.), and increase the risk of bleeding.
- sulfonylureas (see Drug Class, Section Four), and increase the risk of hypoglycemia.

Sulfisoxazole may ***decrease*** the effects of

- penicillins.

▷ *Driving, Hazardous Activities:* This drug may cause dizziness. Restrict activities as necessary.

Aviation Note: The use of this drug ***may be a disqualification*** for piloting. Consult a designated Aviation Medical Examiner.

Exposure to Sun: Use caution until sensitivity has been determined. Some sulfonamide drugs can cause photosensitivity (see Glossary).

SULINDAC
(sul IN dak)

Introduced: 1976

Class: Mild analgesic, anti-inflammatory

Prescription: USA: Yes
Canada: Yes

Controlled Drug: USA: No
Canada: No

Available as Generic: No

Brand Name: Clinoril

BENEFITS versus RISKS

Possible Benefits	*Possible Risks*
EFFECTIVE RELIEF OF MILD TO MODERATE PAIN AND INFLAMMATION	Gastrointestinal pain, ulceration, bleeding (rare) Rare liver damage Rare kidney damage Rare bone marrow depression (aplastic anemia)

▷ **Principal Uses**

As a Single Drug Product: Used primarily to relieve mild to moderately severe pain associated with (1) rheumatoid arthritis and osteoarthritis; (2) acute and chronic gout; and (3) bursitis, tendinitis and related disorders.

How This Drug Works: Not completely established. It is thought that this drug reduces the tissue concentrations of prostaglandins (and related compounds), substances involved in the production of inflammation and pain.

Available Dosage Forms and Strengths
Tablets — 150 mg, 200 mg

▷ **Usual Adult Dosage Range:**   150 to 200 mg twice/day, 12 hours apart. The total daily dosage should not exceed 400 mg. **Note: Actual dosage and administration schedule must be determined by the physician for each patient individually.**

▷ **Dosing Instructions:**   Preferably taken on an empty stomach, 1 hour before or 2 hours after eating. However, it may be taken with or after food if necessary to reduce stomach irritation. Take with a full glass of water and remain upright (do not lie down) for 30 minutes. The tablet may be crushed for administration.

Usual Duration of Use: Continual use on a regular schedule for 2 to 3 weeks is usually necessary to determine this drug's effectiveness in

relieving the discomfort of arthritis. Acute gout usually responds within 7 days. Shoulder bursitis or tendinitis usually responds within 7 to 14 days. Long-term use (months to years) requires supervision and periodic evaluation by your physician. Consult your physician on a regular basis.

▷ **This Drug Should Not Be Taken If**
  • you have had an allergic reaction to it previously.
  • you are subject to asthma or nasal polyps caused by aspirin.
  • you have active peptic ulcer disease or any form of gastrointestinal bleeding.
  • you have a bleeding disorder or a blood cell disorder.
  • you have severe impairment of liver or kidney function.

▷ **Inform Your Physician Before Taking This Drug If**
  • you are allergic to aspirin or to other aspirin substitutes.
  • you have a history of peptic ulcer disease or any type of bleeding disorder.
  • you have impaired liver or kidney function.
  • you have high blood pressure or a history of heart failure.
  • you are taking any of the following: acetaminophen, aspirin or other aspirin substitutes, anticoagulants, oral antidiabetic drugs.

  Possible Side-Effects (natural, expected and unavoidable drug actions)
  Fluid retention (edema).
  Drowsiness in sensitive individuals.

▷ **Possible Adverse Effects** (unusual, unexpected and infrequent reactions)
  If any of the following develop, consult your physician promptly for guidance.
  Mild Adverse Effects
  Allergic Reactions: Skin rash, hives, itching.
  Headache, dizziness, mild numbness and tingling, blurred vision, ringing in the ears.
  Mouth sores, indigestion, nausea, vomiting, constipation, diarrhea.
  Serious Adverse Effects
  Allergic Reactions: Anaphylactic reaction (see Glossary), severe skin reactions.
  Idiosyncratic Reactions: Drug-induced pneumonitis with fever.
  Active peptic ulcer, with or without bleeding.
  Liver damage with jaundice (see Glossary).
  Kidney damage with painful urination, bloody urine, reduced urine formation.
  Rare bone marrow depression (see Glossary): fatigue, weakness, fever, sore throat, abnormal bleeding or bruising.

▷ **Possible Effects on Sexual Function**
  Vaginal bleeding (less than 1%).
  Male breast enlargement (causal relationship not established).

Possible Delayed Adverse Effects: Mild anemia due to "silent" blood loss from the stomach (less than that caused by aspirin).

▷ **Adverse Effects That May Mimic Natural Diseases or Disorders**
Liver reaction may suggest viral hepatitis.

Natural Diseases or Disorders That May Be Activated by This Drug
Peptic ulcer disease, ulcerative colitis.

CAUTION
1. Dosage should always be limited to the smallest amount that produces reasonable improvement.
2. This drug may mask early indications of infection. Inform your physician if you think you are developing an infection of any kind.

Precautions for Use
By Infants and Children: Safety and effectiveness for use by those under 12 years of age have not been established.
By Those over 60 Years of Age: Small doses are advisable until tolerance is determined. Observe for any indications of liver or kidney toxicity, fluid retention, dizziness, confusion, impaired memory, stomach bleeding or constipation.

▷ **Advisability of Use During Pregnancy**
Pregnancy Category: C (tentative). See Pregnancy Code inside back cover.
Animal studies: A low incidence of birth defects has been reported but not confirmed.
Human studies: Information from adequate studies of pregnant women is not available.
The manufacturer does not recommend the use of this drug during pregnancy.

Advisability of Use if Breast-Feeding
Presence of this drug in breast milk: Unknown.
Avoid drug or refrain from nursing.

Habit-Forming Potential: None.

Effects of Overdosage: Stomach irritation, nausea, vomiting, diarrhea.

Possible Effects of Long-Term Use: Fluid retention.

Suggested Periodic Examinations While Taking This Drug (at physician's discretion)
Complete blood cell counts, liver and kidney function tests, complete eye examinations if vision is altered in any way.

▷ **While Taking This Drug, Observe the Following**
Foods: No restrictions.
Beverages: No restrictions. May be taken with milk.

▷ *Alcohol:* Use with caution. The irritant action of alcohol on the stomach lining, added to the irritant action of this drug in sensitive individuals, can increase the risk of stomach ulceration and/or bleeding.

Tobacco Smoking: No interactions expected.

▷ *Other Drugs*

Sulindac may ***increase*** the effects of

- acetaminophen (Tylenol, etc.), and increase the risk of kidney damage; avoid prolonged use of this combination.
- anticoagulants (Coumadin, etc.), and increase the risk of bleeding; monitor prothrombin time, adjust dose accordingly.

Sulindac ***taken concurrently*** with the following drugs may increase the risk of bleeding; avoid these combinations:

- aspirin.
- dipyridamole (Persantine).
- indomethacin (Indocin).
- sulfinpyrazone (Anturane).
- valproic acid (Depakene).

▷ *Driving, Hazardous Activities:* This drug may cause drowsiness or dizziness. Restrict activities as necessary.

Aviation Note: The use of this drug ***may be a disqualification*** for piloting. Consult a designated Aviation Medical Examiner.

Exposure to Sun: No restrictions.

TAMOXIFEN
(ta MOX i fen)

Introduced: 1973

Class: Antiestrogen, anticancer

Prescription: USA: Yes
  Canada: Yes

Controlled Drug: USA: No
  Canada: No

Available as Generic: No

Brand Names: Nolvadex, ✦Nolvadex-D, ✦Tamofen

BENEFITS versus RISKS	
Possible Benefits	***Possible Risks***
EFFECTIVE ADJUNCTIVE TREATMENT IN ADVANCED BREAST CANCER in 30% to 40% of cases	Severe increase in tumor or bone pain, transient Thromophlebitis, pulmonary embolism Abnormally high blood calcium levels Eye changes: corneal opacities, retinal injury

▷ **Principal Uses**

As a Single Drug Product: Used primarily as an alternative to estrogens and androgens (male sex hormones) to treat advanced breast cancer in postmenopausal women. It is also used to stimulate ovulation in premenopausal women with infertility.

How This Drug Works: Not completely established. It is thought that by blocking the uptake of estradiol (estrogen), this drug removes or reduces a stimulus to breast cancer cells.

Available Dosage Forms and Strengths
Tablets — 10 mg, 20 mg (in Canada)

▷ **Usual Adult Dosage Range:** 10 to 20 mg twice/day, morning and evening. **Note: Actual dosage and administration schedule must be determined by the physician for each patient individually.**

▷ **Dosing Instructions:** May be taken either on an empty stomach or with food. The tablet may be crushed for administration.

Usual Duration of Use: Continual use on a regular schedule for 4 to 10 weeks is usually necessary to determine this drug's effectiveness in controlling the growth and spread of advanced breast cancer. In the presence of bone involvement, treatment for several months may be required to evaluate effectiveness. Long-term use (months to years) requires supervision and periodic evaluation by your physician. Consult your physician on a regular basis.

▷ **This Drug Should Not Be Taken If**
- you have had a serious allergic or adverse reaction to it previously.
- you have active phlebitis.
- you have a significant deficiency of white blood cells or blood platelets.

▷ **Inform Your Physician Before Taking This Drug If**
- you have a history of thrombophlebitis or pulmonary embolism.
- you have a history of abnormally high blood calcium levels.
- you have a history of any type of blood cell or bone marrow disorder.
- you have cataracts or other visual impairment.
- you have impaired liver function.
- you plan to have surgery in the near future.

Possible Side-Effects (natural, expected and unavoidable drug actions)
Hot flashes, fluid retention, weight gain.

▷ **Possible Adverse Effects** (unusual, unexpected and infrequent reactions)
If any of the following develop, consult your physician promptly for guidance.
Mild Adverse Effects
Allergic Reaction: Skin rash.
Headache, dizziness, drowsiness, depression, fatigue, confusion.
Nausea, vomiting, itching in genital area, loss of hair.

Serious Adverse Effects

Initial "flare" of severe pain in tumor or involved bone.

Development of thrombophlebitis, risk of pulmonary embolism.

Eye changes: corneal opacities, retinal injury.

Development of abnormally high blood calcium levels.

Transient decreases in white blood cells and blood platelets.

▷ **Possible Effects on Sexual Function**

Premenopausal: altered timing and pattern of menstruation.

Postmenopausal: vaginal bleeding.

This drug may be effective in treating the following conditions:
- male infertility due to abnormally low sperm counts.
- male breast enlargement and tenderness.
- chronic female breast pain (mastalgia).

CAUTION

1. If this drug is used prior to your menopause, it may induce ovulation and predispose to pregnancy. Since this drug should not be used during pregnancy, some method of contraception (other than oral contraceptives) is advised.
2. Do not take any form of estrogen while taking this drug; estrogens can inhibit tamoxifen's effectiveness.

▷ **Advisability of Use During Pregnancy**

Pregnancy Category: X (tentative). See Pregnancy Code inside back cover.

Animal studies: No birth defects due to this drug reported.

Human studies: Information from adequate studies of pregnant women is not available.

This drug can have estrogenic effects. It should not be used during pregnancy.

Advisability of Use if Breast-Feeding

Presence of this drug in breast milk: Unknown.

Avoid drug or refrain from nursing.

Habit-Forming Potential: None.

Effects of Overdosage: No information available.

Possible Effects of Long-Term Use: Development of abnormally high blood calcium levels.

Suggested Periodic Examinations While Taking This Drug (at physician's discretion)

Complete blood cell counts, measurements of blood calcium levels.

Complete eye examinations if impaired vision occurs.

▷ **While Taking This Drug, Observe the Following**

Foods: No restrictions.

Beverages: No restrictions. May be taken with milk.

▷　　*Alcohol:* No interactions expected.

Tobacco Smoking: No interactions expected.
▷   *Other Drugs*
   The following drugs may *decrease* the effects of tamoxifen
   • estrogens.
   • oral contraceptives (those that contain estrogens).
▷   *Driving, Hazardous Activities:* This drug may cause dizziness or drowsiness. Restrict activities as necessary.
   Aviation Note: The use of this drug *may be a disqualification* for piloting. Consult a designated Aviation Medical Examiner.
   Exposure to Sun: No restrictions.

TEMAZEPAM
(tem AZ e pam)

Introduced: 1978

Prescription: USA: Yes
   Canada: Yes

Available as Generic: USA: Yes
   Canada: No

Class: Hypnotic, benzodiazepines

Controlled Drug: USA: C-IV*
   Canada: No

Brand Names: Razepam, Restoril, Temaz

BENEFITS versus RISKS	
Possible Benefits	*Possible Risks*
EFFECTIVE HYPNOTIC after 4 weeks of continual use	Habit-forming potential with long-term use
Wide margin of safety with therapeutic doses	Minor impairment of mental functions ("hangover" effect)

▷ **Principal Uses**
   As a Single Drug Product: This member of the benzodiazepine class of "minor tranquilizers" is used exclusively as a bedtime sedative to induce sleep.

How This Drug Works: It is thought that this drug produces a calming effect by enhancing the action of the nerve transmitter gamma-aminobutyric acid (GABA), which in turn blocks the arousal of higher brain centers and helps to induce sleep.

Available Dosage Forms and Strengths
   Capsules — 15 mg, 30 mg

▷ **Usual Adult Dosage Range:** 15 to 30 mg at bedtime. Total daily dosage should not exceed 90 mg. **Note: Actual dosage and administration**

*See Schedules of Controlled Drugs inside back cover.

schedule must be determined by the physician for each patient individually.

▷ **Dosing Instructions:**   Preferably taken on an empty stomach to hasten absorption and induce sleep rapidly. The capsule may be opened for administration. Do not discontinue this drug abruptly if taken for more than 4 weeks.

Usual Duration of Use: Periods of 3 to 5 nights intermittently, repeated as needed with appropriate dosage adjustment. Avoid uninterrupted and prolonged use. The duration of use should not exceed 2 weeks without reappraisal of continued need.

▷ **This Drug Should Not Be Taken If**
- you have had an allergic reaction to it previously.
- you have acute narrow-angle glaucoma, inadequately treated.

▷ **Inform Your Physician Before Taking This Drug If**
- you are allergic to any benzodiazepine drug (see Drug Class, Section Four).
- you have a history of alcoholism or drug abuse.
- you are pregnant or planning pregnancy.
- you have impaired liver or kidney function.
- you have a history of serious depression or mental disorder.
- you are taking other drugs with sedative effects.
- you have any of the following: asthma, emphysema, epilepsy, myasthenia gravis.

Possible Side-Effects (natural, expected and unavoidable drug actions)
"Hangover" effects on arising: drowsiness, lethargy and unsteadiness.

▷ **Possible Adverse Effects** (unusual, unexpected and infrequent reactions)
If any of the following develop, consult your physician promptly for guidance.
Mild Adverse Effects
Allergic Reactions: Skin rash, hives.
Dizziness, fainting, slurred speech, nausea, indigestion.
Serious Adverse Effects
Idiosyncratic Reactions: Nervousness, talkativeness, irritability, apprehension, euphoria, excitement, hallucinations.

▷ **Possible Effects on Sexual Function:**   None reported.

CAUTION
1. This drug should not be discontinued abruptly if it has been taken continually for more than 4 weeks.
2. The concurrent use of some over-the-counter drug products that contain antihistamines (allergy and cold preparations, sleep aids) can cause excessive sedation in sensitive individuals.
3. Regular nightly use of any hypnotic drug should be avoided.

4. If you experience a "hangover" effect, avoid hazardous activities (driving, etc.) and the use of alcohol.

Precautions for Use
By Infants and Children: Safety and effectiveness for use by those under 18 years of age have not been established.

By Those over 60 Years of Age: It is advisable to use smaller doses (15 mg) at first to determine your response. Observe for the possible development of lethargy, indifference, fatigue, weakness, unsteadiness, disturbing dreams, nightmares and paradoxical reactions of excitement, agitation, anger, hostility and rage.

▷ **Advisability of Use During Pregnancy**
Pregnancy Category: X (tentative). See Pregnancy Code inside back cover.
Animal studies: Rib defects reported in rats; skull and rib defects reported in rabbits.
Human studies: Information from adequate studies of pregnant women is not available.
Avoid use during entire pregnancy.

Advisability of Use if Breast-Feeding
Presence of this drug in breast milk: Probably yes.
Avoid drug or refrain from nursing.

Habit-Forming Potential: This drug can produce psychological and/or physical dependence (see Glossary) if used in large doses for an extended period of time. Avoid continual use.

Effects of Overdosage: Marked drowsiness, weakness, feeling of drunkenness, staggering gait, tremor, stupor progressing to deep sleep or coma.

Possible Effects of Long-Term Use: Psychological and/or physical dependence.

Suggested Periodic Examinations While Taking This Drug (at physician's discretion)
Complete blood cell counts during long-term use.

▷ **While Taking This Drug, Observe the Following**
Foods: No restrictions.
Beverages: Avoid excessive intake of caffeine-containing beverages (coffee, tea, cola) within 4 hours of taking this drug. May be taken with milk.
▷ *Alcohol:* Use with extreme caution until the combined effect has been determined. Alcohol may increase the absorption of this drug and add to its depressant effects on the brain. It is advisable to avoid alcohol completely throughout the day and night if it is necessary to drive or to engage in any hazardous activity.
Tobacco Smoking: Heavy smoking may reduce the hypnotic action of this drug.

Marijuana Smoking: Increased sedation and significant impairment of intellectual and physical performance.

▷ *Other Drugs*

Temazepam may *increase* the effects of
- digoxin (Lanoxin), and cause digoxin toxicity.
- phenytoin (Dilantin), and cause phenytoin toxicity.

Temazepam may *decrease* the effects of
- levodopa (Sinemet, etc.), and reduce its effectiveness in treating Parkinson's disease.

The following drugs may *increase* the effects of temazepam
- cimetidine (Tagamet).
- disulfiram (Antabuse).
- isoniazid (INH, Rifamate, etc.).
- oral contraceptives.
- valproic acid (Depakene).

The following drugs may *decrease* the effects of temazepam
- rifampin (Rimactane, etc.).
- theophylline (Aminophylline, Theo-Dur, etc.).

▷ *Driving, Hazardous Activities:* This drug can impair mental alertness, judgment, physical coordination and reaction time. Avoid hazardous activities accordingly.

Aviation Note: The use of this drug *is a disqualification* for piloting. Consult a designated Aviation Medical Examiner.

Exposure to Sun: No restrictions.

Exposure to Heat: Use caution until the effect of excessive perspiration is determined. Because of reduced urine volume, this drug may accumulate in the body and produce effects of overdosage.

Discontinuation: Avoid sudden discontinuation if this drug has been taken for over 4 weeks without interruption. Dosage should be tapered gradually to prevent a withdrawal syndrome that could include depression, confusion, hallucinations, tremor, seizures, muscle cramping, sweating and vomiting.

TERAZOSIN
(ter AY zoh sin)

Introduced: 1987

Class: Antihypertensive

Prescription: USA: Yes

Controlled Drug: USA: No

Available as Generic: No

Brand Name: Hytrin

BENEFITS versus RISKS

Possible Benefits	*Possible Risks*
EFFECTIVE TREATMENT OF MILD TO MODERATE HYPERTENSION when used alone or in combination with other antihypertensive drugs	"First dose" drop in blood pressure with fainting (1%) Fluid retention (5.5%) Rapid heart rate (1.9%)

▷ **Principal Uses**

As a Single Drug Product: Used primarily as a "step 1" antihypertensive drug to initiate treatment of mild to moderate hypertension. Also used in conjunction with other drugs to treat moderate to severe hypertension.

How This Drug Works: It is thought that by blocking certain actions of the sympathetic nervous system, this drug causes direct relaxation and expansion of blood vessel walls, thus lowering the pressure of the blood within the vessels.

Available Dosage Forms and Strengths
Tablets — 1 mg, 2 mg, 5 mg

▷ **Usual Adult Dosage Range:** Initiate treatment with a "test dose" of 1 mg to determine the patient's response within the first 2 hours. If tolerated satisfactorily, increase dose cautiously (as needed and tolerated) up to 5 mg/24 hours taken as a single dose at bedtime. Total daily dosage should not exceed 20 mg. **Note: Actual dosage and administration schedule must be determined by the physician for each patient individually.**

▷ **Dosing Instructions:** Preferably taken at bedtime to avoid orthostatic hypotension (see Glossary). May be taken without regard to food. The tablet may be crushed for administration.

Usual Duration of Use: Continual use on a regular schedule for 6 to 8 weeks is usually necessary to determine this drug's effectiveness in controlling hypertension. Long-term use (months to years) requires supervision and periodic evaluation by your physician. Consult your physician on a regular basis.

Possible Advantages of This Drug
May be used to initiate treatment.
Usually effective with once-a-day dosage.
Rarely causes depression or impotence.
Does not alter blood cholesterol, potassium or sugar.

▷ **This Drug Should Not Be Taken If**
- you have had an allergic reaction to it previously.
- you are experiencing mental depression.

- you have angina (active coronary artery disease) and you are not taking a beta-blocking drug. (Consult your physician.)

▷ **Inform Your Physician Before Taking This Drug If**
- you have experienced orthostatic hypotension (see Glossary) when using other antihypertensive drugs.
- you have a history of mental depression.
- you have impaired circulation to the brain, or a history of stroke.
- you have coronary artery disease.
- you have active liver disease or impaired liver function.
- you have impaired kidney function.
- you plan to have surgery under general anesthesia in the near future.

Possible Side-Effects (natural, expected and unavoidable drug actions)
Orthostatic hypotension (1.3%), drowsiness (5.4%), salt and water retention (5.5%), dry mouth, nasal congestion (5.9%), constipation.

▷ **Possible Adverse Effects** (unusual, unexpected and infrequent reactions)
If any of the following develop, consult your physician promptly for guidance.
Mild Adverse Effects
Allergic Reaction: Skin rash.
Headache (16.2%), dizziness (19.3%), fatigue (6.9%), weakness (11.3%), nervousness (2.3%), sweating, numbness and tingling (2.9%), blurred vision (1.6%).
Palpitation (4.3%), rapid heart rate (1.9%), shortness of breath (3.1%).
Nausea (4.4%), vomiting, diarrhea, abdominal pain.
Serious Adverse Effects
Mental depression (0.3%).

▷ **Possible Effects on Sexual Function:**   Impotence (1.2%).

Natural Diseases or Disorders That May Be Activated by This Drug
Latent coronary artery insufficiency.

CAUTION
1. Observe for the possible "first dose" response of precipitous drop in blood pressue, with or without fainting; this usually occurs within 30 to 90 minutes. Limit initial doses to 1 mg taken at bedtime for the first 3 days; remain supine after taking these trial doses.
2. Impaired kidney function may increase your sensitivity to this drug and require smaller than usual doses.
3. Consult your physician if you plan to use over-the-counter remedies for allergic rhinitis or head colds; these preparations contain drugs that may interact with terazosin.

Precautions for Use
By Infants and Children: Safety and effectiveness for use by those under 12 years of age have not been established.
By Those over 60 Years of Age: Begin treatment with no more than 1 mg/ day for the first 3 days. Subsequent increases in dose must be very

gradual and carefully supervised by your physician. The occurrence of orthostatic hypotension can cause unexpected falls and injury; sit or lie down promptly if you feel light-headed or dizzy. Report any indications of dizziness or chest pain promptly.

▷ **Advisability of Use During Pregnancy**
Pregnancy Category: C (tentative). See Pregnancy Code inside back cover.
Animal studies: No birth defects found in rat or rabbit studies.
Human studies: Information from adequate studies of pregnant women is not available.
Use this drug only if clearly needed. Ask your physician for guidance.

Advisability of Use if Breast-Feeding
Presence of this drug in breast milk: Unknown.
Monitor nursing infant closely and discontinue drug or nursing if adverse effects develop.

Habit-Forming Potential: None.

Effects of Overdosage: Orthostatic hypotension, headache, generalized flushing, rapid heart rate, extreme weakness, irregular heart rhythm, circulatory collapse.

Possible Effects of Long-Term Use: None reported.

Suggested Periodic Examinations While Taking This Drug (at physician's discretion)
Measurements of blood pressure in lying, sitting and standing positions.
Measurements of body weight to detect fluid retention.

▷ **While Taking This Drug, Observe the Following**
Foods: No restrictions. Avoid excessive salt intake.
Beverages: No restrictions. May be taken with milk.
▷ *Alcohol:* Use with extreme caution until the combined effects have been determined. Alcohol can exaggerate the blood-pressure-lowering actions of this drug and cause excessive reduction.
Tobacco Smoking: Nicotine can contribute significantly to this drug's ability to intensify coronary insufficiency in susceptible individuals. All forms of tobacco should be avoided.
▷ *Other Drugs*
The following drugs may *increase* the effects of terazosin
- beta-adrenergic-blocking drugs (see Drug Class, Section Four); the severity and duration of the "first dose" hypotensive response may be increased.

The following drugs may *decrease* the effects of terazosin
- estrogens.
- indomethacin (Indocin).
▷ *Driving, Hazardous Activities:* This drug may cause dizziness or drowsiness. Restrict activities as necessary.
Aviation Note: The use of this drug *is a disqualification* for piloting. Consult a designated Aviation Medical Examiner.

Exposure to Sun: No restrictions.

Exposure to Cold: Use caution until combined effect has been determined. Cold environments may increase this drug's ability to cause coronary insufficiency (angina) and hypothermia (see Glossary) in susceptible individuals.

Heavy Exercise or Exertion: Excessive exertion can augment this drug's ability to induce angina. See Angina in Section Two.

Discontinuation: If you are taking this drug as part of your treatment program for congestive heart failure, do not discontinue it abruptly. Ask your physician for guidance.

TERBUTALINE
(ter BYU ta leen)

Introduced: 1974

Class: Antiasthmatic, bronchodilator

Prescription: USA: Yes
Canada: Yes

Controlled Drug: USA: No
Canada: No

Available as Generic: No

Brand Names: Brethaire, Brethine, Bricanyl, ✦Bricanyl Spacer

BENEFITS versus RISKS	
Possible Benefits	*Possible Risks*
VERY EFFECTIVE RELIEF OF BRONCHOSPASM	Increased blood pressure
	Fine hand tremor
	Irregular heart rhythm (with excessive use)

▷ **Principal Uses**

As a Single Drug Product: To relieve acute bronchial asthma and to reduce the frequency and severity of chronic, recurrent asthmatic attacks; also used to relieve reversible bronchospasm associated with chronic bronchitis and emphysema.

How This Drug Works: By stimulating certain sympathetic nerve terminals, this drug acts to dilate those bronchial tubes that are in sustained constriction, thereby increasing the size of the airway and improving the ability to breathe.

Available Dosage Forms and Strengths
Aerosol — 0.2 mg/actuation, 0.25 mg/actuation (Canada)
Injection — 1 mg per ml
Tablets — 2.5 mg, 5 mg

▷ **Usual Adult Dosage Range:**   Aerosol: 0.4 mg taken in 2 separate inhalations 1 minute apart; repeat every 4 to 6 hours as needed. Tablets: 2.5 to 5 mg taken 3 times/day, 6 hours apart. The total daily dosage should not exceed 15 mg. **Note: Actual dosage and administration schedule must be determined by the physician for each patient individually.**

▷ **Dosing Instructions:**   May be taken on empty stomach or with food or milk. Tablets may be crushed for administration. For aerosol, follow the written instructions carefully. Do not overuse.

Usual Duration of Use: According to individual requirements. Do not use beyond the time necessary to terminate episodes of asthma.

Possible Advantages of This Drug
Rapid onset of action.
Long duration of action.
Highly effective relief of asthma.

▷ **This Drug Should Not Be Taken If**
- you have had an allergic reaction to any dosage form of it previously.
- you currently have an irregular heart rhythm.
- you are taking, or have taken within the past 2 weeks, any monoamine oxidase (MAO) type A inhibitor drug (see Drug Class, Section Four).

▷ **Inform Your Physician Before Taking This Drug If**
- you are overly sensitive to other drugs that stimulate the sympathetic nervous system.
- you are currently using epinephrine (Adrenalin, Primatene Mist, etc.) to relieve asthmatic breathing.
- you have a seizure disorder.
- you have any type of heart or circulatory disorder, especially high blood pressure or coronary heart disease.
- you have diabetes or an overactive thyroid gland (hyperthyroidism).
- you are taking any form of digitalis or any stimulant drug.

Possible Side-Effects (natural, expected and unavoidable drug actions)
Aerosol: dryness or irritation of mouth or throat, altered taste. Tablet: nervousness, tremor, palpitation.

▷ **Possible Adverse Effects** (unusual, unexpected and infrequent reactions)
If any of the following develop, consult your physician promptly for guidance.
Mild Adverse Effects
Headache, dizziness, drowsiness, restlessness, insomnia.
Rapid, pounding heartbeat; increased sweating; muscle cramps in arms and legs.
Nausea, heartburn, vomiting.

Serious Adverse Effects
Rapid or irregular heart rhythm, intensification of angina, increased blood pressure.

▷ **Possible Effects on Sexual Function:**   None reported.

Natural Diseases or Disorders That May Be Activated By This Drug
Latent coronary artery disease, diabetes or high blood pressure.

CAUTION
1. Concurrent use of this drug by aerosol inhalation with beclomethasone aerosol (Beclovent, Vanceril) may increase the risk of toxicity due to fluorocarbon propellants. It is advisable to use this aerosol 20 to 30 minutes *before* beclomethasone aerosol. This will reduce the risk of toxicity and will enhance the penetration of beclomethasone.
2. ***Avoid excessive use of aerosol inhalation.*** The excessive or prolonged use of this drug by inhalation can reduce its effectiveness and cause serious heart rhythm disturbances, including cardiac arrest.
3. Do not use this drug concurrently with epinephrine. These two drugs may be used alternately if an interval of 4 hours is allowed between doses.
4. If you do not respond to your usually effective dose, ask your physician for guidance. Do not increase the size or frequency of the dose without your physician's approval.

Precautions for Use
By Infants and Children: Safety and effectiveness for use by those under 12 years of age have not been established.
By Those over 60 Years of Age: Avoid excessive and continual use. If acute asthma is not relieved promptly, other drugs will have to be tried. Observe for the development of nervousness, palpitations, irregular heart rhythm and muscle tremors. Use with extreme caution if you have hardening of the arteries, heart disease or high blood pressure.

▷ **Advisability of Use During Pregnancy**
Pregnancy Category: B (tentative). See Pregnancy Code inside back cover.
Animal studies: No significant birth defects reported in mouse and rat studies.
Human studies: Information from adequate studies of pregnant women is not available.
Use only if clearly needed. Ask your physician for guidance.

Advisability of Use if Breast-Feeding
Presence of this drug in breast milk: Yes.
Monitor nursing infant closely and discontinue drug or nursing if adverse effects develop.

Habit-Forming Potential: None.

Effects of Overdosage: Nervousness, palpitation, rapid heart rate, sweating, headache, tremor, vomiting, chest pain.

Possible Effects of Long-Term Use: Loss of effectiveness. See *CAUTION* category above.

Suggested Periodic Examinations While Taking This Drug (at physician's discretion)
Blood pressure measurements, evaluation of heart status.

▷ **While Taking This Drug, Observe the Following**
Foods: No restrictions.
Beverages: Avoid excessive use of caffeine-containing beverages: coffee, tea, cola, chocolate.
▷ *Alcohol:* No interactions expected.
Tobacco Smoking: No interactions expected.
▷ *Other Drugs*
Terbutaline *taken concurrently* with
- monoamine oxidase (MAO) type A inhibitor drugs may cause excessive increase in blood pressure and undesirable heart stimulation (see Drug Class, Section Four).
The following drugs may *decrease* the effects of terbutaline
- beta blocker drugs may impair its effectiveness (see Drug Class, Section Four).
▷ *Driving, Hazardous Activities:* Usually no restrictions. Use caution if excessive nervousness or dizziness occurs.
Aviation Note: The use of this drug *is a disqualification* for piloting. Consult a designated Aviation Medical Examiner.
Exposure to Sun: No restrictions.
Heavy Exercise or Exertion: Use caution. Excessive exercise can induce asthma in sensitive individuals.

TERFENADINE
(ter FEN a deen)

Introduced: 1977

Class: Antihistamines

Prescription: USA: Yes
Canada: No

Controlled Drug: USA: No
Canada: No

Available as Generic: No

Brand Names: Seldane, Seldane-D

```
┌─────────────────────────────────────────────────────────────┐
│                    BENEFITS versus RISKS                     │
│                                                              │
│      Possible Benefits              Possible Risks           │
│   EFFECTIVE RELIEF OF          Infrequent headache           │
│     ALLERGIC RHINITIS AND      Mild fatigue                  │
│     ALLERGIC SKIN DISORDERS    Minor digestive disturbances  │
│                                Slight atropinelike effects   │
└─────────────────────────────────────────────────────────────┘
```

▷ **Principal Uses**

    As a Single Drug Product: Used primarily to provide symptomatic relief in allergic and related disorders: seasonal and perennial allergic rhinitis (hay fever), allergic conjunctivitis and vasomotor rhinitis; also in hives and localized swellings (angioedema) of allergic origin.

How This Drug Works: Antihistamines reduce the intensity of the allergic response by blocking the action of histamine after it has been released from sensitized tissue cells in the eyes, nose and skin.

Available Dosage Forms and Strengths

    Suspension — 30 mg per 5-ml teaspoonful (Canada)

    Tablets — 60 mg

▷ **Usual Adult Dosage Range:** 60 mg every 8 to 12 hours as needed. The total daily dosage should not exceed 360 mg. **Note: Actual dosage and administration schedule must be determined by the physician for each patient individually.**

▷ **Dosing Instructions:** May be taken with food or milk to prevent stomach irritation. The tablet may be crushed for administration.

Usual Duration of Use: Continual use on a regular schedule for 2 to 3 days is usually necessary to determine this drug's effectiveness in relieving the symptoms of allergic rhinitis and dermatosis. It may be necessary to take this drug throughout the entire pollen season, depending upon individual sensitivity. However, antihistamines should not be taken continually (without interruption) for long-term use. Limit their use to periods that require symptomatic relief. Consult your physician on a regular basis.

Possible Advantages of This Drug

    Fast onset of action, relief within one hour.

    No loss of effectiveness with continual use.

    No drowsiness or impaired mental function that is so characteristic of other antihistamines.

▷ **This Drug Should Not Be Taken If**

- you have had an allergic reaction to any dosage form of it previously.
- you are currently undergoing allergy skin tests.

▷ **Inform Your Physician Before Taking This Drug If**

- you have had any allergic reactions or unfavorable responses to the previous use of antihistamines.

Possible Side-Effects (natural, expected and unavoidable drug actions)
Dry nose, mouth or throat.

▷ **Possible Adverse Effects** (unusual, unexpected and infrequent reactions)
If any of the following develop, consult your physician promptly for guidance.
Mild Adverse Effects
Allergic Reactions: Skin rash, itching.
Headache, nervousness, fatigue.
Increased appetite, indigestion, nausea, vomiting.
Serious Adverse Effects
None reported.

▷ **Possible Effects on Sexual Function**
Altered timing and pattern of menstruation.
Female breast enlargement with milk production.

CAUTION
1. Discontinue this drug 4 days before diagnostic skin testing procedures in order to prevent false negative test results.
2. Do not use this drug if you have active bronchial asthma, bronchitis or pneumonia. It may thicken bronchial mucus and make it more difficult to remove (by absorption or coughing).

Precautions for Use
By Infants and Children: Safety and effectiveness for use by those under 12 years of age have not been established.
By Those over 60 Years of Age: You may be more susceptible to the development of headache and fatigue. Use smaller doses at longer intervals if necessary.

▷ **Advisability of Use During Pregnancy**
Pregnancy Category: C (tentative). See Pregnancy Code inside back cover.
Animal studies: No birth defects due to this drug reported.
Human studies: Information from adequate studies of pregnant women is not available.
Use this drug only if clearly needed. Ask your physician for guidance.

Advisability of Use if Breast-Feeding
Presence of this drug in breast milk: Unknown.
Avoid drug or refrain from nursing.

Habit-Forming Potential: None.

Effects of Overdosage: No information available. No serious or threatening effects expected.

Possible Effects of Long-Term Use: None reported.

Suggested Periodic Examinations While Taking This Drug (at physician's discretion)
None required.

▷ **While Taking This Drug, Observe the Following**
  Foods: No restrictions.
  Beverages: No restrictions. May be taken with milk.
▷ *Alcohol:* No interactions expected.
  Tobacco Smoking: No interactions expected.
▷ *Other Drugs:* No significant interactions reported to date.
  Hazardous Activities: No restrictions.
  Aviation Note: The use of this drug **is probably not a disqualification** for piloting. Consult a designated Aviation Medical Examiner.
  Exposure to Sun: No restrictions.

TETRACYCLINE
(te trah SI kleen)

Introduced: 1953

Class: Antibiotic, tetracyclines

Prescription: USA: Yes
  Canada: Yes

Controlled Drug: USA: No
  Canada: No

Available as Generic: Yes

Brand Names: Achromycin, Achromycin V, ✦Apo-Tetra, Cyclopar, ✦Medicycline, Mysteclin-F [CD], ✦Neo-Tetrine, Nor-Tet, ✦Novotetra, Panmycin, Retet, Robitet, Sumycin, Tetra-C, Tetracyn, Tetralan, Tetram, Tropicycline

---

BENEFITS versus RISKS	
Possible Benefits	*Possible Risks*
EFFECTIVE TREATMENT OF INFECTIONS due to susceptible bacteria and protozoa	ALLERGIC REACTIONS, mild to severe: ANAPHYLAXIS, DRUG-INDUCED HEPATITIS (rare)
	Drug-induced colitis
	Superinfections (bacterial or fungal)
	Rare blood cell disorders: hemolytic anemia, abnormally low white cell and platelet counts

---

▷ **Principal Uses**
  As a Single Drug Product: This member of the tetracycline drug class is used primarily to (1) treat a broad range of infections caused by susceptible bacteria and protozoa (short-term use); and (2) treat severe, resistant pustular acne (long-term use).

As a Combination Drug Product [CD]: This drug is available in combination with amphotericin B, an antifungal antibiotic that is provided to reduce the risk of developing an overgrowth of yeast organisms (superinfection) of the gastrointestinal tract.

How This Drug Works: This drug prevents the growth and multiplication of susceptible bacteria by interfering with their formation of essential proteins.

Available Dosage Forms and Strengths

Capsules — 100 mg, 250 mg, 500 mg
Ointment — 3%
Ointment, ophthalmic — 10 mg per gram
Solution, topical — 2.2 mg per ml
Suspension, ophthalmic — 10 mg per ml
Suspension, oral — 125 mg per 5-ml teaspoonful
Tablets — 250 mg, 500 mg

▷ **Usual Adult Dosage Range:** 250 to 500 mg/6 hours, or 500 to 1000 mg/12 hours. The total daily dosage should not exceed 4000 mg (4 grams). **Note: Actual dosage and administration schedule must be determined by the physician for each patient individually.**

▷ **Dosing Instructions:** Preferably taken on an empty stomach, 1 hour before or 2 hours after eating. However, to reduce stomach irritation it may be taken with crackers that contain insignificant amounts of iron, calcium, magnesium or zinc. Avoid all dairy products for 2 hours before and after taking this drug. Take at the same time each day, with a full glass of water. Take the full course prescribed. The tablet may be crushed and the capsule may be opened for administration.

Usual Duration of Use: The time required to control the acute infection and be free of fever and symptoms for 48 hours. This varies with the nature of the infection. Long-term use (months to years, as for treatment of acne) requires supervision and periodic evaluation. Consult your physician on a regular basis.

▷ **This Drug Should Not Be Taken If**
- you are allergic to any tetracycline drug (see Drug Class, Section Four).
- you are pregnant or breast-feeding.

▷ **Inform Your Physician Before Taking This Drug If**
- it is prescribed for a child under 8 years of age.
- you have a history of liver or kidney disease.
- you have systemic lupus erythematosus.
- you are taking any penicillin drug.
- you are taking any anticoagulant drug.
- you plan to have surgery under general anesthesia in the near future.

Possible Side-Effects (natural, expected and unavoidable drug actions)
Superinfections (see Glossary), often due to yeast organisms. These can occur in the mouth, intestinal tract, rectum and/or vagina, resulting in rectal and vaginal itching.

▷ **Possible Adverse Effects** (unusual, unexpected and infrequent reactions)
If any of the following develop, consult your physician promptly for guidance.
Mild Adverse Effects
Allergic Reactions: Skin rash, hives, itching of hands and feet, swelling of face or extremities.
Loss of appetite, stomach irritation, nausea, vomiting, diarrhea.
Irritation of mouth or tongue, "black tongue," sore throat, abdominal cramping or pain.
Serious Adverse Effects
Allergic Reactions: Anaphylactic reaction (see Glossary), asthma, fever, swollen joints and lymph glands.
Drug-induced hepatitis with jaundice.
Permanent discoloration and/or malformation of teeth when taken under 8 years of age, including unborn child and infant.
Impaired vision, increased intracranial pressure.
Drug-induced colitis.
Rare blood cell disorders: hemolytic anemia (see Glossary); abnormally low white blood cell count, causing fever, sore throat and infections; abnormally low blood platelet count, causing abnormal bleeding or bruising.

▷ **Possible Effects on Sexual Function:** Decreased effectiveness of oral contraceptives taken concurrently (several case reports of pregnancy).

▷ **Adverse Effects That May Mimic Natural Diseases or Disorders**
Drug-induced hepatitis may suggest viral hepatitis.

Natural Diseases or Disorders That May Be Activated by This Drug
Systemic lupus erythematosus.

CAUTION
1. Antacids, dairy products and preparations containing aluminum, bismuth, calcium, iron, magnesium or zinc can prevent adequate absorption of this drug and reduce its effectiveness significantly.
2. Troublesome and persistent diarrhea can develop in sensitive individuals. If diarrhea persists for more than 24 hours, discontinue this drug and consult your physician.
3. If surgery under general anesthesia is required while taking this drug, the choice of anesthetic agent must be considered carefully to prevent serious kidney damage.

Precautions for Use
By Infants and Children: If possible, tetracyclines should not be given to children under 8 years of age because of the risk of permanent dis-

coloration and deformity of the teeth. Rarely, young infants may develop increased intracranial pressure within the first 4 days of receiving this drug. Tetracyclines may inhibit normal bone growth and development.

By Those over 60 Years of Age: Dosage must be carefully individualized and based upon determinations of kidney function. Natural skin changes may predispose to severe and prolonged itching reactions in the genital and anal regions.

▷ **Advisability of Use During Pregnancy**

Pregnancy Category: D (tentative). See Pregnancy Code inside back cover.
Animal studies: Tetracycline causes limb defects in rats, rabbits and chickens.
Human studies: Information from studies of pregnant women indicates that this drug can cause impaired development and discoloration of teeth and other developmental defects.
It is advisable to avoid this drug completely during entire pregnancy.

Advisability of Use if Breast-Feeding

Presence of this drug in breast milk: Yes.
Avoid drug or refrain from nursing.

Habit-Forming Potential: None.

Effects of Overdosage: Stomach burning, nausea, vomiting, diarrhea.

Possible Effects of Long-Term Use: Superinfections; rarely, impairment of bone marrow, liver or kidney function.

Suggested Periodic Examinations While Taking This Drug (at physician's discretion)

Complete blood cell counts, liver and kidney function tests.
During extended use, sputum and stool examinations may detect early superinfection due to yeast organisms.

▷ **While Taking This Drug, Observe the Following**

Foods: Avoid cheeses, yogurt, ice cream, iron-fortified cereals and supplements and meats for 2 hours before and after taking this drug. Calcium and iron can combine with this drug and reduce its absorption significantly.

Beverages: Avoid all forms of milk for 2 hours before and after taking this drug.

▷ *Alcohol:* No interactions expected. However, it is best avoided if you have active liver disease.

Tobacco Smoking: No interactions expected.

▷ *Other Drugs*

Tetracyclines may ***increase*** the effects of
- oral anticoagulants, and make it necessary to reduce their dosage.
- digoxin (Lanoxin), and cause digitalis toxicity.
- lithium (Eskalith, Lithane, etc.), and increase the risk of lithium toxicity.

Tetracyclines may *decrease* the effects of
- oral contraceptives, and impair their effectiveness in preventing pregnancy.
- penicillins, and impair their effectiveness in treating infections.

Tetracyclines *taken concurrently* with
- methoxyflurane anesthesia may impair kidney function.

The following drugs may *decrease* the effects of tetracyclines
- antacids (aluminum and magnesium preparations, sodium bicarbonate, etc.) may reduce drug absorption.
- iron and mineral preparations may reduce drug absorption.

▷ *Driving, Hazardous Activities:* Usually no restrictions. However, this drug may cause nausea or diarrhea. Restrict activities as necessary.

Aviation Note: The use of this drug *may be a disqualification* for piloting. Consult a designated Aviation Medical Examiner.

Exposure to Sun: Use caution until sensitivity has been determined. Some tetracyclines can cause photosensitivity (see Glossary).

THEOPHYLLINE
(thee OFF i lin)

Other Names: Aminophylline, oxtriphylline

Introduced: 1929

Class: Antiasthmatic, bronchodilator, xanthines

Prescription: USA: Yes
Canada: No

Controlled Drug: USA: No
Canada: No

Available as Generic: Yes

Brand Names: Accurbron, Amesec [CD], Brondecon [CD], Bronkaid Tablets [CD], Bronkodyl, Bronkolixir [CD], Bronkotabs [CD], Choledyl, Constant-T, Elixicon, Elixophyllin, LaBID, Lodrane, Marax [CD], Marax DF [CD], Mudrane GG Elixir & Tablets [CD], Mudrane Tablets [CD], ✦PMS Theophylline, ✦Pulmophylline, Quadrinal [CD], Quibron [CD], Quibron Plus [CD], Quibron-T Dividose, ✦Quibron-T/SR, Respbid, Slo-bid, Slo-Phyllin, Slo-Phyllin GG [CD], Slo-Phyllin Gyrocaps, Somophyllin-CRT, Somophyllin-DF, Somophyllin-T, ✦Somophyllin-12, Sustaire, ✦Tedral Preparations [CD], Theobid Duracaps, Theo-Dur, Theolair, Theophyl-SR, Theo-24, Theovent

```
┌─────────────────────────────────────────────────────────────────┐
│                    BENEFITS versus RISKS                          │
│                                                                   │
│         Possible Benefits              Possible Risks             │
│   EFFECTIVE RELIEF OF ACUTE      NARROW TREATMENT RANGE           │
│     BRONCHIAL ASTHMA             FREQUENT STOMACH                  │
│   MODERATELY EFFECTIVE             DISTRESS                        │
│     CONTROL OF CHRONIC,          Gastrointestinal bleeding         │
│     RECURRENT BRONCHIAL          Central nervous system toxicity,  │
│     ASTHMA                         seizures                        │
│   Moderately effective symptomatic   Heart rhythm disturbances     │
│     relief in chronic bronchitis and                              │
│     emphysema                                                     │
└─────────────────────────────────────────────────────────────────┘
```

▷ **Principal Uses**

As a Single Drug Product: Used primarily to relieve the shortness of breath and wheezing characteristic of acute bronchial asthma, and to prevent the recurrence of asthmatic episodes. It is also useful in relieving the asthmaticlike symptoms that are associated with some types of chronic bronchitis and emphysema.

As a Combination Drug Product [CD]: This drug is available in combination with several other drugs that are beneficial in the overall management of bronchial asthma and related conditions. Ephedrine is added to enhance the bronchodilator effects; guaifenesin is added to provide an expectorant effect that thins the mucus secretions in the bronchial tubes; mild sedatives such as phenobarbital are added to allay the anxiety that often accompanies acute attacks of asthma.

How This Drug Works: By inhibiting the enzyme phosphodiesterase, this drug produces an increase in the tissue chemical cyclic AMP. This causes relaxation of the muscles in the bronchial tubes and blood vessels of the lung, resulting in relief of bronchospasm, expanded lung capacity and improved lung circulation.

Available Dosage Forms and Strengths

Capsules —	100 mg, 200 mg, 250 mg
Capsules, prolonged-action —	50 mg, 60 mg, 75 mg, 100 mg, 125 mg, 130 mg, 200 mg, 250 mg, 260 mg, 300 mg
Elixir —	80 mg, 150 mg per 15-ml tablespoonful
Oral solution —	80 mg, 160 mg per 15-ml tablespoonful
Oral suspension —	300 mg per 15-ml tablespoonful
Syrup —	80 mg, 150 mg per 15-ml tablespoonful
Tablets —	100 mg, 125 mg, 200 mg, 250 mg, 300 mg
Tablets, prolonged-action —	100 mg, 200 mg, 250 mg, 300 mg, 400 mg, 450 mg, 500 mg

▷ **Usual Adult Dosage Range:** Because of its potential toxicity, this drug is given according to body weight. For acute asthma: Initially, 6 mg/kg as the first dose; then 3 mg/kg every 6 hours for 12 hours; then 3 mg/kg every 8 hours as needed. For maintenance: 16 mg/kg/24 hours, or 400 mg/24 hours, whichever is less, taken in 3 or 4 divided doses at intervals of 6 to 8 hours. The total daily dosage should not exceed 900 mg. **Note: Actual dosage and administration schedule must be determined by the physician for each patient individually.**

▷ **Dosing Instructions:** May be taken with or following food to reduce stomach irritation. The regular capsules may be opened and the regular tablets may be crushed for administration. The prolonged action dosage forms should be swallowed whole and not altered.

Usual Duration of Use: Continual use on a regular schedule for 48 to 72 hours is usually necessary to determine this drug's effectiveness in controlling the breathing impairment associated with bronchial asthma and chronic lung disease. Long-term use (months to years) requires supervision and periodic evaluation by your physician. Consult your physician on a regular basis.

▷ **This Drug Should Not Be Taken If**
- you have had an allergic reaction to it previously.
- you have active peptic ulcer disease.

▷ **Inform Your Physician Before Taking This Drug If**
- you have had an unfavorable reaction to any xanthine drug previously (see Drug Class, Section Four).
- you have a history of peptic ulcer disease.
- you have impaired liver or kidney function.
- you have hypertension, heart disease or any type of heart rhythm disorder.

Possible Side-Effects (natural, expected and unavoidable drug actions)
Nervousness, insomnia, rapid heart rate, increased urine volume.

▷ **Possible Adverse Effects** (unusual, unexpected and infrequent reactions)
If any of the following develop, consult your physician promptly for guidance.
Mild Adverse Effects
Allergic Reactions: Skin rash, hives.
Headache, dizziness, irritability, tremor, fatigue, weakness.
Loss of appetite, nausea, vomiting, abdominal pain, diarrhea, excessive thirst.
Flushing of face.
Serious Adverse Effects
Idiosyncratic Reactions: Marked anxiety, confusion, behavioral disturbances.
Central nervous system toxicity: muscle twitching, seizures.
Heart rhythm abnormalities, rapid breathing, low blood pressure.

Gastrointestinal bleeding.

▷ **Possible Effects on Sexual Function:**   None reported.

Natural Diseases or Disorders That May Be Activated by This Drug
Latent peptic ulcer disease.

CAUTION
1. This drug should not be taken concurrently with other antiasthmatic drugs unless you are directed to do so by your physician. Serious overdosage could result.
2. It has been reported that influenza vaccine may delay the elimination of this drug and cause accumulation to toxic levels.

Precautions for Use
By Infants and Children: Observe for indications of toxicity: irritability, agitation, tremors, lethargy, fever, vomiting, rapid heart rate and breathing, seizures.
By Those over 60 Years of Age: Start treatment with small doses until your tolerance has been determined. You may be more susceptible to the development of stomach irritation, nausea, vomiting or diarrhea. When used concurrently with coffee (caffeine) or with nasal decongestants, this drug may cause excessive stimulation and a hyperactivity syndrome.

▷ **Advisability of Use During Pregnancy**
Pregnancy Category: C (tentative). See Pregnancy Code inside back cover.
Animal studies: Significant birth defects due to this drug reported in mice.
Human studies: Information from adequate studies of pregnant women is not available. No increase in birth defects reported in 394 exposures to this drug.
Avoid this drug during the first 3 months. Use it otherwise only if clearly needed. Ask your physician for guidance.

Advisability of Use if Breast-Feeding
Presence of this drug in breast milk: Yes.
Avoid drug or refrain from nursing.

Habit-Forming Potential: None.

Effects of Overdosage: Nausea, vomiting, restlessness, irritability, confusion, delirium, seizures, high fever, weak pulse, coma.

Possible Effects of Long-Term Use: Gastrointestinal irritation.

Suggested Periodic Examinations While Taking This Drug (at physician's discretion)
Measurement of blood theophylline levels, especially with high dosage or long-term use. (See Therapeutic Drug Monitoring in Section One.)

▷ **While Taking This Drug, Observe the Following**
Foods: No restrictions.
Beverages: Avoid excessive use of caffeine-containing beverages: coffee, tea, cola; this combination could cause nervousness and insomnia.
▷ *Alcohol:* No interactions expected. May have additive effect on stomach irritation.
Tobacco Smoking: May hasten the elimination of this drug and reduce its effectiveness. Higher doses may be necessary to maintain a therapeutic blood level.
▷ *Other Drugs*
Theophylline may ***decrease*** the effects of
• lithium (Lithane, Lithobid, etc.), and reduce its effectiveness.
Theophylline ***taken concurrently*** with
• halothane (anesthesia) may cause heart rhythm abnormalities.
• phenytoin (Dilantin) may cause decreased effects of both drugs.
The following drugs may ***increase*** the effects of theophylline
• cimetidine (Tagamet) may cause theophylline toxicity.
• erythromycin (E-Mycin, Erythrocin, etc.) may cause theophylline toxicity.
• oral contraceptives.
• troleandomycin (TAO).
The following drugs may ***decrease*** the effects of theophylline
• barbiturates (phenobarbital, etc.).
• beta blocker drugs (see Drug Class, Section Four).
• rifampin (Rifadin, Rimactane, etc.).
▷ *Driving, Hazardous Activities:* This drug may cause dizziness. Restrict activities as necessary.
Aviation Note: The use of this drug ***may be a disqualification*** for piloting. Consult a designated Aviation Medical Examiner.
Exposure to Sun: No restrictions.
Occurrence of Unrelated Illness: Acute viral respiratory infections can delay the elimination of this drug significantly. Observe closely for indications of toxicity and the need to reduce dosage or lengthen the dosage interval.
Discontinuation: Avoid prolonged and unnecessary use of this drug. When you have achieved an asthma-free state, withdraw this drug gradually over several days.

THIORIDAZINE
(thi oh RID a zeen)

Introduced: 1959

Prescription: USA: Yes
Canada: Yes

Class: Strong tranquilizer, phenothiazines

Controlled Drug: USA: No
Canada: No

Available as Generic: USA: Yes
           Canada: Yes

Brand Names: ♦Apo-Thioridazine, Mellaril, Mellaril-S, Millazine, ♦Novo-ridazine, ♦PMS Thioridazine

---

BENEFITS versus RISKS

Possible Benefits	*Possible Risks*
EFFECTIVE CONTROL OF ACUTE MENTAL DISORDERS in the majority of patients: beneficial effects on thinking, mood and behavior	SERIOUS TOXIC EFFECTS ON BRAIN with long-term use
Relief of anxiety, agitation and tension	Liver damage with jaundice (infrequent)
Possibly effective in the management of the hyperactivity syndrome in children	Rare blood cell disorders: abnormally low white blood cell count

---

▷ **Principal Uses**

As a Single Drug Product: This antipsychotic drug is used primarily in the management of the following conditions: moderate to marked depression with significant anxiety and nervous tension; agitation, anxiety, depression and exaggerated fears in the elderly; severe behavioral problems in children characterized by hyperexcitability, combativeness, short attention span and rapid swings in mood.

How This Drug Works: Not completely established. Present theory is that by inhibiting the action of dopamine in certain brain centers, this drug acts to correct an imbalance of nerve impulse transmissions that is thought to be responsible for certain mental disorders.

Available Dosage Forms and Strengths
       Concentrate — 30 mg, 100 mg per ml
    Oral suspension — 25 mg, 100 mg per 5-ml teaspoonful
          Tablets — 10 mg, 15 mg, 25 mg, 50 mg, 100 mg, 150 mg, 200 mg

▷ **Usual Adult Dosage Range:**   Initially, 25 to 100 mg 3 times/day. Dose may be increased by 25 to 50 mg at 3- to 4-day intervals as needed and tolerated. Usual dosage range is 200 to 800 mg daily, divided into 2 to 4 doses. The total daily dosage should not exceed 800 mg. **Note: Actual dosage and administration schedule must be determined by the physician for each patient individually.**

▷ **Dosing Instructions:**   May be taken with or following meals to reduce stomach irritation. The tablets may be crushed for administration.

Usual Duration of Use: Continual use on a regular schedule for 3 to 4 weeks is usually necessary to determine this drug's effectiveness in controlling psychotic disorders. If not significantly beneficial within 6 weeks, it should be discontinued. Long-term use (months to years) requires periodic evaluation of response, appropriate dosage adjustment and consideration of continued need. Consult your physician on a regular basis.

▷ **This Drug Should Not Be Taken If**
  • you are allergic to any of the drugs bearing the brand names listed above.
  • you have active liver disease.
  • you have cancer of the breast.
  • you have a current blood cell or bone marrow disorder.

▷ **Inform Your Physician Before Taking This Drug If**
  • you are allergic or abnormally sensitive to any phenothiazine drug (see Drug Class, Section Four).
  • you have impaired liver or kidney function.
  • you have any type of seizure disorder.
  • you have diabetes, glaucoma or heart disease.
  • you have a history of lupus erythematosus.
  • you are taking any drug with sedative effects.
  • you plan to have surgery under general or spinal anesthesia in the near future.

Possible Side-Effects (natural, expected and unavoidable drug actions)
  Drowsiness (usually during the first 2 weeks), orthostatic hypotension (see Glossary), blurred vision, dry mouth, nasal congestion, constipation, impaired urination.
  Pink or purple coloration of urine, of no significance.

▷ **Possible Adverse Effects** (unusual, unexpected and infrequent reactions)
  If any of the following develop, consult your physician promptly for guidance.
  Mild Adverse Effects
  Allergic Reactions: Skin rash, hives, low-grade fever.
  Lowering of body temperature, especially in the elderly. (See Hypothermia in Glossary.)
  Increased appetite and weight gain.
  Weakness, agitation, insomnia, impaired day and night vision.
  Chronic constipation, fecal impaction.
  Serious Adverse Effects
  Allergic Reactions: Hepatitis with jaundice (see Glossary), severe skin reactions.
  Depression, disorientation, seizures, loss of peripheral vision.
  Rapid heart rate, heart rhythm disorders.
  Blood cell disorders: reduced white blood cell count (more common in the elderly).

Nervous system reactions: Parkinson-like disorders (see Glossary), severe restlessness, muscle spasms involving the face and neck, tardive dyskinesia (see Glossary).

▷ **Possible Effects on Sexual Function**
Decreased male and female libido; inhibited ejaculation (49% to 60%); impotence (54%); impaired female orgasm; priapism (see Glossary).
Male breast enlargement and tenderness.
Female breast enlargement with milk production.
Altered timing and pattern of menstruation.
False positive pregnancy test results.

▷ **Adverse Effects That May Mimic Natural Diseases or Disorders**
Nervous system reactions may suggest true Parkinson's disease.
Liver reactions may suggest viral hepatitis.
Reactions resembling systemic lupus erythematosus can occur.

Natural Diseases or Disorders That May Be Activated by This Drug
Latent epilepsy, glaucoma, diabetes mellitus, prostatism (see Glossary).

CAUTION
1. Many over-the-counter medications (see OTC Drugs in Glossary) for allergies, colds and coughs contain drugs that can interact unfavorably with this drug. Ask your physician or pharmacist for guidance before using any such medications.
2. Antacids that contain aluminum and/or magnesium can prevent the absorption of this drug and reduce its effectiveness.
3. Obtain prompt evaluation of any change or disturbance of vision.

Precautions for Use
By Infants and Children: Use of this drug is not recommended in children under 2 years of age. Do not use this drug in the presence of symptoms suggestive of Reye syndrome (see Glossary). Children with acute infectious diseases ("flulike" infections, chicken pox, measles, etc.) are more prone to develop muscular spasms of the face, back and extremities when this drug is given for any reason.
By Those over 60 Years of Age: Small doses are advisable until individual response has been determined. You may be more susceptible to the development of drowsiness, lethargy, constipation, lowering of body temperature (hypothermia) and orthostatic hypotension (see Glossary). This drug can enhance existing prostatism (see Glossary). You may also be more susceptible to the development of Parkinson-like reactions and/or tardive dyskinesia (see discussion of these terms in Glossary). These reactions must be recognized early since they may become unresponsive to treatment and irreversible.

▷ **Advisability of Use During Pregnancy**
Pregnancy Category: C (tentative). See Pregnancy Code inside back cover.
Animal studies: The results of rodent studies are conflicting.

Human studies: No increase in birth defects reported in 23 exposures. Information from adequate studies of pregnant women is not available.

Avoid drug during the first 3 months. Use it otherwise only if clearly needed. Ask your physician for guidance.

Advisability of Use if Breast-Feeding
Presence of this drug in breast milk: Yes, in minute amounts.
Monitor nursing infant closely and discontinue drug or nursing if adverse effects develop.

Habit-Forming Potential: None.

Effects of Overdosage: Marked drowsiness, weakness, tremor, agitation, unsteadiness, deep sleep, coma, convulsions.

Possible Effects of Long-Term Use: Opacities in the cornea or lens of the eye, pigmentation of the retina. Tardive dyskinesia (see Glossary).

Suggested Periodic Examinations While Taking This Drug (at physician's discretion)
Complete blood cell counts, especially between the fourth and tenth weeks of treatment.
Liver function tests, electrocardiograms.
Complete eye examinations—eye structures and vision.
Careful inspection of the tongue for early evidence of fine, involuntary, wavelike movements that could indicate the beginning of tardive dyskinesia.

▷ **While Taking This Drug, Observe the Following**
Foods: No restrictions.
Nutritional Support: A riboflavin (vitamin B-2) supplement should be taken with long-term use.
Beverages: No restrictions. May be taken with milk.
▷ *Alcohol:* Avoid completely. Alcohol can increase the sedative action of phenothiazines and accentuate their depressant effects on brain function and blood pressure. Phenothiazines can increase the intoxicating effects of alcohol.
Tobacco Smoking: Possible reduction of drowsiness from drug.
Marijuana Smoking: Moderate increase in drowsiness; accentuation of orthostatic hypotension; increased risk of precipitating latent psychoses, confusing the interpretation of mental status and drug responses.
▷ *Other Drugs*
Thioridazine may *increase* the effects of
• all sedative drugs, especially meperidine (Demerol), and cause excessive sedation.
• all atropinelike drugs, and cause nervous system toxicity.
Thioridazine may *decrease* the effects of

- guanethidine (Ismelin, Esimil), and reduce its effectiveness in lowering blood pressure.

Thioridazine **taken concurrently** with

- lithium (Lithobid, Lithotabs) may impair the effectiveness of lithium and cause nervous system toxicity.

The following drugs may **decrease** the effects of thioridazine

- antacids containing aluminum and/or magnesium.
- barbiturates (see Drug Class, Section Four).
- benztropine (Cogentin).
- disulfiram (Antabuse).
- trihexyphenidyl (Artane).

▷ *Driving, Hazardous Activities:* This drug can impair mental alertness, judgment and physical coordination. Avoid hazardous activities.

Aviation Note: The use of this drug *is a disqualification* for piloting. Consult a designated Aviation Medical Examiner.

Exposure to Sun: Use caution until sensitivity has been determined. Some phenothiazines can cause photosensitivity (see Glossary).

Exposure to Heat: Use caution and avoid excessive heat as much as possible. This drug may impair the regulation of body temperature and increase the risk of heat stroke.

Exposure to Cold: Use caution and dress warmly. This drug can increase the risk of hypothermia in the elderly.

Discontinuation: After a period of long-term use, do not discontinue this drug suddenly. Gradual withdrawal over 2 to 3 weeks under physician supervision is recommended. Do not discontinue this drug without your physician's knowledge and approval.

THIOTHIXENE
(thi oh THIX een)

Introduced: 1967

Class: Strong tranquilizer, thioxanthenes

Prescription: USA: Yes
Canada: Yes

Controlled Drug: USA: No
Canada: No

Available as Generic: USA: Yes
Canada: No

Brand Name: Navane

BENEFITS versus RISKS	
Possible Benefits	*Possible Risks*
EFFECTIVE CONTROL OF ACUTE MENTAL DISORDERS in the majority of patients: beneficial effects on thinking, mood and behavior	SERIOUS TOXIC EFFECTS ON BRAIN with long-term use Liver damage with jaundice (rare) Rare blood cell disorders: abnormally low white blood cell count

▷ **Principal Uses**

As a Single Drug Product: This antipsychotic drug is used to ameliorate the psychotic thinking and behavior associated with acute psychoses of unknown nature, episodes of mania and paranoia, and acute schizophrenia.

How This Drug Works: Not completely established. Present theory is that, by inhibiting the action of dopamine, this drug acts to correct an imbalance of nerve impulse transmissions that is thought to be responsible for certain mental disorders.

Available Dosage Forms and Strengths
Capsules — 1 mg, 2 mg, 5 mg, 10 mg, 20 mg
Concentrate — 5 mg per ml
Injections — 2 mg, 5 mg per ml

▷ **Usual Adult Dosage Range:**   Initially, 2 to 5 mg 2 or 3 times daily. Dose may be increased by 2 mg at 3- to 4-day intervals as needed and tolerated. Usual dosage range is 20 to 30 mg daily. The total daily dosage should not exceed 60 mg. **Note: Actual dosage and administration schedule must be determined by the physician for each patient individually.**

▷ **Dosing Instructions:**   May be taken with or following meals to reduce stomach irritation. The capsules may be opened for administration. The liquid concentrate must be diluted just before administration by adding it to 8 ounces of water, milk, fruit juice or carbonated beverage.

Usual Duration of Use: Continual use on a regular schedule for several weeks is usually necessary to determine this drug's effectiveness in controlling psychotic disorders. If not significantly beneficial within 6 weeks, it should be discontinued. Long-term use (months to years) requires periodic evaluation of response, appropriate dosage adjustment and consideration of continued need. Consult your physician on a regular basis.

▷ **This Drug Should Not Be Taken If**
- you have had an allergic reaction to it previously.
- you have active liver disease.
- you have cancer of the breast.
- you have a current blood cell or bone marrow disorder.

▷ **Inform Your Physician Before Taking This Drug If**
- you are allergic or abnormally sensitive to other thioxanthene drugs or any phenothiazine drug (see Drug Classes, Section Four).
- you have impaired liver or kidney function.
- you have any type of seizure disorder.
- you have diabetes, glaucoma or heart disease.
- you have a history of lupus erythematosus.
- you are taking any drug with sedative effects.

- you drink alcohol daily.
- you plan to have surgery under general or spinal anesthesia in the near future.

Possible Side-Effects (natural, expected and unavoidable drug actions)
Mild drowsiness (usually during the first 2 weeks), orthostatic hypotension (see Glossary), blurred vision, dry mouth, nasal congestion, constipation, impaired urination.

▷ **Possible Adverse Effects** (unusual, unexpected and infrequent reactions)
If any of the following develop, consult your physician promptly for guidance.
Mild Adverse Effects
Allergic Reactions: Skin rash, hives, itching.
Lowering of body temperature, especially in the elderly. (See Hypothermia in Glossary.)
Fluid retention, weight gain.
Dizziness, weakness, agitation, insomnia, impaired vision.
Nausea, vomiting.
Serious Adverse Effects
Allergic Reactions: Rare hepatitis with jaundice (see Glossary), anaphylactic reaction (see Glossary).
Idiosyncratic Reactions: Paradoxical worsening of psychotic symptoms. Development of the neuroleptic malignant syndrome: high fever, high (or low) blood pressure, severe muscle rigidity, impaired breathing, rapid heart rate, seizures.
Depression, disorientation, seizures, deposits in cornea and lens.
Rapid heart rate, heart rhythm disorders.
Blood cell disorders: reduced white blood cell count.
Nervous system reactions: Parkinson-like disorders (see Glossary), severe restlessness, muscle spasms involving the face and neck, tardive dyskinesia (see Glossary).

▷ **Possible Effects on Sexual Function**
Altered timing and pattern of menstruation.
Impotence (rare).
Male breast enlargement and tenderness.
Female breast enlargement with milk production.

▷ **Adverse Effects That May Mimic Natural Diseases or Disorders**
Nervous system reactions may suggest true Parkinson's disease or Reye syndrome (see Glossary).
Liver reactions may suggest viral hepatitis.

Natural Diseases or Disorders That May Be Activated by This Drug
Latent epilepsy, glaucoma, prostatism (see Glossary).

CAUTION
1. Many over-the-counter medications (see OTC Drugs in Glossary) for allergies, colds and coughs contain drugs that can interact unfa-

vorably with this drug. Ask your physician or pharmacist for guidance before using any such medications.

2. Antacids that contain aluminum and/or magnesium may prevent the absorption of this drug and reduce its effectiveness.
3. Obtain prompt evaluation of any change or disturbance of vision.

Precautions for Use

By Infants and Children: Use of this drug is not recommended in children under 12 years of age. Do not use this drug in the presence of symptoms suggestive of Reye syndrome (see Glossary). Children with acute infectious diseases ("flulike" infections, chicken pox, measles, etc.) are more prone to develop muscular spasms of the face, back and extremities when this drug is given.

By Those over 60 Years of Age: Small doses are advisable until individual response has been determined. You may be more susceptible to the development of drowsiness, lethargy, constipation, lowering of body temperature (hypothermia) and orthostatic hypotension (see Glossary). This drug can enhance existing prostatism (see Glossary). You may also be more susceptible to the development of Parkinson-like reactions and/or tardive dyskinesia (see discussion of these terms in Glossary). These reactions must be recognized early since they may become unresponsive to treatment and irreversible.

▷ ### Advisability of Use During Pregnancy

Pregnancy Category: B (tentative). See Pregnancy Code inside back cover.
Animal studies: No birth defects reported in rats, rabbits or monkeys.
Human studies: Information from adequate studies of pregnant women is not available.

Avoid drug during the first 3 months if possible. Avoid during the last month because of possible effects on the newborn infant.

Advisability of Use if Breast-Feeding

Presence of this drug in breast milk: Unknown.
Avoid drug or refrain from nursing.

Habit-Forming Potential: None.

Effects of Overdosage: Marked drowsiness, weakness, tremor, agitation, unsteadiness, deep sleep, coma, convulsions.

Possible Effects of Long-Term Use: Opacities in the cornea or lens of the eye, pigmentation of the retina. Tardive dyskinesia (see Glossary).

Suggested Periodic Examinations While Taking This Drug (at physician's discretion)

Complete blood cell counts, especially between the fourth and tenth weeks of treatment.
Liver function tests, electrocardiograms.
Complete eye examinations—eye structures and vision.

Careful inspection of the tongue for early evidence of fine, involuntary, wavelike movements that could indicate the beginning of tardive dyskinesia.

▷ **While Taking This Drug, Observe the Following**

Foods: No restrictions.

Beverages: No restrictions. May be taken with milk.

▷   *Alcohol:* Avoid completely. Alcohol can increase the sedative action of thiothixene and accentuate its depressant effects on brain function and blood pressure. Thiothixene can increase the intoxicating effects of alcohol.

Tobacco Smoking: No interactions expected.

Marijuana Smoking: Moderate increase in drowsiness; accentuation of orthostatic hypotension; increased risk of precipitating latent psychoses, confusing the interpretation of mental status and drug responses.

▷   *Other Drugs*

Thiothixene may *increase* the effects of

- all sedative drugs, especially barbiturates and narcotic analgesics, and cause excessive sedation.
- all atropinelike drugs, and cause nervous system toxicity.

Thiothixene may *decrease* the effects of

- guanethidine (Ismelin, Esimil), and reduce its effectiveness in lowering blood pressure.

The following drugs may *decrease* the effects of thiothixene

- antacids containing aluminum and/or magnesium.
- barbiturates (see Drug Class, Section Four).
- benztropine (Cogentin).
- trihexyphenidyl (Artane).

▷   *Driving, Hazardous Activities:* This drug can impair mental alertness, judgment and physical coordination. Avoid hazardous activities.

Aviation Note: The use of this drug **is a disqualification** for piloting. Consult a designated Aviation Medical Examiner.

Exposure to Sun: Use caution until sensitivity has been determined. This drug can cause photosensitivity (see Glossary).

Exposure to Heat: Use caution and avoid excessive heat as much as possible. This drug may impair the regulation of body temperature and increase the risk of heat stroke.

Exposure to Cold: Use caution and dress warmly. This drug can increase the risk of hypothermia in the elderly.

Discontinuation: After a period of long-term use, do not discontinue this drug suddenly. Gradual withdrawal over 2 to 3 weeks under physician supervision is recommended. Do not discontinue this drug without your physician's knowledge and approval. The relapse rate of schizophrenia after discontinuation is 50% to 60%.

THYROID
(THI royd)

Introduced: 1896

Prescription: USA: Yes
    Canada: Yes

Available as Generic: Yes

Class: Thyroid hormones

Controlled Drug: USA: No
    Canada: No

Brand Names: Armour Thyroid, Proloid, S-P-T, Thyrar, Thyroid Strong, Thyroid USP Enseals

---

BENEFITS versus RISKS

Possible Benefits	*Possible Risks*
EFFECTIVE REPLACEMENT THERAPY IN STATES OF THYROID HORMONE DEFICIENCY (HYPOTHYROIDISM) EFFECTIVE TREATMENT OF SIMPLE GOITER AND CHRONIC THYROIDITIS EFFECTIVE TREATMENT OF THYROID GLAND CANCER	Intensification of angina in presence of coronary artery disease

---

▷ **Principal Uses**

As a Single Drug Product: This natural form of thyroid hormones (derived from animal thyroid glands) is used primarily to correct a deficiency of these hormones (hypothyroidism). In the absence of true thyroid deficiency, the use of this drug to treat nonspecific fatigue, obesity, infertility or slow growth is inappropriate and possibly harmful.

How This Drug Works: Not completely established. By altering the processes of cellular chemistry that store energy in an inactive (reserve) form, this drug makes more energy available for biochemical activity and increases the rate of cellular metabolism of all tissues throughout the body.

Available Dosage Forms and Strengths

        Capsules — 65 mg, 130 mg, 195 mg, 325 mg
        Tablets — 16 mg, 32 mg, 65 mg, 98 mg, 100 mg, 130 mg, 195 mg, 200 mg, 260 mg, 325 mg
    Tablets, enteric-coated — 32 mg, 65 mg, 130 mg
    Tablets, sugar-coated — 32 mg, 65 mg, 130 mg, 195 mg

▷ Usual **Adult Dosage Range:**   Initially, 60 mg/day; increase dose by 60 mg at intervals of 1 month as needed and tolerated. The usual maintenance dose is 60 to 180 mg/day. **Note: Actual dosage and administration schedule must be determined by the physician for each patient individually.**

▷ **Dosing Instructions:**   Preferably taken in the morning on an empty stomach to ensure maximal absorption and uniform results. The capsules may be opened and the uncoated tablets may be crushed for administration.

Usual Duration of Use: Continual use on a regular schedule for 4 to 6 weeks is usually necessary to determine this drug's effectiveness in correcting the symptoms of thyroid deficiency. Long-term use (months to years, possibly for life) requires supervision and periodic evaluation by your physician. Consult your physician on a regular basis.

▷ **This Drug Should Not Be Taken If**
- you have had an allergic reaction to it previously.
- you are recovering from a recent heart attack; ask your physician for guidance.
- you are using it to lose weight and your thyroid function is normal (no deficiency).

▷ **Inform Your Physician Before Taking This Drug If**
- you have high blood pressure, any form of heart disease or diabetes.
- you have a history of Addison's disease or adrenal gland deficiency.
- you are taking any antiasthmatic medications.
- you are taking an anticoagulant.

Possible Side-Effects (natural, expected and unavoidable drug actions)
None if dosage is adjusted correctly.

▷ **Possible Adverse Effects** (unusual, unexpected and infrequent reactions)
If any of the following develop, consult your physician promptly for guidance.
Mild Adverse Effects
Allergic Reactions: Skin rash, hives.
Headache in sensitive individuals, even with proper dosage adjustment.
Serious Adverse Effects
Increased frequency or intensity of angina in the presence of coronary artery disease.

▷ **Possible Effects on Sexual Function**
Altered menstrual pattern during dosage adjustments.
Possibly beneficial in treating impaired sexual function that is associated with true hypothyroidism.

Natural Diseases or Disorders That May Be Activated by This Drug
Latent coronary artery disease.

CAUTION

1. The need for and response to thyroid hormone treatment varies greatly from person to person. Careful supervision of individual response is necessary to determine correct dosage. Do not change your dosage schedule without consulting your physician.
2. Thyroid hormonal content of drug products may vary significantly among commercial brands. To ensure consistent results from your medication, it is advisable to continue using the same brand throughout your treatment program.

Precautions for Use

By Infants and Children: This drug is not appropriate for treating hypothyroidism in infants and young children. The drug of choice for this purpose is thyroxine. (See the Drug Profile of Thyroxine that follows.)

By Those over 60 Years of Age: This drug must be used cautiously by this age group. Usually the requirements for thyroid hormone replacement are about 25% lower than in younger adults. Observe closely for any indications that suggest possible overdosage.

▷ **Advisability of Use During Pregnancy**

Pregnancy Category: A (tentative). See Pregnancy Code inside back cover.

Animal studies: No information available.

Human studies: Thyroid hormones do not reach the fetus (cross the placenta) in significant amounts. Clinical experience has shown that appropriate use of thyroid hormones causes no adverse effects on the fetus.

Use this drug only if clearly needed and with carefully adjusted dosage.

Advisability of Use if Breast-Feeding

Presence of this drug in breast milk: Yes.

Breast-feeding is considered safe with correctly adjusted dosage.

Habit-Forming Potential: None.

Effects of Overdosage: Headache, sense of increased body heat, nervousness, increased sweating, hand tremors, insomnia, rapid and irregular heart action, diarrhea, muscle cramping, weight loss.

Possible Effects of Long-Term Use: Bone loss (osteoporosis) in the lumbar vertebrae (spine).

Suggested Periodic Examinations While Taking This Drug (at physician's discretion)

Measurement of thyroid hormone levels in blood.

▷ **While Taking This Drug, Observe the Following**

Foods: No restrictions.

Beverages: No restrictions.

▷   *Alcohol:* No interactions expected.

Tobacco Smoking: No interactions expected.

▷ *Other Drugs*

Thyroid may ***increase*** the effects of
- warfarin (Coumadin), and increase the risk of bleeding; reduction in the dosage of anticoagulant is usually necessary.

Thyroid may ***decrease*** the effects of
- digoxin (Lanoxin), when correcting hypothyroidism; a larger dose of digoxin may be needed.

Thyroid ***taken concurrently*** with
- all antidiabetic drugs (insulin and sulfonylureas) may require an increase in the dosage of the antidiabetic agent to obtain proper control of blood sugar levels. After correct doses of both drugs have been determined, a reduction in the dose of thyroid may require a simultaneous reduction in the dose of the antidiabetic drug to prevent hypoglycemia.
- tricyclic antidepressants (see Drug Class, Section Four) may cause an increase in the activity of both drugs; monitor for indications of overdosage of each drug.

The following drugs may ***decrease*** the effects of thyroid
- cholestyramine (Cuemid, Questran) may reduce its absorption; intake of the two drugs should be separated by 5 hours.

▷ *Driving, Hazardous Activities:* No restrictions.

Aviation Note: The use of this drug ***is probably not a disqualification*** for piloting. Consult a designated Aviation Medical Examiner.

Exposure to Sun: No restrictions.

Exposure to Heat: This drug may decrease individual tolerance to warm environments, increasing discomfort due to heat. Consult your physician if you develop symptoms of overdosage during the warm months of the year.

Heavy Exercise or Exertion: Use caution if you have angina (coronary artery disease). This drug may increase the frequency or severity of angina during physical activity.

Discontinuation: This drug must be taken continually on a regular schedule to correct thyroid deficiency. Do not discontinue it without consulting your physician.

THYROXINE
(thi ROX een)

Other Names: Levothyroxine, L-thyroxine, T-4

Introduced: 1953

Class: Thyroid hormones

Prescription: USA: Yes
Canada: Yes

Controlled Drug: USA: No
Canada: No

Available as Generic: USA: Yes
Canada: No

Brand Names: ◆Eltroxin, Euthroid [CD], Levothroid, Levoxine, Synthroid, Thyrolar [CD]

BENEFITS versus RISKS

Possible Benefits	*Possible Risks*
EFFECTIVE REPLACEMENT THERAPY IN STATES OF THYROID HORMONE DEFICIENCY (HYPOTHYROIDISM) EFFECTIVE TREATMENT OF SIMPLE GOITER AND CHRONIC THYROIDITIS EFFECTIVE TREATMENT OF THYROID GLAND CANCER	Intensification of angina in presence of coronary artery disease Drug-induced hyperthyroidism (with excessive dosage)

▷ **Principal Uses**

As a Single Drug Product: This synthetic thyroid hormone is used primarily to correct thyroid deficiency (hypothyroidism). In addition, it is used to suppress thyroid function in the treatment of simple goiter and the management of Hashimoto's thyroiditis. It is also of value as adjunctive therapy in the management of thyroid gland cancer.

As a Combination Drug Product [CD]: This thyroid hormone is available in combination with the other principal thyroid hormone, liothyronine, in a preparation that resembles the natural hormone material produced by the thyroid gland.

How This Drug Works: Not completely established. By altering the processes of cellular chemistry that store energy in an inactive (reserve) form, this drug makes more energy available for biochemical activity and increases the rate of cellular metabolism of all tissues throughout the body.

Available Dosage Forms and Strengths

Injections — 100 mcg per ml, 200 mcg per vial

Tablets — 0.0125 mg, 0.025 mg, 0.05 mg, 0.075 mg, 0.1 mg, 0.112 mg, 0.125 mg, 0.15 mg, 0.175 mg, 0.2 mg, 0.3 mg

▷ **Usual Adult Dosage Range:** Initially, 0.05 to 0.10 mg/day. The dose may be increased at intervals of 2 to 3 weeks as needed and tolerated. The usual maintenance dose is 0.025 to 0.3 mg/day. The total daily dosage should not exceed 0.4 mg. **Note: Actual dosage and administration schedule must be determined by the physician for each patient individually.**

▷ **Dosing Instructions:** Preferably taken in the morning on an empty stomach to ensure maximal absorption and uniform results. The tablets may be crushed for administration.

Usual Duration of Use: Continual use on a regular schedule for 4 to 6 weeks is usually necessary to determine this drug's effectiveness in correcting the symptoms of thyroid deficiency. Long-term use (months to years, possibly for life) requires supervision and periodic evaluation by your physician. Consult your physician on a regular basis.

▷ **This Drug Should Not Be Taken If**
- you have had an allergic reaction to it previously.
- you are recovering from a recent heart attack; ask your physician for guidance.
- you are using it to lose weight and your thyroid function is normal (no deficiency).

▷ **Inform Your Physician Before Taking This Drug If**
- you have high blood pressure, any form of heart disease or diabetes.
- you have a history of Addison's disease or adrenal gland deficiency.
- you are taking any antiasthmatic medications.
- you are taking an anticoagulant.

Possible Side-Effects (natural, expected and unavoidable drug actions)
None if dosage is adjusted correctly.

▷ **Possible Adverse Effects** (unusual, unexpected and infrequent reactions)
If any of the following develop, consult your physician promptly for guidance.
Mild Adverse Effects
Allergic Reactions: Skin rash, hives.
Headache in sensitive individuals, even with proper dosage adjustment.
Serious Adverse Effects
Increased frequency or intensity of angina in the presence of coronary artery disease.
Note: Other adverse effects are manifestations of excessive dosage. See Effects of Overdosage category.

▷ **Possible Effects on Sexual Function**
Altered menstrual pattern during dosage adjustments.
Possibly beneficial in treating impaired sexual function that is associated with true hypothyroidism.

Natural Diseases or Disorders That May Be Activated by This Drug
Latent coronary artery insufficiency (angina), diabetes.

CAUTION
1. The need for and response to thyroid hormone treatment varies greatly from person to person. Careful supervision of individual response is necessary to determine correct dosage. Do not change your dosage schedule without consulting your physician.
2. In the absence of verified thyroid deficiency, this drug should not be used to treat nonspecific fatigue, obesity, infertility or slow growth. Such use is inappropriate and could be harmful.

Precautions for Use
By Infants and Children: To facilitate normal growth and development, the thyroid-deficient child often requires higher dosage than the

adult. A transient loss of hair may occur during the early months of treatment.

By Those over 60 Years of Age: This drug must be used cautiously by this age group. Usually the requirements for thyroid hormone replacement are about 25% lower than in younger adults. Observe closely for any indications that suggest possible overdosage.

▷ **Advisability of Use During Pregnancy**

Pregnancy Category: A (tentative). See Pregnancy Code inside back cover.

Animal studies: Cataract formation reported in rat studies. Other defects reported in rabbit and guinea pig studies.

Human studies: Thyroid hormones do not reach the fetus (cross the placenta) in significant amounts. Clinical experience has shown that appropriate use of thyroid hormones causes no adverse effects on the fetus.

Use this drug only if clearly needed and with carefully adjusted dosage.

Advisability of Use if Breast-Feeding

Presence of this drug in breast milk: Yes, in minimal amounts.

Breast-feeding is considered safe with correctly adjusted dosage.

Habit-Forming Potential: None.

Effects of Overdosage: Headache, sense of increased body heat, nervousness, increased sweating, hand tremors, insomnia, rapid and irregular heart action, diarrhea, muscle cramping, weight loss.

Possible Effects of Long-Term Use: Bone loss (osteoporosis) in the lumbar vertebrae (spine).

Suggested Periodic Examinations While Taking This Drug (at physician's discretion)

Measurement of thyroid hormone levels in blood.

▷ **While Taking This Drug, Observe the Following**

Foods: No restrictions.

Beverages: No restrictions.

▷ *Alcohol:* No interactions expected.

Tobacco Smoking: No interactions expected.

▷ *Other Drugs*

Thyroxine may *increase* the effects of

• warfarin (Coumadin), and increase the risk of bleeding; reduction in the dosage of anticoagulant is usually necessary.

Thyroxine may *decrease* the effects of

• digoxin (Lanoxin), when correcting hypothyroidism; a larger dose of digoxin may be needed.

Thyroxine *taken concurrently* with

• all antidiabetic drugs (insulin and sulfonylureas) may require an increase in the dosage of the antidiabetic agent to obtain proper control of blood sugar levels. After correct doses of both drugs have been determined, a reduction in the dose of thyroid may require a simultaneous reduction in the dose of the antidiabetic drug to prevent hypoglycemia.

- tricyclic antidepressants (see Drug Class, Section Four) may cause an increase in the activity of both drugs; monitor for indications of overdosage of each drug.

The following drugs may *decrease* the effects of thyroxine

- cholestyramine (Cuemid, Questran) may reduce its absorption; intake of the two drugs should be separated by 5 hours.

▷ *Driving, Hazardous Activities:* No restrictions.

Aviation Note: The use of this drug *is probably not a disqualification* for piloting. Consult a designated Aviation Medical Examiner.

Exposure to Sun: No restrictions.

Exposure to Heat: This drug may decrease individual tolerance to warm environments, increasing discomfort due to heat. Consult your physician if you develop symptoms of overdosage during the warm months of the year.

Heavy Exercise or Exertion: Use caution if you have angina (coronary artery disease). This drug may increase the frequency or severity of angina during physical activity.

Discontinuation: This drug must be taken continually on a regular schedule to correct thyroid deficiency. Do not discontinue it without consulting your physician.

TIMOLOL
(TI moh lohl)

Introduced: 1972

Class: Antianginal, antiglaucoma, antihypertensive, migraine preventive, beta-adrenergic blocker

Prescription: USA: Yes
Canada: Yes

Controlled Drug: USA: No
Canada: No

Available as Generic: USA: No
Canada: No

Brand Names: Blocadren, Timolide [CD], Timoptic

```
┌─────────────────────────────────────────────────────────────────┐
│                   BENEFITS versus RISKS                          │
│                                                                   │
│         Possible Benefits              Possible Risks            │
│    EFFECTIVE, WELL-TOLERATED     CONGESTIVE HEART FAILURE         │
│    AS: ANTIANGINAL DRUG in          in advanced heart disease    │
│    effort-induced angina;         Worsening of angina in coronary│
│    ANTIGLAUCOMA DRUG in              heart disease (if drug is    │
│    open-angle glaucoma;              abruptly withdrawn)          │
│    ANTIHYPERTENSIVE DRUG          Masking of low blood sugar      │
│    in mild to moderate               (hypoglycemia) in drug-treated│
│    hypertension                      diabetes                    │
│    EFFECTIVE PREVENTION OF        Provocation of asthma           │
│    MIGRAINE HEADACHES                                             │
│    Effective adjunct in the                                      │
│    prevention of recurrent heart                                 │
│    attack (myocardial infarction)                                │
└─────────────────────────────────────────────────────────────────┘
```

▷ **Principal Uses**

As a Single Drug Product: This member of the beta blocker drug class is used primarily to treat (1) classical effort-induced angina, certain types of heart rhythm disturbance and high blood pressure; (2) increased internal eye pressure and chronic open-angle glaucoma. It is also beneficial in preventing the recurrence of heart attacks (myocardial infarction). In addition, it is used to reduce the frequency and severity of migraine headaches.

As a Combination Drug Product [CD]: This drug is available in combination with hydrochlorothiazide for the treatment of hypertension. This combination product includes two "step 1" drugs with different mechanisms of action; it is intended to provide greater effectiveness and convenience for long-term use.

How This Drug Works: By blocking certain actions of the sympathetic nervous system, this drug

- reduces the rate and contraction force of the heart, thus lowering the ejection pressure of the blood leaving the heart and reducing the oxygen requirement for heart function.
- reduces the degree of contraction of blood vessel walls, resulting in their relaxation and expansion and consequent lowering of blood pressure.
- prolongs the conduction time of nerve impulses through the heart, of benefit in the management of certain heart rhythm disorders.
- slows the formation of fluid (aqueous humor) in the anterior chamber of the eye and improves its drainage from the eye, thus lowering the internal eye pressure.

Available Dosage Forms and Strengths

Eye solutions — 0.25%, 0.5%

     Tablets — 5 mg, 10 mg, 20 mg

▷ **Usual Adult Dosage Range:** Varies with indication.

Antianginal and antihypertensive: Initially, 10 mg 2 times/day; increase dose gradually every 7 days as needed and tolerated. Usual maintenance dose is 10 to 20 mg twice/day. The total daily dosage should not exceed 60 mg.

Migraine headache prevention: Initially, 10 mg 2 times/day; increase dose as needed to 10 mg in the morning and 20 mg at night.

Recurrent heart attack prevention: 10 mg twice/day.

Antiglaucoma: 1 drop in affected eye every 12 to 24 hours.

Note: Actual dosage and administration schedule must be determined by the physician for each patient individually.

▷ **Dosing Instructions:**   Preferably taken 1 hour before eating to maximize absorption. The tablet may be crushed for administration. Do not discontinue this drug abruptly.

Usual Duration of Use: Continual use on a regular schedule for 10 to 14 days is usually necessary to determine this drug's effectiveness in preventing angina, controlling heart rhythm disorders and lowering blood pressure. Maximal effectiveness may require continual use for 6 to 8 weeks. The long-term use of this drug (months to years) will be determined by the course of your symptoms over time and your response to the overall treatment program (weight reduction, salt restriction, smoking cessation, etc.). Consult your physician on a regular basis.

Currently a "Drug of Choice" for initiating treatment of hypertension with a single drug.

▷ **This Drug Should Not Be Taken If**
- you have had an allergic reaction to it previously.
- you have Prinzmetal's variant angina (coronary artery spasm).
- you have congestive heart failure.
- you have an abnormally slow heart rate or a serious form of heart block.
- you are taking, or have taken within the past 14 days, any monoamine oxidase (MAO) type A inhibitor drug (see Drug Class, Section Four).

▷ **Inform Your Physician Before Taking This Drug If**
- you have had an adverse reaction to any beta blocker drug in the past (see Drug Class, Section Four).
- you have a history of serious heart disease, with or without episodes of heart failure.
- you have a history of hay fever (allergic rhinitis), asthma, chronic bronchitis or emphysema.
- you have a history of overactive thyroid function (hyperthyroidism).
- you have a history of low blood sugar (hypoglycemia).
- you have impaired liver or kidney function.
- you have diabetes or myasthenia gravis.

- you are currently taking any form of digitalis, quinidine or reserpine, or any calcium blocker drug (see Drug Class, Section Four).
- you plan to have surgery under general anesthesia in the near future.

Possible Side-Effects (natural, expected and unavoidable drug actions)
Lethargy and fatigability, cold extremities, slow heart rate, light-headedness in upright position (see Orthostatic Hypotension in Glossary).

▷ **Possible Adverse Effects** (unusual, unexpected and infrequent reactions)
If any of the following develop, consult your physician promptly for guidance.
Mild Adverse Effects
Allergic Reactions: Skin rash, itching.
Headache, dizziness, visual disturbances, vivid dreams.
Indigestion, nausea, vomiting, diarrhea.
Numbness and tingling in extremities.
Serious Adverse Effects
Allergic Reactions: Laryngospasm, severe dermatitis.
Idiosyncratic Reactions: Acute behavioral disturbances: depression, hallucinations.
Chest pain, shortness of breath, precipitation of congestive heart failure.
Induction of bronchial asthma (in asthmatic individuals).
Masking of warning signs of impending low blood sugar (hypoglycemia) in drug-treated diabetes.

▷ **Possible Effects on Sexual Function**
Decreased libido, impaired erection, impotence.
Note: All of these effects can occur with the use of timolol eye drops at recommended dosage.

▷ **Adverse Effects That May Mimic Natural Diseases or Disorders**
Reduced blood flow to extremities may resemble Raynaud's phenomenon (see Glossary).

Natural Diseases or Disorders That May Be Activated by This Drug
Prinzmetal's variant angina, Raynaud's disease, intermittent claudication, myasthenia gravis (questionable).

CAUTION
1. ***Do not discontinue this drug suddenly*** without the knowledge and guidance of your physician. Carry a notation on your person that you are taking this drug.
2. Consult your physician or pharmacist before using nasal decongestants usually present in over-the-counter cold preparations and nose drops. These can cause sudden increases in blood pressure when taken concurrently with beta blocker drugs.
3. Report the development of any tendency to emotional depression (rare with this drug).

Precautions for Use

By Infants and Children: Safety and effectiveness for use by those under 12 years of age have not been established. However, if this drug is used, observe for the development of low blood sugar (hypoglycemia) during periods of reduced food intake.

By Those over 60 Years of Age: Proceed **cautiously** with all antihypertensive drugs. Unacceptably high blood pressure should be reduced without creating the risks associated with excessively low blood pressure. Start treatment with small doses, and monitor the blood pressure response frequently. Sudden, rapid and excessive reduction of blood pressure can predispose to stroke or heart attack. Observe for dizziness, unsteadiness, tendency to fall, confusion, hallucinations, depression or urinary frequency.

▷ **Advisability of Use During Pregnancy**

Pregnancy Category: C (tentative). See Pregnancy Code inside back cover.
Animal studies: No significant increase in birth defects due to this drug.
Human studies: Information from adequate studies of pregnant women is not available.
Avoid use of drug during the first 3 months if possible. Use this drug only if clearly needed. Ask your physician for guidance.

Advisability of Use if Breast-Feeding

Presence of this drug in breast milk: Probably yes.
Monitor nursing infant closely and discontinue drug or nursing if adverse effects develop.

Habit-Forming Potential: None.

Effects of Overdosage: Weakness, slow pulse, low blood pressure, fainting, cold and sweaty skin, congestive heart failure, possible coma and convulsions.

Possible Effects of Long-Term Use: Reduced heart reserve and eventual heart failure in susceptible individuals with advanced heart disease.

Suggested Periodic Examinations While Taking This Drug (at physician's discretion)

Complete blood cell counts (because of adverse effects of other drugs of this class).
Measurements of blood pressure, evaluation of heart function.

▷ **While Taking This Drug, Observe the Following**

Foods: No restrictions. Avoid excessive salt intake.
Beverages: No restrictions. May be taken with milk.
▷   *Alcohol:* Use with caution until the combined effect has been determined. Alcohol may exaggerate this drug's ability to lower the blood pressure and may increase its mild sedative effect.
Tobacco Smoking: Nicotine may reduce this drug's effectiveness in treating angina, heart rhythm disorders and high blood pressure. In ad-

dition, high doses of this drug may potentiate the constriction of the bronchial tubes caused by regular smoking.

▷ *Other Drugs*

Timolol may ***increase*** the effects of

- other antihypertensive drugs, and cause excessive lowering of blood pressure. Dosage adjustments may be necessary.
- lidocaine (Xylocaine, etc.).
- reserpine (Ser-Ap-Es, etc.), and cause sedation, depression, slowing of the heart rate and lowering of the blood pressure.
- verapamil (Calan, Isoptin), and cause excessive depression of heart function; monitor this combination closely.

Timolol may ***decrease*** the effects of

- theophyllines (Aminophyllin, Theo-Dur, etc.), and reduce their antiasthmatic effectiveness.

Timolol ***taken concurrently*** with

- clonidine (Catapres) requires close monitoring for rebound high blood pressure if clonidine is withdrawn while timolol is still being taken.
- epinephrine (Adrenalin, etc.) may cause marked rise in blood pressure and slowing of the heart rate.
- insulin requires close monitoring to avoid undetected hypoglycemia (see Glossary).

The following drugs may ***increase*** the effects of timolol

- chlorpromazine (Thorazine, etc.)
- cimetidine (Tagamet).
- methimazole (Tapazole).
- propylthiouracil (Propacil).

The following drugs may ***decrease*** the effects of timolol

- barbiturates (phenobarbital, etc.).
- indomethacin (Indocin), and possibly other "aspirin substitutes," may impair timolol's antihypertensive effect.
- rifampin (Rifadin, Rimactane).

▷ *Driving, Hazardous Activities:* Use caution until the full extent of dizziness, lethargy and blood pressure change have been determined.

Aviation Note: The use of this drug ***may be a disqualification*** for piloting. Consult a designated Aviation Medical Examiner.

Exposure to Sun: No restrictions.

Exposure to Heat: Caution advised. Hot environments can lower blood pressure and exaggerate the effects of this drug.

Exposure to Cold: Caution advised. Cold environments can enhance the circulatory deficiency in the extremities that may occur with this drug. The elderly should take precautions to prevent hypothermia (see Glossary).

Heavy Exercise or Exertion: It is advisable to avoid exertion that produces light-headedness, excessive fatigue or muscle cramping. The use of this drug may intensify the hypertensive response to isometric exercise.

Occurrence of Unrelated Illness: The fever that accompanies systemic infections can lower blood pressure and require adjustment of dosage. Illnesses that cause nausea or vomiting may interrupt the regular dosage schedule. Ask your physician for guidance.

Discontinuation: It is advisable to avoid sudden discontinuation of this drug in all situations; this is especially true in the presence of coronary artery disease. If possible, gradual reduction of dose over a period of 2 to 3 weeks is recommended. Ask your physician for specific guidance.

TOCAINIDE
(toh KAY nide)

Introduced: 1976

Class: Antiarrhythmic

Prescription: USA: Yes
Canada: Yes

Controlled Drug: USA: No
Canada: No

Available as Generic: USA: No
Canada: No

Brand Name: Tonocard

BENEFITS versus RISKS	
Possible Benefits	*Possible Risks*
EFFECTIVE TREATMENT OF SELECTED HEART RHYTHM DISORDERS (ventricular)	DRUG-INDUCED HEART RHYTHM DISORDERS (10.9%) CONGESTIVE HEART FAILURE (4%) Rare blood cell disorders: aplastic anemia, abnormally low white blood cell and platelet counts Drug-induced lung damage

▷ **Principal Uses**

As a Single Drug Product: This drug is classified as a Type 1 antiarrhythmic agent, similar to procainamide and quinidine in its actions. It is used primarily to correct and prevent the recurrence of (1) abnormally rapid heart rates (tachycardia) that arise in the ventricles (lower heart chambers); and (2) premature beats arising in the ventricles.

How This Drug Works: By slowing the transmission of electrical impulses throughout the conduction system of the heart, this drug assists in restoring normal heart rate and rhythm.

Available Dosage Forms and Strengths
Tablets — 400 mg, 600 mg

▷ **Usual Adult Dosage Range:**   Do not take a loading dose. Initiate treatment with 400 mg/8 hours. If needed and tolerated, the dose may be increased gradually to 600 mg/8 hours. The total daily dosage should not exceed 2400 mg. **Note: Actual dosage and administration schedule must be determined by the physician for each patient individually.**

▷ **Dosing Instructions:**   May be taken without regard to meals, but may be taken with or following food if desired to reduce stomach irritation. Take at same time each day to obtain uniform results. The tablet may be crushed for administration.

Usual Duration of Use: Continual use on a regular schedule for 1 to 2 weeks is usually necessary to determine this drug's effectiveness in correcting or preventing responsive rhythm disorders. Long-term use requires supervision and periodic evaluation by your physician. Consult your physician on a regular basis.

▷ **This Drug Should Not Be Taken If**
• you have had an allergic reaction to it previously.
• you are allergic to local anesthetics of the Novocain type.
• you have second-degree or third-degree heart block (with no pacemaker).

▷ **Inform Your Physician Before Taking This Drug If**
• you have had any unfavorable reactions to other antiarrhythmic drugs in the past.
• you have a history of heart disease of any kind, especially heart block.
• you have impaired liver or kidney function.
• you are taking any form of digitalis, a potassium supplement or any diuretic drug that can cause excessive loss of body potassium (ask physician).

Possible Side-Effects (natural, expected and unavoidable drug actions)
Flushing, increased sweating, light-headedness.
The onset of tremors indicates that the dose is reaching the maximum that can be tolerated.

▷ **Possible Adverse Effects** (unusual, unexpected and infrequent reactions)
If any of the following develop, consult your physician promptly for guidance.
Mild Adverse Effects
Allergic Reactions: Skin rash (8%), hives, itching.
Headache (4%), dizziness (15%), visual disturbance (1.5%), fatigue (0.8%), tremor (8%), numbness (9%).
Loss of appetite, indigestion, nausea (14%), vomiting (4%), diarrhea (4%).

Serious Adverse Effects

Idiosyncratic Reactions: Confusion, disorientation, hallucinations (2.7%).

Drug-induced heart rhythm disorders (10%), congestive heart failure (4%), shortness of breath, palpitations, chest pain.

Drug-induced lung damage: pneumonitis and fibrosis, causing cough and breathing difficulty. (Usually occurs after 3 to 18 weeks of drug use.)

Bone marrow depression (see Glossary): fatigue, weakness, fever, sore throat, abnormal bleeding or bruising. (Usually occurs after 2 to 12 weeks of drug use.)

▷ **Possible Effects on Sexual Function:**   None reported.

▷ **Adverse Effects That May Mimic Natural Diseases or Disorders**

Lung reactions may suggest an infectious bronchitis or pneumonia.

CAUTION

1. Thorough evaluation of your heart function (including electrocardiograms) is necessary prior to using this drug.
2. Periodic evaluation of your heart function is necessary to determine your response to this drug. Some individuals may experience worsening of their heart rhythm disorder and/or deterioration of heart function. Close monitoring of heart rate, rhythm and overall performance is essential.
3. Dosage must be adjusted carefully for each individual. Do not change your dosage without the knowledge and supervision of your physician.
4. Do not take any other antiarrhythmic drug while taking this drug unless directed to do so by your physician.

Precautions for Use

By Infants and Children: Safety and effectiveness for use by those under 12 years of age have not been established. Initial use of this drug requires hospitalization and supervision by a qualified cardiologist.

By Those over 60 Years of Age: Reduced kidney function may require reduction in dosage. Observe carefully for light-headedness, dizziness, unsteadiness and tendency to fall.

▷ **Advisability of Use During Pregnancy**

Pregnancy Category: C (tentative). See Pregnancy Code inside back cover.

Animal studies: No birth defects reported in rat or rabbit studies; however, an increase in fetal resorptions, stillbirths and abortions was reported.

Human studies: Information from adequate studies of pregnant women is not available.

Avoid this drug during first 3 months. Use this drug only if clearly needed. Ask your physician for guidance.

Advisability of Use if Breast-Feeding
Presence of this drug in breast milk: Unknown.
Avoid drug or refrain from nursing.

Habit-Forming Potential: None.

Effects of Overdosage: Impaired urination, constipation, marked drop in blood pressure, abnormal heart rhythms, slow heart rate, congestive heart failure, seizures.

Possible Effects of Long-Term Use: None reported.

Suggested Periodic Examinations While Taking This Drug (at physician's discretion)
Electrocardiograms, complete blood cell counts, measurements of potassium blood levels.

▷ **While Taking This Drug, Observe the Following**
Foods: No restrictions. Ask physician regarding need for salt restriction and advisability of eating potassium-rich foods.
Beverages: No restrictions. May be taken with milk.
▷ *Alcohol:* Use caution until the combined effects have been determined. Alcohol can increase the blood-pressure-lowering effects of this drug.
Tobacco Smoking: Nicotine can cause irritability of the heart and reduce the effectiveness of this drug. Follow physician's advice regarding smoking.
▷ *Other Drugs*
Tocainide may ***increase*** the effects of
• antihypertensive drugs, and cause excessive lowering of blood pressure.
• beta blocker drugs (see Drug Class, Section Four).
The following drugs may ***decrease*** the effects of tocainide
• diuretics that promote potassium loss.
▷ *Driving, Hazardous Activities:* This drug may cause dizziness or blurred vision. Restrict activities as necessary.
Aviation Note: The use of this drug ***may be a disqualification*** for piloting. Consult a designated Aviation Medical Examiner.
Exposure to Sun: No restrictions.
Occurrence of Unrelated Illness: Disorders that cause vomiting, diarrhea or dehydration can affect this drug's action adversely. Report such developments promptly.
Discontinuation: This drug should not be discontinued abruptly following long-term use. Ask your physician for guidance regarding gradual dose reduction.

TOLAZAMIDE
(tohl AZ a mide)

Introduced: 1966   **Class:** Antidiabetic, sulfonylureas
Prescription: USA: Yes   **Controlled Drug:** USA: No

Available as Generic: Yes

Brand Names: Ronase, Tolamide, Tolinase

BENEFITS versus RISKS

Possible Benefits	*Possible Risks*
Assistance in regulating blood sugar in noninsulin-dependent diabetes (adjunctive to appropriate diet and weight control)	HYPOGLYCEMIA, severe and prolonged Drug-induced liver damage Rare bone marrow depression (see Glossary) Hemolytic anemia (see Glossary)

▷ **Principal Uses**

As a Single Drug Product: To assist in the control of mild to moderately severe type II diabetes mellitus (adult, maturity-onset) that does not require insulin, but that cannot be adequately controlled by diet alone.

How This Drug Works: It is thought that this drug (1) stimulates the release of insulin (by a pancreas that is capable of responding to stimulation), and (2) enhances the utilization of insulin by appropriate tissues.

Available Dosage Forms and Strengths

Tablets — 100 mg, 250 mg, 500 mg

▷ **Usual Adult Dosage Range:**   Initially, 100 to 250 mg daily with breakfast. At 7-day intervals, the dose may be increased by increments of 100 to 250 mg daily as needed and tolerated. The total daily dosage should not exceed 1000 mg (1 gram). A "loading" or priming dose is not necessary and should not be given. **Note: Actual dosage and administration schedule must be determined by the physician for each patient individually.**

▷ **Dosing Instructions:**   If the daily maintenance dose is found to be more than 500 mg, the total dose should be divided into 2 equal doses: the first taken with the morning meal, the second with the evening meal. The tablet may be crushed for administration.

Usual Duration of Use: Continual use on a regular schedule for several weeks is usually necessary to determine this drug's effectiveness in controlling diabetes. Failure to respond to maximal doses within 1 month constitutes a primary failure. Up to 10% of those who respond initially may develop secondary failure of the drug later. The duration of effective use can only be determined by periodic measurement of the blood sugar. Consult your physician on a regular basis.

▷ **This Drug Should Not Be Taken If**
- you have had an allergic reaction to it previously.
- you have severe impairment of liver or kidney function.
- you are pregnant.

▷ **Inform Your Physician Before Taking This Drug If**
- you are allergic to other sulfonylurea drugs or to "sulfa" drugs. (See Drug Classes, Section Four).
- your diabetes has been unstable or "brittle" in the past.
- you do not know how to recognize or treat hypoglycemia (see Glossary).
- you have a history of congestive heart failure, peptic ulcer disease, cirrhosis of the liver, hypothyroidism or porphyria.

Possible Side-Effects (natural, expected and unavoidable drug actions)
If drug dosage is excessive or food intake is delayed or inadequate, abnormally low blood sugar (hypoglycemia) will occur as a predictable drug effect.

▷ **Possible Adverse Effects** (unusual, unexpected and infrequent reactions)
If any of the following develop, consult your physician promptly for guidance.
Mild Adverse Effects
Allergic Reactions: Skin rash, hives, itching, drug fever.
Headache, ringing in the ears.
Indigestion, heartburn, nausea, vomiting, diarrhea.
Serious Adverse Effects
Allergic Reactions: Hepatitis with jaundice (see Glossary).
Idiosyncratic Reactions: Hemolytic anemia (see Glossary); disulfiram-like reaction with concurrent use of alcohol (see Glossary), infrequent with this drug.
Bone marrow depression (see Glossary): fatigue, weakness, fever, sore throat, abnormal bleeding or bruising.

▷ **Possible Effects on Sexual Function**   None reported.

▷ **Adverse Effects That May Mimic Natural Diseases or Disorders**
Liver reactions may suggest viral hepatitis.

CAUTION
1. This drug must be regarded as only one part of the total program for the management of your diabetes. It is not a substitute for a properly prescribed diet and regular exercise.
2. Over a period of time (usually several months), this drug may lose its effectiveness in controlling blood sugar levels. Periodic follow-up examinations are necessary to monitor all aspects of response to drug treatment.

Precautions for Use
By Infants and Children: This drug is not effective in type I (juvenile, growth-onset) insulin-dependent diabetes.

By Those over 60 Years of Age: This drug should be used with caution in this age group. Start treatment with 100 mg/day; increase dosage cautiously and monitor closely to prevent hypoglycemic reactions. Repeated episodes of hypoglycemia in the elderly can cause brain damage.

▷ **Advisability of Use During Pregnancy**

Pregnancy Category: C (tentative). See Pregnancy Code inside back cover.

Animal studies: No birth defects due to this drug reported in rats.

Human studies: Information from adequate studies of pregnant women is not available.

Because uncontrolled blood sugar levels during pregnancy are associated with a higher incidence of birth defects, many experts recommend that insulin (instead of an oral agent) be used as necessary to control diabetes during the entire pregnancy.

Use during pregnancy is not recommended by the manufacturer.

Advisability of Use if Breast-Feeding

Presence of this drug in breast milk: Probably yes.

Avoid drug or refrain from nursing.

Habit-Forming Potential: None.

Effects of Overdosage: Symptoms of mild to severe hypoglycemia: headache, light-headedness, faintness, nervousness, confusion, tremor, sweating, heart palpitation, weakness, hunger, nausea, vomiting, stupor progressing to coma.

Possible Effects of Long-Term Use: Reduced function of the thyroid gland (hypothyroidism). Reports of increased frequency and severity of heart and blood vessel diseases associated with long-term use of this class of drugs are highly controversial and inconclusive. A direct cause-and-effect relationship (see Glossary) is tenuous. Ask your physician for guidance.

Suggested Periodic Examinations While Taking This Drug (at physician's discretion)

Complete blood cell counts, liver function tests, thyroid function tests, periodic evaluation of heart and circulatory system.

▷ **While Taking This Drug, Observe the Following**

Foods: Follow the diabetic diet prescribed by your physician.

Beverages: As directed in the diabetic diet. May be taken with milk.

▷   *Alcohol:* Use with extreme caution until the combined effect has been determined. Alcohol can exaggerate this drug's hypoglycemic effect. This drug infrequently causes a marked intolerance of alcohol resulting in a disulfiramlike reaction (see Glossary): facial flushing, sweating, palpitation.

Tobacco Smoking: No interactions expected.

▷ *Other Drugs*

The following drugs may *increase* the effects of tolazamide

- aspirin, and other salicylates.
- cimetidine (Tagamet).
- clofibrate (Atromid S).
- fenfluramine (Pondimin).
- monoamine oxidase (MAO) type A inhibitor drugs (see Drug Class, Section Four).
- phenylbutazone (Butazolidin).
- ranitidine (Zantac).

The following drugs may *decrease* the effects of tolazamide

- beta blocker drugs (see Drug Class, Section Four).
- bumetanide (Bumex).
- diazoxide (Proglycem).
- ethacrynic acid (Edecrin).
- furosemide (Lasix).
- phenytoin (Dilantin).
- thiazide diuretics (see Drug Class, Section Four).

▷ *Driving, Hazardous Activities:* Regulate your dosage schedule, eating schedule and physical activities very carefully to prevent hypoglycemia. Be able to recognize the early symptoms of hypoglycemia so you can avoid hazardous activities and take corrective measures.

Aviation Note: Diabetes *is a disqualification* for piloting. Consult a designated Aviation Medical Examiner.

Exposure to Sun: Use caution until sensitivity has been determined. Some drugs of this class can cause photosensitivity (see Glossary).

Occurrence of Unrelated Illness: Acute infections, illnesses causing vomiting or diarrhea, serious injuries and surgical procedures can interfere with diabetic control and may require the use of insulin. If any of these conditions occur, consult your physician promptly.

Discontinuation: Because of the possibility of secondary failure, it is advisable to evaluate the continued benefit of this drug every 6 months.

TOLBUTAMIDE
(tohl BYU ta mide)

Introduced: 1956

Class: Antidiabetic, sulfonylureas

Prescription: USA: Yes
Canada: Yes

Controlled Drug: USA: No
Canada: No

Available as Generic: Yes

Brand Names: ✦Apo-Tolbutamide, ✦Mobenol, ✦Novobutamide, Oramide, Orinase

```
┌──────────────────────────────────────────────────────────┐
│                  BENEFITS versus RISKS                     │
│                                                            │
│      Possible Benefits            Possible Risks           │
│  Assistance in regulating blood   HYPOGLYCEMIA, severe and │
│    sugar in noninsulin-dependent    prolonged              │
│    diabetes (adjunctive to        Drug-induced liver damage│
│    appropriate diet and weight    Rare bone marrow depression│
│    control)                         (See Glossary)         │
│                                   Hemolytic anemia (See Glossary)│
└──────────────────────────────────────────────────────────┘
```

▷ **Principal Uses**

  As a Single Drug Product: To assist in the control of mild to moderately severe type II diabetes mellitus (adult, maturity-onset) that does not require insulin, but that cannot be adequately controlled by diet alone.

  How This Drug Works: It is thought that this drug (1) stimulates the release of insulin (by a pancreas that is capable of responding to stimulation), and (2) enhances the utilization of insulin by appropriate tissues.

  Available Dosage Forms and Strengths
    Tablets — 250 mg, 500 mg

▷ **Usual Adult Dosage Range:** Initially, 500 mg twice a day. The dose may be increased or decreased every 48 to 72 hours until the minimal amount required for satisfactory control is determined. The usual range is 500 to 2000 mg/24 hours. The total daily dosage should not exceed 3000 mg (3 grams). A "loading" or priming dose is not necessary and should not be given. **Note: Actual dosage and administration schedule must be determined by the physician for each patient individually.**

▷ **Dosing Instructions:** May be taken with food (morning and evening meals) to reduce stomach irritation. The tablet may be crushed for administration.

  Usual Duration of Use: Continual use on a regular schedule for several weeks is usually necessary to determine this drug's effectiveness in controlling diabetes. Failure to respond to maximal doses within 1 month constitutes a primary failure. Up to 15% of those who respond initially may develop secondary failure of the drug within the first year. The duration of effective use can only be determined by periodic measurement of the blood sugar. Consult your physician on a regular basis.

▷ **This Drug Should Not Be Taken If**
  • you have had an allergic reaction to it previously.
  • you have severe impairment of liver or kidney function.
  • you are pregnant.

▷ **Inform Your Physician Before Taking This Drug If**
- you are allergic to other sulfonylurea drugs or to "sulfa" drugs. (See Drug Classes, Section Four).
- your diabetes has been unstable or "brittle" in the past.
- you do not know how to recognize or treat hypoglycemia (see Glossary).
- you have a history of congestive heart failure, peptic ulcer disease, cirrhosis of the liver, hypothyroidism or porphyria.

Possible Side-Effects (natural, expected and unavoidable drug actions)
If drug dosage is excessive or food intake is delayed or inadequate, abnormally low blood sugar (hypoglycemia) will occur as a predictable drug effect.

▷ **Possible Adverse Effects** (unusual, unexpected and infrequent reactions)
If any of the following develop, consult your physician promptly for guidance.
Mild Adverse Effects
Allergic Reactions: Skin rash, hives, itching, drug fever.
Headache, ringing in the ears, weakness.
Indigestion, heartburn, nausea, vomiting.
Serious Adverse Effects
Allergic Reactions: Hepatitis with jaundice (see Glossary).
Idiosyncratic Reactions: Hemolytic anemia (see Glossary); disulfiram-like reaction with concurrent use of alcohol (see Glossary), infrequent with this drug.
Bone marrow depression (see Glossary): fatigue, weakness, fever, sore throat, abnormal bleeding or bruising.

▷ **Possible Effects on Sexual Function**   None reported.

▷ **Adverse Effects That May Mimic Natural Diseases or Disorders**
Liver reactions may suggest viral hepatitis.

Natural Diseases or Disorders That May Be Activated by This Drug
Acute intermittent porphyria (see Glossary).

CAUTION
1. This drug must be regarded as only one part of the total program for the management of your diabetes. It is not a substitute for a properly prescribed diet and regular exercise.
2. Over a period of time (usually several months), this drug may lose its effectiveness in controlling blood sugar levels. Periodic follow-up examinations are necessary to monitor all aspects of response to drug treatment.

Precautions for Use
By Infants and Children: This drug is not effective in type I (juvenile, growth-onset) insulin-dependent diabetes.
By Those over 60 Years of Age: This drug should be used with caution in this age group. Start treatment with 500 mg/day; increase dosage

cautiously and monitor closely to prevent hypoglycemic reactions. Repeated episodes of hypoglycemia in the elderly can cause brain damage.

▷ **Advisability of Use During Pregnancy**
Pregnancy Category: C (tentative). See Pregnancy Code inside back cover.
Animal studies: Ocular and bone birth defects reported in rat studies.
Human studies: Information from adequate studies of pregnant women is not available.
Because uncontrolled blood sugar levels during pregnancy are associated with a higher incidence of birth defects, many experts recommend that insulin (instead of an oral agent) be used as necessary to control diabetes during the entire pregnancy.
Use during pregnancy is not recommended by the manufacturer.

Advisability of Use if Breast-Feeding
Presence of this drug in breast milk: Yes.
Avoid drug or refrain from nursing.

Habit-Forming Potential: None.

Effects of Overdosage: Symptoms of mild to severe hypoglycemia: headache, light-headedness, faintness, nervousness, confusion, tremor, sweating, heart palpitation, weakness, hunger, nausea, vomiting, stupor progressing to coma.

Possible Effects of Long-Term Use: Reduced function of the thyroid gland (hypothyroidism). Reports of increased frequency and severity of heart and blood vessel diseases associated with long-term use of this class of drugs are highly controversial and inconclusive. A direct cause-and-effect relationship (see Glossary) is tenuous. Ask your physician for guidance.

Suggested Periodic Examinations While Taking This Drug (at physician's discretion)
Complete blood cell counts, liver function tests, thyroid function tests, periodic evaluation of heart and circulatory system.

▷ **While Taking This Drug, Observe the Following**
Foods: Follow the diabetic diet prescribed by your physician.
Beverages: As directed in the diabetic diet. May be taken with milk.
▷ *Alcohol:* Use with extreme caution until the combined effect has been determined. Alcohol can exaggerate this drug's hypoglycemic effect. This drug infrequently causes a marked intolerance of alcohol resulting in a disulfiramlike reaction (see Glossary): facial flushing, sweating, palpitation.
Tobacco Smoking: No interactions expected.
▷ *Other Drugs*
The following drugs may ***increase*** the effects of tolbutamide
• aspirin, and other salicylates.

- chloramphenicol (Chloromycetin).
- cimetidine (Tagamet).
- clofibrate (Atromid S).
- fenfluramine (Pondimin).
- monoamine oxidase (MAO) type A inhibitor drugs (see Drug Class, Section Four).
- phenylbutazone (Butazolidin).
- ranitidine (Zantac).
- sulfonamide drugs (see Drug Class, Section Four).

The following drugs may *decrease* the effects of tolbutamide

- beta blocker drugs (see Drug Class, Section Four).
- bumetanide (Bumex).
- diazoxide (Proglycem).
- ethacrynic acid (Edecrin).
- furosemide (Lasix).
- phenytoin (Dilantin).
- rifampin (Rifadin, Rimactane).
- thiazide diuretics (see Drug Class, Section Four).

▷ *Driving, Hazardous Activities:* Regulate your dosage schedule, eating schedule and physical activities very carefully to prevent hypoglycemia. Be able to recognize the early symptoms of hypoglycemia so you can avoid hazardous activities and take corrective measures.

Aviation Note: Diabetes *is a disqualification* for piloting. Consult a designated Aviation Medical Examiner.

Exposure to Sun: Use caution until sensitivity has been determined. Some drugs of this class can cause photosensitivity (see Glossary).

Occurrence of Unrelated Illness: Acute infections, illnesses causing vomiting or diarrhea, serious injuries and surgical procedures can interfere with diabetic control and may require the use of insulin. If any of these conditions occur, consult your physician promptly.

Discontinuation: Because of the possibility of secondary failure, it is advisable to evaluate the continued benefit of this drug every 6 months.

TOLMETIN
(TOHL met in)

Introduced: 1976

Class: Mild analgesic, anti-inflammatory

Prescription: USA: Yes
Canada: Yes

Controlled Drug: USA: No
Canada: No

Available as Generic: No

Brand Names: Tolectin, Tolectin DS

BENEFITS versus RISKS

Possible Benefits	*Possible Risks*
EFFECTIVE RELIEF OF MILD TO MODERATE PAIN AND INFLAMMATION	Gastrointestinal pain, ulceration, bleeding (rare) Rare liver damage Rare kidney damage Rare blood cell disorders: hemolytic anemia, abnormally low white blood cell and platelet counts

---

▷ **Principal Uses**

As a Single Drug Product: Used primarily to relieve mild to moderately severe pain and inflammation associated with (1) acute and chronic rheumatoid arthritis; (2) osteoarthritis; and (3) juvenile rheumatoid arthritis.

How This Drug Works: Not completely established. It is thought that this drug reduces the tissue concentrations of prostaglandins (and related compounds), substances involved in the production of inflammation and pain.

Available Dosage Forms and Strengths
   Capsules — 400 mg
   Tablets — 200 mg

▷ **Usual Adult Dosage Range:**   Initially, 400 mg 3 times/day. For maintenance: adjust dosage from 600 mg to 1600 mg daily as needed, taken in 3 or 4 divided doses. The total daily dosage should not exceed 2000 mg (2.0 grams) for rheumatoid arthritis, or 1600 mg (1.6 grams) for osteoarthritis. **Note: Actual dosage and administration schedule must be determined by the physician for each patient individually.**

▷ **Dosing Instructions:**   Preferably taken on an empty stomach, 1 hour before or 2 hours after eating. However, it may be taken with or after food if necessary to reduce stomach irritation. Take with a full glass of water and remain upright (do not lie down) for 30 minutes. Schedule dosing to include one in the morning and one at bedtime. The capsule may be opened and the tablet may be crushed for administration.

Usual Duration of Use: Continual use on a regular schedule for 1 to 2 weeks is usually necessary to determine this drug's effectiveness in relieving the discomfort of arthritis. Long-term use (months to years) requires supervision and periodic evaluation by your physician. Consult your physician on a regular basis.

▷ **This Drug Should Not Be Taken If**
   • you have had an allergic reaction to it previously.
   • you are subject to asthma or nasal polyps caused by aspirin.

- you have active peptic ulcer disease or any form of gastrointestinal bleeding.
- you have a bleeding disorder or a blood cell disorder.
- you have severe impairment of liver or kidney function.

▷ **Inform Your Physician Before Taking This Drug If**
- you are allergic to aspirin or to other aspirin substitutes.
- you have a history of peptic ulcer disease or any type of bleeding disorder.
- you have impaired liver or kidney function.
- you have high blood pressure or a history of heart failure.
- you are taking any of the following: acetaminophen, aspirin or other aspirin substitutes, anticoagulants, oral antidiabetic drugs.

Possible Side-Effects (natural, expected and unavoidable drug actions)
Fluid retention (edema).
Drowsiness in sensitive individuals.

▷ **Possible Adverse Effects** (unusual, unexpected and infrequent reactions)
If any of the following develop, consult your physician promptly for guidance.
Mild Adverse Effects
Allergic Reactions: Skin rash, hives, itching.
Headache, dizziness, blurred vision, ringing in the ears.
Mouth sores, indigestion, nausea, vomiting, constipation, diarrhea.
Serious Adverse Effects
Allergic Reactions: Anaphylactic reaction (see Glossary), severe skin reactions.
Active peptic ulcer, with or without bleeding.
Liver damage with jaundice (see Glossary).
Kidney damage with painful urination, bloody urine, reduced urine formation.
Abnormally low white blood cell count: fever, sore throat.
Abnormally low blood platelet count: abnormal bleeding or bruising.

▷ **Possible Effects on Sexual Function:**   None reported.

Possible Delayed Adverse Effects: Mild anemia due to "silent" blood loss from the stomach (less than that caused by aspirin).

▷ **Adverse Effects That May Mimic Natural Diseases or Disorders**
Liver reaction may suggest viral hepatitis.

Natural Diseases or Disorders That May Be Activated by This Drug
Peptic ulcer disease, ulcerative colitis.

CAUTION
1. Dosage should always be limited to the smallest amount that produces reasonable improvement.
2. This drug may mask early indications of infection. Inform your physician if you think you are developing an infection of any kind.

Precautions for Use

By Infants and Children: Safety and effectiveness for use by those under 2 years of age have not been established.

By Those over 60 Years of Age: Small doses are advisable until tolerance is determined. Observe for any indications of liver or kidney toxicity, fluid retention, dizziness, confusion, impaired memory, stomach bleeding or constipation.

▷ **Advisability of Use During Pregnancy**

Pregnancy Category: B (tentative). See Pregnancy Code inside back cover.

Animal studies: No birth defects due to this drug reported.

Human studies: Information from adequate studies of pregnant women is not available.

The manufacturer does not recommend the use of this drug during pregnancy.

Advisability of Use if Breast-Feeding

Presence of this drug in breast milk: Unknown.

Avoid drug or refrain from nursing.

Habit-Forming Potential: None.

Effects of Overdosage: Stomach irritation, nausea, vomiting, diarrhea.

Possible Effects of Long-Term Use: Fluid retention.

Suggested Periodic Examinations While Taking This Drug (at physician's discretion)

Complete blood cell counts, liver and kidney function tests, complete eye examinations if vision is altered in any way.

▷ **While Taking This Drug, Observe the Following**

Foods: No restrictions.

Beverages: No restrictions. May be taken with milk.

▷   *Alcohol:* Use with caution. The irritant action of alcohol on the stomach lining, added to the irritant action of this drug in sensitive individuals, can increase the risk of stomach ulceration and/or bleeding.

Tobacco Smoking: No interactions expected.

▷   *Other Drugs*

Tolmetin may ***increase*** the effects of

- acetaminophen (Tylenol, etc.), and increase the risk of kidney damage; avoid prolonged use of this combination.
- anticoagulants (Coumadin, etc.), and increase the risk of bleeding; monitor prothrombin time, adjust dose accordingly.

Tolmetin ***taken concurrently*** with the following drugs may increase the risk of bleeding; avoid these combinations:

- aspirin.
- dipyridamole (Persantine).
- indomethacin (Indocin).
- sulfinpyrazone (Anturane).

- valproic acid (Depakene).

▷ *Driving, Hazardous Activities:* This drug may cause drowsiness or dizziness. Restrict activities as necessary.

Aviation Note: The use of this drug **may be a disqualification** for piloting. Consult a designated Aviation Medical Examiner.

Exposure to Sun: No restrictions.

TRAZODONE
(TRAZ oh dohn)

Introduced: 1967

Prescription: USA: Yes
Canada: Yes

Available as Generic: USA: Yes
Canada: No

Class: Antidepressants

Controlled Drug: USA: No
Canada: No

Brand Name: Desyrel, Trialodine

BENEFITS versus RISKS

Possible Benefits	*Possible Risks*
EFFECTIVE TREATMENT IN ALL TYPES OF DEPRESSIVE ILLNESS, with or without anxiety	Adverse behavioral effects: confusion, disorientation, delusions, hallucinations (all infrequent)
	Potential for inducing heart rhythm disorders (in individuals with heart disease)

▷ **Principal Uses**

As a Single Drug Product: Used to provide symptomatic relief in all types of depression, with or without anxiety or agitation. The primary intent is to initiate restoration of normal mood with a minimum of adverse drug effects.

How This Drug Works: Not completely established. It is thought that this drug increases the availability of the nerve impulse transmitter serotonin within certain brain centers and thereby relieves the symptoms of emotional depression.

Available Dosage Forms and Strengths
Tablets — 50 mg, 100 mg, 150 mg, 300 mg

▷ **Usual Adult Dosage Range:** Initially, 50 mg 3 times/day. The dose may be increased by 50 mg daily at intervals of 3 or 4 days as needed and

tolerated. The total daily dosage should not exceed 400 mg. **Note:
Actual dosage and administration schedule must be determined by
the physician for each patient individually.**

▷ **Dosing Instructions:**   Best taken with food to improve absorption. The tablet may be crushed for administration. If excessive drowsiness or dizziness occurs, it is advisable to take a larger portion of the total daily
dose at bedtime and to divide the remaining amount into 2 or 3
smaller doses to be taken during the day.

Usual Duration of Use: Continual use on a regular schedule for 2 to 4
weeks is usually necessary to determine this drug's effectiveness in
relieving the symptoms of depression. Long-term use (weeks to
months) requires supervision and periodic evaluation by your physician. Consult your physician on a regular basis.

▷ **This Drug Should Not Be Taken If**
  • you have had an allergic reaction to it previously.
  • you are recovering from a recent heart attack (myocardial infarction).
  • you are taking, or have taken within the past 14 days, any monoamine
    oxidase (MAO) type A inhibitor drug (see Drug Class, Section Four).

▷ **Inform Your Physician Before Taking This Drug If**
  • you have a history of any of the following: alcoholism, epilepsy, heart
    disease (especially heart rhythm disorders).
  • you have impaired liver or kidney function.
  • you are taking any antihypertensive drugs.
  • you plan to have surgery under general anesthesia in the near future.

Possible Side-Effects (natural, expected and unavoidable drug actions)
    Drowsiness, light-headedness, blurred vision, dry mouth, constipation.

▷ **Possible Adverse Effects** (unusual, unexpected and infrequent reactions)
    **If any of the following develop, consult your physician promptly for
    guidance.**
    Mild Adverse Effects
    Allergic Reaction: Skin rash.
    Headache, dizziness, fatigue, impaired concentration, nervousness,
      tremors.
    Rapid heart rate, palpitations.
    Peculiar taste, stomach discomfort, nausea, vomiting, diarrhea.
    Muscular aches and pains.
    Serious Adverse Effects
    Behavioral effects: Confusion, anger, hostility, disorientation, impaired
      memory, delusions, hallucinations, nightmares.
    Irregular heart rhythms, low blood pressure, fainting.

▷ **Possible Effects on Sexual Function**
    Decreased male libido; increased female libido.
    Inhibited ejaculation, impotence, priapism (see Glossary).
    Altered timing and pattern of menstruation.

CAUTION
1. If you experience a significant degree of mouth dryness while using this drug, consult your dentist regarding the risk of gum erosion or tooth decay. Ask for his guidance in ways to keep the mouth comfortably moist.
2. It is advisable to withhold this drug if electroconvulsive therapy (ECT) is to be used.

Precautions for Use
By Infants and Children: Safety and effectiveness for use by those under 18 years of age have not been established.

By Those over 60 Years of Age: During the first two weeks of treatment, observe for the development of restlessness, agitation, excitement, forgetfulness, confusion or disorientation. Be aware of possible unsteadiness and incoordination that may predispose to falling. This drug may enhance prostatism (see Glossary).

▷ **Advisability of Use During Pregnancy**
Pregnancy Category: C (tentative). See Pregnancy Code inside back cover.
Animal studies: Fetal deaths and birth defects reported.
Human studies: Information from adequate studies of pregnant women is not available.
Avoid this drug completely during the first 3 months. Use otherwise only if clearly needed. Ask your physician for guidance.

Advisability of Use if Breast-Feeding
Presence of this drug in breast milk: Yes.
Avoid drug or refrain from nursing.

Habit-Forming Potential: None.

Effects of Overdosage: Marked drowsiness, weakness, confusion, tremors, low blood pressure, rapid heart rate, stupor, coma, possible seizures.

Possible Effects of Long-Term Use: None reported.

Suggested Periodic Examinations While Taking This Drug (at physician's discretion)
Complete blood cell counts. (This drug may cause slight reductions in white blood cell counts. This should be monitored closely if infection, sore throat or fever develops.)
Serial blood pressure readings and electrocardiograms.

▷ **While Taking This Drug, Observe the Following**
Foods: No restrictions.
Beverages: No restrictions. May be taken with milk.
▷ *Alcohol:* Avoid completely. This drug can increase markedly the intoxicating effects of alcohol and accentuate its depressant action on brain functions.
Tobacco Smoking: No interactions expected.

▷ *Other Drugs*

Trazodone may *increase* the effects of

- antihypertensive drugs, and cause excessive lowering of blood pressure; dosage adjustments may be necessary.
- drugs with sedative effects, and cause excessive sedation.
- phenytoin (Dilantin), by raising its blood level; observe for phenytoin toxicity.

▷ *Driving, Hazardous Activities:* This drug may cause dizziness or drowsiness. Restrict activities as necessary.

Aviation Note: The use of this drug *is a disqualification* for piloting. Consult a designated Aviation Medical Examiner.

Exposure to Sun: No restrictions.

Discontinuation: It is advisable to discontinue this drug gradually. Ask your physician for guidance in dosage reduction over an appropriate period of time.

TRIAMTERENE
(tri AM ter een)

Introduced: 1964

Class: Diuretic

Prescription: USA: Yes
Canada: Yes

Controlled Drug: USA: No
Canada: No

Available as Generic: No

Brand Names: ✦Apo-Triazide [CD], Dyazide [CD], Dyrenium, Maxzide [CD], Maxzide-25 [CD], ✦Novotriamzide [CD]

BENEFITS versus RISKS	
Possible Benefits	*Possible Risks*
EFFECTIVE PREVENTION OF POTASSIUM LOSS when used adjunctively with other diuretics EFFECTIVE DIURETIC IN REFRACTORY CASES OF FLUID RETENTION when used adjunctively with other diuretics	ABNORMALLY HIGH BLOOD POTASSIUM LEVEL with excessive use Rare blood cell disorders: megaloblastic anemia, abnormally low white blood cell and platelet counts

▷ **Principal Uses**

As a Single Drug Product: This mild diuretic is used as part of the treatment program for the management of congestive heart failure and disorders of the liver and kidney that are accompanied by excessive fluid retention (edema). It is also used in conjunction with other measures to treat high blood pressure. It is used primarily in situations where it is advisable to prevent loss of potassium from the body.

As a Combination Drug Product [CD]: This drug is available in combination with hydrochlorothiazide, a different kind of diuretic that promotes the loss of potassium from the body. Triamterene is used in this combination to counteract the potassium-wasting effect of the thiazide diuretic.

How This Drug Works: Not completely established. It is thought that by inhibiting the enzyme system that initiates the sodium-potassium exchange process, this drug prevents the reabsorption of sodium and the excretion of potassium by the kidney. Thus the drug promotes the excretion of sodium (and water with it) and the retention of potassium.

Available Dosage Forms and Strengths
Capsules — 50 mg, 100 mg

▷ **Usual Adult Dosage Range:**   Initially, 100 mg twice daily. The dose is then adjusted according to individual response. The usual maintenance dose is 100 to 200 mg/day, divided into 2 doses. The total daily dosage should not exceed 300 mg. **Note: Actual dosage and administration schedule must be determined by the physician for each patient individually.**

▷ **Dosing Instructions:**   May be taken with or following meals to promote absorption of the drug and to reduce stomach irritation. The capsule may be opened for administration. Intermittent or alternate-day use is recommended to minimize the possibility of sodium and potassium imbalance.

Usual Duration of Use: Continual use on a regular schedule for 3 to 5 days is usually necessary to determine this drug's effectiveness in clearing edema, and for 2 to 3 weeks to determine its effect on hypertension. Long-term use (months to years) requires supervision and periodic evaluation by your physician. Consult your physician on a regular basis.

▷ **This Drug Should Not Be Taken If**
  • you have had an allergic reaction to it previously.
  • you have severely impaired liver or kidney function.

▷ **Inform Your Physician Before Taking This Drug If**
  • you have a history of liver or kidney disease.
  • you have diabetes or gout.
  • you are taking any of the following: antihypertensives, a digitalis preparation, another diuretic, lithium or a potassium preparation.
  • you plan to have surgery under general anesthesia in the near future.

Possible Side-Effects (natural, expected and unavoidable drug actions)
> With excessive use: abnormally high blood potassium levels, abnormally low blood sodium levels, dehydration.
> Blue coloration of the urine (of no significance).

▷ **Possible Adverse Effects** (unusual, unexpected and infrequent reactions)
> **If any of the following develop, consult your physician promptly for guidance.**

Mild Adverse Effects
Allergic Reactions: Skin rash, itching.
Headache, dizziness, unsteadiness, weakness, drowsiness, lethargy.
Dry mouth, nausea, vomiting, diarrhea.

Serious Adverse Effects
Allergic Reaction: Anaphylactic reaction (see Glossary).
Symptomatic potassium excess: confusion, numbness and tingling in lips and extremities, fatigue, weakness, shortness of breath, slow heart rate, low blood pressure.
Rare blood cell disorders: megaloblastic anemia, causing weakness and fatigue; abnormally low white blood cell count, causing infection, fever or sore throat; abnormally low blood platelet count, causing abnormal bleeding or bruising.

▷ **Possible Effects on Sexual Function:**   None reported.

CAUTION
> 1. Do not take potassium supplements or increase your intake of potassium-rich foods while taking this drug.
> 2. Do not discontinue this drug abruptly unless abnormally high blood levels of potassium develop.
> 3. Avoid the liberal use of salt substitutes that contain potassium; these are a potential cause of potassium excess.

Precautions for Use
By Infants and Children: This drug is not recommended for use in children.
By Those over 60 Years of Age: The natural decline in kidney function may predispose to potassium retention in the body. Limit continual use of this drug to periods of 2 to 3 weeks. Observe for indications of potassium excess: slow heart rate, irregular heart rhythms, low blood pressure, confusion, drowsiness. The excessive use of diuretics can cause harmful loss of body water (dehydration), increased viscosity of the blood and an increased tendency of the blood to clot, predisposing to stroke, heart attack or thrombophlebitis.

▷ **Advisability of Use During Pregnancy**
Pregnancy Category: B (tentative). See Pregnancy Code inside back cover.
Animal studies: No birth defects due to this drug reported.
Human studies: Information from adequate studies of pregnant women is not available.

This drug should not be used during pregnancy unless a very serious complication of pregnancy occurs for which this drug is significantly beneficial.

Advisability of Use if Breast-Feeding
Presence of this drug in breast milk: Yes.
Avoid drug or refrain from nursing.

Habit-Forming Potential: None.

Effects of Overdosage: Thirst, drowsiness, fatigue, weakness, nausea, vomiting, confusion, irregular heart rhythm, low blood pressure.

Possible Effects of Long-Term Use: Potassium accumulation to abnormally high blood levels.

Suggested Periodic Examinations While Taking This Drug (at physician's discretion)
Complete blood cell counts.
Measurements of blood sodium, potassium and chloride levels.
Kidney function tests.

▷ **While Taking This Drug, Observe the Following**
Foods: No restrictions. Avoid excessive restriction of salt.
Beverages: No restrictions. May be taken with milk.
▷ *Alcohol:* Use with caution until the combined effects have been determined. Alcohol may enhance the drowsiness and the blood-pressure-lowering effect of this drug.
Tobacco Smoking: No interactions expected.
▷ *Other Drugs*
Triamterene may ***increase*** the effects of
• amantadine (Symmetrel).
• digoxin (Lanoxin).
Triamterene ***taken concurrently*** with
• captopril (Capoten) may cause excessively high blood potassium levels.
• indomethacin (Indocin) may increase the risk of kidney damage.
• lithium may cause accumulation of lithium to toxic levels.
• potassium preparations may cause excessively high blood potassium levels.
▷ *Driving, Hazardous Activities:* This drug may cause dizziness and drowsiness. Restrict activities as necessary.
Aviation Note: The use of this drug ***may be a disqualification*** for piloting. Consult a designated Aviation Medical Examiner.
Exposure to Sun: Use caution until your sensitivity has been determined. This drug may cause photosensitivity (see Glossary).
Discontinuation: With high dosage or prolonged use, it is advisable to withdraw this drug gradually. Sudden discontinuation may cause rebound potassium excretion and resultant potassium deficiency. Ask your physician for guidance.

TRIAZOLAM
(tri AY zoh lam)

Introduced: 1974

Prescription: USA: Yes
Canada: Yes

Available as Generic: USA: No
Canada: No

Brand Name: Halcion

Class: Hypnotic, benzodiazepines

Controlled Drug: USA: C-IV*
Canada: No

BENEFITS versus RISKS

Possible Benefits	*Possible Risks*
EFFECTIVE HYPNOTIC with short duration of action	Habit-forming potential with long-term use
Wide margin of safety with therapeutic doses	Minor impairment of mental functions ("hangover" effect)

▷ **Principal Uses**

As a Single Drug Product: This member of the benzodiazepine class of "minor tranquilizers" is used exclusively as a bedtime sedative to induce sleep. It is useful in the short-term management of insomnia characterized by difficulty in falling asleep, frequent awakenings during the night and early morning awakening.

How This Drug Works: It is thought that this drug produces a calming effect by enhancing the action of the nerve transmitter gamma-aminobutyric acid (GABA), which in turn blocks the arousal of higher brain centers and helps to induce sleep.

Available Dosage Forms and Strengths

Tablets — 0.125 mg, 0.25 mg, 0.5 mg

▷ **Usual Adult Dosage Range:** 0.125 to 0.5 mg at bedtime. The total daily dosage should not exceed 0.5 mg. **Note: Actual dosage and administration schedule must be determined by the physician for each patient individually.**

▷ **Dosing Instructions:** Preferably taken on an empty stomach to hasten absorption and induce sleep rapidly. The tablet may be crushed for administration. Do not discontinue this drug abruptly if taken for more than 4 weeks.

Usual Duration of Use: Periods of 3 to 5 nights intermittently, repeated as needed with appropriate dosage adjustment. Avoid uninterrupted

*See Schedules of Controlled Drugs inside back cover.

and prolonged use. The duration of use should not exceed 2 weeks without reappraisal of continued need.

▷ **This Drug Should Not Be Taken If**
  • you have had an allergic reaction to it previously.

▷ **Inform Your Physician Before Taking This Drug If**
  • you are allergic to any benzodiazepine drug (see Drug Class, Section Four).
  • you have a history of alcoholism or drug abuse.
  • you are pregnant or planning pregnancy.
  • you have impaired liver or kidney function.
  • you have a history of serious depression or mental disorder.
  • you are taking other drugs with sedative effects.
  • you have any of the following: asthma, emphysema, epilepsy, myasthenia gravis.

Possible Side-Effects (natural, expected and unavoidable drug actions)
  "Hangover" effects on arising: drowsiness (14%), lethargy and unsteadiness (4.6%).

▷ **Possible Adverse Effects** (unusual, unexpected and infrequent reactions)
  If any of the following develop, consult your physician promptly for guidance.
  Mild Adverse Effects
  Allergic Reactions: Skin rash, itching.
  Headache, dizziness, fatigue, blurred vision.
  Nausea, indigestion, constipation, diarrhea.
  Serious Adverse Effects
  Idiosyncratic Reactions: Nervousness, talkativeness, irritability, apprehension, euphoria, excitement, hallucinations.
  Confusion, mental depression.

▷ **Possible Effects on Sexual Function:**   None reported.

CAUTION
  1. This drug should not be discontinued abruptly if it has been taken continually for more than 4 weeks.
  2. The concurrent use of some over-the-counter drug products that contain antihistamines (allergy and cold preparations, sleep aids) can cause excessive sedation in sensitive individuals.
  3. Regular nightly use of any hypnotic drug should be avoided.
  4. If you experience a "hangover" effect, avoid hazardous activities (driving, etc.) and the use of alcohol.

Precautions for Use
  By Infants and Children: Safety and effectiveness for use by those under 18 years of age have not been established.
  By Those over 60 Years of Age: It is advisable to use smaller doses (0.125 mg) at first to determine your response. Observe for the possible de-

velopment of lethargy, indifference, fatigue, weakness, unsteadiness, disturbing dreams, nightmares and paradoxical reactions of excitement, agitation, anger, hostility and rage.

▷ **Advisability of Use During Pregnancy**
Pregnancy Category: X (tentative). See Pregnancy Code inside back cover.
Animal studies: Benzodiazepines cause significant birth defects in test animals.
Human studies: Information from adequate studies of pregnant women is not available.
Avoid use during entire pregnancy.

Advisability of Use if Breast-Feeding
Presence of this drug in breast milk: Probably yes.
Avoid drug or refrain from nursing.

Habit-Forming Potential: This drug can produce psychological and/or physical dependence (see Glossary) if used in large doses for an extended period of time. Avoid continual use.

Effects of Overdosage: Marked drowsiness, weakness, feeling of drunkenness, staggering gait, tremor, stupor progressing to deep sleep or coma.

Possible Effects of Long-Term Use: Psychological and/or physical dependence.

Suggested Periodic Examinations While Taking This Drug (at physician's discretion)
Complete blood cell counts during long-term use.

▷ **While Taking This Drug, Observe the Following**
Foods: No restrictions.
Beverages: Avoid excessive intake of caffeine-containing beverages (coffee, tea, cola) within 4 hours of taking this drug. May be taken with milk.
▷ *Alcohol:* Use with extreme caution until the combined effect has been determined. Alcohol may increase the absorption of this drug and add to its depressant effects on the brain. It is advisable to avoid alcohol completely throughout the day and night if it is necessary to drive or to engage in any hazardous activity.
Tobacco Smoking: Heavy smoking may reduce the hypnotic action of this drug.
Marijuana Smoking: Increased sedation and significant impairment of intellectual and physical performance.
▷ *Other Drugs*
Triazolam may *increase* the effects of
• digoxin (Lanoxin), and cause digoxin toxicity.
• phenytoin (Dilantin), and cause phenytoin toxicity.
Triazolam may *decrease* the effects of
• levodopa (Sinemet, etc.), and reduce its effectiveness in treating Parkinson's disease.

The following drugs may *increase* the effects of triazolam
- cimetidine (Tagamet).
- disulfiram (Antabuse).
- isoniazid (INH, Rifamate, etc.).
- oral contraceptives.
- valproic acid (Depakene).

The following drugs may *decrease* the effects of triazolam
- rifampin (Rimactane, etc.).
- theophylline (Aminophylline, Theo-Dur, etc.).

▷ *Driving, Hazardous Activities:* This drug can impair mental alertness, judgment, physical coordination and reaction time. Avoid hazardous activities accordingly.

Aviation Note: The use of this drug *is a disqualification* for piloting. Consult a designated Aviation Medical Examiner.

Exposure to Sun: No restrictions.

Exposure to Heat: Use caution until the effect of excessive perspiration is determined. Because of reduced urine volume, this drug may accumulate in the body and produce effects of overdosage.

Discontinuation: Avoid sudden discontinuation if this drug has been taken for over 4 weeks without interruption. Dosage should be tapered gradually to prevent a withdrawal syndrome that could include depression, confusion, hallucinations, tremor, seizures, muscle cramping, sweating and vomiting.

TRIFLUOPERAZINE
(tri floo oh PER a zeen)

Introduced: 1958

Class: Strong tranquilizer, phenothiazines

Prescription: USA: Yes
Canada: Yes

Controlled Drug: USA: No
Canada: No

Available as Generic: USA: Yes
Canada: No

Brand Names: ✦Apo-Trifluoperazine, ✦Novoflurazine, ✦Solazine, Stelazine, Suprazine, ✦Terfluzine

---

BENEFITS versus RISKS

Possible Benefits	*Possible Risks*
EFFECTIVE CONTROL OF ACUTE MENTAL DISORDERS in the majority of patients: beneficial effects on thinking, mood and behavior	SERIOUS TOXIC EFFECTS ON BRAIN with long-term use Liver damage with jaundice (infrequent) Rare blood cell disorders: abnormally low red and white blood cell and platelet counts

---

▷ **Principal Uses**

As a Single Drug Product: This antipsychotic drug is used primarily to treat psychotic thinking and behavior associated with acute psychoses of unknown nature, mania, paranoid states and acute schizophrenia. It is most effective in those who are withdrawn and apathetic and in those with agitation, delusions and hallucinations.

How This Drug Works: Not completely established. Present theory is that by inhibiting the action of dopamine, this drug acts to correct an imbalance of nerve impulse transmissions that is thought to be responsible for certain mental disorders.

Available Dosage Forms and Strengths
    Concentrate — 10 mg per ml
      Injection — 2 mg per ml
        Tablets — 1 mg, 2 mg, 5 mg, 10 mg

▷ **Usual Adult Dosage Range:**   Initially, 1 or 2 mg twice daily. The dose may be increased by 1 or 2 mg at 3- to 4-day intervals as needed and tolerated. Usual dosage range is 10 to 30 mg daily. The total daily dosage should not exceed 40 mg. **Note: Actual dosage and administration schedule must be determined by the physician for each patient individually.**

▷ **Dosing Instructions:**   May be taken with or following meals to reduce stomach irritation. The tablets may be crushed for administration.

Usual Duration of Use: Continual use on a regular schedule for several weeks is usually necessary to determine this drug's effectiveness in controlling psychotic disorders. If not significantly beneficial within 6 weeks, it should be discontinued. Long-term use (months to years) requires periodic evaluation of response, appropriate dosage adjustment and consideration of continued need. Consult your physician on a regular basis.

▷ **This Drug Should Not Be Taken If**
  • you are allergic to any of the drugs bearing the brand names listed above.
  • you have active liver disease.
  • you have cancer of the breast.
  • you have a current blood cell or bone marrow disorder.

▷ **Inform Your Physician Before Taking This Drug If**
  • you are allergic or abnormally sensitive to any phenothiazine drug (see Drug Class, Section Four).
  • you have impaired liver or kidney function.
  • you have any type of seizure disorder.
  • you have diabetes, glaucoma or heart disease.
  • you have a history of lupus erythematosus.
  • you are taking any drug with sedative effects.

- you plan to have surgery under general or spinal anesthesia in the near future.

Possible Side-Effects (natural, expected and unavoidable drug actions)
Drowsiness (usually during the first 2 weeks), orthostatic hypotension (see Glossary), blurred vision, dry mouth, nasal congestion, constipation, impaired urination.
Pink or purple coloration of urine, of no significance.

▷ **Possible Adverse Effects** (unusual, unexpected and infrequent reactions)
If any of the following develop, consult your physician promptly for guidance.
Mild Adverse Effects
Allergic Reactions: Skin rash, hives, low-grade fever.
Lowering of body temperature, especially in the elderly. (See Hypothermia in Glossary.)
Increased appetite and weight gain.
Dizziness, weakness, agitation, insomnia, impaired day and night vision.
Chronic constipation, fecal impaction.
Serious Adverse Effects
Allergic Reactions: Hepatitis with jaundice (see Glossary), severe skin reactions, anaphylactic reaction (see Glossary).
Depression, disorientation, seizures, loss of peripheral vision.
Rapid heart rate, heart rhythm disorders.
Blood cell disorders: significant reduction in all cellular elements of the blood (reduced counts of red cells, white cells and blood platelets).
Nervous system reactions: Parkinson-like disorders (see Glossary), severe restlessness, muscle spasms involving the face and neck, tardive dyskinesia (see Glossary) (10% to 20%).

▷ **Possible Effects on Sexual Function**
Altered timing and pattern of menstruation.
Male breast enlargement and tenderness.
Female breast enlargement with milk production.
Spontaneous male orgasm, paradoxical (1 case reported).
Inhibited ejaculation, painful ejaculation, priapism (see Glossary).
Delayed female orgasm.
False positive pregnancy test result.

▷ **Adverse Effects That May Mimic Natural Diseases or Disorders**
Nervous system reactions may suggest true Parkinson's disease.
Liver reactions may suggest viral hepatitis.
Reactions resembling systemic lupus erythematosus may occur.

Natural Diseases or Disorders That May Be Activated by This Drug
Latent epilepsy, glaucoma, diabetes mellitus, prostatism (see Glossary).

CAUTION
1. Many over-the-counter medications (see OTC Drugs in Glossary) for allergies, colds and coughs contain drugs that can interact unfa-

vorably with this drug. Ask your physician or pharmacist for guidance before using any such medications.

2. Antacids that contain aluminum and/or magnesium may prevent the absorption of this drug and reduce its effectiveness.
3. Obtain prompt evaluation of any change or disturbance of vision.

Precautions for Use

By Infants and Children: Use of this drug is not recommended in children under 6 years of age. Do not use this drug in the presence of symptoms suggestive of Reye syndrome (see Glossary). Children with acute infectious diseases ("flulike" infections, chicken pox, measles, etc.) are more prone to develop muscular spasms of the face, back and extremities when this drug is given.

By Those over 60 Years of Age: Small doses are advisable until individual response has been determined. You may be more susceptible to the development of drowsiness, lethargy, constipation, lowering of body temperature (hypothermia) and orthostatic hypotension (see Glossary). This drug may enhance existing prostatism (see Glossary). You may also be more susceptible to the development of Parkinson-like reactions and/or tardive dyskinesia (see discussion of these terms in Glossary). These reactions must be recognized early since they may become unresponsive to treatment and irreversible.

▷ Advisability of Use During Pregnancy

Pregnancy Category: C (tentative). See Pregnancy Code inside back cover.
Animal studies: Significant birth defects reported in mouse and rat studies.
Human studies: No increase in birth defects reported in 700 exposures. Information from adequate studies of pregnant women is not available.
Avoid drug during the first 3 months; avoid during the last month because of possible adverse effects on the newborn infant.

Advisability of Use if Breast-Feeding

Presence of this drug in breast milk: Yes, in minute amounts.
Monitor nursing infant closely and discontinue drug or nursing if adverse effects develop.

Habit-Forming Potential: None.

Effects of Overdosage: Marked drowsiness, weakness, tremor, agitation, unsteadiness, deep sleep, coma, convulsions.

Possible Effects of Long-Term Use: Tardive dyskinesia (see Glossary).

Suggested Periodic Examinations While Taking This Drug (at physician's discretion)

Complete blood cell counts, especially between the fourth and tenth weeks of treatment.
Liver function tests, electrocardiograms.

Complete eye examinations—eye structures and vision.

Careful inspection of the tongue for early evidence of fine, involuntary, wavelike movements that could indicate the beginning of tardive dyskinesia.

▷ **While Taking This Drug, Observe the Following**

Foods: No restrictions.

Nutritional Support: A riboflavin (vitamin B-2) supplement should be taken with long-term use.

Beverages: No restrictions. May be taken with milk.

▷   *Alcohol:* Avoid completely. Alcohol can increase the sedative action of phenothiazines and accentuate their depressant effects on brain function and blood pressure. Phenothiazines can increase the intoxicating effects of alcohol.

Tobacco Smoking: Possible reduction of drowsiness from drug.

Marijuana Smoking: Moderate increase in drowsiness; accentuation of orthostatic hypotension; increased risk of precipitating latent psychoses, confusing the interpretation of mental status and drug responses.

▷   *Other Drugs*

Trifluoperazine may ***increase*** the effects of

* all sedative drugs, especially narcotic analgesics, and cause excessive sedation.
* all atropinelike drugs, and cause nervous system toxicity.

Trifluoperazine may ***decrease*** the effects of

* guanethidine (Ismelin, Esimil), and reduce its effectiveness in lowering blood pressure.

Trifluoperazine ***taken concurrently*** with

* lithium (Lithobid, Lithotabs) may impair the effectiveness of lithium and cause nervous system toxicity.

The following drugs may ***decrease*** the effects of trifluoperazine

* antacids containing aluminum and/or magnesium.
* barbiturates (see Drug Class, Section Four).
* benztropine (Cogentin).
* disulfiram (Antabuse).
* trihexyphenidyl (Artane).

▷   *Driving, Hazardous Activities:* This drug can impair mental alertness, judgment and physical coordination. Avoid hazardous activities.

Aviation Note: The use of this drug ***is a disqualification*** for piloting. Consult a designated Aviation Medical Examiner.

Exposure to Sun: Use caution until sensitivity has been determined. Some phenothiazines can cause photosensitivity (see Glossary).

Exposure to Heat: Use caution and avoid excessive heat as much as possible. This drug may impair the regulation of body temperature and increase the risk of heat stroke.

Exposure to Cold: Use caution and dress warmly. This drug can increase the risk of hypothermia in the elderly.

Discontinuation: After a period of long-term use, do not discontinue this drug suddenly. Gradual withdrawal over 2 to 3 weeks under physician supervision is recommended. Do not discontinue this drug without your physician's knowledge and approval. The relapse rate of schizophrenia after discontinuation is 50% to 60%.

TRIMETHOBENZAMIDE
(tri meth oh BEN za mide)

Introduced: 1959

Class: Antiemetic

Prescription: USA: Yes

Controlled Drug: USA: No

Available as Generic: Yes

Brand Names: Arrestin, Hymetic, T-Gen, Tigan

BENEFITS versus RISKS	
Possible Benefits	*Possible Risks*
Possibly effective prevention and control of nausea and vomiting in selected disorders	TOXIC EFFECTS ON BRAIN: disorientation, Parkinson-like tremors, muscle spasms and rigidity, seizures Rare liver damage Rare blood cell disorders: abnormally low white blood cell count

▷ **Principal Uses**

As a Single Drug Product: Used exclusively for the control of nausea and vomiting associated with motion sickness, inner ear infections, Meniere's syndrome, surgery and radiation therapy. It is not as effective as the phenothiazines in relieving nausea and preventing vomiting, but it is significantly safer to use for long-term therapy.

How This Drug Works: Not completely established. It is thought that this drug relieves nausea and prevents vomiting by suppressing the transmission of nerve impulses to the vomiting centers in the brain.

Available Dosage Forms and Strengths
     Capsules — 100 mg, 250 mg
     Injection — 100 mg per ml
  Suppositories — 100 mg, 200 mg

▷ **Usual Adult Dosage Range:** 250 mg every 4 to 6 hours as needed. The total daily dosage should not exceed 1000 mg. **Note: Actual dosage and**

administration schedule must be determined by the physician for each patient individually.

▷ **Dosing Instructions:** May be taken without regard to food. The capsule may be opened for administration.

Usual Duration of Use: Continual use on a regular schedule for 24 to 48 hours is usually necessary to determine this drug's effectiveness in controlling nausea and vomiting. If this drug is not effective within 3 days, it should be discontinued. Long-term use requires supervision and periodic evaluation by your physician. Consult your physician on a regular basis.

▷ **This Drug Should Not Be Taken If**
- you have had an allergic reaction to it previously.
- you have any symptoms suggestive of Reye syndrome (see Glossary).
- you have active liver disease.
- you have any type of blood cell or bone marrow disorder.

▷ **Inform Your Physician Before Taking This Drug If**
- you have had any unfavorable reactions to antihistamine drugs in the past.
- you have impaired liver or kidney function.
- you have a seizure disorder.
- you have any type of parkinsonism.
- you have a history of blood cell or bone marrow disorders, especially one induced by drugs.

Possible Side-Effects (natural, expected and unavoidable drug actions)
Drowsiness.
Temporary drop in blood pressure when given by injection.

▷ **Possible Adverse Effects** (unusual, unexpected and infrequent reactions)
If any of the following develop, consult your physician promptly for guidance.
Mild Adverse Effects
Allergic Reaction: Skin rash.
Headache, dizziness, blurred vision, muscle spasms.
Diarrhea.
Serious Adverse Effects
Nervous system reactions: mental depression, disorientation, seizures, Parkinson-like syndrome (see Glossary).
Liver damage with jaundice (see Glossary).
Blood cell disorder: abnormally low white blood cell count, causing infections, fever, sore throat.

▷ **Possible Effects on Sexual Function:** None reported.

▷ **Adverse Effects That May Mimic Natural Diseases or Disorders**
Liver reaction may suggest viral hepatitis.

Natural Diseases or Disorders That May Be Activated by This Drug
Reye syndrome (see Glossary).

CAUTION
1. The suppository form of this drug contains 2% benzocaine; it should not be used by anyone who is allergic to benzocaine or related local anesthetics.
2. This drug has a toxicity pattern similar to the phenothiazines. It may lower the seizure threshold in epileptic individuals. Observe closely for any change in seizure patterns.

Precautions for Use
By Infants and Children: Do not use this drug in children of any age with symptoms suggestive of Reye syndrome or with illnesses that predispose to Reye syndrome (see Glossary). Children with "flulike" infections, measles, chicken pox, etc. are very susceptible to adverse effects when this drug is given to control nausea or vomiting.
By Those over 60 Years of Age: Observe closely for excessive sedation, weakness, unsteadiness or tendency to fall. Take precautions to prevent injury.

▷ **Advisability of Use During Pregnancy**
Pregnancy Category: B (tentative). See Pregnancy Code inside back cover.
Animal studies: No birth defects reported in rat and rabbit studies.
Human studies: No increase in birth defects reported in 700 exposures to this drug. Information from adequate studies of pregnant women is not available.
Avoid use of drug during the first 3 months if possible. Use it otherwise only if clearly needed. Ask your physician for guidance.

Advisability of Use if Breast-Feeding
Presence of this drug in breast milk: Unknown.
Avoid drug or refrain from nursing.

Habit-Forming Potential: None.

Effects of Overdosage: Drowsiness, weakness, incoordination, muscle spasms in neck and extremities, confusion, disorientation, seizures, coma.

Possible Effects of Long-Term Use: None reported.

Suggested Periodic Examinations While Taking This Drug (at physician's discretion)
Complete blood cell counts, liver function tests.

▷ **While Taking This Drug, Observe the Following**
Foods: No restrictions.
Beverages: No restrictions. May be taken with milk.
▷   *Alcohol:* Avoid completely. Alcohol may increase the depressant effects of this drug on brain function.

Tobacco Smoking: No interactions expected.

▷ *Other Drugs*
   Trimethobenzamide may ***increase*** the effects of
   • other drugs with sedative effects, and cause excessive sedation; con-
     current use may provoke other reactions of nervous system toxicity:
     severe spasms of neck and back muscles, seizures and coma.

▷ *Driving, Hazardous Activities:* This drug may cause dizziness and drowsiness. Restrict activities as necessary.
   Aviation Note: The use of this drug ***is a disqualification*** for piloting. Consult a designated Aviation Medical Examiner.
   Exposure to Sun: No restrictions.

TRIMETHOPRIM
(tri METH oh prim)

Introduced: 1966

Class: Anti-infective

Prescription: USA: Yes
    Canada: Yes

Controlled Drug: USA: No
    Canada: No

Available as Generic: USA: Yes
    Canada: No

Brand Names: ✦Apo-Sulfatrim [CD], ✦Apo-Sulfatrim DS [CD], Bactrim
[CD], Bactrim DS [CD], Bethaprim [CD], Comoxol [CD], ✦Coptin
[CD], Cotrim [CD], ✦Novotrimel [CD], ✦Novotrimel DS [CD], Prolo-
prim, ✦Protrin [CD], ✦Protrin DF [CD], ✦Roubac [CD], Septra [CD],
Septra DS [CD], Trimpex, Uroplus DS [CD], Uroplus SS [CD]

BENEFITS versus RISKS

Possible Benefits	*Possible Risks*
EFFECTIVE TREATMENT OF INFECTIONS due to susceptible microorganisms	Rare blood cell disorders: megaloblastic anemia, methemoglobinemia, abnormally low white blood cell and platelet counts

---

▷ **Principal Uses**
   As a Single Drug Product: Used primarily to treat the initial episode of
   certain infections of the urinary tract that are not complicated by the
   presence of kidney stones or obstructions to the normal flow of urine.
   It is sometimes used to prevent the recurrence of such infections.

As a Combination Drug Product [CD]: This drug is available in combination with sulfamethoxazole; the generic name co-trimoxazole is used in some countries to identify this combination. It is very effective in the treatment of certain urinary tract infections, middle ear infections, chronic bronchitis, acute enteritis and certain types of pneumonia.

How This Drug Works: This drug prevents the growth and multiplication of susceptible infecting organisms by inactivating the enzyme systems that are necessary for the formation of essential nuclear elements and cell proteins.

Available Dosage Forms and Strengths

        Tablets — 100 mg, 200 mg
        Tablets — 80 mg combined with 400 mg of sulfamethoxazole
        Tablets — 160 mg combined with 800 mg of sulfamethoxazole
  Oral suspension — 40 mg combined with 200 mg of sulfamethoxazole per 5-ml teaspoonful

▷ **Usual Adult Dosage Range:**   100 mg every 12 hours for 10 days. For certain pneumonias, the same dose is given every 6 hours. The total daily dosage should not exceed 640 mg. **Note: Actual dosage and administration schedule must be determined by the physician for each patient individually.**

▷ **Dosing Instructions:**   May be taken without regard to meals. However, it may also be taken with or following food if necessary to reduce stomach irritation. The tablet may be crushed for administration.

Usual Duration of Use: Continual use on a regular schedule for 7 to 14 days is usually necessary to determine this drug's effectiveness in controlling responsive infections. The actual duration of use will depend upon the nature of the infection.

Currently a "Drug of Choice" (when combined with sulfamethoxazole) for preventing pneumonia (due to pneumocystis carinii) in patients with AIDS.

▷ **This Drug Should Not Be Taken If**
  • you have had an allergic reaction to it previously.
  • you have an anemia due to folic acid deficiency.

▷ **Inform Your Physician Before Taking This Drug If**
  • you have a history of folic acid deficiency.
  • you have impaired liver or kidney function.
  • you are pregnant or breast-feeding.

Possible Side-Effects (natural, expected and unavoidable drug actions)
None with short-term use.

▷ **Possible Adverse Effects** (unusual, unexpected and infrequent reactions)
  If any of the following develop, consult your physician promptly for guidance.
  Mild Adverse Effects
    Allergic Reactions: Skin rash (2.9%), itching, drug fever.
    Headache, abnormal taste, sore mouth or tongue, loss of appetite, nausea, vomiting, abdominal cramping, diarrhea.
  Serious Adverse Effects
    Allergic Reactions: Severe dermatitis with peeling of skin.
    Blood cell disorders: megaloblastic anemia, methemoglobinemia, abnormally low white blood cell and platelet counts. (All are rare.)

▷ **Possible Effects on Sexual Function:** None reported.

CAUTION
  1. Certain strains of bacteria that cause urinary tract infections can develop resistance to this drug. If you do not show significant improvement within 10 days, consult your physician.
  2. Comply with your physician's request for periodic blood counts during long-term therapy.

Precautions for Use
  By Infants and Children: Safety and effectiveness for use by those under 2 months of age have not been established.
  By Those over 60 Years of Age: The natural decline in liver and kidney function may require smaller doses. If you develop itching reactions in the genital or anal areas, report this promptly.

▷ **Advisability of Use During Pregnancy**
  Pregnancy Category: C (tentative). See Pregnancy Code inside back cover.
    Animal studies: Birth defects due to this drug reported in rat and rabbit studies.
    Human studies: Information from adequate studies of pregnant women is not available.
    Avoid use of drug during the first 3 months and during the last 2 weeks of pregnancy. Use this drug otherwise only if clearly needed. Ask your physician for guidance.

Advisability of Use if Breast-Feeding
  Presence of this drug in breast milk: Yes.
  Avoid drug or refrain from nursing.

Habit-Forming Potential: None.

Effects of Overdosage: Headache, dizziness, confusion, depression, nausea, vomiting, bone marrow depression, possible liver toxicity with jaundice.

Possible Effects of Long-Term Use: Impaired production of red and white blood cells and blood platelets.

Suggested Periodic Examinations While Taking This Drug (at physician's
discretion)
Complete blood cell counts.

▷ **While Taking This Drug, Observe the Following**
Foods: No restrictions.
Beverages: No restrictions. May be taken with milk.
▷   *Alcohol:* No interactions expected.
Tobacco Smoking: No interactions expected.
▷   *Other Drugs*
Trimethoprim may ***increase*** the effects of
• phenytoin (Dilantin), and cause phenytoin toxicity.
The following drugs may ***decrease*** the effects of trimethoprim
• rifampin (Rifadin, Rimactane).
▷   *Driving, Hazardous Activities:* No restrictions.
Aviation Note: The use of this drug is probably not a disqualification for
piloting. Consult a designated Aviation Medical Examiner.
Exposure to Sun: No restrictions.

VALPROIC ACID
(val PROH ik)

Introduced: 1967   **Class:** Anticonvulsant

Prescription: USA: Yes   **Controlled Drug:** USA: No
Canada: Yes   Canada: No

Available as Generic: USA: Yes
Canada: No

Brand Names: Depa, Depakene, Depakote, Deproic

BENEFITS versus RISKS

Possible Benefits	*Possible Risks*
EFFECTIVE CONTROL OF MULTIPLE SEIZURE TYPES: ABSENCE SEIZURES, TONIC-CLONIC SEIZURES, MYOCLONIC SEIZURES, PSYCHOMOTOR SEIZURES when used adjunctively with other antiseizure drugs	LIVER TOXICITY, infrequent but may be severe Rare reduction of blood platelets and impaired platelet function with risk of bleeding

---

▷ **Principal Uses**
As a Single Drug Product: Used effectively in the management of the following types of epilepsy: simple and complex absence seizures (petit

mal); tonic-clonic seizures (grand mal); myoclonic seizures; complex partial seizures (psychomotor, temporal lobe epilepsy). It is sometimes used adjunctively with other anticonvulsants as needed.

How This Drug Works: Not completely established. It is thought that by increasing the availability of the nerve impulse transmitter gamma-aminobutyric acid (GABA), this drug suppresses the spread of abnormal electrical discharges that cause seizures.

Available Dosage Forms and Strengths
>   Capsules — 250 mg
>   Syrup — 250 mg per 5-ml teaspoonful
> Tablets, enteric-coated — 125 mg, 250 mg, 500 mg

▷ **Usual Adult Dosage Range:**   Initially, 15 mg/kg/24 hours. The dose is increased cautiously by 5 to 10 mg/kg/24 hours every 7 days as needed and tolerated. ***The usual daily dose is from 1000 mg to 1600 mg in divided doses.*** The total daily dosage should not exceed 60 mg/kg. **Note: Actual dosage and administration schedule must be determined by the physician for each patient individually.**

▷ **Dosing Instructions:**   Preferably taken 1 hour before meals. However, it may be taken with or following food if necessary to prevent stomach irritation. The capsule should not be opened and the tablet should not be crushed for administration. Do not administer the syrup in carbonated beverages. It may be diluted in water or milk.

Usual Duration of Use: Continual use on a regular schedule for 2 weeks is usually necessary to determine this drug's effectiveness in reducing the frequency and severity of seizures. Long-term use (months to years) requires supervision and periodic evaluation by your physician. Consult your physician on a regular basis.

▷ **This Drug Should Not Be Taken If**
- you have had an allergic reaction to it previously.
- you have active liver disease.
- you have an active bleeding disorder.

▷ **Inform Your Physician Before Taking This Drug If**
- you have a history of liver disease or impaired liver function.
- you have a history of any type of bleeding disorder.
- you are pregnant or planning pregnancy.
- you have myasthenia gravis.
- you are taking any of the following drugs: anticoagulants; other anticonvulsants; antidepressants, either the tricyclic type or monoamine oxidase (MAO) type A inhibitors (see Drug Classes, Section Four).
- you plan to have surgery or dental extraction in the near future.

Possible Side-Effects (natural, expected and unavoidable drug actions)
Drowsiness and lethargy (5%).

▷ **Possible Adverse Effects** (unusual, unexpected and infrequent reactions)
   If any of the following develop, consult your physician promptly for guidance.
   Mild Adverse Effects
   Allergic Reaction: Skin rash (rare).
   Headache, dizziness, confusion, unsteadiness, slurred speech.
   Nausea, indigestion, stomach cramps, diarrhea.
   Temporary loss of scalp hair.
   Serious Adverse Effects
   Idiosyncratic Reactions: Bizarre behavior, hallucinations.
   Drug-induced hepatitis with jaundice (see Glossary).
   Drug-induced pancreatitis.
   Possible Reye syndrome (see Glossary).
   Reduced formation of blood platelets and impaired function of platelets, with increased risk of abnormal bleeding.

▷ **Possible Effects on Sexual Function**
   Altered timing and pattern of menstruation.
   Female breast enlargement with milk production.
   Decreased libido.
   Decreased effectiveness of oral contraceptives taken concurrently (6%).

▷ **Adverse Effects That May Mimic Natural Diseases or Disorders**
   Liver reactions may suggest viral hepatitis.

   CAUTION
   1. The capsules and tablets should be swallowed whole without alteration to avoid irritation of the mouth and throat.
   2. This drug can impair normal blood clotting mechanisms. In the event of injury, dental extraction, or need for surgery, inform your physician or dentist that you are taking this drug.
   3. Because this drug can impair the normal function of blood platelets, it is advisable to avoid aspirin (which has the same effect).
   4. Over-the-counter drug products that contain antihistamines (allergy and cold remedies, sleep aids) can enhance the sedative effects of this drug.

   Precautions for Use
   By Infants and Children: The concurrent use of aspirin with this drug can cause abnormal bleeding or bruising. Children with mental retardation, organic brain disease or severe seizure disorders may be at increased risk for severe liver toxicity while taking this drug. Observe closely for the development of fever that could indicate the onset of a drug-induced Reye syndrome (see Glossary). Avoid concurrent use of clonazepam (Clonopin); the combined use could result in continuous petit mal episodes.
   By Those over 60 Years of Age: Start treatment with small doses and increase dosage cautiously. Observe closely for excessive sedation, confusion or unsteadiness that could predispose to falling and injury.

▷ **Advisability of Use During Pregnancy**

Pregnancy Category: D (tentative). See Pregnancy Code inside back cover.

Animal studies: Palate and skeletal birth defects reported in mouse, rat and rabbit studies.

Human studies: Information from adequate studies of pregnant women is not available. There have been several reports of birth defects attributed to the use of this drug during early pregnancy.

Consult your physician regarding the advantages and disadvantages of using this drug. If it is used, it is advisable to keep the dose as low as possible.

Advisability of Use if Breast-Feeding

Presence of this drug in breast milk: Yes, in small amounts.

Monitor nursing infant closely and discontinue drug or nursing if adverse effects develop.

Habit-Forming Potential: None.

Effects of Overdosage: Increased drowsiness, weakness, unsteadiness, confusion, stupor progressing to coma.

Possible Effects of Long-Term Use: None reported.

Suggested Periodic Examinations While Taking This Drug (at physician's discretion)

Complete blood cell counts and baseline liver function tests should be done before treatment is started. During treatment, blood counts should be repeated every month and liver function tests repeated every 2 months.

▷ **While Taking This Drug, Observe the Following**

Foods: No restrictions.

Beverages: Do not administer the syrup in carbonated beverages; this could liberate the valproic acid and irritate the mouth and throat. This drug may be taken with milk.

▷ *Alcohol:* Use extreme caution until the combined effects have been determined. Alcohol can increase the sedative effect of this drug. Also, this drug can increase the depressant effects of alcohol on brain function.

Tobacco Smoking: No interactions expected.

▷ *Other Drugs*

Valproic acid may ***increase*** the effects of

- anticoagulants (Coumadin, etc.), and increase the risk of bleeding.
- antidepressants, both monoamine oxidase (MAO) type A inhibitors and tricyclics, and cause toxicity.
- phenobarbital, and cause barbiturate intoxication.
- phenytoin (Dilantin), and cause phenytoin toxicity.

Valproic acid ***taken concurrently*** with

- antiplatelet drugs: aspirin, dipyridamole (Persantine), sulfinpyrazone (Anturane) may enhance the inhibition of platelet function and increase the risk of bleeding.

▷ *Driving, Hazardous Activities:* This drug may cause drowsiness, dizziness or confusion. Restrict activities as necessary.

Aviation Note: The use of this drug *is a disqualification* for piloting. Consult a designated Aviation Medical Examiner.

Exposure to Sun: No restrictions.

Discontinuation: **Do not discontinue this drug suddenly.** Abrupt withdrawal can cause repetitive seizures that are difficult to control.

VERAPAMIL
(ver AP a mil)

Introduced: 1967

Class: Antianginal, antiarrhythmic, antihypertensive, calcium channel blocker

Prescription: USA: Yes
Canada: Yes

Controlled Drug: USA: No
Canada: No

Available as Generic: USA: Yes
Canada: No

Brand Names: Calan, Calan SR, Isoptin, Isoptin SR

BENEFITS versus RISKS

Possible Benefits	*Possible Risks*
EFFECTIVE PREVENTION OF BOTH MAJOR TYPES OF ANGINA	Congestive heart failure
	Low blood pressure (2.9%)
EFFECTIVE CONTROL OF HEART RATE IN CHRONIC ATRIAL FIBRILLATION AND FLUTTER	Heart rhythm disturbance
	Fluid retention (1.7%)
	Liver damage without jaundice (very rare)
EFFECTIVE PREVENTION OF PAROXYSMAL ATRIAL TACHYCARDIA (PAT)	
EFFECTIVE TREATMENT OF HYPERTENSION	

▷ **Principal Uses**

As a Single Drug Product: Used primarily to treat (1) angina pectoris due to coronary artery spasm (Prinzmetal's variant angina) that occurs spontaneously and is not associated with exertion; (2) classical angina-of-effort (due to atherosclerotic disease of the coronary arteries) in individuals who have not responded to or cannot tolerate the nitrates and beta blocker drugs customarily used to treat this disorder; (3) abnormally rapid heart rate due to chronic atrial fibrillation or flutter; (4) recurrent paroxysmal atrial tachycardia; and (5) primary hypertension.

How This Drug Works: Not completely established. It is thought that by blocking the normal passage of calcium through certain cell walls (which is necessary for the function of nerve and muscle tissue), this drug slows the spread of electrical activity through the conduction system of the heart and inhibits the contraction of coronary arteries and peripheral arterioles. As a result of these combined effects, this drug

- prevents spontaneous spasm of the coronary arteries (Prinzmetal's type of angina).
- reduces the rate and contraction force of the heart during exertion, thus lowering the oxygen requirement of the heart muscle; this reduces the occurrence of effort-induced angina (classical angina pectoris).
- reduces the degree of contraction of peripheral arterial walls, resulting in their relaxation and consequent lowering of blood pressure. This further reduces the work load of the heart during exertion and contributes to the prevention of angina.
- slows the rate of electrical impulses through the conduction system of the heart and thereby prevents excessively rapid heart action (tachycardia).

Available Dosage Forms and Strengths
Injection — 5 mg per 2 ml
Tablets — 40 mg, 80 mg, 120 mg
Tablets, prolonged-action — 240 mg

▷ **Usual Adult Dosage Range:**   Initially, 80 mg 3 or 4 times daily. The dose may be increased gradually at 1- to 7-day intervals as needed and tolerated. The usual maintenance dose is from 240 mg to 480 mg daily in 3 or 4 divided doses. The total daily dosage should not exceed 480 mg. **Note: Actual dosage and administration schedule must be determined by the physician for each patient individually.**

▷ **Dosing Instructions:**   Preferably taken before meals and at bedtime. The tablet may be crushed for administration.

Usual Duration of Use: Continual use on a regular schedule for 2 to 4 weeks is usually necessary to determine this drug's effectiveness in reducing the frequency and severity of angina. Reduction of elevated blood pressure may be apparent within the first 1 to 2 weeks. For long-term use (months to years), determine the smallest effective dose; this requires supervision and periodic evaluation by your physician. Consult your physician on a regular basis.

Possible Advantages of This Drug

No adverse effects of blood levels of glucose, potassium or uric acid.
Does not increase blood cholesterol or triglyceride levels.
Does not impair capacity for exercise.

Currently a "Drug of Choice" for initiating treatment of hypertension with a single drug.

▷ This Drug Should Not Be Taken If

- you have had an allergic reaction to it previously.
- you have active liver disease.
- you have a "sick sinus" syndrome (and do not have an artificial pacemaker).
- you have been told that you have a second-degree or third-degree heart block.
- you have low blood pressure—systolic pressure below 90.

▷ Inform Your Physician Before Taking This Drug If

- you have had an unfavorable response to any calcium blocker drug in the past.
- you are currently taking any other drugs, especially digitalis or a beta blocker drug (see Drug Class, Section Four).
- you have had a recent stroke or heart attack.
- you have a history of congestive heart failure or heart rhythm disorders.
- you have impaired liver or kidney function.
- you have a history of drug-induced liver damage.

Possible Side-Effects (natural, expected and unavoidable drug actions)

Low blood pressure (2.9%), fluid retention (1.7%).

▷ Possible Adverse Effects (unusual, unexpected and infrequent reactions)

If any of the following develop, consult your physician promptly for guidance.

Mild Adverse Effects

Allergic Reactions: Skin rash, hives, itching, aching joints.
Headache (1.8%), dizziness (3.6%), fatigue (1.1%).
Nausea (1.6%), indigestion, constipation (6.3%).

Serious Adverse Effects

Serious disturbances of heart rate and/or rhythm, congestive heart failure (0.9%).
Drug-induced liver damage without jaundice (very rare).

▷ Possible Effects on Sexual Function

Altered timing and pattern of menstruation.
Male breast enlargement and tenderness.
Impotence (20%).

CAUTION

1. Be sure to inform all physicians and dentists you consult that you are taking this drug. Note the use of this drug on your card of personal identification.

2. You may use nitroglycerin and other nitrate drugs as needed to relieve acute episodes of angina pain. However, if you detect that your angina attacks are becoming more frequent or intense, notify your physician promptly.
3. If this drug is used concurrently with a beta blocker drug, you may develop excessively low blood pressure.
4. This drug may cause swelling of the feet and ankles. This may not be indicative of either heart or kidney dysfunction.

Precautions for Use

By Infants and Children: Safety and effectiveness for use by those under 12 years of age have not been established.

By Those over 60 Years of Age: You may be more susceptible to the development of weakness, dizziness, fainting and falling. Take necessary precautions to prevent injury. Report promptly any changes in your pattern of thirst and urination.

▷ **Advisability of Use During Pregnancy**

Pregnancy Category: C (tentative). See Pregnancy Code inside back cover.

Animal studies: Toxic effects on the embryo and retarded growth of the fetus (but no birth defects) reported in rat studies.

Human studies: Information from adequate studies of pregnant women is not available.

Avoid this drug during the first 3 months. Use during the last 6 months only if clearly needed. Ask your physician for guidance.

Advisability of Use if Breast-Feeding

Presence of this drug in breast milk: Possibly yes.

Avoid drug or refrain from nursing.

Habit-Forming Potential: None.

Effects of Overdosage: Flushed and warm skin, sweating, light-headedness, irritability, rapid heart rate, low blood pressure, loss of consciousness.

Possible Effects of Long-Term Use: None reported.

Suggested Periodic Examinations While Taking This Drug (at physician's discretion)

Evaluations of heart function, including electrocardiograms; liver and kidney function tests, with long-term use.

▷ **While Taking This Drug, Observe the Following**

Foods: No restrictions. Avoid excessive salt intake.

Beverages: No restrictions. May be taken with milk.

▷ *Alcohol:* Use with caution until combined effects have been determined. Alcohol may exaggerate the drop in blood pressure experienced by some individuals.

Tobacco Smoking: Nicotine can reduce the effectiveness of this drug. Avoid all forms of tobacco.

Marijuana Smoking: Possible reduced effectiveness of this drug; mild to moderate increase in angina; possible changes in electrocardiogram, confusing interpretation.

▷ *Other Drugs*

Verapamil may ***increase*** the effects of

- carbamazepine (Tegretol), and cause carbamazepine toxicity.
- digitoxin and digoxin, and cause digitalis toxicity.

Verapamil ***taken concurrently*** with

- beta blocker drugs (see Drug Class, Section Four) may affect heart rate and rhythm adversely. Careful monitoring by your physician is necessary if these drugs are taken concurrently.

The following drugs may ***increase*** the effects of verapamil

- cimetidine (Tagamet).

▷ *Driving, Hazardous Activities:* Usually no restrictions. This drug may cause dizziness. Restrict activities as necessary.

Aviation Note: Coronary artery disease ***is a disqualification*** for piloting. Consult a designated Aviation Medical Examiner.

Exposure to Sun: Use caution until sensitivity has been determined. This drug may cause photosensitivity (see Glossary).

Exposure to Heat: Caution advised. Hot environments can exaggerate the blood-pressure-lowering effects of this drug. Observe for light-headedness or weakness.

Heavy Exercise or Exertion: This drug may improve your ability to be more active without resulting angina pain. Use caution and avoid excessive exercise that could impair heart function in the absence of warning pain.

Discontinuation: Do not discontinue this drug abruptly. Consult your physician regarding gradual withdrawal to prevent the development of rebound angina.

WARFARIN
(WAR far in)

Introduced: 1941

Class: Anticoagulant, coumarins

Prescription: USA: Yes
Canada: Yes

Controlled Drug: USA: No
Canada: No

Available as Generic: USA: Yes
Canada: No

Brand Names: ✦Athrombin-K, Carfin, Coumadin, Panwarfin, Sofarin, ✦Warfilone

BENEFITS versus RISKS	
Possible Benefits	*Possible Risks*
EFFECTIVE PREVENTION OF BOTH ARTERIAL AND VENOUS THROMBOSIS EFFECTIVE PREVENTION OF EMBOLIZATION IN THROMBOEMBOLIC DISORDERS	NARROW TREATMENT RANGE Dose-related bleeding (5% to 7%) Skin and soft tissue hemorrhage with tissue death (rare)

▷ **Principal Uses**

As a Single Drug Product: Used exclusively for its anticoagulant effect in treating the following conditions: (1) acute thrombosis (clot) or thrombophlebitis of the deep veins; (2) acute pulmonary embolism, resulting from blood clots that originate anywhere in the body; (3) atrial fibrillation, to prevent clotting of blood inside the heart that could result in embolization of small clots to any part of the body; (4) acute myocardial infarction (heart attack), to prevent clotting and embolization; (5) transient ischemic attack (TIA), a temporary reduction of blood flow to a part of the brain; used here to reduce the risk of repeated attacks or possible stroke. Other possible uses include the long-term prevention of recurrent heart attack, and prevention of embolization from the heart in those individuals with artificial heart valves.

How This Drug Works: The coumarin anticoagulants interfere with the production of four essential blood clotting factors by blocking the action of vitamin K. This leads to a deficiency of these clotting factors in circulating blood and inhibits blood clotting mechanisms.

Available Dosage Forms and Strengths
  Injection — 50 mg/vial
  Tablets — 2 mg, 2.5 mg, 5 mg, 7.5 mg, 10 mg

▷ **Usual Adult Dosage Range:** Initially, 10 to 15 mg daily for 2 to 3 days. A large loading dose is inappropriate and may be hazardous. For maintenance, 2 to 10 mg/day. The dosage is adjusted according to the prothrombin time. **Note: Actual dosage and administration schedule must be determined by the physician for each patient individually.**

▷ **Dosing Instructions:** Preferably taken when the stomach is empty, and at the same time each day to ensure uniform results. The tablet may be crushed for administration.

Usual Duration of Use: Continual use on a regular schedule for 3 to 5 days is usually necessary to determine this drug's effectiveness in providing significant anticoagulation. An additional 10 to 14 days is required to determine the optimal maintenance dose for each individual. Long-term use (months to years) requires supervision and periodic evaluation by your physician. Consult your physician on a regular basis.

▷ **This Drug Should Not Be Taken If**
- you have had an allergic reaction to it previously.
- you have an active peptic ulcer or active ulcerative colitis.
- you have had a recent stroke.

▷ **Inform Your Physician Before Taking This Drug If**
- you are now taking **any other drugs,** either prescription drugs or over-the-counter drug products.
- you are pregnant or planning pregnancy.
- you have a history of a bleeding disorder.
- you have high blood pressure.
- you have abnormally heavy or prolonged menstrual bleeding.
- you have diabetes.
- you are using an indwelling catheter.
- you have impaired liver or kidney function.
- you plan to have surgery or dental extraction in the near future.

Possible Side-Effects (natural, expected and unavoidable drug actions)
Minor episodes of bleeding may occur even though dosage and prothrombin times are well within the recommended range.

▷ **Possible Adverse Effects** (unusual, unexpected and infrequent reactions)
If any of the following develop, consult your physician promptly for guidance.
Mild Adverse Effects
Allergic Reactions: Skin rash, hives.
Loss of scalp hair.
Loss of appetite, nausea, vomiting, cramping, diarrhea.
Serious Adverse Effects
Allergic Reaction: Drug fever (see Glossary).
Idiosyncratic Reactions: Bleeding into skin and soft tissues causing gangrene of breast, toes and localized areas anywhere (rare).
Abnormal bleeding from nose, gastrointestinal tract, urinary tract or uterus.

▷ **Possible Effects on Sexual Function:**   None reported.

▷ **Adverse Effects That May Mimic Natural Diseases or Disorders**
Drug-induced fever may suggest infection.

Natural Diseases or Disorders That May Be Activated by This Drug
Bleeding from "silent" peptic ulcer, intestinal or bladder polyp or tumor.

CAUTION
1. Always carry with you a card of personal identification that includes a statement that **you are taking an anticoagulant drug.**

2. While taking this drug, always consult your physician *before* starting any new drug, changing the dosage schedule of any drug or discontinuing any drug.

Precautions for Use

By Those over 60 Years of Age: Small doses are mandatory until your individual sensitivity has been determined. Observe regularly for indications of excessive drug effects: prolonged bleeding from shaving cuts, bleeding gums, bloody urine, rectal bleeding, excessive bruising.

▷ **Advisability of Use During Pregnancy**
Pregnancy Category: X. See Pregnancy Code inside back cover.
Animal studies: Fetal hemorrhage and death due to this drug reported in mice.
Human studies: Information from studies of pregnant women indicates fetal defects and fetal hemorrhage due to this drug.
The manufacturers state that this drug is contraindicated during entire pregnancy.

Advisability of Use if Breast-Feeding

Presence of this drug in breast milk: Yes.
Avoid drug or refrain from nursing.

Habit-Forming Potential: None.

Effects of Overdosage: Episodes of bleeding from minor surface bleeding (nose, gums, small lacerations) to major internal bleeding: vomiting blood, bloody urine or stool.

Possible Effects of Long-Term Use: None reported.

Suggested Periodic Examinations While Taking This Drug (at physician's discretion)
Regular determinations of prothrombin time are essential to safe dosage and proper control.
Urine analyses for blood.

▷ **While Taking This Drug, Observe the Following**
Foods: A larger intake than usual of foods rich in vitamin K may reduce the effectiveness of this drug and make larger doses necessary. Foods rich in vitamin K include: asparagus, bacon, beef liver, cabbage, cauliflower, fish, green leafy vegetables.
Beverages: No restrictions. May be taken with milk.
▷ *Alcohol:* Limit alcohol to one drink daily. Note: Heavy users of alcohol with liver damage may be very sensitive to anticoagulants and require smaller than usual doses.
Tobacco Smoking: Heavy smokers may require relatively larger doses of this drug.
▷ *Other Drugs*
Warfarin may *increase* the effects of
• phenytoin (Dilantin).

The following drugs may *increase* the effects of warfarin
- amiodarone.
- androgens.
- cephalosporins.
- chloral hydrate.
- cimetidine.
- clofibrate.
- dextrothyroxine.
- disulfiram.
- glucagon.
- metronidazole.
- phenylbutazone.
- quinidine.
- salicylates.
- sulfinpyrazone.
- sulfonamides.
- thyroid hormones.

The following drugs may *decrease* the effects of warfarin
- barbiturates.
- carbamazepine.
- cholestyramine.
- ethchlorvynol.
- glutethimide.
- griseofulvin.
- rifampin.
- vitamin K.

▷ *Driving, Hazardous Activities:* No restrictions.

Aviation Note: The use of this drug *is a disqualification* for piloting. Consult a designated Aviation Medical Examiner.

Exposure to Sun: No restrictions.

Discontinuation: Do not discontinue this drug abruptly unless abnormal bleeding occurs. Ask your physician for guidance regarding gradual reduction in dosage over a period of 3 to 4 weeks.

ZIDOVUDINE
(zi DOH vyoo deen)

Other Names: AZT, azidothymidine

Introduced: 1987   **Class:** Antiviral

Prescription: USA: Yes   **Controlled Drug:** USA: No
  Canada: Yes   Canada: No

Available as Generic: USA: No
  Canada: No

Brand Name: Retrovir

<table>
<tr><td colspan="2" align="center">BENEFITS versus RISKS</td></tr>
<tr><td align="center">*Possible Benefits*</td><td align="center">*Possible Risks*</td></tr>
<tr><td>PROLONGATION OF LIFE AND REDUCED INCIDENCE OF INFECTIONS IN TREATING AIDS AND AIDS-RELATED COMPLEX</td><td>SERIOUS BONE MARROW DEPRESSION (see Glossary)
Brain toxicity
Lip, mouth and tongue sores</td></tr>
</table>

▷ **Principal Uses**

As a Single Drug Product: Used primarily to treat selected patients who have acquired immunodeficiency syndrome (AIDS) or acquired immunodeficiency syndrome-related complex (ARC) caused by human immunodeficiency virus (HIV); it is used specifically to treat those with interstitial plasma cell pneumonia or a marked deficiency of helper T-lymphocytes. This drug is not a cure for AIDS, and it does not reduce the risk of transmission of AIDS infection to others through sexual contact or contamination of blood.

How This Drug Works: By interfering with essential enzyme systems, this drug is thought to prevent the growth and reproduction of HIV particles within tissue cells, thus limiting the severity and extent of HIV infection.

Available Dosage Forms and Strengths
Capsules — 100 mg

▷ **Usual Adult Dosage Range:** 200 mg/4 hours throughout the day and night (no omission for activities or sleep). Smaller and larger doses may be used according to individual patient characteristics. **Note: Actual dosage and administration schedule must be determined by the physician for each patient individually.**

▷ **Dosing Instructions:** Preferably taken on an empty stomach, but may be taken with or following food. Take exactly as prescribed. The capsule may be opened and the contents mixed with food just prior to administration.

Usual Duration of Use: Continual use on a regular schedule for 10 to 12 weeks is usually necessary to determine this drug's effectiveness in improving the course of symptomatic AIDS infection. Long-term use requires periodic evaluation of response and dosage adjustment. Consult your physician on a regular basis.

▷ **This Drug Should Not Be Taken If**
- you have had a serious allergic reaction to it previously.
- you have a serious degree of uncorrected bone marrow depression.

▷ **Inform Your Physician Before Taking This Drug If**
- you have a history of either folic acid or vitamin B-12 deficiency.
- you have impaired liver or kidney function.

Possible Side-Effects (natural, expected and unavoidable drug actions)
None reported.

▷ **Possible Adverse Effects** (unusual, unexpected and infrequent reactions)
If any of the following develop, consult your physician promptly for guidance.

Mild Adverse Effects
Allergic Reactions: Skin rash, hives, itching.
Headache (50%), weakness (20%), drowsiness, dizziness, nervousness, insomnia.
Nausea (50%), stomach pain (20%), diarrhea (12%), loss of appetite and vomiting (5% to 11%), altered taste, lip sores, swollen mouth or tongue.
Muscle aches (8%), fever, sweating.

Serious Adverse Effects
Confusion, loss of speech, twitching, tremors, seizures (representing brain toxicity).
Bone marrow depression (see Glossary): fatigue, weakness, fever, sore throat, abnormal bleeding or bruising. Anemia occurs most commonly after 4 to 6 weeks of treatment; abnormally low white blood cell counts occur after 6 to 8 weeks of treatment.

▷ **Possible Effects on Sexual Function:**   None reported.

Possible Delayed Adverse Effects: Significant anemia and deficient white blood cell counts may develop after this drug has been discontinued.

▷ **Adverse Effects That May Mimic Natural Diseases or Disorders**
Seizures may suggest the possibility of epilepsy.

CAUTION
1. This drug is not a cure for AIDS or AIDS-related complex. Nor does it protect completely against other infections or complications. Follow your physician's instructions and take all medications exactly as prescribed.
2. This drug does not reduce the risk of transmitting AIDS to others through sexual contact or contamination of the blood. The use of an effective condom is mandatory. Needles for drug administration should not be shared.

Precautions for Use
By Infants and Children: Safety and effectiveness for use by those under 14 years of age have not been established.
By Those over 60 Years of Age: Impaired kidney function will require dosage reduction.

▷ **Advisability of Use During Pregnancy**
Pregnancy Category: C (tentative). See Pregnancy Code inside back cover.
Animal studies: Rat studies reveal no birth defects.
Human studies: Information from adequate studies of pregnant women is not available.
Consult your physician for specific guidance.

Advisability of Use if Breast-Feeding
Presence of this drug in breast milk: Unknown.
Avoid drug or refrain from nursing.

Habit-Forming Potential: None.

Effects of Overdosage: Nausea, vomiting, diarrhea, bone marrow depression.

Possible Effects of Long-Term Use: Serious anemia and loss of white blood cells.

Suggested Periodic Examinations While Taking This Drug (at physician's discretion)
Complete blood cell counts before starting treatment and weekly thereafter until tolerance is established. Continual monitoring for bone marrow depression is necessary during entire course of treatment.

▷ **While Taking This Drug, Observe the Following**
Foods: No restrictions.
Beverages: No restrictions. May be taken with milk.
▷ *Alcohol:* No interactions expected.
Tobacco Smoking: No interactions expected.
▷ *Other Drugs*
The following drugs may ***increase*** the effects of zidovudine and enhance its toxicity
- acetaminophen.
- acyclovir.
- aspirin.
- benzodiazepines (see Drug Class, Section Four).
- cimetidine.
- indomethacin.
- morphine.
- probenecid.
- sulfonamides (see Drug Class, Section Four).
▷ *Driving, Hazardous Activities:* This drug may cause dizziness or fainting. Restrict activities as necessary.
Aviation Note: The use of this drug ***is a disqualification*** for piloting. Consult a designated Aviation Medical Examiner.
Exposure to Sun: No restrictions.
Discontinuation: Do not discontinue this drug without your physician's knowledge and guidance.

DRUG CLASSES

Drug Classes

Throughout the Drug Profiles in Section Three reference is made to various drug classes. The reader may be advised to consult Section Four to become familiar with the drugs which belong to a particular class of drugs that share important characteristics in their chemical composition or in their actions within the body. Often it is important to know that *any* drug (or *all* drugs) within a given class can be expected to behave in a particular way. Such information may be useful in preventing interactions that could reduce the effectiveness of the drugs in use or result in unanticipated and sometimes hazardous adverse effects.

The presentation of each Drug Class is divided into two listings. The upper list contains the more widely recognized brand names of the drugs within the class; the lower list contains the generic names of the class members. In some instances the number of brand names in use is so large that a complete listing is not possible. In such cases, to be certain that you are consulting the correct drug class, determine the generic name of the drug that concerns you and consult the lower list to see if it is included there. The generic name listing is sufficiently complete to serve the scope of this book.

The following page lists the names of all the Drug Classes included in this section.

LIST OF DRUG CLASSES

Amphetaminelike Drugs
Analgesics, Mild
Analgesics, Strong (Narcotic Drugs)
Antiacne Drugs
Antiallergic Drugs
Antianginal Drugs
Antiarthritic/Anti-inflammatory
  Drugs (Aspirin Substitutes)
Antiasthmatic Drugs
  (Bronchodilators)
Antibiotics
Anticoagulants
Antidepressants
Antidiabetics, Oral (Sulfonylureas)
Antidiarrheal Drugs
Antiepileptic Drugs
  (Anticonvulsants)
Antiglaucoma Drugs
Antigout Drugs
Antihistamines
Antihypertensives
Anti-infective Drugs (Nonantibiotic-
  Antimicrobials)
Anti-itching Drugs (Antipruritics)
Anti-Motion Sickness/Antinausea
  Drugs (Antiemetics)
Antiparkinsonism Drugs
Antispasmodics, Synthetic
Appetite Suppressants
  (Anorexiants)
Atropinelike Drugs
Barbiturates
Benzodiazepines
Beta-Adrenergic-Blocking Drugs
  (Beta Blockers)
Calcium Channel-Blocking Drugs
  (Calcium Blockers)

Cephalosporins
Cholesterol-Reducing Drugs
Cortisonelike Drugs (Adrenocortical
  Steroids)
Cough Suppressants (Antitussives)
Decongestants
Digitalis Preparations
Diuretics
Female Sex Hormones
Fever-Reducing Drugs
  (Antipyretics)
Heart Rhythm Regulators
  (Antiarrhythmic Drugs)
Histamine (H-2)-Blocking Drugs
  (H-2 Blockers)
Male Sex Hormones (Androgens)
Monoamine Oxidase (MAO)
  Inhibitor Drugs
Muscle Relaxants
Nitrates
Penicillins
Phenothiazines
Salicylates
Sedatives/Sleep Inducers,
  Nonbarbiturate (Hypnotics)
Sulfonamides ("Sulfa" Drugs)
Sulfonylureas
Tetracyclines
Thiazide Diuretics
Tranquilizers, Mild (Antianxiety
  Drugs)
Tranquilizers, Strong
  (Antipsychotic Drugs)
Vasodilators
Xanthines

AMPHETAMINELIKE DRUGS

BRAND NAMES

Amodex
Benzedrine
Biphetamine
Desoxyn
Dexatrim
Dexedrine

Didrex
Fastin
Ionamin
Obalan
Plegine
Preludin

Ritalin
Tenuate
Tepanil
Tora
Wilpowr

GENERIC NAMES

amphetamine
benzphetamine
dextroamphetamine
diethylpropion
levamphetamine
methamphetamine

methylphenidate
phendimetrazine
phenmetrazine
phentermine
phenylpropanolamine

ANALGESICS, MILD

BRAND NAMES

Anaprox
A.S.A. Preparations
Darvocet
Darvon
Datril

Hycodan
Indocin
Motrin
Nebs
Percodan

Talwin
Taper
Tempra
Tylenol
Valadol

GENERIC NAMES

acetaminophen
aspirin
codeine
hydrocodone
ibuprofen
indomethacin

naproxen
oxycodone
paregoric
pentazocine
propoxyphene

ANALGESICS, STRONG

(Narcotic Drugs)

BRAND NAMES
Demerol
Dilaudid
Dolophine
Leritine

GENERIC NAMES

anileridine
hydromorphone
meperidine
methadone
morphine

ANTIACNE DRUGS

BRAND NAMES

Accutane
Achromycin V
Eryderm
Lucidol
Retin-A

GENERIC NAMES

benzoyl peroxide
erythromycin
isotretinoin
tetracycline
tretinoin

ANTIALLERGIC DRUGS

See: Antihistamines
Cortisonelike Drugs

ANTIANGINAL DRUGS

BRAND NAMES

Calan	Nitrostat
Cardene	Peritrate
Cardizem	Procardia
Corgard	Tenormin
Inderal	
Isoptin	
Isordil	

GENERIC NAMES

beta blockers (see Class)	nifedipine
diltiazem	nitrates (see Class)
nicardipine	verapamil

ANTIARTHRITIC/ANTI-INFLAMMATORY DRUGS

(Aspirin Substitutes)

BRAND NAMES

Ansaid	Nalfon
Clinoral	Naprosyn
Dolobid	Orudis
Feldene	Suprol
Indocin	Tolectin
Meclomen	Voltaren
Motrin	

GENERIC NAMES

diclofenac	meclofenamate
diflunisal	naproxen
fenoprofen	piroxicam
flurbiprofen	sulindac
ibuprofen	suprofen
indomethacin	tolmetin
ketoprofen	

ANTIASTHMATIC DRUGS

(Bronchodilators)

BRAND NAMES

Aarane
Adrenalin
Alupent
Aminodur
Brethine
Bricanyl
Bronkodyl
Bronkometer
Bronkosol
Bronkotabs

Choledyl
Elixophyllin
Intal
Isuprel
Lufyllin
Medihaler-Epi
Medihaler-Iso
Metaprel
Neothylline
Norisodrine

Proternol
Proventil
Slo-Phyllin
Somophylline
Sus-Phrine
Theolair
Tornalate
Vaponefrin
Ventolin

GENERIC NAMES

albuterol
aminophylline
bitolterol
cromolyn
dyphylline
ephedrine
epinephrine

isoetharine
isoproterenol
metaproterenol
oxtriphylline
terbutaline
theophylline

ANTIBIOTICS

BRAND NAMES

See respective Classes listed under Generic Names.

GENERIC NAMES

cephalosporins
chloramphenicol
clindamycin
erythromycins

lincomycin
penicillins
rifampin
tetacyclines

ANTICOAGULANTS

Coumarin Class

BRAND NAMES

Coumadin
Dicumarol
Liquamar
Panwarfin
Sintrom
Tromexan

GENERIC NAMES

acenocoumarol
dicumarol
phenprocoumon
warfarin

Indandione Class

BRAND NAMES

Danilone
Dipaxin
Eridione
Hedulin
Miradon

GENERIC NAMES

anisindione
diphenadione
phenindione

ANTIDEPRESSANTS

Bicyclic Antidepressants

BRAND NAMES

Prozac

GENERIC NAMES

fluoxetine

Tricyclic Antidepressants

BRAND NAMES

Adapin	Pertofrane
Asendin	Presamine
Aventyl	Sinequan
Elavil	Surmontil
Endep	Tofranil
Norpramin	Vivactil
Pamelor	

GENERIC NAMES

amitriptyline	imipramine
amoxapine	nortriptyline
desipramine	protriptyline
doxepin	trimipramine

Tetracyclic Antidepressants

BRAND NAMES

Ludiomil

GENERIC NAMES

maprotiline

Other Antidepressants

BRAND NAMES
Desyrel

GENERIC NAMES

trazodone

ANTIDIABETICS, ORAL

Sulfonylurea Class

BRAND NAMES

Chloronase	Glucotrol
DiaBeta	Micronase
Diabinese	Mobenol
Dimelor	Orinase
Dymelor	Stabinol
Euglucon	Tolinase

GENERIC NAMES

acetohexamide
chlorpropamide
glipizide
glyburide
tolazamide
tolbutamide

ANTIDIARRHEAL DRUGS

BRAND NAMES

Donnagel
Imodium
Kaopectate
Lomotil
Parepectolin

GENERIC NAMES

atropine
diphenoxylate
kaolin
loperimide
paregoric
pectin

ANTIEPILEPTIC DRUGS

(Anticonvulsants)

BRAND NAMES

Clonopin	Mysoline
Depakene	Tegretol
Diamox	Valium
Dilantin	Zarontin
Luminal	

GENERIC NAMES

acetazolamide	phenobarbital
carbamazepine	phenytoin
clonazepam	primidone
diazepam	valproic acid
ethosuximide	

ANTIGLAUCOMA DRUGS

BRAND NAMES

Diamox
Glaucon
Isopto-carpine
Timoptic

GENERIC NAMES

acetazolamide
epinephrine
pilocarpine
timolol

ANTIGOUT DRUGS

BRAND NAMES

Anaprox
Anturane
Benemid
Clinoril
Naprosyn
Zyloprim

GENERIC NAMES

allopurinol
colchicine
naproxen
probenecid
sulfinpyrazone
sulindac

ANTIHISTAMINES

BRAND NAMES

Actidil
Atarax
Benadryl
Bonine
Chlor-Trimeton
Clistin
Decapryn
Dimetane
Dramamine
Hispril
Histadyl
Histalon
Inhiston
Marezine
Neo-Antergan
Norflex
Optimine
Periactin
Phenergan
Pyribenzamine
Seldane
Tavist
Trimeton
Vistaril

GENERIC NAMES

azatadine
brompheniramine
carbinoxamine
chlorpheniramine
clemastine
cyclizine
cyproheptadine
dimenhydrinate
diphenhydramine
diphenylpyraline
doxylamine
hydroxyzine
meclizine
methapyrilene
orphenadrine
pheniramine
promethazine
pyrilamine
terfenidine
tripelennamine
triprolidine

ANTIHYPERTENSIVES

BRAND NAMES

Aldomet	HydroDiuril	Normodyne
Anhydron	Hygroton	Prinivil
Apresoline	Hytrin	Renese
Blocadren	Inderal	Saluron
Capoten	Inversine	Sectral
Cardene	Ismelin	Serpasil
Catapres	Lasix	Tenex
Corgard	Levatol	Tenormin
Diuril	Loniten	Trandate
Enduron	Lopressor	Vasotec
Esbaloid	Lozol	Visken
Esidrix	Minipress	Zestril
Eutonyl	Naqua	
Exna	Naturetin	

GENERIC NAMES

bendroflumethiazide	enalapril	methyclothiazide
benzthiazide	furosemide	methyldopa
beta blockers (see Class)	guanethidine	minoxidil
	guanfacine	nicardipine
bethanidine	hydralazine	pargyline
captopril	hydrochlorothiazide	penbutolol
chlorothiazide	hydroflumethiazide	polythiazide
chlorthalidone	indapamide	prazosin
clonidine	lisinopril	reserpine
cyclothiazide	mecamylamine	terazosin
		trichlormethiazide

ANTI-INFECTIVE DRUGS
(Nonantibiotic-Antimicrobials)

BRAND NAMES

Bactrim	Macrodantin
Cipro	NegGram
Flagyl	Noroxin
Furadantin	Septra
Gantrisin	

GENERIC NAMES

ciprofloxacin
metronidazole
nalidixic acid
nitrofurantoin
norfloxacin
sulfonamides (see Class)
trimethoprim

ANTI-ITCHING DRUGS
(Antipruritics)

BRAND NAMES

Atarax
Cortaid
Dermolate
Periactin
Temaril
Vistaril

GENERIC NAMES

cortisonelike drugs (see Class)
cyproheptadine
hydroxyzine
trimeprazine

ANTI-MOTION SICKNESS/ANTINAUSEA DRUGS

(Antiemetics)

BRAND NAMES

Antivert	Compazine	Phenergan
Atarax	Dexedrine	Thorazine
Benadryl	Dramamine	Tigan
Bonine	Marezine	Vistaril

GENERIC NAMES

chlorpromazine
cyclizine
dextroamphetamine
dimenhydrinate
diphenhydramine
hydroxyzine

meclizine
prochlorperazine
promethazine
scopolamine
trimethobenzamide

ANTIPARKINSONISM DRUGS

BRAND NAMES

Akineton	Eldepryl	Parsidol
Artane	Kemadrin	Permax
Bendopa	Larodopa	Phenoxene
Biodopa	Levodopa	Pipanol
Cogentin	Norflex	Sinemet
Disipal	Pagitane	Symmetrel
Dopar	Parda	Tremin
	Parlodel	

GENERIC NAMES

amantadine
benztropine
biperiden
bromocriptine
chlorphenoxamine
cycrimine
ethopropazine

levodopa
orphenadrine
pergolide
procyclidine
selegiline
trihexyphenidyl

ANTISPASMODICS, SYNTHETIC

Antrenyl	Nacton	Quarzan
Banthine	Pamine	Robinul
Bentyl	Pathilon	Tral
Cantil	Prantal	Trocinate
Darbid	Pro-Banthine	

clidinium	isopropamide	poldine
dicyclomine	mepenzolate	propantheline
diphemanil	methantheline	thiphenamil
glycopyrrolate	methscopolamine	tridihexethyl
hexocyclium	oxyphenonium	

APPETITE SUPPRESSANTS

(Anorexiants)

Dexedrine	Preludin
Dietac	Pre-Sate
Fastin	Sanorex
Ionamin	Tenuate
Plegine	Tepanil
Pondimin	

chlorphentermine	phendimetrazine
dextroamphetamine	phenmetrazine
diethylpropion	phentermine
fenfluramine	phenylpropanolamine
mazindol	

ATROPINELIKE DRUGS

The drugs included in the following groups may exhibit atropinelike (anticholinergic) action. This can be important in the management of certain diseases and in potential interactions with other drugs used concurrently.

All drugs containing:

atropine	Antidepressants, tricyclic
belladonna	Antihistamines (some)
hyoscyamine	Antiparkinsonism Drugs
scopolamine	(some)
	Antispasmodics, Synthetic
	Muscle Relaxants (some)

BARBITURATES

BRAND NAMES

Alurate	Mebaral
Amytal	Nembutal
Butisol	Sandoptal
Lotusate	Seconal
Luminal	Sombulex

GENERIC NAMES

amobarbital	mephobarbital
aprobarbital	pentobarbital
butabarbital	phenobarbital
butalbital	secobarbital
hexobarbital	talbutal

BENZODIAZEPINES

BRAND NAMES

Ativan	Paxipam
Centrax	Restoril
Clonopin	Serax
Dalmane	Tranxene
Halcion	Valium
Libritabs	Verstran
Librium	Xanax

GENERIC NAMES

alprazolam	halazepam
chlordiazepoxide	lorazepam
clonazepam	oxazepam
clorazepate	prazepam
diazepam	temazepam
flurazepam	triazolam

BETA-ADRENERGIC-BLOCKING DRUGS

(Beta Blockers)

BRAND NAMES

Blocadren	Sectral
Corgard	Tenormin
Inderal	Trandate
Levatol	Visken
Lopressor	
Normodyne	

GENERIC NAMES

acebutolol	penbutolol
atenolol	pindolol
labetalol	propranolol
metoprolol	timolol
nadolol	

CALCIUM CHANNEL-BLOCKING DRUGS

(Calcium Blockers)

BRAND NAMES

Calan
Cardene
Cardizem
Isoptin
Procardia

GENERIC NAMES

diltiazem
nicardipine
nifedipine
verapamil

CEPHALOSPORINS

BRAND NAMES

Anspor
Ceclor
Ceftin
Ceporex
Duricef

Keflex
Novolexin
Ultracef
Velosef

GENERIC NAMES

cefaclor
cefadroxil
cefuroxime
cephalexin
cephradine

CHOLESTEROL-REDUCING DRUGS

BRAND NAMES

Atromid S	Lopid
Choloxin	Lorelco
Colestid	Mevacor
Cytellin	Nicobid
	Questran

GENERIC NAMES

cholestyramine	gemfibrozil
clofibrate	lovastatin
colestipol	niacin
dextrothyroxine	probucol
	sitosterols

CORTISONELIKE DRUGS

(Adrenocortical Steroids)

BRAND NAMES

Aristocort	Dexamethadrone	Meticorten
Colisone	Dexasone	Novadex
Cortef	Gammacorten	Novapred
Cortril	Hexadrol	Paracort
Decadron	Hydeltra	Prednis
Delta-Cortef	Hydrocortone	Servisone
Deltasone	Inflamase	Sterane
Deltra	Kenacort	Valisone
Deronil	Maxidex	Vanceril
Dexameth	Medrol	Wescopred

GENERIC NAMES

beclomethasone	methylprednisolone
betamethasone	prednisolone
cortisone	prednisone
dexamethasone	triamcinolone
hydrocortisone	

COUGH SUPPRESSANTS

(Antitussives)

BRAND NAMES

Benylin
Benylin DM
Dilaudid
Hycodan

Phenergan
Tessalon
Tussionex

GENERIC NAMES

benzonatate
codeine
dextromethorphan
diphenhydramine

hydrocodone
hydromorphone
promethazine

DECONGESTANTS

BRAND NAMES

Afrin
Gluco-Fedrin
Neo-Synephrine
Novafed
Otrivin

Privine
Propadrine
Sudafed
Tyzine

GENERIC NAMES

ephedrine
naphazoline
oxymetazoline
phenylephrine
phenylpropanolamine

pseudoephedrine
tetrahydrozoline
xylometazoline

DIGITALIS PREPARATIONS

BRAND NAMES

Crystodigin   Lanoxicaps
Digifortis   Lanoxin
Digiglusin   Purodigin
Gitaligin

GENERIC NAMES

digitalis   digoxin
digitoxin   gitalin

DIURETICS

BRAND NAMES

Aldactone   Hygroton
Bumex   Lasix
Diamox   Lozol
Diulo   Midamor
Diuril   Zaroxolyn
Dyrenium   (See Thiazide
Edecrin   Brand Names)

GENERIC NAMES

acetazolamide   indapamide
amiloride   metolazone
bumetanide   spironolactone
chlorthalidone   thiazides (see Class)
ethacrynic acid   triamterene
furosemide

FEMALE SEX HORMONES

BRAND NAMES

Estrogens	*Progestogens*
Delestrogen	Amen
DES	Curretab
Estinyl	Megace
Estrace	Micronor
Estrovis	Morlutin
Evex	Ovrette
Feminone	Provera
Ogen	
Premarin	
TACE	

GENERIC NAMES

Estrogens	*Progestogens*
chlorotrianisene	medroxyprogesterone
diethylstilbestrol	megestrol
estradiol	norethindrone
estrogens, conjugated	norgestrel
estrogens, esterified	
estropipate	
ethinyl estradiol	
quinestrol	

FEVER-REDUCING DRUGS

(Antipyretics)

BRAND NAMES

Anaprox	Naprosyn
Clinoril	Ponstel
Indocin	Rufen
Motrin	Tolectin
Nalfon	Tylenol

GENERIC NAMES

acetaminophen	ibuprofen	naproxen
aspirin	indomethacin	sulindac
fenoprofen	mefenamic acid	tolmetin

HEART RHYTHM REGULATORS

(Antiarrhythmic Drugs)

BRAND NAMES

Calan	Pronestyl
Crystodigin	Purodigin
Inderal	Quinaglute
Isoptin	Quinidex
Lanoxin	Quinora
Mexitil	Tambocor
Norpace	Tonocard
Procan SR	

GENERIC NAMES

digitoxin	procainamide
digoxin	propranolol
disopyramide	quinidine
flecainide	tocainide
mexiletine	verapamil

HISTAMINE (H-2)-BLOCKING DRUGS

(H-2 Blockers)

BRAND NAMES

Axid
Pepcid
Tagamet
Zantac

GENERIC NAMES

cimetidine
famotidine
nizatidine
ranitidine

MALE SEX HORMONES

(Androgens)

BRAND NAMES

Android
Android F
Depo-Testosterone
Halotestin
Metandren

Oratestin
Ora-Testryl
Oreton
Oreton Methyl
Testred

GENERIC NAMES

fluoxymesterone
methyltestosterone
testosterone

MONOAMINE OXIDASE (MAO) INHIBITOR DRUGS

MAO Type A Inhibitors

(Food restrictions apply)

BRAND NAMES

Actomol
Catron
Drazine
Eutonyl
Furoxone
Marplan

Marsilid
Nardil
Niamid
Parnate
Tersavid

GENERIC NAMES

furazolidone
iproniazid
isocarboxazid
mebanazine
nialamide
pargyline

phenelzine
pheniprazine
phenoxypropazine
piohydrazine
tranylcypromine

MAO Type B Inhibitors

(Food restrictions do not apply)

<u>BRAND NAMES</u>

Eldepryl

<u>GENERIC NAMES</u>

selegiline

MUSCLE RELAXANTS

<u>BRAND NAMES</u>

Equanil	Rela
Flexeril	Robaxin
Lioresal	Skelaxin
Norflex	Soma
Paraflex	Valium
Parafon Forte	

<u>GENERIC NAMES</u>

baclofen	meprobamate
carisoprodol	metaxalone
chlorzoxazone	methocarbamol
cyclobenzaprine	orphenadrine
diazepam	

NITRATES

<u>BRAND NAMES</u>

Cardilate	Nitro-Bid	Peritrate
Isordil	Nitroglyn	SK-Petn
Laserdil	Nitrospan	Sorbide
Neo-Corovas	Nitrostat	Sorbitrate

<u>GENERIC NAMES</u>

erythrityl tetranitrate
isosorbide dinitrate
nitroglycerin
pentaerythritol tetranitrate

PENICILLINS

BRAND NAMES

Alpen	Omnipen	Principen
Amcill	Orbenin	Prostaphlin
Amoxil	Pathocil	Spectrobid
Bactocil	Penbritin	Tegopen
Dynapen	Pentids	Unipen
Geocillin	Pen-Vee K	V-Cillin K
Geopen	Polycillin	Veracillin
Larotid	Polymox	

GENERIC NAMES

amoxicillin	dicloxacillin
ampicillin	nafcillin
bacampicillin	oxacillin
carbenicillin	penicillin G
cloxacillin	penicillin V

PHENOTHIAZINES

BRAND NAMES

Chlor-PZ	Proketazine	Tacaryl
Compazine	Prolixin	Temaril
Largon	Promatar	Thorazine
Levoprome	Quide	Tindal
Mellaril	Repoise	Torecan
Parsidol	Serentil	Trilafon
Permitil	Sparine	Vesprin
Phenergan	Stelazine	

GENERIC NAMES

acetophenazine	methdilazine	propiomazine
butaperazine	methotrimeprazine	thiethylperazine
carphenazine	perphenazine	thioridazine
chlorpromazine	piperacetazine	trifluoperazine
ethopropazine	procholorperazine	triflupromazine
fluphenazine	promazine	trimeprazine
mesoridazine	promethazine	

SALICYLATES

BRAND NAMES

Arthropan
Bufferin
Causalin
Ecotrin
Empirin
Magan
Neocylate
Uracel

GENERIC NAMES

aspirin
choline salicylate
magnesium salicylate
potassium salicylate
sodium salicylate

SEDATIVES/SLEEP INDUCERS, NONBARBITURATE

(Hypnotics)

BRAND NAMES

Carbrital
Dalmane
Doriden
Dorimide
Felsules
Halcion
Noctec
Noludar
Parest
Placidyl
Restoril
Somnafac
Sopor
Valmid

GENERIC NAMES

carbromal
chloral hydrate
ethchlorvynol
ethinamate
flurazepam
glutethimide
methyprylon
temazepam
triazolam

SULFONAMIDES

("Sulfa" Drugs)

BRAND NAMES

Azulfidine	Gantanol	Sonilyn
Coco-Diazine	Gantrisin	Suladyne
Cosulfa	Kynex	Thiosulfil
Dagenan	Madribon	Triple Sulfas
Diamox	Midicel	Urobiotic
Elkosin	Neotrizine	

GENERIC NAMES

acetazolamide	sulfamethazine	sulfapyridine
sulfachlorpyridazine	sulfamethizole	sulfasalazine
sulfadiazine	sulfamethoxazole	sulfisomidine
sulfadimethoxine	sulfamethoxy-	sulfisoxazole
sulfamerazine	pyridazine	trisulfapyrimidines

SULFONYLUREAS

BRAND NAMES

Chloronase	Micronase
DiaBeta	Mobenol
Diabinese	Novobutamide
Dimelor	Orinase
Dymelor	Tolbutone
Euglucon	Tolinase
Glucotrol	

GENERIC NAMES

acetohexamide
chlorpropamide
glipizide
glyburide
tolazamide
tolbutamide

TETRACYCLINES

BRAND NAMES

Achromycin	Rondomycin	Tetracyn
Aureomycin	Steclin	Vectrin
Declomycin	Sumycin	Velacycline
Minocin	Terramycin	Vibramycin
Panmycin	Tetrachel	

GENERIC NAMES

chlortetracycline	minocycline
demeclocycline	oxytetracycline
doxycycline	rolitetracycline
methacycline	tetracycline

THIAZIDE DIURETICS

BRAND NAMES

Anhydron	Hydrazide	Naqua
Chemhydrazide	Hydrid	Naturetin
Diucardin	Hydrite	Neocodema
Diuchlor	Hydro-Aquil	Novohydrazide
Diuril	Hydrodiuretex	Oretic
Duretic	HydroDiuril	Renese
Edemol	Hydrosaluret	Saluron
Enduron	Hydrozide	Thiuretic
Esidrix	Metahydrin	Urozide
Exna		

GENERIC NAMES

bendroflumethiazide	hydroflumethiazide
benzthiazide	methyclothiazide
chlorothiazide	polythiazide
cyclothiazide	trichlormethiazide
hydrochlorothiazide	

TRANQUILIZERS, MILD

(Antianxiety Drugs)

BRAND NAMES

Atarax	Miltown	Tybatran
Buspar	Paxipam	Ultran
Deprol	Serax	Valium
Equanil	Trancopal	Vistaril
Fenarol	Tranxene	Xanax
Librium		

GENERIC NAMES

alprazolam	halazepam
benactyzine	hydroxyzine
buspirone	meprobamate
chlordiazepoxide	oxazepam
chlormezanone	phenaglycodol
clorazepate	tybamate
diazepam	

TRANQUILIZERS, STRONG

(Antipsychotic Drugs)

BRAND NAMES

Carbolith	Lithotabs	Serpasil
Eskalith	Loxitane	Taractan
Haldol	Moban	(See Phenothiazines,
Lithane	Navane	Brand Names)
Lithonate	Sandril	

GENERIC NAMES

chlorprothixene	phenothiazines (see Class)
haloperidol	reserpine
lithium	thiothixene
loxapine	
molindone	

VASODILATORS

BRAND NAMES

Arlidin   Pavabid
Cerespan   Vasodilan
Cyclospasmol   Vasospan
Ethatab

GENERIC NAMES

cyclandelate
ethaverine
isoxsuprine
nylidrin
papaverine

XANTHINES

BRAND NAMES

Aminodur   Quibron-T
Bronkodyl   Slo-Phyllin
Choledyl   Theo-Dur
Droxine   Theolixir
Elixophylline   Theovent

GENERIC NAMES

aminophylline
dyphylline
oxtriphylline
theophylline

SECTION FIVE

A GLOSSARY
OF
DRUG-RELATED TERMS

Glossary

Addiction The traditional term used to identify the irresistible craving for and compulsive use of habit-forming drugs. The more recent preference for the term *dependence* has served to clarify the distinction between habituation and addiction. Drugs capable of producing addiction do so by interacting with the biochemistry of the brain in such a way that they assume a working role. This physical incorporation of the drug into the fundamental processes of brain tissue function is responsible for the agony of the "withdrawal syndrome"—the intense mental and physical pain experienced by the addict when intake of the drug is stopped abruptly. Thus addiction is a *physical dependence*. (See DEPENDENCE for a further account of physical and psychological dependence.)

Adverse Effect or Reaction An abnormal, unexpected, infrequent and usually unpredictable injurious response to a drug. Used in this restrictive sense, the term *adverse reaction* does *not* include effects of a drug which are normally a part of its pharmacological action, even though such effects may be undesirable and unintended. (See SIDE-EFFECT.) Adverse reactions are of three basic types: those due to drug *allergy*, those caused by individual *idiosyncrasy* and those representing *toxic* effects of drugs on tissue structure and function (see ALLERGY, IDIOSYNCRASY and TOXICITY).

Allergy (Drug) An abnormal mechanism of drug response that occurs in individuals who produce injurious antibodies* that react with foreign substances—in this instance, a drug. The person who is allergic by na-

---

*Antibodies are special tissue proteins that combine with substances foreign to the body. Protective antibodies destroy bacteria and neutralize toxins. Injurious antibodies, reacting with foreign substances, cause the release of histamine, the principal chemical responsible for allergic reactions.

ture and has a history of hay fever, asthma, hives or eczema is more likely to develop drug allergies. Allergic reactions to drugs take many forms: skin eruptions of various kinds, fever, swollen glands, painful joints, jaundice, interference with breathing, acute collapse of circulation, etc. Drug allergies can develop gradually over a long period of time, or they can appear with dramatic suddenness and require life-saving intervention.

Analgesic A drug that is used primarily to relieve pain. Analgesics are of three basic types: (1) Simple, nonnarcotic analgesics that relieve pain by suppressing the local production of prostaglandins and related substances; examples are acetaminophen, aspirin and the large group of nonsteroidal anti-inflammatory drugs known as aspirin substitutes (Motrin, Advil, Naprosyn, etc.). (2) Narcotic analgesics or opioids ("like opium" derivatives) that relieve pain by suppressing its perception in the brain; examples are morphine, codeine and hydrocodone (natural derivatives of opium), and meperidine or pentazocine (synthetic drug products). (3) Local anesthetics that prevent or relieve pain by rendering sensory nerve endings insensitive to painful stimulation; an example is the urinary tract analgesic phenazopyridine (Pyridium).

Anaphylactic (Anaphylactoid) Reaction A group of symptoms which represent (or resemble) a sometimes overwhelming and dangerous allergic reaction due to extreme hypersensitivity to a drug. Anaphylactic reactions, whether mild, moderate or severe, often involve several body systems. Mild symptoms consist of itching, hives, nasal congestion, nausea, abdominal cramping and/or diarrhea. Sometimes these precede more severe symptoms such as choking, shortness of breath and sudden loss of consciousness (usually referred to as anaphylactic shock).

Characteristic features of anaphylactic reaction must be kept in mind. It can result from a very small dose of drug; it develops suddenly, usually within a few minutes after taking the drug; it can be rapidly progressive and can lead to fatal collapse in a short time if not reversed by appropriate treatment. A developing anaphylactic reaction is a true medical emergency. Any adverse effect that appears within 20 minutes after taking a drug should be considered the early manifestation of a possible anaphylactic reaction. Obtain medical attention immediately! (See ALLERGY, DRUG and HYPERSENSITIVITY.)

Antihypertensive A drug used to lower excessively high blood pressure. The term *hypertension* denotes blood pressure above the normal range. It does not refer to excessive nervous or emotional tension. The term *antihypertensive* is sometimes used erroneously as if it had the same meaning as *antianxiety* (or tranquilizing) drug action.

Today there are more than 100 drug products in use for treating hypertension. Those most frequently prescribed for long-term use fall into three major groups:

drugs that increase urine production (the diuretics)
drugs that relax blood vessel walls
drugs that reduce the activity of the sympathetic nervous system

Regardless of their mode of action, all these drugs share an ability to lower the blood pressure. It is important to remember that many other drugs can interact with antihypertensive drugs: some add to their effect and cause excessive reduction in blood pressure; others interfere with their action and reduce their effectiveness. Anyone who is taking medications for hypertension should consult with his or her physician whenever drugs are prescribed for the treatment of other conditions as well.

Antipyretic A drug that is used to treat fever because of its ability to lower body temperature that is elevated above the normal. Antipyretics relieve fever through their effects on the temperature regulating center in the hypothalamus of the brain. Their actions cause dilation of the blood vessels (capillary beds) in the skin, bringing overheated blood to the surface for cooling; in addition, the sweat glands are stimulated to provide copious perspiration that cools the body further through evaporation. An antipyretic drug may also be analgesic (acetaminophen), or analgesic and anti-inflammatory (aspirin).

Aplastic Anemia A form of bone marrow failure in which the production of all 3 types of blood cells is seriously impaired (also known as pancytopenia). Aplastic anemia can occur spontaneously from unknown causes, but about one-half of reported cases are induced by certain drugs or chemicals. The symptoms reflect the consequences of inadequate supplies of all 3 blood cell types: deficiency of red blood cells (anemia) results in fatigue, weakness and pallor; deficiency of white blood cells (leukopenia) predisposes to infections; deficiency of blood platelets (thrombocytopenia) leads to spontaneous bruising and hemorrhage. Treatment is difficult and the outcome unpredictable. Even with the best of care, approximately 50% of cases end fatally.

These drugs and chemicals are known to be capable of inducing aplastic anemia:

acetazolamide	meprobamate
anticancer drugs	methimazole
aspirin	oxyphenbutazone
benzene (solvent)	penicillin
carbamazepine	phenacetin
carbon tetrachloride (solvent)	phenylbutazone
chlordane (insecticide)	phenytoin
chlordiazepoxide	primidone
chloromycetin	promazine
chlorothiazide	quinacrine
chlorpheniramine	sulfonamides
chlorpromazine	tetracyclines
chlorpropamide	thiouracil
colchicine	tolbutamide
DDT (insecticide)	triflupromazine
indomethacin	trimethadione
lithium	tripelennamine
mephenytoin	

Although aplastic anemia is a rare consequence of drug treatment (3 in 100,000 users of quinacrine, for example), anyone taking a drug capable of inducing it should have complete blood cell counts periodically if the drug is to be used over an extended period of time.

Bioavailability The measurable characteristics of a drug product (usually a tablet or a capsule) that represent how rapidly the active drug ingredient is absorbed into the bloodstream and to what extent it is absorbed. Two types of measurements—(1) blood levels of the drug at certain time intervals after administration, and (2) the duration of the drug's presence in the blood—indicate how much of the drug is available for biological activity and for how long.

Another method of determining a drug product's bioavailability is to measure (1) the cumulative amount of the drug (or any breakdown product after transformation) that is excreted in the urine, and (2) the rate of drug accumulation in the urine.

The two major factors that govern a drug product's bioavailability are the chemical and physical characteristics (the formulation) of the dosage form given, and the functional state of the digestive system of the individual who takes it. A drug product that disintegrates rapidly in a normally functioning stomach and small intestine produces blood levels of the absorbed drug quite promptly. Such a drug product can be demonstrated to possess good bioavailability.

Specially designed laboratory tests are now available to evaluate a drug product's potential bioavailability when taken by the "average" individual.

Bioequivalence It is generally accepted that the ability of a drug product to produce its intended therapeutic effect is directly related to its bioavailability. When a particular drug is marketed by several manufacturers, often in a variety of dosage forms, it is critically important that the drug product selected for use be one that possesses the bioavailability necessary to be effective therapeutically. Substantial variations occur among manufacturers in the formulation of their drug products. Although the principal drug ingredient of products from different firms may be identical chemically, it cannot be assumed that these products possess equal bioavailability and are therefore equal therapeutically.

The bioavailability of any drug product is governed to a large extent by the physical characteristics of its formulation; these in turn determine how rapidly and how completely the drug product disintegrates and releases its active drug component(s) for absorption into the bloodstream. Drug products that contain the same principal drug ingredient but are combined with different inert additives, are coated with different substances or are enclosed in capsules of different composition may or may not possess the same bioavailability. Those that do are said to be bioequivalent, and can be relied upon to be equally effective in achieving therapeutic results.

If you consider having your prescription filled with the generic equivalent of a brand name drug product, ask your physician *and* pharmacist for guidance. This decision requires professional judgment in each case. In many treatment situations, reasonable differences in the bioavailability patterns among drug products are acceptable. In some situations, however, because of the serious nature of the illness, or because it is mandatory that blood levels of the drug be maintained within a narrowly defined range, it is essential to use the drug product that has been demonstrated to possess reliable bioavailability.

Blood Platelets The smallest of the three types of blood cells produced by the bone marrow. Platelets are normally present in very large numbers. Their primary function is to assist the process of normal blood clotting so as to prevent excessive bruising and bleeding in the event of injury. When present in proper numbers and functioning normally, platelets preserve the retaining power of the walls of the smaller blood vessels. By initiating appropriate clotting processes in the blood, platelets seal small points of leakage in the vessel walls, thereby preventing spontaneous bruising or bleeding (that which is unprovoked by trauma).

Certain drugs and chemicals may reduce the number of available blood platelets to abnormally low levels. Some of these drugs act by suppressing platelet formation; other drugs hasten their destruction. When the number of functioning platelets falls below a critical level, blood begins to leak through the thin walls of smaller vessels. The outward evidence of this leakage is the spontaneous appearance of scattered bruises in the skin of the thighs and legs. This is referred to as purpura. Bleeding may occur anywhere in the body, internally as well as superficially into the tissues immediately beneath the skin.

Bone Marrow Depression A serious reduction in the ability of the bone marrow to carry on its normal production of blood cells. This can occur as an adverse reaction to the toxic effect of certain drugs and chemicals on bone marrow components. When functioning normally, the bone marrow produces the majority of the body's blood cells. These consist of three types: the red blood cells (erythrocytes), the white blood cells (leukocytes) and the blood platelets (thrombocytes). Each type of cell performs one or more specific functions, all of which are indispensable to the maintenance of life and health.

Drugs that are capable of depressing bone marrow activity can impair the production of all types of blood cells simultaneously or of only one type selectively. Periodic examinations of the blood can reveal significant changes in the structure and number of the blood cells that indicate a possible drug effect on bone marrow activity.

Impairment of the production of red blood cells leads to anemia, a condition of abnormally low red cells and hemoglobin. This causes weakness, loss of energy and stamina, intolerance of cold environments and shortness of breath on physical exertion. A reduction in the formation of white blood cells can impair the body's immunity and lower its resistance to infection. These changes may result in the development of fever, sore throat or pneumonia. When the formation of blood platelets is suppressed to abnormally low levels, the blood loses its ability to quickly seal small points of leakage in blood vessel walls. This may lead to episodes of unusual and abnormal spontaneous bruising or to prolonged bleeding in the event of injury.

Any of these symptoms can occur in the presence of bone marrow depression. They should alert both patient and physician to the need for prompt studies of blood and bone marrow.

Brand Name The registered trade name given to a drug product by its manufacturer. Many drugs are marketed by more than one manufacturer or distributor. Each company adopts a distinctive trade name to distinguish its brand of the generic drug from that of its competitors. Thus a brand name designates a proprietary drug—one that is protected by patent or copyright. Generally brand names are shorter, easier to pronounce and more readily remembered than their generic counterparts.

Cause-and-Effect Relationship A possible causative association between a drug and an observed biologic event—most commonly a side-effect or an adverse effect. Knowledge of a drug's full spectrum of effects (wanted and unwanted) is highly desirable when weighing its benefits and risks in any treatment situation. However, it is often impossible to establish with certainty that a particular drug is the primary agent responsible for a suspected adverse effect. In the evaluation of every cause-and-effect relationship, therefore, meticulous consideration must be given to such factors as the time sequence of drug administration and possible reaction, the use of multiple drugs, possible interactions among these drugs, the effects of the disease under treatment, the physiological and psychological characteristics of the patient and the possible influence of unrecognized disorders and malfunctions.

The majority of adverse drug reactions occur sporadically, unpredictably and infrequently in the general population. A *definite* cause-and-effect relationship between drug and reaction is established when (1) the adverse effect immediately follows administration of the drug; or (2) the adverse effect disappears after the drug is discontinued (dechallenge) and promptly reappears when the drug is used again (rechallenge); or (3) the adverse effects are clearly the expected and predictable toxic consequences of drug overdosage.

In contrast to the obvious "causative" (definite) relationship, there exists a large gray area of "probable," "possible" and "coincidental" associations that are clouded by varying degrees of uncertainty. These classifications usually apply to alleged drug reactions that require a relatively long time to develop, are of low incidence and for which there are no clear-cut objective means of demonstrating a causal mechanism that links drug and reaction. Clarification of cause-and-effect relationships in these uncertain groups requires carefully designed observation over a long period of time, followed by sophisticated statistical analysis. Occasionally the public is alerted to a newly found "relationship" based upon suggestive but incomplete data. Though early warning is clearly in the public interest, such announcements should make clear whether the presumed relationship is based upon definitive criteria or is simply inferred because the use of a drug and an observed event were found to occur together within an appropriate time frame.

The most competent techniques for evaluating cause-and-effect relationships of adverse drug reactions have been devised by the Division of Tissue Reactions to Drugs, a research unit of the Armed Forces Institute of Pathology. Based upon a highly critical examination of all available evidence, the Division's study of 2800 drug-related deaths yielded the following levels of certainty regarding cause-and-effect relationship:

No association	5.0%
Coincidental	14.5%
Possible	33.0%
Probable	30.0%
Causative	17.5%

It is significant that expert evaluation of 2800 drug-related cases concluded that only 47.5% could be substantiated as definitely or probably causative.

Contraindication A condition or disease that precludes the use of a particular drug. Some cointraindications are *absolute*, meaning that the use of the drug would expose the patient to extreme hazard and therefore cannot be justified. Other contraindications are *relative*, meaning that the condition or disease does not entirely bar the use of the drug but requires that, before the decision to use the drug is made, special consideration be given to factors which could aggravate existing disease, interfere with current treatment or produce new injury.

Dependence The preferred term used to identify the drug-dependent states of *psychological dependence* (or *habituation*), and *physical dependence* (or *addiction*). In addition, a third kind of drug-dependence can be included under this term. This might be called *functional dependence*—the need to use a drug continuously in order to sustain a particular body function, the impairment of which causes annoying symptoms of varying degree and significance.

Psychological dependence is a form of neurotic behavior. Its principal characteristic is an obsession to satisfy a particular desire, be it one of self-gratification or one of escape from some real or imagined distress. Psychological dependence is a very human trait that is seen often in many socially acceptable patterns and practices such as entertainment, gambling, sports and collecting. A common form of this dependence in today's culture is the increasing reliance upon drugs to help in coping with the everyday problems of living: pills for frustration, disappointment, nervous stomach, tension headache and insomnia. The 20 million smokers of marijuana have found it to be a drug that eases their stress, one whose effectiveness fosters habit (psychological dependence) but not addiction.

Physical dependence, which is true addiction, includes two elements: habituation and tolerance. Addicting drugs provide relief from anguish and pain swiftly and effectively; they also induce a physiological tolerance that requires increasing dosage or repeated use if they are to remain effective. These two features foster the continued need for the drug and lead to its becoming a functioning component in the biochemistry of the brain. As this occurs, the drug assumes an "essential" role in ongoing chemical processes. (Thus some authorities prefer the term *chemical dependence*.) Sudden removal of the drug from the system causes a major upheaval in body chemistry and provokes a withdrawal syndrome—the intense mental and physical pain experienced by the addict when intake of the drug is stopped abruptly—that is the hallmark of addiction.

    Functional dependence differs significantly from both psychological and physical dependence. It occurs when a drug effectively relieves an annoying or distressing condition and the particular body function involved becomes increasingly dependent upon the action of the drug to provide a sense of well-being. Drugs which are capable of inducing functional dependence are used primarily for the relief of symptoms. They do not act on the brain to produce alteration of mood or consciousness as do those drugs with potential for either psychological or physical dependence. The most familiar example of functional dependence is the "laxative habit." Some types of constipation are made worse by the wrong choice of laxative, and natural function gradually fades as the colon becomes more and more dependent upon the action of certain laxative drugs.

Disulfiramlike (Antabuselike) Reaction The symptoms that result from the interaction of alcohol and any drug that is capable of provoking the pattern of response typical of the "Antabuse effect." The interacting drug interrupts the normal decomposition of alcohol by the liver and thereby permits the accumulation of a toxic by-product that enters the bloodstream. When sufficient levels of both alcohol and drug are present in the blood the reaction occurs. It consists of intense flushing and warming of the face, a severe throbbing headache, shortness of breath, chest pains, nausea, repeated vomiting, sweating and weakness. If the amount of alcohol ingested has been large enough, the reaction may progress to blurred vision, vertigo, confusion, marked drop in blood pressure and loss of consciousness. Severe reactions may lead to convulsions and death. The reaction can last from 30 minutes to several hours, depending upon the amount of alcohol in the body. As the symptoms subside, the individual is exhausted and usually sleeps for several hours.

Diuretic A drug that alters kidney function to increase the volume of urine. Diuretics use several different mechanisms to increase urine volume, and these, in turn, have different effects on body chemistry. Diuretics are used primarily to (1) remove excess water from the body (as in congestive heart failure and some types of liver and kidney disease), and (2) treat hypertension by promoting the excretion of sodium from the body.

Dosage Forms and Strengths This information category in the individual

Drug Profiles (Section Three) uses several abbreviations to designate measurements of weight and volume. These are

mcg = microgram = 1,000,000th of a gram (weight)
mg = milligram = 1000th of a gram (weight)
ml = milliliter = 1000th of a liter (volume)
gm = gram = 1000 milligrams (weight)

There are approximately 65 mg in 1 grain.
There are approximately 5 ml in 1 teaspoonful.
There are approximately 15 ml in 1 tablespoonful.
There are approximately 30 ml in 1 ounce.
1 milliliter of water weighs 1 gram.
There are approximately 454 grams in 1 pound.

Drug, Drug Product Terms often used interchangeably to designate a medicine (in any of its dosage forms) used in medical practice. Strictly speaking, the term *drug* refers to the single chemical entity that provokes a specific response when placed within a biological system—the "active" ingredient. A *drug product* is the manufactured dosage form—tablet, capsule, elixir, etc.—that contains the active drug intermixed with inactive ingredients to provide for convenient administration.

Drug products which contain only one active ingredient are referred to as single entity drugs. Drug products with two or more active ingredients are called combination drugs (designed [CD] in the lists of brand names in the Drug Profiles, Section Three).

Drug Class A group of drugs that are similar in chemistry, method of action and use in treatment. Because of their common characteristics, many drugs within a class will produce the same side-effects and have similar potential for provoking related adverse reactions and interactions. However, significant variations among members within a drug class can occur. This sometimes allows the physician an important degree of selectivity in choosing a drug if certain beneficial actions are desired or particular side-effects are to be minimized.

Examples: Antihistamines, phentothiazines, tetracyclines (see Section Four).

Drug Fever The elevation of body temperature that occurs as an unwanted manifestation of drug action. Drugs can induce fever by several mechanisms; these include allergic reactions, drug-induced tissue damage, acceleration of tissue metabolism, constriction of blood vessels in the skin with resulting decrease in loss of body heat and direct action on the temperature-regulating center in the brain.

The most common form of drug fever is that associated with allergic reactions. It may be the only allergic manifestation apparent, or it may be part of a complex of allergic symptoms that can include skin rash, hives, joint swelling and pain, enlarged lymph glands, hemolytic anemia or hepatitis. The fever usually appears about 7 to 10 days after starting the drug and may vary from low-grade to alarmingly high levels. It may be sustained or intermittent, but it usually persists for as long as the drug is taken. In previously sensitized individuals drug fever may occur within 1 or 2 hours after taking the first dose of medication.

While many drugs are capable of producing fever, the following are more commonly responsible:

allopurinol	novobiocin
antihistamines	para-aminosalicylic acid
atropinelike drugs	penicillin
barbiturates	pentazocine
coumarin anticoagulants	phenytoin
hydralazine	procainamide
iodides	propylthiouracil
isoniazid	quinidine
methyldopa	rifampin
nadalol	sulfonamides

Extension Effect An unwanted but predictable drug response that is a logical consequence of mild to moderate overdosage. An extension effect is an exaggeration of the drug's normal pharmacological action; it can be thought of as a mild form of dose-related toxicity (see OVERDOSAGE and TOXICITY).

Example: The continued "hangover" of drowsiness and mental sluggishness that persists after arising in the morning is a common extension effect of a long-acting sleep-inducing drug (hypnotic) taken the night before.

Example: The persistent intestinal cramping and diarrhea that result from too generous a dose of laxative are extension effects of the drug's anticipated action.

Generic Name The official, common or public name used to designate an active drug entity, whether in pure form or in dosage form. Generic names are coined by committees of officially appointed drug experts and are approved by governmental agencies for national and international use. Thus they are nonproprietary. Many drug products are marketed under the generic name of the principal active ingredient and bear no brand name of the manufacturer.

While the total number of prescriptions written in the United States in 1986 increased by 0.6%, prescriptions specifying the *generic name* of the drug increased by 8.6%. Generically written prescriptions now account for 13.5% of all new prescriptions written in the United States. The drugs most commonly prescribed by generic name are listed below, ranked in descending order of the number of new prescriptions issued.

amoxicillin	erythromycin
penicillin VK	hydrochlorothiazide
ampicillin	acetaminophen/codeine
tetracycline	doxycycline
prednisone	phenobarbital

Habituation A form of drug dependence based upon strong psychological gratification rather than the physical (chemical) dependence of addiction. The habitual use of drugs that alter mood or relieve minor discomforts results from a compulsive need to feel pleasure and satisfaction or to escape the manifestations of emotional distress. The abrupt cessation of habituating drugs does not produce the withdrawal syndrome seen in addiction. Thus habituation is a *psychological dependence*. (See DEPENDENCE for a further account of psychological and physical dependence.)

Hemolytic Anemia A form of anemia (deficient red blood cells and hemoglobin) resulting from the premature destruction (hemolysis) of circulating red blood cells. Several mechanisms can be responsible for the development of hemolytic anemia; among these is the action of certain drugs and chemicals. Some individuals are susceptible to hemolytic anemia because of a genetic deficiency in the makeup of their red blood cells. If such people are given certain antimalarial drugs, sulfa drugs or numerous other drugs, some of their red cells will disintegrate on contact with the drug. (About 10% of American blacks have this genetic trait.)

Another type of drug-induced hemolytic anemia is a form of drug allergy. Many drugs in wide use (including quinidine, methyldopa, levodopa and chlorpromazine) are known to cause hemolytic destruction of red cells as a hypersensitivity (allergic) reaction.

Hemolytic anemia can occur abruptly (with evident symptoms) or silently. The acute form lasts about 7 days and is characterized by fever, pallor, weakness, dark-colored urine and varying degrees of jaundice (yellow coloration of eyes and skin). When drug-induced hemolytic anemia is mild, involving the destruction of only a small number of red blood cells, there may be no symptoms to indicate its presence. Such episodes are detected only by means of laboratory studies (see IDIOSYNCRASY and ALLERGY, DRUG).

Hepatitislike Reaction Changes in the liver, induced by certain drugs, which closely resemble those produced by viral hepatitis. The symptoms of drug-induced hepatitis and virus-induced hepatitis are often so similar that the correct cause cannot be established without precise laboratory studies.

Hepatitis due to drugs may be a form of drug allergy (as in reaction to many of the phenothiazines), or it may represent a toxic adverse effect (as in reaction to some of the monoamine oxidase inhibitor drugs). Liver reactions of significance usually result in jaundice and represent serious adverse effects (see JAUNDICE).

Hypersensitivity A term subject to varying usages for many years. One common use has been to identify the trait of overresponsiveness to drug action, that is, an intolerance to even small doses. Used in this sense, the term indicates that the nature of the response is appropriate but the degree of response is exaggerated.

The term is more widely used today to identify a state of allergy. To have a *hypersensitivity* to a drug is to be *allergic* to it (see ALLERGY, DRUG).

Some individuals develop cross-hypersensitivity. This means that once a person has developed an allergy to a certain drug, that person will experience an allergic reaction to other drugs which are closely related in chemical composition.

Example: The patient was known to be *hypersensitive* by nature, having a history of seasonal hay fever and asthma since childhood. His *allergy* to tetracycline developed after his third course of treatment. This drug *hypersensitivity* manifested itself as a diffuse, measleslike rash.

Hypnotic A drug that is used primarily to induce sleep. There are several classes of drugs that have hypnotic effects: antihistamines, barbiturates, benzodiazepines and several unrelated compounds. Within the past 15 years the benzodiazepines, because of their relative safety and lower potential for inducing dependence, have largely replaced the barbiturates as the most commonly used hypnotics. The body usually develops a tolerance to the hypnotic effect after several weeks of continual use. To maintain their effectiveness, hypnotics should be used intermittently for short periods of time.

Hypoglycemia A condition in which the amount of glucose (a sugar) in the blood is below the normal range. Since normal brain function is dependent upon an adequate supply of glucose, reducing the level of glucose in the blood below a critical point will cause serious impairment of brain activity. The resulting symptoms are characteristic of the hypoglycemic state. Early indications are headache, a sensation resembling mild drunkenness and an inability to think clearly. These may be accompanied by hunger. As the level of blood glucose continues to fall, nervousness and confusion develop. Varying degrees of weakness, numbness, trembling, sweating and rapid heart action follow. If sugar is not provided at this point and the blood glucose level drops further, impaired speech, incoordination and unconsciousness, with or without convulsions, will follow.

Hypoglycemia in any stage requires prompt recognition and treatment. Because of the potential for injury to the brain, the mechanisms and management of hypoglycemia should be understood by all who use drugs capable of producing it.

Hypothermia A state of the body characterized by an unexpected decline of internal body temperature to levels significantly below the norm of 98.6 degrees F or 37 degrees C. By definition, hypothermia means a body temperature of less than 95 degrees F or 35 degrees C. The elderly and debilitated are more prone to develop hypothermia if clothed inadequately and exposed to cool environments. Most episodes are initiated by room temperatures below 65 degrees F or 18.3 degrees C. The condition often develops suddenly, can mimic a stroke and has a mortality rate of 50%. Some drugs, such as phenothiazines, barbiturates and benzodiazepines, are conducive to the development of hypothermia in susceptible individuals.

Idiosyncrasy An abnormal mechanism of drug response that occurs in individuals who have a peculiar defect in their body chemistry (often hereditary) which produces an effect totally unrelated to the drug's normal pharmacological action. Idiosyncrasy is not a form of allergy. The actual chemical defects responsible for certain idiosyncratic drug re-actions are well understood; others are not.

Example: Approximately 100 million people in the world (including 10% of American blacks) have a specific enzyme deficiency in their red blood cells that causes these cells to disintegrate when exposed to drugs such as sulfonamides (Gantrisin, Kynex), nitrofurantoin (Furadantin, Macrodantin), probenecid (Benemid), quinine and quinidine. As a result of this reaction, these drugs (and others) can cause a significant anemia in susceptible individuals.

Example: Approximately 5% of the population of the United States is susceptible to the development of glaucoma on prolonged use of cortisone-related drugs (see Cortisone Drug Class in Section Four).

Immunosuppressive A drug that significantly impairs (suppresses) the functions of the body's immune system. In some instances, immunosuppression is an intended drug effect as in the use of cyclosporine to prevent the immune system from rejecting a transplanted heart or kidney. In other instances, it is an unwanted side-effect as in the long-term use of cortisonelike drugs (to control chronic asthma) that suppresses the immune system sufficiently to permit reactivation of a dormant tuberculosis. Immunosuppressant drugs are being used to treat several chronic disorders that are thought to be autoimmune diseases, notably advanced rheumatoid arthritis, ulcerative colitis and systemic lupus erythematosus.

Interaction An unwanted change in the body's response to a drug that results when a second drug that is capable of altering the action of the first is administered at the same time. Some drug interactions can enhance the effect of either drug, producing an overresponse similar to overdosage. Other interactions may reduce drug effectiveness and cause inadequate response. A third type of interaction can produce a seemingly unrelated toxic response with no associated increase or decrease in the pharmacological actions of the interacting drugs.

Theoretically, many drugs can interact with one another, but in reality drug interactions are comparatively infrequent. Many interactions can be anticipated, and the physician can make appropriate adjustments in dosage to prevent or minimize unintended fluctuations in drug response.

Jaundice A yellow coloration of the skin (and the white portion of the eyes) that occurs when excessive bile pigments accumulate in the blood as a result of impaired liver function. Jaundice can be produced by several mechanisms. It may occur as a manifestation of a wide variety of diseases, or it may represent an adverse reaction to a particular drug. At times it is difficult to distinguish between disease-induced jaundice and drug-induced jaundice.

Jaundice due to a drug is always a serious adverse effect. Anyone taking a drug that is capable of causing jaundice should watch closely for any significant change in the color of urine or feces. Dark discoloration of the urine and paleness (lack of color) of the stool may be early indications of a developing jaundice. Should either of these symptoms occur, it is advisable to discontinue the drug and notify the prescribing physician promptly. Diagnostic tests are available to clarify the nature of the jaundice.

Lupus Erythematosus (LE) A serious disease of unknown cause that occurs in two forms, one limited to the skin (discoid LE) and the other involving several body systems (systemic LE). Both forms occur predominantly in young women. About 5% of cases of the discoid form convert to the systemic form. Basically, systemic LE is a disorder of the body's immune system which may result in chronic, progressive inflammation and destruction of the connective tissue framework of the skin, blood vessels, joints, brain, heart muscle, lungs and kidneys. Altered proteins in the blood lead to the formation of antibodies which react with certain organ tissues to produce the inflammation and destruction characteristic of the disease. A reduction in the number of white blood cells and blood platelets often occurs. The course of systemic LE is usually quite protracted and unpredictable. While no cure is known, satisfactory management may be achieved in some cases by the judicious use of cortisonelike drugs.

Several drugs in wide use are capable of initiating a form of systemic LE quite similar to that which occurs spontaneously. (More than 100 cases due to the use of procainamide have been reported.) Suggestive symptoms may appear as early as 2 weeks or as late as 8 years after starting the responsible drug. The initial symptoms usually consist of low-grade fever, skin rashes of various kinds, aching muscles and multiple joint pains. Chest pains (pleurisy) are fairly common. Enlargement of the lymph glands occurs less frequently. Symptoms usually subside following discontinuation of the responsible drug, but laboratory evidence of the reaction may persist for many months.

Drugs known to induce systemic LE include:

chlorpromazine	phenothiazines (some)
clofibrate	phenylbutazone
hydralazine	phenytoin
isoniazid	practolol
oral contraceptives	procainamide
penicillamine	thiouracil
phenolphthalein	

Orthostatic Hypotension A type of low blood pressure that is related to body position or posture (also called postural hypotension). The individual who is subject to orthostatic hypotension may have a normal blood pressure while lying down, but on sitting upright or standing he will experience sudden sensations of lightheadedness, dizziness and a feeling of impending faint that compel him to return quickly to a lying position. These symptoms are manifestations of inadequate blood flow (oxygen supply) to the brain due to an abnormal delay in the rise in blood pressure that always occurs as the body adjusts the circulation to the erect position.

Many drugs (especially the stronger antihypertensives) may cause orthostatic hypotension. Individuals who experience this drug effect should report it to their physician so that appropriate dosage adjustment can be made to minimize it. Failure to correct or to compensate for these sudden drops in blood pressure can lead to severe falls and injury.

The tendency to orthostatic hypotension can be reduced by avoiding sudden standing, prolonged standing, vigorous exercise and exposure to hot environments. Alcoholic beverages should be used cautiously until their combined effect with the drug in use has been determined.

Overdosage The meaning of this term should not be limited to the concept of doses that clearly exceed the normal dosage range recommended by the manufacturer. The optimal dose of many drugs (that amount which gives the greatest benefit with least distress) varies greatly from person to person. What may be an average dose for the majority of individuals will be an overdose for some and an underdose for others. Numerous factors, such as age, body size, nutritional status and liver and kidney function, have significant influence on dosage requirements. Drugs with narrow safety margins often produce indications of overdosage if something delays the regular elimination of the customary daily dose. In this instance, overdosage results from accumulation of prescribed daily doses. Massive overdosage—as occurs with accidental ingestion of drugs by children or with suicidal intention by adults—is referred to as poisoning.

Over-the-Counter (OTC) Drugs Drug products that can be purchased without prescription. Many are available in food stores, variety stores and newsstands as well as in conventional drug stores. Because of the unrestricted availability of these drugs, many people do not look upon OTC medicines as drugs. But drugs they are! And like the more potent drug products that are sold only on prescription, they are chemicals that are capable of a wide variety of actions on biological systems. Within the last 30 years, many OTC drugs have assumed greater importance because of their ability to interact unfavorably with some widely used prescription drugs. Serious problems in drug management can arise when (1) the patient fails to inform the physician of the OTC drug(s) he is taking ("because they really aren't drugs") and (2) the physician fails to specify that his question about what medicines are being taken currently *includes all OTC drugs*. During any course of treatment, whether medical or surgical, the patient should consult with the physician regarding any OTC drug that he wishes to take.

The major classes of OTC drugs for internal use include:

allergy medicines (antihistamines)	aspirin substitutes
antacids	asthma aids
antiworm medicines	cold medicines (decongestants)
aspirin and aspirin combinations	cough medicines

diarrhea remedies
digestion aids
diuretics
iron preparations
laxatives
menstrual aids
motion sickness remedies
pain relievers

reducing aids
salt substitutes
sedatives and tranquilizers
sleeping pills
stimulants (caffeine)
sugar substitutes (saccharin)
tonics
vitamins

Paradoxical Reaction An unexpected drug response that is not consistent with the known pharmacology of the drug and may in fact be the opposite of the intended and anticipated response. Such reactions are due to individual sensitivity or variability and can occur in any age group. They are seen more commonly, however, in children and the elderly.

Example: An 80-year-old man was admitted to a nursing home following the death of his wife. He had difficulty adjusting to his new environment and was restless, agitated and irritable. He was given a trial of the tranquilizer diazepam (Valium) to relax him, starting with small doses. On the second day of medication he became confused and erratic in behavior. The dose of diazepam was increased. On the third day he began to wander aimlessly, talked incessantly in a loud voice and displayed anger and hostility when attempts were made to help him. Suspecting the possibility of a paradoxical reaction, the diazepam was discontinued. All behavioral disturbances gradually subsided within 3 days.

Parkinson-like Disorders (Parkinsonism) A group of symptoms that resembles those caused by Parkinson's disease, a chronic disorder of the nervous system also known as shaking palsy. The characteristic features of parkinsonism include a fixed, emotionless facial expression (masklike in appearance), a prominent trembling of the hands, arms or legs and stiffness of the extremities that limits movement and produces a rigid posture and gait.

Parkinsonism is a fairly common adverse effect that occurs in about 15% of all patients who take large doses of strong tranquilizers (notably the phenothiazines) or use them over an extended period of time. If recognized early, the Parkinson-like features will lessen or disappear with reduced dosage or change in medication. In some instances, however, Parkinson-like changes may become permanent, requiring appropriate medication for their control.

Peripheral Neuritis (Peripheral Neuropathy) A group of symptoms that results from injury to nerve tissue in the extremities. A variety of drugs and chemicals are capable of inducing changes in nerve structure or function. The characteristic pattern consists of a sensation of numbness and tingling that usually begins in the fingers and toes and is accompanied by an altered sensation to touch and vague discomfort ranging from aching sensations to burning pain. Severe forms of peripheral neuritis may include loss of muscular strength and coordination.

A relatively common form of peripheral neuritis is that seen with the long-term use of isoniazid in the treatment of tuberculosis. If vitamin B-6 (pyridoxine) is not given concurrently with isoniazid, peripheral neuritis may occur in sensitive individuals. Vitamin B-6 can be both preventive and curative in this form of drug-induced peripheral neuritis.

Since peripheral neuritis can also occur as a late complication following many viral infections, care must be taken to avoid assigning a cause-and-effect relationship to a drug which is not responsible for the nerve injury (see CAUSE-AND-EFFECT RELATIONSHIP).

Peyronie's Disease A permanent deformity of the penis caused by the formation of dense fibrous (scarlike) tissue within the system of penile vessels that become engorged with blood during the process of erection. During sexual arousal, this inelastic fibrous tissue causes a painful downward bowing of the penis that hampers or precludes satisfactory intercourse. This condition has been associated with the use of phenytoin (Dilantin, etc.) and with most members of the beta blocker class of drugs (see Drug Class, Section Four).

Pharmacology The medical science that relates to the development and use of medicinal drugs, their composition and action in animals and man. Used in its broadest sense, pharmacology embraces the related sciences of medicinal chemistry, experimental therapeutics and toxicology.

Example: The widely used sulfonylurea drugs (Diabinese, Dymelor, Orinase, Tolinase) are effective in the treatment of some forms of diabetes because of the accidental discovery that some of their parent "sulfa" drugs produced hypoglycemia (low blood sugar) during their early therapeutic trials as anti-infectives. Subsequent investigation of the mechanisms of action (*pharmacology*) of these drugs revealed that they are capable of stimulating the pancreas to release more insulin.

Pharmacological studies on another group of "sulfa"-related drugs— the thiazide diuretics—revealed that they could induce the kidney to excrete more water and salt in the urine. This drug action is of great value in treating high blood pressure and heart failure.

Photosensitivity A drug-induced change in the skin that results in the development of a rash or exaggerated sunburn on exposure to the sun or ultraviolet lamps. The reaction is confined to uncovered areas of skin, providing a clue to the nature of its cause. (See Table 3 in Section Six.)

Porphyria The porphyrias are a group of hereditary disorders characterized by excessive production of prophyrins, essential respiratory pigments of the body. (One porphyrin is a component of hemoglobin, the pigment of red blood cells.) Two forms of porphyria—acute intermittent porphyria and cutaneous porphyria—can be activated by the use of certain drugs. Acute intermittent porphyria involves damage to the nervous system; an acute attack can include fever, rapid heart rate, vomiting, pain in the abdomen and legs, hallucinations, seizures, paralysis and coma. Twenty-three drugs (or drug classes) can induce an acute attack; among these are the barbiturates, "sulfa" drugs, chlordiazepoxide (Librium), chlorpropamide (Diabinese), methyldopa (Aldomet) and phenytoin (Dilantin). Cutaneous porphyria involves damage to the skin and liver. An episode can include reddening and blistering of the skin, followed by crust formation, scarring and excessive hair growth; repeated liver damage can lead to cirrhosis. This form of porphyria can be precipitated by chloroquine, estrogen, oral contraceptives and excessive iron.

Priapism The prolonged, painful erection of the penis usually unassociated with sexual arousal or stimulation. It is caused by obstruction to the outflow (drainage) of blood through the veins at the root of the penis. Erection may persist for 30 minutes to a few hours and then subside spontaneously; or it may persist for up to 30 hours and require surgical drainage of blood from the penis for relief. More than half of the episodes of priapism induced by drugs result in permanent impotence. Sickle cell anemia (or trait) may predispose to priapism; individuals with this disorder should avoid all drugs that may induce priapism.

Drugs reported to induce priapism include the following:

anabolic steroids (male hormone–like drugs: Anadrol, Anavar, Android, Halotestin, Metandren, Oreton, Testred, Winstrol)
chlorpromazine (Thorazine)
cocaine
guanethidine (Ismelin)
haloperidol (Haldol)
heparin
levodopa (Sinemet)
molindone (Moban)
prazosin (Minipress)
prochlorperazine (Compazine)
trazodone (Desyrel)
trifluoperazine (Stelazine)
warfarin (Coumadin)

Prostatism This term refers to the difficulties associated with an enlarged prostate gland. As the prostate enlarges (a natural development in aging men), it constricts the urethra (outflow passage) where it joins the urinary bladder and impedes urination. This causes a reduction in the size and force of the urinary stream, hesitancy in starting the flow of urine, interruption of urination and incomplete emptying of the bladder. Atropine and drugs with atropinelike effects can impair the bladder's ability to compensate for the obstructing prostate gland, thus intensifying all of the above symptoms.

Raynaud's Phenomenon This term refers to intermittent episodes of reduced blood flow into the fingers or toes, with resulting paleness, discomfort, numbness and tingling. It is due to an exaggerated constriction of the small arteries that supply blood to the digits. Characteristically an attack is precipitated either by emotional stress or exposure to cold. It can occur as part of a systemic disorder (lupus erythematosus, scleroderma), or it can occur without apparent cause (Raynaud's disease).

Some widely used drugs, notably beta-adrenergic blockers and products that contain ergotamine, are conducive to the development of Raynaud-like symptoms in predisposed individuals.

Reye (Reye's) Syndrome An acute, often fatal, childhood illness characterized by swelling of the brain and toxic degeneration of the liver. It usually develops during recovery from a flulike infection, measles or chickenpox. Symptoms include fever, headache, delirium, loss of consciousness and seizures. It is one of the 10 major causes of death in children aged 1 to 10 years. Evidence to date suggests that the syndrome may be due to the combined effects of viral infection and chemical toxins (possibly drugs) in a genetically predisposed child. Drugs that have been used just prior to the onset of symptoms include acetaminophen, aspirin, antibiotics and antiemetics (drugs to control nausea and vomiting). Although it has not been definitely established that drugs actually cause Reye syndrome, it is thought that they may contribute to its development or adversely affect its course. Current recommendations are to avoid the use of acetaminophen, aspirin and antiemetic drugs in children with flulike infections, chickenpox or measles.

Secondary Effect A by-product or complication of drug use which does not occur as part of the drug's primary pharmacological activity. Secondary effects are unwanted consequences and may therefore be classified as adverse effects.

Example: The reactivation of dormant tuberculosis can be a *secondary effect* of long-term cortisone administration for arthritis. Cortisone and related drugs (see Drug Class, Section Four) suppress natural immunity and lower resistance to infection.

Example: The cramping of leg muscles can be a *secondary effect* of diuretic (urine-producing) drug treatment for high blood pressure. Excessive loss of potassium through increased urination renders the muscle vulnerable to painful spasm during exercise.

Side-Effect A normal, expected and predictable response to a drug that accompanies the principal (intended) response sought in treatment. Side-effects are part of a drug's pharmacological activity and thus are unavoidable. Most side-effects are undesirable. The majority cause minor annoyance and inconvenience; some may cause serious problems in managing certain diseases; a few can be hazardous.

Example: The drug propantheline (Pro-Banthine) is used to treat peptic ulcer because one of the consequences of its pharmacological action is the reduction of acid formation in the stomach (an intended effect). Other consequences can include blurring of near vision, dryness of the mouth and constipation. These are *side-effects.*

Superinfection (Suprainfection) The development of a second infection that is superimposed upon an initial infection currently under treatment. The superinfection is caused by organisms that are not susceptible to the killing action of the drug(s) used to treat the original (primary) infection. Superinfections usually occur during or immediately following treatment with a broad spectrum antibiotic—one that is capable of altering the customary balance of bacterial populations in various parts of the body. The disturbance of this balance permits the overgrowth of organisms that normally exist in numbers too small to cause disease. The superinfection may also require treatment, using those drugs that are effective against the offending organism.

   Example: Recurrent infections of the kidney and bladder often require repeated courses of treatment with a variety of anti-infective drugs. When these are taken by mouth they can suppress the normally dominant types of bacteria present in the colon and rectum, encouraging the overgrowth of yeast organisms which are capable of causing *colitis.* When this occurs, colitis is a *superinfection.*

Tardive Dyskinesia A late-developing, drug-induced disorder of the nervous system characterized by involuntary bizarre movements of the jaws, lips and tongue. It occurs after long-term treatment with the more potent drugs used in the management of serious mental illness. While it may occur in any age group, it is more common in the middle-aged and the elderly. Older, chronically ill women are particularly susceptible to this adverse drug effect. Once developed, the pattern of uncontrollable chewing, lip puckering and repetitive tongue protruding (fly-catching movement) appears to be irreversible. No consistently satisfactory treatment or cure is available. To date, there is no way of identifying beforehand the individual who may develop this distressing reaction to drug treatment, and there is no known prevention. Fortunately, the persistent dyskinesia (abnormal movement) is not accompanied by further impairment of mental function or deterioration of intelligence. It is ironic, however, that the patient who shows significant improvement in his mental illness but is unfortunate enough to develop tardive dyskinesia may have to remain hospitalized because of a reaction to a drug that was given to make it possible for him to leave the hospital.

Tolerance An adaptation by the body that lessens responsiveness to a drug on continuous administration. Body tissues become accustomed to the drug's presence and react to it less vigorously. Tolerance can be beneficial or harmful in treatment.

   Examples: Beneficial tolerance occurs when the hay fever sufferer finds that the side-effect of drowsiness gradually disappears after 4 or 5 days of continuous use of antihistamines.

   Harmful tolerance occurs when the patient with "shingles" (herpes zoster) finds that the usual dose of codeine is no longer sufficient to relieve pain and that the need for increasing dosage creates a risk of physical dependence or addiction.

Toxicity The capacity of a drug to dangerously impair body functions or to damage body tissues. Most drug toxicity is related to total dosage: the larger the overdose, the greater the toxic effects. Some drugs, however, can produce toxic reactions when used in normal doses. Such adverse effects are not due to allergy or idiosyncrasy; in many instances their mechanisms are not fully understood. Toxic effects due to overdosage are generally a harmful extension of the drug's normal pharmacological actions and—to some extent—are predictable and preventable. Toxic reactions which occur with normal dosage are unrelated to the drug's known pharmacology and for the most part are unpredictable and unexplainable.

Tyramine A chemical present in many common foods and beverages that causes no difficulties to body functioning under normal circumstances. The main pharmacological action of tyramine is to raise the blood pressure. Normally, enzymes present in many body tissues neutralize this action of tyramine in the quantities in which it is consumed in the average diet. The principal enzyme responsible for neutralizing the blood-pressure-elevating action of tyramine (and chemicals related to it) is monoamine oxidase (MAO) type A. Monoamine oxidase type A serves an important regulatory function that helps to balance several of the chemical processes in the body that control certain activities of the nervous system. Stabilization of the blood pressure is one of these activities. If the action of monoamine oxidase type A is blocked, chemical substances like tyramine function unopposed, and relatively small amounts can cause alarming and dangerous elevations of blood pressure.

Several drugs in use today are capable of blocking the action of monoamine oxidase type A. These drugs are commonly referred to as monoamine oxidase (MAO) type A inhibitors (see Drug Class, Section Four). If an individual is taking one of these drugs and his diet includes foods or beverages that contain a significant amount of tyramine, he may experience a sudden increase in blood pressure. Before this interaction of food and drug was understood, several deaths due to brain hemorrhage occurred in persons taking MAO type A inhibitor drugs as a result of an extreme elevation of blood pressure following a meal of tyramine-rich foods.

It should be noted also that MAO inhibitor drugs can interact with many other drugs and cause serious adverse effects. Consult your physician before taking *any* drug concurrently with one that can inhibit the action of monoamine oxidase, type A or B.

Any protein-containing food that has undergone partial decomposition may present a hazard because of its increased tyramine content. The following foods and beverages have been reported to contain varying amounts of tyramine. Unless their tyramine content is known to be insignificant, they should be avoided altogether while taking a MAO type A inhibitor drug. Consult your physician about the advisability of using any of the foods or beverages on these lists if you are taking such drugs.

FOODS	BEVERAGES
Aged cheeses of all kinds*	Beer (unpasteurized)
Avocado	Chianti wine
Banana skins	Sherry wine

*Cottage cheese, cream cheese and processed cheese are safe to eat.

FOODS	BEVERAGES
Beef liver (unless fresh and used at once)	Vermouth
"Bovril" extract	
Broad bean pods	
Chicken liver (unless fresh and used at once)	
Chocolate	
Figs, canned	
Fish, canned	
Fish, dried and salted	
Herring, pickled	
"Marmite" extract	
Meat extracts	
Meat tenderizers	
Raisins	
Raspberries	
Sour cream	
Soy sauce	
Yeast extracts	

NOTE: *Any* high-protein food that is aged or has undergone breakdown by putrefaction probably contains tyramine and could produce a hypertensive crisis in anyone taking MAO type A inhibiting drugs.

TABLES OF DRUG INFORMATION

TABLE 1

Your Drugs and Behavior

In addition to producing side-effects that can alter mood and disturb emotional stability, some drugs are capable of inducing unexpected and unpredictable patterns of abnormal thinking and behavior. Such responses are relatively infrequent, but the nature and degree of mental disturbance can, at times, be quite alarming and potentially dangerous for both patient and family. It is now well recognized that such paradoxical responses are often of an idiosyncratic nature, and that the individual with a history of a serious mental or emotional disorder is more likely to experience bizarre reactions involving disturbed behavior.

It is often difficult to judge whether a particular aberration of thought or behavior is primarily a feature of the disorder under treatment or an effect of one (or more) drugs the patient may be taking at the time. If in doubt, it is advisable to discontinue any drug with potential for such side-effects and observe for changes during a drug-free period.

Drugs reported to impair *concentration* and/or *memory*

antihistamines*
antiparkinsonism drugs*
barbiturates*
benzodiazepines*
isoniazid

monoamine oxidase inhibitor
   drugs*
phenytoin
primidone
scopolamine

Drugs reported to cause *confusion, delirium* or *disorientation*

acetazolamide
aminophylline
antidepressants*
antihistamines*
atropinelike drugs*
barbiturates*
benzodiazepines*
bromides
carbamazepine
chloroquine
cimetidine
cortisonelike drugs*
cycloserine
digitalis

digitoxin
digoxin
disulfiram
ethchlorvynol
ethinamate
fenfluramine
glutethimide
isoniazid
levodopa
meprobamate
para-aminosalicylic acid
phenelzine
phenothiazines*
phenytoin

*See Drug Class, Section Four.

Drugs reported to cause *confusion, delirium* or *disorientation* (cont.)

piperazine
primidone
propranolol

reserpine
scopolamine

Drugs reported to cause *paranoid thinking*

bromides
cortisonelike drugs*
diphenhydramine

disulfiram
isoniazid
levodopa

Drugs reported to cause *schizophreniclike behavior*

amphetamines*
ephedrine
fenfluramine

phenmetrazine
phenylpropanolamine

Drugs reported to cause *maniclike behavior*

antidepressants*
cortisonelike drugs*

levodopa
monoamine oxidase inhibitor
     drugs*

Less apparent—but no less important—are the mood-altering *side-effects* of some drugs which are prescribed primarily for altogether unrelated conditions, with no intention of modifying emotional status. In keeping with the wide variation of individual response to the primary and intended effects of drugs, it is to be expected that the emotional and behavioral secondary effects will also be quite unpredictable and will vary enormously from person to person. However, the following experiences have been observed with sufficient frequency to establish recognizable patterns.

Drugs reported to cause *nervousness* (anxiety and irritability)

amantadine
amphetaminelike drugs* (appetite
   suppressants)
antihistamines*
caffeine

chlorphenesin
cortisonelike drugs*
ephedrine
epinephrine
isoproterenol

*See Drug Class, Section Four.

Drugs reported to cause *nervousness* (cont.)

levodopa
liothyronine (in excessive dosage)
methylphenidate
methysergide
monoamine oxidase inhibitor
  drugs*

nylidrin
oral contraceptives
theophylline
thyroid (in excessive dosage)
thyroxine (in excessive dosage)

Drugs reported to cause *emotional depression*

amantadine
amphetamine* (on withdrawal)
benzodiazepines*
carbamazepine
chloramphenicol
cortisonelike drugs*
cycloserine
digitalis
digitoxin
digoxin
diphenoxylate
estrogens
ethionamide
fenfluramine (on withdrawal)
fluphenazine
guanethidine

haloperidol
indomethacin
isoniazid
levodopa
methsuximide
methyldopa
methysergide
metoprolol
oral contraceptives
phenylbutazone
procainamide
progesterones
propranolol
reserpine
sulfonamides*
vitamin D (in excessive dosage)

Drugs reported to cause *euphoria*

amantadine
aminophylline
amphetamines
antihistamines* (some)
antispasmodics, synthetic*
aspirin
barbiturates*
benzphetamine
chloral hydrate
clorazepate
codeine
cortisonelike drugs*

diethylpropion
diphenoxylate
ethosuximide
flurazepam
haloperidol
levodopa
meprobamate
methysergide
monoamine oxidase inhibitor
  drugs*
morphine
pargyline

*See Drug Class, Section Four.

Drugs reported to cause *euphoria* (cont.)

pentazocine
phenmetrazine
propoxyphene

scopalamine
tybamate

Drugs reported to cause *excitement*

acetazolamide
amantadine
amphetaminelike drugs*
antidepressants*
antihistamines*
atropinelike drugs*
barbiturates* (paradoxical response)
benzodiazepines* (paradoxical response)
cortisonelike drugs
cycloserine
diethylpropion
digitalis
ephedrine
epinephrine

ethinamate (paradoxical response)
ethionamide
glutethimide (paradoxical response)
isoniazid
isoproterenol
levodopa
meperidine and MAO inhibitor drugs*
methyldopa and MAO inhibitor drugs*
methyprylon (paradoxical response)
nalidixic acid
orphenadrine
quinine
scopolamine

*See Drug Class, Section Four.

TABLE 2

Your Drugs and Vision

Approximately 3.5% of all adverse drug effects involve impairment of vision or damage to structures of the eye. Some effects, such as blurring of vision or double vision, may occur shortly after starting a drug. These quickly disappear with adjustment of dosage. More subtle and serious effects, such as the development of cataracts or damage to the retina or optic nerve, may not occur until a drug has been in continuous use for an extended period of time. Some of these changes are irreversible. If you are taking a drug that can affect the eye in any way, you are urged to report promptly any eye discomfort or change in vision so that appropriate evaluation can be made and corrective action taken as soon as possible.

Drugs reported to cause *blurring of vision*

acetazolamide
antiarthritic/anti-inflammatory
  drugs
antidepressants*
antihistamines*
atropinelike drugs*
chlorthalidone
ciprofloxacin
cortisonelike drugs*

diethylstilbestrol
etretinate
fenfluramine
norfloxacin
oral contraceptives
phenytoin
sulfonamides*
tetracyclines*
thiazide diuretics*

Drugs reported to cause *double vision*

antidepressants*
antidiabetic drugs*
antihistamines*
aspirin
barbiturates*
benzodiazepines*
bromides
carbamazepine
carisoprodol
chloroquine
chlorprothixene
ciprofloxacin
clomiphene
colchicine

colistin
cortisonelike drugs*
digitalis
digitoxin
digoxin
ethionamide
ethosuximide
etretinate
guanethidine
hydroxychloroquine
indomethacin
isoniazid
levodopa
mephenesin

*See Drug Class, Section Four.

Drugs reported to cause *double vision* (cont.)

methocarbamol
methsuximide
morphine
nalidixic acid
nitrofurantoin
norfloxacin
oral contraceptives
orphenadrine
oxyphenbutazone
pentazocine

phenothiazines*
phensuximide
phenylbutazone
phenytoin
primidone
propranolol
quinidine
sedatives/sleep inducers*
thiothixene
tranquilizers*

Drugs reported to cause *farsightedness*

ergot
penicillamine

sulfonamides* (possibly)
tolbutamide (possibly)

Drugs reported to cause *nearsightedness*

acetazolamide
aspirin
carbachol
chlorthalidone
codeine
cortisonelike drugs*
ethosuximide
methsuximide
morphine

oral contraceptives
penicillamine
phenothiazines*
phensuximide
spironolactone
sulfonamides*
tetracyclines*
thiazide diuretics*

Drugs reported to *alter color vision*

acetaminophen
amodiaquine
amyl nitrite
aspirin
atropine
barbiturates*
belladonna
chloramphenicol

chloroquine
chlorpromazine
chlortetracycline
cortisonelike drugs*
digitalis
digitoxin
digoxin
disulfiram

*See Drug Class, Section Four.

Drugs reported to *alter color vision* (cont.)

epinephrine
ergotamine
erythromycin
ethchlorvynol
ethionamide
fluphenazine
furosemide
hydroxychloroquine
indomethacin
isocarboxazid
isoniazid
mephenamic acid
mesoridazine
methysergide
nalidixic acid
norfloxacin
oral contraceptives
oxyphenbutazone
paramethadione
pargyline
penicillamine

pentylenetetrazol
perphenazine
phenacetin
phenylbutazone
primidone
prochlorperazine
promazine
promethazine
quinacrine
quinidine
quinine
reserpine
sodium salicylate
streptomycin
sulfonamides*
thioridazine
tranylcypromine
trifluoperazine
triflupromazine
trimeprazine
trimethadione

Drugs reported to cause *sensitivity to light* (photophobia)

antidiabetic drugs*
atropinelike drugs*
bromides
chloraquine
clomiphene
digitoxin
doxepin
ethambutol
ethionamide
ethosuximide
etretinate
hydroxychloroquine
mephenytoin

methsuximide
monoamine oxidase inhibitor
  drugs*
nalidixic acid
norfloxacin
oral contraceptives
paramethadione
phenothiazines*
quinidine
quinine
tetracyclines*
trimethadione

*See Drug Class, Section Four.

Drugs reported to cause *halos around lights*

amyl nitrite
chloroquine
cortisonelike drugs*
digitalis
digitoxin
digoxin
hydrochloroquine

nitroglycerin
norfloxacin
oral contraceptives
paramethadione
phenothiazines*
quinacrine
trimethadione

Drugs reported to cause *visual hallucinations*

amantadine
amphetaminelike drugs*
amyl nitrite
antihistamines*
aspirin
atropinelike drugs*
barbiturates*
benzodiazepines*
bromides
carbamazepine
cephalexin
cephaloglycin
chloroquine
cycloserine
digitalis
digoxin
disulfiram
ephedrine
furosemide
griseofulvin

haloperidol
hydroxychloroquine
indomethacin
isosorbide
levodopa
nialamide
oxyphenbutazone
pargyline
pentazocine
phenothiazines*
phenylbutazone
phenytoin
primidone
propranolol
quinine
sedatives/sleep inducers*
sulfonamides*
tetracyclines*
tricyclic antidepressants*
tripelennamine

Drugs reported to impair the use of *contact lenses*

brompheniramine
carbinoxamine
chlorpheniramine
cyclizine
cyproheptadine
dexbrompheniramine
dexchlorpheniramine

dimethindene
diphenhydramine
diphenpyraline
furosemide
oral contraceptives
terfenadine
tripelennamine

*See Drug Class, Section Four.

Drugs reported to cause *cataracts* or *lens deposits*

allopurinol
busulfan
chlorpromazine
chlorprothixene
cortisonelike drugs*
fluphenazine
mesoridazine
methotrimeprazine
perphenazine
phenmetrazine

pilocarpine
prochlorperazine
promazine
promethazine
thioridazine
thiothixene
trifluoperazine
triflupromazine
trimeprazine

*See Drug Class, Section Four.

TABLE 3
Your Drugs and the Sun: Photosensitivity

Some drugs are capable of sensitizing the skin of some individuals to the action of ultraviolet light. This can cause uncovered areas of the skin to react with a rash or exaggerated burn on exposure to sun or ultraviolet lamps. If you are taking any of the following drugs, ask your physician for guidance and use caution with regard to sun exposure.

acetohexamide
amitriptyline
amoxapine
barbiturates
bendroflumethiazide
carbamazepine
chlordiazepoxide
chloroquine
chlorothiazide
chlorpromazine
chlorpropamide
chlortetracycline
chlorthalidone
clindamycin
cyproheptadine
demeclocycline
desipramine
diethylstilbestrol
diltiazem
diphenhydramine
doxepin
doxycycline
estrogen
fluphenazine
glyburide
gold preparations
griseofulvin
hydrochlorothiazide
hydroflumethiazide
imipramine
isotretinoin

lincomycin
maprotiline
mesoridazine
methacycline
methotrexate
nalidixic acid
nortriptyline
oral contraceptives
oxyphenbutazone
oxytetracycline
perphenazine
phenobarbital
phenylbutazone
phenytoin
prochlorperazine
promazine
promethazine
protriptyline
pyrazinamide
sulfonamides
tetracycline
thioridazine
tolazamide
tolbutamide
tranylcypromine
triamterene
trifluoperazine
trimeprazine
trimipramine
triprolidine

TABLE 4
Your Drugs and Sexuality

It is now well established that certain drugs have the potential for affecting sexual functions in a variety of unintended ways. Many commonly prescribed drugs can cause both obvious and subtle effects on one or more aspects of sexual expression. Patients are usually unaware that changes in sexual performance or response may be related to medications they are taking. If they should suspect it, they are often reluctant to discuss the possible association with their physician. In some situations, the sexual dysfunction may be a natural consequence of the disorder under treatment or of a concurrent and undetected disorder, possibilities often overlooked by both practitioner and patient. It is well known that disorders such as diabetes, kidney failure, hypertension, epression and alcoholism may reduce libido and cause failure of erection. In addition, many of the drugs commonly used to treat these conditions may have the ability to augment a subclinical sexual dysfunction through unavoidable pharmacological activity. Such situations require the closest cooperation between therapist and patient in order to correctly assess the possible cause-and-effect relationships and to modify the treatment program appropriately.

Possible Drug Effects on Male Sexuality

1. Increased libido
     androgens (replacement therapy in deficiency states)
     baclofen (Lioresal)
     chlordiazepoxide (Librium) (antianxiety effect)
     diazepam (Valium) (antianxiety effect)
     haloperidol (Haldol)
     levodopa (Larodopa, Sinemet) (may be an indirect effect due to improved sense of well-being)

2. Decreased libido
     antihistamines
     barbiturates
     chlordiazepoxide (Librium) (sedative effect)
     chlorpromazine (Thorazine) 10% to 20% of users
     cimetidine (Tagamet)
     clofibrate (Atromid-S)
     clonidine (Catapres) 10% to 20% of users
     danazol (Danocrine)
     diazepam (Valium) (sedative effect)
     disulfiram (Antabuse)
     estrogens (therapy for prostatic cancer)
     fenfluramine (Pondimin)
     heroin

licorice
medroxyprogesterone (Provera)
methyldopa (Aldomet) 10% to 15% of users
perhexilene (Pexid)
prazosin (Minipress) 15% of users
propranolol (Inderal) rarely
reserpine (Serpasil, Ser-Ap-Es)
spironolactone (Aldactone)
tricyclic antidepressants (TAD's)

3. Impaired erection (impotence)
anticholinergics
antihistamines
baclofen (Lioresal)
barbiturates (when abused)
beta blockers (see Drug Class, Section Four)
chlordiazepoxide (Librium) (in high dosage)
chlorpromazine (Thorazine)
cimetidine (Tagamet)
clofibrate (Atromid-S)
clonidine (Catapres) 10% to 20% of users
cocaine
diazepam (Valium) (in high dosage)
digitalis and its glycosides
disopyramide (Norpace)
disulfiram (Antabuse) (uncertain)
estrogens (therapy for prostatic cancer)
ethacrynic acid (Edecrin) 5% of users
ethionamide (Trecator-SC)
fenfluramine (Pondimin)
furosemide (Lasix) 5% of users
guanethidine (Ismelin)
haloperidol (Haldol) 10% to 20% of users
heroin
hydroxyprogesterone (therapy for prostatic cancer)
licorice
lithium (Lithonate)
marijuana
mesoridazine (Serentil)
methantheline (Banthine)
methyldopa (Aldomet) 10% to 15% of users
monoamine oxidase (MAO) type A inhibitors, 10% to 15% of users
perhexilene (Pexid)
prazosin (Minipres) infrequently
reserpine (Serpasil, Ser-Ap-Es)
spironolactone (Aldactone)
thiazide diuretics, 5% of users

thioridazine (Mellaril)
tricyclic antidepressants (TAD's)

4. Impaired ejaculation
   anticholinergics
   barbiturates (when abused)
   chlorpromazine (Thorazine)
   clonidine (Catapres)
   estrogens (therapy for prostatic cancer)
   guanethidine (Ismelin)
   heroin
   mesoridazine (Serentil)
   methyldopa (Aldomet)
   monoamine oxidase (MAO) type A inhibitors
   phenoxybenzamine (Dibenzyline)
   phentolamine (Regitine)
   reserpine (Serpasil, Ser-Ap-Es)
   thiazide diuretics
   thioridazine (Mellaril)
   tricyclic antidepressants (TAD's)

5. Decreased testosterone
   adrenocorticotropic hormone (ACTH)
   barbiturates
   digoxin (Lanoxin)
   haloperidol (Haldol)
      increased testosterone with low dosage
      decreased testosterone with high dosage
   lithium (Lithonate)
   marijuana
   medroxyprogesterone (Provera)
   monoamine oxidase (MAO) type A inhibitors
   spironolactone (Aldactone)

6. Impaired spermatogenesis (reduced fertility)
   adrenocorticosteroids (prednisone, etc.)
   androgens (moderate to high dosage, extended use)
   antimalarials
   aspirin (abusive, chronic use)
   chlorambucil (Leukeran)
   cimetidine (Tagamet)
   colchicine
   co-trimoxazole (Bactrim, Septra)
   cyclophosphamide (Cytoxan)
   estrogens (therapy for prostatic cancer)
   marijuana
   medroxyprogesterone (Provera)
   methotrexate
   monoamine oxidase (MAO) type A inhibitors

niridazole (Ambilhar)
nitrofurantoin (Furadantin)
spironolactone (Aldactone)
sulfasalazine (Azulfidine)
testosterone (moderate to high dosage, extended use)
vitamin C (in doses of 1 gram or more)

7. Testicular disorders
   Swelling
   tricyclic antidepressants (TAD's)
   Inflammation
   oxyphenbutazone (Tandearil)
   Atrophy
   androgens (moderate to high dosage, extended use)
   chlorpromazine (Thorazine)
   cyclophosphamide (Cytoxan) (in prepubescent boys)
   spironolactone (Aldactone)

8. Penile disorders
   Priapism (see Glossary)
   anabolic steroids (male hormonelike drugs)
   chlorpromazine (Thorazine)
   cocaine
   guanethidine (Ismelin)
   haloperidol (Haldol)
   heparin
   levodopa (Sinemet)
   molindone (Moban)
   prazosin (Minipress)
   prochlorperazine (Compazine)
   trazodone (Desyrel)
   trifluoperazine (Stelazine)
   warfarin (Coumadin)
   Peyronie's disease (see Glossary)
   beta blocker drugs (see Drug Class, Section Four)
   phenytoin (Dilantin, etc.)

9. Gynecomastia (excessive development of the male breast)
   androgens (partial conversion to estrogen)
   BCNU
   busulfan (Myleran)
   chlormadinone
   chlorpromazine (Thorazine)
   chlortetracycline (Aureomycin)
   cimetidine (Tagamet)
   clonidine (Catapres) (infrequently)
   diethylstilbestrol (DES)
   digitalis and its glycosides
   estrogens (therapy for prostatic cancer)

ethionamide (Trecator-SC)
griseofulvin (Fulvicin, etc.)
haloperidol (Haldol)
heroin
human chorionic gonadotropin
isoniazid (INH, Nydrazid)
marijuana
mestranol
methyldopa (Aldomet)
phenelzine (Nardil)
reserpine (Serpasil, Ser-Ap-Es)
spironolactone (Aldactone)
thioridazine (Mellaril)
tricyclic antidepressants (TAD's)
vincristine (Oncovin)

10. Feminization (loss of libido, impotence, gynecomastia, testicular atrophy)
    conjugated estrogens (Premarin, etc.)

11. Precocious puberty
    anabolic steroids
    androgens
    isoniazid (INH)

Possible Drug Effects on Female Sexuality

1. Increased libido
    androgens
    chlordiazepoxide (Librium) (antianxiety effect)
    diazepam (Valium) (antianxiety effect)
    mazindol (Sanorex)
    oral contraceptives (freedom from fear of pregnancy)

2. Decreased libido
    See list of drug effects on male sexuality. Some of these *may* have
    potential for reducing libido in the female. The literature is sparse
    on this subject.

3. Impaired arousal and orgasm
    anticholinergics
    clonidine (Catapres)
    methyldopa (Aldomet)
    monoamine oxidase inhibitors (MAOI's)
    tricyclic antidepressants (TAD's)

4. Breast enlargement
    penicillamine
    tricyclic antidepressants (TAD's)

5. Galactorrhea (spontaneous flow of milk)
   amphetamine
   chlorpromazine (Thorazine)
   cimetidine (Tagamet)
   haloperidol (Haldol)
   heroin
   methyldopa (Aldomet)
   metoclopramide (Reglan)
   oral contraceptives
   phenothiazines
   reserpine (Serpasil, Ser-Ap-Es)
   sulpiride (Equilid)
   tricyclic antidepressants (TAD's)

6. Ovarian failure (reduced fertility)
   anesthetic gases (operating room staff)
   cyclophosphamide (Cytoxan)
   cytostatic drugs
   danazol (Danacrine)
   medroxyprogesterone (Provera)

7. Altered menstruation (menstrual disorders)
   adrenocorticosteroids (prednisone, etc.)
   androgens
   barbiturates (when abused)
   chlorambucil (Leukeran)
   chlorpromazine (Thorazine)
   cyclophosphamide (Cytoxan)
   danazol (Danocrine)
   estrogens
   ethionamide (Trecator-SC)
   haloperidol (Haldol)
   heroin
   isoniazid (INH, Nydrazid)
   marijuana
   medroxprogesterone (Provera)
   oral contraceptives
   phenothiazines
   progestins
   radioisotopes
   rifampin (Rifadin, Rifamate, Rimactane)
   spironolactone (Aldactone)
   testosterone
   thioridazine (Mellaril)
   vitamin A (in excessive dosage)

8. Virilization (acne, hirsutism, lowering of voice, enlargement of clitoris)
   anabolic drugs
   androgens

haloperidol (Haldol)
oral contraceptives (lowering of voice)

9. Precocious puberty
   estrogens (in hair lotions)
   isoniazid (INH, Nydrazid)

TABLE 5

Your Drugs and Alcohol

Beverages containing alcohol may interact unfavorably with a wide variety of drugs. The most important (and most familiar) interaction occurs when the depressant action on the brain of sedatives, sleep-inducing drugs, tranquilizers and narcotic drugs is intensified by alcohol. Alcohol may also reduce the effectiveness of some drugs, and it can interact with certain other drugs to produce toxic effects. Some drugs may increase the intoxicating effects of alcohol, producing further impairment of mental alertness, judgment, physical coordination and reaction time.

While drug interactions with alcohol are generally predictable, the intensity and significance of these interactions can vary greatly from one individual to another and from one occasion to another. This is because many factors influence what happens when drugs and alcohol interact. These factors include individual variations in sensitivity to drugs (including alcohol), the chemistry and quantity of the drug, the type and amount of alcohol consumed and the sequence in which drug and alcohol are taken. If you need to use any of the drugs listed in the following tables, you should ask your physician for guidance concerning the use of alcohol.

Drugs with which it is advisable to avoid alcohol completely

Drug name or class	Possible interaction with alcohol
amphetamines	excessive rise in blood pressure with alcoholic beverages containing tyramine**
antidepressants*	excessive sedation, increased intoxication
barbiturates*	excessive sedation
bromides	confusion, delirium, increased intoxication
calcium carbamide	disulfiramlike reaction**
carbamazepine	excessive sedation
chlorprothixene	excessive sedation
chlorzoxazone	excessive sedation
disulfiram	disulfiram reaction**
ergotamine	reduced effectiveness of ergotamine
fenfluramine	excessive stimulation of nervous system with some beers and wines
furazolidone	disulfiramlike reaction**

*See Drug Class, Section Four.
**See Glossary.

Drug name or class	Possible interaction with alcohol
haloperidol	excessive sedation
MAO inhibitor drugs*	excessive rise in blood pressure with alcoholic beverages containing tyramine**
meperidine	excessive sedation
meprobamate	excessive sedation
methotrexate	increased liver toxicity and excessive sedation
metronidazole	disulfiramlike reaction**
narcotic drugs	excessive sedation
oxyphenbutazone	increased stomach irritation and/or bleeding
pentazocine	excessive sedation
pethidine	excessive sedation
phenothiazines*	excessive sedation
phenylbutazone	increased stomach irritation and/or bleeding
procarbazine	disulfiramlike reaction**
propoxyphene	excessive sedation
reserpine	excessive sedation, orthostatic hypotension**
sleep-inducing drugs (hypnotics)	excessive sedation
carbromal	
chloral hydrate	
ethchlorvynol	
ethinamate	
glutethimide	
flurazepam	
methaqualone	
methyprylon	
temazepam	
triazolam	
thiothixene	excessive sedation
tricyclic antidepressants*	excessive sedation, increased intoxication
trimethobenzamide	excessive sedation

Drugs with which alcohol should be used only in small amounts (use cautiously until combined effects have been determined)

acetaminophen (Tylenol, etc.)	increased liver toxicity
amantadine	excessive lowering of blood pressure

*See Drug Class, Section Four.
**See Glossary.

Drug name or class	Possible interaction with alcohol
antiarthritic/anti-inflammatory drugs	increased stomach irritation and/or bleeding
anticoagulants (coumarins)*	increased anticoagulant effect
antidiabetic drugs (sulfonylureas)*	increased antidiabetic effect, excessive hypoglycemia**
antihistamines*	excessive sedation
antihypertensives*	excessive orthostatic hypotension**
aspirin (large doses or continuous use)	increased stomach irritation and/or bleeding
benzodiazepines*	excessive sedation
carisoprodol	increased alcoholic intoxication
diethylpropion	excessive nervous system stimulation with alcoholic beverages containing tyramine**
dihydroergotoxine	excessive lowering of blood pressure
diphenoxylate	excessive sedation
dipyridamole	excessive lowering of blood pressure
diuretics*	excessive orthostatic hypotension**
ethionamide	confusion, delirium, psychotic behavior
fenoprofen	increased stomach irritation and/or bleeding
griseofulvin	flushing and rapid heart action
ibuprofen	increased stomach irritation and/or bleeding
indomethacin	increased stomach irritation and/or bleeding
insulin	excessive hypoglycemia**
iron	excessive absorption of iron
isoniazid	decreased effectiveness of isoniazid, increased incidence of hepatitis
lithium	increased confusion and delirium (avoid all alcohol if any indication of lithium overdosage)
methocarbamol	excessive sedation
methotrimeprazine	excessive sedation
methylphenidate	excessive nervous system stimulation with alcoholic beverages containing tyramine**
metoprolol	excessive orthostatic hypotension**
nalidixic acid	increased alcoholic intoxication

*See Drug Class, Section Four.
**See Glossary.

Drug name or class	Possible interaction with alcohol
naproxen	increased stomach irritation and/or bleeding
nicotinic acid	possible orthostatic hypotension**
nitrates* (vasodilators)	possible orthostatic hypotension**
nylidrin	increased stomach irritation
orphenadrine	excessive sedation
phenelzine	increased alcoholic intoxication
phenoxybenzamine	possible orthostatic hypotension**
phentermine	excessive nervous system stimulation with alcoholic beverages containing tyramine**
phenytoin	decreased effect of phenytoin
pilocarpine	prolongation of alcohol effect
prazosin	excessive lowering of blood pressure
primidone	excessive sedation
propranolol	excessive orthostatic hypotension**
sulfonamides*	increased alcoholic intoxication
sulindac	increased stomach irritation and/or bleeding
tolmetin	increased stomach irritation and/or bleeding
tranquilizers (mild)	excessive sedation
chlordiazepoxide	
clorazepate	
diazepam	
hydroxyzine	
meprobamate	
oxazepam	
phenaglycodol	
tybamate	
tranylcypromine	increased alcoholic intoxication

Drugs capable of producing a disulfiramlike reaction** when used concurrently with alcohol

antidiabetic drugs (sulfonylureas)*	nifuroxine
calcium carbamide	nitrofurantoin
chloral hydrate	procarbazine
chloramphenicol	quinacrine
disulfiram	sulfonamides*
furazolidone	tinidazole
metronidazole	tolazoline

*See Drug Class, Section Four.
**See Glossary.

TABLE 6
High-Potassium Foods

Diuretic drugs that cause loss of potassium from the body are often used to treat conditions that also require a reduced intake of sodium. The high-potassium foods listed below have been selected for their compatibility with a sodium restricted diet (500 to 1000 mg of sodium daily).

Beverages

orange juice
prune juice
skim milk
tea
tomato juice
whole milk

Breads and Cereals

brown rice
cornbread
griddle cakes
muffins
oatmeal
shredded wheat
waffles

Fruits

apricot
avocado
banana
fig
honeydew melon
mango
orange
papaya
prune

Meats

beef
chicken
codfish
flounder
haddock
halibut
liver
pork
rockfish
salmon
turkey
veal

Vegetables

baked beans
lima beans
mushrooms
navy beans
parsnips
radishes
squash
sweet potato
tomato
white potato

Sources

The following sources were consulted in the compilation and revision of this book:

Adverse Drug Reaction Bulletin. Edited by D. M. Davies. Newcastle upon Tyne, England: Regional Postgraduate Institute for Medicine and Dentistry, 1989.

AMA Department of Drugs, *AMA Drug Evaluations*, 6th ed. Chicago: American Medical Association, 1986.

Andreoli, T. E., Carpenter, C. C. J., Plum, F., Smith, L. H., eds., *Cecil Essentials of Medicine*. Philadelphia: W. B. Saunders Co., 1986.

Arndt, K. A., *Manual of Dermatologic Therapeutics*, 4th ed. Boston: Little, Brown and Co., 1989.

Atkinson, A. J., Ambre, J. J., *Kalman and Clark's Drug Assay, The Strategy of Therapeutic Drug Monitoring*, 2nd ed. New York: Masson Publishing USA, 1985.

Avery, G. S., ed., *Drug Treatment*, 2nd ed. Sydney, Australia: ADIS Press, 1980.

Berkow, R., ed., *The Merck Manual*, 15th ed. Rahway, New Jersey: Merck Sharp & Dohme Research Laboratories, 1987.

Bevan, J. A., ed., *Essentials of Pharmacology*. Hagerstown, Maryland: Harper & Row, 1976.

Billups, N. F., ed., *American Drug Index 1989*. Philadelphia: J. B. Lippincott Co., 1989.

Branch, W. T., *Office Practice of Medicine*, 2nd ed. Philadelphia: W. B. Saunders Co., 1987.

Briggs, G. G., Bodendorfer, T. W., Freeman, R. K., Yaffee, S. J., *Drugs in Pregnancy and Lactation*. Baltimore: Williams & Wilkins, 1983.

Brooke, M. H., *A Clinician's View of Neuromuscular Diseases*, 2nd ed. Baltimore: Williams & Wilkins, 1986.

Canadian Pharmaceutical Association, *Compendium of Pharmaceuticals and Specialties*, 24th ed. Ottawa: Canadian Pharmaceutical Association, 1989.

Cape, Ronald, *Aging: Its Complex Management*. Hagerstown, Maryland: Harper & Row, 1978.

Clin-Alert. Medford, New Jersey: Clin-Alert, Inc., 1988–1989.

Davies, D. M., ed., *Textbook of Adverse Drug Reactions*, 2nd ed. New York: Oxford University Press, 1981.

Diamond, S., Dalessio, D. J., eds., *The Practicing Physician's Approach to Headache*, 4th ed. Baltimore: Williams & Wilkins, 1986.

Drug Interaction Facts. Edited by R. J. Mangini. St. Louis: Facts and Comparisons Division, J. B. Lippincott Co., 1989.

Drug Interactions Newsletter. Edited by P. D. Hansten, J. R. Horn. Spokane, Washington: Applied Therapeutics, Inc., 1989.

Drug Newsletter. Edited by G. H. Schwach, B. R. Olin. St. Louis: Facts and Comparisons Division, J. B. Lippincott Co., 1989.

Drug Therapy, Clinical Therapeutics for Physicians. New York: Biomedical Information Corporation, 1989.

Dukes, M. N. G., ed., *Meyler's Side Effects of Drugs*, 9th ed. Amsterdam: Excerpta Medica, 1980.

Encyclopedia of Associations, 23rd ed., Vol. 1, Part 2. Detroit: Gale Research, Inc., 1989.

Facts and Comparisons. Edited by B. R. Olin. St. Louis: Facts and Comparisons Division, J. B. Lippincott Co., 1989.

F.D.A. Drug Bulletin. Rockville, Maryland: Department of Health and Human Services, Food and Drug Administration.

Fraunfelder, F. T., *Drug-Induced Ocular Side Effects and Drug Interactions*. Philadelphia: Lea & Febiger, 1976.

Goodman, L. S., Gilman, A., eds., *The Pharmacological Basis of Therapeutics*, 7th ed. New York: Macmillan, 1985.

Greenberger, N. J., Arvanitakis, C., Hurwitz, A., *Drug Treatment of Gastrointestinal Disorders*. New York: Churchill Livingstone, 1978.

Hansten, P. D., *Drug Interactions*, 6th ed. Philadelphia: Lea & Febiger, 1989.

Heinonen, O. P., Slone, D., Shapiro, S., *Birth Defects and Drugs in Pregnancy*. Littleton, Massachusetts: PSG Publishing Co., 1977.

Hollister, L. E., *Clinical Pharmacology of Psychotherapeutic Drugs*, 2nd ed. New York: Churchill Livingstone, 1983.

Huff, B. B., ed., *The Physicians' Desk Reference*, 43rd ed. Oradell, New Jersey: Medical Economics Company, 1989.

International Drug Therapy Newsletter. Edited by F. J. Ayd. Baltimore: Ayd Medical Communications, 1989.

Jefferson, J. W., Greist, J. H., *Primer of Lithium Therapy*. Baltimore: Williams & Wilkens, 1977.

Journal of the American Medical Association. Edited by G. D. Lundberg. Chicago: American Medical Association, 1989.

Koller, W. C., ed., *Handbook of Parkinson's Disease*. New York: Marcel Dekker, 1987.

Kolodny, R. C., Masters, W. H., Johnson, V. E., *Textbook of Sexual Medicine*. Boston: Little, Brown and Co., 1979.

Lawrence, R. A., *Breast-Feeding*. St. Louis: Mosby, 1980.

Lieberman, M. L., *The Sexual Pharmacy*. New York: New American Library, 1988.

Long, J. W., *Clinical Management of Prescription Drugs*. Philadelphia: Harper & Row, 1984.

McEvoy, G. K., ed., *American Hospital Formulary Service, Drug Information 89*. Bethesda, Maryland: American Society of Hospital Pharmacists, 1989.

Maddin, S., ed., *Current Dermatologic Therapy*. Philadelphia: W. B. Saunders Co., 1982.

The Medical Letter on Drugs and Therapeutics. Edited by H. Aaron. New Rochelle, New York: The Medical Letter, Inc., 1989.

Melmon, K. L., Morrelli, H. F., *Clinical Pharmacology*, 2nd ed. New York: Macmillan, 1978.

Messerli, F. H., ed., *Current Clinical Practice*. Philadelphia: W. B. Saunders Co., 1987.

Meyler, L., Herxheimer, A., eds., *Side-Effects of Drugs*, Vol. 8. Amsterdam: Excerpta Medica, 1975.

Mohler, S. R., *Medication and Flying: A Pilot's Guide*. Boston: Boston Publishing Co., 1982.

The New England Journal of Medicine. Edited by A. S. Relman. Boston: The Massachusetts Medical Society, 1989.

Pharmacotherapy, The Journal of Human Pharmacology and Drug Therapy. Edited by R. T. Scheife. Boston: Pharmacotherapy Publications, Inc., 1987.

Postgraduate Medicine, The Journal of Applied Medicine for the Primary Care Physician. Minneapolis: McGraw-Hill, Inc., 1989.

Raj, P. P., *Practical Management of Pain*. Chicago: Year Book Medical Publishers, Inc., 1986.

Rakel, R. E., ed., *Conn's Current Therapy 1989*. Philadelphia: W. B. Saunders Co., 1989.

Rational Drug Therapy, Pharmacology for Physicians. Bethesda, Maryland: American Society for Pharmacology and Experimental Therapeutics, 1989.

Reynolds, J. E. F., ed. *Martindale, The Extra Pharmacopoeia*, 28th ed. London: The Pharmaceutical Press, 1982.

Rodman, M. J., Smith, D. W., *Clinical Pharmacology in Nursing*. Philadelphia: J. B. Lippincott Co., 1984.

Rogers, C. S., McCue, J. D., eds., *Managing Chronic Disease*. Oradell, New Jersey: Medical Economics Books, 1987.

Sauer, G. C., *Manual of Skin Diseases*, 5th ed. Philadelphia: J. B. Lippincott Co., 1985.

Schardein, J. L., *Drugs As Teratogens*. Cleveland: CRC Press, 1976.

Shepard, T. H., *Catalog of Teratogenic Agents*, 3rd ed. Baltimore: Johns Hopkins University Press, 1980.

Smith, L. H., Thier, S. O., *Pathophysiology, The Biological Principles of Disease*, 2nd ed. Philadelphia: W. B. Saunders Co., 1985.

Speight, T. M., ed., *Avery's Drug Treatment*, 3rd ed. Auckland: ADIS Press, 1987.

Swash, M., Schwartz, M. S., *Neuromuscular Diseases*, 2nd ed. Berlin: Springer-Verlag, 1988.

Tuchmann-Duplessis, H., *Drug Effects on the Fetus*. Sydney, Australia: ADIS Press, 1975.

USAN 1989 and the USP Dictionary of Drug Names. Edited by M. C. Griffiths. Rockville, Maryland: United States Pharmacopeial Convention, Inc., 1988.

USP Dispensing Information 1989, 9th ed., Vol. 1, *Drug Information for the Health Care Provider*. Rockville, Maryland: United States Pharmacopeial Convention, 1989.

Utian, W. H., *Menopause in Modern Perspective*. New York: Appleton-Century-Crofts, 1980.

Wartak, J., *Drug Dosage and Administration*. Baltimore: University Park Press, 1983.

Worley, R. J., ed., *Clinical Obstetrics and Gynecology*, Vol. 24, No. 1: *Menopause*. Hagerstown, Maryland: Harper & Row, 1981.

Index

This index contains all the brand and generic drug names included in Section Three and the names and alternative names of the disorders and conditions for which drug management is described in Section Two.

Brand names of drugs appear in italic type and are capitalized.

Each brand name is followed by the generic name of its Drug Profile in Section Three.

The symbol [CD] indicates that the brand name represents a combination drug that contains the generic drug components listed below it. To be fully familiar with any combination drug [CD], it is necessary to read the Drug Profile of each of the components listed. The brand name of a combination drug *may* or *may not* appear in the brand name list of each Drug Profile that is cited in the index as a component of a particular combination drug. The index listing of component drugs for any combination drug product represents the manufacturer's formulation of that brand at the time this information was compiled for publication.

The symbol ✤ before the brand name of a combination drug indicates that the brand name is used in both the United States and Canada, but that the ingredients in the combination product in each country differ. The Canadian drug is marked with the symbol ✤ to distinguish it from the American drug which has the same name.

A generic name with no page designation indicates an active component of a combination drug for which there is no Profile in Section Three. It is included to alert you to its presence, should you wish to consult your physician regarding its significance.

Accurbron, theophylline, 903
Accutane, isotretinoin, 560
acebutolol, 157
acetaminophen, 161
Acetazolam, acetazolamide, 164
acetazolamide, 164
acetylsalicylic acid. *See* aspirin
Achromycin, tetracycline, 899
Achromycin V, tetracycline, 899
acne, 30
acne vulgaris. *See* acne
Actifed-A [CD]
   CONTAINS
   acetaminophen, 161
   pseudoephedrine*
   triprolidine*
Actifed w/Codeine [CD]
   CONTAINS
   codeine, 356
   pseudoephedrine*
   triprolidine*
acyclovir, 168
Adalat, nifedipine, 694
Adapin, doxepin, 433
Adrenalin, epinephrine, 444
adrenaline. *See* epinephrine
Advil, ibuprofen, 536
affective disorder. *See* depression
Afrin, oxymetazoline, 729
Ak-Chlor, chloramphenicol, 292
Ak-Cide [CD]
   CONTAINS
   prednisolone, 798
   sulfacetamide*
Ak-Dex, dexamethasone, 386
Ak-Tate, prednisolone, 798
Ak-Zol, acetazolamide, 164

Alatone, spironolactone, 862
Alazine, hydralazine, 521
albuterol, 170
Aldactazide [CD]
   CONTAINS
   hydrochlorothiazide, 525
   spironolactone, 862
Aldactone, spironolactone, 862
Aldoclor [CD]
   CONTAINS
   chlorothiazide, 300
   methyldopa, 628
Aldomet, methyldopa, 628
Aldoril-15/25 [CD]
   CONTAINS
   hydrochlorothiazide, 525
   methyldopa, 628
Aldoril D30/D50 [CD]
   CONTAINS
   hydrochlorothiazide, 525
   methyldopa, 628
Alka-Mints, calcium carbonate, 263
Alka-Seltzer Effervescent Pain Reliever &
   Antacid [CD]
   CONTAINS
   aspirin, 205
   citric acid*
   sodium bicarbonate*
Alka-Seltzer Plus [CD]
   CONTAINS
   aspirin, 205
   chlorpheniramine, 304
   phenylpropanolamine*
Alkets [CD]
   CONTAINS
   calcium carbonate, 263
   magnesium carbonate*
   magnesium oxide*

*The symbol [CD] indicates that the brand name given is a combination drug consisting of generic drug components listed below it. If there is no page numbering following the name of the generic drug component, there is no Drug Profile for that ingredient in this book.

methyldopa, 628
Apo-Methyldopa, methyldopa, 628
Apo-Metoprolol, metoprolol, 647
Apo-Metronidazole, metronidazole, 652
Apo-Naproxen, naproxen, 679
Apo-Nitrofurantoin, nitrofurantoin, 698
Apo-Oxazepam, oxazepam, 722
Apo-Penicillin VK, penicillin V, 737
Apo-Perphenazine, perphenazine, 750
Apo-Phenylbutazone, phenylbutazone,
    768
Apo-Piroxicam, piroxicam, 784
Apo-Prednisone, prednisone, 803
Apo-Primidone, primidone, 808
Apo-Propranolol, propranolol, 834
Apo-Quinidine, quinidine, 843
Apo-Sulfamethoxazole, sulfamethoxazole,
    868
Apo-Sulfatrim [CD]
    CONTAINS
    sulfamethoxazole, 868
    trimethoprim, 963
Apo-Sulfatrim DS [CD]
    CONTAINS
    sulfamethoxazole, 868
    trimethoprim, 963
Apo-Sulfisoxazole, sulfisoxazole, 876
Apo-Tetra, tetracycline, 899
Apo-Thioridazine, thioridazine, 907
Apo-Tolbutamide, tolbutamide, 937
Apo-Triazide [CD]
    CONTAINS
    hydrochlorothiazide, 525
    triamterene, 948
Apo-Trifluoperazine, trifluoperazine, 955
Apresazide [CD]
    CONTAINS
    hydralazine, 521
    hydrochlorothiazide, 525
Apresoline-Esidrix [CD]
    CONTAINS
    hydralazine, 521
    hydrochlorothiazide, 525
Apresoline, hydralazine, 521
Aquachloral Supprettes, chloral hydrate,
    289
Aquatensen, methyclothiazide, 623
Armour Thyroid, thyroid, 917
Arrestin, trimethobenzamide, 960
arterial hypertension. *See* hypertension
A.S.A. Enseals, aspirin, 205
ASA. *See* aspirin
Asasantine [CD]
    CONTAINS
    aspirin, 205
    dipyridamole, 421

Ascriptin [CD]
    CONTAINS
    aluminum hydroxide*
    aspirin, 205
    calcium carbonate, 263
    magnesium hydroxide*
Ascriptin A/D [CD]
    CONTAINS
    aluminum hydroxide*
    aspirin, 205
    calcium carbonate, 263
    magnesium hydroxide*
Asendin, amoxapine, 195
Aspergum, aspirin, 205
aspirin, 205
Aspirin, aspirin, 205
asthma, 41
Astrin, aspirin, 205
Atarax, hydroxyzine, 533
Atasol, acetaminophen, 161
Atasol-8, -15, -30 [CD]
    CONTAINS
    acetaminophen, 161
    codeine, 356
Atasol Forte, acetaminophen, 161
atenolol, 211
Athrombin-K, warfarin, 974
Ativan, lorazepam, 586
atrophic arthritis. *See* rheumatoid
    arthritis
atropine, 216
Augmentin [CD]
    CONTAINS
    amoxicillin, 199
    clavulanic acid*
auranofin, 220
autoimmune myasthenia gravis. *See*
    myasthenia gravis
Aventyl, nortriptyline, 712
Axid, nizatidine, 706
Axotal [CD]
    CONTAINS
    aspirin, 205
    butalbital, 256
Azaline, sulfasalazine, 872
azatadine, 223
azathioprine, 226
Azdone [CD]
    CONTAINS
    aspirin, 205
    hydrocodone, 530
azidothymidine. *See* zidovudine
Azo Gantanol [CD]
    CONTAINS
    phenazopyridine, 755
    sulfamethoxazole, 868

---

*The symbol [CD] indicates that the brand name given is a combination drug consisting of generic
drug components listed below it. If there is no page numbering following the name of the generic
drug component, there is no Drug Profile for that ingredient in this book.

*The symbol [CD] indicates that the brand name given is a combination drug consisting of generic drug components listed below it. If there is no page numbering following the name of the generic drug component, there is no Drug Profile for that ingredient in this book.

*The symbol [CD] indicates that the brand name given is a combination drug consisting of generic
drug components listed below it. If there is no page numbering following the name of the generic
drug component, there is no Drug Profile for that ingredient in this book.

---

*The symbol [CD] indicates that the brand name given is a combination drug consisting of generic drug components listed below it. If there is no page numbering following the name of the generic drug component, there is no Drug Profile for that ingredient in this book.

*The symbol [CD] indicates that the brand name given is a combination drug consisting of generic drug components listed below it. If there is no page numbering following the name of the generic drug component, there is no Drug Profile for that ingredient in this book.

*The symbol [CD] indicates that the brand name given is a combination drug consisting of generic drug components listed below it. If there is no page numbering following the name of the generic drug component, there is no Drug Profile for that ingredient in this book.

*The symbol [CD] indicates that the brand name given is a combination drug consisting of generic drug components listed below it. If there is no page numbering following the name of the generic drug component, there is no Drug Profile for that ingredient in this book.

*The symbol [CD] indicates that the brand name given is a combination drug consisting of generic drug components listed below it. If there is no page numbering following the name of the generic drug component, there is no Drug Profile for that ingredient in this book.

---

*The symbol [CD] indicates that the brand name given is a combination drug consisting of generic
drug components listed below it. If there is no page numbering following the name of the generic
drug component, there is no Drug Profile for that ingredient in this book.

*The symbol [CD] indicates that the brand name given is a combination drug consisting of generic drug components listed below it. If there is no page numbering following the name of the generic drug component, there is no Drug Profile for that ingredient in this book.

*The symbol [CD] indicates that the brand name given is a combination drug consisting of generic drug components listed below it. If there is no page numbering following the name of the generic drug component, there is no Drug Profile for that ingredient in this book.

About the Author

James W. Long, M.D., was born in Allentown, Pennsylvania. He received his premedical education from the University of Maryland and his medical degree from the George Washington University School of Medicine in Washington, D.C. For twenty years he was in the private practice of internal medicine in the Washington metropolitan area, and for over thirty-five years he was a member of the faculty of the George Washington University School of Medicine. He has served with the Food and Drug Administration, the National Library of Medicine, and the Bureau of Health Manpower of the National Institutes of Health. Prior to his retirement, Dr. Long was director of Health Services for the National Science Foundation in Washington. He lives in Oxford, Maryland.

Dr. Long's involvement in drug information activities includes service on the H.E.W. Task Force on Prescription Drugs, on the F.D.A. Task Force on Adverse Drug Reactions, as a delegate-at-large to the U.S. Pharmacopeial Convention, as editorial consultant for *Hospital Formulary*, as a director of the Drug Information Association, and as a member of the Toxicology Information Program Committee of the National Research Council/National Academy of Sciences. He was consultant to the Food and Drug Administration, serving as advisor to their staff on the development of patient package inserts. He is also the author of numerous articles in professional journals. *The Essential Guide to Prescription Drugs* is an outgrowth of his conviction that the general public needs and is entitled to practical drug information which is the equivalent of the professional "package insert." He believes the patient can be reasonably certain of using medications with the least risk and the greatest benefit only when the patient has all the relevant information about the drugs he or she is taking.

Schedules of Controlled Drugs*

Schedule I: Non-medicinal substances with high abuse potential and dependence liability. Used for research purposes only. Examples: heroin, marijuana, LSD. Not legally available for medicinal use by prescription.

Schedule II: Medicinal drugs in current use that have the highest abuse potential and dependence liability. Examples: opium derivatives (morphine, codeine, etc.), meperidine (Demerol), amphetamines (Dexedrine), short-acting barbiturates (Amytal, Nembutal, Seconal). A written prescription is required. Telephoned prescribing is prohibited. No refills are allowed.

Schedule III: Medicinal drugs with abuse potential and dependence liability less than Schedule II drugs but greater than Schedule IV or V drugs. Examples: codeine, hydrocodone and paregoric in combination with one or more non-narcotic drugs, some hypnotics (Doriden, Noludar), some appetite suppressants (Didrex, Tenuate, Sanorex). A telephoned prescription is permitted, to be converted to written form by the dispensing pharmacist. Prescriptions must be renewed every 6 months. Refills are limited to 5.

Schedule IV: Medicinal drugs with less abuse potential and dependence liability than Schedule III drugs. Examples: pentazocine (Talwin), propoxyphene (Darvon), all benzodiazepines (Librium, Valium, etc.), certain hypnotics (Placidyl, Noctec, Valmid, etc.). Prescription requirements are the same as for Schedule III.

Schedule V: Medicinal drugs with the lowest abuse potential and dependence liability. Examples: diphenoxylate (Lomotil), loperamide (Imodium). Drugs requiring a prescription are handled the same as any non-scheduled prescription drug. Some non-prescription drugs can be sold only with approval of the pharmacist; the buyer is required to sign a log of purchase at the time the drug is dispensed. Examples: codeine and hydrocodone in combination with other active, non-narcotic drugs, sold in preparations that contain limited quantities for control of cough and diarrhea.

*Under jurisdiction of the Controlled Substances Act of 1970.

Advisability of Drug Use During P

Definitions of FDA Pregnancy Categorie

Category A: Adequate and well-controlled studie women are **negative** for fetal abnormalities. Ri is remote.

Category B: Animal reproduction studies are **negativ** normalities. Information from adequate and v studies in pregnant women is not available.

OR

Animal reproduction studies are **positive** for fet ties. Adequate and well-controlled studies in pre are **negative** for fetal abnormalities. Risk to the tively unlikely.

Category C: Animal reproduction studies are **positiv** normalities. Information from adequate and w studies in pregnant women is not available.

OR

Information from animal reproduction studies a quate and well-controlled studies in pregnant w available. Possible benefits of the drug are thoug potential risks to the fetus.

Category D: Studies in pregnant women and/or pre-m vestigational) or post-marketing experience demo **tive** evidence of human fetal risk. The drug is need disease or in life-threatening situations where saf ineffective or cannot be used.

Category X: Animal reproduction studies and/or huma studies are **positive** for fetal abnormalities.

OR

Studies in pregnant women and/or pre-marketing tional) or post-marketing experience demonstrate idence of human fetal risk.

AND

Potential risks to the fetus outweigh possible ben drug. Use is **contraindicated**.

*Adapted from the Federal Register statement in Vol. 44, No. 124, 26, 1979.

About the Author

James W. Long, M.D., was born in Allentown, Pennsylvania. He received his premedical education from the University of Maryland and his medical degree from the George Washington University School of Medicine in Washington, D.C. For twenty years he was in the private practice of internal medicine in the Washington metropolitan area, and for over thirty-five years he was a member of the faculty of the George Washington University School of Medicine. He has served with the Food and Drug Administration, the National Library of Medicine, and the Bureau of Health Manpower of the National Institutes of Health. Prior to his retirement, Dr. Long was director of Health Services for the National Science Foundation in Washington. He lives in Oxford, Maryland.

Dr. Long's involvement in drug information activities includes service on the H.E.W. Task Force on Prescription Drugs, on the F.D.A. Task Force on Adverse Drug Reactions, as a delegate-at-large to the U.S. Pharmacopeial Convention, as editorial consultant for *Hospital Formulary*, as a director of the Drug Information Association, and as a member of the Toxicology Information Program Committee of the National Research Council/National Academy of Sciences. He was consultant to the Food and Drug Administration, serving as advisor to their staff on the development of patient package inserts. He is also the author of numerous articles in professional journals. *The Essential Guide to Prescription Drugs* is an outgrowth of his conviction that the general public needs and is entitled to practical drug information which is the equivalent of the professional "package insert." He believes the patient can be reasonably certain of using medications with the least risk and the greatest benefit only when the patient has all the relevant information about the drugs he or she is taking.

Schedules of Controlled Drugs*

Schedule I: Non-medicinal substances with high abuse potential and dependence liability. Used for research purposes only. Examples: heroin, marijuana, LSD. Not legally available for medicinal use by prescription.

Schedule II: Medicinal drugs in current use that have the highest abuse potential and dependence liability. Examples: opium derivatives (morphine, codeine, etc.), meperidine (Demerol), amphetamines (Dexedrine), short-acting barbiturates (Amytal, Nembutal, Seconal). A written prescription is required. Telephoned prescribing is prohibited. No refills are allowed.

Schedule III: Medicinal drugs with abuse potential and dependence liability less than Schedule II drugs but greater than Schedule IV or V drugs. Examples: codeine, hydrocodone and paregoric in combination with one or more non-narcotic drugs, some hypnotics (Doriden, Noludar), some appetite suppressants (Didrex, Tenuate, Sanorex). A telephoned prescription is permitted, to be converted to written form by the dispensing pharmacist. Prescriptions must be renewed every 6 months. Refills are limited to 5.

Schedule IV: Medicinal drugs with less abuse potential and dependence liability than Schedule III drugs. Examples: pentazocine (Talwin), propoxyphene (Darvon), all benzodiazepines (Librium, Valium, etc.), certain hypnotics (Placidyl, Noctec, Valmid, etc.). Prescription requirements are the same as for Schedule III.

Schedule V: Medicinal drugs with the lowest abuse potential and dependence liability. Examples: diphenoxylate (Lomotil), loperamide (Imodium). Drugs requiring a prescription are handled the same as any non-scheduled prescription drug. Some non-prescription drugs can be sold only with approval of the pharmacist; the buyer is required to sign a log of purchase at the time the drug is dispensed. Examples: codeine and hydrocodone in combination with other active, non-narcotic drugs, sold in preparations that contain limited quantities for control of cough and diarrhea.

*Under jurisdiction of the Controlled Substances Act of 1970.

Advisability of Drug Use During Pregnancy

Definitions of FDA Pregnancy Categories*

Category A: Adequate and well-controlled studies in pregnant women are **negative** for fetal abnormalities. Risk to the fetus is remote.

Category B: Animal reproduction studies are **negative** for fetal abnormalities. Information from adequate and well-controlled studies in pregnant women is not available.

OR

Animal reproduction studies are **positive** for fetal abnormalities. Adequate and well-controlled studies in pregnant women are **negative** for fetal abnormalities. Risk to the fetus is relatively unlikely.

Category C: Animal reproduction studies are **positive** for fetal abnormalities. Information from adequate and well-controlled studies in pregnant women is not available.

OR

Information from animal reproduction studies **and** from adequate and well-controlled studies in pregnant women is not available. Possible benefits of the drug are thought to justify potential risks to the fetus.

Category D: Studies in pregnant women and/or pre-marketing (investigational) or post-marketing experience demonstrate **positive** evidence of human fetal risk. The drug is needed in serious disease or in life-threatening situations where safer drugs are ineffective or cannot be used.

Category X: Animal reproduction studies and/or human pregnancy studies are **positive** for fetal abnormalities.

OR

Studies in pregnant women and/or pre-marketing (investigational) or post-marketing experience demonstrate **positive** evidence of human fetal risk.

AND

Potential risks to the fetus outweigh possible benefits of the drug. Use is **contraindicated**.

*Adapted from the Federal Register statement in Vol. 44, No. 124, Tuesday, June 26, 1979.

U.S. Master Tax Guide®

KEY FIGURES FOR THE 2014 TAX YEAR

To stay current with legislation that may affect these rates and amounts, visit the CCH website at CCHGroup.com/TaxUpdates.

STANDARD DEDUCTIONS

Married, Filing Joint Return (and Surviving Spouse)	$	12,400
Head of Household	$	9,100
Unmarried (Not Surviving Spouse or Head of Household)	$	6,200
Married, Filing Separate Return	$	6,200
Dependent Standard Deduction (Minimum)	$	1,000
Additional Amount for Blindness or Age	$	1,200
Additional Amount as Above if Unmarried and Not S.S.	$	1,550

ITEMIZED DEDUCTIONS

Phaseout of Itemized Deductions (AGI Threshold Starts)		
Married, Filing Joint Return (and Surviving Spouse)	$	305,050
Head of Household	$	279,650
Unmarried (Not Surviving Spouse or Head of Household)	$	254,200
Married, Filing Separate Return	$	152,525
Nonbusiness Casualty Loss (AGI Threshold)		10%
Medical Deduction (AGI Threshold)		
Taxpayers, Generally		10%
Taxpayer or Spouse, Age 65 and Older		7.5%
Miscellaneous Itemized Deduction (AGI Threshold)		2%

EXEMPTIONS

Personal and Dependent Amount	$	3,950
Phaseout of Exemptions (AGI Threshold Starts)		
Married, Filing Joint Return (and Surviving Spouse)	$	305,050
Head of Household	$	279,650
Unmarried (Not Surviving Spouse or Head of Household)	$	254,200
Married, Filing Separate Return	$	152,525

EDUCATION PROVISIONS

American Opportunity (Modified Hope) Credit	$	2,500
Lifetime Learning Credit	$	2,000
Coverdell Education Savings Account Contribution	$	2,000
Student Loan Interest Deduction	$	2,500
Phaseout of U.S. Savings Bond Interest Exclusion (MAGI Threshold Starts)		
Married, Filing Joint Return	$	113,950
Unmarried, Surviving Spouse, or Head of Household	$	76,000

ALTERNATIVE MINIMUM TAX (AMT)

Excess Taxable Income Threshold for 28% Rate		
Individuals, Estates, and Trusts, Generally	$	182,500
Married, Filing Separate Return	$	91,250
Exemption Amounts		
Married, Filing Joint Return (and Surviving Spouse)	$	82,100
Unmarried and Head of Household (not Surviving Spouse)	$	52,800
Married, Filing Separate Return	$	41,050
Estate and Trust	$	23,500
Phaseout of AMT Exemption (AMTI Threshold Starts)		
Married, Filing Joint Return (and Surviving Spouse)	$	156,500
Unmarried and Head of Household (not Surviving Spouse)	$	117,300
Married, Filing Separate Return	$	78,250
Estate and Trust	$	78,250

QUICK TAX FACTS

NET INVESTMENT INCOME

Additional Tax on Net Investment Income of High-Income Taxpayers	3.8%

NET CAPITAL GAINS AND QUALIFIED DIVIDENDS

Taxpayers in 10% or 15% Income Tax Bracket	0%
Taxpayers in 25%, 28%, 33% or 35% Income Tax Bracket	15%
Taxpayers in 39.6% Income Tax Bracket	20%
Unrecaptured Gain on Real Estate (Section 1250 gain)	25%
Collectibles and Qualified Small Business Stock	28%

ESTATE AND GIFT TAXES

Estate & Gift Basic Exclusion Amount	$ 5,340,000
Annual Gift Tax Exclusion (Per Donee)	$ 14,000
Maximum Estate & Gift Tax Rate	40%

CODE SEC. 179 EXPENSE ALLOWANCE

Maximum Deduction	$ 25,000*
Investment Limitation	$ 200,000*

PAYROLL TAXES

FICA or Self-Employed Combined Rate (OASDI + Medicare)	15.3%
FICA (Employer or Employee) Rate (OASDI + Medicare)	7.65%
OASDI (Employer or Employee) Rate	6.2%
OASDI Maximum Base	$ 117,000
Medicare (Employer and Employee) Rate	1.45%
Additional Medicare Rate (High-Income Employees and Self-Employed)	0.9%
FUTA Rate	6.0%
FUTA Wage Base	$ 7,000
Nanny Tax Threshold	$ 1,900

RETIREMENT/PENSION PLANS

Maximum Elective Deferral to 401(k), 403(b), 457, and Thrift Plans	$ 17,500
Maximum Elective Deferral to SIMPLE 401(k) and SIMPLE IRA Plans	$ 12,000
Maximum Contribution Limit to Traditional and Roth IRAs	$ 5,500
Catch-Up Contributions Limits (For Individuals Age 50 and Over)	
401(k), 403(b), 457, and Thrift Plans	$ 5,500
SIMPLE 401(k) and SIMPLE IRA Plans	$ 2,500
Traditional and Roth IRAs	$ 1,000
Limit on Annual Additions to Defined Contribution Plans and SEPs	$ 52,000
Annual Compensation Limit for Determining Contributions	$ 260,000
SEP Minimum Compensation Amount	$ 550
Limit on Annual Benefits Under Defined Benefit Plans	$ 210,000
Highly Compensated Employee Threshold	$ 115,000

HEALTH CARE

Health Savings Account (HSA) Contribution Limit	
Self-Only Coverage	$ 3,300
Family Coverage	$ 6,550
Health Flexible Savings Account (FSA) Contribution Limit	$ 2,500

TRANSPORTATION

Business Mileage Rate	56¢
Medical and Moving Mileage Rate	23.5¢
Charitable Mileage Rate	14¢
Depreciation Component of Standard Mileage Rate	22¢
High/Low Cost Locality Per Diem Travel Rates (after 9/30/13)	High: $251 / Low: $170
High/Low Cost Locality Per Diem Travel Rates (after 9/30/14)	High: $259 / Low: $172

* Visit CCHGroup.com/TaxUpdates for legislative developments that may affect the Code Sec. 179 expense limits for 2014.

2015

U.S. MASTER
TAX GUIDE®

98TH EDITION

Wolters Kluwer, CCH Editorial Staff Publication

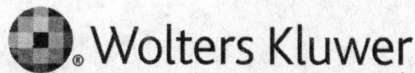

This publication is designed to provide accurate and authoritative information in regard to the subject matter covered. It is sold with the understanding that the publisher is not engaged in rendering legal, accounting, or other professional service. If legal advice or other expert assistance is required, the services of a competent professional person should be sought.

ISBN: 978-0-8080-3873-3 (paperback edition)

ISBN: 978-0-8080-3909-9 (hardbound edition)

4025 W. Peterson Ave.
Chicago, IL 60646-6085
800 248 3248
CCHGroup.com

Printed in the United States of America

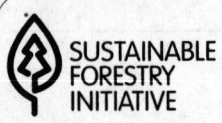

SUSTAINABLE FORESTRY INITIATIVE

Certified Sourcing

www.sfiprogram.org

SFI-01042

Preface

Income taxation in the United States has been around for 100 years. From the very beginning, Wolters Kluwer, CCH was there and is still setting the standard as the number one quick reference resource for tax professionals. Wolters Kluwer, CCH is proud to serve the tax professional community with this new edition of the *U.S. Master Tax Guide* ®. The 98th Edition of this industry standard explains the complex set of tax rules and is designed to provide fast and reliable answers to tax questions affecting individuals and businesses. In all, 29 chapters contain comprehensive, timely, and precise explanation of the ever-changing federal income tax rules for individuals, businesses, estates, and trusts.

The 2015 Edition reflects significant guidance issued by the IRS on the 3.8 percent net investment income (NII) tax on high-income individuals, and the 0.9 percent additional Medicare tax for high-income wage earners and self-employed individuals. Also reflected is additional IRS guidance regarding same-sex couples who were legally married in jurisdictions that recognize these marriages in light of the Supreme Court's decision in *E. S. Windsor*, (2013-1 USTC ¶ 50,400). In addition, the 2015 Edition reflects the final regulations and additional guidance governing when taxpayers must capitalize and when they can deduct business expenses for acquiring, maintaining, repairing, and replacing tangible property. Coverage is also provided on final regulations for individuals to maintain, and employers to provide, minimum essential health care coverage.

In an effort to keep users of the *Guide* current on events taking place after the date of publication, Wolters Kluwer, CCH has established a website at *CCHGroup.com/TaxUpdates* for any late-breaking 2014 year-end tax legislation or for other significant tax developments that might affect the *Guide's* coverage.

As in previous editions, major legislative provisions are highlighted at ¶ 1 and reflected throughout the *Guide*, while important non-legislative tax developments are conveniently highlighted at ¶ 2 and concisely explained for quick reference and understanding. In addition, the *Guide* comes complete with many timesaving features that help practitioners quickly and easily determine how particular tax items and situations should be treated (see the following page for a listing and description of these "Key Features"). The *Guide* also contains a handy Quick Tax Facts card that can be detached for an at-a-glance reference to key tax figures and other often-referenced amounts for the 2014 tax year.

Not only does the *U.S. Master Tax Guide* ® assist in the preparation of 2014 tax returns, it also serves as a reference tool for more comprehensive tax research and tax planning via extensive footnotes and other references to the Internal Revenue Code, Income Tax Regulations, and Wolters Kluwer, CCH's STANDARD FEDERAL TAX REPORTS ®, FEDERAL ESTATE AND GIFT TAX REPORTER, TAX RESEARCH CONSULTANT, and Practical Tax Explanations series.

For additional analysis of new and complex tax issues, and as a way to earn valuable continuing education credits, *Top Federal Tax Issues for 2015* is provided along with the *Guide*. This course provides helpful insights for the practitioner to keep abreast of the most significant new rules and changes by explaining the most important new provisions and developments in 2015 specifically applicable to 2015 and the IRS rules and regulations that go into effect in 2015. It also examines current audit and litigation issues that have developed over the past year that create a new environment for tax strategies initiated in 2014.

Finally, for treatment of state tax topics, please refer to Wolters Kluwer, CCH's *State Tax Guidebooks* (12 states available–CA, CT, FL, IL, MA, MI, NJ, NY, NC, OH, PA and TX) and Wolters Kluwer, CCH's *State Tax Handbook* covering all 50 states and the District of Columbia.

November 2014

Key Features

In addition to 29 chapters of tax law explanations, the *U.S. Master Tax Guide*® provides a wealth of information in the pages that lead up to Chapter 1. Some of these timesaving tools and features are described below, listed by paragraph location.

OVERVIEW (¶ 1-6): The Overview division contains informative features available to facilitate research and dealing with clients, including the following.

- "Tax Legislation," a highlight of provisions from this year's enacted tax legislation.
- "Looking Ahead — Potential Tax Developments for 2015," a look ahead by Wolter Kluwer, CCH's Principal Analyst Mark Luscombe, J.D., LL.M., C.P.A.
- "AGI Phaseout Thresholds," includes a number of tax items subject to phaseout restrictions.
- "Where to File Returns," a listing of income tax return mailing addresses.
- "2015 Tax Calendar," shows the filing dates for 2014 tax returns and tax payments throughout 2015.

TAX RATES (¶ 11-53): This section contains the 2014 and 2015 tax rate schedules for individuals and estates and trusts, the corporate tax rate schedule and related rates, and the estate and gift tax rate schedule, as well as a listing of key excise tax rates.

CHECKLISTS (¶ 55-65): A collection of checklists designed to provide tax return preparers with quick references to assist in answering common questions regarding the inclusion of items in income, the deductibility of certain expenses, the treatment of various medical expenses, the availability of tax credits, and a list of IRS forms to use.

SPECIAL TAX TABLES (¶ 83-88): This is a collection of often-used interest rates and percentages including:

- Applicable Federal Rates (AFRs)
- Adjusted Applicable Federal Rates
- Federal Long-Term Tax-Exempt Rates
- Low-Income Housing Credit percentages

ADDITIONAL FORMATS: To provide flexibility for users, the *Guide* is available in either a softbound or hardbound print edition and an e-Book version. The *Guide* is also available on *IntelliConnect*, Wolter Kluwer, CCH's industry-leading research platform that combines the quick-reference ease and reliability of the *Guide* with current primary sources including the Internal Revenue Code, Income Tax Regulations, cases, IRS rulings, and more.

TAX UPDATE RESOURCE: Wolters Kluwer, CCH has established a website at *CCH-Group.com/TaxUpdates* for users of the *Guide* to visit periodically in order to stay current with post-publication tax legislation and key tax developments.

Wolters Kluwer, CCH Tax and Accounting

EDITORIAL STAFF

DETAILED TABLE OF CONTENTS

Filing 2014 Returns

OVERVIEW

¶ 1 Tax Legislation

Tax Legislation. Only four minor tax-related acts were passed and enacted during the year.

- The *Philippines Charitable Giving Assistance Act* (P.L. 113-92) was enacted on March 25, 2014, which allows a calendar-year taxpayer who made qualified charitable contributions after March 25, 2014, and before April 15, 2014, to relief organizations responding to the tragedy caused by Typhoon Haiyan to be treated as made on December 31, 2013, rather than in 2014.

- The *Cooperative and Small Employer Charity Pension Flexibility Act* (P.L. 113-97) was enacted on April 7, 2014, providing permanent relief to eligible cooperative plans and plans of Code Sec. 501(c)(3) organizations maintained by more than one employer from complying with the defined benefit funding restrictions imposed by the *Pension Protection Act of 2006* (P.L. 109-208). A defined benefit retirement plan that otherwise qualifies as a cooperative and small employer charity (CSEC) plan may elect out of CSEC status and the funding requirements of Code Sec. 433.

- The *Highway and Transportation Funding Act of 2014* (P.L. 113-159) was enacted on August 8, 2014, extending the expenditure authority of the Highway Trust Fund through May, 31, 2015. In addition, the legislation provides funding stabilization for defined benefit pension plans by modifying for plan years beginning after December 31, 2012, the MAP-21 specified percentage ranges for determining whether a segment rate must be adjusted upward or downward.

- The *Tribal General Welfare Exclusion Act of 2014* (P.L. 113-168) was enacted on September 26, 2014, providing an exclusion from gross income under new Code Sec. 139E for the value of any Indian general welfare benefit under an Indian tribal government program. An Indian general welfare benefit is any payment made, or services provided, under an Indian tribal government program to, or on behalf of, a member of an Indian tribe or his or her spouse or dependent.

At the time of publication, Congress has yet to pass any significant tax legislation, including any "tax extender" legislation. Many popular tax credits and deductions expired on December 31, 2013, and therefore may not be claimed for 2014 tax year until legislation, if any, is enacted extending the provisions. For individuals, this includes the deductions for state and local sales taxes, qualified tuition and related expenses, and mortgage insurance premiums among other tax breaks. For businesses, extenders include the increased expensing limits under Code Sec. 179, bonus depreciation, and the research and development credit.

For information on further legislative and other key tax-related developments following publication of the *U.S. Master Tax Guide*®, visit the *U.S. Master Tax Guide*® website at *CCHGroup.com/TaxUpdates*.

¶ 2 What's New on 2014 Returns

The *U.S. Master Tax Guide* ® reflects all of the important administrative and judicial developments of 2014, including final regulations, major court decisions, and important rulings of the Internal Revenue Service. Legislative highlights are at ¶ 1. Below are additional highlights of the changes in 2014 with the greatest impact on individuals and businesses.

OVERVIEW

Retirement and Benefits

Withholding

Estate, Gifts and Generation-Skipping Transfer Tax

¶ 3 Looking Ahead – Potential Tax Developments for 2015

Typical of an election year, the year 2014 has been a fairly quiet one in terms of tax legislation. Funding the Federal government's Highway Trust Fund was supposed to generate a little tax activity but ended up only resulting in some smoothing of funding obligations for defined benefit retirement plans. The regularly expiring tax provisions that expired at the end of 2013 have remained expired through 2014, with no action expected until at least after the November 2014 midterm elections. The last time that these provisions had expired they were not extended until January 1 of the following year. Also caught up in this Congressional inaction on tax legislation is a growing list of technical corrections to prior tax legislation. Other issues expected to be on the agenda for 2015 include the continued roll-out of health care reform, corporate inversions, same-sex marriages, and fundamental tax reform.

The Expired Provisions and Tax Reform

Expired tax provisions have continued to be caught up in the tax reform debate. Both Republicans and Democrats circulated serious and more detailed tax reform proposals during 2014, and the leaders of the tax writing committees toured the country promoting tax reform. However, it appears that tax reform has been put off again until 2015 at least. Some have suggested that perhaps too many details came forward on tax reform this year, and the details dampened support. House Republicans in particular have suggested that the extension of expired provisions should be part of the tax reform debate, but as tax reform looks less likely, another two-year extension of expired provisions is looking more likely—retroactive to January 1, 2014, and through 2015.

Corporate Inversions and Tax Reform

A new tax focus for 2014 was corporate inversions, through which U.S. multinational companies merge with smaller overseas companies and move their official corporate home overseas, often lowering taxes. Several highly publicized proposed inversion deals were criticized by the Obama Administration and members of Congress. Several legislative proposals have been put forward to make corporate inversions less attractive. Republicans have tended to favor addressing corporate inversions as part of tax reform on the basis that it is the high corporate tax rates that are making inversions attractive in the first place. As hope for tax reform in 2014 fades, there may develop some consensus to attack corporate inversions as long as some tax reform elements get included in the legislation. The Administration has acted to limit some of the attractiveness of inversions with tools available in its regulatory arsenal but is still pushing for more complete Congressional action.

Tax Provisions of the Affordable Care Act

The tax provisions of the Affordable Care Act continue to become effective. The year 2014 was the start of the health insurance mandate for individuals requiring them to obtain minimum essential health coverage or face a penalty, i.e., the shared responsibility payment, if they do not qualify for an exemption. The year 2014 also saw the beginning of a refundable health insurance premium assistance credit to help lower income households afford health insurance.

For employers, 2014 saw an enhancement in the small employer health insurance credit. The employer health insurance mandate which requires employers with 50 or more full-time employees to offer health insurance to the employees of face a penalty has been put off until 2015 (2016 if the employer has 50 to 99 full-time employees). Also, many of the reporting requirements imposed on employers with respect to the Affordable Care Act have also been postponed until 2015.

Same-Sex Marriages

The year 2014 saw continuing judicial activity in the aftermath of the Supreme Court decision in *E.S. Windsor* (2013-2 USTC ¶ 50,400) declaring a key provision of the Defense of Marriage Act unconstitutional. A number of courts have found that state constitutional provisions or statutes banning same-sex marriage or barring recognition of same-sex marriages legally performed in other states are unconstitutional. Although a couple of federal district courts have upheld the bans, so far all of the Federal Circuit Courts of Appeals that have addressed the issue have declared the bans unconstitutional. The Supreme Court, just prior to publication, denied all requests for review of the appellate court rulings, thus, lifting the stays on enforcement of their decisions. In the meantime, however, same-sex couples will have to closely monitor developments in their particular state to determine what filing status is appropriate for state income tax filing.

Technical Corrections

Technical corrections are usually noncontroversial minor corrections of errors made when prior tax laws were enacted. Typically, they are attached to other tax legislation when enacted. The lack of recent tax legislation has also meant the lack of a vehicle for enacting these technical corrections. They will likely be attached to any legislation extending expired provisions, when and if those extensions are enacted.

The November 2014 Elections

The outcome of the November 2014 elections could impact tax legislation for the remainder of 2014 and through 2015. If the Republicans retain control of the House and gain control of the Senate, there may be a tendency to try to defer action on tax issues until the new Congress forms in 2015. This could mean that the expired tax provisions would receive at most an extension through 2014 with the new Congress taking up extenders as part of a Republican tax reform agenda in 2015. If the Democrats retain control of the Senate, there may be less inclination to try to put off any tax issues to 2015 and expired provisions and corporate inversions may be more likely to be addressed in the 2014 lame duck session following the November elections.

¶ 4 AGI Phaseout Thresholds

Adjusted gross income (AGI) levels in excess of certain phaseout thresholds limit the following deductions, credits and other tax benefits. This chart provides the beginning point for the 2014 thresholds and the ending point of the phaseout, where applicable.

Tax Item	Taxpayers Affected	Phaseout—Begin	Phaseout—End
Itemized Deductions (Overall Limit)	joint and surviving spouse filers	$305,050	N/A
	head-of-household filers	$279,650	N/A
	single filers	$254,200	N/A
	married individuals filing separately	$152,525	N/A
Floor on Itemized Medical Expenses Deduction	taxpayers under 65	10% of AGI	N/A
	taxpayers 65 or older	7.5% of AGI	N/A
Floor on Miscellaneous Itemized Deductions	all taxpayers	2% of AGI	N/A
Itemized Deduction of Casualty Loss	all taxpayers	10% of AGI	N/A
Personal Exemption	joint or surviving spouse filers	$305,050	$427,550
	head of household filers	$279,650	$402,150
	single filers	$254,200	$376,700
	married individuals filing separately	$152,525	$213,775
Child Tax Credit*	single, head of household	$75,000	phaseout varies by taxpayer
	married filing separately	$55,000	phaseout varies by taxpayer
	joint filers	$110,000	phaseout varies by taxpayer
Dependent Care Credit	single, head of household, joint filers	35% credit if AGI not over $15,000	20% credit if AGI over $43,000
Elderly and Disabled Credit	single, head of household	$7,500	$17,500
	joint filers	$10,000	$20,000 if one qualifying spouse; $25,000 if two qualifying spouses
	married filing separately	$5,000	$12,500
Adoption Credit*	all filers	$197,880	$237,880
Adoption Assistance Programs*	all filers	$197,880	$237,880
Earned Income Credit	single, head of household, surviving spouse, no child	$8,110	$14,590
	single, head of household, surviving spouse, one child	$17,830	$38,511
	single, head of household, surviving spouse, two children	$17,830	$43,756
	single, head of household, surviving spouse, three or more children	$17,830	$46,997
	joint filers, no child	$13,540	$20,020
	joint filers, one child	$23,260	$43,941

Tax Item	Taxpayers Affected	Phaseout—Begin	Phaseout—End
	joint filers, two children	$23,260	$49,186
	joint filers, three or more children	$23,260	$52,427
American Opportunity Credit*	single, head of household	$80,000	$90,000
	joint filers	$160,000	$180,000
Lifetime Learning Credit*	single, head of household	$54,000	$64,000
	joint filers	$108,000	$128,000
Student Loan Interest Deduction*	single, head of household	$65,000	$80,000
	joint filers	$130,000	$160,000
Savings Bonds Interest Exclusion*	single, head of household	$76,000	$91,000
	joint filers	$113,950	$143,950
Coverdell Education Savings Accounts*	single, head of household, married filing separately	$95,000	$110,000
	joint filers	$190,000	$220,000
IRA Deduction* (for taxpayers covered by retirement plan at work)	single, head of household	$60,000	$70,000
	joint filers (contributing spouse covered by retirement plan at work)	$96,000	$116,000
	joint filers (contributing spouse not covered by retirement plan at work; other spouse is covered by retirement plan at work)	$181,000	$191,000
	married filing separately	$0	$10,000
Roth IRA Contribution*	single, head of household	$114,000	$129,000
	joint filers	$181,000	$191,000
	married filing separately	$0	$10,000
Rental Real Estate Passive Losses	single, head of household, joint filers	$100,000	$150,000
	married filing separately	$50,000	$75,000
Mortgage Bond Subsidy Recapture*	all filers	AGI relative to area median income	N/A

* Modified AGI, as defined by the relevant Code sections, is used instead of AGI.

¶ 5 Where to File Returns

Individuals. Listed below are the mailing addresses to use for filing self-prepared individual income tax return and by individuals filing returns prepared by a tax professionals (¶ 111). Individual taxpayers and tax professionals may also consult the IRS website at http://www.irs.gov/uac/Where-To-File-Addresses-for-Tax-Professionals for the most current mailing addresses.

The first line of the address should be Internal Revenue Service, but no street address is needed. To facilitate processing for all taxpayers of the 50 states and the District of Columbia who do not need to enclose a payment with the return, each form (1040, 1040A, 1040EZ) uses a different ZIP+4 ZIP Code extension. If you are filing a client's Form 1040A and are not enclosing a payment, use the address in the middle column with the ZIP Code extension, -0015. If you are filing a client's Form 1040EZ and are not enclosing a payment, use the address in the middle column with the ZIP Code extension, -0014. If a payment is enclosed with the form, each form (1040, 1040A, 1040EZ) uses the same mailing address shown in the last column below.

If you are filing **Form 1040** *and are located in:*	*And are not enclosing a payment, mail your return to:*	*And are enclosing a payment, mail your return to:*
Alabama, Georgia, Kentucky, New Jersey, North Carolina, South Carolina, Tennessee, Virginia	Kansas City, MO 64999-0002	P.O. Box 931000 Louisville, KY 40293-1000
Florida, Louisiana, Mississippi, Texas	Austin, TX 73301-0002	P.O. Box 1214 Charlotte, NC 28201-1214
Alaska, Arizona, California, Colorado, Hawaii, Idaho, Nevada, New Mexico, Oregon, Utah, Washington, Wyoming	Fresno, CA 93888-0002	P.O. Box 7704 San Francisco, CA 94120-7704
Arkansas, Illinois, Indiana, Iowa, Kansas, Michigan, Minnesota, Montana, Nebraska, North Dakota, Ohio, Oklahoma, South Dakota, Wisconsin	Fresno, CA 93888-0002	P.O. Box 802501 Cincinnati, OH 45280-2501
Connecticut, Delaware, District of Columbia, Maine, Maryland, Massachusetts, Missouri, New Hampshire, New York, Pennsylvania, Rhode Island, Vermont, West Virginia	Kansas City, MO 64999-0002	P.O. Box 37008 Hartford, CT 06176-7008
A foreign country, U.S. possession or territory, or use an APO or FPO address, or file Form 2555, 2555-EZ, 4563, or 8891, or are a dual-status alien	Austin, TX 73301-0215 USA	P.O. Box 1303 Charlotte, NC 28201-1303

Guam: citizen of or permanent resident	Department of Revenue and Taxation Government of Guam P.O. Box 23607 GMF, GU 96921
Virgin Islands: bona fide resident	U.S.V.I. Bureau of Internal Revenue 6115 Estate Smith Bay St. Thomas, VI 00802

Corporations and Partnerships. A corporation or partnership should file Form 1120 or Form 1065 in accordance with the "Where to File" addresses listed in the instructions to the forms. A corporation or partnership is "located in" the place where it has its principal place of business or principal office or agency. If a corporation or partnership is without a principal office or agency or principal place of business in the United States, returns are to be filed with the Internal Revenue Service Center in Ogden, Utah.

Estates and Trusts. A fiduciary of an estate or trust, including the fiduciary of a charitable or split interest trust (described in Code Sec. 4947(a)) or of a pooled income fund (described in Code Sec. 642(c)(5), should generally file Form 1041 in accordance with the instructions to the form. A fiduciary is "located in" the place where he (it) resides or has his (its) principal place of business.

Private Delivery Services. Certain private delivery services designated by the IRS are available to meet the "timely mailed as timely filing/paying" rule for tax returns and payments. The designated private delivery services are:

• DHL Express (DHL): DHL Same Day Service.

• Federal Express (FedEx): FedEx Priority Overnight, FedEx Standard Overnight, FedEx 2Day, FedEx International Priority, and FedEx International First.

• United Parcel Service (UPS): UPS Next Day Air, UPS Next Day Air Saver, UPS 2nd Day Air, UPS 2nd Day Air A.M., UPS Worldwide Express Plus, and UPS Worldwide Express.

The private delivery service will provide information for getting written proof of the mailing date.

¶ 6 2015 Tax Calendar

Each date shown below is the last day for filing the return or making the payment of tax indicated. For income tax returns, the due dates apply to calendar-year taxpayers only. Employment tax due dates are determined on a calendar-year basis for all taxpayers. **If any statutory due date falls on a Saturday, Sunday, or legal holiday, the due date is the next succeeding day that is not a Saturday, Sunday, or legal holiday (national, District of Columbia, or statewide in the state where the return is to be filed).**

This day 2015	Tax Return Due Dates
Jan. 15th—	**Estimated Taxes.** Final installment of 2014 estimated tax (Form 1040-ES) by individuals unless income tax return is filed with final payment by February 2, 2015. Payment in full of estimated tax by farmers and fishermen unless income tax returns are filed by March 2, 2015.
	Final installment of 2014 estimated tax (Form 1041-ES) by trusts, calendar-year estates, and certain residuary trusts in existence more than two years, unless Form 1041 is filed and taxes are paid in full by February 2, 2015.
Feb. 2nd—	**Employers' Taxes.** Employers of nonagricultural and nonhousehold employees file return on Form 941 for withheld income and FICA taxes in last quarter of 2014.[1]
	Employers of agricultural workers must file the annual Form 943 to report income and FICA taxes withheld on 2014 wages.[1]
	Employers must file Form 940, annual return of federal unemployment (FUTA) taxes for 2014.[1]
	Withholding. Employees' statements (Form W-2 and Form 1099-R) for amounts withheld in 2014 to be furnished by employer to employees.
	Individuals. Individuals, other than farmers and fishermen, who owed, but did not pay, estimated tax on January 15th must file final 2014 income tax return and pay tax in full to avoid late payment penalty.
	Trusts and Estates. Trusts, as well as estates and certain residuary trusts in existence more than two years, that owed but did not pay estimated tax on January 15th must file final 2014 income tax return and pay tax in full to avoid late payment penalty.
	Information Returns. Annual statements must be furnished to recipients of: dividends and liquidating distributions (Form 1099-DIV); interest, including interest on bearer certificates of deposit (Form 1099-INT); patronage dividends (Form 1099-PATR); original issue discount (Form 1099-OID); certain government payments, including unemployment compensation and state and local tax refunds of $10 or more (Form 1099-G); royalty payments of $10 or more, rent or other business payments of $600 or more, prizes and awards of $600 or more, crop insurance proceeds of $600 or more, fishing boat proceeds, and medical and health care payments of $600 or more (Form 1099-MISC); debt canceled by certain financial entities including financial institutions, credit unions, and Federal Government agencies of $600 or more (Form 1099-C); distributions from retirement or profit-sharing plans, IRAs, SEPs, or insurance contracts (Form 1099-R); payments received from a third party settlement entity (Form 1099-K).
	Business recipients of $600 or more of interest on any mortgage must furnish Form 1098 to payer.
	Information called for on Form 8300 must be provided to each payer in a transaction of more than $10,000 in cash at any time during 2014. (Form 8300 must have been filed with the IRS by the 15th day after the date of the transaction.)

This day 2015	**Tax Return Due Dates**

Partnerships must provide Form 8308 to the transferor and transferee in any exchange of a partnership interest that involved unrealized receivables or substantially appreciated inventory items.

Trustees or issuers of IRAs or SEPs must provide participants with a statement of the account's value.

Feb. 17th— **Individuals.** Last day for filing Form W-4 by employees who wish to claim exemption from withholding of income tax for 2015.

Information Returns. Annual statements must be furnished to recipients of proceeds from broker and barter exchange transactions (Form 1099-B); proceeds from real estate transactions (Form 1099-S); broker payments in lieu of dividends or tax-exempt interest, and gross proceeds paid to an attorney (Form 1099-MISC).

Mar. 2nd— **Information Returns.** Annual 1099 series returns (together with transmittal Form 1096) for paper filings or, if filing electronically, by March 31, must be filed with the IRS to report payments to recipients who received Form 1099 on January 31st, as indicated above.

Business recipients of $600 or more of interest from an individual on any mortgage must file Form 1098 with the IRS (together with transmittal Form 1096) for paper filings or, if filing electronically, by March 31st.

Withholding. Form W-2 "A" copies for 2014 (together with transmittal Form W-3) must be filed with the Social Security Administration. If filing electronically, the due date is extended to March 31st.

Form W-2G and Form 1099-R for 2014 "A" copies (together with transmittal Form 1096) for paper filings or, if filing electronically, by March 31st, must be filed with the IRS.

Individuals. Last day for farmers and fishermen who owed, but did not pay, estimated tax on January 15th to file 2014 calendar-year income tax return and pay tax in full to avoid late payment penalty.

Mar. 16th— **Corporations.** Due date of 2014 income tax returns (Form 1120) for calendar-year U.S. corporations or calendar-year foreign corporations with offices in the United States. Fiscal-year U.S. corporations and foreign corporations with a U.S. office must file by the 15th day of the 3rd month following the close of the tax year.

Last date for filing application (Form 7004) by calendar-year corporations for automatic six-month extension to file 2014 income tax return.

Form 5452 for reporting nontaxable corporate distributions made to shareholders during calendar year 2014 should be filed by calendar-year corporations with income tax return. Fiscal-year corporations file Form 5452 with income tax return for first fiscal year ending after calendar year in which distributions were made.

Calendar-year corporations' 2014 information return (Form 5471) with respect to foreign corporations. (Fiscal-year corporations file form with income tax return.)

Last date for a calendar-year corporation to file an amended income tax return (Form 1120X) for the calendar year 2011.[2]

S Corporations. Due date of 2014 income tax returns for calendar-year S corporations (Form 1120S) and to provide each shareholder with a copy of Schedule K-1.

Last date for filing application (Form 7004) by S corporations for automatic six-month extension to file 2014 income tax return.

Last date for filing Form 2553 to elect to be treated as an S corporation beginning with calendar year 2015. The penalty for filing the election late is to postpone treatment as an S corporation until calendar year 2016.

This day 2015	Tax Return Due Dates

Withholding. File returns on Form 1042 and Form 1042-S to report tax withheld at the source from nonresident aliens, foreign corporations, foreign partnerships and foreign fiduciaries of a trust or estate.

Mar. 31st—

Information Returns—Electronic Filing. Due date for filing Form 1099 series (for reporting certain payments) and Form 1098 (for reporting receipt of mortgage interest) with the IRS electronically.

Withholding—Electronic Filing. Last day for filing Form W-2 with the SSA or Form W-2G with the IRS if filing electronically.

Apr. 15th—

Individuals. Income tax and self-employment tax returns of individuals for calendar year 2014 and income tax returns of calendar-year decedents who died in 2014 (Form 1040, Form 1040A, or Form 1040EZ). Fiscal-year individuals must file returns or requests for extension by the 15th day of the 4th month after the close of the tax year.

Last day for calendar-year individuals to file application (Form 4868) for automatic six-month extension to file 2014 income tax return.

Individuals' information returns (Form 5471) with respect to foreign corporations to be filed with Form 1040.

Last day for individuals to file amended income tax returns (Form 1040X) for the calendar year 2011.

Estimated Tax. Calendar-year corporations pay first installment of 2015 estimated income taxes. Fiscal-year corporations are to make payments on the 15th day of the 4th, 6th, 9th, and 12th months of the tax year.

Payment of first installment of 2015 estimated income taxes (Form 1040-ES) by calendar-year individuals, other than farmers and fishermen. Estimated tax payments for fiscal-year individuals are due on the 15th day of the 4th, 6th, and 9th months of the tax year and the 1st month of the following tax year.

Trusts and calendar-year estates and certain residuary trusts in existence more than two years must make first payment of estimated taxes for 2015 (Form 1041-ES). Fiscal-year estates must make payments on the 15th day of the 4th, 6th, and 9th months of the fiscal year and the 1st month of the following fiscal year.

Trusts and Estates. Fiduciary income tax return (Form 1041) for calendar year 2014. Fiscal-year estates must file by the 15th day of the 4th month following close of the tax year.

Last day for calendar year estates and trusts to file application (Form 7004) for automatic five-month extension of time to file 2014 income tax return.

Last day for estates and trusts to file amended tax returns for calendar year 2011.

Partnerships. Last day for filing income tax return (Form 1065) for calendar year 2014. Returns for fiscal-year partnerships are due on the 15th day of the 4th month after the close of the tax year.

Last day for calendar-year U.S. partnerships to file application (Form 7004) for automatic five-month extension to file 2014 income tax return.

Last day for calendar-year partnerships to file an amended return for 2011.

Information Returns. Annual information return (Form 1041-A) for split-interest trusts and complex trusts claiming charitable deductions under Code Sec. 642(c) and annual information return (Form 5227) for charitable remainder trusts, pooled income funds, and Code Sec. 4947(a)(2) trusts must be filed.

This day 2015	**Tax Return Due Dates**

Apr. 30th—   **Employers' Taxes.** Employers of nonagricultural and nonhousehold employees must file return on Form 941 to report income tax withholding and FICA taxes for the first quarter of 2015.[3]

May 15th—   **Exempt Organizations.** Annual information return (Form 990) for 2014 by calendar-year organizations exempt or claiming exemption from tax under Code Sec. 501 or Code Sec. 4947(a)(1). Fiscal-year organizations must file by 15th day of 5th month after close of the tax year.

Calendar-year private foundations and Code Sec. 4947(a) trusts treated as private foundations must file Form 990-PF, and private foundations must pay the first quarter installment of estimated excise tax on net investment or tax on unrelated business income. Fiscal-year organizations must file by 15th day of 5th month after close of tax year, for both Form 990-PF and estimated taxes referred to above.

Calendar-year Code Sec. 501(a) organizations with unrelated business income must file income tax return on Form 990-T. Fiscal-year organizations must file by 15th day of 5th month following close of tax year.

Exempt organizations requesting an extension of time to file Form 990 may file Form 8868.

June 1st—   **Information Returns.** Annual statement to IRS regarding 2014 account balances for an IRA or SEP (Form 5498). Participants and IRS must be provided with IRA plan contribution information.

June 15th—   **Individuals.** Last day for nonresident alien individuals not subject to withholding to file income tax return for calendar year 2014.

Estimated Tax. Calendar-year corporations must pay second installment of 2015 estimated tax.

Payment of second installment of 2015 estimated tax by individuals (Form 1040-ES), other than farmers and fishermen, by trusts and by estates (Form 1041-ES), and certain residuary trusts in existence more than two years. Nonresident aliens who have no wages subject to U.S. withholding must make first payment (Form 1040-ES (NR)).

Corporations. Last day for foreign corporations that do not maintain an office or place of business in U.S. to file income tax return (Form 1120F) for calendar year 2014.

July 31st—   **Employers' Taxes.** Employers of nonagricultural and nonhousehold employees must file return on Form 941 to report income tax withholding and FICA taxes for the second quarter of 2015.[4]

Sept. 15th—   **Estimated Tax.** Payment of third installment of 2015 estimated tax by calendar-year corporations.

Payment of third installment of 2015 estimated tax by individuals (Form 1040-ES), other than farmers and fishermen, by trusts and by estates (Form 1041-ES), and certain residuary trusts in existence more than two years.

Corporations. Last day for filing 2014 income tax return by calendar-year corporations that obtained automatic six-month filing extension.

Exempt Organizations. Last day for exempt calendar-year farmers' cooperatives to file 2014 income tax returns (Form 1120-C). Fiscal-year cooperatives must file by the 15th day of the 9th month following the close of the tax year. An automatic six-month extension of the filing date may be obtained by filing Form 7004.

Estates and Trusts. Last day for filing 2014 Form 1041 for calendar-year estates and trusts that obtained an automatic five-month filing extension.

This day 2015	**Tax Return Due Dates**
	Partnerships. Last day for filing 2014 Form 1065 for calendar-year partnerships that obtained an automatic five-month filing extension.
October 15th—	**Individuals.** Last day for filing 2014 income tax return (Form 1040) by calendar-year individuals who obtained automatic six-month filing extension.
Nov. 2—	**Employers' Taxes.** Employers of nonagricultural and nonhousehold employees must file return on Form 941 to report income tax withholding and FICA taxes for the third quarter of 2015.[5]
Dec. 15th—	**Estimated Tax.** Payment of last installment of 2015 estimated tax by calendar-year corporations.
This day 2016	
Jan. 15th—	**Estimated Taxes.** Final installment of 2015 estimated tax (Form 1040-ES) by individuals unless income tax return is filed with final payment by February 1, 2016. Payment in full of estimated tax by farmers and fishermen unless income tax returns are filed by March 1, 2015.
	Final installment of 2015 estimated tax (Form 1041-ES) by trusts, calendar-year estates, and certain residuary trusts in existence more than two years, unless Form 1041 is filed and taxes are paid in full by February 1, 2016.
Feb. 1st—	**Individuals.** Final income tax return for 2015 by calendar-year individuals (Form 1040) and by trusts and estates (Form 1041) in existence more than two years who owed but did not pay 2015 estimated tax otherwise due January 15th.

[1] If timely deposits in full payment of tax due were made, the due date for Form 940, Form 941, and Form 943 is February 10, 2015.

[2] Fiscal-year corporations generally must file within three years of the date the original return was due.

[3] If timely deposits in full payment of taxes due were made, the due date for Form 941 is May 10, 2015.

[4] If timely deposits in full payment of taxes due were made, the due date for Form 941 is August 10, 2015.

[5] If timely deposits in full payment of taxes due were made, the due date for Form 941 is November 10, 2015.

EMPLOYMENT TAX DEPOSITS

Income Tax Withholding, FICA Taxes, Backup Withholding. Employment taxes are withheld income tax, FICA contributions, and backup withholding on reportable payments. Generally, an employer must make either MONTHLY or SEMIWEEKLY deposits during a calendar year based upon the aggregate amount of employment taxes paid during the "lookback" period. The lookback period for each calendar year is the 12-month period that ended the preceding June 30. Thus, an employer's obligation to make deposits in 2015 will be based upon the aggregate employment taxes paid during the period July 1, 2013, through June 30, 2014 (¶ 2651). New employers are considered to have an aggregate tax liability of zero for any calendar quarter in which the employer did not exist.

Monthly Deposits. Monthly deposits are required if the aggregate amount of employment taxes reported by the employer for the lookback period is $50,000 or less. Monthly deposits are due on the 15th day of the following month in which the payments were made.

Semiweekly Deposits. An employer is a semiweekly depositor for the entire calendar year if the aggregate amount of employment taxes during the lookback period exceeds $50,000. Further, a monthly depositor will become a semiweekly depositor on the first day after the employer becomes subject to the One-Day Rule, discussed later. Semiweekly deposits are generally due on either Wednesday or Friday—depending upon the timing of the employer's pay period. Employers with payment dates, i.e., paydays, that fall on Wednesday, Thursday, or Friday must deposit the employment taxes on or before the following Wednesday. Employers with payment dates that fall on Saturday, Sunday, Monday, or Tuesday must make their deposit on or before the following Friday. An employer will always have three business days in which to make the deposit. Thus, if any of the three weekdays following the close of a semiweekly period is a holiday, then the employer will have an additional business day in which to make the deposit.

One-Day Rule. If an employer has accumulated $100,000 or more of undeposited employment taxes, then the taxes must be deposited by the close of the next banking day.

Federal Unemployment (FUTA) Taxes. The calendar year is divided into four quarters for purposes of determining when deposits of federal unemployment tax (FUTA) are necessary. The periods end on March 31, June 30, September 30, and December 31. If the employer's FUTA tax liability is $500 or less, then the employer does not have to deposit the tax, instead the amount may be carried forward and added to the liability for the next quarter to determine if a deposit is required. If the employer owes more than $500 in undeposited FUTA tax at the end of a quarter, including any FUTA tax carried forward from an earlier quarter, then the tax owed must be deposited by the end of the next month by either a electronic funds transfer (EFTPS) direct or a EFTPS financial institution.

Schedules and Tables

TAX RATES

TAX RATE SCHEDULES FOR 2014 AND 2015

NOTE. The 2014 Tax Rate Schedules reproduced below are based on the rate changes and inflation adjustments to the tax brackets released by the Internal Revenue Service in Rev. Proc. 2013-35. The 2015 Tax Rate Schedules reproduced below are based on the rate changes and inflation adjustments to the tax brackets released by the IRS in Rev. Proc. 2014-61.

The 2014 and 2015 tax rate schedules for single individuals are at ¶ 11; for married individuals filing jointly and surviving spouses, see ¶ 13; for married individuals filing separately, see ¶ 15; for heads of households, see ¶ 17; and for estates and nongrantor trusts, see ¶ 19.

¶ 11 SCHEDULE X: Single Individuals

2014

Taxable Income Over	But Not Over	Pay	+	% on Excess	of the amount over—
$0—	$9,075	$0		10%	$0
9,075—	36,900	907.50		15	9,075
36,900—	89,350	5,081.25		25	36,900
89,350—	186,350	18,193.75		28	89,350
186,350—	405,100	45,353.75		33	186,350
405,100—	406,750	117,541.25		35	405,100
406,750—	. . . . . .	118,118.75		39.6	406,750

2015

Taxable Income Over	But Not Over	Pay	+	% on Excess	of the amount over—
$0—	$9,225	$0		10%	$0
9,225—	37,450	922.50		15	9,225
37,450—	90,750	5,156.25		25	37,450
90,750—	189,300	18,481.25		28	90,750
189,300—	411,500	46,075.25		33	189,300
411,500—	413,200	119,401.25		35	411,500
413,200—	. . . . . .	119,996.25		39.6	413,200

¶ 13 SCHEDULE Y-1: Married Filing Jointly and Surviving Spouses

2014

Taxable Income Over	But Not Over	Pay	+	% on Excess	of the amount over—
$0—	$18,150	$0		10%	$0
18,150—	73,800	1,815.00		15	18,150
73,800—	148,850	10,162.50		25	73,800
148,850—	226,850	28,925.00		28	148,850
226,850—	405,100	50,765.00		33	226,850
405,100—	457,600	109,587.50		35	405,100
457,600—	. . . . . .	127,962.50		39.6	457,600

2015

Taxable Income Over	But Not Over	Pay	+	% on Excess	of the amount over—
$0—	$18,450	$0		10%	$0
18,450—	74,900	1,845.00		15	18,450
74,900—	151,200	10,312.50		25	74,900
151,200—	230,450	29,387.50		28	151,200
230,450—	411,500	51,577.50		33	230,450
411,500—	464,850	111,324.00		35	411,500
464,850—	. . . . . .	129,996.50		39.6	464,850

¶ 15 SCHEDULE Y-2: Married Individuals Filing Separately

2014

Taxable Income Over	But Not Over	Pay	+	% on Excess	of the amount over—
$0—	$9,075	$0		10%	$0
9,075—	36,900	907.50		15	9,075
36,900—	74,425	5,081.25		25	36,900
74,425—	113,425	14,462.50		28	74,425
113,425—	202,550	25,382.50		33	113,425
202,550—	228,800	54,793.75		35	202,550
228,800—	. . . . . .	63,981.25		39.6	228,800

2015

Taxable Income Over	But Not Over	Pay	+	% on Excess	of the amount over—
$0—	$9,225	$0		10%	$0
9,225—	37,450	922.50		15	9,225
37,450—	75,600	5,156.25		25	37,450
75,600—	115,225	14,693.75		28	75,600
115,225—	205,750	25,788.75		33	115,225
205,750—	232,425	55,662.00		35	205,750
232,425—	. . . . . .	64,998.25		39.6	232,425

TAX RATES

¶ 17 SCHEDULE Z: Heads of Households

2014

Taxable Income Over	But Not Over	Pay	+	% on Excess	of the amount over—
$0—	$12,950	$0		10%	$0
12,950—	49,400	1,295.00		15	12,950
49,400—	127,550	6,762.50		25	49,400
127,550—	206,600	26,300.00		28	127,550
206,600—	405,100	48,434.00		33	206,600
405,100—	432,200	113,939.00		35	405,100
432,200—	. . . . . .	123,424.00		39.6	432,200

2015

Taxable Income Over	But Not Over	Pay	+	% on Excess	of the amount over—
$0—	$13,150	$0		10%	$0
13,150—	50,200	1,315.00		15	13,150
50,200—	129,600	6,872.50		25	50,200
129,600—	209,850	26,722.50		28	129,600
209,850—	411,500	49,192.50		33	209,850
411,500—	439,000	115,737.00		35	411,500
439,000—	. . . . . .	125,362.00		39.6	439,000

¶ 19 INCOME TAX RATE SCHEDULES FOR USE BY ESTATES AND NONGRANTOR TRUSTS

2014

Taxable Income Over	But Not Over	Pay	+	% on Excess	of the amount over—
$0—	$2,500	$0		15%	$0
2,500—	5,800	375.00		25	2,500
5,800—	8,900	1,200.00		28	5,800
8,900—	12,150	2,068.00		33	8,900
12,150—	. . . . . .	3,140.50		39.6	12,150

2015

Taxable Income Over	But Not Over	Pay	+	% on Excess	of the amount over—
$0—	$2,500	$0		15%	$0
2,500—	5,900	375.00		25	2,500
5,900—	9,050	1,225.00		28	5,900
9,050—	12,300	2,107.00		33	9,050
12,300—	. . . . . .	3,179.50		39.6	12,300

➤➤➤ *Caution: This is a draft 2014 Tax Computation Worksheet. At the time of publication, the IRS had not yet released the 2014 Tax Computation Worksheet. For the latest information, see CCHGroup.com/TaxUpdates.*

¶ 20 2014 Tax Computation Worksheet

2014 Tax Computation Worksheet—Line 44

 See the instructions for line 44 to see if you must use the worksheet below to figure your tax.

Note. If you are required to use this worksheet to figure the tax on an amount from another form or worksheet, such as the Qualified Dividends and Capital Gain Tax Worksheet, the Schedule D Tax Worksheet, Schedule J, Form 8615, or the Foreign Earned Income Tax Worksheet, enter the amount from that form or worksheet in column (a) of the row that applies to the amount you are looking up. Enter the result on the appropriate line of the form or worksheet that you are completing.

Section A—Use if your filing status is **Single.** Complete the row below that applies to you.

Taxable income. If line 43 is—	(a) Enter the amount from line 43	(b) Multiplication amount	(c) Multiply (a) by (b)	(d) Subtraction amount	Tax. Subtract (d) from (c). Enter the result here and on Form 1040, line 44
At least $100,000 but not over $186,350	$	× 28% (.28)	$	$ 6,824.25	$
Over $186,350 but not over $405,100	$	× 33% (.33)	$	$ 16,141.75	$
Over $405,100 but not over $406,750	$	× 35% (.35)	$	$ 24,243.75	$
Over $406,750	$	× 39.6% (.396)	$	$ 42,954.25	$

Section B—Use if your filing status is **Married filing jointly** or **Qualifying widow(er).** Complete the row below that applies to you.

Taxable income. If line 43 is—	(a) Enter the amount from line 43	(b) Multiplication amount	(c) Multiply (a) by (b)	(d) Subtraction amount	Tax. Subtract (d) from (c). Enter the result here and on Form 1040, line 44
At least $100,000 but not over $148,850	$	× 25% (.25)	$	$ 8,287.50	$
Over $148,850 but not over $226,850	$	× 28% (.28)	$	$ 12,753.00	$
Over $226,850 but not over $405,100	$	× 33% (.33)	$	$ 24,095.50	$
Over $405,100 but not over $457,600	$	× 35% (.35)	$	$ 32,197.50	$
Over $457,600	$	× 39.6% (.396)	$	$ 53,247.10	$

Section C—Use if your filing status is **Married filing separately.** Complete the row below that applies to you.

Taxable income. If line 43 is—	(a) Enter the amount from line 43	(b) Multiplication amount	(c) Multiply (a) by (b)	(d) Subtraction amount	Tax. Subtract (d) from (c). Enter the result here and on Form 1040, line 44
At least $100,000 but not over $113,425	$	× 28% (.28)	$	$ 6,376.50	$
Over $113,425 but not over $202,550	$	× 33% (.33)	$	$ 12,047.75	$
Over $202,550 but not over $228,800	$	× 35% (.35)	$	$ 16,098.75	$
Over $228,800	$	× 39.6% (.396)	$	$ 26,623.55	$

Section D—Use if your filing status is **Head of household.** Complete the row below that applies to you.

Taxable income. If line 43 is—	(a) Enter the amount from line 43	(b) Multiplication amount	(c) Multiply (a) by (b)	(d) Subtraction amount	Tax. Subtract (d) from (c). Enter the result here and on Form 1040, line 44
At least $100,000 but not over $127,550	$	× 25% (.25)	$	$ 5,587.50	$
Over $127,550 but not over $206,600	$	× 28% (.28)	$	$ 9,414.00	$
Over $206,600 but not over $405,100	$	× 33% (.33)	$	$ 19,744.00	$
Over $405,100 but not over $432,200	$	× 35% (.35)	$	$ 27,846.00	$
Over $432,200	$	× 39.6% (.396)	$	$ 47,727.20	$

¶20

2014 TAX TABLE—INDIVIDUALS

>>>→ *Caution: This is a draft 2014 Tax Table. At the time of publication, the IRS had not yet released the 2014 Tax Table. For the latest information, see CCHGroup.com/TaxUpdates.*

¶ 25 2014 Tax Table for Use with Form 1040

☐ The Tax Table that follows is for use with Form 1040. A similar Tax Table applies to Forms 1040A and 1040EZ.

2014 TAX TABLE   Based on Taxable Income. For persons with taxable incomes of less than $100,000.

Read down the income columns of the tax table until you find the line covering the taxable income shown on line 43 of Form 1040 (line 27 of Form 1040A or line 6 of Form 1040EZ). Then read across that income line until you find the column heading that describes your filing status. Enter the tax found there on line 44 of Form 1040 (line 28 of Form 1040A or line 10 of Form 1040EZ).

»»→ Caution: *This is a draft 2014 Tax Table. At the time of publication, the IRS had not yet released the 2014 Tax Table. For the latest information, see CCHGroup.com/TaxUpdates.*

2014 Tax Table

⚠️ CAUTION — See the instructions for line 44 to see if you must use the Tax Table below to figure your tax.

Example. Mr. and Mrs. Brown are filing a joint return. Their taxable income on Form 1040, line 43, is $25,300. First, they find the $25,300-$25,350 taxable income line. Next, they find the column for married filing jointly and read down the column. The amount shown where the taxable income line and filing status column meet is $2,891. This is the tax amount they should enter on Form 1040, line 44.

Sample Table

At Least	But Less Than	Single	Married filing jointly*	Married filing separately	Head of a household
			Your tax is—		
25,200	25,250	3,330	2,876	3,330	3,136
25,250	25,300	3,338	2,884	3,338	3,144
25,300	25,350	3,345	(2,891)	3,345	3,151
25,350	25,400	3,353	2,899	3,353	3,159

At least	But less than	Single	Married filing jointly*	Married filing separately	Head of a household
			Your tax is—		
0	5	0	0	0	0
5	15	1	1	1	1
15	25	2	2	2	2
25	50	4	4	4	4
50	75	6	6	6	6
75	100	9	9	9	9
100	125	11	11	11	11
125	150	14	14	14	14
150	175	16	16	16	16
175	200	19	19	19	19
200	225	21	21	21	21
225	250	24	24	24	24
250	275	26	26	26	26
275	300	29	29	29	29
300	325	31	31	31	31
325	350	34	34	34	34
350	375	36	36	36	36
375	400	39	39	39	39
400	425	41	41	41	41
425	450	44	44	44	44
450	475	46	46	46	46
475	500	49	49	49	49
500	525	51	51	51	51
525	550	54	54	54	54
550	575	56	56	56	56
575	600	59	59	59	59
600	625	61	61	61	61
625	650	64	64	64	64
650	675	66	66	66	66
675	700	69	69	69	69
700	725	71	71	71	71
725	750	74	74	74	74
750	775	76	76	76	76
775	800	79	79	79	79
800	825	81	81	81	81
825	850	84	84	84	84
850	875	86	86	86	86
875	900	89	89	89	89
900	925	91	91	91	91
925	950	94	94	94	94
950	975	96	96	96	96
975	1,000	99	99	99	99

1,000

At least	But less than	Single	Married filing jointly*	Married filing separately	Head of a household
			Your tax is—		
1,000	1,025	101	101	101	101
1,025	1,050	104	104	104	104
1,050	1,075	106	106	106	106
1,075	1,100	109	109	109	109
1,100	1,125	111	111	111	111
1,125	1,150	114	114	114	114
1,150	1,175	116	116	116	116
1,175	1,200	119	119	119	119
1,200	1,225	121	121	121	121
1,225	1,250	124	124	124	124
1,250	1,275	126	126	126	126
1,275	1,300	129	129	129	129
1,300	1,325	131	131	131	131
1,325	1,350	134	134	134	134
1,350	1,375	136	136	136	136
1,375	1,400	139	139	139	139
1,400	1,425	141	141	141	141
1,425	1,450	144	144	144	144
1,450	1,475	146	146	146	146
1,475	1,500	149	149	149	149
1,500	1,525	151	151	151	151
1,525	1,550	154	154	154	154
1,550	1,575	156	156	156	156
1,575	1,600	159	159	159	159
1,600	1,625	161	161	161	161
1,625	1,650	164	164	164	164
1,650	1,675	166	166	166	166
1,675	1,700	169	169	169	169
1,700	1,725	171	171	171	171
1,725	1,750	174	174	174	174
1,750	1,775	176	176	176	176
1,775	1,800	179	179	179	179
1,800	1,825	181	181	181	181
1,825	1,850	184	184	184	184
1,850	1,875	186	186	186	186
1,875	1,900	189	189	189	189
1,900	1,925	191	191	191	191
1,925	1,950	194	194	194	194
1,950	1,975	196	196	196	196
1,975	2,000	199	199	199	199

2,000

At least	But less than	Single	Married filing jointly*	Married filing separately	Head of a household
			Your tax is—		
2,000	2,025	201	201	201	201
2,025	2,050	204	204	204	204
2,050	2,075	206	206	206	206
2,075	2,100	209	209	209	209
2,100	2,125	211	211	211	211
2,125	2,150	214	214	214	214
2,150	2,175	216	216	216	216
2,175	2,200	219	219	219	219
2,200	2,225	221	221	221	221
2,225	2,250	224	224	224	224
2,250	2,275	226	226	226	226
2,275	2,300	229	229	229	229
2,300	2,325	231	231	231	231
2,325	2,350	234	234	234	234
2,350	2,375	236	236	236	236
2,375	2,400	239	239	239	239
2,400	2,425	241	241	241	241
2,425	2,450	244	244	244	244
2,450	2,475	246	246	246	246
2,475	2,500	249	249	249	249
2,500	2,525	251	251	251	251
2,525	2,550	254	254	254	254
2,550	2,575	256	256	256	256
2,575	2,600	259	259	259	259
2,600	2,625	261	261	261	261
2,625	2,650	264	264	264	264
2,650	2,675	266	266	266	266
2,675	2,700	269	269	269	269
2,700	2,725	271	271	271	271
2,725	2,750	274	274	274	274
2,750	2,775	276	276	276	276
2,775	2,800	279	279	279	279
2,800	2,825	281	281	281	281
2,825	2,850	284	284	284	284
2,850	2,875	286	286	286	286
2,875	2,900	289	289	289	289
2,900	2,925	291	291	291	291
2,925	2,950	294	294	294	294
2,950	2,975	296	296	296	296
2,975	3,000	299	299	299	299

* This column must also be used by a qualifying widow(er).

(Continued)

¶25

>>>→ *Caution: This is a draft 2014 Tax Table. At the time of publication, the IRS had not yet released the 2014 Tax Table. For the latest information, see CCHGroup.com/TaxUpdates.*

If line 43 (taxable income) is—		And you are—			
At least	But less than	Single	Married filing jointly *	Married filing separately	Head of a household
		Your tax is—			

3,000

At least	But less than	Single	Married filing jointly *	Married filing separately	Head of a household
3,000	3,050	303	303	303	303
3,050	3,100	308	308	308	308
3,100	3,150	313	313	313	313
3,150	3,200	318	318	318	318
3,200	3,250	323	323	323	323
3,250	3,300	328	328	328	328
3,300	3,350	333	333	333	333
3,350	3,400	338	338	338	338
3,400	3,450	343	343	343	343
3,450	3,500	348	348	348	348
3,500	3,550	353	353	353	353
3,550	3,600	358	358	358	358
3,600	3,650	363	363	363	363
3,650	3,700	368	368	368	368
3,700	3,750	373	373	373	373
3,750	3,800	378	378	378	378
3,800	3,850	383	383	383	383
3,850	3,900	388	388	388	388
3,900	3,950	393	393	393	393
3,950	4,000	398	398	398	398

4,000

At least	But less than	Single	Married filing jointly *	Married filing separately	Head of a household
4,000	4,050	403	403	403	403
4,050	4,100	408	408	408	408
4,100	4,150	413	413	413	413
4,150	4,200	418	418	418	418
4,200	4,250	423	423	423	423
4,250	4,300	428	428	428	428
4,300	4,350	433	433	433	433
4,350	4,400	438	438	438	438
4,400	4,450	443	443	443	443
4,450	4,500	448	448	448	448
4,500	4,550	453	453	453	453
4,550	4,600	458	458	458	458
4,600	4,650	463	463	463	463
4,650	4,700	468	468	468	468
4,700	4,750	473	473	473	473
4,750	4,800	478	478	478	478
4,800	4,850	483	483	483	483
4,850	4,900	488	488	488	488
4,900	4,950	493	493	493	493
4,950	5,000	498	496	498	498

5,000

At least	But less than	Single	Married filing jointly *	Married filing separately	Head of a household
5,000	5,050	503	503	503	503
5,050	5,100	508	508	508	508
5,100	5,150	513	513	513	513
5,150	5,200	518	518	518	518
5,200	5,250	523	523	523	523
5,250	5,300	528	526	528	528
5,300	5,350	533	533	533	533
5,350	5,400	538	538	538	538
5,400	5,450	543	543	543	543
5,450	5,500	548	548	548	548
5,500	5,550	553	553	553	553
5,550	5,600	558	558	558	558
5,600	5,650	563	563	563	563
5,650	5,700	568	568	568	568
5,700	5,750	573	573	573	573
5,750	5,800	578	578	578	578
5,800	5,850	583	583	583	583
5,850	5,900	588	588	588	588
5,900	5,950	593	593	593	593
5,950	6,000	598	598	598	598

6,000

At least	But less than	Single	Married filing jointly *	Married filing separately	Head of a household
6,000	6,050	603	603	603	603
6,050	6,100	608	608	608	608
6,100	6,150	613	613	613	613
6,150	6,200	618	618	618	618
6,200	6,250	623	623	623	623
6,250	6,300	628	628	628	628
6,300	6,350	633	633	633	633
6,350	6,400	638	638	638	638
6,400	6,450	643	643	643	643
6,450	6,500	648	648	648	648
6,500	6,550	653	653	653	653
6,550	6,600	658	658	658	658
6,600	6,650	663	663	663	663
6,650	6,700	668	668	668	668
6,700	6,750	673	673	673	673
6,750	6,800	678	678	678	678
6,800	6,850	683	683	683	683
6,850	6,900	688	688	688	688
6,900	6,950	693	693	693	693
6,950	7,000	698	698	698	698

7,000

At least	But less than	Single	Married filing jointly *	Married filing separately	Head of a household
7,000	7,050	703	703	703	703
7,050	7,100	708	708	708	708
7,100	7,150	713	713	713	713
7,150	7,200	718	718	718	718
7,200	7,250	723	723	723	723
7,250	7,300	728	728	728	728
7,300	7,350	733	733	733	733
7,350	7,400	738	738	738	738
7,400	7,450	743	743	743	743
7,450	7,500	748	748	748	748
7,500	7,550	753	753	753	753
7,550	7,600	758	758	758	758
7,600	7,650	763	763	763	763
7,650	7,700	768	768	768	768
7,700	7,750	773	773	773	773
7,750	7,800	778	778	778	778
7,800	7,850	783	783	783	783
7,850	7,900	788	788	788	788
7,900	7,950	793	793	793	793
7,950	8,000	798	798	798	798

8,000

At least	But less than	Single	Married filing jointly *	Married filing separately	Head of a household
8,000	8,050	803	803	803	803
8,050	8,100	808	808	808	808
8,100	8,150	813	813	813	813
8,150	8,200	818	818	818	818
8,200	8,250	823	823	823	823
8,250	8,300	828	828	828	828
8,300	8,350	833	833	833	833
8,350	8,400	838	838	838	838
8,400	8,450	843	843	843	843
8,450	8,500	848	848	848	848
8,500	8,550	853	853	853	853
8,550	8,600	858	858	858	858
8,600	8,650	863	863	863	863
8,650	8,700	868	868	868	868
8,700	8,750	873	873	873	873
8,750	8,800	878	878	878	878
8,800	8,850	883	883	883	883
8,850	8,900	888	888	888	888
8,900	8,950	893	893	893	893
8,950	9,000	898	898	898	898

9,000

At least	But less than	Single	Married filing jointly *	Married filing separately	Head of a household
9,000	9,050	903	903	903	903
9,050	9,100	908	908	908	908
9,100	9,150	915	913	915	913
9,150	9,200	923	918	923	918
9,200	9,250	930	923	930	923
9,250	9,300	938	928	938	928
9,300	9,350	945	933	945	933
9,350	9,400	953	938	953	938
9,400	9,450	960	943	960	943
9,450	9,500	968	948	968	948
9,500	9,550	975	953	975	953
9,550	9,600	983	958	983	958
9,600	9,650	990	963	990	963
9,650	9,700	998	968	998	968
9,700	9,750	1,005	973	1,005	973
9,750	9,800	1,013	978	1,013	978
9,800	9,850	1,020	983	1,020	983
9,850	9,900	1,028	988	1,028	988
9,900	9,950	1,035	993	1,035	993
9,950	10,000	1,043	998	1,043	998

10,000

At least	But less than	Single	Married filing jointly *	Married filing separately	Head of a household
10,000	10,050	1,050	1,003	1,050	1,003
10,050	10,100	1,058	1,008	1,058	1,008
10,100	10,150	1,065	1,013	1,065	1,013
10,150	10,200	1,073	1,018	1,073	1,018
10,200	10,250	1,080	1,023	1,080	1,023
10,250	10,300	1,088	1,028	1,088	1,028
10,300	10,350	1,095	1,033	1,095	1,033
10,350	10,400	1,103	1,038	1,103	1,038
10,400	10,450	1,110	1,043	1,110	1,043
10,450	10,500	1,118	1,048	1,118	1,048
10,500	10,550	1,125	1,053	1,125	1,053
10,550	10,600	1,133	1,058	1,133	1,058
10,600	10,650	1,140	1,063	1,140	1,063
10,650	10,700	1,148	1,068	1,148	1,068
10,700	10,750	1,155	1,073	1,155	1,073
10,750	10,800	1,163	1,078	1,163	1,078
10,800	10,850	1,170	1,083	1,170	1,083
10,850	10,900	1,178	1,088	1,178	1,088
10,900	10,950	1,185	1,093	1,185	1,093
10,950	11,000	1,193	1,098	1,193	1,098

11,000

At least	But less than	Single	Married filing jointly *	Married filing separately	Head of a household
11,000	11,050	1,200	1,103	1,200	1,103
11,050	11,100	1,208	1,108	1,208	1,108
11,100	11,150	1,215	1,113	1,215	1,113
11,150	11,200	1,223	1,118	1,223	1,118
11,200	11,250	1,230	1,123	1,230	1,123
11,250	11,300	1,238	1,128	1,238	1,128
11,300	11,350	1,245	1,133	1,245	1,133
11,350	11,400	1,253	1,138	1,253	1,138
11,400	11,450	1,260	1,143	1,260	1,143
11,450	11,500	1,268	1,148	1,268	1,148
11,500	11,550	1,275	1,153	1,275	1,153
11,550	11,600	1,283	1,158	1,283	1,158
11,600	11,650	1,290	1,163	1,290	1,163
11,650	11,700	1,298	1,168	1,298	1,168
11,700	11,750	1,305	1,173	1,305	1,173
11,750	11,800	1,313	1,178	1,313	1,178
11,800	11,850	1,320	1,183	1,320	1,183
11,850	11,900	1,328	1,188	1,328	1,188
11,900	11,950	1,335	1,193	1,335	1,193
11,950	12,000	1,343	1,198	1,343	1,198

(Continued)

* This column must also be used by a qualifying widow(er).

Need more information or forms? Visit IRS.gov.   - 76 -

¶25

»»→ *Caution:* *This is a draft 2014 Tax Table. At the time of publication, the IRS had not yet released the 2014 Tax Table. For the latest information, see CCHGroup.com/TaxUpdates.*

12,000

At least	But less than	Single	Married filing jointly*	Married filing separately	Head of a household
12,000	12,050	1,350	1,203	1,350	1,203
12,050	12,100	1,358	1,208	1,358	1,208
12,100	12,150	1,365	1,213	1,365	1,213
12,150	12,200	1,373	1,218	1,373	1,218
12,200	12,250	1,380	1,223	1,380	1,223
12,250	12,300	1,388	1,228	1,388	1,228
12,300	12,350	1,395	1,233	1,395	1,233
12,350	12,400	1,403	1,238	1,403	1,238
12,400	12,450	1,410	1,243	1,410	1,243
12,450	12,500	1,418	1,248	1,418	1,248
12,500	12,550	1,425	1,253	1,425	1,253
12,550	12,600	1,433	1,258	1,433	1,258
12,600	12,650	1,440	1,263	1,440	1,263
12,650	12,700	1,448	1,268	1,448	1,268
12,700	12,750	1,455	1,273	1,455	1,273
12,750	12,800	1,463	1,278	1,463	1,278
12,800	12,850	1,470	1,283	1,470	1,283
12,850	12,900	1,478	1,288	1,478	1,288
12,900	12,950	1,485	1,293	1,485	1,293
12,950	13,000	1,493	1,298	1,493	1,299

13,000

At least	But less than	Single	Married filing jointly*	Married filing separately	Head of a household
13,000	13,050	1,500	1,303	1,500	1,306
13,050	13,100	1,508	1,308	1,508	1,314
13,100	13,150	1,515	1,313	1,515	1,321
13,150	13,200	1,523	1,318	1,523	1,329
13,200	13,250	1,530	1,323	1,530	1,336
13,250	13,300	1,538	1,328	1,538	1,344
13,300	13,350	1,545	1,333	1,545	1,351
13,350	13,400	1,553	1,338	1,553	1,359
13,400	13,450	1,560	1,343	1,560	1,366
13,450	13,500	1,568	1,348	1,568	1,374
13,500	13,550	1,575	1,353	1,575	1,381
13,550	13,600	1,583	1,358	1,583	1,389
13,600	13,650	1,590	1,363	1,590	1,396
13,650	13,700	1,598	1,368	1,598	1,404
13,700	13,750	1,605	1,373	1,605	1,411
13,750	13,800	1,613	1,378	1,613	1,419
13,800	13,850	1,620	1,383	1,620	1,426
13,850	13,900	1,628	1,388	1,628	1,434
13,900	13,950	1,635	1,393	1,635	1,441
13,950	14,000	1,643	1,398	1,643	1,449

14,000

At least	But less than	Single	Married filing jointly*	Married filing separately	Head of a household
14,000	14,050	1,650	1,403	1,650	1,456
14,050	14,100	1,658	1,408	1,658	1,464
14,100	14,150	1,665	1,413	1,665	1,471
14,150	14,200	1,673	1,418	1,673	1,479
14,200	14,250	1,680	1,423	1,680	1,486
14,250	14,300	1,688	1,428	1,688	1,494
14,300	14,350	1,695	1,433	1,695	1,501
14,350	14,400	1,703	1,438	1,703	1,509
14,400	14,450	1,710	1,443	1,710	1,516
14,450	14,500	1,718	1,448	1,718	1,524
14,500	14,550	1,725	1,453	1,725	1,531
14,550	14,600	1,733	1,458	1,733	1,539
14,600	14,650	1,740	1,463	1,740	1,546
14,650	14,700	1,748	1,468	1,748	1,554
14,700	14,750	1,755	1,473	1,755	1,561
14,750	14,800	1,763	1,478	1,763	1,569
14,800	14,850	1,770	1,483	1,770	1,576
14,850	14,900	1,778	1,488	1,778	1,584
14,900	14,950	1,785	1,493	1,785	1,591
14,950	15,000	1,793	1,498	1,793	1,599

15,000

At least	But less than	Single	Married filing jointly*	Married filing separately	Head of a household
15,000	15,050	1,800	1,503	1,800	1,606
15,050	15,100	1,808	1,508	1,808	1,614
15,100	15,150	1,815	1,513	1,815	1,621
15,150	15,200	1,823	1,518	1,823	1,629
15,200	15,250	1,830	1,523	1,830	1,636
15,250	15,300	1,838	1,528	1,838	1,644
15,300	15,350	1,845	1,533	1,845	1,651
15,350	15,400	1,853	1,538	1,853	1,659
15,400	15,450	1,860	1,543	1,860	1,666
15,450	15,500	1,868	1,548	1,868	1,674
15,500	15,550	1,875	1,553	1,875	1,681
15,550	15,600	1,883	1,558	1,883	1,689
15,600	15,650	1,890	1,563	1,890	1,696
15,650	15,700	1,898	1,568	1,898	1,704
15,700	15,750	1,905	1,573	1,905	1,711
15,750	15,800	1,913	1,578	1,913	1,719
15,800	15,850	1,920	1,583	1,920	1,726
15,850	15,900	1,928	1,588	1,928	1,734
15,900	15,950	1,935	1,593	1,935	1,741
15,950	16,000	1,943	1,598	1,943	1,749

16,000

At least	But less than	Single	Married filing jointly*	Married filing separately	Head of a household
16,000	16,050	1,950	1,603	1,950	1,756
16,050	16,100	1,958	1,608	1,958	1,764
16,100	16,150	1,965	1,613	1,965	1,771
16,150	16,200	1,973	1,618	1,973	1,779
16,200	16,250	1,980	1,623	1,980	1,786
16,250	16,300	1,988	1,628	1,988	1,794
16,300	16,350	1,995	1,633	1,995	1,801
16,350	16,400	2,003	1,638	2,003	1,809
16,400	16,450	2,010	1,643	2,010	1,816
16,450	16,500	2,018	1,648	2,018	1,824
16,500	16,550	2,025	1,653	2,025	1,831
16,550	16,600	2,033	1,658	2,033	1,839
16,600	16,650	2,040	1,663	2,040	1,846
16,650	16,700	2,048	1,668	2,048	1,854
16,700	16,750	2,055	1,673	2,055	1,861
16,750	16,800	2,063	1,678	2,063	1,869
16,800	16,850	2,070	1,683	2,070	1,876
16,850	16,900	2,078	1,688	2,078	1,884
16,900	16,950	2,085	1,693	2,085	1,891
16,950	17,000	2,093	1,698	2,093	1,899

17,000

At least	But less than	Single	Married filing jointly*	Married filing separately	Head of a household
17,000	17,050	2,100	1,703	2,100	1,906
17,050	17,100	2,108	1,708	2,108	1,914
17,100	17,150	2,115	1,713	2,115	1,921
17,150	17,200	2,123	1,718	2,123	1,929
17,200	17,250	2,130	1,723	2,130	1,936
17,250	17,300	2,138	1,728	2,138	1,944
17,300	17,350	2,145	1,733	2,145	1,951
17,350	17,400	2,153	1,738	2,153	1,959
17,400	17,450	2,160	1,743	2,160	1,966
17,450	17,500	2,168	1,748	2,168	1,974
17,500	17,550	2,175	1,753	2,175	1,981
17,550	17,600	2,183	1,758	2,183	1,989
17,600	17,650	2,190	1,763	2,190	1,996
17,650	17,700	2,198	1,768	2,198	2,004
17,700	17,750	2,205	1,773	2,205	2,011
17,750	17,800	2,213	1,778	2,213	2,019
17,800	17,850	2,220	1,783	2,220	2,026
17,850	17,900	2,228	1,788	2,228	2,034
17,900	17,950	2,235	1,793	2,235	2,041
17,950	18,000	2,243	1,798	2,243	2,049

18,000

At least	But less than	Single	Married filing jointly*	Married filing separately	Head of a household
18,000	18,050	2,250	1,803	2,250	2,056
18,050	18,100	2,258	1,808	2,258	2,064
18,100	18,150	2,265	1,813	2,265	2,071
18,150	18,200	2,273	1,819	2,273	2,079
18,200	18,250	2,280	1,826	2,280	2,086
18,250	18,300	2,288	1,834	2,288	2,094
18,300	18,350	2,295	1,841	2,295	2,101
18,350	18,400	2,303	1,849	2,303	2,109
18,400	18,450	2,310	1,856	2,310	2,116
18,450	18,500	2,318	1,864	2,318	2,124
18,500	18,550	2,325	1,871	2,325	2,131
18,550	18,600	2,333	1,879	2,333	2,139
18,600	18,650	2,340	1,886	2,340	2,146
18,650	18,700	2,348	1,894	2,348	2,154
18,700	18,750	2,355	1,901	2,355	2,161
18,750	18,800	2,363	1,909	2,363	2,169
18,800	18,850	2,370	1,916	2,370	2,176
18,850	18,900	2,378	1,924	2,378	2,184
18,900	18,950	2,385	1,931	2,385	2,191
18,950	19,000	2,393	1,939	2,393	2,199

19,000

At least	But less than	Single	Married filing jointly*	Married filing separately	Head of a household
19,000	19,050	2,400	1,946	2,400	2,206
19,050	19,100	2,408	1,954	2,408	2,214
19,100	19,150	2,415	1,961	2,415	2,221
19,150	19,200	2,423	1,969	2,423	2,229
19,200	19,250	2,430	1,976	2,430	2,236
19,250	19,300	2,438	1,984	2,438	2,244
19,300	19,350	2,445	1,991	2,445	2,251
19,350	19,400	2,453	1,999	2,453	2,259
19,400	19,450	2,460	2,006	2,460	2,266
19,450	19,500	2,468	2,014	2,468	2,274
19,500	19,550	2,475	2,021	2,475	2,281
19,550	19,600	2,483	2,029	2,483	2,289
19,600	19,650	2,490	2,036	2,490	2,296
19,650	19,700	2,498	2,044	2,498	2,304
19,700	19,750	2,505	2,051	2,505	2,311
19,750	19,800	2,513	2,059	2,513	2,319
19,800	19,850	2,520	2,066	2,520	2,326
19,850	19,900	2,528	2,074	2,528	2,334
19,900	19,950	2,535	2,081	2,535	2,341
19,950	20,000	2,543	2,089	2,543	2,349

20,000

At least	But less than	Single	Married filing jointly*	Married filing separately	Head of a household
20,000	20,050	2,550	2,096	2,550	2,356
20,050	20,100	2,558	2,104	2,558	2,364
20,100	20,150	2,565	2,111	2,565	2,371
20,150	20,200	2,573	2,119	2,573	2,379
20,200	20,250	2,580	2,126	2,580	2,386
20,250	20,300	2,588	2,134	2,588	2,394
20,300	20,350	2,595	2,141	2,595	2,401
20,350	20,400	2,603	2,149	2,603	2,409
20,400	20,450	2,610	2,156	2,610	2,416
20,450	20,500	2,618	2,164	2,618	2,424
20,500	20,550	2,625	2,171	2,625	2,431
20,550	20,600	2,633	2,179	2,633	2,439
20,600	20,650	2,640	2,186	2,640	2,446
20,650	20,700	2,648	2,194	2,648	2,454
20,700	20,750	2,655	2,201	2,655	2,461
20,750	20,800	2,663	2,209	2,663	2,469
20,800	20,850	2,670	2,216	2,670	2,476
20,850	20,900	2,678	2,224	2,678	2,484
20,900	20,950	2,685	2,231	2,685	2,491
20,950	21,000	2,693	2,239	2,693	2,499

* This column must also be used by a qualifying widow(er).

(Continued)

Need more information or forms? Visit IRS.gov.

¶25

»»→ Caution: *This is a draft 2014 Tax Table. At the time of publication, the IRS had not yet released the 2014 Tax Table. For the latest information, see CCHGroup.com/TaxUpdates.*

21,000 / 22,000 / 23,000

If line 43 (taxable income) is—		And you are—			
At least	But less than	Single	Married filing jointly *	Married filing separately	Head of a household
		Your tax is—			
21,000					
21,000	21,050	2,700	2,246	2,700	2,506
21,050	21,100	2,708	2,254	2,708	2,514
21,100	21,150	2,715	2,261	2,715	2,521
21,150	21,200	2,723	2,269	2,723	2,529
21,200	21,250	2,730	2,276	2,730	2,536
21,250	21,300	2,738	2,284	2,738	2,544
21,300	21,350	2,745	2,291	2,745	2,551
21,350	21,400	2,753	2,299	2,753	2,559
21,400	21,450	2,760	2,306	2,760	2,566
21,450	21,500	2,768	2,314	2,768	2,574
21,500	21,550	2,775	2,321	2,775	2,581
21,550	21,600	2,783	2,329	2,783	2,589
21,600	21,650	2,790	2,336	2,790	2,596
21,650	21,700	2,798	2,344	2,798	2,604
21,700	21,750	2,805	2,351	2,805	2,611
21,750	21,800	2,813	2,359	2,813	2,619
21,800	21,850	2,820	2,366	2,820	2,626
21,850	21,900	2,828	2,374	2,828	2,634
21,900	21,950	2,835	2,381	2,835	2,641
21,950	22,000	2,843	2,389	2,843	2,649
22,000					
22,000	22,050	2,850	2,396	2,850	2,656
22,050	22,100	2,858	2,404	2,858	2,664
22,100	22,150	2,865	2,411	2,865	2,671
22,150	22,200	2,873	2,419	2,873	2,679
22,200	22,250	2,880	2,426	2,880	2,686
22,250	22,300	2,888	2,434	2,888	2,694
22,300	22,350	2,895	2,441	2,895	2,701
22,350	22,400	2,903	2,449	2,903	2,709
22,400	22,450	2,910	2,456	2,910	2,716
22,450	22,500	2,918	2,464	2,918	2,724
22,500	22,550	2,925	2,471	2,925	2,731
22,550	22,600	2,933	2,479	2,933	2,739
22,600	22,650	2,940	2,486	2,940	2,746
22,650	22,700	2,948	2,494	2,948	2,754
22,700	22,750	2,955	2,501	2,955	2,761
22,750	22,800	2,963	2,509	2,963	2,769
22,800	22,850	2,970	2,516	2,970	2,776
22,850	22,900	2,978	2,524	2,978	2,784
22,900	22,950	2,985	2,531	2,985	2,791
22,950	23,000	2,993	2,539	2,993	2,799
23,000					
23,000	23,050	3,000	2,546	3,000	2,806
23,050	23,100	3,008	2,554	3,008	2,814
23,100	23,150	3,015	2,561	3,015	2,821
23,150	23,200	3,023	2,569	3,023	2,829
23,200	23,250	3,030	2,576	3,030	2,836
23,250	23,300	3,038	2,584	3,038	2,844
23,300	23,350	3,045	2,591	3,045	2,851
23,350	23,400	3,053	2,599	3,053	2,859
23,400	23,450	3,060	2,606	3,060	2,866
23,450	23,500	3,068	2,614	3,068	2,874
23,500	23,550	3,075	2,621	3,075	2,881
23,550	23,600	3,083	2,629	3,083	2,889
23,600	23,650	3,090	2,636	3,090	2,896
23,650	23,700	3,098	2,644	3,098	2,904
23,700	23,750	3,105	2,651	3,105	2,911
23,750	23,800	3,113	2,659	3,113	2,919
23,800	23,850	3,120	2,666	3,120	2,926
23,850	23,900	3,128	2,674	3,128	2,934
23,900	23,950	3,135	2,681	3,135	2,941
23,950	24,000	3,143	2,689	3,143	2,949

24,000 / 25,000 / 26,000

If line 43 (taxable income) is—		And you are—			
At least	But less than	Single	Married filing jointly *	Married filing separately	Head of a household
		Your tax is—			
24,000					
24,000	24,050	3,150	2,696	3,150	2,956
24,050	24,100	3,158	2,704	3,158	2,964
24,100	24,150	3,165	2,711	3,165	2,971
24,150	24,200	3,173	2,719	3,173	2,979
24,200	24,250	3,180	2,726	3,180	2,986
24,250	24,300	3,188	2,734	3,188	2,994
24,300	24,350	3,195	2,741	3,195	3,001
24,350	24,400	3,203	2,749	3,203	3,009
24,400	24,450	3,210	2,756	3,210	3,016
24,450	24,500	3,218	2,764	3,218	3,024
24,500	24,550	3,225	2,771	3,225	3,031
24,550	24,600	3,233	2,779	3,233	3,039
24,600	24,650	3,240	2,786	3,240	3,046
24,650	24,700	3,248	2,794	3,248	3,054
24,700	24,750	3,255	2,801	3,255	3,061
24,750	24,800	3,263	2,809	3,263	3,069
24,800	24,850	3,270	2,816	3,270	3,076
24,850	24,900	3,278	2,824	3,278	3,084
24,900	24,950	3,285	2,831	3,285	3,091
24,950	25,000	3,293	2,839	3,293	3,099
25,000					
25,000	25,050	3,300	2,846	3,300	3,106
25,050	25,100	3,308	2,854	3,308	3,114
25,100	25,150	3,315	2,861	3,315	3,121
25,150	25,200	3,323	2,869	3,323	3,129
25,200	25,250	3,330	2,876	3,330	3,136
25,250	25,300	3,338	2,884	3,338	3,144
25,300	25,350	3,345	2,891	3,345	3,151
25,350	25,400	3,353	2,899	3,353	3,159
25,400	25,450	3,360	2,906	3,360	3,166
25,450	25,500	3,368	2,914	3,368	3,174
25,500	25,550	3,375	2,921	3,375	3,181
25,550	25,600	3,383	2,929	3,383	3,189
25,600	25,650	3,390	2,936	3,390	3,196
25,650	25,700	3,398	2,944	3,398	3,204
25,700	25,750	3,405	2,951	3,405	3,211
25,750	25,800	3,413	2,959	3,413	3,219
25,800	25,850	3,420	2,966	3,420	3,226
25,850	25,900	3,428	2,974	3,428	3,234
25,900	25,950	3,435	2,981	3,435	3,241
25,950	26,000	3,443	2,989	3,443	3,249
26,000					
26,000	26,050	3,450	2,996	3,450	3,256
26,050	26,100	3,458	3,004	3,458	3,264
26,100	26,150	3,465	3,011	3,465	3,271
26,150	26,200	3,473	3,019	3,473	3,279
26,200	26,250	3,480	3,026	3,480	3,286
26,250	26,300	3,488	3,034	3,488	3,294
26,300	26,350	3,495	3,041	3,495	3,301
26,350	26,400	3,503	3,049	3,503	3,309
26,400	26,450	3,510	3,056	3,510	3,316
26,450	26,500	3,518	3,064	3,518	3,324
26,500	26,550	3,525	3,071	3,525	3,331
26,550	26,600	3,533	3,079	3,533	3,339
26,600	26,650	3,540	3,086	3,540	3,346
26,650	26,700	3,548	3,094	3,548	3,354
26,700	26,750	3,555	3,101	3,555	3,361
26,750	26,800	3,563	3,109	3,563	3,369
26,800	26,850	3,570	3,116	3,570	3,376
26,850	26,900	3,578	3,124	3,578	3,384
26,900	26,950	3,585	3,131	3,585	3,391
26,950	27,000	3,593	3,139	3,593	3,399

27,000 / 28,000 / 29,000

If line 43 (taxable income) is—		And you are—			
At least	But less than	Single	Married filing jointly *	Married filing separately	Head of a household
		Your tax is—			
27,000					
27,000	27,050	3,600	3,146	3,600	3,406
27,050	27,100	3,608	3,154	3,608	3,414
27,100	27,150	3,615	3,161	3,615	3,421
27,150	27,200	3,623	3,169	3,623	3,429
27,200	27,250	3,630	3,176	3,630	3,436
27,250	27,300	3,638	3,184	3,638	3,444
27,300	27,350	3,645	3,191	3,645	3,451
27,350	27,400	3,653	3,199	3,653	3,459
27,400	27,450	3,660	3,206	3,660	3,466
27,450	27,500	3,668	3,214	3,668	3,474
27,500	27,550	3,675	3,221	3,675	3,481
27,550	27,600	3,683	3,229	3,683	3,489
27,600	27,650	3,690	3,236	3,690	3,496
27,650	27,700	3,698	3,244	3,698	3,504
27,700	27,750	3,705	3,251	3,705	3,511
27,750	27,800	3,713	3,259	3,713	3,519
27,800	27,850	3,720	3,266	3,720	3,528
27,850	27,900	3,728	3,274	3,728	3,534
27,900	27,950	3,735	3,281	3,735	3,541
27,950	28,000	3,743	3,289	3,743	3,549
28,000					
28,000	28,050	3,750	3,296	3,750	3,558
28,050	28,100	3,758	3,304	3,758	3,564
28,100	28,150	3,765	3,311	3,765	3,571
28,150	28,200	3,773	3,319	3,773	3,579
28,200	28,250	3,780	3,326	3,780	3,586
28,250	28,300	3,788	3,334	3,788	3,594
28,300	28,350	3,795	3,341	3,795	3,601
28,350	28,400	3,803	3,349	3,803	3,609
28,400	28,450	3,810	3,356	3,810	3,616
28,450	28,500	3,818	3,364	3,818	3,624
28,500	28,550	3,825	3,371	3,825	3,631
28,550	28,600	3,833	3,379	3,833	3,639
28,600	28,650	3,840	3,386	3,840	3,646
28,650	28,700	3,848	3,394	3,848	3,654
28,700	28,750	3,855	3,401	3,855	3,661
28,750	28,800	3,863	3,409	3,863	3,669
28,800	28,850	3,870	3,416	3,870	3,676
28,850	28,900	3,878	3,424	3,878	3,684
28,900	28,950	3,885	3,431	3,885	3,691
28,950	29,000	3,893	3,439	3,893	3,699
29,000					
29,000	29,050	3,900	3,446	3,900	3,706
29,050	29,100	3,908	3,454	3,908	3,714
29,100	29,150	3,915	3,461	3,915	3,721
29,150	29,200	3,923	3,469	3,923	3,729
29,200	29,250	3,930	3,476	3,930	3,736
29,250	29,300	3,938	3,484	3,938	3,744
29,300	29,350	3,945	3,491	3,945	3,751
29,350	29,400	3,953	3,499	3,953	3,759
29,400	29,450	3,960	3,506	3,960	3,766
29,450	29,500	3,968	3,514	3,968	3,774
29,500	29,550	3,975	3,521	3,975	3,781
29,550	29,600	3,983	3,529	3,983	3,789
29,600	29,650	3,990	3,536	3,990	3,796
29,650	29,700	3,998	3,544	3,998	3,804
29,700	29,750	4,005	3,551	4,005	3,811
29,750	29,800	4,013	3,559	4,013	3,819
29,800	29,850	4,020	3,566	4,020	3,826
29,850	29,900	4,028	3,574	4,028	3,834
29,900	29,950	4,035	3,581	4,035	3,841
29,950	30,000	4,043	3,589	4,043	3,849

(Continued)

* This column must also be used by a qualifying widow(er).

Need more information or forms? Visit IRS.gov.

⋙→ *Caution: This is a draft 2014 Tax Table. At the time of publication, the IRS had not yet released the 2014 Tax Table. For the latest information, see CCHGroup.com/TaxUpdates.*

TAX RATES

30,000

At least	But less than	Single	Married filing jointly *	Married filing separately	Head of a household
30,000	30,050	4,050	3,596	4,050	3,856
30,050	30,100	4,058	3,604	4,058	3,864
30,100	30,150	4,065	3,611	4,065	3,871
30,150	30,200	4,073	3,619	4,073	3,879
30,200	30,250	4,080	3,626	4,080	3,886
30,250	30,300	4,088	3,634	4,088	3,894
30,300	30,350	4,095	3,641	4,095	3,901
30,350	30,400	4,103	3,649	4,103	3,909
30,400	30,450	4,110	3,656	4,110	3,916
30,450	30,500	4,118	3,664	4,118	3,924
30,500	30,550	4,125	3,671	4,125	3,931
30,550	30,600	4,133	3,679	4,133	3,939
30,600	30,650	4,140	3,686	4,140	3,946
30,650	30,700	4,148	3,694	4,148	3,954
30,700	30,750	4,155	3,701	4,155	3,961
30,750	30,800	4,163	3,709	4,163	3,969
30,800	30,850	4,170	3,716	4,170	3,976
30,850	30,900	4,178	3,724	4,178	3,984
30,900	30,950	4,185	3,731	4,185	3,991
30,950	31,000	4,193	3,739	4,193	3,999

31,000

At least	But less than	Single	Married filing jointly *	Married filing separately	Head of a household
31,000	31,050	4,200	3,746	4,200	4,006
31,050	31,100	4,208	3,754	4,208	4,014
31,100	31,150	4,215	3,761	4,215	4,021
31,150	31,200	4,223	3,769	4,223	4,029
31,200	31,250	4,230	3,776	4,230	4,036
31,250	31,300	4,238	3,784	4,238	4,044
31,300	31,350	4,245	3,791	4,245	4,051
31,350	31,400	4,253	3,799	4,253	4,059
31,400	31,450	4,260	3,806	4,260	4,066
31,450	31,500	4,268	3,814	4,268	4,074
31,500	31,550	4,275	3,821	4,275	4,081
31,550	31,600	4,283	3,829	4,283	4,089
31,600	31,650	4,290	3,836	4,290	4,096
31,650	31,700	4,298	3,844	4,298	4,104
31,700	31,750	4,305	3,851	4,305	4,111
31,750	31,800	4,313	3,859	4,313	4,119
31,800	31,850	4,320	3,866	4,320	4,126
31,850	31,900	4,328	3,874	4,328	4,134
31,900	31,950	4,335	3,881	4,335	4,141
31,950	32,000	4,343	3,889	4,343	4,149

32,000

At least	But less than	Single	Married filing jointly *	Married filing separately	Head of a household
32,000	32,050	4,350	3,896	4,350	4,156
32,050	32,100	4,358	3,904	4,358	4,164
32,100	32,150	4,365	3,911	4,365	4,171
32,150	32,200	4,373	3,919	4,373	4,179
32,200	32,250	4,380	3,926	4,380	4,186
32,250	32,300	4,388	3,934	4,388	4,194
32,300	32,350	4,395	3,941	4,395	4,201
32,350	32,400	4,403	3,949	4,403	4,209
32,400	32,450	4,410	3,956	4,410	4,216
32,450	32,500	4,418	3,964	4,418	4,224
32,500	32,550	4,425	3,971	4,425	4,231
32,550	32,600	4,433	3,979	4,433	4,239
32,600	32,650	4,440	3,986	4,440	4,246
32,650	32,700	4,448	3,994	4,448	4,254
32,700	32,750	4,455	4,001	4,455	4,261
32,750	32,800	4,463	4,009	4,463	4,269
32,800	32,850	4,470	4,016	4,470	4,276
32,850	32,900	4,478	4,024	4,478	4,284
32,900	32,950	4,485	4,031	4,485	4,291
32,950	33,000	4,493	4,039	4,493	4,299

33,000

At least	But less than	Single	Married filing jointly *	Married filing separately	Head of a household
33,000	33,050	4,500	4,046	4,500	4,306
33,050	33,100	4,508	4,054	4,508	4,314
33,100	33,150	4,515	4,061	4,515	4,321
33,150	33,200	4,523	4,069	4,523	4,329
33,200	33,250	4,530	4,076	4,530	4,336
33,250	33,300	4,538	4,084	4,538	4,344
33,300	33,350	4,545	4,091	4,545	4,351
33,350	33,400	4,553	4,099	4,553	4,359
33,400	33,450	4,560	4,106	4,560	4,366
33,450	33,500	4,568	4,114	4,568	4,374
33,500	33,550	4,575	4,121	4,575	4,381
33,550	33,600	4,583	4,129	4,583	4,389
33,600	33,650	4,590	4,136	4,590	4,396
33,650	33,700	4,598	4,144	4,598	4,404
33,700	33,750	4,605	4,151	4,605	4,411
33,750	33,800	4,613	4,159	4,613	4,419
33,800	33,850	4,620	4,166	4,620	4,426
33,850	33,900	4,628	4,174	4,628	4,434
33,900	33,950	4,635	4,181	4,635	4,441
33,950	34,000	4,643	4,189	4,643	4,449

34,000

At least	But less than	Single	Married filing jointly *	Married filing separately	Head of a household
34,000	34,050	4,650	4,196	4,650	4,456
34,050	34,100	4,658	4,204	4,658	4,464
34,100	34,150	4,665	4,211	4,665	4,471
34,150	34,200	4,673	4,219	4,673	4,479
34,200	34,250	4,680	4,226	4,680	4,486
34,250	34,300	4,688	4,234	4,688	4,494
34,300	34,350	4,695	4,241	4,695	4,501
34,350	34,400	4,703	4,249	4,703	4,509
34,400	34,450	4,710	4,256	4,710	4,516
34,450	34,500	4,718	4,264	4,718	4,524
34,500	34,550	4,725	4,271	4,725	4,531
34,550	34,600	4,733	4,279	4,733	4,539
34,600	34,650	4,740	4,286	4,740	4,546
34,650	34,700	4,748	4,294	4,748	4,554
34,700	34,750	4,755	4,301	4,755	4,561
34,750	34,800	4,763	4,309	4,763	4,569
34,800	34,850	4,770	4,316	4,770	4,576
34,850	34,900	4,778	4,324	4,778	4,584
34,900	34,950	4,785	4,331	4,785	4,591
34,950	35,000	4,793	4,339	4,793	4,599

35,000

At least	But less than	Single	Married filing jointly *	Married filing separately	Head of a household
35,000	35,050	4,800	4,346	4,800	4,606
35,050	35,100	4,808	4,354	4,808	4,614
35,100	35,150	4,815	4,361	4,815	4,621
35,150	35,200	4,823	4,369	4,823	4,629
35,200	35,250	4,830	4,376	4,830	4,636
35,250	35,300	4,838	4,384	4,838	4,644
35,300	35,350	4,845	4,391	4,845	4,651
35,350	35,400	4,853	4,399	4,853	4,659
35,400	35,450	4,860	4,406	4,860	4,666
35,450	35,500	4,868	4,414	4,868	4,674
35,500	35,550	4,875	4,421	4,875	4,681
35,550	35,600	4,883	4,429	4,883	4,689
35,600	35,650	4,890	4,436	4,890	4,696
35,650	35,700	4,898	4,444	4,898	4,704
35,700	35,750	4,905	4,451	4,905	4,711
35,750	35,800	4,913	4,459	4,913	4,719
35,800	35,850	4,920	4,466	4,920	4,726
35,850	35,900	4,928	4,474	4,928	4,734
35,900	35,950	4,935	4,481	4,935	4,741
35,950	36,000	4,943	4,489	4,943	4,749

36,000

At least	But less than	Single	Married filing jointly *	Married filing separately	Head of a household
36,000	36,050	4,950	4,496	4,950	4,756
36,050	36,100	4,958	4,504	4,958	4,764
36,100	36,150	4,965	4,511	4,965	4,771
36,150	36,200	4,973	4,519	4,973	4,779
36,200	36,250	4,980	4,526	4,980	4,786
36,250	36,300	4,988	4,534	4,988	4,794
36,300	36,350	4,995	4,541	4,995	4,801
36,350	36,400	5,003	4,549	5,003	4,809
36,400	36,450	5,010	4,556	5,010	4,816
36,450	36,500	5,018	4,564	5,018	4,824
36,500	36,550	5,025	4,571	5,025	4,831
36,550	36,600	5,033	4,579	5,033	4,839
36,600	36,650	5,040	4,586	5,040	4,846
36,650	36,700	5,048	4,594	5,048	4,854
36,700	36,750	5,055	4,601	5,055	4,861
36,750	36,800	5,063	4,609	5,063	4,869
36,800	36,850	5,070	4,616	5,070	4,876
36,850	36,900	5,078	4,624	5,078	4,884
36,900	36,950	5,088	4,631	5,088	4,891
36,950	37,000	5,100	4,639	5,100	4,899

37,000

At least	But less than	Single	Married filing jointly *	Married filing separately	Head of a household
37,000	37,050	5,113	4,646	5,113	4,906
37,050	37,100	5,125	4,654	5,125	4,914
37,100	37,150	5,138	4,661	5,138	4,921
37,150	37,200	5,150	4,669	5,150	4,929
37,200	37,250	5,163	4,676	5,163	4,936
37,250	37,300	5,175	4,684	5,175	4,944
37,300	37,350	5,188	4,691	5,188	4,951
37,350	37,400	5,200	4,699	5,200	4,959
37,400	37,450	5,213	4,706	5,213	4,966
37,450	37,500	5,225	4,714	5,225	4,974
37,500	37,550	5,238	4,721	5,238	4,981
37,550	37,600	5,250	4,729	5,250	4,989
37,600	37,650	5,263	4,736	5,263	4,996
37,650	37,700	5,275	4,744	5,275	5,004
37,700	37,750	5,288	4,751	5,288	5,011
37,750	37,800	5,300	4,759	5,300	5,019
37,800	37,850	5,313	4,766	5,313	5,026
37,850	37,900	5,325	4,774	5,325	5,034
37,900	37,950	5,338	4,781	5,338	5,041
37,950	38,000	5,350	4,789	5,350	5,049

38,000

At least	But less than	Single	Married filing jointly *	Married filing separately	Head of a household
38,000	38,050	5,363	4,796	5,363	5,056
38,050	38,100	5,375	4,804	5,375	5,064
38,100	38,150	5,388	4,811	5,388	5,071
38,150	38,200	5,400	4,819	5,400	5,079
38,200	38,250	5,413	4,826	5,413	5,086
38,250	38,300	5,425	4,834	5,425	5,094
38,300	38,350	5,438	4,841	5,438	5,101
38,350	38,400	5,450	4,849	5,450	5,109
38,400	38,450	5,463	4,856	5,463	5,116
38,450	38,500	5,475	4,864	5,475	5,124
38,500	38,550	5,488	4,871	5,488	5,131
38,550	38,600	5,500	4,879	5,500	5,139
38,600	38,650	5,513	4,886	5,513	5,146
38,650	38,700	5,525	4,894	5,525	5,154
38,700	38,750	5,538	4,901	5,538	5,161
38,750	38,800	5,550	4,909	5,550	5,169
38,800	38,850	5,563	4,916	5,563	5,176
38,850	38,900	5,575	4,924	5,575	5,184
38,900	38,950	5,588	4,931	5,588	5,191
38,950	39,000	5,600	4,939	5,600	5,199

* This column must also be used by a qualifying widow(er).

(Continued)

Need more information or forms? Visit IRS.gov.

¶25

>>>→ *Caution: This is a draft 2014 Tax Table. At the time of publication, the IRS had not yet released the 2014 Tax Table. For the latest information, see CCHGroup.com/TaxUpdates.*

If line 43 (taxable income) is—		And you are—			
At least	But less than	Single	Married filing jointly *	Married filing separately	Head of a household
		Your tax is—			

39,000

At least	But less than	Single	MFJ*	MFS	HoH
39,000	39,050	5,613	4,946	5,613	5,206
39,050	39,100	5,625	4,954	5,625	5,214
39,100	39,150	5,638	4,961	5,638	5,221
39,150	39,200	5,650	4,969	5,650	5,229
39,200	39,250	5,663	4,976	5,663	5,236
39,250	39,300	5,675	4,984	5,675	5,244
39,300	39,350	5,688	4,991	5,688	5,251
39,350	39,400	5,700	4,999	5,700	5,259
39,400	39,450	5,713	5,006	5,713	5,266
39,450	39,500	5,725	5,014	5,725	5,274
39,500	39,550	5,738	5,021	5,738	5,281
39,550	39,600	5,750	5,029	5,750	5,289
39,600	39,650	5,763	5,036	5,763	5,296
39,650	39,700	5,775	5,044	5,775	5,304
39,700	39,750	5,788	5,051	5,788	5,311
39,750	39,800	5,800	5,059	5,800	5,319
39,800	39,850	5,813	5,066	5,813	5,326
39,850	39,900	5,825	5,074	5,825	5,334
39,900	39,950	5,838	5,081	5,838	5,341
39,950	40,000	5,850	5,089	5,850	5,349

40,000

At least	But less than	Single	MFJ*	MFS	HoH
40,000	40,050	5,863	5,096	5,863	5,356
40,050	40,100	5,875	5,104	5,875	5,364
40,100	40,150	5,888	5,111	5,888	5,371
40,150	40,200	5,900	5,119	5,900	5,379
40,200	40,250	5,913	5,126	5,913	5,386
40,250	40,300	5,925	5,134	5,925	5,394
40,300	40,350	5,938	5,141	5,938	5,401
40,350	40,400	5,950	5,149	5,950	5,409
40,400	40,450	5,963	5,156	5,963	5,416
40,450	40,500	5,975	5,164	5,975	5,424
40,500	40,550	5,988	5,171	5,988	5,431
40,550	40,600	6,000	5,179	6,000	5,439
40,600	40,650	6,013	5,186	6,013	5,446
40,650	40,700	6,025	5,194	6,025	5,454
40,700	40,750	6,038	5,201	6,038	5,461
40,750	40,800	6,050	5,209	6,050	5,469
40,800	40,850	6,063	5,216	6,063	5,476
40,850	40,900	6,075	5,224	6,075	5,484
40,900	40,950	6,088	5,231	6,088	5,491
40,950	41,000	6,100	5,239	6,100	5,499

41,000

At least	But less than	Single	MFJ*	MFS	HoH
41,000	41,050	6,113	5,246	6,113	5,506
41,050	41,100	6,125	5,254	6,125	5,514
41,100	41,150	6,138	5,261	6,138	5,521
41,150	41,200	6,150	5,269	6,150	5,529
41,200	41,250	6,163	5,276	6,163	5,536
41,250	41,300	6,175	5,284	6,175	5,544
41,300	41,350	6,188	5,291	6,188	5,551
41,350	41,400	6,200	5,299	6,200	5,559
41,400	41,450	6,213	5,306	6,213	5,566
41,450	41,500	6,225	5,314	6,225	5,574
41,500	41,550	6,238	5,321	6,238	5,581
41,550	41,600	6,250	5,329	6,250	5,589
41,600	41,650	6,263	5,336	6,263	5,596
41,650	41,700	6,275	5,344	6,275	5,604
41,700	41,750	6,288	5,351	6,288	5,611
41,750	41,800	6,300	5,359	6,300	5,619
41,800	41,850	6,313	5,366	6,313	5,626
41,850	41,900	6,325	5,374	6,325	5,634
41,900	41,950	6,338	5,381	6,338	5,641
41,950	42,000	6,350	5,389	6,350	5,649

42,000

At least	But less than	Single	MFJ*	MFS	HoH
42,000	42,050	6,363	5,396	6,363	5,656
42,050	42,100	6,375	5,404	6,375	5,664
42,100	42,150	6,388	5,411	6,388	5,671
42,150	42,200	6,400	5,419	6,400	5,679
42,200	42,250	6,413	5,426	6,413	5,686
42,250	42,300	6,425	5,434	6,425	5,694
42,300	42,350	6,438	5,441	6,438	5,701
42,350	42,400	6,450	5,449	6,450	5,709
42,400	42,450	6,463	5,456	6,463	5,716
42,450	42,500	6,475	5,464	6,475	5,724
42,500	42,550	6,488	5,471	6,488	5,731
42,550	42,600	6,500	5,479	6,500	5,739
42,600	42,650	6,513	5,486	6,513	5,746
42,650	42,700	6,525	5,494	6,525	5,754
42,700	42,750	6,538	5,501	6,538	5,761
42,750	42,800	6,550	5,509	6,550	5,769
42,800	42,850	6,563	5,516	6,563	5,776
42,850	42,900	6,575	5,524	6,575	5,784
42,900	42,950	6,588	5,531	6,588	5,791
42,950	43,000	6,600	5,539	6,600	5,799

43,000

At least	But less than	Single	MFJ*	MFS	HoH
43,000	43,050	6,613	5,546	6,613	5,806
43,050	43,100	6,625	5,554	6,625	5,814
43,100	43,150	6,638	5,561	6,638	5,821
43,150	43,200	6,650	5,569	6,650	5,829
43,200	43,250	6,663	5,576	6,663	5,836
43,250	43,300	6,675	5,584	6,675	5,844
43,300	43,350	6,688	5,591	6,688	5,851
43,350	43,400	6,700	5,599	6,700	5,859
43,400	43,450	6,713	5,606	6,713	5,866
43,450	43,500	6,725	5,614	6,725	5,874
43,500	43,550	6,738	5,621	6,738	5,881
43,550	43,600	6,750	5,629	6,750	5,889
43,600	43,650	6,763	5,636	6,763	5,896
43,650	43,700	6,775	5,644	6,775	5,904
43,700	43,750	6,788	5,651	6,788	5,911
43,750	43,800	6,800	5,659	6,800	5,919
43,800	43,850	6,813	5,666	6,813	5,926
43,850	43,900	6,825	5,674	6,825	5,934
43,900	43,950	6,838	5,681	6,838	5,941
43,950	44,000	6,850	5,689	6,850	5,949

44,000

At least	But less than	Single	MFJ*	MFS	HoH
44,000	44,050	6,863	5,696	6,863	5,956
44,050	44,100	6,875	5,704	6,875	5,964
44,100	44,150	6,888	5,711	6,888	5,971
44,150	44,200	6,900	5,719	6,900	5,979
44,200	44,250	6,913	5,726	6,913	5,986
44,250	44,300	6,925	5,734	6,925	5,994
44,300	44,350	6,938	5,741	6,938	6,001
44,350	44,400	6,950	5,749	6,950	6,009
44,400	44,450	6,963	5,756	6,963	6,016
44,450	44,500	6,975	5,764	6,975	6,024
44,500	44,550	6,988	5,771	6,988	6,031
44,550	44,600	7,000	5,779	7,000	6,039
44,600	44,650	7,013	5,786	7,013	6,046
44,650	44,700	7,025	5,794	7,025	6,054
44,700	44,750	7,038	5,801	7,038	6,061
44,750	44,800	7,050	5,809	7,050	6,069
44,800	44,850	7,063	5,816	7,063	6,076
44,850	44,900	7,075	5,824	7,075	6,084
44,900	44,950	7,088	5,831	7,088	6,091
44,950	45,000	7,100	5,839	7,100	6,099

45,000

At least	But less than	Single	MFJ*	MFS	HoH
45,000	45,050	7,113	5,846	7,113	6,106
45,050	45,100	7,125	5,854	7,125	6,114
45,100	45,150	7,138	5,861	7,138	6,121
45,150	45,200	7,150	5,869	7,150	6,129
45,200	45,250	7,163	5,876	7,163	6,136
45,250	45,300	7,175	5,884	7,175	6,144
45,300	45,350	7,188	5,891	7,188	6,151
45,350	45,400	7,200	5,899	7,200	6,159
45,400	45,450	7,213	5,906	7,213	6,166
45,450	45,500	7,225	5,914	7,225	6,174
45,500	45,550	7,238	5,921	7,238	6,181
45,550	45,600	7,250	5,929	7,250	6,189
45,600	45,650	7,263	5,936	7,263	6,196
45,650	45,700	7,275	5,944	7,275	6,204
45,700	45,750	7,288	5,951	7,288	6,211
45,750	45,800	7,300	5,959	7,300	6,219
45,800	45,850	7,313	5,966	7,313	6,226
45,850	45,900	7,325	5,974	7,325	6,234
45,900	45,950	7,338	5,981	7,338	6,241
45,950	46,000	7,350	5,989	7,350	6,249

46,000

At least	But less than	Single	MFJ*	MFS	HoH
46,000	46,050	7,363	5,996	7,363	6,256
46,050	46,100	7,375	6,004	7,375	6,264
46,100	46,150	7,388	6,011	7,388	6,271
46,150	46,200	7,400	6,019	7,400	6,279
46,200	46,250	7,413	6,026	7,413	6,286
46,250	46,300	7,425	6,034	7,425	6,294
46,300	46,350	7,438	6,041	7,438	6,301
46,350	46,400	7,450	6,049	7,450	6,309
46,400	46,450	7,463	6,056	7,463	6,316
46,450	46,500	7,475	6,064	7,475	6,324
46,500	46,550	7,488	6,071	7,488	6,331
46,550	46,600	7,500	6,079	7,500	6,339
46,600	46,650	7,513	6,086	7,513	6,346
46,650	46,700	7,525	6,094	7,525	6,354
46,700	46,750	7,538	6,101	7,538	6,361
46,750	46,800	7,550	6,109	7,550	6,369
46,800	46,850	7,563	6,116	7,563	6,376
46,850	46,900	7,575	6,124	7,575	6,384
46,900	46,950	7,588	6,131	7,588	6,391
46,950	47,000	7,600	6,139	7,600	6,399

47,000

At least	But less than	Single	MFJ*	MFS	HoH
47,000	47,050	7,613	6,146	7,613	6,406
47,050	47,100	7,625	6,154	7,625	6,414
47,100	47,150	7,638	6,161	7,638	6,421
47,150	47,200	7,650	6,169	7,650	6,429
47,200	47,250	7,663	6,176	7,663	6,436
47,250	47,300	7,675	6,184	7,675	6,444
47,300	47,350	7,688	6,191	7,688	6,451
47,350	47,400	7,700	6,199	7,700	6,459
47,400	47,450	7,713	6,206	7,713	6,466
47,450	47,500	7,725	6,214	7,725	6,474
47,500	47,550	7,738	6,221	7,738	6,481
47,550	47,600	7,750	6,229	7,750	6,489
47,600	47,650	7,763	6,236	7,763	6,496
47,650	47,700	7,775	6,244	7,775	6,504
47,700	47,750	7,788	6,251	7,788	6,511
47,750	47,800	7,800	6,259	7,800	6,519
47,800	47,850	7,813	6,266	7,813	6,526
47,850	47,900	7,825	6,274	7,825	6,534
47,900	47,950	7,838	6,281	7,838	6,541
47,950	48,000	7,850	6,289	7,850	6,549

(Continued)

* This column must also be used by a qualifying widow(er).

Need more information or forms? Visit IRS.gov.

¶25

»»→ **Caution: This is a draft 2014 Tax Table. At the time of publication, the IRS had not yet released the 2014 Tax Table. For the latest information, see CCHGroup.com/TaxUpdates.**

48,000 – 50,000

If line 43 (taxable income) is— At least	But less than	Single	Married filing jointly*	Married filing separately	Head of a household
			Your tax is—		
48,000					
48,000	48,050	7,863	6,296	7,863	6,556
48,050	48,100	7,875	6,304	7,875	6,564
48,100	48,150	7,888	6,311	7,888	6,571
48,150	48,200	7,900	6,319	7,900	6,579
48,200	48,250	7,913	6,326	7,913	6,586
48,250	48,300	7,925	6,334	7,925	6,594
48,300	48,350	7,938	6,341	7,938	6,601
48,350	48,400	7,950	6,349	7,950	6,609
48,400	48,450	7,963	6,356	7,963	6,616
48,450	48,500	7,975	6,364	7,975	6,624
48,500	48,550	7,988	6,371	7,988	6,631
48,550	48,600	8,000	6,379	8,000	6,639
48,600	48,650	8,013	6,386	8,013	6,646
48,650	48,700	8,025	6,394	8,025	6,654
48,700	48,750	8,038	6,401	8,038	6,661
48,750	48,800	8,050	6,409	8,050	6,669
48,800	48,850	8,063	6,416	8,063	6,676
48,850	48,900	8,075	6,424	8,075	6,684
48,900	48,950	8,088	6,431	8,088	6,691
48,950	49,000	8,100	6,439	8,100	6,699
49,000					
49,000	49,050	8,113	6,446	8,113	6,706
49,050	49,100	8,125	6,454	8,125	6,714
49,100	49,150	8,138	6,461	8,138	6,721
49,150	49,200	8,150	6,469	8,150	6,729
49,200	49,250	8,163	6,476	8,163	6,736
49,250	49,300	8,175	6,484	8,175	6,744
49,300	49,350	8,188	6,491	8,188	6,751
49,350	49,400	8,200	6,499	8,200	6,759
49,400	49,450	8,213	6,506	8,213	6,769
49,450	49,500	8,225	6,514	8,225	6,781
49,500	49,550	8,238	6,521	8,238	6,794
49,550	49,600	8,250	6,529	8,250	6,806
49,600	49,650	8,263	6,536	8,263	6,819
49,650	49,700	8,275	6,544	8,275	6,831
49,700	49,750	8,288	6,551	8,288	6,844
49,750	49,800	8,300	6,559	8,300	6,856
49,800	49,850	8,313	6,566	8,313	6,869
49,850	49,900	8,325	6,574	8,325	6,881
49,900	49,950	8,338	6,581	8,338	6,894
49,950	50,000	8,350	6,589	8,350	6,906
50,000					
50,000	50,050	8,363	6,596	8,363	6,919
50,050	50,100	8,375	6,604	8,375	6,931
50,100	50,150	8,388	6,611	8,388	6,944
50,150	50,200	8,400	6,619	8,400	6,956
50,200	50,250	8,413	6,626	8,413	6,969
50,250	50,300	8,425	6,634	8,425	6,981
50,300	50,350	8,438	6,641	8,438	6,994
50,350	50,400	8,450	6,649	8,450	7,006
50,400	50,450	8,463	6,656	8,463	7,019
50,450	50,500	8,475	6,664	8,475	7,031
50,500	50,550	8,488	6,671	8,488	7,044
50,550	50,600	8,500	6,679	8,500	7,056
50,600	50,650	8,513	6,686	8,513	7,069
50,650	50,700	8,525	6,694	8,525	7,081
50,700	50,750	8,538	6,701	8,538	7,094
50,750	50,800	8,550	6,709	8,550	7,106
50,800	50,850	8,563	6,716	8,563	7,119
50,850	50,900	8,575	6,724	8,575	7,131
50,900	50,950	8,588	6,731	8,588	7,144
50,950	51,000	8,600	6,739	8,600	7,156

51,000 – 53,000

If line 43 (taxable income) is— At least	But less than	Single	Married filing jointly*	Married filing separately	Head of a household
			Your tax is—		
51,000					
51,000	51,050	8,613	6,746	8,613	7,169
51,050	51,100	8,625	6,754	8,625	7,181
51,100	51,150	8,638	6,761	8,638	7,194
51,150	51,200	8,650	6,769	8,650	7,206
51,200	51,250	8,663	6,776	8,663	7,219
51,250	51,300	8,675	6,784	8,675	7,231
51,300	51,350	8,688	6,791	8,688	7,244
51,350	51,400	8,700	6,799	8,700	7,256
51,400	51,450	8,713	6,806	8,713	7,269
51,450	51,500	8,725	6,814	8,725	7,281
51,500	51,550	8,738	6,821	8,738	7,294
51,550	51,600	8,750	6,829	8,750	7,306
51,600	51,650	8,763	6,836	8,763	7,319
51,650	51,700	8,775	6,844	8,775	7,331
51,700	51,750	8,788	6,851	8,788	7,344
51,750	51,800	8,800	6,859	8,800	7,356
51,800	51,850	8,813	6,866	8,813	7,369
51,850	51,900	8,825	6,874	8,825	7,381
51,900	51,950	8,838	6,881	8,838	7,394
51,950	52,000	8,850	6,889	8,850	7,406
52,000					
52,000	52,050	8,863	6,896	8,863	7,419
52,050	52,100	8,875	6,904	8,875	7,431
52,100	52,150	8,888	6,911	8,888	7,444
52,150	52,200	8,900	6,919	8,900	7,456
52,200	52,250	8,913	6,926	8,913	7,469
52,250	52,300	8,925	6,934	8,925	7,481
52,300	52,350	8,938	6,941	8,938	7,494
52,350	52,400	8,950	6,949	8,950	7,506
52,400	52,450	8,963	6,956	8,963	7,519
52,450	52,500	8,975	6,964	8,975	7,531
52,500	52,550	8,988	6,971	8,988	7,544
52,550	52,600	9,000	6,979	9,000	7,556
52,600	52,650	9,013	6,986	9,013	7,569
52,650	52,700	9,025	6,994	9,025	7,581
52,700	52,750	9,038	7,001	9,038	7,594
52,750	52,800	9,050	7,009	9,050	7,606
52,800	52,850	9,063	7,016	9,063	7,619
52,850	52,900	9,075	7,024	9,075	7,631
52,900	52,950	9,088	7,031	9,088	7,644
52,950	53,000	9,100	7,039	9,100	7,656
53,000					
53,000	53,050	9,113	7,046	9,113	7,669
53,050	53,100	9,125	7,054	9,125	7,681
53,100	53,150	9,138	7,061	9,138	7,694
53,150	53,200	9,150	7,069	9,150	7,706
53,200	53,250	9,163	7,076	9,163	7,719
53,250	53,300	9,175	7,084	9,175	7,731
53,300	53,350	9,188	7,091	9,188	7,744
53,350	53,400	9,200	7,099	9,200	7,756
53,400	53,450	9,213	7,106	9,213	7,769
53,450	53,500	9,225	7,114	9,225	7,781
53,500	53,550	9,238	7,121	9,238	7,794
53,550	53,600	9,250	7,129	9,250	7,806
53,600	53,650	9,263	7,136	9,263	7,819
53,650	53,700	9,275	7,144	9,275	7,831
53,700	53,750	9,288	7,151	9,288	7,844
53,750	53,800	9,300	7,159	9,300	7,856
53,800	53,850	9,313	7,166	9,313	7,869
53,850	53,900	9,325	7,174	9,325	7,881
53,900	53,950	9,338	7,181	9,338	7,894
53,950	54,000	9,350	7,189	9,350	7,906

54,000 – 56,000

If line 43 (taxable income) is— At least	But less than	Single	Married filing jointly*	Married filing separately	Head of a household
			Your tax is—		
54,000					
54,000	54,050	9,363	7,196	9,363	7,919
54,050	54,100	9,375	7,204	9,375	7,931
54,100	54,150	9,388	7,211	9,388	7,944
54,150	54,200	9,400	7,219	9,400	7,956
54,200	54,250	9,413	7,226	9,413	7,969
54,250	54,300	9,425	7,234	9,425	7,981
54,300	54,350	9,438	7,241	9,438	7,994
54,350	54,400	9,450	7,249	9,450	8,006
54,400	54,450	9,463	7,256	9,463	8,019
54,450	54,500	9,475	7,264	9,475	8,031
54,500	54,550	9,488	7,271	9,488	8,044
54,550	54,600	9,500	7,279	9,500	8,056
54,600	54,650	9,513	7,286	9,513	8,069
54,650	54,700	9,525	7,294	9,525	8,081
54,700	54,750	9,538	7,301	9,538	8,094
54,750	54,800	9,550	7,309	9,550	8,106
54,800	54,850	9,563	7,316	9,563	8,119
54,850	54,900	9,575	7,324	9,575	8,131
54,900	54,950	9,588	7,331	9,588	8,144
54,950	55,000	9,600	7,339	9,600	8,156
55,000					
55,000	55,050	9,613	7,346	9,613	8,169
55,050	55,100	9,625	7,354	9,625	8,181
55,100	55,150	9,638	7,361	9,638	8,194
55,150	55,200	9,650	7,369	9,650	8,206
55,200	55,250	9,663	7,376	9,663	8,219
55,250	55,300	9,675	7,384	9,675	8,231
55,300	55,350	9,688	7,391	9,688	8,244
55,350	55,400	9,700	7,399	9,700	8,256
55,400	55,450	9,713	7,406	9,713	8,269
55,450	55,500	9,725	7,414	9,725	8,281
55,500	55,550	9,738	7,421	9,738	8,294
55,550	55,600	9,750	7,429	9,750	8,306
55,600	55,650	9,763	7,436	9,763	8,319
55,650	55,700	9,775	7,444	9,775	8,331
55,700	55,750	9,788	7,451	9,788	8,344
55,750	55,800	9,800	7,459	9,800	8,356
55,800	55,850	9,813	7,466	9,813	8,369
55,850	55,900	9,825	7,474	9,825	8,381
55,900	55,950	9,838	7,481	9,838	8,394
55,950	56,000	9,850	7,489	9,850	8,406
56,000					
56,000	56,050	9,863	7,496	9,863	8,419
56,050	56,100	9,875	7,504	9,875	8,431
56,100	56,150	9,888	7,511	9,888	8,444
56,150	56,200	9,900	7,519	9,900	8,456
56,200	56,250	9,913	7,526	9,913	8,469
56,250	56,300	9,925	7,534	9,925	8,481
56,300	56,350	9,938	7,541	9,938	8,494
56,350	56,400	9,950	7,549	9,950	8,506
56,400	56,450	9,963	7,556	9,963	8,519
56,450	56,500	9,975	7,564	9,975	8,531
56,500	56,550	9,988	7,571	9,988	8,544
56,550	56,600	10,000	7,579	10,000	8,556
56,600	56,650	10,013	7,586	10,013	8,569
56,650	56,700	10,025	7,594	10,025	8,581
56,700	56,750	10,038	7,601	10,038	8,594
56,750	56,800	10,050	7,609	10,050	8,606
56,800	56,850	10,063	7,616	10,063	8,619
56,850	56,900	10,075	7,624	10,075	8,631
56,900	56,950	10,088	7,631	10,088	8,644
56,950	57,000	10,100	7,639	10,100	8,656

(Continued)

* This column must also be used by a qualifying widow(er).

Need more information or forms? Visit IRS.gov.

¶25

>>>→ *Caution: This is a draft 2014 Tax Table. At the time of publication, the IRS had not yet released the 2014 Tax Table. For the latest information, see CCHGroup.com/TaxUpdates.*

57,000

If line 43 (taxable income) is— At least	But less than	Single	Married filing jointly*	Married filing separately	Head of a household
57,000	57,050	10,113	7,646	10,113	8,869
57,050	57,100	10,125	7,654	10,125	8,681
57,100	57,150	10,138	7,661	10,138	8,694
57,150	57,200	10,150	7,669	10,150	8,706
57,200	57,250	10,163	7,676	10,163	8,719
57,250	57,300	10,175	7,684	10,175	8,731
57,300	57,350	10,188	7,691	10,188	8,744
57,350	57,400	10,200	7,699	10,200	8,756
57,400	57,450	10,213	7,706	10,213	8,769
57,450	57,500	10,225	7,714	10,225	8,781
57,500	57,550	10,238	7,721	10,238	8,794
57,550	57,600	10,250	7,729	10,250	8,806
57,600	57,650	10,263	7,736	10,263	8,819
57,650	57,700	10,275	7,744	10,275	8,831
57,700	57,750	10,288	7,751	10,288	8,844
57,750	57,800	10,300	7,759	10,300	8,856
57,800	57,850	10,313	7,766	10,313	8,869
57,850	57,900	10,325	7,774	10,325	8,881
57,900	57,950	10,338	7,781	10,338	8,894
57,950	58,000	10,350	7,789	10,350	8,906

58,000

At least	But less than	Single	Married filing jointly*	Married filing separately	Head of a household
58,000	58,050	10,363	7,796	10,363	8,919
58,050	58,100	10,375	7,804	10,375	8,931
58,100	58,150	10,388	7,811	10,388	8,944
58,150	58,200	10,400	7,819	10,400	8,956
58,200	58,250	10,413	7,826	10,413	8,969
58,250	58,300	10,425	7,834	10,425	8,981
58,300	58,350	10,438	7,841	10,438	8,994
58,350	58,400	10,450	7,849	10,450	9,006
58,400	58,450	10,463	7,856	10,463	9,019
58,450	58,500	10,475	7,864	10,475	9,031
58,500	58,550	10,488	7,871	10,488	9,044
58,550	58,600	10,500	7,879	10,500	9,056
58,600	58,650	10,513	7,886	10,513	9,069
58,650	58,700	10,525	7,894	10,525	9,081
58,700	58,750	10,538	7,901	10,538	9,094
58,750	58,800	10,550	7,909	10,550	9,106
58,800	58,850	10,563	7,916	10,563	9,119
58,850	58,900	10,575	7,924	10,575	9,131
58,900	58,950	10,588	7,931	10,588	9,144
58,950	59,000	10,600	7,939	10,600	9,156

59,000

At least	But less than	Single	Married filing jointly*	Married filing separately	Head of a household
59,000	59,050	10,613	7,946	10,613	9,169
59,050	59,100	10,625	7,954	10,625	9,181
59,100	59,150	10,638	7,961	10,638	9,194
59,150	59,200	10,650	7,969	10,650	9,206
59,200	59,250	10,663	7,976	10,663	9,219
59,250	59,300	10,675	7,984	10,675	9,231
59,300	59,350	10,688	7,991	10,688	9,244
59,350	59,400	10,700	7,999	10,700	9,256
59,400	59,450	10,713	8,006	10,713	9,269
59,450	59,500	10,725	8,014	10,725	9,281
59,500	59,550	10,738	8,021	10,738	9,294
59,550	59,600	10,750	8,029	10,750	9,306
59,600	59,650	10,763	8,036	10,763	9,319
59,650	59,700	10,775	8,044	10,775	9,331
59,700	59,750	10,788	8,051	10,788	9,344
59,750	59,800	10,800	8,059	10,800	9,356
59,800	59,850	10,813	8,066	10,813	9,369
59,850	59,900	10,825	8,074	10,825	9,381
59,900	59,950	10,838	8,081	10,838	9,394
59,950	60,000	10,850	8,089	10,850	9,406

60,000

At least	But less than	Single	Married filing jointly*	Married filing separately	Head of a household
60,000	60,050	10,863	8,096	10,863	9,419
60,050	60,100	10,875	8,104	10,875	9,431
60,100	60,150	10,888	8,111	10,888	9,444
60,150	60,200	10,900	8,119	10,900	9,456
60,200	60,250	10,913	8,126	10,913	9,469
60,250	60,300	10,925	8,134	10,925	9,481
60,300	60,350	10,938	8,141	10,938	9,494
60,350	60,400	10,950	8,149	10,950	9,506
60,400	60,450	10,963	8,156	10,963	9,519
60,450	60,500	10,975	8,164	10,975	9,531
60,500	60,550	10,988	8,171	10,988	9,544
60,550	60,600	11,000	8,179	11,000	9,556
60,600	60,650	11,013	8,186	11,013	9,569
60,650	60,700	11,025	8,194	11,025	9,581
60,700	60,750	11,038	8,201	11,038	9,594
60,750	60,800	11,050	8,209	11,050	9,606
60,800	60,850	11,063	8,216	11,063	9,619
60,850	60,900	11,075	8,224	11,075	9,631
60,900	60,950	11,088	8,231	11,088	9,644
60,950	61,000	11,100	8,239	11,100	9,656

61,000

At least	But less than	Single	Married filing jointly*	Married filing separately	Head of a household
61,000	61,050	11,113	8,248	11,113	9,669
61,050	61,100	11,125	8,254	11,125	9,681
61,100	61,150	11,138	8,261	11,138	9,694
61,150	61,200	11,150	8,269	11,150	9,706
61,200	61,250	11,163	8,276	11,163	9,719
61,250	61,300	11,175	8,284	11,175	9,731
61,300	61,350	11,188	8,291	11,188	9,744
61,350	61,400	11,200	8,299	11,200	9,756
61,400	61,450	11,213	8,306	11,213	9,769
61,450	61,500	11,225	8,314	11,225	9,781
61,500	61,550	11,238	8,321	11,238	9,794
61,550	61,600	11,250	8,329	11,250	9,806
61,600	61,650	11,263	8,336	11,263	9,819
61,650	61,700	11,275	8,344	11,275	9,831
61,700	61,750	11,288	8,351	11,288	9,844
61,750	61,800	11,300	8,359	11,300	9,856
61,800	61,850	11,313	8,366	11,313	9,869
61,850	61,900	11,325	8,374	11,325	9,881
61,900	61,950	11,338	8,381	11,338	9,894
61,950	62,000	11,350	8,389	11,350	9,906

62,000

At least	But less than	Single	Married filing jointly*	Married filing separately	Head of a household
62,000	62,050	11,363	8,396	11,363	9,919
62,050	62,100	11,375	8,404	11,375	9,931
62,100	62,150	11,388	8,411	11,388	9,944
62,150	62,200	11,400	8,419	11,400	9,956
62,200	62,250	11,413	8,426	11,413	9,969
62,250	62,300	11,425	8,434	11,425	9,981
62,300	62,350	11,438	8,441	11,438	9,994
62,350	62,400	11,450	8,449	11,450	10,006
62,400	62,450	11,463	8,456	11,463	10,019
62,450	62,500	11,475	8,464	11,475	10,031
62,500	62,550	11,488	8,471	11,488	10,044
62,550	62,600	11,500	8,479	11,500	10,056
62,600	62,650	11,513	8,486	11,513	10,069
62,650	62,700	11,525	8,494	11,525	10,081
62,700	62,750	11,538	8,501	11,538	10,094
62,750	62,800	11,550	8,509	11,550	10,106
62,800	62,850	11,563	8,516	11,563	10,119
62,850	62,900	11,575	8,524	11,575	10,131
62,900	62,950	11,588	8,531	11,588	10,144
62,950	63,000	11,600	8,539	11,600	10,156

63,000

At least	But less than	Single	Married filing jointly*	Married filing separately	Head of a household
63,000	63,050	11,613	8,546	11,613	10,169
63,050	63,100	11,625	8,554	11,625	10,181
63,100	63,150	11,638	8,561	11,638	10,194
63,150	63,200	11,650	8,569	11,650	10,206
63,200	63,250	11,663	8,576	11,663	10,219
63,250	63,300	11,675	8,584	11,675	10,231
63,300	63,350	11,688	8,591	11,688	10,244
63,350	63,400	11,700	8,599	11,700	10,256
63,400	63,450	11,713	8,606	11,713	10,269
63,450	63,500	11,725	8,614	11,725	10,281
63,500	63,550	11,738	8,621	11,738	10,294
63,550	63,600	11,750	8,629	11,750	10,306
63,600	63,650	11,763	8,636	11,763	10,319
63,650	63,700	11,775	8,644	11,775	10,331
63,700	63,750	11,788	8,651	11,788	10,344
63,750	63,800	11,800	8,659	11,800	10,356
63,800	63,850	11,813	8,666	11,813	10,369
63,850	63,900	11,825	8,674	11,825	10,381
63,900	63,950	11,838	8,681	11,838	10,394
63,950	64,000	11,850	8,689	11,850	10,406

64,000

At least	But less than	Single	Married filing jointly*	Married filing separately	Head of a household
64,000	64,050	11,863	8,696	11,863	10,419
64,050	64,100	11,875	8,704	11,875	10,431
64,100	64,150	11,888	8,711	11,888	10,444
64,150	64,200	11,900	8,719	11,900	10,456
64,200	64,250	11,913	8,726	11,913	10,469
64,250	64,300	11,925	8,734	11,925	10,481
64,300	64,350	11,938	8,741	11,938	10,494
64,350	64,400	11,950	8,749	11,950	10,506
64,400	64,450	11,963	8,756	11,963	10,519
64,450	64,500	11,975	8,764	11,975	10,531
64,500	64,550	11,988	8,771	11,988	10,544
64,550	64,600	12,000	8,779	12,000	10,556
64,600	64,650	12,013	8,786	12,013	10,569
64,650	64,700	12,025	8,794	12,025	10,581
64,700	64,750	12,038	8,801	12,038	10,594
64,750	64,800	12,050	8,809	12,050	10,606
64,800	64,850	12,063	8,816	12,063	10,619
64,850	64,900	12,075	8,824	12,075	10,631
64,900	64,950	12,088	8,831	12,088	10,644
64,950	65,000	12,100	8,839	12,100	10,656

65,000

At least	But less than	Single	Married filing jointly*	Married filing separately	Head of a household
65,000	65,050	12,113	8,846	12,113	10,669
65,050	65,100	12,125	8,854	12,125	10,681
65,100	65,150	12,138	8,861	12,138	10,694
65,150	65,200	12,150	8,869	12,150	10,706
65,200	65,250	12,163	8,876	12,163	10,719
65,250	65,300	12,175	8,884	12,175	10,731
65,300	65,350	12,188	8,891	12,188	10,744
65,350	65,400	12,200	8,899	12,200	10,756
65,400	65,450	12,213	8,906	12,213	10,769
65,450	65,500	12,225	8,914	12,225	10,781
65,500	65,550	12,238	8,921	12,238	10,794
65,550	65,600	12,250	8,929	12,250	10,806
65,600	65,650	12,263	8,936	12,263	10,819
65,650	65,700	12,275	8,944	12,275	10,831
65,700	65,750	12,288	8,951	12,288	10,844
65,750	65,800	12,300	8,959	12,300	10,856
65,800	65,850	12,313	8,966	12,313	10,869
65,850	65,900	12,325	8,974	12,325	10,881
65,900	65,950	12,338	8,981	12,338	10,894
65,950	66,000	12,350	8,989	12,350	10,906

(Continued)

* This column must also be used by a qualifying widow(er).

Need more information or forms? Visit IRS.gov.   - 82 -

¶25

»»→ Caution: This is a draft 2014 Tax Table. At the time of publication, the IRS had not yet released the 2014 Tax Table. For the latest information, see CCHGroup.com/TaxUpdates.

TAX RATES

66,000

At least	But less than	Single	Married filing jointly *	Married filing separately	Head of a household
66,000	66,050	12,363	8,996	12,363	10,919
66,050	66,100	12,375	9,004	12,375	10,931
66,100	66,150	12,388	9,011	12,388	10,944
66,150	66,200	12,400	9,019	12,400	10,956
66,200	66,250	12,413	9,026	12,413	10,969
66,250	66,300	12,425	9,034	12,425	10,981
66,300	66,350	12,438	9,041	12,438	10,994
66,350	66,400	12,450	9,049	12,450	11,006
66,400	66,450	12,463	9,056	12,463	11,019
66,450	66,500	12,475	9,064	12,475	11,031
66,500	66,550	12,488	9,071	12,488	11,044
66,550	66,600	12,500	9,079	12,500	11,056
66,600	66,650	12,513	9,086	12,513	11,069
66,650	66,700	12,525	9,094	12,525	11,081
66,700	66,750	12,538	9,101	12,538	11,094
66,750	66,800	12,550	9,109	12,550	11,106
66,800	66,850	12,563	9,116	12,563	11,119
66,850	66,900	12,575	9,124	12,575	11,131
66,900	66,950	12,588	9,131	12,588	11,144
66,950	67,000	12,600	9,139	12,600	11,156

67,000

At least	But less than	Single	Married filing jointly *	Married filing separately	Head of a household
67,000	67,050	12,613	9,146	12,613	11,169
67,050	67,100	12,625	9,154	12,625	11,181
67,100	67,150	12,638	9,161	12,638	11,194
67,150	67,200	12,650	9,169	12,650	11,206
67,200	67,250	12,663	9,176	12,663	11,219
67,250	67,300	12,675	9,184	12,675	11,231
67,300	67,350	12,688	9,191	12,688	11,244
67,350	67,400	12,700	9,199	12,700	11,256
67,400	67,450	12,713	9,206	12,713	11,269
67,450	67,500	12,725	9,214	12,725	11,281
67,500	67,550	12,738	9,221	12,738	11,294
67,550	67,600	12,750	9,229	12,750	11,306
67,600	67,650	12,763	9,236	12,763	11,319
67,650	67,700	12,775	9,244	12,775	11,331
67,700	67,750	12,788	9,251	12,788	11,344
67,750	67,800	12,800	9,259	12,800	11,356
67,800	67,850	12,813	9,266	12,813	11,369
67,850	67,900	12,825	9,274	12,825	11,381
67,900	67,950	12,838	9,281	12,838	11,394
67,950	68,000	12,850	9,289	12,850	11,406

68,000

At least	But less than	Single	Married filing jointly *	Married filing separately	Head of a household
68,000	68,050	12,863	9,296	12,863	11,419
68,050	68,100	12,875	9,304	12,875	11,431
68,100	68,150	12,888	9,311	12,888	11,444
68,150	68,200	12,900	9,319	12,900	11,456
68,200	68,250	12,913	9,326	12,913	11,469
68,250	68,300	12,925	9,334	12,925	11,481
68,300	68,350	12,938	9,341	12,938	11,494
68,350	68,400	12,950	9,349	12,950	11,506
68,400	68,450	12,963	9,356	12,963	11,519
68,450	68,500	12,975	9,364	12,975	11,531
68,500	68,550	12,988	9,371	12,988	11,544
68,550	68,600	13,000	9,379	13,000	11,556
68,600	68,650	13,013	9,386	13,013	11,569
68,650	68,700	13,025	9,394	13,025	11,581
68,700	68,750	13,038	9,401	13,038	11,594
68,750	68,800	13,050	9,409	13,050	11,606
68,800	68,850	13,063	9,416	13,063	11,619
68,850	68,900	13,075	9,424	13,075	11,631
68,900	68,950	13,088	9,431	13,088	11,644
68,950	69,000	13,100	9,439	13,100	11,656

69,000

At least	But less than	Single	Married filing jointly *	Married filing separately	Head of a household
69,000	69,050	13,113	9,446	13,113	11,669
69,050	69,100	13,125	9,454	13,125	11,681
69,100	69,150	13,138	9,461	13,138	11,694
69,150	69,200	13,150	9,469	13,150	11,706
69,200	69,250	13,163	9,476	13,163	11,719
69,250	69,300	13,175	9,484	13,175	11,731
69,300	69,350	13,188	9,491	13,188	11,744
69,350	69,400	13,200	9,499	13,200	11,756
69,400	69,450	13,213	9,506	13,213	11,769
69,450	69,500	13,225	9,514	13,225	11,781
69,500	69,550	13,238	9,521	13,238	11,794
69,550	69,600	13,250	9,529	13,250	11,806
69,600	69,650	13,263	9,536	13,263	11,819
69,650	69,700	13,275	9,544	13,275	11,831
69,700	69,750	13,288	9,551	13,288	11,844
69,750	69,800	13,300	9,559	13,300	11,856
69,800	69,850	13,313	9,566	13,313	11,869
69,850	69,900	13,325	9,574	13,325	11,881
69,900	69,950	13,338	9,581	13,338	11,894
69,950	70,000	13,350	9,589	13,350	11,906

70,000

At least	But less than	Single	Married filing jointly *	Married filing separately	Head of a household
70,000	70,050	13,363	9,596	13,363	11,919
70,050	70,100	13,375	9,604	13,375	11,931
70,100	70,150	13,388	9,611	13,388	11,944
70,150	70,200	13,400	9,619	13,400	11,956
70,200	70,250	13,413	9,626	13,413	11,969
70,250	70,300	13,425	9,634	13,425	11,981
70,300	70,350	13,438	9,641	13,438	11,994
70,350	70,400	13,450	9,649	13,450	12,006
70,400	70,450	13,463	9,656	13,463	12,019
70,450	70,500	13,475	9,664	13,475	12,031
70,500	70,550	13,488	9,671	13,488	12,044
70,550	70,600	13,500	9,679	13,500	12,056
70,600	70,650	13,513	9,686	13,513	12,069
70,650	70,700	13,525	9,694	13,525	12,081
70,700	70,750	13,538	9,701	13,538	12,094
70,750	70,800	13,550	9,709	13,550	12,106
70,800	70,850	13,563	9,716	13,563	12,119
70,850	70,900	13,575	9,724	13,575	12,131
70,900	70,950	13,588	9,731	13,588	12,144
70,950	71,000	13,600	9,739	13,600	12,156

71,000

At least	But less than	Single	Married filing jointly *	Married filing separately	Head of a household
71,000	71,050	13,613	9,746	13,613	12,169
71,050	71,100	13,625	9,754	13,625	12,181
71,100	71,150	13,638	9,761	13,638	12,194
71,150	71,200	13,650	9,769	13,650	12,206
71,200	71,250	13,663	9,776	13,663	12,219
71,250	71,300	13,675	9,784	13,675	12,231
71,300	71,350	13,688	9,791	13,688	12,244
71,350	71,400	13,700	9,799	13,700	12,256
71,400	71,450	13,713	9,806	13,713	12,269
71,450	71,500	13,725	9,814	13,725	12,281
71,500	71,550	13,738	9,821	13,738	12,294
71,550	71,600	13,750	9,829	13,750	12,306
71,600	71,650	13,763	9,836	13,763	12,319
71,650	71,700	13,775	9,844	13,775	12,331
71,700	71,750	13,788	9,851	13,788	12,344
71,750	71,800	13,800	9,859	13,800	12,356
71,800	71,850	13,813	9,866	13,813	12,369
71,850	71,900	13,825	9,874	13,825	12,381
71,900	71,950	13,838	9,881	13,838	12,394
71,950	72,000	13,850	9,889	13,850	12,406

72,000

At least	But less than	Single	Married filing jointly *	Married filing separately	Head of a household
72,000	72,050	13,863	9,896	13,863	12,419
72,050	72,100	13,875	9,904	13,875	12,431
72,100	72,150	13,888	9,911	13,888	12,444
72,150	72,200	13,900	9,919	13,900	12,456
72,200	72,250	13,913	9,926	13,913	12,469
72,250	72,300	13,925	9,934	13,925	12,481
72,300	72,350	13,938	9,941	13,938	12,494
72,350	72,400	13,950	9,949	13,950	12,506
72,400	72,450	13,963	9,956	13,963	12,519
72,450	72,500	13,975	9,964	13,975	12,531
72,500	72,550	13,988	9,971	13,988	12,544
72,550	72,600	14,000	9,979	14,000	12,556
72,600	72,650	14,013	9,986	14,013	12,569
72,650	72,700	14,025	9,994	14,025	12,581
72,700	72,750	14,038	10,001	14,038	12,594
72,750	72,800	14,050	10,009	14,050	12,606
72,800	72,850	14,063	10,016	14,063	12,619
72,850	72,900	14,075	10,024	14,075	12,631
72,900	72,950	14,088	10,031	14,088	12,644
72,950	73,000	14,100	10,039	14,100	12,656

73,000

At least	But less than	Single	Married filing jointly *	Married filing separately	Head of a household
73,000	73,050	14,113	10,046	14,113	12,669
73,050	73,100	14,125	10,054	14,125	12,681
73,100	73,150	14,138	10,061	14,138	12,694
73,150	73,200	14,150	10,069	14,150	12,706
73,200	73,250	14,163	10,076	14,163	12,719
73,250	73,300	14,175	10,084	14,175	12,731
73,300	73,350	14,188	10,091	14,188	12,744
73,350	73,400	14,200	10,099	14,200	12,756
73,400	73,450	14,213	10,106	14,213	12,769
73,450	73,500	14,225	10,114	14,225	12,781
73,500	73,550	14,238	10,121	14,238	12,794
73,550	73,600	14,250	10,129	14,250	12,806
73,600	73,650	14,263	10,136	14,263	12,819
73,650	73,700	14,275	10,144	14,275	12,831
73,700	73,750	14,288	10,151	14,288	12,844
73,750	73,800	14,300	10,159	14,300	12,856
73,800	73,850	14,313	10,169	14,313	12,869
73,850	73,900	14,325	10,181	14,325	12,881
73,900	73,950	14,338	10,194	14,338	12,894
73,950	74,000	14,350	10,206	14,350	12,906

74,000

At least	But less than	Single	Married filing jointly *	Married filing separately	Head of a household
74,000	74,050	14,363	10,219	14,363	12,919
74,050	74,100	14,375	10,231	14,375	12,931
74,100	74,150	14,388	10,244	14,388	12,944
74,150	74,200	14,400	10,256	14,400	12,956
74,200	74,250	14,413	10,269	14,413	12,969
74,250	74,300	14,425	10,281	14,425	12,981
74,300	74,350	14,438	10,294	14,438	12,994
74,350	74,400	14,450	10,306	14,450	13,006
74,400	74,450	14,463	10,319	14,463	13,019
74,450	74,500	14,475	10,331	14,477	13,031
74,500	74,550	14,488	10,344	14,491	13,044
74,550	74,600	14,500	10,356	14,505	13,056
74,600	74,650	14,513	10,369	14,519	13,069
74,650	74,700	14,525	10,381	14,533	13,081
74,700	74,750	14,538	10,394	14,547	13,094
74,750	74,800	14,550	10,406	14,561	13,106
74,800	74,850	14,563	10,419	14,575	13,119
74,850	74,900	14,575	10,431	14,589	13,131
74,900	74,950	14,588	10,444	14,603	13,144
74,950	75,000	14,600	10,456	14,617	13,156

This column must also be used by a qualifying widow(er).

(Continued)

¶25

⋙→ Caution: This is a draft 2014 Tax Table. At the time of publication, the IRS had not yet released the 2014 Tax Table. For the latest information, see CCHGroup.com/TaxUpdates.

75,000 / 76,000 / 77,000

| If line 43 (taxable income) is— | | And you are— | | | |
At least	But less than	Single	Married filing jointly *	Married filing separately	Head of a household
			Your tax is—		
75,000	75,050	14,613	10,469	14,631	13,169
75,050	75,100	14,625	10,481	14,645	13,181
75,100	75,150	14,638	10,494	14,659	13,194
75,150	75,200	14,650	10,506	14,673	13,206
75,200	75,250	14,663	10,519	14,687	13,219
75,250	75,300	14,675	10,531	14,701	13,231
75,300	75,350	14,688	10,544	14,715	13,244
75,350	75,400	14,700	10,556	14,729	13,256
75,400	75,450	14,713	10,569	14,743	13,269
75,450	75,500	14,725	10,581	14,757	13,281
75,500	75,550	14,738	10,594	14,771	13,294
75,550	75,600	14,750	10,606	14,785	13,306
75,600	75,650	14,763	10,619	14,799	13,319
75,650	75,700	14,775	10,631	14,813	13,331
75,700	75,750	14,788	10,644	14,827	13,344
75,750	75,800	14,800	10,656	14,841	13,356
75,800	75,850	14,813	10,669	14,855	13,369
75,850	75,900	14,825	10,681	14,869	13,381
75,900	75,950	14,838	10,694	14,883	13,394
75,950	76,000	14,850	10,706	14,897	13,406
76,000	76,050	14,863	10,719	14,911	13,419
76,050	76,100	14,875	10,731	14,925	13,431
76,100	76,150	14,888	10,744	14,939	13,444
76,150	76,200	14,900	10,756	14,953	13,456
76,200	76,250	14,913	10,769	14,967	13,469
76,250	76,300	14,925	10,781	14,981	13,481
76,300	76,350	14,938	10,794	14,995	13,494
76,350	76,400	14,950	10,806	15,009	13,506
76,400	76,450	14,963	10,819	15,023	13,519
76,450	76,500	14,975	10,831	15,037	13,531
76,500	76,550	14,988	10,844	15,051	13,544
76,550	76,600	15,000	10,856	15,065	13,556
76,600	76,650	15,013	10,869	15,079	13,569
76,650	76,700	15,025	10,881	15,093	13,581
76,700	76,750	15,038	10,894	15,107	13,594
76,750	76,800	15,050	10,906	15,121	13,606
76,800	76,850	15,063	10,919	15,135	13,619
76,850	76,900	15,075	10,931	15,149	13,631
76,900	76,950	15,088	10,944	15,163	13,644
76,950	77,000	15,100	10,956	15,177	13,656
77,000	77,050	15,113	10,969	15,191	13,669
77,050	77,100	15,125	10,981	15,205	13,681
77,100	77,150	15,138	10,994	15,219	13,694
77,150	77,200	15,150	11,006	15,233	13,706
77,200	77,250	15,163	11,019	15,247	13,719
77,250	77,300	15,175	11,031	15,261	13,731
77,300	77,350	15,188	11,044	15,275	13,744
77,350	77,400	15,200	11,056	15,289	13,756
77,400	77,450	15,213	11,069	15,303	13,769
77,450	77,500	15,225	11,081	15,317	13,781
77,500	77,550	15,238	11,094	15,331	13,794
77,550	77,600	15,250	11,106	15,345	13,806
77,600	77,650	15,263	11,119	15,359	13,819
77,650	77,700	15,275	11,131	15,373	13,831
77,700	77,750	15,288	11,144	15,387	13,844
77,750	77,800	15,300	11,156	15,401	13,856
77,800	77,850	15,313	11,169	15,415	13,869
77,850	77,900	15,325	11,181	15,429	13,881
77,900	77,950	15,338	11,194	15,443	13,894
77,950	78,000	15,350	11,206	15,457	13,906

78,000 / 79,000 / 80,000

| If line 43 (taxable income) is— | | And you are— | | | |
At least	But less than	Single	Married filing jointly *	Married filing separately	Head of a household
			Your tax is—		
78,000	78,050	15,363	11,219	15,471	13,919
78,050	78,100	15,375	11,231	15,485	13,931
78,100	78,150	15,388	11,244	15,499	13,944
78,150	78,200	15,400	11,256	15,513	13,956
78,200	78,250	15,413	11,269	15,527	13,969
78,250	78,300	15,425	11,281	15,541	13,981
78,300	78,350	15,438	11,294	15,555	13,994
78,350	78,400	15,450	11,306	15,569	14,006
78,400	78,450	15,463	11,319	15,583	14,019
78,450	78,500	15,475	11,331	15,597	14,031
78,500	78,550	15,488	11,344	15,611	14,044
78,550	78,600	15,500	11,356	15,625	14,056
78,600	78,650	15,513	11,369	15,639	14,069
78,650	78,700	15,525	11,381	15,653	14,081
78,700	78,750	15,538	11,394	15,667	14,094
78,750	78,800	15,550	11,406	15,681	14,106
78,800	78,850	15,563	11,419	15,695	14,119
78,850	78,900	15,575	11,431	15,709	14,131
78,900	78,950	15,586	11,444	15,723	14,144
78,950	79,000	15,600	11,456	15,737	14,156
79,000	79,050	15,613	11,469	15,751	14,169
79,050	79,100	15,625	11,481	15,765	14,181
79,100	79,150	15,638	11,494	15,779	14,194
79,150	79,200	15,650	11,506	15,793	14,206
79,200	79,250	15,663	11,519	15,807	14,219
79,250	79,300	15,675	11,531	15,821	14,231
79,300	79,350	15,688	11,544	15,835	14,244
79,350	79,400	15,700	11,556	15,849	14,256
79,400	79,450	15,713	11,569	15,863	14,269
79,450	79,500	15,725	11,581	15,877	14,281
79,500	79,550	15,738	11,594	15,891	14,294
79,550	79,600	15,750	11,606	15,905	14,306
79,600	79,650	15,763	11,619	15,919	14,319
79,650	79,700	15,775	11,631	15,933	14,331
79,700	79,750	15,788	11,644	15,947	14,344
79,750	79,800	15,800	11,656	15,961	14,356
79,800	79,850	15,813	11,669	15,975	14,369
79,850	79,900	15,825	11,681	15,989	14,381
79,900	79,950	15,838	11,694	16,003	14,394
79,950	80,000	15,850	11,706	16,017	14,406
80,000	80,050	15,863	11,719	16,031	14,419
80,050	80,100	15,875	11,731	16,045	14,431
80,100	80,150	15,888	11,744	16,059	14,444
80,150	80,200	15,900	11,756	16,073	14,456
80,200	80,250	15,913	11,769	16,087	14,469
80,250	80,300	15,925	11,781	16,101	14,481
80,300	80,350	15,938	11,794	16,115	14,494
80,350	80,400	15,950	11,806	16,129	14,506
80,400	80,450	15,963	11,819	16,143	14,519
80,450	80,500	15,975	11,831	16,157	14,531
80,500	80,550	15,988	11,844	16,171	14,544
80,550	80,600	16,000	11,856	16,185	14,556
80,600	80,650	16,013	11,869	16,199	14,569
80,650	80,700	16,025	11,881	16,213	14,581
80,700	80,750	16,038	11,894	16,227	14,594
80,750	80,800	16,050	11,906	16,241	14,606
80,800	80,850	16,063	11,919	16,255	14,619
80,850	80,900	16,075	11,931	16,269	14,631
80,900	80,950	16,088	11,944	16,283	14,644
80,950	81,000	16,100	11,956	16,297	14,656

81,000 / 82,000 / 83,000

| If line 43 (taxable income) is— | | And you are— | | | |
At least	But less than	Single	Married filing jointly *	Married filing separately	Head of a household
			Your tax is—		
81,000	81,050	16,113	11,969	16,311	14,669
81,050	81,100	16,125	11,981	16,325	14,681
81,100	81,150	16,138	11,994	16,339	14,694
81,150	81,200	16,150	12,006	16,353	14,706
81,200	81,250	16,163	12,019	16,367	14,719
81,250	81,300	16,175	12,031	16,381	14,731
81,300	81,350	16,188	12,044	16,395	14,744
81,350	81,400	16,200	12,056	16,409	14,756
81,400	81,450	16,213	12,069	16,423	14,769
81,450	81,500	16,225	12,081	16,437	14,781
81,500	81,550	16,238	12,094	16,451	14,794
81,550	81,600	16,250	12,106	16,465	14,806
81,600	81,650	16,263	12,119	16,479	14,819
81,650	81,700	16,275	12,131	16,493	14,831
81,700	81,750	16,288	12,144	16,507	14,844
81,750	81,800	16,300	12,156	16,521	14,856
81,800	81,850	16,313	12,169	16,535	14,869
81,850	81,900	16,325	12,181	16,549	14,881
81,900	81,950	16,338	12,194	16,563	14,894
81,950	82,000	16,350	12,206	16,577	14,906
82,000	82,050	16,363	12,219	16,591	14,919
82,050	82,100	16,375	12,231	16,605	14,931
82,100	82,150	16,388	12,244	16,619	14,944
82,150	82,200	16,400	12,256	16,633	14,956
82,200	82,250	16,413	12,269	16,647	14,969
82,250	82,300	16,425	12,281	16,661	14,981
82,300	82,350	16,438	12,294	16,675	14,994
82,350	82,400	16,450	12,306	16,689	15,006
82,400	82,450	16,463	12,319	16,703	15,019
82,450	82,500	16,475	12,331	16,717	15,031
82,500	82,550	16,488	12,344	16,731	15,044
82,550	82,600	16,500	12,356	16,745	15,056
82,600	82,650	16,513	12,369	16,759	15,069
82,650	82,700	16,525	12,381	16,773	15,081
82,700	82,750	16,538	12,394	16,787	15,094
82,750	82,800	16,550	12,406	16,801	15,106
82,800	82,850	16,563	12,419	16,815	15,119
82,850	82,900	16,575	12,431	16,829	15,131
82,900	82,950	16,588	12,444	16,843	15,144
82,950	83,000	16,600	12,456	16,857	15,156
83,000	83,050	16,613	12,469	16,871	15,169
83,050	83,100	16,625	12,481	16,885	15,181
83,100	83,150	16,638	12,494	16,899	15,194
83,150	83,200	16,650	12,506	16,913	15,206
83,200	83,250	16,663	12,519	16,927	15,219
83,250	83,300	16,675	12,531	16,941	15,231
83,300	83,350	16,688	12,544	16,955	15,244
83,350	83,400	16,700	12,556	16,969	15,256
83,400	83,450	16,713	12,569	16,983	15,269
83,450	83,500	16,725	12,581	16,997	15,281
83,500	83,550	16,738	12,594	17,011	15,294
83,550	83,600	16,750	12,606	17,025	15,306
83,600	83,650	16,763	12,619	17,039	15,319
83,650	83,700	16,775	12,631	17,053	15,331
83,700	83,750	16,788	12,644	17,067	15,344
83,750	83,800	16,800	12,656	17,081	15,356
83,800	83,850	16,813	12,669	17,095	15,369
83,850	83,900	16,825	12,681	17,109	15,381
83,900	83,950	16,838	12,694	17,123	15,394
83,950	84,000	16,850	12,706	17,137	15,406

(Continued)

* This column must also be used by a qualifying widow(er).

Need more information or forms? Visit IRS.gov.

¶25

>>>→ *Caution: This is a draft 2014 Tax Table. At the time of publication, the IRS had not yet released the 2014 Tax Table. For the latest information, see CCHGroup.com/TaxUpdates.*

TAX RATES

84,000

If line 43 (taxable income) is— At least	But less than	And you are— Single	Married filing jointly *	Married filing separately	Head of a household
		Your tax is—			
84,000	84,050	16,863	12,719	17,151	15,419
84,050	84,100	16,875	12,731	17,165	15,431
84,100	84,150	16,888	12,744	17,179	15,444
84,150	84,200	16,900	12,756	17,193	15,456
84,200	84,250	16,913	12,769	17,207	15,469
84,250	84,300	16,925	12,781	17,221	15,481
84,300	84,350	16,938	12,794	17,235	15,494
84,350	84,400	16,950	12,806	17,249	15,506
84,400	84,450	16,963	12,819	17,263	15,519
84,450	84,500	16,975	12,831	17,277	15,531
84,500	84,550	16,988	12,844	17,291	15,544
84,550	84,600	17,000	12,856	17,305	15,556
84,600	84,650	17,013	12,869	17,319	15,569
84,650	84,700	17,025	12,881	17,333	15,581
84,700	84,750	17,038	12,894	17,347	15,594
84,750	84,800	17,050	12,906	17,361	15,606
84,800	84,850	17,063	12,919	17,375	15,619
84,850	84,900	17,075	12,931	17,389	15,631
84,900	84,950	17,088	12,944	17,403	15,644
84,950	85,000	17,100	12,956	17,417	15,656

85,000

At least	But less than	Single	Married filing jointly *	Married filing separately	Head of a household
85,000	85,050	17,113	12,969	17,431	15,669
85,050	85,100	17,125	12,981	17,445	15,681
85,100	85,150	17,138	12,994	17,459	15,694
85,150	85,200	17,150	13,006	17,473	15,706
85,200	85,250	17,163	13,019	17,487	15,719
85,250	85,300	17,175	13,031	17,501	15,731
85,300	85,350	17,188	13,044	17,515	15,744
85,350	85,400	17,200	13,056	17,529	15,756
85,400	85,450	17,213	13,069	17,543	15,769
85,450	85,500	17,225	13,081	17,557	15,781
85,500	85,550	17,238	13,094	17,571	15,794
85,550	85,600	17,250	13,106	17,585	15,806
85,600	85,650	17,263	13,119	17,599	15,819
85,650	85,700	17,275	13,131	17,613	15,831
85,700	85,750	17,288	13,144	17,627	15,844
85,750	85,800	17,300	13,156	17,641	15,856
85,800	85,850	17,313	13,169	17,655	15,869
85,850	85,900	17,325	13,181	17,669	15,881
85,900	85,950	17,338	13,194	17,683	15,894
85,950	86,000	17,350	13,206	17,697	15,906

86,000

At least	But less than	Single	Married filing jointly *	Married filing separately	Head of a household
86,000	86,050	17,363	13,219	17,711	15,919
86,050	86,100	17,375	13,231	17,725	15,931
86,100	86,150	17,388	13,244	17,739	15,944
86,150	86,200	17,400	13,256	17,753	15,956
86,200	86,250	17,413	13,269	17,767	15,969
86,250	86,300	17,425	13,281	17,781	15,981
86,300	86,350	17,438	13,294	17,795	15,994
86,350	86,400	17,450	13,306	17,809	16,006
86,400	86,450	17,463	13,319	17,823	16,019
86,450	86,500	17,475	13,331	17,837	16,031
86,500	86,550	17,488	13,344	17,851	16,044
86,550	86,600	17,500	13,356	17,865	16,056
86,600	86,650	17,513	13,369	17,879	16,069
86,650	86,700	17,525	13,381	17,893	16,081
86,700	86,750	17,538	13,394	17,907	16,094
86,750	86,800	17,550	13,406	17,921	16,106
86,800	86,850	17,563	13,419	17,935	16,119
86,850	86,900	17,575	13,431	17,949	16,131
86,900	86,950	17,588	13,444	17,963	16,144
86,950	87,000	17,600	13,456	17,977	16,156

87,000

If line 43 (taxable income) is— At least	But less than	And you are— Single	Married filing jointly *	Married filing separately	Head of a household
		Your tax is—			
87,000	87,050	17,613	13,469	17,991	16,169
87,050	87,100	17,625	13,481	18,005	16,181
87,100	87,150	17,638	13,494	18,019	16,194
87,150	87,200	17,650	13,506	18,033	16,206
87,200	87,250	17,663	13,519	18,047	16,219
87,250	87,300	17,675	13,531	18,061	16,231
87,300	87,350	17,688	13,544	18,075	16,244
87,350	87,400	17,700	13,556	18,089	16,256
87,400	87,450	17,713	13,569	18,103	16,269
87,450	87,500	17,725	13,581	18,117	16,281
87,500	87,550	17,738	13,594	18,131	16,294
87,550	87,600	17,750	13,606	18,145	16,306
87,600	87,650	17,763	13,619	18,159	16,319
87,650	87,700	17,775	13,631	18,173	16,331
87,700	87,750	17,788	13,644	18,187	16,344
87,750	87,800	17,800	13,656	18,201	16,356
87,800	87,850	17,813	13,669	18,215	16,369
87,850	87,900	17,825	13,681	18,229	16,381
87,900	87,950	17,838	13,694	18,243	16,394
87,950	88,000	17,850	13,706	18,257	16,406

88,000

At least	But less than	Single	Married filing jointly *	Married filing separately	Head of a household
88,000	88,050	17,863	13,719	18,271	16,419
88,050	88,100	17,875	13,731	18,285	16,431
88,100	88,150	17,888	13,744	18,299	16,444
88,150	88,200	17,900	13,756	18,313	16,456
88,200	88,250	17,913	13,769	18,327	16,469
88,250	88,300	17,925	13,781	18,341	16,481
88,300	88,350	17,938	13,794	18,355	16,494
88,350	88,400	17,950	13,806	18,369	16,506
88,400	88,450	17,963	13,819	18,383	16,519
88,450	88,500	17,975	13,831	18,397	16,531
88,500	88,550	17,988	13,844	18,411	16,544
88,550	88,600	18,000	13,856	18,425	16,556
88,600	88,650	18,013	13,869	18,439	16,569
88,650	88,700	18,025	13,881	18,453	16,581
88,700	88,750	18,038	13,894	18,467	16,594
88,750	88,800	18,050	13,906	18,481	16,606
88,800	88,850	18,063	13,919	18,495	16,619
88,850	88,900	18,075	13,931	18,509	16,631
88,900	88,950	18,088	13,944	18,523	16,644
88,950	89,000	18,100	13,956	18,537	16,656

89,000

At least	But less than	Single	Married filing jointly *	Married filing separately	Head of a household
89,000	89,050	18,113	13,969	18,551	16,669
89,050	89,100	18,125	13,981	18,565	16,681
89,100	89,150	18,138	13,994	18,579	16,694
89,150	89,200	18,150	14,006	18,593	16,706
89,200	89,250	18,163	14,019	18,607	16,719
89,250	89,300	18,175	14,031	18,621	16,731
89,300	89,350	18,188	14,044	18,635	16,744
89,350	89,400	18,201	14,056	18,649	16,756
89,400	89,450	18,215	14,069	18,663	16,769
89,450	89,500	18,229	14,081	18,677	16,781
89,500	89,550	18,243	14,094	18,691	16,794
89,550	89,600	18,257	14,106	18,705	16,806
89,600	89,650	18,271	14,119	18,719	16,819
89,650	89,700	18,285	14,131	18,733	16,831
89,700	89,750	18,299	14,144	18,747	16,844
89,750	89,800	18,313	14,156	18,761	16,856
89,800	89,850	18,327	14,169	18,775	16,869
89,850	89,900	18,341	14,181	18,789	16,881
89,900	89,950	18,355	14,194	18,803	16,894
89,950	90,000	18,369	14,206	18,817	16,906

90,000

If line 43 (taxable income) is— At least	But less than	And you are— Single	Married filing jointly *	Married filing separately	Head of a household
		Your tax is—			
90,000	90,050	18,383	14,219	18,831	16,919
90,050	90,100	18,397	14,231	18,845	16,931
90,100	90,150	18,411	14,244	18,859	16,944
90,150	90,200	18,425	14,256	18,873	16,956
90,200	90,250	18,439	14,269	18,887	16,969
90,250	90,300	18,453	14,281	18,901	16,981
90,300	90,350	18,467	14,294	18,915	16,994
90,350	90,400	18,481	14,306	18,929	17,006
90,400	90,450	18,495	14,319	18,943	17,019
90,450	90,500	18,509	14,331	18,957	17,031
90,500	90,550	18,523	14,344	18,971	17,044
90,550	90,600	18,537	14,356	18,985	17,056
90,600	90,650	18,551	14,369	18,999	17,069
90,650	90,700	18,565	14,381	19,013	17,081
90,700	90,750	18,579	14,394	19,027	17,094
90,750	90,800	18,593	14,406	19,041	17,106
90,800	90,850	18,607	14,419	19,055	17,119
90,850	90,900	18,621	14,431	19,069	17,131
90,900	90,950	18,635	14,444	19,083	17,144
90,950	91,000	18,649	14,456	19,097	17,156

91,000

At least	But less than	Single	Married filing jointly *	Married filing separately	Head of a household
91,000	91,050	18,663	14,469	19,111	17,169
91,050	91,100	18,677	14,481	19,125	17,181
91,100	91,150	18,691	14,494	19,139	17,194
91,150	91,200	18,705	14,506	19,153	17,206
91,200	91,250	18,719	14,519	19,167	17,219
91,250	91,300	18,733	14,531	19,181	17,231
91,300	91,350	18,747	14,544	19,195	17,244
91,350	91,400	18,761	14,556	19,209	17,256
91,400	91,450	18,775	14,569	19,223	17,269
91,450	91,500	18,789	14,581	19,237	17,281
91,500	91,550	18,803	14,594	19,251	17,294
91,550	91,600	18,817	14,606	19,265	17,306
91,600	91,650	18,831	14,619	19,279	17,319
91,650	91,700	18,845	14,631	19,293	17,331
91,700	91,750	18,859	14,644	19,307	17,344
91,750	91,800	18,873	14,656	19,321	17,356
91,800	91,850	18,887	14,669	19,335	17,369
91,850	91,900	18,901	14,681	19,349	17,381
91,900	91,950	18,915	14,694	19,363	17,394
91,950	92,000	18,929	14,706	19,377	17,406

92,000

At least	But less than	Single	Married filing jointly *	Married filing separately	Head of a household
92,000	92,050	18,943	14,719	19,391	17,419
92,050	92,100	18,957	14,731	19,405	17,431
92,100	92,150	18,971	14,744	19,419	17,444
92,150	92,200	18,985	14,756	19,433	17,456
92,200	92,250	18,999	14,769	19,447	17,469
92,250	92,300	19,013	14,781	19,461	17,481
92,300	92,350	19,027	14,794	19,475	17,494
92,350	92,400	19,041	14,806	19,489	17,506
92,400	92,450	19,055	14,819	19,503	17,519
92,450	92,500	19,069	14,831	19,517	17,531
92,500	92,550	19,083	14,844	19,531	17,544
92,550	92,600	19,097	14,856	19,545	17,556
92,600	92,650	19,111	14,869	19,559	17,569
92,650	92,700	19,125	14,881	19,573	17,581
92,700	92,750	19,139	14,894	19,587	17,594
92,750	92,800	19,153	14,906	19,601	17,606
92,800	92,850	19,167	14,919	19,615	17,619
92,850	92,900	19,181	14,931	19,629	17,631
92,900	92,950	19,195	14,944	19,643	17,644
92,950	93,000	19,209	14,956	19,657	17,656

* This column must also be used by a qualifying widow(er).

(Continued)

¶25

⟫→ *Caution: This is a draft 2014 Tax Table. At the time of publication, the IRS had not yet released the 2014 Tax Table. For the latest information, see CCHGroup.com/TaxUpdates.*

93,000

At least	But less than	Single	Married filing jointly *	Married filing separately	Head of a household
93,000	93,050	19,223	14,969	19,671	17,069
93,050	93,100	19,237	14,981	19,685	17,681
93,100	93,150	19,251	14,994	19,699	17,694
93,150	93,200	19,265	15,006	19,713	17,706
93,200	93,250	19,279	15,019	19,727	17,719
93,250	93,300	19,293	15,031	19,741	17,731
93,300	93,350	19,307	15,044	19,755	17,744
93,350	93,400	19,321	15,056	19,769	17,756
93,400	93,450	19,335	15,069	19,783	17,769
93,450	93,500	19,349	15,081	19,797	17,781
93,500	93,550	19,363	15,094	19,811	17,794
93,550	93,600	19,377	15,106	19,825	17,806
93,600	93,650	19,391	15,119	19,839	17,819
93,650	93,700	19,405	15,131	19,853	17,831
93,700	93,750	19,419	15,144	19,867	17,844
93,750	93,800	19,433	15,156	19,881	17,856
93,800	93,850	19,447	15,169	19,895	17,869
93,850	93,900	19,461	15,181	19,909	17,881
93,900	93,950	19,475	15,194	19,923	17,894
93,950	94,000	19,489	15,206	19,937	17,906

94,000

At least	But less than	Single	Married filing jointly *	Married filing separately	Head of a household
94,000	94,050	19,503	15,219	19,951	17,919
94,050	94,100	19,517	15,231	19,965	17,931
94,100	94,150	19,531	15,244	19,979	17,944
94,150	94,200	19,545	15,256	19,993	17,956
94,200	94,250	19,559	15,269	20,007	17,969
94,250	94,300	19,573	15,281	20,021	17,981
94,300	94,350	19,587	15,294	20,035	17,994
94,350	94,400	19,601	15,306	20,049	18,006
94,400	94,450	19,615	15,319	20,063	18,019
94,450	94,500	19,629	15,331	20,077	18,031
94,500	94,550	19,643	15,344	20,091	18,044
94,550	94,600	19,657	15,356	20,105	18,056
94,600	94,650	19,671	15,369	20,119	18,069
94,650	94,700	19,685	15,381	20,133	18,081
94,700	94,750	19,699	15,394	20,147	18,094
94,750	94,800	19,713	15,406	20,161	18,106
94,800	94,850	19,727	15,419	20,175	18,119
94,850	94,900	19,741	15,431	20,189	18,131
94,900	94,950	19,755	15,444	20,203	18,144
94,950	95,000	19,769	15,456	20,217	18,156

95,000

At least	But less than	Single	Married filing jointly *	Married filing separately	Head of a household
95,000	95,050	19,783	15,469	20,231	18,169
95,050	95,100	19,797	15,481	20,245	18,181
95,100	95,150	19,811	15,494	20,259	18,194
95,150	95,200	19,825	15,506	20,273	18,206
95,200	95,250	19,839	15,519	20,287	18,219
95,250	95,300	19,853	15,531	20,301	18,231
95,300	95,350	19,867	15,544	20,315	18,244
95,350	95,400	19,881	15,556	20,329	18,256
95,400	95,450	19,895	15,569	20,343	18,269
95,450	95,500	19,909	15,581	20,357	18,281
95,500	95,550	19,923	15,594	20,371	18,294
95,550	95,600	19,937	15,606	20,385	18,306
95,600	95,650	19,951	15,619	20,399	18,319
95,650	95,700	19,965	15,631	20,413	18,331
95,700	95,750	19,979	15,644	20,427	18,344
95,750	95,800	19,993	15,656	20,441	18,358
95,800	95,850	20,007	15,669	20,455	18,369
95,850	95,900	20,021	15,681	20,469	18,381
95,900	95,950	20,035	15,694	20,483	18,394
95,950	96,000	20,049	15,706	20,497	18,406

96,000

At least	But less than	Single	Married filing jointly *	Married filing separately	Head of a household
96,000	96,050	20,063	15,719	20,511	18,419
96,050	96,100	20,077	15,731	20,525	18,431
96,100	96,150	20,091	15,744	20,539	18,444
96,150	96,200	20,105	15,756	20,553	18,456
96,200	96,250	20,119	15,769	20,567	18,469
96,250	96,300	20,133	15,781	20,581	18,481
96,300	96,350	20,147	15,794	20,595	18,494
96,350	96,400	20,161	15,806	20,609	18,506
96,400	96,450	20,175	15,819	20,623	18,519
96,450	96,500	20,189	15,831	20,637	18,531
96,500	96,550	20,203	15,844	20,651	18,544
96,550	96,600	20,217	15,856	20,665	18,556
96,600	96,650	20,231	15,869	20,679	18,569
96,650	96,700	20,245	15,881	20,693	18,581
96,700	96,750	20,259	15,894	20,707	18,594
96,750	96,800	20,273	15,906	20,721	18,606
96,800	96,850	20,287	15,919	20,735	18,619
96,850	96,900	20,301	15,931	20,749	18,631
96,900	96,950	20,315	15,944	20,763	18,644
96,950	97,000	20,329	15,956	20,777	18,656

97,000

At least	But less than	Single	Married filing jointly *	Married filing separately	Head of a household
97,000	97,050	20,343	15,969	20,791	18,669
97,050	97,100	20,357	15,981	20,805	18,681
97,100	97,150	20,371	15,994	20,819	18,694
97,150	97,200	20,385	16,006	20,833	18,706
97,200	97,250	20,399	16,019	20,847	18,719
97,250	97,300	20,413	16,031	20,861	18,731
97,300	97,350	20,427	16,044	20,875	18,744
97,350	97,400	20,441	16,056	20,889	18,756
97,400	97,450	20,455	16,069	20,903	18,769
97,450	97,500	20,469	16,081	20,917	18,781
97,500	97,550	20,483	16,094	20,931	18,794
97,550	97,600	20,497	16,106	20,945	18,806
97,600	97,650	20,511	16,119	20,959	18,819
97,650	97,700	20,525	16,131	20,973	18,831
97,700	97,750	20,539	16,144	20,987	18,844
97,750	97,800	20,553	16,156	21,001	18,856
97,800	97,850	20,567	16,169	21,015	18,869
97,850	97,900	20,581	16,181	21,029	18,881
97,900	97,950	20,595	16,194	21,043	18,894
97,950	98,000	20,609	16,206	21,057	18,906

98,000

At least	But less than	Single	Married filing jointly *	Married filing separately	Head of a household
98,000	98,050	20,623	16,219	21,071	18,919
98,050	98,100	20,637	16,231	21,085	18,931
98,100	98,150	20,651	16,244	21,099	18,944
98,150	98,200	20,665	16,256	21,113	18,956
98,200	98,250	20,679	16,269	21,127	18,969
98,250	98,300	20,693	16,281	21,141	18,981
98,300	98,350	20,707	16,294	21,155	18,994
98,350	98,400	20,721	16,306	21,169	19,006
98,400	98,450	20,735	16,319	21,183	19,019
98,450	98,500	20,749	16,331	21,197	19,031
98,500	98,550	20,763	16,344	21,211	19,044
98,550	98,600	20,777	16,356	21,225	19,056
98,600	98,650	20,791	16,369	21,239	19,069
98,650	98,700	20,805	16,381	21,253	19,081
98,700	98,750	20,819	16,394	21,267	19,094
98,750	98,800	20,833	16,406	21,281	19,106
98,800	98,850	20,847	16,419	21,295	19,119
98,850	98,900	20,861	16,431	21,309	19,131
98,900	98,950	20,875	16,444	21,323	19,144
98,950	99,000	20,889	16,456	21,337	19,156

99,000

At least	But less than	Single	Married filing jointly *	Married filing separately	Head of a household
99,000	99,050	20,903	16,469	21,351	19,169
99,050	99,100	20,917	16,481	21,365	19,181
99,100	99,150	20,931	16,494	21,379	19,194
99,150	99,200	20,945	16,506	21,393	19,206
99,200	99,250	20,959	16,519	21,407	19,219
99,250	99,300	20,973	16,531	21,421	19,231
99,300	99,350	20,987	16,544	21,435	19,244
99,350	99,400	21,001	16,556	21,449	19,256
99,400	99,450	21,015	16,569	21,463	19,269
99,450	99,500	21,029	16,581	21,477	19,281
99,500	99,550	21,043	16,594	21,491	19,294
99,550	99,600	21,057	16,606	21,505	19,306
99,600	99,650	21,071	16,619	21,519	19,319
99,650	99,700	21,085	16,631	21,533	19,331
99,700	99,750	21,099	16,644	21,547	19,344
99,750	99,800	21,113	16,656	21,561	19,356
99,800	99,850	21,127	16,669	21,575	19,369
99,850	99,900	21,141	16,681	21,589	19,381
99,900	99,950	21,155	16,694	21,603	19,394
99,950	100,000	21,169	16,706	21,617	19,406

> **$100,000 or over use the Tax Computation Worksheet**

* This column must also be used by a qualifying widow(er).

Need more information or forms? Visit IRS.gov.   - 86 -

¶25

CORPORATION INCOME TAX RATES

¶ 33 Corporations

The corporate tax rates are as follows:

Taxable Income Over	But Not Over	Pay	+	% on Excess	of the amount over—
$0—	$50,000	$0		15%	$0
50,000—	75,000	7,500		25	50,000
75,000—	100,000	13,750		34	75,000
100,000—	335,000	22,250		39	100,000
335,000—	10,000,000	113,900		34	335,000
10,000,000—	15,000,000	3,400,000		35	10,000,000
15,000,000—	18,333,333	5,150,000		38	15,000,000
18,333,333—	. . . .			35	0

Taxable income of certain personal service corporations is taxed at a flat rate of 35 percent (¶ 219).

¶ 34 Controlled Group of Corporations

A controlled group of corporations is subject to the regular corporate income tax rates (¶ 33) as though the group is one corporation (¶ 289).

¶ 35 Personal Holding Companies

In addition to regular corporate income taxes (¶ 33), a special tax is imposed on any corporation which is a personal holding company. For tax years beginning after December 31, 2012, the additional tax is 20 percent of the corporation's undistributed personal holding company income (¶ 275).

¶ 36 Insurance Companies and Regulated Investment Companies

The regular corporate tax rates (¶ 33) apply to an insurance company's taxable income (¶ 2370 and ¶ 2378). In the case of regulated investment companies (RIC or mutual fund), the corporate tax rates apply to investment company taxable income (¶ 2303).

¶ 37 Accumulated Earnings Tax

In addition to regular corporate income taxes (¶ 33), a corporation may be subject to a special tax on its accumulated taxable income. For tax years beginning after December 31, 2012, the tax is 20 percent of the corporation's accumulated taxable income. A corporation is entitled to a $250,000 accumulated earnings credit ($150,000 for personal service corporations) against the tax (¶ 251).

¶ 38 Foreign Corporations

The income of a foreign corporation that is not effectively connected with a U.S. trade or business is taxed at a rate of 30 percent unless a lower tax rate is provided under a income tax treaty (¶ 2431). Domestic corporate rates (¶ 33) apply to the income of a foreign corporation that is effectively connected with a U.S. trade or business (¶ 2425).

¶ 39 Real Estate Investment Trusts

A real estate investment trust (REIT) will be subject to regular corporate income tax rates (¶ 33) on its real estate investment trust taxable income (¶ 2329).

ESTATE AND GIFT TAXES

¶ 40 Unified Transfer Tax Rate Schedules

The basic estate and gift tax rate structure that applied to decedents dying and gifts made during 2010 through 2012 continues to apply for estates of decedents dying and gifts made after December 31, 2012, with the exception of the rates that apply to taxable transfers in excess of $500,000. Accordingly, the maximum tax rate is 40 percent for transfers made after December 31, 2012 (Code Sec. 2001). The unified tax rate schedule for 2013 and later years and 2010—2012 is as follows:

Unified Transfer Tax Rate Schedule, 2013 and Later Years

Column A	Column B	Column C	Column D
Taxable amount over	Taxable amount not over	Tax on amount in column A	Rate of tax on excess over amount in column A Percent
$0	$10,000	$0	18
10,000	20,000	1,800	20
20,000	40,000	3,800	22
40,000	60,000	8,200	24
60,000	80,000	13,000	26
80,000	100,000	18,200	28
100,000	150,000	23,800	30
150,000	250,000	38,800	32
250,000	500,000	70,800	34
500,000	750,000	155,800	37
750,000	1,000,000	248,300	39
1,000,000	. . . .	345,800	40

Unified Transfer Tax Rate Schedule, 2010*—2012

Column A	Column B	Column C	Column D
Taxable amount over	Taxable amount not over	Tax on amount in column A	Rate of tax on excess over amount in column A Percent
$0	$10,000	$0	18
10,000	20,000	1,800	20
20,000	40,000	3,800	22
40,000	60,000	8,200	24
60,000	80,000	13,000	26
80,000	100,000	18,200	28
100,000	150,000	23,800	30
150,000	250,000	38,800	32
250,000	500,000	70,800	34
500,000	. . . .	155,800	35

*The estates of decedents dying in 2010 were allowed to elect out of the estate tax regime, effectively reducing their estate tax rate to zero (Act Sec. 301(c) of the Tax Relief, Unemployment Insurance Reauthorization, and Job Creation Act of 2010 (P.L. 111-312)).

Generation-Skipping Transfer (GST) Tax. All GSTs are subject to tax at a flat rate equal to the product of the maximum federal estate tax rate under the unified rate schedule (40 percent for 2013 and thereafter) and the "inclusion ratio" (¶ 2943).

¶40

Nonresident Aliens. The transfer tax rates that apply to U.S. citizens and resident aliens also apply to nonresident aliens, for certain property situated within the United States (¶ 2903 and ¶ 2940).

¶ 41 Transfer Tax Credits, Exclusions, and Exemptions

Estate Tax Applicable Credit and Exclusion Amounts, 2011—2015

Year	Applicable Credit Amount	Applicable Exclusion Amount
2011	1,730,800	5,000,000
2012	1,772,800	5,120,000
2013	2,045,800	5,250,000
2014	2,081,800	5,340,000
2015	2,117,800	5,430,000

Gift Tax Applicable Credit and Exclusion Amounts, 2011—2015

Year	Applicable Credit Amount	Applicable (Lifetime) Exclusion Amount
2011	1,730,800	5,000,000
2012	1,772,800	5,120,000
2013	2,045,800	5,250,000
2014	2,081,800	5,340,000
2015	2,117,800	5,430,000

Gift Tax Annual Exclusion. There is an annual exclusion of $14,000 per donee for gifts made in 2014 ($14,000 per donee for 2015), with an annual maximum of $28,000 per donee for spouses who use gift-splitting in 2014 ($28,000 per donee in 2015) (¶ 2905).

Generation Skipping Transfer (GST) Exemption Amounts, 2011—2015

Year	Exemption Amount
2011	5,000,000
2012	5,120,000
2013	5,250,000
2014	5,340,000
2015	5,430,000

Nonresident Aliens. The annual gift tax exclusion is available to nonresident alien donors (¶ 2905). Where permitted by treaty, the estate of a nonresident alien is allowed a credit equal to the unified credit available to a U.S. citizen multiplied by the proportion of the decedent's entire gross estate situated in the United States (¶ 2940). In computing the credit, property is not treated as situated in the United States if such property is exempt from tax under any treaty. In other cases, a unified credit of $13,000 is allowed. The estate of a resident of a U.S. possession is entitled to a unified credit equal to the greater of (1) $13,000; or (2) $46,800 multiplied by the percentage of the decedent's gross estate situated in the United States (Code Sec. 2102).

With respect to the gift tax, no portion of the unified credit may be used as a credit against gift taxes payable on a lifetime transfers by a nonresident alien.

¶ 43 State Death Taxes

Estates of decedents may claim a deduction in determining the value of the gross estate for estate, inheritance, legacy, or succession taxes paid to any state or the District of Columbia (¶ 2933).

OTHER TAXES

¶ 47 Self-Employment Taxes

For calendar year 2014, a tax rate of 15.3 percent is imposed on net earnings from self-employment. The rate consists of a 12.4 percent component for Social Security (old-age, survivors, and disability insurance (OASDI)) and a 2.9 percent component for Medicare hospital insurance (HI). The OASDI rate applies only to net earnings from self-employment up to the OASDI wage base of $117,000 in 2014. The Medicare rate applies to all net earnings in 2014 (¶ 2664). The Medicare rate is increased by 0.9 percent to 3.8 percent for net earnings from self-employment in excess of $200,000 ($250,000 in the case of a joint return; $125,000 in the case of a married individual filing separately). In the case of a joint return, the additional 0.9 percent tax for Medicare is imposed on the combined income of both spouses. For 2015, the OASDI rate applies to net earnings from self-employment up to the OASDI wage base of $118,500. The Medicare rate applies to all net earnings in 2015.

¶ 49 Employment Taxes

FICA Taxes. Under the Federal Insurance Contributions Act (FICA), taxes are imposed on both employers and employees on wages paid to the employee for Social Security (old-age, survivors, and disability insurance (OASDI)), and Medicare hospital insurance (HI) (¶ 2648). For calendar year 2014, the tax rate on both the employer's and the employee's portion of wages is 7.65 percent (15.3 percent total), consisting of a 6.2 percent rate for OASDI and a 1.45 percent rate for Medicare. The OASDI rate for employers and employees applies only to wages up to the OASDI wage base of $117,000 in 2014. The Medicare rate applies to all wages in 2014. The Medicare rate on the employee's portion of wages is increased 0.9 percent to 2.35 percent for wages in excess of $200,000 ($250,000 in the case of a joint return; $125,000 in the case of a married individual filing separately). In the case of a joint return, the additional 0.9 percent tax for Medicare is imposed on the combined income of both spouses. For 2015, the OASDI rate applies to wages up to the OASDI wage base of $118,500. The Medicare rate applies to all wages in 2015.

Medicare Payments. Medicare Part B premiums ($104.90 per month in 2014 and 2015) qualify as deductible medical expenses (¶ 1019).

Unemployment Compensation. Under the Federal Unemployment Tax Act (FUTA), a tax is imposed on the first $7,000 of wages paid to a covered employee by an employer who employs one or more persons in covered employment in each of 20 days in a year, each day being in a different week, or who has a payroll for covered employment of at least $1,500 in a calendar quarter in the current or preceding calendar year (¶ 2649). The FUTA tax rate is 6.0 percent for wages paid in 2014. Since employers are allowed credits against the FUTA rate through participation in state unemployment insurance laws, the net FUTA rate actually paid by most employers is 0.6 percent in 2014, except when credit reductions are in effect in a state. The unemployment tax also applies to any person who paid total cash wages of $1,000 or more to a household employee during any calendar quarter in the current or preceding calendar year.

Railroad Retirement Tax. The Railroad Retirement and Survivors' Improvement Act provides benefits similar to those as under Social Security and Medicare. Tier I benefits are financed by taxes on employers and employees equal to those under FICA. The tax rate on the employer's and the employee's portion of wages for calendar year 2014 is 7.65 percent (15.3 percent total), consisting of a 6.2 percent rate for OASDI and a 1.45 percent rate for Medicare. The OASDI rate for employers and employees applies only to wages up to the OASDI wage base of $117,000 in 2014. The Medicare rate applies to all wages in 2014. The Medicare rate on the employee's portion of wages is increased 0.9 percent to 2.35 percent for wages in excess of $200,000 ($250,000 in the case of a joint return; $125,000 in the case of a married individual filing separately). In the case of a joint return, the additional 0.9 percent tax for Medicare is imposed on the combined income of both spouses. For 2015, the OASDI rate applies to wages up to the OASDI wage base of $118,500. The Medicare rate applies to all wages in 2015.

Tier II benefits are also available equivalent to a private pension plan and financed with employers and employees contributing a certain percentage of pay toward to system to finance benefits. For calendar year 2014, a tier II tax rate of 12.6 percent for employers and 4.4 percent for employees is imposed on annual compensation within a compensation base of $87,000. For calendar year 2015, a tier II tax rate of 12.6 percent for employers and 4.4 percent for employees is imposed on annual compensation within a compensation base of $88,200.

¶ 53 Excise Taxes

Identified below are various excise taxes.

FUELS
Gasoline
Gasoline (per gallon) . . . . 18.4¢
Diesel fuel, biodiesel, and kerosene
Diesel fuel (except if used on a farm for farming purposes) (per
    gallon) . . . . 24.4¢
Diesel fuel for use in trains (per gallon) . . . . 0.1¢
Diesel-water fuel emulsions (per gallon) . . . . 19.8¢
Kerosene (except if used in a farm for farming purposes) (per
    gallon) . . . . 24.4¢
B-100 (100 percent biodiesel) (per gallon) . . . . 24.4¢
Special fuels
Special motor fuel (per gallon) . . . . 18.4¢
Liquefied petroleum gas (LPG) . . . . 18.3¢
"P Series" fuels . . . . 18.4¢
Compressed natural gas (CNG) (per energy equivalent of a
    gallon of gasoline) . . . . 18.3¢
Liquefied hydrogen . . . . 18.4¢
Any liquid fuel derived from coal (including peat) through the
    Fischer-Tropsch process (per gallon) . . . . 24.4¢
Liquid fuel derived from biomass (per gallon) . . . . 24.4¢
Liquefied natural gas (LNG) (per gallon) . . . . 24.3¢
Liquefied gas derived from biomass (per gallon) . . . . 18.4¢
Qualified ethanol produced from coal (per gallon) . . . . 18.4¢
Qualified methanol produced from coal (per gallon) . . . . 18.4¢
Partially exempt ethanol produced from natural gas (per gallon) . . . . 11.4¢
Partially exempt methanol produced from natural gas (per
    gallon) . . . . 9.25¢
Fuel used on inland waterways
Inland waterways fuel use tax (per gallon) . . . . 20.1¢
Aviation fuels
Kerosene used in commercial aviation (when removed from a
    refinery or terminal directly into the fuel tank of an aircraft)
    (per gallon) . . . . 4.4¢
Kerosene used in noncommercial aviation (when removed from a
    refinery or terminal directly into the fuel tank of an aircraft)
    (per gallon) . . . . 21.9¢
Noncommercial aviation gasoline (per gallon) . . . . 19.4¢
Fuel used in fractional aircraft ownership program flights (per
    gallon) . . . . 14.1¢ surtax after
                                                        3/31/2012

Fuel credits
Alcohol or alcohol in fuel mixtures if 190 proof or greater (per
    gallon) (ethanol) . . . . 45¢ credit until 2012
Alcohol of 190 proof or greater if benefited from the small
    ethanol producers credit (per gallon) . . . . 55¢ credit until 2012
Alcohol and alcohol in fuel mixtures if less than 190, but at least
    150 proof (per gallon) (ethanol) . . . . 33.33¢ credit
                                                        until 2012
Alcohol if less than 190, but at least 150 proof if benefited from
    the small ethanol producers credit (per gallon) . . . . 43.33¢ credit
                                                        until 2012

¶53

Alcohol if 190 proof or greater (per gallon) (methanol) . . . . .60¢ credit until 2012
Alcohol if at least 150, but less than 190 proof (per gallon)
   (methanol) . . . . .45¢ credit until 2012
Second generation biofuel (per gallon) . . . . $1.01 credit until 2014
Biodiesel and biodiesel mixtures (per gallon) . . . . $1.00 credit until 2014
Agri-biodiesel (per gallon) . . . . $1.00 credit until 2014
Agri-biodiesel if benefited from the small agri-biodiesel producer
   credit (per gallon) . . . . $1.10 credit until 2014
Renewable diesel and renewable diesel mixtures (per gallon) . . . . $1.00 credit until 2014
Alternative fuel (as defined in Code Sec. 6426(d)(2)) (per gallon) . . 50¢ credit until 2014 (but
                                                                          until 9/30/2014 for
                                                                          liquefied hydrogen)

Crude oil
Crude oil (per barrel) . . . . 8¢
HEAVY TRUCKS, TRAILERS
Truck chassis or body (that is suitable for use with a vehicle in
   excess of 33,000 lbs. gross vehicle weight) . . . . 12% of retail price
Trailer and semitrailer chassis or body (that is suitable for use
   with a trailer or semitrailer in excess of 26,000 lbs. gross
   vehicle weight) . . . . 12% of retail price
Parts and accessories installed on taxable vehicles within 6
   months after being placed in service (when cost of parts or
   accessories exceeds $1,000) . . . . 12% of retail price
HIGHWAY-TYPE TIRES
Tires with load capacity of 3,500 lbs. or less . . . . No tax
Tires with load capacity over 3,500 lbs. . . . . .9.45¢ for each 10 lbs. of tire
                                                                   load capacity over 3,500 lbs.
Super single tires designed for steering . . . . .9.45¢ for each 10 lbs. of tire
                                                                   load capacity over 3,500 lbs.
Super single tires not designed for steering . . . . 4.725¢ for each 10 lbs. of
                                                                   tire load capacity over 3,500
                                                                                           lbs.
Biasply tires . . . . 4.725¢ for each 10 lbs. of
                                                                   tire load capacity over 3,500
                                                                                           lbs.

GAS GUZZLER TAX
Mileage ratings per gallon of at least 22.5 . . . . $ 0
Mileage ratings per gallon of at least 21.5 but less than 22.5 1,000
Mileage ratings per gallon of at least 20.5 but less than 21.5 1,300
Mileage ratings per gallon of at least 19.5 but less than 20.5 1,700
Mileage ratings per gallon of at least 18.5 but less than 19.5 2,100
Mileage ratings per gallon of at least 17.5 but less than 18.5 2,600
Mileage ratings per gallon of at least 16.5 but less than 17.5 3,000
Mileage ratings per gallon of at least 15.5 but less than 16.5 3,700
Mileage ratings per gallon of at least 14.5 but less than 15.5 4,500
Mileage ratings per gallon of at least 13.5 but less than 14.5 5,400
Mileage ratings per gallon of at least 12.5 but less than 13.5 6,400
Mileage ratings per gallon of less than 12.5 7,700

¶53

FACILITIES AND SERVICES
Communications
Local telephone service and teletypewriter service 3%
Transportation by air
Domestic passenger tickets . . . . 7.5% plus $4 (from 1/1/14-12/31/14) for each flight segment (excepting segments to or from rural airports)

Alaska and Hawaii passenger tickets (amount per person per
    departure) (from 1/1/14-12/31/14) $8.70
International passenger tickets (amount per person for each
    arrival and for each departure) (from 1/1/14-12/31/14) $17.50
Air freight waybill 6.25%
Transportation by water
Persons $3.00
Port use tax on imports (harbor maintenance tax) . . . . 0.125% of cargo value
ALCOHOL TAXES
Distilled spirits (per gallon) $13.50
Beer (per barrel—31 gallons or less) $18.00
First 60,000 barrels removed during calendar year by U.S.
    brewer producing not more than 2 million barrels during year
    (per barrel) $7.00
Wines
Not more than 14% alcohol (per gallon) $1.07
More than 14 to 21% alcohol (per gallon) $1.57
More than 21 to 24% alcohol (per gallon) $3.15
More than 24% alcohol (per gallon) $13.50
Artificially carbonated wines (per gallon) $3.30
Champagne and other sparkling wines (per gallon) $3.40
Hard cider derived from apples containing at least ½ of 1% and
    less than 7% alcohol (per gallon) $0.226
TOBACCO TAXES
Cigars weighing not more than 3 lbs. (per 1,000) $50.33
Cigars weighing more than 3 lbs. . . . . 52.75% of sales price, not to exceed 40.26 cents per cigar
Cigarettes weighing not more than 3 lbs. (per 1,000) $50.33
Cigarettes weighing more than 3 lbs. (per 1,000) $105.69
Cigarette papers (per 50 papers) . . . . 3.15¢
Cigarette tubes (per 50 tubes) . . . . 6.30¢
Snuff (per pound) $1.51
Chewing tobacco (per pound) . . . . 50.33¢
Pipe tobacco (per pound) . . . . $2.8311 cents
Roll-your-own tobacco (per pound) $24.78
WAGERING TAXES
State authorized wagers placed with bookmakers and lottery
    operators . . . . 0.25% of wager amt.
Unauthorized wagers placed with bookmakers and lottery
    operators . . . . 2% of wager amt.
License fee on state authorized persons accepting wagers (per
    year, per person) $50
License fee on unauthorized persons accepting wagers (per year,
    per person) $500

HIGHWAY MOTOR VEHICLE USE TAX

Vehicles of less than 55,000 lbs. . . . . No tax

Vehicles of 55,000 lbs.—75,000 lbs. (per year) . . . . $100 per year + $22 for
each 1,000 lbs. (or fraction
thereof) over 55,000 lbs.

Vehicles over 75,000 lbs. (per year) $550

FIREARMS

Transfer taxes (per firearm) . . . . $5 (concealable weapons)
or $200

Occupational taxes (per year) . . . . $1,000 (importers or
manufacturers), or $500
(dealers, small importers
and manufacturers)

Pistols and revolvers . . . . .10% of sales price

Firearms other than pistols and revolvers . . . . .11% of sales price

Ammunition (shells and cartridges) . . . . .11% of sales price

OTHER TAXES

Electric outboard motors . . . . 3% of sales price

Fishing tackle boxes . . . . 3% of sales price

Sport fishing equipment . . . . .10% of sales price

Bows with a peak draw weight of at least 30 pounds . . . . .11% of sales price

Quivers, broadheads, points . . . . .11% of sales price

Arrow shafts . . . . .48¢ per shaft

Coal—underground mines . . . . lower of $1.10 per ton or
4.4% of sales price

Coal—surface mines . . . . lower of 55¢ per ton or 4.4%
of sales price

Vaccines . . . . 75¢ per dose on taxable
vaccines

Indoor tanning services . . . . 10% of amount paid

Casualty insurance and indemnity, fidelity and surety bonds (per
dollar of premium paid) . . . . .4¢

Life insurance, sickness and accident policies, and annuity
contracts (per dollar of premium paid) . . . . .1¢

Reinsurance of taxable contracts above (per dollar of premium
paid) . . . . .1¢

Preparing Income Tax Returns

CHECKLISTS

¶ 55 Checklist for Items of Income

The determination of whether an item of income is includible in income and, thus, taxable, or whether it is excludable from income is crucial to the determination of tax liability. An item that is includible increases tax liability, depending on the amount, whereas an excludable item decreases tax liability. The following chart, which is arranged alphabetically by income item, indicates whether the item is includible or excludable from income. A reference to further details in the 2015 *U.S. Master Tax Guide*® is also provided.

Income Item	Includible in Income	Paragraph Reference
Accident and health insurance premiums, employer-paid (except for long-term care benefits provided through flexible spending accounts and subject to limitation as to medical savings accounts and health savings accounts)	No	¶ 2013
Accident and health plans proceeds (under insurance purchased by taxpayer or under employee supported plans) where premiums did not give taxpayer a previous medical expense deduction	No	¶ 2015 ¶ 1288;
Agreement not to compete, payments received for	Yes	¶ 1743
Alaska Permanent Fund dividends	Yes	¶ 105
Alimony, support and separate maintenance payments, receipt of	Yes	¶ 773
Allowances received by dependents of members of the Armed Forces	No	¶ 896
Annuities (amounts in excess of cost)	Yes	¶ 819
Annuities, interest on advance premiums	Yes	¶ 724
Annuity contract, death benefit (amount in excess of cost)	Yes	¶ 817
Antitrust action, punitive damages recovered	Yes	¶ 852
Armed Forces pay (except "combat zone" or "missing" status pay)	Yes	¶ 891
Athletic facilities on employer's premises, value of use . .	No	¶ 2094
Attorney's contingent fee, includible in plaintiff's gross income	Yes	¶ 852
Awards, generally	Yes	¶ 852
Back pay	Yes	¶ 852
Bad debts, prior taxes and interest on taxes, recovery of, provided no tax benefit in prior year	No	¶ 799
Bargain purchases from employer to extent discount exceeds gross profit percentage	Yes	¶ 789

Income Item	Includible in Income	Paragraph Reference
Barter income	Yes	¶ 785
Beauty contest winners, receipt of scholarships and amounts for personal appearances	Yes	¶ 785
Bequests and devises, generally	No	¶ 847
Bonds, state, city, etc., interest on, generally	No	¶ 724
Bonuses	Yes	¶ 713
Buried treasure	Yes	¶ 785
Business interruption insurance proceeds:		
. based on income experience	Yes	¶ 759
. based on per diem idleness	No	¶ 759
Business profits	Yes	¶ 759
Business relocation payments	Yes	¶ 759
Business subsidies for construction or contributions by customer or potential customer	Yes	¶ 759
Cancellation of debt	Yes	¶ 855
Capital contributions to corporation	No	¶ 1660
Car pool receipts by car owner for transportation of other employees	No	¶ 945
Car used for business purposes by full-time car salesperson, value of use	No	¶ 947
Checks, uncashed by payee, for previously deducted items	Yes	¶ 1543
Child or dependent care plan benefits, employer-subsidized, limited	No	¶ 2065
Child support payments	No	¶ 776
Christmas bonuses from employer, based on percentage of salary (aside from token gifts such as hams, turkeys, etc., given for goodwill)	Yes	¶ 713
Civil Rights Act violation, back pay recovery	Yes	¶ 852
Clergy fees and contributions received unless earned as agent of religious order	Yes	¶ 713
COBRA premium assistance	No	¶ 888
"Combat zone" pay, military	No	¶ 895
Commissions	Yes	¶ 713
Commodity credit loans, receipt of (optional)	Yes	¶ 769
Compensated Work Therapy program payments for veterans and their families	No	¶ 891
Compensation, property received, value of	Yes	¶ 1681
Contract cancellation, payments received for	Yes	¶ 1563
Contribution in aid of construction	Yes	¶ 1660
Damages:		
. back pay	Yes	¶ 852
. personal physical injuries or sickness	No	¶ 852
. slander or libel of personal reputation	Yes	¶ 852
Death benefits:		
. employer paid, in general	Yes	¶ 2011
. government plan, public safety officer	No	¶ 813
Debts:		
. cancellation of, related to principal residence, from 2007 through 2013, up to $2,000,000	No	¶ 855
. gratuitous cancellation of	No	¶ 855
. nongratuitous cancellation of	Yes	¶ 855
Defamation damage award, compensating injury to business and professional reputation	Yes	¶ 852
Deferred income under certain nonqualified deferred compensation plans	Yes	¶ 2199

CHECKLISTS

Income Item	Includible in Income	Paragraph Reference
Dependent care assistance program payments, limited . .	No	¶ 2065
Disability payments, other than for loss of wages, all taxpayers, including veterans	No	¶ 891
Disability pensions, Veterans' Administration	No	¶ 891
Disaster unemployment payments	Yes	¶ 722
Discharge of indebtedness:		
. debt on a principal residence, from 2007 through 2013, up to $2,000,000	No	¶ 855
. gratuitous	No	¶ 855
. nongratuitous	Yes	¶ 855
Dividends, stock distributed in lieu of money	Yes	¶ 733
Drawing account, excess cancelled by employer	Yes	¶ 713
Educational assistance, employer-provided under a nondiscriminatory plan	No	¶ 2067
Embezzlement proceeds	Yes	¶ 785
Employee achievement awards, qualified	No	¶ 2069
Employee discount, qualified	No	¶ 2088
Employment contract, amounts received by employee for cancellation	Yes	¶ 713
Endowment policies, generally as to non-annuity payments until cost is recovered	No	¶ 841
Farm income	Yes	¶ 767
Farmers, government payments to offset operating losses or lack of profits	Yes	¶ 767
Fellowships and scholarships, degree programs	No	¶ 865
Financial counseling:		
. fees, employer-paid	Yes	¶ 713
. services, employer-provided, related to a qualified retirement plan	No	¶ 2093
Foreign earned income (limited exclusion)	Yes	¶ 2402
Foster parents, reimbursements for care of a qualified foster child	No	¶ 883
Fringe benefits:		
. athletic facilities	No	¶ 2094
. *de minimis* fringe benefit	No	¶ 2089
. employee discounts	No	¶ 2088
. in general	No	¶ 2085
. military base realignment and closure benefits	No	¶ 2095
. moving expenses reimbursements	No	¶ 2092
. no-additional-cost-services	No	¶ 2087
. retirement planning services	No	¶ 2093
. transportation fringe benefit	No	¶ 2091
. working condition fringe benefits	No	¶ 2090
Future services, prepayment for	Yes	¶ 1537
Gain on sale of personal residence:		
. up to $250,000 ($500,000 for joint filers)	No	¶ 1705
Gains:		
. condemnation of nonresidential property unless award is used for replacement	Yes	¶ 1716
. discount on later sale or redemption of bonds purchased with excess number of interest coupons detached (stripped bonds)	Yes	¶ 1952
. obligations purchased or satisfied for less than face value	Yes	¶ 1958
. partner's sale of asset to partnership	Yes	¶ 443
. sales of depreciable property	Yes	¶ 1780

Income Item	Includible in Income	Paragraph Reference
. sales of goodwill	Yes	¶ 1743
. sales of patents	Yes	¶ 1767
. sales of property, generally	Yes	¶ 1701
. sales of stock in foreign corporations	Yes	¶ 2487
. swap-fund transfers	Yes	¶ 1731
Gambling winnings:		
. illegal	Yes	¶ 785
. legal	Yes	¶ 785
Gifts	No	¶ 849
Government employees, additional compensation as inducement to accept foreign service employment ("post differentials")	Yes	¶ 714
Health insurance proceeds, not paid by the insured's employer or financed by the insured's employer through contributions that were not included in the employee's gross income	No	¶ 851
Health Savings Accounts partner's/shareholder's contributions made by partnership/S corporation	Yes	¶ 2035
Hedging transactions, commodity futures transactions	Yes	¶ 1949
Hobby income (nonprofit activities, deductions limited)	Yes	¶ 1195
Illegal transactions, gains from: gambling, betting, lotteries, illegal businesses, embezzlement, protection money, etc.	Yes	¶ 785
Illness, employee's compensation during, except to extent qualifying as insurance benefits	Yes	¶ 851
Incentive stock options	No	¶ 1923
Income tax refunds:		
. state, to extent of tax benefit from prior deduction	Yes	¶ 799
Inheritances	No	¶ 847
Insider's profits	Yes	¶ 1760
Insurance policy dividends:		
. distributed, up to total of all net premiums paid	No	¶ 2373
. retained by insurer and applied against premium	No	¶ 2373
Insurance proceeds:		
. business interruption insurance, based on lost income	Yes	¶ 759
. use or occupancy, actual loss of net profits	Yes	¶ 759
Interest-free loans:		
. loans in excess of *de minimis* amount, deemed interest	Yes	¶ 795
. loans within *de minimis* amount	No	¶ 795
Interest on:		
. bank deposits or accounts	Yes	¶ 724
. bonds, debentures, or notes	Yes	¶ 724
. claim awarded by judgment	Yes	¶ 852
. condemnation awards	Yes	¶ 1716
. deferred legacies	Yes	¶ 847
. federal obligations	Yes	¶ 2838
. insurance contracts	Yes	¶ 724
. refund of federal taxes	Yes	¶ 2765
Involuntary conversions, gain from, if reinvested	No	¶ 1713
Juror's mileage allowance	No	¶ 713
Jury fees	Yes	¶ 1010
Layoff pay benefits:		
. supplemental unemployment benefit plan, company-financed	Yes	¶ 722

CHECKLISTS

Income Item	Includible in Income	Paragraph Reference
Lease cancellation, payments received for	Yes	¶ 762
Leased retail space, cash or rent reductions received for construction or improvements	No	¶ 676
Legal services plan, employer contributions and value of benefits received	Yes	¶ 713
Lessee's improvements, value of to lessor upon termination of lease	No	¶ 1234
Libel or slander of personal reputation, exemplary damages	Yes	¶ 852
Life insurance contract, distributed from qualified plan . .	Yes	¶ 2055
Life insurance dividends:		
. distributed, up to total of all net premiums paid	No	¶ 2373
. retained by insurer and applied against premium . . .	No	¶ 2373
Life insurance dividends, veterans	No	¶ 891
Life insurance, group-term premiums paid by employer, to extent of employer's cost of $50,000 or less of insurance	No	¶ 2055
Life insurance proceeds, paid on death of the insured . . .	No	¶ 803
Living expenses paid by insurance while damaged home being repaired	No	¶ 877
Lodging and meals, employer provided:		
. furnished on the business premises for the convenience of the employer	No	¶ 2089
. furnished on the business premises for the convenience of the employer and as a condition of employment	No	¶ 2089
Losses, previously deducted, reimbursement for or expense items	Yes	¶ 1127
Meals, cost of, furnished on employer's premises for employer's convenience	No	¶ 2089
Medicaid rebates to drug manufacturers	No	¶ 799
Medical care reimbursements, employer-financed accident and health plan	No	¶ 2015
Medical loss ratio (MLR) rebates:		
. insurance premiums previously deducted	Yes	¶ 2031
. insurance premiums not previously deducted	No	¶ 2031
Military personnel, basic pay	Yes	¶ 895
Military service, employer-payments to employees	Yes	¶ 896
Mortgage indebtedness, prepayment at a discount to the extent of the discount	Yes	¶ 855
Moving expenses, qualified, employer-reimbursement . .	No	¶ 2092
National Labor Relations Board, back-pay award	Yes	¶ 2604
National Service Life Insurance dividends	No	¶ 891
Nobel prize and similar awards if donated by recipient to qualified entity	No	¶ 2069
Nonqualified deferred compensation plan, assets set aside to fund	Yes	¶ 2199
Obligations, federal interest on	Yes	¶ 724
Old age, disability, survivors' benefit payments, Social Security or Railroad Retirement Acts, below base amount	No	¶ 716
Parsonage, rental value of, furnished to a minister or rabbi as part of compensation; rental allowances if used to rent or provide a home	No	¶ 875
Partnership, distributive share of taxable income	Yes	¶ 431
Patents, sale to controlled foreign corporation	Yes	¶ 2491

Income Item	Includible in Income	Paragraph Reference
Pensions:		
. annuities, etc., for personal injuries or sickness	No	¶ 852
. distributions attributable to employer contributions .	Yes	¶ 2127
Personal physical injuries, damages	No	¶ 852
Political campaign contributions, with exceptions	No	¶ 696
Prizes	Yes	¶ 785
Professional fees	Yes	¶ 713
Pulitzer prize and similar awards if donated by recipient to qualified entity	No	¶ 785
Punitive damages	Yes	¶ 852
Purchases, nondiscriminatory employee-discounts	No	¶ 2088
Railroad Retirement Act benefits, below base amount . . .	No	¶ 716
Rebates, credits, price reductions received by customers	No	¶ 759
Rent reductions received by retail tenants for construction or improvements	No	¶ 764
Rents	Yes	¶ 762
Retirement pay attributable to employer contributions other than veterans' disability retirement pay	Yes	¶ 716
Reward, informer's	Yes	¶ 701
Royalties	Yes	¶ 763
Salaries, including those of state and federal employees and amounts employer withholds for income, Social Security, and Railroad Retirement taxes	Yes	¶ 714
Scholarships and fellowships, degree programs, qualified	No	¶ 865
Security deposits, when retained by lessor (advance rent)	Yes	¶ 1537
Sickness and injury benefits:		
. employer's plan, subject to limitations	No	¶ 851
. workers' compensation equivalent	No	¶ 851
Social Security old age, disability and survivor's benefits, below base amount	No	¶ 716
State contracts, profits on	Yes	¶ 759
Stock distributions in general	No	¶ 733A
. convertible preferred stock or debentures	Yes	¶ 1738
. disproportionate distributions	Yes	¶ 1738
. distributions of common and preferred stock	Yes	¶ 1738
. dividends on preferred stock	Yes	¶ 733
. increasing shareholder's proportionate interest	Yes	¶ 1738
. in lieu of money	Yes	¶ 1738
Stock options, incentive	No	¶ 1923
Strike benefits, generally	Yes	¶ 702
Strike benefits, union and non-union employees in need, paid in form of food, clothes, etc.	No	¶ 702
Supper money, employer-paid, occasional due to overtime work	No	¶ 2089
Supplemental security income (SSI) payments	No	¶ 716
Support payment, received from former spouse as alimony	Yes	¶ 772
Surviving spouse, decedent's salary continued, depending on intent as a gift	No	¶ 719
Survivor annuities, paid to family of public safety officer .	No	¶ 813
Taxes:		
. employees', employer-paid	Yes	¶ 713
. refunds of, not previously deducted or deducted without tax benefit	No	¶ 799
Tenancy, payments for surrender of	Yes	¶ 676

CHECKLISTS

Income Item	Includible in Income	Paragraph Reference
Tips	Yes	¶ 717
Treasure trove	Yes	¶ 785
Treaty-exempt income	No	¶ 2450
Tuition, employer-paid under qualified plans	No	¶ 2067
Unemployment benefit plans, supplemental payments . .	Yes	¶ 722
Unemployment benefits	Yes	¶ 722
U.S. Savings Bonds, earned increase during year, if cash-method taxpayer elects	Yes	¶ 730
Use and occupancy insurance proceeds, income experience	Yes	¶ 877
Vacation fund allowance, union agreement	Yes	¶ 713
Veterans Administration payments	No	¶ 893
Veterans' benefits, generally	No	¶ 891
Veterans' bonuses, state	No	¶ 896
Virtual currency, received for goods or services	Yes	¶ 785
Wages	Yes	¶ 713
Workers' Compensation Acts, payments related to occupational injuries	No	¶ 851
"Wrap-around" annuity contracts sold by life insurance companies, interest on	Yes	¶ 817

¶ 57 Checklist for Deductions

The Internal Revenue Code permits a number of wide-ranging deductions that may be taken into account in arriving at taxable income. The Code contains a number of rules and restrictions concerning the expenses that qualify as deductions and the taxpayers who may claim them. Although deductions generally reduce taxable income, deductions from gross income, available to all qualifying taxpayers, must be distinguished from deductions from adjusted gross income (AGI), available only to those taxpayers who itemize. Certain miscellaneous itemized deductions, including unreimbursed employee business expenses and investment expenses, are deductible by an individual only if the aggregate amount of such deductions exceeds two percent of AGI (¶ 1011). In addition, deductions that can be taken currently must be distinguished from those that can be taken over a number of tax years through depreciation or amortization.

The chart below lists a number of expenses that a taxpayer might incur. The chart indicates for each expense a symbol(s) representing the possible availability of a deduction, its timing, and whether it is deductible from gross income or AGI. Many deductions have special rules. The chart also provides the 2015 *U.S. Master Tax Guide* ® paragraph number where further information on the deduction may be found.

The following symbols are used:

D/GI = Deductible from gross income

D/AGI = Deductible from AGI

D/Am = Deductible over a period of time

ND = Nondeductible

Abandonment of business real property	D/GI, ¶ 1109
Accident and health plans	
. employer contributions	D/GI, ¶ 908
Accounting fees	
. business	D/GI, ¶ 901
. capital transactions . . .	D/Am, ¶ 903
. connected with trade or business	D/GI, ¶ 901
. investors	D/AGI, ¶ 1086
. organization of business ($5,000 deduction and excess amortizable over 15 years)	D/GI, D/Am, ¶ 904
. reorganization of business	ND, ¶ 904
Accounting system, installation	D/GI, ¶ 991
Administrative expenses of estate	D/AGI, ¶ 2925
Admissions to political dinners, programs, inaugural balls, etc.	ND, ¶ 976
Advertising expenses	
. business cards	D/GI, ¶ 969
. catalogs	
. . long term	D/Am, ¶ 969
. generally	D/GI, ¶ 969
. home demonstrations .	D/GI, ¶ 969
. package design costs .	D/GI, ¶ 969
. political convention programs and other political publications .	ND, ¶ 969
. prizes and contests . . .	D/GI, ¶ 969

. product launch costs . .	D/GI, ¶ 969
. promotional activities .	D/GI, ¶ 918
Airline pilot, special clothing	D/AGI, ¶ 1083
Airplane, heavy maintenance expenses	D/GI, ¶ 901
Alcohol fuels credit, unused	D/Am, ¶ 1365I
Alimony payments	D/GI, ¶ 1008
Amortization of premium on taxable bonds (optional) .	D/AGI, ¶ 1012
Appraisal fees	
. acquisition of capital asset	ND, ¶ 990
. connection with trade or business	D/AGI, ¶ 1092
Architect's fees (capital expenditure)	D/Am, ¶ 903
Architectural services	
. domestic production activities	D/GI, ¶ 980F
Attorney's and accountant's fees in contesting tax claims (nonbusiness) . . .	D/AGI, ¶ 1092
Attorney's fees	
. accounting suit by former partner, defense of	D/GI, ¶ 1010A
. acquisition of corporate control	ND, ¶ 237
. business debts, collection of	D/GI, ¶ 1093
. civil rights suits	D/GI, ¶ 1010A
. condemnation proceeding, defense of	ND, ¶ 1010A

Clinical testing deduction if
credit is elected . . . . . . ND, ¶ 1365S
Club dues (limited) . . . . . . D/AGI, ¶ 913A
Coal royalty contracts
. expenses related to . . . ND, ¶ 1289
. if there is no production,
or no income, under
contracts . . . . D/AGI, ¶ 1289
Commissions
. paid as compensation . D/GI, ¶ 906
. sale of real estate or
securities
. . dealers . . . . D/GI, ¶ 1983
. . other taxpayers . . . . ND, ¶ 906
Commissions on sale of real
estate and securities, dealer
only (other than taxpayers
deduct from selling price) D/GI, ¶ 1983
Commuting expenses . . . . ND, ¶ 945
Compensation, reasonable . D/GI, ¶ 906
Computer software (business
use)
. development costs . . . D/GI, D/Am,
¶ 980
. leased software . . . . . D/GI, ¶ 980
. purchased software . . D/Am, ¶ 980
Construction
. domestic production
activities . . . . D/GI, ¶ 980F
Contributions by employer to
employer-financed accident
and health plans for benefit
of employees . . . . D/GI, ¶ 908
Contributions by employer to
state unemployment
insurance and state
disability funds . . . . . . D/GI, ¶ 922
Contributions by members to
a labor union (voluntary) ND, ¶ 1080
Contributions paid (within
certain limits) during year
to charitable, etc.,
organizations . . . . D/AGI, ¶ 1058
Convention (political)
programs, cost of
advertising in . . . . ND, ¶ 976
Conventions (see "Business
conventions")
Cooperative housing
corporation, share of taxes
or interest paid by . . . . D/AGI, ¶ 1040
Copyright costs . . . . D/Am, ¶ 1089
Cost recovery, business
property or property held
for the production of
income . . . . D/Am, ¶ 1747
Credit and debit card
convenience fees for paying
taxes . . . . D/AGI, ¶ 1092

Cruise ship business
conventions (limited) . . . D/GI, ¶ 959
Custodian fees . . . . D/AGI, ¶ 1086
Day care providers
. standard meal deduction
. . . . D/GI, ¶ 964
Defending title to property
(capital expenditure) . . . ND, ¶ 1611
Demolition of structure . . . ND, ¶ 1105
Dependents . . . . D/AGI, ¶ 137
Depletion . . . . D/Am, ¶ 1289
Depreciation, business
property or property held
for production of income . D/Am, ¶ 1747
. election to expense
(limited) . . . . D/GI, ¶ 1747
Diaper service . . . . ND, ¶ 1015
Disbarment proceedings,
attorneys' fees and
expenses in defending . . D/GI, ¶ 981
Doctor's staff privilege fees at
hospital (capital
expenditures) . . . . D/Am, ¶ 981
Domestic production
activities . . . . D/GI, ¶ 980A
Dues
. chamber of commerce . D/GI, ¶ 913A
. charitable, religious,
educational
organizations . . . . . . D/AGI, ¶ 1059
. clubs organized for
business, pleasure,
recreation, or any other
social purpose . . . . . ND, ¶ 913
. professional associations
. . . . D/GI, ¶ 981
. union dues . . . . D/AGI, ¶ 1080
Education expenses
. higher education
expenses (through
2013) . . . . D/GI, ¶ 1082
Education expenses
(employee)
. maintaining or improving
required skills . . . . . D/AGI, ¶ 1082
. minimum requirements
for job . . . . ND, ¶ 1082
. new trade or business . ND, ¶ 1082
Educational assistance plan
payments . . . . D/GI, ¶ 2067
Efficiency engineers' fees . . D/GI, ¶ 901
Electricity
. domestic production
activities . . . . D/GI, ¶ 980
Embezzlement loss . . . . . D/GI, ¶ 1123
Employee's expenses
. entertaining customers
. . reimbursed expenses D/GI, ¶ 915
. . unreimbursed
expenses . . . . 50% D/AGI,
¶ 910

. worthless stock and securities	D/GI, ¶ 1916
Lump sum distribution-ordinary income portion .	D/GI, ¶ 2143
Machinery . incidental repairs	D/GI, ¶ 991
Materials and supplies, business (incidentals) . .	D/GI, ¶ 901
Maternity clothes	ND, ¶ 1016
Meals provided for employees . employer's cost of providing meals on premises	D/GI, ¶ 2089
. meals directly related to business	50% D/GI, ¶ 911
Medical, dental and hospital expenses (to the extent exceeding 10% of adjusted gross income; 7.5% of AGI for taxpayers age 65 or older)	D/AGI, ¶ 59; ¶ 1015
Medical savings account . .	D/GI, ¶ 2035; ¶ 2037
Mine development expenditures	D/GI, ¶ 988
Mine exploration expenditures	D/GI, ¶ 987
Mortgages . insurance premiums (through 2013)	D/AGI, ¶ 1048A
. interest	D/AGI, ¶ 1047
Moving expenses . meals	ND, ¶ 1073
. other expenses . . employee, reimbursed	D/GI, ¶ 1076
. . employee, unreimbursed	D/GI ¶ 1073
. . self employed	D/GI, ¶ 1073
Moving machinery	D/GI, ¶ 901
Musician's clothing, used exclusively in business . .	D/AGI, ¶ 1083
National Labor Relations Board award to employees, payment by employer . . .	D/GI, ¶ 2604
Net operating loss deduction	D/GI, ¶ 1430
New business, cost of starting up ($5,000 deduction and excess amortizable over 15 years)	D/GI, D/Am, ¶ 904
Nonbusiness bad debts (limited)	D/GI, ¶ 1007
Nontrade or nonbusiness expenses incurred in preserving income-producing property	D/AGI, ¶ 1085
Nurse's uniform	D/AGI, ¶ 1083
Office in home (limited) . employee	D/AGI, ¶ 965
. principal place of business	D/GI, ¶ 945
Office supplies	D/GI, ¶ 963
Operating loss in prior or subsequent year	D/GI, ¶ 1145
Organization expenses of corporation ($5,000 deduction and excess amortizable over 15 years)	D/GI, D/Am, ¶ 904
Original construction of greens on a golf course .	ND, ¶ 991
Outside salesperson . meals—see Meals, employees' business . moving expenses—see Moving expenses . travel expenses	D/AGI, ¶ 941B; ¶ 1073
Package design costs	D/GI, ¶ 969
Partners' fixed or guaranteed payments for services or for use of capital (allowed as business deduction to partnership)	D/GI, ¶ 421
Partnership organization expenses, unless election to amortize	ND, ¶ 477
Passport fee, business trip .	D/GI, ¶ 955
Passport fee (except for business purposes)	ND, ¶ 955
Penalties	generally ND, ¶ 972
. Environmental Protection Agency: . . Clean Air Act violation	ND, ¶ 972
. . nonconformance penalty	D/GI, ¶ 972
. penalty on early withdrawal of time deposit	D/GI, ¶ 1111
Performing artists (limitation on gross income) . employee business expenses	D/GI, ¶ 941A
Permanent improvements . business property . . .	D/Am, ¶ 1201
. tenants	D/Am, ¶ 764
"Points" on home mortgage (if customarily required in geographic area in which indebtedness was incurred)	D/AGI, ¶ 1055
Police officer's uniform and cost of cleaning	D/AGI, ¶ 1083
Political contributions . corporations, businesses, etc.	ND, ¶ 976
. individuals	ND, ¶ 976

CHECKLISTS

Political publications, cost of
   advertising in . . . .   ND (generally),
                    ¶ 976

Postage costs, business . . .   D/GI, ¶ 901

Premiums paid on a business
   insurance "professional
   overhead expense disability
   policy" . . . .   D/GI, ¶ 908A

Prepaid interest or finance
   charges . . . .   D/Am, ¶ 1055

Prizes and contests—see
   "Promotional activities"

Professional associations,
   dues
   . unreimbursed employee
     expense . . . .   D/AGI, ¶ 981

Professional books and
   journals and information
   services
   . unreimbursed employee
     expense . . . .   D/AGI, ¶ 981

Promotional activities
   . coupons . . . .   D/GI, ¶ 918
   . prizes and contests . . .   D/GI, ¶ 969

Protective clothing . . . . . .   D/AGI, ¶ 1083

Raffle tickets, cost of . . . . .   ND, ¶ 1061

Railroad retirement tax paid
   by employers . . . .   D/GI, ¶ 716

Railway trainman's uniform   D/AGI, ¶ 1083

Real estate impact fees . . .   ND, ¶ 1288A

Reconditioning and health-
   restoring expenses of
   employees paid by
   employers . . . .   D/GI, ¶ 1016

Refinery property (limited) .   D/GI, ¶ 977C

Reforestation costs . . . . . .   D/GI, D/Am,
                    ¶ 530

Reimbursed expenses
   (otherwise deductible) . .   D/GI, ¶ 942

Removal of architectural and
   transportation barriers to
   the handicapped and
   elderly (limited) . . . . . .   D/AGI, ¶ 1365M

Rent, business property . . .   D/GI, ¶ 986

Reorganization expenditures .
   . . . .   ND, ¶ 904

Repairs to business property .
   . . . .   D/GI, D/Am,
                    ¶ 903

Repairs to personal residence
   . . . .   ND, ¶ 966

Research and experimental
   expenditures connected
   with a trade or business .   D/GI, D/Am,
                    ¶ 979

Restaurant smallwares
   (limited) . . . .   D/GI, ¶ 1825

Retirement plans,
   contributions to
   . employer . . . .   D/GI, ¶ 2115

. individuals (limited) . .   D/GI, ¶ 2121;
                    ¶ 2157;
                    ¶ 2171;
                    ¶ 2183; ¶ 2189

. savings incentive match
   plan for employees
   (SIMPLE) . . . .   D/GI, ¶ 2183;
                    ¶ 2185

. self-employed individuals
   . . . .   D/GI, ¶ 2107

. simplified employee
   pension contributions   D/GI, ¶ 2189

Return, federal or state
   income tax, gift tax, etc.,
   cost of having prepared
   (including investor) . . . .   D/AGI, ¶ 973

Safe deposit boxes, rental for
   protection of income
   producing property
   . investor . . . .   D/AGI, ¶ 1085

Salaries
   . bonuses . . . .   D/GI, ¶ 906
   . commissions . . . . . .   D/GI, ¶ 906
   . related parties . . . . . .   D/GI, ¶ 915

Salespersons' expenses
   . reimbursed . . . .   D/GI, ¶ 942
   . unreimbursed . . . . . .   D/AGI ¶ 942
   . . automobile expenses   D/AGI, ¶ 946
   . . entertaining customers,
     reimbursed . . . . . .   D/GI, ¶ 915
   . . entertaining customers,
     unreimbursed . . . . .   50% D/AGI,
                    ¶ 910
   . . gifts to customers (up
     to $25) . . . .   D/AGI, ¶ 918
   . . membership dues in
     business or social clubs
     . . . .   ND, ¶ 981
   . . subscriptions to
     business, professional
     or trade publications, if
     for business reasons .   D/AGI, ¶ 981
   . . transportation
     expenses,
     unreimbursed . . . . .   D/AGI, ¶ 916
   . . travel expenses . . . .   D/AGI, ¶ 949

Sales tax (state) (through
   2013) . . . .   D/AGI, ¶ 1021

Self-employment tax (limited
   to 50%) . . . .   D/GI, ¶ 2664

Servants, social security taxes
   paid for . . . .   ND, ¶ 923

Severance payments . . . . .   D/GI, ¶ 2075

Shareholder's proxy fight
   expenses . . . .   D/AGI, ¶ 309

Smallwares, restaurant
   (limited) . . . .   D/GI, ¶ 1825

Social Security taxes
   . employees . . . .   ND, ¶ 923
   . employers . . . .   D/GI (only as
                    business
                    expense),
                    ¶ 923

Soil and water conservation
expenditures, farmers . .   D/GI, D/Am,
¶ 982

Stamp taxes
. dealers/investors . . . .   D/GI, ¶ 1611
. trade or business . . . .   D/GI, ¶ 1611
. transfer of personal
residence . . . .   ND, ¶ 1611

Start-up expenditures,
business ($5,000 deduction
and excess amortizable
over 15 years) . . . .   D/GI, D/Am,
¶ 904

Stock redemption costs . . .   ND, ¶ 742

Subscriptions, professional
journals (self-employed) .   D/GI, ¶ 981

Supplemental unemployment
compensation benefits,
repayments by recipients   D/GI, ¶ 1009

Surgeon's uniform
(employee) . . . .   D/AGI, ¶ 1083

Tax penalty payments . . . .   ND, ¶ 972

Tax refresher course,
lawyer's . . . .   D/GI, ¶ 981

Tax returns, cost of
preparation
. business . . . .   D/GI, ¶ 1092
. individual . . . .   D/AGI, ¶ 1092

Taxes . . . .   ¶ 1021
. automobile excise taxes .
. . . .   D/Am, ¶ 126

Teachers, classroom
expenses (through 2013)   D/GI, ¶ 1084

Telephone service (as a
business expense) . . . .   D/GI, ¶ 961

Theft loss
. business . . . .   D/GI, ¶ 1123
. nonbusiness . . . .   D/AGI, ¶ 1123

Timber
. reforestation expenses
($10,000 deduction and
excess amortizable over
7 years) . . . .   D/GI, D/Am,
¶ 1287

. post-establishment
fertilization . . . .   D/GI, ¶ 901

Tires (see "Automobile
expenses" and "Truck
tires")

Title costs (perfecting or
defending title to property,
including costs of
defending condemnation
proceedings) (capital
expenditure) . . . .   D/Am, ¶ 1611

Tools, unreimbursed cost,
useful life of one year or
less . . . .   D/AGI, ¶ 901

Trade association dues,
unreimbursed employee
expenses . . . .   D/AGI, ¶ 981

Trade or business expenses
(securities dealers and
traders) . . . .   D/GI, ¶ 1086

Trademark and trade name
expenditures . . . .   D/Am, ¶ 1288

Transfer taxes . . . .   ND, ¶ 41

Travel expenses (employees)
. commuting expenses .   ND, ¶ 945
. reimbursed . . . .   D/GI, ¶ 954
. unreimbursed . . . . . .   D/AGI, ¶ 952
. . baseball players
(including meals and
lodging) . . . .   D/AGI, ¶ 954
. . business and pleasure
trips . . . .   D/AGI, ¶ 952
. . commercial fishing
boat crew members, for
travel, meals, and
lodging away from
home port . . . .   D/AGI, ¶ 952
. . congressmen, up to
$3,000 of living
expenses . . . .   D/AGI, ¶ 950
. . expenses of traveling
from principal place to
minor place of business
. . . .   D/AGI, ¶ 952
. . government
employees, expenses in
excess of per diem
allowances . . . .   D/AGI, ¶ 953
. . lawyers . . . .   D/AGI, ¶ 981
. . meals, reimbursed . .   D/GI, ¶ 954
. . meals, unreimbursed   50% D/AGI,
¶ 952
. . members of Congress,
up to $3,000 of living
expenses . . . .   D/AGI, ¶ 950
. . National Guard and
Military Reserve
members (limited) . .   D/GI, ¶ 950
. . physician, medical
conventions . . . . . .   D/AGI, ¶ 959
. . railroad employees'
meals and lodging while
away from "home
terminal" . . . .   D/AGI, ¶ 916
. . salespersons . . . . . .   D/AGI, ¶ 1011
. . teachers, scientific
meetings and
conventions . . . . . .   D/AGI, ¶ 959
. . truck drivers' (long
line) meals and lodging
while away from "home
terminal" . . . .   D/AGI, ¶ 949

Truck tires
. replacement tires
(limited) . . . .   D/GI, ¶ 946
. with life less than a year .
. . . .   D/GI, ¶ 946

CHECKLISTS

Truck use tax (unless as
  business expense) ....   ND, ¶ 1021
Uncollectible notes (see "Bad
  debts")
Uniform and special clothing
  costs
  . baseball uniforms ....   D/AGI, ¶ 1083
  . clothing required for
    business ....   D/AGI, ¶ 1083
  . employer-reimbursed
    costs ....   D/GI, ¶ 1083
  . jockey's riding apparel .   D/AGI, ¶ 1083
  . nurses' uniforms ....   D/AGI, ¶ 1083
  . protective clothing ...   D/AGI, ¶ 1083

. work shoes, metal tipped
  ....   D/AGI, ¶ 1083
Union payments
  . dues ....   D/AGI, ¶ 1080
  . fines ....   D/AGI, ¶ 972
Utilities, personal ....   ND, ¶ 963
Wages and salaries ......   D/GI, ¶ 906
Waiters, waitresses
  . special uniforms ....   D/AGI, ¶ 1083
Water, potable
  . domestic production
    activities ....   D/GI, ¶ 980D
Work shoes, metal tipped for
  protection of worker ...   D/AGI, ¶ 1083

¶ 59 Checklist for Medical Expenses

Generally, a medical expense deduction is allowed for expenses incurred in the diagnosis, cure, mitigation, treatment or prevention of disease, or for the purpose of affecting any structure or function of the body for the individual or for the individual's spouse or dependents (¶ 1016). The deduction covers expenses that have not been reimbursed by medical insurance or other sources.

Despite the broad scope of medical expenses, not every expense incurred for medical care is deductible. Also, there is a 10-percent-of-adjusted-gross-income floor on the medical expense deduction for most taxpayers (for tax years ending before January 1, 2017, the floor is 7.5 percent if a taxpayer or spouse is age 65 or older before the close of the tax year). The chart, below, lists specific types of expenses and whether or not a deduction for the expense is permitted. The user can easily check whether an official determination has been made as to the deductibility of a particular type of expense.

Medical Expense	Deductible	Authority
Abortion		
. legal	Yes	Rev. Rul. 73-201, 1973-1 CB 140, as clarified by Rev. Rul. 73-603, 1973-2 CB 76, and Rev. Rul. 97-9, 1997-1 CB 77
Accident and health insurance		
. medical care portion separately stated and reasonable in amount	Yes	Code Sec. 213(d)(1)(D) and (d)(6); Reg. § 1.213-1(e)(4)
. medical care portion not separately stated or, if separately stated, not reasonable in amount	No	Code Sec. 213(d)(6)(A); Reg. § 1.213-1(e)(4)
Acupuncture	Yes	Rev. Rul. 72-593, 1972-2 CB 180
Adoption		
. medical costs of adopted child	Yes	Rev. Rul. 60-255, 1960-2 CB 105
. medical costs of natural mother	No	*B.L. Kilpatrick,* 68 TC 469, Dec. 34,493
Air conditioner		
. allergy relief	Yes	Rev. Rul. 55-261, 1955-1 CB 307
. cystic fibrosis relief	Yes	*R. Gerard,* 37 TC 826, Dec. 25,331 (Acq.)
. detachable, for sick person's use only	Yes	Reg. § 1.213-1(e)(1)(iii)
. permanent improvement to property (if not directly related to medical care)	No	Reg. § 1.213-1(e)(1)(iii); *G.W. Wade,* 61-2 USTC ¶ 9709
Alcoholism, treatment of	Yes	Rev. Rul. 73-325, 1973-2 CB 75
Ambulance hire	Yes	Reg. § 1.213-1(e)(1)(ii)
Anticipated medical expenses	No	*W.B. Andrews,* 37 TCM 744, Dec. 35,144(M), TC Memo. 1978-174
Attendant to accompany blind or deaf student	Yes	Rev. Rul. 64-173, 1964-1 CB (Part 1) 121; *R.A. Baer Est.,* 26 TCM 170, Dec. 28,352(M), TC Memo. 1967-34
Automobile (see Car)		
Baby sitting expenses to enable parent to see doctor	No	Rev. Rul. 78-266, 1978-2 CB 123
Birth control pills	Yes	Rev. Rul. 73-200, 1973-1 CB 140
Blind persons		
. attendant to accompany student	Yes	Rev. Rul. 64-173, 1964-1 (Part I) CB 121
. braille books and magazines, excess cost over cost of regular editions	Yes	Rev. Rul. 75-318, 1975-2 CB 88
. seeing-eye dog	Yes	Rev. Rul. 55-261, 1955-1 CB 307

Medical Expense	Deductible	Authority
. special education (see Schools, special)		
. special educational aids to mitigate condition	Yes	Rev. Rul. 58-223, 1958-1 CB 156
Breast pumps and supplies	Yes	Announcement 2011-14, 2011-9 IRB 532
Capital expenditures		
. home modifications for handicapped individual	Yes	Rev. Rul. 87-106, 1987-2 CB 67
. permanent improvement to property, if not directly related to medical care	No	Reg. § 1.213-1(e)(1)(iii)
. primary purpose medical care	Yes	Reg. § 1.213-1(e)(1)(iii)
Car		
. depreciation on	No	*M.S. Gordon,* 37 TC 986, Dec. 25,364; *R.K. Weary,* CA-10, 75-1 USTC ¶ 9173, *cert. denied,* 423 US 838
. equipping to accommodate wheelchair passengers, excess cost of	Yes	Rev. Rul. 70-606, 1970-2 CB 66
. insurance, medical coverage for persons other than taxpayer, spouse and children	No	Rev. Rul. 73-483, 1973-2 CB 75
. special controls for a person with a disability	Yes	Rev. Rul. 66-80, 1966-1 CB 57
Chauffeur, salary of	No	*W.E. Buck,* 47 TC 113, Dec. 28,175
Chemical dependency treatment (see Alcoholism, treatment of, and Drug addiction, recovery from)		
Childbirth preparation classes		
. "coach"	No	IRS Letter Ruling 8919009
. mother, for obstetrical care	Yes	IRS Letter Ruling 8919009
Chiropractors	Yes	Rev. Rul. 55-261, 1955-1 CB 307, as modified by Rev. Rul. 63-91, 1963-1 CB 54
Christian Science practitioners	Yes	Rev. Rul. 55-261, 1955-1 CB 307, as modified by Rev. Rul. 63-91, 1963-1 CB 54
Clarinet and lessons, alleviation of severe teeth malocclusion	Yes	Rev. Rul. 62-210, 1962-2 CB 89
Clothing, suitable for use other than therapy	No	*M.C. Montgomery,* 51 TC 410, Dec. 29,270, aff'd on other issues, CA-6, 70-2 USTC ¶ 9466
Computer data bank, storage and retrieval of medical records	Yes	Rev. Rul. 71-282, 1971-2 CB 166
Contact lenses	Yes	Reg. § 1.213-1(e)(1)(iii); Rev. Rul. 74-429, 1974-2 CB 83
. replacement insurance	Yes	Rev. Rul. 74-429, 1974-2 CB 83
Contraceptives, prescription	Yes	Rev. Rul. 73-200, 1973-1 CB 140
Cosmetic surgery		
. necessary to ameliorate a deformity arising from a congenital abnormality, personal injury, or disfiguring disease	Yes	Code Sec. 213(d)(9); Senate Finance Committee Report to P.L. 101-508
. unnecessary	No	Code Sec. 213(d)(9); Senate Finance Committee Report to P.L. 101-508
Crime victims, compensated medical expenses of	No	Rev. Rul. 74-74, 1974-1 CB 18
Crutches	Yes	Reg. § 1.213-1(e)(1)(iii)

Medical Expense	Deductible	Authority
Dancing lessons	No	*R.C. France,* CA-6, 82-1 USTC ¶ 9225, aff'g 40 TCM 508, Dec. 37,023(M), TC Memo. 1980-215
Deaf persons		
. hearing aid	Yes	Rev. Rul. 55-261, 1955-1 CB 307
. hearing-aid animal	Yes	Rev. Rul. 68-295, 1968-1 CB 92
. lip reading expenses for the deaf	Yes	Rev. Rul. 55-261, 1955-1 CB 307
. notetaker, deaf student	Yes	*R.A. Baer Est.,* 26 TCM 170, Dec. 28,352(M), TC Memo. 1967-34
. special education (see Schools, special)		
. telephone, specially equipped, including repairs	Yes	Rev. Rul. 71-48, 1971-1 CB 99, as amplified by Rev. Rul. 73-53, 1973-1 CB 139
. television, closed-caption decoder	Yes	Rev. Rul. 80-340, 1980-2 CB 81
. visual alert system	Yes	IRS Letter Ruling 8250040
Dental fees	Yes	Reg. § 1.213-1(e)(1)(ii)
Dentures (artificial teeth)	Yes	Reg. § 1.213-1(e)(1)(ii)
Deprogramming services	No	IRS Letter Ruling 8021004
Diagnostic fees	Yes	Reg. § 1.213-1(e)(1)(ii)
Diapers		
. diaper service	No	Rev. Rul. 55-261, 1955-1 CB 307
. disposable, to alleviate severe neurological disease	Yes	IRS Letter Ruling 8137085
Doctors' fees	Yes	Reg. § 1.213-1(e)(1)(i); Rev. Rul. 55-261, 1955-1 CB 307
Domestic aid, for nursing-type service	Yes	Rev. Rul. 58-339, 1958-2 CB 106
Drug addiction, recovery from	Yes	Rev. Rul. 72-226, 1972-1 CB 96
Drugs and medicines		
. illegal/controlled substances, even when prescribed	No	Rev. Rul. 97-9, 1997-1 CB 77
. over-the-counter (non-prescription)	No	Code Sec. 213(b); Rev. Rul. 2003-58, 2003-1 CB 959
. prescription, legal	Yes	Code Sec. 213(b)
Dust elimination system	No	*F.S. Delp,* 30 TC 1230, Dec. 23,167
Dyslexia, language training	Yes	Rev. Rul. 69-607, 1969-2 CB 40
Ear piercing	No	Rev. Rul. 82-111, 1982-1 CB 48
Electrolysis	No	Code Sec. 213(d)(9); Senate Finance Committee Report to P.L. 101-508
Elevator, alleviation of cardiac condition	Yes	Reg. § 1.213-1(e)(1)(iii); *J.E. Berry,* DC Okla., 58-2 USTC ¶ 9870, 174 FSupp 748; Rev. Rul. 59-411, 1959-2 CB 100, as modified by Rev. Rul. 83-33, 1983-1 CB 70
Equipment, supplies, or diagnostic devices for medical care, non-prescription	Yes	Rev. Rul. 2003-58, 2003-1 CB 959
Eye examinations and glasses	Yes	Reg. § 1.213-1(e)(1)(ii) and (iii)
Fallout shelter, prevention of disease	No	*F.H. Daniels,* 41 TC 324, Dec. 26,414
Fertility enhancement	Yes	IRS Letter Ruling 200318017; IRS Pub. 502
Fluoride device; on advice of dentist	Yes	Rev. Rul. 64-267, 1964-2 CB 69
Founder's fee, prepaid, to retirement home; portion attributable to medical care	Yes	Rev. Rul. 76-481, 1976-2 CB 82, as clarified by Rev. Rul. 93-72, 1993-2 CB 77
Funeral expenses	No	*K.P. Carr,* 39 TCM 253, Dec. 36,352(M), TC Memo. 1979-400

CHECKLISTS

Medical Expense	Deductible	Authority
Furnace	No	*J.L. Seymour,* 14 TC 1111, Dec. 17,675
Glasses	Yes	Reg. § 1.213-1(e)(1)(ii)
Gravestone	No	*C.W. Libby Est.,* 14 TCM 699, Dec. 21,110(M), TC Memo. 1955-180
Guide animals (see Service animals)		
Hair transplants, surgical	No	Code Sec. 213(d)(9); Senate Finance Committee Report to P.L. 101-508
Halfway house or specially selected home, for adjustment from mental hospital	Yes	Rev. Rul. 69-499, 1969-2 CB 39; IRS Letter Ruling 7714016
Handicapped persons (see, also, specific handicap or equipment)		
. home modification (see Capital expenses)		
. special training or education (see Schools, special)		
Health club dues		
. not related to a particular medical condition	No	Rev. Rul. 55-261, 1955-1 CB 307
. prescribed by physician for medical condition	Yes	Rev. Rul. 55-261, 1955-1 CB 307
Health Maintenance Organization (HMO)	Yes	Reg. § 1.213-1(e)(4); IRS Pub. 502
Hearing aids (see Deaf persons)		
Hospital care, in-patient	Yes	Reg. § 1.213-1(e)(1)(v)
Hospital services	Yes	Reg. § 1.213-1(e)(1)(ii)
Hygienic supplies	No	Reg. § 1.213-1(e)(2); *O.G. Russell,* 12 TCM 1276, Dec. 19,973(M)
Indian medicine man	Yes	*R.H. Tso,* 40 TCM 1277, Dec. 37,260(M), TC Memo. 1980-339
Insulin	Yes	Code Sec. 213(b)
Insurance		
. accident and health insurance (see Accident and health insurance)		
. hospital insurance (HI) payroll tax paid	No	Rev. Rul. 66-216, 1966-2 CB 100
. long term care insurance (within limits)	Yes	Code Secs. 213(d)(1)(D) and 7702B
. Medicare A premiums (voluntarily enrolled taxpayer)	Yes	Rev. Rul. 79-175, 1979-1 CB 117
. Medicare B premiums	Yes	Reg. § 1.213-1(e)(4)
. premiums for loss of income	No	Reg. § 1.213-1(e)(4)
. premiums for loss of life, limb or sight	No	Reg. § 1.213-1(e)(4)
. premiums for medical care	Yes	Reg. § 1.213-1(e)(4)
. self-employed	Yes	Code Sec. 162(l)
Iron lung	Yes	Rev. Rul. 55-261, 1955-1 CB 307
Laboratory fees	Yes	Reg. § 1.213-1(e)(1)(ii)
Lactation expenses	Yes	Announcement 2011-14, 2011-9 IRB 532
Laetrile, prescribed	No	Rev. Rul. 97-9, 1997-1 CB 77
Lamaze classes (see Childbirth preparation classes)		
Laser eye surgery	Yes	Rev. Rul. 2003-57, 2003-1 CB 959
Lead paint, removal	Yes	Rev. Rul. 79-66, 1979-1 CB 114
Legal expenses		
. authorization of treatment for mental illness	Yes	Rev. Rul. 71-281, 1971-2 CB 165
. divorce upon medical advice	No	*J.H. Jacobs,* 62 TC 813, Dec. 32,773

¶59

Medical Expense	Deductible	Authority
Lifetime medical care fee, prepaid, to retirement home; portion attributable to medical care	Yes	Rev. Rul. 75-302, 1975-2 CB 86, Rev. Rul. 75-303, 1975-2 CB 87, as clarified by Rev. Rul. 93-72, 1993-2 CB 77
Limbs, artificial	Yes	Reg. § 1.213-1(e)(1)(ii)
Lodging		
. care not provided in hospital or equivalent outpatient facility	No	*A.L. Polyak,* 94 TC 337, Dec. ¶ 46,443
. limited to $50 per night per person	Yes	Code Sec. 213(d)(2)
Long term care expenses	Yes	Code Secs. 213(d)(1)(C) and 7702B
Marriage counseling	No	Rev. Rul. 75-319, 1975-2 CB 88
Maternity clothes	No	Rev. Rul. 55-261, 1955-1 CB 307
Mattress, prescribed for alleviation of arthritis	Yes	Rev. Rul. 55-261, 1955-1 CB 307
Nursing home, medical reasons	Yes	*W.B. Counts,* 42 TC 755, Dec. 26,893 (Acq.)
Nursing services (including board and employer's portion of social security tax if paid by taxpayer)	Yes	Reg. § 1.213-1(e)(1)(ii); Rev. Rul. 57-489, 1957-2 CB 207
Obstetrical expenses	Yes	Reg. § 1.213-1(e)(1)(ii)
Operations		
. illegal	No	Reg. § 1.213-1(e)(1)(ii)
. legal	Yes	Reg. § 1.213-1(e)(1)(ii)
Optometrists	Yes	Rev. Rul. 55-261, 1955-1 CB 307
Orthodontia	Yes	Reg. § 1.213-1(e)(1)(ii)
Orthopedic shoes, excess cost	Yes	IRS Letter Ruling 8221118
Osteopaths	Yes	Rev. Rul. 55-261, 1955-1 CB 307, as modified by Rev. Rul. 63-91, 1963-1 CB 54
Oxygen equipment, breathing difficulty	Yes	Rev. Rul. 55-261, 1955-1 CB 307
Patterning exercises, handicapped child	Yes	Rev. Rul. 70-170, 1970-1 CB 51
Plumbing, special fixtures for handicapped	Yes	Rev. Rul. 70-395, 1970-2 CB 65
Pregnancy test kit	Yes	IRS Pub. 502
Prosthesis	Yes	Reg. § 1.213-1(e)(1)(ii)
Psychiatric care	Yes	Rev. Rul. 55-261, 1955-1 CB 307
Psychologists	Yes	Rev. Rul. 63-91, 1963-1 CB 54
Psychotherapists	Yes	Rev. Rul. 63-91, 1963-1 CB 54
Reclining chair for cardiac patient	Yes	Rev. Rul. 58-155, 1958-1 CB 156
Reconstructive surgery, after mastectomy for breast cancer	Yes	Rev. Rul. 2003-57, 2003-1 CB 959
Remedial reading for dyslexic child	Yes	Rev. Rul. 69-607, 1969-2 CB 40
Residence, loss on sale, move medically recommended	No	Rev. Rul. 68-319, 1968-1 CB 92
Retirement home, cost of medical care	Yes	Reg. § 1.213-1(e)(1)(v); *H.W. Smith Est.,* 79 TC 313, Dec. 39,273 (Acq.)
Sanitarium rest home, cost of medical care (and meals and lodging, if warranted by individual's condition)	Yes	Reg. § 1.213-1(e)(1)(v)
Schools, special, relief of handicap	Yes	Reg. § 1.213-1(e)(1)(v); Rev. Rul. 58-533, 1958-2 CB 108; Rev. Rul. 70-285, 1970-1 CB 52; Rev. Rul. 78-340, 1978-2 CB 124
Scientology "audits" and "processing"	No	*D.H. Brown,* CA-8, 75-2 USTC ¶ 9718, *aff'g* 62 TC 551, Dec. 32,701; Rev. Rul. 78-190, 1978-1 CB 74

CHECKLISTS

Medical Expense	*Deductible*	*Authority*
Self-help, medical	No	*B. Doody,* 32 TCM 547, Dec. 32,006(M), TC Memo. 1973-126
Service animals		
. hearing-aid animal	Yes	Rev. Rul. 68-295, 1968-1 CB 92
. other	Yes	Senate Finance Committee Report to P.L. 100-647
. seeing-eye dog	Yes	Reg. § 1.213-1(e)(1)(iii); Rev. Rul. 55-261, 1955-1 CB 307
Sexual dysfunction, therapy for	Yes	Rev. Rul. 75-187, 1975-1 CB 92
Smoking, program to stop	Yes	Rev. Rul. 99-28, 1999-1 CB 1269
Spiritual guidance	No	*M. Miller,* 40 TCM 243, Dec. 36,911(M), TC Memo. 1980-136
Sterilization operation, legal	Yes	Rev. Rul. 73-603, 1973-2 CB 76, clarifying Rev. Rul. 73-201, 1973-1 CB 140
Swimming pool, treatment of polio or arthritis	Yes	*C.B. Mason,* DC Hawaii, 57-2 USTC ¶ 10,012; Rev. Rul. 83-33, 1983-1 CB 70
Tattoos	No	Rev. Rul. 82-111, 1982-1 CB 48
Taxicab to doctor's office	Yes	Rev. Rul. 55-261, 1955-1 CB 307
Teeth		
. artificial	Yes	Reg. § 1.213-1(e)(1)(ii)
. whitening procedure	No	Rev. Rul. 2003-57, 2003-1 CB 959
Telephone, specially equipped		
. deaf persons	Yes	Rev. Rul. 71-48, 1971-1 CB 99, amplified by Rev. Rul. 73-53, 1973-1 CB 139
. modified for person in an iron lung	Yes	Rev. Rul. 55-261, 1955-1 CB 307
Television, closed caption decoder	Yes	Rev. Rul. 80-34, 1980-2 CB 81
Therapy, received as medical treatment	Yes	Reg. § 1.213-1(e)(1)(ii)
Toilet articles	No	Reg. § 1.213-1(e)(2); *O.G. Russell,* 12 TCM 1276, Dec. 19,973(M)
Transplant, donor's costs of	Yes	Rev. Rul. 68-452, 1968-2 CB 111; Rev. Rul. 73-189, 1973-1 CB 139
Transportation, cost incurred essentially and primarily for medical care	Yes	Code Sec. 213(d)(1)(B); Reg. § 1.213-1(e)(1)(iv)
Trips, general health improvement	No	Reg. § 1.213-1(e)(1)(ii) and (iv)
Vacations, health restorative	No	Reg. § 1.213-1(e)(1)(ii) and (iv); Rev. Rul. 57-130, 1957-1 CB 108
Vacuum cleaner, alleviation of dust allergy	No	Rev. Rul. 76-80, 1976-1 CB 71
Vasectomy, legal	Yes	Rev. Rul. 73-201, 1973-1 CB 140, clarified by Rev. Rul. 73-603, 1973-2 CB 76, and Rev. Rul. 97-9, 1997-1 CB 77
Visual alert system for hearing impaired	Yes	IRS Letter Ruling 8250040
Weight loss program		
. for treatment of specific disease	Yes	Rev. Rul. 2002-19, 2002-1 CB 778
. to improve appearance, prescribed	No	Rev. Rul. 79-151, 1979-1 CB 116; IRS Pub. 502
Wheelchair	Yes	Reg. § 1.213-1(e)(1)(iii)
Wig, prescribed to alleviate mental discomfort resulting from disease	Yes	Rev. Rul. 62-189, 1962-2 CB 88
X-rays	Yes	Reg. § 1.213-1(e)(1)(ii)

¶ 61 Checklist for Credits

The Internal Revenue Code provides for a number of credits that may be taken into account when arriving at a tax liability. A tax credit directly reduces a taxpayer's tax liability dollar for dollar, rather than reducing the taxpayer's taxable income as a deduction does. Both individual and business taxpayers are eligible for tax credits, and certain credits are available to both types of taxpayers.

The two charts below show the availability of the nonbusiness and business credits. All paragraph references are to the 2015 *U.S. Master Tax Guide* ®. The date ranges are time periods for which the credits are available for calendar-year taxpayers. Fiscal-year taxpayers should consult the referenced paragraph to determine if any special requirements are applicable.

Nonbusiness Credits

Nonbusiness Credits	Years Available	Paragraph Reference
Adoption credit:		
. nonrefundable	After 12/31/2011	¶ 1307
. refundable	1/1/2010—12/31/2011	¶ 1326A
Alternative fuel vehicle refueling property credit:		
. non-hydrogen property	1/1/2006—12/31/2013	¶ 1355
. hydrogen property	Until 12/31/2014	¶ 1355
Alternative motor vehicle credit:		
. fuel cell motor vehicle credit	Until 12/31/2014	¶ 1346
. plug-in electric motor vehicle conversion credit	2/18/2009—12/31/2011	¶ 1350
Child and dependent care credit	Permanent	¶ 1301
Child tax credit	Permanent	¶ 1305
COBRA premium credit	9/1/2008—8/31/2011	¶ 1391
Earned income credit	Permanent	¶ 1322
Educational credits:		
. American Opportunity credit	1/1/2009—12/31/2017	¶ 1303
. Hope scholarship credit	After 12/31/2017	¶ 1303
. lifetime learning credit	Permanent	¶ 1303
Elderly and permanently and totally disabled credit	Permanent	¶ 1302
First-time homebuyer credit:		
. certain military personnel	1/1/2009—4/30/2011	¶ 1324
First-time homebuyer credit for the District of Columbia	Until 12/31/2011	¶ 1308
Foreign tax credit	Permanent	¶ 2475
Health insurance costs credit:		
. for TAA and/or alternative TAA eligible individuals	Until 12/31/2013	¶ 1332
. for PBGC eligible individuals	Until 12/31/2013	¶ 1332
Health insurance premium assistance credit	After 12/31/2013	¶ 1331
Minimum tax credit:		
. nonrefundable	Permanent	¶ 1309
. refundable	12/20/2006—12/31/2012	¶ 1327
Mortgage interest credit	Permanent	¶ 1306
Mutual fund capital gains credit	Permanent	¶ 1330
Nonbusiness energy property credit:		
. lifetime limit of $500	1/1/2011—12/31/2013	¶ 1341
Plug-in electric drive motor vehicle credit:		
. generally	1/1/2010 until phased out	¶ 1351
. 2- and 3-wheeled vehicles	1/1/2012—12/31/2013	¶ 1351
Plug-in electric vehicle credit for small vehicles	2/18/2009—12/31/2011	¶ 1354

Nonbusiness Credits	*Years Available*	*Paragraph Reference*
Residential energy efficient property credit	Until 12/31/2016	¶ 1342
Retirement savings contributions credit	Permanent	¶ 1304
Tax credit bonds:		
. build America bond credit	Bonds issued between 2/18/2009—12/31/2010	¶ 1378
. new clean renewable energy bond credit	Bonds issued after 10/3/2008	¶ 1374
. qualified energy conservation bond credit	Bonds issued after 10/3/2008	¶ 1375
. qualified forestry conservation bond credit	Bonds issued between 5/23/2008—5/22/2010	¶ 1373
. school construction bond credit .	Bonds issued between 2/18/2009—12/31/2010	¶ 1377
. zone academy bond credit	Bonds issued between 10/4/2008—12/31/2011	¶ 1376
Withheld tax on wages credit	Permanent	¶ 1321

Business Credits

Business Credits	*Years Available*	*Paragraph Reference*
Agricultural chemicals security credit .	5/23/2008—12/31/2012	¶ 1365HH
Alcohol fuels credit:		
. second generation biofuel	1/1/2009—12/31/2013	¶ 1365I
. other alcohol fuels	Until 12/31/2011	¶ 1365I
Alternative fuel vehicle refueling property credit:		
. non-hydrogen property	Until 12/31/2013	¶ 1355
. hydrogen property	Until 12/31/2014	¶ 1355
Alternative motor vehicle credit:		
. fuel cell motor vehicle credit . . .	Until 12/31/2014	¶ 1346
. plug-in electric motor vehicle conversion credit	2/18/2009—12/31/2011	¶ 1350
Biodiesel and renewable diesel fuels credit:		
. small agri-biodiesel producer credit	Until 12/31/2013	¶ 1365X
. renewable biodiesel	Until 12/31/2013	¶ 1365X
. other biodiesel	Until 12/31/2013	¶ 1365X
Carbon dioxide sequestration credit . . .	10/3/2008—until phased out	¶ 1365JJ
Coal production credit	Permanent	¶ 1365D
Disabled access credit	Permanent	¶ 1365M
Distilled spirits excise tax carrying credit	Permanent	¶ 1365Z
Electricity produced from renewable resources credit (available 5 to 10 years after facilities are placed into service):		
. Indian coal production facilities . .	Placed in service before 1/1/2009	¶ 1365N
. refined coal facilities	Placed in service before 12/31/2011	¶ 1365N
. small irrigation power facilities . .	Placed in service before 10/3/2008	¶ 1365N
. all other facilities	Construction begining before 1/1/2014	¶ 1365N

Business Credits	Years Available	Paragraph Reference
Employer credit for differential wage payments to military personnel	Until 12/31/2013	¶ 1365II
Employer credit for providing child care	Permanent	¶ 1365V
Empowerment zone credit	Until 12/31/2013	¶ 1365O
Energy credit	Permanent[1]	¶ 1365C
Energy efficient appliance credit	Until 12/31/2013	¶ 1365DD
Energy efficient home credit	Until 12/31/2013	¶ 1365CC
Energy project credit	After 2/17/2009	¶ 1365F
Federal excise fuel tax credit	Permanent	¶ 1329
FICA tip credit	Permanent	¶ 1365R
Foreign tax credit	Permanent	¶ 2475
Gasification project credit	Permanent	¶ 1365E
General business credit	See specific credit component	¶ 1365
Health insurance credit for small employers	After 12/31/2009	¶ 1333
Indian employment credit	Until 12/31/2013	¶ 1365Q
Investment credit	See specific credit component	¶ 1365A
Low-income housing credit	Permanent	¶ 1365K
Low sulfur diesel fuel production credit	Permanent	¶ 1365Y
Mine rescue team training credit	Until 12/31/2013	¶ 1365GG
Minimum tax credit	Permanent	¶ 1309
New markets tax credit	Until 12/31/2013; carryover amounts until 12/31/2018	¶ 1365T
Nonconventional source fuel production credit	For coke or coke gas produced before 1/1/2010 that is sold no later than four years after the coke or coke gas is first sold	¶ 1365BB
Nuclear power facilities production credit	Until 12/31/2020	¶ 1365AA
Orphan drug credit	Permanent	¶ 1365S
Pension plan startup costs credit for small employers	Permanent	¶ 1365U
Plug-in electric drive motor vehicle credit:		
. generally	1/1/2010 until phased out	¶ 1351
. 2- and 3-wheeled vehicles	1/1/2012—12/31/2013	¶ 1351
Plug-in electric vehicle credit for small vehicles	2/18/2009—12/31/2011	¶ 1354
Puerto Rico and U.S. possessions credit (available only to existent claimants from American Samoan companies) .	Until 12/31/2013	¶ 1362
Railroad track maintenance credit	Until 12/31/2013	¶ 1365W
Rehabilitation credit	Permanent	¶ 1365B
Research credit	Until 12/31/2013	¶ 1365J
Work opportunity credit:		
. generally	Until 12/31/2013	¶ 1365G
. qualified veteran	11/22/2011—12/31/2013	¶ 1365G

[1] Exceptions apply.

¶ 63 Checklist for Forms

The following chart lists key forms in use by the IRS and provides paragraph references to the main discussions of those forms in the 2015 *U.S. Master Tax Guide* ®.

Form	Paragraph reference	Form	Paragraph reference
56	¶ 2747	1040, Schedule B	¶ 105
433-A	¶ 2723	1040, Schedule C	¶ 105
433-B	¶ 2723	1040, Schedule D	¶ 128
656	¶ 2723	1040, Schedule E	¶ 105
706	¶ 2938; ¶ 2944	1040, Schedule EIC	¶ 1322
706, Schedule A	¶ 2912	1040, Schedule F	¶ 767
706, Schedule A-1	¶ 2922	1040, Schedule H	¶ 2652
706, Schedule B	¶ 2912	1040, Schedule J	¶ 767
706, Schedule C	¶ 2912	1040, Schedule R	¶ 1302
706, Schedule D	¶ 2915	1040, Schedule SE	¶ 2664
706, Schedule E	¶ 2919	1040A	¶ 105
706, Schedule F	¶ 2912	1040A, Schedule EIC	¶ 1322
706, Schedule G	¶ 2913; ¶ 2914	1040-C	¶ 2411
706, Schedule H	¶ 2918	1040-ES	¶ 2685
706, Schedule I	¶ 2917	1040-EZ	¶ 105
706, Schedule J	¶ 2925	1040NR	¶ 2425
706, Schedule K	¶ 2925	1040NR-EZ	¶ 2425
706, Schedule L	¶ 2925	1040-PR	¶ 2501
706, Schedule M	¶ 2926	1040-SS	¶ 2501
706, Schedule O	¶ 2932	1040-V	¶ 2525
706, Schedule Q	¶ 2934	1040X	¶ 2505
706, Schedule R	¶ 2944	1041	¶ 510
706, Schedule R-1	¶ 2944	1041, Schedule I	¶ 1401
706-A	¶ 2922	1041, Schedule J	¶ 567
706-CE	¶ 2934	1041, Schedule K-1	¶ 510
706-D	¶ 2937	1041-A	¶ 537
706-GS(D)	¶ 2944	1041-ES	¶ 511
706-GS(T)	¶ 2944	1041-QFT	¶ 575
706-NA	¶ 2940	1041-T	¶ 511
709	¶ 2910	1042	¶ 2455
712	¶ 2915	1042-S	¶ 2455
843	¶ 2813	1042-T	¶ 2455
851	¶ 295	1045	¶ 1145
866	¶ 2721	1065	¶ 406
870	¶ 2712	1065, Schedule D	¶ 1758
906	¶ 2721	1065, Schedule K-1	¶ 406
911	¶ 2707	1066	¶ 2343
940	¶ 2650	1066, Schedule Q	¶ 2344
941	¶ 2650	1098	¶ 2565
943	¶ 2650	1098-C	¶ 1070A
944	¶ 2650	1098-E	¶ 2565
945	¶ 2650	1098-T	¶ 2565
966	¶ 211	1099-A	¶ 2565
970	¶ 1565	1099-B	¶ 2565
972	¶ 259	1099-C	¶ 2565
973	¶ 259	1099-DIV	¶ 2565
976	¶ 2317	1099-G	¶ 2565
982	¶ 855	1099-H	¶ 2565
990	¶ 625	1099-INT	¶ 2565
990, Schedule C	¶ 613	1099-K	¶ 2565
990-BL	¶ 625	1099-MISC	¶ 2565
990-EZ	¶ 625	1099-OID	¶ 1952
990-PF	¶ 625	1099-PATR	¶ 2565
990-T	¶ 658	1099-R	¶ 2565
990-W	¶ 633	1099-S	¶ 2565
1023	¶ 623	1116	¶ 2476
1024	¶ 692	1118	¶ 2476
1028	¶ 698	1120	¶ 211
1040	¶ 105	1120, Schedule PH	¶ 275
1040, Schedule A	¶ 1011	1120, Schedule UTP	¶ 2501

Form	Paragraph reference
1120-C	¶ 698
1120-F	¶ 2425
1120-FSC	¶ 2501
1120-H	¶ 699
1120-IC-DISC	¶ 2501
1120-L	¶ 2370
1120-ND	¶ 2501
1120-PC	¶ 2501
1120-POL	¶ 696
1120-REIT	¶ 2326
1120-RIC	¶ 2301
1120S	¶ 351
1120-SF	¶ 2501
1120X	¶ 2759
1122	¶ 295
1127	¶ 2537
1128	¶ 1513
1138	¶ 1145
1139	¶ 2773
1310	¶ 178
2063	¶ 2411
2106	¶ 942; ¶ 1215
2120	¶ 147
2210	¶ 2875
2210-F	¶ 2875
2220	¶ 241
2350	¶ 2509
2438	¶ 2305; ¶ 2329
2439	¶ 1330; ¶ 2305; ¶ 2329
2441	¶ 1301
2553	¶ 306
2555	¶ 2408
2555-EZ	¶ 2408
2848	¶ 2708A
3115	¶ 1529
3468	¶ 1365A
3520	¶ 588
3520-A	¶ 588
3800	¶ 1365
3903	¶ 1073
3921	¶ 2565
3922	¶ 2565
4070	¶ 2605
4070A	¶ 717
4136	¶ 1329
4137	¶ 717
4255	¶ 1365A
4361	¶ 2667
4466	¶ 247
4562	¶ 1201; ¶ 1208; ¶ 1214
4563	¶ 2414
4626	¶ 1401
4684	¶ 1121; ¶ 1123
4720	¶ 590A; ¶ 610; ¶ 614; ¶ 617; ¶ 635; ¶ 637
4768	¶ 2938
4797	¶ 1208; ¶ 1211; ¶ 1713; ¶ 1747; ¶ 1779
4868	¶ 2509
4876-A	¶ 2498
4952	¶ 1094
4970	¶ 567
4972	¶ 2143
5213	¶ 1195

Form	Paragraph reference
5227	¶ 537
5304-SIMPLE	¶ 2181
5305-SEP	¶ 2189
5305-SIMPLE	¶ 2181
5329	¶ 2127; ¶ 2151; ¶ 2161; ¶ 2169; ¶ 2173
5405	¶ 1324
5471	¶ 2487
5498	¶ 2565
5500	¶ 2137
5500-SF	¶ 2137
5558	¶ 2137
5695	¶ 1341; ¶ 1342
5713	¶ 2496
5735	¶ 1362
5768	¶ 613
5884	¶ 1365G
6198	¶ 1155
6251	¶ 1401
6252	¶ 1801
6478	¶ 1365I
6765	¶ 1365J
6781	¶ 1948
7004	¶ 2509
8027	¶ 2605
8082	¶ 415
8275	¶ 2856; ¶ 2858; ¶ 2863
8275-R	¶ 2856; ¶ 2858; ¶ 2863
8282	¶ 627
8283	¶ 1070A
8288	¶ 2442
8288-A	¶ 2442
8288-B	¶ 2442
8300	¶ 2565
8332	¶ 139A
8379	¶ 163
8396	¶ 1306
8582	¶ 1169
8582-CR	¶ 1169
8586	¶ 1365K
8594	¶ 1620
8596	¶ 2565
8596-A	¶ 2565
8606	¶ 2160; ¶ 2165; ¶ 2173¶ 2173; ¶ 2177
8611	¶ 1365K
8615	¶ 103
8621	¶ 2490
8689	¶ 2416
8716	¶ 1501
8801	¶ 1309; ¶ 1327
8802	¶ 2450
8804	¶ 2503
8809	¶ 2455
8810	¶ 1169
8811	¶ 2343
8812	¶ 1305
8814	¶ 103
8815	¶ 863
8818	¶ 863
8820	¶ 1365S
8822	¶ 2711
8822-B	¶ 2711
8824	¶ 1721; ¶ 1732

Form	Paragraph reference	Form	Paragraph reference
8825	¶ 1169	8907	¶ 1365BB
8826	¶ 1365M	8908	¶ 1365CC
8827	¶ 1309	8909	¶ 1365DD
8828	¶ 105	8910	¶ 1345
8829	¶ 961	8911	¶ 1355
8832	¶ 201	8912	¶ 1371
8833	¶ 2450	8918	¶ 2593
8834	¶ 1354	8919	¶ 105
8835	¶ 1365N	8923	¶ 1365GG
8839	¶ 1307	8925	¶ 804
8840	¶ 2409	8927	¶ 2317
8843	¶ 2409	8928	¶ 2015
8844	¶ 1365O	8930	¶ 2141
8845	¶ 1365Q	8931	¶ 1365HH
8846	¶ 1365R	8932	¶ 1365II
8849	¶ 1329	8933	¶ 1365JJ
8850	¶ 1365G	8936	¶ 1351
8854	¶ 2412	8938	¶ 2572
8855	¶ 516	8940	¶ 623
8857	¶ 162	8941	¶ 1333
8859	¶ 1308	8944	¶ 2503
8863	¶ 1303	8948	¶ 2503
8864	¶ 1365X	8949	¶ 1735
8865	¶ 2487	8955-SSA	¶ 2137
8866	¶ 1229	8959	¶ 2648
8867	¶ 2518	8960	¶ 129
8868	¶ 2509	9465	¶ 2529
8869	¶ 304	HUD-1	¶ 1055
8871	¶ 696	SS-4	¶ 2652
8872	¶ 696	SS-5	¶ 116
8874	¶ 1365T	SS-8	¶ 2602
8875	¶ 2340	T	¶ 1772
8879	¶ 2517	W-2	¶ 2565
8880	¶ 1304	W-2G	¶ 2642
8881	¶ 1365U	W-3	¶ 2650
8882	¶ 1365V	W-4	¶ 2634
8885	¶ 1332	W-4P	¶ 2643
8886	¶ 2592	W-4S	¶ 2604
8886-T	¶ 619	W-4V	¶ 2629
8888	¶ 2155	W-7	¶ 2579
8889	¶ 2035	W-7A	¶ 2579
8898	¶ 2414	W-8BEN	¶ 2455
8899	¶ 627	W-8ECI	¶ 2455
8900	¶ 1365W	W-8EXP	¶ 2455
8903	¶ 980A	W-8IMY	¶ 2455
8906	¶ 1365Z	W-9	¶ 2579

¶ 64 Guide to Information Returns

The following chart lists information returns in use by the IRS. It provides reportable payment types and amounts, as well as the due dates for filing the returns with the IRS and for providing statements to a payee or other person.

(If any date shown falls on a Saturday, Sunday, or legal holiday, the due date is the next business day.)

Form	Title	What To Report	Amounts To Report	To IRS	Due Date — To Recipient (unless indicated otherwise)
1042-S	Foreign Person's U.S. Source Income Subject to Withholding	Income such as interest, dividends, royalties, pensions and annuities, etc., and amounts withheld under Chapter 3 (nonresident aliens and foreign corporations). Also, distributions of effectively connected income by publicly traded partnerships or nominees.	See form instructions	March 15	March 15
1097-BTC	Bond Tax Credit	Tax credit bond credits to shareholders.	All amounts	February 28*	On or before the 15th day of the 2nd calendar month after the close of the calendar month in which the credit is allowed
1098	Mortgage Interest Statement	Mortgage interest (including points) and certain mortgage insurance premiums you received in the course of your trade or business from individuals and reimbursements of overpaid interest.	$600 or more	February 28*	(To Payer/Borrower) January 31
1098-C	Contributions of Motor Vehicles, Boats, and Airplanes	Information regarding a donated motor vehicle, boat, or airplane.	Gross proceeds of more than $500	February 28*	(To Donor) 30 days from date of sale or contribution
1098-E	Student Loan Interest Statement	Student loan interest received in the course of your trade or business.	$600 or more	February 28*	January 31
1098-MA	Mortgage Assistance Payment	Assistance payments paid to homeowners from funds allocated from the Housing Finance Authority Innovation Fund for the Hardest Hit Housing Markets (HFA Hardest Hit Fund) or the Emergency Homeowner's Loan Program.	All amounts	February 28*	January 31
1098-T	Tuition Statement	Qualified tuition and related expenses, reimbursements or refunds, and scholarships or grants (optional).	See instructions	February 28*	January 31
1099-A	Acquisition or Abandonment of Secured Property	Information about the acquisition or abandonment of property that is security for a debt for which you are the lender.	All amounts	February 28*	(To Borrower) January 31

				Due Date	
Form	**Title**	**What To Report**	**Amounts To Report**	**To IRS**	**To Recipient (unless indicated otherwise)**
1099-B	Proceeds From Broker and Barter Exchange Transactions	Sales or redemptions of securities, futures transactions, commodities, and barter exchange transactions.	All amounts	February 28*	February 15**
1099-C	Cancellation of Debt	Cancellation of a debt owed to a financial institution, the Federal Government, a credit union, RTC, FDIC, NCUA, a military department, the U.S. Postal Service, the Postal Rate Commission, or any organization having a significant trade or business of lending money.	$600 or more	February 28*	January 31
1099-CAP	Changes in Corporate Control and Capital Structure	Information about cash, stock, or other property from an acquisition of control or the substantial change in capital structure of a corporation.	Over $1000	February 28*	(To Shareholders) January 31
1099-DIV	Dividends and Distributions	Distributions, such as dividends, capital gain distributions, or nontaxable distributions, that were paid on stock and liquidation distributions.	$10 or more, except $600 or more for liquidations	February 28*	January 31**
1099-G	Certain Government Payments	Unemployment compensation, state and local income tax refunds, agricultural payments, and taxable grants.	$10 or more for refunds and unemployment	February 28*	January 31
1099-H⁺	Health Coverage Tax Credit (HCTC) Advance Payments	Health insurance premiums paid on behalf of certain individuals.	All amounts	February 28*	January 31
1099-INT	Interest Income	Interest income.	$10 or more ($600 or more in some cases)	February 28*	January 31**
1099-K	Payment Card and Third Party Network Transactions	Payment card transactions.	All amounts	February 28*	January 31
		Third party network transactions.	$20,000 or more **and** 200 or more transactions	February 28*	January 31
1099-LTC	Long-Term Care and Accelerated Death Benefits	Payments under a long-term care insurance contract and accelerated death benefits paid under a life insurance contract or by a viatical settlement provider.	All amounts	February 28*	January 31

Form	Title	What To Report	Amounts To Report	Due Date	
				To IRS	To Recipient (unless indicated otherwise)
1099-MISC	Miscellaneous Income	Rent or royalty payments; prizes and awards that are not for services, such as winnings on TV or radio shows (including payments reported pursuant to an election described in Reg. § 1.1471-4(d)(5)(i)(A) or reported as described in Reg. § 1.1471-4(d)(2)(iii)(A)).	$600 or more, except $10 or more for royalties	February 28*	January 31**
	(Also, use to report direct sales of $5,000 or more of consumer goods for resale.)	Payments to crew members by owners or operators of fishing boats including payments of proceeds from sale of catch.	All amounts	February 28*	January 31**
		Code Sec. 409A income from nonqualified deferred compensation plans (NQDCs).	All amounts	February 28*	January 31**
		Payments to a physician, physicians' corporation, or other supplier of health and medical services. Issued mainly by medical assistance programs or health and accident insurance plans.	$600 or more	February 28*	January 31**
		Payments for services performed for a trade or business by people not treated as its employees (including payments reported pursuant to an election described in Reg. § 1.1471-4(d)(5)(i)(A) or reported as described in Reg. § 1.1471-4(d)(2)(iii)(A)). Examples: fees to subcontractors or directors and golden parachute payments.	$600 or more	February 28*	January 31**
		Fish purchases paid in cash for resale.	$600 or more	February 28*	January 31**
		Crop insurance proceeds.	$600 or more	February 28*	January 31**
		Substitute dividends and tax-exempt interest payments reportable by brokers.	$10 or more	February 28*	February 15**
		Gross proceeds paid to attorneys.	$600 or more	February 28*	February 15**
		A U.S. account for Chapter 4 purposes (FATCA) to which you made no payments during the year that are reportable on any applicable Form 1099 (or a U.S. account to which you made payments during the year that do not reach the applicable reporting threshold for any applicable Form 1099) reported pursuant to an election described in Reg. § 1.1471-4(d)(5)(i)(A).	All amounts (including $0)	February 28*	January 31**

¶64

Form	Title	What To Report	Amounts To Report	Due Date To IRS	Due Date To Recipient (unless indicated otherwise)
1099-OID	Original Issue Discount	Original issue discount including amounts reported pursuant to an election described in Reg. § 1.1471-4(d)(5)(i)(A) or reported as described in Reg. § 1.1471-4(d)(2)(iii)(A)).	$10 or more	February 28*	January 31**
1099-PATR	Taxable Distributions Received From Cooperatives	Distributions from cooperatives passed through to their patrons including any domestic production activities deduction and certain pass-through credits.	$10 or more	February 28*	January 31
1099-Q	Payments From Qualified Education Programs (Under Sections 529 and 530)	Earnings from qualified tuition programs and Coverdell ESAs.	All amounts	February 28*	January 31
1099-R	Distributions From Pensions, Annuities, Retirement or Profit-Sharing Plans, IRAs, Insurance Contracts, etc.	Distributions from retirement or profit-sharing plans, any IRA, insurance contracts, and IRA recharacterizations (including payments reported pursuant to an election described in Reg. § 1.1471-4(d)(5)(i)(B) or reported as described in Reg. § 1.1471-4(d)(2)(iii)(A)).	$10 or more	February 28*	January 31
1099-S	Proceeds From Real Estate Transactions	Gross proceeds from the sale or exchange of real estate and certain royalty payments.	Generally, $600 or more	February 28*	February 15
1099-SA	Distributions From an HSA, Archer MSA, or Medicare Advantage MSA	Distributions from an HSA, Archer MSA, or Medicare Advantage MSA.	All amounts	February 28*	January 31
3921	Exercise of an Incentive Stock Option Under Section 422(b)	Transfer of stock pursuant to the exercise of an incentive stock option under Code Sec. 422(b).	All amounts	February 28*	January 31
3922	Transfer of Stock Acquired Through an Employee Stock Purchase Plan Under Section 423(c)	Transfer of stock acquired through an employee stock purchase plan under Code Sec. 423(c).	All amounts	February 28*	January 31
5498	IRA Contribution Information	Contributions (including rollover contributions) to any individual retirement arrangement (IRA) including a SEP, SIMPLE, and Roth IRA; Roth conversions; IRA recharacterizations; and the fair market value (FMV) of the account.	All amounts	May 31	(To Participant) For FMV/RMD Jan 31; For contributions, May 31

Form	Title	What To Report	Amounts To Report	Due Date To IRS	To Recipient (unless indicated otherwise)
5498-A	Qualified Longevity Anuity Contract Information	Status of a contract purchased or held under any plan, annuity, or account described in Code Sec. 401(a), 403(b), 408 (other than a Roth IRA), or eligible governmental plan under Code Sec. 457(b) intended to be a qualifying longevity annuity contract (QLAC) defined in A-17 of Reg. § 1.401(a)(9)-6.	All amounts	May 31	May 31
5498-ESA	Coverdell ESA Contribution Information	Contributions (including rollover contributions) to a Coverdell ESA.	All amounts	May 31	April 30
5498-SA	HSA, Archer MSA, or Medicare Advantage MSA Information	Contributions to an HSA (including transfers and rollovers) or Archer MSA and the FMV of an HSA, Archer MSA, or Medicare Advantage MSA.	All amounts	May 31	(To Participant) May 31
W-2G	Certain Gambling Winnings	Gambling winnings from horse racing, dog racing, jai alai, lotteries, keno, bingo, slot machines, sweepstakes, wagering pools, poker tournaments, etc.	Generally, $600 or more; $1,200 or more from bingo or slot machines; $1,500 or more from keno	February 28*	January 31
W-2	Wage and Tax Statement	Wages, tips, other compensation; Social Security, Medicare, and withheld income taxes. Include bonuses, vacation allowances, severance pay, certain moving expense payments, some kinds of travel allowances, and third-party payments of sick pay.	See separate instructions	(TO SSA) Last day of February*	(To Recipient) January 31

* The due date is March 31 if filed electronically.
** The due date is March 15 for reporting by trustees and middlemen of WHFITs.
⁺ Absent further legislation, the HCTC Advance Payment expired on 12/31/2013.

CHECKLISTS

¶64

¶ 65 Checklist for Types of Payments

The following chart lists common payments and the forms used to file and report them. It is not a complete list of all payments, and the absence of a payment from the list does not indicate that the payment is not reportable.

Type of Payment	Report on Form	Type of Payment	Report on Form
Abandonment	1099-A	Exercise of incentive stock option	
Accelerated death benefits	1099-LTC	under Code Sec. 422(b)	3921
Acquisition of control	1099-CAP	Fees, employee	W-2
Advance health insurance payments		Fees, nonemployee	1099-MISC
(expired 12/31/2013 absent further		Fishing boat crew members proceeds .	
legislation)	1099-H		1099-MISC
Agriculture payments	1099-G	Fish purchases for cash	1099-MISC
Allocated tips	W-2	Foreclosures	1099-A
Alternate TAA payments	1099-G	Foreign persons' income	1042-S
Annuities	1099-R	401(k) contributions	W-2
Archer MSAs:		404(k) dividend	1099-DIV
Contributions	5498-SA	Gambling winnings	W-2G
Distributions	1099-SA	Golden parachute, employee	W-2
Attorney, fees and gross proceeds	1099-MISC	Golden parachute, nonemployee	1099-MISC
Auto reimbursements, employee	W-2	Grants, taxable	1099-G
Auto reimbursements, nonemployee	1099-MISC	Health care services	1099-MISC
Awards, employee	W-2	Health insurance advance payments	
Awards, nonemployee	1099-MISC	(expired 12/31/2013 absent further	
Barter exchange income	1099-B	legislation)	1099-H
Bond tax credit	1097-BTC	Health savings accounts:	
Bonuses, employee	W-2	Contributions	5498-SA
Bonuses, nonemployee	1099-MISC	Distributions	1099-SA
Broker transactions	1099-B	Income attributable to domestic	
Cancellation of debt	1099-C	production activities, deduction for	1099-PATR
Capital gain distributions	1099-DIV	Income tax refunds, state and local .	1099-G
Car expense, employee	W-2	Indian gaming profits paid to tribal	
Car expense, nonemployee	1099-MISC	members	1099-MISC
Changes in capital structure	1099-CAP	Interest income	1099-INT
Charitable gift annuities	1099-R	Tax-exempt	1099-INT
Commissions, employee	W-2	Interest, mortgage	1098
Commissions, nonemployee	1099-MISC	IRA contributions	5498
Commodities transactions	1099-B	IRA distributions	1099-R
Compensation, employee	W-2	Life insurance contract distributions	1099-R,
Compensation, nonemployee	1099-MISC		1099-LTC
Contributions of motor vehicles, boats,		Liquidation, distributions in	1099-DIV
and airplanes	1098-C	Loans, distribution from pension plan	1099-R
Cost of current life insurance protection		Long-term care benefits	1099-LTC
	1099-R	Medicare Advantage MSAs:	
Coverdell Educational Savings Accounts (ESAs):		Contributions	5498-SA
Contributions	5498-ESA	Distributions	1099-SA
Distributions	1099-Q	Medical services	1099-MISC
Crop insurance proceeds	1099-MISC	Mileage, employee	W-2
Damages	1099-MISC	Mileage, nonemployee	1099-MISC
Death benefits	1099-R	Military retirement	1099-R
Accelerated	1099-LTC	Mortgage assistance payments	1098-MA
Debt cancellation	1099-C	Mortgage interest	1098
Dependent care payments	W-2	Moving expense	W-2
Direct rollovers	1099-Q,	Nonemployee compensation	1099-MISC
	1099-R,	Nonqualified deferred compensation:	
	5498	Beneficiary	1099-R
Direct sales of consumer products for		Employee	W-2
resale	1099-MISC	Nonemployee	1099-MISC
Directors' fees	1099-MISC	Original issue discount (OID)	1099-OID
Discharge of indebtedness	1099-C	Patronage dividends	1099-PATR
Dividends	1099-DIV	Payment card transactions	1099-K
Donation of motor vehicle	1098-C	Pensions	1099-R
Education loan interest	1098-E	Points	1098
Employee business expense		Prizes, employee	W-2
reimbursement	W-2	Prizes, nonemployee	1099-MISC
Employee compensation	W-2	Profit-sharing plan	1099-R
Excess deferrals, excess contributions,		Punitive damages	1099-MISC
distributions of	1099-R		

Type of Payment	Report on Form
Qualified longevity annuity contract information	5498-A
Qualified plan distributions	1099-R
Qualified tuition program payments .	1099-Q
Real estate transactions	1099-S
Recharacterized IRA contributions ..	1099-R, 5498
Refund, state and local tax	1099-G
Rents	1099-MISC
Retirement	1099-R
Roth conversion IRAs:	
Contributions	5498
Distributions	1099-R
Roth IRAs:	
Contributions	5498
Distributions	1099-R
Royalties	1099-MISC
Timber, pay-as-cut contract	1099-S
Sales:	
Real estate	1099-S
Securities	1099-B
Code Sec. 1035 exchange	1099-R

Type of Payment	Report on Form
SEPs:	
Contributions	W-2, 5498
Distributions	1099-R
Severance pay	W-2
Sick pay	W-2
SIMPLEs:	
Contributions	W-2, 5498
Distributions	1099-R
Student loan interest	1098-E
Substitute payments in lieu of dividends or tax-exempt interest	1099-MISC
Supplemental unemployment	W-2
Tax refunds, state and local	1099-G
Third-party network payments	1099-K
Tips	W-2
Transfer of stock acquired through an employee stock purchase plan under Code Sec. 423(c)	3922
Tuition	1098-T
Unemployment benefits	1099-G
Vacation allowance, employee	W-2
Vacation allowance, nonemployee ..	1099-MISC
Wages	W-2

SPECIAL TAX TABLES

¶ 83 Applicable Federal Rates

Following are the monthly applicable federal interest rates for January 2014 through November 2014 published by the IRS for purposes of testing imputed interest in below-market interest loans (¶ 795) and debt-for-property transactions (¶ 1954). The rates are also relevant under the golden parachute rules (¶ 907) and for testing interest in connection with deferred payments for the use of property (¶ 1859).

In the case of below-market interest loans that are demand or gift loans, an amount deemed the "foregone" interest is treated as transferred from the lender to the borrower and retransferred by the borrower to the lender as interest. In order to simplify the computation of such foregone interest, the IRS prescribes a "blended annual rate," which is 0.28% on loans for the calendar year 2014.

		Period for Compounding			
		Annual	Semiannual	Quarterly	Monthly
January 2014					
	Short-Term				
	AFR	.25	.25	.25	.25
110%	AFR	.28	.28	.28	.28
120%	AFR	.30	.30	.30	.30
130%	AFR	.33	.33	.33	.33
	Mid-Term				
	AFR	1.75	1.74	1.74	1.73
110%	AFR	1.92	1.91	1.91	1.90
120%	AFR	2.10	2.09	2.08	2.08
130%	AFR	2.27	2.26	2.25	2.25
150%	AFR	2.63	2.61	2.60	2.60
175%	AFR	3.07	3.05	3.04	3.03
	Long-Term				
	AFR	3.49	3.46	3.45	3.44
110%	AFR	3.85	3.81	3.79	3.78
120%	AFR	4.19	4.15	4.13	4.11
130%	AFR	4.55	4.50	4.47	4.46

		Period for Compounding			
		Annual	Semiannual	Quarterly	Monthly
February 2014					
	Short-Term				
	AFR	.30	.30	.30	.30
110%	AFR	.33	.33	.33	.33
120%	AFR	.36	.36	.36	.36
130%	AFR	.39	.39	.39	.39
	Mid-Term				
	AFR	1.97	1.96	1.96	1.95
110%	AFR	2.17	2.16	2.15	2.15
120%	AFR	2.36	2.35	2.34	2.34
130%	AFR	2.57	2.55	2.54	2.54
150%	AFR	2.96	2.94	2.93	2.92
175%	AFR	3.46	3.43	3.42	3.41
	Long-Term				
	AFR	3.56	3.53	3.51	3.50
110%	AFR	3.92	3.88	3.86	3.85
120%	AFR	4.28	4.24	4.22	4.20
130%	AFR	4.64	4.59	4.56	4.55
March 2014					
	Short-Term				
	AFR	.28	.28	.28	.28
110%	AFR	.31	.31	.31	.31
120%	AFR	.34	.34	.34	.34
130%	AFR	.36	.36	.36	.36
	Mid-Term				
	AFR	1.84	1.83	1.83	1.82
110%	AFR	2.02	2.01	2.00	2.00
120%	AFR	2.21	2.20	2.19	2.19
130%	AFR	2.39	2.38	2.37	2.37
150%	AFR	2.77	2.75	2.74	2.73
175%	AFR	3.23	3.20	3.19	3.18
	Long-Term				
	AFR	3.36	3.33	3.32	3.31
110%	AFR	3.69	3.66	3.64	3.63
120%	AFR	4.04	4.00	3.98	3.97
130%	AFR	4.38	4.33	4.31	4.29
April 2014					
	Short-Term				
	AFR	.28	.28	.28	.28
110%	AFR	.31	.31	.31	.31
120%	AFR	.34	.34	.34	.34
130%	AFR	.36	.36	.36	.36
	Mid-Term				
	AFR	1.81	1.80	1.80	1.79
110%	AFR	1.99	1.98	1.98	1.97
120%	AFR	2.17	2.16	2.15	2.15
130%	AFR	2.35	2.34	2.33	2.33
150%	AFR	2.72	2.70	2.69	2.68
175%	AFR	3.17	3.15	3.14	3.13
	Long-Term				
	AFR	3.32	3.29	3.28	3.27
110%	AFR	3.65	3.62	3.60	3.59
120%	AFR	3.99	3.95	3.93	3.92
130%	AFR	4.33	4.28	4.26	4.24

SPECIAL TABLES

	Period for Compounding			
	Annual	*Semiannual*	*Quarterly*	*Monthly*
May 2014				
Short-Term				
AFR	.33	.33	.33	.33
110% AFR	.36	.36	.36	.36
120% AFR	.40	.40	.40	.40
130% AFR	.43	.43	.43	.43
Mid-Term				
AFR	1.93	1.92	1.92	1.91
110% AFR	2.12	2.11	2.10	2.10
120% AFR	2.31	2.30	2.29	2.29
130% AFR	2.52	2.50	2.49	2.49
150% AFR	2.90	2.88	2.87	2.86
175% AFR	3.39	3.36	3.35	3.34
Long-Term				
AFR	3.27	3.24	3.23	3.22
110% AFR	3.59	3.56	3.54	3.53
120% AFR	3.93	3.89	3.87	3.86
130% AFR	4.25	4.21	4.19	4.17
June 2014				
Short-Term				
AFR	.32	.32	.32	.32
110% AFR	.35	.35	.35	.35
120% AFR	.38	.38	.38	.38
130% AFR	.42	.42	.42	.42
Mid-Term				
AFR	1.91	1.90	1.90	1.89
110% AFR	2.10	2.09	2.08	2.08
120% AFR	2.29	2.28	2.27	2.27
130% AFR	2.49	2.47	2.46	2.46
150% AFR	2.87	2.85	2.84	2.83
175% AFR	3.36	3.33	3.32	3.31
Long-Term				
AFR	3.14	3.12	3.11	3.10
110% AFR	3.46	3.43	3.42	3.41
120% AFR	3.77	3.74	3.72	3.71
130% AFR	4.10	4.06	4.04	4.03
July 2014				
Short-Term				
AFR	.31	.31	.31	.31
110% AFR	.34	.34	.34	.34
120% AFR	.37	.37	.37	.37
130% AFR	.40	.40	.40	.40
Mid-Term				
AFR	1.82	1.81	1.81	1.80
110% AFR	2.00	1.99	1.99	1.98
120% AFR	2.18	2.17	2.16	2.16
130% AFR	2.36	2.35	2.34	2.34
150% AFR	2.74	2.72	2.71	2.70
175% AFR	3.20	3.17	3.16	3.15
Long-Term				
AFR	3.06	3.04	3.03	3.02
110% AFR	3.37	3.34	3.33	3.32
120% AFR	3.68	3.65	3.63	3.62
130% AFR	3.99	3.95	3.93	3.92

		Period for Compounding			
		Annual	*Semiannual*	*Quarterly*	*Monthly*
August 2014					
	Short-Term				
	AFR	.36	.36	.36	.36
110%	AFR	.40	.40	.40	.40
120%	AFR	.43	.43	.43	.43
130%	AFR	.47	.47	.47	.47
	Mid-Term				
	AFR	1.89	1.88	1.88	1.87
110%	AFR	2.08	2.07	2.06	2.06
120%	AFR	2.27	2.26	2.25	2.25
130%	AFR	2.45	2.44	2.43	2.43
150%	AFR	2.84	2.82	2.81	2.80
175%	AFR	3.32	3.29	3.28	3.27
	Long-Term				
	AFR	3.09	3.07	3.06	3.05
110%	AFR	3.41	3.38	3.37	3.36
120%	AFR	3.71	3.68	3.66	3.65
130%	AFR	4.03	3.99	3.97	3.96
September 2014					
	Short-Term				
	AFR	.36	.36	.36	.36
110%	AFR	.40	.40	.40	.40
120%	AFR	.43	.43	.43	.43
130%	AFR	.47	.47	.47	.47
	Mid-Term				
	AFR	1.86	1.85	1.85	1.84
110%	AFR	2.05	2.04	2.03	2.03
120%	AFR	2.23	2.22	2.21	2.21
130%	AFR	2.42	2.41	2.40	2.40
150%	AFR	2.80	2.78	2.77	2.76
175%	AFR	3.27	3.24	3.23	3.22
	Long-Term				
	AFR	2.97	2.95	2.94	2.93
110%	AFR	3.28	3.25	3.24	3.23
120%	AFR	3.57	3.54	3.52	3.51
130%	AFR	3.88	3.84	3.82	3.81
October 2014					
	Short-Term				
	AFR	.38	.38	.38	.38
110%	AFR	.42	.42	.42	.42
120%	AFR	.46	.46	.46	.46
130%	AFR	.49	.49	.49	.49
	Mid-Term				
	AFR	1.85	1.84	1.84	1.83
110%	AFR	2.03	2.02	2.01	2.01
120%	AFR	2.22	2.21	2.20	2.20
130%	AFR	2.40	2.39	2.38	2.38
150%	AFR	2.78	2.76	2.75	2.74
175%	AFR	3.25	3.22	3.21	3.20
	Long-Term				
	AFR	2.89	2.87	2.86	2.85
110%	AFR	3.18	3.16	3.15	3.14
120%	AFR	3.47	3.44	3.43	3.42
130%	AFR	3.76	3.73	3.71	3.70

SPECIAL TABLES

Period for Compounding				
	Annual	Semiannual	Quarterly	Monthly
November 2014				
Short-Term				
AFR	.39	.39	.39	.39
110% AFR	.43	.43	.43	.43
120% AFR	.47	.47	.47	.47
130% AFR	.51	.51	.51	.51
Mid-Term				
AFR	1.90	1.89	1.89	1.88
110% AFR	2.09	2.08	2.07	2.07
120% AFR	2.28	2.27	2.26	2.26
130% AFR	2.48	2.46	2.45	2.45
150% AFR	2.86	2.84	2.83	2.82
175% AFR	3.34	3.31	3.30	3.29
Long-Term				
AFR	2.91	2.89	2.88	2.87
110% AFR	3.21	3.18	3.17	3.16
120% AFR	3.50	3.47	3.46	3.45
130% AFR	3.80	3.76	3.74	3.73

¶ 84 Adjusted Applicable Federal Rates

Code Sec. 1288 provides that, in determining original issue discount on tax-exempt obligations, an adjustment must be made to the applicable federal rates (¶ 83) to take into account the tax exemption for interest on the obligations.

Adjusted Applicable Federal Rates

January 2014

	Annual Compounding	SemiAnnual Compounding	Quarterly Compounding	Monthly Compounding
Short-term rate	.25%	.25%	.25%	.25%
Mid-term rate	1.56%	1.55%	1.55%	1.55%
Long-term rate	3.49%	3.46%	3.45%	3.44%

February 2014

	Annual Compounding	SemiAnnual Compounding	Quarterly Compounding	Monthly Compounding
Short-term rate	.30%	.30%	.30%	.30%
Mid-term rate	1.56%	1.55%	1.55%	1.55%
Long-term rate	3.56%	3.53%	3.51%	3.50%

March 2014

	Annual Compounding	SemiAnnual Compounding	Quarterly Compounding	Monthly Compounding
Short-term rate	.28%	.28%	.28%	.28%
Mid-term rate	1.84%	1.83%	1.83%	1.82%
Long-term rate	3.36%	3.33%	3.32%	3.31%

April 2014

	Annual Compounding	SemiAnnual Compounding	Quarterly Compounding	Monthly Compounding
Short-term rate	.26%	.26%	.26%	.26%
Mid-term rate	1.35%	1.35%	1.35%	1.35%
Long-term rate	3.32%	3.29%	3.28%	3.27%

May 2014

	Annual Compounding	SemiAnnual Compounding	Quarterly Compounding	Monthly Compounding
Short-term rate	.33%	.33%	.33%	.33%
Mid-term rate	1.41%	1.41%	1.41%	1.41%
Long-term rate	3.27%	3.24%	3.23%	3.22%

June 2014

	Annual Compounding	SemiAnnual Compounding	Quarterly Compounding	Monthly Compounding
Short-term rate	.32%	.32%	.32%	.32%
Mid-term rate	1.37%	1.37%	1.37%	1.37%
Long-term rate	3.14%	3.12%	3.11%	3.10%

July 2014

	Annual Compounding	SemiAnnual Compounding	Quarterly Compounding	Monthly Compounding
Short-term rate	.31%	.31%	.31%	.31%
Mid-term rate	1.40%	1.40%	1.40%	1.40%
Long-term rate	3.06%	3.04%	3.03%	3.02%

August 2014

	Annual Compounding	SemiAnnual Compounding	Quarterly Compounding	Monthly Compounding
Short-term rate	.36%	.36%	.36%	.36%
Mid-term rate	1.38%	1.38%	1.38%	1.38%
Long-term rate	3.05%	3.03%	3.02%	3.01%

September 2014

	Annual Compounding	SemiAnnual Compounding	Quarterly Compounding	Monthly Compounding
Short-term rate	.36%	.36%	.36%	.36%
Mid-term rate	1.35%	1.35%	1.35%	1.35%
Long-term rate	2.94%	2.92%	2.91%	2.90%

SPECIAL TABLES

	Annual Compounding	SemiAnnual Compounding	Quarterly Compounding	Monthly Compounding
		October 2014		
Short-term rate 38%		.38%	.38%	.38%
Mid-term rate 1.27%		1.27%	1.27%	1.27%
Long-term rate 2.77%		2.75%	2.74%	2.73%
		November 2014		
	Annual Compounding	SemiAnnual Compounding	Quarterly Compounding	Monthly Compounding
Short-term rate 39%		.39%	.39%	.39%
Mid-term rate 1.31%		1.31%	1.31%	1.31%
Long-term rate 2.80%		2.78%	2.77%	2.76%

¶ 85 Federal Long-Term Tax-Exempt Rates

Code Sec. 382 provides that the long-term tax-exempt rate for purposes of net operating loss carryforwards shall be the highest of the adjusted federal long-term rates (¶ 84) for the three months ending with the month in which the particular ownership change occurs. Each rate below is the highest for the 3-month period.

Long-Term Tax-Exempt Rates

Month	Rate
January 2014	3.49%
February 2014	3.56%
March 2014	3.56%
April 2014	3.56%
May 2014	3.36%
June 2014	3.32%
July 2014	3.27%
August 2014	3.14%
September 2014	3.06%
October 2014	3.05%
November 2014	2.94%

¶ 86 Applicable Credit Percentages for Low-Income Housing

Code Sec. 42 provides that applicable credit percentages for low-income housing are to be computed so that the present value of the 10 annual credit amounts at the beginning of the 10-year credit period equals either 70% or 30% of the qualified basis of the low-income units in a project. The discount rate for determining the present value in these computations is a rate equal to 72% of the average of the month's AFR for mid-term and long-term obligations. The applicable credit percentage for new construction or rehabilitation expenditures not federally subsidized is indicated under the 70% rate column. The applicable credit percentage for subsidized construction or rehabilitation expenditures and the acquisition of existing housing is indicated under the 30% rate column. See ¶ 1365K.

Applicable Credit Percentages for Low-Income Housing

Month	70% Rate	30% Rate
January 2014	7.60%	3.26%
February 2014	7.64%	3.27%
March 2014	7.60%	3.26%
April 2014	7.59%	3.25%
May 2014	7.60%	3.26%
June 2014	7.58%	3.25%
July 2014	7.56%	3.24%
August 2014	7.57%	3.25%
September 2014	7.56%	3.24%
October 2014	7.54%	3.23%
November 2014	7.55%	3.24%

SPECIAL TABLES

⫸→ *Caution: This is a draft 2014 Earned Income Credit (EIC) Table. At the time of publication, the IRS had not yet released the 2014 Earned Income Credit (EIC) Table. For the latest information, see CCHGroup.com/TaxUpdates.*

¶ 87 Earned Income Credit

The earned income credit tables are used in conjunction with the Form 1040 or Form 1040A, and Schedule EIC. The Schedule EIC must be filed with the taxpayer's tax return in order to claim the earned income credit. The credit, as computed on the EIC Worksheet found in the Form 1040 instructions, is entered on the appropriate line of Form 1040 or Form 1040A. Form 1040EZ may be used to claim the earned income credit in limited circumstances.

>>>→ *Caution: This is a draft 2014 Earned Income Credit (EIC) Table. At the time of publication, the IRS had not yet released the 2014 Earned Income Credit (EIC) Table. For the latest information, see CCHGroup.com/TaxUpdates.*

2014 Earned Income Credit (EIC) Table
Caution. This is **not** a tax table.

1. To find your credit, read down the "At least - But less than" columns and find the line that includes the amount you were told to look up from your EIC Worksheet.

2. Then, go to the column that includes your filing status and the number of qualifying children you have. Enter the credit from that column on your EIC Worksheet.

Example. If your filing status is single, you have one qualifying child, and the amount you are looking up from your EIC Worksheet is $2,455, you would enter $842.

If the amount you are looking up from the worksheet is—		And your filing status is—			
		Single, head of household, or qualifying widow(er) and the number of children you have is—			
At least	But less than	0	1	2	3
		Your credit is—			
2,400	2,450	186	825	970	1,091
2,450	2,500	189	842	990	1,114

If the amount you are looking up from the worksheet is—		Single, head of household, or qualifying widow(er) and the number of children you have is—				Married filing jointly and the number of children you have is—			
At least	But less than	0	1	2	3	0	1	2	3
		Your credit is—				Your credit is—			
$1	$50	$2	$9	$10	$11	$2	$9	$10	$11
50	100	6	26	30	34	6	26	30	34
100	150	10	43	50	56	10	43	50	56
150	200	13	60	70	79	13	60	70	79
200	250	17	77	90	101	17	77	90	101
250	300	21	94	110	124	21	94	110	124
300	350	25	111	130	146	25	111	130	146
350	400	29	128	150	169	29	128	150	169
400	450	33	145	170	191	33	145	170	191
450	500	36	162	190	214	36	162	190	214
500	550	40	179	210	236	40	179	210	236
550	600	44	196	230	259	44	196	230	259
600	650	48	213	250	281	48	213	250	281
650	700	52	230	270	304	52	230	270	304
700	750	55	247	290	326	55	247	290	326
750	800	59	264	310	349	59	264	310	349
800	850	63	281	330	371	63	281	330	371
850	900	67	298	350	394	67	298	350	394
900	950	71	315	370	416	71	315	370	416
950	1,000	75	332	390	439	75	332	390	439
1,000	1,050	78	349	410	461	78	349	410	461
1,050	1,100	82	366	430	484	82	366	430	484
1,100	1,150	86	383	450	506	86	383	450	506
1,150	1,200	90	400	470	529	90	400	470	529
1,200	1,250	94	417	490	551	94	417	490	551
1,250	1,300	98	434	510	574	98	434	510	574
1,300	1,350	101	451	530	596	101	451	530	596
1,350	1,400	105	468	550	619	105	468	550	619
1,400	1,450	109	485	570	641	109	485	570	641
1,450	1,500	113	502	590	664	113	502	590	664
1,500	1,550	117	519	610	686	117	519	610	686
1,550	1,600	120	536	630	709	120	536	630	709
1,600	1,650	124	553	650	731	124	553	650	731
1,650	1,700	128	570	670	754	128	570	670	754
1,700	1,750	132	587	690	776	132	587	690	776
1,750	1,800	136	604	710	799	136	604	710	799
1,800	1,850	140	621	730	821	140	621	730	821
1,850	1,900	143	638	750	844	143	638	750	844
1,900	1,950	147	655	770	866	147	655	770	866
1,950	2,000	151	672	790	889	151	672	790	889
2,000	2,050	155	689	810	911	155	689	810	911
2,050	2,100	159	706	830	934	159	706	830	934
2,100	2,150	163	723	850	956	163	723	850	956
2,150	2,200	166	740	870	979	166	740	870	979
2,200	2,250	170	757	890	1,001	170	757	890	1,001
2,250	2,300	174	774	910	1,024	174	774	910	1,024
2,300	2,350	178	791	930	1,046	178	791	930	1,046
2,350	2,400	182	808	950	1,069	182	808	950	1,069
2,400	2,450	186	825	970	1,091	186	825	970	1,091
2,450	2,500	189	842	990	1,114	189	842	990	1,114
2,500	2,550	193	859	1,010	1,136	193	859	1,010	1,136
2,550	2,600	197	876	1,030	1,159	197	876	1,030	1,159
2,600	2,650	201	893	1,050	1,181	201	893	1,050	1,181
2,650	2,700	205	910	1,070	1,204	205	910	1,070	1,204
2,700	2,750	208	927	1,090	1,226	208	927	1,090	1,226
2,750	2,800	212	944	1,110	1,249	212	944	1,110	1,249

If the amount you are looking up from the worksheet is—		Single, head of household, or qualifying widow(er) and the number of children you have is—				Married filing jointly and the number of children you have is—			
At least	But less than	0	1	2	3	0	1	2	3
		Your credit is—				Your credit is—			
2,800	2,850	216	961	1,130	1,271	216	961	1,130	1,271
2,850	2,900	220	978	1,150	1,294	220	978	1,150	1,294
2,900	2,950	224	995	1,170	1,316	224	995	1,170	1,316
2,950	3,000	228	1,012	1,190	1,339	228	1,012	1,190	1,339
3,000	3,050	231	1,029	1,210	1,361	231	1,029	1,210	1,361
3,050	3,100	235	1,046	1,230	1,384	235	1,046	1,230	1,384
3,100	3,150	239	1,063	1,250	1,406	239	1,063	1,250	1,406
3,150	3,200	243	1,080	1,270	1,429	243	1,080	1,270	1,429
3,200	3,250	247	1,097	1,290	1,451	247	1,097	1,290	1,451
3,250	3,300	251	1,114	1,310	1,474	251	1,114	1,310	1,474
3,300	3,350	254	1,131	1,330	1,496	254	1,131	1,330	1,496
3,350	3,400	258	1,148	1,350	1,519	258	1,148	1,350	1,519
3,400	3,450	262	1,165	1,370	1,541	262	1,165	1,370	1,541
3,450	3,500	266	1,182	1,390	1,564	266	1,182	1,390	1,564
3,500	3,550	270	1,199	1,410	1,586	270	1,199	1,410	1,586
3,550	3,600	273	1,216	1,430	1,609	273	1,216	1,430	1,609
3,600	3,650	277	1,233	1,450	1,631	277	1,233	1,450	1,631
3,650	3,700	281	1,250	1,470	1,654	281	1,250	1,470	1,654
3,700	3,750	285	1,267	1,490	1,676	285	1,267	1,490	1,676
3,750	3,800	289	1,284	1,510	1,699	289	1,284	1,510	1,699
3,800	3,850	293	1,301	1,530	1,721	293	1,301	1,530	1,721
3,850	3,900	296	1,318	1,550	1,744	296	1,318	1,550	1,744
3,900	3,950	300	1,335	1,570	1,766	300	1,335	1,570	1,766
3,950	4,000	304	1,352	1,590	1,789	304	1,352	1,590	1,789
4,000	4,050	308	1,369	1,610	1,811	308	1,369	1,610	1,811
4,050	4,100	312	1,386	1,630	1,834	312	1,386	1,630	1,834
4,100	4,150	316	1,403	1,650	1,856	316	1,403	1,650	1,856
4,150	4,200	319	1,420	1,670	1,879	319	1,420	1,670	1,879
4,200	4,250	323	1,437	1,690	1,901	323	1,437	1,690	1,901
4,250	4,300	327	1,454	1,710	1,924	327	1,454	1,710	1,924
4,300	4,350	331	1,471	1,730	1,946	331	1,471	1,730	1,946
4,350	4,400	335	1,488	1,750	1,969	335	1,488	1,750	1,969
4,400	4,450	339	1,505	1,770	1,991	339	1,505	1,770	1,991
4,450	4,500	342	1,522	1,790	2,014	342	1,522	1,790	2,014
4,500	4,550	346	1,539	1,810	2,036	346	1,539	1,810	2,036
4,550	4,600	350	1,556	1,830	2,059	350	1,556	1,830	2,059
4,600	4,650	354	1,573	1,850	2,081	354	1,573	1,850	2,081
4,650	4,700	358	1,590	1,870	2,104	358	1,590	1,870	2,104
4,700	4,750	361	1,607	1,890	2,126	361	1,607	1,890	2,126
4,750	4,800	365	1,624	1,910	2,149	365	1,624	1,910	2,149
4,800	4,850	369	1,641	1,930	2,171	369	1,641	1,930	2,171
4,850	4,900	373	1,658	1,950	2,194	373	1,658	1,950	2,194
4,900	4,950	377	1,675	1,970	2,216	377	1,675	1,970	2,216
4,950	5,000	381	1,692	1,990	2,239	381	1,692	1,990	2,239
5,000	5,050	384	1,709	2,010	2,261	384	1,709	2,010	2,261
5,050	5,100	388	1,726	2,030	2,284	388	1,726	2,030	2,284
5,100	5,150	392	1,743	2,050	2,306	392	1,743	2,050	2,306
5,150	5,200	396	1,760	2,070	2,329	396	1,760	2,070	2,329
5,200	5,250	400	1,777	2,090	2,351	400	1,777	2,090	2,351
5,250	5,300	404	1,794	2,110	2,374	404	1,794	2,110	2,374
5,300	5,350	407	1,811	2,130	2,396	407	1,811	2,130	2,396
5,350	5,400	411	1,828	2,150	2,419	411	1,828	2,150	2,419
5,400	5,450	415	1,845	2,170	2,441	415	1,845	2,170	2,441
5,450	5,500	419	1,862	2,190	2,464	419	1,862	2,190	2,464
5,500	5,550	423	1,879	2,210	2,486	423	1,879	2,210	2,486
5,550	5,600	426	1,896	2,230	2,509	426	1,896	2,230	2,509

(Continued)

Need more information or forms? Visit IRS.gov.

SPECIAL TABLES

¶87

»»→ Caution: This is a draft 2014 Earned Income Credit (EIC) Table. At the time of publication, the IRS had not yet released the 2014 Earned Income Credit (EIC) Table. For the latest information, see CCHGroup.com/TaxUpdates.

Earned Income Credit (EIC) Table - *Continued* (**Caution.** This is **not** a tax table.)

If the amount you are looking up from the worksheet is–		And your filing status is– Single, head of household, or qualifying widow(er) and the number of children you have is–				Married filing jointly and the number of children you have is–			
		0	1	2	3	0	1	2	3
At least	But less than	Your credit is–				Your credit is–			
5,600	5,650	430	1,913	2,250	2,531	430	1,913	2,250	2,531
5,650	5,700	434	1,930	2,270	2,554	434	1,930	2,270	2,554
5,700	5,750	438	1,947	2,290	2,576	438	1,947	2,290	2,576
5,750	5,800	442	1,964	2,310	2,599	442	1,964	2,310	2,599
5,800	5,850	446	1,981	2,330	2,621	446	1,981	2,330	2,621
5,850	5,900	449	1,998	2,350	2,644	449	1,998	2,350	2,644
5,900	5,950	453	2,015	2,370	2,666	453	2,015	2,370	2,666
5,950	6,000	457	2,032	2,390	2,689	457	2,032	2,390	2,689
6,000	6,050	461	2,049	2,410	2,711	461	2,049	2,410	2,711
6,050	6,100	465	2,066	2,430	2,734	465	2,066	2,430	2,734
6,100	6,150	469	2,083	2,450	2,756	469	2,083	2,450	2,756
6,150	6,200	472	2,100	2,470	2,779	472	2,100	2,470	2,779
6,200	6,250	476	2,117	2,490	2,801	476	2,117	2,490	2,801
6,250	6,300	480	2,134	2,510	2,824	480	2,134	2,510	2,824
6,300	6,350	484	2,151	2,530	2,846	484	2,151	2,530	2,846
6,350	6,400	488	2,168	2,550	2,869	488	2,168	2,550	2,869
6,400	6,450	492	2,185	2,570	2,891	492	2,185	2,570	2,891
6,450	6,500	496	2,202	2,590	2,914	496	2,202	2,590	2,914
6,500	6,550	496	2,219	2,610	2,936	496	2,219	2,610	2,936
6,550	6,600	496	2,236	2,630	2,959	496	2,236	2,630	2,959
6,600	6,650	496	2,253	2,650	2,981	496	2,253	2,650	2,981
6,650	6,700	496	2,270	2,670	3,004	496	2,270	2,670	3,004
6,700	6,750	496	2,287	2,690	3,026	496	2,287	2,690	3,026
6,750	6,800	496	2,304	2,710	3,049	496	2,304	2,710	3,049
6,800	6,850	496	2,321	2,730	3,071	496	2,321	2,730	3,071
6,850	6,900	496	2,338	2,750	3,094	496	2,338	2,750	3,094
6,900	6,950	496	2,355	2,770	3,116	496	2,355	2,770	3,116
6,950	7,000	496	2,372	2,790	3,139	496	2,372	2,790	3,139
7,000	7,050	496	2,389	2,810	3,161	496	2,389	2,810	3,161
7,050	7,100	496	2,406	2,830	3,184	496	2,406	2,830	3,184
7,100	7,150	496	2,423	2,850	3,206	496	2,423	2,850	3,206
7,150	7,200	496	2,440	2,870	3,229	496	2,440	2,870	3,229
7,200	7,250	496	2,457	2,890	3,251	496	2,457	2,890	3,251
7,250	7,300	496	2,474	2,910	3,274	496	2,474	2,910	3,274
7,300	7,350	496	2,491	2,930	3,296	496	2,491	2,930	3,296
7,350	7,400	496	2,508	2,950	3,319	496	2,508	2,950	3,319
7,400	7,450	496	2,525	2,970	3,341	496	2,525	2,970	3,341
7,450	7,500	496	2,542	2,990	3,364	496	2,542	2,990	3,364
7,500	7,550	496	2,559	3,010	3,386	496	2,559	3,010	3,386
7,550	7,600	496	2,576	3,030	3,409	496	2,576	3,030	3,409
7,600	7,650	496	2,593	3,050	3,431	496	2,593	3,050	3,431
7,650	7,700	496	2,610	3,070	3,454	496	2,610	3,070	3,454
7,700	7,750	496	2,627	3,090	3,476	496	2,627	3,090	3,476
7,750	7,800	496	2,644	3,110	3,499	496	2,644	3,110	3,499
7,800	7,850	496	2,661	3,130	3,521	496	2,661	3,130	3,521
7,850	7,900	496	2,678	3,150	3,544	496	2,678	3,150	3,544
7,900	7,950	496	2,695	3,170	3,566	496	2,695	3,170	3,566
7,950	8,000	496	2,712	3,190	3,589	496	2,712	3,190	3,589
8,000	8,050	496	2,729	3,210	3,611	496	2,729	3,210	3,611
8,050	8,100	496	2,746	3,230	3,634	496	2,746	3,230	3,634
8,100	8,150	496	2,763	3,250	3,656	496	2,763	3,250	3,656
8,150	8,200	491	2,780	3,270	3,679	496	2,780	3,270	3,679
8,200	8,250	487	2,797	3,290	3,701	496	2,797	3,290	3,701
8,250	8,300	483	2,814	3,310	3,724	496	2,814	3,310	3,724
8,300	8,350	479	2,831	3,330	3,746	496	2,831	3,330	3,746
8,350	8,400	475	2,848	3,350	3,769	496	2,848	3,350	3,769
8,400	8,450	472	2,865	3,370	3,791	496	2,865	3,370	3,791
8,450	8,500	468	2,882	3,390	3,814	496	2,882	3,390	3,814
8,500	8,550	464	2,899	3,410	3,836	496	2,899	3,410	3,836
8,550	8,600	460	2,916	3,430	3,859	496	2,916	3,430	3,859
8,600	8,650	456	2,933	3,450	3,881	496	2,933	3,450	3,881
8,650	8,700	452	2,950	3,470	3,904	496	2,950	3,470	3,904
8,700	8,750	449	2,967	3,490	3,926	496	2,967	3,490	3,926
8,750	8,800	445	2,984	3,510	3,949	496	2,984	3,510	3,949
8,800	8,850	441	3,001	3,530	3,971	496	3,001	3,530	3,971
8,850	8,900	437	3,018	3,550	3,994	496	3,018	3,550	3,994
8,900	8,950	433	3,035	3,570	4,016	496	3,035	3,570	4,016
8,950	9,000	430	3,052	3,590	4,039	496	3,052	3,590	4,039
9,000	9,050	426	3,069	3,610	4,061	496	3,069	3,610	4,061
9,050	9,100	422	3,086	3,630	4,084	496	3,086	3,630	4,084
9,100	9,150	418	3,103	3,650	4,106	496	3,103	3,650	4,106
9,150	9,200	414	3,120	3,670	4,129	496	3,120	3,670	4,129
9,200	9,250	410	3,137	3,690	4,151	496	3,137	3,690	4,151
9,250	9,300	407	3,154	3,710	4,174	496	3,154	3,710	4,174
9,300	9,350	403	3,171	3,730	4,196	496	3,171	3,730	4,196
9,350	9,400	399	3,188	3,750	4,219	496	3,188	3,750	4,219
9,400	9,450	395	3,205	3,770	4,241	496	3,205	3,770	4,241
9,450	9,500	391	3,222	3,790	4,264	496	3,222	3,790	4,264
9,500	9,550	387	3,239	3,810	4,286	496	3,239	3,810	4,286
9,550	9,600	384	3,256	3,830	4,309	496	3,256	3,830	4,309
9,600	9,650	380	3,273	3,850	4,331	496	3,273	3,850	4,331
9,650	9,700	376	3,290	3,870	4,354	496	3,290	3,870	4,354
9,700	9,750	372	3,305	3,890	4,376	496	3,305	3,890	4,376
9,750	9,800	368	3,305	3,910	4,399	496	3,305	3,910	4,399
9,800	9,850	365	3,305	3,930	4,421	496	3,305	3,930	4,421
9,850	9,900	361	3,305	3,950	4,444	496	3,305	3,950	4,444
9,900	9,950	357	3,305	3,970	4,466	496	3,305	3,970	4,466
9,950	10,000	353	3,305	3,990	4,489	496	3,305	3,990	4,489
10,000	10,050	349	3,305	4,010	4,511	496	3,305	4,010	4,511
10,050	10,100	345	3,305	4,030	4,534	496	3,305	4,030	4,534
10,100	10,150	342	3,305	4,050	4,556	496	3,305	4,050	4,556
10,150	10,200	338	3,305	4,070	4,579	496	3,305	4,070	4,579
10,200	10,250	334	3,305	4,090	4,601	496	3,305	4,090	4,601
10,250	10,300	330	3,305	4,110	4,624	496	3,305	4,110	4,624
10,300	10,350	326	3,305	4,130	4,646	496	3,305	4,130	4,646
10,350	10,400	322	3,305	4,150	4,669	496	3,305	4,150	4,669
10,400	10,450	319	3,305	4,170	4,691	496	3,305	4,170	4,691
10,450	10,500	315	3,305	4,190	4,714	496	3,305	4,190	4,714
10,500	10,550	311	3,305	4,210	4,736	496	3,305	4,210	4,736
10,550	10,600	307	3,305	4,230	4,759	496	3,305	4,230	4,759
10,600	10,650	303	3,305	4,250	4,781	496	3,305	4,250	4,781
10,650	10,700	299	3,305	4,270	4,804	496	3,305	4,270	4,804
10,700	10,750	296	3,305	4,290	4,826	496	3,305	4,290	4,826
10,750	10,800	292	3,305	4,310	4,849	496	3,305	4,310	4,849
10,800	10,850	288	3,305	4,330	4,871	496	3,305	4,330	4,871
10,850	10,900	284	3,305	4,350	4,894	496	3,305	4,350	4,894
10,900	10,950	280	3,305	4,370	4,916	496	3,305	4,370	4,916
10,950	11,000	277	3,305	4,390	4,939	496	3,305	4,390	4,939
11,000	11,050	273	3,305	4,410	4,961	496	3,305	4,410	4,961
11,050	11,100	269	3,305	4,430	4,984	496	3,305	4,430	4,984
11,100	11,150	265	3,305	4,450	5,006	496	3,305	4,450	5,006
11,150	11,200	261	3,305	4,470	5,029	496	3,305	4,470	5,029
11,200	11,250	257	3,305	4,490	5,051	496	3,305	4,490	5,051
11,250	11,300	254	3,305	4,510	5,074	496	3,305	4,510	5,074
11,300	11,350	250	3,305	4,530	5,096	496	3,305	4,530	5,096
11,350	11,400	246	3,305	4,550	5,119	496	3,305	4,550	5,119
11,400	11,450	242	3,305	4,570	5,141	496	3,305	4,570	5,141
11,450	11,500	238	3,305	4,590	5,164	496	3,305	4,590	5,164
11,500	11,550	234	3,305	4,610	5,186	496	3,305	4,610	5,186
11,550	11,600	231	3,305	4,630	5,209	496	3,305	4,630	5,209
11,600	11,650	227	3,305	4,650	5,231	496	3,305	4,650	5,231
11,650	11,700	223	3,305	4,670	5,254	496	3,305	4,670	5,254
11,700	11,750	219	3,305	4,690	5,276	496	3,305	4,690	5,276
11,750	11,800	215	3,305	4,710	5,299	496	3,305	4,710	5,299
11,800	11,850	212	3,305	4,730	5,321	496	3,305	4,730	5,321
11,850	11,900	208	3,305	4,750	5,344	496	3,305	4,750	5,344
11,900	11,950	204	3,305	4,770	5,366	496	3,305	4,770	5,366
11,950	12,000	200	3,305	4,790	5,389	496	3,305	4,790	5,389
12,000	12,050	196	3,305	4,810	5,411	496	3,305	4,810	5,411
12,050	12,100	192	3,305	4,830	5,434	496	3,305	4,830	5,434
12,100	12,150	189	3,305	4,850	5,456	496	3,305	4,850	5,456
12,150	12,200	185	3,305	4,870	5,479	496	3,305	4,870	5,479
12,200	12,250	181	3,305	4,890	5,501	496	3,305	4,890	5,501
12,250	12,300	177	3,305	4,910	5,524	496	3,305	4,910	5,524
12,300	12,350	173	3,305	4,930	5,546	496	3,305	4,930	5,546
12,350	12,400	169	3,305	4,950	5,569	496	3,305	4,950	5,569
12,400	12,450	166	3,305	4,970	5,591	496	3,305	4,970	5,591
12,450	12,500	162	3,305	4,990	5,614	496	3,305	4,990	5,614
12,500	12,550	158	3,305	5,010	5,636	496	3,305	5,010	5,636
12,550	12,600	154	3,305	5,030	5,659	496	3,305	5,030	5,659
12,600	12,650	150	3,305	5,050	5,681	496	3,305	5,050	5,681
12,650	12,700	146	3,305	5,070	5,704	496	3,305	5,070	5,704
12,700	12,750	143	3,305	5,090	5,726	496	3,305	5,090	5,726
12,750	12,800	139	3,305	5,110	5,749	496	3,305	5,110	5,749

(Continued)

Need more information or forms? Visit IRS.gov. - 61 -

¶87

»»→ *Caution:* **This is a draft 2014 Earned Income Credit (EIC) Table. At the time of publication, the IRS had not yet released the 2014 Earned Income Credit (EIC) Table. For the latest information, see CCHGroup.com/TaxUpdates.**

Earned Income Credit (EIC) Table - Continued   (**Caution.** This is **not** a tax table.)

If the amount you are looking up from the worksheet is–		Single, head of household, or qualifying widow(er) and the number of children you have is–				Married filing jointly and the number of children you have is–			
At least	But less than	0	1	2	3	0	1	2	3
		Your credit is–				Your credit is–			
12,800	12,850	135	3,305	5,130	5,771	496	3,305	5,130	5,771
12,850	12,900	131	3,305	5,150	5,794	496	3,305	5,150	5,794
12,900	12,950	127	3,305	5,170	5,816	496	3,305	5,170	5,816
12,950	13,000	124	3,305	5,190	5,839	496	3,305	5,190	5,839
13,000	13,050	120	3,305	5,210	5,861	496	3,305	5,210	5,861
13,050	13,100	116	3,305	5,230	5,884	496	3,305	5,230	5,884
13,100	13,150	112	3,305	5,250	5,906	496	3,305	5,250	5,906
13,150	13,200	108	3,305	5,270	5,929	496	3,305	5,270	5,929
13,200	13,250	104	3,305	5,290	5,951	496	3,305	5,290	5,951
13,250	13,300	101	3,305	5,310	5,974	496	3,305	5,310	5,974
13,300	13,350	97	3,305	5,330	5,996	496	3,305	5,330	5,996
13,350	13,400	93	3,305	5,350	6,019	496	3,305	5,350	6,019
13,400	13,450	89	3,305	5,370	6,041	496	3,305	5,370	6,041
13,450	13,500	85	3,305	5,390	6,064	496	3,305	5,390	6,064
13,500	13,550	81	3,305	5,410	6,086	496	3,305	5,410	6,086
13,550	13,600	78	3,305	5,430	6,109	493	3,305	5,430	6,109
13,600	13,650	74	3,305	5,450	6,131	489	3,305	5,450	6,131
13,650	13,700	70	3,305	5,460	6,143	485	3,305	5,460	6,143
13,700	13,750	66	3,305	5,460	6,143	482	3,305	5,460	6,143
13,750	13,800	62	3,305	5,460	6,143	478	3,305	5,460	6,143
13,800	13,850	59	3,305	5,460	6,143	474	3,305	5,460	6,143
13,850	13,900	55	3,305	5,460	6,143	470	3,305	5,460	6,143
13,900	13,950	51	3,305	5,460	6,143	466	3,305	5,460	6,143
13,950	14,000	47	3,305	5,460	6,143	462	3,305	5,460	6,143
14,000	14,050	43	3,305	5,460	6,143	459	3,305	5,460	6,143
14,050	14,100	39	3,305	5,460	6,143	455	3,305	5,460	6,143
14,100	14,150	36	3,305	5,460	6,143	451	3,305	5,460	6,143
14,150	14,200	32	3,305	5,460	6,143	447	3,305	5,460	6,143
14,200	14,250	28	3,305	5,460	6,143	443	3,305	5,460	6,143
14,250	14,300	24	3,305	5,460	6,143	439	3,305	5,460	6,143
14,300	14,350	20	3,305	5,460	6,143	436	3,305	5,460	6,143
14,350	14,400	16	3,305	5,460	6,143	432	3,305	5,460	6,143
14,400	14,450	13	3,305	5,460	6,143	428	3,305	5,460	6,143
14,450	14,500	9	3,305	5,460	6,143	424	3,305	5,460	6,143
14,500	14,550	5	3,305	5,460	6,143	420	3,305	5,460	6,143
14,550	14,600	*	3,305	5,460	6,143	417	3,305	5,460	6,143
14,600	14,650	0	3,305	5,460	6,143	413	3,305	5,460	6,143
14,650	14,700	0	3,305	5,460	6,143	409	3,305	5,460	6,143
14,700	14,750	0	3,305	5,460	6,143	405	3,305	5,460	6,143
14,750	14,800	0	3,305	5,460	6,143	401	3,305	5,460	6,143
14,800	14,850	0	3,305	5,460	6,143	397	3,305	5,460	6,143
14,850	14,900	0	3,305	5,460	6,143	394	3,305	5,460	6,143
14,900	14,950	0	3,305	5,460	6,143	390	3,305	5,460	6,143
14,950	15,000	0	3,305	5,460	6,143	386	3,305	5,460	6,143
15,000	15,050	0	3,305	5,460	6,143	382	3,305	5,460	6,143
15,050	15,100	0	3,305	5,460	6,143	378	3,305	5,460	6,143
15,100	15,150	0	3,305	5,460	6,143	374	3,305	5,460	6,143
15,150	15,200	0	3,305	5,460	6,143	371	3,305	5,460	6,143
15,200	15,250	0	3,305	5,460	6,143	367	3,305	5,460	6,143
15,250	15,300	0	3,305	5,460	6,143	363	3,305	5,460	6,143
15,300	15,350	0	3,305	5,460	6,143	359	3,305	5,460	6,143
15,350	15,400	0	3,305	5,460	6,143	355	3,305	5,460	6,143
15,400	15,450	0	3,305	5,460	6,143	352	3,305	5,460	6,143
15,450	15,500	0	3,305	5,460	6,143	348	3,305	5,460	6,143
15,500	15,550	0	3,305	5,460	6,143	344	3,305	5,460	6,143
15,550	15,600	0	3,305	5,460	6,143	340	3,305	5,460	6,143
15,600	15,650	0	3,305	5,460	6,143	336	3,305	5,460	6,143
15,650	15,700	0	3,305	5,460	6,143	332	3,305	5,460	6,143
15,700	15,750	0	3,305	5,460	6,143	329	3,305	5,460	6,143
15,750	15,800	0	3,305	5,460	6,143	325	3,305	5,460	6,143
15,800	15,850	0	3,305	5,460	6,143	321	3,305	5,460	6,143
15,850	15,900	0	3,305	5,460	6,143	317	3,305	5,460	6,143
15,900	15,950	0	3,305	5,460	6,143	313	3,305	5,460	6,143
15,950	16,000	0	3,305	5,460	6,143	309	3,305	5,460	6,143

If the amount you are looking up from the worksheet is–		Single, head of household, or qualifying widow(er) and the number of children you have is–				Married filing jointly and the number of children you have is–			
At least	But less than	0	1	2	3	0	1	2	3
		Your credit is–				Your credit is–			
16,000	16,050	0	3,305	5,460	6,143	306	3,305	5,460	6,143
16,050	16,100	0	3,305	5,460	6,143	302	3,305	5,460	6,143
16,100	16,150	0	3,305	5,460	6,143	298	3,305	5,460	6,143
16,150	16,200	0	3,305	5,460	6,143	294	3,305	5,460	6,143
16,200	16,250	0	3,305	5,460	6,143	290	3,305	5,460	6,143
16,250	16,300	0	3,305	5,460	6,143	286	3,305	5,460	6,143
16,300	16,350	0	3,305	5,460	6,143	283	3,305	5,460	6,143
16,350	16,400	0	3,305	5,460	6,143	279	3,305	5,460	6,143
16,400	16,450	0	3,305	5,460	6,143	275	3,305	5,460	6,143
16,450	16,500	0	3,305	5,460	6,143	271	3,305	5,460	6,143
16,500	16,550	0	3,305	5,460	6,143	267	3,305	5,460	6,143
16,550	16,600	0	3,305	5,460	6,143	264	3,305	5,460	6,143
16,600	16,650	0	3,305	5,460	6,143	260	3,305	5,460	6,143
16,650	16,700	0	3,305	5,460	6,143	256	3,305	5,460	6,143
16,700	16,750	0	3,305	5,460	6,143	252	3,305	5,460	6,143
16,750	16,800	0	3,305	5,460	6,143	248	3,305	5,460	6,143
16,800	16,850	0	3,305	5,460	6,143	244	3,305	5,460	6,143
16,850	16,900	0	3,305	5,460	6,143	241	3,305	5,460	6,143
16,900	16,950	0	3,305	5,460	6,143	237	3,305	5,460	6,143
16,950	17,000	0	3,305	5,460	6,143	233	3,305	5,460	6,143
17,000	17,050	0	3,305	5,460	6,143	229	3,305	5,460	6,143
17,050	17,100	0	3,305	5,460	6,143	225	3,305	5,460	6,143
17,100	17,150	0	3,305	5,460	6,143	221	3,305	5,460	6,143
17,150	17,200	0	3,305	5,460	6,143	218	3,305	5,460	6,143
17,200	17,250	0	3,305	5,460	6,143	214	3,305	5,460	6,143
17,250	17,300	0	3,305	5,460	6,143	210	3,305	5,460	6,143
17,300	17,350	0	3,305	5,460	6,143	206	3,305	5,460	6,143
17,350	17,400	0	3,305	5,460	6,143	202	3,305	5,460	6,143
17,400	17,450	0	3,305	5,460	6,143	199	3,305	5,460	6,143
17,450	17,500	0	3,305	5,460	6,143	195	3,305	5,460	6,143
17,500	17,550	0	3,305	5,460	6,143	191	3,305	5,460	6,143
17,550	17,600	0	3,305	5,460	6,143	187	3,305	5,460	6,143
17,600	17,650	0	3,305	5,460	6,143	183	3,305	5,460	6,143
17,650	17,700	0	3,305	5,460	6,143	179	3,305	5,460	6,143
17,700	17,750	0	3,305	5,460	6,143	176	3,305	5,460	6,143
17,750	17,800	0	3,305	5,460	6,143	172	3,305	5,460	6,143
17,800	17,850	0	3,305	5,460	6,143	168	3,305	5,460	6,143
17,850	17,900	0	3,298	5,451	6,133	164	3,305	5,460	6,143
17,900	17,950	0	3,290	5,440	6,122	160	3,305	5,460	6,143
17,950	18,000	0	3,282	5,429	6,112	156	3,305	5,460	6,143
18,000	18,050	0	3,274	5,419	6,101	153	3,305	5,460	6,143
18,050	18,100	0	3,266	5,408	6,091	149	3,305	5,460	6,143
18,100	18,150	0	3,258	5,398	6,080	145	3,305	5,460	6,143
18,150	18,200	0	3,250	5,387	6,070	141	3,305	5,460	6,143
18,200	18,250	0	3,242	5,377	6,059	137	3,305	5,460	6,143
18,250	18,300	0	3,234	5,366	6,049	133	3,305	5,460	6,143
18,300	18,350	0	3,226	5,356	6,038	130	3,305	5,460	6,143
18,350	18,400	0	3,218	5,345	6,028	126	3,305	5,460	6,143
18,400	18,450	0	3,210	5,335	6,017	122	3,305	5,460	6,143
18,450	18,500	0	3,202	5,324	6,007	118	3,305	5,460	6,143
18,500	18,550	0	3,194	5,314	5,996	114	3,305	5,460	6,143
18,550	18,600	0	3,186	5,303	5,986	111	3,305	5,460	6,143
18,600	18,650	0	3,178	5,293	5,975	107	3,305	5,460	6,143
18,650	18,700	0	3,170	5,282	5,965	103	3,305	5,460	6,143
18,700	18,750	0	3,162	5,272	5,954	99	3,305	5,460	6,143
18,750	18,800	0	3,154	5,261	5,943	95	3,305	5,460	6,143
18,800	18,850	0	3,146	5,250	5,933	91	3,305	5,460	6,143
18,850	18,900	0	3,138	5,240	5,922	88	3,305	5,460	6,143
18,900	18,950	0	3,130	5,229	5,912	84	3,305	5,460	6,143
18,950	19,000	0	3,122	5,219	5,901	80	3,305	5,460	6,143
19,000	19,050	0	3,114	5,208	5,891	76	3,305	5,460	6,143
19,050	19,100	0	3,106	5,198	5,880	72	3,305	5,460	6,143
19,100	19,150	0	3,098	5,187	5,870	68	3,305	5,460	6,143
19,150	19,200	0	3,090	5,177	5,859	65	3,305	5,460	6,143

* If the amount you are looking up from the worksheet is at least $14,550 but less than $14,590, and you have no qualifying children, your credit is $2.
If the amount you are looking up from the worksheet is $14,590 or more, and you have no qualifying children, you cannot take the credit.

(Continued)

Need more information or forms? Visit IRS.gov.

¶87

»»→ Caution: This is a draft 2014 Earned Income Credit (EIC) Table. At the time of publication, the IRS had not yet released the 2014 Earned Income Credit (EIC) Table. For the latest information, see CCHGroup.com/TaxUpdates.

Earned Income Credit (EIC) Table - Continued   (**Caution.** This is **not** a tax table.)

The "Single, head of household, or qualifying widow(er)" and "Married filing jointly" credit columns give the credit for 0, 1, 2, and 3 children.

At least	But less than	Single/HoH/QW 0	1	2	3	MFJ 0	1	2	3
19,200	19,250	0	3,082	5,166	5,849	61	3,305	5,460	6,143
19,250	19,300	0	3,074	5,156	5,838	57	3,305	5,460	6,143
19,300	19,350	0	3,066	5,145	5,828	53	3,305	5,460	6,143
19,350	19,400	0	3,058	5,135	5,817	49	3,305	5,460	6,143
19,400	19,450	0	3,050	5,124	5,807	46	3,305	5,460	6,143
19,450	19,500	0	3,042	5,114	5,796	42	3,305	5,460	6,143
19,500	19,550	0	3,034	5,103	5,786	38	3,305	5,460	6,143
19,550	19,600	0	3,026	5,093	5,775	34	3,305	5,460	6,143
19,600	19,650	0	3,018	5,082	5,764	30	3,305	5,460	6,143
19,650	19,700	0	3,010	5,071	5,754	26	3,305	5,460	6,143
19,700	19,750	0	3,002	5,061	5,743	23	3,305	5,460	6,143
19,750	19,800	0	2,994	5,050	5,733	19	3,305	5,460	6,143
19,800	19,850	0	2,986	5,040	5,722	15	3,305	5,460	6,143
19,850	19,900	0	2,978	5,029	5,712	11	3,305	5,460	6,143
19,900	19,950	0	2,970	5,019	5,701	7	3,305	5,460	6,143
19,950	20,000	0	2,962	5,008	5,691	3	3,305	5,460	6,143
20,000	20,050	0	2,954	4,998	5,680	*	3,305	5,460	6,143
20,050	20,100	0	2,946	4,987	5,670	0	3,305	5,460	6,143
20,100	20,150	0	2,938	4,977	5,659	0	3,305	5,460	6,143
20,150	20,200	0	2,930	4,966	5,649	0	3,305	5,460	6,143
20,200	20,250	0	2,922	4,956	5,638	0	3,305	5,460	6,143
20,250	20,300	0	2,914	4,945	5,628	0	3,305	5,460	6,143
20,300	20,350	0	2,906	4,935	5,617	0	3,305	5,460	6,143
20,350	20,400	0	2,898	4,924	5,607	0	3,305	5,460	6,143
20,400	20,450	0	2,890	4,913	5,596	0	3,305	5,460	6,143
20,450	20,500	0	2,882	4,903	5,585	0	3,305	5,460	6,143
20,500	20,550	0	2,874	4,892	5,575	0	3,305	5,460	6,143
20,550	20,600	0	2,866	4,882	5,564	0	3,305	5,460	6,143
20,600	20,650	0	2,858	4,871	5,554	0	3,305	5,460	6,143
20,650	20,700	0	2,850	4,861	5,543	0	3,305	5,460	6,143
20,700	20,750	0	2,842	4,850	5,533	0	3,305	5,460	6,143
20,750	20,800	0	2,834	4,840	5,522	0	3,305	5,460	6,143
20,800	20,850	0	2,826	4,829	5,512	0	3,305	5,460	6,143
20,850	20,900	0	2,818	4,819	5,501	0	3,305	5,460	6,143
20,900	20,950	0	2,810	4,808	5,491	0	3,305	5,460	6,143
20,950	21,000	0	2,802	4,798	5,480	0	3,305	5,460	6,143
21,000	21,050	0	2,794	4,787	5,470	0	3,305	5,460	6,143
21,050	21,100	0	2,786	4,777	5,459	0	3,305	5,460	6,143
21,100	21,150	0	2,778	4,766	5,449	0	3,305	5,460	6,143
21,150	21,200	0	2,770	4,756	5,438	0	3,305	5,460	6,143
21,200	21,250	0	2,762	4,745	5,428	0	3,305	5,460	6,143
21,250	21,300	0	2,754	4,734	5,417	0	3,305	5,460	6,143
21,300	21,350	0	2,746	4,724	5,406	0	3,305	5,460	6,143
21,350	21,400	0	2,738	4,713	5,396	0	3,305	5,460	6,143
21,400	21,450	0	2,730	4,703	5,385	0	3,305	5,460	6,143
21,450	21,500	0	2,722	4,692	5,375	0	3,305	5,460	6,143
21,500	21,550	0	2,714	4,682	5,364	0	3,305	5,460	6,143
21,550	21,600	0	2,706	4,671	5,354	0	3,305	5,460	6,143
21,600	21,650	0	2,698	4,661	5,343	0	3,305	5,460	6,143
21,650	21,700	0	2,690	4,650	5,333	0	3,305	5,460	6,143
21,700	21,750	0	2,682	4,640	5,322	0	3,305	5,460	6,143
21,750	21,800	0	2,674	4,629	5,312	0	3,305	5,460	6,143
21,800	21,850	0	2,666	4,619	5,301	0	3,305	5,460	6,143
21,850	21,900	0	2,658	4,608	5,291	0	3,305	5,460	6,143
21,900	21,950	0	2,650	4,598	5,280	0	3,305	5,460	6,143
21,950	22,000	0	2,642	4,587	5,270	0	3,305	5,460	6,143
22,000	22,050	0	2,634	4,577	5,259	0	3,305	5,460	6,143
22,050	22,100	0	2,626	4,566	5,249	0	3,305	5,460	6,143
22,100	22,150	0	2,618	4,555	5,238	0	3,305	5,460	6,143
22,150	22,200	0	2,610	4,545	5,227	0	3,305	5,460	6,143
22,200	22,250	0	2,602	4,534	5,217	0	3,305	5,460	6,143
22,250	22,300	0	2,594	4,524	5,206	0	3,305	5,460	6,143
22,300	22,350	0	2,586	4,513	5,196	0	3,305	5,460	6,143
22,350	22,400	0	2,579	4,503	5,185	0	3,305	5,460	6,143
22,400	22,450	0	2,571	4,492	5,175	0	3,305	5,460	6,143
22,450	22,500	0	2,563	4,482	5,164	0	3,305	5,460	6,143
22,500	22,550	0	2,555	4,471	5,154	0	3,305	5,460	6,143
22,550	22,600	0	2,547	4,461	5,143	0	3,305	5,460	6,143
22,600	22,650	0	2,539	4,450	5,133	0	3,305	5,460	6,143
22,650	22,700	0	2,531	4,440	5,122	0	3,305	5,460	6,143
22,700	22,750	0	2,523	4,429	5,112	0	3,305	5,460	6,143
22,750	22,800	0	2,515	4,419	5,101	0	3,305	5,460	6,143
22,800	22,850	0	2,507	4,408	5,091	0	3,305	5,460	6,143
22,850	22,900	0	2,499	4,398	5,080	0	3,305	5,460	6,143
22,900	22,950	0	2,491	4,387	5,069	0	3,305	5,460	6,143
22,950	23,000	0	2,483	4,376	5,059	0	3,305	5,460	6,143
23,000	23,050	0	2,475	4,366	5,048	0	3,305	5,460	6,143
23,050	23,100	0	2,467	4,355	5,038	0	3,305	5,460	6,143
23,100	23,150	0	2,459	4,345	5,027	0	3,305	5,460	6,143
23,150	23,200	0	2,451	4,334	5,017	0	3,305	5,460	6,143
23,200	23,250	0	2,443	4,324	5,006	0	3,305	5,460	6,143
23,250	23,300	0	2,435	4,313	4,996	0	3,305	5,460	6,143
23,300	23,350	0	2,427	4,303	4,985	0	3,294	5,446	6,129
23,350	23,400	0	2,419	4,292	4,975	0	3,286	5,436	6,118
23,400	23,450	0	2,411	4,282	4,964	0	3,278	5,425	6,108
23,450	23,500	0	2,403	4,271	4,954	0	3,270	5,415	6,097
23,500	23,550	0	2,395	4,261	4,943	0	3,262	5,404	6,087
23,550	23,600	0	2,387	4,250	4,933	0	3,254	5,394	6,076
23,600	23,650	0	2,379	4,240	4,922	0	3,246	5,383	6,066
23,650	23,700	0	2,371	4,229	4,912	0	3,238	5,373	6,055
23,700	23,750	0	2,363	4,219	4,901	0	3,230	5,362	6,045
23,750	23,800	0	2,355	4,208	4,890	0	3,223	5,352	6,034
23,800	23,850	0	2,347	4,197	4,880	0	3,215	5,341	6,024
23,850	23,900	0	2,339	4,187	4,869	0	3,207	5,330	6,013
23,900	23,950	0	2,331	4,176	4,859	0	3,199	5,320	6,002
23,950	24,000	0	2,323	4,166	4,848	0	3,191	5,309	5,992
24,000	24,050	0	2,315	4,155	4,838	0	3,183	5,299	5,981
24,050	24,100	0	2,307	4,145	4,827	0	3,175	5,288	5,971
24,100	24,150	0	2,299	4,134	4,817	0	3,167	5,278	5,960
24,150	24,200	0	2,291	4,124	4,806	0	3,159	5,267	5,950
24,200	24,250	0	2,283	4,113	4,796	0	3,151	5,257	5,939
24,250	24,300	0	2,275	4,103	4,785	0	3,143	5,246	5,929
24,300	24,350	0	2,267	4,092	4,775	0	3,135	5,236	5,918
24,350	24,400	0	2,259	4,082	4,764	0	3,127	5,225	5,908
24,400	24,450	0	2,251	4,071	4,754	0	3,119	5,215	5,897
24,450	24,500	0	2,243	4,061	4,743	0	3,111	5,204	5,887
24,500	24,550	0	2,235	4,050	4,733	0	3,103	5,194	5,876
24,550	24,600	0	2,227	4,040	4,722	0	3,095	5,183	5,866
24,600	24,650	0	2,219	4,029	4,711	0	3,087	5,173	5,855
24,650	24,700	0	2,211	4,018	4,701	0	3,079	5,162	5,845
24,700	24,750	0	2,203	4,008	4,690	0	3,071	5,151	5,834
24,750	24,800	0	2,195	3,997	4,680	0	3,063	5,141	5,823
24,800	24,850	0	2,187	3,987	4,669	0	3,055	5,130	5,813
24,850	24,900	0	2,179	3,976	4,659	0	3,047	5,120	5,802
24,900	24,950	0	2,171	3,966	4,648	0	3,039	5,109	5,792
24,950	25,000	0	2,163	3,955	4,638	0	3,031	5,099	5,781
25,000	25,050	0	2,155	3,945	4,627	0	3,023	5,088	5,771
25,050	25,100	0	2,147	3,934	4,617	0	3,015	5,078	5,760
25,100	25,150	0	2,139	3,924	4,606	0	3,007	5,067	5,750
25,150	25,200	0	2,131	3,913	4,596	0	2,999	5,057	5,739
25,200	25,250	0	2,123	3,903	4,585	0	2,991	5,046	5,729
25,250	25,300	0	2,115	3,892	4,575	0	2,983	5,036	5,718
25,300	25,350	0	2,107	3,882	4,564	0	2,975	5,025	5,708
25,350	25,400	0	2,099	3,871	4,554	0	2,967	5,015	5,697
25,400	25,450	0	2,091	3,860	4,543	0	2,959	5,004	5,687
25,450	25,500	0	2,083	3,850	4,532	0	2,951	4,994	5,676
25,500	25,550	0	2,075	3,839	4,522	0	2,943	4,983	5,665
25,550	25,600	0	2,067	3,829	4,511	0	2,935	4,972	5,655

* If the amount you are looking up from the worksheet is at least $20,000 but less than $20,020, and you have no qualifying children, your credit is $1.
If the amount you are looking up from the worksheet is $20,020 or more, and you have no qualifying children, you cannot take the credit.

(Continued)

¶87

>>> *Caution: This is a draft 2014 Earned Income Credit (EIC) Table. At the time of publication, the IRS had not yet released the 2014 Earned Income Credit (EIC) Table. For the latest information, see CCHGroup.com/TaxUpdates.*

Earned Income Credit (EIC) Table - *Continued*   (**Caution. This is not** a tax table.)

If the amount you are looking up from the worksheet is–		Single, head of household, or qualifying widow(er) and the number of children you have is–				Married filing jointly and the number of children you have is–				If the amount you are looking up from the worksheet is–		Single, head of household, or qualifying widow(er) and the number of children you have is–				Married filing jointly and the number of children you have is–			
		0	1	2	3	0	1	2	3			0	1	2	3	0	1	2	3
At least	But less than	Your credit is–				Your credit is–				At least	But less than	Your credit is–				Your credit is–			
25,600	25,650	0	2,059	3,818	4,501	0	2,927	4,962	5,644	29,200	29,250	0	1,484	3,060	3,743	0	2,352	4,204	4,886
25,650	25,700	0	2,051	3,808	4,490	0	2,919	4,951	5,634	29,250	29,300	0	1,476	3,050	3,732	0	2,344	4,193	4,876
25,700	25,750	0	2,043	3,797	4,480	0	2,911	4,941	5,623	29,300	29,350	0	1,468	3,039	3,722	0	2,336	4,183	4,865
25,750	25,800	0	2,035	3,787	4,469	0	2,903	4,930	5,613	29,350	29,400	0	1,460	3,029	3,711	0	2,328	4,172	4,855
25,800	25,850	0	2,027	3,776	4,459	0	2,895	4,920	5,602	29,400	29,450	0	1,452	3,018	3,701	0	2,320	4,162	4,844
25,850	25,900	0	2,019	3,766	4,448	0	2,887	4,909	5,592	29,450	29,500	0	1,444	3,008	3,690	0	2,312	4,151	4,834
25,900	25,950	0	2,011	3,755	4,438	0	2,879	4,899	5,581	29,500	29,550	0	1,436	2,997	3,680	0	2,304	4,141	4,823
25,950	26,000	0	2,003	3,745	4,427	0	2,871	4,888	5,571	29,550	29,600	0	1,428	2,987	3,669	0	2,296	4,130	4,813
26,000	26,050	0	1,995	3,734	4,417	0	2,863	4,878	5,560	29,600	29,650	0	1,420	2,976	3,658	0	2,298	4,120	4,802
26,050	26,100	0	1,987	3,724	4,406	0	2,855	4,867	5,550	29,650	29,700	0	1,412	2,965	3,648	0	2,280	4,109	4,792
26,100	26,150	0	1,979	3,713	4,396	0	2,847	4,857	5,539	29,700	29,750	0	1,404	2,955	3,637	0	2,272	4,098	4,781
26,150	26,200	0	1,971	3,703	4,385	0	2,839	4,846	5,529	29,750	29,800	0	1,396	2,944	3,627	0	2,264	4,088	4,770
26,200	26,250	0	1,963	3,692	4,375	0	2,831	4,836	5,518	29,800	29,850	0	1,388	2,934	3,616	0	2,256	4,077	4,760
26,250	26,300	0	1,955	3,681	4,364	0	2,823	4,825	5,508	29,850	29,900	0	1,380	2,923	3,606	0	2,248	4,067	4,749
26,300	26,350	0	1,947	3,671	4,353	0	2,815	4,815	5,497	29,900	29,950	0	1,372	2,913	3,595	0	2,240	4,056	4,739
26,350	26,400	0	1,939	3,660	4,343	0	2,807	4,804	5,486	29,950	30,000	0	1,364	2,902	3,585	0	2,232	4,046	4,728
26,400	26,450	0	1,931	3,650	4,332	0	2,799	4,793	5,476	30,000	30,050	0	1,356	2,892	3,574	0	2,224	4,035	4,718
26,450	26,500	0	1,923	3,639	4,322	0	2,791	4,783	5,465	30,050	30,100	0	1,348	2,881	3,564	0	2,216	4,025	4,707
26,500	26,550	0	1,915	3,629	4,311	0	2,783	4,772	5,455	30,100	30,150	0	1,340	2,871	3,553	0	2,208	4,014	4,697
26,550	26,600	0	1,907	3,618	4,301	0	2,775	4,762	5,444	30,150	30,200	0	1,332	2,860	3,543	0	2,200	4,004	4,686
26,600	26,650	0	1,899	3,608	4,290	0	2,767	4,751	5,434	30,200	30,250	0	1,324	2,850	3,532	0	2,192	3,993	4,676
26,650	26,700	0	1,891	3,597	4,280	0	2,759	4,741	5,423	30,250	30,300	0	1,316	2,839	3,522	0	2,184	3,983	4,665
26,700	26,750	0	1,883	3,587	4,269	0	2,751	4,730	5,413	30,300	30,350	0	1,308	2,829	3,511	0	2,176	3,972	4,655
26,750	26,800	0	1,875	3,576	4,259	0	2,743	4,720	5,402	30,350	30,400	0	1,300	2,818	3,501	0	2,168	3,962	4,644
26,800	26,850	0	1,867	3,566	4,248	0	2,735	4,709	5,392	30,400	30,450	0	1,292	2,807	3,490	0	2,160	3,951	4,634
26,850	26,900	0	1,859	3,555	4,238	0	2,727	4,699	5,381	30,450	30,500	0	1,284	2,797	3,479	0	2,152	3,941	4,623
26,900	26,950	0	1,851	3,545	4,227	0	2,719	4,688	5,371	30,500	30,550	0	1,276	2,786	3,469	0	2,144	3,930	4,612
26,950	27,000	0	1,843	3,534	4,217	0	2,711	4,678	5,360	30,550	30,600	0	1,268	2,776	3,458	0	2,136	3,919	4,602
27,000	27,050	0	1,835	3,524	4,206	0	2,703	4,667	5,350	30,600	30,650	0	1,260	2,765	3,448	0	2,128	3,909	4,591
27,050	27,100	0	1,827	3,513	4,196	0	2,695	4,657	5,339	30,650	30,700	0	1,252	2,755	3,437	0	2,120	3,898	4,581
27,100	27,150	0	1,819	3,502	4,185	0	2,687	4,646	5,329	30,700	30,750	0	1,244	2,744	3,427	0	2,112	3,888	4,570
27,150	27,200	0	1,811	3,492	4,174	0	2,679	4,636	5,318	30,750	30,800	0	1,236	2,734	3,416	0	2,104	3,877	4,560
27,200	27,250	0	1,803	3,481	4,164	0	2,671	4,625	5,307	30,800	30,850	0	1,228	2,723	3,406	0	2,096	3,867	4,549
27,250	27,300	0	1,795	3,471	4,153	0	2,663	4,614	5,297	30,850	30,900	0	1,220	2,713	3,395	0	2,088	3,856	4,539
27,300	27,350	0	1,787	3,460	4,143	0	2,655	4,604	5,286	30,900	30,950	0	1,212	2,702	3,385	0	2,080	3,846	4,528
27,350	27,400	0	1,780	3,450	4,132	0	2,647	4,593	5,276	30,950	31,000	0	1,204	2,692	3,374	0	2,072	3,835	4,518
27,400	27,450	0	1,772	3,439	4,122	0	2,639	4,583	5,265	31,000	31,050	0	1,196	2,681	3,364	0	2,064	3,825	4,507
27,450	27,500	0	1,764	3,429	4,111	0	2,631	4,572	5,255	31,050	31,100	0	1,188	2,671	3,353	0	2,056	3,814	4,497
27,500	27,550	0	1,756	3,418	4,101	0	2,623	4,562	5,244	31,100	31,150	0	1,180	2,660	3,343	0	2,048	3,804	4,486
27,550	27,600	0	1,748	3,408	4,090	0	2,615	4,551	5,234	31,150	31,200	0	1,172	2,650	3,332	0	2,040	3,793	4,476
27,600	27,650	0	1,740	3,397	4,080	0	2,607	4,541	5,223	31,200	31,250	0	1,164	2,639	3,322	0	2,032	3,783	4,465
27,650	27,700	0	1,732	3,387	4,069	0	2,599	4,530	5,213	31,250	31,300	0	1,156	2,628	3,311	0	2,024	3,772	4,455
27,700	27,750	0	1,724	3,376	4,059	0	2,591	4,520	5,202	31,300	31,350	0	1,148	2,618	3,300	0	2,016	3,762	4,444
27,750	27,800	0	1,716	3,366	4,048	0	2,583	4,509	5,192	31,350	31,400	0	1,140	2,607	3,290	0	2,008	3,751	4,433
27,800	27,850	0	1,708	3,355	4,038	0	2,575	4,499	5,181	31,400	31,450	0	1,132	2,597	3,279	0	2,000	3,740	4,423
27,850	27,900	0	1,700	3,345	4,027	0	2,567	4,488	5,171	31,450	31,500	0	1,124	2,586	3,269	0	1,992	3,730	4,412
27,900	27,950	0	1,692	3,334	4,016	0	2,559	4,478	5,160	31,500	31,550	0	1,116	2,576	3,258	0	1,984	3,719	4,402
27,950	28,000	0	1,684	3,323	4,006	0	2,551	4,467	5,150	31,550	31,600	0	1,108	2,565	3,248	0	1,976	3,709	4,391
28,000	28,050	0	1,676	3,313	3,995	0	2,543	4,456	5,139	31,600	31,650	0	1,100	2,555	3,237	0	1,968	3,698	4,381
28,050	28,100	0	1,668	3,302	3,985	0	2,535	4,446	5,128	31,650	31,700	0	1,092	2,544	3,227	0	1,960	3,688	4,370
28,100	28,150	0	1,660	3,292	3,974	0	2,527	4,435	5,118	31,700	31,750	0	1,084	2,534	3,216	0	1,952	3,677	4,360
28,150	28,200	0	1,652	3,281	3,964	0	2,519	4,425	5,107	31,750	31,800	0	1,076	2,523	3,206	0	1,944	3,667	4,349
28,200	28,250	0	1,644	3,271	3,953	0	2,511	4,414	5,097	31,800	31,850	0	1,068	2,513	3,195	0	1,936	3,656	4,339
28,250	28,300	0	1,636	3,260	3,943	0	2,503	4,404	5,086	31,850	31,900	0	1,060	2,502	3,185	0	1,928	3,646	4,328
28,300	28,350	0	1,628	3,250	3,932	0	2,495	4,383	5,076	31,900	31,950	0	1,052	2,492	3,174	0	1,920	3,635	4,318
28,350	28,400	0	1,620	3,239	3,922	0	2,487	4,383	5,065	31,950	32,000	0	1,044	2,481	3,164	0	1,912	3,625	4,307
28,400	28,450	0	1,612	3,229	3,911	0	2,479	4,372	5,055	32,000	32,050	0	1,036	2,471	3,153	0	1,904	3,614	4,297
28,450	28,500	0	1,604	3,218	3,901	0	2,471	4,362	5,044	32,050	32,100	0	1,028	2,460	3,143	0	1,896	3,604	4,286
28,500	28,550	0	1,596	3,208	3,890	0	2,463	4,351	5,034	32,100	32,150	0	1,020	2,449	3,132	0	1,888	3,593	4,276
28,550	28,600	0	1,588	3,197	3,880	0	2,455	4,341	5,023	32,150	32,200	0	1,012	2,439	3,121	0	1,880	3,583	4,265
28,600	28,650	0	1,580	3,187	3,869	0	2,447	4,330	5,013	32,200	32,250	0	1,004	2,428	3,111	0	1,872	3,572	4,254
28,650	28,700	0	1,572	3,176	3,859	0	2,439	4,320	5,002	32,250	32,300	0	996	2,418	3,100	0	1,864	3,561	4,244
28,700	28,750	0	1,564	3,166	3,848	0	2,431	4,309	4,992	32,300	32,350	0	988	2,407	3,090	0	1,856	3,551	4,233
28,750	28,800	0	1,556	3,155	3,837	0	2,424	4,299	4,981	32,350	32,400	0	981	2,397	3,079	0	1,848	3,540	4,223
28,800	28,850	0	1,548	3,144	3,827	0	2,416	4,288	4,971	32,400	32,450	0	973	2,386	3,069	0	1,840	3,530	4,212
28,850	28,900	0	1,540	3,134	3,816	0	2,408	4,277	4,960	32,450	32,500	0	965	2,376	3,058	0	1,832	3,519	4,202
28,900	28,950	0	1,532	3,123	3,806	0	2,400	4,267	4,949	32,500	32,550	0	957	2,365	3,048	0	1,824	3,509	4,191
28,950	29,000	0	1,524	3,113	3,795	0	2,392	4,256	4,939	32,550	32,600	0	949	2,355	3,037	0	1,816	3,498	4,181
29,000	29,050	0	1,516	3,102	3,785	0	2,384	4,246	4,928	32,600	32,650	0	941	2,344	3,027	0	1,808	3,488	4,170
29,050	29,100	0	1,508	3,092	3,774	0	2,376	4,235	4,918	32,650	32,700	0	933	2,334	3,016	0	1,800	3,477	4,160
29,100	29,150	0	1,500	3,081	3,764	0	2,368	4,225	4,907	32,700	32,750	0	925	2,323	3,006	0	1,792	3,467	4,149
29,150	29,200	0	1,492	3,071	3,753	0	2,360	4,214	4,897	32,750	32,800	0	917	2,313	2,995	0	1,784	3,456	4,139

(Continued)

Need more information or forms? Visit IRS.gov.

¶87

»»→ Caution: *This is a draft 2014 Earned Income Credit (EIC) Table. At the time of publication, the IRS had not yet released the 2014 Earned Income Credit (EIC) Table. For the latest information, see CCHGroup.com/TaxUpdates.*

Earned Income Credit (EIC) Table - Continued   (Caution. This is **not** a tax table.)

At least	But less than	Single, head of household, or qualifying widow(er) and the number of children you have is— 0	1	2	3	Married filing jointly and the number of children you have is— 0	1	2	3
32,800	32,850	0	909	2,302	2,985	0	1,776	3,446	4,128
32,850	32,900	0	901	2,292	2,974	0	1,768	3,435	4,118
32,900	32,950	0	893	2,281	2,963	0	1,760	3,425	4,107
32,950	33,000	0	885	2,270	2,953	0	1,752	3,414	4,097
33,000	33,050	0	877	2,260	2,942	0	1,744	3,403	4,086
33,050	33,100	0	869	2,249	2,932	0	1,736	3,393	4,075
33,100	33,150	0	861	2,239	2,921	0	1,728	3,382	4,065
33,150	33,200	0	853	2,228	2,911	0	1,720	3,372	4,054
33,200	33,250	0	845	2,218	2,900	0	1,712	3,361	4,044
33,250	33,300	0	837	2,207	2,890	0	1,704	3,351	4,033
33,300	33,350	0	829	2,197	2,879	0	1,696	3,340	4,023
33,350	33,400	0	821	2,186	2,869	0	1,688	3,330	4,012
33,400	33,450	0	813	2,176	2,858	0	1,680	3,319	4,002
33,450	33,500	0	805	2,165	2,848	0	1,672	3,309	3,991
33,500	33,550	0	797	2,155	2,837	0	1,664	3,298	3,981
33,550	33,600	0	789	2,144	2,827	0	1,656	3,288	3,970
33,600	33,650	0	781	2,134	2,816	0	1,648	3,277	3,960
33,650	33,700	0	773	2,123	2,806	0	1,640	3,267	3,949
33,700	33,750	0	765	2,113	2,795	0	1,632	3,256	3,939
33,750	33,800	0	757	2,102	2,784	0	1,625	3,246	3,928
33,800	33,850	0	749	2,091	2,774	0	1,617	3,235	3,918
33,850	33,900	0	741	2,081	2,763	0	1,609	3,224	3,907
33,900	33,950	0	733	2,070	2,753	0	1,601	3,214	3,896
33,950	34,000	0	725	2,060	2,742	0	1,593	3,203	3,886
34,000	34,050	0	717	2,049	2,732	0	1,585	3,193	3,875
34,050	34,100	0	709	2,039	2,721	0	1,577	3,182	3,865
34,100	34,150	0	701	2,028	2,711	0	1,569	3,172	3,854
34,150	34,200	0	693	2,018	2,700	0	1,561	3,161	3,844
34,200	34,250	0	685	2,007	2,690	0	1,553	3,151	3,833
34,250	34,300	0	677	1,997	2,679	0	1,545	3,140	3,823
34,300	34,350	0	669	1,986	2,669	0	1,537	3,130	3,812
34,350	34,400	0	661	1,976	2,658	0	1,529	3,119	3,802
34,400	34,450	0	653	1,965	2,648	0	1,521	3,109	3,791
34,450	34,500	0	645	1,955	2,637	0	1,513	3,098	3,781
34,500	34,550	0	637	1,944	2,627	0	1,505	3,088	3,770
34,550	34,600	0	629	1,934	2,616	0	1,497	3,077	3,760
34,600	34,650	0	621	1,923	2,605	0	1,489	3,067	3,749
34,650	34,700	0	613	1,912	2,595	0	1,481	3,056	3,739
34,700	34,750	0	605	1,902	2,584	0	1,473	3,045	3,728
34,750	34,800	0	597	1,891	2,574	0	1,465	3,035	3,717
34,800	34,850	0	589	1,881	2,563	0	1,457	3,024	3,707
34,850	34,900	0	581	1,870	2,553	0	1,449	3,014	3,696
34,900	34,950	0	573	1,860	2,542	0	1,441	3,003	3,686
34,950	35,000	0	565	1,849	2,532	0	1,433	2,993	3,675
35,000	35,050	0	557	1,839	2,521	0	1,425	2,982	3,665
35,050	35,100	0	549	1,828	2,511	0	1,417	2,972	3,654
35,100	35,150	0	541	1,818	2,500	0	1,409	2,961	3,644
35,150	35,200	0	533	1,807	2,490	0	1,401	2,951	3,633
35,200	35,250	0	525	1,797	2,479	0	1,393	2,940	3,623
35,250	35,300	0	517	1,786	2,469	0	1,385	2,930	3,612
35,300	35,350	0	509	1,776	2,458	0	1,377	2,919	3,602
35,350	35,400	0	501	1,765	2,448	0	1,369	2,909	3,591
35,400	35,450	0	493	1,754	2,437	0	1,361	2,898	3,581
35,450	35,500	0	485	1,744	2,426	0	1,353	2,888	3,570
35,500	35,550	0	477	1,733	2,416	0	1,345	2,877	3,559
35,550	35,600	0	469	1,723	2,405	0	1,337	2,866	3,549
35,600	35,650	0	461	1,712	2,395	0	1,329	2,856	3,538
35,650	35,700	0	453	1,702	2,384	0	1,321	2,845	3,528
35,700	35,750	0	445	1,691	2,374	0	1,313	2,835	3,517
35,750	35,800	0	437	1,681	2,363	0	1,305	2,824	3,507
35,800	35,850	0	429	1,670	2,353	0	1,297	2,814	3,496
35,850	35,900	0	421	1,660	2,342	0	1,289	2,803	3,486
35,900	35,950	0	413	1,649	2,332	0	1,281	2,793	3,475
35,950	36,000	0	405	1,639	2,321	0	1,273	2,782	3,465

At least	But less than	Single, head of household, or qualifying widow(er) and the number of children you have is— 0	1	2	3	Married filing jointly and the number of children you have is— 0	1	2	3
36,000	36,050	0	397	1,628	2,311	0	1,265	2,772	3,454
36,050	36,100	0	389	1,618	2,300	0	1,257	2,761	3,444
36,100	36,150	0	381	1,607	2,290	0	1,249	2,751	3,433
36,150	36,200	0	373	1,597	2,279	0	1,241	2,740	3,423
36,200	36,250	0	365	1,586	2,269	0	1,233	2,730	3,412
36,250	36,300	0	357	1,575	2,258	0	1,225	2,719	3,402
36,300	36,350	0	349	1,565	2,247	0	1,217	2,709	3,391
36,350	36,400	0	341	1,554	2,237	0	1,209	2,698	3,380
36,400	36,450	0	333	1,544	2,226	0	1,201	2,687	3,370
36,450	36,500	0	325	1,533	2,216	0	1,193	2,677	3,359
36,500	36,550	0	317	1,523	2,205	0	1,185	2,666	3,349
36,550	36,600	0	309	1,512	2,195	0	1,177	2,656	3,338
36,600	36,650	0	301	1,502	2,184	0	1,169	2,645	3,328
36,650	36,700	0	293	1,491	2,174	0	1,161	2,635	3,317
36,700	36,750	0	285	1,481	2,163	0	1,153	2,624	3,307
36,750	36,800	0	277	1,470	2,153	0	1,145	2,614	3,296
36,800	36,850	0	269	1,460	2,142	0	1,137	2,603	3,286
36,850	36,900	0	261	1,449	2,132	0	1,129	2,593	3,275
36,900	36,950	0	253	1,439	2,121	0	1,121	2,582	3,265
36,950	37,000	0	245	1,428	2,111	0	1,113	2,572	3,254
37,000	37,050	0	237	1,418	2,100	0	1,105	2,561	3,244
37,050	37,100	0	229	1,407	2,090	0	1,097	2,551	3,233
37,100	37,150	0	221	1,396	2,079	0	1,089	2,540	3,223
37,150	37,200	0	213	1,386	2,068	0	1,081	2,530	3,212
37,200	37,250	0	205	1,375	2,058	0	1,073	2,519	3,201
37,250	37,300	0	197	1,365	2,047	0	1,065	2,508	3,191
37,300	37,350	0	189	1,354	2,037	0	1,057	2,498	3,180
37,350	37,400	0	182	1,344	2,026	0	1,049	2,487	3,170
37,400	37,450	0	174	1,333	2,016	0	1,041	2,477	3,159
37,450	37,500	0	166	1,323	2,005	0	1,033	2,466	3,149
37,500	37,550	0	158	1,312	1,995	0	1,025	2,456	3,138
37,550	37,600	0	150	1,302	1,984	0	1,017	2,445	3,128
37,600	37,650	0	142	1,291	1,974	0	1,009	2,435	3,117
37,650	37,700	0	134	1,281	1,963	0	1,001	2,424	3,107
37,700	37,750	0	126	1,270	1,953	0	993	2,414	3,096
37,750	37,800	0	118	1,260	1,942	0	985	2,403	3,086
37,800	37,850	0	110	1,249	1,932	0	977	2,393	3,075
37,850	37,900	0	102	1,239	1,921	0	969	2,382	3,065
37,900	37,950	0	94	1,228	1,910	0	961	2,372	3,054
37,950	38,000	0	86	1,217	1,900	0	953	2,361	3,044
38,000	38,050	0	78	1,207	1,889	0	945	2,350	3,033
38,050	38,100	0	70	1,196	1,879	0	937	2,340	3,022
38,100	38,150	0	62	1,186	1,868	0	929	2,329	3,012
38,150	38,200	0	54	1,175	1,858	0	921	2,319	3,001
38,200	38,250	0	46	1,165	1,847	0	913	2,308	2,991
38,250	38,300	0	38	1,154	1,837	0	905	2,298	2,980
38,300	38,350	0	30	1,144	1,826	0	897	2,287	2,970
38,350	38,400	0	22	1,133	1,816	0	889	2,277	2,959
38,400	38,450	0	14	1,123	1,805	0	881	2,266	2,949
38,450	38,500	0	6	1,112	1,795	0	873	2,256	2,938
38,500	38,550	0	*	1,102	1,784	0	865	2,245	2,928
38,550	38,600	0	0	1,091	1,774	0	857	2,235	2,917
38,600	38,650	0	0	1,081	1,763	0	849	2,224	2,907
38,650	38,700	0	0	1,070	1,753	0	841	2,214	2,896
38,700	38,750	0	0	1,060	1,742	0	833	2,203	2,886
38,750	38,800	0	0	1,049	1,731	0	826	2,193	2,875
38,800	38,850	0	0	1,038	1,721	0	818	2,182	2,865
38,850	38,900	0	0	1,028	1,710	0	810	2,171	2,854
38,900	38,950	0	0	1,017	1,700	0	802	2,161	2,843
38,950	39,000	0	0	1,007	1,689	0	794	2,150	2,833
39,000	39,050	0	0	996	1,679	0	786	2,140	2,822
39,050	39,100	0	0	986	1,668	0	778	2,129	2,812
39,100	39,150	0	0	975	1,658	0	770	2,119	2,801
39,150	39,200	0	0	965	1,647	0	762	2,108	2,791

* If the amount you are looking up from the worksheet is at least $38,500 but less than $38,511, and you have one qualifying child, your credit is $1.
If the amount you are looking up from the worksheet is $38,511 or more, and you have one qualifying child, you cannot take the credit.

(Continued)

¶87

>>>→ *Caution: This is a draft 2014 Earned Income Credit (EIC) Table. At the time of publication, the IRS had not yet released the 2014 Earned Income Credit (EIC) Table. For the latest information, see CCHGroup.com/TaxUpdates.*

Earned Income Credit (EIC) Table - Continued (Caution. This is **not** a tax table.)

At least	But less than	Single, HoH, QW — 0	1	2	3	MFJ — 0	1	2	3
39,200	39,250	0	0	954	1,637	0	754	2,098	2,780
39,250	39,300	0	0	944	1,626	0	746	2,087	2,770
39,300	39,350	0	0	933	1,616	0	738	2,077	2,759
39,350	39,400	0	0	923	1,605	0	730	2,066	2,749
39,400	39,450	0	0	912	1,595	0	722	2,056	2,738
39,450	39,500	0	0	902	1,584	0	714	2,045	2,728
39,500	39,550	0	0	891	1,574	0	706	2,035	2,717
39,550	39,600	0	0	881	1,563	0	698	2,024	2,707
39,600	39,650	0	0	870	1,552	0	690	2,014	2,696
39,650	39,700	0	0	859	1,542	0	682	2,003	2,686
39,700	39,750	0	0	849	1,531	0	674	1,992	2,675
39,750	39,800	0	0	838	1,521	0	666	1,982	2,664
39,800	39,850	0	0	828	1,510	0	658	1,971	2,654
39,850	39,900	0	0	817	1,500	0	650	1,961	2,643
39,900	39,950	0	0	807	1,489	0	642	1,950	2,633
39,950	40,000	0	0	796	1,479	0	634	1,940	2,622
40,000	40,050	0	0	786	1,468	0	626	1,929	2,612
40,050	40,100	0	0	775	1,458	0	618	1,919	2,601
40,100	40,150	0	0	765	1,447	0	610	1,908	2,591
40,150	40,200	0	0	754	1,437	0	602	1,898	2,580
40,200	40,250	0	0	744	1,426	0	594	1,887	2,570
40,250	40,300	0	0	733	1,416	0	586	1,877	2,559
40,300	40,350	0	0	723	1,405	0	578	1,866	2,549
40,350	40,400	0	0	712	1,395	0	570	1,856	2,538
40,400	40,450	0	0	701	1,384	0	562	1,845	2,528
40,450	40,500	0	0	691	1,373	0	554	1,835	2,517
40,500	40,550	0	0	680	1,363	0	546	1,824	2,506
40,550	40,600	0	0	670	1,352	0	538	1,813	2,496
40,600	40,650	0	0	659	1,342	0	530	1,803	2,485
40,650	40,700	0	0	649	1,331	0	522	1,792	2,475
40,700	40,750	0	0	638	1,321	0	514	1,782	2,464
40,750	40,800	0	0	628	1,310	0	506	1,771	2,454
40,800	40,850	0	0	617	1,300	0	498	1,761	2,443
40,850	40,900	0	0	607	1,289	0	490	1,750	2,433
40,900	40,950	0	0	596	1,279	0	482	1,740	2,422
40,950	41,000	0	0	586	1,268	0	474	1,729	2,412
41,000	41,050	0	0	575	1,258	0	466	1,719	2,401
41,050	41,100	0	0	565	1,247	0	458	1,708	2,391
41,100	41,150	0	0	554	1,237	0	450	1,698	2,380
41,150	41,200	0	0	544	1,226	0	442	1,687	2,370
41,200	41,250	0	0	533	1,216	0	434	1,677	2,359
41,250	41,300	0	0	522	1,205	0	426	1,666	2,349
41,300	41,350	0	0	512	1,194	0	418	1,656	2,338
41,350	41,400	0	0	501	1,184	0	410	1,645	2,327
41,400	41,450	0	0	491	1,173	0	402	1,634	2,317
41,450	41,500	0	0	480	1,163	0	394	1,624	2,306
41,500	41,550	0	0	470	1,152	0	386	1,613	2,296
41,550	41,600	0	0	459	1,142	0	378	1,603	2,285
41,600	41,650	0	0	449	1,131	0	370	1,592	2,275
41,650	41,700	0	0	438	1,121	0	362	1,582	2,264
41,700	41,750	0	0	428	1,110	0	354	1,571	2,254
41,750	41,800	0	0	417	1,100	0	346	1,561	2,243
41,800	41,850	0	0	407	1,089	0	338	1,550	2,233
41,850	41,900	0	0	396	1,079	0	330	1,540	2,222
41,900	41,950	0	0	386	1,068	0	322	1,529	2,212
41,950	42,000	0	0	375	1,058	0	314	1,519	2,201
42,000	42,050	0	0	365	1,047	0	306	1,508	2,191
42,050	42,100	0	0	354	1,037	0	298	1,498	2,180
42,100	42,150	0	0	343	1,026	0	290	1,487	2,170
42,150	42,200	0	0	333	1,015	0	282	1,477	2,159
42,200	42,250	0	0	322	1,005	0	274	1,466	2,148
42,250	42,300	0	0	312	994	0	266	1,455	2,138
42,300	42,350	0	0	301	984	0	258	1,445	2,127
42,350	42,400	0	0	291	973	0	250	1,434	2,117
42,400	42,450	0	0	280	963	0	242	1,424	2,106
42,450	42,500	0	0	270	952	0	234	1,413	2,096
42,500	42,550	0	0	259	942	0	226	1,403	2,085
42,550	42,600	0	0	249	931	0	218	1,392	2,075
42,600	42,650	0	0	238	921	0	210	1,382	2,064
42,650	42,700	0	0	228	910	0	202	1,371	2,054
42,700	42,750	0	0	217	900	0	194	1,361	2,043
42,750	42,800	0	0	207	889	0	186	1,350	2,033
42,800	42,850	0	0	196	879	0	178	1,340	2,022
42,850	42,900	0	0	186	868	0	170	1,329	2,012
42,900	42,950	0	0	175	857	0	162	1,319	2,001
42,950	43,000	0	0	164	847	0	154	1,308	1,991
43,000	43,050	0	0	154	836	0	146	1,297	1,980
43,050	43,100	0	0	143	826	0	138	1,287	1,969
43,100	43,150	0	0	133	815	0	130	1,276	1,959
43,150	43,200	0	0	122	805	0	122	1,266	1,948
43,200	43,250	0	0	112	794	0	114	1,255	1,938
43,250	43,300	0	0	101	784	0	106	1,245	1,927
43,300	43,350	0	0	91	773	0	98	1,234	1,917
43,350	43,400	0	0	80	763	0	90	1,224	1,906
43,400	43,450	0	0	70	752	0	82	1,213	1,896
43,450	43,500	0	0	59	742	0	74	1,203	1,885
43,500	43,550	0	0	49	731	0	66	1,192	1,875
43,550	43,600	0	0	38	721	0	58	1,182	1,864
43,600	43,650	0	0	28	710	0	50	1,171	1,854
43,650	43,700	0	0	17	700	0	42	1,161	1,843
43,700	43,750	0	0	7	689	0	34	1,150	1,833
43,750	43,800	0	0	*	678	0	27	1,140	1,822
43,800	43,850	0	0	0	668	0	19	1,129	1,812
43,850	43,900	0	0	0	657	0	11	1,118	1,801
43,900	43,950	0	0	0	647	0	**	1,108	1,790
43,950	44,000	0	0	0	636	0	0	1,097	1,780
44,000	44,050	0	0	0	626	0	0	1,087	1,769
44,050	44,100	0	0	0	615	0	0	1,076	1,759
44,100	44,150	0	0	0	605	0	0	1,066	1,748
44,150	44,200	0	0	0	594	0	0	1,055	1,738
44,200	44,250	0	0	0	584	0	0	1,045	1,727
44,250	44,300	0	0	0	573	0	0	1,034	1,717
44,300	44,350	0	0	0	563	0	0	1,024	1,706
44,350	44,400	0	0	0	552	0	0	1,013	1,696
44,400	44,450	0	0	0	542	0	0	1,003	1,685
44,450	44,500	0	0	0	531	0	0	992	1,675
44,500	44,550	0	0	0	521	0	0	982	1,664
44,550	44,600	0	0	0	510	0	0	971	1,654
44,600	44,650	0	0	0	499	0	0	961	1,643
44,650	44,700	0	0	0	489	0	0	950	1,633
44,700	44,750	0	0	0	478	0	0	939	1,622
44,750	44,800	0	0	0	468	0	0	929	1,611
44,800	44,850	0	0	0	457	0	0	918	1,601
44,850	44,900	0	0	0	447	0	0	908	1,590
44,900	44,950	0	0	0	436	0	0	897	1,580
44,950	45,000	0	0	0	426	0	0	887	1,569
45,000	45,050	0	0	0	415	0	0	876	1,559
45,050	45,100	0	0	0	405	0	0	866	1,548
45,100	45,150	0	0	0	394	0	0	855	1,538
45,150	45,200	0	0	0	384	0	0	845	1,527
45,200	45,250	0	0	0	373	0	0	834	1,517
45,250	45,300	0	0	0	363	0	0	824	1,506
45,300	45,350	0	0	0	352	0	0	813	1,496
45,350	45,400	0	0	0	342	0	0	803	1,485
45,400	45,450	0	0	0	331	0	0	792	1,475
45,450	45,500	0	0	0	320	0	0	782	1,464
45,500	45,550	0	0	0	310	0	0	771	1,453
45,550	45,600	0	0	0	299	0	0	760	1,443

* If the amount you are looking up from the worksheet is at least $43,750 but less than $43,756, and you have two qualifying children, your credit is $1.
If the amount you are looking up from the worksheet is $43,756 or more, and you have two qualifying children, you cannot take the credit.

** If the amount you are looking up from the worksheet is at least $43,900 but less than $43,941, and you have one qualifying child, your credit is $3.
If the amount you are looking up from the worksheet is $43,941 or more, and you have one qualifying child, you cannot take the credit.

(Continued)

Need more information or forms? Visit IRS.gov.

¶87

➤➤➤ *Caution: This is a draft 2014 Earned Income Credit (EIC) Table. At the time of publication, the IRS had not yet released the 2014 Earned Income Credit (EIC) Table. For the latest information, see CCHGroup.com/TaxUpdates.*

Earned Income Credit (EIC) Table - Continued   (**Caution.** This is **not** a tax table.)

If the amount you are looking up from the worksheet is—		Single, head of household, or qualifying widow(er) and the number of children you have is—				Married filing jointly and the number of children you have is—			
At least	But less than	0	1	2	3	0	1	2	3
		Your credit is—				Your credit is—			
45,600	45,650	0	0	0	289	0	0	750	1,432
45,650	45,700	0	0	0	278	0	0	739	1,422
45,700	45,750	0	0	0	268	0	0	729	1,411
45,750	45,800	0	0	0	257	0	0	718	1,401
45,800	45,850	0	0	0	247	0	0	708	1,390
45,850	45,900	0	0	0	236	0	0	697	1,380
45,900	45,950	0	0	0	226	0	0	687	1,369
45,950	46,000	0	0	0	215	0	0	676	1,359
46,000	46,050	0	0	0	205	0	0	666	1,348
46,050	46,100	0	0	0	194	0	0	655	1,338
46,100	46,150	0	0	0	184	0	0	645	1,327
46,150	46,200	0	0	0	173	0	0	634	1,317
46,200	46,250	0	0	0	163	0	0	624	1,306
46,250	46,300	0	0	0	152	0	0	613	1,296
46,300	46,350	0	0	0	141	0	0	603	1,285
46,350	46,400	0	0	0	131	0	0	592	1,274
46,400	46,450	0	0	0	120	0	0	581	1,264
46,450	46,500	0	0	0	110	0	0	571	1,253
46,500	46,550	0	0	0	99	0	0	560	1,243
46,550	46,600	0	0	0	89	0	0	550	1,232
46,600	46,650	0	0	0	78	0	0	539	1,222
46,650	46,700	0	0	0	68	0	0	529	1,211
46,700	46,750	0	0	0	57	0	0	518	1,201
46,750	46,800	0	0	0	47	0	0	508	1,190
46,800	46,850	0	0	0	36	0	0	497	1,180
46,850	46,900	0	0	0	26	0	0	487	1,169
46,900	46,950	0	0	0	15	0	0	476	1,159
46,950	47,000	0	0	0	*	0	0	466	1,148
47,000	47,050	0	0	0	0	0	0	455	1,138
47,050	47,100	0	0	0	0	0	0	445	1,127
47,100	47,150	0	0	0	0	0	0	434	1,117
47,150	47,200	0	0	0	0	0	0	424	1,108
47,200	47,250	0	0	0	0	0	0	413	1,095
47,250	47,300	0	0	0	0	0	0	402	1,085
47,300	47,350	0	0	0	0	0	0	392	1,074
47,350	47,400	0	0	0	0	0	0	381	1,064
47,400	47,450	0	0	0	0	0	0	371	1,053
47,450	47,500	0	0	0	0	0	0	360	1,043
47,500	47,550	0	0	0	0	0	0	350	1,032
47,550	47,600	0	0	0	0	0	0	339	1,022
47,600	47,650	0	0	0	0	0	0	329	1,011
47,650	47,700	0	0	0	0	0	0	318	1,001
47,700	47,750	0	0	0	0	0	0	308	990
47,750	47,800	0	0	0	0	0	0	297	980
47,800	47,850	0	0	0	0	0	0	287	969
47,850	47,900	0	0	0	0	0	0	276	959
47,900	47,950	0	0	0	0	0	0	266	948
47,950	48,000	0	0	0	0	0	0	255	938
48,000	48,050	0	0	0	0	0	0	244	927
48,050	48,100	0	0	0	0	0	0	234	916
48,100	48,150	0	0	0	0	0	0	223	906
48,150	48,200	0	0	0	0	0	0	213	895
48,200	48,250	0	0	0	0	0	0	202	885
48,250	48,300	0	0	0	0	0	0	192	874
48,300	48,350	0	0	0	0	0	0	181	864
48,350	48,400	0	0	0	0	0	0	171	853
48,400	48,450	0	0	0	0	0	0	160	843
48,450	48,500	0	0	0	0	0	0	150	832
48,500	48,550	0	0	0	0	0	0	139	822
48,550	48,600	0	0	0	0	0	0	129	811
48,600	48,650	0	0	0	0	0	0	118	801
48,650	48,700	0	0	0	0	0	0	108	790
48,700	48,750	0	0	0	0	0	0	97	780
48,750	48,800	0	0	0	0	0	0	87	769

If the amount you are looking up from the worksheet is—		Single, head of household, or qualifying widow(er) and the number of children you have is—				Married filing jointly and the number of children you have is—			
At least	But less than	0	1	2	3	0	1	2	3
		Your credit is—				Your credit is—			
48,800	48,850	0	0	0	0	0	0	76	759
48,850	48,900	0	0	0	0	0	0	65	748
48,900	48,950	0	0	0	0	0	0	55	737
48,950	49,000	0	0	0	0	0	0	44	727
49,000	49,050	0	0	0	0	0	0	34	716
49,050	49,100	0	0	0	0	0	0	23	706
49,100	49,150	0	0	0	0	0	0	13	695
49,150	49,200	0	0	0	0	0	0	**	685
49,200	49,250	0	0	0	0	0	0	0	674
49,250	49,300	0	0	0	0	0	0	0	664
49,300	49,350	0	0	0	0	0	0	0	653
49,350	49,400	0	0	0	0	0	0	0	643
49,400	49,450	0	0	0	0	0	0	0	632
49,450	49,500	0	0	0	0	0	0	0	622
49,500	49,550	0	0	0	0	0	0	0	611
49,550	49,600	0	0	0	0	0	0	0	601
49,600	49,650	0	0	0	0	0	0	0	590
49,650	49,700	0	0	0	0	0	0	0	580
49,700	49,750	0	0	0	0	0	0	0	569
49,750	49,800	0	0	0	0	0	0	0	558
49,800	49,850	0	0	0	0	0	0	0	548
49,850	49,900	0	0	0	0	0	0	0	537
49,900	49,950	0	0	0	0	0	0	0	527
49,950	50,000	0	0	0	0	0	0	0	516
50,000	50,050	0	0	0	0	0	0	0	506
50,050	50,100	0	0	0	0	0	0	0	495
50,100	50,150	0	0	0	0	0	0	0	485
50,150	50,200	0	0	0	0	0	0	0	474
50,200	50,250	0	0	0	0	0	0	0	464
50,250	50,300	0	0	0	0	0	0	0	453
50,300	50,350	0	0	0	0	0	0	0	443
50,350	50,400	0	0	0	0	0	0	0	432
50,400	50,450	0	0	0	0	0	0	0	422
50,450	50,500	0	0	0	0	0	0	0	411
50,500	50,550	0	0	0	0	0	0	0	400
50,550	50,600	0	0	0	0	0	0	0	390
50,600	50,650	0	0	0	0	0	0	0	379
50,650	50,700	0	0	0	0	0	0	0	369
50,700	50,750	0	0	0	0	0	0	0	358
50,750	50,800	0	0	0	0	0	0	0	348
50,800	50,850	0	0	0	0	0	0	0	337
50,850	50,900	0	0	0	0	0	0	0	327
50,900	50,950	0	0	0	0	0	0	0	316
50,950	51,000	0	0	0	0	0	0	0	306
51,000	51,050	0	0	0	0	0	0	0	295
51,050	51,100	0	0	0	0	0	0	0	285
51,100	51,150	0	0	0	0	0	0	0	274
51,150	51,200	0	0	0	0	0	0	0	264
51,200	51,250	0	0	0	0	0	0	0	253
51,250	51,300	0	0	0	0	0	0	0	243
51,300	51,350	0	0	0	0	0	0	0	232
51,350	51,400	0	0	0	0	0	0	0	221
51,400	51,450	0	0	0	0	0	0	0	211
51,450	51,500	0	0	0	0	0	0	0	200
51,500	51,550	0	0	0	0	0	0	0	190
51,550	51,600	0	0	0	0	0	0	0	179
51,600	51,650	0	0	0	0	0	0	0	169
51,650	51,700	0	0	0	0	0	0	0	158
51,700	51,750	0	0	0	0	0	0	0	148
51,750	51,800	0	0	0	0	0	0	0	137
51,800	51,850	0	0	0	0	0	0	0	127
51,850	51,900	0	0	0	0	0	0	0	116
51,900	51,950	0	0	0	0	0	0	0	106
51,950	52,000	0	0	0	0	0	0	0	95

* If the amount you are looking up from the worksheet is at least $46,950 but less than $46,997, and you have three qualifying children, your credit is $5.
If the amount you are looking up from the worksheet is $46,997 or more, and you have three qualifying children, you cannot take the credit.

** If the amount you are looking up from the worksheet is at least $49,150 but less than $49,186, and you have two qualifying children, your credit is $4.
If the amount you are looking up from the worksheet is $49,186 or more, and you have two qualifying children, you cannot take the credit.

(Continued)

Need more information or forms? Visit IRS.gov.   - 67 -

➤➤➤→ *Caution: This is a draft 2014 Earned Income Credit (EIC) Table. At the time of publication, the IRS had not yet released the 2014 Earned Income Credit (EIC) Table. For the latest information, see CCHGroup.com/TaxUpdates.*

Earned Income Credit (EIC) Table - *Continued*   (**Caution**. This is **not** a tax table.)

If the amount you are looking up from the worksheet is—		Single, head of household, or qualifying widow(er) and the number of children you have is—				Married filing jointly and the number of children you have is—				If the amount you are looking up from the worksheet is—		Single, head of household, or qualifying widow(er) and the number of children you have is—				Married filing jointly and the number of children you have is—			
		0	1	2	3	0	1	2	3			0	1	2	3	0	1	2	3
At least	But less than	Your credit is—				Your credit is—				At least	But less than	Your credit is—				Your credit is—			
52,000	52,050	0	0	0	0	0	0	0	85	52,400	52,427	0	0	0	0	0	0	0	3
52,050	52,100	0	0	0	0	0	0	0	74										
52,100	52,150	0	0	0	0	0	0	0	64										
52,150	52,200	0	0	0	0	0	0	0	53										
52,200	52,250	0	0	0	0	0	0	0	42										
52,250	52,300	0	0	0	0	0	0	0	32										
52,300	52,350	0	0	0	0	0	0	0	21										
52,350	52,400	0	0	0	0	0	0	0	11										

Need more information or forms? Visit IRS.gov.

SPECIAL TABLES

¶87

¶ 88 Average Itemized Deductions

For those taxpayers who itemize their deductions on Schedule A of Form 1040, the following chart should be of special interest. Based on preliminary statistics for 2012 returns, the chart shows the average deductions of taxpayers for tax year 2012 for interest (¶ 1043), taxes (¶ 1021), medical and dental expenses (¶ 1015), and charitable contributions (¶ 1058). While it may be interesting for those who itemize their deductions to compare them with these average figures, the chart should *not* be considered as indicating amounts that would be allowed by the IRS. In any case, taxpayers must be able to substantiate claimed itemized deductions.

Individual Income Tax Returns, Preliminary Data, 2012, Table 1 (Source: *Winter 2014 Statistics of Income (SOI) Bulletin*).

PRELIMINARY AVERAGE ITEMIZED DEDUCTIONS FOR TAX YEAR 2012 BY ADJUSTED GROSS INCOME RANGES

Adjusted Gross Income Ranges	Medical Expenses	Taxes	Interest	Charitable Contributions
Under $ 15,000	$8,675	$3,231	$6,979	$1,501
$ 15,000 to $ 30,000	7,688	3,310	7,190	2,184
$ 30,000 to $ 50,000	6,939	3,932	7,047	2,404
$ 50,000 to $ 100,000	7,988	6,201	8,310	2,990
$ 100,000 to $ 200,000	9,634	10,848	10,399	3,939
$ 200,000 to $ 250,000	17,667	17,556	13,344	5,667
$ 250,000 or more	33,521	49,986	18,786	22,001

Chapter 1

INDIVIDUALS

Filing of Tax Returns

101. Who Must File an Individual Tax Return. All U.S. citizens and resident aliens (¶ 2409) are liable for federal income tax on their worldwide income, without regard to whether the income arose from sources within or outside of the United States (Code Sec. 1; Reg. § 1.1-1(b)).[1] For each tax year, a return (¶ 105) must be filed by a U.S. citizen or a resident alien who has at least a specified minimum amount of gross income.

Filing Thresholds. The filing threshold for most individuals is the sum of the applicable exemption amount (¶ 133) and the applicable standard deduction amount (¶ 126) for the tax year (Code Sec. 6012).[2] The additional standard deduction for taxpayers age 65 or older at the end of the tax year is also taken into account for determining the filing threshold amount; the additional standard deduction for taxpayers who are blind at the end of the tax year is *not* considered. A taxpayer's gross income for this purpose is computed without regard to the exclusion of gain from the sale of a personal residence (¶ 1705) and the exclusion of foreign earned income and housing expenses for U.S. citizens and residents living abroad (¶ 2402).

Generally, the gross income levels at which individuals must file income tax returns for 2014 are:

Single individual (including individuals treated as unmarried for tax purposes; see ¶ 173)	$10,150
Single individual, 65 or older	11,700
Married individual, separate return	3,950
Married couple, joint return	20,300
Married couple, joint return, one spouse 65 or older	21,500
Married couple, joint return, both spouses 65 or older	22,700
Head of household	13,050
Head of household, 65 or older	14,600
Qualifying widow(er) (surviving spouse)	16,350
Qualifying widow(er) (surviving spouse), 65 or older	17,550

Generally, the gross income levels at which individuals must file income tax returns for 2015:

Single individual (including individuals treated as unmarried for tax purposes; see ¶ 173)	$10,300
Single individual, 65 or older	11,850
Married individual, separate return	4,000
Married couple, joint return	20,600
Married couple, joint return, one spouse 65 or older	21,850
Married couple, joint return, both spouses 65 or older	23,100
Head of household	13,250
Head of household, 65 or older	14,800
Qualifying widow(er) (surviving spouse)	16,600
Qualifying widow(er) (surviving spouse), 65 or older	17,850

References are to Standard Federal Tax Reports; Tax Research Consultant; and Practical Tax Explanations.

[1] ¶ 3260, ¶ 3265; INDIV: 100; § 1,001   [2] ¶ 35,142; FILEIND: 15,152; § 1,305.05

The above income levels for a married couple filing a joint return are not applicable if, at the close of their tax year, the couple does not share the same household or if some other taxpayer is entitled to claim a dependency exemption for either spouse, e.g., a married student who is supported by a parent. In this case, a return for 2014 must be filed if gross income equals $3,950 or more ($4,000 or more for 2015).

Dependents. A child or other individual who can be claimed as a dependent on another person's tax return must file a return if that individual's income exceeds certain threshold amounts for earned or unearned income (Code Sec. 6012(a)(1)(C)).[3] Earned income includes salaries, wages, tips, professional fees, and taxable scholarship and fellowship grants. Unearned income includes investment-type income such as taxable interest, ordinary dividends, capital gain distributions, unemployment compensation, Social Security benefits, pensions, annuities, cancellation of debt income, and distributions of unearned income from a trust. The parent of a child who is subject to the kiddie tax and who has income only from interest or dividends may elect to report the child's income on the parent's return (¶ 103). The child will then *not* have to file a return.

With respect to a dependent child or other individual who is *neither* age 65 or older, or blind, at the end of 2014 and for whom a dependency exemption is allowable to another taxpayer (¶ 137), a return must be filed for the 2014 tax year if the individual has:

- over $1,000 of unearned income (over $1,050 for 2015);

- over $6,200 of earned income (over $6,300 for 2015); or

- a total of unearned and earned income which exceeds the larger of $1,000 or earned income (up to $5,850; $5,950 for 2015) plus $350.

All married dependents under age 65 with gross income of at least $5 whose spouse files a separate return on Form 1040 and itemizes deductions on Schedule A must file a return.

With respect to a dependent child or other individual who is *either* age 65 or older, or blind, at the end of 2014, and for whom a dependency exemption is allowed to another taxpayer (¶ 137), a return must be filed if the dependent's:

- earned income exceeds the basic standard deduction amount for an unmarried individual plus the additional standard deduction amounts to which he or she is entitled;

- unearned income exceeds the sum of $1,000 plus the additional standard deduction amounts to which he or she is entitled; or

- gross income exceeds the greater of (1) the total of earned income plus $350 (but not to exceed the basic standard deduction amount for an unmarried individual) plus the additional standard deduction amounts to which he or she is entitled; or (2) $1,000 plus the additional standard deduction amounts to which he or she is entitled (¶ 126).

If a guardian or other person is charged with the care of a minor individual or the minor individual's property, or a person under a disability, the return for the individual should be filed by the responsible person, unless already filed by the individual or some other person (¶ 504).

Return Requirement. If the applicable gross income test for the filing threshold is met, then a return must still be filed even though the individual's exemptions and deductions are such that no tax would be due. If the gross income test is *not* met, then a return should be filed whenever a refund of tax or any refundable credit, i.e., the earned income credit, is available. A return is also required if:

References are to Standard Federal Tax Reports; Tax Research Consultant; and Practical Tax Explanations.

[3] ¶ 35,142; FILEIND: 15,152; § 1,305.05

- net earnings from self-employment in 2014 are at least $400 (¶ 2664);
- Social Security and/or Medicare (commonly referred to as FICA) taxes are due on tip income not reported to an employer (¶ 717) or on wages received from an employer who did not withhold the taxes;
- uncollected Social Security, Medicare, or Railroad Retirement Tax Act (RRTA) taxes are due on tips reported to an employer or on group-term life insurance;
- liability for alternative minimum tax is incurred (¶ 1401);
- additional tax on a qualified retirement plan or individual retirement account (IRA) is due as calculated on Form 5329 (¶ 2169);
- additional tax on a health savings account (HSA) (¶ 2035) or Archer medical savings account (MSA) (¶ 2037) is due as calculated on Form 5329;
- household employment taxes are due (¶ 2652);
- tax is due from the recapture of any of the following: the first-time homebuyer credit (¶ 1324); the investment credit (¶ 1365A); the low-income housing credit (¶ 1365K); the new markets credit (¶ 1365T); the qualified plug-in electric drive motor vehicle credit (¶ 1351); the Indian employment credit (¶ 1365Q); the alternative motor vehicle credit (¶ 1345); the employer-provided child care credit (¶ 1365V); the alternative fuel vehicle refueling property credit (¶ 1355); the qualified plug-in electric and electric drive motor vehicle credit (¶ 1354); the education credits (¶ 1303); the COBRA premium assistance credit (¶ 1391); or on the disposition of a home purchased with a federally subsidized mortgage; or
- wages of $108.28 or more were earned from a church or qualified church-controlled organization that is exempt from employer FICA taxes (¶ 2601).

Any person who is required to file an income tax return must report on that return the amount of tax-exempt interest received or accrued during the tax year (¶ 724) (Code Sec. 6012(d)).

103. Returns of Children or Dependents. A child or dependent is generally taxed in the same manner as any other taxpayer on income, including wages, income from property, and trust income (¶ 554). Special rules, however, apply for calculating a child's tax liability if he or she is required to file a return (¶ 101). First, no personal exemption is allowed to an individual eligible to be claimed as a dependent on another taxpayer's return (¶ 135) (Code Sec. 151(d)(2)).[4] Second, the basic standard deduction for dependents in 2014 is limited to the greater of $1,000 or the sum of $350 plus earned income, but not in excess of $6,200, the standard deduction amount for unmarried individuals ($1,050, $350, and $6,300, respectively, for 2015) (¶ 126) (Code Sec. 63(c)(5); Rev. Proc. 2013-35; Rev. Proc. 2014-61).[5] Finally, if a child's income tax is not paid, an assessment made against the child will be treated as if it were made against the child's parent to the extent that the tax is attributable to amounts received for the child's services (Code Sec. 6201(c)).[6]

Kiddie Tax. Ordinarily, a child's tax liability is computed in the same manner as any other taxpayer after taking into account the limits on the personal exemption and standard deduction, if applicable (¶ 123). Certain children with investment income may be subject to tax on that income at the parent's top marginal rate if this results in a higher tax than would apply at the child's rate (Code Sec. 1(g)).[7] This is commonly referred to as the "kiddie tax," and it applies if:

- the child is required to file a tax return;
- the child does not file a joint return for the tax year;
- the child's investment income is more than $2,000 for 2014 (more than $2,100 for 2015);

References are to Standard Federal Tax Reports; Tax Research Consultant; and Practical Tax Explanations.

[4] ¶ 8000; FILEIND: 15,152.25; § 1,505

[5] ¶ 6020; FILEIND: 15,152.25; § 1,505

[6] ¶ 37,502; INDIV: 18,156.10; § 3,005.30

[7] ¶ 3260; INDIV: 18,154; § 1,510.05

INDIVIDUALS

- either parent of the child is alive at the end of the year; and
- the child is:
  - under the age of 18 at the end of the tax year;
  - under the age of 19 at the end of the tax year and does not provide more than half of his or her own support with earned income; or
  - under the age of 24 at the end of the tax year, a full-time student, and does not provide more than half of his or her own support with earned income.

The kiddie tax applies to the child's net unearned income, which is the portion of the child's adjusted gross income (AGI) for the tax year that is not attributable to earned income. This amount is further reduced by the limitation on the dependent standard deduction amount ($1,000 for 2014; $1,050 for 2015) and by the greater of either $1,000 in 2014 ($1,050 for 2015) or the child's itemized deductions relating to the production of the unearned income (Code Sec. 1(g)(4)). Even though, under state law, compensation for a child's personal services may be treated as belonging to the parent, and even though the money is not retained by the child, it is considered gross income of the child for federal income tax purposes (Reg. § 1.73-1).[8]

The marginal tax rate of the parent with the greater amount of taxable income applies in the case of married individuals filing separately. If the child's parents are divorced or legally separated and the custodial parent has not remarried, the return of the custodial parent should be used. If the custodial parent has remarried, the stepparent is treated as the child's parent for purposes of determining the marginal tax rate. Form 8615 is used to figure the kiddie tax.

Parent's Election. The parents of a child may elect to include on their return the unearned income of a child to avoid the kiddie tax (Code Sec. 1(g)(7); Rev. Proc. 2013-35; Rev. Proc. 2014-61). The election can only be made if all of the following requirements are met:

- the child is required to file a tax return and would otherwise be subject to the kiddie tax;
- the child's only income for the tax year is from interest and dividends, including Alaska Permanent Fund dividends;
- the income was more than $1,000 but less than $10,000 for 2014 ($1,050 and $10,500 in 2015, respectively);
- no estimated tax payments were made for the year in the child's name and Social Security number, including any overpayment of tax from the previous tax year; and
- the child is not subject to backup withholding.

The election is made by filing Form 8814. Electing parents are then taxed on their child's income in excess of $2,000 for the 2014 tax year (in excess of $2,100 for 2015). They must also report an additional tax liability of either $100 ($105 for 2015) if the child's taxable income is more than $1,000 (more than $1,050 for 2015) or 10 percent of the child's income if it is less than $1,000 (less than $1,050 for 2015).

105. Forms in Use for 2014. Three principal forms are available for use by the majority of individuals for filing income tax returns. These forms include Form 1040, a shorter return form, Form 1040A, and for certain taxpayers with no dependents, Form 1040EZ. If the applicable filing conditions are met, any of the forms in the 1040 series may serve as a separate return or as a joint return. If a married person's filing status is married filing separately and the taxpayer uses Form 1040 and itemizes deductions, then his or her spouse can file Form 1040 and either itemize deductions or claim a standard deduction of zero. If the individual decides to claim a standard deduction of zero, he or she may choose to file Form 1040A. These rules do not apply to a spouse who is eligible to file as unmarried or as head of household (¶ 173).

References are to Standard Federal Tax Reports; Tax Research Consultant; and Practical Tax Explanations.

[8] ¶ 6150; INDIV: 18,152; § 3,005.30

Form 1040EZ. For the 2014 tax year, the simplified income tax return, Form 1040EZ, may be used by a taxpayer who:

- is filing as single or married filing jointly (a taxpayer who was a nonresident alien at any time during the year may file Form 1040EZ *only* if his or her filing status is married filing jointly);

- does not claim any dependents (¶ 137);

- does not claim any adjustments to income (¶ 1005);

- does not claim any tax credits other than the earned income tax credit (¶ 1322);

- is under age 65 and not blind, including the spouse if filing a joint return, at the end of 2014;

- has taxable income of less than $100,000 (¶ 123);

- has income from *only* wages, salaries, tips, unemployment compensation, taxable scholarships and/or fellowship grants, Alaska Permanent Fund dividends, and taxable interest income not exceeding $1,500;

- has his or her earned tips included in boxes 5 and 7 of Form W-2;

- does not owe household employment taxes on wages paid to a household employee; and

- is not a debtor in a chapter 11 bankruptcy case filed after October 16, 2005.

If the taxpayer does *not* meet *all* the requirements, then he or she must use either Form 1040 or Form 1040A.

Form 1040A. For the 2014 tax year, Form 1040A may be used by an unmarried individual filing as single, a married couple filing jointly or separately, an individual filing as head of household (¶ 173), or a qualifying widow(er) with a dependent child (a surviving spouse) (¶ 175) if the taxpayer:

- has gross income only from: wages, salaries, and tips; interest and ordinary dividends (including Alaska Permanent Fund dividends); capital gains distributions; taxable scholarship and fellowship grants; taxable distributions from IRAs, pensions and annuities; unemployment compensation; and taxable Social Security or railroad retirement benefits;

- has only adjustments to gross income for the deduction of educator expenses (¶ 1084), IRA contributions (¶ 2157), student loan interest paid (¶ 1082), or tuition and fees paid (¶ 1082);

- does not itemize deductions (¶ 1011);

- has taxable income of less than $100,000;

- does not claim any tax credits other than the child tax credit (¶ 1305), the additional child tax credit, the educational credits (¶ 1303), the earned income credit (¶ 1322), the child and dependent care credit (¶ 1301), the elderly and disabled credit (¶ 1302), or the retirement savings contributions credit (¶ 1304); and

- does not have an alternative minimum tax (AMT) adjustment on stock acquired from the exercise of an incentive stock option (¶ 1435).

Comment: Absent further legislation, the deduction for educator expenses has expired for tax years beginning after December 31, 2013. For the latest legislative updates, visit our website www.CCHGroup.com/TaxUpdates.

Form 1040A may also be used by taxpayers who received dependent care benefits (¶ 2065) or owe tax from the recapture of an education credit (¶ 1303) or the AMT (¶ 1401).

Form 1040. For the 2014 tax year, Form 1040 must be used by a taxpayer if he or she:

- has taxable income of $100,000 or more;
- itemizes deductions;

¶105

• has income that cannot be reported on Form 1040EZ or 1040A, including tax-exempt interest from private activity bonds issued after August 7, 1986 (¶ 729), self-employment (net earnings of at least $400) (¶ 2667), rents and royalties (¶ 762 and ¶ 763), taxable state and local income tax refunds (¶ 799), alimony received (¶ 771), capital gains (¶ 1735), business income (¶ 759), or farm income (¶ 767);

• claims any credit against tax other than those credits which may be claimed on Form 1040A;

• claims any adjustments to income other than the adjustments listed for Form 1040A;

• receives in any month tips of $20 or more that are not reported fully to the employer, has a Form W-2 that shows allocated tips that must be reported in income, owes Social Security or Medicare tax on tips not reported to the employer, or has a Form W-2 that shows any uncollected Social Security, Medicare, or Railroad Retirement Tax Act (RRTA) taxes on tips or on group-term life insurance;

• owes or claims any of the items set out as *Other Taxes* in the discussion following, with the exception of the alternative minimum tax;

• is the grantor of, or transferor to, a foreign trust (¶ 588);

• can exclude foreign earned income received as a U.S. citizen (¶ 2402) or resident alien, certain income received from sources in Puerto Rico due to being a bona fide resident of Puerto Rico, or certain income received from sources in a U.S. possession while a resident of American Samoa (¶ 2414);

• receives or pays accrued interest on securities transferred between interest payment dates (¶ 728);

• earns wages of $108.28 or more from a church or church-controlled organization that is exempt from employer social security taxes;

• receives any nontaxable dividends or capital gain distributions;

• is reporting original issue discount in an amount more or less than that shown on Form 1099-OID;

• receives income as a partner (¶ 415 and ¶ 431), an S corporation shareholder (¶ 309), or a beneficiary of an estate or trust (¶ 554);

• has financial accounts in foreign countries (exceptions apply if the combined value of the accounts was $10,000 or less or if the accounts were with a U.S. military banking facility operated by a U.S. financial institution) (¶ 2570);

• is reporting household employment taxes (¶ 2652);

• receives a health savings account (HSA) funding distribution from his or her individual retirement account (IRA) (¶ 2035);

• is a debtor in a bankruptcy case filed after October 16, 2005; or

• must repay the first-time homebuyer credit (¶ 1324).

Calculating Taxable Income. The basic Form 1040 is a single-sheet, two-page form. To it are added any necessary supporting schedules or forms, depending upon the particular circumstances of the individual taxpayer. Adjustments to gross income on the bottom of page 1 of Form 1040 (commonly referred to as above-the-line deductions) are principally those deductions that may be taken whether or not the standard deduction is employed. They include the deductions for:

• educator expenses (¶ 1084);

• employee business expenses of certain fee-basis state or local government officials (¶ 941), performing artists (¶ 941A), and reservist's business expenses (¶ 941E);

• health savings accounts (HSAs) and Archer medical savings accounts (MSAs) (¶ 2035 and ¶ 2037);

• moving expenses (¶ 1073);

• one-half of self-employment tax (¶ 2664);

• contributions to self-employed retirement plans (¶ 2107);

- health insurance premiums paid by self-employed individuals (¶ 908);
- the forfeited interest penalty for premature withdrawals from a time savings account (¶ 1111);
- alimony paid (¶ 771);
- contributions to individual retirement arrangements (IRAs) (¶ 2157);
- student loan interest (¶ 1082);
- qualified tuition and fees (¶ 1082);
- the domestic production activities deduction (¶ 980A);
- jury duty pay given to an employer (¶ 941 and ¶ 1010);
- amortization of forestation or reforestation expenses (¶ 1287);
- repayment of supplemental unemployment benefits (¶ 1009);
- contributions to Code Sec. 501(c)(18) pension plans (¶ 602);
- contributions by certain chaplains to Code Sec. 403(b) plans (¶ 2191);
- expenses incurred with respect to the rental of personal property (¶ 1085);
- attorney's fees and court costs for certain federal claims (¶ 1093); and
- attorney fees and court costs paid in connection with an award from the IRS for information that significantly contributed to the detection of tax law violations (¶ 1010A).

Comment: Absent further legislation, the above-the-line deductions for educator expenses and for qualified tuition and fees have expired for tax years beginning after December 31, 2013. For the latest legislative updates, visit our website www.CCHGroup.com/TaxUpdates.

Once adjusted gross income (AGI) is determined, the appropriate personal exemption amount, and either itemized deductions or the standard deduction amount, are subtracted from AGI to calculate taxable income.

Credits. A number of credits whose excess over tax liability is not refundable in the current year are subtracted from the resulting tax in the following order:

- foreign tax credit (¶ 2475);
- credit for child and dependent care expenses (¶ 1301);
- education credits (¶ 1303);
- retirement savings contributions credit (¶ 1304);
- child tax credit (¶ 1305);
- residential energy credit (¶ 1341);
- credit for the elderly or for the permanently and totally disabled (¶ 1302);
- mortgage interest credit (¶ 1306);
- alternative fuel vehicle refueling property credit (personal use) (¶ 1355);
- general business credit (¶ 1365);
- credit for prior year alternative minimum tax (¶ 1309);
- the new clean renewable energy bond credit (¶ 1374); and
- the qualified plug-in electric drive motor vehicle credit (personal use) (¶ 1351).

Comment: Absent further legislation, the residential energy credit, the alternative fuel vehicle refueling property credit, and the qualified plug-in electric drive motor vehicle credit have expired for tax years beginning after December 31, 2013. For the latest legislative updates, visit our website www.CCHGroup.com/TaxUpdates.

Other Taxes. The following taxes are then added:

- alternative minimum tax (¶ 1401);
- self-employment tax (¶ 2664);

• Social Security, Medicare, and/or RRTA tax owing on tip income not reported to the employer, computed on Form 4137, and employee FICA, Medicare, and/or RRTA tax on tips where the employer did not withhold proper amounts, computed on Form 8919 (¶ 2606);

• excess contribution, excess distribution, and premature distribution taxes for IRAs and qualified pension or annuity plans, excess accumulations in qualified pension plans (including IRAs), Archer MSAs and HSAs, or early distribution tax for a modified endowment contract entered into after June 20, 1988, computed on Form 5329 (¶ 2035, ¶ 2037, ¶ 2151, ¶ 2161, and ¶ 2197);

• household employment taxes (¶ 2652);

• recapture of any of the following: the first-time homebuyer credit (¶ 1324); the investment credit (¶ 1365A); the low-income housing credit (¶ 1365K); the new markets credit (¶ 1365T); the qualified plug-in electric drive motor vehicle credit (¶ 1351); the Indian employment credit (¶ 1365Q); the alternative motor vehicle credit (¶ 1345); the employer-provided child care credit (¶ 1365V); the alternative fuel vehicle refueling property credit (¶ 1355); the qualified plug-in electric and electric motor vehicle credit (¶ 1354); education credits (¶ 1303); household employment taxes (¶ 2650); COBRA premium assistance credit (¶ 1391); or on the disposition of a home purchased with a federally subsidized mortgage;

• the "Section 72(m)(5) excess benefits tax" imposed on a five-percent owner of a business who receives a distribution of excess benefits from a qualified pension or annuity plan;

• uncollected Social Security, Medicare, and/or RRTA tax on tips with respect to employees who received wages that were insufficient to cover the Social Security, Medicare, and RRTA tax due on tips reported to their employers;

• uncollected Social Security, Medicare, and/or RRTA tax on group-term life insurance (¶ 2055);

• the additional 0.9-percent Medicare tax on high-income wage earners (¶ 2648);

• the 3.8-percent net investment income tax on high-income individuals (¶ 129);

• any excise tax due on "golden parachute" payments (¶ 907); and

• tax on accumulated distribution of trusts.

Payments. To arrive at final tax due or refund owed, the taxpayer subtracts from the above balance the following:

• federal income tax withheld (¶ 2601);

• 2014 estimated tax payments and amounts applied from 2013 return;

• earned income credit (¶ 1322);

• amounts paid with the application for automatic filing extension (¶ 2509);

• additional child tax credit (¶ 1305);

• refundable portion of the American Opportunity (modified Hope) credit (¶ 1303);

• excess Social Security tax and/or Tier 1 railroad retirement (RRTA) tax withheld from individuals paid more than a total of $117,000 in wages in 2014 by two or more employers (excess Tier 2 RRTA tax withheld from individuals paid more than a total of $87,000 by two or more employers is claimed on Form 843, not Form 1040) (¶ 2648);

• health insurance costs credit (¶ 1332);

• credit for excise tax on gasoline and special fuels used in business and credit on certain diesel-powered vehicles (¶ 1329);

• a shareholder's share of capital gains tax paid by a regulated investment company (mutual fund) (¶ 2305); and

- the refundable portion of long-term unused prior year minimum tax credit (expired) (¶ 1327).

Comment: Absent further legislation, the health insurance costs credit has expired for tax years beginning after December 31, 2013. For the latest legislative updates, visit our website www.CCHGroup.com/TaxUpdates.

Schedules and Supporting Documents. The following schedules and forms are filed with the basic Form 1040 as needed:

- Schedule A for itemizing deductions;

- Schedule B for reporting (a) more than $1,500 of ordinary dividend income and/or other stock distributions, (b) more than $1,500 of taxable interest income or claiming the exclusion of interest from series EE U.S. savings bonds issued after 1989 used for higher educational expenses, and (c) any interests in foreign accounts and trusts;

- Schedule C or Schedule C-EZ for claiming profit or loss from a sole proprietorship;

- Schedule D for reporting a summary of capital gains and losses;

- Schedule E for reporting income or loss from (a) rents and royalties, (b) partnerships and S corporations, (c) estates and trusts, and (d) real estate mortgage investment conduits (REMICs);

- Schedule EIC for providing information regarding the earned income credit;

- Schedule F for computing income and expenses from farming;

- Schedule H for reporting employment taxes for domestic workers paid $1,900 or more during 2014;

- Schedule J for reporting farm income averaging;

- Schedule R for claiming the tax credit for the elderly or the disabled;

- Schedule SE for computing the tax due on income from self-employment;

- Form 2106 or 2106-EZ for computing employee business expenses;

- Form 3903 for calculating moving expenses;

- Form 4562 for reporting depreciation and amortization;

- Form 4684 for reporting personal casualty or theft losses;

- Form 4797 for reporting gains and losses from sales of business assets or from involuntary conversions other than casualty or theft losses (business casualty and theft losses are reported on Form 4684, Section B);

- Form 6251 for computing the alternative minimum tax;

- Form 8283 for claiming a deduction for a noncash charitable contribution where the total claimed value of the contributed property exceeds $500;

- Form 8582 for computing the amount of passive activity loss;

- Form 8606 for reporting nondeductible IRA contributions, for figuring the basis of an IRA, and for calculating nontaxable distributions;

- Form 8615 for computing the tax for certain children who have investment income in excess of $2,000 in 2014;

- Form 8814 for electing to report a child's unearned income on the parents' income tax return;

- Form 8829 for figuring allowable expenses for business use of a home;

- Form 8834 for figuring the personal credit amount for the purchase of a qualified plug-in electric or electric vehicle credit;

- Form 8853 for figuring the allowable deduction for contributions to an Archer Medical Savings Account (Archer MSA);

- Form 8888 for direct deposit of income tax refunds into more than one account including, but not limited to, individual retirement accounts;

- Form 8889 for figuring the allowable deduction for contributions to a Health Savings Account (HSA);
- Form 8919, for reporting uncollected Social Security and Medicare taxes on wages;
- Form 8949 for reporting sales and exchanges of capital assets;
- Form 8959, for reporting additional Medicare tax on high-income wage earners; and
- Form 8960, for reporting the net investment income tax by high-income individuals.

The following forms are for computing and claiming credits:

- Form 1116 to compute the foreign tax credit for individuals, estates or trusts;
- Form 2441 to figure the child and dependent care credit;
- Form 3800 if any of the components of the general business credit are claimed;
- Form 5405 for calculating the amount of the credit recapture for first-time homebuyer claims (¶ 1324);
- Form 5884 to calculate the work opportunity credit;
- Form 8396 to figure the mortgage interest credit and any carryforwards;
- Form 8801 to compute the credit for prior year alternative minimum tax including the refundable portion;
- Form 8812 to claim the additional child tax credit;
- Form 8828 to compute the recapture of a federal mortgage subsidy;
- Form 8834 to determine the amount of qualified electric vehicle passive activity credits from prior years;
- Form 8839 to claim the adoption credit;
- Form 8863 to claim the education credits;
- Form 8880 to claim the credit for qualified retirement savings contributions;
- Form 8882 to claim the credit for employer-provided child care facilities and services;
- Form 8885 to claim the health insurance costs credit;
- Form 8903 to claim the deduction for domestic production activity;
- Form 8910 to claim the alternative motor vehicle credit;
- Form 8911 to claim the alternative fuel vehicle refueling property credit; and
- Form 8912 to claim the credit for holders of tax credit bonds;

IRS Computation of Tax. Any taxpayer who files an individual tax return by the due date, April 15, 2015, can have the IRS compute the tax under certain conditions on Form 1040, Form 1040A, and Form 1040EZ. The IRS may also figure the credit for the elderly or the disabled and the earned income credit. See IRS Pub. 17 for the requirements to have the IRS compute a taxpayer's tax liability or these credits. These returns must have all applicable lines completed, be signed (by both spouses if filing jointly) and dated. If taxpayers want to designate a friend, family member or any other person to be allowed to discuss their 2014 tax return with the IRS, they must check the Yes box in the Third Party Designee area and provide the necessary information. Inclusion of a daytime telephone number of the taxpayer will speed the process should any questions arise. Form W-2 and any other required forms necessary to complete the return should be attached. If the taxpayer overpaid his or her taxes for the year, the IRS will refund that amount. If an amount is due, the taxpayer must pay the amount no later than 30 days from the billing date or due date of the return; failure to do so may result in penalties and interest.

Rounding Off Amounts. Dollar amounts on the return and accompanying schedules and forms may be rounded off to the nearest whole dollar.

¶105

107. Due Date for Individual Returns. Individual income tax returns are generally due on or before the 15th day of the 4th month following the close of the tax year (April 15 in the case of a calendar-year taxpayer) (¶ 2505) (Code Sec. 6072; Reg. § 1.6072-1).[9] U.S. citizens and resident aliens living outside the country have an additional two months to file their returns (June 15 in the case of a calendar-year taxpayer). Similarly, a nonresident alien who has wages *not* subject to withholding generally may also file a return as late as the 15th day of the 6th month after the close of the tax year. A nonresident alien who has wages subject to withholding, however, must file a return by the 15th day of the 4th month following the close of the tax year. If any due date falls on a Saturday, Sunday, or legal holiday, the return may be filed on the next succeeding day that is not a Saturday, Sunday, or legal holiday (Code Sec. 7503; Reg. § 301.7503-1).[10] An individual taxpayer can obtain—without seeking IRS approval—an automatic six-month extension of time to file his or her tax return (¶ 109).

An individual may correct an error in a return, without incurring interest or penalties, by filing an amended return (Form 1040X) and paying any additional tax due on or before the last day prescribed for filing the original return. For further information regarding amended returns, see ¶ 2505.

109. Extension for Filing. An individual may obtain an automatic six month extension for filing Forms 1040, 1040A or 1040EZ by filing Form 4868 before the due date of the return, accompanied by a reasonable estimate of tax due for the year (¶ 2509) (Reg. § 1.6081-4).[11] U.S. citizens or residents who live and have a main place of business or post of duty outside the U.S. and Puerto Rico, or who are in military or naval service on duty outside the U.S. and Puerto Rico, generally file their income tax return by the 15th of the sixth month after the close of the tax year (June 15 in the case of a calendar-year taxpayer). These individuals, upon filing of Form 4868, are given an automatic additional four-month extension for the filing of their return (Reg. § 1.6081-5).[12] An automatic extension of time for filing a return will not extend the time for payment of any tax due, and interest and penalties may apply. Finally, interest will be charged on any unpaid tax from the original due date of the return.

111. Where to File Returns. The IRS strongly encourages all taxpayers to file their returns electronically through the IRS's e-file system. For individuals who prefer to mail their income tax returns, the returns are filed with the Internal Revenue Service Center for the region in which the individual's residence or principal place of business is located (Code Sec. 6091; Reg. § 1.6091-2).[13] Taxpayers must be aware that income tax returns which include a tax payment are mailed to a different address than returns showing a refund or no tax liability. U.S. citizens living abroad, nonresident aliens, and certain other taxpayers must file their income tax returns if no payment of tax is required at the IRS Service Center located in Austin, Texas. If a payment is required, the return should be filed at the IRS Service Center in Charlotte, North Carolina. For a list of addresses of filing locations, see ¶ 5.

116. Identifying Number. Every taxpayer must record his or her taxpayer identification number (TIN) on the income tax return (Code Sec. 6109(a); Reg. § 301.6109-1).[14] This is either the taxpayer's Social Security number, Individual Taxpayer Identification Number (ITIN) (for use by resident or nonresident aliens who do not qualify for a Social Security number), or Adoption Taxpayer Identification Number (ATIN) (a temporary taxpayer identification number for use by individuals in the process of adopting a child for whom they are unable to obtain a Social Security number until the adoption is final) (¶ 2579). If a taxpayer does not have a TIN, he or she should apply for either a Social Security number using Form SS-5, an ITIN using Form W-7, or an ATIN using Form W-7A. Taxpayers must provide TINs for dependents and qualifying children for the purpose of claiming a dependency exemption (¶ 133), the earned income tax credit (¶ 1322), the child care credit (¶ 1301), the adoption credit (¶ 1307), and the child tax

---

References are to Standard Federal Tax Reports; Tax Research Consultant; and Practical Tax Explanations.

[9] ¶ 36,720, ¶ 36,721; FILEIND: 18,052.20; § 1,325.05

[10] ¶ 42,630, ¶ 42,631; FILEBUS: 15,056; § 1,325.05

[11] ¶ 36,793; FILEBUS: 15,104; § 1,325.10

[12] ¶ 36,795; FILEBUS: 15,104.15; § 1,325.10

[13] ¶ 36,800, ¶ 36,808; FILEBUS: 12,150; § 1,325.20

[14] ¶ 36,960, ¶ 36,961; FILEBUS: 12,106; § 1,335

credit (¶ 1305). An ATIN, however, cannot be used for purposes of claiming the earned income tax credit. Individuals claiming the earned income tax credit must also include TINs for themselves and their spouses, if married. Failure to include a correct TIN will be treated as a mathematical or clerical error, as will instances when the information provided differs from the information on file with the IRS that is obtained from the Social Security Administration (Code Sec. 6213(g)(2)(F)).[15] The parent of any child to whom the rules governing taxation of unearned income of minor children apply must provide his or her TIN to the child for inclusion on the child's tax return (¶ 103).

117. Estimated Taxes. Individuals are required to make estimated tax payments if the amount of tax they pay through withholding on wages and other payments will not adequately cover their tax liability for the year (¶ 2875). As 2014 ends, the first responsibility of the calendar-year taxpayer is to review payments of estimated tax for 2014 to make sure that these tax payments and the income tax withheld from wages during the year are sufficient to avoid penalties on the last installment, which is due January 15, 2015. The 2014 estimated tax payments, plus income tax withheld from wages, are credited against tax due for 2014. Any underpayment of tax must be made up by a payment with the final return, and any overpayment is either refunded or credited against the estimated tax for the next year, whichever the taxpayer elects on the return (¶ 2682). For the special rules related to estimated tax payments for farmers and fishermen, see ¶ 2691.

Overpayment. An individual who has been making payments of estimated tax for 2014, and who finds that by paying the installment scheduled for January 15, 2015, he or she will overpay the 2014 tax, may:

- make the payment as scheduled on or before January 15, 2015, file the return on or before April 15, 2015, and direct whether the overpayment should be refunded or credited toward the 2015 estimated tax;

- reduce the payment due on or before January 15, 2015, so that the estimated tax payments plus withholding will meet the tax liability that will be shown on the return to be filed on or before April 15, 2015;

- pay enough estimated tax to cover the minimum requirement as described at ¶ 2875 in order to avoid a penalty on the January 15, 2015, payment and then pay any difference on the final return, filed on or before April 15, 2015; or

- file the final return on or before February 2, 2015 (January 31, 2015, is a Saturday), add up all payments of estimated tax plus any withholding, and use this return for a final accounting of 2014 tax liability.

Underpayment. The law provides a penalty for underpayment of estimated tax. A taxpayer can avoid this penalty by paying the minimum installment authorized under one of the exceptions described at ¶ 2682. The taxpayer may file the tax return for calendar year 2014 on or before February 2, 2015 (January 31, 2015, is a Saturday), and pay any balance of tax that may still be due for 2014. Under this method, no penalty will apply for failure to make the last quarterly installment, and any penalty for underpayment of any of the three earlier installments will not be increased (¶ 2688).

Computation of Tax Liability

123. Taxable Income of Individuals. An individual computes his or her tax liability for a tax year by multiplying taxable income by the applicable tax rate, subtracting allowable credits, and adding other taxes. The computation of taxable income starts with gross income (¶ 701), from which certain deductions (commonly referred to as either adjustments to gross income or the above-the-line deductions) are subtracted to determine the taxpayer's adjusted gross income (AGI) (¶ 1005). After AGI is determined, certain other deductions are subtracted from a taxpayer's AGI to determine his or her taxable income. These include the deduction for personal and dependency exemptions (¶ 133), the standard deduction (¶ 126), or, in lieu of the standard deduction, the taxpayer's itemized deductions (¶ 1011). Once taxable income is determined, the tax-

---

References are to Standard Federal Tax Reports; Tax Research Consultant; and Practical Tax Explanations.

[15] ¶ 37,545; FILEBUS: 12,106;
§ 1,335

payer's tax liability is generally computed by applying the appropriate tax rates based on the taxpayer's filing status (single, married filing jointly, head of household, surviving spouse, or married filing separately). Subject to certain exceptions, taxpayers *must* use either the tax rate tables or tax schedules issued by the IRS to compute their income tax. See ¶ 128 for a discussion of the tax rate tables and tax schedules.

126. Standard Deduction. An individual taxpayer who does not elect to itemize deductions (¶ 1014) computes taxable income by subtracting from adjusted gross income (AGI) the standard deduction and the deduction for personal exemptions (¶ 133). Taxpayers have a choice of itemizing deductions or claiming the standard deduction, whichever will result in a higher deduction. The standard deduction amount is the sum of the basic standard deduction, plus the additional standard deduction amounts for aged and blind taxpayers.[16]

Basic Standard Deduction. The basic standard deduction amount varies according to the taxpayer's filing status and is adjusted annually for inflation. The basic standard deduction amounts available to individuals in 2014 are (Code Sec. 63(c)(2); Rev. Proc. 2013-35; Rev. Proc. 2014-61):

Filing status	2014 standard deduction amount
Married filing jointly and surviving spouses	$12,400
Married filing separately	6,200
Head of household filers	9,100
Single filers	6,200

The basic standard deduction amounts available to individuals in 2015 are:

Filing status	2015 standard deduction amount
Married filing jointly and surviving spouses	$12,600
Married filing separately	6,300
Head of household filers	9,250
Single filers	6,300

A taxpayer who can be claimed as a dependent on another taxpayer's return is limited to a smaller standard deduction regardless of whether the individual actually is claimed as a dependent. The dependent's basic standard deduction may not exceed the greater of $1,000 ($1,050 for 2015) or the sum of $350 and the individual's earned income, up to the applicable standard deduction amount (for single taxpayers: $6,200 for 2014; $6,300 for 2015) (Code Sec. 63(c)(5); Rev. Proc. 2013-35; Rev. Proc. 2014-61).[17] The limit applies to the basic standard deduction and not to any additional amount such as for elderly or blind taxpayers. A scholarship or fellowship grant that is *not* excludable from the dependent's gross income (¶ 865) is considered earned income for this purpose (IRS Pub. 501).

Elderly and/or Blind Taxpayers. Taxpayers who are age 65 or older, or blind, or both, at the end of the tax year receive an additional standard deduction amount that is added to the basic standard deduction shown in the table above. The additional amount is $1,200 for tax years beginning in 2014 for married individuals, whether filing jointly or separately, and surviving spouses ($1,250 for 2015). The additional amount is $1,550 for tax years beginning in 2014 for unmarried individuals, whether filing as single or as head of household ($1,550 for 2015) (Code Sec. 63(f), Reg. § 1.151-1; Rev. Proc. 2013-35; Rev. Proc. 2014-61).[18] Two additional standard deduction amounts are allowed to an individual who is both over 65 and blind at the end of the tax year. Thus, married taxpayers filing jointly, both of whom are over 65 and blind, would claim four of the additional standard deduction amounts.

A taxpayer claiming the additional standard deduction must be either age 65 or blind, or both, before the close of the tax year. An individual who reaches age 65 on January 1st of any year is deemed to have reached that age on the preceding December 31st. A taxpayer claiming the additional amount for blindness must obtain a certified

[16] ¶ 6020, ¶ 6023.10; FILEIND: 12,100; § 1,010.15

[17] ¶ 6020; FILEIND: 12,106; § 1,010.15

[18] ¶ 6020, ¶ 8001; FILEIND: 12,104; § 1,010.15

statement from a doctor or registered optometrist. The statement, which should be kept with the taxpayer's records, must state either that: (1) the individual cannot see better than 20/200 in the better eye with glasses or contact lenses; or (2) the individual's field of vision is 20 degrees or less.

A married taxpayer filing separately may claim the additional amounts for a spouse who had no gross income for the year and was not claimed as a dependent by another taxpayer (Code Sec. 151(b)). A taxpayer who claims a dependency exemption for an individual who is either age 65 or older, blind, or both may *not* claim the additional standard deduction amounts for that individual.

Taxpayers Ineligible for Standard Deduction. When married taxpayers file separate returns, both spouses should either itemize their deductions or claim the standard deduction. This is because if one spouse itemizes and the other does not, the non-itemizing spouse's standard deduction amount will be zero, even if such spouse is age 65 or older, or blind, or both. This rule does not apply if one spouse qualifies to file as head-of-household. A zero standard deduction amount also applies to nonresident aliens, estates or trusts, common trust funds, or partnerships, and to individuals with short tax years due to a change in their annual accounting period (Code Sec. 63(c)(6)).[19] Taxpayers who itemize even though their itemized deductions are less than the standard deduction must check the box on the last line of Schedule A of Form 1040 to make this election.

128. Tax Rates and Tables for Individuals. Most individuals determine their income tax liability by applying the appropriate tax rate to their taxable income (¶ 123) based on their filing status (¶ 152 and ¶ 173). There are seven tax rates for individuals for 2013 and thereafter, which are 10, 15, 25, 28, 33, 35, and, for individuals with taxable income in excess of the applicable threshold amount, 39.6 percent (Code Sec. 1(i)).[20] All threshold amounts are subject to inflation adjustment. The applicable threshold amounts for 2014 are $457,600 for married taxpayers filing jointly or surviving spouse filers, $432,200 for head of household filers, $406,750 for unmarried individuals other than head of household and surviving spouse filers, and $228,800 for married taxpayers filing separately. The applicable threshold amounts for 2015 are $464,850 for married taxpayers filing jointly or surviving spouse filers, $439,000 for head of household filers, $413,200 for unmarried individuals other than head of household and surviving spouse filers, and $232,425 for married taxpayers filing separately.

For 2014, the 10-percent bracket applies to the first $9,075 of taxable income for single filers and married taxpayers filing separately ($9,225 for 2015), the first $12,950 of taxable income for head-of-household filers ($13,150 for 2015), and the first $18,150 of taxable income for married taxpayers filing jointly and surviving spouses ($18,450 for 2015) (Rev. Proc. 2013-35; Rev. Proc. 2014-61). The upper limit of the 15-percent tax bracket for joint filers is 200 percent of the upper limit of the 15-percent tax bracket for single filers (Code Sec. 1(f)(8)).

Subject to certain exceptions listed below, individuals *must* use either the tax rate tables or tax schedules issued by the IRS to compute their income tax (Code Sec. 3).[21] Taxpayers whose taxable income is less than $100,000 must use the tax tables reproduced at ¶ 25. Taxpayers whose taxable income is $100,000 or more must use the Tax Computation Worksheet in the Form 1040 Instructions (reproduced at ¶ 20), which is based on the tax rate schedules at ¶ 11 for single taxpayers, ¶ 13 for married individuals filing jointly and surviving spouses, ¶ 15 for married individuals filing separately, and ¶ 17 for heads of households, in order to compute their tax. Taxpayers may *not* use the table if they file short-period returns because of a change in their annual accounting periods (¶ 1507).

Tax Calculation on Form 8615. Form 8615 must be used to figure the tax of a child subject to the "kiddie tax" rules (¶ 103). Taxpayers required to calculate their tax on Form 8615 may compute taxable income using Form 1040 or Form 1040A. Form 8615 is

---

References are to Standard Federal Tax Reports; Tax Research Consultant; and Practical Tax Explanations.

[19] ¶ 6020; FILEIND: 12,108;   [20] ¶ 3260; FILEIND: 15,054;   [21] ¶ 3345; FILEIND: 15,054.10;
§ 1,010.15   § 1,015   § 1,015

not filed if the child's parent elects to include the child's unearned income on the parent's return.

Capital Gain Tax Calculation. Taxpayers who had a net capital gain from a sale or exchange (¶ 1736) use Form 1040, Schedule D, Part III, to determine which of the capital gains tax worksheets to use to calculate the amount of tax on the capital gains. Taxpayers with sales or exchanges of assets taxed at the 28-percent rate or with unrecaptured Code Sec. 1250 gains, or both, complete the "Schedule D Tax Worksheet" in the Instructions to Schedule D of Form 1040. All other taxpayers, including those with only qualified dividends and net capital gains from a distribution of a regulated investment company (RIC/mutual fund), complete the "Qualified Dividends and Capital Gains Tax Worksheet" in the Form 1040 or 1040A instructions.

129. Net Investment Income Tax. An individual is subject to an additional 3.8 percent tax for tax years beginning after December 31, 2012, on the lesser of net investment income for the tax year or the excess modified adjusted gross income (MAGI) for the tax year over a threshold amount (Code Sec. 1411; Reg. § 1.1411-2).[22] The net investment tax is determined using Form 8960. Although the tax is an addition to the regular income tax liability, it is taken into account for purposes of calculating estimated tax payments and underpayment penalties (Code Sec. 6654(a) and (f)). The tax also applies to the net investment income of estates and trusts (¶ 517).

For individuals, the net investment income tax (previously referred to as the unearned income Medicare contribution tax) is 3.8 percent of the lesser of (1) the taxpayer's net investment income for the tax year, or (2) the excess of MAGI for the tax year over the threshold amount of $200,000 ($250,000 for married taxpayers filing jointly and surviving spouses, and $125,000 for a married taxpayer filing separately). MAGI is the taxpayer's adjusted gross income (AGI) increased by any foreign income excluded from gross income for the year under Code Sec. 911 less any deductions, exclusions, or credits properly allocable to such foreign income.

The net investment income tax applies to all individuals subject to U.S. taxation other than nonresident aliens (Reg. § 1.1411-2). Special rules apply to U.S. citizens or residents married to a nonresident alien. The default position is that these couples are treated as married filing separately for purposes of the tax. If they elect to file jointly under Code Sec. 6013(g) (¶ 152), however, these couples may also make a separate election to apply the joint return election for net investment income tax purposes, so that the tax applies to their combined investment income.

Net investment income is the excess of the sum of the following items, less any otherwise allowable deductions properly allocable to such income or gain (Reg. § 1.1411-4):

(a) gross income from interest, dividends, annuities, royalties, rents, and substitute interest and dividend payments, but not to the extent this income is derived in the ordinary course of an active trade or business;

(b) other gross income (not described in (a)) from a passive activity under Code Sec. 469 (¶ 1169), or from a trade or business of a trader trading in financial instruments or commodities; and

(c) net gain included in computing taxable income that is attributable to the disposition of property, but not to the extent the property was held in an active trade or business.

Any item that is excluded from gross income for regular income tax purposes is also excluded from net investment income and MAGI (Reg. § 1.1411-1(d)(4)). Some examples of such items are: excludable gain on the sale of a taxpayer's personal residence; veterans' benefits; and tax-exempt bond interest (Joint Committee on Taxation, Technical Explanation of the Revenue Provisions of the "Reconciliation Act of 2010," as amended, in combination with the "Patient Protection and Affordable Care Act" (JCX 18-10)).

References are to Standard Federal Tax Reports; Tax Research Consultant; and Practical Tax Explanations.

[22] ¶ 32,602, ¶ 32,603H; INDIV: 69,150; § 1,022.10

Net investment income generally does not include income and gain derived in the ordinary course of a trade or business, unless the trade or business is a passive activity or that of a trader trading in financial instruments or commodities. If an individual owns or engages in a trade or business directly (or indirectly through owning a disregarded entity), the determination of whether gross income is derived in a trade or business is made at the individual level. If an individual owns an interest in a trade or business through one or more passthrough entities, e.g., a partnership or S corporation, the determination of whether gross income is derived in a passive activity is made at the owner level, and the determination of whether gross income is derived in the trade or business of a trader trading in financial instruments or commodities is made at the entity level (Reg. § 1.1411-4(b)). Similar rules apply for determining whether net gain is attributable to property held in a trade or business. For purposes of determining net gain, a disposition is a sale, exchange, transfer, conversion, cash settlement, cancellation, termination, lapse, expiration, or other disposition. Net gain cannot be less than zero, and losses from dispositions of capital assets are allowed to offset gains, unless the asset's disposition is subject to the net investment income tax. The $3,000 deduction ($1,500 for married individuals filing separate returns) under Code Sec. 1211 (¶ 1752) may not be taken against losses on capital assets but may be taken against other net investment income (Reg. § 1.1411-4). Losses deductible under Code Sec. 165, including losses attributable to casualty, theft, and abandonment or other worthlessness (¶ 1101), are applied to calculate net gains, and then any excess losses are applied as properly allocable deductions against investment income (Reg. § 1.1411-4(d)).

Property held in a trade or business does not generally include an interest in a partnership or stock in an S corporation, so gain from the disposition of such an interest or stock is usually treated as net gain. However, special rules apply upon the disposition of an active interest in a partnership or S corporation (Prop. Reg. § 1.1411-7).

The net investment income tax rules might cause taxpayers to reconsider the way they have previously grouped activities for passive activity loss purposes under Code Sec. 469. In light of this concern, taxpayers subject to the net investment income tax are provided with a one-time election to regroup activities under Code Sec. 469 to allow for realignment of grouped activities to properly reflect the interaction of the Code Sec. 469 rules and income for net investment income tax purposes. Further, regrouping may be done on an amended return if the taxpayer was not subject to net investment income tax on the original return (Reg. § 1.469-11(b)(3)(iv)).[23]

Net investment income includes any income, gain, or loss that is attributable to an investment of working capital (Reg. § 1.1411-6). Net investment income does not include a distribution from qualified employee benefit plans or arrangements, including: a qualified pension, profit sharing, and stock-bonus plan; qualified annuity plan under Code Sec. 403(a) or (b); a traditional or Roth IRA; or a Code Sec. 457 plan of a government or tax-exempt organization (Reg. § 1.1411-8). However, a distribution from a qualified plan or arrangement that is includible in gross income is taken into account for determining the taxpayer's MAGI in the net investment income tax calculation.

Special rules are provided for self-employed individuals (Reg. § 1.1411-9) and controlled foreign corporations and passive foreign investment companies (Reg. § 1.1411-10).

131. Individual Health Care Coverage Mandate. Effective for tax years beginning after December 31, 2013, an individual is required to either maintain minimum essential health care coverage or make a shared responsibility payment, i.e., a penalty payment for failure to maintain minimum essential health care coverage (Code Sec. 5000A; Reg. § § 1.5000A-1—1.5000A-5).[24] The shared responsibility payment (i.e., the penalty) is imposed on an applicable individual for each month he or she fails to maintain minimum essential health care coverage for him- or herself, or his or her dependents.

References are to Standard Federal Tax Reports; Tax Research Consultant; and Practical Tax Explanations.

[23] ¶ 21,965F; INDIV: 69,160.20; § 17,415.05

[24] ¶ 34,962, ¶ 34,962D— ¶ 34,962L; HEALTH: 3,050; § 42,001

If the taxpayer qualifies to claim an individual as a dependent on his or her income tax return (¶ 137), then the taxpayer, rather than the dependent, is liable for the shared responsibility payment that would otherwise be imposed on the dependent during the taxpayer's tax year, regardless of whether the taxpayer actually claims the dependency exemption (Reg. § 1.5000A-1(c)). If an individual qualifies as a dependent of more than one taxpayer, the taxpayer who properly claims the dependency exemption is liable for the penalty. If no one claims the dependency exemption, the taxpayer with priority under the rules of Code Sec. 152 will be liable for the penalty. Special rules govern who is responsible for dependents that are placed for adoption, adopted, or placed in foster care. Married taxpayers who file a joint return are jointly liable for the penalty that is imposed on either one of them for any month during the tax year.

The penalty is included on the taxpayer's income tax return for the tax year that includes the month for which the penalty is imposed (Code Sec. 5000A(b)(2)). It must be paid upon notice and demand by the IRS, and is assessed and collected in the same manner as other tax imposed under the Code (Reg. § 1.5000A-5). A taxpayer, however, will not be subject to any criminal prosecution or criminal penalty for failing to timely pay the penalty. In addition, the IRS cannot file a notice of lien or levy on any property to collect any unpaid penalty but they may use any overpayment due the taxpayer to offset any liability for the penalty.

Applicable Individuals. Every individual is an applicable individual subject to the penalty for failure to maintain minimum health care coverage, unless he or she is a member of a specific group whose members are not considered applicable individuals (Code Sec. 5000A(d); Reg. § 1.5000A-3). Members of these groups include:

- individuals who have obtained a religious conscience exemption as a member of a recognized religious sect or division described in Code Sec. 1402(g)(1), i.e., groups objecting to private and public insurance, and who adhere to the established tenets or teachings of the sect or division;

- individuals who are members of a health care sharing ministry, which is an organization described under Code Sec. 501(c)(3), and tax exempt under Code Sec. 501(a), whose members share the same ethical and religious beliefs and share medical expenses among themselves, that retains members even after they develop a medical condition, that has been in existence since December 31, 1999, whose members have shared all medical expenses continuously since then, and that conducts an annual audit that is performed by an independent certified public accountant and made public upon request;

- individuals who are not U.S. citizens or nationals, or are not lawfully present in the United States; and

- individuals who are incarcerated, except for those incarcerated while waiting for disposition of their charges.

There are also a number of exemptions from maintaining minimal health care coverage (Code Sec. 5000A(e)). An individual who is otherwise an applicable individual may be exempt from the penalty if he or she:

- cannot afford health care coverage, meaning that the individual's required contribution exceeds eight percent of his or her household income;

- has household income below his or her income thresholds for filing an income tax return for the tax year (¶ 101);

- lacked minimum essential coverage for a continuous period of less than three months;

- is a member of an Indian tribe as defined for purposes of the Indian employment credit under Code Sec. 45A; or

- experiences a hardship with respect to the capability to obtain coverage under a qualified health plan.

A taxpayer's minimum required contribution for purposes of the unaffordable coverage exemption is either (1) the annual premium for self-only minimum essential coverage of an employer-sponsored plan, or (2) the annual premium of the single lowest cost bronze plan available in the individual market through a Health Benefit Exchange, reduced by the health care credit under Code Sec. 36B (¶ 1331) (Code Sec. 5000A(e)(1)(B)). For 2014, this annual premium cannot exceed eight percent of a taxpayer's household income; for calendar years after 2014, the required contribution percentage is indexed to premium costs. For 2015, the required contribution percentage is 8.05 percent (Rev. Proc. 2014-37).

The taxpayer's household income for this purpose is the sum of his or her modified adjusted gross income (MAGI), plus the MAGI of all other individuals in the taxpayer's family for whom the taxpayer is allowed a dependency exemption deduction and who were required to file an income tax return for the tax year (Code Sec. 5000A(c)(4)). MAGI is the taxpayer's adjusted gross income (AGI) increased by any exclusion from gross income under Code Sec. 911, foreign earned income and housing costs, plus any tax-exempt interest received during the tax year. Household income must be increased by any required contribution made through a salary reduction agreement and excluded from the individual's gross income, e.g., health insurance premiums paid through a cafeteria plan.

> **Example 1:** Susanna is an unmarried individual with no dependents. In November 2015, Susanna is eligible to enroll in self-only coverage under a plan offered by her employer for calendar year 2016. If she enrolls in this plan, she is required to pay $5,000 of the total annual premium. In 2016, Susanna's annual income is $60,000. Her minimum required contribution is $5,000, the portion of the annual premium that she pays for self-only coverage. However, assuming no increase in the contribution percentage after 2014, Susanna will be considered to lack affordable coverage for 2016 because her required contribution ($5,000) is greater than eight percent of her household income ($60,000 x 8% = $4,800) (Reg. § 1.5000A-3(e)(3)(iii), Ex. 1).

> **Example 2:** Bill and Kate are married and file a joint return for 2016. They have two children. In November 2015, Bill is eligible to enroll in self-only coverage in his employer's sponsored plan for calendar year 2016, with his total annual premium being $5,000. Kate and the children are eligible for family coverage under the same plan, at a total annual premium of $20,000. The family's total household income for 2016 is $90,000. Bill's minimum required contribution is equal to his premium for self-only coverage ($5,000). Bill has affordable coverage available for himself, because the annual premium for self-only coverage ($5,000) is less than eight percent of his household income ($90,000 x 8% = $7,200). The required minimum contribution for Kate and the two children is Bill's share of the cost for family coverage ($20,000). Assuming no increase in the contribution percentage after 2014, Kate and the two children lack affordable health care coverage, because their required minimum contribution ($20,000) exceeds eight percent of their household income ($90,000 x 8% = $7,200) (Reg. § 1.5000A-3(e)(3)(iii), Ex. 2).

A short lapse of minimum essential coverage, i.e., short coverage gap, is defined as a continuous period of less than three months. The continuous period is determined without regard to the calendar year. If the taxpayer has more than one continuous lapse of coverage, only the first lapsed period will be counted for this exception (Code Sec. 5000A(e)(4); Reg. § 1.5000A-3(j)).

> **Example 3:** Dave has minimum essential coverage in the current year from January 1 through March 2. After March 2, he does not have minimum essential coverage until he enrolls in an employer sponsored plan effective on June 15. Dave has minimum essential coverage for January, February and March, and June through December. Coverage on the first day of the month qualifies the entire month to be considered a coverage month. Dave is considered without minimum essential coverage for April and May, a continuous period of only two months. Dave will qualify for the short term coverage gap exemption (Reg. § 1.5000A-3(j)(4), Ex. 1).

Hardship exemption certificates are issued by an Exchange and certify that an individual has suffered a hardship as defined in 45 CFR 166.605(g) with respect to obtaining minimum essential coverage (Reg. § 1.5000A-3(h)(2)).

Minimum Essential Coverage. Minimum essential coverage means health care coverage under a government-sponsored program (Medicare, Medicaid, CHIP, etc.), an eligible employer-sponsored plan, a health insurance plan offered in the individual market, a group health plan in which the individual was enrolled on March 23, 2010, or any other coverage recognized by the IRS (Code Sec. 5000A(f); Reg. § 1.5000A-2). Minimum essential coverage does not include health insurance coverage that consists of excepted benefits, such as accident or disability benefits, liability insurance, workers compensation, credit-only insurance, automobile medical payments, or coverage for on-site medical clinics. Under proposed regulations, which would apply to tax years beginning after December 31, 2013, certain government-sponsored limited benefit coverage (line of duty coverage for inactive service members, Medicaid coverage for the medically needy, etc.) would not constitute minimum essential coverage (Prop. Reg. § 1.5000A-2); however, relief is provided for months in 2014 in which an individual has such coverage so that shared responsibility payments would not be imposed (Notice 2014-10).

If benefits are provided under a separate policy, certificate, or insurance contract, then excepted benefits also include: (1) limited scope dental or vision benefits, benefits for long-term care, nursing home care, home health care, community-based care, or any combination thereof, and other similar limited benefits; (2) coverage only for a specified disease or illness; (3) hospital indemnity or other fixed indemnity insurance; and (4) Medicare supplemental health insurance, coverage supplemental to the medical and dental coverage provided to military personnel, and similar supplemental coverage provided to coverage under a group health plan.

Amount of Penalty. The penalty for failing to maintain minimum essential health care coverage, i.e., the shared responsibility payment, for any month is the lesser of:

- the national average premium for a bronze-level coverage plan offered through an Exchange for the tax year for a family that is the size of the taxpayer's family; or

- the sum of a "monthly penalty" amounts for each individual in the taxpayer's family (Code Sec. 5000A(c)(1); Reg. § 1.5000A-4).

The monthly national average premium for qualified health plans that have a bronze level of coverage and are offered through Exchanges in 2014 is $204 per individual and $1,020 for a shared responsibility family with five or more members (Rev. Proc. 2014-46).

The monthly penalty amount is equal to $1/12$ multiplied by the greater of:

- the flat dollar amount, or
- the excess income amount.

The flat dollar amount is the lesser of:

- the sum of the applicable dollar amounts for all applicable individuals in the taxpayer's family who lack minimum essential coverage and whom the taxpayer is required to insure, or

- 300 percent of the applicable dollar amount for the calendar year with or within which the tax year ends.

The applicable dollar amount is $95 for 2014, $325 for 2015, and $695 for 2016. The applicable dollar amount will be inflation-adjusted for tax years after 2016. Any adjustment that is not a multiple of $50 is to be rounded down to the next lowest $50 increment. Special rules apply for individuals under the age of 18 (Reg. § 1.5000A-4(b)(2)).

The excess income amount is the product of the income percentage times the excess of the taxpayer's household income over the taxpayer's applicable filing threshold (¶ 101). The income percentage is one percent for 2014; two percent for 2015, and two and one-half percent for 2016 and thereafter.

> **Example 4:** George is an unmarried individual with no dependents. He does not have minimum essential health care coverage for any month during 2014, and does not qualify for an exemption. For 2014, his household income is $40,000, and his applicable filing threshold is $10,150. George's flat dollar amount is $95. To determine his payment using the income formula, he must subtract $10,150 (filing threshold) from $40,000 (2014 household income). The result is $29,850. One percent of $29,850 equals $298.50. The annual national average premium for bronze level coverage for 2014 is $2,448 ($204 x 12). Because $298.50 is greater

than $95 and less than $2,448, George's shared responsibility payment for 2014 is $298.50, or $24.87 for each month he is uninsured and subject to penalty in 2014 (1/12 x $298.50).

Personal and Dependency Exemptions

133. Exemption Amount. An individual may claim a personal exemption deduction (¶ 135) and an exemption deduction for each person he or she claims as a dependent (¶ 137) on his or her tax return. The amount of a personal exemption (for the taxpayer and spouse) and of a dependency exemption (for each of the taxpayer's dependents) is adjusted annually for inflation. The exemption amount is $3,950 for 2014 ($4,000 for 2015) (Code Sec. 151(d); Rev. Proc. 2013-35; Rev. Proc. 2014-61).[25] The dependency exemption is denied to claimants who fail to provide the dependent's correct taxpayer identification number on the return claiming the dependency exemption (Code Sec. 151(e)).

Taxpayers whose adjusted gross income (AGI) exceeds an applicable threshold amount based on filing status must reduce the amount of their otherwise allowable exemption deduction for tax years beginning after December 31, 2012 (Code Sec. 151(d)(3)).[26] The applicable threshold amounts for 2014 are:

- $305,050 for married individuals filing a joint return and surviving spouses ($309,900 for 2015);
- $279,650 for heads of households ($284,050 for 2015);
- $254,200 for single individuals ($258,250 for 2015); and
- $152,525 for married individuals filing a separate return ($154,950 for 2015).

The threshold amounts are subject to inflation adjustment for tax years beginning after 2013. The taxpayer's deduction for personal and dependency exemptions is reduced by two percent for each $2,500 or fraction thereof by which the AGI exceeds the threshold amount. In the case of a married individual filing separately, the exemption reduction will be reduced by two percent for each $1,250 or fraction thereof by which AGI exceeds the threshold amount. In no case will the deduction for exemptions be reduced by more than 100 percent.

For tax years beginning in 2010 through 2012, the deduction for personal and dependency exemptions was *not* reduced or eliminated for higher-income taxpayers.

135. Personal Exemptions. An individual may generally claim a personal exemption deduction for himself or herself equal to the exemption amount for the year ($3,950 for 2014; $4,000 for 2015) (¶ 133) on his or her tax return, plus any exemptions for dependents (¶ 137) (Code Sec. 151(b); Reg. § 1.151-1; Rev. Proc. 2013-35; Rev. Proc. 2014-61).[27] *No* exemption, however, is allowed to an individual who is eligible to be claimed as a dependent on another taxpayer's return. Thus, students who work part-time during the year or for the summer may *not* claim a personal exemption on their own return if their parents, or any other taxpayers, are *entitled* to claim them on their return. If dependents who are not allowed their own exemptions have gross income in an amount not exceeding $1,000 in 2014 ($1,050 for 2015), they will *not* be taxed on that amount and need *not* file income tax returns (¶ 101).

A husband and wife are allowed at least two personal exemptions when filing a joint return, even if one spouse has no income. If a husband and wife file a joint return, neither can be claimed as a dependent on the return of any other taxpayer. If a husband and wife file separate returns, each must take his or her own exemption on their respective return. If a husband or wife file separate returns and one of the spouses has no gross income and is *not* the dependent of another taxpayer, then the spouse with gross income may claim the personal exemption for the other spouse on his or her separate return. A married taxpayer who files a separate return may *not* claim two exemptions for his or her spouse, one as a spouse and one as a dependent.

References are to Standard Federal Tax Reports; Tax Research Consultant; and Practical Tax Explanations.

[25] ¶ 8000, ¶ 8005.12; FILEIND: 6,050; § 1,205

[26] ¶ 8000; FILEIND: 6,052; § 1,205

[27] ¶ 8000, ¶ 8001; FILEIND: 6,104; § 1,210.05

A resident alien may claim his or her own personal exemption and, if he or she files a joint return, may claim a similar exemption for his or her spouse. However, unless one of the elections noted at ¶ 2410 applies, the filing of a joint return is *not* permissible if either spouse was a nonresident alien at any time during the tax year (Code Sec. 6013(a)(1); Reg. § 1.6013-1(b)).[28]

137. Exemption for Dependent. A taxpayer may claim an exemption deduction ($3,950 for 2014; $4,000 for 2015) for each person he or she claims as a dependent that is a qualifying child (¶ 137A) or qualifying relative (¶ 137B), in addition to his or her personal exemption deduction (¶ 135) (Code Secs. 151(c) and 152; Rev. Proc. 2013-35; Rev. Proc. 2014-61).[29] Anyone claimed as a dependent, or the taxpayer's spouse if filing a joint return, by another taxpayer, however, is barred from claiming another individual as a dependent (Code Sec. 152(b)(1)). Thus, an individual cannot be claimed as a dependent if he or she files a joint return with his or her spouse for the same tax year, unless the return was filed as a claim for refund (¶ 138). The individual to be claimed as a dependent must also be a U.S. citizen, national, or resident of the United States or a contiguous country.

137A. Qualifying Child Definition. A individual taxpayer is allowed to claim a dependency exemption (¶ 137) for each person who is a qualifying child (Code Sec. 152(c)).[30] The following five requirements must all be met for an individual to be considered a qualifying child.

- *Relationship.* The individual must bear one of the following relationships to the taxpayer:

    — a son, daughter, stepson, stepdaughter, or a descendant of such child; or

    — a brother, sister, stepbrother, stepsister, or a descendant of such relative (Code Sec. 152(c)(2) and (f)(1)).

The relationship test includes foster and adopted children. An eligible foster child is a child who is placed with the taxpayer by an authorized placement agency or by a decree issued by the courts. An eligible adopted child includes both a legally adopted child and a child legally placed for adoption.

- *Age.* The individual must be younger than the taxpayer, and either under the age of 19 at the end of the calendar year, or under the age of 24 at the end of the calendar year and a full-time student. An individual who is totally and permanently disabled (¶ 1302) at any time during the year satisfies the age requirement regardless of his or her age (Code Sec. 152(c)(3)). An individual is a full-time student if enrolled or registered for at least part of five calendar months in a year at a qualified educational institution or a qualified on-farm training program (Code Sec. 152(f)(2); Reg. § 1.151-3(b)).

- *Principal Place of Abode.* The individual must have the same principal place of abode as the taxpayer for more than one-half of the year (Code Sec. 152(c)(1)(B)). Temporary absences for illness, school, vacation, or military service may count as time living with the taxpayer. Special rules apply in the case of children of divorced or separated parents (¶ 139A). A child who is born or dies during the tax year is considered as living with the taxpayer for the entire year if the taxpayer's home was the child's home for the entire time he or she was alive (Rev. Rul. 73-156).

- *Support.* The individual must *not* provide more than one-half of his or her own support for the year (Code Sec. 152(c)(1)(D) and (f)(5)). For this purpose, if the individual is the taxpayer's child and is a full-time student, amounts received as scholarships are not considered support.

- *Joint Return.* The individual cannot have filed a joint return with his or her spouse except as a claim for refund (¶ 138) (Code Sec. 152(c)(1)(E)).

References are to Standard Federal Tax Reports; Tax Research Consultant; and Practical Tax Explanations.

[28] ¶ 35,160, ¶ 35,161; FILEIND: 3,250; § 37,125.15

[29] ¶ 8000, ¶ 8007; FILEIND: 6,150; § 1,201

[30] ¶ 8007; FILEIND: 6,154; § 1,215.05

¶137A

In the event that an individual may be claimed as the qualifying child by two or more taxpayers, the taxpayers may decide between themselves who will claim the individual as a qualifying child. If the taxpayers cannot agree and more than one taxpayer is entitled to claim the individual as a qualifying child, regardless of whether they file a return and actually claim the qualifying child, the IRS will disallow all but one of the claims based on the tie-breaking rules discussed at ¶ 139.

If the child or individual fails to meet all the requirements to be considered a qualifying child, the individual may still be claimed as a dependent if he or she meets all the requirements for a qualifying relative (¶ 137B).

137B. Qualifying Relative Definition. An individual taxpayer is allowed to claim a dependency exemption (¶ 137) for each individual who is a qualifying relative and who fails to meet the requirements to be considered a qualifying child (¶ 137A). The following four requirements must all be met for an individual to be considered a qualifying relative (Code Sec. 152(d)).[31]

- *Relationship.* The individual must bear one of the following relationships to the taxpayer:

    — a child, stepchild, adopted child, eligible foster child, or a descendant of such child (see ¶ 137A for the definition of adopted and foster child);

    — a brother, sister, stepbrother, stepsister, half brother, or half sister;

    — a parent, grandparent, or other direct ancestor (other than foster parent), as well as any stepparent;

    — a brother or sister of the taxpayer's parent (aunt or uncle), and any son or daughter of the taxpayer's brother or sister (niece or nephew);

    — a son-in-law, daughter-in-law, father-in-law, mother-in-law, brother-in-law or sister-in-law; or

    — an individual who, for the entire year, has the same principal place of abode as the taxpayer and is a member of the taxpayer's household (temporary absences for illness, school, vacation, or military service are permitted) (Code Sec. 152(d)(2)).

    Once established, a relationship does not terminate due to divorce or death of a spouse.

- *Gross Income.* The individual's gross income for the calendar year (¶ 143) in which the taxpayer's tax year begins must be less than the exemption amount for the year (¶ 133) ($3,950 for 2014; $4,000 for 2015) (Code Sec. 152(d)(1)(B); Rev. Proc. 2013-35; Rev. Proc. 2014-61).

- *Support.* Over half of the individual's total support for that calendar year must have been furnished by the taxpayer (¶ 147) (Code Sec. 152(d)(1)(C)).

- *Not A Qualifying Child.* The individual must *not* be the qualifying child of the taxpayer or of any other taxpayer for the tax year (¶ 137A) (Code Sec. 152(d)(1)(D)).

For purposes of the requirement that an individual not be the qualifying child of another taxpayer, an unrelated child that lives with and is supported by a taxpayer may be claimed as a qualifying relative if the other individual for whom the child is a qualifying child does not file a return or files a return solely to claim a refund of withheld taxes (Notice 2008-5). For example, a boyfriend would be allowed to claim a dependency exemption for his girlfriend's unrelated child provided she is not required to file a return under Code Sec. 6012 or, if she files a return, it is only for the purpose of claiming a refund. If she files a return to claim the earned income credit, then she is considered to have filed a return and the boyfriend is denied the dependency exemption.

In the event that an individual can be claimed as the qualifying relative by two or more taxpayers, the taxpayers may decide between themselves who will claim the

---

References are to Standard Federal Tax Reports; Tax Research Consultant; and Practical Tax Explanations.

[31] ¶ 8007; FILEIND: 6,156; § 1,220.05

¶137B

individual as a qualifying relative. If the taxpayers cannot agree and more than one taxpayer is entitled to claim the individual as a qualifying relative, regardless of whether they file a return and actually claim the qualifying relative, the IRS will disallow all but one of the claims based on the tie-breaking rules discussed at ¶ 139.

138. Married Dependents. A married individual cannot be claimed as a dependent (¶ 133) if he or she joins with his or her spouse to file a joint return (¶ 154) (Code Sec. 152(b)(2)).[32] Thus, a parent cannot claim a married child as a dependent if the child has filed a joint return with his or her spouse. The only exception to this rule is if the sole purpose for filing the joint return was to obtain a refund and neither the dependent nor the spouse would have a tax liability if they had filed separately (Rev. Rul. 65-34, affirming Rev. Rul. 54-567). In this situation, the IRS views the return as simply a claim for refund.

139. Two or More Taxpayers Claiming the Same Qualifying Child. An individual may meet the requirements to be a qualifying child or qualifying relative of more than one taxpayer. Only one taxpayer, however, can claim the individual for purposes of claiming the dependency exemption (¶ 137). Generally, if an individual may be claimed as a qualifying child by two or more taxpayers, the taxpayers may decide between themselves who will treat the child as a qualifying child, subject to the tie-breaking rules. If the taxpayers cannot agree and more than one taxpayer is entitled to claim the individual as a qualifying child, regardless of whether a return is filed and the qualifying child is claimed, the IRS will disallow all but one of the claims based on the following tie-breaking rules (Code Sec. 152(c)(4); Notice 2006-86):[33]

- If only one of the taxpayers is the child's parent, then the child is the qualifying child for that parent.

- If the child's parents do not file a joint return, then the child is the qualifying child of the parent with whom the child lived with the longest during the year.

- If the child resided with both parents equally during the year and the parents do not file a joint return, then the child is the qualifying child of the parent with the highest adjusted gross income (AGI).

- If none of the taxpayers claiming the child are the child's parent, then the child is the qualifying child of the person with the highest AGI.

- If the parents may claim the child as a qualifying child, but do not actually do so, then the child may be the qualifying child of any other taxpayer but only if the other taxpayer's AGI is higher than the AGI of either parent.

When applying the tie-breaking rules above, the taxpayer is allowed to claim the child as a qualifying child for purposes of the dependency exemption (¶ 137), head-of-household filing status (¶ 173), the child tax credit (¶ 1305), the dependent care credit (¶ 1301), the exclusion for dependent care benefits (¶ 2065), and the earned income credit (¶ 1322).

For a discussion of the separate tie-breaker rules for divorced and separated parents, see ¶ 139A.

139A. Exemptions for Children of Divorced Parents. The dependency exemption for a child who is a qualifying child or qualifying relative of divorced or separated parents usually will go to the parent who has primary custody of the child for the calendar year. The custodial parent is determined by the number of nights in which the child resided with the parent (Code Sec. 152(e); Reg. § 1.152-4).[34] When the child spends an equal amount of time with each parent, the parent with the higher adjusted gross income (AGI) is allowed to claim the dependency exemption.

The custodial parent, however, can waive the dependency exemption and the child may be treated as the qualifying child or qualifying relative of the noncustodial parent if all of the following requirements are met:

References are to Standard Federal Tax Reports; Tax Research Consultant; and Practical Tax Explanations.

[32] ¶ 8005.56, ¶ 8007; FILEIND: 6,152; § 1,210.05

[33] ¶ 8007; FILEIND: 6,154.25; § 1,215.35

[34] ¶ 8007, ¶ 8150; FILEIND: 6,158.05; § 1,215.40

• the parents are divorced or legally separated under a decree of divorce or separate maintenance, separated under a written separation agreement, or lived apart at all times during the last six months of the calendar year, including parents who were never married and who do not live together;

• one or both parents provided more than half of the child's total support for the calendar year determined without regard to any multiple support agreement (¶ 147); however, when a parent has remarried, support received from the parent's spouse is treated as received from the parent (Code Sec. 152(d)(5)(B));

• one or both parents have legal custody of the child for more than half of the calendar year; and

• the custodial parent makes a written declaration on Form 8332 that he or she will not claim the exemption and the noncustodial parent attaches the declaration to his or her tax return for each year the exemption is claimed.

If all of the above requirements are met, the noncustodial parent may claim the child as a qualifying child for purposes of the dependency exemption (¶ 137), the child tax credit (¶ 1305), and any education credits attributable to educational expenses made for the child by the noncustodial parent (¶ 1303). Even if the dependency exemption is released, the custodial parent may still claim the child as a qualifying child for purposes of the head of household filing status (¶ 173), dependent care credit (¶ 1301), exclusion of dependent care benefits (¶ 2065), and earned income tax credit (¶ 1322) (Notice 2006-86).

Moreover, so long as the first three requirements listed above are met, regardless of whether the custodial parent releases the claim to an exemption, if the child is the qualifying child or qualifying relative of one of the parents, he or she can be treated as a dependent of both parents for purposes of:

(1) the child's receipt of benefits under a parent's employer-provided health care plan (¶ 2015);

(2) contributions to an accident or health plan by a parent's employer on behalf of the child (¶ 2013);

(3) the child's use of a fringe benefit that qualifies as a no-additional-cost service or qualified employee discount (¶ 2087 and ¶ 2088, respectively);

(4) the child's deductible medical expense (¶ 1015); and

(5) the child's qualified medical expenses paid from distributions from a health savings account (HSA) or Archer medical savings account (MSA) that are excludable from gross income (¶ 2035 and ¶ 2037, respectively) (Rev. Proc. 2008-48).

141. Claiming the Dependency Exemption. Personal exemptions are claimed on Form 1040 or 1040A. The taxpayer, spouse, and dependents are listed in the "Exemptions" section on page 1 of either form. The total number of exemptions is then multiplied by the exemption amount ($3,950 for 2014; $4,000 for 2015) and used to figure taxable income (¶ 133). On a joint return, the dependency exemption is allowed if the dependent is the qualifying child or qualifying relative of one of the spouses (¶ 137) (Reg. § 1.152-2(d); Rev. Proc. 2013-35; Rev. Proc. 2014-61).[35]

If a parent is barred from claiming an exemption for a child because that child fails to meet either the qualifying child (¶ 137A) or qualifying relative (¶ 137B) requirements, the child may claim a personal exemption on his or her own return. Also a dependent, whether a qualifying child or a qualifying relative, who has earned income on which tax has been withheld should file a return even though he or she is claimed as a dependent by another. The return will serve as a claim for refund of the tax withheld if the dependent incurs no tax liability. If a dependent child of the taxpayer has only earned income in excess of the standard deduction amount for the year (¶ 126), unearned income in excess of $1,000, gross income exceeding the larger of $1,000 or the standard deduction amount for the year, or self-employment income of $400 or more, a return must be filed whether or not the child is claimed as a dependent (¶ 101 and ¶ 2670).

References are to Standard Federal Tax Reports; Tax Research Consultant; and Practical Tax Explanations.

[35] ¶ 8050; FILEIND: 6,152; § 1,201

In a community property state (¶ 710), if a child's support is derived from community income, some or all of the exemptions may, by agreement, be taken by either the husband or wife on a separate return. A single exemption amount, however, may *not* be divided between them.[36]

143. Gross Income of a Qualifying Relative Dependent. For an individual to be a qualifying relative for purposes of the dependency exemption (¶ 137B), his or her gross income for the calendar year in which the taxpayer's tax year begins must be less than the exemption amount for that year ($3,950 for 2014; $4,000 for 2015) (Rev. Proc. 2013-35; Rev. Proc. 2014-61) (¶ 133). In determining whether a dependent has gross income in excess of the exemption amount, it is statutory gross income, not gross sales, adjusted gross, net or any other amount of income, that is counted. Thus, gross income is taken into account without deductions. For example, gross rents are counted, without reduction for rental expenses or depreciation. A partner's share of partnership gross income, rather than net income, is counted. Any income excludable from the claimed dependent's gross income, i.e., exempt interest, disability, or Social Security, however, is disregarded, as well as income received by a permanently and totally disabled individual at a sheltered workshop school (Code Sec. 152(d)(4); IRS Pub. 17).[37] Excludable income is counted in determining whether the taxpayer has furnished over half of the dependent's support (¶ 147).

> **Example:** Paul's mother, who lived in his home, earned $500 in 2014 from baby-sitting. She was injured in an accident and received $2,650 in compensatory damages. Paul contributed $2,000 for her support in 2014. The damage award is not taxable income and is not counted for purposes of the $3,950 gross income test, but if Paul's mother spent at least $1,500 of this amount (plus the $500 she received for baby-sitting) in 2014 for her own support, Paul could *not* claim her as a dependent because he would not have furnished *more* than one-half of her support. If less than $2,000 was spent by Paul's mother for her own support, Paul would be entitled to the dependency exemption.

147. Support of a Qualifying Relative Dependent. For an individual to be a qualifying relative for purposes of the dependency exemption (¶ 137B), a taxpayer must furnish more than one-half of the *total* support for the individual for the tax year. See, however, the special rule for children of divorced parents at ¶ 139A (Code Sec. 152(d)(1); Reg. § 1.152-1).[38] Thus, if an individual provides more than one-half of his or her own support for the tax year, then generally no other taxpayer can meet the support test and no one can claim that individual as a qualifying relative. If any other individual taxpayer provides more than one-half of a person's support, only that other taxpayer can meet the support test, except in the case of certain divorced parents (¶ 139A).

Multiple Support Agreement. If no one taxpayer provides more than one-half of the support for an individual, any taxpayer who actually provides more than 10 percent of the individual's support can be treated as having met the support test if a multiple support agreement is filed (Code Sec. 152(d)(3); Reg. § 1.152-3).[39] To be eligible to use a multiple support agreement, more than one-half of the individual's support must be received from a group of persons including the taxpayer, each of whom would otherwise have been entitled to claim the individual as a dependent if they each had furnished more than one-half of the individual's support, and no one taxpayer furnished more than one-half of that support. The person claiming the dependency exemption completes Form 2120 verifying that each person who contributed more than 10 percent of the support signed a written declaration stating that he or she will not claim the exemption. The statement must include the calendar year for which the waiver for claiming the dependency exemption applies, the name of the qualifying relative, and the name, address and Social Security number of the person waiving the exemption claim. These

---

References are to Standard Federal Tax Reports; Tax Research Consultant; and Practical Tax Explanations.

[36] ¶ 8005.23; INDIV: 24,160; § 1,201

[37] ¶ 8007; FILEIND: 6,156.20; § 1,220.15

[38] ¶ 8007, ¶ 8008; FILEIND: 6,156.15; § 1,220.20

[39] ¶ 8007, ¶ 8100; FILEIND: 6,156.15; § 1,220.20

statements must be retained with the taxpayer's records in the event the taxpayer is called upon to justify claiming the dependency exemption.

Support Defined. The support test is applied by comparing the amount of support provided by the taxpayer with the total amount of support received by the dependent from all sources during the calendar year in which the taxpayer's tax year begins. "Total" support is the sum of:

- the fair rental value of lodging furnished to a qualifying relative dependent;

- the costs of all items of expense paid out directly by or for the benefit of the qualifying relative dependent, such as clothing, education, medical and dental care, gifts, transportation, church contributions, and entertainment and recreation; and

- a proportionate share of the expenses incurred in supporting the whole household that cannot be directly attributed to each individual, such as food.[40]

The proportionate share of household expenses does not include items that represent the cost of maintaining a house, such as heat, electricity, repairs, taxes, etc., because these costs are accounted for in the fair rental value of the lodging furnished to the dependent. Medical care includes the premiums paid on a medical care policy, but not the benefits provided by the policy. Medicare benefits, both basic and supplementary, as well as Medicaid, are also disregarded in determining support.

Certain capital expenditures qualify as items of support, such as the cost of an automobile purchased for a qualifying relative dependent and the cost of furniture and appliances. However, the following have been held not to be items of support: (1) income and Social Security taxes paid by a dependent child from his own income; (2) funeral expenses of a qualifying relative dependent; (3) costs incurred by a parent in exercising visitation rights, and (4) life insurance premium costs.[41]

In determining whether a taxpayer furnished more than one-half of a qualifying relative dependent's total support, the support provided by the taxpayer, by the dependent, and by third parties must be taken into account. In addition, only the amount of the cash actually expended for items of support is taken into account. The source and tax status of money used to provide support is, generally, not controlling. It may come from taxable income, tax-exempt receipts, and loans. Furthermore, the year in which the support is received, and not the year of payment of the indebtedness incurred, is controlling in determining whether over one-half of the support is furnished by the taxpayer, regardless of his or her method of tax accounting.[42]

In the case of the taxpayer's child (¶ 137), or stepchild who is a student, any amounts received as scholarships do not have to be taken into account (Reg. § 1.152-1(c)).[43] Educational benefits received under the U.S. Navy's educational assistance program are *not* considered to be scholarships.[44]

Survivor and old-age insurance benefits received under the Social Security Act and used for support are considered as having been contributed by the recipient to his or her own support.[45] Benefit payments made to an individual under state public assistance laws and measured solely by the needs of the recipient are considered as having been used entirely by that individual for his or her own support unless it is shown otherwise.[46] Amounts expended by a state for the training and education of handicapped children, including mentally retarded children who qualify as "students" and are in a state institution that qualifies as an "educational institution," are not considered to constitute support, except where the state assumes custody of the child involved.[47] Aid to Families with Dependent Children (AFDC) payments are considered support by the state and not by the parent.[48]

References are to Standard Federal Tax Reports; Tax Research Consultant; and Practical Tax Explanations.

[40] ¶ 8005.54, ¶ 8005.80; FILEIND: 6,160; § 1,220.20

[41] ¶ 8005.38, ¶ 8005.80; FILEIND: 6,152.05; § 1,220.20

[42] ¶ 8005.81; FILEIND: 6,160.10; § 1,220.20

[43] ¶ 8008; FILEIND: 6,158.20; § 1,220.20

[44] ¶ 8005.62; FILEIND: 6,158.20; § 1,220.20

[45] ¶ 8005.71; FILEIND: 6,160.25; § 1,220.20

[46] ¶ 8005.60; FILEIND: 6,160.25; § 1,220.20

[47] ¶ 8005.72; FILEIND: 6,160.25; § 1,220.20

[48] ¶ 8005.60; FILEIND: 6,160.25; § 1,220.20

149. Effect of Death on Exemption. The personal or dependency exemption amount claimed by a taxpayer (¶ 133) is not reduced because of the death of a taxpayer, his or her spouse, or a dependent during the tax year (Reg. § 1.152-1(b)).[49]

> **Example 1:** A child is born on December 31, 2014, and dies in January 2015. A full exemption is allowed for the child in both years.

The death of one spouse will also *not* deprive the survivor of the right to claim the exemptions of the deceased. The crucial date for determining marital status is the last day of the tax year. If a spouse dies during the tax year, however, this determination is made as of the date of death (Code Sec. 7703(a)).[50]

On the final separate return of a decedent, in addition to the deceased's own personal exemption, the exemptions for the surviving spouse may be taken if the surviving spouse had no gross income and was not a dependent of anyone else (¶ 135). Further, since the dependency exemption is based upon furnishing over half the support during the calendar year in which the tax year of the taxpayer begins, a decedent who furnished over half the support to a person otherwise qualifying as a dependent would be entitled to the full exemption for such dependent, without proration.

> **Example 2:** Allen furnishes the full support for his aged father up to the date of Allen's death on September 1, 2014, and over one-half of the total support for the year. A $3,950 exemption is allowed for the father on Allen's final return. But if Allen died on April 1 and his brother, Bob, supported their father for the balance of the year, incurring a larger expense than Allen did during the first part of the year, Bob would be entitled to the exemption. If the support in the latter case was furnished equally by Bob and another brother, Carl, from April 1 on, and if none of the three brothers furnished over half of the father's support for the calendar year, any one of them, including the executor of Allen's estate (on Allen's final return), could take the exemption if the other two brothers renounced their right to the exemption for that year (¶ 147). Regardless of the amount of support, no exemption is allowed to any of the three brothers for their father if the father had gross income of $3,950 or more during calendar year 2014 (¶ 137B).

150. Missing and/or Kidnapped Children. A dependency exemption may be claimed for any child of the taxpayer, regardless of whether the child qualifies as a qualifying child or qualifying relative, if the child is presumed by a law enforcement agency to have been kidnapped by someone other than a member of the family and had resided at the taxpayer's principal place of abode for more than one-half of the year before the kidnapping (Code Sec. 152(f)(6)).[51]

Filing Status

152. Joint Return—Who May File. Married taxpayers may elect to file a joint return or file as married persons filing separately. In most cases, it is more beneficial for married taxpayers to file a joint return (¶ 156). A husband and wife may file a joint return even though one spouse has no income or deductions (Code Sec. 6013; Reg. § 1.6013-1),[52] but only if:

- their tax years begin on the same date;
- they are not legally separated under a decree of divorce or separate maintenance on the last day of the tax year; and
- neither is a nonresident alien at any time during the year.

Marital status for federal tax purposes depends on state law. Taxpayers married in compliance with the laws of one state remain married regardless of where they reside. Recognition of this principal has been extended to common-law marriages (Rev. Rul. 58-66) and to same-sex couples (Rev. Rul. 2013-17).[53] Same-sex married couples may elect to amend any prior open tax years under this ruling. However, couples in registered domestic partnerships, civil unions, and any other similar formal relationship

---

References are to Standard Federal Tax Reports; Tax Research Consultant; and Practical Tax Explanations.

[49] ¶ 8008; FILEIND: 6,158.10; § 1,220.10

[50] ¶ 43,170; FILEIND: 3,202; § 1,210.10

[51] ¶ 8007; FILEIND: 6,158.15; § 1,215.10

[52] ¶ 35,160, ¶ 35,161; FILEIND: 18,056; § 1,320.05

[53] ¶ 35,171.0223; FILEIND: 18,056; § 1,105, § 46,951

¶152

that is *not* denominated as a marriage under the laws of the state cannot use either married filing jointly or married filing separately status for federal tax purposes, even if the laws of the state of celebration grant them all the same benefits and privileges as a married couple.

A U.S. citizen or resident and his or her nonresident alien spouse, however, can elect to file a joint return if they agree to be taxed on their worldwide income and supply all necessary books and records and other information pertinent to the determination of tax liability (¶ 2410) (Code Sec. 6013(g)). Further, a one-time election to file a joint return is available in the year in which a nonresident alien spouse becomes a resident (Code Sec. 6013(h)).

If a husband and wife are on a calendar-year basis or have fiscal years that begin on the same date, then they can file a joint return. However, if they have different tax years for some reason other than the intervention of death (¶ 164), then they cannot file a joint return. If newly married spouses with different tax years want to change the year of one spouse to coincide with that of the other so as to be able to file jointly, then they may do so by following the rules described at ¶ 1513. A husband and wife may file a joint return even though they have different accounting methods, e.g., one is on the cash basis and the other is on the accrual basis, if such methods clearly reflect their income.

Even though a husband and wife are not living together on the last day of the tax year, they may still file a joint return if they are *not* legally separated under a decree of divorce or separate maintenance on that date (Reg. § 1.6013-4).[54] Spouses who are separated under an interlocutory decree of divorce are considered husband and wife and are entitled to file a joint return until the decree becomes final. However, certain married individuals living apart may file separate returns as heads of households (¶ 173).

Spouses of military personnel serving in a combat zone and missing in action may file a joint return for any tax year until the tax year beginning two years after the termination of combat activities in that zone (Code Sec. 6013(f)).[55]

154. Joint Return—Election to File. When married individuals file separate returns for a tax year, they can elect to make a joint return for that year after the period for timely filing has expired. This change of filing status is usually achieved by the filing of an amended return on Form 1040X within three years of the last date prescribed by law for the filing of the separate return or returns, without taking into account any extension of time granted to either spouse (Code Sec. 6013(b)(2)).[56] However, the change to a joint return cannot be made:

- after either spouse timely files a petition with the Tax Court pursuant to a notice of deficiency which was mailed to either spouse for the tax year;

- after either spouse commences a suit in any court for the recovery of any part of the tax for such tax year;

- after either spouse enters into a closing agreement with respect to such tax year; or

- after either spouse has compromised any civil or criminal case arising with respect to such tax year.

Once a joint return has been filed for a tax year, the spouses may *not* thereafter file separate returns after the time for filing the return of either spouse has expired (Reg. § 1.6013-1(a)).[57] The exception being if either spouse dies during the tax year, then only the executor or administrator of the estate of the deceased spouse may elect to change from a joint to a separate return (¶ 168).

References are to Standard Federal Tax Reports; Tax Research Consultant; and Practical Tax Explanations.

[54] ¶ 35,165; FILEIND: 18,056.10; § 1,320.10

[55] ¶ 35,160; FILEIND: 18,056.30; § 1,320.10

[56] ¶ 35,160; FILEIND: 18,056.05; § 1,320.25

[57] ¶ 35,161; FILEIND: 18,056.05; § 1,320.25

The Tax Court has ruled that a couple could elect to file a joint return even though the IRS had previously prepared and filed returns for the husband with a status of married filing separately (*J.V. Millsap*, Dec. 45,179, 91 TC 926). The IRS's filing of substitute returns did not bar the taxpayer from contesting either the deficiency or the IRS's choice of his filing status. The former standard that the IRS's choice precludes taxpayers from selecting a different filing status will be applied only when the issue is appealable to the U.S. Court of Appeals for the Tenth Circuit (*R.E. Smalldridge*, CA-10, 86-2 USTC ¶ 9764).

156. Joint Return v. Separate Return. It is generally more beneficial for married taxpayers to file a joint return (¶ 152). The filing of a joint return will result in a savings of tax in those instances in which differences in the tax rate brackets for joint and separate returns result in higher tax rates for married individuals filing separately. Unlike with separate returns, taxable income (¶ 123) on a joint return is the entire taxable income amount of the couple. Although there are two taxpayers on the joint return, there is only one taxable income amount and only one adjusted gross income (AGI) amount (Reg. § 1.6013-4).[58] In addition, the total exemptions (¶ 135) of a husband and wife are subtracted in determining taxable income.

> **Example:** For 2014, Joe has taxable income in the amount of $14,500, and his wife, Trisha, has taxable income in the amount of $37,550. If they elect to file a joint return, they will not be subject to the 25-percent tax rate because their combined taxable income of $52,050 does not exceed the $73,800 threshold amount for 2014 (¶ 13). If they elect to file separate returns, however, $650, which represents the portion of Trisha's income that exceeds the $36,900 threshold, falls within the 25-percent tax bracket for the year (¶ 15).

Also, if only one spouse has income, it would be impractical for the income earner to use married filing separately status. This filing status carries a basic standard deduction of $6,200 for 2014, whereas joint filers have a basic standard deduction of $12,400 for 2014 (¶ 126). It should be noted that a married individual generally may *not* claim the credit for the elderly or permanently disabled (¶ 1302), the child and dependent care credit (¶ 1301), the earned income credit (¶ 1322), or the educational credits (¶ 1303) unless he or she files a joint return with his or her spouse.

There are circumstances under which married taxpayers might reduce their tax liability by filing separate returns. For example, a spouse whose medical expenses are high, but not high enough to exceed 10 percent of the AGI reported on a joint return (7.5 percent of AGI for tax years ending before January 1, 2017, for individuals age 65 or older by the end of the tax year), may exceed the AGI threshold on a separate return (¶ 1015). In light of the two-percent-of-AGI floor on miscellaneous itemized deductions (¶ 1011), a spouse who incurs substantial unreimbursed employee business or investment expenses might be better off filing separately. The same rationale holds true for casualty and disaster loss deductions, which are subject to a 10-percent-of-AGI floor (¶ 1131).

Actual tax comparisons should be made using both joint and separate returns if there is doubt as to which method produces a more favorable result. Considerations other than tax savings might enter into the decision to file a separate, rather than a joint return. For example, one spouse may wish to avoid a tax deficiency liability assessed against the other spouse (¶ 162).

162. Joint Return—Liability for Taxes. A husband and wife are liable jointly and individually for the entire amount of tax, penalties, and interest arising out of a joint return (Code Sec. 6013(d)(3)).[59] Relief is available under certain circumstances, commonly referred to as "innocent spouse relief" (Code Sec. 6015).[60] Three types of innocent spouse relief are available to the electing spouse: liability relief (commonly referred to as innocent spouse relief) (Code Sec. 6015(b)), separation of liability relief (Code Sec. 6015(c)), or equitable relief (Code Sec. 6015(f)). A spouse must generally request one of these types of relief on Form 8857 within two years of the IRS beginning

---

References are to Standard Federal Tax Reports; Tax Research Consultant; and Practical Tax Explanations.

[58] ¶ 35,165; FILEIND: 18,056.35; § 1,320.05

[59] ¶ 35,160; FILEIND: 18,056.40; § 1,320.30

[60] ¶ 35,185; INDIV: 18,050; § 39,040.05

collection of a tax deficiency or assessment. Equitable relief requests on or after July 25, 2011, however, may be requested within the limitations period for filing any claim for refund (¶ 2763) or for the collection of tax (¶ 2735) (Notice 2011-70). Transitional rules also apply for individuals in various stages of seeking, or having been denied, equitable innocent spouse relief.

Any determination by the IRS regarding any type of innocent spouse relief is reviewable in the Tax Court.[61] Notice of the election for relief is required to be given to the non-electing spouse, who may participate in any hearings on the relief requested (Code Sec. 6015(h)(2); Reg. § 1.6015-6(a)(1)).[62] The Tax Court has held that the non-electing spouse has the right to a "stand-alone" hearing regarding the appropriateness of granting relief to the electing spouse (*T. Corson*, Dec. 53,882, 114 TC 354); *K.A. King*, Dec. 53,994, 115 TC 118). However, the appellate courts have limited the jurisdiction of the Tax Court with regard to spousal relief. The Tax Court has no jurisdiction to make any spousal relief determination unless the IRS has issued a deficiency notice to the taxpayer (*G.A. Ewing*, CA-9, 2006-1 USTC ¶ 50,191; *T.E. Bartman*, CA-8, 2006-1 USTC ¶ 50,298). There are additional requirements for jurisdictions located in community property states (IRS Pub. 555).

Liability Relief (Innocent Spouse Relief). To qualify for liability relief (commonly referred to as innocent spouse relief), the requesting taxpayer must meet *all* the following requirements:

- filed a joint return for the tax year which has an *understatement of tax* due to *erroneous items* of the other spouse;

- establish that at the time of signing the tax return the taxpayer did not know, or have reason to know, there was an understatement of tax; and

- show that it would be unfair to hold the innocent spouse liable for the understatement of tax, taking into account all the facts and circumstances (Code Sec. 6015(b)).[63]

A key element for the IRS will be whether the electing spouse received any substantial benefits, or later was divorced or separated from, or deserted by, the other spouse.

Separation of Liability Relief. Alternatively, the taxpayer may elect to obtain relief by separation of liabilities (Code Sec. 6015(c)).[64] To qualify, an individual must have filed a joint return, and either:

- be no longer married to, or be legally separated from, the spouse with whom the joint return was filed, or

- must *not* have been a member of the same household with the other spouse for a 12-month period ending on the date of the filing of Form 8857.

The burden of proof on income and deductions is on the taxpayer who elects relief under separation of liability.

Equitable Relief. Should an individual fail to qualify for either of the first two types of relief, he or she may still obtain relief from the tax liabilities, interest and penalties by electing equitable relief (Code Sec. 6015(f)).[65] The taxpayer must show that, under *all* facts and circumstances, it would be unfair to be held liable for the understatement or underpayment of taxes. The IRS has issued guidance for taxpayers seeking equitable relief (Rev. Proc. 2013-34).

163. Joint Return—Injured Spouse Claim. When married taxpayers file a joint return and one spouse has not paid child or spousal support, or certain federal debts, e.g., student loans, all or part of the tax overpayment shown on the joint return may be used to satisfy the past-due debt of the delinquent spouse. The nonobligated spouse may, however, be entitled to a refund of his or her part of the overpayment if that individual:

References are to Standard Federal Tax Reports; Tax Research Consultant; and Practical Tax Explanations.

[61] ¶ 35,192.815; INDIV: 18,052.20; § 39,040.05

[62] ¶ 35,185, ¶ 35,187E; INDIV: 18,052.15; § 39,040.25

[63] ¶ 35,185; INDIV: 18,054; § 39,040.10

[64] ¶ 35,185; INDIV: 18,056; § 39,040.15

[65] ¶ 35,185; INDIV: 18,058; § 39,040.20

- is not required to pay the past-due amount;

- received and reported income, i.e., wages, taxable interest, etc., on the joint return; and

- made and reported payments, i.e., withheld federal income taxes or estimated taxes, on the joint return (Financial Management Service Reg. § 285.3).[66]

To make this type of claim, the nonobligated spouse can either write "Injured Spouse" in the upper left corner of the jointly-filed Form 1040 and attach Form 8379, or file Form 8379 by itself after filing the joint return.

164. Joint Return—Effect of Death. A joint return may be filed when one or both spouses died during the year, and the tax year of both began on the same day, whether this year is a fiscal or calendar year. When a joint return is filed, it is treated as if the tax years of both spouses ended on the closing date of the surviving spouse's tax year (Reg. § 1.6013-3).[67]

166. Joint Return—Surviving Spouse. A surviving spouse who is a widow(er) with dependent children may continue to use the tax rates for married taxpayers filing jointly for two tax years immediately following the year of death of his or her spouse (¶ 175). A surviving spouse may *not* file a joint return in the year the other spouse dies if the surviving spouse remarries before the close of the tax year. The surviving spouse may, however, file a joint return with his or her new spouse for that year if all other requirements are met. The surviving spouse may not file a joint return with the deceased spouse if the tax year of either spouse is a fractional part of a year resulting from a change of accounting period (Reg. § 1.6013-1(d)).[68]

> **Example:** Stan and Tracy file joint returns on a calendar-year basis. Tracy dies on March 1, 2014. Thereafter, Stan receives permission to change his accounting period to a fiscal year beginning July 1, 2014. A joint return cannot be filed for the short tax year ending June 30, 2014.

168. Joint Return—Return with a Deceased Spouse. Generally, where one spouse dies, a joint return can be filed only by the executor or administrator and the survivor (¶ 178). The surviving spouse, alone, however, may file a joint return if:

- no return was filed by the decedent for the tax year at issue;

- no executor or administrator was appointed; and

- no executor or administrator was appointed before the last day for filing the return of the surviving spouse, including any extensions of time for filing.

Even if all of the above tests are met, an administrator or executor, subsequently appointed, may disaffirm a joint return made by the surviving spouse by filing a separate return for the decedent. This disaffirmance must be made within one year after the last day allowed for filing the return of the surviving spouse including extensions. If a disaffirmance is made, then the already filed joint return will be considered the survivor's separate return. The survivor's tax will be figured by excluding all of the items properly includible in the return of the deceased spouse (Reg. § 1.6013-1(d)).[69]

173. Head of Household Filing Status. Individuals who qualify to file as head of household are generally entitled to a higher standard deduction (¶ 126) and lower tax rates than single individuals. See Tax Rate Schedule Z (¶ 17) or the Tax Computation Worksheet (¶ 20) and the "Head of a Household" column in the Tax Table (¶ 25). In order to qualify for head of household status, an individual must be unmarried or considered unmarried, and not a surviving spouse (¶ 175) at the close of the tax year (Code Sec. 2(b)).[70] In addition, the taxpayer must maintain a household which, for more than one-half of the tax year, is the principal place of abode of a qualifying individual who is a member of the household.

References are to Standard Federal Tax Reports; Tax Research Consultant; and Practical Tax Explanations.

[66] ¶ 38,527; INDIV: 18,062, IRS: 33,102; § 40,015.15

[67] ¶ 35,164; FILEIND: 18,056.25; § 1,320.05

[68] ¶ 35,161; FILEIND: 18,056.20, FILEIND: 18,056.25; § 38,145.05

[69] ¶ 35,161; FILEIND: 18,056.25; § 1,320.20

[70] ¶ 3310; FILEIND: 3,150; § 1,115.05

A qualifying individual includes a qualifying child of the taxpayer for dependency exemption purposes (¶ 137A) determined without regard to the rules for divorced parents (¶ 139A). A child is not a qualifying individual for head-of-household status purposes, however, if the child is married at the close of the taxpayer's tax year and (i) files a joint return with his or her spouse (Code Sec. 152(b)(2)), or (ii) is not a U.S. citizen, a U.S. national, or a resident of the United States, Canada, or Mexico (Code Sec. 152(b)(3)). For purposes of this requirement, an adopted child or a foster child, as defined under the qualifying child rules, is treated as the taxpayer's child by blood.

A qualifying individual also includes any other person who is a dependent of the taxpayer if the taxpayer is entitled to claim a dependency deduction for that person (¶ 137). A taxpayer, however, cannot claim head-of-household status if the only reason for being able to claim an individual as a dependent is based on either the individual living as a member of the taxpayer's household for the full year as a qualifying relative (¶ 137B), or claiming the dependency exemption under a multiple support agreement (¶ 147).

An individual qualifies for head of household status if a *separate* household is maintained for a parent for the tax year. The separate household must be the parent's principal place of abode, and the parent must qualify as the child's dependent (¶ 137). A parent's principal place of abode can include residence in a rest home or home for the aged. An institutionalized or hospitalized dependent, other than a parent, may also qualify a taxpayer as head of a household if the taxpayer can prove that the taxpayer's home was the "principal" place of abode of the dependent, even though the dependent may never return home because of the nature of the infirmity (Code Sec. 2(b)(1)(B); Reg. § 1.2-2(b)(4)).[71]

Marital Status. The marital status of an individual for the purpose of applying the head of household rates is determined at the end of a tax year. A taxpayer is considered to be unmarried at the end of a tax year if his or her spouse was a nonresident alien at any time during the tax year, or if he or she is legally separated from his or her spouse under a decree of divorce or separate maintenance at the close of the tax year. A taxpayer under an interlocutory decree of divorce is not legally separated. A widow or widower may not use the head of household rates in those tax years in which he or she is eligible to use the joint tax rates under the surviving spouse rules discussed at ¶ 175.

A married taxpayer will be considered unmarried and eligible for head of household status if the taxpayer's spouse was not a member of the household for the last six months of the year and if the household is the principal place of abode of a child for whom the taxpayer is entitled to a dependency exemption (¶ 137) (Code Secs. 2(c) and 7703(b)).[72] The taxpayer, however, will still be eligible for head-of-household status even if no dependency exemption is available for a child because the taxpayer waived the exemption (¶ 139A). A nonresident alien who is considered unmarried may not use the head of household tax rate but must use the tax rate schedule for single individuals (Reg. § 1.2-2(b)(6)).[73]

Maintains Household. An individual taxpayer "maintains a household" if (1) the taxpayer furnishes, with funds attributable to him or her, more than one-half the cost of maintaining the home during the tax year and (2) at least one of the qualifying individuals described previously lives there for more than one-half of the year except for temporary absence. An exemption is made for institutionalized or hospitalized dependents. Birth or death of a qualifying individual during the year will not disqualify the taxpayer as the head of a household if the individual lived in the household during the part of the year when he or she was alive (Code Sec. 2(b)(1); Reg. § 1.2-2(c)).[74]

The cost of maintaining a household includes the expenses incurred for the mutual benefit of the occupants by reason of its use as the principal place of abode. These expenses include property taxes, mortgage interest, rent, utility charges, upkeep and

References are to Standard Federal Tax Reports; Tax Research Consultant; and Practical Tax Explanations.

[71] ¶ 3310, ¶ 3325; FILEIND: 3,154; § 1,115.30

[72] ¶ 3310, ¶ 43,170; FILEIND: 3,204; § 1,115.10

[73] ¶ 3325; FILEIND: 3,250; § 1,115.10

[74] ¶ 3310, ¶ 3325; FILEIND: 3,154.05; § 1,115.15

repairs, property insurance, food consumed on the premises, and other household expenses. They do *not* include the cost of clothing, education, medical treatment, vacations, life insurance, transportation, food consumed off the premises, or the value of services rendered by the taxpayer or by any person who qualifies the taxpayer as head of a household (Reg. § 1.2-2(d)).[75]

175. Surviving Spouse Filing Status. A surviving spouse (qualifying widow(er)) may use the joint return tax rates for two tax years following the year of death of the husband or wife, but *only* if the survivor remains unmarried and maintains a household (¶ 173) that, for the entire tax year, is the principal place of abode of a child, adopted child, foster child, or stepchild for whom the taxpayer is entitled to the dependency exemption (¶ 137) (Code Sec. 2(a); Reg. § 1.2-2(a)).[76] See ¶ 164 for a discussion of filing a joint return for the year of death of one spouse.

A widow(er) who qualifies as a surviving spouse uses the joint return rate schedule (Schedule Y-1) at ¶ 13, the Tax Computation Worksheet at ¶ 20 or the Tax Table at ¶ 25 and must use either Form 1040 or Form 1040A. This benefit is afforded a surviving spouse only if he or she was entitled to file a joint return with the deceased spouse for the tax year in which the deceased spouse died.

It should be emphasized that the benefit entitles the survivor only to the joint return tax rates; it does not authorize him or her to file a joint return or claim any personal exemptions other than his or her own and those of the dependent or dependents for whom the household is maintained. For 2014, a qualifying widow(er) (surviving spouse) with dependent children is generally entitled to joint return rate benefits if the spouse died at any time during 2012 or 2013 (Code Sec. 2(a)(1)(A)).

In determining eligibility for filing as a surviving spouse, the date of death of a person serving in a combat zone who was missing in action is considered to be two years after the termination of combat activities in that zone, unless death has been established at an earlier time (Code Sec. 2(a)(3)).

176. Single Filing Status. Unmarried individuals who do not qualify to file their returns as a married individual (¶ 152), as a surviving spouse (¶ 175), or as a head of household (¶ 173) must file their returns as a single taxpayer (Code Sec. 1(c)).[77] See ¶ 103 for a discussion on the filing requirements for a child with earned and unearned income.

Tax Treatment of Decedent's Final Return

178. Who Must File for a Decedent. An income tax return must be filed for a deceased person who would have been required to file a return if he or she were still alive during the tax year (¶ 101) (Code Sec. 6012). This final return covers a short year, including the part of the year up to the date of death. A decedent's final return is due at the same time his or her return would have been due had he or she lived (¶ 107).[78] The final return is filed on Form 1040, 1040A, or 1040EZ if the decedent met the gross income filing test for the short period, or otherwise would have been required to file a return, e.g., the decedent had more than $400 of self-employment earnings. The word "DECEASED," the decedent's name, and the date of death should be written across the top of page 1 of the return.

The return for the decedent must be filed by his or her administrator, executor, or any other person charged with responsibility for the decedent's affairs. The surviving spouse should, however, file the decedent's final return if there is no executor or administrator. A surviving spouse may also file a joint return for the decedent's final year (¶ 168). Whoever files the return for the decedent may file a separate return or a joint return (¶ 164). All personal exemptions to which the decedent was entitled while he or she was alive may be claimed. If a refund is due, the personal representative must attach

References are to Standard Federal Tax Reports; Tax Research Consultant; and Practical Tax Explanations.

[75] ¶ 3325; FILEIND: 3,154.10; § 1,115.15
[76] ¶ 3310, ¶ 3325; FILEIND: 3,100; § 1,120
[77] ¶ 3,260; FILEIND: 3,050; § 1,110
[78] ¶ 35,142; ACCTNG: 24,256; § 1,305.10

to the return either Form 1310 or a copy of the court certificate showing his or her appointment. A surviving spouse filing a joint return with the decedent can claim the refund without attaching Form 1310.

180. Due Date. The final return of a decedent is due by the date on which the return would have been due had death not occurred (¶ 107). Thus, for a calendar-year taxpayer who died in 2014, the final return is due by April 15, 2015 (Reg. § 1.6072-1(a)).[79]

182. How Income Is Treated. When a cash-basis taxpayer dies, only income actually or constructively received up to the date of death is included in the final return. If the decedent was on the accrual basis of accounting, income accrued up to the date of death is included in the final return. Income that accrues *only because of death*, however, is not included (Code Sec. 451; Reg. § 1.451-1(b)).[80] These rules also apply to successive decedents as rights to receive "income in respect of a prior decedent" (Reg. § 1.691(a)-1(c)).[81]

Any amount of gross income *not* reported on the return of the decedent is, when received, includible in the income of the person receiving such amounts by inheritance or survivorship as "income in respect of a decedent." The person receiving the income may be the decedent's estate or, if the estate does not collect an item of income but distributes the right to receive it to a testamentary trust or to the heir, next of kin, legatee, or devisee, it is included in the income of such trust, heir, next of kin, legatee, or devisee (Code Sec. 691(a); Reg. § 1.691(a)-2).[82]

The depreciation recapture rules under Code Secs. 1245 and 1250 apply to sales or other dispositions of property subject to those rules where the income therefrom is treated as income on the decedent's final return or as income in respect of a decedent under Code Sec. 691. See ¶ 1779 and following for a complete discussion. These rules, however, do not apply to transfers of depreciable property at death (Code Secs. 1245(b)(2) and 1250(d)(2)).[83]

184. Installment Obligation. Collections on an installment obligation acquired from a decedent are treated as items of income in respect of a decedent (¶ 182) if the decedent had been reporting the profit on the installment basis (Code Sec. 691(a)(4); Reg. § 1.691(a)-5).[84] If, however, the obligor of the installment obligation acquires the uncollected obligation, then the decedent's estate is considered to have made a taxable disposition of the installment obligation. Thus, any previously unreported gain will be recognized by the estate. This rule also applies if the obligation is canceled because of the death of the payee or if the estate allows the obligation to become unenforceable because it is canceled by the executor.

187. Deductions for Decedents. Deductible expenses and other items are not accrued on the final return of a decedent unless his or her accounting method requires it, but are deductible instead by the estate or person who pays them or is liable for their payment (Code Sec. 461; Reg. § 1.461-1(b)).[85] Similar treatment is given to the foreign tax credit (Code Sec. 691(b); Reg. § 1.691(b)-1).[86]

Expenses for medical care of the decedent, paid out of his or her estate within one year from the date of death, are deductible on the decedent's final income tax return (Reg. § 1.213-1(d)).[87] However, the estate must attach a statement, in duplicate, to the decedent's return waiving the right to claim the deduction on the estate tax return.

Business expenses, income-producing expenses, interest, and taxes for which the decedent was liable but which were not properly allowable as a deduction on his or her last return will be allowed when paid as a deduction by the estate or, if the estate was not liable, then as a deduction by the person who by reason of the decedent's death

References are to Standard Federal Tax Reports; Tax Research Consultant; and Practical Tax Explanations.

[79] ¶ 36,721; ACCTNG: 24,256.05; § 1,305.10

[80] ¶ 21,002, ¶ 21,003; ACCTNG: 9,408; § 38,145.05

[81] ¶ 24,901; ESTTRST: 6,060; § 38,145.05

[82] ¶ 24,900, ¶ 24,902; EST-TRST: 6,054; § 38,145.05

[83] ¶ 30,902, ¶ 31,000; DEPR: 18,104; § 38,145.05

[84] ¶ 24,900, ¶ 24,905; EST-TRST: 6,056, ESTTRST: 6,116; § 18,370

[85] ¶ 21,802, ¶ 21,805; EST-TRST: 6,206, ESTTRST: 6,208; § 38,145.05

[86] ¶ 24,900, ¶ 24,907; EST-TRST: 6,206.30; § 3,050

[87] ¶ 12,541; ESTTRST: 6,208.05; § 7,220

acquires—subject to such obligation—an interest in property of the decedent (Reg. § 1.691(b)-1(a)).[88] The percentage depletion deduction is allowed only to the person who receives the income in respect of the decedent to which the deduction relates (Reg. § 1.691(b)-1(b)).

189. How Recipient Treats Decedent's Income. A decedent's income that is to be accounted for by the recipient retains the same character it would have had in the hands of the decedent (Code Sec. 691(a)(3); Reg. § 1.691(a)-3).[89] Thus, if the income would have been earned income, exempt income, or interest to the decedent, it is the same kind of income to the recipient.

191. Deduction of Estate Taxes. If a person includes in gross income an item of income that had accrued as of the date of death of a decedent or prior successive decedents, so that it was included in the valuation of the estate for estate tax purposes, that person may take a corresponding deduction based on the estate tax attributable to the net value of the income item (Code Sec. 691(c); Reg. § 1.691(c)-1).[90] This deduction is taken by individuals on Form 1040 and by estates and trusts on Form 1041. In the case of individuals, it may be taken only if deductions are itemized on Schedule A. For individuals, as well as for estates and trusts, the deduction is not subject to the two-percent-of-adjusted-gross-income floor on miscellaneous deductions (Code Sec. 67(b)(7)).[91] In the case of any generation-skipping transfer tax imposed on a taxable termination or a direct skip as a result of the death of the transferor, a deduction is available for the portion of this tax attributable to items of gross income that were not properly includible in the gross income of the trust before the date of such termination (Code Sec. 691(c)(3)).[92]

References are to Standard Federal Tax Reports; Tax Research Consultant; and Practical Tax Explanations.

[88] ¶ 24,907; ESTTRST: 6,206.05; § 32,925.05

[89] ¶ 24,900, ¶ 24,901; ESTTRST: 6,056; § 32,910

[90] ¶ 24,900, ¶ 24,909; ESTTRST: 6,156; § 32,925.10

[91] ¶ 6060; FILEIND: 12,054; § 7,110.10

[92] ¶ 24,900; ESTTRST: 6,158; § 32,925.10

Chapter 2

CORPORATIONS

Corporate Formation

201. How Organizations Are Taxed. A corporation, like any business entity, is formed by one or more persons to conduct a business venture and divide profits among investors (Reg. §§ 301.7701-2, 301.7701-3).[1] A corporation files a charter or articles of incorporation in a state, in a U.S. possession, with a foreign government (¶ 2425), or (in certain cases) with the U.S. government. It prepares bylaws, has its business affairs overseen by a board of directors, and issues stock. Under the check-the-box regulations, entities formed under a corporation statute are automatically classified as corporations and may not elect to be treated as any other kind of entity; other entities are allowed to elect corporate status on Form 8832. Thus, an entity that is a partnership or limited liability company (¶ 402B) under the laws of the state in which it is formed may elect to be taxed as a C corporation or an S corporation under the Code. However, partnerships that are publicly traded are taxed as corporations unless 90 percent or more of the gross income consists of qualifying passive-type income (Code Sec. 7704; Reg. §§ 1.7704-1 and 1.7704-3).[2]

For tax purposes, the predominant forms of business enterprises are C corporations, S corporations (¶ 301), partnerships (¶ 401), and sole proprietorships. These different forms are treated differently under federal tax law and care should be taken in choosing the appropriate entity for the business. Although many of the Code's provisions apply to all of these entities, some areas of the law are specially tailored for each type. The classification of an entity will have a lingering tax impact throughout the entity's existence.

Of the types of business organization, income earned in a C corporation is generally subject to the toughest tax bite, as the earnings are taxed twice. First, a *corporate* income tax is imposed on the corporation's net earnings (¶ 219). Then, after the earnings are distributed to shareholders as dividends, each shareholder must pay taxes separately on its share of the dividends (¶ 733–¶ 740). A corporation can reduce, or even eliminate, its federal income tax liability by distributing its income as salary to shareholder-employees who actually perform valuable services for the corporation (¶ 713). Although this can reduce taxation at the corporate level, employees who receive payments from a corporation in exchange for services must still pay tax on the amount received, which is treated as salary.

This scheme of taxation differs radically from that applied to partnerships, limited liability companies, S corporations, and sole proprietorships. These entities do not pay

---

References are to Standard Federal Tax Reports; Tax Research Consultant; and Practical Tax Explanations.

[1] ¶ 43,082, ¶ 43,083; CCORP: 100, PART: 3,102; § 30,015.05, § 30,015.10

[2] ¶ 43,180, ¶ 43,180B, ¶ 43,181D; PART: 3,250

an entity-level tax on their earnings. There is no income tax on partnerships (¶ 404), or on limited liability companies (¶ 402B) treated as partnerships for federal tax purposes. Nor (in most cases) is there an S corporation income tax (¶ 319) or sole proprietorship income tax. Rather, the owners or members of these entities are taxed on their share of the entity's earnings.

203. Tax-Free Contributions in Exchange for Stock. A corporation is formed by the transfer of money or property from shareholders to the corporate entity in return for corporate stock. If one or more shareholders transfer money or property to a corporation solely in exchange for stock of that corporation, and if the shareholders control the corporation immediately after the exchange, neither the shareholders nor the corporation recognizes any gain or loss (Code Secs. 351(a) and 1032).[3] To be considered in "control," the transferring shareholders—as a group—must own, immediately after the exchange: (1) at least 80 percent of the total combined voting power of all classes of stock entitled to vote, and (2) at least 80 percent of the total number of shares of all other classes of stock (Code Sec. 368(c)).[4] The exchanges need not actually be simultaneous to avoid nonrecognition of gain (Reg. § 1.351-1(a)(1)).[5] Rather, all that is required is a situation where the rights of the parties have been previously defined and the execution of the agreement proceeds in an orderly manner.

Money or property transferred to a controlled corporation generally includes all property, tangible or intangible, with certain limitations (Code Sec. 351(d)).[6] Stock issued for services, indebtedness of the corporation that is not evidenced by a security, or interest on indebtedness of the corporation that accrued on or after the beginning of the transferor's holding period for the debt are not considered issued in return for property.

Shareholders can be individuals, estates, trusts, partnerships, or other corporations (Reg. § 1.351-1(a)(1)).[7] However, the rules permitting tax-free transfers to a corporation in exchange for corporate stock do not apply if the transferee corporation is an investment company (Code Sec. 351(e)(1)).[8]

If the transferor owners receive additional property along with the stock when they transfer property to the corporation, the transfer can still qualify as a contribution to a controlled corporation described in Code Sec. 351 (Code Sec. 351(b); Reg. § 1.351-2(a)).[9] The shareholders are taxed on any additional property received ("boot"). Thus, gain is recognized, but only to the extent of the cash received plus the fair market value of the additional property received. No loss is recognized on the transfer.

Assumption of Liabilities. If property transferred in what would otherwise be a Code Sec. 351 tax-free transaction is subject to liabilities, the acceptance of the transfer or the assumption of the liabilities does not prevent the transaction from being tax free (Code Sec. 357).[10] This rule does not apply if the principal purpose of the transfer is tax avoidance or if liabilities assumed by the transferee exceed the transferor's basis in the property.

Bankruptcy. A debtor must recognize gain or loss upon its transfer of assets to a controlled corporation pursuant to a plan approved by a bankruptcy court (other than a reorganization plan) in which the stock is exchanged (Code Sec. 351(e)(2)).[11] Essentially, the transaction is treated as if the property had first been transferred to the creditors and then transferred by them to the controlled corporation. If less than all the stock is transferred to creditors, only a proportionate share of the gain or loss must be recognized. Both the basis of the stock and of the assets are adjusted for the gain or loss recognized on the transfer to the corporation. Note that this rule does not apply to a transfer by one corporation to another corporation in a bankruptcy case. Instead, such a transfer is considered a Code Sec. 368(a)(1)(G) reorganization and its tax consequences are determined accordingly (¶ 2247).

References are to Standard Federal Tax Reports; Tax Research Consultant; and Practical Tax Explanations.

[3] ¶ 16,402, ¶ 29,622; CCORP: 3,050; § 26,101

[4] ¶ 16,750; CCORP: 3,054; § 26,105.05

[5] ¶ 16,403; CCORP: 3,054.05; § 26,105.05

[6] ¶ 16,402; CCORP: 3,052; § 26,110.05

[7] ¶ 16,403; CCORP: 3,050; § 26,101

[8] ¶ 16,402; CCORP: 3,062

[9] ¶ 16,402, ¶ 16,404B; CCORP: 3,102.10; § 26,120

[10] ¶ 16,520; CCORP: 3,106; § 26,125.05

[11] ¶ 16,402; CCORP: 3,114

Reporting Requirements. If a person receives stock of a corporation in exchange for property in a Code Sec. 351 transaction and that person is a significant transferor (that is, the person owns, immediately after the exchange, at least five percent of the corporation's outstanding stock if the stock owned is publicly traded, or at least one percent of the corporation's outstanding stock if the stock owned is not publicly traded), then the person and the corporation must each attach to their tax returns a complete statement of all the facts pertinent to the exchange, including (Reg. § 1.351-3):[12]

(1) the name and employer identification number (if any) of the transferee corporation (for the statement filed by the significant transferor), or the name and taxpayer identification number (if any) of every significant transferor (for the statement filed by the transferee corporation);

(2) the date(s) of the transfer(s) of assets;

(3) the aggregate fair market value and basis, determined immediately before the exchange, of the property transferred by the significant transferor, or received by the transferee corporation, as applicable, in the exchange; and

(4) the date and control number of any private letter ruling(s) issued by the IRS in connection with the Code Sec. 351 exchange.

However, the transferee corporation does not have to file a statement if a significant transferor's statement that includes the required information is attached to the same return for the same Code Sec. 351 exchange.

Return and Payment of Tax

211. Annual and Short-Period Corporate Returns. A corporation must file an income tax return, even if it has no income or if no tax is due (Code Sec. 6012(a)(2); Reg. § 1.6012-2).[13] Form 1120 must be filed on or before the 15th day of the third month that follows the close of its tax year (Code Sec. 6072(b); Reg. § 1.6072-2).[14] If the last day of a corporation's tax year does not end on the last day of a month (as in the case of a dissolved corporation whose tax year ends on the date of dissolution), the return is due on or before the 15th day of the third full month following the date of dissolution. If the due date for filing a return falls on a Saturday, Sunday, or legal holiday, the return must be filed by the first following business day (¶ 2549). Timely mailing generally is regarded as timely filing (¶ 2553).

A corporation's tax year generally may be a calendar year or a fiscal year (¶ 1501). Restrictions apply, however, to the choice of tax years by S corporations, personal service corporations, and REITs or REMICs. A corporation's return may not cover a period of more than a year. In a slight exception to this rule, a corporation may elect to use an annual filing period that fluctuates between 52 and 53 weeks (¶ 1505). A return may cover less than a year if a corporation was formed during the year or dissolved during the year. For example, if a corporation elects the calendar year method but starts operations on August 1, it must report income from August 1 to December 31. If a calendar-year corporation dissolves on June 30, it must file a short-period return covering the period from January 1 to June 30. In addition to filing its regular income tax return, a corporation that has adopted a resolution to dissolve itself or liquidate all or part of its stock must file Form 966 (Code Sec. 6043; Reg. § 1.6043-1).[15]

215. Due Date for Corporate Taxes. The due date for the payment of a corporation's taxes is generally the same as the due date for the filing of a return, without regard to filing extensions—the 15th day of the third month that follows the close of its tax year (Code Sec. 6151).[16] A corporation that anticipates a tax liability of $500 or more must estimate its taxes and make quarterly estimated tax payments (including estimated payments of the alternative minimum tax) using electronic fund transfers. If the liability

---

References are to Standard Federal Tax Reports; Tax Research Consultant; and Practical Tax Explanations.

[12] ¶ 16,404C; CCORP: 3,404; § 26,165

[13] ¶ 35,142, ¶ 35,145; FILEBUS: 3,052.05; § 39,025

[14] ¶ 36,720, ¶ 36,724; FILEBUS: 3,052.05; § 26,030.05

[15] ¶ 35,880, ¶ 35,881; FILEBUS: 9,352, CCORP: 27,054; § 38,145.10

[16] ¶ 37,080; FILEBUS: 6,102.05; § 39,305.05

exceeds the total estimated payments, the corporation must pay the remaining amount by the due date of its return. Failure to pay estimated taxes may be penalized (¶ 241). Corporations may file for an extension of time to file returns or to pay taxes (¶ 2509 and ¶ 2537).

Computation of Tax Liability

219. Corporate Tax Rates. Corporations are subject to the following tax rates on their taxable income (Code Secs. 11 and 1201):[17]

If taxable income is:				Of the amt. over—
Over—	But not over—	Tax is—		
$0	$50,000		15%	$0
50,000	75,000	$7,500	+ 25%	50,000
75,000	100,000	13,750	+ 34%	75,000
100,000	335,000	22,250	+ 39%	100,000
335,000	10,000,000	113,900	+ 34%	335,000
10,000,000	15,000,000	3,400,000	+ 35%	10,000,000
15,000,000	18,333,333	5,150,000	+ 38%	15,000,000
18,333,333	—		35%	0

Qualified Personal Service Corporations. The corporate graduated rates do not apply to qualified personal service corporations. Such corporations are instead taxed at a flat rate of 35 percent of taxable income (¶ 273). Qualified personal service corporations perform services in the fields of health, law, engineering, architecture, accounting (including the preparation of tax returns), actuarial science, the performing arts, or consulting. Substantially all of the stock of a personal service corporation is held by employees, retired employees, or their estates (Code Secs. 11(b)(2) and 448(d)(2)).[18]

Foreign Corporations. Foreign corporations are taxed at regular U.S. corporate rates on most income that is effectively connected with a U.S. trade or business (¶ 2429) and are subject to a flat 30-percent withholding tax on U.S.-source fixed or determinable income that is not effectively connected (¶ 2431). Tax treaties between the U.S. and foreign countries may provide for lower rates or exemptions from taxation.

Additional Taxes. In addition to the regular corporate income tax, the alternative minimum tax (AMT) may be imposed on a corporation having tax preference items (¶ 1401). A corporation is exempt from the AMT if it is the corporation's first year or it is a small corporation with average annual gross receipts for the three-tax-year period (or portion thereof) ending before the current tax year not in excess of $7.5 million (¶ 1415). The $7.5-million amount is reduced to $5 million for the corporation's first three-tax-year period. Certain corporations used by their shareholders for the purpose of avoiding taxes might also be subject to the accumulated earnings tax (¶ 251–¶ 269) or the personal holding company tax (¶ 275–¶ 287).

221. Corporate Taxable Income. The corporate tax rates (¶ 219) are applied to a corporation's "taxable income" (Code Sec. 11).[19] Taxable income is the corporation's gross income for the year minus allowable deductions. The principal items of corporation income include gross sales receipts, dividends and interest received, rent and royalty income, and capital gains. The common deductions for a corporation in computing its taxable income include compensation paid to officers and workers, expenses for repairs and maintenance of property, taxes, licenses, interest paid, depreciation and depletion, advertising, and deductible amounts paid to pension and profit-sharing plans and employee benefit programs. In addition, a corporation may be entitled to special deductions for dividends received from other corporations (¶ 223), affiliates (¶ 229), and foreign corporations (¶ 231), as well as deductions for organizational expenses (¶ 237) and domestic production activities (¶ 980A).

References are to Standard Federal Tax Reports; Tax Research Consultant; and Practical Tax Explanations.

[17] ¶ 3365, ¶ 30,352; CCORP: 100, SALES: 15,210; § 16,527.10, § 26,010

[18] ¶ 3365, ¶ 20,800; CCORP: 100; § 27,110

[19] ¶ 3365; CCORP: 100; § 26,001

A corporation generally must use the accrual method of accounting to determine when income and expenses are reported (¶ 1515). The cash basis of accounting may be used, however, by a qualified personal service corporation (¶ 219), a corporation engaged in a farming business (¶ 1519), or a corporation whose average annual gross receipts do not exceed $5 million for the three tax years preceding the current tax year (Code Sec. 448).[20] Securities dealers must use the mark-to-market method of accounting (¶ 1903).

223. Dividends Received from Other Corporations. A corporation is entitled to a special deduction from gross income for dividends received from a domestic corporation that is subject to income tax (Code Sec. 243).[21] The deduction is: (1) 70 percent of dividends received from corporations owned less than 20 percent (by stock vote and value) by the recipient corporation; (2) 80 percent of dividends received from a 20-percent-owned corporation—a corporation having at least 20 percent (but generally less than 80 percent) of its stock owned by the recipient corporation; (3) 100 percent of qualifying dividends received from members of the same affiliated group (generally, 80-percent-or-more common ownership) to which the recipient corporation belongs; and (4) 100 percent of dividends received by a small business investment company (¶ 2392). These rules also apply to dividends received from a foreign corporation that are paid out of the earnings and profits of a taxable domestic predecessor corporation.

The aggregate amount of dividends-received deductions that may be taken by a corporation is limited to 70 percent (80 percent in the case of 20-percent-owned corporations) of its taxable income, computed without regard to any net operating loss deduction, the domestic production activities deduction, dividends-received deduction, dividends-paid deduction in the case of public utilities, the deduction for the U.S.-source portion of dividends from 10-percent-owned foreign corporations, the deduction for certain dividends received from wholly owned foreign subsidiaries, capital loss carryback, or adjustment for nontaxed portions of extraordinary dividends received. This limitation is applied first with respect to any 80-percent-deductible dividends and then separately for 70-percent-deductible dividends (after reducing taxable income by the 80-percent-deductible dividends), but it does not apply for the year if the full deduction results in a net operating loss (Code Sec. 246(b)).[22] Further, it does not apply in the case of dividends received by a small business investment company.

The dividends-received deduction is not allowed in computing the accumulated earnings tax (¶ 251) or the tax on personal holding companies (¶ 275). The deduction is allowed to a resident foreign corporation, as well as to a domestic corporation. No deduction is allowed for dividends received from a corporation exempt from income tax (including an exempt farmers' cooperative) during the tax year or the preceding year (Code Sec. 246(a)).[23]

Holding Period. The dividends-received deduction is only allowed if the underlying stock is held for at least 46 days during the 91-day period beginning on the date 45 days before the ex-dividend date of the stock (Code Sec. 246(c)).[24] If the stock is cumulative preferred stock with an arrearage of dividends, it must be held at least 91 days during the 181-day period beginning on the date 90 days before the ex-dividend date. The ex-dividend date is the first day the stock trades without a buyer having a right to an announced dividend and, to account for the delay needed to accommodate settlement, is normally two business days before the record date (the day when the company determines who is the record owner of the stock). A person who buys stock on the trading day before the ex-dividend date will receive a dividend, while a person who buys the stock on the ex-dividend date will not.

References are to Standard Federal Tax Reports; Tax Research Consultant; and Practical Tax Explanations.

[20] ¶ 20,800; ACCTNG: 6,050; § 38,215.05

[21] ¶ 13,051; CCORP: 9,050; § 26,501

[22] ¶ 13,200; CCORP: 9,212; § 26,510.15

[23] ¶ 13,200; CCORP: 9,062; § 26,510.10

[24] ¶ 13,200; CCORP: 9,204; § 26,510.20

¶223

The holding period is reduced for any period during which the taxpayer's risk of loss with respect to the stock is diminished because the taxpayer has (1) an option to sell, is under an obligation to sell, or has made (and not closed) a short sale of substantially identical stock or securities; (2) granted an option to purchase substantially identical stock or securities; or (3) reduced the risk by virtue of holding one or more other positions with respect to substantially similar or related property.

Debt-Financed Portfolio Stock. The dividends-received deduction is reduced for dividends received from debt-financed portfolio stock by a percentage related to the amount of debt incurred to purchase such stock. The deduction is calculated by multiplying the difference between 100 percent and the average portfolio indebtedness by 70 percent (80 percent in the case of 20-percent-owned corporations) (Code Sec. 246A).[25] However, any required reduction is limited to the amount of the interest deduction allocable to the related dividend. In addition, the reduction does not apply to dividends that are eligible for 100-percent dividends-received deduction for (1) qualifying dividends received from a member of an affiliated group and (2) dividends received from a small business investment company.

Other Limitations. Capital gain dividends from a regulated investment company (mutual fund) or a real estate investment trust, and distributions that are a return of capital, do not qualify for the dividends-received deduction (Code Sec. 243(d)).[26] Additionally, the deduction is not allowed to the extent that the taxpayer is under an obligation (pursuant to a short sale or otherwise) to make related payments with respect to positions in substantially similar or related property (Code Sec. 246(c)(1)(B)).[27]

The deduction for dividends received on certain preferred stock of a public utility is reduced to the extent the public utility was allowed a dividends-paid deduction (Code Secs. 244 and 247).[28]

227. Debt-Equity Rule. For instruments issued by corporations and advances made to corporations, a question can arise as to whether such instruments and advances are treated as bona fide debt of the corporation or as an equity interest in the corporation. If they are treated as a bona fide debt of the corporation, it can deduct interest payments as a business expense, and the shareholders can receive principal payments as a tax-free return of capital. However, if they are treated as stock, the corporation cannot deduct payments made with respect to such instruments.

The Code lists five factors that may be considered in making the debt-equity determination (Code Sec. 385):[29]

> (1) whether there is a written, unconditional promise to pay on demand or on a specified date a sum certain in money in return for an adequate consideration in money or money's worth, and to pay a fixed rate of interest;

> (2) whether there is subordination to or preference over any indebtedness of the corporation;

> (3) the ratio of debt to equity of the corporation;

> (4) whether there is convertibility into the stock of the corporation; and

> (5) the relationship between holdings of stock in the corporation and holdings of the interest in question.

The courts have developed other guidelines to be used in making a debt-equity determination.[30]

229. 100-Percent Dividends-Received Deduction for Affiliates. Affiliated corporations are allowed a 100-percent dividends-received deduction for qualifying dividends received from members of the affiliated group (Code Sec. 243).[31] A qualifying dividend is any dividend received by a corporation that is a member of the same affiliated group as the corporation distributing it.

References are to Standard Federal Tax Reports; Tax Research Consultant; and Practical Tax Explanations.

[25] ¶ 13,250; CCORP: 9,208

[26] ¶ 13,051; CCORP: 9,062; § 26,510.10

[27] ¶ 13,200; CCORP: 9,206

[28] ¶ 13,100, ¶ 13,300; CCORP: 9,210, CCORP: 9,250

[29] ¶ 17,340; CCORP: 3,302

[30] ¶ 15,704.264; CCORP: 3,304

[31] ¶ 13,051; CCORP: 9,100; § 26,505

2 | CORPORATIONS

If the affiliated group includes at least one life insurance company, no dividend by any member of the group will be treated as qualified unless a special election is in effect for the tax year in which the dividend is received. If any member of an affiliated group elects the foreign tax credit, then all members of the group that pay or accrue foreign taxes must elect the credit in order for any dividend paid by a member of the group to qualify for the 100-percent dividends-received deduction.

231. Dividends from Foreign Corporations. A domestic corporation is entitled to a 70-percent (80-percent in the case of 20-percent-owned corporations (¶ 223)) deduction of the U.S.-source portion of dividends received from a foreign corporation that is at least 10 percent owned, by vote and value, by the domestic corporation (Code Sec. 245(a)).[32] The U.S.-source portion of a dividend is the amount that bears the same ratio to the dividend as undistributed U.S. earnings bear to total undistributed earnings.

A 100-percent dividends-received deduction is allowed to a domestic corporation for dividends paid by a wholly owned foreign subsidiary out of its earnings and profits for the tax year (Code Sec. 245(b)).[33] All of the foreign subsidiary's gross income must be effectively connected with a U.S. trade or business.

Debt-Financed Portfolio Stock. Any reduction in the dividends-received deduction resulting from the rules concerning debt-financed portfolio stock (¶ 223) must be computed before applying the above ratios.

237. Organizational Expenditures. A corporation may elect to deduct up to $5,000 of any organizational expenses it incurs in the tax year in which it begins business (Code Sec. 248; Reg. § 1.248-1).[34] A taxpayer is deemed to have made an election to deduct and amortize organizational expenses in the tax year in which the active trade or business to which the expenditures relate begins. A taxpayer may choose to forego the deemed election by clearly electing to capitalize its organizational expenditures on a timely filed federal income tax return, including extensions, for the tax year in which the active trade or business to which the expenditures relate begins. The $5,000 deducted for organizational expenses must be reduced by the amount by which the expenses exceed $50,000. Any remaining balance of organizational expenditures that are not immediately deductible must be amortized over a 180-month period.

Organizational expenditures are those that are (1) connected directly with the creation of the corporation, (2) chargeable to capital account, and (3) of a character that would be amortizable over the life of the corporation if its life were limited by its charter. They include expenses of temporary directors and organizational meetings, state fees for incorporation privileges, accounting service costs incident to organization, and legal service expenditures, such as for drafting of documents, minutes of organizational meetings, and terms of the original stock certificates.

Expenditures connected with issuing or selling stock or with the transfer of assets to a corporation are not amortizable. Instead, such costs must be netted against the proceeds of the stock sale. Pre-opening or start-up expenses, such as employee training, advertising, and expenses of lining up suppliers or potential customers, are not organizational expenses, but may be amortizable as start-up expenditures (¶ 904). Likewise, corporate expenditures that are incurred in investigating the creation or acquisition of an active trade or business or in creating such a trade or business do not qualify for amortization as organizational expenses, but may qualify as start-up expenses (Rev. Rul. 99-23).[35]

References are to Standard Federal Tax Reports; Tax Research Consultant; and Practical Tax Explanations.

[32] ¶ 13,150; CCORP: 9,152; § 26,510.10

[33] ¶ 13,150; CCORP: 9,154; § 26,510.10

[34] ¶ 13,350, ¶ 13,351; BUSEXP: 9,452.05; § 9,210.05

[35] ¶ 12,371.25; DEPR: 21,404.10; § 9,205.10

239. Domestic Production Activities. A corporation may claim a deduction against gross income equal to the applicable percentage of its qualified production activities income (QPAI) or its taxable income (whichever is less) (i.e., manufacturer's deduction (¶ 980A)). The amount of the deduction for any tax year, however, may not exceed 50 percent of the W-2 wages the taxpayer deducts in calculating its QPAI.

Estimated Tax

241. Penalty for Underpayment of Corporate Estimated Tax. A corporation that anticipates a tax bill of $500 or more must estimate its income tax liability for the current tax year and pay four quarterly estimated tax installments (using electronic funds transfers) during that year (Code Sec. 6655).[36] Any underpayment of a required install-ment results in an addition to tax on the amount of the underpayment for the period of underpayment. The addition to tax is based on current interest rates (¶ 2838).

The period of underpayment begins with the due date of the underpaid installment and ends with the earlier of (1) the date that the underpayment is satisfied or (2) the 15th day of the third month after the close of the tax year. Each estimated tax payment is credited against unpaid installments in the order in which they are required to be paid.

No addition to tax applies if the tax shown on the return (or the actual tax if no return is filed) is less than $500. If there is an underpayment, the taxpayer may use Form 2220 to determine whether the addition to tax applies and, if so, the amount of the penalty. However, a corporation is not required to file the form, as the IRS will determine any penalty owed and notify the corporation of the amount due (Instructions to Form 2220).

What is the Tax? The tax liabilities to which corporate estimated tax applies are: (1) the corporate income tax (¶ 219), the alternative tax on corporate capital gains (¶ 1738), or the income tax imposed on insurance companies (¶ 2370), whichever applies; (2) the alternative minimum tax (¶ 1401); and (3) the tax on gross transportation income of foreign corporations (Code Sec. 887).[37] For this purpose, the 30-percent tax on fixed, determinable, annual or periodic income of a foreign corporation not effectively con-nected with a U.S. business is considered a corporate income tax (¶ 2431). The total expected tax liability is reduced by the sum of the credits against tax. Special rules apply for estimating the book income adjustment by corporations that use the annualization method to calculate estimated tax liability (¶ 245).

243. Time and Amount of Corporate Estimated Tax Payments. For calendar-year corporations, estimated tax installments are due on April 15, June 15, September 15, and December 15. Installments of fiscal-year corporations are due on the 15th day of the fourth, sixth, ninth, and twelfth months of the tax year (Code Sec. 6655).[38] If any due date falls on a Saturday, Sunday, or legal holiday, the payment is due on the first following business day. Corporations required to deposit taxes must transfer their tax deposits electronically from their accounts to the IRS's general account (Reg. § 31.6302-1(h)).[39]

To avoid a penalty for underpayment of estimated taxes (¶ 241), each installment must equal at least 25 percent of the lesser of:

(1) 100 percent of the tax shown on the current year's tax return (or of the actual tax if no return is filed), or

(2) 100 percent of the tax shown on the corporation's return for the preced-ing tax year, provided a positive tax liability was shown and the preceding tax year consisted of 12 months (Code Sec. 6655(d))[40] (but see special limitation on *"Large Corporations,"* below).

References are to Standard Federal Tax Reports; Tax Research Consultant; and Practical Tax Explanations.

[36] ¶ 39,565; FILEBUS: 6,050, FILEBUS: 6,056, FILEBUS: 6,058; § 26,015.05, § 26,015.10

[37] ¶ 27,580; INTL: 3,602

[38] ¶ 39,565; FILEBUS: 6,054.05; § 26,015.10

[39] ¶ 38,055B; FILEBUS: 6,106.10; § 39,320.20

[40] ¶ 39,565; FILEBUS: 6,052.05; § 26,015.05, § 26,015.15

A lower installment amount may be paid if it is shown that use of an annualized income method or, for corporations with seasonal incomes, an adjusted seasonal method would result in a lower required installment (¶ 245).

Example: The X Corporation, a calendar-year taxpayer, estimates at the end of March that its federal income tax for the current tax year would be $800,000. Accordingly, it pays $200,000 [25% of ($800,000 × 100%)] of estimated tax by April 15, and another $200,000 by June 15. At the end of August, a recalculation shows that its tax for the year is expected to be $1 million. Assuming that there is no later change in the estimated tax, the estimated tax installments for September and December are computed as follows:

Estimated tax required to be paid by 9/15 [75% of ($1 million × 100%)]	$750,000
Less payments made in April and June	$400,000
Payment due in September	$350,000
Payment due in December [25% of ($1 million × 100%)]	$250,000
Total estimated tax payments	$1,000,000

Large Corporations. A "large corporation"—one with taxable income of at least $1 million in any one of the three immediately preceding tax years—is prohibited from using its prior year's tax liability (method (2), above), *except* in determining the first installment of its tax year (Code Sec. 6655(d)(2) and (g)(2)).[41] Any reduction in a large corporation's first installment as a result of using the prior year's tax must be recaptured in the corporation's second installment. In applying the $1-million test, taxable income is computed without regard to net operating loss carryovers or capital loss carrybacks. Also, a controlled group of corporations (¶ 291) must divide a single $1-million amount among its members.

Corporations with $1 Billion in Assets. Corporations with $1 billion or more in assets are required to make larger and smaller estimated tax payments in certain months in 2017 (Act Sec. 4 of Amendment to Africa Growth and Opportunity Act (P.L. 112-163)). Specifically, for a payment due in July, August, or September of 2017, the amount due is 100.25 percent of the estimated tax the taxpayer would otherwise be required to pay. For a payment in October, November, or December of 2017, the amount due is 99.75 percent of the amount that would otherwise be due.

245. Annualization and Seasonal Income Methods. A corporation may make a lower required installment payment of estimated taxes (¶ 243) where its annualized income installment or adjusted seasonal installment is less than the regular amount of the required installment. The annualized income installment is the product of the tax on the corporation's taxable income (including alternative minimum taxable income and modified alternative minimum taxable income) for the corresponding portion of the tax year on an annualized basis, and reduced by all prior required installments for the tax year (Code Sec. 6655(e); Reg. § 1.6655-2).[42] A corporation can choose between using the standard monthly periods or either of two optional monthly periods. An election to use either of the two optional monthly periods is effective only for the year of election. The election must be made on or before the date required for the first installment payment.

Installment	Standard Monthly Periods	Optional Monthly Periods #1	Optional Monthly Periods #2
1st	first 3 months	first 2 months	first 3 months
2nd	first 3 months	first 4 months	first 5 months
3rd	first 6 months	first 7 months	first 8 months
4th	first 9 months	first 10 months	first 11 months

To annualize income, multiply the income for the applicable period by 12 and divide by the number of months in the period. A corporation that uses the annualization

---

References are to Standard Federal Tax Reports; Tax Research Consultant; and Practical Tax Explanations.

[41] ¶ 39,565; FILEBUS: 6,052.05; § 26,015.05

[42] ¶ 39,565, ¶ 39,568; FILEBUS: 6,052.10; § 26,015.10

method and switches to another method during the same tax year must, in its first installment under the new method, recapture 100 percent of any reduction achieved in the earlier installments.

Adjusted Seasonal Installments. Adjusted seasonal installments may be used only if the average of the corporation's taxable income for the same six-month period in the three preceding years was 70 percent or more of annual taxable income. An adjusted seasonal installment is the excess (if any) of (a) 100 percent of the amount determined by following the four steps set forth below, over (b) the aggregate amount of all prior required installments for the tax year. The steps are as follows:

(1) take the taxable income for the portion of the tax year up to the month in which the installment is due (filing month);

(2) divide this amount by the "base period percentage" for such months;

(3) determine the tax on the result; and

(4) multiply the tax by the base period percentage for the filing month and all preceding months during the tax year.

For any period of months, the "base period percentage" is the average percentage that the taxable income for the corresponding months in each of the three preceding tax years bears to the taxable income for those years (Code Sec. 6655(e)(3); Reg. § 1.6655-3).[43]

247. Quick Refund for Estimated Tax Overpayment. A corporation may apply for a refund of an overpayment of estimated tax immediately after the close of its tax year if its overpayment is at least 10 percent of the expected tax liability and amounts to at least $500. Overpayment, for this purpose, is the excess of the estimated tax paid over what the corporation expects its final income tax liability to be at the time the application is filed. The application must be filed by the 15th day of the 3rd month after the close of the tax year and before the day on which the corporation files its income tax return for the tax year for which a quick refund is requested (Code Sec. 6425; Reg. §§ 1.6425-1— 1.6425-3).[44] The taxpayer should file Form 4466. An extension of time to file Form 1120 will not extend the time for filing Form 4466.

Accumulated Earnings Tax

251. Accumulated Earnings Tax. In addition to being liable for regular income taxes, every corporation (other than personal holding companies (¶ 277), tax-exempt organizations (¶ 601), or passive foreign investment companies (¶ 2490)) may be liable for the accumulated earnings tax. The tax is in the form of a penalty and applies if a corporation is formed or used for the purpose of avoiding the imposition of income tax upon its shareholders by permitting its earnings or profits to accumulate instead of being distributed (Code Secs. 531 and 532).[45] A corporation is presumed to be availed of for a tax avoidance purpose if its earnings are accumulated beyond the reasonable needs of its business (¶ 265). The tax may be imposed on a corporation without regard to the number of shareholders, so it applies to both closely held and publicly held corporations.

For tax years beginning after December 31, 2012, the accumulated earnings tax is 20 percent of the corporation's accumulated taxable income (¶ 253) (Code Sec. 531).[46] For tax years beginning before January 1, 2013, the rate is 15 percent. There is no particular form that a corporation files to compute the tax. Instead, the IRS enforces the tax by reaching a conclusion whether enough dividends were paid during the tax year based on the corporation's filed income tax return. Interest on any underpayment is computed from the date the corporation's tax return is due without regard to extensions (Code Sec. 6601(b)(4)).[47]

References are to Standard Federal Tax Reports; Tax Research Consultant; and Practical Tax Explanations.

[43] ¶ 39,565, ¶ 39,570; FILEBUS: 6,052.10; § 26,015.10

[44] ¶ 38,840—¶ 38,843; IRS: 33,358; § 26,015.20

[45] ¶ 23,001, ¶ 23,010; CCORP: 18,250; § 26,901

[46] ¶ 23,001; CCORP: 18,250; § 26,901

[47] ¶ 39,410; PENALTY: 9,054.05; § 40,105.15

2 CORPORATIONS

253. Accumulated Taxable Income. The accumulated earnings tax (¶ 251) is imposed on a corporation's accumulated taxable income for the tax year. Accumulated taxable income is the corporation's taxable income with certain adjustments, and minus the sum of the dividends-paid deduction (¶ 259) and the accumulated earnings credit (¶ 261). The adjustments to taxable income include the following (Code Sec. 535; Reg. § 1.535-2):[48]

(1) A deduction is allowed for federal income taxes, as well as for income, war, and excess profits taxes of foreign countries and U.S. possessions (to the extent not allowed as deductions in computing taxable income) accrued during the tax year, regardless of the accounting method used. The deduction will not include any accumulated earnings tax or personal holding company tax paid.

(2) Charitable contributions for the tax year are deductible without regard to the 10-percent-of-taxable-income limitation (¶ 927).

(3) No deduction is allowed for dividends received or for dividends paid by public utilities on certain preferred stock.

(4) The net operating loss deduction is not allowed.

(5) A corporation (other than a mere holding company or investment company) is allowed a deduction for net capital losses incurred for the tax year determined without regard to capital loss carryovers. However, the deduction is reduced by the lesser of the (1) capital gains deducted in earlier years that have not already been used in a previous year to reduce the capital loss reduction, or (2) the corporation's accumulated earnings and profits at the close of the preceding year.

(6) A deduction is allowed for net capital gains for the year taking into account capital loss carryovers, reduced by the taxes attributable to them. In the case of a foreign corporation, only net capital gains that are effectively connected with the conduct of a trade or business within the United States and that are not exempt under treaty are taken into account.

(7) No capital loss carryback or carryover is allowed.

(8) A controlled foreign corporation (CFC) is allowed to deduct the amount of its subpart F income that is required to be included in the income of its U.S. shareholders (¶ 2488). However, if the corporation would otherwise calculate its accumulated taxable income on a gross basis, then the corporation's deduction must be reduced by any deduction that may have reduced a U.S. shareholder's income inclusion.

Although exempt interest income is excludable from accumulated taxable income for purposes of determining the accumulated earnings tax base, it is considered for purposes of determining whether earnings and profits have been accumulated beyond the reasonable needs of the business (¶ 265) (Rev. Rul. 70-497).[49]

Holding or Investment Companies. If a corporation is a mere holding or investment company, then in determining its accumulated taxable income: (1) net capital losses may not be deducted, (2) net short-term capital gains are deductible only to the extent of any capital loss carryovers, and (3) accumulated earnings and profits cannot be less than they would have been had the rules in (1) and (2) been applied in computing earnings and profits (Code Sec. 535(b)(8)).[50]

Foreign Corporations. A foreign corporation is subject to U.S. income tax on U.S. source income, including the accumulated earnings tax (¶ 2425). Thus, foreign source income is generally excluded from accumulated taxable income. However, if 10 percent or more of the earnings and profits of any foreign corporation is derived from U.S. sources, then any distribution out of such earnings and profits (and any interest payment) retains its character as U.S.-source income upon receipt by a U.S.-owned

References are to Standard Federal Tax Reports; Tax Research Consultant; and Practical Tax Explanations.

[48] ¶ 23,040, ¶ 23,042; CCORP: 18,252; § 26,905.10   [49] ¶ 23,018.897; CCORP: 18,150; § 26,910.10   [50] ¶ 23,040; CCORP: 18,104

foreign corporation (Code Sec. 535(d)).[51] A U.S.-owned foreign corporation is any foreign corporation in which 50 percent or more of voting power or total value is held directly or indirectly by U.S. persons.

259. Dividends-Paid Deduction. Dividends paid by regulated investment companies (mutual funds), real estate investment trusts (REITs), personal holding companies, and corporations subject to the accumulated earnings tax are deductible in determining accumulated taxable income (¶ 253) (Code Sec. 561).[52] The deduction is the sum of dividends paid during the tax year, consent dividends, and, in the case of a personal holding company, dividends carried over from the two preceding tax years (¶ 275). The deduction is unaffected by the taxpayer's accounting method, but rather is based upon the amount of dividends actually paid by the corporation and received by the shareholder. A corporation subject to the accumulated earnings tax is required, and a personal holding company may elect, to deduct dividends paid within 2½ months of the end of the tax year (Code Sec. 563).[53]

The dividends-paid deduction may be claimed for any payment that is a distribution of property to shareholders with respect to their stock and paid out of earnings and profits (¶ 747) (Code Sec. 562).[54] For a personal holding company, however, the deduction is up to the amount of undistributed personal holding company income, regardless of its earnings and profits (Code Sec. 316(b)(2)(A)). No deduction is allowed for preferential dividends. On the other hand, distributions in complete liquidation of a corporation other than a personal holding company are included as part of the deduction. Distributions in complete liquidation of a personal holding company can be included depending on whether the distributee is a noncorporate or corporate shareholder. For a regulated investment company, the deduction is computed without regard to capital gain dividends and exempt-interest dividends (¶ 2303). For a REIT, the deduction is computed without regard to excluded net income from foreclosure property (¶ 2329).

Consent Dividend. A consent dividend is any dividend that a shareholder agrees to include in taxable income, even though the corporation does not make an actual distribution (Code Sec. 565).[55] The consent dividend is treated as paid by the corporation on the last day of its tax year and immediately contributed as paid-in capital by the shareholder. A consent dividend may be paid only with respect to consent stock, which is either common stock or preferred stock with unlimited participation; thus, the consent dividend must not be a preferential dividend. Shareholders consent on Form 972 that the corporation includes with Form 973 when filing its return to claim the dividends-paid deduction for consent dividends.

261. Accumulated Earnings Credit. For a corporation other than a holding or investment company, the accumulated earnings credit allowed in computing accumulated taxable income (¶ 253) is an amount equal to the part of the earnings and profits of the tax year retained for the reasonable needs of the business, reduced by the net capital gain (which is itself reduced by the amount of income tax attributable to it). A minimum amount of $250,000 ($150,000 for personal service corporations (¶ 219)) may be accumulated from past and present earnings combined by all corporations, including holding or investment companies. This minimum amount is the only credit allowable to a holding or investment company (Code Sec. 535(c)).[56] Only one $250,000 accumulated earnings credit is allowed to a controlled group of corporations (¶ 291) (Code Sec. 1561(a)(2)).[57] The single credit is to be divided equally among the corporations.

263. Basis of Liability for Accumulated Earnings Tax. Although the accumulated earnings tax is computed as a percentage of the corporation's accumulated taxable income (¶ 253), liability for the tax hinges on whether the corporation was formed or

---

References are to Standard Federal Tax Reports; Tax Research Consultant; and Practical Tax Explanations.

[51] ¶ 23,040; CCORP: 18,052

[52] ¶ 23,450; CCORP: 9,300; § 26,905.15

[53] ¶ 23,490; CCORP: 9,308; § 26,905.15

[54] ¶ 23,470; CCORP: 9,304; § 26,905.15

[55] ¶ 23,530; CCORP: 9,316; § 26,905.15

[56] ¶ 23,040; CCORP: 18,254; § 26,905.20

[57] ¶ 33,340; CCORP: 18,254, CCORP: 42,054

availed of to avoid the income tax on income otherwise receivable by its shareholders. A corporation can be subject to the accumulated earnings tax for a year in which it has accumulated taxable income on hand even though, because of a stock redemption, no earnings and profits were accumulated for the tax year (*GPD, Inc.*, CA-6, 75-1 USTC ¶ 9142).[58]

The courts have shifted the focus of attention from earnings and profits to liquidity.[59] The reason for this change in emphasis is that the earnings-and-profits figure often is no indication of the funds available to the corporation to meet its business needs and pay dividends to its shareholders. Whether a corporation can be subjected to the accumulated earnings tax is therefore determined by comparing the reasonable needs of its business (¶ 265) to its total liquid assets at the end of the year. Liquid assets include the corporation's cash and marketable securities.

265. Reasonable Needs of the Business. In order to justify an accumulation of income, there must be a reasonable business need for it and a definite plan for its use. Since a corporation is given a credit (¶ 261) for its reasonable business needs (including reasonably anticipated needs) in figuring the accumulated earnings tax, the resolution of most disputes hinges on this issue.

The Code does not contain a comprehensive definition of reasonable business needs. However, a number of acceptable and unacceptable grounds for accumulating income are listed in the regulations (Code Sec. 537(b); Reg. § 1.537-2).[60] Acceptable grounds include: (1) business expansion and plant replacement; (2) acquisition of a business through purchase of stock or assets; (3) debt retirement; (4) working capital; and (5) investments or loans to suppliers or customers necessary to the maintenance of the corporation's business. The self-insurance of product liability risks is also a business need for which earnings and profits may be accumulated to a reasonable extent.

Unacceptable grounds include: (1) loans to shareholders and expenditures for their personal benefit; (2) loans to relatives or friends of shareholders or to others who have no reasonable connection with the business; (3) loans to a commonly controlled corporation; (4) investments that are not related to the business; and (5) accumulations to provide against unrealistic hazards.

Courts have used an operating-cycle approach to determine the amount of working capital a corporation needs. An operating cycle consists of (1) an inventory cycle (conversion of cash and raw materials into inventory), (2) a receivables cycle (conversion of inventory into accounts receivable and cash), and, possibly, (3) a credit cycle (accounts payable turnover).[61]

A stock redemption under Code Sec. 303 to pay death taxes and expenses (¶ 745) and a redemption of stock in order to bring a private foundation within the 20-percent excess business holdings limit (¶ 640) are good cause for an accumulation of income (Code Sec. 537(a)).[62] Although other types of stock redemptions are not accorded this certainty, accumulations to redeem a minority interest (or the interest of one of two 50-percent stockholders) have been approved where they would eliminate dissent, would prevent the minority interest from falling into hostile hands, or were an essential ingredient of an employee incentive plan. Court decisions in this area show that except in rare circumstances, the redemption of a majority interest is not good cause for accumulating income.[63]

267. Burden of Proof of Reasonable Business Needs. On the issue of whether a corporation has accumulated income in excess of the reasonable needs of its business (¶ 265), the burden of proof in the Tax Court is on the government in two instances (Code Sec. 534; Reg. § 1.534-2).[64] First, the burden is on the government if, in advance of

References are to Standard Federal Tax Reports; Tax Research Consultant; and Practical Tax Explanations.

[58] ¶ 23,045.37; CCORP: 18,100
[59] ¶ 23,045.65, ¶ 23,074.36; CCORP: 18,170; § 26,910.10
[60] ¶ 23,070, ¶ 23,072; CCORP: 18,154; § 26,910.10
[61] ¶ 23,074.625; CCORP: 18,158
[62] ¶ 23,070; CCORP: 18,168; § 26,910.10
[63] ¶ 23,018.895; CCORP: 18,168.15
[64] ¶ 23,020, ¶ 23,022; CCORP: 18,200

a formal deficiency notice, it does not notify the corporation by certified or registered mail of its intention to assess a deficiency based in whole or in part on the accumulated earnings tax or fails to state the tax years at issue. Second, in the event of such notification, the burden falls on the government if the corporation responds within 60 days with a statement of the grounds on which it relies to establish the reasonableness of all or any part of its accumulation of income. In other courts, the burden of proof is wholly on the corporation.

269. Tax Avoidance Intent for Accumulated Earnings Tax. One of the conditions that must exist before a corporation can be subject to the accumulated earnings tax is an intent to avoid the income tax on its shareholders (Code Sec. 533).[65] If the corporation accumulates income beyond the reasonable needs of its business (or if it is a mere holding or investment company), a presumption of tax avoidance intent arises. This presumption can be overcome by showing that tax avoidance was not one of the purposes of the accumulation of income (*Donruss Co.*, 69-1 USTC ¶ 9167; *Shaw-Walker*, 69-1 USTC ¶ 9198).[66]

Personal Service Corporations

273. Personal Service Corporations. A personal service corporation (PSC) is one that furnishes personal services performed by employee-owners (Code Secs. 269A and 280H; Proposed Reg. § 1.269A-1(a)).[67] An "employee-owner" is an employee who owns, directly or indirectly, more than 10 percent of the outstanding stock of the corporation on any day during the corporation's tax year. If (1) substantially all of the services of a PSC are performed for, or on behalf of, one other corporation, partnership, or other entity, and (2) the principal purpose for forming or using the PSC is the avoidance or evasion of income tax by reducing the income of any employee-owner or securing the benefit of any expense, deduction, credit, exclusion or other allowance for any employee-owner that would not otherwise be available, then the IRS may allocate income, deductions, credits, exclusions, or other allowances between the PSC and its employee-owners in order to prevent tax evasion or avoidance or to clearly reflect the income of both. The purpose of evading or avoiding income tax can be shown by a reduction in the tax liability of, or the increase of tax benefits to, an employee-owner or by any other increase in tax benefits. Code Sec. 280H restricts the amount that can be deducted by a PSC for amounts paid to owners if the corporation has elected a noncalendar tax year.

Personal Holding Companies

275. Tax on Personal Holding Companies. In addition to being liable for regular income taxes, a corporation that is a personal holding company (¶ 277) will be liable for a separate tax on its "undistributed personal holding company income." The personal holding company tax was enacted when the highest corporate income tax rate was well below the highest individual income tax rate. It was designed to prevent individuals from establishing a corporation to receive and hold investment income or compensation so that it would be taxed at a lower rate (i.e., "incorporated pocketbooks"). Even though the corporate and individual income tax rates have somewhat equalized, the personal holding company tax still applies.

Effective for tax years beginning after December 31, 2012, the personal holding company tax is 20 percent of a corporation's undistributed personal holding company income (Code Sec. 541; Reg. § 1.541-1).[68] Effective for tax years beginning before January 1, 2013, the tax rate is 15 percent. Undistributed personal holding company income is computed by making the following adjustments to the corporation's taxable income, not just its personal holding company income (Code Sec. 545):[69]

(1) A deduction is allowed for federal income taxes, as well as for income, war, and excess profits taxes of foreign countries and U.S. possessions (to the

References are to Standard Federal Tax Reports; Tax Research Consultant; and Practical Tax Explanations.

[65] ¶ 23,015; CCORP: 18,100; § 26,910.05
[66] ¶ 23,018.26; CCORP: 18,102; § 26,910.05
[67] ¶ 14,300, ¶ 14,301, ¶ 15,160; ACCTNG: 24,550, ACCTNG: 30,150; § 27,101
[68] ¶ 23,152, ¶ 23,153; CCORP: 36,250; § 27,001
[69] ¶ 23,250; CCORP: 36,250; § 27,010.20

extent not allowed as deductions in computing taxable income) accrued during the tax year, regardless of the accounting method used.

(2) Charitable contributions for the tax year are deductible but the 20-to-50-percent contribution base for individuals (¶ 1059) must be used, rather than the 10-percent base normally allowed to corporations (¶ 927).

(3) No deduction is allowed for dividends received or for dividends paid by public utilities on certain preferred stock.

(4) The net operating loss deduction is not allowed.

(5) A deduction is allowed for net capital gains for the year, reduced by the taxes attributable to them. In the case of a foreign corporation, only net capital gains that are effectively connected with the conduct of a trade or business within the United States and that are not exempt under treaty are taken into account.

(6) Any deduction for ordinary and necessary business expenses, as well as depreciation, attributable to the operation and maintenance of property owned or operated by the corporation is limited to the aggregate rental income or other compensation earned from the property, unless the corporation shows that the compensation received was the highest available, the property was held in a bona fide business operated for profit, and either there was a reasonable expectation of a profit or the property was necessary for carrying on the corporation's business.

After these adjustments are made, the dividends-paid deduction is deducted from the adjusted taxable income (¶ 259). The amount of deduction for a personal holding company includes a dividend carryover from the two preceding tax years (Code Sec. 564).[70] The carryover is the excess of the dividends paid in the two preceding years over the income for such years. Any remaining balance is the corporation's undistributed personal holding company income.

Personal holding company taxes are computed and reported on Schedule PH, which is attached to the corporation's Form 1120.

277. Personal Holding Company Defined. A personal holding company is any corporation in which at least 60 percent of adjusted ordinary gross income for the tax year is personal holding company income (¶ 281), and at any time during the last half of the tax year more than 50 percent in value of its outstanding stock is owned, directly or indirectly, by or for not more than five individuals (¶ 285) (Code Sec. 542; Reg. §§ 1.542-1—1.542-3).[71] For this purpose, individuals include: a qualified pension, profit-sharing, or stock bonus plan (¶ 2101); a supplemental unemployment benefit (SUB) trust (¶ 692); a private foundation (¶ 631); or part of a trust permanently set aside or used exclusively for charitable purposes (¶ 537).

Certain corporations are exempt from the personal holding company tax, even though they meet the income and stock ownership qualifications (Code Sec. 542(c)). These include tax-exempt corporations (¶ 601); banks or domestic building and loan associations (¶ 2383); certain lending and finance companies that meet gross income, deduction, and loan tests; life insurance companies (¶ 2370); surety companies; corporations in bankruptcy or similar proceedings (unless the purpose of the case is to avoid the personal holding company tax); and foreign corporations. A small business investment company (¶ 2392) is exempt from personal holding company tax if it is licensed by the Small Business Administration, but not if any shareholder of the company owns directly or indirectly a five-percent-or-more proprietary interest in a small business concern to which the investment company provides funds, or five percent or more in value of outstanding stock of such a concern.

281. Personal Holding Company Income. The term "personal holding company income" for purposes of the personal holding company tax (¶ 275) means the portion of the adjusted ordinary gross income that consists of (Code Sec. 543):[72]

References are to Standard Federal Tax Reports; Tax Research Consultant; and Practical Tax Explanations.

[70] ¶ 23,510; CCORP: 9,314; § 27,010.20

[71] ¶ 23,190—¶ 23,193; CCORP: 36,000; § 27,001

[72] ¶ 23,210; CCORP: 36,150; § 27,010.15

(1) dividends, interest, royalties (other than mineral, oil and gas, copyright, or computer software royalties), and annuities (however, such income does not include interest received by a broker or dealer in connection with any securities or money market instruments held as inventory or primarily for sale to customers, margin accounts, or any financing for a customer secured by securities or money market instruments);

(2) rents, unless they constitute 50 percent or more of the adjusted ordinary gross income, and unless the sum of dividends paid during the tax year, dividends paid after the close of the tax year but considered paid on the last day of the year, and consent dividends (¶ 259), equals or exceeds the amount by which personal holding company income exceeds 10 percent of the ordinary gross income;

(3) mineral, oil, and gas royalties, unless (a) they constitute 50 percent or more of the adjusted ordinary gross income, (b) the other personal holding company income for the tax year is not more than 10 percent of the ordinary gross income, and (c) the ordinary and necessary business expense deductions, other than compensation for personal services rendered by shareholders, are 15 percent or more of adjusted ordinary gross income;

(4) copyright royalties, unless (a) apart from royalties derived from the works of shareholders, they make up 50 percent or more of the ordinary gross income, (b) personal holding company income for the tax year (not taking into account copyright royalties and dividends in any corporation in which the taxpayer owns at least 50 percent of all classes of voting stock and at least 50 percent of the value of all classes of stock) is 10 percent or less of the ordinary gross income, and (c) ordinary and necessary business expense deductions, other than compensation for personal services rendered by shareholders and deductions for royalties, equal or exceed 25 percent of the amount by which the ordinary gross income exceeds the sum of royalties paid or accrued and depreciation allowed;

(5) rents from the distribution and exhibition of produced films (that is, rents from a film interest acquired before the film production was substantially complete) unless such rents are 50 percent or more of the ordinary gross income;

(6) amounts received as compensation for the use of, or right to use, tangible property of the corporation where, at any time during the tax year, 25 percent or more in value of the outstanding stock of the corporation is owned, directly or indirectly, by or for an individual entitled to the use of the property, whether such right is obtained directly from the corporation or by means of a sublease or other arrangement (but this paragraph applies only if the corporation's other personal holding company income, computed with certain adjustments, for the tax year is more than 10 percent of its ordinary gross income);

(7) amounts received by a corporation from contracts for personal services, including gain from the sale or other disposition thereof, if (a) some person other than the corporation has the right to designate (by name or by description) the individual who is to perform the services or if the individual who is to perform the services is designated (by name or by description) in the contract and (b) at some time during the tax year 25 percent or more in value of the outstanding stock of the corporation is owned, directly or indirectly, by or for the individual who has performed, is to perform, or may be designated (by name or by description) as the one to perform such services; and

(8) income required to be reported by a corporate beneficiary under the income tax provisions relating to estates and trusts.

Active Business Computer Software Royalties. Active business computer software royalties received in connection with the licensing of computer software are excluded from personal holding company income (Code Sec. 543(d)).[73] To qualify for the exclusion: (1) the royalties must be derived by a corporation actively engaged in the trade or

---

References are to Standard Federal Tax Reports; Tax Research Consultant; and Practical Tax Explanations.

[73] ¶ 23,210; CCORP: 36,156.15

business of developing, manufacturing, or producing computer software; (2) the royalties must make up at least 50 percent of the corporation's gross income; (3) business and research expenses relating to the royalties must equal or exceed 25 percent of ordinary gross income; and (4) dividends must equal or exceed the excess of personal holding company income over 10 percent of ordinary gross income. If one member of an affiliated group receives software royalties, it will be treated as having met the above requirements if another member meets the requirements.

283. Adjusted Ordinary Gross Income. In determining whether 60 percent or more of a corporation's "adjusted ordinary gross income" is personal holding company income (¶ 281), the following adjustments must be made to ordinary gross income (Code Sec. 543(b)(2)):[74]

(1) Rental income must be reduced by deductions for depreciation and amortization, property taxes, interest, and rents paid that are attributable to such income.

(2) Income from mineral, oil, and gas royalties and from working interests in oil and gas wells must be reduced by deductions for depreciation, amortization and depletion, property and severance taxes, interest, and rents paid that are attributable to such income.

(3) Interest on U.S. bonds held for sale by a dealer who is making a primary market for these obligations, and interest on condemnation awards, judgments, and tax refunds, must be excluded.

(4) Rent received from the lease of tangible personal property manufactured by a taxpayer engaged in substantial manufacturing or production of property of the same type must be reduced by deductions for depreciation and amortization, taxes, rent, and interest paid that are attributable to such income.

All capital gains are excluded in determining whether the 60-percent test has been met because it is based on adjusted ordinary gross income.

285. Constructive Ownership of Personal Holding Company. The following constructive ownership rules apply in determining whether (1) a corporation is a personal holding company (¶ 277), (2) amounts received under a personal service contract are personal holding company income (¶ 281), (3) copyright royalties are personal holding company income, or (4) compensation for the use of property is personal holding company income (Code Sec. 544; Reg. § 1.544-1):[75]

(1) Stock owned, directly or indirectly, by or for a corporation, partnership, estate, or trust is considered owned proportionately by its shareholders, partners, or beneficiaries.

(2) An individual is considered to own the stock owned, directly or indirectly, by or for his or her family (brothers and sisters (whole or half blood), spouse, ancestors, and lineal descendants), or by or for his or her partner.

(3) If any person has an option to acquire stock, such stock is considered owned by such person. An option to acquire an option, and each one of a series of such options, is regarded as an option to acquire stock. This rule is applied in preference to rule (2), above, when both rules apply.

(4) Stock constructively owned by a corporation, partnership, estate, or trust will be reattributed to its owners or beneficiaries so that they are treated as constructive owners of the stock. However, stock constructively and not actually owned by an individual will not be reattributed.

(5) Outstanding securities convertible into stock (whether or not during the tax year) are considered outstanding stock, but only if the effect of the inclusion of all such securities is to make the corporation a personal holding company.

References are to Standard Federal Tax Reports; Tax Research Consultant; and Practical Tax Explanations.

[74] ¶ 23,210; CCORP: 36,106; § 27,010.10

[75] ¶ 23,230, ¶ 23,231; CCORP: 36,058

¶283

287. Deficiency Dividend Deduction. If a deficiency is determined in the personal holding company tax (¶ 275), the corporation may then distribute dividends and, in redetermining the undistributed personal holding company income, reduce or eliminate the deficiency by means of a deduction for "deficiency dividends" in the amount of the dividends so paid (Code Sec. 547; Reg. §§ 1.547-1—1.547-7).[76] The distribution must be made within 90 days after the deficiency determination. Claim for the deduction must be filed within 120 days of the determination.

Controlled Corporate Groups

289. Allocation of Tax Benefits. A controlled group of corporations (¶ 291) is allowed only one set of graduated income tax brackets for regular income tax purposes (¶ 219) and one $250,000 accumulated earnings credit for the accumulated earning tax (¶ 261). Controlled groups are also allowed one $40,000 exemption amount for alternative minimum tax purposes (¶ 1410). Each of these items is to be allocated equally among the members of the group unless they all consent to a different apportionment (Code Sec. 1561).[77]

Dividends-Received Deduction. Since a parent-subsidiary controlled group is also an affiliated group, a 100-percent dividends-received deduction may be taken with respect to dividends paid from one member to another (¶ 223). A 70-percent deduction is allowed for distributions between members of a brother-sister controlled group.

291. What Is a Controlled Group. There are three types of controlled corporate groups—parent-subsidiary, brother-sister, and combined groups (Code Sec. 1563(a)).[78] A parent-subsidiary controlled group exists if: (1) one or more chains of corporations are connected through stock ownership with a common parent corporation; (2) 80 percent or more of the voting power or value of the stock of each corporation in the group other than the parent is owned by one or more corporations in the group; and (3) the common parent owns at least 80 percent of the voting power or value of the stock of one of the other corporations in the group (not counting stock owned directly by other members).

A brother-sister controlled group exists if five or fewer persons (individuals, estates, or trusts) own stock possessing more than 50 percent of the total combined voting power of all classes of stock entitled to vote, or more than 50 percent of the total value of all stock, taking into account the stock ownership of each person only to the extent the person owns stock in each corporation.

A combined group consists of three or more corporations, each of which is a member of either a parent-subsidiary controlled group or a brother-sister controlled group, and at least one of which is the common parent of a parent-subsidiary group and also is a member of a brother-sister group.

293. Controlled Corporations—Expenses, Interest, and Losses. Controlled groups of corporations are subject to the related-party transaction rules of Code Sec. 267 (¶ 1717), under which controlled members must use a matching rule that defers the deductibility of an expense or interest by a payor until the payment is included in the payee's income (Code Sec. 267(a)(2)).[79] Also, losses on sales between members of a controlled group must be deferred until the property is sold to an unrelated person (Code Sec. 267(f)).[80] The loss-deferral rule does not apply, however, to sales to a domestic international sales corporation (DISC) (¶ 2498), to sales of inventory in the ordinary course of business if one of the parties is a foreign corporation, or to loan repayment losses attributable to foreign currency value reductions.

References are to Standard Federal Tax Reports; Tax Research Consultant; and Practical Tax Explanations.

[76] ¶ 23,290—¶ 23,297; CCORP: 36,300; § 27,015

[77] ¶ 33,340; CCORP: 42,050

[78] ¶ 33,360; CCORP: 42,102, CCORP: 42,104, CCORP: 42,106

[79] ¶ 14,150; BUSEXP: 21,160; § 17,605

[80] ¶ 14,150; CCORP: 42,260, SALES: 39,112

Consolidated Returns

295. Consolidated Returns. An affiliated group of corporations may file a consolidated income tax return for the tax year instead of filing separate returns (Code Sec. 1501).[81] An "affiliated group" is one or more chains of includible corporations connected through stock ownership with a common parent that is an includible corporation if (1) the common parent directly owns stock possessing at least 80 percent of the total voting power of at least one of the other includible corporations and has a value equal to at least 80 percent of the total value of the stock of the corporation, and (2) stock meeting the 80-percent test in each includible corporation other than the common parent is owned directly by one or more of the other includible corporations (Code Sec. 1504(a)).[82]

A consolidated return may be filed only if all corporations that were members of the affiliated group *at any time* during the tax year consent prior to the last day for filing the return. The making of a consolidated return is such consent. The common parent corporation, when filing a consolidated return, must attach Form 851. In addition, for the first year a consolidated return is filed, each subsidiary must attach a Form 1122 (consent to be included in the consolidated return) (Code Sec. 1501; Reg. § 1.1502-75(b)).[83]

The following corporations may not file consolidated returns (Code Sec. 1504(b)):[84]

(1) tax-exempt corporations (¶ 601), except that such organizations may be affiliated with other such organizations at least one of which is organized only to hold title for exempt organizations and from which the others derive income;

(2) life insurance companies (¶ 2370), except for those included in the group at the election of the common parent (Code Sec. 1504(c));[85]

(3) foreign corporations, except for Canadian or Mexican subsidiaries for which the common parent makes an election to treat them as domestic corporations includible in the consolidated group (Code Sec. 1504(d));[86]

(4) corporations electing the Code Sec. 936 possessions tax credit (¶ 1362);

(5) regulated investment companies (mutual funds) and real estate investment trusts (but see ¶ 2340 for circumstances in which a REIT may treat income and deductions of a qualified subsidiary as its own);

(6) domestic international sales corporations (DISCs); and

(7) S corporations.

297. Advantages and Disadvantages. The advantages of filing a consolidated income tax return (¶ 295) include: (1) offsetting operating losses of one company against the profits of another (see the rule for dual resident companies below); (2) offsetting capital losses of one company against the capital gains of another (see ¶ 2285 on newly acquired corporations); (3) avoidance of tax on intercompany distributions; (4) deferral of income on intercompany transactions; (5) use by the corporate group of the excess of one member's foreign tax credit over its limitation; and (6) designation of the parent corporation as agent of the group for all tax purposes.

The disadvantages include: (1) the effect on later years' returns; (2) deferral of losses on intercompany transactions; (3) additional bookkeeping required to keep track of deferred intercompany transactions; (4) intercompany profit in inventories still within the group must be reflected in annual inventory adjustments; (5) possible elimination of foreign tax credits when the limiting fraction is diminished because of lack of foreign income on the part of some members; and (6) possible accumulated earnings tax liability when the consolidated accumulated earnings and profits of the group exceed the minimum credit amount.

References are to Standard Federal Tax Reports; Tax Research Consultant; and Practical Tax Explanations.

[81] ¶ 33,121; CCORP: 45,050, CONSOL: 7,000

[82] ¶ 33,260; CCORP: 45,052, CONSOL: 7,050

[83] ¶ 33,121, ¶ 33,195; CCORP: 45,102, CONSOL: 9,100

[84] ¶ 33,260; CCORP: 45,054, CONSOL: 7,100

[85] ¶ 33,260; CCORP: 45,054.10, CONSOL: 7,106

[86] ¶ 33,260; CCORP: 45,054.05, CONSOL: 7,108.05

Dual Resident Companies. If a U.S. corporation is subject to foreign tax on its worldwide income, or on a residence basis as opposed to a source basis, any net operating loss it incurs in a year cannot reduce the taxable income of any other member of a U.S. affiliated group for any tax year (Reg. § 1.1503-2).[87] The IRS has issued regulations addressing the losses of dual resident companies filing consolidated returns (Reg. § § 1.1503(d)-1—1.1503(d)-8).[88]

Preferred Dividends. Income out of which a member of an affiliated group, other than a common parent, distributes preferred dividends to a nonmember may not be offset by the group's net operating losses or capital losses (Code Sec. 1503(f)).[89] Taxes on that income may not be offset by most group tax credits.

Golden Parachutes. All members of an affiliated group are treated as a single corporation when determining excessive payments that are contingent on a change in corporate control (¶ 907) (Code Sec. 280G(d)(5)).[90]

References are to Standard Federal Tax Reports; Tax Research Consultant; and Practical Tax Explanations.

[87] ¶ 33,242; CCORP: 45,264, CONSOL: 63,000

[88] ¶ 33,245—¶ 33,252; CCORP: 45,264, CONSOL: 63,400—CONSOL: 64,100

[89] ¶ 33,240; CCORP: 45,318, CONSOL: 75,100

[90] ¶ 15,150; COMPEN: 30,050; § 45,020.05

Chapter 3
S CORPORATIONS

S Corporation Status

301. Introduction—S Corporation Status. An S corporation is a corporation that elects and is eligible to choose S corporation status (¶ 303–¶ 305) and whose shareholders at the time consent to the corporation's choice (¶ 306). In general, an S corporation does not pay any income tax (with exceptions discussed in ¶ 335 and following). Instead, the corporation's income and deductions are passed through to its shareholders. The shareholders must then report the income and deductions on their own income tax returns.

To the extent the special S corporation rules (found in Code Sec. 1361 and following) do not apply, S corporations are governed by the "regular" (C corporation) corporate tax rules. Thus, while the taxation of income earned by, and the allocation of losses incurred by, S corporations closely parallel the taxation of partnerships with respect to items of partnership income and loss, S corporations generally are treated as regular corporations for purposes of the rules relating to corporate distributions, redemptions, liquidations, and reorganizations, as well as contributions of capital by S corporation shareholders (Code Sec. 1371).[1]

303. Corporations Eligible to Elect S Corporation Status. To become an S corporation, an organization must be a "small business corporation" (Code Sec. 1361; Reg. § 1.1361-1(b)).[2] All the following requirements must be met:

(1) The entity must be a domestic corporation that is organized under the laws of any state or U.S. territory or a domestic eligible entity (like a partnership or limited liability company) that elects to be taxed as a corporation under the check-the-box rules (Reg. § § 1.1361-1(c), 301.7701-3).[3]

(2) The corporation may have as shareholders only individuals, estates, certain trusts, and certain tax-exempt organizations (¶ 304). Partnerships and corporations cannot be shareholders.

(3) Only U.S. citizens or residents can be shareholders.

(4) The corporation can have only one class of stock (¶ 305).

A few limited types of corporations are ineligible to be small business corporations (Code Sec. 1361(b)(2)):[4]

- a financial institution that uses the reserve method of accounting;
- an insurance company taxed under subchapter L of the Code (¶ 2370);
- a corporation that has elected to take the Puerto Rico and possessions tax credit (¶ 1362); or
- a DISC or former DISC.

References are to Standard Federal Tax Reports; Tax Research Consultant; and Practical Tax Explanations.

[1] ¶ 32,140; SCORP: 368; § 28,901

[2] ¶ 32,021, ¶ 32,024A; SCORP: 150; § 28,001

[3] ¶ 32,024A, ¶ 43,083; PART: 3,102, SCORP: 152

[4] ¶ 32,021; SCORP: 154; § 28,001

An existing domestic eligible entity that is treated as a partnership for tax purposes is allowed to change its tax status and elect to be taxed as an S corporation. In other words, provided requirements applicable to check-the-box elections and S corporations are met, the entity may elect to change its tax status from partnership to corporation and also file an S election. There will be no intervening C year between the partnership tax year and the S tax year, so long as the check-the-box and S elections are effective on the same date and both sets of deadlines are met (Rev. Rul. 2009-15).[5]

100-Shareholder Limitation. A qualifying S corporation can have no more than 100 shareholders (Code Sec. 1361(b)(1)(A) and (c)).[6] In certain cases, two or more shareholders can be counted as only one shareholder for this purpose if they have one of several relationships to one another. For example, two spouses (and their estates) are counted as a single shareholder. In addition, all qualifying members of a family who hold corporation stock are treated as one shareholder of the S corporation. A family is defined as a common ancestor, the lineal descendants of the common ancestor, and the spouses (or former spouses) of the common ancestor and the descendants. The common ancestor can be no more than six generations removed from the youngest shareholder who is treated as a member of the family on the latest of: (1) the date the S corporation election is made (¶ 306); (2) the earliest date that a family member first holds stock in the corporation; or (3) October 22, 2004. Additionally, in determining whether certain children are lineal descendants and members of a family, any legally adopted child, any child lawfully placed with the individual for legal adoption, and any eligible foster child are treated as a child by blood. The estate of a family member is treated as a member of the family for purposes of determining the number of shareholders.

304. Eligible S Corporation Shareholders. All shareholders of an S corporation must be individuals, estates, certain specified trusts, or certain tax-exempt organizations (Code Sec. 1361(b)(1)(B)).[7] Partnerships and C corporations are not eligible to hold stock in an S corporation. The prohibition on a partnership holding S corporation stock does not extend to a limited liability company (LLC) with a single, individual member that is taxed as a disregarded entity. The owner of the single-member LLC is treated as the owner of the S corporation stock. Single-member LLCs that "check the box" to be taxed as C corporations may not hold stock in an S corporation. Taxpayers who only hold restricted bank director stock are not considered shareholders for determining whether an S corporation has an ineligible shareholder (Code Sec. 1361(f)).

Trusts. Trusts eligible to hold S corporation shares include grantor trusts (where the grantor is regarded as the shareholder) and voting trusts (where each beneficiary is treated as a shareholder) (Code Sec. 1361(c)(2); Reg. § 1.1361-1(h)).[8]

A trust that qualifies as a traditional or Roth individual retirement arrangement (IRA) is generally not an eligible S corporation shareholder (*Taproot Administrative Services, Inc.*, Dec. 57,950, 133 TC 202 (2009), aff'd, CA-9, 2012-1 USTC ¶ 50,256; Rev. Rul. 92-73).[9] An IRA, however, may hold stock in a bank or depository holding company that is an S corporation if the IRA held the stock as of October 22, 2004 (Code Sec. 1361(c)(2)(A)(vi)).[10] If the IRA decides to sell bank stock held as of October 22, 2004, it can sell the stock to the IRA beneficiary within 120 days after the corporation made the S corporation election without violating the prohibited transaction rules.

Any testamentary trust that receives S corporation stock is an eligible S corporation shareholder unless the trust is treated as an eligible shareholder only for two years after the deemed owner's death. The IRS may extend the two-year limit under an extension for estate tax payments. A charitable remainder trust is not an eligible S corporation shareholder (Rev. Rul. 92-48).[11]

References are to Standard Federal Tax Reports; Tax Research Consultant; and Practical Tax Explanations.

[5] ¶ 32,053.36; LLC: 18,200; § 28,010.05

[6] ¶ 32,021; SCORP: 156; § 28,005.05

[7] ¶ 32,021; SCORP: 158; § 28,010.05

[8] ¶ 32,021, ¶ 32,024A; SCORP: 158.20; § 28,010.10, § 28,010.20

[9] ¶ 32,026.815; SCORP: 158.35; § 28,010.40

[10] ¶ 32,021; SCORP: 158.35; § 28,010.40

[11] ¶ 24,468.22; SCORP: 160.05; § 28,715.05

ESBTs. An electing small business trust (ESBT) can be an S corporation shareholder (Code Sec. 1361(c)(2)(A)(v), (c)(2)(B)(v), and (e)).[12] An ESBT is a trust that does not have as a beneficiary any person other than an individual, estate, or organization eligible to accept charitable contributions under Code Sec. 170 (other than a political entity). Any portion of an ESBT that consists of S corporation stock is treated as a separate trust and will be taxed at the highest rate of tax for estates and trusts with limited deductions and credits, and no exemption amount for alternative minimum tax purposes.

Also, an ESBT cannot have any interest acquired by purchase, and a specific election to be treated as an electing trust must have been filed by the trustee. This election is irrevocable without the consent of the IRS. This type of trust does not include a qualified subchapter S trust (see below) or a trust that is exempt from income tax.

In the case of an ESBT, each potential current beneficiary of the trust is treated as a shareholder, except that for any period if there is no potential current beneficiary of the trust, the trust itself is treated as the shareholder. A potential current beneficiary is a person who is entitled to a distribution from the trust or who may receive a distribution at the discretion of any person. Any person who may benefit from a power of appointment is not a potential current beneficiary if the power has not been exercised. If the potential current beneficiaries of an ESBT would disqualify an S corporation, the ESBT has a grace period of one year to dispose of its stock in the S corporation, thereby avoiding disqualification.

QSSTs. A qualified subchapter S trust (QSST) whose beneficiary chooses to be treated as owner of the S corporation stock held by the trust also may hold stock in an S corporation (Code Sec. 1361(d); Reg. § 1.1361-1(j)).[13] A QSST must own stock in at least one S corporation and must distribute all of its income to one individual who is a U.S. citizen or resident. The QSST beneficiary is taxed on all items of income, loss, deduction, and credit attributable to the S corporation stock held by the QSST. However, the QSST, not the beneficiary, is treated as the owner of the S corporation stock for purposes of determining the tax consequences of the trust's disposition of the S corporation stock. In addition, the terms of the QSST must provide:

(1) there may be only one income beneficiary at any time;

(2) trust corpus may be distributed only to the income beneficiary;

(3) each income interest must end no later than the death of the income beneficiary; and

(4) if the trust ends at any time during the life of the income beneficiary, it must distribute all of its assets to the beneficiary.

Successive income beneficiaries are permitted. The income beneficiary's election to treat the trust as a QSST may be revoked only with the consent of the IRS. The election is effective for up to two months and 15 days before the election date. A separate election must be made with respect to each corporation the stock of which is held by the trust and must be made by each successive income beneficiary.

Exempt Organizations as Shareholders. Certain tax-exempt organizations can be S corporation shareholders. These are qualified pension, profit-sharing, and stock bonus plans; charitable organizations; and Code Sec. 501(c)(3) organizations.

QSSS. Even though a corporation generally cannot be an S corporation shareholder, an S corporation is permitted to own a qualified subchapter S subsidiary (QSSS or QSub) (Code Sec. 1361(b)(3)).[14] This includes any domestic corporation that qualifies as an S corporation and is 100 percent owned by an S corporation parent that elects to treat it as a QSSS. A QSSS is not taxed as a separate corporation, and all its tax items are treated as belonging to the parent. Form 8869 should be used by all S corporations to elect QSub treatment for wholly owned corporate subsidiaries.

References are to Standard Federal Tax Reports; Tax Research Consultant; and Practical Tax Explanations.

[12] ¶ 32,021; SCORP: 158.30; § 28,010.30

[13] ¶ 32,021, ¶ 32,024A; SCORP: 160; § 28,010.25

[14] ¶ 32,021; SCORP: 550; § 28,020.05

305. Single Class of Stock Requirement. A qualifying S corporation may have only one class of stock outstanding. These shares must confer identical rights to distribution and liquidation proceeds (Code Sec. 1361(b)(1)(D) and (c)(5); Reg. §1.1361-1(l)).[15] Differences in voting rights, however, are permitted. A corporate obligation that qualifies as "straight debt" is not considered a second class of stock. Buy-sell and redemption agreements restricting transferability of the stock are generally disregarded in determining whether the corporation has a single class of stock.

Stock of an S corporation does not include stock received for the performance of services that is substantially nonvested, unless the holder has made a Code Sec. 83(b) election to include the value of the stock in income (Reg. §1.1361-1(b)(3)).[16] However, stock warrants, call options, or other similar stock rights to purchase stock (collectively, "options") generally are treated as stock of the corporation if the options are substantially certain to be exercised at a strike price substantially below fair market value. This rule does not apply if the option was issued:

(1) to a commercial lender;

(2) in connection with the performance of services, provided the option is nontransferable and does not have a readily ascertainable fair market value when issued (¶ 713); or

(3) at a strike price that is at least 90 percent of the stock's fair market value (Reg. §1.1361-1(l)(4)(iii)).[17]

In addition, restricted bank director stock is not taken into account as outstanding stock in applying the provisions of subchapter S (Code Sec. 1361(f)(1)).[18] Accordingly, it is not treated as a second class of stock in the S corporation.

306. How to Make an S Election. The election of S corporation status must be made by a qualified corporation (¶ 303–¶ 305), with the unanimous consent of the shareholders, on or before the 15th day of the 3rd month of its tax year in order for the election to be effective beginning with the year when made (Code Sec. 1362(a), (b), and (c); Reg. §1.1362-6).[19] The election is made on Form 2553. The corporation must meet all of the eligibility requirements for the pre-election portion of the tax year, and all persons who were shareholders during the pre-election portion also must consent to the election. If these requirements are not met during the pre-election period, the election becomes effective the following year.

A "domestic eligible entity" (¶ 402A) may file both its check-the-box and S elections simply by filing Form 2553. It does not need to file Form 8832. The two elections will apply as of the same effective date (Reg. §301.7701-3(c)(1)(v)(C)).[20]

Late Elections. The IRS has provided a simplified procedure for obtaining relief from a late or invalid S corporation election, electing small business trust election, qualified subchapter S trust (QSST) election, or qualified subchapter S subsidiary (QSub) election (¶ 304). Relief is generally available if the request for relief is filed within three years and 75 days after the date on which the election is intended to be effective (Rev. Proc. 2013-30).[21] An entity may request relief for a late S corporation election by filing with the applicable IRS Service Center: (1) a properly completed Form 2553 with Form 1120S for the corporation's current tax year; (2) properly completed Form 2553 with a Form 1120S for one of the corporation's late-filed prior-year Forms 1120S; or (3) a properly completed Form 2553 submitted independently of Form 1120S.

The simplified procedure requesting late-election relief also applies where a domestic eligible entity has failed to timely file both its S corporation election and its election to be treated as a corporation under the check-the-box rules (¶ 402A). An entity that obtains relief under the simplified procedure is treated as having made both an election

---

References are to Standard Federal Tax Reports; Tax Research Consultant; and Practical Tax Explanations.

[15] ¶ 32,021, ¶ 32,024A; SCORP: 162; §28,015.05

[16] ¶ 32,024A; SCORP: 162.05

[17] ¶ 32,024A; SCORP: 162.15; §28,015.10

[18] ¶ 32,021; SCORP: 162.05

[19] ¶ 32,040, ¶ 32,047; SCORP: 200; §28,105.05

[20] ¶ 43,083; STAGES: 6,154.10; §28,125

[21] ¶ 32,053.41; SCORP: 206; §28,140.05

to be classified as an association taxable as a corporation and an S corporation election as of the same date.

Prior to September 3, 2013, two simplified methods were available for shareholders to request relief for late filing of an S election (Rev. Procs. 2003-43 and 2007-62).[22] Under Rev. Proc. 2003-43, certain eligible entities would be granted relief for failing to timely file these elections if the request for relief was filed within 24 months of the due date of the election. Relief would be granted under Rev. Proc. 2007-62 where the application for relief was filed no later than six months after the due date (with extensions) of the S corporation's tax return for such year. These procedures were to be followed in lieu of the letter ruling process. Therefore, user fees did not apply to corrective actions under these procedures. Prior to September 3, 2013, Rev. Procs. 2004-48 and 2007-62[23] applied to an eligible entity that failed to timely elect S corporation status and to be treated as a corporation under the check-the-box rules.

Community Property. Shareholders in community property states are also eligible for automatic relief for late S elections if their spouses did not file timely shareholder consents (Rev. Proc. 2004-35).[24] To qualify for relief, the S corporation election must be invalid solely because the spouse's signature is missing from the election form. Shareholders must alert the IRS that they are seeking relief under Rev. Proc. 2004-35 and identify the number of shares they own as of the date of the election. Each spouse must sign a separate statement indicating his or her consent to the election.

307. Termination of S Election. S corporation status is automatically terminated if any event occurs that would prohibit the corporation from making the election in the first place (Code Sec. 1362(d)(2); Reg. § 1.1362-2(b)).[25] The election is ended as of the date on which the disqualifying event occurs. Also, if a corporation has accumulated earnings and profits as of the end of three consecutive years, and the corporation's passive investment income exceeds 25 percent of its gross receipts in each of those three years, its election is ended beginning with the following tax year (Code Sec. 1362(d)(3); Reg. § 1.1362-2(c)).[26] For this purpose, dividends received by an S corporation from a C corporation subsidiary of which the S corporation owns 80 percent or more of stock are not treated as passive investment income to the extent the dividends are attributable to the earnings and profits derived from the active conduct of a trade or business.

An S corporation election may be revoked with the consent of shareholders holding more than 50 percent of the outstanding shares of stock (voting and nonvoting) on the day the revocation is made. A revocation may designate a prospective effective date (Code Sec. 1362(d)(1); Reg. § 1.1362-2(a)).[27] If no date is specified, a revocation made on or before the 15th day of the 3rd month of a corporation's tax year is effective on the first day of the tax year. A revocation made after this date is effective on the first day of the following tax year.

If an election is ended or revoked, the corporation may not reelect S corporation status without IRS consent until the 5th year after the year in which the termination or revocation became effective (Code Sec. 1362(g); Reg. § 1.1362-5).[28] An S corporation whose status as a qualified subchapter S subsidiary (QSSS or QSub) (¶ 304) has ended also cannot elect to be treated as a qualified subchapter S subsidiary until the 5th year after the year in which the termination was effective (Code Sec. 1361(b)(3)(D)).[29]

In addition to formally filing an election to end S corporation status, an S corporation can simply create a situation that bars it from being an S corporation. For example, an election to revoke S corporation status relates back to the beginning of the tax year only if the election is made before the 16th day of the third month of the corporation's tax year. Elections made after that date apply to the next tax year. However, if an S

References are to Standard Federal Tax Reports; Tax Research Consultant; and Practical Tax Explanations.

[22] ¶ 32,053.41; SCORP: 206; § 28,140.10

[23] ¶ 32,053.41; SCORP: 206; § 28,140.20

[24] ¶ 32,053.41; SCORP: 206; § 28,115.10

[25] ¶ 32,040, ¶ 32,043; SCORP: 304; § 28,210

[26] ¶ 32,040, ¶ 32,043; SCORP: 306; § 28,215.05

[27] ¶ 32,040, ¶ 32,043; SCORP: 302; § 28,205.05

[28] ¶ 32,040, ¶ 32,046; SCORP: 312; § 28,130

[29] ¶ 32,021; SCORP: 558; § 28,020.10

¶307

corporation wants to end S status immediately, an S corporation can create a situation where S status will immediately be ended. For example, the S corporation's shareholders can create another corporation and transfer one share of S corporation stock to the new corporation. Because corporations cannot be S corporation shareholders, the S corporation status ends on the date the share of stock is transferred to a disqualified shareholder and it is not necessary to wait until the next tax year for the revocation of the S corporation election to become effective.

Reorganizations. A corporation's Subchapter S election does not terminate merely because it is a party to a reorganization if it continues to meet the S corporation eligibility requirements.[30] Typically, this issue arises because the reorganization results in an ineligible shareholder owning stock of the S corporation. For example, the IRS ruled that the S election of a corporation that was acquired by another corporation in a stock-for-stock B reorganization terminated on the date of acquisition. On the other hand, the IRS has ruled that A, C, and F reorganizations did not cause the S elections of the respective corporations to terminate when all owners of the corporations after the transaction were eligible S corporation shareholders.

Frequently, reorganizations can involve transfers of the same corporate stock several different times to different parties as part of the transaction. The intermediate parties may be deemed to hold the stock only for an instant before transferring it to its ultimate holder. There is a question as to whether a corporation's Subchapter S election terminates where one or more of these intermediate parties is not an eligible S corporation shareholder. This issue is not addressed by the Code or regulations; however, the IRS has privately ruled that having such shareholders, who acquire a corporation's stock only to immediately transfer it to another party, does not cause the corporation's S election to terminate (LTRs 200453007 and 9010042).

Correction of Inadvertent Terminations. If a corporation's S election is inadvertently terminated or invalid when made, and the corporation makes a timely correction, the IRS can waive the termination or can permit the election (Code Sec. 1362(f); Reg. § 1.1362-4).[31] The IRS is also authorized to provide a waiver where an election to treat family members as one shareholder or to treat a corporation as a QSub is invalid when made or inadvertently terminated. To obtain a waiver, the corporation must correct any condition that barred it from qualifying as an S corporation, or otherwise made an election invalid, and must obtain any required shareholder consents. All shareholders must agree to make such adjustments as may be required by the IRS.

Election to End Tax Year. If a shareholder disposes of his or her interest in an S corporation and all "affected" shareholders consent to the termination, the tax year can be treated as two tax years, the first of which ends on the date of termination (Code Sec. 1377(a)(2)).[32] Affected shareholders include the shareholder whose interest is terminated and all shareholders to whom such shareholder has transferred shares during the tax year.

Taxation of Shareholders

309. Taxation of S Corporation Shareholders. Each shareholder of an S corporation separately accounts for his or her pro rata share of corporate items of income, deduction, loss, and credit in his or her tax year in which the corporation's tax year ends (Code Sec. 1366(a); Reg. §§1.1366-1(a) and 1.1377-1).[33] Certain items must be separately stated whenever they could affect the shareholder's individual tax liability (¶320). A shareholder's share of each item generally is computed based on the number of shares he held on each day of the corporation's tax year.

The character of an item included in a shareholder's pro rata share of S corporation income is generally determined as if the item was realized directly from the source from which the corporation realized it or was incurred in the same manner in which the

---

References are to Standard Federal Tax Reports; Tax Research Consultant; and Practical Tax Explanations.

[30] ¶ 32,053.69; SCORP: 304.10; §28,920

[31] ¶ 32,040, ¶ 32,045; SCORP: 308; §28,220

[32] ¶ 32,240; SCORP: 402.15; §28,445.10, §28,445.15

[33] ¶ 32,080, ¶ 32,081, ¶ 32,240C; SCORP: 402; §28,405

corporation incurred it, subject to exceptions (Code Sec. 1366(b); Reg. § 1.1366-1(b)).[34] Thus, when income passes through from the S corporation to the shareholder, the character of that income passes through as well. For example, if an S corporation makes a charitable contribution to a qualifying organization, a shareholder's pro rata share of the S corporation's charitable contribution is characterized as made to a qualifying organization.

Similarly, if an S corporation has capital gain on the sale or exchange of a capital asset, a shareholder's pro rata share of that gain is also characterized as a capital gain regardless of whether the shareholder is otherwise a dealer in that type of property. However, this rule does not apply when the S corporation is formed or availed of for a principal purpose of selling or exchanging contributed property that, in the hands of the shareholder, would not have produced capital gain if sold or exchanged by the shareholder. The same exception applies when the S corporation is formed or availed of for a principal purpose of selling or exchanging contributed property that, in the hands of a shareholder, would have produced capital loss if sold or exchanged by the shareholder. Any loss recognized by the corporation is treated as a capital loss to the extent that, immediately before the contribution, the adjusted basis of the property in the hands of the shareholder exceeded the fair market value of the property.

Duty of Consistency. A shareholder of an S corporation must treat a Subchapter S item in a manner consistent with the treatment of that item on the S corporation's return (Code Sec. 6037).[35] Any shareholder who does not treat the item consistently must file a statement identifying the inconsistency.

At-Risk and Passive Activity Rules. The at-risk rules disallow losses that exceed an investor's amount at risk (¶ 1155). Generally, the amount at risk is the amount of investment that an investor could lose. The at-risk rules apply to all individuals, including S corporation shareholders, and are applied at the shareholder level (Code Sec. 465).[36] The at-risk amount is determined at the close of the S corporation's tax year. Thus, an S corporation shareholder who realizes that his or her at-risk amount is low, and wishes to deduct an anticipated S corporation net loss, can make additional contributions to the entity.

Likewise, passive activity loss (PAL) rules generally are applied at the shareholder level (¶ 1169) (Code Sec. 469).[37] However, several determinations that affect the application of the PAL rules must be made at the corporate level. For example, the determination of whether an activity constitutes a trade or business, as opposed to a rental activity, is made at the corporate level. The distinction between portfolio and nonportfolio income is also made at the corporate level. This information is conveyed via the Schedule K-1 (Form 1120S) that is provided to the shareholder by the corporation. The shareholder then uses the information to apply the PAL and at-risk limitations when preparing his or her individual tax return.

Since a qualified subchapter S trust (QSST) (¶ 304) is treated as the shareholder when it disposes of S corporation stock, the application of the at-risk and PAL rules would normally be determined at the trust level, not the beneficiary level. To ensure that the beneficiary can take disallowed losses on the QSST's disposition of the stock, the at-risk and passive activity loss rules apply as if the beneficiary disposed of the stock (Code Sec. 1361(d)(1)(C)).[38]

Small Business Stock. Because S corporations are not entitled to ordinary loss treatment from the sale of qualified small business stock under Code Sec. 1244 (¶ 1911), and because the character of loss items passes through to shareholders, S corporation shareholders cannot claim ordinary losses incurred by the S corporation from the sale of qualified small business stock (*V.D. Rath*, Dec. 49,266, 101 TC 196 (1993)).[39] However, when the S corporation stock itself is qualified small business stock, shareholders may claim ordinary loss deductions if all the requirements are met.

References are to Standard Federal Tax Reports; Tax Research Consultant; and Practical Tax Explanations.

[34] ¶ 32,080, ¶ 32,081; SCORP: 402.05; § 28,420

[35] ¶ 35,520; PART: 60,402, SCORP: 402.05; § 28,425

[36] ¶ 21,850; SCORP: 406; § 28,430.30

[37] ¶ 21,960; BUSEXP: 33,050; § 28,430.35

[38] ¶ 32,021; SCORP: 160; § 17,435.20

[39] ¶ 30,800.59; SALES: 18,154; § 28,440.25

¶309

312. Domestic Production Activities of S Corporation Shareholders. An S corporation cannot claim the domestic production activities deduction (DPAD) (¶ 980A). Instead, the deduction is determined at the shareholder level (Code Sec. 199(d)(1); Reg. § 1.199-5(c)).[40] Generally, each shareholder computes its deduction separately on Form 8903 by aggregating its pro rata share of qualified production activity (QPA) items of the S corporation (i.e., income, expenses) with its share of QPA items from other sources. The shareholder does not have to be directly engaged in the S corporation's trade or business to claim the deduction on the basis of its share of QPA items.

For purposes of determining the deduction, the activities of an S corporation are not attributed to its shareholders (or vice-versa) (Reg. § 1.199-5(g)). For example, if the S corporation manufactures qualified production property within the United States and then distributes the property to the shareholder who subsequently sells, licenses, leases, or otherwise disposes of the property, then the income derived by the shareholder will not qualify as domestic production gross receipts (DPGR). A limited exception is provided for expanded affiliated groups.

Allocation of Items. A shareholder's pro rata share of expenses allocable to the S corporation's QPA is taken into account even if the corporation has no taxable income. If the shareholder is unable to claim a loss or deduction of the corporation for regular tax purposes (i.e., at-risk, passive loss, or basis limitations), then such loss or deduction cannot be used when computing the DPAD. The amount of any loss or deduction is subject to proportionate reduction if it is only partially allowed for regular tax purposes. Also, a loss or deduction that is temporarily disallowed for regular tax purposes may be taken into account in computing the DPAD in the tax year that it is allowed for regular tax purposes.

Instead of taking into account its pro rata share of each QPA item of the S corporation, a shareholder may compute his or her deduction by combining its pro rata share of the S corporation's qualified productions activities income (QPAI) and W-2 wages with his or her QPAI and W-2 wages from other sources. This option only applies if the S corporation has elected to use the small business overall method for allocating costs, expenses, and other deductions to its DPGR. Special rules apply to 20-percent shareholders of S corporations engaged in film or television production.

Sale of Stock. Gain or loss recognized on the sale of S corporation stock will not be taken into account by a shareholder in computing its QPAI (Reg. § 1.199-5(f)). This is because the sale of an interest in the corporation does not reflect the realization of DPGR by the entity.

W-2 Wage Limitation. A shareholder of an S corporation computes the W-2 wage limitation for the DPAD by aggregating its share of W-2 wages from the S corporation allocable to DPGR with W-2 wages allocable to DPGR from other sources.

314. S Corporations and the Net Investment Income Tax. Effective for tax years beginning after December 31, 2012, individuals, trusts, and estates are subject to a 3.8-percent tax on the lesser of their net investment income for the tax year or the excess of their modified adjusted gross income (MAGI) for the tax year over a threshold amount (¶ 129). S corporations are not subject to the net investment income (NII) tax, but S corporation shareholders may be subject to the tax on income items related to their investments in the corporation.

Allocations of Net Investment Income. Net investment income generally includes income and gain from passive activities. It generally does not include gross income derived in the ordinary course of a trade or business. Thus, income from a trade or business conducted by the S corporation in which the shareholder actively participates is not considered net investment income to the shareholder (Reg. § 1.1411-4(b)(2)).[41] However, income from a trade or business that is a passive activity with respect to the shareholder is included in the shareholder's net investment income. In other words, the shareholder's distributive share of income earned by the S corporation that would be net

---

References are to Standard Federal Tax Reports; Tax Research Consultant; and Practical Tax Explanations.

[40] ¶ 12,468, ¶ 12,472D; BUSEXP: 6,214; § 6,020.05

[41] ¶ 32,604; INDIV: 69,160.15, ESTTRST: 12,256

investment income had it been earned directly by the shareholder is considered net investment income to the shareholder. In addition, if the S corporation is engaged in the trade or business of a trader trading in financial instruments or commodities, the income or loss from that trade or business is excluded from the shareholder's NII without regard to whether the shareholder is himself engaged in the trade or business.

Dispositions of S Corporation Stock. Net gain or loss upon the disposition of S corporation stock is considered net investment income only to the extent it would be taken into account as such by the shareholder if all S corporation property were sold at fair market value immediately before the disposition (Code Sec. 1411(c)(4); Proposed Reg. §1.1411-7).[42] Specifically, gain or loss from property used in the S corporation's trade or business is excluded from NII for purposes of the tax, unless the trade or business is a passive activity with respect to the shareholder or involves trading in financial instruments or commodities.

315. Basis in S Corporation Stock. An S corporation shareholder's basis in his or her stock is determined under the same rules that apply to C corporation shareholders. Thus, the original basis of the shareholder's stock is the purchase price for the stock (money or the fair market value of any property given in exchange for the stock) (Code Sec. 1012).[43] Stock acquired by gift normally carries over the donor's basis (¶1630). The basis of stock acquired from a decedent is its fair market value on the date of the decedent's death or on the alternate valuation date, if elected (¶1633). During the time the corporation is an S corporation, each shareholder must make adjustment to his or her stock (¶317).

Similarly, the rules providing for contributions to controlled corporations under Code Sec. 351 (¶203) and tax-free corporate reorganizations under Code Sec. 368 (¶2209) are generally applicable to S corporations (Code Sec. 1371).[44] Thus, the basis of stock received under a tax-free reorganization is equal to the transferor's basis in the property transferred, plus any gain, minus the fair market value of the boot received, and minus any loss recognized in the transaction.

Stock for Services. An S corporation may grant stock to an employee or other service provider as part of a compensation package. Typically, in a stock-for-services arrangement, S corporation stock may be transferred to an employee at a particular price or for nothing, with the rights to the stock becoming vested only after a number of years of employment. The value of the S stock at that vesting point has usually appreciated from its value at the time of transfer. The difference between the amount that the employee pays for the S stock and the fair market value of the stock at the time the employee's rights to the stock are vested must be included in the employee's ordinary gross income (¶713). The S corporation gets a compensation deduction for the amount the employee includes in income in the year the employee includes it in income.

317. Adjustments to Basis in S Corporation Stock. The stock basis of each S corporation shareholder (¶315) is *increased* by the shareholder's portion of:

(1) all income items of the corporation (including tax-exempt income) that are separately computed and passed through to shareholders;

(2) the income of the corporation that is not separately computed; and

(3) the excess of the corporation's deductions for depletion (¶1289) over the basis of the property subject to depletion (Code Sec. 1367(a)(1); Reg. §1.1367-1(b)).[45]

References are to Standard Federal Tax Reports; Tax Research Consultant; and Practical Tax Explanations.

[42] ¶32,602, ¶32,604N; INDIV: 69,160.40; §1,022.15

[43] ¶29,330; SALES: 6,050; §28,605.10

[44] ¶32,140; CCORP: 3,202, CCORP: 39,256; §26,130

[45] ¶32,100, ¶32,100B; SCORP: 410.05; §28,610.05

A shareholder's basis is *decreased* by the portion of:

    (1) distributions that are not includible in the shareholder's income (¶ 309);

    (2) all loss and deduction items of the corporation that are separately stated and passed through to shareholders (but see the discussion below with respect to charitable contributions of appreciated property);

    (3) the nonseparately computed loss of the corporation;

    (4) any expense of the corporation not deductible in computing its taxable income and not properly chargeable to capital account; and

    (5) the amount of the shareholder's deduction for depletion with respect to oil and gas wells to the extent that it does not exceed his or her proportionate share of the adjusted basis of such property (Code Sec. 1367(a)(2); Reg. § 1.1367-1(c)).[46]

If a shareholder's stock basis is reduced to zero, the remaining net decrease attributable to losses and deductions is applied to reduce any basis in debt owed to the shareholder by the corporation (¶ 318). Distributions may not be applied against basis in debt. Any net increase in basis in a subsequent year is applied to restore the basis of indebtedness before it may be applied to increase the shareholder's stock basis.

Generally, stock basis adjustments are determined as of the close of the corporation's tax year, and the adjustments are effective as of that date. However, if a shareholder disposes of stock during the corporation's tax year, the adjustments with respect to that stock are effective immediately before the disposition (Reg. § 1.1367-1(d)).[47] An adjustment for a nontaxable item is determined for the tax year in which the item would have been includible or deductible under the corporation's method of accounting for federal income tax purposes if the item had been subject to federal income taxation.

Charitable Deductions. For tax years beginning before January 1, 2014, the amount of a shareholder's basis reduction in the stock of an S corporation by reason of a charitable contribution of property made by the corporation equals the shareholder's pro rata share of the adjusted basis of the contributed property (Code Sec. 1367(a)(2)).

    Planning Note: Absent further legislation, the reduction of an S corporation shareholder's outside basis by the shareholder's pro rata share of the basis of contributed property will not apply for contributions made in tax years beginning after December 31, 2013. For the latest legislative updates, visit our website, www.CCHGroup.com/TaxUpdates.

Cancellation of Indebtedness. Discharge of indebtedness income of an S corporation that is excluded from the corporation's income (¶ 855) is not taken into account as an item of income that flows through to any shareholder (¶ 309) and so does not increase a shareholder's basis in S corporation stock (Code Sec. 108(d)(7)(A); Reg. § 1.108-7(d)).[48]

318. Basis in S Corporation Debt. For purposes of deducting S corporation losses, a shareholder has basis in certain debts of the S corporation to the shareholder (Code Sec. 1366(d)(1)(B); Reg. § 1.1366-2(a)(2)).[49] Under final regulations that apply to indebtedness between an S corporation and its shareholder resulting from any transaction occurring on or after July 22, 2014, the debt in question must run directly to the shareholder and represent a bona fide indebtedness of the S corporation. Federal tax principles generally determine whether indebtedness is bona fide, based on all relevant facts and circumstances. Unlike a partner in a partnership, an S corporation shareholder does not receive basis or an increase in basis for debt of the S corporation to an outside lender. A mere guaranty by the shareholder of the S corporation's debt to a third party also does not qualify for an increase in the shareholder's basis, including acting as a surety, accommodation party, or in any similar capacity relating to the loan.

References are to Standard Federal Tax Reports; Tax Research Consultant; and Practical Tax Explanations.

[46] ¶ 32,100, ¶ 32,100B; SCORP: 410.05; § 28,615

[47] ¶ 32,100B; SCORP: 410.05; § 28,620

[48] ¶ 7002, ¶ 7006; SALES: 12,212.10, SCORP: 404.10; § 28,610.10

[49] ¶ 32,080, ¶ 32,082; SCORP: 404.05; § 28,630.05, § 28,630.10

The courts have held that, in order for a shareholder to have basis in debt owed to that shareholder by an S corporation, there must be an actual economic outlay by the shareholder to the corporation (*M.G. Underwood*, Dec. 33,016, 63 TC 468 (1975), aff'd, CA-5, 76-2 USTC ¶ 9557).[50] In other words, only the kind of debt that proves an actual investment by the shareholder, not merely one given in return for a promise by the shareholder for some future outlay, gives rise to or increases basis. The IRS rejected the "actual economic outlay" test in the regulations discussed above and substituted the bona fide indebtedness requirement. Both the courts and the IRS agree, however, that the S corporation's indebtedness must run directly to the shareholder, not merely to an entity in which he is an owner. Thus, indebtedness running from the S corporation to a passthrough entity in which the shareholder has an interest will not be attributed to the shareholder for this purpose.

The basis that a shareholder has in debt owed to that shareholder by the S corporation must be adjusted like the shareholder's basis in stock. Adjustments are calculated before the basis in indebtedness is affected (Code Sec. 1367(b)(2); Reg. § 1.1367-2).[51] When decreases relating to losses, deductions, noncapital, nondeductible expenses, and certain oil and gas depletion deductions have reduced stock basis to zero, any excess is applied to reduce debt basis. Any indebtedness by the corporation to the shareholder that has been satisfied by the corporation or disposed of or forgiven by the shareholder during the tax year is not held by the shareholder at the close of that year and is not subject to basis reduction. Generally, the adjustments to debt basis are made as of the close of the tax year. If the shareholder terminates his or her interest in the corporation during the tax year, however, the adjustments in basis to debt are applied with respect to any S corporation debt held by the shareholder immediately before the termination of the shareholder's interest in the corporation. If there is a reduction in the shareholder's basis in S corporation debt, any net increase in any subsequent tax year is applied first to the restoration of that reduction before any increase is applied to stock basis.

319. S Corporation's Taxable Income. An S corporation must compute its taxable income for purposes of determining the amount of income, gain, loss, deduction and credit passed through to its shareholders (¶ 309). Computation of an S corporation's taxable income parallels the computation of the taxable income of an individual, except that organizational expenditures may be amortized (¶ 237) and the reduction in certain corporate tax benefits (¶ 1445) is applied if the S corporation was a C corporation for any of its three immediately preceding tax years. Moreover, certain deductions allowed to individuals, such as those for personal exemptions, charitable contributions, medical expenses, alimony, and net operating losses, are not allowed to the S corporation when calculating taxable income (Code Sec. 1363(b)).[52] Certain items must be separately stated when passed through to shareholders (¶ 320).

An S corporation cannot carry over or carry back any item from a year that the corporation is not an S corporation to a year that the corporation is an S corporation (Code Sec. 1371(b)).[53] Thus, no carryforward or carryback, such as a net operating loss, arising from a tax year for which a corporation is a C corporation may be carried to a tax year for which the corporation is an S corporation. No carryforward or carryback arises at the corporate level in a tax year for which a corporation is an S corporation. However, a tax year for which a corporation is an S corporation is treated as a tax year for purposes of determining the number of tax years to which an item may be carried back or carried forward. Thus, while the item remains intact during the time the corporation is an S corporation, those years count for any carryforward period applicable to the item.

320. Separately Stated Items of S Corporation Income. Certain items of the taxable income of an S corporation (¶ 319) must be separately stated (Code Sec. 1363(b)).[54] These items must be reported and computed separately from items that can be combined. Items that must be separately stated include, but are not limited to:

References are to Standard Federal Tax Reports; Tax Research Consultant; and Practical Tax Explanations.

[50] ¶ 32,084.325; SCORP: 404.05; § 28,630.10
[51] ¶ 32,100, ¶ 32,100C; SCORP: 410.10; § 28,630.15

[52] ¶ 32,060; SCORP: 352; § 28,401
[53] ¶ 32,140; SCORP: 354; § 28,415

[54] ¶ 32,060; SCORP: 352; § 28,405

¶319

(1) net income or loss from rental activities, including rental real estate activities;

(2) portfolio income or loss and expenses related to portfolio income or loss;

(3) Code Sec. 1231 net gain or loss;

(4) charitable contributions, grouped by the percentage limitations of Code Sec. 170(b);

(5) Code Sec. 179 expense deductions;

(6) the low-income housing credit;

(7) investment interest expense;

(8) tax preference and adjustment items needed to compute shareholders' alternative minimum tax;

(9) gains and losses from wagering transactions;

(10) medical, dental, etc., expenses;

(11) itemized deductions;

(12) capital gain or loss grouped by applicable holding periods;

(13) foreign taxes paid or accrued;

(14) tax-exempt income; and

(15) passive activity items for each of the corporation's activities (Code Sec. 1366(a)(1)(A); Reg. § 1.1366-1(a)).[55]

Each shareholder must take also into account the shareholder's pro rata share of the nonseparately computed income or loss of the S corporation. Nonseparately computed income or loss is the corporation's gross income less the deductions allowed to the corporation, determined by excluding any item requiring separate computation.

Nonbusiness Bad Debts. An S corporation may claim a nonbusiness bad debt deduction (¶ 1143) in the same manner as an individual when computing an S corporation's taxable income. Accordingly, an S corporation that incurs a nonbusiness bad debt must separately state the debt as a short-term capital loss (Rev. Rul. 93-36). Partially or wholly worthless business debts, on the other hand, are included in nonseparately stated S corporation income or loss (¶ 1135).

321. Limits on S Corporation Deductions. A shareholder's currently deductible share of the corporation's losses and deductions for any tax year is limited to the total of his or her adjusted basis in the corporation's stock (¶ 315) and any bona fide debt of the S corporation owed to the shareholder (¶ 318) (Code Sec. 1366(d)).[56]

An S corporation's itemized deductions are separately stated items (¶ 320). Thus, the 2-percent floor on miscellaneous itemized deductions (¶ 1011) is applied at the shareholder level rather than at the S corporation level (Temp. Reg. § 1.67-2T(b)(1)).[57] Shareholders of an S corporation take into account separately their pro rata share of the corporation's miscellaneous itemized deductions, add them to their other individual miscellaneous deductions, and can deduct them to the extent they exceed 2 percent of their individual adjusted gross income.

The election to expense the cost of Code Sec. 179 property (¶ 1208) is made at the S corporation level (Reg. § 1.179-1(h)).[58] The dollar, investment, and taxable income limitations apply at both the S corporation and shareholder levels (Code Sec. 179(d)(8); Reg. § 1.179-2).[59]

Charitable Deductions. For tax years beginning before January 1, 2014, the basis limitation does not apply to a charitable contribution of appreciated property to the extent the shareholder's pro rata share of the contribution exceeds the shareholder's pro rata share of the adjusted basis of the property (Code Sec. 1366(d)(4); Rev. Rul. 2008-16).[60]

References are to Standard Federal Tax Reports; Tax Research Consultant; and Practical Tax Explanations.

[55] ¶ 32,080, ¶ 32,081; SCORP: 352.05; § 28,405

[56] ¶ 32,080; SCORP: 404; § 28,430.15

[57] ¶ 6062; INDIV: 39,102.05; § 28,440.45

[58] ¶ 12,121; DEPR: 12,156; § 28,440.15

[59] ¶ 12,120, ¶ 12,122; DEPR: 12,112; § 9,815.15, § 28,440.15

[60] ¶ 32,080, ¶ 32,101.27; SCORP: 402.10; § 28,440.10

Planning Note: Absent further legislation, the reduction of an S corporation shareholder's outside basis by the shareholder's pro rata share of the basis of contributed property will not apply for contributions made in tax years beginning after December 31, 2013. For the latest legislative updates, visit our website, www.CCHGroup.com/TaxUpdates.

Suspended Losses and Deductions. If the amount of the loss or deduction of a shareholder is limited for a tax year, the excess is treated as incurred by the corporation in the next tax year for that individual shareholder and may be carried forward until used by that shareholder (Code Sec. 1366(d)(2)).[61] Disallowed losses and deductions may be transferred only to a current or former spouse of the shareholder when the S corporation stock is transferred between spouses or incident to divorce in a nontaxable transaction (¶ 1734).

If the shareholder's losses or deductions are limited for the last tax year in which the corporation is an S corporation, the excess is treated as incurred by the shareholder on the last day of the corporation's post-termination transition period (¶ 329) (Code Sec. 1366(d)(3)). The excess amount cannot exceed the shareholder's adjusted basis of the stock in the corporation, determined at the close of the last day of the post-termination transition period. The losses or deductions taken into account during this period reduce the shareholder's basis in the stock of the corporation. Losses of an S corporation that are suspended under the at-risk rules (¶ 1155) are carried forward to the post-termination period.

322. Employee Benefits Provided to S Corporation Shareholders. The tax treatment of fringe benefits (¶ 2085) paid to employees of an S corporation is different for owner-employees than for other employees (Code Sec. 1372).[62] Fringe benefits paid to S corporation employees who are not shareholders, or who own 2 percent or less of the outstanding S corporation stock, are tax free. They can be excluded from the employees' taxable wages and are deductible as fringe benefits by the corporation. Employee-owners owning more than 2 percent of the S corporation stock, on the other hand, are not treated as employees for fringe benefit purposes, and their fringe benefits may not be tax free. More-than-2-percent owners are treated in the same manner as partners in a partnership (¶ 421).

Health Insurance Expenses. An owner-employee who owns more than 2 percent of the S corporation stock can deduct 100 percent of the amount paid for medical insurance for himself, his spouse and dependents under a plan established by the S corporation (Code Sec. 162(l)(1) and (5); Notice 2008-1).[63] The S corporation must either pay the plan's premium payments itself or must reimburse the shareholder for the payments.

For purposes of the deduction, a more-than-2-percent shareholder's wages from the S corporation are treated as the shareholder's earned income. No deduction is allowed in excess of an individual's earned income within the meaning of Code Sec. 401(c) derived from the trade or business with respect to which the plan providing the health insurance is established.

Tax Treatment of Distributions

323. S Corporation Distributions. Distributions of cash or property received by a shareholder from an S corporation are taxed accordingly depending on whether the corporation has earnings and profits. An S corporation generally has no earnings and profits unless attributable to tax years when the corporation was not an S corporation. An S corporation may also succeed to the earnings and profits of an acquired or merged corporation.

For an S corporation without earnings and profits, distributions are treated first as a nontaxable return of capital to the extent of the shareholder's basis in stock and then as a gain from the sale or exchange of property (Code Sec. 1368(b); Reg. § 1.1368-1(c)).[64]

References are to Standard Federal Tax Reports; Tax Research Consultant; and Practical Tax Explanations.

[61] ¶ 32,080; SCORP: 404; § 28,430.25

[62] ¶ 32,160; SCORP: 352.20; § 28,801

[63] ¶ 8500, ¶ 32,161.50; SCORP: 352.20; § 28,815

[64] ¶ 32,120, ¶ 32,120B; SCORP: 452; § 28,505

For an S corporation with earnings and profits, unless an election is made to distribute the earnings and profits as dividends (¶ 333), distributions are treated as:

(1) a nontaxable return of capital, to the extent of the corporation's "accumulated adjustments account" (AAA) (¶ 325);

(2) dividends, to the extent of the S corporation's accumulated earnings and profits;

(3) a nontaxable return of capital, to the extent of the shareholder's remaining stock basis; and

(4) gain from the sale or exchange of property (Code Sec. 1368(c); Reg. § 1.1368-1(d)).[65]

Before applying these rules, the shareholder's stock basis and the AAA are adjusted for the corporate items passed through from the corporate tax year during which the distribution is made.

If an employee stock ownership plan (ESOP) holds S corporation shares that are employer securities, and the ESOP took out a loan to purchase the employer securities, the prohibited transaction rules will not apply to distributions by the S corporation that are used to repay the loan, and the plan's status as an ESOP will not be jeopardized (Code Sec. 4975(f)(7)).[66]

325. Accumulated Adjustments Account. The accumulated adjustments account (AAA) is used to compute the tax effect of distributions made by an S corporation with accumulated earnings and profits (¶ 323) (Code Sec. 1368(e); Reg. § 1.1368-2).[67] The AAA is generally a measure of the corporation's accumulated gross income, less expenses, that has not been distributed. The AAA is zero on the first day of a corporation's first S corporation tax year. It is *increased* by:

(1) all corporate income items (excluding tax-exempt income items) that are separately stated and passed through to shareholders (¶ 320);

(2) nonseparately computed corporate income; and

(3) the excess of deductions for depletion over the basis of the property subject to depletion.

The AAA is *decreased* by:

(1) certain nontaxable corporate distributions;

(2) all loss and deduction items of the corporation that are separately stated and passed through (other than items that are not deductible in computing taxable income and not properly chargeable to capital account);

(3) the nonseparately computed loss of the corporation;

(4) the nondeductible amounts that are unrelated to the production of tax-exempt income; and

(5) the amount of the shareholder's deduction for oil and gas depletion.

As indicated, an S corporation's AAA is not increased by tax-exempt income, and it is not decreased by an expense related to the tax-exempt income. For example, premiums paid by an S corporation on an employer-owned life insurance contract (COLI), of which the S corporation is a beneficiary, do not reduce the S corporation's AAA. Nor is the AAA increased by death benefits received by the corporation under the policy that meets one of the exceptions for COLI (¶ 804) (Rev. Rul. 2008-42).[68]

No adjustment is made for federal taxes arising when the corporation was a C corporation. Because the AAA may become negative, the account becomes positive only after the negative balance is restored by later income (Code Sec. 1368(e)(1)(A); Reg. § 1.1368-2).[69] The amount in the AAA as of the close of a tax year is determined without regard to any net negative adjustment for the tax year. A negative adjustment occurs in

---

[65] ¶ 32,120, ¶ 32,120B; SCORP: 454; § 28,510.05, § 28,510.20
[66] ¶ 34,400; RETIRE: 75,302

[67] ¶ 32,120, ¶ 32,120C; SCORP: 458; § 28,510.10
[68] ¶ 32,121.20; SCORP: 458.05; § 28,510.10

[69] ¶ 32,120, ¶ 32,120C; SCORP: 458.05, SCORP: 458.10; § 28,510.10

any tax year in which negative adjustments to the account exceed increases to the account.

Distributions received by an S corporation shareholder in a stock redemption that is treated as a Code Sec. 301 distribution are treated as distributions that reduce the S corporation's AAA (Rev. Rul. 95-14).[70] For a distribution in redemption of an S corporation's stock, if the redemption is treated as an exchange under Code Sec. 302 or 303, the AAA is decreased by an amount determined by multiplying the account balance by the number of shares redeemed and dividing the product by the total number of shares outstanding. This adjustment is made before the distribution rules are applied (Code Sec. 1368(e)(1)(B)).

The AAA relates only to the most recent continuous period in which the corporation has been an S corporation. However, the period does not include tax years beginning before January 1, 1983 (Code Sec. 1368(e)(2); Reg. § 1.1368-2(a)).[71] If corporate distributions during a tax year exceed the amount in the AAA at the end of that year, the balance of the account is allocated among distributions in proportion to their respective sizes (¶ 329) (Code Sec. 1368(c)).[72]

329. Post-Termination Distributions by S Corporations. If an S corporation ends its election, the corporation has the opportunity for a limited period of time to unfreeze the income that was previously taxed to shareholders under the passthrough rules but that was not actually distributed by the corporation. Specifically, any cash distribution by the corporation with respect to its stock during the post-termination transition period is applied against and reduces the adjusted basis of the stock to the extent that the amount of the distribution does not exceed the AAA (Code Secs. 1371(e) and 1377(b)).[73]

The term "post-termination transition period" is:

(1) the period beginning on the day after the last day of the corporation's last tax year as an S corporation and ending on the later of: (a) the day which is one year after such last day or (b) the due date for filing the return for the last tax year as an S corporation (including extensions);

(2) the 120-day period beginning on the date of any determination pursuant to an audit of the taxpayer which follows the termination of the corporation's election and which adjusts a subchapter S item of income, loss, or deduction of the corporation arising during the S period (Code Sec. 1368(e)(2));[74] or

(3) the 120-day period beginning on the date of a determination that the corporation's election had ended for a previous tax year.

If the AAA is not exhausted by the end of the post-termination transition period, it disappears. Any distributions made thereafter are taxed under the usual subchapter C rules—first, as a distribution of current earnings and profits; next, as a distribution of accumulated earnings and profits; then, as a return of capital to the extent of the shareholder's basis; and, finally, as a capital gain. Because the AAA is always reflected in the basis of the shareholder's stock, failure to exhaust it during the transition period moves it, in effect, below current and accumulated earnings and profits in the priority system for distributions. The grace period for post-termination distributions applies only to cash distributions. It does not apply to noncash distributions. A noncash distribution is taxed under the usual subchapter C rules.

333. S Corporation Election to Distribute Earnings. An S corporation can avoid the priority system (¶ 323) for treatment of distributions by electing to treat distributions as dividends (Code Sec. 1368(e)(3); Reg. § 1.1368-1(f)(2)).[75] An S corporation might elect to treat a distribution as taxable dividends if it wants to avoid a termination of its Subchapter S status on account of excess passive investment income. However, all shareholders who receive a distribution during the tax year must consent to such treatment. If the election is made, the corporation is not required to distribute its entire AAA (¶ 325) at the end of its tax year before it can pay a dividend.

References are to Standard Federal Tax Reports; Tax Research Consultant; and Practical Tax Explanations.

[70] ¶ 32,121.20; SCORP: 458.15; § 28,510.10

[71] ¶ 32,120, ¶ 32,120C; SCORP: 458.05; § 28,510.10

[72] ¶ 32,120; SCORP: 454; § 28,510.10

[73] ¶ 32,140, ¶ 32,240; SCORP: 462; § 28,515

[74] ¶ 32,120; SCORP: 462; § 28,515

[75] ¶ 32,120, ¶ 32,120B; SCORP: 456; § 28,510.25

Taxation of Corporation

335. Taxation of S Corporation. Since an S corporation is a passthrough entity (¶ 301 and ¶ 309), it is generally not subject to federal income taxes. However, an S corporation may be liable for the following corporate-level tax liabilities and is required to make estimated tax payments attributable to them:

(1) the tax imposed on built-in gains or capital gains (¶ 337);

(2) the tax on excess net passive income (¶ 341);

(3) the recapture of the investment credit on the disposition of property placed in service before 1985; and

(4) the recapture of LIFO benefits upon conversion to an S corporation (¶ 339) (Code Sec. 6655(g)(4)).[76]

If the S corporation was incorporated after 1982, immediately became an S corporation, and has no earnings or profits, only the capital gains tax applies. If the S corporation was incorporated and elected S corporation status before 1987, the tax on built-in gains does not apply.

337. Tax on Built-In Gains of S Corporation. A corporate-level tax ("built-in gains tax") is imposed on S corporations that dispose of assets that appreciated in value during tax years when the corporation was a C corporation (Code Sec. 1374).[77] The built-in gains tax applies only to corporations that made S corporation elections after 1986. A tax imposed on certain capital gains of S corporations continues to apply to corporations that made S elections before 1987.

An S corporation may be liable for tax on its built-in gains if:

(1) it was a C corporation prior to making its S corporation election;

(2) it has a net recognized built-in gain within the recognition period; and

(3) the net recognized built-in gain for the tax year does not exceed the net unrealized built-in gain minus the net recognized built-in gain for prior years in the recognition period, to the extent that such gains were subject to tax.

A recognized built-in loss is any loss recognized during the recognition period on the disposition of any asset to the extent that the S corporation establishes that: (1) the asset was held by the S corporation at the beginning of its first tax year as an S corporation, and (2) the loss is not greater than the excess of (a) the adjusted basis of the asset at the beginning of the corporation's first tax year as an S corporation, over (b) the fair market value of the asset at that time.

Recognition Period. For assets disposed of during an S corporation's tax year beginning after December 31, 2013, the recognition period for net built-in gain is the ten-year period beginning on the first day on which the corporation is an S corporation or acquires C corporation assets in a carryover basis transaction (Code Sec. 1374(d)(7); Reg. § 1.1374-1(d)).[78] For example, if the first day of the recognition period is July 12, 2004, the last day of the recognition period is July 11, 2014.

For assets disposed of during an S corporation's tax year beginning in 2011, 2012, or 2013, the recognition period for net built-in gain is reduced to five years. For example, if the first day of the recognition period is July 12, 2008, the last day of the recognition period will be July 11, 2013. The reduction in the recognition period for 2011 through 2013 applies separately with respect to any asset acquired in a carryover basis transaction.

> **Planning Note:** Absent further legislation, the reduction of the recognition period for build-in gains to five years has expired for assets disposed of during an S corporation's tax year beginning after December 31, 2013. For the latest legislative updates, visit our website www.CCHGroup.com/TaxUpdates.

Amount of Tax. The tax is computed by applying the highest corporate income tax rate to the S corporation's net recognized built-in gain for the tax year. The amount of

---

References are to Standard Federal Tax Reports; Tax Research Consultant; and Practical Tax Explanations.

[76] ¶ 39,565; SCORP: 362, SCORP: 370; § 28,315.05, § 29,020.15

[77] ¶ 32,201; SCORP: 356; § 28,305.05

[78] ¶ 32,201, ¶ 32,201C; SCORP: 356.05; § 28,305.15

the net recognized built-in gain is taxable income. However, any net operating loss carryforward arising in a tax year in which the corporation was a C corporation is allowed as a deduction against the net recognized built-in gain of the S corporation. Capital loss carryforwards may also be used to offset recognized built-in gains (Code Sec. 1374(b) and (d); Reg. § 1.1374-5).[79] Furthermore, business tax credit carryovers of an S corporation, arising in a tax year in which the corporation was a C corporation, can offset the built-in gains tax of the S corporation (Code Sec. 1374(b)(3)(B); Reg. § 1.1374-6).[80]

Installment Sales. If an S corporation sells an asset within the recognition period and reports the sale under the installment method (¶ 1801), the payments received, whether within the recognition period or not, are subject to the built-in gains tax to the extent they are built-in gains (Code Sec. 1374(d)(7)(E)).[81]

The term "net recognized built-in gain" means the lesser of (1) the amount that would be the taxable income of the S corporation if only recognized built-in gains and recognized built-in losses were taken into account, or (2) the corporation's taxable income (Code Sec. 1374(d)(2); Reg. § 1.1374-2).[82] In the case of a corporation that made its S corporation election on or after March 31, 1988, any net recognized built-in gain that is not subject to the built-in gains tax due to the net income limitation is carried forward. The amount of recognized built-in gain passed through and taxed to shareholders is reduced by the tax imposed on the built-in gain and paid by the S corporation (Code Sec. 1366(f)(2)).[83]

339. LIFO Recapture by S Corporation. A C corporation that maintains its inventory using the last-in, first-out (LIFO) method (¶ 1565) for its last tax year before an S corporation election becomes effective must include in gross income a LIFO recapture amount when it converts to S corporation status. LIFO recapture is also required for transfers of inventory from a C corporation to an S corporation in a tax-free reorganization (Code Sec. 1363(d); Reg. § 1.1363-2).[84] The LIFO recapture amount is the amount, if any, by which the amount of the inventory assets using the first-in, first-out (FIFO) method (¶ 1564) exceeds the inventory amount of such assets under the LIFO method.

The tax attributable to the inclusion in income of any LIFO recapture amount is payable by the corporation in four equal installments. The first payment is due on or before the due date of the corporate tax return for the electing corporation's last tax year as a C corporation. The three subsequent installments are due on or before the respective due dates of the S corporation's returns for the three succeeding tax years. No interest is payable on these installments if they are paid by the respective due dates.

341. Passive Investment Income of S Corporation. S corporations with Subchapter C earnings and profits and with total passive investment income totaling more than 25 percent of gross receipts are subject to an income tax computed by multiplying the corporation's excess net passive income by the highest corporate income tax rate (Code Sec. 1375; Reg. § 1.1375-1).[85] Passive investment income is gross receipts derived from royalties, rents, dividends, interest (excluding interest on installment sales of inventory to customers and income of certain lending and financing businesses), and annuities (Code Sec. 1362(d)(3)(C); Reg. § 1.1362-2(c)(5)).[86] However, such income derived by an S corporation in the ordinary course of its trade or business is generally excluded from the definition of passive investment income. In the case of an S corporation bank (including a bank holding company and a depository institution holding company), passive investment income does not include interest earned by the bank and any dividends received on assets that the bank is required to hold. The exception for assets applies to stock in the Federal Reserve Bank, Federal Home Loan Bank, or Federal Agriculture Mortgage Bank, and participation certificates issued by a Federal Intermediate Credit Bank.

References are to Standard Federal Tax Reports; Tax Research Consultant; and Practical Tax Explanations.

[79] ¶ 32,201, ¶ 32,202H; SCORP: 356.10, SCORP: 356.25; § 28,305.40

[80] ¶ 32,201, ¶ 32,202J; SCORP: 356.30; § 28,305.45

[81] ¶ 32,201; SCORP: 356.55

[82] ¶ 32,201, ¶ 32,202B; SCORP: 356.05; § 28,305.20

[83] ¶ 32,080; SCORP: 402.05; § 28,305.65

[84] ¶ 32,060, ¶ 32,061B; SCORP: 352.35; § 28,315.05

[85] ¶ 32,220, ¶ 32,221; SCORP: 360; § 28,310.05

[86] ¶ 32,040, ¶ 32,043; SCORP: 360; § 28,310.20

Excess net passive income is the amount that bears the same ratio to net passive income as the amount of passive investment income that exceeds 25 percent of gross receipts bears to passive investment income (Code Sec. 1375(b); Reg. § 1.1375-1(b)).[87] Net passive income is passive investment income reduced by any allowable deduction directly connected with the production of such income except for the net operating loss deduction (¶ 1145) and the special deductions allowed to corporations in computing taxable income (¶ 221—¶ 237). Excess net passive income cannot exceed the corporation's taxable income for the tax year computed without regard to any net operating loss deduction and without regard to the special deductions allowed to corporations, other than the deduction for organizational expenditures (¶ 237). Passive investment income is determined without taking into account any recognized built-in gain or loss during the recognition period (¶ 337). This means that S corporations without earnings and profits cannot be taxed on excess net passive income if they have no taxable income. This can happen if the corporation has net operating losses and income from passive investments. The tax is not merely carried over; there is no tax due if during the year the corporation did not have taxable income.

The tax on excess net passive income reduces each item of passive income by the amount of tax attributable to it and thereby reduces the amount of passive investment income that each shareholder must take into account in computing gross income (Code Sec. 1366(f)(3)).[88]

The only credits allowable against the passive investment income tax are those for certain uses of gasoline and special fuels (¶ 1329) (Code Sec. 1375(c); Reg. § 1.1375-1(c)).[89]

The IRS may waive the tax on excess net passive income if the S corporation establishes that it made a good-faith determination at the close of the tax year that it had no C corporation earnings and profits and that it distributed such earnings and profits within a reasonable time after determining that they existed (Code Sec. 1375(d); Reg. § 1.1375-1(d)).[90]

349. Foreign Income of S Corporation. Foreign taxes paid by an S corporation pass through to shareholders who can elect to treat them as deductions or credits on their individual returns (Code Sec. 1373).[91] Since an S corporation is treated as a partnership (rather than a corporation) for purposes of the foreign tax credit provisions of the Code, neither it nor its shareholders may claim the indirect foreign tax credit (¶ 2475) for taxes paid by a foreign corporation in which the S corporation is a shareholder. The foreign loss recapture rules apply to an S corporation that previously passed foreign losses through to the shareholders and subsequently terminates its S corporation status. For the purpose of computing the amount of foreign losses that must be recaptured, the making or termination of an S corporation election is treated as a disposition of the business.

Returns and Tax Year

351. S Corporation Returns. An S corporation is required to file Form 1120S for each tax year that the election to be treated as an S corporation is in effect (¶ 303), regardless of whether the corporation has taxable income for that year (Reg. § 1.6012-2(h)).[92] An S corporation's return is due on or before the 15th day of the third month following the close of the tax year (Reg. § 1.6037-1(b)).[93] An automatic six-month extension of time to file the S corporation's return may be obtained by filing Form 7004 on or before the due date of its Form 1120S (Reg. § 1.6081-3(a)).[94]

References are to Standard Federal Tax Reports; Tax Research Consultant; and Practical Tax Explanations.

[87] ¶ 32,220, ¶ 32,221; SCORP: 358; § 28,310.10
[88] ¶ 32,080; SCORP: 356, SCORP: 402.05; § 28,310.05, § 28,310.30
[89] ¶ 32,220, ¶ 32,221; SCORP: 360; § 28,310.05
[90] ¶ 32,220, ¶ 32,221; SCORP: 360; § 28,310.25
[91] ¶ 32,180; SCORP: 364; § 13,405.20, § 28,410.05
[92] ¶ 35,145; SCORP: 500; § 29,010.10
[93] ¶ 35,521; SCORP: 500; § 29,010.10
[94] ¶ 36,790; FILEBUS: 15,104.10; § 29,010.10

An S corporation is required to provide to each shareholder a copy of the information shown on Schedule K-1 that is attached to Form 1120S. The information must be provided on or before the day the corporation files Form 1120S (Code Sec. 6037(b)).[95]

An S corporation that fails to timely file any required return may be subject to penalties (¶ 353).

353. Failure to File Penalties for S Corporations. An S corporation that fails to timely file Form 1120S (¶ 351) (or files an incomplete return) is liable for a penalty of $195 per shareholder, per month for a maximum of twelve months, unless reasonable cause is shown (Code Sec. 6699).[96] An S corporation may not contest the penalty assessment in the Tax Court but can pay the entire penalty and then sue for a refund.

An S corporation may also be subject to penalties for failure to furnish Schedules K-1 to its shareholders (Code Sec. 6722).[97] For each failure to furnish Schedule K-1 to a shareholder when due and each failure to include on Schedule K-1 all the information required to be shown (or the inclusion of incorrect information), a $100 penalty may be imposed with regard to each Schedule K-1 for which a failure occurs. If the requirement to report correct information is intentionally disregarded, each penalty is increased to the greater of $250 or 10 percent of the aggregate amount of items required to be reported.

355. Tax Year of S Corporation. The tax year of an S corporation must be a permitted year. Permitted years include the calendar year, a tax year elected under Code Sec. 444 (¶ 1501), a 52-53 week tax year ending with reference to the calendar year or a tax year elected under Code Sec. 444, or any other tax year for which the corporation establishes a business purpose to the satisfaction of the IRS (Reg. § 1.1378-1(a)).[98] The procedures for an S corporation to establish a business purpose are contained in Rev. Proc. 2006-46.[99]

An S corporation may elect to have a tax year other than its required tax year. Generally, this election may be made only if the deferral period of the tax year elected is not longer than three months. The S corporation makes this election by filing Form 8716 (¶ 1501). If such an election is made, the S corporation may be required to make certain tax payments.

References are to Standard Federal Tax Reports; Tax Research Consultant; and Practical Tax Explanations.

[95] ¶ 35,520; SCORP: 500; § 29,010.10

[96] ¶ 40,023; PENALTY: 3,208.45; § 29,010.20

[97] ¶ 40,230; PENALTY: 3,204.05; § 29,010.20

[98] ¶ 32,261; SCORP: 252, SCORP: 258; § 28,410.15

[99] ¶ 32,262.10; SCORP: 256; § 28,410.15

Chapter 4

PARTNERSHIPS

Choice of Entity

401. Partnership Defined. A partnership includes a syndicate, group, pool, joint venture, or other unincorporated organization that carries on any business, financial operation, or venture, and that is not, within the meaning of the Code, a trust, estate, or corporation (Code Sec. 761).[1] A noncorporate entity with at least two members can be classified under the check-the-box rules (¶ 402A) either as a partnership or as an association taxable as a corporation. A noncorporate entity with one member can be taxed either as a corporation or as a sole proprietorship (Reg. § 301.7701-3).[2]

401A. Limited Partnerships. A limited partnership is a partnership (¶ 401) that has one or more general partners and one or more limited partners. Limited partnerships are formed under the limited partnership laws of each state. Unlike general partnerships in which all the partners are responsible for partnership liabilities, limited partners are not responsible for partnership liabilities beyond the amount of their investments. In addition, under state law, limited partners cannot participate in partnership management.

401B. Limited Liability Partnerships. Limited liability partnerships (LLPs) are partnerships (¶ 401) that are generally used by professionals such as accountants or attorneys. An LLP is a general partnership in which each individual partner remains liable for his or her own malpractice as well as the liabilities arising out of the wrongful acts or omissions of those over whom the partner has supervisory duties. The increasing use of LLPs reflects changed perceptions as to the traditional concepts of joint and several liability for large professional partnerships with hundreds of partners scattered over the country or even on different continents.

Each state and the District of Columbia have LLP-enabling legislation. Some states offer members of LLPs limited protection from partnership liabilities, such as limiting the protection to malpractice claims against other partners. Other states offer full protection from liabilities, including the partnership's contractual liabilities. These are called "full shield" states.

As a practical matter, LLPs are most likely to be used to give liability protection to partners in an existing partnership. This conversion does not create a new partnership, as the IRS has ruled that the registration of a general partnership as a registered limited liability partnership does not cause a termination of the partnership for purposes of Code

---

References are to Standard Federal Tax Reports; Tax Research Consultant; and Practical Tax Explanations.

[1] ¶ 25,600; PART: 3,100; § 30,015.05

[2] ¶ 43,083; PART: 3,102; § 30,015.10

¶401B

Sec. 708(b) (Rev. Rul. 95-55).[3] In such a case, the partnership is required to continue to use the same method of accounting used before its registration. Each partners total percentage interest in the partnership's profits, losses, and capital remains the same after the registration as an LLP.

Limited Liability Limited Partnerships. Some states have passed legislation allowing limited liability limited partnerships (LLLPs). These entities operate like a traditional limited partnership, but the general partner also has the limitations on personal liability of a partner in a limited liability partnership.

402. Exclusion from Partnership Provisions. In two different sets of circumstances, entities that would otherwise be considered partnerships (¶ 401) may elect to not have all or part of Subchapter K apply or to not be treated as partnerships for federal income tax purposes. Application of the partnership tax rules can be avoided in certain cases where the income of the partners can be adequately determined without partnership-level computation and in the case of certain husband-wife partnerships.

Unincorporated organizations may elect not to be taxed as partnerships if they are used either for investment purposes only or for the joint production, extraction, or use— but not the sale—of property under an operating agreement (Code Sec. 761(a)).[4] The exclusion also can be used by securities dealers for a short period for the purpose of underwriting, selling, or distributing a particular issue of securities. The exclusion can be elected only if the partners' incomes can be determined without computing the entity's income first.

An unincorporated organization may choose to be completely or only partially excluded from the partnership provisions. However, the IRS does not allow an organization making the partial election to be excluded from the tax-year conformity rules of Code Sec. 706 or from the limitations on the allowance of losses (¶ 416 and ¶ 425) (Rev. Rul. 57-215).[5] This election removes the entity from all or a portion of the subchapter K partnership provisions.

Qualified Joint Ventures. A business co-owned by a husband and wife who file a joint return may elect to be taxed as a qualified joint venture instead of a partnership for federal tax purposes (Code Sec. 761(f)).[6] A qualified joint venture is a joint venture involving the conduct of a trade or business if (1) the only members of the joint venture are a husband and wife, (2) both spouses materially participate in the trade or business, and (3) both spouses elect to have the provision apply. The IRS takes the position that qualified joint ventures include only businesses that are owned and operated by spouses as co-owners, and do not include businesses that are run as a state law entity, such as a limited liability company (IRS Pub. 1635).

All items of income, gain, loss, deduction, and credit from a qualified joint venture are divided between the spouses in accordance with their respective interests in the venture. Each spouse takes into account his or her respective share of these items as a sole proprietor. Each spouse should account for his or her respective share on the appropriate form (Schedule C or Schedule F of Form 1040).

402A. Check-the-Box Regulations. Most entities that qualify for partnership treatment also qualify for electing out of partnership treatment under the check-the-box regulations. Any business entity not required to be treated as a corporation for federal tax purposes may choose its own classification (Reg. § 301.7701-3).[7] An entity with two or more members can be classified either as a partnership or as an association taxed as a corporation. An entity with only one member can choose to be taxed as a corporation or can be disregarded as an entity separate from its owner. A single-member limited liability company (SMLLC) cannot elect partnership status because a partnership, by definition, has two or more partners.

References are to Standard Federal Tax Reports; Tax Research Consultant; and Practical Tax Explanations.

[3] ¶ 25,202.27; PART: 3,108; § 30,005.15

[4] ¶ 25,600; PART: 3,350; § 30,015.20

[5] ¶ 25,602.11; PART: 3,356.15; § 30,015.20

[6] ¶ 25,600; PART: 3,358; § 30,015.20

[7] ¶ 43,083; PART: 3,102; § 30,015.10

Domestic entities with two or more members that do not file an election have a default classification of partnership. A domestic entity with one member that does not elect to be taxed as a corporation is considered a disregarded entity—i.e., it is ignored, and the taxpayer is treated as a sole proprietorship. Thus, a domestic LLC will be taxed as a partnership or disregarded entity unless it files an election to be taxed as a corporation.

The check-the-box rules apply somewhat differently to foreign business organizations. Entities listed in Reg. § 301.7701-2(b)(8) are considered corporations and are not eligible to be partnerships under the check-the-box rules. Any other foreign entity may be taxed as either a corporation or partnership (or a disregarded entity if it has one owner). A foreign business entity where all owners have limited liability will generally be treated as a corporation unless it elects to be taxed as a partnership. A foreign business entity where one or more owners has unlimited liability will generally be taxed as a partnership unless it elects to be taxed as a corporation. Thus, the foreign equivalent of an LLC (such as a German *GmbH*), where all members have limited liability, will be taxed as a corporation unless it elects to be taxed as a partnership. The default classification for foreign and domestic entities existing before January 1, 1997, is the classification the entity claimed immediately prior to that date.

Note that the term "limited liability" is not precisely defined by the regulations, and it may be uncertain whether the IRS would consider a given foreign law to provide for limited liability for all members of an entity. It will usually be easier and safer for practitioners to file an election under the check-the-box rules for a foreign entity rather than to determine what its default classification would be.

An election not to be taxed as a partnership under the check-the-box regulations is filed on Form 8832 and applies to all Code provisions. This is different from an election under Code Sec. 761 (¶ 402), which removes a partnership only from the provisions of subchapter K (Code Secs. 701—777).[8]

402B. Limited Liability Companies. A state-registered limited liability company (LLC) can be taxed as a partnership for federal income tax purposes. However, its members, like corporate shareholders, are not personally liable for the entity's debts or liabilities. Under the check-the-box rules, an LLC can choose partnership status to avoid taxation at the entity level as an association taxed as a corporation.

Unlike limited partners, LLC members may participate in management without risking personal liability for company debts. In addition, no limitations are placed on the number of owners as compared to a maximum limit on the number of S corporation shareholders. There is also no limitation on the different types of owners of an LLC compared with S corporations which may generally only have U.S. resident individuals or certain types of trusts as shareholders. Additional advantages over S corporations include the ability to make disproportionate allocations and distributions (Code Sec. 704)[9] and to distribute appreciated property to members without the recognition of gain (Code Sec. 731(b)).[10] Members may also exchange appreciated property for membership interests without the recognition of gain or loss (Code Sec. 721).[11]

Conversion from Partnership to LLC. A conversion of a partnership into an LLC that is taxed as a partnership for federal income tax purposes is treated as a nontaxable partnership-to-partnership conversion (Rev. Rul. 95-37).[12] The conversion is treated as a contribution of assets to the new partnership under Code Sec. 721 and does not result in gain or loss to the partners. The tax results are the same whether the LLC is formed in the same state as the former partnership or in a different state. Upon such a conversion, the tax year of the converting partnership does not close with respect to any of the partners, and the resulting LLC does not need to obtain a new taxpayer identification number.

References are to Standard Federal Tax Reports; Tax Research Consultant; and Practical Tax Explanations.

[8] ¶ 25,060—¶ 25,628; PART: 100; § 30,001

[9] ¶ 25,120; PART: 30,000; § 30,501

[10] ¶ 25,320; PART: 33,152; § 30,530.05

[11] ¶ 25,240; PART: 9,050; § 30,105.10

[12] ¶ 25,243.13; PART: 3,106.10; § 30,930.20

Conversion from C Corporation to LLC. The conversion of an existing C corporation into an LLC taxed as a partnership is generally treated as a liquidation of the corporation and thus a taxable event for both the corporation and the shareholders (Code Sec. 7701; LTR 9701029).[13] The possible tax hit diminishes the attractiveness of existing corporate entities converting to LLCs. This is especially true if the corporation holds appreciated property. Only a corporation with little or no net worth and shareholders with bases exceeding the amount of any distribution can escape this tax result. The conversion can be accomplished in one of two ways: (1) the assets of the corporation can be contributed to the LLC in return for membership interests which are then distributed to the shareholders in liquidation of the corporation; or (2) the corporation can distribute its assets in complete liquidation, and the shareholders can then contribute their undivided interests in the assets to the LLC in exchange for the membership interests.

Conversion from S Corporation to LLC. For an S corporation to convert to an LLC taxed as a partnership, it must undergo the same process as a C corporation discussed above. However, unlike a C corporation, when an S corporation distributes appreciated assets to its shareholders in exchange for their stock, there is no double tax. Because the S corporation is a flowthrough entity, the gain incurred at the corporate level passes through to the shareholders and is generally included in income on the shareholder's individual tax return.

Any gain recognized by the shareholder as a result of the gain attributable to the liquidating distribution increases the shareholder's stock basis. The shareholder's increased basis then reduces the amount of gain recognized or increases the amount of loss recognized. Thus, with one exception relating to the built-in gains tax (¶ 337), there is a single level of taxation. Although, with an S corporation, there is usually only this one level of taxation, rather than the two levels of taxation inherent with the C corporation, this single level of taxation may still be enough to dissuade an S corporation from converting to an LLC.

Series LLCs. Several states, including Delaware, permit the creation of separate series within an LLC. The debts and other liabilities of each series are only enforceable against that series. Each series is recognized as a distinct entity for state law purposes and each series can have its own separate business purposes. A series can be terminated without affecting the other series of the LLC. Under proposed regulations, effective when they are published as final, each series of a series organization (such as a series LLC) would be treated for federal tax purposes as an entity formed under local law, regardless of whether local law actually treats the series as a separate entity (Prop. Reg. § 301.7701-1(a)(5)).[14]

Publicly Traded Partnerships

403. Publicly Traded Partnerships. A publicly traded partnership (PTP) is taxed as a corporation unless 90 percent or more of its gross income is derived from qualifying passive income sources—interest, dividends, real property rents, gain from the disposition of real property, mining and natural resource income, and gain from the disposition of capital assets or Code Sec. 1231(b) property held for the production of such income (Code Sec. 7704).[15] A PTP is a partnership with interests traded on an established securities market or readily tradable on a secondary market (or its substantial equivalent), including master limited partnerships. A partnership that was publicly traded on December 17, 1987, continues to be treated as a partnership rather than a corporation if it meets certain conditions (Code Sec. 7704(g); Reg. § 1.7704-2(a)(1)).[16]

A grandfather rule exempts electing 1987 partnerships from corporate treatment if the partnership existed as a PTP or was treated as having existed as a PTP on December 17, 1987, elected to continue its partnership status, and does not add a substantial new line of business. A grandfathered electing 1987 partnership must pay an annual 3.5-percent tax on any income from the conduct of an active business.

References are to Standard Federal Tax Reports; Tax Research Consultant; and Practical Tax Explanations.

[13] ¶ 43,080; LLC: 18,150   [15] ¶ 43,180; PART: 3,250   [16] ¶ 43,180, ¶ 43,181; PART: 3,256
[14] ¶ 43,081A; STAGES: 24,200

¶403

Partnership-Level Issues

404. Partners Taxation Principals. A partnership does not pay federal income tax; rather, items of partnership income, gain, loss, deduction, and credit flow through to the partners, who are taxed in their individual capacities on their distributive shares of partnership taxable income. However, a partnership is a tax-reporting entity that must file an annual partnership return (¶ 406). In determining federal income tax, a partner must take into account his or her distributive share of partnership income or loss for the year, as well as his or her distributive share of certain separately stated items (¶ 431) of partnership income, gain, loss, deduction, or credit. A partner's distributive share of partnership items is includible on his or her individual income tax return (or corporate income tax return for corporate partners) for his or her tax year in which the partnership tax year ends (Code Sec. 706(a)).[17]

A partner is generally not taxed on distributions of cash (including marketable securities) or property received from the partnership, except to the extent that any money (including marketable securities) distributed exceeds the partner's adjusted basis in his or her partnership interest immediately before the distribution (¶ 453). Taxable gain can also result from distributions of property that were contributed to a partnership with a built-in gain (if property has a fair market value in excess of its adjusted basis) and from property distributions that are characterized as sales and exchanges (¶ 432).

A 3.8-percent net investment income tax is applicable to individuals, estates, and trusts, but not to partnerships (¶ 129) (Code Sec. 1411).[18] Income from trades or businesses conducted by partnerships is not considered net investment income. However, income from a trade or business that is a passive activity with respect to the partner is included in the partner's net investment income. Thus, the partner's distributive share of income earned by a partnership that would otherwise be net investment income in the hands of the partner is considered net investment income to the partner.

406. Partnership Return (Form 1065). Annual information reporting on Form 1065 is required by a partnership regardless of whether or not the partnership has taxable income for the tax year. Although Code Sec. 6063[19] states that the return may be signed by any one of the partners, the instructions to Form 1065 indicate that the form must be signed by one of the partnership's general partners or, in the case of an LLC, by one of the member managers (¶ 415). A U.S. partnership's return on Form 1065 is due on or before the 15th day of the fourth month following the close of the tax year. A foreign partnership that does not have U.S.-source income is not required to file a partnership return if the partnership has no income effectively connected with U.S. trade or business, and no U.S. partners at any time during the partnership's tax year (Reg. § 1.6031(a)-1(b)(3)(ii)).[20] Form 7004 should be used to apply for an automatic five-month filing extension (Reg. § 1.6081-2).[21]

If a partnership that is required to file a return for any tax year fails to file a return on time or fails to include all the information required to be shown on the return, the partnership is subject to a penalty for each month or fraction of a month the failure continues, up to a maximum of twelve months, unless the partnership shows that the failure is due to reasonable cause. The penalty generally is $195, multiplied by the number of persons who were partners in the partnership during any part of the tax year. Reasonable cause exists only if significant mitigating factors are present, or the failure to file arose from factors beyond the filer's control, and the filer establishes that it acted in a responsible manner both before and after the failure. A partnership may not contest the penalty assessment in the Tax Court but must pay the entire penalty and then sue for a refund (Code Sec. 6698).[22] Certain domestic partnerships with 10 or fewer partners

---

References are to Standard Federal Tax Reports; Tax Research Consultant; and Practical Tax Explanations.

[17] ¶ 25,160; PART: 6,052; § 30,125

[18] ¶ 32,602; INDIV: 69,160.60; § 1,022.15

[19] ¶ 36,640; PART: 18,160.05; § 30,435

[20] ¶ 35,383; PART: 18,160.15; § 39,205.15

[21] ¶ 36,788; PART: 18,160.05; § 39,215.20

[22] ¶ 39,995; PART: 18,162.10; § 30,435

do not have to pay the penalty if all partners have fully reported their distributive shares on timely filed income tax returns (Rev. Proc. 84-35).[23]

A partnership that is required to file a Form 1065 generally must furnish each partner with a Schedule K-1 that provides the partner's distributive share of partnership income, gain, loss, deduction, or credit, and any additional information that is necessary to enable the partner to determine the correct income tax treatment of a partnership item (Temp. Reg. § 1.6031(b)-1T(a)(3); Rev. Proc. 2012-17).[24] Effective February 13, 2012, in order to provide Schedule K-1 to partners in an electronic format, a partnership must obtain their consent. IRS approval to use a substitute K-1 is not required if the electronic copy furnished is an exact copy of the official Schedule K-1.

410. Changes in Partnership Membership. The tax year of a partnership closes with respect to a partner whose entire interest in the partnership ends, whether by a sale of the entire interest or otherwise (Code Sec. 706(c)(2)(A)).[25] The sale of a portion of a partnership interest does not result in the closing of the partnership's tax year with respect to the selling partner.

In the case of a sale, exchange, gift, or liquidation of a partner's entire interest in a partnership, the partnership "closes the books" as to that partner (Code Sec. 706(c)(2)(A); Reg. § 1.706-1(c)(2)).[26] In this case, the date of the disposition of the partnership interest is treated *as to the withdrawing partner* as if it is the close of the tax year. That partner's share of the partnership tax items is then determined as of that date, and the partner must include his or her share of partnership tax items in income for the tax year in which his or her partnership interest ends. However, a partnership does not have to make an interim closing of the books. Instead, a retiring partner's share of income may, by agreement among the partners, be estimated by taking a pro rata portion of the amount of such items the partner would have included in income had he or she remained a partner until the end of the partnership tax year. The prorated amount may be based on the portion of the tax year that has elapsed prior to the sale, exchange, or liquidation, or may be determined under any other method that is reasonable.

Technical Termination. A partnership is considered to terminate if, within a 12-month period, there is a sale or exchange of 50 percent or more of the total interest in partnership capital and profits (Code Sec. 708(b)(1)(B)).[27]

Changes in Partnership Interests During Tax Year. If there is a change in any partner's interest in the partnership (for instance, because of the retirement of a partner, entry of a new partner, or simply a change in the allocations of partnership items), each remaining partner's distributive share must take into account the varying interests during the partnership tax year (Code Sec. 706(d); Reg. § 1.706-1).[28] This rule generally may be satisfied either by using an interim closing of the books or by pro rating income, losses, etc., for the entire year. However, special rules apply with respect to cash-basis items and tiered partnerships.

If there is a change in any partner's interest in the partnership, the distributive shares of certain cash-method items are determined by assigning the appropriate portion of each item to each day to which it is attributable and then by allocating the daily portions among the partners in proportion to their interests in the partnership at the close of each day. For this purpose, cash-method items are interest, taxes, payments for services or for the use of property, and any other item specified in the regulations. Cash-method items deductible or includible within the tax year but attributable to a time period before the beginning of the tax year (for example, payment during the tax year for services performed in the prior tax year) are assigned to the first day of the tax year. If persons to whom such items are allocable are no longer partners on the first day of the

---

References are to Standard Federal Tax Reports; Tax Research Consultant; and Practical Tax Explanations.

[23] ¶ 40,000.10; PART: 18,162.10; § 30,435

[24] ¶ 35,385, ¶ 35,389.16; PART: 18,162.15; § 30,435

[25] ¶ 25,160; PART: 6,154; § 38,145.15

[26] ¶ 25,160, ¶ 25,161; PART: 24,112; § 30,910.05

[27] ¶ 25,200; PART: 51,100; § 31,010.05

[28] ¶ 25,160, ¶ 25,161; PART: 24,114, PART: 24,116; § 30,425.10, § 30,910.05

tax year, then their portion of the items must be capitalized by the partnership and allocated to the basis of partnership assets pursuant to Code Sec. 755. Cash-method items attributable to periods following the close of the tax year (for example, properly deductible prepaid expenses) are assigned to the last day of the tax year.

In the case of changes in a partner's interest in an upper-tier partnership that has an ownership interest in a lower-tier partnership, each partner's distributive share of any items of the upper-tier partnership attributable to the lower-tier partnership is determined by: (1) assigning the appropriate portion of each such item to the appropriate days of the upper-tier partnership's tax year on which the upper-tier partnership is a partner in the lower-tier partnership; and (2) allocating the assigned portion among the partners in proportion to their interests in the upper-tier partnership as of the close of each day (Code Sec. 706(d)(3)).[29]

415. Administrative and Judicial Proceedings at Partnership Level. The determination of the tax treatment of partnership items is generally made at the partnership level in a single administrative partnership proceeding rather than in separate proceedings with each partner. Rules from the Tax Equity and Fiscal Responsibility Act of 1982 (P.L. 97-248) (or TEFRA audit rules) govern proceedings that must be conducted at the partnership level for the assessment and collection of tax deficiencies or for tax refunds arising out of the partners' distributive shares of income, deductions, credits, and other partnership items (Code Secs. 6221—6233).[30] See also ¶ 482 for special rules applying to electing large partnerships.

Notice of the beginning of administrative proceedings and the resulting final partnership administrative adjustment (FPAA) must be given to all partners whose names and addresses are furnished to the IRS, except those with less than a 1-percent interest in partnerships that have more than 100 partners (Code Sec. 6223).[31] However, a group of partners having an aggregate profits interest of 5 percent or more may request notice to be mailed to a designated partner. Each partnership should have a tax matters partner who is to receive notice on behalf of small partners not entitled to notice and to keep all of the partners informed of all administrative and judicial proceedings at the partnership level (Code Sec. 6231).[32] The tax matters partner is either the general partner designated as such by the partnership or, in the absence of a designation, the general partner with the largest interest in partnership profits for the relevant tax year. Settlement agreements may be entered into between the tax matters partner and the IRS that bind the parties to the agreement and may extend to other partners who request to enter into consistent settlement agreements (Code Sec. 6224).[33]

Consistency Requirement. Each partner is required to treat partnership items on his or her return in a manner consistent with the treatment of such items on the partnership return (Code Sec. 6222).[34] A partner may be penalized for intentional disregard of this requirement. The consistency requirement may be waived if the partner files a statement (Form 8082) identifying the inconsistency or shows that it resulted from an incorrect schedule furnished by the partnership.

The IRS may apply entity-level audit procedures when it appears from the return that such procedures should apply. The IRS's determination will stand even if it later proves to be erroneous (Code Sec. 6231(g)).[35]

References are to Standard Federal Tax Reports; Tax Research Consultant; and Practical Tax Explanations.

[29] ¶ 25,160; PART: 24,114; §30,910.05

[30] ¶ 37,565—¶ 37,900; PART: 60,050; §31,105

[31] ¶ 37,590; PART: 60,150; §31,110.15

[32] ¶ 37,770; PART: 60,100; §31,110.10

[33] ¶ 37,640; PART: 60,200; §31,110.10

[34] ¶ 37,570; PART: 60,058; §31,115

[35] ¶ 37,770; PART: 60,054; §31,105

Innocent Spouse Relief. Innocent spouse relief is available with respect to partnership-level proceedings (Code Sec. 6230).[36]

If the spouse of a partner in a partnership subject to the TEFRA audit rules asserts that the innocent spouse rules apply with respect to a liability attributable to any adjustment to a partnership item, the spouse may file a request for an abatement of the assessment with the IRS. The spouse must file the request within 60 days after the notice of a computational adjustment has been mailed by the IRS. Upon receipt of the request, the IRS must abate the assessment. If the IRS chooses to reassess the abated tax, it then has 60 days after the date of the abatement in which to make any reassessment. In such a scenario, the regular deficiency procedures apply.

If the taxpayer claiming innocent spouse relief files a Tax Court petition under Code Sec. 6213 with respect to the request for abatement, the Tax Court can determine only whether the innocent spouse requirements have in fact been satisfied. For purposes of this determination, the treatment of the TEFRA partnership items under the settlement, the final partnership administrative adjustment (FPAA), or the court decision (whichever is appropriate) that gave rise to the liability in question is conclusive.

Small Partnership Exception. The TEFRA audit rules do not apply to partnerships with 10 or fewer partners if each partner is an individual U.S. resident, a C corporation, or estate, and each partner's share of any partnership item is the same as his or her distributive share of every other partnership item. However, these small partnerships may elect to have the TEFRA audit rules apply (Code Sec. 6231(a)(1)(B)).[37] The partnership also can specially allocate items without jeopardizing its exception from TEFRA audit rules. Once a small partnership elects to have the TEFRA rules apply, the election cannot be revoked without IRS consent.

416. Partnership's Required Tax Year. A partnership generally cannot have a tax year other than its majority-interest taxable year (Code Sec. 706(b)).[38] This is the tax year that, on each testing day, constitutes the tax year of one or more partners having an aggregate interest in partnership profits and capital of more than 50 percent. The testing day is the first day of the partnership's tax year (determined without regard to the majority interest rule). A partnership that changes to a majority-interest tax year is generally not required to change to another tax year for the two tax years following the year of change.

If the partnership has no majority-interest tax year, then its tax year must be the same as the tax year of all of the partnership's principal partners (partners who individually own five percent or more of the partnership's profits or capital) (Code Sec. 706(b)(1)(B)(ii)).[39] Partnerships that are unable to determine a tax year under either of the foregoing methods must adopt a tax year that results in the least aggregate deferral of income to the partners (Reg. § 1.706-1).[40] A partnership may avoid the tax year rules if it can establish a business purpose for selecting a different tax year (Code Sec. 706(b)(1)(C); Reg. § 1.706-1(b)(2)).[41]

Code Sec. 444 Election. Certain partnerships are permitted to make an election to have a tax year other than the normally required tax year (Code Sec. 444).[42] For any tax year for which an election is made, a partnership generally must make a required payment that is intended to represent the tax on the income deferred through the use of a tax year other than a required year. The payment is due on May 15 of the calendar year following the calendar year in which the Code Sec. 444 election year begins (¶ 1501) (Code Sec. 7519; Temp. Reg. § 1.7519-2T(a)(4)(ii)).[43]

References are to Standard Federal Tax Reports; Tax Research Consultant; and Practical Tax Explanations.

[36] ¶ 37,750; PART: 60,312

[37] ¶ 37,770; PART: 60,054; § 31,105

[38] ¶ 25,160; PART: 6,102; § 30,120.10

[39] ¶ 25,160; PART: 6,104; § 30,120.15

[40] ¶ 25,161; PART: 6,106; § 30,120.20

[41] ¶ 25,160, ¶ 25,161; PART: 6,108

[42] ¶ 20,600; PART: 6,110; § 30,120.30

[43] ¶ 42,770, ¶ 42,773; PART: 6,110; § 30,120.05

417. Partnership Taxable Income. While a partnership is not subject to tax (¶ 404), its taxable income is the key feature by which the partnership passes through its income or loss to its partners (Code Sec. 701).[44] Each partner generally must account for his or her distributive share of partnership taxable income in computing income tax. The partner's share of partnership tax items is reported to him or her by the partnership on Schedule K-1 of Form 1065. A partner's basis in his or her partnership interest is increased by his or her distributive share of partnership taxable income, while the partner's basis generally decreases by the amount distributed to the partner by the partnership. Thus, if a partnership distributes all of its taxable income by the end of the partnership tax year, the basis of each partner's interest in the partnership does not change (Code Secs. 705 and 731(a)).[45]

The taxable income of a partnership is computed in the same manner as that of an individual except that the following deductions and carryovers are not allowed to a partnership:

     (1) the deduction for personal exemptions (¶ 133);

     (2) the deduction for foreign taxes (note that the taxes are allocated to the partners as separately stated items);

     (3) the net operating loss deduction (which is determined at the partner level, not the partnership level) (¶ 1145);

     (4) the deduction for charitable contributions (which is allocated to the partners as a separately stated item) (¶ 1058);

     (5) individuals' itemized deductions (medical expenses, etc.);

     (6) the capital loss carryover (which is determined at the partner level, not the partnership level) (¶ 1754);

     (7) the domestic production activities deduction (which is determined at the partner level, not the partnership level) (¶ 980A), and

     (8) depletion deductions with respect to oil and gas wells (which are allocated to the partners as separately stated items) (¶ 1289) (Code Sec. 703(a); Reg. § 1.703-1).[46]

In addition, certain items of gain, loss, etc. must be separately stated (¶ 431).

418. Partnership Anti-Abuse Regulations. Regulations give the IRS the power to recast transactions that attempt to use the partnership provisions for tax-avoidance purposes (Reg. § 1.701-2).[47] Under the rules, a partnership must be *bona fide* and each partnership transaction must be entered into for a substantial business purpose. The form of each transaction must be respected under substance-over-form rules. Finally, the tax consequences to each partner of partnership operations and transactions must accurately reflect the partners' economic agreement and clearly reflect each partner's income. Whether there is a principal purpose of substantially reducing the present value of the partners' aggregate tax liability is determined at the partnership level.

In abusive situations, the IRS can treat a partnership as the aggregate of its partners, in whole or in part, as appropriate to carry out the purpose of any Code or regulation provision. However, to the extent that a Code or regulation provision prescribes treatment of the partnership as an entity and the treatment and ultimate tax results are clearly contemplated by the provision, the IRS will not recast a transaction.

419. Elections by Partnerships. Most elections affecting the computation of income derived from a partnership must be made by the partnership. Thus, elections as to methods of accounting, methods of computing depreciation, the Code Sec. 179 expensing election, the election not to use the installment sales provision, the option to expense

---

References are to Standard Federal Tax Reports; Tax Research Consultant; and Practical Tax Explanations.

[44] ¶ 25,060; PART: 18,050; § 30,401

[45] ¶ 25,140, ¶ 25,320; PART: 15,056, PART: 15,058; § 30,210.15

[46] ¶ 25,100, ¶ 25,101; PART: 18,052; § 30,405

[47] ¶ 25,061B; PART: 3,110; § 30,130

intangible drilling and development costs, and similar elections must be made by the partnership and must apply to all partners, insofar as the partnership transactions are concerned (Reg. § 1.703-1(b)).[48] In the case of an involuntary conversion of partnership property, the partnership also must purchase replacement property and elect nonrecognition of gain treatment (Rev. Rul. 66-191).[49]

Individual partners may make elections to (1) use as a credit or as a deduction their distributive shares of foreign taxes of the partnership, (2) deduct or capitalize their shares of the partnership's mining exploration expenditures, or (3) reduce basis in connection with discharge of indebtedness under Code Sec. 108 (Code Sec. 703(b)).[50]

Regulations provide for an automatic six-month extension for making elections if the time for making the election also is the due date of the return for which the election is made (Reg. §§ 301.9100-1, 301.9100-2, and 301.9100-3).[51]

421. Guaranteed Payments to Partners. Any fixed payments to partners for services or for the use of capital made without regard to partnership income are treated as though paid to a nonpartner for purposes of computing partnership gross income and business expense deductions (¶ 432). Thus, guaranteed payments are regarded as ordinary income to the recipient and deductible by the partnership if they are ordinary and necessary business expenses (¶ 901) (Code Sec. 707(c); Reg. § 1.707-1(c)).[52] This rule applies only to the extent that the amounts paid are in fact guaranteed payments determined without regard to the income of the partnership (Code Sec. 707(c); Reg. § 1.707-4).[53] The partner must report the payments on his or her return for the tax year within or with which ends the partnership year in which the partnership deducted the payments as paid or accrued under its method of accounting.

> **Example 1:** In the AB partnership, Ann is the managing partner and is entitled to receive a fixed annual payment of $100,000 for her services, without regard to the income of the partnership. Her distributive share of partnership profit and loss is 10 percent. After deducting her guaranteed payment, the partnership has $300,000 ordinary income. Ann must include $130,000 ($100,000 guaranteed payment plus $30,000 distributive share) as ordinary income for her tax year within or with which the partnership tax year ends. If the partnership had shown a $100,000 loss after deduction of Ann's guaranteed payment, her guaranteed payment ($100,000) would be reported as income and her $10,000 distributive share of the loss, subject to the loss limitations of Code Sec. 704(d) (¶ 425), would be taken into account on her individual tax return.

If a partner is entitled to a minimum payment and the percentage of profits is less than the minimum payment, the guaranteed payment is the difference between the minimum payment and the distributive share of the profits determined before the deduction of the minimum payment (Reg. § 1.707-1(c)).[54] Only the amount of the guaranteed payment may qualify as a deductible business expense of the partnership.

> **Example 2:** The AB partnership agreement provides that Ann is to receive 30% of partnership income before taking into account any guaranteed payments, but not less than $100,000. The income of the partnership is $600,000, and Ann is entitled to $180,000 (30% of $600,000) as her distributive share. Because her distributive share exceeds the minimum amount that was guaranteed, no part of the $180,000 is a guaranteed payment. If the partnership had income of only $200,000, Ann's distributive share would have been $60,000 (30% of $200,000), and the remaining $40,000 payable to Ann would have been a guaranteed payment.

A partner who receives a guaranteed salary payment is not regarded as an employee of the partnership for the purpose of withholding of income or Social Security

---

References are to Standard Federal Tax Reports; Tax Research Consultant; and Practical Tax Explanations.

[48] ¶ 25,101; PART: 18,152; § 30,301

[49] ¶ 29,650.704; SALES: 27,166.10; § 30,301

[50] ¶ 25,100; PART: 18,154; § 30,301

[51] ¶ 44,014, ¶ 44,014AE, ¶ 44,014AG; FILEBUS: 15,150; § 39,220

[52] ¶ 25,180, ¶ 25,181; PART: 27,100; § 30,735.05

[53] ¶ 25,180, ¶ 25,181C; PART: 27,102; § 30,735.10

[54] ¶ 25,181; PART: 27,110; § 30,735.15

¶421

taxes, or for pension plans. The guaranteed salary is includible in self-employment income for the purpose of the self-employment tax along with the partner's share of ordinary income or loss of the partnership (Reg. § 1.707-1(c); Rev. Rul. 56-675).[55]

Fringe Benefits. The value of fringe benefits (¶ 2085) provided to a partner for services rendered in the capacity as a partner is generally treated as a guaranteed payment (Code Sec. 162(l); Rev. Rul. 91-26).[56] As such, the value of the benefit is generally deductible by the partnership as an ordinary and necessary business expense; the value of the benefit is included in the partner's gross income, unless a Code provision allowing exclusion of the benefit specifically provides that the exclusion applies to partners. Thus, a payment of premiums by a partnership for a partner's health or accident insurance is generally deductible by the partnership and included in the partner's gross income. As an alternative, a partnership may choose to account for premiums paid for a partner's insurance by reducing that partner's distributions. In this case, the premiums are not deductible by the partnership and all partners' distributive shares are unaffected by payment of the premiums. A partner can deduct 100 percent of the cost of the health insurance premiums paid on his or her behalf.

Partner Loss Deductions

425. Partnership Loss Limited to Partner's Basis. The amount of partnership loss (including capital loss) that may be recognized by a partner is limited to the amount of the adjusted basis (before reduction by the current year's loss) of his or her interest in the partnership at the end of the partnership tax year in which the loss occurred. Any disallowed loss is carried forward to, and may be deducted by the partner in, subsequent partnership tax years (to the extent that his or her basis exceeds zero before deducting the loss) (Reg. § 1.704-1(d)).[57] Techniques that have been used to increase a partner's basis so that he or she can deduct losses that otherwise would be unavailable include making additional contributions to the capital of the partnership (¶ 443) and increasing the partner's share of partnership liabilities (¶ 447).

426. Partners and the At-Risk Rules. The rules limiting a partner's deduction for any tax year to the amount the partner has at risk in the partnership for that year (¶ 1155) apply at the partner level, not the partnership level (Code Sec. 465; Temp. Reg. § 1.469-2T(d)(6)).[58] A partner is not at risk for any portion of a partnership liability for which he or she has no personal liability. The at-risk loss limitation rules are applied after taking into account the basis limitation for partners' losses but before the limitations applicable to computing any passive activity loss for the year.

Real Estate Exception. The at-risk rules generally apply to the holding of property in the same manner as they apply to other activities (Code Sec. 465(b)(6)).[59] However, an exception applies to the holding of real estate. A taxpayer is at risk with respect to qualified nonrecourse financing that is secured by the real property used in the activity of holding real estate. Thus, lending provided by any person actively and regularly engaged in the business of lending money is qualified nonrecourse financing. Such lenders generally include banks, savings and loan associations, credit unions, insurance companies regulated under federal, state, or local law, or pension trusts. Further, qualified nonrecourse financing includes a loan made by any federal, state, or local government or a governmental entity or a loan that is guaranteed by any federal, state, or local government. Convertible debt cannot be treated as qualified nonrecourse financing.

Qualified nonrecourse financing can be provided by a related person (generally, family members, fiduciaries, and corporations, or partnerships in which a person has at least a 10-percent interest) if the financing from the related person is commercially reasonable and on substantially the same terms as loans involving unrelated persons.

References are to Standard Federal Tax Reports; Tax Research Consultant; and Practical Tax Explanations.

[55] ¶ 25,181, ¶ 25,183.30; PART: 27,112; § 30,735.20

[56] ¶ 8500, ¶ 25,183.16; PART: 27,104; § 21,225, § 30,735.10

[57] ¶ 25,121; PART: 15,202; § 30,430.10

[58] ¶ 21,850, ¶ 21,963; PART: 15,204; § 17,301

[59] ¶ 21,850; BUSEXP: 42,160; § 17,305.10

427. Partnerships and the Passive Activity Loss Rules. The passive activity loss limitations (¶ 1169) apply at the partner level to each partner's share of any loss or credit attributable to a passive activity of the partnership (Code Sec. 469).[60] A partnership may engage in both passive and nonpassive activities. For example, a partnership may engage in business that is a passive activity of its limited partners (who normally do not participate in the management of a limited partnership), and it may also have investment assets that produce portfolio income (not a passive activity). Thus, a partner who disposes of his or her interest in a partnership must allocate any gain or loss among the various activities of the partnership in order to determine the amount that is passive gain or loss and the amount that is nonpassive gain or loss. In general, the allocation is made in accordance with the relative value of the partnership's assets.

To allow a partner to make these calculations, a partnership must report separately a partner's share of income or losses and credits from each of its trade or business activities, rental real estate activities, and rental activities other than rental real estate. The separate activities must be reported on a statement attached to the Schedule K-1 provided to the partner (Instructions to Form 1065). A partnership's portfolio income, which is excluded from passive income, must also be separately reported.

A passive activity of a partner generally is: (1) a trade or business activity in which the partner does not materially participate, or (2) any rental activity. Except as otherwise provided (Temp. Reg. § 1.469-5T(e)(2)),[61] an interest in an activity as a limited partner in a limited partnership is not one in which the partner materially participates. If a partnership reports amounts from more than one activity on a partner's Schedule K-1 and one or more of the activities is passive to the partner, the partnership must attach a statement detailing the income, losses, deductions, and credits from each passive activity and the line of Schedule K-1 on which that amount is included.

427A. Net Operating Loss Deduction of Partners. The benefit of the net operating loss deduction (¶ 1145) is not allowed to the partnership but instead to its partners (Reg. § 1.702-2).[62] For purposes of determining his or her individual net operating loss, each partner takes into account his or her distributive share of income, gain, loss, deduction, or credit of the partnership as if each item were realized directly from the source from which it was realized by the partnership or incurred in the same manner as it was incurred by the partnership.

Partner's Distributive Share of Partnership Items

428. Allocations of Partnership Items Under Partnership Agreement. A partner's distributive share of income, gain, loss, deduction, or credit is generally determined by the partnership agreement. Allocations of any partnership item must have substantial economic effect if they are to be recognized for Code purposes (Code Sec. 704(b); Reg. § 1.704-1(b)).[63] If a partnership agreement does not provide for the allocation of partnership items or if partnership allocations lack substantial economic effect, the partner's distributive share is determined according to his or her interest in the partnership.

Economic Effect. Allocations have economic effect if they are consistent with the underlying economic arrangement of the partners (Reg. § 1.704-1(b)(2)(ii)).[64] For instance, a limited partner who has no risk under the partnership agreement other than his or her initial capital contribution ordinarily may not be allocated losses attributable to a partnership recourse liability to the extent such losses exceed his or her capital contribution. These recourse losses ordinarily must be allocated to the partners (usually the general partners) who bear the ultimate burden of discharging the partnership's liability. A partnership's nonrecourse deductions—those attributable to those liabilities of the partnership for which no partner bears personal liability (for example, a mortgage secured only by a building and the land on which it is located)—are deemed to lack

---

References are to Standard Federal Tax Reports; Tax Research Consultant; and Practical Tax Explanations.

[60] ¶ 21,960; PART: 15,206; § 30,430.05, § 30,430.20

[61] ¶ 21,965; PART: 15,206; § 17,435.20

[62] ¶ 25,084; PART: 18,306; § 30,405

[63] ¶ 25,120, ¶ 25,121; PART: 21,100; § 30,610.05

[64] ¶ 25,121; PART: 21,150; § 30,610.05

economic effect and must be allocated according to the partners' interests in the partnership (¶ 448).

Partnership allocations may be deemed to have substantial economic effect if the requirements of *optional* safe harbor provisions are met (Reg. § 1.704-1(b)(2)).[65] Generally, to satisfy the safe harbor, a partnership must maintain its "book" capital accounts as set out by Reg. § 1.704-1 and make tax allocations consistent with the capital accounts. A second safe harbor in Reg. § 1.704-2 applies to the allocation of nonrecourse deductions.

Substantiality. The economic effect of an allocation is generally considered substantial if there is a reasonable possibility that the allocation will substantially affect the dollar amounts to be received by the partners from the partnership, independent of tax consequences (Reg. § 1.704-1(b)(2)(iii)).[66]

Contributed Property. Income, gain, loss, and deductions attributable to property contributed to a partnership by a partner must be allocated among the partners to take into account the variation between the property's fair market value and its basis to the partnership at the time of contribution (Code Sec. 704(c)).[67] The partnership's basis in the contributed property at the time of contribution in exchange for a partnership interest is the basis of the property in the hands of the contributing partner. The potential gain or loss (built-in gain or loss) with respect to the contributed property must be allocated to the contributing partner. A similar rule applies to contributions by cash-method partners of accounts payable and other accrued but unpaid items.

Special rules prevent use of allocations to improperly shift the tax consequences associated with contributed property among partners in a partnership (Reg. § 1.704-3(a)(10)).[68] Under the Code Sec. 704(c) anti-abuse rule, an allocation method is not reasonable if the property contribution and the corresponding allocation of tax items regarding the property are made with a view to shifting the tax consequences of built-in gain or loss among the partners in a manner that substantially reduced the present value of the partners' aggregate tax liability (¶ 418). Also, the distribution of built-in gain or loss property to partners other than the contributing partner within seven years of its contribution to the partnership may result in the recognition of gain or loss to the contributing partner if distributed to the other partners (¶ 453).

430. Disproportionate Partnership Distributions. Disproportionate distribution rules apply if an actual or constructive distribution to a partner changes his or her proportionate interest in a partnership's unrealized receivables or inventory. The purpose of these rules is to prevent conversion of ordinary income to capital gain on the distribution or a change in share of unrealized receivables or substantially appreciated inventory.

A disproportionate distribution is treated as a sale or exchange of the receivables or inventory items from the partnership to the partner (Code Sec. 751(b)).[69] This results in ordinary income rather than capital gain. Under Code Sec. 751(f), these rules cannot be avoided through the use of tiered partnerships. Sale or exchange treatment does not apply to a distribution of property that the distributee contributed to the partnership or to payments to a retiring partner or a successor in interest of a deceased partner.

Although the substantially appreciated inventory test was dropped for most appreciated inventory in the case of a sale or exchange of a partnership interest (¶ 434), it remains in effect for disproportionate distributions from a partnership to its partners. Inventory is considered to be substantially appreciated if its fair market value exceeds the partnership's basis in the property by 120 percent or more. The inventory need not appreciate in value after the partnership acquired it to satisfy the 120-percent test.

References are to Standard Federal Tax Reports; Tax Research Consultant; and Practical Tax Explanations.

[65] ¶ 25,121; PART: 21,150, PART: 21,358; § 30,610.10

[66] ¶ 25,121; PART: 21,200; § 30,615.05

[67] ¶ 25,120; PART: 9,150; § 30,625.05

[68] ¶ 25,134; PART: 9,152.05; § 30,625.05

[69] ¶ 25,500; PART: 30,100; § 30,540.10

431. Separate Reporting of Partnership Items. In determining tax, each partner must account separately for his or her distributive share of the following partnership items (Code Sec. 702):[70]

(1) short-term capital gains and losses,

(2) long-term capital gains and losses,

(3) gains and losses from sales or exchanges of property used in a trade or business or subject to involuntary conversion (¶ 1747),

(4) charitable contributions (¶ 1061),

(5) dividends for which there is a dividends-received deduction (¶ 223),

(6) taxes paid or accrued to foreign countries and to U.S. possessions (¶ 2475),

(7) taxable income or loss, exclusive of items requiring separate computation, and

(8) other items required to be stated separately either by Reg. § 1.702-1[71] or because separate statement could affect the income tax liability of any partner, including:

- recovery of bad debts, prior taxes, and delinquency amounts,

- gains and losses from wagering transactions (¶ 785),

- soil and water conservation expenditures (¶ 982),

- deductible investment expenses (¶ 1085),

- medical and dental expenses (¶ 1015),

- alimony payments (¶ 771),

- amounts paid to cooperative housing corporations (¶ 1040),

- intangible drilling and development costs (¶ 989),

- alternative minimum tax adjustments and tax preference items (¶ 1425 and ¶ 1430),

- investment tax credit recapture (¶ 1365A),

- recapture of mining exploration expenditures (¶ 987),

- information necessary for partners to compute oil and gas depletion allowances (¶ 1289),

- cost of recovery property being currently expensed (¶ 1208),

- work opportunity tax credit (¶ 1365G),

- alcohol fuels credit (¶ 1365I),

- net earnings from self-employment (¶ 2670),

- investment interest (¶ 1094),

- income or loss to the partnership on certain distributions of unrealized receivables and inventory items to a partner (¶ 453),

- any items subject to a special allocation under the partnership agreement (¶ 428),

- contributions (and the deductions for contributions) made on a partner's behalf to qualified retirement plans (¶ 2115 and ¶ 2117), and

- domestic production activities income and expenses (¶ 431A).

The need for a separate statement of various partnership items gives rise to the separate reporting of these items on Form 1065 and Schedules K and K-1.

References are to Standard Federal Tax Reports; Tax Research Consultant; and Practical Tax Explanations.

[70] ¶ 25,080; PART: 18,054; § 30,410

[71] ¶ 25,081; PART: 18,054; § 30,410

¶431

Partnerships that regularly carry on a trade or business are required to furnish to tax-exempt partners a separate statement of items of unrelated business taxable income (Code Sec. 6031(d)).[72]

431A. Domestic Production Activities by Partnerships. A partnership cannot claim the deduction for qualified production activities (¶ 980A and following). Instead, the deduction is determined at the partner level (Code Sec. 199(d)(1); Reg. § 1.199-5(b)(1)).[73] Each partner generally computes its deduction separately on Form 8903 by aggregating its proportionate share of qualified production activity (QPA) items of the partnership (i.e., income, expenses) with its share of QPA items from other sources. The partner does not have to be directly engaged in the partnership's trade or business to claim the deduction on the basis of its share of QPA items.

A partner will not be treated as directly conducting the QPA of the partnership (and vice versa) with respect to property transferred between the parties (Reg. § 1.199-5(g)).[74] For example, if a partner manufactures qualified production property within the United States and then contributes the property to the partnership which subsequently sells, licenses, leases, or otherwise disposes of the property, then the income derived by the partnership will not qualify as domestic production gross receipts (DPGR). A limited exception is provided for certain qualifying oil and gas partnerships and expanded affiliated groups.

Allocation of Items. QPA items of a partnership are allocated to each partner as any other tax item (¶ 428). This includes special allocations of QPA items, subject to the rules of Reg. § 1.704-1(b), including the rules for determining substantial economic effect (¶ 428). A partner's distributive share of expenses allocable to the partnership's QPA must be taken into account even if the partnership has no taxable income. If a partner is unable to claim a loss or deduction for regular tax purposes (i.e., at-risk, passive loss, or basis limitations), then the loss or deduction cannot be taken into account in computing the Code Sec. 199 deduction. The amount of any loss or deduction is subject to proportionate reduction if it is only partially allowed for regular tax purposes. Also, a loss or deduction that is temporarily disallowed for regular tax purposes may be used in computing the Code Sec. 199 deduction in the tax year that it is allowed for regular tax purposes.

Instead of taking into account its distributive share of each QPA item of the partnership, a partner may compute its deduction by combining its distributive share of the partnership's qualified production activities income (QPAI) and W-2 wages with its QPAI and W-2 wages from other sources. This option only applies if the partnership has elected to use the small business overall method for allocating costs, expenses, and other deductions to its DPGR (¶ 980A and following). A partner's share of QPAI from a partnership may be less than zero under this method.

Special rules apply to 20-percent partners of partnerships engaged in film or television production (Code Sec. 199(d)(1)(A)(iv)).[75]

Sale of Partnership Interest. Gain or loss recognized on the sale of a partnership interest will not be taken into account by a partner in computing its QPAI (Reg. § 1.199-5(f)).[76] This is because the sale of the partnership interest does not reflect the realization of DPGR by the entity. However, if the taxpayer receives a distribution of unrealized receivables or partnership inventory for its entire partnership interest (Code Sec. 751 property (¶ 434 and ¶ 436)), then any gain or loss which would be attributable to the sale or other disposition of such assets which would give rise to QPAI may be taken into account by the partner.

References are to Standard Federal Tax Reports; Tax Research Consultant; and Practical Tax Explanations.

[72] ¶ 35,381; PART: 18,162.15; § 30,410

[73] ¶ 12,468, ¶ 12,472D; BUSEXP: 6,212.05, BUSEXP: 6,212.10; § 30,415.05

[74] ¶ 12,472D; BUSEXP: 6,212.10; § 30,415.05

[75] ¶ 12,468; BUSEXP: 6,152.05

[76] ¶ 12,472D; BUSEXP: 6,212.05, BUSEXP: 6,212.10

¶431A

W-2 Wage Limitation. A partner computes the W-2 wage limitation for the Code Sec. 199 deduction by aggregating its share of W-2 wages from the partnership allocable to DPGR with its W-2 wages allocable to DPGR from other sources.

432. Members' Dealings with Own Partnership. Transactions between a partnership and partner may be deemed to be between a partnership and a nonpartner under certain circumstances (Code Sec. 707(a)).[77] This rule prevents the use of disguised payments to circumvent the requirement that a partnership capitalize certain expenses (such as syndication and organization expenses).

Disguised Sales. In order to prevent such manipulation, the Code provides that if:

> (1) a partner performs services for a partnership or transfers property to a partnership,

> (2) there is a related direct or indirect allocation and distribution to the partner, and

> (3) the performance of the partner's service (or the partner's transfer of property) and the allocation and distribution, when viewed together, are properly characterized as a transaction that occurred between the partnership and the partner acting as a nonpartner,

then, for income tax purposes, the transaction is treated as if it occurred between the partnership and a nonpartner (Code Sec. 707).[78]

If this provision applies to a transaction, then the allocation and distribution made by the partnership to the partner is recharacterized as a payment for services or property and, where required, the payment must be capitalized or otherwise treated in a manner consistent with its recharacterization. The partners' shares of taxable income or loss must then be redetermined.

Whether a transfer constitutes a disguised sale is based on facts and circumstances. However, contributions and distributions made within a two-year period are presumed to be a sale, while such transactions occurring more than two years apart are presumed not to be a sale (Reg. § 1.707-3(c) and (d)).[79] Exceptions to these presumptions are provided for guaranteed payments for capital, reasonable preferred returns, and operating cash flow distributions (Reg. § 1.707-4).[80]

Transactions Between Controlled Partnerships. Special rules also apply to controlled partnerships. Loss is not allowed from a sale or exchange of property (other than an interest in the partnership) between a partnership and a person whose interest in the partnership's capital *or* profits is more than 50 percent. Loss is also not allowed if the sale or exchange is between two partnerships in which the same persons own more than 50 percent of the capital or profits interests (Code Sec. 707(b)(1)).[81] In either case, if one of the purchasers or transferees realizes gain on a later sale, the gain is taxable only to the extent it exceeds the amount of the disallowed loss attributable to the property sold. Gain recognized on transactions involving controlled partnerships is treated as ordinary income if the property sold or exchanged is not a capital asset in the hands of the transferee (Code Sec. 707(b)(2)).[82]

Code Sec. 267(a)(1) disallows deductions for losses from the sale or exchange of property between related persons described in Code Sec. 267(b), including a partnership and a corporation controlled by the same persons (¶ 1717). Although this loss-denial rule does not apply to a transaction between a partnership and a partner, it does apply to a transaction between a partnership and a person who has a relationship with a partner that is otherwise specified in Code Sec. 267(b) (Reg. § 1.267(b)-1(b)).[83] Under Code Sec. 267(a)(2), accrued interest and expense deductions are not deductible until paid if the

---

References are to Standard Federal Tax Reports; Tax Research Consultant; and Practical Tax Explanations.

[77] ¶ 25,180; PART: 27,050; § 30,701

[78] ¶ 25,180; PART: 27,058; § 30,715.05

[79] ¶ 25,181B; PART: 27,058.05; § 30,715.15, § 30,715.20

[80] ¶ 25,181C; PART: 27,058.10; § 30,715.25

[81] ¶ 25,180; PART: 27,152; § 30,720.10

[82] ¶ 25,180; PART: 27,154; § 30,720.15

[83] ¶ 14,153; PART: 27,152; § 30,720.10

¶432

amount giving rise to the deduction is owed to a related cash-method taxpayer. For purposes of this rule, a partnership and persons holding interests in the partnership (actually or constructively) or persons related (under Code Sec. 267(b) or 707(b)(1)) to actual or constructive partners are treated as related persons (¶ 905 and ¶ 1540B) (Code Sec. 267(e)(1)).[84]

Sale and Liquidation of Partner's Interest

434. Purchase or Sale of a Partnership Interest. The sale or exchange of a partnership interest generally is treated as the sale of a single capital asset rather than a sale of each of the underlying partnership properties (Code Sec. 741).[85] The amount of gain or loss is based on the partner's basis in his or her partnership interest and the amount realized on the sale (Code Sec. 721).[86] The sale of a partnership interest to a partner or to a nonpartner should be distinguished from the redemption of a partner's interest by the partnership (¶ 435).

Despite the general rule that the gain or loss on the sale of a partnership interest is a capital gain or loss, a partner may recognize ordinary income or loss under the constructive sale rules if he or she receives a disproportionate distribution of partnership unrealized receivables or inventory (¶ 430).

If a partner abandons or forfeits his or her partnership interest, the partner recognizes a loss equal to their basis in the partnership interest. Thus, a partner with a zero basis in its partnership interest is not allowed an abandonment loss (*E.J. LeBlanc*, FedCl, 2010-1 USTC ¶ 50,104). If the partnership has liabilities, the abandoning partner is deemed to have received a distribution from the partnership when he or she is relieved of the liabilities. In such a case, the partner's loss is the basis in his or her interest less any liabilities of which the partner is relieved. An abandonment of a partnership interest, if there are no partnership liabilities from which the partner is relieved, results in an ordinary loss because no sale or exchange has taken place (*P.B. Citron*, Dec. 97 TC 200 (1991); *G.G. Gannon*, Dec. 16 TC 1134 (1951)).[87] If there are partnership liabilities of which the abandoning partner is relieved, the resulting gain or loss is a capital gain or loss (*A.O. Stilwell*, Dec. 46 TC 247 (1966)).[88] Even a *de minimis* actual or deemed distribution generally results in a capital loss treatment to the partner. Capital loss is also mandated if the transaction is, in substance, a sale or exchange (Rev. Rul. 93-80).[89]

For purposes of the 3.8-percent net investment income tax, net gain or loss upon the disposition of a partnership interest is considered net investment income only to the extent it would be taken into account by the partner if all partnership property were sold at fair market value immediately before the disposition (¶ 129) (Code Sec. 1411).[90]

Unrealized Receivables and Inventory. A partner recognizes ordinary income or loss on any portion of a sale of a partnership interest that is attributable to his or her share of the partnership's unrealized receivables and inventory (¶ 436) (Code Sec. 751(a)).[91] The gain is measured by the portion of the selling price attributable to unrealized receivables and inventory and the partner's basis in these assets. The partner's basis is the basis the partner's share of partnership unrealized receivables and inventory would have if these assets were distributed to the partner in a current distribution (Reg. § 1.751-1(a)(2)).[92] Capital gain or loss is determined by subtracting the partner's remaining basis from the rest of the amount realized (Reg. § 1.741-1(a)).[93]

References are to Standard Federal Tax Reports; Tax Research Consultant; and Practical Tax Explanations.

[84] ¶ 14,150; PART: 27,160; § 30,730.05

[85] ¶ 25,440; PART: 39,050; § 30,905.05

[86] ¶ 25,240; PART: 39,052, PART: 39,054; § 30,905.05

[87] ¶ 25,442.12, ¶ 25,422.545; PART: 39,058.05; § 30,905.45, § 30,905.50

[88] ¶ 25,422.545; PART: 39,058.10; § 30,905.10

[89] ¶ 25,442.12; PART: 36,104.15; § 30,905.45

[90] ¶ 32,602; INDIV: 69,156; § 1,022.10

[91] ¶ 25,500; PART: 42,050; § 30,905.25

[92] ¶ 25,501; PART: 42,054; § 30,905.25

[93] ¶ 25,441; PART: 42,052; § 30,905.25

435. Partnership Interest Redeemed by Partnership. If a partner's interest is liquidated solely through a distribution of partnership property other than money (including marketable securities), no gain is recognized (Code Sec. 731(a)).[94] The partner's basis in his or her partnership interest is transferred to the distributed assets, and any gain is recognized when the assets are disposed of by the former partner.

If a partner receives money or marketable securities as all or part of a liquidating distribution, he or she recognizes gain to the extent that the value of the cash or marketable securities exceeds his or her basis in the partnership interest (Code Secs. 731(c) and 732(b)).[95] A partner recognizes loss if no property other than money, unrealized receivables, and inventory items is distributed to the partner, and his or her basis in their partnership interest exceeds the amount of money plus the basis of the distributed receivables and inventory (Code Sec. 731(a)).[96] However, if the partner is relieved of any or all of his or her share of partnership liabilities, the relief from liability is treated the same as a cash distribution (Reg. § 1.731-1(a)(1)).[97]

If a partner receives cash and unrealized receivables and inventory for his or her partnership interest, loss can be recognized in the amount by which the basis in the partnership interest exceeds the amount of money, plus the basis of the distributed receivables and inventory (Code Sec. 731(a)(2)).[98]

> **Example:** Martin has an adjusted basis in his partnership interest of $100,000. He retires from the partnership and receives as a distribution in liquidation of his interest his share of partnership property. This share is $50,000 cash and inventory with a basis to him of $30,000. Martin can recognize a loss of $20,000, his basis minus the money received and his basis in the inventory distributed to him ($100,000 – ($50,000 + $30,000) = $20,000).

If a partner receives money or property in exchange for any part of his or her partnership interest, the amount attributable to the partner's share of the partnership's unrealized receivables or inventory items results in ordinary income or loss. This treatment applies to the unrealized receivables portion of the payments to a retiring partner or successor in interest of a deceased partner only if that part is not treated as paid in exchange for partnership property. The rationale behind this rule is that the inventory or the accounts receivable would give rise to ordinary income had the partnership interest not been sold. However, if the partner does not sell the distributed inventory items within five years from the date of distribution, the gain can be recognized as a capital gain (Code Sec. 735(a)(2)).[99] For this purpose, inventory does not include real estate or depreciable trade or business property (¶ 436) (Code Sec. 735(c)(1)).[100]

For exchanges of partnership interests involving unrealized receivables or inventory, the partnership must file an information return describing the exchange and furnish statements to each party (Reg. § 1.6050K-1).[101]

436. Unrealized Receivables and Inventory Items of Partnerships. Unrealized receivables of a partnership includes any rights to income for services or goods that are not capital assets that have not been included in gross income under the method of accounting employed by the partnership (Code Sec. 751(c); Reg. § 1.751-1(c)).[102] This classification generally relates to cash-method partnerships that have acquired a contractual or legal right to income for goods or services. It usually does not apply to an accrual-method partnership because it has already included unrealized receivables in gross income.

References are to Standard Federal Tax Reports; Tax Research Consultant; and Practical Tax Explanations.

[94] ¶ 25,320; PART: 36,102; § 30,910.05

[95] ¶ 25,320, ¶ 25,340; PART: 36,102; § 30,515.10

[96] ¶ 25,320; PART: 36,104.05; § 30,515.15

[97] ¶ 25,321; PART: 36,102; § 30,515.20

[98] ¶ 25,320; PART: 36,104.10; § 30,515.40, § 30,910.05

[99] ¶ 25,400; PART: 36,202; § 30,915.10

[100] ¶ 25,400; PART: 36,202; § 30,915.05

[101] ¶ 36,241; PART: 42,058; § 30,915.20

[102] ¶ 25,500, ¶ 25,501; PART: 42,100; § 30,540.15

Unrealized receivables also includes certain property to the extent of the amount of gain that would have been realized and recharacterized or recaptured as ordinary income by the partnership if it had sold the property at its fair market value at the time of the sale or exchange of the partnership interest being considered. The types of property covered, which include depreciable personal property and real property, are listed in the flush language of Code Sec. 751(c). This property is not treated as an unrealized receivable for purposes of Code Sec. 736, relating to payments in liquidation of a retiring or deceased partner's interest.

Inventory items of a partnership is defined broader than the term itself might suggest (Code Sec. 751(d); Reg. § 1.751-1(d)(2)).[103] It includes not only inventory, but also any other assets that would not be treated either as capital assets or section 1231 assets (generally, depreciable property and land used in a trade or business) if they were sold by the partnership (or by the partner, if he or she had held them). Thus, the term might include a copyright or artistic work, accounts receivable for services and inventory, or any unrealized receivables.

Distributions of inventory made in exchange for all or a part of a partner's interest in other partnership property, including money, are governed by the "substantially appreciated" rule (¶ 430) (Code Sec. 751(b); Reg. § 1.751-1(d)).[104] Thus, gain from such distributions is taxed as ordinary income if the fair market value of the partnership's inventory exceeds 120 percent of its adjusted basis.

438. Retiring Partner's or Successor's Shares. Payments made in liquidation of the interest of a retiring or deceased partner are considered distributions by the partnership to the extent that the payments are in exchange for the partner's interest in partnership property; otherwise they are considered a distributive share of partnership income or guaranteed payment (Code Secs. 736 and 761(d)).[105] This provision does not apply if the estate or other successor in interest of a deceased partner continues as a partner in its own right under local law (Reg. § 1.736-1(a)(1)).[106] In addition, it applies only to payments made by the partnership and not to transactions, such as the sale of a partnership interest, between the partners.

Under Code Sec. 731, distributions are generally nontaxable except to the extent that money distributed exceeds the partner's adjusted basis for his or her partnership interest (¶ 453); the excess is treated as capital gain. However, all gain relating to inventory is treated as being from the sale of a noncapital asset (Code Sec. 751(b)).[107] The partners' valuation in an arm's-length agreement of a retiring or deceased partner's interest in partnership property is presumptively correct, but that presumption may be rebutted (Reg. § 1.736-1(b)(1)).[108]

Payments for unrealized receivables and goodwill are treated as distributive shares of partnership income or as guaranteed payments if capital is not a material income-producing factor and the retiring or deceased partner was a general partner (Code Sec. 736(b)(2) and (3)).[109] Such payments are deductible by the partnership. If these two requirements are not met, payments for goodwill are treated as payments for partnership property and do not create a deduction for the partnership. However, payments for goodwill can be treated as payments for property if: (1) the goodwill was originally purchased by the partnership or otherwise acquired in a transaction resulting in a cash basis to the partnership, *or* (2) the partnership agreement calls for a reasonable payment for goodwill.

Such payments result in capital gain or loss to the extent of the partnership's basis in the goodwill. In fixing the amount attributable to goodwill, an amount arrived at under

---

References are to Standard Federal Tax Reports; Tax Research Consultant; and Practical Tax Explanations.

[103] ¶ 25,500, ¶ 25,501; PART: 42,152; § 30,540.20

[104] ¶ 25,500, ¶ 25,501; PART: 30,050; § 30,915.05

[105] ¶ 25,420, ¶ 25,600; PART: 48,050; § 30,560.05

[106] ¶ 25,421; PART: 48,050; § 30,560.05

[107] ¶ 25,500; PART: 48,050; § 30,575

[108] ¶ 25,421; PART: 48,050; § 30,565.10

[109] ¶ 25,420; PART: 48,150; § 30,565.05, § 30,575

an arm's-length agreement generally is accepted by the IRS. A formula approach involving the capitalization of earnings in excess of a fair market rate of return on the partnership's net tangible assets may be used, but only where there is no better basis for making such a determination (Rev. Rul. 68-609).[110]

These excluded amounts and other payments made for an interest in the partnership property are treated as either distributive shares of partnership income or as guaranteed payments (Code Sec. 736(a)).[111] If the payments are determined by reference to partnership income, they are taxed as a distributive share to the recipient; if not, they are treated as guaranteed payments (¶ 421). Accordingly, if the payments consist of a percentage of partnership profits, they reduce the distributive shares of income of the remaining partners. If they are guaranteed payments, the effect is the same because they are deductible as business expenses in determining partnership taxable income. In either event, the payments are treated as ordinary income in the hands of the recipient partner.

Example 1: Partnership ABC is a personal service partnership and its balance sheet is as follows:

Assets	Adjusted basis	Market value	Liabilities and Capital	Adjusted basis	Market value
Cash	$130,000	$130,000	Liabilities .	$30,000	$30,000
Accounts			Capital:		
receivable . .	0	300,000	A	100,000	210,000
Capital and Sec.			B	100,000	210,000
1231 assets .	200,000	230,000	C	100,000	210,000
Total	$330,000	$660,000	Total .	$330,000	$660,000

General Partner A retires from the partnership in accordance with an agreement whereby his share of liabilities (⅓ of $30,000) is assumed. In addition, he is to receive $90,000 in the year of retirement, plus $100,000 in each of the two succeeding years, for a total of $300,000 (including his $10,000 share of liabilities) for his partnership interest. The value of A's interest in the partnership's section 736(b) property is $120,000 (⅓ of $360,000, the sum of $130,000 cash and $230,000, the fair market value of Code Sec. 1231 assets). The accounts receivable are not included in A's interest in partnership property because A is a general partner in a partnership in which capital is not a material income-producing factor. Assuming that the basis of A's interest is $110,000 ($100,000, the basis of his capital investment, plus $10,000, his share of partnership liabilities), he realizes a capital gain of $10,000 on the sale of his interest in partnership property. The $180,000 balance to be received by him is treated as guaranteed payments taxable to A as ordinary income.

The $100,000 that A receives in each of the three years would ordinarily be allocated as follows: $40,000 as payments for A's interest in section 736(b) property ($120,000/$300,000 × $100,000) and the balance of $60,000 as guaranteed payments. While the $10,000 capital gain is normally recognized in the first year, A may elect to prorate the gain over the three-year period.

Example 2: Assume the same facts as in Example 1, above, except that the agreement provides for payments to A for three years of a percentage of annual income instead of a fixed amount. In such case, all payments received by A are treated as payments for A's interest in partnership property until he has received $120,000. Thereafter, the payments are treated as a distributive share of partnership income to A (Reg. § 1.736-1(b)(7)).

References are to Standard Federal Tax Reports; Tax Research Consultant; and Practical Tax Explanations.

[110] ¶ 25,422.51; PART: 48,308, VALUE: 12,050; § 30,565.05, § 30,575

[111] ¶ 25,420; PART: 48,150; § 30,910.10

¶438

For income tax purposes, a retired partner or a deceased partner's successor is treated as a partner until his or her interest has been completely liquidated (Reg. § 1.736-1(a)(6)).[112]

440. Partner Receiving Income In Respect of a Decedent. All payments to the successor of a deceased partner under Code Sec. 736(a), relating to payments made in liquidation of a deceased partner's interest and considered as a distributive share or guaranteed payment (¶ 438), are income in respect of a decedent (Code Sec. 753; Reg. § 1.753-1).[113] Under Code Sec. 691, the payments are taxed to the recipient when received to the extent that they are not properly includible in the short tax year ending with the decedent's death. The estate or heir of a deceased partner is also treated as receiving income in respect of a decedent to the extent that amounts are received from an outsider in exchange for rights to future payments by the partnership representing distributive shares or guaranteed payments.

Partnership Contributions, Distributions, and Basis

443. Contribution to Partnership. No gain or loss is recognized by either a partnership or any of its partners upon a contribution of property to the partnership in exchange for a partnership interest (Code Sec. 721(a); Reg. § 1.721-1).[114] This is true whether the contribution is made to an existing partnership or to a newly formed partnership. However, a partner must recognize any gain realized on the transfer of appreciated property to a partnership that would be treated as an investment company if the partnership were incorporated (Code Secs. 707(c) and 721(b)).[115] Further, the value of a capital interest in a partnership that is transferred to a partner in exchange for his or her services is taxable to him or her as ordinary income, provided that the interest is not subject to a substantial risk of forfeiture (¶ 713) (Reg. § 1.721-1(b)).[116] The receipt of a profits interest in exchange for services rendered is not taxable as ordinary income (Rev. Proc. 93-27, clarified by Rev. Proc. 2001-43).[117]

The basis of a partner's interest acquired in exchange for his or her contribution to the partnership is the amount of the money contributed plus the adjusted basis to the contributing partner of any property contributed (Code Sec. 722).[118] If a partner receives a partnership interest as compensation for services rendered or to be rendered, resulting in taxable income to the incoming partner, that income is added to the basis of the partnership interest (Reg. § 1.722-1).[119] If the contributed property is subject to debt, or if liabilities of the partner are assumed by the partnership, the basis of the contributing partner's interest is reduced by the portion of the indebtedness assumed by the other partners (¶ 447) (Code Sec. 752).[120] The assumption of the partner's debt by others is treated as a distribution of money to the partner and as a contribution of money by those assuming the debt.

The basis to the partnership of property contributed by a partner is the adjusted basis of such property in the hands of the contributing partner at the time of the contribution and any gain the partner recognized on the transfer (Code Sec. 723).[121] However, it has been held that the basis of a nonbusiness asset (for example, a personal automobile) converted to a business asset upon contribution to a partnership was its fair market value at the time of contribution (*L.Y.S. Au*, CA-9, 64-1 USTC ¶ 9447).[122] The holding period of a contributed asset includes the period during which it was held by the contributing partner (Reg. § 1.723-1).[123]

References are to Standard Federal Tax Reports; Tax Research Consultant; and Practical Tax Explanations.

[112] ¶ 25,421; PART: 48,050; § 31,005.10, § 31,005.15

[113] ¶ 25,540, ¶ 25,541; PART: 48,304; § 32,901

[114] ¶ 25,240, ¶ 25,241; PART: 9,050; § 30,105.05

[115] ¶ 25,180, ¶ 25,240; PART: 9,058; § 30,105.10

[116] ¶ 25,241; PART: 12,050; § 30,115.15

[117] ¶ 25,243.12; PART: 12,100; § 30,115.15

[118] ¶ 25,260; PART: 15,050; § 30,205.05

[119] ¶ 25,261; PART: 12,152; § 30,205.15

[120] ¶ 25,520; PART: 9,100; § 30,220.10

[121] ¶ 25,280; PART: 9,056; § 30,105.10

[122] ¶ 25,282.02; PART: 9,056

[123] ¶ 25,281; PART: 9,056; § 30,105.20

¶443

Only the contributing partner may take into account any built-in loss. In determining items allocated to the noncontributing partners, the basis of the contributed property is the property's fair market value at the time of contribution (Code Sec. 704(c)(1)(C)).[124] Proposed regulations effective for partnership contributions occurring on or after the date the regulations are published as final, would clarify that the Code Sec. 704(c)(1)(C) basis adjustment is initially equal to the built-in loss associated with the property and then is adjusted in a generally similar manner to basis adjustments required by the Code Sec. 743 regulations (Proposed Reg. § 1.704-3(f)).[125]

Unrealized receivables and inventory items contributed by the partner to the partnership retain their ordinary income character in the hands of the partnership (Code Sec. 724).[126] That is, unrealized receivables remain ordinary income property up to the time of disposal by the partnership and inventory items remain ordinary income property for the five-year period beginning on the date of contribution. In addition, a partner's contribution of property with a built-in capital loss results in retention of the property's capital loss status in the hands of the partnership to the extent of built-in loss for the five-year period beginning on the date of contribution.

To prevent avoidance of these rules through the partnership's exchange of contributed unrealized receivables, inventory items, or capital loss property in a nonrecognition transaction (or series of transactions), the rule applies to any substituted basis property resulting from the exchange. It does not apply, however, to any stock in a C corporation received in an exchange of property for stock if the contributor is in control following the exchange (Code Secs. 351 and 735(c)(2)).[127] For this purpose, control is at least 80 percent of the total combined voting power of all classes of stock entitled to vote and at least 80 percent of the total number of shares of all other classes of stock of the corporation (Code Sec. 368(c)).[128]

445. Increases and Decreases in Basis of Partner's Interest. The basis of a partner's interest is *increased* by his or her distributive share of partnership taxable income, the partnership's tax-exempt income, and the excess of the partnership deductions for depletion over the basis to the partnership of the depletable property (Code Sec. 705).[129] The basis of the partner's interest is *decreased* (but not below zero) by distributions to the partner from the partnership (¶ 453) and by the sum of the partners's share of partnership losses and partnership expenditures not deductible in computing its taxable income and not chargeable to capital account, and the partner's depletion deduction for oil and gas wells. Distributions are to be taken into account before losses in adjusting the partner's interest basis (Rev. Rul. 66-94).[130]

> **Example:** Partner A of ABC partnership has an $80,000 basis for her partnership interest. During the tax year, she receives cash distributions of $50,000, and her share of the partnership's losses is $40,000. Her interest is adjusted as follows:

Basis at beginning of year	$80,000	
Less cash distributions	50,000	$30,000
Less share of losses ($40,000) but only to the extent that the basis is not reduced below zero		30,000
Adjusted basis for interest		0

Because basis is decreased by distributions received before reduction by A's share of partnership losses, no gain is recognized under Code Sec. 731 on the cash distribution. However, $10,000 of A's share of partnership loss is disallowed and carried forward to subsequent tax years (¶ 425).

The basis of partnership interests may also be determined by reference to proportionate shares of the adjusted basis of partnership property that would be distributable if

---

References are to Standard Federal Tax Reports; Tax Research Consultant; and Practical Tax Explanations.

[124] ¶ 25,120; PART: 45,112; § 30,625.05

[125] ¶ 25,134BB; PART: 45,112

[126] ¶ 25,300; PART: 9,250; § 30,105.20

[127] ¶ 16,402, ¶ 25,400; PART: 36,202; § 30,105.20

[128] ¶ 16,750; CCORP: 3,054; § 26,105.10

[129] ¶ 25,140; PART: 15,056, PART: 15,058; § 30,210.10, § 30,210.15

[130] ¶ 25,144.12; PART: 15,060; § 30,210.20

¶445

the partnership were to be terminated. This alternative rule is available only in limited circumstances if a partner cannot practically apply the general rule or when the IRS approves (Code Sec. 705(b); Reg. § 1.705-1(b)).[131]

For purposes of determining a partner's basis in his or her partnership interest, or for figuring gain or loss on a distribution, advances or drawings of money or property against a partner's distributive share of income are treated as current distributions made on the last day of the partnership's tax year (Reg. § 1.731-1(a)(1)(ii)).[132] Money received by a partner under an obligation to repay the partnership is not a distribution but is a loan that is treated as a transaction between the partnership and a nonpartner (Reg. §§ 1.707-1(a) and 1.731-1(c)(2)).[133]

447. Partnership Liabilities Treated as Distributions or Contributions. Any increase in a partner's share of partnership liabilities, including a partner's assumption of partnership liabilities or receipt of partnership property subject to a liability (limited to the fair market value of the encumbered property), is treated as a contribution of money that increases a partner's basis in his or her interest (Code Secs. 722 and 752(a)).[134] A decrease in a partner's share of partnership liabilities is treated as a distribution of money by the partnership, which decreases the distributee partner's basis in his or her partnership interest (but not below zero) (Code Secs. 733 and 752(b)).[135] When a partner's basis has been reduced to zero, such deemed distributions can result in a taxable gain (¶ 453).

448. Allocation of Partnership Liabilities. Partners' shares of partnership liabilities (and corresponding allocations of basis) depend upon whether the liability is "recourse" or "nonrecourse." In addition, separate rules apply in the case of nonrecourse debts of the partnership if a partner is the lender or has guaranteed repayment of the debt.

Recourse Liabilities. Liabilities are recourse to the extent that a partner bears the economic risk of loss if the liability is not satisfied by the partnership. Recourse liabilities are allocated in accordance with the partners' economic risk of loss (Reg. § 1.752-2(a)).[136] Economic risk of loss is generally borne by a partner to the extent that he or she must make a contribution to the partnership (including the obligation to restore a deficit capital account) or pay a creditor if all partnership assets, including money, were deemed worthless and all partnership liabilities were due and payable (Reg. § 1.752-2(b)(1)).[137] Thus, a limited partner cannot be allocated recourse liabilities in excess of his or her capital contribution and future contribution obligations unless he or she has agreed to restore any deficit in his or her capital account or to indemnify other partners for their debts with respect to a liability. A partner does not bear the economic risk of loss if he or she is entitled to reimbursement from other partners or the partnership—for example, through an indemnification agreement or a state law right to subrogation (Reg. § 1.752-2(b)(5)).[138] Recourse liabilities must be allocated to a partner if a related person bears the risk of loss for the liability (Reg. § 1.752-4(b)).[139]

Nonrecourse Liabilities. Nonrecourse liabilities are those for which no partner bears the economic risk of loss—for example, a mortgage on an office building that is secured only by a lien on the building and on the rents, but with no personal obligation to repay the loan on the part of any of the owners. Such liabilities are generally shared by the partners in a manner that correlates with their allocations of deductions attributable to the liabilities (¶ 428).[140] A partner's share of nonrecourse liabilities of a partnership equals the sum of: (1) the partner's share of partnership minimum gain, (2) the amount

---

References are to Standard Federal Tax Reports; Tax Research Consultant; and Practical Tax Explanations.

[131] ¶ 25,140, ¶ 25,141; PART: 15,100; § 30,210.25

[132] ¶ 25,321; PART: 33,052.10; § 30,210.20

[133] ¶ 25,181, ¶ 25,321; PART: 33,052.05; § 30,210.20

[134] ¶ 25,260, ¶ 25,520; PART: 9,100; § 30,215.05

[135] ¶ 25,360, ¶ 25,520; PART: 9,100; § 30,215.05

[136] ¶ 25,523; PART: 15,254; § 30,215.15

[137] ¶ 25,523; PART: 15,254.10; § 30,215.15

[138] ¶ 25,523; PART: 15,254.25; § 30,215.15

[139] ¶ 25,525; PART: 15,254.20; § 30,215.35

[140] ¶ 25,120; PART: 15,254.10; § 30,215.20

of any taxable gain under Code Sec. 704(c) that would be allocated to the partner if the partnership disposed of all partnership property subject to one or more nonrecourse liabilities of the partnership in full satisfaction of the liabilities and no other consideration, and (3) the partner's share of the excess nonrecourse liabilities as determined in accordance with the partner's share of partnership profits (Reg. § 1.752-3(a)).[141]

Although excess nonrecourse liabilities are allocated in accordance with the partners' respective profits interests, the partnership agreement may state their profits interests for purposes of sharing nonrecourse liabilities, provided that the stated sharing ratios are reasonably consistent with the allocation of some significant item of partnership income or gain among the partners. Because no partner bears the economic risk of loss for nonrecourse liabilities, limited partners may be allocated shares of such liabilities (and the basis in such liabilities) in amounts exceeding their total capital contribution obligations.

Partner Nonrecourse Loans and Guarantees. A partner who lends money to the partnership on a nonrecourse basis bears the economic risk of loss for the liability. Likewise, a partner who guarantees an otherwise nonrecourse liability bears the risk of loss to the extent of his or her guarantee (Reg. § 1.752-2(d)(2)).[142]

A loss incurred on the abandonment or worthlessness of a partnership interest is an ordinary loss if sale or exchange treatment does not apply. If there is an actual or deemed distribution to the partner, or if the transaction is otherwise in substance a sale or exchange, the partner's loss is capital except as provided in Code Sec. 751(b).[143] A deemed distribution includes the relief from partnership debts in which the abandoning partner shares. As with other losses, the partners must establish the finality and uncollectability of the loss (Reg. § 1.165-1(d)).[144]

453. Gain or Loss on Distribution to Partners. The income of a partnership is taxable to the partners in accordance with their distributive shares of partnership taxable income (¶ 428). It does not matter when or if the income is actually distributed to the partners. However, distributions to partners decrease the partners' bases for their partnership interests (¶ 445).

> **Example 1:** A partner contributes $100,000 to the capital of a partnership. During the first year, his share of the partnership taxable income is $25,000, but only $10,000 of this amount is actually distributed to him. The $25,000 taxable income increases his basis to $125,000, and the $10,000 distribution decreases it to $115,000.

No gain or loss is recognized by a partnership on a distribution of property to a partner, including money, except to the extent that any money distributed exceeds the adjusted basis of the partner's interest in the partnership immediately before the distribution (Code Sec. 731(b)).[145] Loss is not recognized by the partner, except upon a distribution in liquidation of a partner's interest in a partnership. If no property other than money and certain securities is distributed to the partner, loss is recognized to the extent of the excess of the adjusted basis of the partner's interest in the partnership over the sum of any money distributed and the basis to the partner of any unrealized receivables and inventory (¶ 436).[146]

If a distribution of money exceeds a partner's basis for his or her interest, gain is recognized by the partner as though the partner had sold or exchanged the partnership interest (Code Sec. 731(a)).[147] This applies both to current distributions and distributions in liquidation of a partner's entire interest in a partnership (Reg. § 1.731-1(a)).[148]

References are to Standard Federal Tax Reports; Tax Research Consultant; and Practical Tax Explanations.

[141] ¶ 25,524; PART: 21,358; § 30,215.20

[142] ¶ 25,523; PART: 15,254.20; § 30,215.25

[143] ¶ 25,500; PART: 39,050; § 30,905.45

[144] ¶ 9803; INDIV: 54,256; § 16,905.20

[145] ¶ 25,320; PART: 33,000, PART: 36,000; § 30,530.05

[146] **MTG: ¶ 25,500**; PART: 36,104; § 30,515.15

[147] ¶ 25,320; PART: 36,102; § 30,515.10

[148] ¶ 25,321; PART: 33,050, PART: 36,050; § 30,515.05

> **Example 2:** Partner A purchases a partnership interest for $100,000. During the first year, A receives a cash distribution of $100,000 and a distribution of property with a fair market value of $30,000. He recognizes no gain on the distributions since the amount of money distributed does not exceed A's basis for his partnership interest ($100,000). If he had received a cash distribution of $130,000, a $30,000 gain would have been recognized.

Distribution of marketable securities generally is treated the same as a distribution of money (Code Sec. 731(c); Reg. § 1.731-2).[149] The securities are valued at their fair market value on the date of the distribution.

Gain is determined only by reference to *money* (including marketable securities) distributed. A partner generally recognizes no gain on a distribution of property until the partner sells or otherwise disposes of the distributed property. Thus, if the taxpayer in Example 2 had received property in kind rather than cash or marketable securities, no gain would have been realized (Reg. § 1.731-1(a)).[150]

A distribution of property encumbered by a liability, however, may cause a partner's share of partnership liabilities to decrease, resulting in a deemed distribution of money to that partner (¶ 447) (Code Sec. 752(b)).[151] For instance, if a partner receives a distribution of property subject to a secured liability, the liability becomes a personal liability of the distributee partner, and there is a decrease in the liabilities of all other partners who had been allocated a share of the liability. These partners must decrease the bases in their partnership interests in the amount of their deemed distributions (but not below zero), and any amounts deemed distributed in excess of their respective bases are taxable as capital gain.

The nonrecognition rules of Code Sec. 731 may not apply if, within a short period before or after property is contributed to a partnership, there is a distribution of either (1) other partnership property to the contributing partner, or (2) the contributed property to another partner (Code Sec. 707(a)(2)(B); Reg. § 1.731-1(c)(3)).[152] If the distribution is made in order to effect an exchange of property between the partnership and a partner, or between two or more partners, then the transaction is treated as an exchange and the disguised sale rules (¶ 432) may apply. There is a presumption that distributions made within two years of a contribution are made as part of a sale arrangement (Reg. § 1.707-3(c)).[153] The presumption can be rebutted if the facts and circumstances clearly establish that there is no sale (Reg. § 1.707-4).[154]

Loss is recognized only if the distribution terminates the partner's interest—and then only if the distribution is limited to money, unrealized receivables, or inventory items (¶ 436) (Code Sec. 731(a)(2)).[155] The amount of the recognized loss is the excess of the adjusted basis of the partner's interest over the sum of any money distributed and the basis to him or her, which is ordinarily the same as the basis to the partnership (¶ 456) of any unrealized receivables or inventory items.

> **Example 3:** A partner whose basis for his partnership interest is $100,000 retires from the partnership, receiving $50,000 in cash and inventory items having a basis to the partnership of $30,000. The taxpayer has a capital loss of $20,000.

These provisions do not apply to the extent that payments are made in liquidation to a retiring or deceased partner and are treated as a distributive share or guaranteed payment (¶ 438), to a distribution for unrealized receivables or appreciated inventory items (¶ 436) (Code Sec. 731(d)),[156] or if the rules governing precontribution gain (¶ 454) are called into play.

References are to Standard Federal Tax Reports; Tax Research Consultant; and Practical Tax Explanations.

[149] ¶ 25,320, ¶ 25,321B; PART: 33,104; § 30,515.10

[150] ¶ 25,321; PART: 33,150; § 30,515.10

[151] ¶ 25,520; PART: 33,204; § 30,515.05

[152] ¶ 25,180, ¶ 25,321; PART: 27,058; § 30,595.05

[153] ¶ 25,181B; PART: 27,058.05; § 30,715.15

[154] ¶ 25,181C; PART: 27,058.05; § 30,715.05

[155] ¶ 25,320; PART: 36,104; § 30,510.20

[156] ¶ 25,320; PART: 45,060; § 30,515.05

454. Partnership Distribution of Contributed Property. A partner who contributes property to a partnership may have to recognize gain or loss if the contributed property is distributed by the partnership to another partner within seven years (Code Sec. 704(c)).[157] The gain or loss recognized under this rule is limited to the difference between the property's tax basis and its fair market value at the time of contribution. Upon distribution of the property within the seven-year period, the precontributed gain or loss recognized is equal to the amount that would have been allocated to the contributing partner had the partnership sold the property rather than distributed it to a partner. Appropriate adjustments must be made to the basis of the contributing partner's partnership interest and to the basis of the distributed property to reflect any gain or loss recognized (¶ 445 and ¶ 456).

The recognition rule does not apply if the property is distributed to the contributing partner (or its successor). Also, the rule does not apply with respect to certain distributions made as part of an exchange of like-kind property.

A similar rule may cause a partner contributing appreciated property to recognize precontribution gain if the partner receives a distribution of other partnership property (except money or marketable securities) within a seven-year period (Code Sec. 737(b)).[158] Precontribution gain must be recognized to the extent that it exceeds the partner's basis for his or her partnership interest at the time the distribution is received.

456. Basis of Property Distributed to Partner. The basis of property received in a distribution from a partnership other than in liquidation of a partner's interest is ordinarily the same as the basis in the hands of the partnership immediately prior to distribution (Code Sec. 732(a)).[159] In no case may the basis of property in the hands of the distributee exceed the basis of his or her partnership interest reduced by the amount of money distributed to the partner in the same transaction.

> **Example 1:** Taxpayer has a basis of $100,000 for his partnership interest. He receives a nonliquidating distribution of $40,000 in cash and property with a basis to the partnership of $80,000. The basis to the partner of the distributed property is $60,000 ($100,000 minus $40,000). The partnership can recover the $20,000 difference by making the election described at ¶ 459.

The basis of property distributed *in liquidation* of a partner's interest is the basis of the distributee's partnership interest less any money received in the same transaction (Code Sec. 732(b)).[160]

A distributee partner's basis adjustment is allocated among distributed assets, first to unrealized receivables and inventory items in an amount equal to the partnership's basis in each such property (Code Sec. 732(c)).[161] For this purpose, unrealized receivables includes any property the sale of which would create ordinary income (Code Sec. 751(c)).[162] For example, this would include depreciation-recapture property. However, the amount of unrealized receivables is limited to that amount that would be treated as ordinary income if the property were sold at fair market value.

Basis is allocated first to the extent of each distributed property's adjusted basis to the partnership. Any remaining basis adjustment that is an increase is allocated among properties with unrealized appreciation in proportion to their respective amounts of unrealized appreciation (to the extent of each property's appreciation) and then in proportion to their respective fair market values.

> **Example 2:** A partnership has two assets, a tractor and a steam shovel. Both assets are distributed to a partner whose adjusted basis in his partnership interest is $550,000. The tractor has a basis to the partnership of $50,000 and a fair market value of $400,000. The steam shovel has a basis to the partnership of $100,000 and a fair market value of $100,000. Basis is first allocated to the tractor in the amount

---

References are to Standard Federal Tax Reports; Tax Research Consultant; and Practical Tax Explanations.

[157] ¶ 25,120; PART: 33,156; § 30,590.05

[158] ¶ 25,425; PART: 33,154; § 30,595.05

[159] ¶ 25,340; PART: 33,162; § 30,510.30

[160] ¶ 25,340; PART: 36,150; § 30,510.30

[161] ¶ 25,340; PART: 33,162.15; § 30,510.35

[162] ¶ 25,500; PART: 42,106; § 30,540.15

of $50,000 and to the steam shovel in the amount of $100,000 (their adjusted bases to the partnership). The remaining basis adjustment is an increase of $400,000 (the partner's $550,000 basis minus the partnership's total basis of $150,000 in the distributed assets). Basis is then allocated to the tractor in the amount of $350,000, its unrealized appreciation, with no allocation to the steam shovel attributable to unrealized appreciation because its fair market value equals the partnership's adjusted basis. The remaining basis adjustment of $50,000 is allocated in the ratio of the assets' fair market values, which are $40,000 to the tractor (for a total basis of $440,000) and $10,000 to the steam shovel (for a total basis of $110,000).

If the remaining basis adjustment is a decrease, it is allocated among properties with unrealized depreciation in proportion to their respective amounts of unrealized depreciation (to the extent of each property's depreciation), and then in proportion to their respective adjusted bases, taking into account the adjustments already made. Accordingly, a partner's substituted basis in distributed partnership property is allocated among multiple properties based on the fair market value of the distributed properties.

Optional Basis Adjustments. If a partner has acquired his or her partnership interest (1) by purchase from a former partner or another partner or (2) from a deceased partner, then the partner can elect to have a special basis adjustment for property other than money received in a distribution from the partnership within two years after the partnership interest was acquired (Code Sec. 732(d)).[163] This can be done if the partnership has not made an election to have the special basis adjustment apply to its assets. The partner's election accomplishes substantially the same result as if the partnership had made the election. The special basis adjustment is the difference between the amount paid for the partnership interest, and the partner's share of the adjusted basis of the partnership assets.

The special basis adjustment applies to property received in current distributions as well as to distributions in complete liquidation of the partner's interest. If the partner makes the election when a distribution of depreciable or depletable property is received, the special basis adjustment is not diminished by any depletion or depreciation on that portion of the basis of partnership property that arises from the special basis adjustment (Reg. § 1.732-1(d)(1)(iv)). Depletion or depreciation on that portion for the period before distribution is allowed or allowable only if the partnership made the election.

If a transferee-partner wishes to make the election, it must be made on his or her tax return for the year of the distribution if the distribution includes any property subject to depreciation, depletion, or amortization. If it does not include any such property, the election may be made with the return for any tax year not later than the first tax year in which the basis of the distributed property is pertinent in determining income tax.

459. Optional Adjustment to Basis of Partnership Assets. If the basis of distributed assets in the hands of the distributee partner is less than the basis of the assets in the hands of the partnership, there may be an "unused" basis. The partnership may elect to adjust the basis of its remaining assets to take up this unused basis (¶ 470) (Code Secs. 734, 754, and 755).[164]

If gain is recognized by a partner because of a distribution of money (¶ 453), a similar increase in the partnership's basis of its remaining assets may be made. If an election is made, the partnership may have to decrease the basis of its remaining assets. The decrease would be required for the excess of the basis of distributed assets to the partner over the basis that the partnership had for those assets, in the event of a distribution in liquidation of a partner's interest. Decrease would also be required to the extent that any distribution to a partner resulted in loss to the partner. Loss results to the partner only if the distribution terminates the partner's interest and generally consists only of money, unrealized receivables, and inventories (¶ 453).

References are to Standard Federal Tax Reports; Tax Research Consultant; and Practical Tax Explanations.

[163] ¶ 25,340; PART: 45,100; § 30,520.05

[164] ¶ 25,380, ¶ 25,560, ¶ 25,580; PART: 45,050; § 30,805.05

Example: An equal three-person partnership has the following assets:

	Partnership's Basis	Fair Market Value
Cash	$120,000	$120,000
Land	60,000	120,000
Securities	90,000	120,000
Total	$270,000	$360,000

If a partner retires and the partnership pays him $120,000 for the fair market value of his partnership interest, the partnership is really distributing $40,000 as his pro rata share of the partnership's cash and paying him $80,000 for his ⅓ interest in the land and in the securities. However, the retiring partner's share of the partnership's basis for these properties totals only $50,000. Therefore, the partnership, if it wishes to reflect the $30,000 excess cost, may elect to adjust the basis of the land and securities.

A partnership is barred from increasing the adjusted basis of remaining property following a distribution of an interest in another partnership if the other partnership has not made a consistent Code Sec. 754 election. In other words, tiered partnerships must make consistent elections.

The allocation of any increase or decrease in basis is made among the various partnership assets or categories of assets (Code Sec. 755).[165] These rules contemplate generally that the allocation will be made first to like-kind assets and will reduce the difference between fair market value and basis of each asset adjusted.

No allocation of basis decrease may be made to stock of a corporate partner. The basis decrease must be allocated to other partnership property. The partnership recognizes gain to the extent the decrease in basis exceeds the basis of the other partnership assets.

462. Character of Gain or Loss on Disposition of Distributed Property. A partner recognizes ordinary gain or loss on the disposition of unrealized receivables or inventory items distributed by the partnership (¶ 436), regardless of whether the inventory has substantially appreciated in value (Code Sec. 735; Reg. § 1.735-1).[166] In the case of inventory items, this rule applies only if the sale takes place within five years of the date of distribution. If the sale takes place after the five-year period, gain may be treated as capital gain if the assets are capital assets in the hands of the partner at that time.

If a partner disposes of distributed unrealized receivables or inventory items in a nonrecognition transaction (or series of transactions), these rules apply to treat gain or loss on the substituted basis property as ordinary income or loss, except in the case of stock in a C corporation received in a Code Sec. 351 exchange. The House Committee Report to the Deficit Reduction Act of 1984 (P.L. 98-369) states that it is intended that the basis tainting rules regarding distributed property apply only for the period during which the underlying rules as to character of gain or loss under Code Sec. 735 would apply if the property were not disposed of in a nonrecognition transaction. For example, if an inventory item was distributed by the partnership, and the partner subsequently disposed of it in a nonrecognition transaction, ordinary income treatment would apply to any substitute basis property only for the duration of the five-year period beginning on the date of the original distribution.

467. Adjustment of Basis on Sale of Partnership Interest. The transfer of a partnership interest by a partner generally does not affect the basis of partnership assets. However, the partnership may elect to adjust the basis of partnership assets to reflect the difference between the transferee's basis for his or her partnership interest (generally, the purchase price) and his or her proportionate share of the adjusted basis

---

References are to Standard Federal Tax Reports; Tax Research Consultant; and Practical Tax Explanations.

[165] ¶ 25,580; PART: 45,150; § 30,520.05

[166] ¶ 25,400, ¶ 25,401; PART: 33,166.05, PART: 36,202; § 30,535.05

of all partnership property (his or her share of the partnership's adjusted basis in the partnership property). The election applies only to the transferee partner and applies where there is a transfer of an interest in a partnership by sale or exchange or upon the death of a partner and not upon the contribution of property (including money) to the partnership (Code Sec. 743; Reg. § 1.743-1(a)).[167]

Basis adjustments must be made to undistributed partnership property any time there is a transfer of a partnership interest and immediately after the transfer the partnership has a substantial built-in loss (more than $250,000), whether or not the partnership has a Code Sec. 754 election in effect (Code Sec. 743(a) and (d)).[168]

The amount of the increase or decrease is an adjustment affecting the transferee partner only (Code Sec. 743(b)).[169] In addition, a partner's proportionate share of the adjusted basis of partnership property is determined in accordance with his or her interest in partnership capital. Where, however, an agreement on contributed property is in effect, the agreement must be taken into account in determining a partner's proportionate share.

A Code Sec. 743 basis adjustment is mandatory in the case of a transferred partnership interest with a substantial built-in loss. A substantial built-in loss exists if the partnership's adjusted basis in the property is more than $250,000 of the fair market value. An electing investment partnership is excepted from this rule. It will not be treated as having a substantial built-in loss and therefore it is not required to make basis adjustments to partnership property (Code Sec. 743(e)(1)).[170]

The basis adjustment must be allocated among the partnership assets in accordance with the rules set out in Code Sec. 755 (¶ 459).[171]

470. Election for Partnership Basis Adjustment. An election to make the basis adjustments described at ¶ 459 and ¶ 467 is made in a written statement filed with the partnership return for the first year to be covered by the election (Reg. § 1.754-1).[172] The election applies to all property distributions and transfers of partnership interests taking place in the year of the election and in all later partnership tax years until revoked..

An automatic extension of 12 months from the original deadline for making the Code Sec. 754 basis adjustment election is generally available, provided the taxpayer takes corrective action within that 12-month extension period (Reg. § 301.9100-2).[173]

Family Partnerships

474. Family Partnerships. The family partnership is a common device for splitting income among family members and having more income taxed in the lower tax brackets. A family member is recognized as a partner for income tax purposes if he or she owns a capital interest in a partnership in which capital is a material income-producing factor, whether or not he or she purchased the interest (Code Sec. 704(e); Reg. § 1.704-1(e)).[174] If capital is *not* a material income-producing factor, a partnership resulting from a gift of an interest might be disregarded as an invalid attempt to assign income. In any event, if all the income is attributable to the personal efforts of the donor, the donor is taxed on the entire income. In addition, the donee's distributive share of income must be proportionate to his or her capital interest, and his or her control over the partnership must be consistent with his or her status as partner.

Family limited partnerships are also used for estate planning purposes (¶ 2903).

References are to Standard Federal Tax Reports; Tax Research Consultant; and Practical Tax Explanations.

[167] ¶ 25,480, ¶ 25,481; PART: 45,100; § 30,810

[168] ¶ 25,480; PART: 45,112; § 30,810

[169] ¶ 25,480; PART: 45,100; § 30,810

[170] ¶ 25,480; PART: 45,112; § 30,810

[171] ¶ 25,580; PART: 45,150; § 30,810

[172] ¶ 25,561; PART: 45,250; § 30,825

[173] ¶ 44,014AE; PART: 45,256; § 30,825

[174] ¶ 25,120, ¶ 25,121; PART: 54,100; § 31,301

Organization, Syndication, Start-Up Costs

477. Partnership Syndication and Organization Fees. Except as provided in Code Sec. 709(b), no deduction is allowed a partnership or a partner for the costs of organizing a partnership (organization fees) or of selling partnership interests (syndication fees) (¶ 481) (Code Sec. 709; Reg. § 1.709-1).[175] Guaranteed payments (¶ 421) made to partners for their services in organizing a partnership are capital expenditures and are not deductible by the partnership.

A partnership may elect to deduct up to $5,000 in organizational expenses, generally in the same manner as start-up expenditures (¶ 481) Code Sec. 709(b).[176] The $5,000 amount is reduced (but not below zero) by the amount by which the organizational expenditures exceed $50,000. The remainder of the organizational expenditures may be amortized ratably over a 180-month period, beginning with the month the active trade or business begins. The partnership is deemed to have made an election to deduct and amortize such expenses for the tax year in which the active trade or business to which the expenditures relate begins. For expenditures paid or incurred after August 16, 2011, a taxpayer may choose to forego the deemed election by affirmatively electing to capitalize its organizational expenditures on a timely filed federal income tax return, including extensions, for the tax year in which the active trade or business to which the expenditures relate begins (Reg. § 1.709-1(b)(2)).[177]

A new partnership formed after a technical termination under Code Sec. 708(b)(1)(B) (¶ 410) (occurring on or after December 9, 2013), must continue amortizing start-up expenses (as provided in Code Sec. 195) over the remainder of the amortization period originally established by the terminating partnership (Reg. § 1.708-1(b)(6)).[178]

481. Partnership Start-Up Expenditures. Taxpayers who pay or incur start-up costs for a trade or business and who subsequently enter the trade or business can elect to expense up to $5,000 of the costs (¶ 904). The $5,000 deduction amount is reduced dollar for dollar when the start-up expenses exceed $50,000. The balance of start-up expenses (if any) are amortized over a period of not less than 180 months, starting with the month in which the business begins (Code Sec. 195).[179] The election must be made on Form 4562 no later than the date (including extensions) for filing the return for the tax year in which the business begins or is acquired (Reg. § 1.195-1(b)).[180] A taxpayer who does not make the election must capitalize the expenses.

In the case of start-up expenses incurred by the partnership itself and for which an election is made, the amortization deduction is taken into account in computing partnership income. In the case of qualifying investigatory expenses incurred in connection with acquiring a partnership interest, the deduction is taken by the partner who has incurred the expenses. A new partnership formed after a technical termination under Code Sec. 708(b)(1)(B) (¶ 410) (occurring on or after December 9, 2013) must continue amortizing start-up expenses (as provided in Code Sec. 195) over the remainder of the amortization period originally established by the terminating partnership (Reg. § 1.708-1(b)(6)).[181]

Electing Large Partnerships

482. Simplified Reporting for Electing Large Partnerships. Partnerships with 100 or more members in the preceding tax year may elect large partnership status (Code Secs. 771—777).[182] An electing large partnership combines most items of partnership income, deduction, credit, and loss at the partnership level and passes through net amounts to the partners. Special rules apply to partnerships engaging in oil and gas activities and to partnerships with residual interests in real estate mortgage investment conduits (REMICs). Service partnerships and commodity pools generally are unable to elect large partnership treatment.

References are to Standard Federal Tax Reports; Tax Research Consultant; and Practical Tax Explanations.

[175] ¶ 25,220, ¶ 25,221C; PART: 18,200; § 9,210.15

[176] ¶ 25,220; PART: 18,200; § 9,210.15

[177] ¶ 25,221C; PART: 18,206.05; § 9,215

[178] ¶ 25,201; PART: 51,256.45; § 31,020.05

[179] ¶ 12,370; PART: 18,104.10; § 9,205.05

[180] ¶ 12,370F; DEPR: 21,406

[181] ¶ 25,201; PART: 51,256.45; § 31,020.05

[182] ¶ 25,604—¶ 25,628; PART: 3,450

A partnership may lose its large partnership status if the number of partners falls below 100 during any partnership tax year. Rules for determining the treatment of a partnership whose membership falls below 100 have not been provided by the IRS.

An electing large partnership does not terminate for tax purposes solely because 50 percent or more of its interests are sold or exchanged within a 12-month period.

484. Deductions and Credits of Electing Large Partnerships. The taxable income of an electing large partnership (¶ 482) is computed in the same manner as in the case of an individual, except that certain items are separately stated, and specified modifications apply (Code Sec. 773).[183] For example, miscellaneous itemized deductions are not separately reported to the partners. In place of applying the 2-percent floor for itemized deductions, 70 percent of the itemized deductions are disallowed at the partnership level. The 70-percent cut is designed to approximate the amount of the deduction that would be lost to the individual partners under the 2-percent floor. The remaining 30 percent is allowed at the partnership level in determining the large partnership's taxable income and is not subject to the 2-percent floor at the partner level.

Tax credits other than the low-income housing credit, the rehabilitation credit, and the credit for producing fuel from nonconventional sources are reported as a single item. Credit recapture also is recognized at the partnership level.

485. Gains and Losses of Electing Large Partnerships. For electing large partnerships (¶ 482), the netting of capital gains and losses occurs at the partnership level (Code Sec. 773).[184] Passive activity items are separated from capital gains stemming from partnership portfolio income. Each partner separately takes into account the partner's distributive shares of net capital gain or net capital loss for passive activity and portfolio items.

Any partnership gains and losses under Code Sec. 1231 (¶ 1747) are netted at the partnership level. Net gain is treated as long-term capital gain and is subject to the rules described above, and any net loss is treated as ordinary loss and consolidated with the partnership's other taxable income.

488. Audit Procedures for Electing Large Partnerships. The TEFRA partnership audit rules normally applicable to partnerships do not apply to electing large partnerships. An electing large partnership, like other partnerships, appoints a representative to handle IRS matters (Code Sec. 6255(b)).[185] Unlike under the TEFRA rules, the representative does not have to be a partner. Only the partnership, and not the individual partners, receives notice of partnership adjustments (Code Sec. 6245(b)).[186] Only the partnership has the right to appeal the adjustment (Code Sec. 6247(a)).[187] After a partnership-level adjustment, prior-year partners and prior tax years generally are not affected. However, prior years can be affected if there has been a partnership dissolution or a finding that the shares of a distribution to partners were erroneous. Instead, the adjustments generally are passed through to current partners.

References are to Standard Federal Tax Reports; Tax Research Consultant; and Practical Tax Explanations.

[183] ¶ 25,612; PART: 18,452, PART: 18,454

[184] ¶ 25,612; PART: 18,452, PART: 18,454

[185] ¶ 37,949Q; PART: 60,652

[186] ¶ 37,937; PART: 60,660

[187] ¶ 37,949D; PART: 60,662

Chapter 5

TRUSTS □ ESTATES

Estates and Trusts as Taxable Entities

501. Trust, Estate, and Fiduciary Defined. A trust is a separate taxable entity for federal income tax purposes. A trust usually involves an arrangement created either by a will upon the creator's death or by a trust instrument that may take effect during the creator's life (Reg. §301.7701-4(a)).[1] Under either arrangement, a trustee takes title to the property in order to protect or conserve it for beneficiaries. Usually, the beneficiaries merely accept the trust's benefits. However, even if the beneficiaries are the persons who planned or created it, the trust will still be recognized as a separate taxable entity if its purpose is to vest the trustee with the responsibility to protect and preserve property on behalf of beneficiaries who cannot share in the discharge of this responsibility. Federal tax law provides specific guidelines for what constitutes a business trust or investment trust (¶ 502) and a liquidating trust (¶ 503). Some types of trusts are governed by special tax rules, such as grantor trusts (¶ 571), charitable trusts (¶ 590), and common trust funds (¶ 595).

Decedents' estates are also considered separate taxable entities for income tax purposes during the period of administration (¶ 507). Other types of estates are discussed at ¶ 504—¶ 506.

Trustees, executors, and certain receivers are considered fiduciaries. A fiduciary is a person who occupies a position of special confidence toward another, who holds in trust property in which another person has the beneficial title or interest, or who receives and controls income of another (Reg. §301.7701-6).[2] However, a person who is an agent of another person is not necessarily a fiduciary for federal income tax purposes, even though a fiduciary relationship may be said to exist for state law purposes. For example, when a person receives income as an agent, intermediary debtor, or conduit, and the income is paid over to another, the agent is not considered a fiduciary for tax purposes. The fiduciary is responsible for computing the entity's income tax liability and paying the resulting tax (¶ 510), and may be personally liable for any tax delinquencies if others are paid in preference to the IRS (¶ 512).

Small Business Trusts. An electing small business trust (ESBT) is a special kind of trust permitted to be a shareholder in an S corporation. An ESBT has no beneficiaries other than individuals or estates eligible to be S corporation shareholders, except that charitable organizations may hold contingent remainder interests. The portion of any ESBT that consists of stock in one or more S corporations is treated as a separate trust (¶ 304 and ¶ 516).

Qualified Domestic Trusts. A qualified domestic trust (QDOT) is a trust that meets certain requirements and is subject to a special estate tax. Property that is transferred

---

References are to Standard Federal Tax Reports; Tax Research Consultant; and Practical Tax Explanations.

[1] ¶ 43,090; ESTTRST: 3,050; §32,005.05   [2] ¶ 43,094; ESTTRST: 100; §32,030.05

¶501

from a citizen decedent to a nonresident alien spouse will not qualify for the usual estate tax marital deduction unless it is transferred from the decedent to a QDOT (¶ 2926).

Foreign Trusts and Estates. A foreign trust is a trust in which (1) no court within the United States can exercise primary supervision over the trust's administration (court test), and (2) no U.S. person has the authority to control all of the trust's substantial decisions (control test). A foreign estate is an estate whose income, from non-U.S. sources which is not effectively connected with the conduct of a trade or business in the United States (¶ 2431), is not includible in gross income for federal income tax purposes (Code Sec. 7701(a)(30) and (31); Reg. § 301.7701-7).[3]

502. Business and Investment Trusts. A business or commercial trust is a trust created as a means of carrying on a profit-making business, usually using capital or property supplied by the beneficiaries (Reg. § 301.7701-4(b)).[4] The trustees or other designated persons are, in effect, managers of the undertaking, whether appointed or controlled by the beneficiaries. This arrangement is treated for federal tax purposes as an association which may be taxed as a corporation or partnership, and is distinguishable from the type of trust discussed at ¶ 501. The fact that the trust property is not supplied by beneficiaries is not sufficient in itself to avoid the trust being classified and taxed as a business entity.

An investment trust may also be taxed as an association, rather than a trust, if there is a power under the trust agreement to vary the investment of the certificate holders (Reg. § 301.7701-4(c)).[5] However, if this power is lacking, the arrangement is taxed as a trust. Unit investment trusts, as defined in the Investment Company Act of 1940, that are set up to hold mutual fund shares for investors are also not taxed as trusts. Instead, their income is taxed directly to the investors (Reg. § 1.851-7).[6]

503. Liquidating Trusts. A liquidating trust formed for the primary purpose of liquidating and distributing the assets transferred to it is taxed as a trust, and not as an association, despite the possibility of profit (Reg. § 301.7701-4(d)).[7] All activities of the trust must be reasonably necessary to, and consistent with, accomplishing the primary purpose of liquidation and distribution. If the liquidation is unreasonably prolonged, or if the liquidation purpose becomes so obscured by business activities that the declared purpose of liquidation can be said to have been lost or abandoned, the arrangement is no longer a liquidating trust.

504. Estate of Minor, Incompetent, or Person Under a Disability. The estate of an infant, incompetent person, or other person under a disability is not a taxable entity separate from the person for whom the fiduciary (¶ 501) is acting (Reg. § 1.641(b)-2(b)).[8] Therefore, the estate of such a person is not required to file a fiduciary return on Form 1041.

A guardian is generally required to file a tax return as an agent for a minor or legally disabled person if the individual would otherwise be required to file a return (Code Sec. 6012(b)(2); Reg. § 1.6012-3(b)(3)).[9] However, a minor can file a return for himself or herself or have someone else file it, relieving the guardian of this obligation. For the tax year during which an incompetent person is declared competent and the fiduciary is discharged, the former incompetent person must file the tax return. An agent filing a return for another person should file Form 2848, granting power of attorney, with the taxpayer's return (Reg. § 1.6012-1(a)(5)).[10] If an agent is used, both the agent and the taxpayer for whom the return is made may be liable for penalties for erroneous, false, or fraudulent returns. One spouse may execute a valid return on behalf of his or her mentally incompetent or disabled spouse prior to appointment of a legal guardian without a formal power of attorney (Rev. Rul. 56-22).[11]

References are to Standard Federal Tax Reports; Tax Research Consultant; and Practical Tax Explanations.

[3] ¶ 43,080, ¶ 43,097; INTL: 3,552.15; § 32,190, § 32,610.30

[4] ¶ 43,090; ESTTRST: 3,102; § 30,005.35

[5] ¶ 43,090; ESTTRST: 3,154; § 30,005.35

[6] ¶ 26,407; RIC: 3,150; § 45,430.05

[7] ¶ 43,090; ESTTRST: 3,158; § 32,125

[8] ¶ 24,265; FILEIND: 18,064; § 39,030.25

[9] ¶ 35,142, ¶ 35,146; FILEIND: 18,064; § 1,305.25, § 39,020.05

[10] ¶ 35,143; FILEBUS: 12,102; § 41,205.05

[11] ¶ 35,150.734; FILEIND: 18,064; § 39,020.05

505. Bankruptcy Estate of Individual Debtor. Property held by a trustee in bankruptcy for an individual under Chapter 7 (liquidation) or Chapter 11 (business reorganization) of the Bankruptcy Code is considered the estate of the debtor (Code Sec. 1398).[12] The estate is treated as a separate taxable entity unless the bankruptcy case is dismissed. The fiduciary of a Chapter 7 or Chapter 11 bankruptcy estate is obligated to file the estate's return. If the bankruptcy plan creates a liquidating trust, the fiduciary must file the trust's return (Code Sec. 6012(b)(4)).[13] The bankruptcy trustee must file a Form 1041 for the bankruptcy estate for any tax year in which the estate in bankruptcy has gross income that equals or exceeds the sum of the personal exemption amount (¶ 133), plus the basic standard deduction for married persons filing separately (¶ 126) for the year ($10,150 for 2014; $10,300 for 2015) (Code Sec. 6012(a)(8)). The tax year for which the fiduciary files a return begins on the date of the bankruptcy petition filing. The return may be for a calendar year or a fiscal year. A trustee in bankruptcy has no authority to file a return on Form 1040 for a bankrupt individual; the individual must file an individual return.

Taxable income for bankruptcy estates is computed in the same manner as for individuals, including the right to a personal exemption, but the tax rates for married persons filing separately apply (¶ 15) (Code Sec. 1398(c); Instructions to Form 1041). If a bankruptcy estate does not itemize deductions, it can claim the standard deduction available for a married person filing separately (¶ 126).

A separate taxable entity is not created when a case is brought under Chapter 13 of the Bankruptcy Code, which involves adjustment of debts of an individual with regular income. A separate taxable entity also is not created when an individual is in receivership (Reg. § 1.641(b)-2(b)).[14]

506. Bankruptcy Estate of Partnership or Corporate Debtor. The commencement of bankruptcy proceedings for a partnership or corporation does not create a separate taxable entity (Code Sec. 1399).[15] Thus, there is no obligation imposed upon the bankruptcy trustee to file a Form 1041 on behalf of the estate. However, a receiver, trustee in dissolution, trustee in bankruptcy, or assignee who, by order of a court, has possession of or holds title to all or substantially all the property or business of a corporation must file the income tax return for the corporation on Form 1120 (Reg. § 1.6012-3(b)(4)).[16] The receiver, trustee, or assignee must file the return whether or not it is operating the property or business of the corporation. A receiver in charge of only *a small part* of the property of a corporation, such as a receiver in mortgage foreclosure proceedings, need not file the return. Bankrupt partnerships must file their returns on Form 1065.

507. Termination of Estates and Trusts. An estate is recognized as a taxable entity only during the period of administration or settlement (i.e., the period actually required by the executor or administrator to perform the ordinary duties of administration, such as collection of assets, payment of debts and legacies, etc.) (Reg. § 1.641(b)-3(a)).[17] This is true whether the period is longer or shorter than that specified under local law for estate settlement. However, estate administration may not be unduly prolonged. For federal tax purposes, the estate is considered terminated after the expiration of a reasonable period for the performance of administration duties, or when all estate assets have been distributed except for a reasonable amount set aside in good faith for the payment of contingent liabilities and expenses. If the estate has joined in making a valid election to treat a qualified revocable trust as part of the estate (¶ 516), then it does not terminate prior to the end of the election period.

A trust is recognized as a taxable entity until the trust property has been distributed to successors, plus a reasonable time after this event as is necessary for the trustee to

---

References are to Standard Federal Tax Reports; Tax Research Consultant; and Practical Tax Explanations.

[12] ¶ 32,410; INDIV: 66,050, INDIV: 66,066

[13] ¶ 35,142; INDIV: 66,066.05; § 32,030.05

[14] ¶ 24,265; INDIV: 66,052.10

[15] ¶ 32,420; INDIV: 66,150

[16] ¶ 35,146; FILEBUS: 3,068

[17] ¶ 24,266; ESTTRST: 9,054, ACCTNG: 24,256.10; § 32,005.10, § 38,145.20

complete trust administration (Reg. § 1.641(b)-3(b)).[18] A trust is also considered terminated when all the assets have been distributed except for a reasonable amount set aside in good faith to pay contingent liabilities and expenses (other than a claim by a beneficiary in that capacity).

Once an estate or trust is considered terminated for tax purposes, its gross income, deductions, and credits subsequent to termination are considered to be the gross income, deductions, and credits of the persons who succeed to the property (Reg. § 1.641(b)-3(d)).

Fiduciary Return and Payment of Tax

510. Return of Estate or Trust by Fiduciary. A fiduciary must file a return on Form 1041 for an estate or trust if: (1) the estate has gross income of $600 or more for the tax year; (2) the trust (other than a trust exempt under Code Sec. 501(a)) has for the tax year any taxable income, or gross income of $600 or more regardless of the amount of taxable income; (3) any beneficiary of the estate or trust is a nonresident alien (unless the trust is exempt under Code Sec. 501(a)); or (4) an individual's bankruptcy estate under Chapter 7 or Chapter 11 of the Bankruptcy Code has gross income equal to or greater than the sum of the personal exemption amount, plus the basic standard deduction amount for married individuals filing separately (¶ 505) (Code Sec. 6012(a); Reg. § 1.6012-3).[19] A foreign estate or foreign trust (¶ 501) generally must file Form 1040NR (Instructions to Form 1041).

When there is more than one fiduciary, the return can be filed by any one of them. However, when an estate has both domiciliary and ancillary representatives, each representative must file a return (Reg. § 1.6012-3(a)(1) and (3)). A trustee of two or more trusts must file a separate return for each trust, even though the trusts were created by the same grantor for the same beneficiaries (Reg. § 1.6012-3(a)(4)). Two or more trusts may be treated as one trust under certain circumstances (¶ 515).

The return must be filed on or before the 15th day of the fourth month following the close of the tax year (Code Sec. 6072(a)).[20] An estate or trust can apply for an automatic five-month extension of time for filing the fiduciary return by filing Form 7004 on or before the due date for filing Form 1041, and making a proper estimate of the amount of tax due for the tax year (Reg. § 1.6081-6; Instructions to Form 7004).[21] The automatic extension period is six months for an individual's Chapter 7 or 11 bankruptcy estate (¶ 505) or for a qualified funeral trust (¶ 575). The automatic extension does not extend the time for payment of any tax due on the return. In addition, the extension to file does not extend the time for a beneficiary of the estate or trust to file its income tax return or to pay any tax on the beneficiary's return.

The fiduciary of an estate or trust need not file a copy of the will or trust instrument with the estate or trust income tax return unless requested by the IRS (Reg. § 1.6012-3(a)(2)).[22] If requested, the fiduciary should file a copy (including any amendments), accompanied by a written declaration of truth and completeness and a statement indicating the provisions of the will or trust instrument that determine the extent to which estate or trust income is taxable to the estate or trust, the beneficiaries, or the grantor.

An estate or trust that is obligated to file an income tax return must furnish a copy of Schedule K-1 of Form 1041 to each beneficiary (1) who receives a distribution from the estate or trust for the year, or (2) to whom any item with respect to the tax year is allocated (Code Sec. 6034A).[23] This statement must contain the information required to be shown on the return and be furnished on or before the date on which the return is to be filed. In addition, a copy must be attached to Form 1041 (Instructions to Form 1041).

References are to Standard Federal Tax Reports; Tax Research Consultant; and Practical Tax Explanations.

[18] ¶ 24,266; ESTTRST: 9,054, ACCTNG: 24,256.10; § 32,005.15, § 38,145.20

[19] ¶ 35,142, ¶ 35,146; IRS: 30,256.10, IRS: 66,152.05; § 32,610.05, § 39,030.10

[20] ¶ 36,720; FILEIND: 18,052.20; § 32,610.15, § 39,205.25

[21] ¶ 36,797; FILEBUS: 15,104.20; § 32,610.15, § 39,215.20

[22] ¶ 35,146; IRS: 30,256.10, IRS: 66,152.05; § 32,610.15

[23] ¶ 35,460; ESTTRST: 100; § 32,610.20, § 39,155.35

A penalty may be assessed for each failure to file or furnish a correct information return (¶ 2816) or payee statement (¶ 2823).

Accounting Period. When filing its first return, an estate may choose the same accounting period as the decedent, or it may choose a calendar tax year or any fiscal tax year. If it chooses the decedent's accounting period, its first return will be for a short period to cover the unexpired term of the decedent's regular tax year (Code Secs. 441 and 443).[24] An exemption of $600 is allowed on a short-period return, without proration (¶ 534) (Reg. § 1.443-1(a)(2)).[25] However, if the estate gets approval from the IRS to change the accounting period, the exemption on the short-period return must be prorated (Reg. § 1.443-1(b)(1)(v)).

Trusts (other than trusts exempt from tax under Code Sec. 501 and wholly charitable trusts under Code Sec. 4947(a)) must adopt a calendar tax year (Code Sec. 644).[26] Thus, a trust must generally file Form 1041 on or before April 15 following the close of the tax year. If April 15 falls on a weekend or holiday, the due date is the next day that is not a Saturday, Sunday, or legal holiday (¶ 2549). An existing trust that is required to change its tax year must annualize any income earned in the short year. A trust must obtain IRS approval to change its annual accounting period to its required (calendar) tax year (¶ 1513).

Payment of Tax. The entire income tax liability of an estate or trust must be paid on or before the due date for its return (Code Sec. 6151).[27] In addition, estates that have been in existence for more than two years and both new and existing trusts must pay estimated tax in the same manner as individuals (¶ 511).

511. Payment of Estimated Tax by Estate or Trust. Estates and trusts are generally required to make quarterly estimated tax payments in the same manner as individuals (¶ 2682). However, estates and grantor trusts that receive the residue of a probate estate under the grantor's will are only required to make estimated tax payments for tax years that end two or more years after the decedent's death (Code Sec. 6654(l)).[28]

Estates or trusts with a short tax year must pay installments of tax on or before the 15th day of the fourth, sixth and ninth months of the tax year, and the 15th day of the first month of the following tax year (¶ 2685). The amount of each installment in a short tax year is determined by dividing the required annual payment by the number of payments required for that year (Notice 87-32).[29]

Estates and trusts generally have 45 days (rather than the 15 days allowed individuals) to compute the payments under the estimated tax annualization rules. The payment due dates are unchanged (Code Sec. 6654(l)).[30] First-time filers must file Form 1041-ES, which includes vouchers to be included with quarterly payments. After the first payment, the IRS should provide pre-printed vouchers. A fiduciary paying estimated tax for more than one trust should submit a separate Form 1041-ES and a separate check for each trust. However, a fiduciary may submit a single check for multiple trusts if a separate estimated tax voucher is submitted for each trust (Announcement 87-32).[31]

The trustee of a trust, or the fiduciary of an estate whose tax year is reasonably expected to be its last tax year, may elect to treat any or all of an estimated tax payment as a payment made by the beneficiary and credited toward the beneficiary's tax liability (Code Sec. 643(g)).[32] If elected, the payment is not treated as an estimated tax payment made by the estate or trust. The election is made on Form 1041-T and must be filed on or before the 65th day after the close of the tax year (March 6, 2015, for calendar year 2014).

References are to Standard Federal Tax Reports; Tax Research Consultant; and Practical Tax Explanations.

[24] ¶ 20,302, ¶ 20,500; ACCTNG: 24,252; § 32,025, § 38,140.05, § 38,145.20

[25] ¶ 20,501; ESTTRST: 12,052; § 32,350, § 38,140.05

[26] ¶ 24,350; ACCTNG: 24,104, ACCTNG: 24,252.25; § 32,025, § 32,610.15

[27] ¶ 37,080; ESTTRST: 100, FILEBUS: 6,102; § 39,305.05

[28] ¶ 39,550; FILEIND: 21,058; § 32,615.05

[29] ¶ 39,560.82; FILEIND: 21,058; § 32,615.05

[30] ¶ 39,550; FILEIND: 21,050; § 1,410, § 32,615.05, § 40,225.10

[31] ¶ 39,560.82; FILEIND: 21,058; § 32,615.05

[32] ¶ 24,320; ESTTRST: 27,054, FILEIND: 21,054.10; § 1,410, § 32,615.10

512. Personal Liability of Fiduciary. Any fiduciary (other than a trustee acting under the Bankruptcy Code) who pays any debt due by the decedent or the estate, in whole or in part, before federal tax obligations are satisfied becomes personally liable for the tax of the estate to the extent of such payments (Reg. §1.641(b)-2; 31 U.S.C. §3713).[33] However, the fiduciary is not liable for amounts paid out for debts that have priority over the federal taxes due and owing on the estate, such as a decedent's funeral expenses or probate administration costs. Further, an executor or administrator who pays other debts is not personally liable unless the executor or administrator has either personal knowledge of a tax due the United States or knowledge that would put a reasonably prudent person on notice that such tax debts exist.[34] Discharge of the fiduciary does not terminate the fiduciary's personal liability for the payment of other debts of the estate without satisfying prior tax claims.

Taxation of Estates and Trusts

514. Taxation of Estates and Trusts—Introduction. An estate or trust is a separate taxable entity (¶ 501). Its entire income for its tax year generally must be reported on Form 1041, which must be filed by the fiduciary (¶ 510). If income is required to be distributed currently or is properly distributed to a beneficiary, the estate or trust is regarded as a conduit with respect to that income. It is allowed a deduction for the portion of gross income that is currently distributable to the beneficiaries or is properly paid or credited to them (¶ 542—¶ 545). The beneficiaries are generally taxed on the part of the income currently distributed, and the estate or trust is taxed on the portion that it has accumulated. The income allocated to a beneficiary retains the same character in the beneficiary's hands that it had in the hands of the estate or trust (Reg. §§1.652(b)-1 and 1.662(b)-1).[35]

For purposes of the income taxation of estates and nongrantor trusts, the term income (without specifying gross income, taxable income, undistributed net income, or distributable net income) refers to income of the estate or trust for the tax year determined under the terms of its governing instrument and applicable local law—that is, income as it would be computed in an accounting to the court having jurisdiction over the estate or trust (Code Sec. 643(b); Reg. §1.643(b)-1).[36] Trust provisions that depart fundamentally from concepts of income and principal are not recognized for tax purposes. However, an allocation of amounts between income and principal pursuant to applicable local law will be respected if local law provides for a reasonable apportionment between the income and remainder beneficiaries of the trust's total return for the year, including ordinary income, tax-exempt income, capital gains, and appreciation.

Income items of an estate or trust are discussed at ¶ 520—¶ 527. Ordinary deductions of an estate or trust are discussed at ¶ 528—¶ 536. The charitable contribution deduction is discussed at ¶ 537—¶ 538. The deduction for distributions to beneficiaries and the concept of distributable net income (DNI) are discussed at ¶ 542—¶ 549. The treatment of tax credits of an estate or trust is discussed at ¶ 540.

515. Multiple Trusts. One grantor may create several trusts, and the income may be taxed separately for each trust. When there is intent to create separate trusts for multiple beneficiaries, the fact that the corpus of each trust is kept in one fund will not necessarily defeat the grantor's intent. Although it is not necessary to divide the corpus physically in order to carry out the intent of the parties, it is necessary to comply literally with the terms of the trust instrument in other respects.[37]

Two or more trusts, however, will be treated as one trust if (1) the trusts have substantially the same grantor or grantors and substantially the same primary beneficiary or beneficiaries, and (2) a principal purpose of the trusts is the avoidance of income tax (Code Sec. 643(f)).[38] A special safe-harbor provision applies to any trust that was

---

References are to Standard Federal Tax Reports; Tax Research Consultant; and Practical Tax Explanations.

[33] ¶ 24,265, ¶ 40,730; IRS: 60,202; §32,030.10, §34,410.07, §39,545

[34] ¶ 40,735.25; IRS: 60,206; §32,030.10, §34,410.07, §39,545

[35] ¶ 24,383, ¶ 24,425; EST-TRST: 24,154, ESTTRST: 30,106; §32,005.05, §32,501, §32,701

[36] ¶ 24,320, ¶ 24,329; EST-TRST: 18,050; §32,010.10

[37] ¶ 24,267.67; ESTTRST: 3,202; §32,185

[38] ¶ 24,320; ESTTRST: 3,204; §32,185

irrevocable on March 1, 1984, except to the extent that corpus is contributed to the trust after that date.

516. Computation of Tax for Estates and Trusts. An estate or trust computes its tax liability by using the separate estate and trust income tax rate schedule at ¶ 19. The taxable income of an estate or trust for purposes of regular income tax is determined by subtracting from its gross income (¶ 520) allowable deductions (¶ 528), amounts distributable to beneficiaries (to the extent of distributable net income (DNI)) (¶ 543), and the proper exemption (¶ 534) (Code Sec. 641; Reg. §§ 1.641(a)-1 and 1.641(b)-1).[39]

The alternative minimum tax (AMT) of an estate or trust is computed by determining DNI under the general rules (¶ 543), subject to further adjustments under the minimum tax rules. The AMT is computed on Part III of Schedule I, Form 1041 (¶ 1401).

Grantor trusts and employees' trusts are subject to special tax treatment (¶ 571 and ¶ 2101).

Qualified Revocable Trusts. A trustee of a qualified revocable trust (QRT) and the executor, if any, of a decedent's estate may join in an election to treat the revocable trust as part of the estate (Code Sec. 645; Reg. § 1.645-1).[40] The election allows the revocable trust to enjoy certain income tax treatment that would otherwise be accorded only to the decedent's estate, such as claiming the unlimited deduction for amounts permanently set aside for charity without first actually paying the amount (¶ 537), waiving the active participation requirement under the passive loss rules for two years after the decedent's death (¶ 1165), and qualifying for amortization of reforestation expenditures (¶ 530). A QRT is any trust or portion of a trust that, on the date of the decedent's death, is treated as owned by the decedent as grantor by reason of a power to revoke the trust (¶ 582), but without regard to powers held by the decedent's spouse (¶ 578). The election is made on Form 8855 which must be filed by the due date (including extensions) of the Form 1041 for the first tax year of the related estate or filing trust. The election period begins on the date of the decedent's death, and ends on the earlier of the day on which both the trust and related estate have distributed all of their assets, or the day before the applicable date, which is either (1) two years after the date of death, if no federal estate tax return is required, or (2) six months after the final determination of estate tax liability, if a federal estate tax return must be filed.

Electing Small Business Trust. An electing small business trust (ESBT) (¶ 501) is taxed in a different manner than other trusts (Code Sec. 641(c); Reg. § 1.641(c)-1).[41] First, the portion of the ESBT that consists of stock in one or more S corporations is treated as a separate trust for purposes of computing the income tax attributable to the S corporation stock held by the trust. This portion of the trust's income is taxed at the highest rate imposed on estates and trusts, and includes:

(1) the items of income, loss, deduction, or credit allocated to the trust as an S corporation shareholder;

(2) gain or loss from the sale of the S corporation stock;

(3) any state or local income taxes and administrative expenses of the trust properly allocable to the S corporation stock; and

(4) any interest expense paid or accrued on debt incurred to acquire S corporation stock.

Capital losses are allowed in computing an ESBT's income only to the extent of capital gains. Moreover, no deduction is allowed for amounts distributed to beneficiaries and, except as described above, no additional deductions or credits are allowed. Also, the ESBT's income is not included in the DNI of the trust and, therefore, is not included in the beneficiaries' income. Furthermore, no item relating to the S corporation stock is apportioned to any beneficiary. The trust's AMT exemption amount is zero. Special rules apply upon termination of all or a part of the ESBT (¶ 304).

References are to Standard Federal Tax Reports; Tax Research Consultant; and Practical Tax Explanations.

[39] ¶ 24,260, ¶ 24,262, ¶ 24,264; ESTTRST: 100; § 32,005.05, § 32,010, § 32,015, § 32,020

[40] ¶ 24,355, ¶ 24,356; EST-TRST: 39,300; § 32,105.10

[41] ¶ 24,260, ¶ 24,266F; SCORP: 166.35; § 32,165

Special rules apply for calculating the 3.8-percent net investment income tax (¶ 517) of an ESBT (Reg. § 1.1411-3(c)).[42]

Gifts from Expatriates. A domestic trust that receives property, directly or indirectly, by gift, devise, bequest, or inheritance from a covered expatriate (¶ 2412) after the date of expatriation must pay a tax equal to the value of such covered gift or bequest multiplied by the greater of the highest federal estate tax rate or the highest federal gift tax rate in effect. Similarly, a covered gift or bequest made to a foreign trust (¶ 501) is subject to the tax, but only at the time a distribution of income or principal is made to a U.S. citizen or resident from the trust that is attributable to the covered gift or bequest. A foreign trust can elect to be treated as a domestic trust for these purposes; the election can be revoked with IRS consent (¶ 2948).

517. Net Investment Income Tax of Estates and Trusts. Effective for tax years beginning after December 31, 2012, an estate or trust is liable for a 3.8-percent net investment income tax on the lesser of: (1) its undistributed net investment income for the tax year, or (2) any excess of its adjusted gross income determined under Code Sec. 67(e) (¶ 528) over the dollar amount at which the highest tax bracket for estates and trusts begins for the tax year ($12,150 for 2014; $12,300 for 2015; ¶ 19) (Code Sec. 1411(a)(2); Reg. § 1.1411-3).[43] An estate or trust's undistributed net investment income is its net investment income (¶ 129) reduced by distributions of net investment income to beneficiaries, and by deductions for amounts of net investment income paid or permanently set aside for a charitable purpose (¶ 537) (Reg. § 1.1411-3(e)).

The tax does not apply to several types of trusts, including (1) trusts that are exempt from federal income taxes; (2) trusts whose unexpired interests are devoted to one or more charitable purposes described in Code Sec. 170(c)(2)(B); (3) grantor trusts (¶ 571); (4) Electing Alaska Native Settlement Trusts; (5) cemetery perpetual care funds under Code Sec. 642(i); and (6) any other trust, fund, or account that is statutorily exempt from federal income tax (Code Sec. 1411(e)(2); Reg. § 1.1411-3(b)). The tax applies to individual debtors' Chapter 7 and Chapter 11 bankruptcy estates (¶ 505). The tax does not apply to foreign trusts or foreign estates (¶ 501), but does apply to distributions of current year income by foreign trusts or foreign estates to their U.S. beneficiaries (Reg. § 1.1411-3(e)(3)).

520. Gross Income of Estates and Trusts. The gross income of an estate or trust is generally determined in the same manner as that of an individual (Code Sec. 641(b); Reg. § 1.641(a)-2).[44] It includes all items of income received during the tax year, including:

    (1) income accumulated in trust for the benefit of unborn or unascertained persons or persons with contingent interests;

    (2) income accumulated or held for future distribution under the terms of the will or trust;

    (3) income that is to be distributed currently by the fiduciary to the beneficiaries, and income collected by the guardian of an infant that is to be held or distributed as the court may direct;

    (4) income received by the estate of a deceased person during the period of administration or settlement of the estate; and

    (5) income that, at the discretion of the fiduciary, may be either distributed to the beneficiaries or accumulated.

Although all the items above are includible in gross income, the tax liability may rest on either the estate or trust as a separate entity or on the beneficiary (¶ 542).

References are to Standard Federal Tax Reports; Tax Research Consultant; and Practical Tax Explanations.

[42] ¶ 32,603L; ESTTRST: 12,256.20

[43] ¶ 32,602, ¶ 32,603L; EST-TRST: 12,256; § 32,022

[44] ¶ 24,260, ¶ 24,263; EST-TRST: 9,052, ESTTRST: 24,100; § 32,201

The allocation of income and deductions between a decedent's estate and the surviving spouse in community property states depends on state community property laws. In most states, the surviving spouse is taxed on one-half of the income flowing from the community property of the estate.[45]

522. Real Estate Income of Estates. State law determines whether income from real estate during the period of administration is taxable to the decedent's estate or to the heirs or devisees (¶ 520). The IRS has ruled that if state law provides that real property is subject to administration, income derived from the property is taxable to the estate even though legal title may pass directly to the heirs or devisees. However, if the administrator is not entitled to possession or control of real property, income from the property is taxable to the heirs or devisees and not to the estate. Even if the property is not subject to the administrator's control, all or a part of the gain from a sale of property is taxable to the estate to the extent that the property was sold, under state law, to raise funds for its administration (Rev. Rul. 57-133; Rev. Rul. 59-375).[46]

523. Personal Property Income of Estates. Income from personal property, including a gain from the sale or exchange of such property, is taxable to the estate (¶ 520). This is because title to personal property vests in the administrator or executor immediately upon appointment and does not pass to the heirs or legatees until the estate is fully administered and distribution is ordered or approved by the courts, and notwithstanding the fact that the basis of the property distributed relates back to the date of the decedent's death.[47]

524. Sale of Property by Estates and Trusts. The gain or loss realized on the sale of property acquired by an estate, trust, or beneficiary is determined under special basis rules, the applicability of which depends on how the property was acquired and the nature of the property sold (¶ 1601 and ¶ 1701).

For estates of decedents dying in 2010, if the executor elected *not* to have the federal estate tax apply to the estate (¶ 2901), then the decedent's estate, a qualified revocable trust (¶ 516), or an heir may be able to exclude from gross income the gain on the sale of the decedent's personal residence (Code Sec. 121(d)(11), prior to repeal by the Tax Relief, Unemployment Insurance Reauthorization, and Job Creation Act of 2010 (P.L. 111-312); Act Sec. 301 of P.L. 111-312).[48] The general rules for the personal residence gain exclusion are discussed at ¶ 1705. This exclusion is not available for estates of 2010 decedents whose executors did not make the special election, or for estates of decedents dying after 2010.

526. Gain on Transfer of Property to Beneficiary. Gain or loss is generally realized by an estate or trust, or by the other beneficiaries, on the distribution of property in kind that satisfies a beneficiary's right to receive a specific dollar amount, specific property other than the property distributed, or other income if income is required to be distributed currently (Reg. § 1.661(a)-2(f)).[49] A special rule generally limits gain recognized on transfers to qualified heirs of property for which a special use valuation election under Code Sec. 2032A was made (¶ 2922) (Code Sec. 1040).[50] However, for estates of decedents dying in 2010 for which the executor elected *not* to have the federal estate tax apply (¶ 2901), this rule limits gain on exchanges that satisfy pecuniary bequests with appreciated property (former Code Sec. 1040, prior to repeal by the Tax Relief, Unemployment Insurance Reauthorization, and Job Creation Act of 2010 (P.L. 111-312); Act Sec. 301 of P.L. 111-312).

For purposes of the rule limiting gain on transfers to qualified heirs of special use valuation property, a marital deduction trust (¶ 2926) comprising a portion of the residuary estate and measured by a percentage of the value of the adjusted gross estate is considered as being provided for in a fixed dollar amount (Rev. Rul. 60-87).[51] Upon a

---

References are to Standard Federal Tax Reports; Tax Research Consultant; and Practical Tax Explanations.

[45] ¶ 2350.2473; INDIV: 24,200, ESTTRST: 9,108; § 32,205.25

[46] ¶ 24,267.5204; ESTTRST: 9,102; § 32,205.30

[47] ¶ 24,267.515; ESTTRST: 9,052; § 32,210.05

[48] ¶ 7260; REAL: 15,150; § 1,610.30, § 34,901

[49] ¶ 24,402; ESTTRST: 21,150; § 32,215, § 32,520

[50] ¶ 29,779, ¶ 29,780; EST-TRST: 21,252; § 18,225

[51] ¶ 24,267.5281; ESTTRST: 21,158; § 32,520

distribution of property to such a trust, the estate realizes gain or loss equal to the difference between the property's fair market value at the distribution date and its federal estate tax value.

Distribution of a stated percentage of trust corpus to the beneficiary before termination of the trust is not considered a satisfaction of a trust obligation for a definite amount of cash or equivalent value in property. Instead, it is treated as a partial distribution of a share of the trust principal. Thus, there is no sale or exchange, and neither the trustee nor the beneficiary realizes taxable income (Rev. Rul. 55-117).[52] However, a trustee or executor may elect to recognize gain or loss on the distribution of noncash property to a beneficiary as if the property had been sold to the beneficiary at its fair market value (Code Sec. 643(e)(3)).[53] The election is made on the return for the year of distribution and applies to all distributions made by the estate or trust during its entire tax year. Thus, an election to recognize gain or loss cannot be made separately for each distribution.

In the event the election is made, the beneficiary's basis in the distributed property is the estate's or trust's adjusted basis just prior to the distribution, adjusted by the gain or loss recognized by the estate or trust. If the election is not made, the beneficiary's basis is the same as the trust's or estate's, and any gain or loss is recognized by the beneficiary when the beneficiary disposes of the property.

Gain recognition on certain property distributions to expatriates is discussed at ¶ 566.

527. Income of Foreign Estates and Trusts. For purposes of computing the taxable income of a foreign estate or foreign trust (¶ 501), the estate or trust is treated as a nonresident alien individual who is not present in the United States at any time (¶ 2409 and ¶ 2425) (Code Sec. 641(b)).[54]

The estate of a nonresident alien is taxed on its income received from U.S. sources, including capital gains and dividends (Rev. Rul. 68-621).[55] The estate is allowed a deduction for distributions to both nonresident aliens and U.S. beneficiaries to the extent that these distributions are not in excess of its distributable net income (¶ 545). The portion of the distribution allocated to capital gains is not includible in the gross income of nonresident alien beneficiaries if they have not resided in the United States for a period of at least 183 days (¶ 2435). However, the portion of a distribution that represents dividends is includible in the gross income of nonresident alien beneficiaries. The fiduciary must withhold U.S. taxes from these dividend distributions at the statutory rate or the applicable treaty rate.

528. Deductions of Estates and Trusts—Generally. Estates and trusts are generally allowed the same deductions as individuals in computing taxable income (Code Sec. 641(b); Reg. § 1.641(b)-1).[56] However, the standard deduction available to estates and trusts is zero (Code Sec. 63(c)(6)(D)).[57] In addition, special rules govern the computation of certain deductions and the allocation of deductions between the beneficiaries and the estate or trust (¶ 529—¶ 538). Further, the estate or trust is permitted to claim a deduction for certain distributions to beneficiaries (¶ 544 and ¶ 545). The limitation on the amount of allowable itemized deductions for higher-income individuals (¶ 1014) does not apply to estates and trusts (Code Sec. 68(e)).[58]

Two-Percent Floor on Itemized Deductions. An estate or trust is generally subject to the two-percent-of-adjusted-gross-income (AGI) floor on miscellaneous itemized deductions (¶ 1011) (Code Sec. 67(e)).[59] The AGI of an estate or trust is computed in the same manner as it is for an individual (¶ 1005), except that the following deductions are allowed from gross income: (1) deductions for expenses paid or incurred in connection with the administration of the estate or trust that would not have been incurred had the

---

References are to Standard Federal Tax Reports; Tax Research Consultant; and Practical Tax Explanations.

[52] ¶ 24,267.5281; ESTTRST: 21,158; § 32,505.15, § 32,520

[53] ¶ 24,320; ESTTRST: 21,102; § 32,505.15, § 32,520

[54] ¶ 24,260; ESTTRST:100; § 32,005.05

[55] ¶ 24,267.4985; ESTTRST: 30,106; § 32,005.05, § 37,005

[56] ¶ 24,260, ¶ 24,264; EST-TRST: 12,000; § 32,301

[57] ¶ 6020; ESTTRST: 12,050; § 32,301

[58] ¶ 6080; ESTTRST: 12,054; § 32,301

[59] ¶ 6060; ESTTRST: 12,054; § 32,345

property not been so held; (2) the personal exemption deduction allowed to estates and trusts (¶ 534); and (3) the deduction for distribution to beneficiaries (¶ 544 and ¶ 545). The IRS has regulatory authority to apply the two-percent floor at the beneficiary level, rather than the entity level, with respect to simple trusts.

The U.S. Supreme Court has ruled that only estate or trust expenses that would be uncommon, unusual, or unlikely for a hypothetical individual to incur are not subject to the two-percent floor (*M.J. Knight, Trustee,* SCt, 2008-1 USTC ¶ 50,132).[60] These types of costs would not "commonly" or "customarily" be incurred by individuals. Hence, investment advisory fees incurred by an estate or trust are generally subject to the two-percent floor. Expenses incurred in administering a bankruptcy estate are fully deductible from gross income (CCA 200630016).

Regulations consistent with *Knight* provide that a cost is subject to the two-percent floor to the extent that it commonly or customarily would be incurred by a hypothetical individual holding the same property (Reg. § 1.67-4(a)).[61] Rules are provided for four specific categories of costs: ownership costs, tax preparation fees, investment advisory fees, and appraisal fees. Fees for investment advice are generally subject to the two-percent floor, but certain incremental costs of investment advice beyond the amount normally charged to an individual investor are not. A single fee or commission (a "bundled fee") paid by an estate or nongrantor trust must be allocated between the costs that are subject to the two-percent floor and those that are not. The allocation can be made using any reasonable method. However, for tax years beginning before January 1, 2015, taxpayers are not required to determine the portion of a bundled fiduciary fee that is subject to the two-percent floor. Instead, taxpayers may deduct 100 percent of the bundled fiduciary fee without regard to the two-percent floor (Reg. § 1.67-4(d); Notice 2011-37).[62]

529. Deductible Expenses of Estates and Trusts. An estate or trust is generally allowed deductions for any ordinary and necessary expenses incurred in carrying on a trade or business (¶ 901), in the production of income or the management or conservation of income-producing property (¶ 1085), or in connection with the determination, collection, or refund of any tax (¶ 1092). Reasonable amounts paid or incurred by a fiduciary on account of administration, including fiduciary fees and litigation expenses, are deductible as well. Such expenses are deductible even if the estate or trust is not engaged in a trade or business, unless the expenses were for the production or collection of tax-exempt income (Reg. § 1.212-1(i)).[63]

Deductions are not allowed for: (1) expenses that are allocable to one or more classes of income exempt from tax (other than interest income); or (2) any amount relating to expenses for the production of income that is allocable to tax-exempt interest income (¶ 970). The IRS allows a deduction for an executor's or administrator's commissions, as paid or accrued, except the portion allocable to tax-exempt income.[64]

Alimony Payments. An estate can deduct the value of periodic alimony payments it makes under the rules regarding deductions for distributions to beneficiaries.[65]

Double Deductions Prohibited. Amounts deductible as administration expenses or losses for estate tax (¶ 2925) or generation-skipping transfer tax (¶ 2942) purposes may not also be deducted, or offset against the sales price of property in determining gain or loss (i.e., selling expenses) for income tax purposes by the estate or any other person (Code Sec. 642(g); Reg. § 1.642(g)-1).[66] However, the estate can deduct such items for income tax purposes if it files a statement (in duplicate) that the items have not been claimed as deductions for estate tax purposes and that all rights to deduct them for such purposes are waived.

References are to Standard Federal Tax Reports; Tax Research Consultant; and Practical Tax Explanations.

[60] ¶ 6064.75; ESTTRST: 12,054; § 32,345

[61] ¶ 6063C; ESTTRST: 12,054; § 32,345

[62] ¶ 6063C, ¶ 6064.75; EST-TRST: 12,054; § 32,345

[63] ¶ 12,521; ESTTRST: 12,054, ESTTRST: 12,056; § 32,315.05

[64] ¶ 12,523.51, ¶ 24,686.80; ESTTRST: 12,058; § 32,315.15

[65] ¶ 6094.31, ¶ 24,267.403, ¶ 24,407.56; ESTTRST: 27,052.10; § 1,905.20, § 32,310

[66] ¶ 24,280, ¶ 24,299; EST-TRST: 9,200, ESTTRST: 9,202; § 32,310

Note that one deduction or portion of a deduction may be allowed for income tax purposes if the appropriate statement is filed, while another deduction or portion is allowed for estate tax purposes (Reg. § 1.642(g)-2).[67] Deductions for taxes, interest, business expenses, and other items accrued *at the decedent's date of death* are allowed as a deduction for estate tax purposes as claims against the estate, and are also allowed as a deduction in respect of a decedent for income tax purposes. However, the estate cannot take an income tax deduction for the decedent's medical and dental expenses that it has paid. These expenses can only be claimed on the estate tax return or the decedent's final income tax return (¶ 1018).

530. Depreciation and Depletion Deductions of Estates and Trusts. Depreciation and depletion deductions must be apportioned between an estate or trust and its beneficiaries (Code Secs. 167(d), 611(b), and 642(e); Reg. §§ 1.167(h)-1, 1.611-1(c), and 1.642(e)-1).[68] Different rules govern estates and trusts.

For a trust, the allowable deduction for depreciation or depletion is apportioned between the income beneficiaries and the trustee on the basis of the trust income allocable to each. However, if the trust instrument or local law requires or permits the trustee to maintain a reserve for depreciation or depletion, the deduction is first allocated to the trustee to the extent that income is set aside for the reserve. Any part of the deduction in excess of the income set aside for the reserve is then apportioned between the income beneficiaries and the trust on the basis of the trust income allocable to each. No effect is given to any allocation that gives any beneficiary or trustee a share of the deduction greater than a pro rata share of the trust income. The allocation is disregarded despite any provisions in the trust instrument, unless the trust instrument or local law requires or permits the trustee to maintain a reserve for depreciation or depletion.

For an estate, the depreciation or depletion allowance is apportioned between the estate and the heirs, legatees, and devisees on the basis of the income from the property allocable to each.

Section 179 Election. Although an estate or trust is entitled to take MACRS depreciation on qualified assets, neither can make a Code Sec. 179 election to expense depreciable business assets (¶ 1208) (Code Sec. 179(d)(4)).[69]

Reforestation Expenditures. Estates can elect to expense reforestation expenditures and amortize any excess expenditures (¶ 1287) (Code Sec. 194).[70] Trusts cannot elect the expense deduction but can elect to amortize such expenditures. Total reforestation expenditures incurred must be apportioned between the income beneficiaries and the fiduciary. Amounts apportioned to a beneficiary must be taken into account in determining the dollar limit on the reforestation expenditures that the beneficiary can expense.

531. Losses and Bad Debt Deductions of Estate and Trusts. An estate or trust can deduct losses from a trade or business or from transactions entered into for profit (¶ 1101). Similarly, the rules governing nonbusiness casualty and theft losses (¶ 1121) apply to an estate or trust. Thus, after the $100-per-occurrence floor has been satisfied, losses in excess of nonbusiness casualty and theft gains are deductible to the extent that they exceed 10 percent of the adjusted gross income (AGI) of the estate or trust. For this purpose, an estate's or trust's administration expenses are allowable as a deduction in computing its AGI (Code Sec. 165(h)(5)(C)).[71]

A nonbusiness casualty or theft loss sustained or discovered during the settlement of an estate is deductible on the estate's income tax return only if it has not been allowed for estate tax purposes (Code Sec. 165(h)(5)(D); Reg. §§ 1.165-7(c) and 1.165-8(b)).[72] A statement to this effect should be filed with the return for the year for which the deduction is claimed.

References are to Standard Federal Tax Reports; Tax Research Consultant; and Practical Tax Explanations.

[67] ¶ 24,300; ESTTRST: 9,202; § 32,310

[68] ¶ 11,002, ¶ 11,048, ¶ 23,920, ¶ 23,922, ¶ 24,280, ¶ 24,297; ESTTRST: 12,102; § 32,335.05

[69] ¶ 12,120; DEPR: 12,050; § 32,335.05

[70] ¶ 12,330; FARM: 24,112; § 32,335.15

[71] ¶ 9802; ESTTRST: 12,060.10; § 7,705.10, § 32,401

[72] ¶ 9802, ¶ 10,004, ¶ 10,100; ESTTRST: 12,060.10; § 7,705.15, § 32,401

Net Operating Losses. An estate or trust is allowed a deduction for net operating losses (NOLs) (¶ 1145) (Reg. § 1.642(d)-1).[73] However, an estate cannot deduct an NOL (or a capital loss (¶ 1752)) sustained by a decedent during the decedent's last tax year. These losses must be deducted on the decedent's final return.[74] In addition, in computing gross income and deductions for the NOL calculation, a trust must not take into account income and deductions attributable to the grantor or any substantial owner under the grantor trusts rules (¶ 571). Also, an estate or trust cannot claim the deductions for charitable contributions (¶ 537) and distributions to beneficiaries (¶ 544 and ¶ 545) in calculating NOLs.

Bad Debts. An estate or trust is entitled to claim bad debt deductions under the rules governing individuals (¶ 1135).

Passive Losses. The passive activity loss rules (¶ 1165) apply to estates and trusts, but not grantor trusts (¶ 1173).

532. Deduction of Taxes by Estates and Trusts. An estate or trust is entitled to the same deductions for taxes as individuals (¶ 1021). In addition, an estate or trust is permitted an offset of the allocable federal estate tax against income in respect of a decedent (¶ 191). The portion of state income taxes allocable to exempt income, other than exempt interest income, is not deductible (¶ 970). The portion of state income taxes attributable to exempt interest income and to income subject to federal income tax is deductible (Rev. Rul. 61-86).[75]

533. Deduction of Interest by Estates and Trusts. Interest paid or accrued during the tax year is deductible by an estate or trust under the same rules that apply to individuals (¶ 1043) (Code Sec. 163).[76] However, there are a number of important differences. For example, interest owed and accrued at the death of the decedent can be deducted on the estate's income tax return as a deduction in respect of the decedent for the tax year in which the interest is paid. If the interest accrues after the decedent's death, it may be claimed as either an estate tax deduction or an income tax deduction (¶ 529). In addition, interest is not deductible by an estate or trust on a debt incurred, or continued, to purchase or carry obligations the interest on which is wholly exempt from federal income taxes (¶ 970). Personal interest of an estate or trust is also nondeductible (¶ 1045). Further, the deduction for investment interest may not exceed net investment income for the tax year (Code Sec. 163(d)).[77] Net capital gain attributable to the disposition of property held for investment is generally excluded from investment income for purposes of computing this limitation. However, a special election is available to increase net capital gain includible in investment income by reducing the amount eligible for capital gain treatment (¶ 1094).

534. Personal Exemption Amount of Estates and Trusts. An estate can claim a personal exemption of $600 in determining its taxable income (Code Sec. 642(b); Reg. § 1.642(b)-1).[78] A simple trust (¶ 542)—one that is required to distribute all of its income currently—is allowed an exemption of $300. A complex trust is entitled to a $100 exemption. If a final distribution of assets has been made during the year, all income of the estate or trust must be reported as distributed to the beneficiaries, without reduction for the amount claimed for the exemption (¶ 535).

A qualified disability trust, whether taxed as a simple or complex trust, can claim an exemption in the amount available to an unmarried individual who is not a surviving spouse or head of a household (¶ 133) (Code Sec. 642(b)(2)(C)). For tax years beginning after December 31, 2012, the exemption for a qualified disability trust is subject to phase-out.

References are to Standard Federal Tax Reports; Tax Research Consultant; and Practical Tax Explanations.

[73] ¶ 24,296; ESTTRST: 12,062; § 32,401, § 32,410

[74] ¶ 24,267.451; ESTTRST: 6,208.15, ESTTRST: 12,062; § 32,401

[75] ¶ 9502.453; ESTTRST: 12,064; § 32,325

[76] ¶ 9102; ESTTRST: 12,064; § 32,320

[77] ¶ 9102; ESTTRST: 12,064; § 7,414, § 7,420.05, § 32,320

[78] ¶ 24,280, ¶ 24,286; ESTTRST: 12,052; § 32,350

535. Loss Carryovers and Excess Deductions of Estates and Trusts. A beneficiary succeeding to the property of an estate or trust can deduct a net operating loss (NOL) carryover (¶ 1149 and ¶ 1153), a capital loss carryover (¶ 562 and ¶ 1754), and deductions in excess of gross income for the year in which the estate or trust terminates (Code Sec. 642(h); Reg. §§ 1.642(h)-1—1.642(h)-5).[79] Excess deductions on termination of an estate or trust are allowed only in computing taxable income and must be taken into account in computing the beneficiary's tax preference items. Such deductions may not be used in computing adjusted gross income. In computing excess deductions, the deductions for personal exemptions and amounts set aside for charitable purposes are disregarded. The deduction is claimed as an itemized deduction or capital loss (depending on its nature) on the beneficiary's tax return filed for the year in which the estate or trust terminates.

An individual debtor's bankruptcy estate (¶ 505) succeeds to certain tax attributes of the debtor, including any NOL carryover (Code Sec. 1398(g)).[80] The tax attributes that become part of the estate are determined as of the first day of the debtor's tax year in which the bankruptcy case commences. If any carryback year of the estate is a tax year before the estate's first tax year, the carryback is taken into account in the tax year of the debtor that corresponds to such carryback year and may offset the pre-bankruptcy income of the debtor (Code Sec. 1398(j)(2)(A)). When the estate closes upon the issuance of a final decree, the debtor succeeds to the same attributes as the estate, including any unused NOL carryover (Code Sec. 1398(i)). The debtor, however, cannot carry an unused NOL carryback from a tax year that ended after commencement of the bankruptcy case to a tax year that precedes the tax year in which the bankruptcy case was commenced (Code Sec. 1398(j)(2)(B)).

536. Domestic Production Activities Deduction of Estates and Trusts. An estate or a nongrantor trust, and the beneficiaries of the estate or trust, may claim the deduction for domestic production activities (¶ 980A) (Code Sec. 199(d)(1)(B); Reg. § 1.199-5(e)).[81] In computing the deduction, an estate or trust apportions W-2 wages, domestic production gross receipts (DPGR), cost of goods sold allocable to DPGR, and expenses, losses and deductions properly allocable to DPGR between the beneficiaries and the fiduciary, and among the beneficiaries. The nine-percent applicable percentage limitation on the deduction is applied to the lesser of the estate's or trust's qualified production activities income (QPAI) or its adjusted gross income (AGI), as determined under the AGI computation rules for estates and trusts (¶ 528).

The estate or trust calculates each beneficiary's share (as well as the estate's or trust's own share, if any) of the estate's or trust's QPAI and W-2 wages at the estate or trust level. The QPAI and W-2 wages are allocated to each beneficiary and to the estate or trust based on the relative proportion of the estate's or trust's distributable net income (DNI) for the tax year that is distributed or required to be distributed to the beneficiary or is retained by the estate or trust (¶ 542 and ¶ 543). If the estate or trust has no DNI for the tax year, QPAI and W-2 wages are allocated entirely to the estate or trust.

Each beneficiary computes his or her Code Sec. 199 deduction by combining their share of QPAI and W-2 wages from the estate or trust with their share of QPAI and W-2 wages from other sources. When determining its total QPAI and W-2 wages from such other sources, the beneficiary does not take into account the items allocated from the estate or trust. The beneficiary's share of W-2 wages from the estate or trust is determined under the law applicable to pass-through entities based on the beginning date of the estate's or trust's tax year, not the beneficiary's tax year (Reg. § 1.199-5(e)(3)).

References are to Standard Federal Tax Reports; Tax Research Consultant; and Practical Tax Explanations.

[79] ¶ 24,280, ¶ 24,301— ¶ 24,305; ESTTRST: 12,150; § 32,415

[80] ¶ 32,410; INDIV: 66,106, INDIV: 66,108; § 3,420.10, § 17,010.05

[81] ¶ 12,468, ¶ 12,472D; BUSEXP: 6,216; § 6,020.20, § 32,355

Grantor Trust. For a grantor trust (¶ 571), the owner computes its QPAI with respect to the owned portion of the trust as if that QPAI had been generated by activities performed directly by the owner (Reg. § 1.199-5(d)). Similarly, for purposes of the wage limitation (¶ 980C), the owner takes into account its share of the trust's W-2 wages that are attributable to the owned portion of the trust. The nongrantor trust provisions (discussed above) do not apply to the owned portion of the trust.

537. Charitable Deductions of Estates and Trusts—Generally. Estates and complex trusts are allowed an unlimited charitable deduction for amounts paid to recognized charities (¶ 1061) out of gross income (other than unrelated business income of a trust (¶ 538)) under the terms of the governing instrument during the tax year (Code Sec. 642(c)).[82] For example, amounts bequeathed to charity that are paid out of corpus under state law are not deductible from income as charitable contributions or as distributions to beneficiaries.[83] However, payments in compromise of bequests to charity are deductible.[84] Limitations on the charitable deduction for estates and trusts are discussed at ¶ 538.

The trustee or administrator may elect to treat charitable payments made during the year following the close of a tax year as having been paid in the earlier year for deduction purposes (Code Sec. 642(c)(1); Reg. § 1.642(c)-1(b)).[85] The election must be made no later than the time, including extensions, prescribed by law for filing the income tax return for the tax year in which payment is made. The election is binding for the tax year for which it is made and may not be revoked after the time for making the election has expired.

Estates may also claim an unlimited deduction for amounts of gross income permanently set aside for charitable purposes (Reg. § 1.642(c)-2).[86] The income must be permanently set aside for a purpose specified in Code Sec. 170(c) or it must be used exclusively for: (1) religious, charitable, scientific, literary, or educational purposes; (2) the prevention of cruelty to children or animals; or (3) the establishment, acquisition, maintenance, or operation of a nonprofit public cemetery. For most complex trusts, the unlimited deduction for gross income that is permanently set aside for charitable purposes does not apply.

A provision in a governing instrument or local law that specifically identifies the source out of which amounts are to be paid, permanently set aside, or used for charitable purposes must have economic effect independent of income tax consequences in order to be respected for federal tax purposes (Reg. § 1.642(c)-3(b)(2)).[87]

Pooled income funds (¶ 593) may claim a set-aside deduction only for gross income attributable to gain from the sale of a long-term capital asset that is permanently set aside for the benefit of the charity (Reg. § 1.642(c)-2(c)).[88] No deduction is allowed with respect to gross income of the fund that is (1) attributable to income other than net long-term capital gains or (2) earned with respect to amounts transferred to the fund before August 1, 1969. The investment and accounting requirements applicable to trusts also apply to pooled income funds.

The charitable deduction is normally computed on Schedule A of Form 1041. However, pooled income funds claiming the set-aside deduction for long-term capital gain and nonexempt charitable trusts under Code Sec. 4947(a)(1) treated as private foundations (¶ 631) must compute their deduction on a separate schedule, rather than Schedule A. Also, a nonexempt charitable trust not treated as a private foundation must file Form 990 or Form 990-EZ in addition to Form 1041 if its gross receipts are normally more than $50,000. However, the trust may file Form 990 or Form 990-EZ to satisfy its Form 1041 filing requirement if it has zero taxable income (¶ 625).

References are to Standard Federal Tax Reports; Tax Research Consultant; and Practical Tax Explanations.

[82] ¶ 24,280, ¶ 24,308.1135; ESTTRST: 15,050; § 32,340.05

[83] ¶ 24,308.115; ESTTRST: 15,050; § 32,340.05, § 32,340.20

[84] ¶ 24,308.105; ESTTRST: 15,260; § 32,340.20

[85] ¶ 24,280, ¶ 24,288; ESTTRST: 15,200; § 32,340.05

[86] ¶ 24,290; ESTTRST: 15,250, ESTTRST: 15,252; § 32,340.15

[87] ¶ 24,291; ESTTRST: 15,064; § 32,340.20

[88] ¶ 24,290; ESTGIFT: 45,252.45; § 32,340.30

¶537

Every trust claiming a charitable deduction for amounts permanently set aside (other than nonexempt charitable trusts under Code Sec. 4947(a)(1), and split-interest trusts under Code Sec. 4947(a)(2)) is required to file an information return on Form 1041-A generally by April 15 following the close of the trust's calendar year (Code Sec. 6034).[89] Form 1041-A does not have to be filed if the trust must distribute all of its income for the tax year (a simple trust). Split-interest trusts (pooled income funds (¶ 593), charitable remainder trusts (¶ 590), and charitable lead trusts (¶ 2932)) file their information return on Form 5227.

Both the trust and the trustee can be liable for a penalty of $10 per day up to a maximum of $5,000 for failure to timely file Form 1041-A (Code Sec. 6652(c)(2)(A) and (C)).[90] A split-interest trust that fails to file or to provide the required information on Form 5227 can be liable for a penalty of $20 per day, up to a maximum of $10,000. If the split-interest trust's gross income exceeds $250,000, the penalty is $100 per day, up to a $50,000 maximum. An additional penalty may be assessed against the person required to file the return if he or she knowingly fails to file or provide the information. Criminal penalties also apply for willful failure to file a return and filing a false or fraudulent return (Reg. § 1.6034-1(d)).[91]

538. Limitations on Charitable Deductions of Trusts. A trust is not entitled to an unlimited charitable deduction (¶ 537) for income that is allocable to its unrelated business income for the tax year (Code Secs. 642(c)(4) and 681(a); Reg. § § 1.642(c)-3(d), 1.681(a)-1, and 1.681(a)-2).[92] The unrelated business income of a trust is computed in much the same manner as the unrelated business taxable income (UBTI) of a tax-exempt organization (¶ 655 and ¶ 687). However, in computing unrelated business income, a trust can claim deductions for payments to charities, subject to the percentage limitations applicable to individuals' charitable deductions (¶ 1058).

Charitable deductions are not allowed for otherwise deductible gifts to an organization upon which a tax has been imposed for termination of private foundation status, unless the IRS has abated the tax (¶ 649) (Code Sec. 508(d)(1) and (3)).[93] General contributors will be denied deductions after the organization is notified of the loss of its private foundation status. Substantial contributors (¶ 635) will be denied deductions in the year in which action is taken to terminate the organization's private foundation status.

If a charitable contribution consists of gain from the sale of qualified small business stock (section 1202 stock) held for more than five years (¶ 1905), the charitable deduction amount must be adjusted for any gain excluded from gross income (Code Sec. 642(c)(4)).[94]

Deductions are also denied for contributions to any private foundation, nonexempt charitable trust, or split-interest trust, as defined in Code Sec. 4947, that fails to meet the governing instrument requirements for private foundations (Code Sec. 508(d)(2)).[95] Deductions for gifts and bequests to any organization are disallowed during the period that the organization fails to notify the IRS that it is claiming exempt status as a charitable organization (¶ 623). Churches, organizations with gross receipts of $5,000 or less, and certain other organizations designated by the IRS are exempt from the notification requirements. Charitable deductions are also disallowed for bequests and gifts to a foreign private foundation after the IRS notifies it that it has engaged in a prohibited transaction, or for a year in which such an organization loses its exempt status for engaging in such a transaction (Code Sec. 4948(c)(4)).[96]

540. Estate and Trust Income Tax Credits. The tax credits allowed to individuals (¶ 1301—¶ 1391) are generally allowed to estates and trusts in computing income tax liability (Reg. § 1.641(b)-1).[97] The credits typically must be apportioned between the

---

References are to Standard Federal Tax Reports; Tax Research Consultant; and Practical Tax Explanations.

[89] ¶ 35,440; ESTTRST: 15,360; § 39,155.30

[90] ¶ 39,480; PENALTY: 3,208; § 33,605.05, § 39,155.30

[91] ¶ 35,441; IRS: 66,150, IRS: 66,200; § 40,245.05, § 41,625.25

[92] ¶ 24,280, ¶ 24,291, ¶ 24,840, ¶ 24,841, ¶ 24,842; ESTTRST: 15,352; § 32,340.05, § 33,901

[93] ¶ 22,790; EXEMPT: 21,502; § 33,240.05

[94] ¶ 24,280; ESTTRST: 15,304; § 16,605.05

[95] ¶ 22,790; EXEMPT: 21,504; § 33,205.20

[96] ¶ 34,160; EXEMPT: 21,352; § 33,205.10, § 33,240.15

[97] ¶ 24,264; ESTTRST: 12,200, ESTTRST: 12,204; § 32,305

estate or trust and the beneficiaries on the basis of the income allocable to each. However, the foreign tax credit (¶ 1361) is allocated according to the proportionate share of the foreign taxes (Code Sec. 642(a); Reg. § 1.642(a)(2)-1).[98]

The general business tax credit is a limited nonrefundable credit against income tax that is claimed after all other nonrefundable credits are claimed (¶ 1365). The amount of the general business tax credit may not exceed the net income tax minus the greater of the tentative minimum tax or 25 percent of the net regular tax liability over $25,000. For estates and trusts, the $25,000 amount must be reduced to an amount that bears the same ratio to $25,000 as the portion of the income of the estate or trust that is not allocated to the beneficiaries bears to the total income of the estate or trust (Code Sec. 38(c)(6)(D)).[99] Any unused credit can be carried back one year and forward 20 years (carryback is three years and carryforward is 15 years for credits that arose in tax years before 1998) (Code Sec. 39).[100]

Estates and trusts are also entitled to claim various refundable tax credits, including the credit for federal income tax withheld on wages and backup withholding (¶ 1321 and ¶ 2645), the credit for taxes paid on undistributed capital gain of a regulated investment company credit (¶ 1330), and the credit for federal excise taxes paid on fuels (¶ 1329).

Income Distribution Deduction

542. Simple v. Complex Trust. The deduction allowed to simple trusts (¶ 544) and to estates and complex trusts (¶ 545) for distributions to beneficiaries is determined by reference to distributable net income (DNI) (¶ 543).

A simple trust is a trust that: (1) is required to distribute all of its income currently whether or not distributions of current income are in fact made; and (2) does not allow any amount to be paid or set aside for charitable contributions (Code Sec. 651; Reg. § 1.651(a)-1).[101] A trust may be a simple trust even though, under local law or the governing trust instrument, capital gains must be allocated to corpus. The income required to be distributed in order for the trust to qualify as a simple trust is the income determined under local law and the governing instrument (Code Sec. 643(b); Reg. § 1.643(b)-1).[102] This will generally include only ordinary income because capital gains under most trust instruments and state laws are considered corpus. A trust will lose its classification as a simple trust (but not its $300 exemption) for any year during which it distributes corpus (¶ 544). Thus, a trust can never be a simple trust during the year of termination or in a year of partial liquidation (Reg. § 1.651(a)-3).[103]

A complex trust is any trust other than a simple trusts described above (Reg. § 1.661(a)-1).[104] The same rules that apply to complex trusts generally also apply to estates.

Loans by Foreign Trusts. A foreign trust (¶ 501) will not be treated as a simple trust if it makes a loan of cash, cash equivalents, or marketable securities to, or permits the uncompensated use of any other trust property by, a grantor or beneficiary who is a U.S. person or a party related to the grantor or beneficiary (Code Sec. 643(i)).[105] The amount of the loan or the fair market value of the property's use is treated as a distribution by the trust for purposes of the distribution deduction (¶ 545), the gross income of trust beneficiaries (¶ 556), and the treatment of excess trust distributions (¶ 567). For trust property other than a loan of cash or marketable securities, distribution treatment does not apply if the trust is paid the fair market value for the property's use within a reasonable time period. Any subsequent transaction between the trust and the original borrower regarding the loan principal—such as the complete or partial repayment, satisfaction, cancellation, or discharge of the loan—or the return of the property used is disregarded.

References are to Standard Federal Tax Reports; Tax Research Consultant; and Practical Tax Explanations.

[98] ¶ 24,280, ¶ 24,282; EST-TRST: 12,202; § 13,405.20, § 32,305

[99] ¶ 4250; ESTTRST: 12,204; BUSEXP: 54,056; § 13,605.10

[100] ¶ 4300; BUSEXP: 54,056, BUSEXP: 54,058; § 13,605.15

[101] ¶ 24,360, ¶ 24,361; EST-TRST: 24,050; § 32,501, § 32,510

[102] ¶ 24,320, ¶ 24,329; EST-TRST: 24,052; § 32,010.10

[103] ¶ 24,363; ESTTRST: 24,056; § 32,501

[104] ¶ 24,401; ESTTRST: 24,050; § 32,501, § 32,515.05

[105] ¶ 24,320; ESTTRST: 18,200; § 32,501

543. Distributable Net Income (DNI). The deductions allowable to an estate or trust for amounts paid or credited to beneficiaries (¶ 544 and ¶ 545) are limited to the entity's distributable net income (DNI). The entity's DNI may also limit the amount of the distribution taxable to the beneficiary (¶ 554) and it is a factor in applying the conduit rule (¶ 559).

The DNI of an estate or trust generally consists of the same items of gross income and deductions that make up the taxable income of the estate or trust. However, there are important modifications: (1) no deduction is allowed for distributions to beneficiaries; (2) the deduction for the personal exemption is disallowed (¶ 534); (3) tax-exempt interest on state and local bonds is included, reduced by amounts which would be deductible but for the disallowance of deductions on expenses and interest related to tax-exempt income; (4) for a foreign trust (¶ 501), gross income from outside the United States (reduced by amounts which would be deductible but for the disallowance of deductions on expenses related to tax-exempt income) and within the United States is included; (5) capital gains are excluded if they are allocable to corpus and are not (a) paid, credited, or required to be distributed to any beneficiary during the tax year, or (b) paid, permanently set aside, or to be used for a charitable purpose (¶ 537); (6) capital losses are excluded except to the extent of their use in determining the amount of capital gains paid, credited, or required to be distributed to any beneficiary during the tax year; and (7) in the case of a simple trust, extraordinary dividends or taxable stock dividends that the fiduciary, acting in good faith, allocates to corpus are excluded (Code Sec. 643(a); Reg. §§ 1.643(a)-0—1.643(a)-7).[106] The DNI of the estate or trust is determined by taking into account a net operating loss (NOL) deduction (¶ 531 and ¶ 556).[107] However, the exclusion of gain from the sale or exchange of qualified small business stock (section 1202 stock) held for more than five years (¶ 1905) is not taken into account in determining DNI (Code Sec. 643(a)(3)).[108]

544. Deduction for Distributions to Beneficiaries of a Simple Trust. A simple trust (¶ 542) may deduct the amount of income that the trustee is under a duty to distribute currently to beneficiaries, even if the trustee makes the actual distribution after the close of the tax year (Code Sec. 651; Reg. §§ 1.651(a)-2 and 1.651(b)-1).[109] If other amounts are distributed—such as a payment from corpus to meet the terms of an annuity payable from income or corpus—the complex trust rules apply for that year, except that the $300 personal exemption (¶ 534) is still allowed (Reg. § 1.642(b)-1).[110] If the income required to be distributed exceeds distributable net income (DNI), the distribution deduction is limited to DNI (¶ 543), computed without including tax-exempt income and related deductions.

545. Deduction for Distributions to Beneficiaries of Complex Trust or Estate. An estate or complex trust (¶ 542) may deduct any amount of income for the tax year that is required to be distributed currently to beneficiaries (Code Sec. 661(a); Reg. § 1.661(a)-2).[111] This includes any amount required to be distributed that may be paid out of income or corpus, to the extent that it is in fact paid out of income. An estate or complex trust may also deduct any other amounts properly paid or credited or required to be distributed in the tax year, including amounts distributable at the discretion of the fiduciary and a distribution in kind. The amount to be taken into account in determining the deduction depends on whether the estate or trust elected to recognize gain on a noncash distribution of property in kind (¶ 526). In no case may the deduction exceed the distributable net income (DNI) of the estate or trust (¶ 543).

References are to Standard Federal Tax Reports; Tax Research Consultant; and Practical Tax Explanations.

[106] ¶ 24,320, ¶ 24,321—¶ 24,328; ESTTRST: 18,050; § 32,505.05

[107] ¶ 24,296, ¶ 24,431.493; ESTTRST: 12,062; § 32,410, § 32,505.05

[108] ¶ 24,320; ESTTRST: 18,056; § 16,605, § 32,505.05

[109] ¶ 24,360, ¶ 24,362, ¶ 24,366; ESTTRST: 24,102; § 32,510

[110] ¶ 24,286; ESTTRST: 24,100; § 32,510

[111] ¶ 24,400, ¶ 24,402; ESTTRST: 27,056; § 32,515.05

Special provisions exclude from the estate or trust's distribution deduction any unlimited charitable contribution (¶ 537), and certain gifts or bequests of a specific sum of money or specific property if paid or distributed all at once or in not more than three installments (¶ 556 and ¶ 564) (Code Sec. 663(a); Reg. § § 1.663(a)-1 and 1.663(a)-2).[112] Also, an estate or trust cannot include in the distribution deduction for the current tax year an amount deemed distributed to a beneficiary in a prior tax year (Reg. § 1.663(a)-3).[113]

Where a will is silent, state law determines whether income or gain during the period of estate administration is properly paid or credited to a legatee (Rev. Rul. 71-335).[114] Also, a testamentary trustee can be a legatee or beneficiary for the purpose of a taxable distribution.[115]

When estate or trust income is of varying types, the distribution deduction is treated as consisting of the same proportion of each class of items entering into the DNI calculation as the total of each class bears to total DNI (Code Sec. 661(b); Reg. § 1.661(b)-1).[116] However, items will be allocated in accordance with a trust instrument or local law providing for a different method of allocation. No deduction is allowed to the estate or trust for the part of a beneficiary's distribution that consists of DNI that is not included in the gross income of the estate or trust, such as tax-exempt interest income (Code Sec. 661(c); Reg. § 1.661(c)-1).[117]

In applying the above rule, all deductions entering into the computation of DNI (including charitable contributions) are allocated among the different types of income that make up the DNI in the following manner (Reg. § § 1.652(b)-3 and 1.661(b)-2):[118]

(1) The deductions *directly* attributable to an income class are allocated to that income. For example, real estate taxes, repairs, the trustee's share of depreciation, fire insurance premiums, etc., would be allocated to rental income.

(2) The deductions *not directly* attributable to a specific income class (such as trustee's commissions, safe deposit box rental, and state income and personal property taxes) may be allocated to any income item (including capital gains) included in computing DNI. However, a trust with nontaxable income must allocate a portion of these deductions to nontaxable income.

(3) Any excess deductions from step (1) may be assigned to any other class of income (including capital gains) in the manner described in step (2). However, excess deductions attributable to tax-exempt income may not be offset against any other class of income. Also, excess deductions from a passive activity (¶ 1169) cannot be allocated to income from a nonpassive activity, or to portfolio income earned by the estate or trust (Instructions to Form 1041).

For purposes of the computation, the unlimited charitable deduction (¶ 537) is first allocated ratably among all classes of income entering into DNI before any other expenses, unless a different allocation is specified by the governing instrument or local law (Reg. § § 1.643(a)-5 and 1.661(b)-2).[119] The charitable deduction is allocated by multiplying it by a ratio: the numerator is the amount of each single class of income, and the denominator is the total of all income classes.

Examples illustrating the allocations are provided at ¶ 559.

References are to Standard Federal Tax Reports; Tax Research Consultant; and Practical Tax Explanations.

[112] ¶ 24,440, ¶ 24,441, ¶ 24,442; ESTTRST: 27,102, EST-TRST: 27,104; § 32,515.05

[113] ¶ 24,443; ESTTRST: 27,106; § 32,515.05

[114] ¶ 24,407.78; ESTTRST: 27,054; § 32,515.05

[115] ¶ 24,407.7951; ESTTRST: 30,050

[116] ¶ 24,400, ¶ 24,403; EST-TRST: 27,056; § 32,515.05, § 32,515.10

[117] ¶ 24,400, ¶ 24,405; EST-TRST: 27,056; § 32,515.05

[118] ¶ 24,386, ¶ 24,404; EST-TRST: 27,056, ESTTRST: 30,250; § 32,515.10

[119] ¶ 24,326, ¶ 24,404; EST-TRST: 27,056, ESTTRST: 30,256; § 32,515.05, § 32,515.10

¶545

546. Estate or Complex Trust's 65-Day Election. The fiduciary of an estate or complex trust can elect annually to treat any distribution or any portion of a distribution to a beneficiary made within the first 65 days following the end of a tax year as having been distributed in the prior year (Code Sec. 663(b); Reg. §§ 1.663(b)-1 and 1.663(b)-2).[120] The election is made on Form 1041, is irrevocable for the year involved, and is binding for that year only. The amount to which the election can apply is the greater of: (1) the estate or trust's income (¶ 514); or (2) distributable net income (DNI) (¶ 543) for the tax year, reduced by any amounts paid, credited, or required to be distributed during the tax year other than those amounts that are subject to the 65-day election. There is no 65-day election for distributions of accumulated income (¶ 567).

548. Annuities Distributable from Income or Corpus. In the case of recurring distributions, payments by an estate or trust (where the amounts to be distributed, paid, or credited are a charge upon the corpus *or* the income) are usually taxable to the beneficiary and deductible by the estate or trust, to the extent that they are made from income (Code Sec. 661(a)(1); Reg. § 1.661(a)-2(b)).[121]

549. Widow(er)'s Allowance. A widow(er)'s or dependent's statutory allowance or award for support during administration of the estate is deductible by an estate if it is paid pursuant to a court order or decree or under local law (Reg. § 1.661(a)-2(e)).[122] The allowance can be paid from either income or principal, but the deduction is limited to the estate's distributable net income (DNI) for the year (¶ 543). Such payments are includible in the recipient's income to the extent of his or her share of the estate's DNI (Reg. §§ 1.662(a)-2(c) and 1.662(a)-3(b)).[123] The allowance is treated as a distribution to a beneficiary, even if it is considered to be a debt of the estate rather than a payment to a beneficiary under local law (Rev. Rul. 75-124).[124]

Taxation of Beneficiaries

554. Taxation of Simple Trust Beneficiary. A beneficiary of a simple trust (¶ 542) must include in gross income the income that is required to be distributed currently to the beneficiary (¶ 514), whether or not it is actually distributed during the tax year, up to the amount of distributable net income (DNI) (¶ 543) (Code Sec. 652; Reg. §§ 1.652(a)-1—1.652(b)-3).[125] If the income required to be distributed exceeds DNI, only a proportionate share of each item is includible in the beneficiary's income. Each income item retains the same character (such as rent, dividends, etc.) that it had in the hands of the trust, and is treated as consisting of the same proportion of each class of items entering into the DNI calculation as the total of each class bears to total DNI, unless the trust instrument specifically allocates a particular type of income to a particular beneficiary. Deductions reflected in the computation of DNI are allocated among the various types of income (¶ 545). On termination of a trust, unused loss carryovers and excess deductions of the trust are allowed to certain beneficiaries (¶ 535). The amounts reported on the beneficiary's return must be consistent with the amounts reported on the trust return (¶ 2823) (Code Sec. 6034A(c)).[126]

Net Investment Income Tax. For purposes of determining the 3.8-percent net investment income tax (¶ 129), net investment income includes a beneficiary's share of DNI to the extent that the character of such income constitutes gross income from certain income items (e.g., interest, dividends, annuities, royalties, rents, gross income from a passive trade or business or from a trader's financial instrument trading business, etc.) or net gain attributable to the disposition of certain property, with further computations for the trust's undistributed net investment income (¶ 517) (Reg. § 1.1411-4(e)(1)).[127]

References are to Standard Federal Tax Reports; Tax Research Consultant; and Practical Tax Explanations.

[120] ¶ 24,440, ¶ 24,444, ¶ 24,445; ESTTRST: 30,304; § 32,515.30

[121] ¶ 24,400, ¶ 24,402; EST-TRST: 27,052; § 32,515.05

[122] ¶ 24,402; ESTTRST: 27,052.10; § 32,525.10

[123] ¶ 24,422, ¶ 24,423; EST-TRST: 27,052.10; § 32,710.05

[124] ¶ 24,431.84; ESTTRST: 27,052.10; § 32,525.10

[125] ¶ 24,380—¶ 24,386; EST-TRST: 24,150; § 32,705.05

[126] ¶ 35,460; ESTTRST: 100; § 32,701

[127] ¶ 32,604; ESTTRST: 12,256.10; § 32,705.05

556. Taxation of Beneficiary of Estate or Complex Trust. A beneficiary of a complex trust (¶ 542) or a decedent's estate must include in gross income the income that is required to be distributed currently to the beneficiary (¶ 514), whether or not it is actually distributed during the tax year, plus any other amounts that are properly paid, credited, or required to be distributed to the beneficiary for the year (Code Sec. 662; Reg. § 1.662(a)-1).[128] For example, income of a trust is taxable to the beneficiaries even where there is no direction as to distribution or accumulation and state law requires distribution.[129] If a fiduciary elects to treat a distribution to a beneficiary made in the year as an amount paid in a prior year (¶ 546), the amount covered by the election is included in the beneficiary's income for the year for which the trust takes the deduction. Special rules also apply to distributions by certain trusts out of accumulated income (¶ 567).

If the amount of income required to be distributed currently to all beneficiaries exceeds distributable net income (DNI) (¶ 543) (computed without the charitable deduction (¶ 537)), then each beneficiary includes in income an amount that bears the same ratio to DNI as the amount of income required to be distributed currently to the beneficiary bears to the amount required to be distributed currently to all beneficiaries (Reg. § 1.662(a)-2(b)).[130]

If the sum of income required to be distributed currently, plus other amounts properly paid, credited, or required to be distributed, exceeds DNI, then the beneficiary includes such other amounts in gross income only to the extent that DNI exceeds income required to be distributed currently (Reg. § 1.662(a)-3(c)).[131] If the other amounts are paid, credited, or required to be distributed to more than one beneficiary, each beneficiary includes in gross income his or her proportionate share of such other amounts includible in gross income. The beneficiary's proportionate share is the amount which bears the same ratio to DNI (after subtracting income required to be distributed currently) as the other amounts distributed to the beneficiary bear to the other amounts distributed to all beneficiaries. The amount to be used in determining the beneficiary's share of estate or trust income depends on whether the estate or trust elected to recognize gain on the distribution (¶ 526).

Any amount which, under a will or trust instrument, is used in full or partial discharge or satisfaction of a legal obligation of any person is included in that person's gross income as though the amount was directly distributed to him or her as a beneficiary (Reg. § 1.662(a)-4).[132] A legal obligation includes an obligation to support another person only if it is not affected by the adequacy of the dependent's own resources. The amount of trust income included in the gross income of a person obligated to support a dependent is limited by the extent of the person's legal obligation under local law. For example, in the case of a parent's obligation to support his or her child, to the extent that the support obligation (including education) is determined under local law by the family's station in life and the means of the parent, it is determined without consideration of the trust income in question. This rule does not pertain to alimony payments or income of an alimony trust (¶ 771).

If a net operating loss carryback of the estate or trust (¶ 531) reduces the DNI of the estate or trust for the prior tax year to which the NOL is carried, the beneficiary's tax liability for the prior year may be recomputed based upon the revised DNI of the estate or trust (Rev. Rul. 61-20).[133]

In allocating the various types of income to the beneficiaries so as to give effect to these tax rules, the amount reflected in the trust's or estate's DNI is determined first. It is charged with directly related expenses and a proportionate part of other expenses, including the unlimited charitable deduction (¶ 537) to the extent it is chargeable to

References are to Standard Federal Tax Reports; Tax Research Consultant; and Practical Tax Explanations.

[128] ¶ 24,420, ¶ 24,421; EST-TRST: 30,000; § 32,710.05
[129] ¶ 24,431.65; ESTTRST: 24,052.05; § 32,710.05
[130] ¶ 24,422; ESTTRST: 30,108; § 32,710.05
[131] ¶ 24,423; ESTTRST: 30,154; § 32,710.05
[132] ¶ 24,424; ESTTRST: 30,052; § 32,710.05
[133] ¶ 24,431.493; ESTTRST: 12,062; § 32,410

income of the current year (Reg. §§ 1.662(b)-1 and 1.662(b)-2).[134] Each beneficiary's share of income paid, credited, or required to be distributed to the beneficiary is then multiplied by fractions, for each class of income, in which the numerator is the amount of such income included in DNI (whether the aggregate is more or less than the DNI), and the denominator is the total DNI (¶ 545). However, if the governing instrument specifies or local law requires a different allocation, such allocation is to be followed. These computations are illustrated at ¶ 559.

Special provisions exclude certain amounts from the beneficiary's gross income (and from the estate or trust's distribution deduction) (Code Sec. 663(a); Reg. §§ 1.663(a)-1, 1.663(a)-2, and 1.663(a)-3).[135] Any amount paid, permanently set aside, or to be used for charitable purposes and allowable for the unlimited charitable deduction (¶ 537) cannot be part of the distribution deduction or treated as an amount distributed for purposes of determining the beneficiary's gross income. Additionally, amounts deemed to be distributed to a beneficiary in a *prior* tax year cannot be deducted by the estate or trust, and are not included in the beneficiary's gross income for the current tax year. Certain gifts or bequests of a specific sum of money or specific property if paid or distributed all at once or in not more than three installments are also excluded (¶ 564).

On termination of an estate or trust, unused loss carryovers and excess deductions of the estate or trust are allowed to certain beneficiaries (¶ 535).

The amounts reported on the beneficiary's return must be consistent with the amounts reported on the estate or trust return (¶ 2823) (Code Sec. 6034A(c)).[136]

Net Investment Income Tax. For purposes of determining the 3.8-percent net investment income tax (¶ 129), net investment income includes a beneficiary's share of DNI to the extent that the character of such income constitutes gross income from certain income items (e.g., interest, dividends, annuities, royalties, rents, gross income from a passive trade or business or from a trader's financial instrument trading business, etc.) or net gain attributable to the disposition of certain property, with further computations for the estate's or trust's undistributed net investment income (¶ 517) (Reg. § 1.1411-4(e)(1)).[137]

557. Separate Shares as Separate Estates or Trusts. Where an estate or trust has two or more beneficiaries and is to be administered in well-defined and separate shares, the shares must be treated as separate estates or trusts in determining the amount of distributable net income (DNI) allocable to the beneficiaries (¶ 554 and ¶ 556) (Code Sec. 663(c); Reg. §§ 1.663(c)-1—1.663(c)-5).[138] This rule limits the tax liability of a beneficiary on a distribution of income and corpus where the income is being accumulated for the benefit of another beneficiary. The separate-share treatment is mandatory, not elective. A trustee or an executor must apply it even if separate and independent accounts are not maintained for each share, or if assets are not physically segregated.

The separate-share rule does not affect situations in which a single trust instrument creates not one, but several separate trusts, as opposed to separate shares in the same trust. It also does not apply to trusts that provide for successive interests (e.g., a trust that provides a life estate to A and remainder to B).

The treatment of separate shares as separate estates or trusts applies *only* for determining DNI in computing the distribution deduction allowable to the estate or trust and the amount includible in the income of the beneficiary. It cannot be applied to obtain more than one deduction for the personal exemption or to split the income of the estate or trust into several shares so as to be taxed at a lower-bracket rate.

559. How the Complex Trust Rules Operate. The examples below illustrate computations of distributable net income (DNI) (¶ 543), the distributive share of a beneficiary (¶ 544 and ¶ 545), and the taxable income of a complex trust. No "throwback" distributions (¶ 567) are involved.

References are to Standard Federal Tax Reports; Tax Research Consultant; and Practical Tax Explanations.

[134] ¶ 24,425, ¶ 24,426; EST-TRST: 30,106; § 32,710.05

[135] ¶ 24,440—¶ 24,443; EST-TRST: 27,100; § 32,710.05, § 32,710.15

[136] ¶ 35,460; ESTTRST: 100; § 32,701

[137] ¶ 32,604; ESTTRST: 12,256.10; § 32,710.05

[138] ¶ 24,440, ¶ 24,446—¶ 24,449; ESTTRST: 27,200; § 32,515.20

Example 1: Trust income: A complex trust has the following items of income in 2014:

Dividends	$16,000
Taxable interest	10,000
Exempt interest	10,000
Rent	4,000
Long-term capital gain allocable to corpus	6,000

The trust has expenses as follows:

Expenses directly allocable to rent	$2,000
Commissions allocable to income	3,000
Commissions allocable to corpus	1,500

On these facts, the trust would have income of $40,000 (¶ 514). The income items consist of dividends, taxable interest, exempt interest and rent. No expenses or charges against income or corpus are subtracted; only receipts treated as income under local law and the governing instrument are counted (e.g., rent). Also, the long-term capital gain is excluded from this income in order to apply the conduit rule (as illustrated in Example 3) because it is not income under local law. It is, however, included in the taxable income computation.

Example 2: Distributable net income: In computing the trust's DNI, the net amount of tax-exempt interest is added to the net income of the trust (after subtracting any charitable contribution). The net amount of tax-exempt interest is the full amount of such interest minus any expenses directly allocable to it and a proportionate part of all general expenses such as commissions. As indicated in Example 1, there are $4,500 in general expenses (i.e., expenses not directly allocable to rental income), so 25 percent ($10,000/$40,000) of $4,500, or $1,125, is allocated to the exempt interest ($10,000), leaving a net of $8,875. This $1,125 must also be excluded from the deductions claimed by the trust as an expense indirectly related to the production of exempt interest income and therefore disallowed by Code Sec. 265 (¶ 970). Accordingly, DNI is $33,500, computed as follows:

Dividends		$16,000
Taxable interest		10,000
Exempt interest ($10,000 less $1,125 allocable to exempt interest)		8,875
Rent		4,000
Total		$38,875
Deductions:		
Rent expense	$2,000	
Commissions ($4,500 less $1,125 allocable to exempt interest)	3,375	5,375
Distributable net income		$33,500

Example 3: Taxable income of beneficiary: There is one beneficiary to whom the trustee must distribute $20,000 under the terms of the trust instrument. The first step in computing the amount taxable to the beneficiary is to determine the extent to which each income item is reflected in DNI, allocating expenses to the various items. Those allocable to exempt interest have already been reflected in the $8,875 figure carried into DNI in Example 2, so no further allocation of that item is needed. Allocation is needed for dividends, rent, and taxable interest income, but this allocation does not have to be proportionate. Expenses directly related to any source or type of income must be allocated directly to that income, but general expenses can be allocated to any taxable income the taxpayer wishes when computing DNI as long as no deficit is created for any item. In this example, it is assumed the trustee allocates all general expenses to taxable interest. Accordingly, the trustee charges the entire $3,375 of general expenses to the taxable interest ($10,000) so that the $33,500 DNI, for the purpose of applying the conduit rule, is deemed to have been derived from:

Rent	$2,000
Taxable interest	6,625
Dividends	16,000
Tax-exempt interest	8,875
	$33,500

The total corresponds to the DNI and is only an intermediate or identification step. Because the amounts actually distributable are less than the amount of DNI, the next step is to multiply each of the above amounts by $20,000/$33,500 to determine what part of each is taxable to the beneficiary and deductible by the trust. Using these figures (the same result could be obtained by determining $2,000/$33,500 of $20,000, $6,625/$33,500 of $20,000, and so on), the apportionment is as follows:

Rent	$1,194.03
Taxable interest	3,955.22
Dividends	9,552.24
Tax-exempt interest	5,298.51
	$20,000.00

The beneficiary's share of income and deductions is reported on Schedule K-1 of Form 1041. The beneficiary will omit the $5,298.51 tax-exempt interest in reporting income from the trust. The $1,194.03 rent, $9,552.24 dividend, and $3,955.22 taxable interest income should be reported on the beneficiary's Form 1040.

Example 4: Taxable income of the trust: The trust is allowed a deduction for the amount required to be distributed currently up to the amount of its DNI, but not for any portion that consists of tax-exempt income. The deduction for distributions, therefore, is $14,701.49 ($20,000 minus $5,298.51). Taxable income of the trust is then computed as follows:

Dividends	$16,000.00	
Taxable Interest	10,000.00	
Rent	4,000.00	
Long-term capital gain	6,000.00	$36,000.00
Less:		
Expenses allocable to rent	$2,000.00	
Commissions allocable to income ($3,000 minus the 25% [$750] allocable to exempt interest)	2,250.00	
Commissions allocable to corpus ($1,500 minus the 25% [$375] allocable to exempt interest)	1,125.00	
Distribution to beneficiary	14,701.49	
Exemption	100.00	20,176.49
Taxable income		$15,823.51

562. Capital Gain or Loss of Estate or Trust. Capital gains, whether long or short term, are generally excluded from distributable net income (DNI) (i.e., are taxed to an estate or trust) to the extent allocated to corpus and not (1) paid, credited, or required to be distributed to any beneficiary during the tax year, or (2) paid, permanently set aside, or to be used for a charitable purpose (Code Sec. 643(a)(3); Reg. § 1.643(a)-3).[139] Capital gains are included in DNI, however, to the extent they are: (1) allocated to income; (2) allocated to corpus but consistently treated by the fiduciary as part of a distribution to a beneficiary; or (3) allocated to corpus but actually distributed to a beneficiary or used by the fiduciary in determining the amount that is distributed or required to be distributed to a beneficiary (¶ 543).

A net capital loss of an estate or trust will reduce the taxable income of the estate or trust, but no part of the loss is deductible by the beneficiaries. If the estate or trust distributes all of its income, the capital loss will not result in a tax benefit for the year of the loss. Losses from the sale or exchange of capital assets are first netted at the trust level against any capital gains, except for capital gains utilized by the fiduciary in determining the amount to be distributed to a particular beneficiary (Reg. § 1.643(a)-3(d)).[140] On termination of an estate or trust, any unused capital loss carryover of the estate or trust is available to the beneficiaries (¶ 535).

References are to Standard Federal Tax Reports; Tax Research Consultant; and Practical Tax Explanations.

[139] ¶ 24,320, ¶ 24,324; EST-TRST: 18,056; § 32,505.10

[140] ¶ 24,324; ESTTRST: 18,058; § 32,505.10

564. Gift or Bequest by Estates and Trusts. An estate or trust may not deduct as a distribution to a beneficiary, and a beneficiary does not include in income, a gift or bequest of a specific sum of money or specific property that is paid or credited in three installments or less (Code Sec. 663(a)(1); Reg. § 1.663(a)-1).[141] However, an amount will *not* be treated as an excluded gift or bequest if the governing instrument provides that the specific sum is payable only from the income of the estate or trust. The following are also *not* treated as an excluded gift or bequest of a sum of money or specific property: (1) an annuity, or periodic gifts of specific property in lieu of or having the effect of an annuity; (2) a residuary estate or the corpus of a trust; or (3) a gift or bequest paid in a lump sum or in three installments or less, if required by the governing instrument to be paid in more than three installments. In determining the number of installments, gifts or bequests of articles of personal use (e.g., personal and household effects, cars, etc.) are disregarded. Also disregarded are transfers of specific real estate, title to which passes directly from the decedent to the devisee under local law.

565. Beneficiary's Tax Year Different From Estate's or Trust's. If a beneficiary has a different tax year from that of an estate or complex trust (¶ 542), the amount to be included in the beneficiary's gross income must be based on the distributable net income (DNI) of the estate or trust (¶ 543) and the amounts paid, credited, or required to be distributed to the beneficiary for any tax year or years of the estate or trust ending with or within his or her tax year (Code Sec. 662(c); Reg. § 1.662(c)-1).[142] Similarly, if a beneficiary of a simple trust has a tax year different from that of the trust, the amount that the beneficiary includes in gross income must be based on the amount of the trust's income for any tax year or years ending with or within his or her tax year (Code Sec. 652(c); Reg. § 1.652(c)-1).[143]

566. Distributions to Expatriates by Nongrantor Trusts. If a covered expatriate (¶ 2412) is a beneficiary of a nongrantor trust on the day before the individual's expatriation date, and receives a direct or indirect distribution of any property from the trust, the trustee must deduct and withhold 30 percent of the taxable portion of the distribution (Code Sec. 877A(f)).[144] Additionally, if the fair market value of the property distributed exceeds the adjusted basis in the hands of the trust, the trust must recognize gain as if the property were sold to the expatriate at its fair market value.

The taxable portion of the distribution is that portion which would be includible in the covered expatriate's gross income had the expatriate continued to be subject to tax as a U.S. citizen or resident. A nongrantor trust is the portion of any trust of which the individual is not considered the owner under the grantor trust rules (¶ 571) as determined immediately before the beneficiary's expatriation date.

The withholding rules apply in a manner similar to those that apply to nonresident aliens (¶ 2455), but the distribution item is not subject to the nonresident alien withholding tax itself or the withholding tax on wages (¶ 2601). Further, the covered expatriate is treated as having waived any claim to a withholding reduction under any treaty with the United States, unless the expatriate agrees to other treatment that the IRS deems appropriate. Items subject to withholding are taxed according to the rules that apply to nonresident aliens (¶ 2429 and ¶ 2431).

567. "Throwback" of Accumulated Income. Special "throwback rules" generally apply to trust distributions made in tax years beginning before August 6, 1997 (Code Secs. 665—668).[145] Although the throwback rules have been repealed for most trusts, they continue to apply to trusts created before March 1, 1984, that would be treated as multiple trusts under Code Sec. 643(f), and to foreign trusts (¶ 501) and domestic trusts that were once treated as foreign trusts.

The throwback rules are designed to prevent the accumulation of trust income by a complex or accumulation trust over a period of years with a distribution to a beneficiary

---

References are to Standard Federal Tax Reports; Tax Research Consultant; and Practical Tax Explanations.

[141] ¶ 24,440, ¶ 24,441; EST-TRST: 27,102; § 32,710.15

[142] ¶ 24,420, ¶ 24,427; EST-TRST: 30,306; § 32,710.10

[143] ¶ 24,380, ¶ 24,387; EST-TRST: 24,158; § 32,705.15

[144] ¶ 27,430; EXPAT: 3,320; § 37,135

[145] ¶ 24,480, ¶ 24,500, ¶ 24,520, ¶ 24,540; ESTTRST: 33,000; § 32,715.05

¶564

only in low-income years. The rules have the effect of carrying back to preceding years any distributions in excess of distributable net income (DNI) (¶ 543) for the distribution year and taxing them to the beneficiaries as if they were distributed in the year the income was accumulated by the trust. This additional income is taxed to the beneficiary in the year that the beneficiary receives the accumulation distribution, but the beneficiary's tax liability is computed on Form 4970 under special rules. Beneficiaries who receive the accumulation distribution from a foreign trust report it and the partial tax on Form 3520. Schedule J of Form 1041 is used to determine the amount, the year, and the character of the additional distributions taxable to beneficiaries under the throwback rules; the trustee must give a copy of Part IV of Schedule J to each beneficiary. The beneficiary is allowed an offset or credit against the partial tax for the proportionate part of the trust's tax for the prior year, thus eliminating any double tax on the income. Beneficiaries of estates are not subject to the throwback rules.

Grantor Trusts

571. Overview of Grantor Trust Rules. Under the grantor trust rules, a person (i.e., the grantor) who transfers property to a trust and retains certain powers or interests (¶ 576—¶ 584) is treated as the owner of the trust property for income tax purposes (Code Sec. 671).[146] As a result, the income, deductions, and credits attributable to the trust are included in determining the grantor's taxable income to the extent of the owned portion of the trust. For income tax purposes, conversion of a nongrantor trust to a grantor trust is not a transfer of the property held by the nongrantor trust to the owner of the grantor trust, so the owner is not required to recognize gain (CCA 200923024).

Family Trusts. Income-producing property is often conveyed in trust for the benefit of a family member in an effort to split any income generated by the property or to otherwise lessen the original owner's tax liability. However, there must be an actual transfer of property to accomplish the desired tax savings; it is not enough to transfer income generated by the property.

In addition, the limitations of the grantor trust rules prevent a taxpayer from escaping tax on the income from property where the taxpayer in effect remains the property owner by retaining control over the trust. For example, a family estate trust "" (i.e., a trust to which an individual transfers personal assets and the right to income in exchange for the beneficial enjoyment of such assets and compensation) is taxed as a grantor trust (Rev. Rul. 75-257).[147] The grantor's assignment of lifetime services or salary to the trust is not recognized for income tax purposes. Such trusts are deemed a "nullity" for income tax purposes and their income is taxable to the persons who created them. Acceptance of this broad economic principle deprives a grantor of any possible refuge in the technicalities of the grantor trust provisions. Expenses incurred in setting up family estate trusts are not deductible under Code Sec. 212.[148] Intra-family transfers of income-producing property cannot also be used to reduce income tax liability by shifting income from the parents' higher tax bracket to their child's generally lower tax bracket. Under the kiddie tax rules, if the net unearned income of the child exceeds an annual inflation-adjusted amount, it is taxed at the parents' top marginal rate (¶ 143).

Net Investment Income Tax. A grantor trust is not subject to the 3.8-percent net investment income tax (¶ 129 and ¶ 517) (Reg. § 1.1411-3(b)(1)).[149] Instead, for purposes of calculating the net investment income of the grantor or other person who is taxable on trust income (¶ 585), each item of income or deduction included in computing his or her taxable income under the grantor trust rules must be treated as if it had been received by, or paid to, the grantor or other person.

575. Funeral Trusts. A qualified funeral trust (QFT) is a nonforeign funeral trust that elects not to be treated as a grantor trust (¶ 571), so that the income tax on the

---

References are to Standard Federal Tax Reports; Tax Research Consultant; and Practical Tax Explanations.

[146] ¶ 24,680; ESTTRST: 36,000; § 32,801

[147] ¶ 24,783.1973; ESTTRST: 3,116; § 46,530.10

[148] ¶ 12,523.50; BUSEXP: 12,064.40; § 46,530.10

[149] ¶ 32,603L; ESTTRST: 12,256.05; § 32,801

annual earnings of the trust is payable by the trustee (Code Sec. 685).[150] A QFT is generally an arrangement that would otherwise be treated as a grantor trust, under which an individual purchases funeral services or necessary property for himself or herself, or for another individual, from a funeral home prior to death and funds the purchase via contributions. There are no dollar limitations on contributions to a QFT, but the contributions must be held, invested, and reinvested by the trust solely to make payments for funeral services or property upon the individual's or the other trust beneficiaries' death.

If the election is made, the income tax rate schedule generally applicable to estates and trusts (¶ 19) is applied to the trust by treating each beneficiary's interest as a separate trust. However, the trust is not entitled to a personal exemption (¶ 534). The trustee's election must be made separately for each such separate trust. No gain or loss is recognized to a purchaser of a funeral trust contract as a result of any payment from the trust to the purchaser due to the cancellation of the contract.

The trustee elects QFT status by filing Form 1041-QFT. The election must be filed no later than the due date (with extensions) for filing the trust income tax return for the year of election. The election applies to each trust reported in the QFT return. The trustee can use the form to file for a single QFT or multiple QFTs having the same trustee. The election may be made for the trust's first eligible year or for any subsequent year. Once made, the election cannot be revoked without IRS consent.

576. Trusts With Reversionary Interest in Grantor. A grantor is considered to be the owner of any portion of a trust (¶ 571) in which the grantor or the grantor's spouse (¶ 578) has a reversionary interest in either the trust corpus or income if the value of the interest exceeds five percent of the value of that portion of the trust (Code Sec. 673).[151] The value of the interest is measured as of the inception of the portion of the trust in which the grantor holds an interest. In determining whether the grantor's reversionary interest exceeds the five-percent threshold, the maximum exercise of discretion in the grantor's favor is assumed. Any postponement of the reacquisition or enjoyment of the interest is considered to be a new transfer in trust. However, no trust income is included in the grantor's income that would not have been included absent postponement. In addition, a grantor is exempt from the reversionary interest rule if the interest takes effect only upon the death of a beneficiary who is a minor lineal descendant of the grantor (under age 21) and if the beneficiary has the entire present interest in all or part of the trust.

578. Powers Held by Grantor's Spouse. A grantor is treated as holding any power or interest in a trust (¶ 571) that is held by a person who was the grantor's spouse at the time the power or interest was created, or who became the grantor's spouse after creation of the power or interest (but only with respect to periods that the individual was the grantor's spouse) (Code Sec. 672(e)).[152] Thus, the grantor trust provisions cannot be avoided by having the spouse of the grantor possess prohibited powers or interests (e.g., spousal remainder trusts). Individuals who are legally separated under a decree of divorce or separate maintenance are not considered to be married for this purpose.

579. Power to Control Beneficial Enjoyment. A grantor of a trust (¶ 571) is taxed on trust income if the grantor or the grantor's spouse (¶ 578) retains the power to control the beneficial enjoyment of trust property or income without the consent of an adverse party (e.g., power to change beneficiaries or to change remainder interests) (Code Sec. 674; Reg. § 1.674(a)-1).[153] There are a number of exceptions to this rules including, but not limited to: (1) an unexercised power to apply income to support a dependent (¶ 137); (2) power to allocate income among charitable beneficiaries; (3) power to distribute corpus limited by a reasonably definite standard; and (4) power to withhold income temporarily (Reg. §§ 1.674(b)-1—1.674(d)-2).[154]

References are to Standard Federal Tax Reports; Tax Research Consultant; and Practical Tax Explanations.

[150] ¶ 24,895; ESTTRST: 39,350; § 32,175

[151] ¶ 24,710; ESTTRST: 39,050; § 32,810

[152] ¶ 24,700; ESTTRST: 36,054; § 32,805.20

[153] ¶ 24,720, ¶ 24,721; EST-TRST: 45,050; § 32,815.05

[154] ¶ 24,722—¶ 24,725; EST-TRST: 45,050, ESTTRST: 45,052; § 32,815.10

581. Retention of Administrative Powers. The grantor of a trust (¶ 571) is taxed on trust income if the grantor or the grantor's spouse (¶ 578) retains administrative powers enabling the grantor to obtain, by dealings with the trust, financial benefits that would not be available in an arm's-length transaction (Code Sec. 675; Reg. § 1.675-1).[155] For example, if the grantor or his or her spouse borrows trust corpus or income at any time during a tax year, the grantor is taxed on the trust income for that entire year, even if the grantor repays the loan with interest during the same year (Rev. Rul. 86-82).[156]

582. Power to Revoke Trust. If a grantor creates a trust (¶ 571) and reserves a right to revoke it, the income of the trust is treated as the grantor's income (Code Sec. 676; Reg. § § 1.676(a)-1 and 1.676(b)-1).[157] The trust income is not taxed to the grantor if the power can only affect the beneficial enjoyment of the income after the occurrence of an event such that the grantor would not be treated as the owner if the power were a reversionary interest (¶ 576). However, the grantor may be treated as the owner after the event occurs unless the power to revoke is then relinquished.

584. Income for Grantor's Benefit. The grantor of a trust (¶ 571) is taxed on trust income that is or may be accumulated for or distributed to the grantor or the grantor's spouse, or used to pay life insurance premiums on either the grantor's or the spouse's life (except for policies irrevocably payable to charities) (Code Sec. 677; Reg. § § 1.677(a)-1 and 1.677(b)-1).[158] To the extent that trust income may be used in satisfaction of the grantor's legal obligation to support a beneficiary (such as a child, but not a spouse), it is regarded as distributable to the grantor. If the discretion to so use the income is not in the grantor acting as such, but in another person (for example, the trustee or the grantor acting as trustee or co-trustee), then that income is includible in the grantor's gross income only to the extent that it is actually used for the beneficiary's support or maintenance. In addition, any capital gain under state law that is added to trust corpus is taxable to the grantor if the corpus reverts to the grantor upon termination of the trust (Reg. § § 1.671-3(b)(2) and 1.677(a)-1(f); Rev. Rul. 58-242; Rev. Rul. 75-267).[159]

585. Income Taxable to Person Other Than Grantor. A person other than the grantor of a trust ¶ (571), including a beneficiary, may be taxed on the trust's income if that person has a power, exercisable alone, to vest trust corpus or income in himself or herself (Code Sec. 678; Reg. § § 1.678(a)-1—1.678(d)-1).[160] For example, if a father establishes a trust for the benefit of his children, but the trust provides that the grantor's brother may take trust property at any time, the brother is treated as the owner and trust income is taxed to him. This rule does not apply if the power is renounced or disclaimed within a reasonable period. This rule also does not apply to a power over income as originally granted or later modified, if the grantor of the trust or a transferor to a foreign trust (¶ 588) is treated as the trust owner under the other grantor trust rules.

A U.S. person who is a beneficiary of a trust is treated as the grantor to the extent that the beneficiary transferred property, directly or indirectly and for less than adequate consideration, to a foreign person who otherwise would have been treated as the owner under the grantor trust rules (Code Sec. 672(f)(5)).[161]

586. Return for Grantor Trust. Items of income, deduction, or credit that are treated as belonging to a trust grantor or another person (¶ 571) are generally not reported by the trust on Form 1041 (Reg. § 1.671-4).[162] Instead, these items are reflected on the income tax return of the grantor (or other person who is taxable on the trust income). A separate statement should be attached to Form 1041 stating the name, taxpayer identification number, and address of the person to whom the income is

---

References are to Standard Federal Tax Reports; Tax Research Consultant; and Practical Tax Explanations.

[155] ¶ 24,740, ¶ 24,741; EST-TRST: 45,100; § 32,820.05

[156] ¶ 24,742.10; ESTTRST: 45,106; § 32,820.10

[157] ¶ 24,760, ¶ 24,761, ¶ 24,762; ESTTRST: 39,250; § 32,825

[158] ¶ 24,780—¶ 24,782; EST-TRST: 42,000; § 32,830.05, § 32,830.10, § 32,830.15

[159] ¶ 24,684, ¶ 24,781, ¶ 24,783.101, ¶ 24,783.34; EST-TRST: 39,150, ESTTRST: 42,054; § 32,830.40

[160] ¶ 24,800—¶ 24,804; EST-TRST: 36,200; § 32,805.10

[161] ¶ 24,700; ESTTRST: 36,056.05; § 32,801

[162] ¶ 24,685; ESTTRST: 36,104; § 32,610.25

taxable, and setting forth the income, deductions, and credits; however, there are other optional reporting methods available to certain types of grantor trusts. Widely held fixed investment trusts have specific information reporting requirements (Reg. § 1.671-5).[163]

588. Foreign Grantor Trust Rules. Any U.S. person transferring property to a foreign trust (¶ 501) (other than certain employee benefits plans and charitable trusts) that has a U.S. beneficiary will be treated as the owner of that portion of the trust attributable to the property transferred (Code Sec. 679).[164] The IRS can presume that the trust has a U.S. beneficiary unless the transferor submits to the IRS any information that the IRS requires regarding the transfer, and demonstrates to the IRS's satisfaction that: (1) under the terms of the trust, no part of the trust's income or corpus may be paid or accumulated during the tax year to or for the benefit of a U.S. person, even if that person's interest is contingent on a future event; and (2) no part of the trust's income or corpus could be paid to or for the benefit of a U.S. person if the trust were terminated at any time during the tax year. The transferor must ensure that the trust satisfies certain reporting requirements, and submit any information the IRS may require regarding the foreign trust (Code Secs. 6048(b) and 6677(a)).[165] A foreign trust with at least one U.S. owner must file Form 3520-A in order for the U.S. owner to satisfy its annual information reporting requirements. The U.S. grantor trust rules (¶ 571) generally do not apply to any portion of a trust that would otherwise be deemed to be owned by a foreign person (Code Sec. 672(f)).[166]

U.S. persons who are treated as owners of foreign trusts under the grantor trust rules (¶ 571) must file Form 3520.

Other Special Trusts

590. Charitable Remainder Trusts. Whenever there is a noncharitable income beneficiary of a trust, gifts of remainder interests qualify for a charitable contribution deduction only if the trust is a charitable remainder annuity trust (CRAT) or a charitable remainder unitrust (CRUT) (Code Sec. 664; Reg. §§ 1.664-1, 1.664-2 and 1.664-3).[167] Charitable contribution deductions are denied for gifts of remainder interests in all other types of trusts. However, if the donor gives *all* the interests in a trust to charity, the above rules do not apply, and a deduction is allowable (¶ 1070).

Qualification. An *annuity trust* is a trust from which a sum certain or a specified amount is to be paid to the income beneficiary (Code Sec. 664(d)(1); Reg. §§ 1.664-1 and 1.664-2). The specified amount cannot be less than five percent or more than 50 percent of the initial net fair market value of all property placed in trust, and it must be paid at least annually to the income beneficiary. Furthermore, the value of the charitable remainder interest must be at least 10 percent of the initial net fair market value of all of the property placed in trust. There are several provisions designed to provide relief to trusts that do not meet the 10-percent test. No contributions can be made to a CRAT after the initial contribution, and the governing instrument must contain a prohibition against future contributions.

A *unitrust* is a trust that specifies that the income beneficiary is to receive annual payments based on a fixed percentage of the net fair market value of the trust's assets as determined each year (Code Sec. 664(d)(2); Reg. §§ 1.664-1 and 1.664-3). The fixed percentage cannot be less than five percent or more than 50 percent of the net fair market value of the trust's assets for the year. However, a qualified CRUT may provide for the distribution each year of five percent of the net fair market value of its assets or the amount of the trust income, whichever is lower. For this purpose, trust income excludes capital gains, and trust assets must be valued annually. The payment requirement may not be discretionary with the trustee. Additional contributions can be made to a unitrust. For most transfers in trust, the value of the charitable remainder interest with respect to each contribution to the unitrust must be at least 10 percent of the net fair

---

References are to Standard Federal Tax Reports; Tax Research Consultant; and Practical Tax Explanations.

[163] ¶ 24,685K; ESTTRST: 36,300

[164] ¶ 24,820; ESTTRST: 36,250; § 32,801, § 32,805.10

[165] ¶ 36,000, ¶ 39,815; ESTTRST: 36,258; § 39,135.15

[166] ¶ 24,700; ESTTRST: 36,056.05; § 32,801

[167] ¶ 24,460, ¶ 24,461, ¶ 24,464, ¶ 24,465; ESTGIFT: 45,200; § 32,150

market value of such contributed property as of the date the property is contributed to the trust. If an additional contribution would cause the trust to fail the 10-percent remainder test, then the contribution will be treated as a transfer to a separate trust under regulations. Other provisions may provide relief to trusts that fail to meet the 10-percent test.

CRATs and CRUTs cannot have noncharitable remainder interests. The remainder interests generally must pass to a charity upon the termination of the last income interest, and the trust instrument must contain a provision that determines how the final payment of a specified distribution is to be made. However, a charitable trust may make certain limited qualified gratuitous transfers of qualified employer securities to an employee stock ownership plan (ESOP) without adversely affecting the status of the charitable remainder trust.

To avoid the possible disqualification of a charitable remainder trust due to a surviving spouse's right of election against the grantor spouse's estate under state law, the IRS created a safe harbor requiring the surviving spouse to irrevocably waive the right (Rev. Proc. 2005-24). Until further guidance is published, the IRS will disregard the existence of a right of election *without* requiring a waiver, but only if the surviving spouse does not exercise the right (Notice 2006-15).[168]

There may be more than one noncharitable income beneficiary, either concurrently or successively, and the income interest may be a life estate or for a term of years not in excess of 20 years. However, a contingency clause may be placed in the trust instrument providing that the noncharitable interest is to terminate and the charitable remainder interest is to be accelerated upon the happening of an event, such as the remarriage of the noncharitable beneficiary (Code Sec. 664(f)).[169] The income beneficiary can receive only a specified or fixed amount from the trust, and the trustee cannot have additional power to invade corpus or to alter, amend, or revoke the trust for the benefit of the noncharitable income beneficiary. The trustee cannot be restricted from investing in income-producing assets (Reg. § 1.664-1(a)(3)).[170]

Division of Trust. The IRS has provided guidelines for dividing a CRAT or a CRUT into two or more separate and equal trusts without violating the charitable remainder trust requirements (Rev. Rul. 2008-41).[171]

Reporting. A CRAT or CRUT does not file Form 1041, but instead is required to file Form 5227. In addition, the fiduciary of a CRAT or CRUT may be required to file other returns regarding the excise tax on unrelated business taxable income (¶ 590A), and the excise taxes on private foundations that apply to charitable remainder trusts (¶ 591). Form 5227 must generally be filed on or before the 15th day of the fourth month following the close of the tax year of the trust (Rev. Proc. 83-32).[172]

590A. Taxation of Charitable Remainder Trust. A charitable remainder annuity trust (CRAT) or a charitable remainder unitrust (CRUT) (¶ 590) is generally exempt from income tax (Code Sec. 664(c); Reg. § 1.664-1).[173] However, if a CRAT or CRUT has unrelated business taxable income (UBTI) (¶ 670), it is subject to a 100-percent excise tax on its UBTI, but will retain its tax-exempt status. The excise tax is treated as paid from corpus, and trust income that is UBTI is income of the trust for purposes of determining the character of distributions made to beneficiaries (¶ 590B). The tax is reported on Form 4720, which must be filed by the due date for Form 5227 (¶ 590). The rule preventing the IRS from filing an additional deficiency notice once a taxpayer files a Tax Court petition challenging the deficiency also applies to this tax. In addition to the tax on UBTI, a charitable remainder trust may be subject to the income and excise taxes imposed on private foundations (¶ 591).

---

[168] ¶ 24,468.18; ESTGIFT: 45,202.15, ESTGIFT: 45,204.05; § 32,150.25
[169] ¶ 24,460; ESTGIFT: 45,202.20, ESTGIFT: 45,204.20; § 32,150.25

[170] ¶ 24,461; ESTGIFT: 45,200; § 32,150.25
[171] ¶ 24,468.12; ESTTRST: 15,354; § 32,150.25

[172] ¶ 24,468.20; ESTTRST: 15,360; § 32,150.25
[173] ¶ 24,460, ¶ 24,461; ESTTRST: 15,354, ESTGIFT: 45,200; § 32,150, § 32,601, § 33,901

590B. Treatment of Charitable Remainder Trust Beneficiaries. Under either a charitable remainder annuity trust (CRAT) or a charitable remainder unitrust (CRUT) (¶ 590), the amount paid to a beneficiary is considered as having the following characteristics in the beneficiary's hands: (1) ordinary income to the extent of the trust's ordinary income for the tax year and its undistributed ordinary income from prior years; (2) capital gains to the extent of the trust's capital gains for the tax year and its undistributed capital gains, determined on a cumulative net basis, for prior years; (3) other income (including tax-exempt interest) to the extent of the trust's other income for the tax year and its undistributed other income from prior years; and (4) a distribution of trust corpus (Code Sec. 664(b); Reg. § § 1.664-1—1.664-4).[174] Items within the ordinary income and capital gains categories are assigned to different subcategories based on the federal income tax rate applicable to each type of income within the category. Categories of income that are taxed at the same rate can be combined into a single class if the tax rate will not change in the future. If the tax rate is temporary, then the categories must be maintained as separate groups (Reg. § 1.664-1(d)(1)(i)).[175]

The characterizations of income items distributed or deemed distributed at any time during the tax year of the charitable remainder trust are determined as of the end of the tax year. Distributions are subject to the tax rate applicable to the income class from which the distribution is derived, not the tax rate applicable when the income was received by the trust (Reg. § 1.664-1(d)(1)(ii)(a)). Gains and losses of long-term capital gain classes are netted prior to netting short-term capital loss against any class of long-term capital gain (Reg. § 1.664-1(d)(1)(iv)).

Net Investment Income Tax. While CRATs and CRUTs are not subject to the 3.8-percent net investment income tax (¶ 129 and ¶ 517), special rules apply for calculating the tax applicable to CRAT and CRUT distributions to beneficiaries (Reg. § 1.1411-3(d)).[176]

591. Private Foundation Rules Applicable to Charitable Trusts. The income and excise taxes imposed on private foundations extend to all nonexempt charitable trusts with certain modifications (Code Sec. 4947).[177] First, a nonexempt trust that devotes all of its unexpired interests to charitable, religious, educational, and other purposes that enable contributors to obtain a charitable deduction is treated as a private foundation (¶ 631). Thus, it may be subject to the excise taxes on: investment income (¶ 633), self-dealing (¶ 635), failure to distribute income (¶ 637), excess business holdings (¶ 640), investments that jeopardize charitable purposes (¶ 642), and certain taxable expenditures (lobbying, electioneering, etc.; ¶ 644). For this purpose, unexpired interests include life or term income interests, interests in trust corpus, and remainder interests.

Second, a nonexempt trust that does not devote all of its unexpired interests to charitable purposes (split-interest trust) is subject to the excise taxes on self-dealing, excess business holdings, investments that jeopardize charitable purposes, and certain taxable expenditures (lobbying, electioneering, etc.) as if it were a private foundation. However, the taxes apply to income to be paid to trust beneficiaries under the terms of the trust instrument only if the trust was a charitable remainder annuity trust (CRAT) or charitable remainder unitrust (CRUT) (¶ 590). The taxes do not, in any event, apply to amounts in trust for which a deduction is not allowable if segregated from deductible amounts.

In addition, the taxes on excess business holdings and investments that jeopardize charitable purposes do not apply to a split-interest trust if: (1) the charity is only an income beneficiary and its beneficial interest is no more than 60 percent of the value of the trust property; or (2) the charity's only interest in the trust is as a remainderman. Split-interest trusts are treated like private foundations with regard to the rules on

---

References are to Standard Federal Tax Reports; Tax Research Consultant; and Practical Tax Explanations.

[174] ¶ 24,460—¶ 24,466; ES-TGIFT: 45,210; § 32,150

[175] ¶ 24,461; ESTGIFT: 45,210; § 32,150

[176] ¶ 32,603L; ESTTRST: 12,256.25

[177] ¶ 34,140; EXEMPT: 21,300; § 33,201

governing instruments and the tax on involuntary termination of status for repeated or willful violations (¶ 631 and ¶ 649).

The excise tax on investment income and failure to distribute income do not apply to split-interest trusts under any circumstances.

593. Pooled Fund Arrangements. A pooled income fund is generally a trust to which a person transfers an irrevocable remainder interest in property for the benefit of a public charity while retaining an income interest in the property for the life of one or more beneficiaries living at the time of the transfer (Code Sec. 642(c)(5); Reg. § 1.642(c)-5).[178] Income, estate, and gift tax charitable contribution deductions are allowed for the value of remainder interests in property transferred to a pooled income fund (Code Sec. 642(c)(3)). To protect the value of depreciable property that will pass to the charitable remainderman, the governing instrument of the pooled income fund must provide for the creation of a depreciation reserve.[179] In addition, the fund: (1) must commingle all property contributed to it; (2) cannot invest in tax-exempt securities; and (3) must be maintained by the recipient charity with no donor or income beneficiary acting as a trustee. The charity does not have to act as trustee of the fund.

Each person who has an income interest resulting from a transfer of property to the fund must be paid an annual income based on the fund's yearly rate of return (i.e., the trust cannot accumulate income for any beneficiary). A pooled income fund's method of calculating its yearly rate of return must be supported by a full statement attached to the fund's annual income tax return. The fund and its beneficiaries are taxable under the rules applicable to trusts, except that the grantor trust rules (¶ 571) do not apply. In addition to its income tax return, a pooled income fund must file an annual information return on Form 5227 regarding its charitable deductions (¶ 537).

595. Common Trust Fund. Each participant in a common trust fund (¶ 2389) must report its share of the taxable income of the fund, whether or not distributed or distributable. The taxable income of a common trust fund is computed in much the same manner as an individual's taxable income, except for the exclusion of capital gains and losses and the deduction for charitable contributions (Code Sec. 584).[180]

References are to Standard Federal Tax Reports; Tax Research Consultant; and Practical Tax Explanations.

[178] ¶ 24,280, ¶ 24,293; ES-TGIFT: 45,252; § 32,340.30

[179] ¶ 24,308.1877, ¶ 24,308.1880; ESTGIFT: 45,252; § 32,340.30

[180] ¶ 23,630; RIC: 12,300

Chapter 6

EXEMPT ORGANIZATIONS

Overview

601. Overview of Tax-Exempt Organizations. A variety of organizations may qualify for exemption from federal income taxation. The most common basis for exempt status is as a charitable organization under Code Sec. 501(c)(3) (¶ 602). Generally, charitable organizations can be either publicly supported or private foundations. While all charitable organizations are subject to limitations on how they operate, private foundations may be subject to excise taxes for engaging in prohibited activities (¶ 631). In addition to charitable organizations under Code Sec. 501(c)(3), there are also a number of organizations that qualify for exempt status if they have a socially beneficial purpose (¶ 692). Regardless of how an entity qualifies as a tax-exempt organization, it may still be subject to federal income tax on any business income not related to its exempt purpose (¶ 655) and any income arising from debt-financed property (¶ 687). All tax-exempt organizations are also subject to various reporting requirements, such as annual information reporting (¶ 625), involvement in tax shelter transactions (¶ 619), and other disclosure requirements (¶ 627).

Code Sec. 501(c)(3) Organizations

602. Charitable Organizations Under Code Sec. 501(c)(3). Code Sec. 501 provides that various classes of nonprofit organizations may be exempt from federal income tax unless they are deemed to be feeder organizations (¶ 694)[1] or they engage in certain prohibited transactions.[2] The most common basis for invoking tax-exempt status falls under Code Sec. 501(c)(3)'s broad exemption for religious, charitable, scientific, literary, and educational organizations (collectively referred to as charitable organizations).[3] Charitable organizations are generally either public charities or private foundations (¶ 631). Among other benefits, exempt status conferred by Code Sec. 501(c)(3) allows a public charity to receive tax-deductible contributions from its donors (¶ 627 and ¶ 1061). Any corporation, community chest, fund, trust, or foundation may qualify for the exemption. Application for recognition of Code Sec. 501(c)(3) federal tax-exempt status is made on Form 1023 or Form 1023-EZ (¶ 623).

To qualify for tax-exempt status under Code Sec. 501(c)(3), the entity must be organized and operated exclusively for religious (¶ 604), charitable, scientific, educational, or literary purposes; prevention of cruelty to children or animals; promotion of amateur sports competition; or testing for public safety. What constitutes a charitable purpose is interpreted broadly and may include purposes beyond those explicitly stated in Code Sec. 501(c)(3). For example, a charitable purpose can include: providing relief to the poor or disadvantaged; the advancement of education, religion, or science; or lessening the burdens of government through the promotion of social welfare or other

---

References are to Standard Federal Tax Reports; Tax Research Consultant; and Practical Tax Explanations.

[1] ¶ 22,670; EXEMPT: 15,350; § 33,001

[2] ¶ 22,680; EXEMPT: 12,208; § 33,825.15

[3] ¶ 22,602; EXEMPT: 3,000, EXEMPT: 9,000; § 33,005.05

¶601

community development (Reg. § 1.501(c)(3)-1(d)).[4] An educational organization can include a child-care center whose services are available to the general public and whose purpose is to enable individuals to be gainfully employed (Code Sec. 501(k)).[5] Regardless of an entity's charitable purpose, it must meet certain organizational, operational, and private benefit tests to qualify as a tax-exempt charitable organization.

Organizational Test. The organizational test requires that the entity's articles of organization specifically limit its purpose to one or more exempt purposes, including that its assets are dedicated to an exempt purpose (Reg. § 1.501(c)(3)-1(b)).[6] The articles of organization also must not expressly permit the organization to carry on activities that do not further the organization's exempt purpose, except where the nonexempt activities are an insubstantial part of the organization's activities. For example, the articles of organization must not allow more than an insubstantial part of the organization's activities to consist of carrying on propaganda or attempting to influence legislation (¶ 613); or authorize the organization to directly or indirectly participate or intervene in any political campaign on behalf of or in opposition to any candidate for public office (¶ 614). Whether an organization meets the organizational requirement is determined exclusively from the language of the articles of organization and not from the activities conducted by the organization. For this purpose, "articles of organization" include trust instruments, corporate charters, articles of association, or any other written instrument by which an organization is created.

Operational Test. The operational test requires that an entity must be operated exclusively for one or more exempt purposes. This means the organization engages primarily in activities that accomplish one or more of its exempt purposes (Reg. § 1.501(c)(3)-1(c)).[7] Only an insubstantial part of the entity's activities may be in the furtherance of nonexempt purposes. Whether an organization has a substantial nonexempt purpose is determined by taking into account all facts and circumstances, including the size and extent of all of the organization's activities. If the entity is an action organization, then it will *not* be considered as operated exclusively for an exempt purpose. An entity is an action organization if it devotes a substantial part of its activities to attempting to influence legislation or if it participates in political campaigns. However, if an organization fails the operational test because it is an action organization, it may still qualify for tax-exempt status as a social welfare organization under Code Sec. 501(c)(4) (¶ 692). If a charitable organization provides commercial-type insurance as an insubstantial part of its activities, then the insurance activity will be treated as an unrelated trade or business (¶ 655) (Code Sec. 501(m) and (n)).[8]

An entity will not be considered as operating exclusively for exempt purposes if any of its net earnings inure in whole or in part to the benefit of private shareholders or individuals. A "private shareholder or individual" is any person having a personal and private interest in the activities of the organization, such as founders of the organization, employees, board members, or family members of officers, employees, etc. The inurement prohibition does not prohibit all payments to a private shareholder or individual but instead is directed at payments that are made for purposes other than as reasonable compensation for goods or services (¶ 617).

Private Benefit Test. An organization is not organized or operated exclusively for charitable purposes unless it serves a public rather than a private interest (outside interests, as opposed to inside interests addressed by the inurement prohibition under the operation test). The question of private benefit often arises in situations in which a charitable organization enters into partnerships and other joint ventures with for-profit entities. The charitable organization can form such ventures and still satisfy the operational test only if it is permitted to act exclusively in furtherance of its exempt purpose and only incidentally for the benefit of the for-profit partners (Rev. Rul. 98-15).[9] In

---

References are to Standard Federal Tax Reports; Tax Research Consultant; and Practical Tax Explanations.

[4] ¶ 22,608; EXEMPT: 3,150; § 33,105

[5] ¶ 22,602; EXEMPT: 3,300; § 33,105

[6] ¶ 22,608; EXEMPT: 3,050; § 33,115

[7] ¶ 22,608; EXEMPT: 3,100; § 33,120

[8] ¶ 22,602; EXEMPT: 15,160

[9] ¶ 22,609.411; EXEMPT: 15,452, EXEMPT: 15,458; § 33,125

addition, the for-profit party cannot be allowed to control or use the charitable organization's activities or assets for its own benefit unless the control or use is incidental.

Charitable Hospitals. In addition to the requirements that apply to all Code Sec. 501(c)(3) organizations, each hospital facility operated by a charitable organization is subject to four additional requirements: (1) each facility must conduct and implement a community health needs assessment; (2) each facility must adopt, implement, and widely publicize a written financial assistance policy; (3) each facility may not bill patients who qualify for financial assistance more than the amount generally billed to insured patients; and (4) the facility (or affiliates) may not undertake extraordinary collection actions against patients (Code Sec. 501(r); Prop. Reg. §§ 1.501(r)–0— 1.501(r)–7).[10] If a hospital organization fails to meet the community health needs assessment requirement, an excise tax of $50,000 for any applicable year is imposed on the hospital (Code Sec. 4959).[11]

604. Churches and Religious Organizations. A church or religious organization is exempt from federal income tax and eligible to receive tax-deductible contributions if it meets the Code Sec. 501(c)(3) requirements (¶ 602). The term "church" is not specifically defined in the Code but generally is used in its generic sense as a place of worship including, for example, mosques and synagogues. It also includes conventions or associations of churches, as well as integrated auxiliaries of a church. For this purpose, a convention or association of churches is a cooperative undertaking by churches of the same or differing denominations (Rev. Rul. 74-224).[12] The fact that the convention or association may extend membership to individuals and those individuals have voting rights will not cause it to lose exempt status (Code Sec. 7701(n)).[13]

It is important to distinguish churches from other religious organizations. To balance the need for the IRS to combat efforts on the part of some individuals and organizations to use churches to avoid taxes, and the equally important need to protect legitimate churches from undue IRS interference in their activities, the Code and regulations contain detailed rules governing when the IRS may inquire into or examine the activities of a "church" (Code Sec. 7611; Reg. § 301.7611-1; Prop. Reg. § 301.7611-1).[14] Religious organizations that are not churches may still be eligible for tax-exempt status, including nondenominational ministries, interdenominational and ecumenical organizations, and other entities whose principal purpose is the study or advancement of religion (IRS Pub. 1828). Unlike churches, however, religious organizations that want to be tax exempt must apply to the IRS for tax-exempt status by filing Form 1023 or Form 1023-EZ (¶ 623).

A religious or apostolic association that does not meet the requirements to be a Code Sec. 501(c)(3) organization may nonetheless qualify as exempt from federal income taxation if it has a common or community treasury. The exemption applies even if the association engages in business for the common good of its members, provided that the members include in their gross income their pro rata share of the association's taxable income as dividends received, whether distributed or not (Code Sec. 501(d); Reg. § 1.501(d)-1).[15] There is no official exemption application form for this purpose. However, the association must file Form 1065 each tax year for information purposes (Reg. § 1.6033-2(e)).[16]

607. Supporting Organizations. A charitable organization under Code Sec. 501(c)(3) that carries out its exempt purpose by providing support to other tax-exempt organizations (usually public charities) (¶ 602) is considered a public charity rather than a private foundation (¶ 631). To qualify as a supporting organization, an organization must not only meet the requirements to be a charitable organization under Code Sec. 501(c)(3) but must also be:

References are to Standard Federal Tax Reports; Tax Research Consultant; and Practical Tax Explanations.

[10] ¶ 22,602, ¶ 22,608C— ¶ 22,608Y; EXEMPT: 3,154

[11] ¶ 34,256; EXEMPT: 3,154

[12] ¶ 11,620.205; EXEMPT: 21,052

[13] ¶ 43,080; EXEMPT: 21,052

[14] ¶ 42,910, ¶ 42,912, ¶ 42,912C; IRS: 18,406

[15] ¶ 22,602, ¶ 22,659; EXEMPT: 3,202; § 33,005.05

[16] ¶ 35,422; EXEMPT: 12,054.20; § 33,005.05

- organized and operated exclusively for the benefit of, to perform the functions of, or to carry out the purposes of a public charity (organizational and operational tests);
  - operated or controlled by a public charity (relationship test); and
  - not controlled either directly or indirectly by a disqualified person (¶ 635), other than a foundation manager or publicly supported charity (lack of control test) (Code Sec. 509(a)(3)).[17]

To satisfy the relationship test, a supporting organization must hold one of three close relationships with the supported organization (Reg. §1.509(a)-4; Temp. Reg. §1.509(a)-4T).[18] In a Type I relationship, the supported organization must exercise a substantial degree of control over the programs, activities, and policies of the supporting organization (comparable to a parent-subsidiary relationship). In a Type II relationship, there must be common control or supervision by persons controlling or supervising both the supporting organization and the supported organization (comparable to brother-sister corporations). In a Type III relationship, the supporting organization must be operated in connection with the supported organization by being responsive to its needs and demands, and by being significantly involved in its operations to the point that the supported organization is dependent upon the supporting organization for the type of support it provides. Regardless of whether these relationship requirements are met, if a Type I or Type III organization supports an organization that is controlled by a donor, then the supporting organization will be treated as a private foundation rather than as a public charity (Code Sec. 509(f)(2)).

A number of special rules also apply to Type III supporting organizations. Each tax year, a Type III organization must provide each supported organization with any information that may be required by the IRS to ensure that the relationship requirements of being a Type III organization are met (Code Sec. 509(f)(1)). This may include the Type III organization's annual information return (Form 990), any tax return filed (Form 990-T), and any annual report. In addition, a Type III organization may not be operated in connection with any public charity that is organized outside the United States. Similarly, a trust will not be considered to be a Type III organization *solely* based on the facts that it is a charitable trust under state law, the public charity is a beneficiary of the trust, and the public charity has the power to enforce the trust terms (Act Sec. 1241(c) of P.L. 109-280).

Tax-exempt organizations use Form 8940 to request determinations about a change in type of supporting organization.

610. Donor Advised Funds. A Code Sec. 501(c)(3) charitable organization (other than a private foundation) may establish a donor advised fund that is a separate account where contributions made by a donor to the organization under which the donor (or person appointed by the donor) reasonably expects to provide nonbinding advice regarding distributions or investments (Code Sec. 4966(d)(2)).[19] The donor may be entitled to a charitable deduction for contributions to a donor advised fund (¶ 1061), but only if the sponsoring organization legally owns and controls the contributions. For this purpose, a donor advised fund does not include any fund that only makes distributions to a single identified organization or governmental entity. It also does not include a fund that allows the donor to provide advice as to which individuals receive grants for travel, study, or similar purposes through a committee that is appointed by the sponsoring organization that is not controlled by a donor or group of donors with advisory privileges and under which all grants are made on an objective and nondiscriminatory basis. The IRS has discretionary authority to exempt a fund or account from treatment as a donor advised fund. The charitable organization must provide information to the IRS when it applies for tax-exempt status (¶ 623) whether it maintains or intends to maintain the donor advised fund, and the manner in which it plans to operate those funds (Code Sec. 508(f)).[20]

References are to Standard Federal Tax Reports; Tax Research Consultant; and Practical Tax Explanations.

[17] ¶ 22,800; EXEMPT: 21,200; §33,020.05

[18] ¶ 22,804, ¶ 22,804H; EXEMPT: 21,200; §33,020.10

[19] ¶ 34,317; EXEMPT: 33,000; §33,720.05

[20] ¶ 22,790; EXEMPT: 33,056; §33,720.05

An excise tax is imposed on any "taxable distribution" from a donor advised fund which is any distribution to a natural person or to any other person if the distribution is for any purpose other than an exempt purpose under Code Sec. 501(c)(3) (¶ 602) (Code Sec. 4966).[21] It also includes any distribution to a disqualified supporting organization (¶ 607), unless the sponsoring organization exercises responsibility for the distribution (Notice 2006-109). A taxable distribution does not include any distribution to a 50-percent organization (¶ 1059), to the sponsoring organization, or to another donor advised fund. The excise tax is 20 percent of the distribution and is imposed on the sponsoring organization. A separate five-percent excise tax is imposed on any fund manager who knowingly agrees to the distribution (up to $10,000 per distribution). A fund manager includes any officer, director, or trustee of the sponsoring organization, as well as an employee having authority with respect to the distribution. Fund managers who knowingly participate in the transaction are jointly and severally liable for the five-percent tax. The taxes on both the sponsoring organization and the fund manager are reported on Form 4720. The IRS has discretionary authority to abate both taxes (¶ 647).

An excise tax is also imposed if a donor advised fund makes a distribution to any person that results in (directly or indirectly) a more-than-incidental benefit to the donor, donor advisor, member of the donor's family, or any entity in which the donor holds more than a 35-percent ownership interest (Code Sec. 4967).[22] The tax is 125 percent of the benefit received and is imposed on the donor, donor advisor, and related persons who recommended the distribution or received the prohibited benefit. A tax of 10 percent of the benefit (up to $10,000) is also imposed on fund managers who agreed to the making of a distribution knowing it would confer a more-than-incidental benefit. All persons liable for the taxes are jointly and severally liable. If the taxes are imposed, the IRS has discretionary authority to abate them (¶ 647). However, neither tax will be imposed if the distribution is subject to tax as an excess benefit transaction (¶ 617). Also, a donor advised fund will be treated as a private foundation for purposes of the excise tax on excess business holdings (¶ 640).

613. Limitations on Lobbying Activities. An organization that otherwise qualifies as a Code Sec. 501(c)(3) charitable organization will be denied tax-exempt status if: (1) a *substantial* part of its activities consists of carrying on propaganda or attempting to influence legislation, or (2) it participates or intervenes in any political campaign on behalf of, or in opposition to, any candidate for public office (Code Sec. 501(h); Reg. § 1.501(h)-1).[23] If a charitable organization engages in substantial legislative activity or participates in any political campaign, then it is an action organization (¶ 602) and not operated exclusively for one or more exempt purposes (Reg. § 1.501(c)(3)-1(c)(3)).[24] There are no specific guidelines as to what constitutes *substantial* legislative activities for this purpose; instead it is determined on the facts and circumstances of each case. However, the IRS has issued guidance for the facts and circumstances to be evaluated in determining whether or not a Code Sec. 501(c)(3) organization has participated or intervened in a political campaign for public office (Rev. Rul. 2007-41).[25] If the organization has made a political expenditure, it will be subject to an excise tax (¶ 614).

As an alternative to the substantial part test, many charitable organizations may elect on Form 5768 a sliding scale limitation on expenditures to objectively determine their permissible level of lobbying activities (Code Sec. 501(h); Reg. § 1.501(h)-2).[26] The election can be made at any time during the organization's tax year. It is effective for the entire tax year and all succeeding years until revoked. Organizations that may not make this election include: churches or a convention or association of churches (¶ 604), private foundations (¶ 631), and supporting organizations (¶ 607) for social welfare organizations, labor unions, trade associations, and organizations that test for public safety (¶ 692).

References are to Standard Federal Tax Reports; Tax Research Consultant; and Practical Tax Explanations.

[21] ¶ 34,317; EXEMPT: 33,150; § 33,720.10

[22] ¶ 34,319; EXEMPT: 33,200; § 33,720.15

[23] ¶ 22,602, ¶ 22,663; EXEMPT: 6,100; § 33,710.05

[24] ¶ 22,608; EXEMPT: 6,102; § 33,710.05

[25] ¶ 22,609.103; EXEMPT: 6,104; § 33,710.05

[26] ¶ 22,602, ¶ 22,664; EXEMPT: 6,150; § 33,710.05

The basic permitted level for lobbying expenditures (but not grassroots lobbying) is 20 percent of the first $500,000 of the electing organization's exempt-purpose expenditures for the year, 15 percent of the second $500,000, 10 percent of the third $500,000, and five percent of any additional expenditures with a maximum annual limitation of $1 million (Code Sec. 4911).[27] In the case of so-called grassroots lobbying—attempts to influence the general public on legislative matters—the basic permitted level is limited to 25 percent of the general lobbying level described above. An excise tax of 25 percent is imposed on any excess lobbying expenditures above these limits. In addition, if an organization's lobbying expenditures normally—on an average over a four-year period— exceed 150 percent of these limits (computed on Schedule C of Form 990), the organization will lose its tax-exempt status (Reg. § 1.501(h)-3).[28]

614. Excise Tax on Political Expenditures. A 10-percent excise tax is imposed on a Code Sec. 501(c)(3) organization for each political expenditure made during the tax year (Code Sec. 4955).[29] For this purpose, a political expenditure is generally defined as any amount paid or incurred by the organization in connection with any participation or intervention in any political campaign on behalf of (or in opposition to) any candidate for public office (¶ 613). A separate 2.5-percent excise tax (up to $5,000) is imposed on any organization manager who agrees to the making of the expenditure if the manager knows that it is a political expenditure, unless the agreement is not willful and due to reasonable cause. An organization manager includes a director, officer, trustee, or any individual with comparable responsibilities.

If the political expenditure is not corrected within a "taxable period," then a second-tier excise tax is imposed on the organization equal to 100 percent of the amount of the expenditure. Organization managers who refuse to agree to all or part of the correction are also subject to a second-tier tax of 50 percent of the amount of the expenditure (up to $10,000). If more than one manager is liable for either the first- or second-tier taxes, then each manager is jointly and severally liable for them. The "taxable period," is the period beginning on the date on which the taxable expenditure is made and ending on the earlier of the date on which a deficiency notice for the first-tier tax is mailed or the date it is assessed. A correction of a political expenditure means the foundation takes all reasonable means to recover the expenditure to the extent possible and establishes safeguards to prevent future political expenditures. If full recovery is not possible, then the foundation must take whatever corrective action is prescribed by the IRS. Both the first and second levels of taxes may be abated under certain circumstances (¶ 647). The organization's taxes are reported on Form 4720.

617. Excess Benefit Transactions. An excise tax is imposed on any "excess benefit transaction" involving a charitable organization under Code Sec. 501(c)(3) (other than a private foundation (¶ 631)), a social welfare organization under Code Sec. 501(c)(4) (¶ 692), or a qualified nonprofit health insurance issuer under Code Sec. 501(c)(29) (Code Sec. 4958).[30] The tax may be applied instead of, or in addition to, the organization being disqualified as an exempt organization due to the prohibition on private inurement (¶ 602). An excess benefit transaction is any transaction in which an economic benefit is provided to a "disqualified person" by the organization that exceeds any consideration given. It also includes any grant, loan, or other payment from a donor advised fund (¶ 610) or a qualified supporting organization (¶ 607) to a disqualified person.

The tax is imposed on the disqualified person and is 25 percent of the amount of the excess benefit or the amount of the grant, loan, or other compensation received from a donor advised fund or qualified supporting organization. A manager of the exempt organization who knowingly participates in the transaction is subject to a separate excise tax of 10 percent, up to $20,000 per act. Managers who knowingly participate in the transaction are jointly and severally liable for the 10-percent tax. However, a manager

---

References are to Standard Federal Tax Reports; Tax Research Consultant; and Practical Tax Explanations.

[27] ¶ 33,960; EXEMPT: 6,156.05; § 33,710.05

[28] ¶ 22,665; EXEMPT: 6,160; § 33,710.05

[29] ¶ 34,240; EXEMPT: 6,106; § 33,710.10

[30] ¶ 34,250; EXEMPT: 6,056; § 33,705.30

will not be liable if participation is not willful and due to reasonable cause. For this purpose, a manager includes a director, officer, trustee, and any other individual of the exempt organization with comparable responsibilities.

If the excess benefit is not corrected within the "taxable period" (¶ 614), then a second-tier excise tax is imposed on the disqualified person equal to 200 percent of the amount of the excess benefit, grant, loan, or other payment. If more than one person is liable for either the first- or second-tier taxes on disqualified persons, then such persons are jointly and severally liable for them. The taxes on disqualified persons and organization managers are reported on Form 4720. However, both levels of taxes may be abated under certain circumstances (¶ 647). In addition, private foundations are subject to different sanctions (¶ 635).

Disqualified Persons. For this purpose, a disqualified person is generally a person who is in a position to exercise substantial influence over the affairs of the exempt organization (including a qualified supporting organization), regardless of the individual's title. Certain family members and entities in which a disqualified person holds at least a 35-percent ownership interest are also treated as disqualified persons. In the case of any donor advised fund, a disqualified person includes any donor, donor advisor, and investment advisor to the fund, as well as any family member or any entity controlled by such persons. A disqualified person with respect to a qualified supporting organization includes any substantial contributor (¶ 635), family member of a substantial contributor, or a 35-percent controlled entity.

619. Involvement in Tax Shelter Transactions. Generally, a tax-exempt entity that is a party to a prohibited tax shelter transaction (¶ 2591), or which becomes a party to a subsequently listed transaction at any time during the tax year, is subject to an excise tax on a percentage of the entity's net income or proceeds attributable to the prohibited transaction. The rate of tax depends on whether the exempt entity *knew or had reason to know* that the transaction was a prohibited tax shelter transaction at the time it became a party to the transaction (Code Sec. 4965).[31] In addition, any manager of a tax-exempt entity who approves or otherwise causes the exempt entity to be a party to a prohibited tax shelter transaction at any time during the tax year, and knew or had reason to know that the transaction was a prohibited tax shelter transaction, must pay a separate excise tax for each approval. For this purpose, a tax-exempt entity includes any tax-exempt organization under Code Sec. 501(c) or religious organization under Code Sec. 501(d), including any charitable organization and any qualified retirement plan, as well as individual retirement accounts (IRA), health savings accounts (HSA), Archer medical savings accounts (MSA), and qualified tuition plans. The tax-exempt entity must file a disclosure of its being a party to a prohibited tax shelter transaction on Form 8886-T and the identity of any other party (including both taxable and tax-exempt parties) to the transaction which is known by the entity (Code Sec. 6033(a)(2); Reg. § 1.6033-5).[32]

623. Application and Modification of Exempt Status. Charitable organizations seeking exempt status under Code Sec. 501(c)(3) must file an application for exemption on Form 1023 or Form 1023-EZ within 15 months (or 27 months with an automatic 12-month extension) from the end of the month in which they are organized (Code Sec. 508; Reg. § 1.508-1; Temp. Reg. § 1.508-1T).[33] Form 1023-EZ, which can only be filed electronically, is meant for organizations with gross receipts of $50,000 or less and assets of $250,000 or less (Rev. Proc. 2014-40). An organization that fails to file a timely notice will not qualify for exempt status for any period prior to the date actual notice is given. A second notification is required to be included on the application if the organization wants to claim public charity status. An organization that fails to notify the IRS of

---

References are to Standard Federal Tax Reports; Tax Research Consultant; and Practical Tax Explanations.

[31] ¶ 34,305; EXEMPT: 6,252; § 33,715

[32] ¶ 35,420, ¶ 35,424E; EXEMPT: 6,254; § 33,715

[33] ¶ 22,790, ¶ 22,791, ¶ 22,791F; EXEMPT: 12,054; § 33,505

public charity status will be presumed to be a private foundation (¶ 631). An organization will be a publicly supported organization qualifying for public charity status in its first five years if it can reasonably be expected to receive the requisite public support during the period (Reg. § 1.170A-9(f)(4)(v)).

Organizations that are not required to file an application for exempt status or notification of public charity status include: (1) any organization (other than a private foundation) whose annual gross receipts normally do not exceed $5,000; (2) churches and their affiliates; (3) any subordinate organization (other than a private foundation) covered by a group exemption of a parent; and (4) certain nonexempt charitable trusts (¶ 591) (Reg. § 1.508-1(a)(3)). However, for such an organization to establish its exemption with the IRS and receive a determination letter, it should file the appropriate information return as proof of its exemption (¶ 625) (Reg. § 1.508-1(a)(4)).

The IRS will issue a favorable determination letter or exemption ruling if the organization's application and supporting documents establish that it meets the particular requirements under which it is claiming tax-exempt status (Rev. Proc. 2014-9).[34] A ruling may also be modified or revoked by the IRS at any time (Reg. § 601.201(n)(6)).[35] Generally, revocations occur prospectively, however, a retroactive revocation may occur where: (1) the IRS was not fully or correctly informed as to the material facts on which the exemption ruling was based, or (2) there have been material changes in law or fact after the original ruling was issued.

If an organization receives an unfavorable exemption ruling, or its exempt status is revoked, it may seek judicial review only after it has exhausted all administrative remedies with the IRS. If an adverse ruling is issued (or if the IRS fails to issue a ruling), the organization can seek a declaratory judgment that it qualifies for exempt status (Code Sec. 7428).[36] If the organization has actually begun operations before it receives an adverse ruling (or its exempt status is revoked retroactively), it may either pay the taxes on its activities it thought were exempt and file for a refund or it can protest the assessment of any taxes in the Tax Court. An organization whose tax-exempt status has been revoked because it did not file annual information returns for three consecutive years (¶ 625) can apply for reinstatement of its status (Rev. Proc. 2014-11; Rev. Proc. 2014-40).[37]

Tax-exempt organizations use Form 8940 to request determinations (other than initial exemption applications) about their tax-exempt status. These determinations include advance approval for foundation set-asides and scholarship approvals, change in type of supporting organization, and termination of foundation status.

625. Annual Information Return. All tax-exempt organizations are generally required to file an annual information return with the IRS, including organizations whose application for exemption is pending, as well as nonexempt charitable trusts (¶ 591) (Code Sec. 6033; Reg. § 1.6033-2).[38] For most organizations, the return is filed on or before the 15th day of the fifth month following the close of the organization's tax year on Form 990, Form 990-EZ, or Form 990-N, depending on its gross receipts and total assets. However, other forms may be required for certain organizations. For example, private foundations file Form 990-PF (¶ 631), farmers' cooperatives file Form 1120-C (¶ 698), religious and apostolic organizations file Form 1065 (¶ 604), and black lung benefits trusts file Form 990-BL. Organizations that exclude exempt function income from their gross income may be required to file a variation of Form 1120 in lieu of, or in addition to, Form 990 or Form 990-EZ, such as political organizations, which file Form 1120-POL (¶ 696), and certain homeowner associations, which file Form 1120-H (¶ 699).

Exempt organizations that are not required to file Form 990 or Form 990-EZ, regardless of gross receipts and total assets, include: any organization (other than a private foundation or supporting organization (¶ 607)) that has annual gross receipts of

---

References are to Standard Federal Tax Reports; Tax Research Consultant; and Practical Tax Explanations.

[34] ¶ 22,604.10; EXEMPT: 12,054; § 33,535

[35] ¶ 43,356; EXEMPT: 12,104; § 33,801

[36] ¶ 41,720; EXEMPT: 12,150; § 33,801

[37] ¶ 43,360.173; EXEMPT: 12,054; § 33,605.20

[38] ¶ 35,420, ¶ 35,422; EXEMPT: 12,252; § 33,605.05

$50,000 or less; any church (including its integrated auxiliary) and convention or association of churches (¶ 604); an exclusively religious activity of a religious order; church-sponsored mission societies; governmental units exempt from taxation; corporations organized under an act of Congress; certain schools affiliated with a church or religious order; and certain foreign or U.S. possession organizations (Code Sec. 6033(a)(3); Reg. § 1.6033-2(g)(1); Rev. Proc. 2011-15).[39] An exempt organization that is not required to file Form 990 or Form 990-EZ because its annual gross receipts normally do not exceed $50,000 is still required to file an annual information return electronically on Form 990-N (Code Sec. 6033(i); Reg. § 1.6033-6; Rev. Proc. 2011-15).[40]

Information Required. Form 990 and Form 990-EZ require an exempt organization to provide information on its finances, governance, compliance with certain federal tax filings and requirements, compensation paid to certain persons, exempt and nonexempt activities, and, in the case of a charitable hospital, the needs identified in its community health needs assessments and a copy of its audited financial statements (Code Sec. 6033(b)). Additional schedules and information are required to be completed depending upon the activities and type of the organization. For example, a charitable organization under Code Sec. 501(c)(3) must include information on its lobbying activities (¶ 613) and any donor advised funds (¶ 610) it sponsors (Code Sec. 6033(e) and (k)). A qualified nonprofit health insurance issuer under Code Sec. 501(c)(29) must include information on the amount of reserves on hand, and the amount of reserves required by each state in which the issuer is licensed to issue qualified health plans (Code Sec. 6033(m)). If an organization was tax-exempt for any of its last five tax years preceding its dissolution, liquidation, termination, or substantial contraction, then it must also include on Form 990 or Form 990-EZ information relating to that event (Code Sec. 6043(b); Reg. § 1.6043-3(b)).[41] Organizations exempt from reporting information on their dissolution or termination include churches, organizations other than private foundations with $5,000 or less in annual gross receipts, and other organizations specified in the regulations.

Disclosure. Tax-exempt organizations, including private foundations, must make available for public inspection, at the organization's principal, regional, and district offices (having three or more employees) during regular business hours, its three most recent annual information returns, as well as a copy of its application for exemption. Charitable organizations must also make available for public inspection any returns related to the organization's unrelated business taxable income (¶ 670) filed in the previous three tax years (Code Sec. 6104; Reg. § 301.6104(d)-3).[42] Organizations do not have to honor requests if they reasonably believe that the request is part of a harassment campaign. Requests may be made either in person or in writing. Copies of an organization's Form 990 must be furnished immediately for requests made in person and within 30 days for written requests. Organizations are permitted to charge a reasonable fee for reproduction and mailing costs. An exempt organization can comply with these disclosure requirements by posting information on its website.

Penalties. A penalty of $20 per day (up to a maximum for any return of $10,000 or five percent of the organization's gross receipts, whichever is less) is imposed on each tax-exempt organization that fails to file an annual information return, files a late return without reasonable cause, or fails to file the information return on dissolution or substantial contraction (Code Sec. 6652(c)).[43] For organizations with gross receipts in excess of $1 million for any year, the penalty increases to $100 per day (up to a maximum for any return of $50,000 or five percent of gross receipts). An additional penalty of $10 a day (up to a maximum $5,000 on any return) is imposed on any officer, trustee, employee, etc., who fails to file the return without reasonable cause after requested by the IRS. There is no monetary penalty on an organization that is required

---

References are to Standard Federal Tax Reports; Tax Research Consultant; and Practical Tax Explanations.

[39] ¶ 35,420, ¶ 35,422, ¶ 35,425.24; EXEMPT: 12,252.05; § 33,605.05

[40] ¶ 35,420, ¶ 35,424J, ¶ 35,425.33; EXEMPT: 12,252.05; § 33,605.15

[41] ¶ 35,880, ¶ 35,885; EXEMPT: 12,252.30; § 33,605.05

[42] ¶ 36,900, ¶ 36,910E; EXEMPT: 12,258; § 33,615

[43] ¶ 39,480; PENALTY: 3,208.15; § 33,615

to file Form 990-N but fails to do so. However, if an organization fails to file an annual return for three consecutive years, its exempt status is automatically revoked (Code Sec. 6033(j)).[44] An organization whose tax-exempt status has been revoked because it did not file annual information returns for three consecutive years can apply for reinstatement of its status (Rev. Proc. 2014-11; Rev. Proc. 2014-40).[45]

Failure to comply with the public disclosure requirements results in a penalty of $20 per day, with a maximum of $10,000 for any annual return. The penalty for a willful failure to comply with the public disclosure requirements is $5,000 for each return or application (Code Sec. 6685).[46] There is no maximum penalty for failure to disclose the organization's exemption application.

627. Other Reporting and Disclosure Requirements. In addition to filing an application for exempt status (¶ 623) and annual information returns (¶ 625), exempt organizations (other than private foundations) have a number of other filing requirements.

Nondeductible Contributions. All tax-exempt organizations that are not eligible to receive deductible charitable contributions (such as lobbying groups, political action committees, labor unions, trade associations, social clubs, and political organizations (¶ 692 and ¶ 1061)) must disclose this fact in a conspicuous and easily recognizable format in their fundraising solicitations (Code Sec. 6113).[47] Violation of this requirement without reasonable cause will subject an organization to a penalty of $1,000 per day of solicitation (up to $10,000 for any calendar year); a higher penalty will apply if the failure was intentional (Code Sec. 6710).[48]

Quid Pro Quo Contributions. Charitable organizations are required to inform donors in a written statement that quid pro quo contributions in excess of $75 are deductible only to the extent that the contributions exceed the value of goods or services provided by the organization (Code Sec. 6115).[49] Failure to make the required disclosure subjects the organization to a penalty of $10 per contribution unless due to reasonable cause (Code Sec. 6714).[50] A quid pro quo contribution is any payment made partly as a contribution to the organization and partly in consideration for goods or services provided by the organization (fundraising dinners and auctions).

Donated Vehicles. A charitable organization is required to provide a donor of a motor vehicle, boat, or airplane with a contemporaneous written acknowledgment of the donation using Form 1098-C, including a certification of the organization's use or sale of the vehicle (¶ 1070A). A donee organization that fails to provide the acknowledgment or that provides a fraudulent acknowledgment will be subject to a penalty (Code Sec. 6720).[51]

Donated Intellectual Property. A charitable organization that receives or accrues net income during a tax year from a qualified intellectual property contribution must file an information return on Form 8899 and provide a copy to the donor (¶ 1062A). The return is required for any tax year that occurs during the 10-year period beginning on the date of the contribution and if the legal life of the donated property has not expired. The organization will be subject to a penalty for failure to file the return (¶ 2816).

Dispositions of Donated Property. A charitable organization is required to file a donee information return on Form 8282 if it sells or otherwise disposes of any charitable deduction property within three years after donated to the organization (Code Sec. 6050L(a)).[52] Charitable donation property is any property (other than cash or public securities) for which the donor claims a charitable contribution deduction of at least $5,000 and for which the organization signed an acknowledgment on Form 8283. The organization will be subject to a penalty for failure to file the return (¶ 2816).

6 | EXEMPT ORGS

References are to Standard Federal Tax Reports; Tax Research Consultant; and Practical Tax Explanations.

[44] ¶ 35,420; EXEMPT: 12,252.05; § 33,605.05

[45] ¶ 43,360.173; EXEMPT: 12,054; § 33,605.20

[46] ¶ 39,871; EXEMPT: 12,258; § 33,615

[47] ¶ 37,040; EXEMPT: 12,302; § 33,620.15

[48] ¶ 40,115; EXEMPT: 12,302.25; § 33,620.15

[49] ¶ 37,065; EXEMPT: 12,306; § 33,620.05

[50] ¶ 40,180; EXEMPT: 12,306.20; § 33,620.05

[51] ¶ 40,207; INDIV: 51,462; § 33,610.35

[52] ¶ 36,260; EXEMPT: 12,262; § 33,610.10

Private Foundations

631. Private Foundations. Charitable organizations under Code Sec. 501(c)(3) are either public charities or private foundations (¶ 602). Public charities generally are organizations that have broad public support or that actively function in a supporting relationship to such organizations. On the other hand, a private foundation typically is funded by one individual, family, or corporation. Thus, a private foundation is any Code Sec. 501(c)(3) organization *other than*:

- a charitable deduction donee listed in Code Sec. 170(b)(1)(A) (¶ 1059);

- a publicly supported organization receiving more than ⅓ of its annual support from members and the public, and not more than ⅓ of its support from investment income and unrelated business income (¶ 655);

- a qualified supporting organization (¶ 607); or

- an organization operated for public safety testing (Code Sec. 509).[53]

An organization that fails a public support test for two consecutive years will be treated as a private foundation as of the beginning of the second year of failure for certain purposes. The organization will be treated as a private foundation for all purposes beginning the first day of the third consecutive year (Reg. § 1.509(a)-3(c)(1)(i)).

Like all Code Sec. 501(c)(3) organizations, a private foundation must provide notice to the IRS for it to be exempt from taxation (¶ 623). However, even if notice is provided, a private foundation will be denied tax-exempt status unless its governing instrument specifically prohibits it from accumulating income (¶ 637), engaging in certain prohibited activities including acts of self-dealing (¶ 635), retaining excess business holdings (¶ 640), making investments which jeopardize its charitable purpose (¶ 642), or making certain taxable expenditures (¶ 644) (Code Sec. 508(e)).[54] All private foundations must also file an annual information return on Form 990-PF reporting gross income, receipts, disbursements, etc. (¶ 625). If at any time during the tax year the foundation has at least $5,000 of assets, it must also include information on its assets, managers, and grants or contributions made during the year (Code Sec. 6033(c); Reg. § 1.6033-3).[55]

633. Investment Income of Private Foundations. A two-percent excise tax is imposed on the "net investment income" of a private foundation (¶ 631) for each tax year (Code Sec. 4940).[56] The tax is reduced to one percent if the foundation satisfies certain requirements as to the amount of charitable distributions it made during the year and if it was not liable for the excise tax on undistributed income (¶ 637) in any of the preceding five tax years. The excise tax is reported on the foundation's annual return, Form 990-PF. Estimated payments of the foundation's liability for the tax (as well as its unrelated business taxable income (UBTI) (¶ 670)) are computed on Form 990-W and the first-quarter installment is due by the 15th day of the fifth month following the foundation's tax year (May 15 for calendar year foundations) (Code Sec. 6655(g)(3)).[57] The net investment income of a private foundation generally includes the foundation's gross investment income and net capital gain, less the ordinary and necessary business expenses incurred for the production or collection of gross investment income. Gross investment income includes interest, dividends, rents, royalties, and payments with respect to securities loans, as well as any similar source of income such as income from annuities and notional principal contracts. It does not include income to the extent it is taken into account as UBTI including any gain or loss from the sale or disposition of property (no capital loss carryovers or carrybacks are allowed).

The tax on investment income will not apply to an exempt "operating foundation," which is any operating foundation that has been publicly supported for at least 10 years, at all times during the tax year it is governed by representatives at least 75 percent of whom represent the general public, and at no time during the tax year does it have an

---

References are to Standard Federal Tax Reports; Tax Research Consultant; and Practical Tax Explanations.

[53] ¶ 22,800; EXEMPT: 21,000; § 33,205.05

[54] ¶ 22,790; EXEMPT: 21,450; § 33,205.20

[55] ¶ 35,420, ¶ 35,423; EXEMPT: 21,552; § 33,205.15

[56] ¶ 34,000; EXEMPT: 24,050; § 33,210.05

[57] ¶ 39,565; EXEMPT: 15,204; § 33,210.10

officer who is a disqualified individual. For this purpose, a disqualified individual is a substantial contributor to the foundation, an owner of more than 20 percent of a business or trust which is a substantial contributor, or a member of the family of any of the preceding. An operating foundation is a foundation that spends at least 85 percent of the lesser of its adjusted net income or its minimum investment return in carrying on its exempt activities (Code Sec. 4942(j)(3); Reg. § 53.4942(b)-1).[58] A nonoperating private foundation is generally a grantmaking organization that does not operate its own charitable program.

635. Prohibitions on Self-Dealing by Private Foundations. Certain acts of self-dealing are prohibited between a disqualified person and a private foundation (¶ 631) (Code Sec. 4941).[59] This includes the sale or exchange of property, loans or other extensions of credit, the furnishing of goods or services, payments of compensation, or the transfer of income or assets to the disqualified person. It does not include the pro rata division of a trust that qualifies as a charitable remainder trust (¶ 590) into two separate trusts (Rev. Rul. 2008-41).[60] For this purpose, a disqualified person includes:

- a substantial contributor (any person who contributes more than $5,000 if that amount is more than two percent of the total contributions received by the foundation before the end of its tax year);

- a foundation manager, including an officer, director, or trustee;

- the owner of more than 20 percent of a corporation, partnership, trust, or other enterprise that is a substantial contributor;

- a member of the family of any of the preceding (including spouse, ancestor, child, grandchild, great grandchild, or spouse of any of these descendants);

- a corporation, trust, estate, or partnership more than 35 percent of which is owned or held by any of the preceding; and

- a government official (Code Sec. 4946).[61]

The disqualified person is subject to a 10-percent excise tax on the amount involved in any act of self-dealing for each year in the taxable period. Any foundation manager who knowingly participates in the self-dealing act is subject to a five-percent excise tax on the amount involved but only if participation was willful and not due to reasonable cause. A second-level tax of 200 percent (50 percent on the manager) applies if the prohibited act is not corrected within the taxable period. For this purpose, the taxable period begins on the date the self-dealing act occurs and ends on the earliest of: (1) the date the deficiency notice for the first-level tax is mailed; (2) the date the first-level tax is assessed; or (3) the date the act of self-dealing is completely corrected (Code Sec. 4941(e)).[62] The maximum tax imposed on a foundation manager is $20,000 per act for each level of tax. The IRS has discretionary authority to abate both levels of tax for the manager and the disqualified person (¶ 647). However, the IRS also has the authority to impose a third-level tax or terminate the foundation's status (¶ 649) if there are repeated or flagrant acts of self-dealing (Code Sec. 6684).[63] The initial excise tax on an act of self-dealing is reported on Form 4720.

637. Undistributed Income of Private Foundations. A private foundation (¶ 631) other than an operating foundation (¶ 633) is required to distribute annually its minimum investment return for the tax year, which generally equals five percent of the foundation's net investment assets (adjusted for certain taxes and loan repayments). Failure to do so will cause the foundation to be subject to an excise tax of 30 percent of any undistributed income (Code Sec. 4942).[64] Undistributed income is the amount the minimum investment return of the foundation exceeds the amount of qualifying distribu-

---

References are to Standard Federal Tax Reports; Tax Research Consultant; and Practical Tax Explanations.

[58] ¶ 34,040, ¶ 34,044; EXEMPT: 24,450; § 33,210.10

[59] ¶ 34,020; EXEMPT: 24,150; § 33,215.05

[60] ¶ 34,031.65; EXEMPT: 24,200

[61] ¶ 34,120; EXEMPT: 24,700; § 33,205.25

[62] ¶ 34,020; EXEMPT: 24,150; § 33,215.05

[63] ¶ 39,865; EXEMPT: 24,162; § 33,215.05

[64] ¶ 34,040; EXEMPT: 24,300; § 33,220.05

6

EXEMPT ORGS

tions made during the tax year. Qualifying distributions include distributions to public charities and private operating foundations, and payments for expenses and assets used for charitable purposes. It does not generally include payments made by the nonoperating private foundation to a supporting organization (¶ 607).

If the foundation fails to make the necessary distributions within the taxable period, then a second-level tax will be imposed equal to 100 percent of the undistributed income. For this purpose, the "taxable period" is the period that begins on the first day of the tax year, and ends on the earlier of the date the deficiency notice for the initial tax is mailed or the date it is assessed. The IRS has discretionary authority to abate both levels of tax (¶ 647). However, a third-level tax may be imposed if there are repeated or flagrant acts of failure to distribute income (Code Sec. 6684).[65] The initial excise tax on undistributed income is reported on Form 4720.

640. Excess Business Holdings of Private Foundations. A private foundation (¶ 631) is allowed to own a certain amount of business enterprises jointly with disqualified persons (¶ 635). However, to curb any abuses, the foundation is subject to a 10-percent excise tax on any "excess business holdings" during the tax year (Code Sec. 4943).[66] If the excess business holdings are not divested within the taxable period (¶ 637), then a second-level tax of 200 percent is imposed. In general, the permitted amount of business ownership that a private foundation and disqualified person may have in any enterprise that is not substantially related to the exempt purposes of the foundation is 20 percent. If third parties have effective control of the business enterprise, then the limit is 35 percent. Special rules apply to certain grandfathered holdings. The IRS has discretionary authority to abate both levels of tax (¶ 647). However, a third-level tax may be imposed if there are repeated or flagrant acts of excess business holdings (Code Sec. 6684).[67]

The excise tax on excess business holdings will apply to donor advised funds (¶ 610) and certain qualified supporting organizations (¶ 607). In applying the tax to donor advised funds, a disqualified person is defined as any donor, a member of the donor's family, or a 35-percent controlled entity (Code Sec. 4943(e)). A qualified supporting organization will be subject to the excess business holdings tax only if it is a Type III supporting organization, or a Code Sec. 501(c)(3) organization that meets the organizational and operational test of a qualified supporting organization and it is not controlled by a disqualified person (Code Sec. 4943(f)). For this purpose, a disqualified person with respect to the supporting organization is any person with substantial influence over the organization (or any family member of such a person), as well as any substantial contributor, family member of a substantial contributor, or 35-percent controlled entity.

642. Investments Jeopardizing Exempt Purpose of Private Foundations. A 10-percent excise tax is imposed on any investment of a private foundation (¶ 631) that jeopardizes the foundation's exempt status (Code Sec. 4944; Reg. § 53.4944-1).[68] A "jeopardizing" investment is generally one that shows a lack of reasonable business care and prudence in providing for the foundation's short- and long-term financial needs. Examples of investments that will be closely scrutinized include trading in securities on margin, trading in commodity futures, investing in working interests in oil and gas wells, and selling short. A 10-percent excise tax is also imposed on any foundation manager who knowingly participates in such an investment (up to $10,000 per investment), unless the participation is not willful but due to a reasonable cause. A second-level tax of 25 percent is imposed on the foundation if the jeopardy situation is not corrected within the taxable period (¶ 637). Any foundation manager who refuses to agree to part or all of the correction will be subject to a second-level tax of five percent of the investment (up to $20,000). If more than one foundation manager is liable for either level of tax, then all

---

References are to Standard Federal Tax Reports; Tax Research Consultant; and Practical Tax Explanations.

[65] ¶ 39,865; EXEMPT: 24,162; § 33,220.05

[66] ¶ 34,060; EXEMPT: 24,500; § 33,225.05

[67] ¶ 39,865; EXEMPT: 24,162; § 33,225.05

[68] ¶ 34,080, ¶ 34,081; EXEMPT: 24,600; § 33,230.05

such managers are jointly and severally liable for them. The IRS has discretionary authority to abate both levels of tax (¶ 647). However, a third-level tax may be imposed on either the foundation or a manager if there are repeated or flagrant acts of jeopardizing investments (Code Sec. 6684).[69]

644. Lobbying and Other Prohibited Expenditures of Private Foundations. A private foundation (¶ 631) is subject to a 20-percent excise tax on the amount of any "taxable expenditure" made during the tax year. Any foundation manager who, without reasonable cause, willfully agrees to the expenditure knowing it is improper, is subject to a five-percent excise tax on the expenditure (up to $10,000) (Code Sec. 4945).[70] A taxable expenditure generally includes any amount paid by the foundation for legislative or political purposes, or any grant to an individual for travel, study, or other similar purpose (unless made under objective standards). It also includes any grant to any organization unless the grantee organization is a public charity, qualified supporting organization (¶ 607), exempt operating foundation (¶ 633), or the nonoperating private foundation exercises responsibility for the expenditure of the grant. A taxable expenditure does not include the pro rata division of a trust that qualifies as a charitable remainder trust (¶ 590) into two separate trusts (Rev. Rul. 2008-41).[71] A second-level tax of 100 percent is imposed on the foundation if the taxable expenditure is not corrected within the taxable period (¶ 637). Any foundation manager who refuses to agree to part or all of the correction will be subject to a second-level tax of 50 percent of the investment (up to $20,000). If more than one foundation manager is liable for either level of tax, then all such managers are jointly and severally liable for them. The IRS has discretionary authority to abate both levels of tax for the foundation or the manager (¶ 647). However, a third-level tax may be imposed if there are repeated or flagrant acts of taxable expenditures (Code Sec. 6684).[72]

647. Abatement of Certain Taxes on Tax-Exempt Organizations. The IRS has discretionary authority not to assess certain first-tier excise taxes imposed on tax-exempt organizations, or to abate such taxes if already assessed, or to provide a credit or refund if the tax is already collected. The IRS will exercise this authority only if the violation giving rise to the imposition of the excise tax in question was due to reasonable cause and not willful neglect, and is corrected within the "correction period" (Code Sec. 4962).[73] First-tier excise taxes to which this relief may apply include: all of the excise taxes imposed on private foundations and disqualified persons (¶ 631), except for the tax on acts of self-dealing (¶ 635); the excise tax on the lobbying and political activities of public charities (¶ 614); the excise tax on excess benefit transactions (¶ 617); and the excise taxes on taxable distributions and prohibited benefits from donor advised funds (¶ 610). The IRS may withhold or abate an assessment of any second-tier excise taxes if the taxable event in question is corrected voluntarily during the correction period (Code Sec. 4961).[74] For this purpose, the correction period is the period beginning on the date of the taxable event and ending 90 days after the deficiency notice for the second-tier tax is mailed (Code Sec. 4963).[75]

649. Termination of Private Foundation Status. The status of any organization as a private foundation (¶ 631) may be terminated voluntarily or involuntarily (Code Sec. 507).[76] A voluntary termination requires the foundation to notify the IRS of its plan to terminate. An involuntary termination occurs when the IRS notifies the foundation of the intent to terminate its status because of willful repeated violations or a willful and flagrant violation giving rise to excise taxes on the foundation. In either case, the private foundation must pay a termination tax equal to the lesser of: (1) the aggregate amount of tax benefits received by the foundation and any of its substantial contributors (¶ 635) since its inception resulting from its exempt status under Code Sec. 501(c)(3); or (2) the

References are to Standard Federal Tax Reports; Tax Research Consultant; and Practical Tax Explanations.

[69] ¶ 39,865; EXEMPT: 24,162; § 33,230.05

[70] ¶ 34,100; EXEMPT: 24,650; § 33,235.05

[71] ¶ 34,031.65; EXEMPT: 24,650

[72] ¶ 39,865; EXEMPT: 24,162; § 33,235.05

[73] ¶ 34,280; EXEMPT: 24,750; § 33,220.10

[74] ¶ 34,260; EXEMPT: 24,750; § 33,220.10

[75] ¶ 34,300; EXEMPT: 24,756; § 33,220.10

[76] ¶ 22,771; EXEMPT: 27,000; § 33,240.05

6

EXEMPT ORGS

value of its net assets. The pro rata division of a trust that qualifies as a charitable remainder trust (¶ 590) into two separate trusts does not terminate private foundation status or cause the termination tax to apply (Rev. Rul. 2008-41).[77]

The IRS may abate a portion or all of the termination tax if, prior to providing notice to the IRS of its voluntary termination, the foundation distributes all of its net assets to another private foundation or public charity described in Code Sec. 170(b)(1)(A) (¶ 1059) that has been in existence for at least five years immediately before the distribution. Under these circumstances, the transfer of assets is not a termination of the foundation's status. Instead, the foundation retains its status until it gives actual notice of its termination to the IRS. When notice is provided after all net assets are transferred, then the termination tax will be zero (but the distributions may give rise to excise taxes). The termination tax may also be abated if the foundation becomes a public charity within 12 months or it actually operates as a public charity for at least five years. However, notice of termination must be provided to the IRS prior to the beginning of the 12-month or five-year termination period.

Tax-exempt organizations use Form 8940 to request determinations about termination of foundation status.

Unrelated Business Taxable Income

655. Tax-Exempt Organizations Subject to Unrelated Business Income Tax. Although a variety of nonprofit organizations with charitable or socially beneficial purposes may be granted tax-exempt status under Code Sec. 501, they are still subject to an unrelated business income tax (¶ 658) (Code Sec. 511).[78] Unrelated business income is income from a trade or business regularly carried on by the exempt organization (¶ 664) that is not substantially related (¶ 667) to the organization's exempt purposes (Code Sec. 512).[79] All types of exempt organizations are subject to the tax except government instrumentalities (other than colleges or universities) and federally licensed businesses or educational institutions sponsored by a religious order (Reg. § 1.511-2).[80] Additionally, title-holding companies may be exempt from tax on unrelated business income if the holding corporation and the payee organization file a consolidated return.

658. Unrelated Business Income Tax Rate and Payment. Tax-exempt organizations subject to the unrelated business income tax (¶ 655) are taxed on their unrelated business taxable income (UBTI) (¶ 670) at ordinary corporate income tax rates (¶ 219 and ¶ 1401) or, if the organization is not incorporated, at trust income tax rates (¶ 19) (Code Sec. 511(a)).[81] Returns are made on Form 990-T and filed at the same time as the organization's annual information return (¶ 625) (Reg. § 1.6012-2(e)).[82] Estimated payments of the exempt organization's liability for UBTI are computed on Form 990-W. The first-quarter installment is due by the 15th day of the fifth month following the organization's tax year (May 15 for calendar year organizations) (Code Sec. 6655(g)(3)).[83]

664. Business Regularly Carried on by Tax-Exempt Organizations. The unrelated business taxable income (UBTI) of a tax-exempt organization (¶ 670) is its gross income from any unrelated trade or business *regularly* carried on by the organization, minus any deductions for expenses related to the trade or business (¶ 682) (Code Sec. 512(a); Reg. § § 1.512(a)-1 and 1.513-1(c)).[84] A trade or business generally includes any activity carried on for the production of income from selling goods or performing services. In determining whether a trade or business is regularly carried on, the frequency and continuity with which an activity is pursued is judged with comparable commercial activities of nonexempt organizations. In the case of a social club, voluntary employees' beneficiary association (VEBA), or an organization for the payment of supplemental

---

References are to Standard Federal Tax Reports; Tax Research Consultant; and Practical Tax Explanations.

[77] ¶ 34,031.65; EXEMPT: 27,000

[78] ¶ 22,820; EXEMPT: 15,000; § 33,905

[79] ¶ 22,830; EXEMPT: 15,050; § 33,910

[80] ¶ 22,822; EXEMPT: 15,058; § 33,905

[81] ¶ 22,820; EXEMPT: 15,202; § 33,901

[82] ¶ 35,145; EXEMPT: 15,204; § 33,901

[83] ¶ 39,565; EXEMPT: 15,204; § 33,901

[84] ¶ 22,830, ¶ 22,831, ¶ 22,841; EXEMPT: 15,054, EXEMPT: 15,252; § 33,910, § 33,915

unemployment benefits (SUB) (¶ 692), UBTI is subject to tax only to the extent that it is not set aside for the purposes that constitute the basis for the organization's exemption (Code Sec. 512(a)(3); Temp. Reg. § 1.512(a)-5T).[85]

667. Business Unrelated to Exempt Function of Tax-Exempt Organizations. The unrelated business taxable income (UBTI) of a tax-exempt organization (¶ 670) includes any income from a business *not substantially related* to the organization's exempt purpose (Code Sec. 513; Reg. § 1.513-1).[86] A business activity is not substantially related to an organization's exempt purpose if it does not contribute importantly to accomplishing that purpose (other than through the production of funds). Whether an activity contributes importantly depends on the facts, including the size and extent of the activities involved in relation to the exempt function they serve. A number of activities will *not* be considered an unrelated trade or business, including any trade or business that:

- has substantially all the work in carrying on the business performed for the organization without compensation;

- is carried on by a Code Sec. 501(c)(3) organization or governmental college or university primarily for the convenience of its members, students, etc.;

- consists of selling merchandise, substantially all of which has been received by the organization as gifts or contributions;

- is a qualified entertainment activity or a qualified convention and trade show activity (¶ 685) (Code Sec. 513(d));

- in the case of a public charity hospital, performs services that a tax-exempt cooperative hospital organization may perform (¶ 699) (Code Sec. 513(e));

- consists of conducting any bingo games if the games are conducted in accordance with local law and do not compete with profit-making businesses (Code Sec. 513(f));

- in the case of a mutual or cooperative telephone or electric company, engages in qualified pole rentals (Code Sec. 513(g));

- includes the exchanging or renting of member donor lists between exempt organizations or the distribution of low-cost articles ($10.40 for 2014; $10.50 for 2015) incidental to the solicitation of charitable contributions (Code Sec. 513(h); Rev. Proc. 2013-35; Rev. Proc. 2014-61); or

- involves the soliciting and receiving of qualified sponsorship payment (Code Sec. 513(i)) (¶ 685).

670. Unrelated Business Taxable Income Defined. The unrelated business taxable income (UBTI) of a tax-exempt organization is its gross income from any unrelated trade or business regularly carried on (¶ 664 and ¶ 667), less the deductions directly connected with the trade or business (¶ 682) (Code Sec. 512).[87] The following income items (and any related deductions) are generally excluded from the calculation of UBTI: dividends, interest, annuities and royalties (¶ 673); rents from real property or incidental rents from personal property leased with real property (¶ 676); gains or losses from the disposition of property other than stock in trade (¶ 679); certain research income; certain amounts received from controlled entities and foreign corporations; income of a mutual or cooperative electric company derived from the sale of electricity from its members; and gains or losses on the disposition of qualified brownfield sites. Annual dues not exceeding $158 for 2014 ($160 for 2015) that are paid to an exempt agricultural or horticultural organization will also be excluded from UBTI (Code Sec. 512(d); Rev. Proc. 2013-35; Rev. Proc. 2014-61).

An exempt organization's calculation of UBTI must include its share of income and deductions from an unrelated trade or business conducted by a partnership (including a

---

References are to Standard Federal Tax Reports; Tax Research Consultant; and Practical Tax Explanations.

[85] ¶ 22,830, ¶ 22,834; EXEMPT: 15,206, EXEMPT: 15,208; § 33,910, § 33,915

[86] ¶ 22,840, ¶ 22,841; EXEMPT: 15,056; § 33,920

[87] ¶ 22,830; EXEMPT: 15,200, EXEMPT: 15,300; § 33,935.05

publicly traded partnership) or S corporation in which it is a partner or shareholder (Code Sec. 512(c) and (e)). However, if the tax year of the organization differs from the partnership's, then the amounts used to calculate UBTI will be based on the income and deductions of the partnership in the tax year that ends within the tax year of the exempt organization. In addition, the organization's share of S corporation income and deductions must be included regardless of whether they would normally be excluded from UBTI (dividends, interest, royalties, etc.).

673. Unrelated Business Taxable Income—Investment Income. Generally, the unrelated business taxable income (UBTI) of a tax-exempt organization (¶ 670) will *not* include investment income such as dividends, interest, annuities, royalties, payments with respect to securities loans, amounts received or accrued as consideration for entering into agreements to make loans, and income derived from notional principal contracts (as well as income from ordinary investments that are substantially similar) (Code Sec. 512(b); Reg. § 1.512(b)-1(a)).[88] Royalties for this purpose include amounts paid to an exempt organization for use of its name, trademarks, and other intellectual property rights in connection with the sale of merchandise or services.[89] However, where an exempt organization provides active services in relation to the marketing of products or services associated with its name or other rights, the income may not be excluded as royalty income. The exclusion for investment income also does not apply to income derived from debt-financed property (¶ 687).

Membership Organizations. Special rules apply to certain membership organizations including a social and recreational club, voluntary employees' beneficiary association (VEBA), or a supplemental unemployment compensation benefit trust (SUB) (¶ 692). Unlike other exempt organizations, these organizations cannot exclude investment income from UBTI and losses from nonexempt activities cannot generally be used to offset investment income. However, gross income does not include exempt function income, which is income from dues, fees, and charges for providing facilities and services for members, dependents, and guests, as well as income set aside for charitable purposes or by a VEBA to provide insurance benefits (Code Sec. 512(a)(3)).[90] An exclusion also applies for gain such organizations realize on the sale of assets used in pursuing their exempt function to the extent the proceeds are reinvested (within a four-year period) in other assets for such purposes. For this purpose, a title-holding corporation whose income is payable to a membership organization will be treated as the exempt organization. To prevent bypassing these limitations through termination of tax-exempt status, a *nonexempt* social club or other membership organization operated primarily to furnish goods or services to members may deduct the cost of furnishing these goods, services, insurance, etc., only to the extent of membership-related income (Code Sec. 277).[91] A nonexempt social club or VEBA is also not allowed to claim the corporate dividends-received deduction (¶ 221).

Look-Through Rules. If an exempt organization receives or accrues a payment of interest, annuity, royalty or rent (but not a dividend) from an entity that it controls, then the payment is includible in the organization's UBTI to the extent it either reduces the net unrelated business income of the controlled entity or increases its net unrelated losses (Code Sec. 512(b)(13)).[92] However, any payment received or accrued after 2005 and before 2014 under a binding written contract in effect on August 17, 2006, is included in the exempt organization's UBTI only to the extent it exceeds the amount that would have been paid if the payment met the requirements for related parties under the transfer pricing rules of Code Sec. 482.

> **Comment:** Absent further legislation, the exclusion of qualifying payments by a controlled entity to a tax-exempt organization from the organization's UBTI has expired for payments received after December 31, 2013. For the latest legislative updates, visit our website www.CCHGroup.com/TaxUpdates.

References are to Standard Federal Tax Reports; Tax Research Consultant; and Practical Tax Explanations.

[88] ¶ 22,830, ¶ 22,835; EXEMPT: 15,302; § 33,935.05

[89] ¶ 22,837.83; EXEMPT: 15,310; § 33,935.05

[90] ¶ 22,830; COMPEN: 54,350, EXEMPT: 15,206, EXEMPT: 15,208; § 33,935.05

[91] ¶ 14,600; ACCTNG: 12,216; § 33,420.25

[92] ¶ 22,830; EXEMPT: 15,304; § 33,935.05

A valuation misstatement penalty applies to excess payments that are included in UBTI. In addition, the exempt organization must report the payments from a controlled entity on its annual return (Code Sec. 6033(h)).[93] The threshold of control of a subsidiary which triggers UBTI is having more than 50-percent ownership (more than 50 percent of stock by vote or value in a corporation, or more than 50 percent of a profits, capital, or beneficial interest of a partnership or other entity). The constructive ownership rules of Code Sec. 318 apply for this purpose (¶ 743).

676. Unrelated Business Taxable Income—Rents. Excluded from the unrelated business taxable income (UBTI) of a tax-exempt organization (¶ 670) are amounts received from the rental of real property, including those rents from personal property leased with real property so long as they are incidental in relation to the total amount of rents under the lease (10 percent or less of total rents from all leased property) (Code Sec. 512(b)(3); Reg. § 1.512(b)-1(c)).[94] However, payments for the use or occupancy of rooms and other space (for example, in a hotel, boarding house, storage facility) where services are also provided primarily for the occupant's convenience and are not those customarily rendered in rental for occupancy only (such as maid service) are not rents from real property. Rents are taxable if they are: (1) rents from real property leased with personal property where more than 50 percent of the rent is attributable to the personal property; (2) rents from both the real and the personal property if the amount of the rents depends on the income or profits derived by any person from the leased property (other than an amount based on a fixed percentage of gross receipts or sales); and (3) unrelated income from debt-financed property (¶ 687).

679. Unrelated Business Taxable Income—Gains and Losses. Excluded from the unrelated business taxable income (UBTI) of a tax-exempt organization (¶ 670) are all gains or losses from the sale, exchange or other disposition (including involuntary conversions and casualties) of property *other than*: (1) stock in trade or other property of a kind properly includible in inventory; (2) property held primarily for sale to customers in the ordinary course of a trade or business; or (3) timber cutting that the organization has elected to consider as a sale or exchange (Code Sec. 512(b)(5); Reg. § 1.512(b)-1(d)).[95] The exclusion also applies to all gains or losses recognized in connection with the organization's investment activities from the lapse or termination of options to buy and sell securities (whether or not written by the organization), as well as options to buy or sell real property. The exclusion does not apply to gains from the sale or other disposition of debt-financed property (¶ 687). Gains from certain pension plan investments in property of troubled financial institutions are also excluded (Code Sec. 512(b)(16)).

682. Unrelated Business Taxable Income—Deductions. In computing unrelated business taxable income (UBTI) (¶ 670), a tax-exempt organization is entitled to deduct all ordinary and necessary business expenses *directly connected* with carrying on the unrelated trade or business (¶ 667). To be directly connected with the conduct of an unrelated business, deductions must have a proximate and primary relationship to carrying on the business. Expenses attributable to an exempt activity are generally not deductible unless: (1) the unrelated business exploits the exempt activity; (2) the business is of a type normally carried on for profit by a taxable organization; and (3) the exempt activity is of a type normally carried on by a taxable organization in carrying on its business. If facilities or personnel are used for both exempt functions and the conduct of an unrelated business, expenses are allocated on a reasonable basis (Code Sec. 512(a) and (b)(12); Reg. § 1.512(a)-1).[96]

In addition to deduction of ordinary and necessary business expenses, an exempt organization is allowed a specific deduction of $1,000, as well as the deduction for charitable contributions allowed to corporations (¶ 927), net operating losses (NOLs) (¶ 1145), and domestic production activities (equal to the appropriate percentage of the

References are to Standard Federal Tax Reports; Tax Research Consultant; and Practical Tax Explanations.

[93] ¶ 35,420; EXEMPT: 15,304; § 33,935.05

[94] ¶ 22,830, ¶ 22,835; EXEMPT: 15,306; § 33,935.05

[95] ¶ 22,830, ¶ 22,835; EXEMPT: 15,302; § 33,935.05

[96] ¶ 22,830, ¶ 22,831; EXEMPT: 15,250; § 33,930

¶682

lesser of qualified production activities income or unrelated business taxable income, rather than taxable income (¶ 980A)). The charitable contribution deduction is allowed whether or not directly connected with the carrying on of the trade or business but is limited to 10 percent of the organization's UBTI, computed without regard to the contributions deduction (Code Sec. 512(b)(10)). An exempt trust that is subject to the unrelated business income tax at trust rates generally is allowed a deduction for charitable contributions in the same amounts as allowed for individuals (¶ 1058). With respect to the NOL deduction, the deduction must only reflect taxable "business income" and carryovers and items attributable to exempt income and expenses are disregarded (Code Sec. 512(b)(6)).

685. Advertising, Sponsorships, and Trade Shows. The sale of advertising in a periodical, journal, or magazine of a tax-exempt organization is considered an unrelated business of the organization (¶ 667) that exploits an exempt activity when the advertising activity is regularly carried on (¶ 664) (Reg. § 1.512(a)-1(d) and (f)).[97] An activity such as advertising does not lose its identity as a trade or business merely because it is carried on within a larger complex of other activities which may or may not be related to the organization's exempt purpose (Reg. § 1.513-1(b)).[98] As a result, advertising revenue is used in computing the organization's unrelated business taxable income (UBTI) (¶ 670) but may be offset by the expenses directly related to the advertising business activity. If facilities and personnel are both used to carry on exempt activities and unrelated advertising, the expenses must be allocated on a reasonable basis.

For this purpose, income realized by an exempt organization from the sponsorship of a public event will generally constitute advertising services. However, the solicitation and receipt of qualified sponsorship payments by an exempt organization is not an unrelated business, and the payments are excluded from computing UBTI (Code Sec. 513(i); Reg. § 1.513-4).[99] A qualified sponsorship payment is any payment by a payor engaged in a trade or business that does not expect any substantial return from the exempt organization other than the use or acknowledgment of the payor's name, logo, or product lines in connection with the activities of the tax-exempt organization. A qualified sponsorship payment does *not* include any payment:

- for advertising the payor's product or services, including messages that contain qualitative or comparative language, price information, an endorsement, or an inducement to purchase, sell or use the payor's products and services;

- contingent upon factors indicating the degree of public exposure at one or more events (attendance, broadcast ratings);

- that entitles the payor to the use or acknowledgment of the business name, logo, or product lines in the exempt organization's publication; or

- made in connection with a qualified convention or trade show activity (a convention or trade show conducted by a charitable organization (¶ 602), social welfare program, labor organization, or business league (¶ 692) that has as one of its purposes the promotion of interest in the products and services of the industry in general, or the education of the attendees regarding new developments or products and services related to the exempt activities of the organizations (Reg. § 1.513-3)).[100]

Taxable Income from Debt-Financed Property

687. Unrelated Debt-Financed Income. A percentage of income from debt-financed property must be included in a tax-exempt organization's unrelated business taxable income (UBTI) (¶ 670) regardless of whether the organization is engaged in a trade or business (Code Sec. 514(a); Reg. § 1.514(a)-1).[101] The percentage included in UBTI is the same percentage (not to exceed 100 percent) as the "average acquisition indebtedness" on the property (¶ 689) for the tax year divided by the "average amount

---

References are to Standard Federal Tax Reports; Tax Research Consultant; and Practical Tax Explanations.

[97] ¶ 22,831; EXEMPT: 15,158; § 33,925.05

[98] ¶ 22,841; EXEMPT: 15,158; § 33,925.05

[99] ¶ 22,840, ¶ 22,843G; EXEMPT: 15,122; § 33,925.05

[100] ¶ 22,843; EXEMPT: 15,112; § 33,925.05

[101] ¶ 22,850, ¶ 22,851; EXEMPT: 18,050; § 33,940.05

of the adjusted basis" of the property. Deductions with respect to each debt-financed property are allowed by applying the same percentage to expenses related to the property, except for any deduction resulting from the carryback or carryover of net capital losses (¶ 1752). For this purpose, debt-financed property generally means any property held to produce income, including gain from its disposition (for example, rental real estate, corporate stock, etc.) on which there is an acquisition indebtedness at any time during the tax year (or preceding 12 months if the property is disposed of during the tax year) (Code Sec. 514(b); Reg. § 1.514(b)-1(a)).[102] Certain property, however, is not debt-financed property even if it is held to produce income (¶ 691).

689. Acquisition Indebtedness on Debt-Financed Property. For any debt-financed property of a tax-exempt organization (¶ 687), "acquisition indebtedness" is the outstanding amount of principal debt: (1) incurred to acquire or improve property; (2) incurred before the acquisition or improvement if it would not have been incurred but for the acquisition or improvement; and (3) incurred after acquisition or improvement if it would not have been incurred but for the acquisition or improvement and was reasonably foreseeable at the time (Code Sec. 514(c); Reg. § 1.514(c)-1).[103]

If property is acquired subject to a mortgage, the amount of the mortgage (or similar lien) is considered acquisition indebtedness, even if the organization does not assume or agree to pay the debt. However, when mortgaged property is received by bequest or devise (or by gift under certain circumstances), the debt will not be treated as an acquisition indebtedness for 10 years from the date of acquisition. A lien for taxes or assessments under state law will be treated similar to a mortgage to the extent the amount becomes due and the organization has an opportunity to pay it.

Acquisition indebtedness does not include debt that was incurred by an exempt organization in the exercise of its exempt purpose. Generally, it also does not include debt incurred by certain qualified organizations (qualified employee benefits trust; an exempt school; exempt title-holding company; retirement income account of church plan) in acquiring or improving real property. Annuities may be excluded from the definition of acquisition indebtedness, as well as certain obligations insured by the Federal Housing Administration or incurred by a small business investment company (¶ 2392).

691. Exceptions to Debt-Financed Property. The following types of property are excluded from the definition of debt-financed property of a tax-exempt organization (¶ 687):

(1) property substantially all the use of which (85 percent or more) is related to the exercise or performance of the organization's tax-exempt function (special rules apply to real property used as a medical clinic);

(2) property to the extent that its income is subject to tax as income from carrying on an unrelated trade or business (however, if any gain on disposition of the property is not included in unrelated business taxable income (¶ 655), it may be income from debt-financed property (¶ 679));

(3) property to the extent that its income is from certain research activities and is excluded from gross income of an unrelated trade or business;

(4) property to the extent it is used in a business where substantially all of the work of carrying on the business is performed without compensation, the Code Sec. 501(c)(3) organization carrying on the business does so primarily for the convenience of members, students, patients, etc., or the business consists of selling merchandise substantially all of which has been received as contributions; and

---

References are to Standard Federal Tax Reports; Tax Research Consultant; and Practical Tax Explanations.

[102] ¶ 22,850, ¶ 22,853; EX-EMPT: 18,100; § 33,940.05

[103] ¶ 22,850, ¶ 22,854; EX-EMPT: 18,200; § 33,940.15

(5) certain brownfield site property to the extent the gain or loss from its sale or exchange would be excluded from gross income of an unrelated trade or business (Code Sec. 514(b); Reg. § 1.514(b)-1).[104]

For (1), (3), and (4) above, use of property by a related organization is taken into account in determining use of an tax-exempt organization. In addition, special rules apply to life income contracts and real property located in the neighborhood of other property owned and used for exempt purposes by the tax-exempt organization.

Other Tax-Exempt Organizations

692. Other Tax-Exempt Organizations under Code Sec. 501(c). In addition to charitable organizations (¶ 602), Code Sec. 501 exempts other types of nonprofit organizations from federal income tax unless they are deemed to be feeder organizations (¶ 694). Among the most common are civic leagues and social welfare organizations, business leagues, social and recreation clubs, and fraternal beneficiary societies. Contributions to these organizations are generally *not* deductible as charitable contributions. An organization described in this section generally files an application for exemption on Form 1024 and an annual information return on Form 990 (¶ 625).

Social Welfare Organizations and Civic Leagues. A civic league or organization is exempt from federal income taxes if it is not organized for profit and is operated *exclusively* for the promotion of social welfare (Code Sec. 501(c)(4)).[105] This includes a local association of employees if the membership is limited to the employees of a designated employer in a particular municipality and whose net earnings are devoted exclusively to charitable, educational, or recreational purposes. An exemption is not allowed if any part of the net earnings of the civic league or organization inures to the benefit of any private shareholder or individual (¶ 602). If the organization provides an excess benefit to certain persons, an excise tax may be imposed (¶ 617).

A civic league or organization will be considered to be operated exclusively for the promotion of social welfare if it *primarily* engages in promoting the common good and general welfare of the community (for example, volunteer fire departments or community association) (¶ 699). Promoting social welfare does not include participation or intervention in the political campaign of any candidate for office. In addition, the promotion of social welfare does not include the operation of a social club for the benefit of its members or carrying on a business similar to for-profit organizations (Reg. § 1.501(c)(4)-1).[106] This includes providing commercial-type insurance unless it is an insubstantial part of the organization's activities, in which case the activity will be treated as an unrelated trade or business (¶ 655) (Code Sec. 501(m) and (n)).[107]

Labor, Agricultural, and Horticultural Organizations. A qualifying labor, agricultural, or horticultural organization is tax-exempt if: (1) no net earnings of the organization inure to the benefit of any member; and (2) it has as its objective the betterment of the conditions of those engaged in such pursuits, the improvement of the grade of their products, and the development of a higher degree of efficiency in their respective occupations (Code Sec. 501(c)(5); Reg. § 1.501(c)(5)-1).[108] This does not include administration of any type of retirement plan. Generally, a qualifying labor organization is an association of workers such as a labor union. An agricultural and horticultural organization is involved with raising livestock, forestry, harvesting crops or aquatic resources, the cultivation of useful or ornamental plants, and similar pursuits (Code Sec. 501(g); IRS Pub. 557).

Business Leagues. A business league, chamber of commerce, real estate board, board of trade, or professional football league is tax-exempt if it is not organized for profit and no part of its net earnings inures to the benefit of any private shareholder or individual (Code Sec. 501(c)(6); Reg. § 1.501(c)(6)-1).[109] A business league is an associa-

---

References are to Standard Federal Tax Reports; Tax Research Consultant; and Practical Tax Explanations.

[104] ¶ 22,850, ¶ 22,853; EXEMPT: 18,100; § 33,940.10

[105] ¶ 22,602; EXEMPT: 9,300; § 33,405.05

[106] ¶ 22,610; EXEMPT: 9,300; § 33,405.05

[107] ¶ 22,602; EXEMPT: 15,160.10, EXEMPT: 15,160.15; § 33,405.05

[108] ¶ 22,602, ¶ 22,612; EXEMPT: 9,050; § 33,410.05

[109] ¶ 22,602, ¶ 22,614; EXEMPT: 9,100; § 33,415.05

tion of persons having some common business interest, a purpose to promote such common interest and not engaging in a regular business of a kind ordinarily carried on for profit. For example, an association engaged in furnishing information to prospective investors is not a business league since its activities do not further any common business interest.

Social Clubs. A social club or similar organization is exempt from federal income taxes if it is organized and operated exclusively for pleasure, recreation, and other nonprofitable purposes and no part of its net earnings inures to the benefit of any person having an interest in the activities of the organization (Code Sec. 501(c)(7); Reg. § 1.501(c)(7)-1; IRS Pub. 557).[110] Membership in the club must be limited, but personal contact, commingling and fellowship must exist between the members. In addition, the club's charter, bylaws, or other governing instrument, or any written policy statement must not provide for discrimination against any person on the basis of race, color, or religion (Code Sec. 501(i)). A club that in good faith limits its membership to the members of a particular religion to further the teachings or principles of that religion will not be considered as discriminating on the basis of religion. Also, the restriction on religious discrimination does not apply to a club that is an auxiliary of a fraternal beneficiary society if that society limits its membership to the members of a particular religion.

A social club is generally only exempt if it is supported solely by membership fees, dues, and assessments. Thus, the club cannot be engaged in any business activities, such as making its facilities available to the public or by selling real estate, timber, or other products. However, a club may receive up to 35 percent of its gross income, including investment income, from sources outside of its membership. Up to 15 percent of the gross receipts may be derived from the use of the club's facilities or services by the public or from other activities not furthering social or recreational purposes for members. If an organization has outside income that is more than these limits, all the facts and circumstances will be taken into account in determining whether the organization qualifies for exempt status (IRS Pub. 557).

Fraternal Beneficiary Societies. A fraternal beneficiary society, order, or association is exempt from federal income taxes if: (1) it operates under the lodge system for the exclusive benefit of the members of a fraternity itself operating under the lodge system; and (2) it provides for the payment of life, sickness, accident, or other benefits to the members of such society, order, or association or their dependents (Code Sec. 501(c)(8)).[111] Contributions by an individual to such societies are deductible as charitable contributions if the gift is to be used exclusively for religious, charitable, scientific, literary, or educational purposes, or for the prevention of cruelty to children or animals (¶ 1061). A domestic fraternal society, order, or association that operates under the lodge system but does not provide for the payment of life, sickness, accident, or other benefits may nonetheless qualify for exemption if its net earnings are devoted exclusively to religious, charitable, scientific, literary, educational, and fraternal purposes (Code Sec. 501(c)(10)).

Other Nonprofit Organizations. Other nonprofit organizations that may be exempt from federal income taxes under Code Sec. 501(c) include:

- corporations organized under an Act of Congress (Code Sec. 501(c)(1));

- title holding corporations for exempt organizations (Code Sec. 501(c)(2) and (25));

- voluntary employees' beneficiary associations (VEBAs) providing life, sickness, accident, and other benefits to members or their dependents or beneficiaries (Code Secs. 501(c)(9) and 505);

- local teachers' retirement fund associations (Code Sec. 501(c)(11));

- local benevolent life insurance associations (Code Sec. 501(c)(12));

References are to Standard Federal Tax Reports; Tax Research Consultant; and Practical Tax Explanations.

[110] ¶ 22,602, ¶ 22,616; EXEMPT: 9,400; § 33,415.05

[111] ¶ 22,602; EXEMPT: 9,150; § 33,425.05

- cemetery companies (Code Sec. 501(c)(13));
- state-chartered credit unions and mutual reserve funds (Code Sec. 501(c)(14));
- mutual insurance companies or associations (other than life insurance) (Code Sec. 501(c)(15));
- corporations used to finance crop operations (¶ 698) (Code Sec. 501(c)(16));
- supplemental unemployment benefit (SUB) trusts (Code Sec. 501(c)(17));
- employee funded pension trusts created before June 25, 1959 (Code Sec. 501(c)(18));
- posts or organizations for veterans, members of the armed services, and their families (Code Sec. 501(c)(19));
- black lung benefit trusts (Code Sec. 501(c)(21));
- domestic trusts set up to pay for withdrawal liability from multi-employer pension plans under ERISA (Code Sec. 501(c)(22));
- veterans organizations created before 1880 (Code Sec. 501(c)(23));
- trusts set up by a corporation in connection with the termination of its pension, profit sharing, or stock bonus plan (Code Sec. 501(c)(24));
- state-sponsored high-risk health coverage organizations (Code Sec. 501(c)(26));
- state-sponsored workers' compensation reinsurance organizations (Code Sec. 501(c)(27));
- national railroad retirement investment trust (Code Sec. 501(c)(28));
- a qualified nonprofit health insurance issuer under the Consumer Operated and Oriented Plan (CO-OP) program established by the Secretary of Health and Human Services (Code Sec. 501(c)(29)); and
- a reinsurance entity established or entered into a contract with by a state government to collect payments and make payments to the health insurance issuers that cover high-risk individuals in the individual market during the three-year period beginning January 1, 2014 (Act Sec. 1341(a) of the Patient Protection and Affordable Care Act of 2010 (P.L. 111-148)).

694. Feeder Organizations. An organization whose primary purpose is to operate a trade or business, with all the profits paid to one or more tax-exempt entities, is known as a feeder organization (Code Sec. 502; Reg. §1.502-1).[112] The fact that the income is turned over to a tax-exempt organization does not entitle the feeder organization to tax-exempt status. A feeder organization is subject to tax unless its activities are an integral part of the exempt activities of the parent organization. For this purpose, a trade or business of a feeder organization does *not* include: (1) rentals if the rents received would not be subject to the unrelated business income tax (¶ 655); (2) any trade or business if substantially all the work of carrying on the trade or business is performed by unpaid individuals or volunteers; or (3) any trade or business that sells merchandise, substantially all of which has been donated or contributed.

696. Political Organizations. A political organization is generally considered tax exempt to the extent that it is organized and operated to accept contributions and make expenditures for influencing the selection, nomination, election, or appointment of any individual to public office (Code Sec. 527).[113] Examples of political organizations include political parties; federal, state, or local candidate committees; other political action committees (PACs); and certain newsletters and segregated funds. The exempt function income of a political organization consists solely of: (1) contributions of money or property; (2) membership dues or fees; or (3) proceeds from a political fundraising

---

References are to Standard Federal Tax Reports; Tax Research Consultant; and Practical Tax Explanations.

[112] ¶ 22,670, ¶ 22,671; EX-EMPT: 15,350; § 33,301

[113] ¶ 22,900; EXEMPT: 9,850; § 33,428.05

event or the sale of political campaign materials. Any other income received (less deductions not related to exempt functions) is taxed at the highest income tax rate for corporations and capital gains. In calculating its taxable income, a political organization is permitted a $100 deduction, but it will not be allowed a net operating loss deduction (¶ 1145), the dividends received deduction (¶ 223), and other special deductions allowed to corporations (¶ 221).

Political organizations with taxable income must determine and report their tax on Form 1120-POL. Political organizations with $25,000 or more of gross receipts ($100,000 for certain state or local organizations) must also file an annual information return on Form 990 or 990-EZ (Code Sec. 6033(g)).[114] All political organizations must notify the IRS (electronically on Form 8871) of their existence within 24 hours of establishment (Code Sec. 527(i)). They must also provide periodic reports on Form 8872 of the contributions they receive and their expenditures (Code Sec. 527(j)). Organizations do not have to meet these two requirements if they have gross receipts of less than $25,000, are already required to file similar reports with the Federal Election Commission, or are certain state or local political organizations. Failure to provide notification will result in all income (including exempt function income) being taxed. In addition, failure to provide periodic reports will result in all undisclosed contributions and expenditures being taxed. A safe harbor is provided that waives the amounts due for failing to comply with the reporting requirements due to reasonable cause but not willful neglect (Rev. Proc. 2007-27).[115] The public disclosure of all returns and forms filed by a political organization is required (Code Sec. 6104).[116]

698. Farmers' Cooperatives. A cooperative (or federation of cooperatives) of farmers, fruit growers, and persons engaged in similar pursuits may qualify for tax-exempt status if the cooperative is organized and operated to market the members' products and return to them net proceeds, or purchase supplies and equipment for the use of members at cost plus expenses (Code Sec. 521; Reg. § 1.521-1).[117] The cooperative can deal with nonmembers, so long as the business does not account for more than 15 percent of all of its business. Application for exemption is filed on Form 1028. A farmers' association that has capital stock will not be denied exemption if: (1) the dividend rate is fixed at the legal rate of interest for the state of incorporation or eight percent (whichever is greater), and (2) substantially all of the stock is owned by producers who market their products or purchase their supplies through the association. A farmers' cooperative will also not be denied exemption if it computes its net earnings by offsetting certain earnings and losses in determining any amount available for distribution to patrons (Code Sec. 1388(j)(1)).[118]

Exempt farmers' cooperatives, and nonexempt corporations operating on a cooperative basis, are subject to regular corporate income and capital gain taxes and must file Form 1120-C to report taxable income (Code Secs. 1381 and 1382; Reg. § 1.1382-3).[119] However, in computing taxable income, all cooperatives are allowed certain deductions from gross income in addition to other deductions allowed to corporations (¶ 221). For example, an exempt farmers' cooperative is permitted a deduction for any dividends paid on capital stock, for amounts paid on a patronage basis arising from certain nonpatronage earnings, and for amounts paid in redemption of certain nonqualified written notices of allocation. In addition, all cooperatives are allowed a deduction for any "patronage dividend" paid or allocated to its members during the tax year. A patronage dividend is an amount paid to a member:

- on the basis of quantity or value of business done with the cooperative;

- under an obligation of the cooperative to pay such amount, where the obligation existed before the cooperative received the amount paid; and

---

References are to Standard Federal Tax Reports; Tax Research Consultant; and Practical Tax Explanations.

[114] ¶ 35,420; EXEMPT: 9,864; § 33,428.30

[115] ¶ 22,911.70; EXEMPT: 9,864; § 33,428.30

[116] ¶ 36,900; EXEMPT: 9,864; § 33,428.30

[117] ¶ 22,880, ¶ 22,881; FARM: 12,200

[118] ¶ 32,380; FARM: 12,250

[119] ¶ 32,300, ¶ 32,320, ¶ 32,323; FARM: 12,100, FARM: 12,150, FARM: 12,200; § 36,040

- which is determined by reference to the net earnings of the cooperative from business done with or for its members. However, net earnings will not be reduced by amounts paid as dividends on capital stock to the extent that the dividends are in addition to amounts otherwise payable to patrons (Code Sec. 1388(a)).[120]

699. Additional Exempt Organizations. There are a number of organizations other than charitable (¶ 602) and social (¶ 692) that may be exempt from federal income taxes, including homeowners' associations, credit counseling organizations, and cooperative service organizations.

Homeowners' Association. A homeowners' association formed to own and maintain common areas and enforce covenants to preserve the appearance of a development may qualify as a tax-exempt social welfare organization under Code Sec. 501(c)(4) (¶ 692). A homeowners' association that is not exempt as a social welfare organization and that is either a condominium management, real estate management, or timeshare association, may nonetheless elect to exclude certain exempt function income from its gross income, including membership dues, fees, and assessments from member-owners. Electing associations are taxed at a flat rate of 30 percent (32 percent for timeshare associations) on both ordinary income and capital gains which are nonexempt. Form 1120-H is used by the association to make the election for each tax year and to report annual taxable income (Code Sec. 528).[121]

Credit Counseling Organizations. An organization that provides credit counseling services as a substantial purpose may not qualify as a tax-exempt organization unless it qualifies as a Code Sec. 501(c)(3) charitable or educational organization (¶ 602), or as a Code Sec. 501(c)(4) social welfare organization (¶ 692) (Code Sec. 501(q)).[122] In addition, the organization: (1) must provide services tailored to customers' specific needs; (2) must not refuse to provide services to customers due to inability to pay or ineligibility for debt management plan enrollment; (3) make no loans to customers; (4) have a reasonable fee policy and must not pay or receive referral fees; (5) have limited ownership of related service providers; and (6) have independent board members with public interests.

Cooperative Service Organizations. A cooperative hospital service organization is exempt from federal income taxation if it performs specifically listed services for two or more patron hospitals that are tax exempt under Code Sec. 501(c)(3) or if it is owned and operated by the federal government or by a state or local government (Code Sec. 501(e)).[123] Services that may be performed include data processing, purchasing (including purchasing insurance on a group basis, such as malpractice and general liability insurance), laboratory, billing and collection (including the purchase of patron accounts receivable on a recourse basis), food, personnel, and clinical services. It does not include laundry services.[124] A cooperative arrangement formed and controlled by a group of exempt educational organizations for the collective investment of their funds may also qualify for tax-exempt status (Code Sec. 501(f)).[125] These organizations qualify for exemption only if all of the relevant requirements of Code Sec. 501(c)(3) are also satisfied.

References are to Standard Federal Tax Reports; Tax Research Consultant; and Practical Tax Explanations.

[120] ¶ 32,380; FARM: 12,104; § 36,040

[121] ¶ 22,920; EXEMPT: 9,500; § 33,429.05

[122] ¶ 22,602; EXEMPT: 10,050; § 33,105

[123] ¶ 22,602; EXEMPT: 3,154

[124] ¶ 22,662.30; EXEMPT: 3,154

[125] ¶ 22,602; EXEMPT: 3,300

Chapter 7

INCOME

What Is "Income"

701. Gross Income Defined. Gross income for federal income tax purposes means all income from whatever source, except for those items specifically excluded by the Code (Code Sec. 61; Reg. § 1.61-1).[1]

Code Sec. 61 lists some of the more common types of gross income. This nonexclusive list includes:

(1) compensation for services, including fees, commissions, fringe benefits, and similar items (¶ 713);

(2) gross income from business (¶ 759, ¶ 767);

(3) gains from dealings in property (¶ 1701);

(4) interest (¶ 724);

(5) rents (¶ 762);

(6) royalties (¶ 763);

(7) dividends (¶ 733);

(8) alimony and separate maintenance payments (¶ 771);

(9) annuities (¶ 817);

(10) income from life insurance and endowment contracts (Reg. § 1.61-10);[2]

(11) pensions (¶ 718);

(12) income from the discharge of indebtedness (¶ 885);

(13) a partner's share of partnership income (¶ 404);

(14) income in respect of a decedent (¶ 182); and

(15) income from an interest in an estate or trust (¶ 554, ¶ 556).

References are to Standard Federal Tax Reports; Tax Research Consultant; and Practical Tax Explanations.

[1] ¶ 5502, ¶ 5503; INDIV: 6,050; § 3,001

[2] ¶ 5708; INDIV: 30,350; § 46,615.20

Although nearly every type of accession to wealth appears to fall within this comprehensive definition, income items should be checked against the specific exclusions in Code Secs. 101—140 (¶ 801). For special rules relating to foreign income, see ¶ 2401. For a detailed list of income items and exclusions, see the Checklist for Items of Income at ¶ 55. For a discussion of the income tax treatment of gifts and inheritances of property, see ¶ 847 and ¶ 849.

702. Determining Income. Court decisions have developed a concept of the term "income" that is quite different from the layman's concept. The U.S. Supreme Court has defined income as an undeniable accession to wealth, clearly realized, and over which the taxpayer has complete dominion (*Glenshaw Glass Co.*, SCt, 55-1 USTC ¶ 9308).[3] Further, the Supreme Court pointed out that it has repeatedly given a liberal construction to this broad definition of what constitutes gross income in recognition of Congress's intent to tax all gain unless specifically exempted. In addition to those items specifically excludable from gross income by law (¶ 801), certain other items are not considered income.

Return of Capital. A return of capital, such as repayment of a loan, is not income unless the loan has been previously deducted as a bad debt, resulting in a tax benefit.[4] Similarly, car pool reimbursements are not income even if only one person provides the car and does the driving.[5]

Damages. Damages, other than punitive damages, that compensate an injured person for personal physical injuries or physical sickness are excludable from gross income (¶ 852). Damages received for personal nonphysical injuries, such as employment discrimination or injury to reputation, are generally taxable.[6]

Interest on a judgment, including mandatory prejudgment interest, is generally includible in income.[7]

See ¶ 759 for treatment of damages awarded for business claims.

Attorney Fees and Court Costs. Court costs and attorney fees paid in connection with an action based on unlawful discrimination under federal law, as well as certain other claims (i.e., whistleblower actions), are deductible from gross income in the determination of adjusted gross income (¶ 1010A).

Governmental Assistance. Many types of government assistance payments are not included in income if they are in the nature of general welfare. For example, rental assistance payments made by the Department of Housing and Urban Development under the National Housing Act and relocation payments made under the Housing and Community Development Act of 1974 are nontaxable.[8] However, payments made by individuals or other nongovernmental entities are not considered payments for the general welfare, and thus are taxable.[9]

Gift v. Income. The characterization of a payment or transfer as either a gift or as taxable income must be made on a case-by-case basis.[10] The U.S. Supreme Court, for example, has held that the value of a "gift" transferred to a business friend for furnishing the names of potential customers is taxable compensation (¶ 849).[11]

Strike and Lockout Benefits. Strike benefits received from a labor union may be treated as nontaxable gifts when the benefits paid in the form of food, clothing, and rent are: (1) given to both member and nonmember strikers, (2) dependent upon individual need, (3) dependent on the unavailability of unemployment compensation or local public

---

References are to Standard Federal Tax Reports; Tax Research Consultant; and Practical Tax Explanations.

[3] ¶ 5900.51; INDIV: 6,052; § 3,001

[4] ¶ 5504.103, ¶ 5504.6305; IN-DIV: 6,058; § 17,101

[5] ¶ 5504.144; INDIV: 33,554; § 4,015

[6] ¶ 5900.14, ¶ 5900.49, ¶ 5900.57; INDIV: 6,354; § 3,810.05

[7] ¶ 6662.513; INDIV: 12,112; § 3,805.35

[8] ¶ 5504.184; INDIV: 33,354; § 4,050

[9] ¶ 5504.193; INDIV: 6,368

[10] ¶ 6553.115; INDIV: 33,100; § 3,615

[11] ¶ 5507.294; INDIV: 33,102; § 3,605.05

¶702

assistance, and (4) given without condition. The fact that benefits are paid only to union members is not, of itself, determinative as to taxability.[12]

Unrealized Appreciation. Unrealized appreciation in the value of property is not income.[13]

Ownership of Income

704. Tax Liability. In the vast majority of cases, the identity of the taxpayer is clear. The taxpayer is simply the person who is legally entitled to receive income. Thus, an individual who receives wages for services is obviously the person who must pay income tax on the wages. However, under certain circumstances, a person may be taxed on income even though, at the time of payment, another receives it because of an anticipatory assignment of income (¶ 705). Special rules also affect the treatment of unearned income of a minor (¶ 706), income from property held in joint tenancy (¶ 709), and income of taxpayers living in community property states (¶ 710).

705. Assignment of Income. Generally, an individual can escape tax on income from property only if the individual makes a valid gift or assignment of the income-producing property itself, as distinguished from an assignment of the income. The U.S. Supreme Court has held that an individual who gave his wife the legally enforceable right to receive the future income generated by his law practice was still taxable on that income (*G.C. Earl*, SCt, 2 USTC ¶ 496).[14] In another case, the Court ruled that an individual who gave his son interest coupons, which were detached from bonds that he owned, was liable for the tax on the interest accrued before the gift and later paid to his son (*P.R.G. Horst*, SCt, 40-2 USTC ¶ 9787).[15] See ¶ 706 for the taxation of the unearned income of minor and certain dependent children.

706. Unearned Income of Minor Child. The amount of net unearned income of a child meeting certain statutory requirements that exceeds an annual inflation-adjusted amount ($2,000 for 2014; $2,100 for 2015) generally is taxed at the parents' highest marginal federal income tax rate. This is referred to as the "kiddie tax." It is designed to lessen the effectiveness of intra-family transfers of income-producing property that would shift income from the parents' higher marginal tax rate to the child's generally lower tax rate, to reduce a family's overall income tax liability. The kiddie tax applies to a child's unearned income regardless of source, and requires a calculation of the parents' allocable tax, which is the increase in the parents' tax liability that results from adding the net unearned income of all of the parents' children meeting the kiddie tax requirements to the parents' taxable income (Code Sec. 1(g)).[16]

See ¶ 103 for more details on the kiddie tax, as well as the parents' election to include a child's unearned income on their return. See ¶ 143 for discussion of dependents with earned income.

709. Joint Tenancy and Tenancy in Common. When property is held in joint tenancy with a right of survivorship, income from the property, including gain or loss upon its sale, is divided between the owners to the extent that each is entitled, under state law, to share in the income. There must be evidence that the joint ownership was bona fide and not used merely as a tax-avoidance scheme. These rules also apply to tenants in common.[17]

710. Community Property Income. In community property states (Arizona, California, Idaho, Louisiana, Nevada, New Mexico, Texas, Washington, and Wisconsin), property acquired by a husband and wife during their marriage while they reside in the community property state is generally regarded as owned by them together, each owning an undivided interest in the whole property. Similarly, income from the property is divided equally between them. Although each state has exceptions in classifying

References are to Standard Federal Tax Reports; Tax Research Consultant; and Practical Tax Explanations.

[12] ¶ 6553.46; COMPEN: 6,068; § 22,110.40

[13] ¶ 5504.119; INDIV: 6,052; § 3,001

[14] ¶ 6553.74; INDIV: 27,052; § 4,110

[15] ¶ 2150.64; INDIV: 27,052; § 4,135.05

[16] ¶ 3260; INDIV: 18,154; § 1,510.05

[17] ¶ 2250.35; INDIV: 18,100

7 | INCOME

income as separate income or community income, the general rule is that salaries, wages, and other compensation for the services of either or both the husband and wife, as well as income from community real and personal property, are community income; but it does not follow in every state that income from separate property is separate income. The states also differ in their treatment of property acquired by inheritance or intestate succession. However, the IRS can disallow the benefits of any community property law to a spouse for any income that the spouse treats as his or hers alone if that spouse fails to notify the other spouse of the nature and amount of the income before the due date, including extensions, for filing the return for the tax year in which the income was derived (Code Sec. 66(b); Reg. § 1.66-3).[18]

Registered Domestic Partners and Same Sex Married Couples. The IRS extended recognition of community property laws to registered domestic partners domiciled in Nevada, Washington, or California, as well as same sex married couples in California, beginning in 2010 (CCA 201021050; IRS Pub. 555).[19] Thus, each partner or spouse must report one-half of the combined community income on their federal income tax return.

In response to the U.S. Supreme Court decision in *E.S. Windsor* (SCt, 2013-2 USTC ¶ 50,400), the IRS will recognize the marriage of same-sex individuals for federal tax purposes if the marriage was validly entered into in a state or foreign country that recognizes same-sex marriages (Rev. Rul. 2013-17).[20] Further, under the "place of celebration rule," the IRS will recognize a marriage for federal tax purposes even if the couple resides in a jurisdiction that does not recognize same-sex marriages. However, a domestic partnership, civil union, or other similar formal relationship will not be treated as a marriage for federal tax purposes if the relationship is not called a "marriage" under state or foreign law. See ¶ 152.

711. Joint v. Separate Return in Community Property States. If separate returns are filed by a married couple residing in a community property state (¶ 710), each spouse must report one-half of the community income (Reg. § 1.66-1).[21] In Idaho, Louisiana, Texas, and Wisconsin, income from the separate property of a spouse is community income, with one-half being allocable to each spouse. In the other community property states, income from separate property is separate income.[22] Each spouse filing a separate return must use Form 8958 to allocate income, deductions, credits, and other return amounts between the spouses.

It is usually more beneficial to file a joint return. There are some situations, however, when filing separate returns may be beneficial for married spouses (¶ 156). See ¶ 152 for more details on filing joint returns.

Nonresident Alien Spouse. A U.S. citizen or resident who is married to a nonresident alien may elect to file a joint return if both agree to be taxed on their worldwide income (¶ 2410). If the couple does not make this election and has community income, any community income that is earned income, trade or business income, partnership income, or income from separate property is basically treated as the separate income of the spouse to whom the particular income item is associated (¶ 2438) (Code Sec. 879).[23]

Separated Spouses. The usual community property rules do not apply to spouses living apart from each other if: (1) they are separated for the entire calendar year; (2) they file separate returns; (3) either or both spouses have community earned income; and (4) they do not transfer between each other more than a *de minimis* amount of the earned income before the end of the calendar year (Code Sec. 66(a); Reg. § 1.66-2).[24] Instead, their community income is treated as if one of the spouses is a nonresident alien and they did not elect to file a joint return (see *Nonresident Alien Spouse,* previously).

References are to Standard Federal Tax Reports; Tax Research Consultant; and Practical Tax Explanations.

[18] ¶ 6050, ¶ 6050F; INDIV: 24,050, INDIV: 24,152; § 39,035.45

[19] ¶ 6051.60; FILEIND: 3,202; § 45,922

[20] ¶ 6051.62; FILEIND: 3,202; § 45,901

[21] ¶ 6050B; FILEIND: 3,212.05; § 45,910.20

[22] ¶ 2350.2475; INDIV: 24,050; § 45,915.20

[23] ¶ 27,460; INDIV: 24,156; § 45,925

[24] ¶ 6050, ¶ 6050D; INDIV: 24,060.05; § 45,920.05

¶711

Innocent Spouse Relief. A requesting spouse may receive relief from federal income tax liability for an item of community income that would be properly treated as the income of the nonrequesting spouse under the Code Sec. 879(a) rules (¶ 2438) if: (1) the requesting spouse does not file a joint return for the tax year in question, and does not include the community income item in his or her gross income; (2) the requesting spouse establishes that he or she did not know and had no reason to know of the item; and (3) under the facts and circumstances, it would be inequitable to include the item in the requesting spouse's gross income. If these requirements are not met, the IRS may still provide relief from a tax liability or deficiency arising from the community income item if failure to do so would be inequitable (Code Sec. 66(c), Reg. § 1.66-4).[25] The IRS has issued guidance for taxpayers seeking equitable relief (Rev. Proc. 2013-34).[26]

Salaries, Wages, and Benefits

713. Compensation for Personal Services. All compensation for personal services, no matter what the form of payment, must be included in gross income (Reg. § 1.61-2).[27] Wages, salaries, commissions, bonuses, fringe benefits that do not qualify for statutory exclusions, tips, payments based on a percentage of profits, rewards, directors' fees, jury fees, election officials' fees, retirement pay and pensions, and other forms of compensation are income in the year received, and not in the year earned, unless the taxpayer reports income on an accrual basis (¶ 1515).

> **Example:** A cash-method salesperson who receives commissions in January 2015 for sales made in 2014 must include those amounts on the 2015 return.

Under the claim-of-right doctrine (¶ 1543), a taxpayer receiving income under a claim of right and without restrictions on its use or disposition is taxed on that income in the year received even though the right to retain the income is not yet fixed or the taxpayer may later be required to return it.[28]

Compensation is income even though the amount is not fixed in advance, as in the case of marriage fees, baptismal offerings, and similar sums received by a member of the clergy.[29] A year-end bonus is usually taxable, particularly if based on salary or length of service. Severance pay and vacation pay are also taxable as compensation. The value of a turkey, ham, or other nominally valued item distributed to an employee on holidays is *not* reportable income even though the employer is entitled to deduct the cost as a business expense. However, a distribution of cash, a gift certificate or gift card, or a similar item of value readily convertible to cash, must be included in the employee's income.[30]

The amount of compensation reported on the return is the gross amount before any reductions for withheld income tax or social security taxes, union dues, insurance, or other deductions by the employer.

Child's Earned Income. Compensation for the services of a child are included in the child's gross income, even if the compensation is or must be received by the parent rather than the child (¶ 103).

Restricted Property Transfers. If stock or other property is given as compensation for services instead of cash, the fair market value (FMV) of the property is included in income unless the property is subject to a substantial risk of forfeiture. (Code Sec. 83; Reg. § 1.83-1).[31] The FMV of the property included in income becomes its basis to the employee. If the property is sold to the employee for less than its market value, the difference between the amount paid and the value of the property is also income.

References are to Standard Federal Tax Reports; Tax Research Consultant; and Practical Tax Explanations.

[25] ¶ 6050, ¶ 6050H; INDIV: 24,154; § 45,920.10

[26] ¶ 6051.20; INDIV: 18,060; § 45,920.10

[27] ¶ 5506; COMPEN: 6,050; § 3,005.05

[28] ¶ 21,005.122; ACCTNG: 27,050; § 4,225.05

[29] ¶ 5507.141; COMPEN: 6,050; § 3,005.05

[30] ¶ 5507.2942; COMPEN: 6,350; § 21,120

[31] ¶ 6380, ¶ 6381; COMPEN: 18,050; § 21,401

If the stock or other property is subject to a substantial risk of forfeiture, no amount is included in income until the year that the property becomes substantially vested as the result of the removal of the risk of forfeiture (Code Sec. 83(a); Reg. § 1.83-1(a)(1)).[32] However, any income (e.g., a dividend) from property that is subject to a substantial risk of forfeiture, or from the right to use such property, is included in income as compensation when received (Rev. Procs. 80-11 and 83-38).[33] Property is considered substantially vested when it is either (1) transferable to another person who is not required to give up the property or its value if the substantial risk of forfeiture occurs or (2) no longer subject to a substantial risk of forfeiture (Code Sec. 83(c)(1); Reg. § 1.83-3).[34]

A substantial risk of forfeiture exists if the right to the property is conditioned on (1) the future performance, or refraining from performance, of substantial services by any person, or (2) the occurrence of a condition related to a purpose of the transfer if the possibility of forfeiture is substantial (Code Sec. 83(c)(1); Reg. § 1.83-3(c)). For property transferred on or after January 1, 2013: (1) a substantial risk of forfeiture may be established *only* by the two conditions described above; (2) in determining whether a substantial risk of forfeiture exists due to a condition related to the purpose of the transfer, the likelihood that the forfeiture event will occur and that the forfeiture will be enforced must both be considered; and (3) except as provided in Reg. § 1.83-3(j) or (k), transfer restrictions do not create a substantial risk of forfeiture if the restriction is violated, even if the violation results in forfeiture of property or in liability for damages, penalties or fees.

A taxpayer who receives property subject to a substantial risk of forfeiture may elect to include in gross income, in the year the property is received, the FMV of the property less any amount paid for the property (Code Sec. 83(b); Reg. § 1.83-2).[35] The election can only be revoked with the consent of the IRS. Once the value of the property is included in income, any subsequent appreciation is not taxed as compensation to the person who performed the services. If the property is forfeited after the election is made and before it is substantially vested, the forfeiture is treated as a sale or exchange on which a loss is realized, equal to any excess of the amount paid for the property minus any amount realized upon the forfeiture. The taxpayer makes the election by attaching to his or her return a statement containing certain required information. The IRS has provided sample language that may be used for making the election, as well as examples of the tax consequences of the election (Rev. Proc. 2012-29).[36]

Stock Options. Nonstatutory stock options (NSOs) are discussed at ¶ 1923. Incentive stock options (ISOs) are discussed at ¶ 1925 and ¶ 1927. Employee stock purchase plans (ESPPs) are discussed at ¶ 1929 and ¶ 1931.

Employee Benefits. Compensation for personal services includes any benefits an employer provides to employee which are not otherwise excludable from income (Reg. § 1.61-21).[37] Excludable employee benefits include:

- amounts received under employer-financed accident and health plans (¶ 2015);

- employer contributions to provide the accident and health benefits (¶ 2013);

- employer contributions to a health savings account (HSA) (¶ 2035), Archer medical savings account (MSA) (¶ 2037), health reimbursement arrangement (HRA) (¶ 2039), or flexible spending arrangement (FSA) (¶ 2041);

- premiums for group-term life insurance to the extent coverage does not exceed $50,000 (¶ 2055);

- qualified adoption expenses reimbursed under an employer adoption assistance program (¶ 2063);

- child and dependent care assistance benefits (¶ 2065);

References are to Standard Federal Tax Reports; Tax Research Consultant; and Practical Tax Explanations.

[32] ¶ 6380, ¶ 6381; COMPEN: 6,104; § 21,430.05

[33] ¶ 6390.63; COMPEN: 18,550; § 21,435

[34] ¶ 6380, ¶ 6383; COMPEN: 18,202, COMPEN: 18,210; § 21,415.05

[35] ¶ 6380, ¶ 6382; COMPEN: 18,300; § 21,475.05

[36] ¶ 6390.77; COMPEN: 18,304; § 21,475.20

[37] ¶ 5906; COMPEN: 33,000; § 3,005.05

¶713

- educational assistance benefits (¶ 2067);
- employee achievement awards to the extent deductible by the employer (¶ 2069);
- qualified moving expense reimbursements (¶ 2092); and
- certain other fringe benefits (¶ 2085).

Some excludable employee benefits may be provided to an employee through the employer's cafeteria plan (¶ 2045).

Employer-Provided Vehicle. An employee who uses an employer-provided vehicle for more than *de minimis* personal use receives a taxable fringe benefit from his or her employer. The amount includible in an employee's wages is determined by the fair market value of its availability (¶ 2059).

Vacation and Club Expenses. The portion of an employee's vacation, athletic club, or health resort expenses that is paid by the employer is taxable to the employee.[38]

Occupational Disability or Insurance Benefit. Compensation received under a workers' compensation act for personal injuries or sickness and amounts received by a taxpayer under a policy of accident and health insurance are excludable from gross income (¶ 851).

714. Compensation of Federal or State Employee. The salaries of all employees or officials of the United States government are taxed the same as those of other individuals (Code Sec. 3401(c)). This is also true for state and local government employees.[39]

715. Treatment of Excessive Salaries. Although an employer is denied a deduction for compensation paid to the extent that the payment is unreasonable (¶ 906), the full amount of the payment is includible in the recipient's income. In the case of an employee-shareholder, excessive compensation may be treated as dividend income. Excessive salaries are taxed only to the extent of the gain if the excess amounts are determined to be payments to the recipient for property rather than compensation (Reg. § 1.162-8).[40]

716. Social Security and Equivalent Railroad Retirement Benefits. A portion of a taxpayer's social security benefits or an equivalent portion of tier 1 railroad retirement benefits may be taxable (Code Sec. 86).[41] The amount includible in gross income is the lesser of one-half of the annual benefits received or one-half of the excess of the taxpayer's provisional income over a specified base amount. If the taxpayer's provisional income exceeds an adjusted base amount, however, up to 85 percent of the benefits may be included (see *85-Percent Inclusion*, following). The Form 1040 Instructions contain a worksheet for computing the taxable amount.

Provisional income is the taxpayer's modified adjusted gross income (MAGI) plus one-half of the social security or tier 1 railroad retirement benefits received. MAGI is the taxpayer's adjusted gross income (¶ 1005) plus any tax-exempt interest received. Adjusted gross income is determined without including any social security benefits or equivalent railroad retirement benefits, and without subtracting the following items from gross income: interest income from savings bonds used to finance higher education (¶ 863), amounts paid under an employer's adoption assistance program (¶ 2063), deductible domestic production activities income (¶ 980A), deductible education loan interest (¶ 1082), deductible tuition and related expenses (in tax years before 2014) (¶ 1082), foreign earned income and foreign housing expenses attributable to living and working abroad (¶ 2402), and certain income of bona fide residents of U.S. possessions (¶ 2414) or Puerto Rico (¶ 2415). The base amount is: (1) $32,000 for joint filers; (2) $0 if married filing separately and the taxpayer lived with his or her spouse at any time during the tax year; and (3) $25,000 for married individuals filing separately who live apart from their spouse for the entire year and individuals filing as single or head-of-household.

References are to Standard Federal Tax Reports; Tax Research Consultant; and Practical Tax Explanations.

[38] ¶ 5507.47; COMPEN: 33,104; § 3,005.05

[39] ¶ 33,502; COMPEN: 6,650; § 22,005.15

[40] ¶ 8639; COMPEN: 6,074; § 9,301

[41] ¶ 6420; INDIV: 6,200; § 3,301

7 INCOME

Example 1: John and Jane Mapes have an adjusted gross income of $24,000 for 2014. John, who is retired, receives social security benefits of $7,200 per year. The couple also receives $6,000 a year from a mutual fund that invests solely in tax-exempt municipal bonds. On their joint return for 2014, the Mapeses would make the following computation to determine how much, if any, of John's social security benefits must be included in their gross income:

(1) Adjusted gross income	$24,000
(2) Plus: All tax-exempt interest	6,000
(3) Modified adjusted gross income	30,000
(4) Plus: One-half of social security benefits	3,600
(5) Provisional income	33,600
(6) Less: Base amount	32,000
(7) Excess above base amount	1,600
(8) One-half of excess above base amount	800
(9) One-half of social security benefits	3,600
(10) Amount includible in gross income (lesser of (8) or (9)) . .	800

Social security benefits are the monthly benefits under Title II of the Social Security Act (Code Sec. 86(d)(1)).[42] Supplemental security income (SSI) payments are authorized by Title XVI of the Social Security Act, and thus are *not* are not included in gross income. Although tier 2 railroad retirement benefits are not taken into account under the above rules, these benefits are taxed in the same manner as benefits paid under qualified retirement plans (Code Sec. 72(r)).[43]

85-Percent Inclusion. Up to 85 percent of an individual's social security benefits or tier 1 railroad retirement benefits may be includible in gross income. This affects taxpayers whose provisional income exceeds the adjusted base amount, which is: (1) $44,000 for married taxpayers filing jointly; (2) $0 for married taxpayers filing separately and not living apart during the entire tax year; and (3) $34,000 for all other taxpayers (Code Sec. 86(c)(2)).

Those who exceed the appropriate adjusted base amount must include in gross income the lesser of: (1) 85 percent of social security benefits or (2) the sum of 85 percent of the excess of provisional income over the adjusted base amount, plus the smaller of: (a) the amount that would otherwise be includible if the second threshold did not apply (i.e., the amount calculated under the 50-percent rules discussed previously), or (b) one-half of the difference of the adjusted base amount over the base amount (i.e., $6,000 for joint filers; $0 for married filing separately and not living apart from their spouse; $4,500 for all other taxpayers).

Example 2: Assume the same facts as in Example 1 above, except that the Mapes' provisional income is increased from $33,600 to $53,600. The includible amount is determined as follows:

(1) Provisional income	$53,600
(2) Adjusted base amount	44,000
(3) Excess of (1) over (2)	9,600
(4) 85% of amount in (3)	8,160
(5) Amount otherwise includible: lesser of (a) ½ of benefits received ($3,600) or (b) ½ of the excess of provisional income minus base amount ($10,800)	3,600
(6) One-half of adjusted base amount minus base amount (for joint filers)	6,000
(7) Lesser of (5) or (6)	3,600
(8) Sum of amounts in (4) and (7)	11,760
(9) 85% of social security benefits	6,120
(10) Amount includible in gross income (lesser of (8) or (9)) . .	6,120

References are to Standard Federal Tax Reports; Tax Research Consultant; and Practical Tax Explanations.

[42] ¶ 6420; INDIV: 6,204; §3,305   [43] ¶ 6102; INDIV: 6,204; §24,101

¶716

Individual Retirement Account (IRA) Contributions. Employed individuals who are covered by a retirement plan and receiving social security benefits must make a special computation to determine the allowable IRA deduction amount (¶ 2157).

717. Tips. Tips received by cab drivers, waiters, barbers, hotel, railroad and cruise ship employees, etc., are taxable (Reg. § 1.61-2(a)(1)).[44] In the absence of proof of the actual amount of tips received, tip income may be reconstructed on the basis of average tips in a given locality for a given type of service.[45]

Tipped employees may use Form 4070A, which should be retained with the individual's tax records, to maintain a daily record of their tips. Cash, check, and credit card tips totalling $20 or more per month are reported to the employer on Form 4070 or a similar statement by the 10th day of the following month (IRS Pub. 531). An employer may also allow tips to be reported electronically (Reg. § 31.6053-1).[46]

Form 4137 is used to compute an employee's liability for social security and Medicare taxes on monthly tips of $20 or more that were not reported to the employer or on tips allocated by a large food and beverage establishment. If an employer was unable to withhold social security and Medicare taxes on reported tip income, the uncollected taxes are shown on Form W-2 and reported as an additional tax on the tipped employee's income tax return. Noncash tips and tips of less than $20 per month are not subject to social security and Medicare tax. These amounts, however, are subject to income tax and must be reported on the employee's return.

See ¶ 2605 regarding duty to report tips monthly to employer on Form 4070, ¶ 2606 regarding employer's withholding requirements, and ¶ 1365R regarding an employer credit for its portion of social security taxes on employee cash tips.

718. Pension. A pension paid to a retired employee is usually taxable compensation (¶ 2101) (Reg. § 1.61-11).[47]

719. Salary Payments to Employee's Survivor. The IRS and the Tax Court have generally taken the position that salary payments made to the surviving spouse of a deceased employee are taxable income, while several U.S. Courts of Appeal have viewed the payments as tax-free gifts.[48] Unpaid salary owed to a taxpayer at the time of his or her death is typically treated as income in respect of a decedent (¶ 182).

720. Compensation Other Than in Cash. When compensation for services is paid for in property, the fair market value (FMV) of the property at the time of receipt must be included in gross income (Reg. § 1.61-2(d)).[49] A note received in payment for services, and not merely as security for the payment, comes within this rule and its FMV must be included in income. A portion of each payment received under the note is excludable from gross income as a recovery of capital (Reg. § 1.61-2(d)(4)).[50]

722. Unemployment Compensation. Recipients of unemployment compensation benefits must include in income the entire annual amount of benefits received (Code Sec. 85; Reg. § 1.85-1).[51] If an employee contributes to a governmental unemployment compensation program but is not allowed to deduct his or her contributions, amounts the employee receives under the program are not unemployment compensation until he or she has recovered the total amount of nondeductible contributions. Payments to laid-off employees from company-financed supplemental unemployment benefit plans (also referred to as "guaranteed annual wage" plans) constitute taxable income to the employees in the year received.[52] Payors report unemployment compensation on Form 1099-G.

723. Deferred Compensation. Not all compensation is paid in the year when services are rendered. Some may be deferred to a later year. There are two types of deferred compensation arrangements—funded and unfunded.

References are to Standard Federal Tax Reports; Tax Research Consultant; and Practical Tax Explanations.

[44] ¶ 5506; COMPEN: 6,058; § 21,301

[45] ¶ 5507.4651, ¶ 35,111.58; ACCTNG: 3,168; § 21,325.05

[46] ¶ 36,461; PAYROLL: 3,406; § 21,305.10

[47] ¶ 5710; RETIRE: 42,300; § 3,040

[48] ¶ 5507.4741, ¶ 6507.83; COMPEN: 48,206; § 3,605.05

[49] ¶ 5506; SALES: 6,062, COMPEN: 6,104; § 3,005.10

[50] ¶ 5506, ¶ 5508.35; COMPEN: 6,106; § 3,005.10

[51] ¶ 6410, ¶ 6411; INDIV: 6,208; § 3,075

[52] ¶ 5507.60; INDIV: 6,208

Funded Arrangements. If deferred compensation is contributed to a trust or is used to purchase an annuity or other insurance contract, the arrangement is funded and a participant may be subject to tax on the trust's income (¶ 2199).

Unfunded Arrangements. If the deferral takes the form of an employer's unsecured promise (i.e., not represented by a note) to pay compensation for current services at some time in the future, and if the employee uses the cash method of accounting, the amount promised is not includible in the employee's gross income until it is received or made available (¶ 906) (Rev. Rul. 60-31, modified by Rev. Rul. 64-279 and Rev. Rul. 70-435).[53] This rule is not altered merely because the employee agrees with the employer in advance to receive compensation on a deferred basis, so long as the agreement is made before the taxpayer obtains an unqualified and unconditional right to the compensation (*J.F. Oates,* CA-7, 53-2 USTC ¶ 9596).[54]

Unfunded Plans of State and Local Governments and Other Tax-Exempt Organizations. The above-described treatment of unfunded deferred compensation plans is modified for participants in plans maintained by state and local governments and other tax-exempt organizations, except for churches and qualified church-controlled organizations (Code Sec. 457).[55] For distributions from an eligible nongovernment plan, the deferred compensation is includible in income only when received by, or unconditionally made available to, a participant. For distributions from an eligible government plan, the deferred compensation is included in gross income only when actually paid. If a plan is not an eligible plan, the present value of the deferred compensation is includible in gross income for the first tax year in which there is no substantial risk of forfeiture, and the tax treatment of any amount made available to a participant is determined under the annuity rules. See ¶ 2193 for further discussion of 457 plans.

Unfunded Plans of Taxable Employers. An unfunded plan of a taxable employer is not subject to limitations similar to those that apply to a tax-exempt employer. As a practical matter, however, such a plan is limited to providing benefits in excess of those permitted under qualified plans or benefits for highly compensated and managerial employees. This is because any other unfunded deferred compensation plan of a taxable employer would be subject to participation, vesting, funding, and fiduciary standards of Employee Retirement Income Security Act of 1974 (ERISA) (P.L. 93-406) (ERISA Secs. 4(b)(5), 201(2), 301(a)(3), and 401(a)(1)). See ¶ 2197 and ¶ 2199 for a discussion of nonqualified deferred compensation plans.

Interest

724. Interest Generally. All interest received or accrued is fully taxable (Reg. § 1.61-7),[56] except interest on tax-exempt state or municipal bonds, including qualified private activity bonds (¶ 729), and interest on U.S. savings bonds used to pay qualified educational expenses (¶ 863). A cash-basis taxpayer is taxed on interest when received. Interest on bank deposits, coupons payable on bonds, etc., is considered available and taxed to a cash-basis taxpayer under the doctrine of constructive receipt and is taxed when credited or due (¶ 1533).

Interest earned on corporate obligations is generally taxed when actually received by, or credited to, a cash-basis taxpayer (Reg. § 1.61-7(a)). The same rule applies to interest on certificates of deposit, time obligations, and similar deposit arrangements on which interest is credited periodically and can be withdrawn without penalty even though the principal cannot be withdrawn without penalty prior to maturity. However, interest on a six-month certificate that is not credited or made available to the holder without penalty before maturity is not includible in the holder's income until the certificate is redeemed or matures (Rev. Rul. 80-157, amplified by Rev. Rul. 82-42).[57]

References are to Standard Federal Tax Reports; Tax Research Consultant; and Practical Tax Explanations.

[53] ¶ 21,009.1967; COMPEN: 15,202; § 25,610.15

[54] ¶ 21,009.135; COMPEN: 15,202; § 25,610.15

[55] ¶ 21,531; COMPEN: 15,150; § 25,310.10 , § 25,315.05

[56] ¶ 5702; INDIV: 12,052; § 3,101

[57] ¶ 21,009.3247; INDIV: 12,102, INDIV: 12,110.10; § 3,101

¶724

Increments in value on growth savings certificates are taxable in the year that the increase occurs because the certificate holder has a present right to redeem the certificate (Rev. Rul. 66-44).[58] Any increment in the value of life insurance or annuity prepaid premiums or premium deposits is income when made available to the policyholder for withdrawal or when credited against premiums payable.[59] Interest on a judgment is taxable even if the underlying award is nontaxable.[60]

When a bond with defaulted interest coupons is bought "flat" (i.e., the price covers both principal and unpaid interest), any interest received that was in default on the date of purchase is not taxable but is a return of capital. If the bond is sold, this amount must be applied to reduce the basis, in turn increasing the gain or reducing the loss. If interest is received for a period which *follows* the date of purchase, it is taxable in full (Reg. § 1.61-7(c)).[61]

Under the accrual method, interest is taxable as it accrues even though it is payable later. An exception to this rule applies when it is discovered before the close of the tax year that the interest owed to the taxpayer will not be collected.[62]

State and Local Bonds; Tax Credit Bonds. The federal government provides financial assistance to state and local governmental agencies by excluding from the gross income of the recipient the interest on certain tax-exempt state and local bonds. Bond interest is not tax free, however, when it is derived from certain state or local bonds that are private activity bonds (¶ 729), bonds that have not been issued in registered form, arbitrage bonds, hedge bonds, or federally guaranteed bonds (Code Secs. 103, 148 and 149).[63]

The federal government also authorizes the issuers of such bonds to issue tax credit bonds. A tax credit bond essentially provides the issuer with a tax-free loan. The bond holders receive a tax credit on their federal income tax at the specified credit rate, instead of interest payments, and the issuer only has to repay the principal. The bond holders must include the credit amount in income, then claim the credit against tax on their return. In effect, the holders will usually receive the same net amount from the credit as they would receive in interest from a conventional state or local bond. See ¶ 1371 for discussion of tax credit bonds.

726. Mortgage Interest. The U.S. Supreme Court held that when a taxpayer forecloses on a mortgage and purchases the property at a foreclosure sale by bidding on the property for the full amount of the mortgage plus accrued unpaid interest, taxable income is realized in the amount of the accrued interest even if the fair market value (FMV) of the property bid on is less than the principal due on the mortgage (*Midland Mutual Life Ins. Co.*, SCt, 37-1 USTC ¶ 9114). Other courts have applied the same rule to *voluntary* conveyances by the mortgagor in consideration for the cancellation of the principal and interest of the mortgage. There is no interest income, however, in the case of such a conveyance if the property is worth less than the principal of the loan.[64] Nor is any taxable income realized if only the principal of the mortgage is bid. For repossessions of real property, see ¶ 1841.

If a creditor bids on a property for a debt, a loss may be deductible if the property is worth less than the debt.[65] Any such loss must take into account the basis and FMV of the property bid on, and therefore a loss may exist even though the creditor bid on the property for more than the debt (*Hadley Falls Trust Co.*, CA-1, 40-1 USTC ¶ 9352).[66] The FMV of the mortgaged property is presumed to be the amount bid in the absence of clear and convincing proof to the contrary (Reg. § 1.166-6). See ¶ 1135 for a discussion of the bad debt deduction, and ¶ 1139 for discussion of secured bad debt.

[58] ¶ 21,009.1142; INDIV: 12,102, INDIV: 12,110.10; § 38,315.15

[59] ¶ 5504.2665; INDIV: 12,118, INDIV: 30,352; § 3,101

[60] ¶ 30,575.166; INDIV: 12,112; § 3,805.35

[61] ¶ 5702, ¶ 5704.3062; INDIV: 12,252.25; § 45,415.15

[62] ¶ 5704.32; INDIV: 12,254; § 3,101

[63] ¶ 6600, ¶ 7870, ¶ 7900; SALES: 51,050; § 3,105

[64] ¶ 5704.338; REAL: 6,154

[65] ¶ 10,750.10; BUSEXP: 48,204

[66] ¶ 10,670.123; BUSEXP: 48,204, REAL: 6,152.10

Seller-Provided Financing. A taxpayer who receives or accrues qualified residence interest from seller-provided financing must include on his or her income tax return the name, address and taxpayer identification number of the person from whom the interest was received or accrued (¶ 1047). Failure to provide this required information will expose the taxpayer to information reporting penalties (¶ 2833).

727. Imputed Interest. Holders of bonds or other obligations issued at a discount may be required to include in gross income a portion of the discount as imputed interest in each year the obligation is held, even though no interest corresponding to this amount is paid or accrued during the period (¶ 1952). Holders of notes or other debt instruments that were issued in exchange for property or services may be required to include in gross income imputed interest if no interest is provided in the debt instrument or the rate of interest is less than the applicable federal rate (AFR) (¶ 1954). Other loans bearing interest at less than the AFR may also result in imputed interest income to the lender (¶ 795).

728. Bond Transaction Between Interest Dates. When a bond is sold between interest dates, part of the sales price represents the interest earned up to the date of sale. The seller reports that portion as interest income in the year of the sale (Reg. § 1.61-7(d)).[67] Because the buyer has paid for the accrued interest as part of the sales price, the interest is a return of capital if it is later paid, which reduces his or her basis in the bond, rather than taxable interest income, except to the extent it exceeds the amount paid the seller (Reg. § 1.61-7(c)). This interest adjustment has no effect on the cost of the bond and apparently has no connection with the adjustment for amortizable bond premium (¶ 1967).

729. Private Activity Bonds. Although interest on obligations of a state or local government is generally excludable from gross income (¶ 724), bond interest is generally not tax free when it is derived from a private activity bond that does not qualify for tax exemption (Code Sec. 103(b)).[68] A private activity bond is part of a state or local government bond issue in which: (1) more than 10 percent of the bond proceeds is to be used for a private business use; and (2) more than 10 percent of the payment of principal or interest is secured by an interest in property to be used for a private business use or payments for such property, or is to be derived from payments for property, or borrowed money, used for a private business use. Alternatively, part of an issue may instead qualify as a private activity bond if the amount of the bond proceeds to be used to make or finance loans to persons other than government units exceeds the lesser of (1) five percent of the proceeds, or (2) $5 million (Code Sec. 141).[69] Bonds issued by a governmental unit to fund the acquisition of existing electric and gas generating and transmission systems are generally treated as private activity bonds (Code Sec. 141(d)).

Private activity bonds that *do* qualify for tax exemption include exempt facility bonds, qualified veterans' mortgage bonds, qualified student loan bonds, qualified redevelopment bonds, qualified Code Sec. 501(c)(3) bonds, qualified mortgage bonds and qualified small-issue bonds (Code Secs. 141—145; IRS Pub. 550).[70] Qualified private activity bonds must meet the applicable volume cap requirements of Code Sec. 146 and the applicable requirements of Code Sec. 147 (Code Sec. 141(e)).

Exempt facility bonds may include certain enterprise zone facility bonds, New York Liberty bonds, Gulf Opportunity Zone (GO Zone) bonds, and recovery zone facility bonds, as well as Midwestern disaster area bonds and Hurricane Ike disaster area bonds (Code Secs. 1394, 1400L(d), 1400N(a)(1), and 1400U-3; Act Secs. 702 and 704, Emergency Economic Stabilization Act of 2008 (P.L. 110-343)).[71] Qualified mortgage bonds

---

References are to Standard Federal Tax Reports; Tax Research Consultant; and Practical Tax Explanations.

[67] ¶ 5702; INDIV: 12,252.20; § 3,101

[68] ¶ 6600; SALES: 51,100; § 3,105.10

[69] ¶ 7702; SALES: 51,100; § 3,105.10

[70] ¶ 7702, ¶ 7740, ¶ 7780, ¶ 7810, ¶ 7821; SALES: 51,150; § 3,105.10

[71] ¶ 32,391, ¶ 32,473, ¶ 32,483, ¶ 32,524; SALES: 51,200, SALES: 51,350; § 3,105.10

may include certain GO Zone bonds, Midwestern disaster area bonds, and Hurricane Ike disaster area bonds. Qualified small issue bonds include tribal manufacturing facility bonds (Code Sec. 7871(c)(3)).[72]

Tax Preference Items. Tax-exempt interest on private activity bonds is ordinarily considered a tax preference for purposes of the alternative minimum tax (AMT) (Code Sec. 57(a)(5)).[73] Thus, the amount of interest received is taken into account in computing alternative minimum taxable income (AMTI) for AMT purposes (¶ 1425). However, exempt interest is *not* a tax preference item on qualified 501(c)(3) bonds, New York Liberty bonds, GO Zone bonds, Midwestern disaster area bonds, or Hurricane Ike disaster area bonds, as well as the following bonds if issued after July 30, 2008: certain exempt facility bonds, qualified mortgage bonds, or qualified veterans' mortgage bonds. Additionally, exempt interest on private activity bonds issued in 2009 or 2010 is *not* treated as a tax preference item.

730. United States Savings Bonds. Interest on U.S. savings bonds is fully taxable (¶ 731). An accrual basis taxpayer reports interest on U.S. savings bonds each year as it accrues. A cash basis taxpayer generally reports U.S. savings bond interest when he or she receives it (¶ 1515). Series HH and H bonds, which the U.S. Treasury no longer issues, were issued at face value, and interest was paid every six months. Paper Series EE and Series E bonds are issued at a discount, and interest is payable on redemption. Electronic Series EE bonds and inflation-indexed Series I bonds are issued at face value, and accrued interest is payable at maturity (IRS Pub. 550).

For a cash basis taxpayer, none of the interest on Series EE, E, or I bonds is taxable until the earlier of (1) the year the bonds are cashed in or disposed of, or (2) the year in which they mature. The taxpayer *may,* however, elect to report the interest income on these bonds each year as it accrues (Code Sec. 454; Reg. § 1.454-1(a); IRS Pub. 550).[74]

Taxable income was not recognized if Series EE or E bonds on which interest reporting was postponed were traded for Series HH or H bonds unless cash was received in the trade. Trades for Series HH bonds are not allowed after August 31, 2004. Any cash received is taxed to the extent of interest earned on the Series EE or E bonds. When the Series HH or H bonds mature, or, if earlier, when they are disposed of, the difference between their redemption value and cost is reported as interest income. Cost is the amount paid for the Series EE or E bonds plus any additional amount paid for the Series HH or H bonds. A taxpayer could have elected to treat all previously unreported accrued interest on Series EE or E bonds traded for Series HH bonds as income in the year of the trade (IRS Pub. 550).

Interest income from U.S. savings bonds is generally reported on Schedule B of the taxpayer's Form 1040 or Form 1040A.

An individual who redeems qualified a U.S. savings bond and uses the interest to pay certain higher education expenses may be able to exclude from gross income some or all of the interest redeemed (¶ 863).

731. Issues of U.S. Obligations. Interest on all obligations of the United States and its agencies and instrumentalities (i.e., U.S. Treasury bills, notes, and bonds) issued after February 28, 1941, is subject to federal taxes to the same extent as private obligations (Reg. § § 1.61-7(b)(2) and (3), and 1.103-4).[75]

References are to Standard Federal Tax Reports; Tax Research Consultant; and Practical Tax Explanations.

[72] ¶ 43,944; SALES: 51,056.15   [74] ¶ 21,500, ¶ 21,501; INDIV: [75] ¶ 5702, ¶ 6606; SALES:
[73] ¶ 5300; FILEIND: 30,252;   12,150; § 3,115.10   51,052; § 3,115.05
§ 15,315

Dividends

733. Dividends. Ordinary dividends are fully includible in gross income. The term "dividend" or "ordinary dividend" for income tax purposes means any distribution made by a corporation to its shareholders, whether in money or other property, out of its earnings and profits accumulated after February 28, 1913, or out of earnings and profits of the tax year (¶ 747) (Code Sec. 316(a); Reg. § 1.316-1).[76] If a dividend is in cash, the amount of the dividend is the amount of the cash. If the dividend is in both cash and noncash property, the amount of the dividend is the amount of the cash plus the fair market value (FMV) of the property distributed (¶ 735). Special rules apply to distributions received by 20-percent corporate shareholders (Code Sec. 301(e)).[77]

Dividends are generally taxed as ordinary income. However, qualified dividend income received by an individual, estate, or trust is taxed at capital gains rates. Qualified dividend income is defined as dividends received during the tax year from a domestic corporation or a qualified foreign corporation (Code Sec. 1(h)(11)).[78] For tax years beginning after December 31, 2012, the capital gains rates for noncorporate taxpayers are 20 percent for individuals, estates, and trusts in the 39.6-percent income tax bracket, 15 percent for most individuals, estates, and trusts, 0 percent for individuals in the 10- or 15-percent income tax brackets, and 0 percent for estates and trusts in the 15-percent income tax bracket. Individuals, estates, and trusts subject to the 20-percent capital gains rate may also be subject to the net investment income tax of 3.8 percent, which brings the capital gains rate for higher-income taxpayers to 23.8 percent. See ¶ 129 for discussion of the net investment income tax and ¶ 1736 for discussion of capital gains rates.

Corporate stock dividends passed through to investors by a mutual fund or other regulated investment company (RIC), partnership, real estate investment trust (REIT), or held by a common trust fund are also eligible for the reduced rate assuming the distribution would otherwise be classified as qualified dividend income.

Investments in tax-deferred retirement vehicles such as regular IRAs, 401(k)s and deferred annuities receive no benefit from the rate reduction. Distributions from these accounts are taxed at ordinary income tax rates even if the funds represent dividends paid on the stocks held in the account.

The reduced tax rates also do not apply to dividends paid by corporations such as credit unions, mutual insurance companies, farmers' cooperatives, nonprofit voluntary employee benefit associations (VEBAs), mutual savings banks, building and loan associations, and certain stock owned for short terms (Code Sec. 1(h)(11)(B)(ii)).[79] Special rules apply to Code Sec. 306 stock, which includes: (1) stock other than common stock received as a tax-free stock dividend, (2) stock other than common stock received in certain tax-free divisions or reorganizations, and (3) stock, including common stock, with a substituted or carryover basis determined by reference to other Code Sec. 306 stock.[80] Special rules also apply to dividends received from foreign corporations (Code Sec. 1(h)(11)(C)).

Holding Period. To qualify for the lower rates, investors are required to hold the stock from which the dividend is paid for more than 60 days in the 121-day period beginning 60 days before the ex-dividend date. The ex-dividend date is the date following the record date on which the corporation finalizes the list of shareholders who will receive the dividend (Code Sec. 1(h)(11)(B)(iii)).[81]

References are to Standard Federal Tax Reports; Tax Research Consultant; and Practical Tax Explanations.

[76] ¶ 15,702, ¶ 15,703; CCORP: 6,050; § 26,201

[77] ¶ 15,302; CCORP: 12,160; § 26,601

[78] ¶ 3260; CCORP: 6,062, SALES: 15,202.55; § 26,230

[79] ¶ 3260; SALES: 15,202.55; § 26,230

[80] ¶ 15,450; CCORP: 24,152; § 26,235.25

[81] ¶ 3260; CCORP: 6,062; § 26,230

733A. Stock Dividends and Stock Rights. Generally, a stockholder need not include in gross income the value of stock received as a stock dividend (Code Sec. 305(a); Reg. §§ 1.305-1—1.305-8).[82] However, the following distributions by a corporation of its stock or stock rights are taxed as a dividend under the rules discussed at ¶ 733. These exceptions include:

(1) distributions in lieu of money (Reg. § 1.305-2);

(2) disproportionate distributions (Reg. § 1.305-3);

(3) convertible preferred stock and debentures (Reg. § 1.305-6);

(4) distributions of common and preferred stock (Reg. § 1.305-4);

(5) certain transactions increasing a shareholder's proportionate interest (Reg. § 1.305-7); and

(6) dividends on preferred stock, unless the limited exception applies (Reg. § 1.305-5).

An increase in the conversion ratio of convertible preferred stock made solely to take account of stock dividends or stock splits on the stock into which the convertible stock can be converted is tax free.

The basis of the stock, stock rights, or fractional shares acquired in a nontaxable distribution is an allocable portion of the basis of the stock on which the distribution was made. To determine the basis of the stock received in a tax-free distribution, the shareholder allocates a part of the basis of the stock previously held to the new stock or stock rights. The basis allocation is made in the proportion of the fair market value of the old stock to the fair market value of the new stock or stock rights on the date of the distribution; not the record date (Code Sec. 307; Reg. § 1.307-1).[83] If the fair market value of rights received in the distribution is less than 15 percent of the fair market value of the old stock, the shareholder takes a basis of zero in the stock rights unless the shareholder elects to allocate a portion of the basis of the old stock in a timely filed return for the year in which the rights were received. An election, once made, is irrevocable (Reg. § 1.307-2).[84]

Any corporation that receives an extraordinary dividend with respect to any share of stock that the corporation has not held for more than two years before the dividend announcement date must reduce its basis in such stock, but not below zero, by the untaxed portion of the extraordinary dividend received. A dividend is extraordinary under the two-year rule if it equals or exceeds 10 percent (5 percent in the case of stock preferred as to dividends) of the shareholder's adjusted basis in the stock (Code Sec. 1059).[85]

733B. Corporate Debt v. Equity. The determination of whether an instrument issued by a corporation is to be treated as stock or as evidence of indebtedness for federal income tax purposes, including whether a distribution is a dividend, is resolved by weighing various factors, such as the source of the payments made to the holder and whether there is an unconditional promise to pay a sum certain together with a fixed rate of interest. For instruments issued after October 24, 1992, the corporate issuer's characterization of the nature of the instrument, made at the time of issuance, is binding upon the corporation and all the holders, but not the IRS. Interest holders are not bound, however, by the issuer's characterization if they disclose any inconsistent treatment on their tax returns (Code Sec. 385(c)).[86]

The IRS closely scrutinizes instruments containing a combination of debt and equity characteristics which are designed to be treated as debt for federal income tax purposes (Notice 94-47). Of particular interest are instruments that contain such equity features as an unreasonably long maturity or an ability to repay principal with the issuer's stock. No

---

References are to Standard Federal Tax Reports; Tax Research Consultant; and Practical Tax Explanations.

[82] ¶ 15,400, ¶ 15,401— ¶ 15,401H, ¶ 15,402; CCORP: 6,252; § 26,235.05

[83] ¶ 15,500, ¶ 15,501; SALES: 6,302, CCORP: 6,250; § 26,235.10

[84] ¶ 15,501B; SALES: 6,302; § 26,235.10

[85] ¶ 30,020, ¶ 30,021; SALES: 6,358; § 26,201, § 26,245

[86] ¶ 17,340, ¶ 17,351.01; CCORP: 3,300; § 26,201

¶733B

deduction is allowed for any interest paid or accrued on a disqualified debt instrument issued after June 8, 1997 (Code Sec. 163(l)). The term "disqualified debt instrument" means any debt that is payable in equity of the issuer or a related party or equity held by the issuer, or any related party, in any other person, specifically if: (1) a substantial portion of the principal or interest is required to be paid or converted, or at the issuer's or related party's option is payable in, or convertible into, equity of the issuer or a related party; (2) a substantial portion of the principal or interest is required to be determined, or may be determined at the option of the issuer or related party, by reference to the value of equity of the issuer or related party; or (3) the debt is part of an arrangement designed to result in payment of the instrument with or by reference to the equity. An exception to the no deduction rule applies for certain instruments issued by dealers in securities (Code Sec. 165(l)(5)).

In addition, the IRS examines corporate transactions designed to produce interest deductions with respect to a related issuance of stock and to provide companies with significant tax advantages in satisfying their equity capital requirements (Notice 94-48). The overall substance of an arrangement whereby a corporation creates a partnership that issues notes to investors and uses most of its capital to buy stock of the corporation is viewed by the IRS as merely an issuance of preferred stock by the corporation. Thus, such a corporation could not deduct an allocable portion of interest expense on the note without an offsetting inclusion of dividend income.

734. When Is a Dividend Received. A dividend on corporate stock is taxable when, in an unqualified manner, it is made subject to the demand of the shareholder (Code Sec. 301; Reg. § 1.301-1(b)).[87] For cash-method shareholders, this generally occurs when payment is actually received. For accrual-method shareholders, this generally occurs when the dividend is constructively received or at the time of declaration. As an exception to the constructive receipt rule, a dividend is taxable when the check is actually received, even though it may be dated and mailed in an earlier tax year, unless the recipient requested delivery by mail in order to delay recognition of income. Therefore, both accrual and cash basis taxpayers essentially may use the cash method for including dividends in income and must report the income as received.[88]

Voluntary repayment of a dividend legally declared and distributed does not negate the receipt of dividend income by a shareholder.[89]

Dividends paid by regulated investment companies (RICs) (i.e., mutual funds) are not always taxable when received (¶ 2303).

Dividends and interest in excess of $1,500 must be reported on Schedule B of the taxpayer's Form 1040 or Form 1040A.

735. Dividend Paid in Property. If any part of a dividend is paid in a form other than cash, the property received must be included in gross income at its fair market value (FMV) at the date of distribution, regardless of whether this date is the same as that on which the distribution is includible in gross income (Code Sec. 301(b)(1) and (3)).[90] When property is distributed to a corporate shareholder, the adjusted basis of the property in the hands of the distributing corporation at the time of the distribution, plus any gain recognized by the distributing corporation, is substituted for the FMV of the property if the adjusted basis is less than the FMV.

The amount of income realized on a distribution is reduced, but not below zero, by the amount of any liability to which property is subject or which is assumed (Code Sec. 301(b)(2); Reg. § 1.301-1).[91] The basis of property received in a distribution is the fair market value of such property (Code Sec. 301(d)).

References are to Standard Federal Tax Reports; Tax Research Consultant; and Practical Tax Explanations.

[87] ¶ 15,302, ¶ 15,303; CCORP: 6,060; § 3,030.05

[88] ¶ 21,009.1235; CCORP: 6,060; § 3,030.05

[89] ¶ 15,704.46, ¶ 15,704.473; CCORP: 6,058; § 3,030.05

[90] ¶ 15,302; CCORP: 6,150; § 26,205

[91] ¶ 15,302, ¶ 15,303; CCORP: 6,154; § 26,205

If a distribution is paid in property having a FMV in excess of the corporation's earnings and profits (¶ 747), the dividend is limited to earnings and profits, accumulated and current. The portion of the distribution that is not a dividend is applied to reduce the basis of the stock. If the amount of the nondividend distribution exceeds the basis of the stock, the excess is treated as a gain from the sale or exchange of the stock (Code Sec. 301(c)).

736. Gain or Loss to Corporation on Nonliquidating Distributions. A corporation does not recognize a gain or loss on the distribution of its stock, or rights to its stock, to shareholders. Similarly, a corporation generally does not recognize gain or loss on the distribution to its shareholders of corporate property (Code Sec. 311(a)).[92] A corporation generally must recognize gain, however, when it distributes appreciated property to its shareholders in any ordinary, nonliquidating distribution to the extent that the fair market value (FMV) of the property exceeds its adjusted basis (Code Sec. 311(b)).[93] Gain or loss rules applicable to corporations on liquidating distributions are discussed at ¶ 2257.

739. Disposition of Section 306 Stock. Code Sec. 306 is designed to prevent a stockholder from receiving a nontaxable stock dividend, other than common on common, or from receiving a stock distribution, other than common stock, in connection with a reorganization, and disposing of it to avoid reporting dividend income.[94]

If Code Sec. 306 stock (¶ 733) is redeemed by a corporation, the amount realized is treated as a distribution of property to which Code Sec. 301 applies and, therefore, will be treated as ordinary income or as a taxable distribution to the extent that it is made out of earnings and profits (¶ 733, ¶ 742, and ¶ 747). If the stock is disposed of otherwise than by a redemption, the amount realized is treated as ordinary income to the extent that the amount realized is not more than the amount that would have been realized as a dividend if, instead of the stock, the corporation had distributed cash in an amount equal to the fair market value of the stock. Therefore, it would be ordinary income up to the stockholder's share of the amount of earnings and profits of the corporation available for distribution.

A shareholder who received a preferred stock dividend on common stock and who donated the dividend to a tax-exempt charitable foundation realized no income on the stock transfer. In addition, the donor would not realize any income from the later sale of the Code Sec. 306 stock by the foundation.[95]

740. Special Rules and Exceptions for Code Sec. 306 Stock. A holder of Code Sec. 306 stock (¶ 733) is not subject to the ordinary income recognition rule for a transfer of Code Sec. 306 stock if the disposition occurs as part of a transaction that cannot be used to bail out earnings and profits. The rules governing gain realized on Code Sec. 306 stock do not apply to a disposition:[96]

    (1) if it is not a redemption,

        (a) is not made, directly or indirectly, to a related person under the constructive ownership rules, and

        (b) terminates the entire stock interest of the shareholder in the corporation, including stock constructively owned;

    (2) if it is a complete redemption of all the stock held in the corporation by the shareholder or in redemption of stock held by a shareholder who is not a corporation and in partial liquidation of the distributing corporation;

    (3) if it is redeemed in a complete liquidation of the corporation;

References are to Standard Federal Tax Reports; Tax Research Consultant; and Practical Tax Explanations.

[92] ¶ 15,550; CCORP: 6,100; § 26,235.10

[93] ¶ 15,550; CCORP: 6,152; § 26,210

[94] ¶ 15,450, ¶ 15,452; CCORP: 24,050; § 26,235.25

[95] ¶ 15,452.19; CCORP: 24,150; § 26,235.25

[96] ¶ 15,450; CCORP: 24,200; § 26,235.25

¶740

(4) to the extent that gain or loss is not recognized with respect to the disposition; or

(5) if the IRS is satisfied that the distribution of the stock and the disposition or redemption, simultaneously or previously, of the stock on which the distribution was made were not in pursuance of a plan having as one of its principal purposes the avoidance of income tax.

The sale of new preferred stock to an employees' trust, however, was held not to be within the scope of Code Sec. 306(a).[97]

Dividends: Distribution in Redemption of Stock

742. Redemption of Stock as a Dividend. If a corporation cancels or redeems its stock in such a manner as to make the distribution equivalent to a dividend distribution, the amount received by the shareholder, to the extent that it is paid out of earnings and profits, is a taxable dividend (Reg. § 1.302-1).[98]

Whether a distribution in connection with a cancellation or redemption of stock is equivalent to a taxable dividend depends on the facts in each case. A cancellation or redemption of a part of the stock, pro rata among all the shareholders, will generally be considered as resulting in a dividend distribution (Reg. § 1.302-2).[99] A redemption can be treated as an exchange of stock, rather than as a dividend, if one of the following four tests is met (Code Sec. 302(b)):[100] (1) the redemption is substantially disproportionate with respect to the shareholder; (2) the redemption terminates the shareholder's entire interest in the corporation; (3) the redemption is not substantially equivalent to a dividend; or (4) the redemption is of stock held by a noncorporate shareholder and is made in partial liquidation of the redeeming corporation. Amounts received by a shareholder in a distribution in complete liquidation of a corporation are not equivalent to the distribution of a taxable dividend (Code Sec. 331).[101]

A distribution is substantially disproportionate as to a shareholder if, after the redemption, the shareholder owns less than 50 percent of the combined voting power of all classes of voting stock and there is an exchange of stock but not of a dividend. Further, the ratio of the shareholder's holdings of voting stock after the redemption to all the voting stock must be less than 80 percent of the ratio of the voting stock the shareholder owned immediately before the redemption to the entire voting stock in the corporation. In addition, a distribution is not substantially disproportionate unless the stockholder's ownership of common stock, whether voting or nonvoting, after and before redemption also meets the 80-percent test (Reg. § 1.302-3).[102]

If a shareholder is entirely bought out, the transaction is treated as an exchange of the stock, and no part of the distribution is taxed as a dividend (Reg. § 1.302-4).[103]

A distribution that is in redemption of stock held by a noncorporate shareholder in partial liquidation of the distributing corporation is a distribution in exchange for the stock and is not taxed as a dividend (Code Sec. 302(b)(4)).[104]

Stock Redemption Expenses. A corporation is not allowed a deduction for any amount paid or incurred in connection with any redemption of its stock or the stock of any related person. This restriction does not apply to deductions for interest paid or accrued within the tax year on indebtedness, deductions for dividends paid in connection with the redemption of stock in a regulated investment company (a mutual fund or RIC), or deductions for amounts properly allocable to indebtedness and amortized over the term of the debt (Code Sec. 162(k)).[105]

References are to Standard Federal Tax Reports; Tax Research Consultant; and Practical Tax Explanations.

[97] ¶ 15,452.21; CCORP: 24,200; § 26,235.25

[98] ¶ 15,326 ; CCORP: 21,102; § 26,305.05

[99] ¶ 15,327; CCORP: 21,250; § 26,305.05

[100] ¶ 15,325; CCORP: 21,150; § 26,301

[101] ¶ 16,002; CCORP: 27,050; § 26,320.05

[102] ¶ 15,328; CCORP: 21,150; § 26,315.05

[103] ¶ 15,329; CCORP: 21,204; § 26,320.05

[104] ¶ 15,325; CCORP: 21,700; § 26,330

[105] ¶ 8500; BUSEXP: 9,412.05; § 26,365

743. Constructive Ownership of Stock. Certain provisions relating to corporate distributions and adjustments, such as distributions in redemption of stock noted at ¶ 742, treat an individual as constructively owning stock held by a related person. Under these constructive ownership rules an individual is treated as owning stock owned, directly or indirectly, by a spouse, if not legally separated under a decree of divorce or separate maintenance, children, including adopted children, grandchildren, and parents (Code Sec. 318(a)(1)).

Stock constructively owned by an individual under the family attribution rule is not treated as owned by that individual for the purpose of applying the constructive stock ownership rule to make another the owner of such stock (Reg. § 1.318-4).[106]

Stock owned, directly or indirectly, by or for a partnership, S corporation, or estate is considered as being owned proportionately by the partners, S corporation shareholders, or beneficiaries. Stock owned, directly or indirectly, by or for a partner, S corporation shareholder, or beneficiary is treated as being owned by the partnership, S corporation, or estate.

Stock owned, directly or indirectly, by or for a trust is considered as being owned by its beneficiaries in proportion to their actuarial interests in the trust. Stock owned, directly or indirectly, by or for a beneficiary of a trust is considered as being owned by the trust. However, a contingent beneficial interest of not more than 5 percent of the value of the trust property is not to be taken into account (Code Sec. 318(a)(2) and (3); Reg. § 1.318-2).[107]

If 50 percent or more in value of the stock in a corporation is owned, directly or indirectly, by or for any person, that person is considered as owning the stock owned, directly or indirectly, by or for the corporation in the proportion that the value of the stock the person owns bears to the value of all the stock in the corporation. The corporation, on the other hand, is considered as owning the stock owned, directly or indirectly, by or for any person holding 50 percent or more in value of its stock, directly or indirectly (Code Sec. 318(a)(2)(C) and (a)(3)(C)).[108]

744. Redemption of Stock Through Use of Related Corporations. If stock of an issuing corporation is acquired by a corporation that is controlled by the issuing corporation, the amount paid for the stock will be a dividend by the issuing corporation, provided that, under the rules outlined at ¶ 742, this amount would be considered a taxable dividend. Also, when the stock of one corporation is sold to a related corporation (i.e., brother-sister corporations), the sale proceeds are considered as distributed in redemption of the stock of the corporation which bought it, governed by the rules at ¶ 742. If the sales are related, it is immaterial whether they are made simultaneously (Reg. § 1.304-2).[109] Whether the sales are related is determined upon the facts and circumstances surrounding all the sales. To the extent that a redemption involving related corporations is treated as a distribution under Code Sec. 301, the transferor and the acquiring corporation are treated as if the transferor had transferred the stock involved to the acquiring corporation in exchange for stock of the acquiring corporation, in a Code Sec. 351(a) nontaxable contribution of capital, and then the acquiring corporation had redeemed the stock it was deemed to have issued (Code Sec. 304(a)(1)).

745. Redemption of Stock to Pay Estate Taxes and Expenses. A distribution of property by a corporation in redemption of its stock that has been included in the gross estate of a decedent for estate tax purposes can qualify as an exchange to the extent that the amount of the distribution does not exceed the sum of the estate, generation-skipping transfer, inheritance, legacy, and succession taxes, including interest, on the estate, plus the funeral and administration expenses allowable as deductions from the

---

References are to Standard Federal Tax Reports; Tax Research Consultant; and Practical Tax Explanations.

[106] ¶ 15,905; CCORP: 21,502; § 26,310.30

[107] ¶ 15,900, ¶ 15,902; CCORP: 21,508; § 26,310.20

[108] ¶ 15,900; CCORP: 21,510; § 26,310.15

[109] ¶ 15,377; CCORP: 21,450; § 26,340

gross estate for federal estate tax purposes (Code Sec. 303(a) and (d)).[110] For discussion of the estate tax, see ¶ 2901 and following.

To qualify for this treatment, the redemption must have been made not later than 90 days after the period of limitations on assessment of the federal estate tax, which is three years after the return is filed (Code Sec. 303(b)(1)(A)). When a petition for redetermination of an estate tax deficiency has been filed with the Tax Court, the redemption period is extended to any time before the expiration of 60 days after the decision of the Tax Court becomes final. A distribution made more than 60 days after the decision of the Tax Court becomes final can be timely, providing it is made within 90 days after expiration of the three-year period.[111]

In order for the redemption not to be treated as a taxable dividend, the value of the decedent's stock in a closely held company must exceed 35 percent of the gross estate, after the deductions for allowable funeral and administration expenses and losses (Code Sec. 302(b)(2)). The shares must be redeemed from a person whose interest in the estate is reduced by payment of estate, generation-skipping transfer, inheritance, and succession taxes or funeral and administration expenses. The value of these redeemed shares is limited to the sum of these deductible expenses.[112]

If stock in a corporation is the subject of a generation-skipping transfer occurring at the same time and as a result of the death of an individual, the tax imposed is treated as an estate tax for purposes of the redemption rules. The period of distribution is measured from the date of the generation-skipping transfer, and the relationship of stock to the decedent's estate is measured with reference solely to the amount of the generation-skipping transfer (Code Sec. 303(d)).[113]

Dividends: Earnings and Profits

747. Sources of Distributions. To be subject to income tax as a dividend (¶ 733), a distribution received by a shareholder must be paid out of earnings and profits of the distributing corporation. A dividend is any distribution made by a corporation to its shareholders out of its earnings and profits accumulated after February 28, 1913, or out of the earnings and profits of the current tax year, computed as of the close of the tax year without diminution by reason of any distributions made during the tax year, without regard to the amount of the earnings and profits at the time the distribution was made (Code Sec. 316; Reg. § 1.316-1).[114]

In order to determine the source of a distribution, consideration should be given first, to the earnings and profits of the tax year; second, to the earnings and profits accumulated since February 28, 1913, but only in the case when, and to the extent that, the distributions made during the tax year are not regarded as out of the earnings and profits of that year; third, to the earnings and profits accumulated before March 1, 1913, only after all of the earnings and profits of the tax year and all the earnings and profits accumulated since February 28, 1913, have been distributed; and fourth, to sources other than earnings and profits only after the earnings and profits have been distributed (Reg. § 1.316-2).[115]

If the current year's earnings and profits are sufficient to cover all distributions made during the year, each distribution is a taxable dividend. If the year's cash distributions, however, exceed current earnings and profits, a part of the earnings and profits must be allocated proportionately to each distribution, on the basis of the following formula: distribution × (current earnings and profits ÷ total distributions). The remaining portion of each distribution not covered by current earnings and profits is then treated as a taxable dividend to the extent of accumulated earnings and profits. If these are not sufficient to cover the remaining portion of any distribution, they are to be applied against each distribution in chronological order until exhausted.

References are to Standard Federal Tax Reports; Tax Research Consultant; and Practical Tax Explanations.

[110] ¶ 15,350; CCORP: 21,650; § 26,340.05

[111] ¶ 15,353.80; CCORP: 21,650; § 26,340.25

[112] ¶ 15,353.30; CCORP: 21,650; § 26,340.15

[113] ¶ 15,350; CCORP: 21,662; § 26,340.05

[114] ¶ 15,702, ¶ 15,703; CCORP: 12,050; § 26,215

[115] ¶ 15,703B; CCORP: 12,050; § 26,215

748. Computation of Earnings and Profits. In computing earnings and profits, all income that is exempt from tax must be included, as well as all items includible in gross income under Code Sec. 61 (Reg. § 1.312-6).[116] Thus, exempt income such as life insurance proceeds and fully tax-exempt interest on state or municipal obligations is included. Similarly, cancellation of indebtedness income and intercorporate dividends are included. The starting point for the computation of earnings and profits is the corporation's taxable income, which is then adjusted to more accurately reflect true economic income available for distribution. This involves the different treatment of certain items from their treatment for tax purposes, including depreciation, depletion, certain reserves, and other items. In many cases, gain or loss from a sale or other disposition will be included in earnings and profits at the time and to the extent that it is recognized for tax purposes (Reg. § 1.312-6).[117] However, there are exceptions to this general rule, and the corporation's earnings and profits are very unlikely to be the same as the corporation's taxable income. As one example, income from installment sales is treated differently than earnings and profits (¶ 756). As another example, some items that are required to be capitalized for income tax purposes are deducted in the computation of earnings and profits (Rev. Rul. 60-123).

The general rule on the distribution of property, including cash, by a corporation is that the earnings and profits for future distributions are reduced by the amount of money distributed, the principal amount of any obligations of the corporation distributed, and the adjusted basis of any other property distributed (Reg. § 1.312-1).[118] If appreciated property is distributed with respect to stock, earnings and profits must be increased by the amount of the gain realized upon the distribution even if the gain is not recognized for purposes of computing taxable income. There are special rules for distributions to 20-percent corporate shareholders (¶ 733).

749. Effect of Deficit on Earnings and Profits. Even if there is an operating deficit at the beginning of the year, total dividends paid are taxable to the extent of profits for the *entire* year (¶ 747) (Reg. § 1.316-1(e)).[119]

750. Effect of Loss on Earnings and Profits. A loss for a preceding year cannot be used to decrease the earnings and profits of the tax year (Reg. § 1.312-6(d)).[120]

751. Redemptions and Earnings and Profits. A corporation that distributes amounts in redemption of its stock can reduce its post-February 28, 1913, accumulated earnings and profits only by the ratable share of those earnings and profits attributable to the redeemed stock (Code Sec. 312(n)(7)).[121]

752. Effect of Reorganization on Earnings and Profits. When a corporate reorganization results in no recognized gain or loss, the company's life as a continuing venture does not stop, so that what were earnings and profits of the original company remain, for purposes of distribution, earnings and profits of the continuing corporation.[122]

753. Effect of Nontaxable Distribution on Earnings and Profits. Nontaxable stock dividends or stock rights do not reduce earnings and profits. The same rule applies to distributions of the stock or securities, or rights to acquire stock or securities, of other corporations and distributions of property or money when they were nontaxable to the recipient when made (Code Sec. 312(d)).[123]

754. Distribution Other Than a Dividend. Any distribution that is a dividend is included in gross income. The portion of a distribution that is not a dividend reduces the adjusted basis of the stock. Any excess of distributions over the basis is treated as a gain from the sale or exchange of property (Code Sec. 301(c)).[124]

References are to Standard Federal Tax Reports; Tax Research Consultant; and Practical Tax Explanations.

[116] ¶ 15,611; CCORP: 12,102; § 26,601

[117] ¶ 15,611; CCORP: 12,100; § 26,610

[118] ¶ 15,601; CCORP: 12,152; § 26,615.05

[119] ¶ 15,703; CCORP: 12,050; § 26,605.05

[120] ¶ 15,611, ¶ 15,612.45; CCORP: 12,050; § 26,605.10

[121] ¶ 15,600; CCORP: 12,210; § 26,305.05

[122] ¶ 17,031.21; CCORP: 12,200; § 26,601

[123] ¶ 15,600; CCORP: 12,156; § 26,235.10

[124] ¶ 15,302; CCORP: 12,050; § 26,215

755. Effect of Depreciation on Earnings and Profits. Depreciation claimed on the corporation's income tax return that is in excess of the straight-line method increases the corporation's current earnings and profits (Code Sec. 312(k)).[125] For tangible property placed in service in tax years beginning after 1986, the alternative MACRS method is used to compute depreciation in order to determine the corporation's earnings and profits (¶ 1247). For depreciable assets first placed in service after 1980, but before 1987, the adjustment to earnings and profits for depreciation is determined under the straight-line ACRS, using extended recovery periods (¶ 1252).[126] For assets placed in service before 1981, the amount of the depreciation deduction for the purpose of computing earnings and profits is generally the amount allowable under the traditional straight-line method, although a corporation that uses the permissible non-accelerated depreciation method (e.g., the machine-hour method) can use that method for earnings and profits purposes.

Also, in computing the earnings and profits of a corporation, any amount that can be deducted under certain provisions, listed later, can be deducted ratably over a period of five years, beginning with the year the amount is deductible under Code Sec. 179 or one of the other relevant sections (Code Sec. 312(k)(3)(B)).[127] This includes property that can be deducted under Code Sec. 179, or Code Sec. 179A for certain clean-fuel vehicles and refueling property placed in service before December 31, 2005, or Code Sec. 179B for certain environmental expenses paid or incurred after December 31, 2002, but not later than December 31, 2009, or Code Sec. 179C for certain refinery property placed in service after August 8, 2005, or Code Sec. 179D for certain energy-efficient property placed into service after December 31, 2005, but before January 1, 2014, or Code Sec. 179E(g) for 50 percent of the cost of advanced mine safety equipment placed in service after December 20, 2006, and before January 1, 2014.[128]

756. Effect of Installment Sales on Earnings and Profits. A corporation that sells property on the installment basis is treated for earnings and profits purposes as if it had not used the installment method (Code Sec. 312(n)(5)).[129]

757. Effect of LIFO Reserve Changes on Earnings and Profits. A corporation's earnings and profits generally must be increased or decreased by the amount of any change in the corporation's "LIFO recapture amount" at the end of each tax year (Code Sec. 312(n)(4)).[130] The term "LIFO recapture amount" means the amount, if any, by which the inventory amount of the inventory assets under the first-in, first-out (FIFO) method exceeds the inventory amount of the assets under the last-in, first-out (LIFO) method.

Business Income

759. Business Profit. Gross income includes "gross income derived from business," which is usually the same as gross profit, *not* gross receipts (Code Sec. 61(a)(2); Reg. § 1.61-3(a)).[131] Gross profit is the total receipts from sales minus the cost of the goods sold, plus investment income and income from other sources. In the case of most mercantile businesses, cost of goods sold includes the purchase price of the article sold plus delivery costs, warehousing, etc. In a manufacturing firm it includes the entire factory cost—materials, direct labor, and factory overhead, including depreciation attributable to manufacturing processes—applicable to goods manufactured and sold. Gross income derived from business is determined without subtracting selling expenses, losses, or other items not ordinarily used in computing costs of goods sold, as well as amounts paid for bribes, kickbacks, fines or penalties for which a business deduction would not be allowed (¶ 972). Cost of goods sold should be determined according to the accounting method consistently used by the taxpayer (¶ 1515).

References are to Standard Federal Tax Reports; Tax Research Consultant; and Practical Tax Explanations.

[125] ¶ 15,600; CCORP: 12,108; § 26,625.15

[126] ¶ 15,612.31; CCORP: 12,108; § 11,001, § 26,625.15

[127] ¶ 15,600; DEPR: 3,452; § 26,625.10

[128] ¶ 12,120, ¶ 12,130; DEPR: 12,050; § 26,625.10

[129] ¶ 15,600; CCORP: 12,106; § 26,625.25

[130] ¶ 15,600; CCORP: 12,106; § 26,625.45

[131] ¶ 5502, ¶ 5511; INDIV: 6,050; § 3,010

Damages for Lost Profit or Capital. Damage awards and amounts received in settlement of claims for business injuries that represent compensation for lost profits are taxable as ordinary income. This rule applies to proceeds from business interruption insurance, liquidated damages, and awards for breach of contract. Damages received for injury to goodwill are a nontaxable return of capital to the extent that the amounts received do not exceed the taxpayer's basis in goodwill. Similarly, compensation for injury to or loss of capital is treated as a nontaxable return of capital to the extent of basis; any excess is treated as a capital gain if received for damage to a capital asset.[132] Punitive damages, such as treble damages under antitrust laws, constitute taxable ordinary income (Reg. § 1.61-14(a)).[133]

See ¶ 852 for damages arising out of employment discrimination claims.

760. Credits Included in Income. If the taxpayer claims a credit for gasoline and special fuels on Form 4136 (¶ 1329), the amount of the credit must be included in gross income to the extent that a business deduction for the products was taken.[134] A cash-basis taxpayer must claim the credit and include the amount in gross income in the same tax year. An accrual-basis taxpayer should include the credit in the gross income for the tax year in which the fuel was actually used (IRS Pub. 510).

A taxpayer who was eligible for the alcohol fuels and biodiesel fuels credits (¶ 1365I; ¶ 1365X) was required to include the allowable credit in gross income for the tax year in which the credit was earned (Code Sec. 87).[135] The total credit allowable was included even though the taxpayer could not use the credit currently because of the credit limitation based on tax liability.

Rents and Royalties

762. Rents. Amounts received or accrued as rents in payment for the use of property must be included in gross income (Code Sec. 61(a)(5); Reg. § 1.61-8).[136] The payment by a lessee of any expenses of a lessor is generally considered additional rental income to the lessor (¶ 765). Consideration received by the lessor for cancellation of a lease is in substitution for rental payments and, thus, not a return of capital. Any reduction in the value of property due to cancellation of a lease is a deductible loss only when fixed by a closed transaction.[137]

Rental activities are generally treated as passive activities (¶ 1181).

Expenses attributable to property held for the production of rents or royalties are deductible in computing adjusted gross income (¶ 1089). An individual lessor reports rental personal property income and expenses on Schedule C or Schedule C-EZ (Form 1040) if he or she is in the personal property rental business, and directly on Form 1040 if not in such business. An individual lessor generally reports rental real estate income and expenses on Part I of Schedule E of Form 1040. The lessor must instead use Schedule C or Schedule C-EZ (Form 1040), however, if he or she provided significant services to the real property lessee.

See ¶ 966 for special rules affecting a taxpayer's rental of his or her residence or vacation home.

763. Royalties. Royalties from copyrights on literary, musical, or artistic works and similar property or from a patent on an invention are includible in gross income (Code Sec. 61(a)(6); Reg. § 1.61-8(a)).[138] Royalties received from oil, gas, or other mineral properties are also includible in gross income. For the treatment of royalties on the disposition of an interest in timber, coal and iron ore, see ¶ 1772. For the depletion allowance for royalties, see ¶ 1289.

References are to Standard Federal Tax Reports; Tax Research Consultant; and Practical Tax Explanations.

[132] ¶ 5900.14, ¶ 5900.15, ¶ 5900.26; INDIV: 6,354; § 3,810.10, § 3,810.20

[133] ¶ 5815; INDIV: 6,356; § 3,810.25

[134] ¶ 4150, ¶ 5602.35; INDIV: 6,376; § 13,540

[135] ¶ 6430; INDIV: 6,376

[136] ¶ 5502, ¶ 5705; REAL: 12,050; § 3,020

[137] ¶ 5706.5162; REAL: 12,252; § 3,020, § 18,630

[138] ¶ 5502, ¶ 5705; SALES: 24,250, FARM: 18,150; § 3,025

Royalties are generally reported on Part I of Schedule E (Form 1040). However, Schedule C or Schedule C-EZ (Form 1040) is used to report royalties received by the holder of an operating oil, gas, or mineral interest, and by self-employed writers, inventors, artists, etc.

764. Improvements by Lessee. Ordinarily, on the termination of a lease, a lessor of real property excludes any income derived from improvements made on the property by the lessee (Code Sec. 109; Reg. § 1.109-1).[139] This exclusion applies to improvements that revert to the lessor upon expiration of a lease as well as to those acquired by the lessor upon forfeiture of a lease prior to the end of the full term. If the improvements represent a liquidation-in-kind of lease rentals, the exclusion does not apply to the extent that the improvements represent such liquidation.

If the lessee makes improvements in lieu of paying rent during the lease term, the lessor has rental income to the extent of the fair market value of the improvements in the year they were made (Reg. §§ 1.61-8(c) and 1.109-1).[140] This treatment of lessee improvements depends on the parties' intention, which may be indicated by the lease terms or the surrounding circumstances.

Construction Allowances. A retail tenant that receives cash or rent reductions from a lessor of retail space with respect to a lease of 15 years or less entered into after August 5, 1997, does not include that amount in gross income, if the tenant uses the amounts for construction or improvement of nonresidential real property that is part of the retail space and used in the tenant's trade or business (Code Sec. 110(a); Reg. § 1.110-1).[141] The lessor must depreciate the improvement as MACRS nonresidential real property (¶ 1234 and ¶ 1240). If the improvement is disposed of or abandoned at the termination of the lease, the lessor must continue to depreciate after the improvement was disposed of or abandoned and may claim a gain or loss by reference to the remaining adjusted basis of the improvement (¶ 1109).

765. Lessor's Obligations Paid by Lessee. If a lessee pays any of the lessor's expenses, such as property taxes, the payment is additional rental income to the lessor (Reg. § 1.61-8(c)).[142] When the taxes paid are income to the lessor, they may be treated as if paid by the lessor in determining their deductibility (¶ 986). If a lessee agrees to pay, in lieu of rent, a dividend on the lessor's stock or interest on its mortgages, the payments will result in rental income to the lessor.[143]

Farming Income

767. Farming As a Business. Income from farming is treated in the same way as income from any other business (¶ 759). Every individual, partnership, or corporation which cultivates, operates, or manages a farm for gain or profit, either as owner or tenant, is designated as a farmer (Reg. § 1.61-4(d)).[144] A person who cultivates or operates a farm for recreation or pleasure, and who experiences a continual net loss from year to year, generally lacks a profit motive and may not deduct the losses (¶ 1195).

In addition to filing Form 1040, an individual engaged in farming for profit must file a Schedule F (Form 1040). Partnerships engaged in farming must file Schedule F (Form 1040) along with Form 1065, and estates and trusts engaged in farming must file Schedule F along with Form 1041. Corporations engaged in farming must file the appropriate Form 1120. An individual farmer must also file Schedule SE (Form 1040) for computing earnings from self-employment (¶ 2676).

References are to Standard Federal Tax Reports; Tax Research Consultant; and Practical Tax Explanations.

[139] ¶ 7020, ¶ 7021; SALES: 42,252, REAL: 12,304; § 18,625

[140] ¶ 5705, ¶ 7021; SALES: 42,252; § 18,625

[141] ¶ 7030, ¶ 7032; REAL: 12,312; § 4,035

[142] ¶ 5705; REAL: 12,066, REAL: 12,070; § 18,610.20

[143] ¶ 5706.564; REAL: 12,070; § 18,610.20

[144] ¶ 5601; FARM: 3,052; § 36,305

Cash Basis. The general rules for all cash-basis taxpayers also apply to a farmer on the cash basis (¶ 1515). A cash-basis farmer does not use inventories, and includes in gross income all cash or the value of merchandise or other property received from the sale of livestock and produce that have been raised, profits from the sale of livestock or other items that have been purchased, and income received from all other sources (Reg. § 1.61-4).[145] A cash-basis farmer may defer recognition of gain from the sale of a crop delivered in one year until the following year if a valid contract with the purchaser or the purchaser's agent prohibits payment until the following year, but not if the payment is deferred merely at the seller's request. If the sales contract states that the farmer has the right to the proceeds of the sale from the purchaser at any time after delivery of the item, the farmer must include the sales price in his or her gross income in the year of the sale, regardless of when payment is received.[146]

Profit from the sale of livestock or other items purchased by a farmer is computed by deducting the cost from the sales price. For the sale of animals that originally were purchased as draft or work animals, or for breeding or dairy purposes and not for resale, the profit is the difference between the sale price and the depreciated basis of the animal sold (Reg. § 1.61-4(a)).

A cash-basis farmer who receives insurance proceeds as a result of destruction or damage to crops may elect to include the proceeds in income in the year after the year of damage if the farmer can show that the income from the crops would normally have been reported in the following year. This includes payments received under the Agricultural Act of 1949, Title II of the Disaster Assistance Act of 1988, or Title I of the Disaster Assistance Act of 1989 as a result of damage to crops caused by drought, flood, or other natural disaster, or the inability to plant crops because of such a natural disaster (Code Sec. 451(d); Reg. § 1.451-6; Rev. Rul. 91-55).[147]

A cash-method farmer who is forced to sell more livestock than usual in the current year due to drought, flood, or other weather-related conditions, in an area designated as eligible for assistance by the federal government, may elect to be taxed on the forced sale income (gain that normally would not have been realized in the year of the forced sale) in the following year if the farmer can show that, under usual business practices, the additional animals would not have been sold in the current year except for the weather-related condition (Code Sec. 451(e); Reg. § 1.451-7).[148]

Accrual Method. A farmer on the accrual method must use inventories taken at the start and the end of the tax year (Reg. § 1.61-4(b)).[149]

Although many farmers may use the cash method, the accrual method of accounting is required for certain farming corporations and partnerships (¶ 1519), and for all farming tax shelters including farming syndicates (¶ 1521) (Code Sec. 447).[150]

Gross profit of a farmer on the accrual basis is calculated by: (1) adding the inventory value of livestock and other products on hand at the end of the year, plus the amount received from the sale of livestock and other products during the year, miscellaneous income items (i.e., breeding fees, rental fees, other incidental farm income), all subsidy or conservation payments treated as income, and gross income from all other sources, and then (2) subtracting from that total the sum of the inventory value of livestock and products on hand at the beginning of the year and the cost of livestock and products purchased during the year, but not livestock held for draft, dairy, or breeding purposes, unless they are included in inventory (Reg. § 1.61-4(b)).

Livestock raised or purchased for sale must be inventoried (¶ 1569). Livestock purchased for draft, breeding or dairy purposes and not for sale may be inventoried, or instead may be treated as capital assets subject to depreciation, if the method used is

---

References are to Standard Federal Tax Reports; Tax Research Consultant; and Practical Tax Explanations.

[145] ¶ 5601; FARM: 3,056; § 36,310.05

[146] ¶ 21,009.453; FARM: 3,056; § 36,035

[147] ¶ 21,002, ¶ 21,018, ¶ 21,021.28; FARM: 3,202; § 36,020

[148] ¶ 21,002, ¶ 21,020; FARM: 3,204; § 36,035

[149] ¶ 5601; FARM: 3,058, FARM: 3,100; § 36,315

[150] ¶ 20,700; FARM: 3,058; § 36,315.10

consistently followed from year to year. If inventoried livestock is sold, its cost must not be taken as an additional deduction in computing taxable income, because the cost is reflected in the inventory (Reg. § 1.61-4(b)). Sales of this livestock are generally reported on Form 4797.

Other Methods. Two other inventory methods are available to farmers—the farm-price method and the unit-livestock-price method (¶ 1569).

Income Averaging. An individual engaged in a farming business or fishing business may elect to average farm income over three years (Code Sec. 1301; Reg. § 1.1301-1).[151] The tax imposed in any tax year equals the sum of the tax computed on taxable income reduced by the amount of farm income elected for averaging plus the increase in tax that would result if taxable income for each of the three prior tax years were increased by an amount equal to one-third of the elected farm income. Schedule J (Form 1040) is used to report the income averaging.

For income from the sale of farm property other than inventory, see the discussion beginning at ¶ 1701. For tax shelter farming operations, see ¶ 1521.

For expenses of a farmer, see ¶ 982–¶ 985. For the application of the uniform capitalization rules to a farming business, see ¶ 999.

768. Patronage Dividend. A cooperative and its patrons are taxed in a way that the business earnings of the cooperative are taxable currently either to the cooperative or, through patronage dividends, to the patrons (¶ 698) (Code Secs. 1382 and 1385).[152]

769. Commodity Credit Corporation Loan. Income from the sale of a crop is normally reported in the year of the sale. If the farmer has pledged all or part of the crop production to secure a Commodity Credit Corporation (CCC) loan, however, the farmer may elect to report the loan proceeds as income in the year received rather than reporting the income in the year of the sale. IRS permission is not required to begin reporting CCC loans in this manner, but once a loan has been reported in income in the year received, all succeeding loans must be reported in the same way unless the IRS grants permission to change the reporting method. The election is made on Schedule F (Form 1040). The amount reported as income becomes the farmer's basis in the commodity and is used to determine gain or loss upon the ultimate disposition of the commodity (Code Sec. 77; Reg. §§ 1.77-1 and 1.77-2).[153] The IRS has adopted procedures for automatic approval of an accounting method change to report CCC loans as loans rather than as income (Rev. Proc. 2011-14).[154]

The repayment amount for a loan secured by an eligible commodity is generally based on the lower of the original loan rate or the alternative repayment rate, as determined by the CCC, for the commodity as of the repayment date. On repayment, therefore, a market gain may be realized if the loan is repaid when the alternative rate is lower than the original rate (Notice 2007-63).[155] When a CCC loan is repaid, regardless of the manner of repayment, the CCC is required to file an information return reporting market gain associated with the repayment (Code Sec. 6039J(a)).[156] The CCC is to report market gain from the repayment of a CCC loan on Form 1099-G.

Alimony Payments

771. Classification. Alimony and separate maintenance payments are income to the recipient/payee and are deductible by the payor if certain requirements are met (¶ 772) (Code Secs. 61(a)(8), 62(a)(10), 71 and 215).[157]

References are to Standard Federal Tax Reports; Tax Research Consultant; and Practical Tax Explanations.

[151] ¶ 31,787, ¶ 31,789; FARM: 3,300; § 36,401

[152] ¶ 32,320, ¶ 32,360; FARM: 12,102; § 36,040

[153] ¶ 6300, ¶ 6301, ¶ 6302; FARM: 3,170; § 36,005.15

[154] ¶ 6304.20; ACCTNG: 21,302.10; § 36,005.15

[155] ¶ 6304.50; FARM: 3,170.20; § 36,005.15

[156] ¶ 35,699G; FILEBUS: 9,378; § 36,005.15

[157] ¶ 5502, ¶ 6002, ¶ 6090, ¶ 12,570; INDIV: 21,150; § 1,901

Alimony payments are taken as a deduction from gross income in arriving at the payor's adjusted gross income and therefore may be claimed by taxpayers regardless of whether they itemize.

772. Divorce and Separation Instruments. Payments made under a divorce or separation instrument are includible in the gross income of the recipient/payee and deductible by the payor as alimony or separate maintenance payments if the following requirements are met:

(1) the payment is in cash, including checks and money orders payable on demand;

(2) the payment is received by or on behalf of a spouse under a divorce or separation instrument;

(3) the instrument does not designate the payment as being not includible in the recipient/payee's gross income and not deductible by the payor;

(4) spouses who are legally separated under a decree of divorce or separate maintenance cannot be members of the same household at the time the payment is made;

(5) there is no liability to make any payment for any period after the death of the payee spouse, or to make any payment, either in cash or property, as a substitute for such payments after the death of the payee spouse;

(6) the spouses must not file joint returns with each other; and

(7) the payment is not fixed by the instrument as child support (¶ 776) (Code Sec. 71(b), (c), and (e); Temp. Reg. § 1.71-1T).[158]

A divorce or separation instrument is defined as: (1) a divorce or separate maintenance decree or a written instrument incident to such a decree, (2) a written separation agreement, or (3) a decree that is not a divorce or separate maintenance decree but requires a spouse to make payments for the support or maintenance of the other spouse (Code Sec. 71(b)(2)).[159]

773. Year of Taxability or Deductibility. Alimony payments are generally includible in the recipient/payee's gross income in the year received (Code Sec. 71(a); Reg. § 1.71-1)[160] and are deductible by the payor in the year paid (Code Sec. 215; Reg. § 1.215-1),[161] regardless of whether the taxpayer employs the cash method or the accrual method of accounting. A recapture rule prevents the front-loading of alimony payments (¶ 774).

774. Three-Year Recapture of Excess Alimony Payments. A special recapture rule applies to *excess* alimony and separate maintenance payments (Code Sec. 71(f)).[162] Its purpose is to prevent property settlement payments from qualifying for alimony treatment. The rule requires the recapture of excess amounts that have been treated as alimony or separate maintenance either during the calendar year in which payments began (the first post-separation year) or in the next succeeding calendar year (the second post-separation year). Excess alimony payments are recaptured in the payor-spouse's tax year beginning in the third post-separation year by requiring the payor-spouse to include the excess in gross income that year. The payee, who previously included the payments in gross income, is entitled to deduct the amount recaptured from gross income in his or her tax year beginning in the third post-separation year.

Excess alimony payments are equal to the sum of the excess payments made in the first post-separation year plus the excess payments made in the second post-separation year.

7 | INCOME

References are to Standard Federal Tax Reports; Tax Research Consultant; and Practical Tax Explanations.

[158] ¶ 6090, ¶ 6092; INDIV: 21,200; § 1,905.05

[159] ¶ 6090; INDIV: 21,204, IN-DIV: 21,300; § 1,905.15

[160] ¶ 6090, ¶ 6091; INDIV: 21,156; § 1,901

[161] ¶ 12,570, ¶ 12,571; INDIV: 21,156; § 1,901

[162] ¶ 6090; INDIV: 21,350; § 1,910.05

The amount of excess payments in the first and second post-separation years is determined under a statutory formula. For the first recapture year, the excess payment amount is the excess, if any, of the total alimony paid in the first post-separation year minus the sum of (1) $15,000 plus (2) the average of the amount of alimony paid in the second post-separation year minus excess payments for that year plus the amount of alimony paid in the third post-separation year. Thus, for the first post-separation year, the following formula is used:

$$\text{1st year excess payments} = \text{alimony paid in 1st year} - \left(\$15,000 + \frac{\left(\substack{\text{alimony} \\ \text{paid in} \\ \text{2nd} \\ \text{year}} - \substack{\text{excess} \\ \text{payments} \\ \text{in 2nd} \\ \text{year}} \right) + \substack{\text{alimony} \\ \text{paid in} \\ \text{3rd} \\ \text{year}}}{2} \right)$$

To calculate the excess payments for the first year, it is necessary to determine the excess payments for the second year. The amount of excess payments for the second year is the excess, if any, of the amount of alimony paid during the second year minus the sum of (1) $15,000 plus (2) the amount of alimony paid in the third year. Thus, for the second post-separation year, the following formula is used:

$$\text{2nd year excess payments} = \text{alimony paid in 2nd year} - \left(\text{alimony paid in 3rd year} + \$15,000 \right)$$

Once the excess payments for both the first and second post-separation years have been determined, the results are added together to determine the amount that must be recaptured in the third post-separation year.

> **Example 1:** In 2012, Mr. Black makes payments totalling $50,000 to his ex-wife. He makes no payments in either 2013 or 2014. Assuming none of the exceptions set forth below apply, $35,000 will be recaptured in 2014. Mr. Black will have to report an additional $35,000 in income, while his ex-wife will be entitled to a $35,000 reduction in income.

> **Example 2:** In 2012, Ms. Gold makes payments totalling $50,000 to her ex-husband. In 2013, she makes $20,000 in payments, but in 2014 she makes no payments. Assuming that none of the exceptions set forth below apply, the total amount that must be recaptured in the third year is $32,500. This represents $5,000 from the second year ($20,000 minus $15,000) and $27,500 from the first year. The amount recaptured from the first year equals the excess of $50,000 over the sum of $15,000 plus $7,500. The $7,500 is the average of the payments for years two and three after reducing the payments by the $5,000 recaptured for year two ($20,000 payment in year two plus $0 payment in year three minus the $5,000 that was required to be recaptured equals $15,000; divided by two equals $7,500).

IRS Pub. 504 contains a worksheet for computing alimony recapture.

Exceptions to Recapture Rule. There are several exceptions to the recapture rule (Code Sec. 71(f)(5)).[163] Recapture is not required if, before the end of the third post-separation year, the alimony or separate maintenance payments terminate because either party dies or the payee-spouse remarries. The recapture rule also does not apply to temporary support payments received under an instrument described in Code Sec. 71(b)(2)(C). Recapture is not required if the alimony or separate maintenance payments fluctuate because of a continuing liability—over at least a three-year period—to pay a fixed portion of income from the earnings of a business or property or from compensation from employment or self-employment. Additionally, the recapture rule does not apply if alimony or separate maintenance payments decline by $15,000 or less over the three-year period.

References are to Standard Federal Tax Reports; Tax Research Consultant; and Practical Tax Explanations.

[163] ¶ 6090; INDIV: 21,356; § 1,910.10

¶774

775. Indirect Alimony Payments. Only a trust under Code Sec. 682 is contemplated in connection with divorce or separate maintenance under instruments executed or modified after 1984. When a beneficial interest in a trust is transferred or created incident to a divorce or separation, the beneficiary-spouse is entitled to the same treatment as the beneficiary of a regular trust, notwithstanding that the payments by the trust qualify as alimony or otherwise discharge a support obligation (Code Sec. 682; Reg. § § 1.682(a)-1, 1.682(b)-1).[164] The payor spouse cannot claim a deduction for a trust distribution to the payee spouse if the distribution is not includible in the payor's gross income (Code Sec. 215(d)).[165]

776. Child Support. Payments that a divorce or separation instrument fixes as payable to support the payor's child are not considered alimony or separate maintenance payments, and thus are not deductible by the payor or taxable to the payee (Code Sec. 71(c); Reg. § 1.71-1(e); Temp. Reg. § 1.71-1T(c)).[166] If any amount specified in the instrument is to be reduced based on a contingency set out in the instrument relating to a child—such as attaining a specified age, dying, leaving school, or marrying—the amount of the specified reduction is treated as child support from the outset. The same rule applies if the reduction called for by the instrument is to occur at a time that can clearly be associated with such contingency. Thus, payments that vary with the status of a child are not deductible.

> **Example:** A divorce instrument provides that alimony payments will be reduced by $500 per month when a child reaches age 18. Under these circumstances, $500 of each payment is treated as child support.

778. Property Transfers Between Spouses or Former Spouses Incident to Divorce. No gain or loss is recognized to the transferor on a transfer of property, either outright or in trust, between spouses or between former spouses incident to divorce (Code Sec. 1041(a); Temp. Reg. § 1.1041-1T).[167] The transfer is treated as a gift to the transferee, and thus the property's value is not includible in the transferee's gross income. The transferee's basis in the property is equal to the transferor's adjusted basis (Code Sec. 1041(b)). A transfer between former spouses is incident to divorce if it occurs within one year after the marriage ceases or is related to the cessation of the marriage (Code Sec. 1041(c)).

Nonrecognition of gain or loss is not available to the transferor if the transferee is a nonresident alien (Code Sec. 1041(d)), or if there is a transfer in trust to the extent that liabilities assumed by the transferee, including liabilities to which the property is subject, exceed the transferor's adjusted basis in the property (Code Sec. 1041(e)). The transferee's basis is increased for any such gain recognized by the transferor.

Other Income

785. Taxation of Miscellaneous or Other Income. Several income items are considered miscellaneous or other income (IRS Pub. 525; Instructions for Form 1040).

Prizes and Awards. Prizes and awards, other than certain types of fellowship grants and scholarships (¶ 865) and limited employee achievement awards, are generally includible in gross income (Code Sec. 74).[168] Awards for religious, charitable, scientific, educational, artistic, literary, or civic achievement are excludable from the recipient's income, but only if (1) the award is transferred unused by the payor to a governmental unit or a tax-exempt religious, charitable, scientific, etc., organization designated by the recipient; (2) the recipient is selected without any action on his or her part to enter the contest or proceeding; and (3) the recipient is not required to render substantial future services as a condition to receiving the prize or award. Thus, Nobel and Pulitzer prize recipients may not exclude from income the value of their awards unless these conditions are met.

References are to Standard Federal Tax Reports; Tax Research Consultant; and Practical Tax Explanations.

[164] ¶ 24,860, ¶ 24,861, ¶ 24,862; INDIV: 21,214; § 2,210.10

[165] ¶ 12,570; INDIV: 21,214; § 2,210.10

[166] ¶ 6090, ¶ 6091, ¶ 6092; INDIV: 21,450; § 2,001

[167] ¶ 29,800, ¶ 29,801; INDIV: 21,050; § 2,101, § 18,230

[168] ¶ 6200; INDIV: 33,150; § 3,060

Employee achievement awards—i.e., items of tangible personal property awarded to an employee by an employer for length of service or safety achievement—are excludable from the employee's gross income only to the extent that the cost of the award is deductible by the employer. The awards cannot represent disguised compensation, and the excludable amount can total no more than $400 for nonqualified awards or $1,600 for qualified awards (¶ 919) (Code Sec. 74(c)).

Gambling Income and Illegal Gains. Gain arising from gambling, betting and lotteries is includible in gross income. A gain from an illegal transaction, such as bootlegging, extortion, embezzlement or fraud, is also includible.[169] Gambling losses are discussed at ¶ 1113.

Bartering. The value of bartered services is includible in gross income, usually on Schedule C (Form 1040) or C-EZ (Form 1040). If the barter involves an exchange of property, a different form may be required for reporting purposes. For example, if the owner of an apartment building permitted an artist to use an apartment in exchange for works of art created by the artist, the building owner reports the fair market value of the art as rental income on Schedule E (Form 1040), and the artist reports the fair rental value of the apartment as income on Schedule C or C-EZ (IRS Pub. 525).[170]

If two individuals are members of a barter club and each agrees to exchange services, the value of the services received by each is includible in gross income. Barter clubs must report exchanges on Form 1099-B in accordance with the rules under Code Sec. 6045 (¶ 2565).[171] Trade or credit units used by a barter club to account for transactions are also includible in gross income when credited to the taxpayer's account.[172]

Cancelled Debt. If a debt is canceled or forgiven, other than as a gift or bequest, the canceled amount generally must be included in gross income (Code Sec. 61(a)(12); Reg. § 1.61-12).[173] Cancelled nonbusiness debt income is usually reported on Form 1040. Whether or not the interest portion of the canceled debt must be included in income depends on whether the interest would be deductible if paid. Exclusions of discharged debt are discussed in ¶ 855.

Insurance. Life insurance proceeds are generally excludable (¶ 803—¶ 809). However, if dividends received exceed the total net premiums paid for the contract, this is reportable income.

Recoveries. The recovery of an amount for which the taxpayer claimed a deduction or credit in an earlier tax year is generally reported as other income on Form 1040 in the tax year of the recovery (¶ 799).

Jury Duty Pay. Jury pay is reportable as other income on Form 1040 (Reg. § 1.61-2(a)(1)).[174] It may be deductible, however, by an employee required to surrender it to his or her employer (¶ 1010).

Certain Taxable Distributions. Distributions from a Coverdell education savings account (¶ 867) or a qualified tuition program (¶ 869) that exceed the amount used to pay for qualified education expenses and are not part of a qualified rollover are includible in income. A similar rule applies to distributions from health savings accounts (¶ 2035) and Archer MSAs (¶ 2037). If an individual fails to remain eligible for a health saving account, he or she may have to include a portion of amounts contributed to the account in gross income (¶ 2035).

References are to Standard Federal Tax Reports; Tax Research Consultant; and Practical Tax Explanations.

[169] ¶ 5504.22, ¶ 5901.25, ¶ 5901.30, ¶ 5901.35, ¶ 5901.40; INDIV: 6,250; § 3,085

[170] ¶ 5508.15; INDIV: 6,378; COMPEN: 6,110; § 3,085

[171] ¶ 35,920; FILEBUS: 9,260; § 3,085

[172] ¶ 5508.15; INDIV: 6,378; § 3,085

[173] ¶ 5502, ¶ 5801; SALES: 12,150; § 3,401

[174] ¶ 5506; COMPEN: 6,102; § 3,005.05

Below-Market Loans. If a below-market gift or demand loan is made, the forgone interest (at the federal rate) is interest income (¶ 795).

Income From the Rental of Personal Property. If the taxpayer rents personal property for purposes of generating profit, but is not in the business of renting personal property, any rental income is considered other income. Allowable deductions for expenses attributable to the property may be deducted in determining adjusted gross income (¶ 1089). If personal property is rented but not for purposes of generating profit, the rental income is treated as other income but expenses are deductible only up to the amount of income (¶ 1195) (IRS Pub. 535).

Hobbies. Income from an activity not engaged for profit is considered other income. Losses and expenses are generally deductible (¶ 1195).

Recapture of Charitable Tax Benefits. The recapture of the charitable contribution deduction for property disposed of within three years of contribution (¶ 1062) or the recapture of a charitable contribution deduction relating to the contribution of a partial interest (¶ 1063) is considered other income.

Treasure Trove. Treasure trove or other found property is gross income for the tax year in which it is reduced to undisputed possession, to the extent of its value in U.S. currency (Reg. § 1.61-14).[175]

Virtual Currency. Virtual currency is a digital representation of value that functions as a medium of exchange, a unit of account, or a store of value. Convertible virtual currency (e.g., Bitcoin), which has an equivalent value in or acts as a substitute for real currency, is treated as property for federal tax purposes. Transactions using convertible virtual currency are subject to the general tax principles that apply to property transactions. A taxpayer who receives convertible virtual currency as payment for goods or services must include in gross income the currency's fair market value, measured in U.S. dollars, as of the date it was received. If a taxpayer successfully "mines" convertible virtual currency (e.g., uses computer resources to validate Bitcoin transactions and maintain the public Bitcoin transaction ledger), the currency's fair market value is includible in gross income as of the date of receipt (Notice 2014-21).[176]

Shareholder's or Employee's Bargain Purchase

789. Bargain Purchase. If an employer transfers property to an employee or an independent contractor at less than its fair market value (FMV), whether or not the transfer is in the form of a sale or exchange, the difference between the amount paid for the property and its FMV at the time of the transfer is income to the purchaser as compensation for personal services (Reg. § 1.61-2(d)(2)).[177] Note, however, that qualified employee discounts are excludable from income (¶ 2088). See ¶ 713 for discussion of restricted property transferred in connection with the performance of services.

If a corporation transfers property to a shareholder at less than the property's FMV, the shareholder is treated as having received a distribution from the transferor-corporation and is subject to the general tax rules for including it in income (¶ 733, ¶ 735) (Reg. § 1.301-1(j)).[178] For treatment of securities transactions as potential income, see ¶ 1901.

In computing the gain or loss on a later sale of the property, its basis is the amount paid for the property, increased by the amount previously included in income in the case of the employee or independent contractor, or by the amount of the distribution in the case of the shareholder.

References are to Standard Federal Tax Reports; Tax Research Consultant; and Practical Tax Explanations.

[175] ¶ 5815; INDIV: 6,360; § 3,085

[176] ¶ 5508.20; INDIV: 6,054; § 19,601

[177] ¶ 5506; COMPEN: 6,150; § 3,005.05

[178] ¶ 15,303; CCORP: 6,060, CCORP: 6,312.05; § 3,030.05, § 26,225.05

Creditor's Financial Income

793. Creditor's Financial Income. A cash-basis creditor reports interest on loans or obligations as it is received. An accrual-basis creditor reports this type of interest as it is earned (i.e., over the term of the loan, as installment payments are due, etc.), or when it is received if payment is received earlier than when due (¶ 724).

Rule of 78s. The IRS will *not* give any tax effect to a provision in a loan agreement that provides interest must be allocated in accordance with the Rule of 78s, because that method of allocating interest does not accurately reflect the true cost of borrowing.[179]

Loan Commission. A loan commission is taxed to an accrual-basis lender in the year the loan is made. A commission deducted from the face amount of the loan is taxed to a cash-basis lender only when received upon payment of the loan or sale of the obligation.[180]

Below-Market Interest Loans

795. Imputed Interest on Below-Market Interest Loans. Loans that carry little or no interest are generally recharacterized as arm's-length transactions in which the lender is treated as having made to the borrower a demand loan bearing an interest rate that is less than the statutory federal rate of interest, or a term loan in which the loan amount is more than the present value of all payments due under the loan (Code Sec. 7872).[181] Concurrently, there is deemed to be a transfer in the form of gift, dividend, contribution to capital, compensation, or other manner of payment, depending upon the nature of the loan, from the lender to the borrower which, in turn, is retransferred by the borrower to the lender to satisfy the accruing interest. These rules apply to: (1) gift loans, (2) corporation-shareholder loans, (3) compensation loans between employer and employee or between independent contractor and client, (4) tax-avoidance loans, (5) any below-market interest loans in which the interest arrangement has a significant effect on either the lender's or borrower's tax liability, and (6) loans to certain continuing care facilities that are not exempt from the rules.

In the case of a demand loan or a gift loan, the imputed interest amount is deemed to be transferred from the lender to the borrower on the last day of the calendar year of the loan. As for a term loan, other than a gift loan, the imputed amount is deemed to have been transferred on the date the loan was made.

Exceptions. A *de minimis* exception applies to gift loans totalling $10,000 or less between individuals if the loan is not directly attributable to the purchase or carrying of income-producing assets (Code Sec. 7872(c)(2)). There is also a $10,000 *de minimis* exception for compensation-related or corporation-shareholder loans that do not have tax avoidance as a principal purpose (Code Sec. 7872(c)(3)). Further, in the case of gift loans between individuals where the total amount outstanding does not exceed $100,000, the amount deemed transferred from the borrower to the lender at the end of the year will be imputed to the lender only to the extent of the borrower's annual net investment income (Code Sec. 7872(d)). For this purpose, net investment income is the excess of investment income minus investment expenses, as under the noncorporate deduction for interest paid on investment debt (¶ 1094). If such income does not exceed $1,000, no imputed interest is deemed transferred to the lender.

The below-market interest rate rules also do not apply to below-market loans owed by a facility which, on the last day of the year in which the loan is made, is a qualified continuing care facility, if the loan was made pursuant to a continuing care contract, and if the lender or the lender's spouse reaches the age of 62 before the close of the tax year (Code Sec. 7872(h)).[182]

References are to Standard Federal Tax Reports; Tax Research Consultant; and Practical Tax Explanations.

[179] ¶ 9104.62; INDIV: 48,264; § 7,405.20

[180] ¶ 20,620.214; COMPEN: 6,302; § 18,510

[181] ¶ 43,956; INDIV: 12,200; § 19,401

[182] ¶ 43,956; INDIV: 12,208.20; § 19,430.15

Employee Relocation Loans. In the case of an employer loan to an employee made in connection with the purchase of a principal residence at a new place of work, the applicable federal rate (AFR) for testing the loan is the rate as of the date the written contract to purchase the residence was entered into (Code Sec. 7872(f)(11); Temp. Reg. § 1.7872-5T(c)(1)).[183] Additionally, employee relocation loans meeting certain requirements are exempt from the below-market interest loan rules. The special treatment for employee relocation loans applies only under circumstances in which the moving expense deduction would be allowed (¶ 1073, ¶ 1075).

Recoveries

799. Tax Treatment of Recoveries. The receipt of an amount that was part of a deduction or credit taken in an earlier tax year is considered a recovery and generally must be included, partially or totally, in income in the year of receipt (Code Sec. 111; Reg. § 1.111-1).[184] Common types of recoveries are refunds, reimbursements, and rebates. Refunds of federal income taxes are not included in income because the taxes are not allowed as a deduction from income. Interest on amounts recovered is income in the year of the recovery.

When the refund or other recovery is for amounts that were paid in separate years, the recovery must be allocated between these years.

> **Example 1:** Marcia VanNauker paid her 2014 estimated state income tax liability of $4,000 in four equal installments in April, June, and September of 2014 and in January of 2015. In May of 2015, she received a $400 refund based on her 2014 state income tax return. Because the tax liability was paid in two years, the amount recovered must be allocated pro rata between the years in which the liability was paid. Since 75 percent of the liability was paid in 2014, 75 percent of the $400 refund ($300) is for amounts paid in 2014 and is a recovery item in 2015 when received. The remaining $100 is offset against the otherwise deductible state tax payments made in 2015.

Itemized Deduction Recoveries. Recoveries of amounts that may be claimed only as itemized deductions are not includible if the taxpayer did not itemize in the prior tax year for which the recovery was received. If a deduction was taken, the includible amount is limited to the amount of the deduction. Thus, the amount of the recovery included in income is the lesser of the amount deducted or the amount recovered.

> **Example 2:** Brent Martin receives a $1,500 medical expense reimbursement in 2014 for expenses incurred in 2013. However, due to the threshold on medical expenses, he was able to claim only a $450 deduction in 2013. The amount that he must include in income in 2014 is $450.

For situations in which a high-income individual's itemized deductions for the prior tax year were reduced because his or her adjusted gross income exceeded a threshold amount (¶ 1014), and the taxpayer recovers all or a portion of the previously deducted amount in a later tax year, the amount includible in income in the year of receipt is the difference between (1) the amount of the prior year's itemized deductions (after the overall limitation has been applied) minus (2) the deductions that would have been claimed (i.e., the greater of (a) itemized deductions after the overall limitation, or (b) standard deduction) had the individual paid the proper amount in the prior year and not received a recovery or refund in the later year (Rev. Rul. 93-75).[185]

A taxpayer who recovers any itemized deduction claimed in a prior tax year must generally include in gross income the entire recovered amount in the tax year it is received if, in the prior tax year: (1) itemized deductions exceeded the standard deduction by at least the recovered amount, and were not subject to the overall limitation (¶ 1014); (2) the deduction for the recovered item equals or exceeds the recovered amount; and (3) the taxpayer had taxable income, had no unused tax credits, and was not subject to the alternative minimum tax. If a taxpayer receives a refund of

---

References are to Standard Federal Tax Reports; Tax Research Consultant; and Practical Tax Explanations.

[183] ¶ 43,956, ¶ 43,957D; IN-DIV: 12,210.05; § 19,430.10

[184] ¶ 7060, ¶ 7061; INDIV: 6,300; § 4,210

[185] ¶ 7062.63; INDIV: 6,302.15; § 4,215

¶799

state or local income tax or state or local general sales tax (see *Special Rules for Recovery of State Tax Refunds,* following), the entire refund amount must be recovered if, in addition to the three requirements listed above, the excess of the state or local tax that the taxpayer elected to deduct minus the state or local tax that the taxpayer elected not to deduct is more than the refund amount of the tax deducted (IRS Pub. 525).

IRS Pub. 525 contains a worksheet for computing the amount of a taxable itemized deduction recovery.

Special Rules for Recovery of State Tax Refunds. For tax years beginning after December 31, 2003, but before January 1, 2014, taxpayers may elect to deduct state and local sales taxes instead of state and local income taxes (¶ 1021). If a taxpayer makes this choice, the maximum state and local tax refund amount that he or she may have to include in income in the year the refund is received is limited to the excess of the tax that the taxpayer chose to deduct for the prior tax year minus the tax he or she did not choose to deduct for the prior year (IRS Pub. 525).

If the taxpayer pays state income taxes in Year 1, and then in Year 2 receives a refund of the state income taxes that were paid in Year 1, the refund is not taxable if, in Year 1, the taxpayer (a) did not itemize his deductions, or (b) elected to deduct state and local general sales taxes instead of state and local income taxes (Instructions to Form 1040).

Nonitemized Deduction Recoveries. A taxpayer that receives a recovery of a prior year deduction amount which was not required to be itemized must include the recovery amount in income in the year of receipt, but only up to the amount of the deduction that reduced the taxpayer's income tax in the prior year. If the taxpayer has both itemized and nonitemized recoveries, the amount includible in income is determined by first figuring the amount of the nonitemized recovery to include in income, adding that amount to adjusted gross income, then determining the amount of the itemized recovery to include in income (IRS Pub. 525).

Amounts Recovered for Credits. If a taxpayer claims a tax credit in a prior tax year, other than the foreign tax credit (¶ 2475) or investment tax credit (¶ 1365A), and during the current tax year there is a downward price adjustment or a similar adjustment on the item for which the credit was claimed, the taxpayer's income tax for the current year is increased by the amount of the credit that is attributable to the adjustment (Code Sec. 111(b)). There is no tax increase, however, if the credit did not reduce income tax in the prior year.

Chapter 8

EXCLUSIONS FROM GROSS INCOME

Exclusions from Gross Income

801. Exclusions from Gross Income. Gross income includes all income that is not specifically excludable by statute or administrative and judicial decisions. In addition to the items listed in Code Secs. 101—140, the following are excludable from gross income:

(1) items of income that, under the U.S. Constitution, are not taxable by the federal government;

(2) items of income that are exempt from tax under the provisions of any act of Congress not inconsistent with, or repealed by, the revenue acts; and

(3) items that are nontaxable under the provisions of foreign tax treaties designed to prevent double taxation.

These exclusions and exemptions should not be confused with deductions from gross income, i.e., losses, expenses, bad debts, etc., which must be shown on a tax return. An exclusion generally does *not* have to be shown on a return.

Life Insurance and Death Benefits

803. Life Insurance Proceeds. Life insurance contract proceeds paid by reason of the death of the insured are generally excluded from gross income regardless of whether they represent the return of premiums paid, the increased value of the policy due to investment, or the death benefit feature, i.e., the policy proceeds exceeding the value of the contract immediately prior to the death of the insured.

It is immaterial whether the proceeds are received in a single sum or otherwise. However, if the proceeds are left with the insurer under an agreement to pay interest, any interest earned and paid is income to the recipient (Code Sec. 101; Reg. §§ 1.101-1(a) and 1.101-3).[1]

A contract must qualify as a life insurance contract under applicable state or foreign law and meet either a cash value accumulation test or a guideline premium/cash value corridor test (Code Sec. 7702).[2] If a contract does not satisfy at least one of these tests, it will be treated as a combination of term insurance and a currently taxable deposit fund, and the policyholder must treat income on the contract as ordinary income in any year paid or accrued (Code Sec. 7702(g)).

Amounts received before the insured's death under a life insurance contract on the life of a terminally or chronically ill individual are also excludable from gross income.

References are to Standard Federal Tax Reports; Tax Research Consultant; and Practical Tax Explanations.

[1] ¶ 6502, ¶ 6503, ¶ 6508; IN-DIV: 30,302, INDIV: 30,306; § 3,515.05

[2] ¶ 43,150; INDIV: 30,400; § 3,505

For chronically, but not terminally, ill individuals, the exclusion is subject to a maximum amount per day, adjusted for inflation, under policies that pay a set amount each day known as per diem policies. If a portion of a life insurance contract benefit is assigned or sold to a viatical settlement provider, any amount received from the sale or assignment is generally excludable (Code Sec. 101(g)).[3]

804. Company-Owned Life Insurance (COLI). In the case of a company-owned life insurance (COLI) contract issued after August 17, 2006, there is a limit on the amount of proceeds paid by reason of the death of the employee that may be excludable from gross income (Code Sec. 101(j)).[4] The applicable policyholder, the employer, or a related person generally may only exclude an amount not exceeding the total of the premiums and other amounts paid by the policyholder, with any excess death benefits being includible in gross income.

Exceptions. The income inclusion rule does not apply to an amount received by reason of the death of certain insured individuals if notice and consent requirements are satisfied. This exception applies if the insured:

- was an employee of the applicable policyholder at any time during the 12-month period before the insured's death; or

- at the time the contract was issued with respect to the policyholder, was (a) a director, (b) a highly compensated employee under Code Sec. 414(q), determined without regard to the election regarding the top-paid 20 percent of the employees (¶ 2114), or (c) a highly compensated individual under Code Sec. 105(h)(5), who is in the group of the highest paid 35 percent of employees (¶ 2017).

The inclusion rule also does not apply if certain notice and consent requirements are satisfied with respect to proceeds that are paid: to a member of the insured's family, as defined in Code Sec. 267(c)(4); to any individual who is the designated beneficiary of the insured under the contract, other than the applicable policyholder; to a trust established for the benefit of the insured's family or a designated beneficiary; or to the estate of the insured. In addition, the rule does not apply to proceeds that are used to buy an equity, capital or profits interest in the policyholder from the insured's heir.

An officer, director, or highly compensated employee within the meaning of Code Sec. 414(q) is an employee for these purposes. The exceptions to the inclusion rule apply only if the insured is a U.S. citizen or resident.

Notice and Consent. To keep excess benefits from being included in income, the policyholder must satisfy the following notice and consent requirements before the issuance of the insurance contract:

- the employee must be notified in writing that the policyholder intends to insure the life of the employee and of the maximum face amount for which the employee can be insured;

- the employee must provide written consent to being insured under the contract and acknowledge that such coverage may continue after the insured terminates employment; and

- the employee must be informed in writing that an applicable policyholder will be a beneficiary of any proceeds payable upon death of the employee.

Annual Reporting. The policyholder of the contract must also satisfy annual reporting and record retention requirements (Code Sec. 6039I; Reg. § 1.6039I-1).[5] A policyholder satisfies the reporting requirements by attaching Form 8925 to the policyholder's tax return.

805. Installment Options for Life Insurance Proceeds. If the beneficiary of a life insurance policy receives the proceeds in installments, any interest element in the life

---

References are to Standard Federal Tax Reports; Tax Research Consultant; and Practical Tax Explanations.

[3] ¶ 6502; INDIV: 30,350; § 3,515.10

[4] ¶ 6502; INDIV: 30,304; § 3,515.15

[5] ¶ 35,699C, ¶ 35,699D; FILEBUS: 9,376; § 3,515.15

¶804

insurance proceeds accruing after the date of the insured's death is included in the income of the beneficiary (Code Sec. 101(d); Reg. § 1.101-4).[6]

807. Transfer of Life Insurance Policy. If a life insurance policy is transferred for valuable consideration, payments on account of the death of the insured are income to the transferee to the extent that they exceed the premiums and other consideration given for the life insurance policy (¶ 845). If the policy was transferred as a tax-free exchange or gift, however, the donor's investment basis in the contract is carried over to the donee, and the death benefits are excludable from gross income. The benefits are also excludable if such a transfer of the contract was to the insured, a partner of the insured, a partnership including the insured, or a corporation of which the insured was a shareholder or officer (Code Sec. 101(a)(2); Reg. § 1.101-1(b)).[7]

809. Life Insurance Dividends. Amounts received from an annuity policy prior to the annuity starting date in the nature of dividends, or return of premiums or other consideration, are not taxable until the amounts received exceed the aggregate of premiums or other consideration paid or deemed to have been paid for the annuity. However, amounts received in the nature of dividends after the start date of the annuity may be fully taxable (¶ 823) (Code Sec. 72(e); Reg. § 1.72-11(b)).[8]

813. Death Benefits of Public Safety Officers. The amount paid as a survivor annuity to the spouse, former spouse, or child of a public safety officer killed in the line of duty is excludable from the recipient's gross income if the annuity is provided under a governmental plan (Code Sec. 101(h)).[9]

Gross income also does not include amounts paid by an employer by reason of the death of an employee who is a specified terrorist victim or an astronaut killed in the line of duty. The exclusion applies to death benefits from a qualified plan that satisfy the incidental death benefit rule (Code Sec. 101(i)).[10]

Annuities

817. Exclusion Ratio for Annuities. Amounts received as an annuity under any annuity, endowment, or life insurance contract, and paid out for reasons other than death of the insured, are excludable from income to the extent of the taxpayer's basis in the contract. The tax-free portion of the income is spread evenly over the annuitant's life expectancy. For contracts with an annuity starting date before 1987, the exclusion remains the same, however, no matter how long the annuitant lives. These annuity rules also apply to contracts whose payments are made over a prescribed number of years (Code Sec. 72; Reg. § § 1.72-1—1.72-11).[11] For Armed Forces personnel annuities, see ¶ 891.

A contract, with certain exceptions, will not be treated as an annuity contract unless it provides that: (1) if the contract holder dies on or after the annuity starting date, but before the entire interest in the contract is distributed, the remainder must be distributed at least as rapidly as under the method used as of the day the holder died, and (2) the entire interest in the contract must be distributed within five years of the holder's death (Code Sec. 72(s)).[12]

To determine the portion of the annuity that is excludable from the recipient's gross income, an "exclusion ratio" is to be determined for each contract (¶ 819). This ratio is usually determined by dividing the "investment in the contract" by the "expected return" (Code Sec. 72(b); Reg. § 1.72-2).[13] The exclusion ratio is then applied to the total amount received as an annuity during the tax year. Any excess amount over the portion determined by the application of the exclusion ratio is includible in the recipient's gross income (Reg. § 1.72-4). In the case of distributions from an individual retirement

References are to Standard Federal Tax Reports; Tax Research Consultant; and Practical Tax Explanations.

[6] ¶ 6502, ¶ 6510; INDIV: 30,308; § 3,515.05
[7] ¶ 6502, ¶ 6503; INDIV: 30,310; § 3,515.05
[8] ¶ 6102, ¶ 6113; COMPEN: 48,058; § 3,510
[9] ¶ 6502; INDIV: 33,560; § 3,530.05
[10] ¶ 6502; INDIV: 33,562; § 3,530.10
[11] ¶ 6102; ¶ 6102B–¶ 6113; INDIV: 30,056; § 3,210
[12] ¶ 6102; INDIV: 30,206; § 3,260.05
[13] ¶ 6102, ¶ 6102D; INDIV: 30,050; § 3,210

arrangement (IRA), the exclusion ratio is determined by dividing the employee's total nondeductible contributions by the balance of the account. All of an individual's IRAs and distributions during a year must be aggregated (¶ 2165). A nontaxable distribution of IRA assets is reported on Form 8606 (Instructions to Form 8606; IRS Pub. 590).

For annuities with a starting date *after* 1986, the exclusion of a portion of each annuity payment cannot be continued indefinitely. Once the total of all exclusions taken for payments under the annuity contract equals the investment in the contract, all subsequent payments are included in income in full (Code Sec. 72(b)(2)). On the other hand, if the annuitant dies before the investment in the contract is fully recovered tax free through the annuity exclusion, a deduction is provided for the annuitant's last year in an amount equal to the unrecovered portion of the investment (Code Sec. 72(b)(3)).

Partial Annuitization of Annuity Contracts. For amounts received in tax years beginning after December 31, 2010, if any amount is received as an annuity for a period of 10 years or more, or for the lives of one or more individuals, under any portion of an annuity, endowment, or life insurance contract, then that portion of the contract is treated as a separate contract (Code Sec. 72(a)(2)). Thus, a portion of the contract may be annuitized, while the balance is not annuitized. In these cases, the investment in the contract is allocated on a pro rata basis between each portion of the contract from which amounts are received as an annuity and the portion of the contract from which amounts are not received as an annuity. The allocation is made for purposes of applying:

(1) the rules relating to the exclusion ratio;

(2) the definitions of the investment in the contract, the expected return, and the annuity starting date; and

(3) the rules for amounts not received as an annuity.

In addition, a separate annuity starting date is determined with respect to each portion of the contract from which amounts are received as an annuity.

819. The "Exclusion Ratio" Formula. The excludable portion of an annuity payment is the annuity payment multiplied by the "exclusion ratio" (¶ 817). The remainder is taxable to the recipient, whether it is the primary annuitant or a secondary annuitant under a joint annuity or joint and survivor annuity. The exclusion ratio is the "investment in the contract" (¶ 821) divided by the "expected return" (¶ 825) under the contract as of the "annuity starting date" (¶ 823). For example, if, as of the annuity starting date, a taxpayer's investment in an annuity contract is $6,000 and his expected return is $10,000, his exclusion ratio is $6,000/$10,000, or 60 percent. If the taxpayer receives a monthly annuity payment of $200, the monthly exclusion is $120 ($200 × 60 percent).

821. "Investment in the Contract" Defined. In determining the exclusion ratio for an annuity (¶ 819), the "investment in the contract" generally is the total amount of premiums or other consideration paid for the contract, less amounts, if any, received before the "annuity starting date" and not included in gross income (Code Sec. 72(c)(1); Reg. § 1.72-6).[14] However, owner-employees may not include the deductible costs of purchasing insurance as part of their investment in the contract (Code Sec. 72(m)(2); Reg. § 1.72-17A(c)). A special adjustment is provided for a refund annuity (¶ 837). For special rules for computing an employee's investment in an annuity received through an employer, see ¶ 2143.

Nonresident Aliens. Certain employer or employee contributions made by or on behalf of nonresident aliens are not considered part of the individual's investment in the contract. The excluded contributions are those:

(1) made with respect to compensation for labor or services by an employee who was a nonresident alien at the time the labor or services were performed and treated as from sources outside the United States; and

(2) that were not subject to tax by the United States or a foreign country but would have been subject to tax if paid in cash.

References are to Standard Federal Tax Reports; Tax Research Consultant; and Practical Tax Explanations.

[14] ¶ 6102, ¶ 6107; INDIV: 30,060; § 3,220.05

Thus, contributions to a foreign pension plan are included in the calculation of the participant's basis only if the participant has been subject to tax on the contribution by the United States or a foreign country (Code Sec. 72(w)).[15]

823. "Annuity Starting Date" Defined. In determining the exclusion ratio for an annuity (¶ 819), the "annuity starting date" is the first day of the first period for which an amount is received as an annuity under the contract. This is the later of:

(1) the date upon which the obligations of the contract become fixed; or

(2) the first day of the period (year, half-year, quarter, or month, depending on whether the payments are made annually, semi-annually, quarterly, or monthly) that ends on the date of the first annuity payment (Code Sec. 72(c)(4); Reg. § 1.72-4(b)).[16]

825. "Expected Return" Computation. In determining the exclusion ratio for an annuity (¶ 819), the "expected return" under the contract is limited to amounts receivable as an annuity or as annuities. If no life expectancy is involved, as in the case of installment payments for a fixed number of years, the expected return is found by totaling the amounts to be received (Code Sec. 72(c)(3); Reg. § 1.72-5(a) and (c)).[17] To determine the expected return under contracts involving life expectancy, actuarial tables prescribed by the IRS must be used. The tables provide a multiplier, based on life expectancy, that is applied to the annual payment to obtain the expected return under the contract (Reg. § 1.72-9).

The expected return will vary, depending on when contributions were made and when amounts were received as an annuity. Gender-neutral tables must be used if the total investment in the contract is made after June 30, 1986. If there was an investment in the contract as of June 30, 1986, and there has been a further investment in the contract after that date, an individual may, instead of using the gender-neutral tables, elect to calculate the exclusion under a special rule. Under this rule, an exclusion amount is calculated using the gender-based tables—as if the investment in the contract as of June 30, 1986, were the only investment in the contract. Then a second exclusion is calculated, using the gender-neutral tables, as if the post-June 30, 1986, investment were the only investment. The two exclusion amounts are then added together to produce the final exclusion. Although, generally, the gender-based annuity tables formerly in effect must still be used if all contributions were made prior to June 30, 1986, an election may be made to use the updated tables if the annuity payments are received after June 30, 1986 (Reg. §§ 1.72-5 and 1.72-6).[18]

For use in the following examples, a portion of Table V (gender-neutral for post-June 30, 1986, investment in the contract (Reg. § 1.72-9))[19] for ordinary life annuities for one life is reproduced below:

TABLE V.—ORDINARY LIFE ANNUITIES—ONE LIFE—EXPECTED RETURN MULTIPLES

Age	Multiple	Age	Multiple
55	28.6	64	20.8
56	27.7	65	20.0
57	26.8	66	19.2
58	25.9	67	18.4
59	25.0	68	17.6
60	24.2	69	16.8
61	23.3	70	16.0
62	22.5	71	15.3
63	21.6	72	14.6

References are to Standard Federal Tax Reports; Tax Research Consultant; and Practical Tax Explanations.

[15] ¶ 6102; RETIRE: 42,304.05; § 3,220.05

[16] ¶ 6102, ¶ 6104; INDIV: 30,054.15; § 3,205

[17] ¶ 6102, ¶ 6106; INDIV: 30,058; § 3,215.05

[18] ¶ 6106, ¶ 6107; INDIV: 30,058; § 3,215.05

[19] ¶ 165; INDIV: 30,058.05; § 910

Example 1: In 2014, X purchases for $8,000 an annuity that provides for payments to him of $50 per month for life. At the annuity starting date, his age at his nearest birthday is 64 years. Table V (gender-neutral) must be used since all his investment in the contract is post-June 1986. Table V shows that for an individual of X's age, the multiple to be used in computing the expected return is 20.8. X's expected return and annual exclusion, therefore, are computed as follows:

Annual payment ($50 per month × 12 months)	$600
Table V multiple	20.8
Expected return ($600 × 20.8)	$12,480
Exclusion ratio . . . . $\frac{8,000}{12,480}$, or 64.10%	
Annual exclusion (64.10% of $600)	$384.60

If payments under the contract are made quarterly, semiannually, or annually, or if the interval between the annuity starting date and the date of the first payment is less than the interval between future payments, an adjustment of the multiple found in the actuarial tables may be required (Reg. § 1.72-5).[20] The amount of the adjustment is found in the following table:

If the number of whole months from the annuity starting date to the first payment date is	0-1	2	3	4	5	6	7	8	9	10	11	12
And payments under the contract are to be made:												
Annually	+.5	+.4	+.3	+.2	+.1	0	0	–.1	–.2	–.3	–.4	–.5
Semiannually	+.2	+.1	0	0	–.1	–.2	..	..	..	..	..	..
Quarterly	+.1	0	–.1	..	..	..	..	..	..	..	..	..

Example 2: Assume the same facts as in Example 1 above, except that the payments under the contract are to be made semiannually in the amount of $300, the first payment being made six full months from the annuity starting date. The table shows the adjustment to be "–.2". Therefore, X's multiple from Table V, 20.8, is adjusted by subtracting 0.2. His adjusted multiple then is 20.6, and his expected return and semiannual exclusion are computed as follows:

Annual payment ($300 × 2)	$600
Table V adjusted multiple	20.6
Expected return ($600 × 20.6)	$12,360
Exclusion ratio . . . . $\frac{8,000}{12,360}$, or 64.72%	
Semiannual exclusion (64.72% of $300)	$194.16

There is a simpler computation, illustrated in Example 3, but it may be used only if the annuity amount does not vary from year to year. This computation determines the annual exclusion by dividing the taxpayer's investment in the contract, i.e., the taxpayer's cost, by the appropriate multiple from the actuarial tables.

Example 3: Assume the same facts as in Example 1. X's annual exclusion is computed as follows:

Cost of annuity	$8,000
Annual payment ($50 per month × 12 months) . . .	$600
Table V multiple	20.8
Annual exclusion . . . . $\frac{8,000}{20.8}$	$385
Annual taxable income ($600 less $385)	$215

References are to Standard Federal Tax Reports; Tax Research Consultant; and Practical Tax Explanations.

[20] ¶ 6106; INDIV: 30,058.10; § 3,215.10

827. Joint and Survivor Annuities and Joint Annuities. In the case of a joint and survivor annuity contract that provides the first annuitant with a fixed monthly income for life and, after his or her death, provides an identical monthly income for life to the second annuitant, the multiple used in computing expected return is found in Table II (gender-based) or Table VI (gender-neutral) under the ages of the living annuitants as of the annuity starting date (Reg. § 1.72-5(b)).[21] For use in the following example, a portion of Table VI (gender-neutral for post-June 30, 1986, investment in the contract) providing expected return multiples for ordinary joint life and last survivor annuities for two lives is reproduced below.

TABLE VI.—ORDINARY JOINT LIFE AND LAST SURVIVOR ANNUITIES—TWO LIVES— EXPECTED RETURN MULTIPLES

Ages	65	66	67	68	69	70	71	72
65	25.0	24.6	24.2	23.8	23.4	23.1	22.8	22.5
66	24.6	24.1	23.7	23.3	22.9	22.5	22.2	21.9
67	24.2	23.7	23.2	22.8	22.4	22.0	21.7	21.3
68	23.8	23.3	22.8	22.3	21.9	21.5	21.2	20.8
69	23.4	22.9	22.4	21.9	21.5	21.1	20.7	20.3
70	23.1	22.5	22.0	21.5	21.1	20.6	20.2	19.8
71	22.8	22.2	21.7	21.2	20.7	20.2	19.8	19.4
72	22.5	21.9	21.3	20.8	20.3	19.8	19.4	18.9

Example: In 2014, Y purchased a joint and survivor annuity providing for payments of $200 a month to be made to Y for life and, upon his death, to his wife, Z, during her lifetime. At the annuity starting date Y's age at his nearest birthday is 68 and Z's is 66. The annuity cost is $44,710. The expected return is as follows:

Annual payment ($200 × 12)	$2,400
Table VI multiple (age 68; age 66)	23.3
Expected return ($2,400 × 23.3)	$55,920

The annual exclusion for both Y and Z is computed as follows:

Exclusion ratio . . . . $\frac{44,710}{55,920}$, or 79.95%

Annual exclusion (79.95% of $2,400) $1,918.80

If a joint and survivor annuity provides for a different monthly income, rather than an identical monthly income, payable to the second annuitant, there is a special computation of expected return that involves the use of both Table I and Table II or Table V and Table VI, whichever are applicable. If a contract involving two annuitants provides for fixed monthly payments to be made as a joint life annuity until the death of the first annuitant, in other words, only as long as both remain alive, the expected return for such a contract is determined under either Table IIA or Table VIA, whichever is applicable. Adjustment of the multiple obtained from the annuity tables, as explained at ¶ 825 for single life annuities, may also be necessary for joint and survivor annuities and joint annuities if payments are made less often than monthly or if the first payment is accelerated.

829. Special Types of Annuities. To compute the exclusion ratio (¶ 819) for a contract that is acquired for a single consideration and that provides for the payment of two or more annuity obligations or elements, the investment in the contract is divided by the aggregate of the expected returns under all the annuity elements (Reg. §§ 1.72-4(e), 1.72-5(e), and 1.72-6(b)).[22] In the case of variable annuities, a special rule is provided for determining the portion of each payment to be "an amount received as an annuity" and excludable from gross income each year (Reg. § 1.72-2(b)(3)).[23] The computation of the expected return for temporary life annuities is determined by multiplying the total of the

---

References are to Standard Federal Tax Reports; Tax Research Consultant; and Practical Tax Explanations.

[21] ¶ 6106; INDIV: 30,066; §3,215.15

[22] ¶ 6104, ¶ 6106, ¶ 6107; INDIV: 30,070; §3,205

[23] ¶ 6102D; INDIV: 30,068; §3,235

annuity payments to be received annually by the multiple shown in Table IV or Table VIII, whichever is applicable, under the annuitant's age as of the annuity starting date and, if applicable, the annuitant's gender, and the nearest whole number of years in the specified period (Reg. § 1.72-5(a)(3)—(5)).[24]

835. Exclusion for Year Annuity Begins. If the first payment an annuitant receives is for a fractional part of a year, the annuitant need only determine the exclusion ratio (¶ 819) as a percentage and apply it to the payment received for the fractional part of the payment period, resulting in the amount of the annuitant's exclusion for the tax year (Reg. § 1.72-4(a)).[25]

> **Example:** John purchased an annuity that provides for semiannual payments of $3,000. The annuity starting date is November 1, and on December 31, John received $1,000 as his first payment under the contract. John's exclusion percentage is 70 percent. He may exclude 70 percent of $1,000, or $700, from his calendar-year income.

837. Refund Annuity. If an annuity contract has a refund feature, including a contract for a life annuity with a minimum period of payments certain, an adjustment must be made to the original investment in the contract when determining the exclusion ratio (¶ 819). The original investment in the contract must be reduced by the value of the refund payment or payment certain as of the annuity starting date (Code Sec. 72(b)(4) and (c); Reg. § 1.72-7).[26] The computation of the adjustment is detailed and involves the use of Table III (gender-based) or Table VII (gender-neutral) of Reg. § 1.72-9.[27]

Generally, an annuity contract contains a refund feature if:

> (1) the annuity payments depend, in whole or in part, upon the continuing life of one or more persons;

> (2) there are payments on or after the death of the annuitant if a specified amount or a stated number of payments has not been made prior to death; and

> (3) the payments are in the nature of a refund of the consideration paid (Code Sec. 72(c)(2); Reg. § 1.72-7).[28]

839. Employee's Annuity. Amounts received as an annuity from qualified employee plans under Code Sec. 401(a), employee annuities under Code Sec. 403(a), and annuity contracts under Code Sec. 403(b) are subject to a simplified method for computing the taxable and tax-free portion of the distributions (Code Sec. 72(d); Notice 98-2).[29]

Post-November 18, 1996, Annuities. Under the simplified method for annuity starting dates beginning after November 18, 1996, but before January 1, 1998, the total number of monthly annuity payments expected to be received is based on the primary annuitant's age at the annuity starting date. The same expected number of payments applies to a single life annuity or a joint and survivor annuity. The expected number of payments is set forth in the following table:

References are to Standard Federal Tax Reports; Tax Research Consultant; and Practical Tax Explanations.

[24] ¶ 6106; INDIV: 30,058.15; § 3,215.05

[25] ¶ 6104; INDIV: 30,056; § 3,210

[26] ¶ 6102, ¶ 6108; INDIV: 30,068; § 3,220.05

[27] ¶ 165; INDIV: 30,062; § 3,220.10

[28] ¶ 6102, ¶ 6108; INDIV: 30,062, RETIRE: 42,304; § 3,220.10

[29] ¶ 17,502, ¶ 18,270, ¶ 6102, ¶ 6140.82; RETIRE: 42,304.10; § 24,405.10

Age of Primary Annuitant on the Annuity Starting Date	Number of Anticipated Payments
55 and under	360
56-60	310
61-65	260
66-70	210
71 and over	160

For annuity starting dates after December 31, 1997, annuities paid over the life of a single individual have anticipated payments as listed in the table above. If, however, the annuity is payable over the lives of more than one individual, the number of anticipated payments is listed in the table below:

Combined Age of Annuitants	Number of Anticipated Payments
110 and under	410
More than 110 but not more than 120	360
More than 120 but not more than 130	310
More than 130 but not more than 140	260
More than 140	210

The number of anticipated payments listed in the table above is based on the employee's age on the annuity starting date. If the number of payments is fixed under the terms of the annuity, that number is to be used rather than the number of anticipated payments listed in the table.

Example 1: At retirement, Jeff Anderson, age 65, begins receiving retirement benefits in the form of a joint and 50-percent survivor annuity to be paid for the joint lives of Jeff and his wife, Jan, age 59. Jeff's annuity starting date is January 1, 2014. Jeff contributed $24,000 to the plan and has received no distributions prior to the annuity starting date. He will receive a monthly retirement benefit of $1,000, and his wife Jan will receive a monthly survivor benefit of $500 upon his death. Jeff's investment in the contract is $24,000 (the after-tax contributions to the plan). The set number of monthly payments will be 310 (Jeff's age, 65, plus Jan's age, 59, at the starting date of the annuity equals 124). The tax-free portion of each $1,000 monthly annuity payment to Jeff is now $77.42, determined by dividing Jeff's investment ($24,000) by the number of monthly payments (310). If Jeff has not recovered the full $24,000 investment at his death, Jan will exclude $77.42 from each $500 monthly annuity payment. Any annuity payments received after 310 payments have been made will be includible in gross income. If Jeff and his wife die before 310 payments have been made, a deduction is allowed on the survivor's last income tax return in the amount of the unrecovered investment.

The simplified method does not apply if the primary annuitant has attained age 75 on the annuity starting date unless there are fewer than five years of guaranteed payments under the annuity (Code Sec. 72(d)(1)(E)). Also, if in connection with commencement of annuity payments, the recipient receives a lump-sum payment that is not part of the annuity stream, then the payment is taxed under the annuity rules of Code Sec. 72(e) as if received before the annuity starting date and the investment in the contract used to calculate the simplified exclusion ratio for the annuity payments is reduced by the amount of the payment (Code Sec. 72(d)(1)(D)).

Pre-November 19, 1996, Annuities. The IRS provided an elective alternative to application of the usual annuity rules for distributions from qualified plans when the annuity starting date was before November 19, 1996. This is a simplified safe-harbor method for determining the tax-free and taxable portions of certain annuity payments made from qualified employee plans, employee annuities, and annuity contracts (Notice 88-118).[30] Distributees who elected to use this method are considered to have complied with Code Sec. 72(b). Payors may also use this method to report the taxable portion of

References are to Standard Federal Tax Reports; Tax Research Consultant; and Practical Tax Explanations.

[30] ¶ 6140.82; RETIRE: 42,304.15; § 24,405.10

the annuity payments on Form 1099-R. The safe-harbor method may be used *only* if the following three conditions are met:

(1) the annuity payments depend upon the life of the distributee or the joint lives of the distributee and beneficiary;

(2) the annuity payments are made from an employee plan qualified under Code Sec. 401(a), an employee annuity under Code Sec. 403(a), or an annuity contract under Code Sec. 403(b); and

(3) the distributee is less than age 75 when annuity payments commence or, if the distributee is age 75 or older, there are fewer than five years of guaranteed payments.

Under the safe-harbor method, the total number of monthly annuity payments expected to be received is based on the distributee's age at the annuity starting date rather than on the life expectancy tables in Reg. § 1.72-9. The same expected number of payments applies to a distributee whether the individual is receiving a single life annuity or a joint and survivor annuity. These payments are set forth in the following table:

Age of Distributee	*Number of Payments*
55 and under	300
56-60	260
61-65	240
66-70	170
71 and over	120

Under the safe-harbor method, the distributee recovers the investment in the contract in level amounts over the number of monthly payments determined from the above table. The portion of each monthly annuity payment that is excluded from gross income by a distributee who uses the safe-harbor method for income tax purposes is a level dollar amount determined by dividing the investment in the contract, including any applicable death benefit exclusion, by the set number of annuity payments from the above table as follows:

$$\frac{\text{Investment}}{\text{Number of monthly payments}} = \begin{array}{c}\text{Tax-free}\\\text{portion of}\\\text{monthly annuity}\end{array}$$

For distributees with annuity starting dates after 1986, annuity payments received after the investment is recovered, usually after the set number of payments has been received, are fully includible in gross income.

Example 2: Assume the same facts as in Example 1 above, except Jeff's annuity start date was January 1, 1996. Under the safe-harbor method, Jeff's investment in the contract is $24,000 (the after-tax contributions to the plan). The set number of monthly payments for a distributee who is age 65 is 240. The tax-free portion of each $1,000 monthly annuity payment to Jeff is $100, determined by dividing Jeff's investment ($24,000) by the number of monthly payments (240). If Jeff has not recovered the full $24,000 investment at his death, Jan will also exclude $100 from each $500 monthly annuity payment. Any annuity payments received after 240 payments have been made will be fully includible in gross income. If Jeff and his wife die before 240 payments have been made, a deduction is allowed on the survivor's last income tax return in the amount of the unrecovered investment.

The dollar amount is excluded from each monthly payment even if the annuity payment amount changes. If the amount excluded is greater than the amount of the monthly annuity, because of decreased survivor payments, each monthly annuity payment is excluded completely until the entire investment is recovered. If annuity payments cease before the set number of payments has been made, a deduction for the unrecovered investment is allowed on the distributee's last tax return. If payments are made to multiple beneficiaries, the excludable amount is based on the oldest beneficiary's age. A pro rata portion is excluded by each beneficiary.

General Rules. For purposes of these rules, the investment in the contract (¶ 821) is determined without regard to the adjustment made for a refund feature (Code Sec. 72(d)(1)(C)).

¶839

In any case where the annuity payments are not made on a monthly basis, appropriate adjustments must be made to take into account the basis on which the payments are actually made (Code Sec. 72(d)(1)(F)).

Employee contributions under a defined contribution plan may be treated as a separate contract (Code Sec. 72(d)(2)).

Railroad Retirement Act Tier 2 benefits received by retired railroad workers and their survivors are subject to federal income tax in the same manner as pension plan benefits paid by private employers (Code Sec. 72(r)).[31]

841. Discharge of Annuity Obligation. Any amount received, whether in a single sum or otherwise, under an annuity, endowment, or life insurance contract in full discharge of the obligation under the contract as a refund of the consideration paid for the contract or any amount received under such contract on its complete surrender, redemption, or maturity is includible in gross income to the extent the amounts exceed the investment in the contract (Code Sec. 72(e); Reg. § 1.72-11).[32] The remainder is taxable to the recipient, whether the recipient is the primary annuitant or a secondary annuitant under a joint annuity or joint and survivor annuity. A penalty is imposed on a policyholder who receives a premature distribution, e.g., before age 59½, unless one of a number of exceptions, such as death or disability, applies (Code Sec. 72(q)).[33]

843. Installment Options for Annuities. If an insured elects under an option in an insurance contract to receive the proceeds as an annuity, instead of a lump sum, and the election is made within 60 days after the day on which the lump sum first became payable, no part of it is taxable under the doctrine of constructive receipt (Code Sec. 72(h); Reg. § 1.72-12).[34] The installment payments are taxed in accordance with the annuity rules.

845. Transfer of Annuities. If a life insurance, endowment, or annuity contract is transferred for a valuable consideration, and the proceeds of the contract are paid to the transferee for reasons other than the death of the insured, e.g., on surrender, redemption, or maturity of the contract, the transferee, including a beneficiary of, or the estate of, a transferee, is taxed as follows:

(1) if the proceeds are received as an annuity or in installments for a fixed period, the transferee computes the tax under the exclusion ratio formula (¶ 819); or

(2) if the proceeds are received in a lump sum, the transferee includes in income only that portion of the proceeds in excess of the consideration paid.

Regardless of how the proceeds are received and taxed, the transferee's consideration paid consists of the actual value of the consideration paid for the transfer, plus the amount of premiums or other consideration paid after the transfer. This transferee rule, however, does not apply if the transferred contract has a basis for gain or loss in the hands of the transferee determined by reference to the transferor's basis, as in the case of a gift or tax-free exchange (Code Sec. 72(g); Reg. § 1.72-10).[35]

A loss realized upon the surrender or forfeiture of an annuity contract by the original purchaser is deductible as an ordinary loss under Code Sec. 165, the basis of the contract being its cost less the amounts previously excluded from gross income (Rev. Rul. 61-201).[36] The IRS maintains that the loss is deducted on Form 1040, Schedule A as a miscellaneous itemized deduction subject to the two-percent-of-adjusted-gross-income floor (IRS Pub. 575).

References are to Standard Federal Tax Reports; Tax Research Consultant; and Practical Tax Explanations.

[31] ¶ 6102; INDIV: 33,358

[32] ¶ 6102, ¶ 6113; INDIV: 30,102.10; § 3,230.10

[33] ¶ 6102; INDIV: 30,204; § 3,255

[34] ¶ 6102, ¶ 6117; INDIV: 30,208; § 3,265.35

[35] ¶ 6102, ¶ 6112; INDIV: 30,064; § 3,220.05

[36] ¶ 9900.111; INDIV: 30,216; § 3,245.10

8

EXCLUSIONS

¶845

Bequests and Gifts

847. Bequests Excluded from Gross Income. The value of property acquired by bequest, devise, or inheritance is excludable from gross income (Code Sec. 102; Reg. § 1.102-1).[37] The *income* flowing from the property, however, is *not* exempt, as, for example, amounts received as investment income from the property or as profit from a sale of the property. The exclusion also does not apply if the bequest consists of income from property. Thus, a bequest of annual rent from the testator's property for 10 years is taxable income to the beneficiary. The beneficiary is required to include in gross income each year the amount of the annual rent. For the basis of inherited property, see ¶ 1633—¶ 1639.

A bequest of a specific sum of money or of specific property from an estate or trust may be exempt from tax if it is paid or credited all at once or in not more than three installments (Code Sec. 663(a)(1); Reg. § 1.663(a)-1).[38] An amount which is paid from the estate or trust income may qualify as a bequest for this purpose if the amount could have been paid from either income or principal. An amount that can only be paid from the estate or trust income, however, will not be treated as a bequest and, thus, will *not* be exempt even when paid in less than four installments.

849. Gifts Excluded from Gross Income. The value of a gift is excludable from gross income, but *any income* from the gift, including profit upon sale, is taxable (Code Sec. 102).[39] A gift of income from the property of an estate or trust is not exempt except in the case of a gift of a specific sum or of specific property paid or credited all at once or in not more than three installments (¶ 847). For a donee's basis for gift property, see ¶ 1630.

Tips are not gifts and are therefore taxable (¶ 717). Food, clothing, and rent payments furnished as strike benefits by a labor union to a needy worker participating in a strike may be considered gifts. In determining whether a gift was made, the fact that benefits were paid only to union members is not controlling.[40]

The exclusion from gross income applicable to the value of property acquired by gift does not apply to any amount transferred by or for an employer to, or for the benefit of, an employee (Code Sec. 102(c)).[41] However, certain employee achievement awards (¶ 2069) and certain fringe benefits provided by employers are excludable (¶ 2085).

Personal Injury and Disability Proceeds

851. Occupational Disability or Insurance Benefit. Compensation received under a workers' compensation act for personal injuries or sickness and amounts received by a taxpayer under a policy of accident and health insurance are excludable from gross income (Code Sec. 104(a)(1); Reg. § 1.104-1).[42] The exclusion also applies to benefits having the characteristics of life insurance proceeds paid under a workers' compensation act to the survivor or survivors of a deceased employee (Reg. § 1.101-1(a)).[43] For a discussion of disability income plans, see ¶ 2025.

Amounts received as a pension, annuity, or similar allowance for personal injuries or sickness resulting from active service in the armed forces of any country or in the Coast and Geodetic Survey or the Public Health Service, or as a disability annuity payable under section 808 of the Foreign Service Act of 1980, are also excludable from gross income (Code Sec. 104(a)(4); Reg. § 1.104-1).[44] The exclusion generally is limited to amounts received for combat-related injury or illness. However, the exclusion will not be less than the maximum amount of disability compensation from the Veterans Administration to which the individual is, or would be, entitled upon application (Code Sec. 104(b)).

References are to Standard Federal Tax Reports; Tax Research Consultant; and Practical Tax Explanations.

[37] ¶ 6550, ¶ 6551; INDIV: 33,102, INDIV: 33,104; § 3,601

[38] ¶ 24,440, ¶ 24,441; INDIV: 33,104; § 32,710.05g

[39] ¶ 6550; INDIV: 33,102, INDIV: 33,104; § 3,601, § 3,615

[40] ¶ 6553.46; COMPEN: 6,068; § 22,110.40

[41] ¶ 6550; INDIV: 33,102.05; § 3,605.10

[42] ¶ 6660, ¶ 6661; INDIV: 33,406, HEALTH: 12,200; § 3,705.10

[43] ¶ 6503; INDIV: 30,302.05

[44] ¶ 6660, ¶ 6661; INDIV: 33,410; § 42,210

Benefits that are payable under state law for occupational injury or illness arising out of employment are nontaxable if the benefits are in the nature of workers' compensation payments (Reg. § 1.104-1(b)).[45] No fault insurance disability benefits received by a passenger injured in an automobile accident under the automobile owner's policy as compensation for loss of income or earning capacity are also excludable from gross income.[46]

If an otherwise excludable amount is for reimbursement of medical expenses previously deducted for tax purposes, the amount must be included in gross income to the extent of the prior deduction. If a portion of an award is specifically allocated to future injury-related medical expenses, the future expenses must be offset by the awarded portion and are not deductible to that extent.[47]

Terrorist Attacks. Disability income received by an individual for injuries received in a terrorist attack while the individual was performing services as a U.S. employee outside the United States is also excludable from gross income (Code Sec. 104(a)(5)).[48]

852. Damages for Personal Injuries or Sickness. Amounts received as damages, other than punitive damages, on account of *personal physical injuries or sickness* are excludable from income (Code Sec. 104(a)(2)).[49] Damages for emotional distress, including the physical symptoms of emotional distress, may not be treated as damages on account of a personal physical injury or sickness, except to the extent of amounts paid for medical care attributable to emotional distress. Accordingly, back pay received in satisfaction of a claim for denial of a promotion due to employment discrimination is not excludable because it is "completely independent of," and thus is *not* "damages received on account of," personal physical injuries or sickness (Rev. Rul. 96-65).

Interest and Punitive Damage Awards. Interest included in an award of damages for personal injury is includible in gross income.[50] Also, punitive damages arising out of personal physical injury action are includible in gross income (Code Sec. 104(a)(2)).[51] Punitive damages may be excludable from income, however, if received in a civil action for wrongful death and the applicable state law provides that *only* punitive damages may be awarded (Code Sec. 104(c)).

Attorney's Fees. The full amount of a litigant's award, including the attorney's contingent fee, regardless of whether paid directly to the attorney or to the individual, is includible in the litigant's gross income under the anticipatory assignment of income theory (*J.W. Banks II*, SCt, 2005-1 USTC ¶ 50,155).[52] For a discussion of the deduction of legal fees and court costs as a miscellaneous deduction, see ¶ 1093. However, attorneys' fees and court costs paid in prosecuting claims based on unlawful discrimination and certain other federal claims, including but not limited to whistleblower actions, are deductible from gross income as an above-the-line deduction (¶ 1010A) (Code Sec. 62(a)).

Cancellation of Debt

855. Discharge of Debt. Income from the discharge of indebtedness is includible in gross income unless it is excludable under Code Sec. 108 or other applicable legislative provision. Five types of exclusions are provided:

(1) a debt discharge in a bankruptcy action under Title 11 of the U.S. Code in which the taxpayer is under the jurisdiction of the court and the discharge is either granted by or is under a plan approved by the court;

References are to Standard Federal Tax Reports; Tax Research Consultant; and Practical Tax Explanations.

[45] ¶ 6661; INDIV: 33,406; § 3,705.05

[46] ¶ 6662.24; INDIV: 33,408; § 42,205

[47] ¶ 6662.41; INDIV: 33,402.10; § 7,210.05

[48] ¶ 6660; HEALTH: 12,256; § 3,710

[49] ¶ 6660; INDIV: 33,402; § 3,805.05

[50] ¶ 6662.513; INDIV: 12,112; § 3,805.35

[51] ¶ 6660; INDIV: 33,402.05; § 3,805.30

[52] ¶ 6662.515; INDIV: 6,358.05; § 3,805.40

¶855

(2) a discharge when the taxpayer is insolvent outside bankruptcy;

(3) a discharge of qualified farm indebtedness;

(4) a discharge of qualified real property business indebtedness, and

(5) a discharge of qualified principal residence indebtedness occurring before January 1, 2014 (Code Sec. 108).[53]

Under certain circumstances, income from the cancellation of student loans is also excludable (see *Student Loans*, following). Form 982 is filed with a debtor's income tax return to report excludable income from the discharge of indebtedness.

A corporation that satisfies a debt by transferring corporate stock to its creditor, or a partnership that transfers a capital or profits interest in the partnership to a creditor, is treated as if it has paid the creditor with money equal to the fair market value of the stock or interest. The corporation or partnership will thus have income from discharge of indebtedness to the extent that the principal of the debt exceeds the value of the stock or partnership interest and any other property transferred (Code Sec. 108(e)(8)).[54] A similar rule applies to debtors, corporate or noncorporate, issuing debt instruments in satisfaction of indebtedness (Code Sec. 108(e)(10)).

Discharge of indebtedness income can result even if the cancelled debt is nonrecourse, i.e., no individual is personally liable for repayment of the debt. Thus, where property securing a nonrecourse debt is transferred in exchange for cancellation of the debt, such as a foreclosure sale, the amount realized from the sale or exchange includes the principal amount of the debt discharged. The IRS has ruled that the writedown of the principal amount of a nonrecourse note by a holder who was not the seller of the property results in the realization of discharge of indebtedness income, even if there is no disposition of the property (Rev. Rul. 91-31).[55]

Effect of Exclusion on Tax Attributes. When an amount is excluded from gross income as the result of a discharge of indebtedness in a Title 11 bankruptcy case, a discharge of indebtedness during insolvency, or a discharge of qualified farm indebtedness, a taxpayer is required to reduce its tax attributes. The reduction in the foreign tax credit, minimum tax credit, passive activity credit, and general business credit carryovers is to be made at a rate of $33\frac{1}{3}$ cents per dollar of excluded income (Code Sec. 108(b)(3)(B)).[56]

Insolvency. The term "insolvent" refers to an excess of liabilities over the fair market value of assets immediately prior to discharge. This exclusion is limited to the amount by which the taxpayer is insolvent. The taxpayer's insolvent amount includes the amount by which a nonrecourse debt exceeds the fair market value of the property securing the debt, but only to the extent that the excess nonrecourse debt is discharged.[57]

Nonrecourse debt in excess of the property's fair market value is separated into two components for purposes of the insolvency exception. First, the excess nonrecourse debt that is forgiven is treated as a liability for purposes of the insolvency exception. Otherwise, the debt discharge could result in a tax when the debtor lacks the ability to pay it. Second, the excess of nonrecourse debt that is not forgiven is not treated as a liability for purposes of the insolvency exception. The IRS's reasoning is that nondischarged debt does not directly impede the taxpayer's ability to pay tax on discharge of recourse or nonrecourse debt, and thus, is not relevant in determining the extent of his insolvency (Rev. Rul. 92-53). The IRS has extended these principles to determine the extent a partner may be insolvent under Code Sec. 108(d)(3) due to the partnership's discharged nonrecourse debt, as determined for each partner under the rules of Code Sec. 704(b) (Rev. Rul. 2012-14, amplifying Rev. Rul. 92-53).

References are to Standard Federal Tax Reports; Tax Research Consultant; and Practical Tax Explanations.

[53] ¶ 7002; SALES: 12,152, SALES: 12,202; §3,420.05

[54] ¶ 7002; SALES: 12,254; §3,401

[55] ¶ 5802.34; SALES: 12,154; §3,415

[56] ¶ 7002; SALES: 12,206; §3,420.05

[57] ¶ 7010.38; SALES: 12,200; §3,420.15

Farmers. Income arising from the discharge of qualified farm indebtedness owed to an unrelated lender, including a federal, state, or local government or agency, or instrumentality of such an agency, may be excluded from a taxpayer's income if certain requirements are met. The debt must be incurred directly in connection with the operation by the taxpayer of the trade or business of farming. Also, at least 50 percent of the taxpayer's aggregate gross receipts for the three tax years preceding the tax year in which the discharge of indebtedness occurs must be attributable to the trade or business of farming. The discharge of indebtedness income is excludable only to the extent absorbed by tax attributes (credits are reduced at a rate of 33⅓ cents per dollar of excluded income) and the adjusted bases of qualified property, i.e., any property held or used in a trade or business or for the production of income (Code Sec. 108(g)). Basis reduction occurs first with respect to depreciable property, then with respect to land used in the business of farming, and finally with respect to other qualified property (Code Sec. 1017(b)(4)).[58]

Qualified Real Property Business Indebtedness. A taxpayer other than a C corporation may elect to exclude from gross income amounts realized from the discharge of debt incurred or assumed in connection with real property used in a trade or business and secured by that property (Code Sec. 108(a)(1)(D) and (c)).[59] If the debt is incurred or assumed after 1992, it must be incurred or assumed to acquire, construct, reconstruct, or substantially improve the real property. The excludable amount is limited to the excess of the outstanding principal amount of the debt over the fair market value of the business real property reduced by the outstanding principal amount of any other qualified business indebtedness secured by the property. Also, the exclusion may not exceed the aggregate adjusted bases of depreciable real property held by the taxpayer immediately before discharge. The excluded amount reduces the basis of depreciable real property.

The election to treat debt as qualified real property business indebtedness must be filed with the taxpayer's timely income tax return, including extensions, for the tax year in which the discharge occurs (Reg. § 1.108-5(b)). The election, which is revocable with the consent of the IRS, is made on Form 982. A taxpayer who fails to make a timely election must request consent to file a late election under Reg. § 301.9100-3.

Qualified Principal Residence Indebtedness. Excludable from gross income is any amount of income from the discharge, in whole or in part, of "qualified principal residence indebtedness" which occurs on or after January 1, 2007, but on or before December 31, 2013. The debt referred to is acquisition indebtedness, as defined in the home mortgage interest deduction provisions of Code Sec. 163(h), but with a $2 million limit ($1 million for a married taxpayer filing a separate return) (Code Sec. 108(a)(1)(E) and (h)(2)).[60]

An individual's acquisition indebtedness is indebtedness with respect to his or her principal residence if it is incurred in the acquisition, construction, or substantial improvement of that residence, and the debt is secured by the residence (¶ 1048). Qualified principal residence interest also includes refinancing of the indebtedness, but only to the extent of the amount of the refinanced indebtedness. Principal residence has the same meaning for purposes of the exclusion as it does for purposes of Code Sec. 121 (¶ 1705) (Code Sec. 108(h)(5)).

Several provisions are included to prevent the abuse of the exclusion of income from the discharge of qualified principal residence indebtedness. The discharge of a loan will not be excludable from gross income if it is as a result of (1) services performed for the lender, or (2) other factors unrelated to either the financial condition of the taxpayer or a decline in value of the residence. In addition, if only a portion of discharged indebtedness is qualified principal residence indebtedness, the exclusion applies only to the amount of discharged debt that exceeds the portion of the debt that is not qualified principal residence indebtedness. The basis of the taxpayer's principal

---

References are to Standard Federal Tax Reports; Tax Research Consultant; and Practical Tax Explanations.

[58] ¶ 7002; SALES: 12,152.15; § 3,420.20

[59] ¶ 7002; SALES: 12,152.20; § 3,420.30

[60] ¶ 7002; SALES: 12,152.25; § 3,420.35

residence is reduced, but not below zero, by the amount of qualified principal residence interest that is excluded from income (Code Sec. 108(h)).

Student Loans. A special income exclusion applies to the discharge of all or part of a student loan if, pursuant to the loan agreement, the discharge is made because the individual works for a specified period of time in certain professions for any of a broad class of employers, e.g., as a doctor or nurse in an underserved rural area (Code Sec. 108(f)).[61] The loan must be made by: (1) a federal, state, or local government or instrumentality, agency, or subdivision of that government; (2) a tax-exempt public benefit corporation that has assumed control of a public hospital with public employees; or (3) an educational institution if (a) it received funds to loan from an entity described in (1) or (2), above, or (b) the student serves, pursuant to a program of the institution, in an occupation or area with unmet needs under the direction of a governmental unit or a tax-exempt Code Sec. 501(c)(3) organization, e.g., charitable, religious, educational, or scientific organization. Loans refinanced through such a program by the institution or certain tax-exempt organizations also qualify for the exclusion.

Deferral of Discharge of Indebtedness Income Resulting from Reacquisition of Business Indebtedness. A taxpayer could elect to include income arising from the discharge through reacquisition of certain indebtedness in gross income ratably over a five-tax-year period (Code Sec. 108(i)).[62] This applied to indebtedness discharged in connection with the reacquisition in 2009 or 2010 of a corporate or business debt instrument. The discharge of indebtedness income is included in the taxpayer's income ratably over a five-year period beginning with the fifth tax year after the year of reacquisition if the reacquisition occurred in 2009, or the fourth tax year after reacquisition if the reacquisition occurred in 2010.

If the taxpayer issued a new debt instrument for the debt instrument being reacquired, and there is original issue discount (OID) with respect to the original instrument, the taxpayer can deduct the OID ratably over the same period as that for which the discharge of indebtedness income is deferred. If a debt instrument was issued by the taxpayer and the proceeds were used to reacquire a debt instrument also issued by the taxpayer, the new instrument is treated as being issued for the instrument being reacquired. The election to defer OID income is made on an instrument-by-instrument basis, and is irrevocable once made.

Special rules address the application of Code Sec. 108(i) to C corporations, S corporations, and partnerships, including, under certain circumstances, a required acceleration of any remaining items of a C corporation's deferred cancellation of indebtedness income (Reg. § § 1.108(i)-0—1.108(i)-3).[63]

Education Benefits

863. U.S. Savings Bond Income Used for Higher Education Expenses. An individual who redeems any qualified U.S. savings bond during the year in order to pay qualified higher education expenses may exclude from income amounts received, provided certain requirements are met (Code Sec. 135).[64] A qualified U.S. savings bond is any such bond issued after 1989 to an individual who has reached age 24 before the date of issuance and which was issued at a discount under 31 U.S.C. § 3105 (Series I or EE bonds). Qualified higher education expenses include tuition and fees required for enrollment or attendance at an eligible educational institution of either a taxpayer, the taxpayer's spouse, or any dependent of the taxpayer for whom the taxpayer is allowed a deduction (Code Sec. 135(c)(2)). Also, taxpayers are entitled to the exclusion if the redemption proceeds are contributed to a qualified tuition program or 529 plan (¶ 869).

A taxpayer must be able to verify the amount of interest excluded. Therefore, the following records should be kept:

References are to Standard Federal Tax Reports; Tax Research Consultant; and Practical Tax Explanations.

[61] ¶ 7002; SALES: 12,152.10; § 3,420.25

[62] ¶ 7002; SALES: 12,252; § 3,420.40

[63] ¶ 7009C—¶ 7009N; SALES: 12,252; § 3,420.40

[64] ¶ 7550; INDIV: 12,162; § 3,120.05

¶863

- A written record of each post-1989 Series EE U.S. savings bond that is cashed in. It must include the serial number, issue date, face value, and total redemption proceeds (principal and interest) of each bond. Form 8818 may be used for this purpose.

- Some form of documentation to show that qualified higher education expenses were paid during the year. This could include canceled checks, credit card receipts or bills from the educational institution.

The amount that may be excludable is limited when the aggregate proceeds of qualified U.S. savings bonds redeemed by a taxpayer during a tax year exceed the qualified higher education expenses paid during that year (Code Sec. 135(b)(1)). Qualified higher education expenses must be reduced by the sum of: any qualified scholarship that is not includible in gross income (¶ 865) as an educational assistance allowance under certain chapters of title 38 of the United States Code; payment other than a gift or inheritance that is exempt from tax, i.e., employer-provided educational assistance (¶ 2067); or as a payment, waiver, or reimbursement under a qualified tuition program (¶ 869) Code Sec. 135(d)(1)). The amount must be further reduced by expenses taken into account for the American opportunity credit or lifetime learning credit (¶ 1303), as well as amounts taken into account in determining the exclusion for distributions from a qualified tuition program or the exclusion for distributions from an Coverdell education savings account (¶ 867) (Code Sec. 135(d)(2)).

The exclusion is subject to a phaseout in the years in which the bonds are cashed and the tuition is paid (Code Sec. 135(b)(2)(B)).[65] For 2014, the phaseout range is $113,950—$143,950 for joint filers and $76,000—$91,000 for all other filers (Rev. Proc. 2013-35). For 2015, the phaseout range is $115,750—$145,750 for joint filers and $77,200—$92,200 for all other filers (Rev. Proc. 2014-61).

Below the phaseout threshold, taxpayers may exclude bond interest up to the amount of qualified higher education expenses. Above the upper phaseout limit, no exclusion is allowed. For those falling within the ranges, the amount of interest excludable from income is reduced, depending on the taxpayer's modified adjusted gross income (AGI). Modified AGI (MAGI) is adjusted gross income *after* applying the partial exclusion for Social Security and tier 1 railroad retirement benefits (¶ 716), the deduction for contributions to a traditional IRA (¶ 2157), and adjustments for limitations on passive activity losses and credits (¶ 1169). In addition, MAGI is calculated *before* the exclusion of interest from U.S. Savings bonds, the exclusion for qualified adoption expenses (¶ 2063), the domestic production activities deduction (¶ 980A), the deduction for interest paid on qualified education loans (¶ 1082), the deduction for qualified tuition and related expenses (¶ 1082), the foreign income exclusion (¶ 2402), and the exclusion for income from sources within Puerto Rico and the U.S. possessions (¶ 2414 and ¶ 2415) (Code Sec. 135(c)(4)). This exclusion is not available to married individuals who file separate returns. The amount of excludable savings bond interest is determined using Form 8815, which is then filed with the taxpayer's Form 1040 or Form 1040A.

865. Scholarships and Fellowship Grants. Any amount received as a qualified scholarship by an individual who is a candidate for a degree at a qualified educational organization, which normally maintains a regular faculty and curriculum and normally has a regularly enrolled body of students in attendance where its educational activities are regularly carried on, is excluded from that individual's gross income (Code Sec. 117; Reg. § 1.117-1).[66] A qualified scholarship includes any amount received by an individual as a scholarship or fellowship grant so long as the amount was used for qualified tuition and related expenses, which are (1) tuition and fees required for enrollment or attendance at a qualified educational organization, and (2) fees, books, supplies, and equipment required for courses of instruction at such an organization. A qualified scholarship does not include amounts used for incidental expenses, e.g., room and board, travel,

---

References are to Standard Federal Tax Reports; Tax Research Consultant; and Practical Tax Explanations.

[65] ¶ 7550; INDIV: 12,162; § 3,120.15

[66] ¶ 7170, ¶ 7172; INDIV: 60,060; § 3,905.05

research, clerical help, and equipment and other expenses that are *not* required for either enrollment or attendance, or in a course of instruction at an educational organization (Prop. Reg. § 1.117-6(c)(2)).

Tuition Reduction. The amount of any qualified tuition reduction to employees of educational institutions is similarly excludable from gross income (Code Sec. 117(d)).[67] The tuition reduction must be provided to an employee of a qualified educational organization as defined under Code Sec. 170(b)(1)(A)(ii). The reduction can be for education provided by the employer or by another qualified educational organization. Moreover, it can be for education provided to the employee, the employee's spouse, dependent child, or other person treated as an employee under Code Sec. 132(h). However, it can only be used for education below the graduate level unless it is for the education of an employee who is a graduate student and who is engaged in teaching or research activities for the employer. Benefits under a qualified tuition reduction program may be excludable only if the program does not discriminate in favor of highly compensated employees.

Employer-Related Grants. Employer-related grants are *not* excludable from gross income if they are considered to be compensation or an incentive to employees (Rev. Proc. 76-47).[68] When educational scholarships are made available to or for the benefit of employees on a preferential basis, such preferential grants suggest an intent to provide additional compensation or an employment incentive and are included in gross income unless they are shown to fall outside the pattern of employment. This is true even if the grants are made by an independent third party, such as a private foundation or a voluntary employees' beneficiary association (VEBA). Educational grants are considered to fall outside the pattern of employment only if seven conditions and at least one of two percentage tests are satisfied. The seven conditions are:

(1) The programs must not be used by the employer, the private foundation, or the organizer to recruit or to induce employees to continue their employment or otherwise follow a course of action sought by the employer.

(2) Selection of grant recipients must be made by a committee consisting wholly of individuals totally independent, except for participation on this committee, and separate from the private foundation, its organizer, and the employer concerned.

(3) The program must impose identifiable minimum requirements for grant eligibility, and these requirements must be related to the purpose of the program.

(4) Selection of grant recipients must be based solely upon substantial objective standards that are completely unrelated to the employment of the recipients or their parents and to the employer's line of business.

(5) A grant may not be terminated because the recipient or the recipient's parent terminates employment with the employer subsequent to the awarding of the grant regardless of the reason for the termination of employment. If a grant is awarded for one academic year and the recipient must reapply for a grant for a subsequent year, the recipient may *not* be considered ineligible for a further grant simply because that individual or the individual's parent is no longer employed by the employer.

(6) The courses of study for which grants are available must not be limited to those that would be of particular benefit to the employer or to the foundation.

(7) The terms of the grant and the courses of study for which grants are available must meet all other requirements for the exclusion and must be consistent with a disinterested purpose of enabling the recipients to obtain an education in their individual capacities solely for their personal benefit and must not include any commitments, understandings or obligations, conditional or unconditional, suggesting that the studies are undertaken by the recipients for the benefit of the

---

References are to Standard Federal Tax Reports; Tax Research Consultant; and Practical Tax Explanations.

[67] ¶ 7170; INDIV: 60,060.10; § 3,910

[68] ¶ 7183.29; INDIV: 60,060.10; § 3,905.15, § 3,910

employer or the foundation, or have as their objective the accomplishment of any purpose of the employer or the foundation, even though consistent with its exempt status, other than enabling the recipients to obtain an education in their individual capacities and solely for their personal benefit.

Under the percentage tests, the number of grants awarded under the program to children of employees must not exceed either (1) 25 percent of the children who were eligible for such grants, were applicants for the grants, and were considered by the selection committee making such grants; or (2) 10 percent of the number of employees' children who can be shown to be eligible for grants in that year, whether or not they submitted an application.

Compensation for Teaching, Research, or Other Services Performed. The exclusions for qualified scholarships and qualified tuition reductions do not apply to amounts representing payments for teaching, research, or other services performed by the student that are required as a condition for receiving the qualified scholarship or qualified tuition reduction (Code Sec. 117(c)).[69] Athletic scholarships awarded to students who are expected, but not required, to participate in sports qualify for exclusion (Rev. Rul. 77-263). The IRS reiterated in response to a Senator's inquiry that it will follow Rev. Rul. 77-263 regardless of the any decision of the National Labor Relation Board (NLRB) in respect to employment status of student athletes (INFO 2014-0016).

Under an exception, amounts received by degree candidates from the National Health Service Corps (NHSC) Scholarship Program or the Armed Forces Health Professions Scholarship and Financial Assistance Program for tuition, fees, books, supplies, and required equipment are excluded from the recipient's gross income even though there is a future service obligation connected to these qualified scholarships (Code Sec. 117(c)(2)). Amounts received by health care professionals under the NHSC Loan Repayment Program are excludable from gross income and employment taxes (Code Sec. 108(f)(4)). This provision also extends to loan repayments received under similar state programs qualified for funding under the Public Health Service Act and repayments under other state loan repayment or forgiveness programs that are intended to provide for increased availability of health care services in underserved or health professional shortage areas.

867. Coverdell Education Savings Accounts. Individuals may open a Coverdell Education Savings Account (Coverdell ESA), formerly called an education IRA, which is created exclusively to help pay for the qualified education expenses of a designated beneficiary (Code Sec. 530).[70] A Coverdell ESA is a tax-exempt trust or custodial account organized in the United States. At the time it is organized the trust must be designated as a Coverdell ESA and the designated beneficiary must be under age 18 or a special needs individual. Contributions to a Coverdell ESA must be made in cash and are *not* deductible. In addition, the maximum annual contribution that can be made is limited to $2,000 a year excluding rollovers. The annual contribution is phased out for joint filers with modified adjusted gross income (MAGI) at or above $190,000 and less than $220,000 (at or above $95,000 and less than $110,000 for single filers). The reduction in permitted contributions based on MAGI applies only to individual contributors. Thus, contributions made by entities, such as a corporation or tax-exempt organization, are not subject to the phaseout rules. Amounts remaining in the account must be distributed within: (1) 30 days after the beneficiary reaches age 30 or (2) 30 days after the death of the beneficiary (see *Rollovers,* following).

Coordination with Other Educational Benefits. Qualified expenses will first be reduced for tax-exempt scholarships or fellowship grants (¶ 865) and any other tax-free educational benefits. Expenses will then be reduced for amounts taken into account in determining the American Opportunity (modified Hope) and lifetime learning credits (¶ 1303). Where a student receives distributions from both a Coverdell ESA and a

---

References are to Standard Federal Tax Reports; Tax Research Consultant; and Practical Tax Explanations.

[69] ¶ 7170; INDIV: 60,060.15; § 3,905.10

[70] ¶ 22,950; INDIV: 60,202; § 1,810.05

qualified tuition plan (¶ 869) that together exceed these remaining expenses, the expenses must be allocated between the distributions (Code Sec. 530(d)(2)(C)).

Distributions. Contributions to Coverdell ESAs are generally treated as gifts to the beneficiaries. Distributions from Coverdell ESAs are excludable from gross income to the extent that the distribution does not exceed the qualified higher education expenses incurred by the designated beneficiary during the year in which the distribution is made (Code Sec. 530(d)(2)(A)). Qualified distributions are tax exempt regardless of whether the designated beneficiary attends an eligible educational institution on a full-time, half-time, or less than half-time basis. However, room and board expenses constitute qualified higher education expenses only if the student is enrolled at an eligible institution on at least a half-time basis (see *Qualifying Education Expenses*, following).

Distributions are deemed paid from both contributions, which are always tax free, and earnings, which may be excludable. The amount of contributions distributed is determined by multiplying the distribution by the ratio that the aggregate amount of contributions bears to the total balance of the account at the time the distribution is made (Code Sec. 530(d)(1)).

If aggregate distributions exceed expenses during the tax year, qualified education expenses are deemed to be paid from a pro rata share of both principal and interest. Thus, the portion of earnings excludable from gross income is based on the ratio that the qualified higher education expenses bear to the total amount of the distribution. The remaining portion of earnings are included in the income of the distributee.

Distributions Not Used for Education. The tax imposed on any taxpayer who receives a payment or distribution from a Coverdell ESA that is includible in gross income will be increased by an additional 10 percent (Code Sec. 530(d)(4)(A)). The additional 10-percent penalty does not apply to distributions: (1) made to a designated beneficiary or the estate of a designated beneficiary after the designated beneficiary's death; (2) attributable to the designated beneficiary being disabled as defined under Code Sec. 72(m)(7); (3) made on account of a scholarship or allowance, as defined under Code Sec. 25A(g)(2), received by the account holder to the extent the amount of the distribution does not exceed the amount of the scholarship or allowance; or (4) that constitute the return of excess contributions and earnings thereon, although earnings are includible in income (Code Sec. 530(d)(2)(A)).

Military Academy Attendance. Since recipients of appointments to military academies are required to fulfill service obligations, the appointments are generally not considered scholarships and the 10-percent penalty applies. Withdrawals from Coverdell ESAs made on account of the beneficiary's attendance at a service academy are not subject to the penalty to the extent the distribution is used for the costs of advanced education (Code Sec. 530(d)(4)). The penalty waiver covers appointments to the United States Military, Navy, Air Force, Coast Guard, and Merchant Marine Academies.

Rollovers. Amounts held in a Coverdell ESA may be distributed and put into a Coverdell ESA for a member of the designated beneficiary's family. These distributions will not be included in the distributee's gross income provided the rollover occurs within 60 days of the distribution. Similarly, any change in the beneficiary of a Coverdell ESA does not constitute a distribution for gross income purposes if the new beneficiary is a member of the family of the original beneficiary and of the same or higher generation. A person's family members are determined under the qualified tuition program rules of Code Sec. 529(e)(2) (Code Sec. 530(d)). Amounts held in a Coverdell ESA may also be rolled over into another Coverdell ESA for the benefit of the same beneficiary.

Qualified Education Expenses. Qualified education expenses include expenses for elementary, secondary, undergraduate, and graduate level education. Tuition, fees, books, supplies, equipment, and special needs services, if required, fall under the definition of education expenses for the designated beneficiary to attend undergraduate or graduate level courses at an eligible education institution. The term also includes room and board provided that the student incurring the expense is enrolled at an eligible education institution on at least a halftime basis. In 2009 and 2010 only, expenses incurred for computer technology or equipment, including Internet access charges, were also qualified expenses for post-secondary students.

¶867

Qualified elementary and secondary expenses also include expenses for academic tutoring, the purchase of computer technology or equipment, or Internet access or related services, room and board, uniforms, transportation, and supplementary items and services such as extended day programs as required or provided by the school (Code Secs. 529(e)(3)(A) and 530(b)(3)).[71] Computer expenses do *not* include software designed for sports, games, or hobbies unless the nature of the software is predominately educational.

Eligible Educational Institution. An eligible educational institution is generally an accredited post-secondary educational institution offering credit toward a bachelor's degree, an associate's degree, a graduate-level or professional degree, or other recognized post-secondary credential. Generally, proprietary and post-secondary vocational institutions are eligible educational institutions (Code Sec. 530(b)(3)). Elementary and secondary schools, i.e., kindergarten through grade 12, are also eligible institutions. Schools may be public, private or religious.

Prohibited Uses of Accounts. A Coverdell ESA will lose its tax-exempt status if it engages in a prohibited transaction or is pledged as security for a loan. Prohibited transactions include loans and use of account assets by the beneficiary or a fiduciary (Code Sec. 4975(c)).[72]

Transfers Upon Death or Divorce. Death or divorce of the designated beneficiary need not cause a taxable distribution to the spouse or ex-spouse. The transfer of a beneficiary's interest in a Coverdell ESA to a spouse or ex-spouse under a divorce or separation agreement is not a taxable transfer, and after the transfer the interest in the account is treated as belonging to the spouse or ex-spouse (Code Sec. 530(d)(7)).[73]

Estate and Gift Tax Treatment. Any contribution to a Coverdell ESA is treated as a completed gift of a present interest from the contributor to the beneficiary at the time of the contribution. Contributions are eligible for the annual gift tax exclusion (¶ 2905) and are excludable for purposes of the generation-skipping transfer tax (Code Sec. 530(d)(3)).[74]

Military Death Benefits as Contributions. An individual who receives a military death gratuity or Servicemembers' Group Life Insurance payment may contribute up to the full amount of such gratuity or payment into a Coverdell ESA, without regard to the annual contribution limit and the income phase-out of the limit that would otherwise apply. A military death benefit contribution to a Coverdell ESA will be considered a tax-free rollover contribution if it is made within one year of the date on which the amount is received, and does not exceed the total amount of gratuity and life insurance payments received, less the amount of such payments contributed to a Roth IRA or to another Coverdell ESA. Such rollovers will be disregarded for purposes of the limit on the number of tax-free rollovers per year (Code Sec. 530(d)(9)).

869. Qualified Tuition Programs (529 Plans). Distributions from a qualified tuition program (QTP, also known as a qualified tuition plan, Code Sec. 529 plan, or 529 plan) are generally not included in the income of the donor or the designated beneficiary, as long as the distributions do not exceed the beneficiary's qualified higher education expenses (Code Sec. 529(c)(3)(B)). A QTP is a program under which an individual may prepay tuition credits or make cash contributions to an account on behalf of a beneficiary for payment of qualified higher education expenses. The program must be established and maintained by a state, state agency, or by an eligible educational institution, i.e., virtually any accredited public, nonprofit, or private college or university. Eligible schools generally include any accredited post-secondary educational institution, so long as contributions made to the program are held in a qualified trust, i.e., one which meets the requirements under Code Sec. 408(a)(2) and (5).[75] A QTP is exempt from all

---

References are to Standard Federal Tax Reports; Tax Research Consultant; and Practical Tax Explanations.

[71] ¶ 22,950; INDIV: 60,206; § 1,810.25

[72] ¶ 34,400; INDIV: 60,202.35; § 24,020.10

[73] ¶ 22,950; INDIV: 60,202.30; § 1,810.40

[74] ¶ 22,950; INDIV: 60,202.10; § 1,810.15

[75] ¶ 18,902; INDIV: 60,204, RETIRE: 66,100; § 1,805.10

federal income taxation, except for the tax imposed on unrelated business income (¶ 655 and following) (Code Sec. 529).[76]

Form 990-T. Colleges and universities of states and other governmental units, as well as subsidiary corporations wholly owned by such colleges and universities, are subject to the Form 990-T filing requirements, unless otherwise exempted as a Code Sec. 501(c)(1) corporation.

Contributions. Contributions to a QTP on behalf of any beneficiary cannot exceed the necessary amount of qualified higher education expenses (QHEEs) for the beneficiary. There are no adjusted gross income phaseout limits. In addition, a taxpayer can contribute to both a QTP and a Coverdell account (¶ 867) in the same year for the same beneficiary.

Qualified Higher Education Expenses (QHEEs). For this purpose, QHEEs include tuition, fees, books, supplies, and equipment required by an educational institution for enrollment or attendance. They also include the reasonable cost of room and board if the beneficiary is enrolled at least half-time (Code Sec. 529(e)(3)).[77] Certain expenses of special needs beneficiaries may also be considered QHEEs. The amount of QHEEs must be reduced by the amount of any other tax free benefits, i.e., scholarship or fellowship grants excluded from gross income (¶ 865), or the education credits (¶ 1303).

Distributions. The part of a distribution representing the amount paid or contributed to a QTP is excludable from gross income to the extent that the distribution is used to pay for QHEEs. The designated beneficiary generally does not have to include in income any earnings distributed from a QTP, if the total distribution is less than or equal to adjusted qualified education expenses (Code Sec. 529(c)(3)). Distributions that exceed the beneficiary's qualified higher education expenses are generally taxed under the Code Sec. 72 annuity rules (¶ 817). The part of any distribution from a QTP that represents amounts paid or contributed to the account represent a return of the investment in the account. Distributions of program earnings in excess of the beneficiary's qualified higher education expenses are includable in income and subject to an additional 10-percent tax, i.e., a penalty (Code Sec. 529(c)(6)).[78]

Rollovers and Transfers. Generally, amounts can be rolled over from one qualified tuition program to another for the benefit of the same designated beneficiary, or another beneficiary who is a member of the same family, without tax consequences. In order to qualify for rollover treatment, a distribution from the first QTP must be paid into the second QTP no later than the 60th day after the payment or distribution is made. If the rollover is made to another QTP of the same beneficiary, then only one such transfer is permitted within 12 months of the previous transfer to any QTP for that designated beneficiary (Code Sec. 529(c)(3)).[79]

Estate and Gift Tax Treatment. A contribution to a QTP is treated as a completed gift of a present interest for gift tax purposes (Code Sec. 529(c)(2)). Thus, the contribution qualifies for the annual gift tax exclusion (¶ 2905). If a donor's contribution exceeds the annual exclusion amount, then he or she may elect to take the excess into account ratably over five years. A QTP contribution does not qualify for the unlimited gift tax exclusion for money used to pay educational expenses (¶ 2907). No portion of a contribution is generally includible in the estate of a donor who dies after June 8, 1997, unless the donor dies during the five-year period in which excess contributions to a QTP are being ratably taken into account.

References are to Standard Federal Tax Reports; Tax Research Consultant; and Practical Tax Explanations.

[76] ¶ 22,940; INDIV: 60,204, EXEMPT: 9,950; § 1,805.05

[77] ¶ 22,940; INDIV: 60,206; § 1,805.20

[78] ¶ 22,940; INDIV: 60,204.15; § 1,805.35

[79] ¶ 22,940; INDIV: 60,204.20; § 1,805.45

¶869

Other Exclusions from Gross Income

871. Exclusion or Rollover of Certain Stock Gains. Noncorporate taxpayers may exclude from gross income a certain percentage of capital gain from the sale or exchange of qualified small business stock held for more than five years and issued after August 10, 1993 (¶ 1905). Noncorporate taxpayers may also elect to roll over capital gain from the sale of qualified business stock held for more than six months if other qualified small business stock is purchased during the 60-day period beginning on the date of sale (¶ 1907). Individuals and C corporations may elect to defer recognition of capital gain realized upon the sale of publicly traded securities if the sale proceeds are used within 60 days to purchase common stock or a partnership interest in a specialized small business investment company (SSBIC) (¶ 1909).

873. Employee Benefits. Compensation for personal services includes any benefits an employer provides to employee which are not otherwise excludable from income (Reg. § 1.61-2(a)).[80] Excludable employee benefits include:

• amounts received under employer-financed accident and health plans (¶ 2015);

• employer contributions to provide the accident and health benefits (¶ 2013);

• employer contributions to a health savings account (HSA) (¶ 2035), Archer medical savings account (MSA) (¶ 2037), health reimbursement arrangement (HRA) (¶ 2039), or flexible spending arrangement (FSA) (¶ 2041);

• premiums for group-term life insurance to the extent coverage does not exceed $50,000 (¶ 2055);

• qualified adoption expenses reimbursed under an employer adoption assistance program (¶ 2063);

• child and dependent care assistance benefits (¶ 2065);

• educational assistance benefits (¶ 2067);

• employee achievement awards to the extent deductible by the employer (¶ 2069); and

• certain other fringe benefits (¶ 2085).

Some excludable employee benefits may be provided to an employee through the employer's cafeteria plan (¶ 2045).

875. Minister's Home or Rental Allowance. Ministers of the gospel may exclude from gross income the rental value of homes furnished by churches as part of their compensation (Code Sec. 107; Reg. § 1.107-1).[81] This includes the portion of a retired minister's pension designated as a rental allowance by the national governing body of a religious denomination having complete control over the retirement fund.[82] The exemption also applies to the rental value of a residence furnished to a retired minister but not a widow.[83]

A minister is entitled to deduct mortgage interest and real property taxes paid on a personal residence even if the amounts expended are derived from a rental allowance that is excludable from the minister's gross income (Code Sec. 265(a)(6)).[84]

877. Reimbursed Living Expenses. A taxpayer whose principal residence is damaged or destroyed by fire, storm, or other casualty and who must temporarily occupy another residence during the repair can exclude from gross income any insurance payments received as reimbursement for *increased* living expenses during such period. This also applies to a person who is denied access to his principal residence by governmental authorities because of the occurrence or threat of occurrence of a casualty (Code Sec. 123; Reg. § 1.123-1).[85]

References are to Standard Federal Tax Reports; Tax Research Consultant; and Practical Tax Explanations.

[80] ¶ 5506; COMPEN: 6,050; § 3,005.05

[81] ¶ 6850, ¶ 6851; COMPEN: 6,554; § 3,005.20

[82] ¶ 6852.12; COMPEN: 6,556; § 3,005.20

[83] ¶ 6852.31; COMPEN: 6,556; § 3,005.20

[84] ¶ 14,050; INDIV: 48,554.05; § 46,110.10

[85] ¶ 7300, ¶ 7301; INDIV: 33,450; § 4,005.10

¶877

The exclusion is limited to the excess of actual living expenses incurred by the taxpayer and members of the household over the normal living expenses they would have incurred during the period. The exclusion covers additional costs incurred in renting suitable housing and any extraordinary expenses for transportation, food, utilities, and miscellaneous items.

881. Government Cost-Sharing Payments. Agricultural and forestry cost-sharing payments made by state or federal governments may be excluded from gross income if:

(1) the Secretary of Agriculture determines that the payments were made primarily for soil and water conservation, environmental protection or restoration, wildlife habitat development, or forest improvement, and

(2) the Treasury Department determines that the payments do not result in a substantial increase in the annual income derived from the property with respect to which the payments were made.

No adjustment to the basis of the property involved is made for the payments and, therefore, no income tax deduction or credit may be taken with respect to them (Code Sec. 126).[86] Further, if the property or improvement purchased with the payments is disposed of within 20 years, the payment amounts are recaptured as ordinary income. A 100-percent recapture rate applies if disposition occurs within the first 10 years, with an annual decrease of 10 percent thereafter (Code Sec. 1255; Temp. Reg. §§16A.1255-1 and 16A.1255-2).[87]

883. Foster Care Payments. Amounts received by a foster care provider from a state or qualified foster care placement agency are excludable from gross income if received for providing care for a qualified foster individual placed in the taxpayer's home or received as a difficulty of care payment (Code Sec. 131).[88] A qualified foster care placement agency is an placement agency that is licensed or certified by a state or local government, or an entity designated by such a government, to make foster care payments to foster care providers. A difficulty of care payment is a payment for the additional care required because the qualified foster individual placed in the taxpayer's home has a physical, mental, or emotional handicap. Effective for payments received on or after January 3, 2014, the IRS will treat qualified Medicaid waiver payments as difficulty of care payments excludable from gross income, regardless of whether the care provider is related or unrelated to the eligible individual (Notice 2014-7). Regular foster care payments are *not* excludable to the extent they are made for more than five individuals in the home who have attained age 19. In the case of difficulty of care payments, payments are *not* excludable to the extent they are made for more than 10 individuals under age 19 and more than five individuals who have attained 19 years of age.

885. Benefits for Volunteer Emergency Responders. For tax years beginning before January 1, 2011, members of qualified volunteer emergency response organizations may generally exclude from gross income certain qualified state and local tax benefits (Code Sec. 139B).[89] The exclusion is subject to an annual limitation of $30 multiplied by the number of months during the tax year in which the volunteer performs such services.

A qualified volunteer emergency response organization is any volunteer organization that provides firefighting or emergency medical services and is required by the state or political subdivision, under a written agreement, to provide such services. A qualified state and local tax benefit is any reduction or rebate of state or local real property taxes, state or local personal property taxes, or state or local income taxes. Any deduction under Code Sec. 164 for state and local taxes is determined with regard to the reduction or rebate (Code Sec. 139B(b)(1)). Expenses paid or incurred by the taxpayer in connection with the performance of services are taken into account as a charitable

---

References are to Standard Federal Tax Reports; Tax Research Consultant; and Practical Tax Explanations.

[86] ¶ 7330; FARM: 3,168; §36,005.10

[87] ¶ 31,080, ¶ 31,081, ¶ 31,082; FARM: 3,168.15; §16,715.05

[88] ¶ 7400; INDIV: 33,250, INDIV: 33,252; §4,010.05

[89] ¶ 7649J; INDIV: 33,312; §4,080

deduction under Code Sec. 170 only to the extent the expenses exceed the amount excluded from income as calculated under the annual limitation (Code Sec. 139B(b)(2)).

Employment Tax Treatment. The excluded benefits and payments under Code Sec. 139B are *not* wages for purposes of federal income tax withholding, FICA, and FUTA (Code Secs. 3121(a)(23), 3306(b)(20), and 3401(a)(23)).

887. Disaster Relief Payments. Individuals who are the victims of a disaster are provided an exclusion from gross income for qualified disaster relief payments, as well as for payments received under Section 406 of the Air Transportation Safety and System Stabilization Act (Code Sec. 139).[90] This exclusion also applies to self-employment and employment taxes, and thus, no withholding is required for qualified disaster relief payments. However, the exclusion does not apply to any individual, or a representative, identified by the Attorney General to have been a participant or conspirator in a terrorist action.

Disaster Relief Payments Defined. Qualified disaster relief payments include payments, from any source, made to or for the benefit of an individual:

    (1) to reimburse or pay reasonable and necessary personal, family, living, or funeral expenses incurred as a result of a qualified disaster;

    (2) to reimburse or pay reasonable and necessary expenses incurred for the repair or rehabilitation of a personal residence or for the repair, rehabilitation, or replacement of its contents to the extent attributable to a qualified disaster;

    (3) by a common carrier that sells or furnishes transportation, e.g. a commercial airlines, for death or personal physical injuries as a result of a qualified disaster; or

    (4) if such amount is paid by a federal, state, or local government in connection with a qualified disaster to promote the general welfare.

Taxpayers in a federally declared disaster (formerly known as a presidentially declared disaster) area who receive grants from state programs, charitable organizations or employers to cover medical, transportation, or temporary housing expenses do not include these grants in gross income (Rev. Rul. 2003-12). However, qualified disaster relief payments do not include payments for any expense compensated for by insurance or otherwise, or payments in the nature of income replacement, such as payments to individuals of lost wages, unemployment compensation, or payments in the nature of business income replacement.

A qualified disaster is:

    (1) a disaster that results from a terroristic or military action as defined under Code Sec. 692(c)(2);

    (2) a federally declared disaster as defined under Code Sec. 165(h)(3)(c)(i);

    (3) a disaster that results from an accident involving a common carrier, or from any other event, which is determined by the IRS to be of a catastrophic nature; or

    (4) a disaster determined by an applicable federal, state or local authority, as determined by the IRS, to warrant assistance.

Air Transportation Safety Act. Taxpayers who are eligible to receive payments under Section 406 of the Air Transportation Safety and System Stabilization Act as a result of physical harm or death incurred from the terrorist-related aircraft crashes on or after September 11, 2001, can exclude these amounts (Code Sec. 139(f)).

References are to Standard Federal Tax Reports; Tax Research Consultant; and Practical Tax Explanations.

[90] ¶ 7646; INDIV: 33,310.05; § 4,055.10

EXCLUSIONS

888. COBRA Premium Assistance. Assistance eligible individuals who became eligible to elect COBRA continuation health care coverage under their employer's plan as a result of an involuntary termination of their employment during the period beginning September 1, 2008, and ending May 31, 2010, were required to pay only 35 percent of the premiums for the coverage. The individual's gross income did *not* include the amount of the premium reduction (Code Sec. 139C).[91] Premium assistance for eligible unemployed individuals terminated on August 31, 2011. See ¶ 2653 for further discussion of COBRA premium assistance.

889. Other Excluded Income. Several other items of income are excluded from gross income.

Holocaust Reparation Payments. Restitution or reparation payments received by persons who suffered Nazi persecution and survived the Holocaust are excludable from gross income (Act Sec. 2 of the Holocaust Restitution Tax Fairness Act of 2002 (P.L. 107-358)).[92] The exclusion extends to any interest earned on these payments. These excludable payments are also *not* included when applying any tax provision that takes into account excluded income in computing modified adjusted gross income, such as the taxation of Social Security benefits.

Native American Health Care Benefits. The amount of qualified health care benefits provided after March 23, 2010, by Indian tribal governments to a member of an Indian tribe or a member's spouse or dependents are excludable from the beneficiary's gross income (Code Sec. 139D).[93] See ¶ 2027 for further discussion of Indian health care benefits.

Energy Conservation Subsidies. The value of any subsidy provided, directly or indirectly, by a public utility to a customer for the purchase or installation of energy conservation measures for a dwelling unit is excludable from the customer's gross income (Code Sec. 136).[94] Energy conservation measures are any installations or modifications designed to reduce the consumption of electricity or natural gas or to improve management of energy demand.

Other Exclusions. Exclusions are also available to human trafficking victims (Notice 2012-12) and certain settlements received by Native Americans (Notice 2013-1, appendix modified by Notice 2014-38).

The IRS has provided guidance on whether a medical loss ratio (MLR) rebate paid to a health insurance policyholder is excludable from the policyholder's taxable income as a returned premium (¶ 2031).

Excludable Military Benefits

891. Armed Forces Benefits. Amounts received from a pension, annuity, or similar payment for *personal injuries* or *sickness* that resulted from combat-related service in the armed forces of *any* country, the National Oceanic and Atmospheric Administration, or the Public Health Service, or from a disability annuity under the provisions of section 808 of the Foreign Service Act of 1980, are excludable from gross income (¶ 851) (Code Sec. 104(a)(4); Reg. § 1.104-1(e)).[95]

Retirement pay received from the government by Armed Service members is *not* excludable from gross income (Code Sec. 61(a)(11)).[96] Disability retirement pay that is computed on the basis of the percentage of disability is fully excludable from gross income, but disability retirement pay that is computed by reference to years of service is excludable only to the extent allowed under the percentage-of-disability method (Reg. § 1.104-1(e)).[97]

References are to Standard Federal Tax Reports; Tax Research Consultant; and Practical Tax Explanations.

[91] ¶ 7649L; HEALTH: 24,118; § 4,085
[92] ¶ 5502; INDIV: 33,308; § 3,835
[93] ¶ 7649N; INDIV: 33,512; § 3,715
[94] ¶ 7560; INDIV: 33,552; § 4,001
[95] ¶ 6660, ¶ 6661; INDIV: 33,410; § 42,210
[96] ¶ 5502, ¶ 5507.121; HEALTH: 12,254; § 45,805.40
[97] ¶ 6661, ¶ 6662.79; HEALTH: 12,252; § 45,805.35

Dividends and proceeds from maturing government endowment insurance contracts under the National Service Life Insurance Act of 1940 and all other acts relating to veterans are excludable from gross income.[98] Interest on dividends left on deposit with the Department of Veterans Affairs is also excludable. If an individual uses accumulated dividends to buy additional paid-up National Service Life Insurance, neither the dividends nor the paid-up insurance is taxable (Rev. Rul. 91-14).

Veterans' benefits under any law administered by the Department of Veterans Affairs are excludable from gross income.[99] This includes amounts paid to veterans or their families in the form of economic recovery payments under the American Recovery and Reinvestment Act of 2009 (P.L. 111-5); educational, training, or subsistence allowances; disability compensation and pension payments for disabilities; compensation for participation in a work therapy program; grants for homes designed for wheelchair living; grants for motor vehicles for veterans who lost their sight or the use of their limbs; and veterans' pensions (38 USC § 5301 and following).

893. Armed Forces Allowances. Allowances for subsistence, uniforms, quarters, travel, and moving furnished to a commissioned officer, chief warrant officer, warrant officer, or enlisted personnel of the Armed Forces, National Oceanic and Atmospheric Administration, or Public Health Service are excludable from gross income (Reg. § 1.61-2(b)).[100]

Housing and cost-of-living allowances received by Armed Forces members to cover the excess cost of quarters and subsistence while on permanent duty at a post outside the United States are also excludable from gross income (Rev. Rul. 61-5).[101] The same rule applies to family separation allowances received on account of overseas assignment.[102] The fact that a member of the military service, National Oceanic and Atmospheric Administration, or Public Health Service receives a tax-free housing allowance will not bar a deduction for mortgage interest or real property taxes on the member's home (Code Sec. 265(a)(6)).[103]

895. Combat Zone Compensation. Enlisted members of the Armed Forces and warrant officers, both commissioned and noncommissioned, may exclude from gross income all pay received for any month during any part of which they served in a combat zone or were hospitalized as a result of wounds, disease, or injury incurred while serving in a combat zone. The exclusion for months of hospitalization does not apply for any month beginning more than two years after the termination of combatant activities in the zone. The same exclusion applies to commissioned officers, but it is limited to the maximum enlisted amount. This amount is the highest rate of basic pay at the highest pay grade that enlisted personnel may receive plus the amount of hostile fire/imminent danger pay that the officer receives (Code Sec. 112; Reg. § 1.112-1).[104]

The following areas, among others, have been designated combat zones qualifying American military personnel serving in these areas for special tax benefits:

(1) the Persian Gulf, the Red Sea, the Gulf of Oman, part of the Arabian Sea, the Gulf of Aden and the geographic areas of Iraq, Kuwait, Saudi Arabia, Oman, Bahrain, Qatar, and the United Arab Emirates, including the airspace above, effective on January 17, 1991 (Executive Order No. 12744; Notice 2003-21);

(2) Bosnia, Herzegovina, Croatia, and Macedonia, effective on November 21, 1995 (P.L. 104-117; Notice 96-34);

(3) the Federal Republic of Yugoslavia (Serbia/Montenegro), Albania, the Adriatic Sea, and the Ionian Sea above the 39th parallel, effective on March 24, 1999 (Executive Order 13119; Notice 99-30, supplementing Notice 96-34);

References are to Standard Federal Tax Reports; Tax Research Consultant; and Practical Tax Explanations.

[98] ¶ 5504.74; ESTGIFT: 21,164

[99] ¶ 5504.785; HEALTH: 12,254; § 4,065.30

[100] ¶ 5506, ¶ 7222.79; COMPEN: 6,606; § 45,805.25

[101] ¶ 5507.111; COMPEN: 33,110

[102] ¶ 5507.110; COMPEN: 33,110

[103] ¶ 14,050; INDIV: 48,554; § 7,420.05

[104] ¶ 7080, ¶ 7081; COMPEN: 6,604; § 3,005.15a

(4) Afghanistan and its airspace, including Jordan, Pakistan, and Tajikistan, effective on September 19, 2001 (Executive Order No. 13239; Notice 2002-17);

(5) Kyrgyzstan and Uzbekistan, effective on October 1, 2001 (Notice 2002-17); and

(6) areas supporting Operation Iraqi Freedom, effective on April 10, 2003.

For a complete list of designated combat zones, see IRS Pub. 3.

Combat pay excludable from gross income may nevertheless be included in earned income for purposes of the earned income tax credit (¶ 1322) and calculating the refundable portion of the child tax credit (¶ 1305). Similarly, combat pay may be treated as compensation in determining the amount military personnel can contribute to their individual retirement accounts (IRAs) (¶ 2153).

896. Qualified Military Benefits. A variety of benefits for military personnel were excludable from gross income under a variety of statutes, regulations, and long-standing administrative practices prior to enactment of the Tax Reform Act of 1986 (P.L. 99-514). In the 1986 Act, it was determined that, in the future, no such exclusions would be permitted except under some provision of the Internal Revenue Code. However, the Act added to the Code a provision that, in effect, grandfathered all of the previous non-Code exclusions (Code Sec. 134).[105] Under this provision, all such exclusions that were in effect on September 9, 1986, continue to be in effect. If a benefit in effect on September 9, 1986, is thereafter modified or adjusted for increases in the cost of living or the like under authority existing on that date, the adjustments are also excludable. Benefits not otherwise categorized as qualified military benefits but provided in connection with an individual's status or service as a member of the uniformed services may be excluded from gross income under other Code sections if their requirements for exclusion are met.

Death Gratuity Payments. Section 1478, Title 10, of the U.S. Code provides that upon notification of the death of military personnel on active duty or combat-related activities, i.e., duty training, a death gratuity will be paid to or for the survivor of the service member. The death gratuity payment effective for death occurring on or after October 7, 2001, is $100,000 (National Defense Authorization Act for Fiscal Year 2006, (P.L. 109-163)). The exclusion from gross income is also allowed for any adjustment in the amount of the death gratuity payments. The limitation on post-September 9, 1986, modifications does not apply to this benefit. Thus, cost-of-living adjustments or other increases in the gratuity amount will not be subject to tax.

Dependent Care Assistance Program. Qualified military benefits include dependent care assistance provided under a dependent care assistance program (¶ 2065) for a current or former uniformed forces service member or for a dependent (Code Sec. 134(b)(4)).

Veterans' Bonuses and Payments. The definition of qualified military benefit includes bonus payments by a state or local government entity to a member or former member of the military, or to any dependents of such a member. The payment must be made "only by reason of" the member's service in a combat zone. Thus, the state or local program under which the bonus is paid must specify that the bonus is *only* available with respect to members who served in a combat zone (Code Sec. 134(b)(6)).

References are to Standard Federal Tax Reports; Tax Research Consultant; and Practical Tax Explanations.

[105] ¶ 7500; COMPEN: 6,606, COMPEN: 6,608; § 4,065.20

Chapter 9

BUSINESS EXPENSES

Trade or Business Expenses

901. Deductibility of Business Expenses—Generally. A taxpayer, whether a corporation, an individual, a partnership, a trust, or an estate, generally may deduct from gross income the ordinary and necessary expenses of carrying on a trade or business that are paid or incurred during the tax year (Code Sec. 162; Reg. § 1.162-1).[1] Business expenses incurred by a cash-basis taxpayer while conducting a business but paid in a year after terminating the business are deductible as business expenses in the year paid (Rev. Rul. 67-12).[2] However, a deduction is not permitted for any expenditure that is a capital expense (¶ 903). Expenses for property used for both business and personal activities must be allocated between the different activities. The origin and character of a claim control whether an expense is a deductible business expense or a nondeductible personal expense.

Ordinary and Necessary. Whether a business expense is ordinary and necessary is based on the facts surrounding the expense. An expense is necessary if it is appropriate and helpful to the taxpayer's business (*S.B. Heininger*, SCt, 44-1 USTC ¶ 9109).[3] An expense is ordinary if it is one that is common and accepted in the particular business activity.

Trade or Business. A "trade or business," although not defined in the tax law, has been characterized as an activity carried on for a livelihood or for profit. A profit motive must be present and some type of economic activity must be conducted. In determining whether an activity is engaged in for profit, all facts and circumstances with respect to the activity are taken into account (Reg. § 1.183-2(b)).[4] No one factor is conclusive in making this determination. In addition, it is not intended that only the factors described below are to be taken into account in making the determination, or that a determination

---

References are to Standard Federal Tax Reports; Tax Research Consultant; and Practical Tax Explanations.

[1] ¶ 8500, ¶ 8501; BUSEXP: 3,100; § 9,001

[2] ¶ 8520.1546; BUSEXP: 3,058.20; § 9,001

[3] ¶ 8520.517; BUSEXP: 3,100; § 9,010.05

[4] ¶ 12,173; BUSEXP: 15,150; § 17,210.05

is to be made on the basis that the number of factors, whether or not listed in the regulations, indicating a lack of profit objective exceeds the number of factors indicating a profit objective, or vice versa. Among the factors that should normally be taken into account are the following: the manner in which the taxpayer carries on the activity; the expertise of the taxpayer or his or her advisors; the time and effort expended by the taxpayer in carrying on the activity; the expectation that assets used in the activity may appreciate in value; the success of the taxpayer in carrying on other similar or dissimilar activities; the taxpayer's history of income or losses with respect to the activity; the amount of occasional profits, if any, that are earned; the financial status of the taxpayer; and elements of personal pleasure or recreation.

903. Capital Expenditures. A taxpayer may not currently deduct a capital expenditure. Broadly defined, a capital expenditure is (1) any amount paid out for new buildings or permanent improvements or betterments made to increase the value of any property or estate, or (2) any amount expended in restoring property or in making good the exhaustion thereof for which an allowance has been made (Code Sec. 263; Reg. § 1.263(a)-1; Temp. Reg. § 1.263(a)-1T).[5] Capital expenditures are included in basis (¶ 1611) and are generally recovered through depreciation, amortization or depletion (¶ 1201). Amounts paid or incurred for incidental repairs and maintenance of property are not capital expenditures.

Capital expenses include amounts paid to produce or acquire tangible or intangible property, to improve tangible property, to facilitate the acquisition of a trade or business or a change in a business entity's capital structure, or to acquire or create an interest in land. They also include amounts paid in corporate financings and restructurings, such as amounts paid by bondholders and shareholders to be used in corporate reorganizations, voluntary contributions by shareholders to a corporation, and amounts paid by a holding company to carry out a guaranty of dividends on the stock of a subsidiary corporation in certain circumstances (Reg. § 1.263(a)-1(d); Temp. Reg. § 1.263(a)-1T(c)).

Taxpayers may elect to treat certain capital expenditures as deductible or deferred expenses, or treat certain deductible expenses as capital expenditures, as provided by the Code (Reg. § 1.263(a)-6; Temp. Reg. § 1.263(a)-6T).[6] These include expenses related to newspaper or magazine circulation (¶ 971); research and experiments (¶ 979); soil and water conservation (¶ 982); Code Sec. 179 property (¶ 1208); clean-fuel vehicles and refueling property; sulfur regulation compliance (¶ 1285); refineries (¶ 1285A); energy efficient commercial buildings (¶ 1286); advanced mine safety equipment (¶ 989A); fertilizer (¶ 985); film and television production (¶ 977B); removal of barriers to the handicapped and elderly (¶ 1287); tertiary injectants; reforestation (¶ 1287); business start-up (¶ 904); environmental remediation (¶ 977); certain disaster expenses; corporate organization (¶ 237); carrying charges (¶ 1614); mine development (¶ 988); and partnership organization and syndication (¶ 477).

Repair Regulations—Effective Date and Accounting Method Changes. The IRS has issued final "repair" regulations relating to amounts paid to acquire, produce, or improve tangible property, which apply to tax years beginning on or after January 1, 2014 (T.D. 9636). The IRS previously issued comprehensive temporary regulations (T.D. 9564). A taxpayer could, but was not required to, apply either the temporary or final regulations to tax years beginning on or after January 1, 2012, and before January 1, 2014. Certain rules, however, apply only to "amounts paid or incurred" in tax years beginning on or after January 1, 2014 or on or after January 1, 2012, if a taxpayer chose early application. Taxpayers who apply the final regulations may rely on Rev. Proc. 2014-16, effective January 24, 2014, for automatic change of accounting method guidance. Rev. Proc. 2014-16 also provides automatic change guidance for taxpayers who applied the temporary regulations in tax years that began on or after January 1, 2012, and before January 1, 2014, effective for change of accounting method applications filed after January 24, 2014. For earlier-filed applications, Rev. Proc. 2012-19 provides the applicable change of accounting method procedures for the temporary regulations.[7]

References are to Standard Federal Tax Reports; Tax Research Consultant; and Practical Tax Explanations.

[5] ¶ 13,700, ¶ 13,701, ¶ 13,702BC; BUSEXP: 9,000; § 10,201

[6] ¶ 13,704J, ¶ 13,704K; BUSEXP: 9,102; § 10,201

[7] ¶ 13,709.105; BUSEXP: 9,099; § 9,930.05

Acquired or Produced Tangible Property. Taxpayers are required to capitalize amounts paid or incurred to produce or acquire a unit of tangible real or personal property, including leasehold improvement property, land and land improvements, buildings, machinery, equipment, furniture, and fixtures unless a current deduction is allowed under the *de minimis* safe harbor (see later) or the rules that apply to materials and supplies (see later). Capitalized amounts include the invoice price, amounts that facilitate the acquisition of the property (i.e., transactions costs), and costs for work performed before the taxpayer places the property in service (e.g., repairs). Amounts paid to acquire real or personal property for resale are also capitalized (Reg. § 1.263(a)-2; Temp. Reg. § 1.263(a)-2T).[8]

An amount facilitates the acquisition of property if the amount is paid in the process of investigating or otherwise pursuing the acquisition or production of the property. Inherently facilitative costs of acquiring or producing property that must be capitalized are amounts paid for: (a) transporting the property, e.g., shipping fees and moving costs; (b) appraisals and valuations; (c) negotiating the terms or structure of the acquisition; (d) tax advice on the acquisition; (e) application fees, bidding costs, or similar expenses; (f) preparing and reviewing the documents that effectuate the acquisition of the property, e.g., preparing the bid, offer, sales contract, or purchase agreement; (g) title examination and evaluation; (h) obtaining regulatory approval of the acquisition; (i) securing permits related to the acquisition, including application fees; (j) conveying property between the parties, including sales and transfer taxes, and title registration costs; (k) finders' fees or brokers' commissions, including contingency fees; (l) architectural, geological, survey, engineering, environmental, or inspection services pertaining to particular properties; and (m) services provided by a qualified intermediary or other facilitator of a like-kind exchange (Reg. § 1.263(a)-2(f); Temp. Reg. § 1.263(a)-2T(f)).

Activities performed in the process of determining whether to acquire real property and which real property to acquire are currently deductible. However, inherently facilitative amounts are capitalized even if paid or incurred during the "whether and which" process (Reg. § 1.263(a)-2(f)(2)(iii); Temp. Reg. § 1.263(a)-2T(f)(2)(iii)).

Employee compensation and overhead do not facilitate the acquisition of real or personal property but may need to be capitalized under the Code Sec. 263A uniform capitalization rules to property produced by the taxpayer or to property acquired for resale (¶ 990). However, a taxpayer may elect to capitalize employee compensation and overhead on a timely filed original federal tax return, including extensions, for the tax year during which the amounts are paid or incurred (Reg. § 1.263(a)-2(f)(2)(iv); Temp. Reg. § 1.263(a)-2T(f)(2)(iv)).

De Minimis Expensing Safe Harbor. Under the final regulations, a taxpayer who meets certain requirements may make an annual *de minimis* safe harbor expensing election on a timely filed (including extensions) income tax return (Reg. § 1.263(a)-1(f)).[9] A taxpayer electing the safe harbor may not capitalize any amount paid in the tax year for the acquisition or production of a unit of tangible property nor treat as a material or supply an amount paid for tangible property if the amount paid for the property costs no more than a specified amount: up to $5,000 for a taxpayer with an applicable financial statement (AFS), and up to $500 for a taxpayer without an AFS. The uniform capitalization rules (¶ 990) may, however, require a taxpayer to capitalize amounts that are deductible under the safe harbor as a direct and allocable indirect cost of property produced by the taxpayer (for example, amounts that improve property) or property acquired for resale.

A taxpayer with an AFS may elect the *de minimis* expensing safe harbor for a tax year if (1) it has at the beginning of the tax year written accounting procedures treating as an expense for non-tax purposes amounts paid or incurred for property that cost less than a certain dollar amount or that has an economic useful life of 12 months or less and (2) it treats such amounts paid or incurred during the tax year as an expense on the

---

References are to Standard Federal Tax Reports; Tax Research Consultant; and Practical Tax Explanations.

[8] ¶ 13,703, ¶ 13,703L; BUSEXP: 9,080; § 10,215.05

[9] ¶ 13,701; BUSEXP: 9,080; § 10,215.15

AFS. If the taxpayer does not have an AFS, the accounting procedures in effect at the beginning of the tax year do not need to be written. However, the taxpayer must expense on its books and records the applicable dollar amount that applies under its accounting procedures.

Under the *de minimis* rule in the temporary regulations, a taxpayer with an AFS who meets requirements similar to those in the final regulations can deduct for tax purposes during the tax year qualifying amounts not in excess of the greater of: (1) one-tenth of one percent of the taxpayer's gross receipts for the tax year as determined for federal income tax purposes; or (2) two percent of the taxpayer's total depreciation and amortization expense for the tax year as determined on its AFS (Temp. Reg. § 1.263(a)-2T(g)).[10] Taxpayers without an AFS cannot deduct amounts under the *de minimis* rule in the temporary regulations. The temporary regulations also differ from the final regulations in that the *de minimis* rule is considered an accounting method, whereas the *de minimis* safe harbor in the final regulations is not an accounting method and only applies if the taxpayer makes the election to apply it.

Repairs. Expenses that keep tangible property in an ordinarily efficient operating condition and do not add to its value or appreciably prolong its useful life are generally deductible as repairs and maintenance costs (Reg. § 1.162-4; Temp. Reg. § 1.162-4T).[11] Taxpayers may elect to capitalize certain repair expenses (see *Election to Capitalize Repair and Maintenance Costs,* following).

Improvements. Expenses that improve a unit of property are capitalized (Reg. § 1.263(a)-3; Temp. Reg. § 1.263(a)-3T).[12] For this purpose, a unit of property is improved if the amounts paid for activities performed after the property is placed in service by the taxpayer either result in a betterment to the unit of property, restore the unit of property, or adapt the unit of property to a new or different use. A taxpayer generally must capitalize all the direct costs of an improvement, as well as all the indirect costs, such as otherwise deductible repair costs, that directly benefit or are incurred by reason of an improvement. Indirect costs that do not directly benefit and are not incurred by reason of an improvement generally are not capital improvements, regardless of whether they are paid or incurred at the same time as a capital improvement.

A betterment is an expenditure that:

- ameliorates a material condition or defect that existed prior to the taxpayer's acquisition of the unit of property or arose during the production of the property, whether or not the taxpayer was aware of the condition or defect at the time of acquisition;

- is for a material addition to the unit of property, such as a physical enlargement, expansion, extension, or addition of a new major component;

- is for a material increase in the capacity of the unit of property, such as additional cubic or linear space; or

- is reasonably expected to materially increase the productivity, efficiency, strength, quality, or output of the unit of property (Reg. § 1.263(a)-3(j)(1); Temp. Reg. § 1.263(a)-3T(h)).

An amount is paid to restore a unit of property if:

- the taxpayer replaces a component of a unit of property and deducts a loss for that component, other than a casualty loss, for example, by making a partial disposition election under Reg. § 1.168(i)-8(d);

- the taxpayer replaces a component of a unit of property and realizes gain or loss by selling or exchanging the component;

- the expenditure is for the restoration of damage to a unit of property caused by a casualty and the taxpayer is required to make a basis adjustment to the unit of property on account of a casualty loss or the receipt of insurance;

References are to Standard Federal Tax Reports; Tax Research Consultant; and Practical Tax Explanations.

[10] ¶ 13,703L; BUSEXP: 9,080; § 10,215.15

[11] ¶ 8620, ¶ 8627AC; BUSEXP: 9,150; § 9,930.05

[12] ¶ 13,704, ¶ 13,704BC; BUSEXP: 9,090; § 10,215.12

- the expenditures return a unit of property to its ordinary efficient operating condition after the property has deteriorated to a state of disrepair and is no longer functional for its intended use;

- the expenditures rebuild a unit of property to a like-new condition after the end of its class life (i.e., its MACRS alternative depreciation system recovery period); or

- the expenditures are for the replacement of a part or a combination of parts that comprise a major component or a substantial structural part of a unit of property (Reg. § 1.263(a)-3(k)(1); Temp. Reg. § 1.263(a)-3T(i)).

Repair expenditures paid in connection with a casualty are currently deductible if the capitalized restoration expenditures exceed the adjusted basis of the property prior to reduction by the casualty loss deduction or insurance reimbursement. If the capitalized restoration expenditures do not exceed the adjusted basis, but the sum of the capitalized restoration expenditures and repair expenditures exceed the adjusted basis, then the repair expenditures not used to offset the adjusted basis may be deducted (Reg. §§ 1.263(a)-3(k)(4)(i) and (k)(7), Example 5). Under the temporary regulations, repair expenditures are not deductible if a basis adjustment is made to a property on account of a casualty loss or event, such as the receipt of insurance (Temp. Reg. § 1.263(a)-3T(i)(1)(iii)).

An adaptation to a new or different use is a type of improvement that is capitalized. In general, an amount is paid to adapt a unit of property to a new or different use if the adaptation is not consistent with the taxpayer's ordinary use of the unit of property at the time it was originally placed in service by the taxpayer (Reg. § 1.263(a)-3(l); Temp. Reg. § 1.263(a)-3T(j)).

Removal Costs. If a taxpayer disposes of a depreciable asset, including a partial disposition under Reg. §§ 1.168(i)-1(e)(1)(ii) or 1.168(i)-8(d), and has taken into account the adjusted basis of the asset or component of the asset in realizing gain or loss, then the costs of removing the asset or component are deductible. If a taxpayer disposes of a component of a unit of property, but the disposal of the component is not a disposition, then the taxpayer must capitalize the removal cost if it directly benefits or is incurred by reason of an improvement to the unit of property (Reg. § 1.263(a)-3(g)(2)). For example, the cost of removing shingles on a roof is deductible if the replacement costs are a deductible repair. However, if the entire roof is replaced and the replacement costs are capitalized, then the removal costs are capitalized provided no loss deduction is claimed on the replaced roof by making the partial disposition election. Special rules apply to demolitions (¶ 1105).

Routine Maintenance Safe Harbor. Both the final and temporary regulations contain a safe harbor rule for routine maintenance activities (Reg. § 1.263(a)-3(i); Temp. Reg. § 1.263(a)-3T(g)).[13] Routine maintenance activities are the recurring activities expected to be performed to keep a unit of property in ordinarily efficient operating order. The activities are considered routine only if at the time the unit of property is placed in service the taxpayer reasonably expects to perform the activities more than once during the class life (i.e., MACRS alternative depreciation system recovery period) of the unit of property.

Routine maintenance *does not* include amounts paid or incurred for a betterment or adaptation. The following types of restorations also do not qualify: the cost of replacing components if a retirement loss is claimed or gain or loss is realized upon a sale of the replaced component; amounts paid for the restoration of damage to a unit of property for which a basis adjustment as a result of a casualty loss or casualty event is required; and the cost of restoring deteriorated and nonfunctional property to its ordinarily efficient operating condition. In addition, routine maintenance does not include amounts paid for repairs, maintenance, or improvement of rotable and temporary spare parts to which the taxpayer applies the optional method of accounting for rotable and temporary spare

---

References are to Standard Federal Tax Reports; Tax Research Consultant; and Practical Tax Explanations.

[13] ¶ 13,704, ¶ 13,704BC;
BUSEXP: 9,096.10; § 10,215.40

parts. Routine maintenance may include the replacement of a major component or substantial structural part of a unit of property.

Under the final regulations, routine maintenance performed on a building structure or any of its building systems qualifies for the routine maintenance safe harbor. The final regulations also disqualify network assets, e.g., railroad track, oil and gas pipelines, water and sewage pipelines, power transmission and distribution lines, and telephone and cable lines, from the safe harbor.

The routine maintenance safe harbor is an accounting method and not an election.

Building Improvements Safe Harbor for Small Taxpayers. A taxpayer with $10 million or less of average annual gross receipts in the three preceding tax years may elect not to capitalize improvements on a building, condominium, or cooperative that has an unadjusted basis, i.e., generally cost, of $1 million or less if the total amount paid or incurred for repairs, maintenance, and improvements for the tax year of the election does not exceed the lesser of (1) $10,000 or (2) two percent of the unadjusted basis of the building. Amounts deducted under the *de minimis* safe harbor or the safe harbor for routine maintenance are counted toward the $10,000 limit. This election is only available under the final regulations and must be made by the due date of the return, including extensions, for the year of the election. The improvements safe harbor for small taxpayers is applied separately to each eligible building owned or leased by the taxpayer. In the case of a lessee, the unadjusted basis of a leased building or leased building space is equal to the total amount of undiscounted rent paid or expected to be paid over the entire lease term, including expected renewal periods (Reg. § 1.263(a)-3(h)).[14]

Election to Capitalize Repair and Maintenance Costs. Under the final regulations only, a taxpayer may elect on a timely filed original return, including extensions, to capitalize as improvements all amounts paid during the tax year for repair and maintenance of tangible property, if the taxpayer incurs these amounts in carrying on its trade or business and treats them as capital expenditures on its books and records for the tax year covered by the election. If the election is made, the taxpayer cannot currently deduct the repair and maintenance amounts affected by the election. The election does not apply to amounts paid for repairs or maintenance of rotable or temporary spare parts to which the optional method of accounting under Reg. § 1.162-3(e) is applied (Reg. § 1.263(a)-3(n)).[15]

Unit of Property. All components that are functionally interdependent comprise a single unit of property. Components are functionally interdependent if the placing in service of one component is dependent on the placing in service the other components (Reg. § 1.263(a)-3(e); Temp. Reg. § 1.263(a)-3T(e)).[16] Although a building, including its structural components, is a unit of property, the improvement rules are applied separately to each building system and the building structure. A building structure consists of a building as defined in Reg. § 1.48-1(e)(1) and its structural components as defined in Reg. § 1.48-1(e)(2), *other than* those designated as building systems. Designated building systems, including their components, that are separate from the building structure are:

    (1) heating, ventilation, and air conditioning (HVAC) systems, including motors, compressors, boilers, furnace, chillers, pipes, ducts, and radiators;

    (2) plumbing systems, including pipes, drains, values, sinks, bathtubs, toilets, water and sanitary sewer collection equipment, and site utility equipment;

    (3) electrical systems, including wiring, outlets, junction boxes, lighting fixtures and associated connectors, and site utility equipment;

    (4) all escalators;

    (5) all elevators;

    (6) fire-protection and alarm systems, including sensing devices, computer controls, sprinkler heads, sprinkler mains, associated pipes or plumbing, pumps,

---

References are to Standard Federal Tax Reports; Tax Research Consultant; and Practical Tax Explanations.

[14] ¶ 13,704; BUSEXP: 9,096.20; § 10,215.12b

[15] ¶ 13,704; BUSEXP: 9,096.25; § 9,930.05.

[16] ¶ 13,704, ¶ 13,704BC; BUSEXP: 9,094; § 10,215.12.

visual and audible alarms, alarms control panels, heat and smoke detection devices, fire escapes, fire doors, emergency exit lighting and signage, and fire fighting equipment;

(7) security systems for the protection of the building and it occupants, including windows and door locks, security cameras, recorders, monitors, motion detectors, security lighting, alarm systems, entry and access systems, and related junction boxes, wiring and conduits;

(8) gas distribution systems, including associated pipes and equipment used to distribute gas to and from the property line and between buildings; and

(9) any other structural components designated as a building system by the IRS in published guidance

Example: A taxpayer replaces the steps on the sole escalator in a building. The improvement rules are applied separately to the escalator because it is a building system. Since the steps are a major component of the escalator, the cost of replacing the steps is for a restoration and must be capitalized. If the improvement rules applied to the entire building, including its building systems, then the steps might not be considered a major component of the building and a repair deduction could be claimed. Generally, the larger the unit of property the more likely an expenditure is for a repair.

Materials and Supplies. The cost of nonincidental materials and supplies are deducted in the tax year they are first used or consumed, while the cost of incidental materials and supplies for which no inventories or records of consumption are kept is deductible in the tax year when paid or incurred if taxable income is clearly reflected (Reg. § 1.162-3(a); Temp. Reg. § 1.162-3T(a)).[17] However, materials and supplies that improve tangible property are capitalized (Reg. § 1.263(a)-3(c); Temp. Reg. § 1.263(a)-3T(c)). In addition, the uniform capitalization rules (¶ 990) require taxpayers to capitalize the direct and allocable indirect costs, including the cost of materials and supplies, of property produced by the taxpayer and property acquired for resale. Taxpayers may also be required to include in inventory certain materials and supplies (Reg. § 1.471-1) (Reg. § 1.162-3(b); Temp. Reg. § 1.162-3T(b)). Finally, the cost of materials and supplies that meet the requirements of the *de minimis* safe harbor are deductible in the year paid or incurred if a taxpayer makes the *de minimis* safe harbor election.

"Materials and supplies" mean tangible property that is used or consumed in the taxpayer's business operations, is not inventory, and is:

- a component that is acquired to maintain, repair, or improve a unit of tangible property owned, leased, or serviced by the taxpayer, but is not acquired as part of any single unit of tangible property;

- fuel, lubricants, water, and similar items that are reasonably expected to be consumed in 12 months or less, beginning when used in a taxpayer's operations;

- a unit of property that has an economic useful life of 12 months or less, beginning when the property is used or consumed in the taxpayer's operations;

- a unit of property with an acquisition or production cost of $200 or less ($100 or less if the taxpayer applies the temporary regulations); or

- identified as a material or supply by the IRS in published guidance (Reg. § 1.162-3(c)(1); Temp. Reg. § 1.162-3T(c)(1)).

Rotable, Temporary, and Standby Emergency Parts. Rotable and temporary spare parts are materials and supplies and their cost is deducted in the year used or consumed unless the taxpayer uses the optional method of accounting to deduct their cost in the year of installation (Reg. § 1.162-3(c)(2); Temp. Reg. § 1.162-3T(c)(2)).[18] If the election is not made rotable and temporary spare parts are treated as used or consumed in the year they are discarded (Reg. § 1.162-3(a)(3); Temp. Reg. § 1.162-3T(a)(3)).

References are to Standard Federal Tax Reports; Tax Research Consultant; and Practical Tax Explanations.

[17] ¶ 8600, ¶ 8605AC;
BUSEXP: 18,558; § 9,935.05

[18] ¶ 8600, ¶ 8605AC;
BUSEXP: 18,558; § 9,935.05

Rotable spare parts are parts that are acquired for installation on a unit of property, removable from that unit of property, generally repaired or improved, and either reinstalled on the same or other property or stored for later installation. Temporary spare parts are parts that are used temporarily until a new or repaired part can be installed and then are removed and stored for later installation (Reg. § 1.162-3(c)(2); Temp. Reg. § 1.162-3T(c)(2)).

A taxpayer may elect to capitalize and depreciate the cost of rotable, temporary, and standby emergency spare parts. The election does not apply to rotable and temporary spare parts for which the optional method of accounting is used (Reg. § 1.162-3(d)).

The *de minimis* safe harbor election under the final regulations does not apply to rotable, temporary, or standby emergency spare parts that a taxpayer elects to capitalize and depreciate or to rotable and temporary spare parts that are accounted for under the optional method (Reg. § 1.162-3(f)).

Intangible Property. Amounts must be capitalized if they are paid or incurred for: (1) specific categories of expenditures that are incurred in acquiring, creating, or enhancing, or that facilitate the acquisition or creation of, an intangible that is acquired from another person in a purchase or similar transaction; (2) certain rights, privileges, or benefits that are created or originated by the taxpayer; (3) a separate and distinct intangible asset; or (4) a future benefit that the IRS identifies in published guidance (Reg. § 1.263(a)-4).[19]

904. Business Start-Up Costs. Taxpayers who pay or incur start-up costs for a trade or business and who subsequently enter the trade or business can elect to expense up to $5,000 of the costs. The $5,000 deduction amount is reduced dollar for dollar when the start-up expenses exceed $50,000. The balance of start-up expenses, if any, are amortized over the 180-month period starting with the month in which the business begins (Code Sec. 195).[20] The election must be made no later than the date, including extensions, for filing the return for the tax year in which the business begins or is acquired. The election is made by completing Part VI of Form 4562. A taxpayer who does not make the election must capitalize the expenses.

A taxpayer is deemed to have made an election to deduct and amortize start-up expenses for the tax year in which the active trade or business to which the expenses relate begins. A taxpayer may choose to forego the deemed election by affirmatively electing to capitalize its start-up costs on a timely filed federal income tax return, including extensions, for the tax year in which the active trade or business begins. The election either to deduct and amortize start-up costs, or capitalize them, applies to all start-up expenses that are related to the active trade or business (Reg. § 1.195-1).[21]

Start-up expenses are those paid or incurred in connection with:

- investigating the creation or acquisition of an active trade or business;
- creating an active trade or business; or
- any activity engaged in for profit or for the production of income before the day on which the active trade or business begins, in anticipation of that activity becoming an active trade or business.

In addition, the start-up expense must be a cost that would be allowable as a deduction if it were paid or incurred in connection with an existing active business in the same field as that entered into by the taxpayer (Code Sec. 195(c)).[22]

Start-up costs do not include any amount with respect to which a deduction is allowed for interest on indebtedness (¶ 1043), taxes (¶ 1021), or research and experimental expenses (¶ 979). If the trade or business is disposed of completely by the taxpayer before the end of the 180-month period, any remaining deferred expenses may be deductible as a loss (¶ 1101) (Code Sec. 195(b)(2)).[23]

References are to Standard Federal Tax Reports; Tax Research Consultant; and Practical Tax Explanations.

[19] ¶ 13,704C; BUSEXP: 9,104.20; § 10,210.05

[20] ¶ 12,370; DEPR: 21,400; § 9,201

[21] ¶ 12,370F; BUSEXP: 12,252; § 9,215

[22] ¶ 12,370; DEPR: 21,400; § 9,205.10

[23] ¶ 12,370; DEPR: 21,450; § 9,205.05

The organizational costs of business entities are a separate class of expense from start-up expenses, though subject to similar rules. Corporate organization fees are discussed at ¶ 237. Costs of organizing a partnership are discussed at ¶ 477 and ¶ 481.

905. Expenses, Interest Deductions, and Losses—Related Taxpayers. When the payor and payee are related taxpayers (¶ 1717), and the payor is on the accrual method of accounting and the payee is on the cash method, no deduction will be allowed for any trade or business expense or interest payable to the payee until the payee includes the payment in income (Code Sec. 267(a)(2)).[24] A similar rule denies a deduction for a loss (except for a loss from a distribution in corporate liquidation) for property sold or exchanged between related taxpayers (Code Sec. 267(a) and (d)).[25] However, upon later sale or exchange of the property by the transferee at a gain, the gain is recognized only to the extent that it exceeds the previously disallowed loss.

Compensation Paid

906. Compensation for Personal Service. A taxpayer carrying on a trade or business is entitled to deduct a reasonable allowance for salaries or other compensation for personal services. The deduction is allowable for the year in which the salary is paid or incurred (Code Sec. 162(a)(1); Reg. § 1.162-7).[26]

Publicly held corporations are generally not able to deduct compensation paid to certain covered employees to the extent that the compensation exceeds $1 million per tax year (Code Sec. 162(m); Reg. § 1.162-27).[27] A "covered employee" is any employee of the taxpayer who, as of the close of the tax year, is:

- the principal executive officer of the taxpayer;
- an individual acting in a capacity as principal executive officer; or
- required to have his or her compensation reported to shareholders under SEC rules by reason of the individual's being among the three highest compensated officers for the tax year (Notice 2007-49).[28]

The $1 million limit does not apply to certain "performance-based compensation" payable solely on account of attaining one or more performance goals (Code Sec. 162(m)(4)(C); Reg. § 1.162-27(e); Prop. Reg. § 1.162-27(e)(2)(vi)(A)).[29] Performance-based compensation can include compensation issued in the form of stock rights and options exercised when the plan specifies the maximum number of shares that may be granted to all employees in the aggregate. Under proposed regulations applicable to tax years ending on or after the date of their publication as final regulations, performance-based compensation attributable to stock rights or stock options must include a specific per-employee limitation on the amount granted.

Awards paid under a corporate bonus plan are not qualified performance-based compensation if the plan allows payments to be made, even if the specified performance goals have not been met, upon the employee's retirement, termination without cause, or voluntary termination of employment for good reason (Rev. Rul. 2008-13).[30] If the bonus was paid solely for attaining a performance goal, the goal must be determined by a compensation committee consisting solely of two or more outside directors. An outside director cannot be a current employee, a former employee who receives compensation during the year, or a current or former officer (Rev. Rul. 2008-32).[31]

Reasonable compensation is the amount that would ordinarily be paid for like services by like enterprises in like circumstances (Reg. § 1.162-7(b)(3)).[32] Thus, whether compensation is reasonable in a given situation depends on the relevant facts and circumstances. Some factors considered include personal ability, responsibility of the position, and economic conditions in the locality. The U.S. Court of Appeals for the

---

References are to Standard Federal Tax Reports; Tax Research Consultant; and Practical Tax Explanations.

[24] ¶ 14,150; ACCTNG: 12,150; § 17,601

[25] ¶ 14,150; SALES: 39,100; § 17,605

[26] ¶ 8500, ¶ 8635; COMPEN: 9,050; § 9,305.05

[27] ¶ 8500, ¶ 9051B; COMPEN: 12,350; § 9,310

[28] ¶ 8636.2763; COMPEN: 12,354

[29] ¶ 8500, ¶ 9051B, ¶ 9051BB; COMPEN: 12,356; § 9,310

[30] ¶ 8636.2768; COMPEN: 12,356.10

[31] ¶ 8636.2764; COMPEN: 12,356.10; § 9,310.15

[32] ¶ 8635; COMPEN: 9,100; § 9,305.10

Seventh Circuit has used an independent-investor test. This test presumes that compensation is reasonable if the company's investors earn their expected rate of return (*Exacto Spring Corporation*, CA-7, 99-2 USTC ¶ 50,964).[33] A bonus is deductible if paid for services performed, and if, when added to other salaries, it does not exceed reasonable compensation (Reg. § 1.162-9).[34] Compensation paid to a relative is deductible if the relative performs needed services that would otherwise be performed by an unrelated party. The deduction is limited to the amount that would have been paid to a third party (*Transport Mfg. & Equip. Co.*, CA-8, 70-2 USTC ¶ 9627).[35]

Officer-Stockholders of Closely Held Corporations. Officer-stockholders of closely held corporations may deduct repayments of salary to their corporation that are made pursuant to an agreement requiring such repayments in the event that the IRS determines the salaries to be excessive (Rev. Rul. 69-115).[36] However, the officer-stockholders may claim the deduction only if the agreement is legally enforceable and was in existence *before* the payment of the amounts.

Deferred Compensation Plans. For unfunded deferred compensation plans, the employer's deduction for compensation is claimed when the compensation, or amount attributable to it, is included in the gross income of the recipient (Code Sec. 404(a)(5) and (b)(1)).[37] For the time of inclusion, see ¶ 723. Other benefits that are excluded from the recipient's gross income are deductible when they otherwise would have been includible in the recipient's gross income but for the exclusion (Code Sec. 404(b)(2)).[38] This rule also applies to compensation paid to independent contractors (Code Sec. 404(d)).[39]

A plan is unfunded if it consists of an unsecured promise to pay compensation at some time in the future. If the employer sets aside a reserve for the future obligation, the plan is unfunded if the employee has no rights in the reserve or its earnings and if the reserve remains solely the property of the employer or other payor, subject to the claims of creditors (Rev. Rul. 55-525).[40]

A plan is presumed to defer compensation if the compensation is received after the 15th day of the third calendar month after the end of the employer's tax year in which the related services are rendered. This presumption may be overcome if the employer establishes that it was administratively or economically impractical to avoid the deferral of compensation beyond the 2½-month period. Payments within the 2½-month period are not treated as deferred compensation and may be accrued by an accrual-method employer in the year earned by the employee (Temp. Reg. § 1.404(b)-1T, Q&A-2).[41]

For a discussion of rules governing the employer's deduction for compensation for deferred compensation plans, see ¶ 2117 and ¶ 2199.

Health Insurance Providers. The deduction for compensation or remuneration paid to officers, directors, or employees of covered health insurance providers, including those that provide services for or on behalf of covered health insurance providers, is limited to $500,000 for disqualified tax years beginning after December 31, 2012 (Code Sec. 162(m)(6); Reg. § 1.162-31).[42] A disqualified tax year is any tax year in which the employer is a covered health insurance provider that receives premiums from providing health insurance coverage for years beginning after December 31, 2009, and before January 1, 2013. For tax years after December 31, 2012, a covered health insurance provider is a health insurance issuer, as defined under Code Sec. 9832(b)(2), for any tax year during which at least 25 percent of the gross premiums it receives from providing health insurance coverage is from providing minimum essential coverage (¶ 131). A *de minimis* rule allows employers that meet the definition of covered health insurance provider to avoid the limitation if premiums received for providing health insurance coverage are less than two percent of gross revenues.

References are to Standard Federal Tax Reports; Tax Research Consultant; and Practical Tax Explanations.

[33] ¶ 8637.227, ¶ 8637.57; COMPEN: 9,114; § 9,305.10

[34] ¶ 8641; COMPEN: 9,054; § 9,335

[35] ¶ 8637.752; COMPEN: 9,202; § 9,305.20

[36] ¶ 8640.165; COMPEN: 9,456; § 7,101

[37] ¶ 18,330; COMPEN: 15,250; § 25,605

[38] ¶ 18,330; COMPEN: 12,108.10; § 25,605

[39] ¶ 18,330; COMPEN: 15,252; § 25,605

[40] ¶ 18,352.48; COMPEN: 15,050; § 25,610.15

[41] ¶ 18,354; COMPEN: 15,254; § 24,005

[42] ¶ 8500, ¶ 9051I; COMPEN: 12,360; § 9,310.05

Deduction Limit for TARP Recipients. Under the Troubled Asset Relief Program (TARP) established pursuant to the Emergency Economic Stabilization Act of 2008 (P.L. 110-343), the federal government is authorized to purchase troubled assets from financial institutions, either through a public auction or directly from the institution. During the period in which financial assistance under TARP remains outstanding, each TARP recipient will be subject to a $500,000 compensation deduction limit (Code Sec. 162(m)(5)).[43] The deduction limit applies during the period that the TARP obligation remains outstanding. There is no threshold amount of assistance an entity must receive to qualify for TARP recipient treatment for these purposes.

907. Golden Parachutes. A corporation that enters into a contract agreeing to pay an employee additional compensation in the event that control or ownership of the corporation changes is barred from taking a deduction for an "excess parachute payment" made to a "disqualified individual" (Code Sec. 280G).[44] A disqualified individual is an employee or independent contractor who performs personal services for any corporation and is an officer, shareholder, or highly compensated person. A personal service corporation is treated as an individual. The disqualified individual is subject to an excise tax of 20 percent of the excess parachute payment in addition to the income tax due (Code Sec. 4999(a)).[45]

Parachute Payment Defined. A parachute payment is any payment in the nature of compensation to a disqualified individual if:

- the payment is contingent on a change in the ownership or effective control of the corporation or a substantial portion of the assets of the corporation; and

- the aggregate present value of such contingent payments equals or exceeds three times an individual's base amount.

Any payment in the nature of compensation to a disqualified individual made under an agreement that violates any securities law or regulations is also considered a parachute payment. Reasonable compensation for personal services to be rendered on or after the date of change or for personal services actually rendered before the date of change are not treated as parachute payments. Additionally, parachute payments do not include payments to or from certain qualified plans (Code Sec. 280G(b)).[46]

Base Amount. The base amount is the individual's annualized includible compensation for the base period (the most recent five tax years ending before the date on which the ownership of control changed, or that portion of the period during which the disqualified individual performed personal services for the corporation) (Code Sec. 280G(b)(3)(A) and (d)(2)).[47]

Exceptions. Generally, a parachute payment does not include any payment made to a disqualified individual by a small business corporation. It also does not include a payment from a corporation, if, immediately before the change in ownership or control, none of the corporation's stock was readily tradable on an established securities market and shareholder approval requirements were met (Code Sec. 280G(b)(5)).[48]

Excess Parachute Payment. An excess parachute payment is an amount equal to the excess of any parachute payment over the portion of the base amount allocated to the payment. The allocable base amount is subtracted from the parachute payment, and the remainder is the excess parachute payment (Code Sec. 280G(b)).[49]

908. Contributions for Employee Benefits and Health Insurance. An employer's deduction for contributions to a funded welfare benefit plan for sickness, accident, hospitalization, or medical benefits is governed by Code Sec. 419 (¶ 2011) (Temp. Reg. § 1.162-10T).[50] Although amounts that are added to a self-insurance reserve account are

---

References are to Standard Federal Tax Reports; Tax Research Consultant; and Practical Tax Explanations.

[43] ¶ 8500; COMPEN: 12,358; § 9,310.05

[44] ¶ 15,150; COMPEN: 30,050; § 21,805.15

[45] ¶ 34,940; COMPEN: 30,250; § 21,820

[46] ¶ 15,150; COMPEN: 30,100; § 21,815.05

[47] ¶ 15,150; COMPEN: 30,150; § 21,805.25

[48] ¶ 15,150; COMPEN: 30,110; § 21,815.15

[49] ¶ 15,150; COMPEN: 30,150; § 21,805.25

[50] ¶ 8751; COMPEN: 42,100; § 9,345

not currently deductible, actual claims charged to the account are deductible (*General Dynamics Corp.*, SCt, 87-1 USTC ¶ 9280).[51] Group health plans that fail to provide COBRA continuing coverage to qualified beneficiaries may subject employers to an excise tax (Code Sec. 4980B).[52]

Self-Employed Persons. Self-employed persons may deduct from gross income 100 percent of amounts paid during the year for health insurance for themselves, spouses, and dependents (Code Sec. 162(l)).[53] The deduction cannot exceed the taxpayer's net earned income derived from the trade or business for which the insurance plan was established, minus the deductions for 50 percent of the self-employment tax and/or the deduction for contributions to qualified retirement plans, self-employed pensions (SEPs), or SIMPLE plans. Amounts eligible for the deduction do not include amounts paid during any month, or part of a month, that the self-employed individual was able to participate in a subsidized health plan maintained by his or her employer or spouses' employer. The IRS has issued guidance providing optional calculation methods to resolve the circular relationship between the health insurance premium assistance credit (¶ 1331) and the self-employed health insurance deduction (Rev. Proc. 2014-41).[54]

Children Under the Age of 27. Children under the age of 27 are considered dependents of a taxpayer for purposes of the deduction for the health insurance costs of a self-employed person, spouse, and dependents. A child includes: a son, daughter, stepson, or stepdaughter of the taxpayer; a foster child placed with the taxpayer by an authorized placement agency or by judgment, decree, or other order of any court of competent jurisdiction; and a legally adopted child of the taxpayer or a child who has been lawfully placed with the taxpayer for legal adoption (Code Sec. 152(f)(1)).[55]

Excise Tax on High-Cost Employer-Provided Insurance. A 40-percent excise tax will be imposed on health coverage providers starting in 2018 to the extent that the aggregate value of employer-sponsored health coverage for an employee exceeds a threshold amount (Code Sec. 4980I).[56]

908A. Disability Payments. A business or professional person may deduct premiums on a policy that pays overhead expenses during a period of disability, but the proceeds under such a policy are includible in gross income (Rev. Rul. 55-264).[57] When an insurance premium is paid in advance for more than one year, only a pro rata portion of the premium is deductible for each year, regardless of the taxpayer's method of accounting (Reg. § 1.461-1; Rev. Rul. 70-413).[58]

908B. Employer-Provided Daycare. Payments to a daycare center are a deductible business expense where the purpose of providing the availability of the day care center is:

- to provide an employee with a place to send his or her child while at work, so that the employee can be reassured that the child is receiving proper care;

- to reduce absenteeism, increase productivity, and reduce company training costs; and

- to reduce employee turnover (Rev. Rul. 73-348).[59]

An S corporation, however, was not allowed to deduct amounts it paid for daycare for its sole shareholder's preschool children where there was no direct relationship to the taxpayer's business, and, despite the S corporation employing over 20 individuals, the S corporation only paid daycare expenses for the taxpayer's children (*F.M. Settimo*, Dec. 56,694(M), 92 TCM 473 (2006)).[60]

References are to Standard Federal Tax Reports; Tax Research Consultant; and Practical Tax Explanations.

[51] ¶ 8522.3947; BUSEXP: 18,210; § 9405.30, § 9,345

[52] ¶ 34,600; HEALTH: 24,100; § 42,850.05

[53] ¶ 8500; HEALTH: 15,100; § 5,401

[54] ¶ 8522.405; HEALTH: 3,322; § 42,015.20

[55] ¶ 8007; FILEIND: 6,154.05; § 1,215.10

[56] ¶ 34,619ZE; HEALTH: 9,302

[57] ¶ 8522.385; BUSEXP: 18,220; § 9,415.05

[58] ¶ 21,805, ¶ 21,817.21; BUSEXP: 18,216; § 9,420.05

[59] ¶ 8752.21; BUSEXP: 3,104; § 9,010.15

[60] ¶ 8520.517; BUSEXP: 3,104; § 9,010.15

Up to $5,000 of child or dependent care assistance services provided to an employee may be excluded from the employee's gross income (¶ 2065).

909. Life Insurance Premiums. Premiums paid by an employer for insurance on the life of an officer or employee are deductible only if it can be shown that:

- premium payments are in the nature of additional compensation;

- total compensation, including premiums, is not unreasonable; and

- the employer is not directly or indirectly a beneficiary under the policy (*L. Hyman & Co.*, Dec. 6447, 21 BTA 159; *Brown Agency, Inc.*, Dec. 6615, 21 BTA 1111).[61]

However, no deduction is allowed an employer for premiums paid under a split dollar arrangement (¶ 2057).

Premiums on group-term life insurance covering the lives of employees are deductible by the employer only if the employer is not a direct or indirect beneficiary (Code Sec. 264(a)(1); Reg. § 1.264-1).[62] The payment of such premiums generally represents income to the employee to the extent that the coverage provided exceeds $50,000 (¶ 2055).

Generally, no deduction is allowed for interest paid or accrued on a debt incurred or continued to purchase or carry any single premium life insurance, endowment or annuity contract. If substantially all the premiums on a life insurance or endowment contract are paid within four years from date of purchase, or if an amount is deposited with the insurer for payment of a substantial number of future premiums on the contract, it is regarded as a single premium contract (Code Sec. 264(a)(2) and (c)).[63]

Interest on a debt incurred to purchase or continue a life insurance, endowment, or annuity contract pursuant to a plan of purchase contemplating the systematic borrowing of part or all of the increases in cash value is not deductible (Code Sec. 264(a)(3)).[64] However, an interest deduction is allowed in limited situations (Code Sec. 264(d)). Special rules may permit the deduction of interest incurred for key person policies owned by corporations (Code Sec. 264(e)).[65]

Entertainment, Meal, and Gift Expenses

910. Entertainment Expenses. Special limits are imposed by Code Sec. 274 on the deduction of business-related entertainment, meals, and gift expenses in addition to those imposed by other Code sections. Specifically, no deduction is allowed for the cost of entertainment, amusement, or recreation unless that cost is either (1) *directly related* to the active conduct of a trade or business (¶ 911), or (2) for entertainment directly before or after a substantial and bona fide business discussion *associated with* the conduct of that trade or business (¶ 912) (Code Sec. 274(a)(1)).

Specific exceptions to these general requirements are discussed at ¶ 915. Entertainment includes entertaining guests at nightclubs, sporting events, theaters, etc. A taxpayer's trade or business is considered in applying an objective test as to what constitutes entertainment. For example, if an appliance distributor conducts a fashion show for the spouses of retailers, the show would generally be considered entertainment (Code Sec. 274(a)(1)(A); Reg. § 1.274-2(b)(1)(ii)).[66] The amount allowable as a business deduction for meal and entertainment expenses is generally limited to 50 percent of these expenses (¶ 916). There are numerous exceptions to the 50-percent limitation rule, which are discussed at ¶ 917.

References are to Standard Federal Tax Reports; Tax Research Consultant; and Practical Tax Explanations.

[61] ¶ 8522.386, ¶ 8636.27; BUSEXP: 18,154.05; § 9405.05

[62] ¶ 14,002, ¶ 14,003; COMPEN: 48,100; § 21,005.05

[63] ¶ 14,002; INDIV: 48,556; § 9405.05

[64] ¶ 14,002; INDIV: 48,556; § 9,405.15

[65] ¶ 14,002; COMPEN: 48,062; § 9,405.15

[66] ¶ 14,402, ¶ 14,405; BUSEXP: 24,550; § 9,610.05, § 9,635.05

Two-Percent-of-AGI Floor. In most situations, an employee's unreimbursed business expenses must be claimed as a miscellaneous itemized deduction, subject to the two-percent-of-adjusted-gross-income (AGI) floor, on Schedule A of Form 1040 (¶ 1011). Any percentage limit, e.g., 50 percent on meal and entertainment expenses, must be taken into account prior to application of the two-percent-of-AGI floor (¶ 942) (Code Sec. 67; Temp. Reg. § 1.67-1T(a)).[67] Certain employees defined by the Code may deduct their unreimbursed expenses directly from gross income (¶ 941B).

911. Directly Related Test. For an entertainment expense to meet the directly related test in order to be deducted as a business expense (¶ 910), the taxpayer must have had more than a general expectation of deriving income, or some other specific business benefit, at some indefinite future time. The taxpayer must engage in the active conduct of business with the person being entertained. In addition, the active conduct of business must be the principal aspect of the combined business and entertainment (Reg. § 1.274-2(c)).[68]

912. Associated Entertainment. Entertainment expenses associated with the active conduct of the taxpayer's business are deductible if they directly precede or follow a bona fide and substantial business discussion (¶ 910). This includes goodwill expenditures to obtain new business or encourage continuation of existing business relationships. The business discussion must be the principal aspect of the combined entertainment and business and must represent an active effort by the taxpayer to obtain income or other specific business benefit (Reg. § 1.274-2(d)).[69]

913. Entertainment Facility. No business deduction is generally allowed for any expense for entertainment facilities, such as yachts, hunting lodges, swimming pools, tennis courts, or bowling alleys (¶ 910) (Code Sec. 274(a)(1)(B)).[70] However, expenses for recreational facilities primarily for the benefit of employees generally are deductible (Reg. § 1.274-2(f)(2)(v)).[71]

913A. Club Dues. As a general rule, no business deduction is permitted for club dues. This rule extends to business, social, athletic, luncheon, sporting, airline, and hotel clubs (Code Sec. 274(a)(3); Reg. § 1.274-2(a)(2)(iii)).[72] However, dues paid to professional or public service organizations (e.g., accounting associations, or Kiwanis and Rotary clubs) are deductible if they are paid for business reasons and the organization's principal purpose is *not* to conduct entertainment activities for members or their guests or to provide those parties with access to entertainment facilities.

914. Entertainment-Related Meals. Generally, an entertainment-related meal expense is *not* deductible unless the taxpayer establishes that the expense is directly related to the active conduct of a trade or business. However, if a meal expense directly precedes or follows a substantial and bona fide business discussion, including a business meeting at a convention, then it is deductible if it is established that the expense was associated with the active conduct of a trade or business. The taxpayer must be able to substantiate the expense (¶ 953) (Code Sec. 274(d); Temp. Reg. § 1.274-5T(c) and (f)).[73]

There are two additional restrictions placed on the deduction of meal expenses: (1) meal expenses generally are not deductible if neither the taxpayer nor the taxpayer's employee is present at the meal, and (2) a deduction will not be allowed for food and beverages to the extent that such expense is lavish or extravagant under the circumstances. These restrictions do not apply to the expenses described in exceptions (2), (3), (4), (7), (8), and (9) at ¶ 915 (Code Sec. 274(k)).[74]

915. Exceptions to Entertainment Rules. The following entertainment expenses are not subject to the special rules for the deduction of entertainment expenses (¶ 912, ¶ 913, and ¶ 914). They are deductible provided that they meet the ordinary and

References are to Standard Federal Tax Reports; Tax Research Consultant; and Practical Tax Explanations.

[67] ¶ 6060, ¶ 6061; BUSEXP: 12,102, FILEIND: 12,054; § 9,635.05
[68] ¶ 14,405; BUSEXP: 24,558; § 9,615
[69] ¶ 14,405; BUSEXP: 24,560; § 9,615
[70] ¶ 14,402; BUSEXP: 24,650; § 9,625.10
[71] ¶ 14,405; BUSEXP: 24,562.20; § 9,630.25
[72] ¶ 14,402, ¶ 14,405; BUSEXP: 24,658; § 9,625.15
[73] ¶ 14,402, ¶ 14,410; BUSEXP: 24,810; § 10,105
[74] ¶ 14,402; BUSEXP: 24,562; § 9,601

necessary requirements and are properly substantiated (Code Sec. 274(e); Reg. § 1.274-2(f)(2)).[75] However, they may be subject to the 50-percent limit rule (¶ 916 and ¶ 917). The exceptions are:

(1) food and beverages for employees furnished on the business premises;

(2) expenses for services, goods, and facilities that are treated as compensation and as wages for withholding tax purposes (however, if the recipient is a specified individual such as an officer, director, or 10-percent shareholder or related person, then the employer's deduction cannot exceed the amount of compensation reported);

(3) reimbursed expenses, but only:

(a) if the services relating to the expenses for which reimbursement is made are performed for an employer and the employer has not treated the expenses as wages subject to withholding; or

(b) if the services are performed for a person other than an employer and the taxpayer incurring the reimbursed expenses accounts to that person;

(4) recreational expenses primarily for employees who are not highly compensated (¶ 2114) (e.g., a company picnic);

(5) expenses of employees', stockholders', agents', or directors' business meetings;

(6) expenses directly related and necessary to attendance at a business meeting of a tax-exempt business league, including a real estate board, chamber of commerce or board of trade;

(7) expenses for goods, services, and facilities made available to the public;

(8) expenses for entertainment sold to customers in a bona fide transaction for adequate consideration; and

(9) expenses for goods, services, and facilities that are furnished to a nonemployee as entertainment, amusement or recreation and are includible in the recipient's income as compensation for services (¶ 713) or as a taxable prize or award (¶ 785).

916. 50-Percent Limit for Meal and Entertainment Expenses. The amount allowable as a business deduction for meal and entertainment expenses is generally limited to 50 percent of such expenses. Food and beverage costs incurred in the course of travel away from home fall within the scope of this rule (Code Sec. 274(n)).[76] The 50-percent limit is applied only after determining the amount of the otherwise allowable deductions. For instance, the portion of a travel meal that is lavish and extravagant must first be subtracted from the meal cost before the 50-percent limit is applied. Related expenses, such as taxes and tips in the case of meals and other charges, and room rental and parking fees in the case of entertainment expenses, must be included in the total expense before applying the 50-percent limit. Allowable deductions for transportation costs to and from a business meal are not reduced.

Transportation Workers. The deductible percentage of the cost of meals consumed while away from home by individuals subject to Department of Transportation hours of service rules (e.g., interstate truck and bus drivers and certain railroad, airline, and merchant marine employees) is 80 percent (Code Sec. 274(n)(3)).[77]

Leased Employees. If an employee or independent contractor incurs meal and incidental expenses (M&IE) in connection with the performance of services for another person and is not reimbursed, then the 50-percent limit applies to any deduction claimed by the employee or independent contractor (Reg. § 1.274-2(f)(2)(iv)).[78] However, if an employee or independent contractor accounts for the expenses to a leasing company

---

References are to Standard Federal Tax Reports; Tax Research Consultant; and Practical Tax Explanations.

[75] ¶ 14,402, ¶ 14,405; BUSEXP: 24,562; § 9,630.10

[76] ¶ 14,402; BUSEXP: 24,600; § 9,635

[77] ¶ 14,402; BUSEXP: 24,606; § 9,640.60

[78] ¶ 49,544; BUSEXP: 24,604; § 9,635.05

and is reimbursed under an allowance arrangement, and the payment is treated as compensation, then he or she is not subject to the 50-percent limit. Instead, the leasing company bears the expense and is subject to the 50-percent limit.

On the other hand, a leasing company will not be subject to the 50-percent limit if, in connection with its performance of services for a third party, it is reimbursed under an allowance arrangement with the third party, and it accounts to the third party in the same manner that the employee accounted for the expenses. In such circumstances, the third party bears the expenses and is subject to the 50-percent limit for the deduction that it claims.

917. Exceptions to 50-Percent Limit for Meal and Entertainment Expenses. The following expenses are *not* subject to the 50-percent limit on meal and entertainment expense deductions (80-percent limit for certain transportations workers) (¶ 916):

(1) expenses described in categories (2), (3), (4), (7), (8), and (9) at ¶ 915;

(2) food and beverage expenses associated with benefits that are excludable from the recipient's gross income as a *de minimis* fringe benefit (¶ 2089);

(3) the cost of a ticket package to a sporting event and related expenses if the event is organized to benefit a tax-exempt organization, all net proceeds of the event are contributed to such organization, and volunteers perform substantially all of the work in carrying out the event; in other situations, a deduction for a ticket may not exceed the ticket's face value;

(4) an employee's meal expenses incurred while moving that are reimbursed by the employer and includible in the employee's gross income (¶ 1076); these expenses are not deductible (¶ 1073); and

(5) expenses for food and beverages provided to employees on certain (a) vessels and (b) oil or gas platforms and drilling rigs and their support camps (Code Sec. 274(l)(1) and (n)).[79]

Skyboxes. When a skybox is rented for more than one event, the deduction may not exceed the price of non-luxury box seats (subject to the usual 50-percent limit) (Code Sec. 274(l)(2)).[80]

Tickets to Collegiate Sporting Events. For any payment to or for an institution of higher education that would be allowable as a charitable deduction but for the fact that the taxpayer thereby receives (directly or indirectly) the right to purchase tickets for seating at an athletic event in an athletic stadium of the institution, 80 percent of that payment is treated as a charitable contribution (Code Sec. 170(l)).[81]

918. Business Gifts. Deductions for business gifts, whether made directly or indirectly, are limited to $25 per recipient per year (Code Sec. 274(b)(1); Reg. § 1.274-3).[82] Items clearly of an advertising nature that cost $4 or less and signs, display racks, or other promotional materials given for use on business premises are not gifts.

919. Employee Achievement Awards. An employer may deduct up to $400 of the cost of an employee achievement award for all nonqualified plan awards to each employee (Code Sec. 274(j)).[83] The employer's deduction for the cost of qualified plan award made to a particular employee is limited to $1,600 per year, taking into account all other qualified and nonqualified awards made to that employee during the tax year.

An employee achievement award is an item of tangible personal property awarded to an employee as part of a meaningful presentation for length-of-service or safety achievements and under circumstances that do not create a significant likelihood of disguised compensation (¶ 2069). It does not apply to awards of cash, gift certificates, or other intangible property such as vacations, meals, lodging, tickets to events, stocks, bond, and other securities.

References are to Standard Federal Tax Reports; Tax Research Consultant; and Practical Tax Explanations.

[79] ¶ 14,402; BUSEXP: 24,604; § 9,640.05

[80] ¶ 14,402; BUSEXP: 24,662; § 9,650

[81] ¶ 11,600; INDIV: 51,052.40; § 7,510.75

[82] ¶ 14,402, ¶ 14,406; BUSEXP: 24,706; § 9,945.05

[83] ¶ 14,402; BUSEXP: 24,714, BUSEXP: 24,716; § 9,340.10

A qualified plan award is an employee achievement award provided under an established written plan or program that does not discriminate in favor of highly compensated employees (¶ 2114) as to eligibility or benefits. An employee achievement award is not a qualified plan award if the average cost of all employee achievement awards under the plan exceeds $400. This average cost calculation includes the entire cost of all qualified plan awards, ignoring employee achievement awards of nominal value.

A length of service award will not qualify if it is received during the employee's first five years of service or if the employee has received another length of service award (other than an award excludable as a *de minimis* fringe benefit (¶ 2089)) during the year or within the last four years. An award will not be considered a safety achievement award if made to a manager, administrator, clerical employee, or other professional employee, or if, during the tax year, awards for safety achievement previously have been made to more than 10 percent of the employees, excluding managers, administrators, clerical employees, or other professional employees.

Taxes

920. Taxes Directly Attributable to Business. Business taxpayers can deduct the taxes listed at ¶ 1021 and any other state, local, and foreign taxes paid or accrued within the tax year to the extent that they are directly attributable to a trade or business or to property held for the production of rents or royalties (Code Sec. 164(a)).[84] Any tax not listed at ¶ 1021 that is paid or accrued by the taxpayer in connection with the acquisition of property is treated as part of the cost of the acquired property or, if in connection with the disposition of property, as a reduction in the amount realized.

The uniform capitalization rules require some taxpayers to capitalize certain taxes that would otherwise be deductible (¶ 990–¶ 999).

921. Business Deduction for Federal Unemployment Insurance Tax. The Federal Unemployment Tax Act (FUTA) tax (¶ 2649) is an *excise* tax, so the employer may deduct it as a business expense if it represents an ordinary and necessary expense paid or incurred during the tax year in the conduct of a trade or business (Reg. § 1.164-2(f)).[85] The FUTA tax is deductible as a business expense after application of credits for the employer's contributions to the state unemployment fund. On the cash basis (¶ 1515), the tax is deductible when paid. On the accrual basis (¶ 1540), the deduction may be accrued for the calendar year in which the wages were paid even though payment of the tax is not due until the following year.

922. Business Deduction for State Unemployment Insurance and Disability Fund Contributions. An employer covered by state unemployment insurance laws is entitled to deduct as taxes only those contributions that are classified as taxes under state law and are incurred in carrying on a trade or business or the production of income.[86] If the state does not classify the contributions as taxes, the employer may be able to deduct them as business expenses. Similar treatment applies to employer contributions to state disability funds.[87] In states that require employees to contribute to state unemployment compensation funds, an employee may claim an itemized deduction for such contributions as state income taxes.[88] Also, compulsory employee contributions to state disability funds are deductible as itemized deductions for state income taxes. However, employee contributions to private disability benefit plans are not deductible by employees. See also the checklist at ¶ 57.

923. Business Deduction for FICA Taxes. An employer's share of the Federal Insurance Contributions Act (FICA) tax for Social Security and Medicare (¶ 2648) is an *excise* tax, so the employer may deduct it as a business expense if it represents an ordinary and necessary expense paid or incurred during the tax year in the conduct of a

---

References are to Standard Federal Tax Reports; Tax Research Consultant; and Practical Tax Explanations.

[84] ¶ 9500; BUSEXP: 21,454; § 16,415, § 16,425
[85] ¶ 9503; INDIV: 45,112.35; § 9,365
[86] ¶ 8752.692—¶ 8752.694, ¶ 9502.31; BUSEXP: 21,506.05; § 9,415.05
[87] ¶ 8752.2959; BUSEXP: 21,506.05
[88] ¶ 9502.31; INDIV: 45,112.20, BUSEXP: 21,506.10; § 22,301

trade or business (Reg. § 1.164-2(f)).[89] The contribution of an employer on wages paid to a domestic worker is not deductible unless it is classified as a business expense (*R.A. Biggs*, CA-6, 71-1 USTC ¶ 9306).[90]

An employee's portion of FICA taxes on his or her wages is not deductible (¶ 1025). However, if the employer pays the employee's portion of the tax without deduction from the employee's wages under an agreement with the employee, the amount is deductible by the employer as a business expense, and is wage income to the employee (Rev. Rul. 86-14).[91]

A self-employed individual may deduct from gross income 50 percent of the self-employment tax imposed for the tax year, other than the additional 0.9-percent Medicare tax on incomes over a certain threshold (¶ 2664) (Code Sec. 164(f)).[92] However, for any tax year that begins in 2011 or 2012, the self-employment tax liability deduction equals the sum of 59.6 percent of the applicable Social Security taxes and 50 percent of the applicable Medicare taxes (Act Sec. 601 of the Tax Relief, Unemployment Insurance Reauthorization, and Job Creation Act of 2010 (P.L. 111-312), amended by Act Sec. 1001 of the Middle Class Tax Relief and Job Creation Act of 2012 (P.L. 112-96)).

Qualified employers did not have to pay their share of Social Security or Railroad Retirement Act taxes on wages or compensation paid after March 18, 2010, and prior to January 1, 2011, to newly hired qualified individuals who were formerly unemployed (¶ 2648).

924. Deduction for Federal and State Income Tax. Federal income taxes are not deductible in determining taxable income (Code Sec. 275).[93] However, they are deductible in determining the amount of a corporation's income subject to the accumulated earnings tax (¶ 251) and the personal holding company tax (¶ 275) (Reg. § § 1.535-2 and 1.545-2).[94] Corporations and partnerships may deduct their state income taxes as business expenses. State income taxes that are based on net business income may only be deducted by self-employed individuals on Schedule A of Form 1040 as an itemized deduction. However, if the state income tax is based on gross business income, the tax may be deducted as a business expense (Temp. Reg. § 1.62-1T(d)).[95]

Charitable Contributions

927. Charitable Deduction Limits for Corporations. The deduction by a corporation for charitable contributions is limited to 10 percent of its taxable income for the year, computed without regard to:

- the deduction for charitable contributions;

- the corporate deductions for dividends received and for dividends paid on certain preferred stock of public utilities;

- the limitation on the deduction for bond premium;

- any net operating loss carryback to the tax year;

- the deduction for domestic production activities; and

- any capital loss carryback to the tax year (Code Sec. 170(b)(2); Reg. § 1.170A-11).[96]

For tax years beginning before January 1, 2014, corporate donors that qualify as farmers or ranchers are allowed deductions for certain qualified conservation contributions of real property interests, up to the difference of 100 percent of the donor's taxable income (computed without regard to the items listed above) minus all other allowable charitable contributions (Code Sec. 170(b)(2)(B)).

References are to Standard Federal Tax Reports; Tax Research Consultant; and Practical Tax Explanations.

[89] ¶ 9503; INDIV: 45,112.35; § 9,365

[90] ¶ 9502.30; INDIV: 45,152.10, PAYROLL: 9,050; § 22,210.60

[91] ¶ 8636.49; INDIV: 45,112.35; § 9,005.20, § 22,210.45

[92] ¶ 9500; BUSEXP: 21,504; § 7,340

[93] ¶ 14,500; BUSEXP: 21,350; § 7,345

[94] ¶ 23,042, ¶ 23,252; CCORP: 18,252, CCORP: 36,254; § 26,905.05, § 27,001

[95] ¶ 6003; INDIV: 45,100; § 9,940.10

[96] ¶ 11,600, ¶ 11,672; CCORP: 9,350; § 7,575.05

Comment: Absent further legislation, the special conservation contribution for qualified corporate farmers and ranchers has expired for contributions made in tax years beginning after December 31, 2013. For the latest legislative updates, visit our website www.CCHGroup.com/TaxUpdates.

A corporation is permitted to carry over to the five succeeding tax years charitable contributions that exceed the 10-percent limit, but deductions in those years are also subject to the maximum limitation (Code Sec. 170(d)(2)). Excess qualified conservation contributions by qualified corporate farmers and ranchers are carried over to the 15 succeeding tax years (Code Sec. 170(b)(2)(B)). Except for the carryover rule, a deduction is allowed only for a charitable contribution paid during the tax year. An accrual-basis corporation, however, may elect to treat as paid during the tax year all or a portion of a contribution that is actually paid within two-and-one-half months after the close of the tax year if it was authorized by the board of directors during the year (Code Sec. 170(a)(2)).

930. Charitable Contributions of Inventory or Scientific Property. Generally, the deduction for a charitable contribution of ordinary income property is the fair market value of that property less the amount that would have been ordinary income if the property had been sold at its fair market value on the date of the contribution (¶ 1062). There are exceptions to this rule in the case of certain contributions by corporations.

Inventory-Type Property. If a corporation, other than an S corporation, makes a gift of inventory, property held for sale to customers in the ordinary course of business, or depreciable or real property used in the trade or business, it may deduct its basis for the property, plus one-half of the property's unrealized appreciation. The claimed deduction, however, may not exceed twice the basis of the property (Code Sec. 170(e)(3)).[97] Moreover, no deduction is allowed for any part of the appreciation that would be ordinary income resulting from recapture. To qualify, the gift must be made to a qualified public charity or a private operating foundation, and the donee's use of the property must be for the care of infants or the ill or needy.

Book Inventory (Expired). C corporations could claim a similar enhanced deduction for donations of book inventories to public schools made through December 31, 2011 (Code Sec. 170(e)(3)(D)). The enhanced deduction generally increased the deductible amount from the donated inventory item's basis to the lesser of (1) the donated inventory item's basis plus one-half of the item's appreciation, or (2) two times the donated inventory item's basis.

Scientific Research Property. A corporation, other than an S corporation, a personal holding company, or a service organization, is entitled to the same deduction for a contribution of certain ordinary income property to an institution of higher education or to an exempt scientific research organization for research purposes as that for inventory-type property (Code Sec. 170(e)(4)).[98] To qualify as a research contribution:

- the contributed property must have been constructed or assembled by the donor;
- the contribution must be made within two years of construction or assembly; and
- the original use of the property must be by the donee.

Several additional requirements must also be satisfied.

Computer Equipment (Expired). A C corporation was entitled to an enhanced deduction for a charitable contribution of computer technology or equipment to an elementary or secondary school or public library through December 31, 2011 (Code Sec. 170(e)(6)).[99] The amount of the deduction was equal to the taxpayer's basis in the donated property plus one-half of the amount of ordinary income that would have been realized if the property had been sold. The deduction could not exceed twice the taxpayer's basis in the donated property. The contribution was to be made within three years of the property's acquisition or substantial completion of its construction or assembly, and the original use of the property must have been by the donor or the donee.

References are to Standard Federal Tax Reports; Tax Research Consultant; and Practical Tax Explanations.

[97] ¶ 11,600; CCORP: 9,354; §7,575.25

[98] ¶ 11,600; CCORP: 9,354; §7,575.25

[99] ¶ 11,600; CCORP: 9,358; §7,575.25

930A. Charitable Contributions of Food. Corporate and noncorporate taxpayers are entitled to an enhanced deduction for charitable donations of food inventory through December 31, 2013 (Code Sec. 170(e)(3)(C)(iv)).[100] The food inventory has to consist of items fit for human consumption and be contributed to a qualified charity or private operating foundation for use in the care of the ill, the needy, or infants. Charitable donations of food after December 31, 2013, are subject to the 10-percent-of-taxable-income limitation (¶ 927).

> **Comment:** Absent further legislation, the enhanced deduction for contributions of food inventory has expired for contributions made after December 31, 2013. For the latest legislative updates, visit our website www.CCHGroup.com/TaxUpdates.

931. Contribution Rules for Corporations. The rules concerning a deduction for the following charitable contributions are the same regardless of whether the contribution is made by a corporate or a noncorporate taxpayer:

- gifts of appreciated property (¶ 1062),
- use of property—partial interests (¶ 1063),
- reduction for interest (¶ 1065),
- gift of future interest in tangible personal property (¶ 1069),
- transfers in trust (¶ 1070),
- appraisals (¶ 1071), and
- denial of deduction (¶ 1068).

See ¶ 1070A for discussion of the reporting, recordkeeping, and substantiation rules for charitable contributions.

Interest

937. Business Deduction for Interest. Interest expense or other borrowing costs incurred in a trade or business or in the production of rental or royalty income is generally deductible from gross income (Code Sec. 163).[101] However, interest paid on debt that is allocable to the production of certain property must be capitalized rather than deducted in the year paid (¶ 993). Special rules also apply for prepaid interest (¶ 1055 and ¶ 1056), investment interest paid by noncorporate taxpayers (¶ 1094), a debt instrument that has original issue discount (¶ 1952), and a debt obligation that is required to be in registered form (¶ 1963).

Interest on debt incurred to purchase or carry commodity investments that are part of a straddle is not currently deductible. The interest must be added to the basis of the commodity. Hedging transactions, however, are exempted from this capitalization rule (¶ 1948 and ¶ 1949).

Earnings Stripping. A corporation is not allowed a deduction for excessive interest paid if the interest will not be taxed as income to the recipient (Code Sec. 163(j)).[102] A corporate partner's share of interest paid or accrued to or by the partnership is treated as paid or accrued by or to the corporation directly.

Corporate Indebtedness Incurred to Acquire Another Corporation's Stock. Generally, there is a $5 million annual limit on the interest deductible by a corporation on a debt incurred to acquire stock or two-thirds of the operating assets of another corporation (Code Sec. 279).[103]

937A. Interest on Income Tax Liability. Interest paid or accrued on income tax assessed on an individual's federal, state, or local income tax liability is *not* a business deduction even though the tax due is related to income from a trade or business (Temp. Reg. § 1.163-9T(b)(2)(i)(A)).[104] This rule also applies to an individual's partnership and S corporation activities. See ¶ 2723 and ¶ 2724 for interest allocations pursuant to compromise and partial payments. Penalties on deficiencies and underestimated tax cannot be deducted.

References are to Standard Federal Tax Reports; Tax Research Consultant; and Practical Tax Explanations.

[100] ¶ 11,600; INDIV: 51,152.15; § 7,525.20

[101] ¶ 9102; BUSEXP: 21,000; § 9,915

[102] ¶ 9102; BUSEXP: 21,210; § 26,201

[103] ¶ 14,700; CCORP: 9,400; § 7,405.10

[104] ¶ 9400; INDIV: 48,350; § 7,345

Employee's Expenses

941. Employee Business Expenses. The performance of services as an employee is considered to be a trade or business. Thus, employee business expenses are generally deductible. *Reimbursed* employee business expenses are deductible from gross income (Code Sec. 62(a)(2)(A)).[105] However, reimbursements that are paid under an accountable plan are excluded from the employee's gross income, and the employee may not deduct reimbursed costs as a business expense (¶ 942). *Unreimbursed* employee business expenses are deductible as miscellaneous itemized deductions, subject to the two-percent-of-adjusted-gross-income (AGI) floor (¶ 1011) and the 50-percent limit for meal and entertainment expenses (80 percent for employees subject to the Department of Transportation's hours of service limitations) (¶ 916), if applicable. Special rules apply to qualified performing artists (¶ 941A), statutory employees (¶ 941B), impairment-related work expenses (¶ 1013), fee-based government employees (¶ 941D), schoolteachers (¶ 941C), and members of the National Guard or Armed Forces Reserves (¶ 941E). An employee is also allowed a deduction from gross income for jury duty pay surrendered to an employer in exchange for regular salary (¶ 1010).

941A. Performing Artist. A qualified performing artist may deduct business expenses in arriving at adjusted gross income on Form 2106 or Form 2106-EZ. Generally, to qualify for this deduction an individual must:

- render services in the performing arts during the tax year for at least two employers;

- have total business deductions attributable to the performance of such services that exceed 10 percent of the income received from such services; and

- have adjusted gross income of $16,000 or less (Code Sec. 62(b)).[106]

941B. Statutory Employees. Individuals who are considered to be statutory employees may deduct their allowable business expenses from gross income (Code Sec. 3121(d); Rev. Rul. 90-93).[107] A statutory employee includes:

- a full-time traveling or city salesperson who solicits orders from wholesalers, restaurants, or similar establishments on behalf of a principal where the merchandise sold is for resale (e.g., food sold to a restaurant) or for supplies used in the buyer's business;

- a full-time life insurance agent whose principal business activity is selling life insurance and/or annuity contracts for one life insurance company;

- an agent-driver or commission-driver engaged in distributing meat, vegetables, bakery goods, beverages (other than milk), or laundry or dry cleaning services; and

- a home worker performing work on material or goods furnished by the employer.

An employer should indicate on the worker's Form W-2 whether the worker is classified as a statutory employee. Statutory employees report their wages, income, and allowable expenses on Schedule C or C-EZ of Form 1040. Statutory employees are not liable for self-employment tax because their employers are obligated to treat such individuals as employees for FICA and FUTA purposes (except for full-time life insurance agents and home workers, who are not considered employees for FUTA purposes).

941C. School Teachers. For tax years beginning before January 1, 2014, eligible educators can deduct up to $250 of the expenses paid or incurred as an above-the-line adjustment to gross income (¶ 1084) (Code Sec. 62(a)(2)(D)).[108] For tax years beginning after 2013, school teachers may deduct expenses paid or incurred for the purchase of school supplies only as miscellaneous itemized deductions subject to the two-percent-of-adjusted-gross-income floor.

References are to Standard Federal Tax Reports; Tax Research Consultant; and Practical Tax Explanations.

[105] ¶ 6002; INDIV: 36,050; § 5,310

[106] ¶ 6002; INDIV: 36,058; § 5,315

[107] ¶ 8524.2547; INDIV: 63,154; § 5,305

[108] ¶ 6002; INDIV: 36,364; § 5,325

Comment: Absent further legislation, the above-the-line deduction allowed to teachers for certain classroom expenses has expired for tax years beginning after December 31, 2013. For the latest legislative updates, visit our website www.CCHGroup.com/TaxUpdates.

941D. Fee-Based Government Officials. Expenses paid or incurred with respect to services performed by an official as an employee of a state or local government are deductible in computing adjusted gross income (Code Sec. 62(a)(2)(C)).[109] The employee must be compensated in whole or in part on a fee basis.

941E. National Guard and Reserve Members. Members of the National Guard and the U.S. Armed Forces Reserves are allowed to deduct travel expenses while away from home to attend meetings and training sessions as an above-the-line deduction (Code Secs. 62(a)(2)(E) and 162(p)).[110] This type of travel has been deemed to be travel away from home in the pursuit of a trade or business when an individual is away from home overnight in connection with his or her service as a member of the guard or reserves. Expenses incurred in connection with the performance of such service are deductible as an above-the-line deduction only when the taxpayer is more than 100 miles away from home. The amount of deductible expenses is limited to the federal per diem rate for the locality of the meeting or training session.

942. Reimbursed and Unreimbursed Employee Business Expenses. The tax treatment of an employee's reimbursed business expenses depends on whether the employer's reimbursement or expense allowance arrangement is an accountable or nonaccountable plan (¶ 952A) (Code Sec. 62; Reg. § 1.62-2).[111] If expenses are reimbursed under an *accountable* plan, the reimbursement is not reported as income on the employee's Form W-2 and the expense may not be claimed as a deduction on the employee's tax return. In this situation, the 50-percent limit on deductions for meals and entertainment applies to the employer (¶ 916). If the employee's deductible business expenses exceed the amounts paid by the accountable plan, and these expenses are adequately substantiated (¶ 943), then the excess expenses are deductible as miscellaneous itemized deductions, subject to the two-percent-of-adjusted-gross-income (AGI) floor (¶ 1011) and the 50-percent limit for meals and entertainment. If expenses are reimbursed under a *nonaccountable* plan, the reimbursements are included in the employee's income. Business expenses that are reimbursed under a nonaccountable plan or not reimbursed at all can be deducted, to the extent they can be adequately substantiated, as miscellaneous itemized deductions, subject to the two-percent-of-AGI floor, and the 50-percent limit for meals and entertainment. The employee reports the expenses on Form 2106 or Form 2106-EZ.

943. Substantiation for Employees' Returns. Business expenses that exceed the reimbursements received under an accountable plan (¶ 952A), that are reimbursed under a nonaccountable plan, or that are not reimbursed at all may be deducted by an employee (¶ 942). As with any other deductible expense, the employee must adequately substantiate business expenses in order to deduct them.

More specific substantiation requirements apply with respect to the following expenses, which are deemed particularly susceptible to abuse: expenses with respect to travel away from home (including meals and lodging), entertainment expenses, business gifts, and expenses in connection with the use of "listed property" (¶ 1211). These expenses must generally be substantiated by adequate records or other sufficient evidence corroborating the taxpayer's own statement (Code Sec. 274(d); Temp. Reg. § 1.274-5T).[112] The expenses must be substantiated as to amount, time, place, and business purpose. For entertainment and gift expenses, the business relationship of the person being entertained or receiving the gift must also be substantiated.

References are to Standard Federal Tax Reports; Tax Research Consultant; and Practical Tax Explanations.

[109] ¶ 6002; INDIV: 36,050; § 5,320

[110] ¶ 6002, ¶ 8500; FILEIND: 9,054.25; § 5,330

[111] ¶ 6002, ¶ 6004; INDIV: 36,054; § 10,120.05

[112] ¶ 14,402, ¶ 14,410; BUSEXP: 24,800; § 10,105.05, § 10,110.05

Substantiation by Adequate Records. A contemporaneous log is not required, but a record of the elements of the expense or use of the listed property made at or near the time of the expenditure or use, supported by sufficient documentary evidence, has a high degree of credibility. Adequate accounting generally requires the submission of an account book, expense diary or log, or similar record maintained by the employee and recorded at or near the time of incurrence of the expense. Documentary evidence, such as receipts or paid bills, is not generally required for expenses that are less than $75. Documentary evidence is required, however, for all lodging expenses (Reg. § 1.274-5(c)(2)(iii)).[113] The employee should also maintain a record of any amounts charged to the employer.

Substantiation of Amount of Meal and Incidental Expenses. The amount of meal and/or incidental expenses (M&IE) deducted by an employee can be substantiated either by retaining evidence of the actual expenses or by use of the standard meal allowance (¶ 954B). The amount of the standard meal allowance varies by location, and for some locations, by the time of year. An individual using the standard meal allowance must still keep records, such as a daily planner or log, to prove the time, place, and business purpose of the expenses. There is no standard lodging amount similar to the standard meal allowance. Employees must be able to substantiate the actual cost of their lodging in order to deduct it.

Transportation and Car Expenses

945. Local Transportation Expenses. A taxpayer's local transportation costs (including self-employed persons and statutory employees) for travel between two specific business locations, whether in the same or different businesses, are deductible from gross income as an ordinary and necessary business expense (Reg. § 1.162-1(a)).[114] The manner of an employee's deduction for transportation expenses generally depends on whether the employee is reimbursed under an accountable plan (¶ 942). Local transportation expenses are generally those incurred for the business use of a car. However, they also include the cost of travel by rail, bus, or taxi.

Commuting Expenses. Commuting expenses between a taxpayer's residence and a business location within the area of the taxpayer's tax home generally are not deductible (Reg. §§ 1.162-2(e) and 1.262-1(b)(5)).[115] However, a deduction is allowed for expenses incurred in excess of ordinary commuting expenses for transporting job-related tools and materials (*D. Fausner*, SCt, 73-2 USTC ¶ 9515).[116] An individual who works at two or more different places in a day may deduct the costs of getting from one place to the other (Rev. Rul. 55-109, modified by Rev. Rul. 90-23).[117]

There is an exception to the general rule that commuting expenses are not deductible. If a taxpayer has at least one regular place of business away from home, then daily transportation expenses for commuting between the taxpayer's residence and a temporary work location in the same trade or business can be deducted (¶ 951) (Rev. Rul. 99-7).[118] For this purpose, a temporary work location is defined using a one-year standard. If employment at a work location is realistically expected to last (and does in fact last) for one year or less, the employment is temporary, absent facts and circumstances to the contrary. Employment at a work location is not temporary if it is realistically expected to last for more than one year, or if there is no realistic expectation that it will last for one year or less, regardless of whether it in fact lasts for more than one year. A taxpayer may at first realistically expect that employment at a work location will last one year or less, but, at a later date, realistically expect that the work will last for more than one year. In this situation, the employment will be treated as temporary, unless facts and circumstances indicate otherwise, until the date that the taxpayer's realistic expectation changes. After that date, the employment will be treated as not temporary.

References are to Standard Federal Tax Reports; Tax Research Consultant; and Practical Tax Explanations.

[113] ¶ 14,408F; BUSEXP: 24,806.15; § 10,105.15
[114] ¶ 8501; BUSEXP: 24,450; § 8,005
[115] ¶ 8527, ¶ 13,601; BUSEXP: 24,458; § 8,010.05
[116] ¶ 8590.25; BUSEXP: 24,460; § 8,010.05
[117] ¶ 8570.175; BUSEXP: 24,454; § 8,010.05
[118] ¶ 8570.143; BUSEXP: 24,458; § 8,010.15

Travel from a Home Office. An individual who uses his or her home as his or her principal place of business (¶ 961) is permitted to deduct transportation expenses between the home and another work location in the same trade or business (Rev. Rul. 99-7).[119] This rule applies regardless of whether the work location is temporary or regular and regardless of the distance.

946. Car Expense. Expenses for gasoline, oil, tires, repairs, insurance, depreciation, parking fees and tolls, licenses, and garage rent incurred for cars used in a trade or business are deductible (¶ 947). The deduction is allowed only for that part of the expenses that is attributable to business (Code Sec. 162; Reg. § 1.162-1).[120] Generally, an employee's unreimbursed expenses can be deducted only as a miscellaneous itemized deduction subject to the two-percent-of-adjusted-gross-income (AGI) floor (¶ 941). See ¶ 1208–¶ 1215 concerning the expensing election and depreciation of a car.

947. Substantiation of Car Expenses. A taxpayer can substantiate car expenses by keeping an exact record of the amount paid for gasoline, insurance, and other costs. However, the standard mileage rate method is a simplified method available to both employees and self-employed persons in computing deductions for car expenses in lieu of calculating the operating and fixed costs allocable to business purposes (Code Sec. 274(d); Temp. Reg. § 1.274-5T).[121]

Standard Mileage Rate. Under the standard mileage method, the taxpayer determines the amount of the allowable deduction by multiplying all the business miles driven during the year by the standard mileage rate. The business portion of parking fees and tolls may be deducted in addition to the standard mileage rate. The standard mileage rate is 56 cents per mile for 2014 (Rev. Proc. 2010-51; Notice 2013-80).[122]

Rural mail carriers receive a qualified reimbursement for expenses incurred for the use of their vehicles for performing the collection and delivery of mail in a rural route. They are allowed a miscellaneous itemized deduction, subject to the two-percent-of-adjusted-gross-income limitation, for their automobile expenses that exceed their qualified reimbursement (Code Sec. 162(o)).[123] Qualified reimbursements in excess of actual automobile expenses continue to be excluded from gross income (H.R. Conf. Rep. No. 108-755).

The standard mileage rate method may be used by businesses, self-employed individuals, or employees in computing the deductible costs of operating automobiles they own or lease for business purposes. The business standard mileage rate may not be used to compute the deductible expenses of five or more automobiles owned or leased by a taxpayer and used simultaneously (i.e., a fleet operation). Using the standard mileage rate in the first year of business use is considered an election to exclude the car from MACRS depreciation (¶ 1236).

For automobiles owned by a taxpayer and used in a trade or business, and for which the business standard mileage rate is used, depreciation is considered to have been allowed at the rate of 22 cents per mile for 2014 (Rev. Proc. 2010-51; Notice 2013-80).[124] The depreciation reduces the basis of the automobile (but not below zero) in determining adjusted basis.

Fixed and Variable Rate (FAVR) Method. The fixed and variable rate allowance (FAVR) also can be used to substantiate automobile expenses. The maximum standard automobile cost for purposes of the FAVR allowance is $28,200 for 2014 ($30,400 for trucks and vans) (Rev. Proc. 2010-51; Notice 2013-80).[125] Under the FAVR method, an employer reimburses its employee's expenses with a mileage allowance using a flat rate or a stated schedule that combines periodic fixed and variable payments. At least five employees must be covered by such an arrangement at all times during the calendar

---

References are to Standard Federal Tax Reports; Tax Research Consultant; and Practical Tax Explanations.

[119] ¶ 8570.143; BUSEXP: 24,456; § 8,010.20
[120] ¶ 8500, ¶ 8501; BUSEXP: 24,500; § 9,005
[121] ¶ 14,402, ¶ 14,410; BUSEXP: 24,502; § 8,065
[122] ¶ 8590.55; BUSEXP: 24,502; § 8,065
[123] ¶ 8500; BUSEXP: 24,506.15; § 8,050
[124] ¶ 14,417.50; BUSEXP: 24,506.05; § 10,125.15
[125] ¶ 8590.55; BUSEXP: 24,912.106; § 10,125.20

year, and at no time can the majority of covered employees be management employees. Additional requirements must also be met.

948. Interest on Car Loans. Interest paid by an employee on a car loan is nondeductible personal interest (¶ 1045). A self-employed taxpayer may claim the interest paid on the business portion of a car as a business expense. The nonbusiness portion is nondeductible personal interest (Code Sec. 163(a)).[126]

Traveling Expenses Away from Home

949. Traveling Expenses Generally. A deduction is allowed for ordinary and necessary traveling expenses incurred by a taxpayer while away from home in the conduct of a trade or business (Code Sec. 162(a)(2); Reg. § 1.162-2).[127] An individual is not away from home unless his or her duties require the individual to be away from the general area of his or her tax home for a period substantially longer than an ordinary workday and it is reasonable for the individual to need to sleep or rest. In some cases, travel expenses may be deductible even though the taxpayer is away from home for a period of less than 24 hours.

Local Lodging. Expenses paid or incurred for local lodging may be deductible as ordinary and necessary expenses of a taxpayer's trade or business, including the trade or business of being an employee (Reg. § 1.162-32).[128] The IRS has provided a safe harbor for certain local lodging at a business meeting, conference, or other activity or function. Other local lodging expenses may be deductible as business expenses depending on the relevant facts and circumstances. The rule applies to lodging provided by the employer or lodging that the employer requires the employee to obtain. The following conditions must be met:

(1) The lodging must be necessary for the individual to participate in a meeting or other business function.

(2) The lodging must not be provided for more than five calendar days and must not recur more frequently than once per calendar quarter.

(3) The employer must require the employee to remain at the meeting or function overnight.

(4) The lodging is not lavish or extravagant and does not provide any significant element of personal pleasure, recreation, or benefit.

950. Tax Home Defined. A individual's tax home for purposes of deducting travel expenses (¶ 949) is considered to be: (1) the taxpayer's regular or principal (if there is more than one regular) place of business, or (2) if the taxpayer has no regular or principal place of business because of the nature of the work, the taxpayer's regular place of abode in a real and substantial sense (Rev. Rul. 75-432).[129] If a taxpayer fails to fall within either category, the taxpayer is an itinerant or someone who has a home wherever he or she happens to be working. Thus, the taxpayer is never away from home for purposes of deducting traveling expenses.

When there are multiple areas of business activity or places of regular employment, the principal place of business is treated as the tax home. In determining the principal place of an individual's business, the following factors are considered:

(1) the time spent on business activity in each area;

(2) the amount of business activity in each area; and

(3) the amount of the resulting financial return in each area (Rev. Rul. 54-147).

Business travel expenses incurred while away from the principal place of business are deductible.[130]

References are to Standard Federal Tax Reports; Tax Research Consultant; and Practical Tax Explanations.

[126] ¶ 9102; INDIV: 48,350; § 8,205

[127] ¶ 8500, ¶ 8527; BUSEXP: 24,050; § 9,510.05

[128] ¶ 9051J; INDIV: 36,306; § 9,505

[129] ¶ 8550.269; BUSEXP: 24,100; § 9,510.05

[130] ¶ 8570.175; BUSEXP: 24,104; § 9,510.15

The tax home of a member of the U.S. Congress is the member's residence in the state or district that the member represents. However, deduction for meals and lodging while in Washington, DC, are limited to $3,000 per year, after applying the two-percent-of-adjusted-gross-income (AGI) floor for miscellaneous itemized deductions (Code Sec. 162(a)).[131]

A member of the U.S. Armed Forces is not away from home while at the individual's permanent duty station (*H.A. Stidger*, SCt, 67-1 USTC ¶ 9309).[132] However, members of the National Guard and Reserves can deduct qualifying expenses as an above-the-line deduction when attending meetings or training sessions (¶ 941E).

951. Temporary v. Indefinite Test. In determining when an individual is away from home for purposes of deducting travel expenses (¶ 949), the nature of the stay and the length of time away from the individual's principal place of business are of prime importance. If the assignment is temporary in nature, the taxpayer is considered away from home and a travel expense deduction is allowed. If the assignment is for an indefinite period of time, the location of the assignment becomes the individual's new tax home, and the individual may not deduct traveling expenses while there. When an individual works away from home at a single location for more than one year, the employment will be treated as indefinite, and related travel expenses will not be deductible (Code Sec. 162(a); Rev. Rul. 93-86; Rev. Rul. 99-7).[133] Employment expected to last more than one year is classified as indefinite, regardless of whether the work actually exceeds a year. Employment that is expected to, and does in fact, last for one year or less is temporary.

The one-year rule does not apply to federal employees certified by the Attorney General as traveling on behalf of the United States in temporary duty status to investigate or prosecute, or to provide support services for the investigation or prosecution of, a federal crime. Such employees may deduct their travel expenses even if their assignment is expected to last for more than one year.

952. Deductible Travel Expenses. The costs of the following items are ordinarily deductible, if paid or incurred while a business owner or employee is traveling away from home on business (¶ 949): meals and lodging; transportation, including a reasonable amount for baggage; necessary samples and display materials; hotel rooms, sample rooms, telephone and fax services, and public stenographers; and the costs, including depreciation (¶ 1211), of maintaining and operating a car for business purposes (Reg. § 1.162-2).[134]

No deduction is allowed for the travel expenses of a spouse, dependent, or other individual who accompanies the taxpayer or employee on a business trip unless such person is an employee of the person who is paying or reimbursing the expenses, the travel of such person serves a bona fide business purpose, and the expenses of such person are otherwise deductible (Code Sec. 274(m)(3)).[135]

A taxpayer may deduct traveling expenses between the principal place of business and place of business at a temporary or minor post of duty. When the taxpayer's family lives at the temporary or minor post of duty, the taxpayer may still claim travel expenses. However, the deduction for meals and lodging is limited to the portion of the taxpayer's expenses that are allocable to the taxpayer's presence there in the actual performance of the taxpayer's duties (Rev. Rul. 55-604).[136]

References are to Standard Federal Tax Reports; Tax Research Consultant; and Practical Tax Explanations.

[131] ¶ 8500; BUSEXP: 24,120; § 9,510.10

[132] ¶ 8570.1236; BUSEXP: 24,120.20; § 9,505

[133] ¶ 8500, ¶ 8570.1327, ¶ 8570.143; BUSEXP: 24,110; § 9,510.25

[134] ¶ 8527; BUSEXP: 24,052; § 9,501

[135] ¶ 14,402; BUSEXP: 24,200; § 9,530

[136] ¶ 8570.175; BUSEXP: 24,104; § 9,505

The deduction for the cost of meals and lodging while away from home on business is limited to amounts that are not lavish or extravagant under the circumstances (Code Sec. 162(a)(2)).[137] The deduction for meals is limited to 50 percent of the total expenses (¶ 916).

952A. Accountable v. Nonaccountable Plans. The arrangement under which an employer reimburses business expenses incurred by employees or provides advances to cover such expenses is either an accountable plan or a nonaccountable plan. Amounts paid under an accountable plan are deductible by the employer and not reported as income to the employee. Amounts paid under a nonaccountable plan are deductible by the employer as compensation reportable on the employee's Form W-2 and subject to withholding requirements. Withholding rules relating to employee expense reimbursements are explained at ¶ 2607 and ¶ 2608. The tax treatment of an employee's business expenses and reimbursements under each type of plan is explained at ¶ 942.

A plan is an accountable plan only if it satisfies the following three conditions:

    (1) the expenses covered under the plan must have a business connection;

    (2) the plan must require employees to substantiate the covered expenses; and

    (3) the plan must require employees who receive advances to return any amounts in excess of their substantiated expenses (Reg. § 1.62-2(c)).[138]

If a plan satisfies these requirements, but an employee fails to return an excess advance to the employer within a reasonable period, only the amount of the substantiated expenses is treated as paid under an accountable plan. The retained excess is treated as paid under a nonaccountable plan. If a plan does not satisfy these requirements, an employee cannot force the employer to treat it as an accountable plan by substantiating the expenses and returning the excess.

Business Connection. The business connection requirement is satisfied if the expenses are deductible business expenses of the employer, paid or incurred in connection with the performance of services as an employee. If a plan also covers bona fide expenses that are related to the employer's business but not deductible, such as travel that is not away from home, the plan is treated as two separate arrangements, one accountable, the other nonaccountable (Reg. § 1.62-2(d)).[139]

Substantiation. The substantiation an accountable plan must require for the expenses it covers must be sufficient to substantiate the expense under the general substantiation rules, which vary depending on the type of expense (Reg. § 1.62-2(e)).[140] If the expense is for travel, meals, lodging, entertainment, gifts, or attributable to the use of listed property (¶ 1211), the substantiation requirement is satisfied if enough information is submitted to the employer to satisfy substantiation requirements (¶ 953), including travel and car expenses deemed substantiated.

If the expense is not in one of the categories stated above, such as expenses for printing a report, then the expense is considered substantiated if enough information is submitted to the employer to enable the employer to identify the specific nature of each expense and to conclude that the expense was attributable to the employer's business activities. The elements of each expense should be substantiated, including the amount, place, time or date, and business purpose.

Deemed Substantiation of Employee's Reimbursed Expenses. An employee's expenses are deemed to be substantiated, for purposes of the accountable plan requirements, if the employee provides an adequate accounting of the expenses to the employer in the form of adequate records (Reg. § 1.274-5(f)(4)).[141] The adequate accounting requirement can be satisfied as to the amount of car expenses and lodging and/or meals and incidental expenses by using the per diem allowances discussed at ¶ 947 and ¶ 954–¶ 954B. Note that in order to deduct unreimbursed expenses for lodging on his or her own return, an employee or self-employed individual must have evidence of the actual costs.

References are to Standard Federal Tax Reports; Tax Research Consultant; and Practical Tax Explanations.

[137] ¶ 8500; BUSEXP: 24,556; § 9,635

[138] ¶ 6004; INDIV: 36,056; § 10,120.10

[139] ¶ 6004; INDIV: 36,056.05; § 10,120.10

[140] ¶ 6004; INDIV: 36,056.10; § 10,120.10

[141] ¶ 14,408F; BUSEXP: 24,800; § 10,115.10

Return of Excess Advances. The return-of-excess-advances requirement is satisfied if employees are required to return amounts received in excess of the expenses that are substantiated or deemed substantiated within a reasonable period of time (Reg. § 1.62-2(f)).[142] Advances must be provided within a reasonable period before the covered expenses are anticipated to be paid or incurred and must be reasonably calculated not to exceed the anticipated expenses. If an employee fails to return the excess within a reasonable period of time, only amounts paid that are not in excess of the amounts substantiated will be treated as paid under an accountable plan. Excess amounts retained will be treated as paid under a nonaccountable plan and must be included in income by the employee. An accountable plan that reimburses expenses pursuant to an IRS-approved mileage (¶ 947) or per diem allowance (¶ 954–¶ 954B) must require the return of the portion that relates to days or miles of travel not substantiated.

Reasonable Period of Time. The provision of advances, the substantiation of expenses, and the return of excess advances must each take place within a reasonable period of time. A reasonable period depends on facts and circumstances, but the IRS has provided two safe harbor methods: the fixed date method and the periodic statement method (Reg. § 1.62-2(g)).[143] Under the fixed date method, the following are treated as occurring within a reasonable period of time:

> (1) advance payments made within 30 days of when an expense is paid or incurred;

> (2) substantiation provided within 60 days after expenses are paid or incurred; or

> (3) return of excess amounts within 120 days after expenses are paid or incurred.

The periodic statement method is a safe harbor for determining reasonable time for the provision of substantiation and the return of excess advances. Under this method, the employer must:

> (1) give each employee periodic statements (no less than quarterly) that set forth the amounts paid under the reimbursement arrangement in excess of the substantiated amount and

> (2) request that the employee either substantiate or return the excess amounts within 120 days of the statement date.

An expense substantiated or amount returned within that period will satisfy the reasonable period requirement.

953. Substantiation Requirements for Business Expenses. In order to claim any deduction, a taxpayer must be able to prove, if the return is audited, that the expenses were in fact paid or incurred. Small expenses and those that are clearly related to the business may be substantiated by the taxpayer's statement or by keeping receipts, sales slips, invoices, cancelled checks, or other evidence of payments. The following expenses, which are deemed particularly susceptible to abuse, must generally be substantiated by adequate records or sufficient evidence corroborating the taxpayer's own statement: expenses with respect to travel away from home (including meals and lodging), entertainment expenses, business gifts, and expenses in connection with the use of listed property such as cars and computers (¶ 1211) (Code Sec. 274(d); Temp. Reg. § 1.274-5T).[144] The expenses must be substantiated as to amount, time, place, and business purpose. For entertainment and gift expenses, the business relationship of the person being entertained or receiving the gift must also be substantiated. An employer's reimbursement arrangement must require employees to satisfy these substantiation requirements in order to be treated as an accountable plan (¶ 952A).

References are to Standard Federal Tax Reports; Tax Research Consultant; and Practical Tax Explanations.

[142] ¶ 6004; INDIV: 36,056.15; § 10,120.10

[143] ¶ 6004; INDIV: 36,056.10; § 10,120.15

[144] ¶ 14,402, ¶ 14,410; BUSEXP: 24,800; § 10,105

Substantiation by Adequate Records. A contemporaneous log is not required, but a record of the elements of the expense or use of the listed property made at or near the time of the expenditure or use, supported by sufficient documentary evidence, has a high degree of credibility. Adequate accounting generally requires the submission of an account book, expense diary or log, or similar record maintained by the employee and recorded at or near the time of incurrence of the expense. Documentary evidence, such as receipts or paid bills, is not generally required for expenses that are less than $75. However, documentary evidence is required for all lodging expenses (Reg. § 1.274-5(c)(2)(iii)).[145] The employee should also maintain a record of any amounts charged to the employer.

The *Cohan* rule, which allows the courts to estimate the amount of a taxpayer's expenses when adequate records do not exist, does not apply for the expenses covered by the substantiation rules of Code Sec. 274(d) (Temp. Reg. § 1.274-5T(a)(1)).[146] However, if a taxpayer has established that the records have been lost due to circumstances beyond the taxpayer's control, such as destruction by fire or flood, then the taxpayer has a right to substantiate claimed deductions by a reasonable construction of the expenditures or use (Temp. Reg. § 1.274-5T(c)(5)).[147]

Employees of the executive and judicial branches and certain employees of the legislative branch of the federal government may substantiate their requests for reimbursement of ordinary and necessary business expenses with an account book or expense log instead of submitting documentary evidence (e.g., receipts or bills) (Rev. Proc. 97-45).[148]

954. Per Diem Methods for Substantiating Employers' Meals and Lodging Expenses. A taxpayer must substantiate the amount, time, place, and business purpose of expenses paid or incurred in traveling away from home (¶ 953). Although the taxpayer has the option of keeping the actual records of travel expenses, the IRS has provided per diem allowances under which the amount of away-from-home meals and incidental expenses (M&IE) may be deemed to be substantiated. These per diem allowances eliminate the need for substantiating actual costs (Rev. Proc. 2011-47).[149] If per diem allowances are used to calculate the deductible amount, the time, place, and business purpose of the travel must still be substantiated by adequate records or other evidence.

Although most frequently used in the employer-employee relationship, per diem allowances may be used in connection with arrangements between any payor and payee, such as between independent contractors and those contracting with them. However, employees related to the payor within the related party rules of Code Sec. 267(b) (using a 10-percent common ownership standard (¶ 1717)) cannot use per diem substantiation methods.

Employees. The per diem method can be used to substantiate an employee's reimbursed expenses (for purposes of the employer's return) only if the arrangement is considered an accountable plan (¶ 952A) and the allowance:

(1) is paid with respect to ordinary and necessary expenses incurred or that the employer reasonably expects to be incurred by an employee for lodging and/or M&IE expenses while traveling away from home in connection with the performance of services as an employee;

(2) is reasonably calculated not to exceed the amount of the expense or the anticipated expenses; and

(3) is paid at the applicable federal per diem rate, a flat rate, or stated schedule.

Types of Per Diem Allowances. There are three types of per diem allowances:

(1) lodging plus M&IE, which provides a per diem allowance to cover lodging as well as meals and incidental expenses (¶ 954A);

References are to Standard Federal Tax Reports; Tax Research Consultant; and Practical Tax Explanations.

[145] ¶ 14,408F; BUSEXP: 24,806.15; § 10,105.15

[146] ¶ 14,410; BUSEXP: 24,802; § 10,105.05

[147] ¶ 14,410; BUSEXP: 24,806; § 10,105.25

[148] ¶ 14,417.38; BUSEXP: 24,906.106; § 10,105.05

[149] ¶ 14,417.421; BUSEXP: 24,808; § 10,125.10

(2) M&IE only, which provides a per diem allowance for meals and incidental expenses only (¶ 954B); and

(3) incidental expenses only, to be used when no meal or lodging expenses are incurred (¶ 954B) (Rev. Proc. 2011-47).[150]

"Incidental expenses" has the same meaning as in the Federal Travel Regulations (41 C.F.R. 300-3.1). Under those regulations, incidental expenses include *only* fees and tips given to porters, baggage carriers, hotel staff, and staff on ships. Transportation between places of lodging or business and places where meals are taken, and the mailing cost of filing travel vouchers and paying employer-sponsored charge card billings, are *no longer* included in the definition of incidental expenses. Taxpayers using per diem rates may separately deduct or be reimbursed for such transportation and mailing expenses (Notice 2014-57).[151]

Expenses of laundry, lodging taxes, and telephone calls are not incidental expenses (IRS Pub. 463). Lodging taxes for travel within the continental United States and for nonforeign travel outside the continental United States are not considered incidental expenses but rather reimbursable miscellaneous expenses. However, lodging taxes have not been removed from the foreign per diem rates set by the U.S. State Department (41 C.F.R. 301-11.27).

Allowances Exceeding Federal Rates. If expenses are substantiated using a per diem amount, regardless of whether it covers lodging plus M&IE or only M&IE, and the reimbursement exceeds the relevant federal per diem rates for that type of allowance, then the employee (or independent contractor) is required to include the excess in gross income. The excess portion is treated as paid under a nonaccountable plan; thus, it must be reported on the employee's Form W-2 and is subject to withholding (Reg. § 1.62-2(h)(2)(i)(B)(1)).[152]

954A. Lodging Plus Meals and Incidental Expenses Per Diem. Under the lodging plus meals and incidental expenses (M&IE) per diem method (¶ 954), the amount of an employee's (or other payee's) reimbursed expenses that is deemed substantiated (for purposes of the employer's return) is equal to the lesser of the employer's per diem allowance or the federal per diem amount for the locality of travel for the period in which the employee is away from home (Rev. Proc. 2011-47).[153] The employer is not required to produce lodging receipts if per diem allowances are used to substantiate such expenses. The locality of travel is the place where the employee stops for sleep or rest. Employees and self-employed individuals may determine their allowable deductions for unreimbursed M&IE while away from home by using the applicable federal M&IE rate (¶ 954B). However, unreimbursed lodging costs must be substantiated by required records, e.g., hotel receipts.

Per Diem Rates. The federal per diem rate for lodging plus M&IE depends upon the locality of travel. For various geographic areas within the continental United States (the 48 contiguous states plus the District of Columbia) (CONUS), the federal per diem rate for a given locality is equal to the sum of a maximum lodging amount and the M&IE rate for that locality. Federal per diem rates have also been established for nonforeign localities outside of the continental United States (OCONUS). These areas include Alaska, Hawaii, Puerto Rico, and possessions of the United States. Rates are also established for foreign travel (foreign OCONUS).

Rates for CONUS, OCONUS, and foreign travel are published under the Federal Travel Regulations for government travel and are updated periodically (Rev. Proc. 2011-47).[154] The travel rates are issued to coincide with the government's fiscal year of October to September.

High-Low Method. In lieu of using the maximum per diem rates from the CONUS table, the high-low method, which is a simplified method for determining a lodging plus

---

References are to Standard Federal Tax Reports; Tax Research Consultant; and Practical Tax Explanations.

[150] ¶ 14,417.421; BUSEXP: 24,912.05; § 10,125.10
[151] ¶ 14,417.421; BUSEXP: 24,912.05; § 10,125.10
[152] ¶ 6004; BUSEXP: 24,904; § 10,125.10
[153] ¶ 14,417.421; BUSEXP: 24,912.05; § 10,125.10
[154] ¶ 14,417.421; BUSEXP: 24,912; § 660, § 670, § 680, § 690

¶954A

M&IE per diem, can be used to compute per diem allowances for travel within the continental United States. This method divides all CONUS localities into two categories: low-cost or high-cost localities (Rev. Proc. 2011-47).[155]

For travel on or after October 1, 2014, through September 30, 2015, the following per diem rates for lodging expenses and M&IE were set by the IRS for high-cost and low-cost localities (Notice 2014-57):

	Lodging expense rate	M&IE rate	Maximum per diem rate
High-cost locality	$194	$65	$259
Low-cost locality	120	52	172

For travel on or after October 1, 2013, through September 30, 2014, the following per diem rates for lodging expenses and M&IE were set by the IRS for high-cost and low-cost localities (Notice 2013-65):

	Lodging expense rate	M&IE rate	Maximum per diem rate
High-cost locality	$186	$65	$251
Low-cost locality	118	52	170

Certain areas are treated as high-cost only during periods of the year (e.g., peak tourist season) and as low-cost during other periods of time. Thus, employers who use the high-low method must determine whether the employee traveled in a high-cost area and if the area was classified as high-cost during the actual period of travel.

If the high-low method is used for an employee, then the payor may not use the actual federal maximum per diem rates for that employee during the calendar year for travel within the continental United States. However, the applicable federal rates for travel outside the continental United States (OCONUS rates) may be used, and the M&IE-only rate may be used or the reimbursement of actual expenses may be made.

Proration of M&IE Allowance. If an individual is traveling away from home for only a portion of the day, there are two alternative methods that may be used to prorate the per diem rate or the M&IE rate. Under the first method, 75 percent of the M&IE rate (or the M&IE portion of the per diem rate) is allowed for each partial day during which an employee or self-employed individual is traveling on business. Under the second method, referred to as the reasonable business practice method, the M&IE rate may be prorated using any method that is consistently applied and in accordance with reasonable business practice. For example, if an employee travels from 9 a.m. one day until 5 p.m. the next day, a proration method that gives an amount equal to two times the M&IE rate will be treated as in accordance with reasonable business practice (Rev. Proc. 2011-47).[156]

Transition Rules. Taxpayers are allowed to continue to use the per diem rates effective prior to October 1, 2014, for the remainder of 2014, or they may begin to use the new per diem rates for reimbursement for travel, as long as they use either the pre-October 1 rates or the updated rates for the October 1 through December 31 period consistently. Taxpayers who used the per diem method or the high-low substantiation method for reimbursement of an individual's travel expenses during the first nine months of calendar-year 2014 must continue to use that method for the remainder of calendar-year 2014. However, taxpayers who use the high-low method during the first nine months of calendar-year 2014 have the option of either continuing to use the rates and localities in effect prior to October 1, 2014, or using the updated rates and localities in effect for travel on and after October 1, 2014, as long as they use the same rates and localities consistently for all employees reimbursed under the high-low method.

954B. Meals-and-Incidental-Expense-Only Per Diem Allowances. A meals-and-incidental-expenses–only per diem allowance may be used to substantiate an employee's or other payee's meal and incidental expenses (M&IEs) for purposes of the employer's return (Rev. Proc. 2011-47).[157] The amount that is deemed substantiated is equal to the

---

References are to Standard Federal Tax Reports; Tax Research Consultant; and Practical Tax Explanations.

[155] ¶ 14,417.421; BUSEXP: 24,912.05; § 10,125.10

[156] ¶ 14,417.421; BUSEXP: 24,808; § 10,125.10

[157] ¶ 14,417.421; BUSEXP: 24,808; § 10,125.10

lesser of the per diem allowance or the amount computed at the federal M&IE rate for the locality of travel for the period that the employee is away from home. If M&IEs are substantiated using a per diem allowance, the entire amount is treated as a food and beverage expense subject to the 50-percent limitation on meal and entertainment expenses (¶ 916).

The M&IE rate must be prorated for partial days of travel away from home (¶ 954A). If an employee's meals are provided by his or her employer, even though the employee may be working from home, the employee is only entitled to deduct the incidental expense portion of the applicable federal per diem M&IE rates (*R.J. Zbylut*, Dec. 57,348(M), 95 TCM 1172 (2008)).[158]

Self-Employed Persons and Employees. Self-employed individuals and employees whose expenses are not reimbursed may also use the M&IE-only rate to substantiate M&IEs while traveling away from home. The taxpayer must actually prove (through adequate records or sufficient corroborative evidence (¶ 953)) the time, place, and business purpose of the travel. While the M&IE rate may be used by an employee or self-employed person to substantiate M&IEs, the amount of lodging costs must be proven by documentary evidence (e.g., a receipt).

Optional Method for Incidental-Expenses-Only Deduction. Taxpayers have available an optional method for claiming the deduction for only incidental expenses in lieu of using actual expenses. Taxpayers who do not incur any meal expenses may deduct $5 per calendar day (or partial day) as ordinary and necessary incidental expenses, paid or incurred, while traveling to any CONUS or OCONUS localities (Notice 2014-57; Notice 2013-65).[159] The optional method is subject to the proration rules for partial days and substantiation requirements for taxpayers who use the per diem method for substantiation (Rev. Proc. 2011-47).[160] The optional method for incidental expenses only cannot also be used by taxpayers already using the following per diem methods:

    (1) the lodging plus M&IE per diem method;

    (2) the M&IE-only method; or

    (3) the high-low method and the optional M&IE-only method (¶ 954A).

Transportation Workers. The M&IE rates for travel away from home for both self-employed persons and employees in the transportation industry are $59 for CONUS localities and $65 for OCONUS localities (Notice 2014-57; Notice 2013-65).[161] An individual is in the transportation industry only if the individual's work: (1) directly involves moving people or goods by airplane, barge, bus, ship, train, or truck, and (2) regularly requires travel away from home that involves travel to localities with differing federal M&IE rates during a single trip.

Transition Rules. Taxpayers under the calendar-year convention for the transportation industry, who used the federal M&IE rates during the first nine months of calendar year 2014 to substantiate the amount of an individual's travel expense, may not use the special transportation industry rates until January 1, 2015 (Rev. Proc. 2011-47).[162] Likewise, taxpayers who used the special transportation industry rates for the first nine months of calendar year 2014 to substantiate the amount of an individual's travel expenses may not use the federal M&IE rates until January 1, 2015.

955. Foreign Travel. Generally, traveling expenses (including meals and lodging) of a taxpayer who travels outside of the United States away from home must be allocated between time spent on the trip for business and time spent for pleasure (¶ 949) (Code Sec. 274(c); Reg. § 1.274-4).[163] When the trip is for not more than one week or when the time spent on personal activities on the trip is less than 25 percent of the total time away from home, no allocation is required and all expenses are deductible. Travel outside the United States does not include any travel within the United States. However, travel that is not from one point in the United States to another point in the United States is considered travel outside the United States.

References are to Standard Federal Tax Reports; Tax Research Consultant; and Practical Tax Explanations.

[158] ¶ 14,417.421; BUSEXP: 24,808; § 10,125.10

[159] ¶ 14,417.421; BUSEXP: 24,912; § 10,125.10

[160] ¶ 14,417.421; BUSEXP: 24,808; § 10,125.10

[161] ¶ 14,417.421; BUSEXP: 24,912; § 10,125.10

[162] ¶ 14,417.28; BUSEXP: 24,808; § 10,125.10

[163] ¶ 14,402, ¶ 14,408; BUSEXP: 24,300; § 9,535.05

When the foreign trip is longer than a week (seven consecutive days counting the day of return but not the day of departure) or 25 percent or more of the time away from home is spent for personal reasons, a deduction for travel expenses will be denied to the extent that they are not allocable to the taxpayer's business or the taxpayer's management of income-producing property.

No allocation is required on a foreign trip when (1) the individual traveling had no substantial control over the arranging of the business trip, or (2) a personal vacation was not a major consideration in making the trip. An employee traveling under a reimbursement or expense account allowance arrangement is not considered as having substantial control over the arranging of a business trip unless the employee is a managing executive (an employee who can, without being vetoed, decide on whether and when to make the trip) or is a 10-percent-or-more owner of the employer.

For special rules governing expenses of attending foreign conventions, seminars, and other similar meetings, see ¶ 959 and ¶ 960.

956. Travel Expenses of State Legislators. A state legislator whose residence is further than 50 miles from the state capitol building may elect to be deemed to be away from home in the pursuit of a trade or business on any day that the legislature is in session (including periods of up to four consecutive days when the legislature is not in session) or on any day when the legislature is not in session but the legislator's presence is formally recorded at a committee meeting (Code Sec. 162(h)).[164]

957. Luxury Water Travel. A deduction for transportation by ocean liner, cruise ship, or other form of water transportation is limited to a daily amount equal to twice the highest per diem travel amount allowable to employees of the federal government while on official business away from home but within the United States. The limitation does not apply to any expense allocable to a convention, seminar, or other meeting that is held on a cruise ship (¶ 959). Separately stated meal and entertainment expenses are subject to the 50-percent limitation rule (¶ 916), prior to the application of the per diem limitation. Statutory exceptions to the 50-percent limit apply (¶ 917) (Code Sec. 274(m)(1)).[165]

958. Travel as a Form of Education. A deduction for travel expenses is not allowed if the expense would be deductible only on the basis that the travel itself constitutes a form of education (Code Sec. 274(m)(2)).[166] See, also, ¶ 1082.

959. Convention Expenses. Deductible travel expenses include those incurred in attending a convention related to the taxpayer's business, even though the taxpayer is an employee (Code Sec. 274(h); Reg. § 1.162-2(d)).[167] The fact that an employee uses vacation or leave time or that attendance at the convention is voluntary will not necessarily negate the deduction. For the rules applicable to foreign conventions, see ¶ 960. Expenses for a convention or meeting in connection with investments, financial planning, or other income-producing property are not deductible.

Cruise Ships. A limited deduction is available for expenses incurred for conventions on U.S. cruise ships (Code Sec. 274(h)(2)).[168] This deduction (limited to $2,000 with respect to all cruises beginning in any calendar year) applies only if:

(1) all ports of such cruise ship are located in the United States or in U.S. possessions;

(2) the taxpayer establishes that the convention is directly related to the active conduct of his or her trade or business; and

(3) the taxpayer includes certain specified information in the return on which the deduction is claimed.

960. Foreign Conventions. No deduction is allowed for expenses allocable to a convention, seminar, or meeting held outside the North American area unless the

---

References are to Standard Federal Tax Reports; Tax Research Consultant; and Practical Tax Explanations.

[164] ¶ 8500; BUSEXP: 24,120; § 9,510

[165] ¶ 14,402; BUSEXP: 24,400; § 9,545.10

[166] ¶ 14,402; INDIV: 60,122.20; § 9,501

[167] ¶ 8527, ¶ 14,402; BUSEXP: 24,160; § 9,515

[168] ¶ 14,402; BUSEXP: 24,162; § 9,545.05

taxpayer establishes that the meeting is directly related to the active conduct of his or her trade or business and that it is as reasonable for the meeting to be held outside the North American area (Code Sec. 274(h)).[169] The factors to be taken into account are:

(1) the purpose of the meeting and the activities taking place at such meeting;

(2) the purposes and activities of the sponsoring organization or group;

(3) the places of residence of the active members of the sponsoring organization or group and the places at which other meetings of the organization or group have been held or will be held; and

(4) such other relevant factors as the taxpayer may present.

The North American area means the 50 states of the United States and the District of Columbia, U.S. possessions, Canada, Mexico, the Republic of the Marshall Islands, the Federated States of Micronesia, and the Republic of Palau. Costs incurred in attending conventions held in the Caribbean or on certain Pacific Islands may also be deductible if the host country is a designated beneficiary country, there is a bilateral or multilateral agreement in effect providing for the exchange of tax information with the United States, and the country has not been found to discriminate in its tax laws against conventions held in the United States. A list of qualifying countries is provided in Rev. Rul. 2011-26.[170] Expenses for foreign conventions on cruise ships are not deductible.

Home Office and Vacation Home Expenses

961. Home Office Deduction. Taxpayers are not entitled to deduct any expenses for using their homes for business purposes unless the expenses are attributable to a portion of the home, or a separate structure, used exclusively on a regular basis:

(1) as the principal place of any business carried on by the taxpayer;

(2) as a place of business that is used by patients, clients, or customers in meeting or dealing with the taxpayer in the normal course of business; or

(3) in connection with the taxpayer's business, if the taxpayer is using a separate structure that is appurtenant to, but not attached to, the home (Code Sec. 280A(c)).[171]

If the taxpayer is an employee, the business use of the home must be for the convenience of the employer (¶ 965). The allowable deduction is computed on Form 8829. The amount deductible is limited to either the taxpayer's actual expenses related to the office or an amount determined under a safe harbor method (¶ 963).

Generally, a specific portion of the taxpayer's home must be used solely for the purpose of carrying on a trade or business in order to satisfy the exclusive use test. This requirement is not met if the portion is used for both business and personal purposes. However, an exception is provided for a wholesale or retail seller whose dwelling unit is the sole fixed location of the trade or business. In this situation, the ordinary and necessary expenses allocable to space within the dwelling unit that is used as a storage unit for inventory or product samples are deductible, provided that the space is used on a regular basis and is a separately identifiable space suitable for storage. Another special exception applies to licensed day care operators (¶ 964).

A taxpayer's principal place of business for this purpose includes a place of business that is used by the taxpayer for the administrative or management activities of any trade or business of the taxpayer if there is no other fixed location where the taxpayer conducts substantial administrative or management activities. Taxpayers who perform administrative or management activities for their trade or business at places other than the home office are not automatically prohibited from taking the deduction based on failure to meet the principal place of business requirement. The following taxpayers are *not* prevented from taking a home office deduction:

References are to Standard Federal Tax Reports; Tax Research Consultant; and Practical Tax Explanations.

[169] ¶ 14,402; BUSEXP: 24,350; § 9,540

[170] ¶ 14,408A.62; BUSEXP: 24,350; § 9,540

[171] ¶ 14,850; BUSEXP: 27,150; § 8,101

(1) taxpayers who have others conduct the taxpayer's administrative or management activities at locations other than the taxpayer's home office (e.g., billing activities);

(2) taxpayers who carry out administrative and management activities at sites that are not fixed locations of the business (e.g., cars or hotel rooms) in addition to performing the activities at the home office;

(3) taxpayers who conduct an insubstantial amount of administrative and management activities at a fixed location other than the home office (e.g., occasionally doing minimal paperwork at another fixed location); and

(4) taxpayers who conduct substantial nonadministrative and nonmanagement business activities at a fixed location other than the home office (e.g., meeting with, or providing services to customers, clients, or patients at a fixed location other than the home office) (Instructions to Form 8829; IRS Pub. 587).[172]

Auction and Consignment Sellers. Auction and consignment sellers may compute their deduction to the extent of expenses allocable to space in the residence used on a regular basis to store inventory and/or product samples if the residence is the sole fixed location of the auction or consignment business (IRS Fact Sheet FS-2007-23).[173]

Residential Telephone. Basic local telephone service charges on the first line in a residence are not deductible as business expenses. Additional charges for long-distance calls, equipment, optional services (e.g., call waiting), or additional telephone lines may be deductible (Code Sec. 262(b)).[174]

963. Limitation on Home Office Deductions. The home office deduction (¶ 961) cannot exceed the gross income from the activity, reduced by the home expenses that would be deductible in the absence of any business use, e.g., mortgage interest, property taxes, etc., and the business expenses not related to the use of the home (Code Sec. 280A(c)(5)).[175] The business related expenses are deducted in a specific order, as follows:

(1) expenses that are required by the business but not allocable to the use of the home (such as office supplies);

(2) expenses that would be deductible even if the home was not used as a place of business (such as mortgage interest and real estate taxes);

(3) expenses related to the household that are allocable to the business use, i.e., utilities and insurance; and

(4) the allocable depreciation expenses.

The deduction of the expenses under items (3) and (4) above cannot create a loss. Unused expenses under items (3) and (4) are carried over to the next year but are still subject to the same limitation rules.

Optional Safe Harbor. A taxpayer may elect to compute the home office deduction by using a simplified safe harbor method effective for tax years beginning on or after January 1, 2013, without having to substantiate, calculate, and allocate deductible home office expenses (Rev. Proc. 2013-13).[176] Under the safe harbor, a taxpayer may claim a home office deduction equal to $5 times the number of square feet of the home office. This rate may be adjusted by the IRS as warranted. However, no more than 300 square feet may be taken into account, limiting the safe-harbor deduction to $1,500. The deduction may also not exceed the taxpayer's gross income from the business. If the safe harbor deduction exceeds the income limit, the excess cannot be carried forward to the next year. A taxpayer cannot use the safe harbor if he or she is reimbursed by an

---

References are to Standard Federal Tax Reports; Tax Research Consultant; and Practical Tax Explanations.

[172] ¶ 14,850.017; BUSEXP: 27,152.05; § 8,120.10

[173] ¶ 8521.112; BUSEXP: 27,158; § 8,125

[174] ¶ 13,600; BUSEXP: 27,056.15; § 8,205

[175] ¶ 14,850; BUSEXP: 27,300; § 8,140

[176] ¶ 14,854.62; BUSEXP: 27,172; § 8,140

employer for the home office expenses. If the safe harbor is used, actual home office expenses *cannot* be deducted, though business expenses unrelated to the business use of the home may still be deducted.

964. Home Office Deduction for Day Care Services. Taxpayers who use their personal residences on a regular basis in the trade or business of providing qualifying day care services (for the care of children, handicapped persons, or the elderly) do not have to meet the exclusive use test under the home office deduction rules (¶ 961) in order to deduct business-related expenses (Code Sec. 280A(c)(4)).[177] However, the deduction is available only if the taxpayer has applied for, has been granted, or is exempt from having a license, certification, or approval as a day care center or as a family or group day care home under the provisions of applicable state law. The deduction of expenses allocable to day care use is limited as described at ¶ 963, and the taxpayer must file Form 8829.

965. Home Office Deduction by Employees. In order for employees to qualify for the home office deduction (¶ 961), they must not only meet the exclusive use requirement, but the exclusive use of the home office must be for the convenience of their employers (Code Sec. 280A(c)(1) and (6)).[178] However, regardless of whether or not an employee meets the exclusive use requirements, an employee is denied a home office deduction for any portion of the home rented to the employer, except for expenses such as home mortgage interest and real property taxes that are deductible absent business use. Generally, an employee's home office expenses must be taken as a miscellaneous itemized deduction, subject to the two-percent-of-adjusted-gross-income floor on Schedule A of Form 1040 (¶ 1011). Statutory employees (¶ 941B) claim home office deductions on Schedule C of Form 1040.

966. Deductions on Rental Residence or Vacation Home. Special rules limit the amount of deductions that may be taken by an individual or an S corporation in connection with the rental of a residence or vacation home, or a portion thereof, that is also used as the taxpayer's residence (Code Sec. 280A).[179] A vacation home includes a dwelling unit, including a house, apartment, condominium, house trailer, boat, or similar property. Deductions that may be claimed without regard to whether or not the home is used for trade or business or for the production of income, e.g., mortgage interest, property taxes, or a casualty loss, are not limited.

Personal Usage Defined. A vacation home is deemed to have been used by the taxpayer for personal purposes on a particular day if, for any part of the day, the home is used:

(1) for personal purposes by the taxpayer, any other person who owns an interest in the home, or the relatives (spouses, brothers, sisters, ancestors, lineal descendants, and spouses of lineal descendants) of either;

(2) by any individual who uses the home under a reciprocal arrangement, whether or not a rental is charged; and

(3) by any other individual who uses the home unless a fair rental is charged.

If the taxpayer rents the home at a fair rental value to any person, including a relative, for use as that person's principal residence, the use by that person is not considered personal use by the taxpayer. This exception applies to a person who owns an interest in the home only if the rental is under a shared equity financing agreement.

Rental Use of Fewer Than 15 Days. If the property is rented for fewer than 15 days during the year, no deductions attributable to such rental are allowable and no rental income is includible in gross income.

Rental Use Exceeding 14 Days. If the property is rented for more than 14 days during the year, deductions are available. If the home is used as a personal residence for more

---

References are to Standard Federal Tax Reports; Tax Research Consultant; and Practical Tax Explanations.

[177] ¶ 14,850; BUSEXP: 27,160; § 46,710.15

[178] ¶ 14,850; BUSEXP: 27,166; § 8,130.05, § 8,130.10

[179] ¶ 14,850; BUSEXP: 27,100, BUSEXP: 27,200; § 1,701, § 1,720.05

than the greater of 14 days or 10 percent of the number of days during the year for which the home is rented at a fair market rental, rental deductions are limited to the gross rental income. If the home is not used as a personal residence by the taxpayer, the rental deductions are not limited to the rental income. The deduction may also be reduced or eliminated under the passive activity loss rules (¶ 1169) or the hobby loss rules if the rental of the residence is not engaged in for profit (¶ 1195).

Ordering of Deduction. Rental expenses are deducted in a specific order from gross rental income. Mortgage interest, real property taxes, and casualty losses attributable to the rental use are deducted first. Next, operating expenses other than depreciation attributable to the rental use are deducted. Last, depreciation and other basis adjustments attributable to rental income are deducted. To determine the amount of these expenses attributable to rental use, the expenses are allocated based on a ratio that the total number of rental days bears to the total days used for all purposes during the year. When the personal usage exceeds the greater of either 14 days or 10 percent of the rental days, according to the IRS, expenses attributable to the use of the rental unit are limited in the same manner as that prescribed under the hobby loss rules at ¶ 1195 (i.e., the total deductions may not exceed the gross rental income, as well as the expenses being limited to a percentage that represents the total days rented divided by the total days used).

The Tax Court, however, has rejected this formula (*D.D. Bolton*, Dec. 38,075, 77 TC 104 (1981); *E.G. McKinney*, Dec. 38,077(M), 42 TCM 467 (1981)).[180] Its position is that mortgage interest and real estate taxes are not subject to the same percentage limitations as are other expenses because they are assessed on an annual basis without regard to the number of days that the property is used. As a result, the percentage limitation for interest and taxes is computed by dividing the total days rented by the total days in the year. This creates the potential of leaving more gross rental income to offset allocated rental expenses.

Example: During the year an individual rents out his vacation home for 91 days and uses the home for personal purposes for 30 days. The gross rental income from the unit is $2,700 for the year. He pays $621 of real property taxes and $2,854 of mortgage interest on the property for the year. The additional expenses for maintenance, repair, and utilities total $2,693.

The IRS allocation of all expenses would be based on 75 percent (91 days rented ÷ 121 days used). In contrast, the Tax Court would allocate taxes and interest based on 25 percent (91 days rented ÷ 365 days) and use the 75-percent limitation for the additional expenses for maintenance, repair, etc.

	IRS	Tax Court
1. Gross rental income	$2,700	$2,700
2. Less: Interest ($2,854)	– 2,141	– 714
Property tax ($621)	– 466	– 155
3. Remaining available income	$93	$1,831
4. Utilities, maintenance, etc.	– 93	– 1,831
5. Net income	$0	$0
6. Unused expense allowable as itemized deductions:		
Interest	$713	$2,140
Property tax	155	466
7. Total allowable deductions	$3,568	$5,306

Bed and Breakfast Inns. The special restrictions on deductions related to a residence used for business and personal purposes do not apply to the portion of the residence used exclusively as a bed and breakfast inn. Expenses related to that portion of a residence may be limited under the hobby loss rules (¶ 1195) (Code Sec. 280A(f)).[181]

References are to Standard Federal Tax Reports; Tax Research Consultant; and Practical Tax Explanations.

[180] ¶ 14,858.15; BUSEXP: 27,304; § 1,720.10　　[181] ¶ 14,850; BUSEXP: 27,054.15; § 1,705

967. Conversion of Property. Individuals who convert their principal residences into rental units (or vice versa) will not be considered to have used the unit for personal purposes for any day during the tax year that occurs before (or after) a qualified rental period for purposes of applying the deduction limitation (¶ 966) allocable to the qualified rental period (Code Sec. 280A(d)(4)).[182] The expenses, however, must be allocated between the periods of rental and personal use. A qualified rental period is a consecutive period of 12 or more months, beginning (or ending) during the tax year, during which the unit is rented or held for rental at its fair market value. The 12-month rental requirement does not apply if the residence is sold or exchanged before it has been rented or held for rental for the full 12 months.

> **Example:** A taxpayer moved out of his principal residence on February 28, 2013, to accept employment in another town. The house was rented at its fair market value from March 15, 2013, through May 14, 2014. The use of the house as a principal residence from January 1 through February 28, 2013, is not counted as personal use. If the taxpayer moved back and reoccupied the home on June 1, 2014, the use of the house as a principal residence from June 1 through December 31, 2014, is not counted as personal use.

Other Business Expenses

968. Fire and Casualty Insurance Premiums. A premium paid for insurance against losses from fire, accident, storm, theft, or other casualty is deductible if it is an ordinary and necessary expense of a business (Reg. § 1.162-1).[183] However, the uniform capitalization rules may require that insurance costs on real or tangible personal property produced or acquired for resale be included in inventory or capitalized, rather than being deducted (¶ 990–¶ 999).

An arrangement between a business and an insurance company that provides for the reimbursement of future remediation costs the business is certain to incur does not constitute an insurance contract for federal income tax purposes, the IRS has determined. The arrangement does not involve the requisite risk shifting to constitute insurance and, therefore, payments made by the business are not deductible as insurance premiums (Rev. Rul. 2007-47, amplifying Rev. Rul. 89-96).[184]

969. Advertising Expenses. Advertising expenses are deductible if they are reasonable in amount and bear a reasonable relation to the business. Deductible expenses may be for the purpose of developing goodwill as well as gaining immediate sales. The cost of advertising is deductible when paid or incurred, even though the advertising program extends over several years or is expected to result in benefits extending over a period of years (Rev. Rul. 92-80).[185] The Tax Court and the IRS require that the cost of printing a catalog that is not replaced annually be amortized over the expected life of the catalog. However, some courts have held to the contrary, taking the view that catalog costs are in the nature of an advertising expense (*Sheldon & Co.*, CA-6, 54-2 USTC ¶ 9526).[186] The costs of public service or other impartial advertising, such as advertising designed to encourage the public to register and to vote, are deductible (Rev. Rul. 62-156).[187]

No deduction may be claimed for expenses of advertising in political programs or for admission to political fund-raising or inaugural functions and similar events (Code Sec. 276).[188] This includes admission to any dinner or program if any part of the proceeds of the event directly or indirectly inures to or for the use of a political party or a political candidate.

Package Design Costs. Package design costs include the graphic arrangement or design of shapes, colors, words, pictures, lettering, and other elements on a given

---

References are to Standard Federal Tax Reports; Tax Research Consultant; and Practical Tax Explanations.

[182] ¶ 14,850; BUSEXP: 27,208; § 1,715.20

[183] ¶ 8501; BUSEXP: 18,202; § 9,415.05

[184] ¶ 8522.3915; BUSEXP: 18,200; § 9,415.05

[185] ¶ 8851.152; BUSEXP: 18,252; § 9,901

[186] ¶ 21,817.2075; BUSEXP: 18,260; § 9,901

[187] ¶ 8952.40; BUSEXP: 18,252; § 9,901

[188] ¶ 14,550; BUSEXP: 18,310; § 9,120.05

product package, or the design of a container with respect to its shape or function (Reg. § 1.263(a)-4(b)(3)(v)).[189] The Tax Court has held that packaging design costs were a deductible advertising expense even though the design provided the company with significant future benefits (*RJR Nabisco*, Dec. 52,786(M), 76 TCM 71 (1998) (Nonacq.)).[190]

970. Expenses of Earning Tax-Exempt Income. No deduction is allowed for any expense allocable to the earning of tax-exempt income (Code Sec. 265; Reg. § 1.265-1).[191] No deduction is allowed for interest paid on a debt incurred or continued in order to purchase or carry tax-exempt bonds or other obligations, regardless of whether the interest expense was incurred in business, in a profit-inspired transaction, or in any other connection.

Generally, banks, thrift institutions, and all other financial institutions may not deduct any portion of their interest expenses allocable to tax-exempt interest on obligations acquired after August 7, 1986. This includes amounts paid in respect of deposits, investment certificates, or withdrawable or repurchasable shares. There is a *de minimis* safe harbor exception to the 100-percent disallowance rule, however, for bonds issued in 2009 and 2010.

Qualified tax-exempt obligations that are issued by a qualified small issuer are not taken into account as investments in tax-exempt bonds and, therefore, are not subject to the 100-percent disallowance rule. Instead, only 20 percent of the interest expense allocable to qualified tax-exempt obligations is disallowed. A qualified small issuer is an issuer that reasonably anticipates that the amount of its tax-exempt obligations, other than certain private activity bonds, will not exceed $10 million during the calendar year. A qualified tax-exempt obligation is a tax-exempt obligation that (1) is issued after August 7, 1986, by a qualified small issuer; (2) is not a private activity bond; and (3) is designated by the issuer as qualifying for the exception from the general rule.

971. Circulation Expenses. Any expenditure to establish, maintain, or increase the circulation of a newspaper, magazine, or other periodical may be deducted in the year paid or incurred even though the taxpayer reports only an allocable portion of the subscription income for each year of the subscription period (¶ 1537) (Code Sec. 173; Reg. § 1.173-1).[192] Taxpayers may also elect to capitalize circulation expenses and amortize them over a three-year period (¶ 1450).

972. Fines, Penalties, Kickbacks, Drug Trafficking. A fine or a penalty paid to a government for the violation of any law is not a deductible business expense (Code Sec. 162(f)).[193] Any illegal bribe or kickback paid directly or indirectly to a domestic government official or employee is not deductible. Bribes and kickbacks paid directly or indirectly to an employee or official of a foreign government are not deductible if they are unlawful under the federal Foreign Corrupt Practices Act of 1977. No deduction is allowed for any payment made directly or indirectly to any person if the payment is a bribe, kickback, or other illegal payment under any U.S. law or under any generally enforced state law that subjects the payor to a criminal penalty or to the loss of license or privilege to engage in a trade or business (Code Sec. 162(c)(2) and (3); Reg. § 1.162-18).[194] A deduction is also denied for any kickback, rebate, or bribe made by any provider of services, supplier, physician, or other person who furnished items or services for which payment is or may be made under Medicare or Medicaid, or in whole or in part out of federal funds under a state plan approved under Medicare or Medicaid, if the kickback, rebate, or bribe is made in connection with the furnishing of such items or services or the making or receiving of such payments. For all the above purposes, a kickback includes a payment in consideration of the referral of a client, patient, or customer.

References are to Standard Federal Tax Reports; Tax Research Consultant; and Practical Tax Explanations.

[189] ¶ 13,704C; BUSEXP: 9,104.10; § 9,970

[190] ¶ 8851.1338; BUSEXP: 18,252.10; § 9,970

[191] ¶ 14,050, ¶ 14,051; BUSEXP: 18,600, RIC: 12,204.20; § 7,420.05, § 9,001

[192] ¶ 12,030, ¶ 12,031; DEPR: 21,252; § 11,520

[193] ¶ 8500; BUSEXP: 18,800; § 9,105, § 9,115

[194] ¶ 8500, ¶ 8857; BUSEXP: 18,800; § 9,105

If a taxpayer is convicted of a criminal violation of the antitrust laws, which contain a treble damage provision, or enters a plea of guilty or no contest to a charged violation, no deduction is allowed for two-thirds of the amount paid to satisfy the judgment or in settlement of a suit brought under section 4 of the Clayton Act (Code Sec. 162(g); Reg. § 1.162-22).[195]

No deduction is allowed for a federal tax penalty (Reg. § 1.162-21(b)(1)(ii)).[196] No deduction or credit is allowed for amounts paid or incurred in the illegal trafficking in drugs listed in the federal Controlled Substances Act. However, an adjustment to gross receipts for the cost of goods sold is permitted (Code Sec. 280E).[197] Damage awards paid in connection with the violation of a federal civil statute and similar penalties may be deductible if they are compensatory, rather than punitive, in nature (Reg. § 1.162-21(b)(2)).[198]

973. Legal Expenses. Legal expenses paid or incurred in connection with a business transaction or primarily for the purpose of preserving existing business reputation and goodwill are ordinarily deductible (*F.W. Staudt*, Dec. 20,040(M), 12 TCM 1417 (1953)).[199] It is not necessary that litigation be involved for legal fees to be deductible. In addition to attorney fees, legal expenses include fees or expenses of accountants and expert witnesses, as well as court stenographic and printing charges.

The deductibility tests are substantially the same as those for other business expenses and preclude a current deduction for a legal expense incurred in the acquisition of capital assets (Reg. § 1.263(a)-2).[200] Litigation costs have to be capitalized when, under the origin of the claim test (or the nature of the claim leading to the payments), they are considered to be incurred to acquire a capital asset.

A taxpayer may deduct, as a business expense, that part of the cost of tax return preparation that is properly allocable to the business, as well as expenses incurred in resolving asserted tax deficiencies relating to the business (*D. Pistoresi*, Dec. 53,243(M), 77 TCM 1368 (1999); *C. Wood*, Dec. 25,086, 37 TC 70 (1961) (Acq.).[201]

For the deductibility of legal expenses arising from the determination of nonbusiness taxes or income-producing property, see ¶ 1092 and ¶ 1093.

974. Lobbying Expenses. Lobbying expenses directed towards influencing federal or state legislation are generally not deductible (Code Sec. 162(e); Reg. § 1.162-20(c)).[202] The prohibition does not generally apply to in-house expenses that do not exceed $2,000 for a tax year. Lobbying expenses pertaining to local legislation are deductible.

975. Federal National Mortgage Association Stock. Initial holders of stock issued by the Federal National Mortgage Association may deduct, as a business expense, the excess of the price paid over the market price of the stock on the date of issuance (Code Sec. 162(d); Reg. § 1.162-19(a)).[203] The basis in the stock is reduced to reflect the deduction.

976. Political Contributions. Contributions made to a political candidate or party are not deductible as a business expense (Code Sec. 162(e)(1)(B)).[204]

977. Environmental Clean-Up Costs (Expired). For expenses paid or incurred before January 1, 2012, a taxpayer could elect to deduct certain environmental cleanup costs in the year in which they occurred, rather than to treat them as a capital expense (Code Sec. 198).[205] The deduction only pertains to the cleanup of hazardous substances located on sites within areas that meet specific requirements. The IRS provided guidance for taxpayers to make this election (Rev. Proc. 98-47).[206]

References are to Standard Federal Tax Reports; Tax Research Consultant; and Practical Tax Explanations.

[195] ¶ 8500, ¶ 8955; BUSEXP: 18,800; § 9,125

[196] ¶ 8953; INDIV: 45,060; § 9,115

[197] ¶ 15,050, ¶ 15,050.25; BUSEXP: 18,808; § 9,110

[198] ¶ 8953; BUSEXP: 18,650; § 9,115

[199] ¶ 8526.4503; BUSEXP: 18,052.05; § 9,920.05

[200] ¶ 8526.4162, ¶ 13,703; BUSEXP: 18,054.05; § 9,920.05

[201] ¶ 8520.73; BUSEXP: 18,050; § 9,920.05

[202] ¶ 8500, ¶ 8951; BUSEXP: 18,302; § 9,120.05, § 9,120.10

[203] ¶ 8500, ¶ 8859; SALES: 6,372.35; § 7,405

[204] ¶ 8500; BUSEXP: 18,310; § 9,120.05

[205] ¶ 12,460; BUSEXP: 18,750; BUSEXP: 18,756; § 10,230

[206] ¶ 12,465.30; BUSEXP: 18,756; § 10,230

977A. Small Refiners' Deduction for Upgrades to Produce Low Sulfur Fuels. Small refiners that invest in upgrading their facilities to produce low-sulfur fuels are allowed to elect to deduct a portion of the costs (Code Sec. 179B).[207] Qualified small refiners may deduct up to 75 percent of the capital costs paid or incurred for the purposes of complying with the Highway Diesel Fuel Sulfur Control Requirements of the Environmental Protection Agency (¶ 1285).

977B. Domestic Film and Television Productions Deduction. A taxpayer may elect to deduct the cost of any qualified film or television production commenced before January 1, 2014 (Code Sec. 181).[208] The maximum deduction is $15 million ($20 million for films produced in certain low-income or distressed communities). See ¶ 1229 for general discussion of the amortization of film and television production costs.

> **Comment:** Absent further legislation, the domestic film and television productions deduction has expired for productions beginning after December 31, 2013. For the latest legislative updates, visit our website www.CCHGroup.com/TaxUpdates.

977C. New Refinery Property Deduction. The builders of new liquid fuel refineries may elect to deduct up to 50 percent of the cost of building a qualified refinery property in the year it is placed in service (Code Sec. 179C).[209] The deduction is available to taxpayers who place a qualified refinery property in service after August 8, 2005, and before January 1, 2014. The expensing deduction is also available with respect to refineries processing liquid fuel directly from shale or tar sands (¶ 1285A).

> **Comment:** Absent further legislation, the partial deduction for the cost of building qualified refinery property has expired for property placed in service after December 31, 2013. For the latest legislative updates, visit our website www.CCHGroup.com/TaxUpdates.

977D. Energy-Efficient Commercial Buildings Deduction. Taxpayers may deduct a portion of the costs of installation of energy-efficient systems into commercial buildings (Code Sec. 179D).[210] The maximum deduction is generally $1.80 per square foot of a qualified commercial property, less the total amount of deductions under this provision taken in prior tax years. Qualified systems include interior lighting, heating, cooling, ventilation, hot water systems, and the building envelope. The deduction is available for qualified commercial property placed in service after December 31, 2005, but before January 1, 2014 (¶ 1286).

> **Comment:** Absent further legislation, the partial deduction for the cost of installing energy-efficient systems into commercial buildings has expired for property placed in service after December 31, 2013. For the latest legislative updates, visit our website www.CCHGroup.com/TaxUpdates.

978. Expenses of Mercantile and Manufacturing Businesses. Merchants and manufacturers generally are subject to the uniform capitalization rules. See the discussion at ¶ 990–¶ 999. However, ordinary and necessary business expenses not covered by such rules may be currently deducted (Reg. § 1.162-1).[211]

979. Research and Experimental Expenses. A taxpayer may elect to deduct certain research and experimental expenses by claiming the deduction on the income tax return for the first tax year in which the costs are paid or incurred in connection with its business (Code Sec. 174; Reg. § 1.174-2).[212] Only costs of research in the laboratory or for experimental purposes, whether carried on by the taxpayer or on behalf of the taxpayer by a third party, are deductible. Market research and normal product testing costs are not considered research expenditures. Once made, the election is applicable to all research costs incurred in the project for the current and all subsequent years.

References are to Standard Federal Tax Reports; Tax Research Consultant; and Practical Tax Explanations.

[207] ¶ 12,134; BUSEXP: 18,908

[208] ¶ 12,144; DEPR: 12,300; § 10,235

[209] ¶ 12,137; BUSEXP: 18,900; § 10,245

[210] ¶ 12,138; BUSEXP: 18,950; § 10,250

[211] ¶ 8501; BUSEXP: 3,050; § 10,310.05

[212] ¶ 12,040, ¶ 12,043; BUSEXP: 9,102.10; § 9,705.05

The costs of obtaining a patent, including attorneys' fees paid or incurred in making and perfecting a patent application, qualify as research or experimental expenditures, but the costs of acquiring another's patent, model, production, or process do not qualify (Reg. § 1.174-2(a)(1)).[213] When the election to defer expenses has been made, the right to amortize ceases when the patent issues. Unrecovered expenditures are recovered through depreciation over the life of the patent (Reg. § 1.174-4(a)(4)).[214] A credit was allowed for increased research and experimental expenses paid or incurred before January 1, 2014 (¶ 1365J). A purchased patent may qualify as a section 197 intangible to be amortized over 15 years (¶ 1288).

980. Computer Software Costs. The tax treatment of computer software used in a trade or business depends on whether the taxpayer has leased the software, developed it internally, or purchased it (Code Sec. 162; Reg. § 1.162-11; Rev. Proc. 2000-50).[215]

Generally, rental payments for leased software are deductible as business expenses over the term of the lease in the same manner as any other rental payments (Rev. Proc. 2000-50).[216] However, acquired computer software is amortizable over 15 years if it is a section 197 intangible (¶ 1288). Software that is not a section 197 intangible is amortized using the straight-line method over a period of 36 months beginning on the first day of the month that the software is placed in service.

Costs incurred by a taxpayer to develop software for sale to others or for internal use may be treated like research and experimental expenses (¶ 979) and may be deducted currently, amortized over a 60-month period (or shorter if established as appropriate), or amortized over a 36-month period, so long as such costs are treated consistently (Rev. Proc. 2000-50).[217]

Computer software is any program designed to cause a computer to perform a desired function (Code Secs. 167(f)(1)(B) and 197(e)(3)(B); Rev. Proc. 2000-50).[218] It does not include any database or similar item unless the database or item is in the public domain and is incidental to the operation of otherwise qualifying computer software.

Software Bundled with Hardware. Software costs that are included, but not separately stated, in the cost of computer hardware are capitalized and depreciated as part of the hardware (Reg. § 1.167(a)-14(b)(2)).[219] In other words, the entire amount is treated as the cost of hardware (tangible property) and is depreciable under MACRS over a five-year recovery period.

Web Site Development Costs. The IRS has yet to issue formal guidance on the treatment of web site development costs.

Domestic Production Activities

980A. Deduction for Domestic Production Activities. A taxpayer may claim a deduction against gross income equal to nine percent of its qualified production activities income (QPAI) (¶ 980B) or its taxable income without regard to the deduction (whichever is less) (Code Sec. 199).[220] In the case of an individual, estate, or trust, QPAI or adjusted gross income (rather than taxable income), figured without regard to the deduction, is used to calculate the deduction. Form 8903 is used to calculate the deduction. In the case of corporate taxpayers, the deduction against gross income is equal to nine percent of its QPAI or its alternative minimum taxable income.

The amount of the domestic production activities deduction for any tax year, however, may not exceed 50 percent of the W-2 wages paid by the taxpayer (¶ 980C) that are allocable to the taxpayer's domestic production gross receipts (¶ 980D).

References are to Standard Federal Tax Reports; Tax Research Consultant; and Practical Tax Explanations.

[213] ¶ 12,043; DEPR: 21,300; § 9,705.10

[214] ¶ 12,046; DEPR: 21,300; § 9,710

[215] ¶ 8500, ¶ 8753, ¶ 8754.1695; DEPR: 15,162.85; § 11,535.05

[216] ¶ 8754.1695; BUSEXP: 18,856.106; § 11,535.15

[217] ¶ 8754.1695; DEPR: 21,308.20; § 11,535.25

[218] ¶ 8500, ¶ 11,030D, ¶ 8754.1695; DEPR: 21,054.15; § 11,410.25

[219] ¶ 11,030D; DEPR: 15,162.85; § 11,535.20

[220] ¶ 12,468; BUSEXP: 6,000; § 6,001

980B. Qualified Production Activities Income. A taxpayer's qualified production activities income (QPAI) is its domestic production gross receipts (DPGR) attributable to the actual conduct of a trade or business during the tax year (¶ 980D), reduced by: (1) the cost of goods sold allocable to DPGR; and (2) other deductions, expenses, and losses that are properly allocable to DPGR (Code Sec. 199(c)(1); Reg. § § 1.199-1(c) and 1.199-4).[221]

Limited Deduction for Oil-Related QPAI. A taxpayer having oil-related qualified production activities income must reduce the domestic production activities deduction by three percent of the least of:

(1) the taxpayer's oil-related qualified production activities income for the tax year;

(2) the taxpayer's qualified production activities income for the tax year; or

(3) taxable income (determined without regard to the domestic production activities deduction) (Code Sec. 199(d)(9)(A)).[222]

If the taxpayer entitled to the deduction is an individual, then modified adjusted gross income (AGI) is substituted for taxable income (Code Sec. 199(d)(2)).

980C. W-2 Wage Limitation. The deduction for domestic production activities (¶ 980A) may not exceed 50 percent of the W-2 wages paid by the taxpayer to its employees for the calendar year ending during the tax year that are properly allocable to the taxpayer's domestic gross production receipts (the wages that the taxpayer deducts in calculating its qualified production activities income (¶ 980B)) (Code Sec. 199(b)(2); Reg. § 1.199-2(a)).[223]

W-2 wages are defined as amounts required to be reported for wages and compensation on Form W-2, plus compensation deferred under Code Sec. 457 plans and elective deferrals under other employer plans (i.e., 401(k)s, 403(b)s, SIMPLEs, and SEPs, as well as designated Roth contributions) (Reg. § 1.199-2(e)).[224] While all of these payments are reported on Form W-2, no single box includes all types of payments. Thus, taxpayers may use one of three methods for computing W-2 wages (Rev. Proc. 2006-47):[225]

(1) *Unmodified box method:* Under the unmodified box method, W-2 wages are the lesser of: (a) the total amount entered for all employees in Box 1 (wages, tips, other compensation) or (b) the total amount entered for all employees in Box 5 (Medicare wages and tips).

(2) *Modified Box 1 method:* Under the modified Box 1 method, the total amount reported in Box 1 for all employees is reduced by (a) amounts included in Box 1 that are not wages subject to federal income tax withholding and (b) amounts included in Box 1 that are not wages but the taxpayer has elected to withhold income on (e.g., supplemental unemployment compensation benefits and certain sick pay). The result is then increased by the total amount reported in Box 12 for all employees that are coded D, E, F, G, or S to arrive at the taxpayer's W-2 wages.

(3) *Tracking wages method:* Under the tracking wages method, the taxpayer actually tracks total wages paid to its employees that are subject to federal income tax withholding and that are reported on Form W-2 (not including supplemental unemployment benefits). The result is then increased by the amount reported in Box 12 and coded D, E, F, G, or S to arrive at the taxpayer's W-2 wages.

Amounts that are treated by a taxpayer as W-2 wages in one tax year (e.g., nonqualified deferred compensation) may not be treated as W-2 wages in another tax year or as W-2 wages of another taxpayer. In addition, an employer with a short tax year must use a modified version of the tracking wages method (Reg. § 1.199-2(b); Rev. Proc. 2006-22). A taxpayer that acquires a major portion of a trade or business may not take

---

References are to Standard Federal Tax Reports; Tax Research Consultant; and Practical Tax Explanations.

[221] ¶ 12,468, ¶ 12,472, ¶ 12,472C; BUSEXP: 6,000; § 6,015.05

[222] ¶ 12,468; BUSEXP: 6,052.10; § 6,010

[223] ¶ 12,468, ¶ 12,472A; BUSEXP: 6,054; § 6,010

[224] ¶ 12,472A; BUSEXP: 6,054; § 6,010

[225] ¶ 12,476.75; BUSEXP: 6,054; § 6,010

into account wages paid to common law employees of the predecessor employer for services rendered to the predecessor employer, even if those wages are reported on Forms W-2 furnished by the taxpayer.

980D. Domestic Production Gross Receipts. Domestic production gross receipts (DPGR) are the gross receipts of the taxpayer that are derived from:

(1) the lease, rental, license, sale, exchange, or other disposition of:

(a) qualifying production property (generally, tangible personal property, computer software, and sound recordings) manufactured, produced, grown, or extracted by the taxpayer in whole or in significant part within the United States;

(b) any qualified film produced by the taxpayer in the United States; or

(c) electricity, natural gas, or potable water produced by the taxpayer in the United States;

(2) construction performed within the United States; and

(3) engineering or architectural services performed in the United States for construction projects located in the United States (Code Sec. 199(c)(4)).[226]

DPGR does not include gross receipts from:

(1) the sale of food and beverages prepared by the taxpayer at a retail establishment;

(2) transmission or distribution of electricity, natural gas, or potable water; or

(3) the lease, rental, license, sale, exchange, or other disposition of land.

For this purpose, the United States is defined as including all 50 states and the District of Columbia, as well as the territorial waters of the United States, and the seabed and subsoil of those submarine areas that are adjacent to the territorial waters of the United States and over which it has exclusive rights, in accordance with international law, with respect to the exploration and exploitation of natural resources (Reg. § 1.199-3(h)).[227] The United States generally does not include possessions and territories of the United States or the airspace or space over the United States and these areas. However, for tax years beginning before January 1, 2014, a taxpayer can take into account its Puerto Rico business activity for its first eight tax years in calculating its DPGR and qualified production activities income (QPAI), if all of the taxpayer's gross receipts from Puerto Rican sources were subject to U.S. income taxation (Code Sec. 199(d)(8)).[228] For purposes of the 50-percent-of-W-2-wages limitation, those taxpayers can take into account wages paid to U.S. citizens who were bona fide residents of Puerto Rico.

> **Comment:** Absent further legislation, the temporary inclusion of Puerto Rico business activity in DPGR has expired for tax years beginning after December 31, 2013. For the latest legislative updates, visit our website www.CCHGroup.com/TaxUpdates.

Generally, a taxpayer may allocate which of its gross receipts are DPGR and non-DPGR using any reasonable method. A specific identification method must be used if the information is readily available and it can be used without undue burden or expense (Reg. § 1.199-1(d)).[229] If a taxpayer has a *de minimis* amount, less than five percent of total gross receipts, of non-DPGR, then all of the taxpayer's gross receipts may be treated as DPGR.

DPGR must be determined on an item-by-item basis (Reg. § 1.199-3(d)).[230] Thus, a taxpayer cannot determine DPGR on a division-by-division, product-line-by-product-line, or transaction-by-transaction basis. This prevents a taxpayer from isolating loss activities from other activities in order to maximize its deduction. An "item" is defined as property,

---

References are to Standard Federal Tax Reports; Tax Research Consultant; and Practical Tax Explanations.

[226] ¶ 12,468; BUSEXP: 6,100; § 6,015.10

[227] ¶ 12,472B; BUSEXP: 6,150; § 6,015.10

[228] ¶ 12,468; BUSEXP: 6,104.05; § 6,015.10

[229] ¶ 12,472; BUSEXP: 6,102.05; § 6,015.20

[230] ¶ 12,472B; BUSEXP: 6,100; § 6,015.05

¶980D

or any portion of property, that is offered to sale to customers and that meets all of the requirements of the manufacturer's deduction.

Generally, gross receipts derived from the performance of a service other than construction, engineering, and architectural activities do not qualify as DPGR (Reg. § 1.199-3(i)).[231] There are several exceptions to this rule. A taxpayer may include in DPGR the gross receipts derived from a qualified warranty, a qualified delivery, distribution, or installation, and provision of a qualified operating manual, as well as a *de minimis* amount, less than five percent of the gross receipts, of embedded services with respect to an underlying item of qualifying property, and services provided under a qualified computer software maintenance agreement. A service is considered embedded if its price is not separately stated from the amount charged for the qualified property.

If a taxpayer exchanges qualified production property it manufactured, produced, etc., for other property in a taxable or nontaxable exchange, the value of the property received may be treated as DPGR. However, unless the taxpayer further manufactures, produces, etc., the property received, any gross receipts from the subsequent sale will not be DPGR even if the property was qualified property in the hands of the other person. Generally, DPGR will also not include any gross receipts derived by the taxpayer from the lease, rental, or license of qualified production property for use by any related person (Code Sec. 199(c)(7)).[232]

980E. Qualified Production Property. Generally, only one taxpayer may claim the domestic production activities deduction with respect to the manufacture, production, growth, or extraction (MPGE) of qualifying production property (QPP) (i.e., tangible personal property, computer software, and sound recordings), as well as the disposition of electricity, natural gas, potable water, or a qualified film (Reg. § 1.199-3(f)(1)).[233] The deduction is claimed by the taxpayer who has the benefits and burdens of ownership of the property under federal income tax principles during the period that the qualifying activity occurs.

The QPP must be MPGE by the taxpayer in whole or in significant part within the United States. QPP will be treated as having been MPGE in significant part in the United States if the MPGE activity performed within the United States is substantial in nature. This is determined on a facts-and-circumstances basis taking into account the nature and relative value added by the taxpayer's U.S. activity (Reg. § 1.199-3(e) and (g)).[234] A safe harbor provides that the significant part requirement will be satisfied if conversion costs, i.e., direct labor and related factory expenses, to MPGE the property are incurred by the taxpayer within the United States and such costs account for 20 percent or more of the total cost of goods sold of the property. For this purpose, packaging, repackaging, labeling, and minor assembly operations are not considered so substantial in nature as to qualify as the MPGE of QPP. In addition, research and experimental activities and the creation of intangibles (other than computer software and sound recordings) do not qualify as substantial activities and may be excluded in calculating the safe harbor.

980F. Construction, Engineering, or Architectural Activities. The domestic production gross receipts (DPGR) of a taxpayer includes the proceeds from the sale, exchange, or other disposition of real property constructed by the taxpayer in the United States (whether or not sold or completed), including compensation for the performance of construction services by the taxpayer and any qualified construction warranty (Reg. § 1.199-3(m)).[235] It also includes proceeds derived from engineering or architectural services performed in the United States for real property construction projects. DPGR does not include proceeds from the lease or rental of real property constructed by the taxpayer. Nor does it include gross receipts attributable to the sale or other disposition of land (though the taxpayer may reduce its cost related to DPGR by the cost of the land).

References are to Standard Federal Tax Reports; Tax Research Consultant; and Practical Tax Explanations.

[231] ¶ 12,472B; BUSEXP: 6,160; § 6,015.10

[232] ¶ 12,468; BUSEXP: 6,104; § 6,015.15

[233] ¶ 12,472B; BUSEXP: 6,160.25; § 6,015.10

[234] ¶ 12,472B; BUSEXP: 6,160.25; § 6,015.10

[235] ¶ 12,472B; BUSEXP: 6,156; § 6,015.10

980G. Allocation of Costs and Deductions. To allocate cost of goods sold (CGS) between domestic production gross receipts (DPGR) and non-DPGR, a taxpayer must use a reasonable method that is satisfactory to the IRS based on all facts and circumstances, including factors set forth in the Regulations (Reg. § 1.199-4(b)).[236] Depending on the facts and circumstances, reasonable methods may include methods based on gross receipts, number of units sold, number of units produced, or total production costs. Ordinarily, it will not be reasonable for a taxpayer to use one method to allocate gross receipts between DPGR and non-DPGR and a different method to allocate CGS that is not demonstrably more accurate than the method used to allocate gross receipts, unless the taxpayer has information readily available to specifically identify CGS allocable to DPGR and can specifically identify that amount without undue burden or expense. If a taxpayer that does not have such information readily available and cannot specifically identify that amount without undue burden or expense, the taxpayer is not required to use a method that specifically identifies CGS allocable to DPGR.

Three methods are provided for apportioning deductions properly allocable to DPGR. For purposes of all three methods, net operating losses (NOLs) and deductions not attributable to the actual conduct of a trade or business (i.e., the standard deduction or personal exemptions) may not be allocated or apportioned to DPGR (Reg. §§ 1.199-4(c) and 1.199-8(c)):[237]

(1) The *Section 861* method is required to be used by a taxpayer unless it is eligible and chooses to use one of the other methods. Under the Section 861 method, a taxpayer must allocate a deduction to the relevant class of gross income to which the deduction relates and then apportion the deduction within each class between DPGR and non-DPGR (Reg. § 1.199-4(d)).[238] If non-DPGR is treated as DPGR by reason of a safe harbor or *de minimis* rule, then deductions related to such non-DPGR must be apportioned to DPGR.

(2) Under the *simplified deduction method*, deductions other than CGS may be ratably apportioned between DPGR and non-DPGR based on relative gross receipts (Reg. § 1.199-4(e)).[239] A taxpayer is eligible to use this method at any time if: (a) its average annual gross receipts during the three-year period prior to the tax year is $100 million or less or (b) its total assets at the end of the tax year attributable to its trade or business are $10 million or less. In the case of a pass-through entity, eligibility to use this method is determined at the owner level. The method is also applied at the owner level, except for trusts and estates.

(3) Under the *small business simplified overall method*, a qualifying small taxpayer may ratably apportion its total costs for the tax year (including CGS and other deductions) between DPGR and non-DPGR based on relative gross receipts (Reg. § 1.199-4(f)).[240] A taxpayer is eligible to use this method if: (a) its average annual gross receipts during the three-year period prior to the tax year is $5 million or less; (b) it is engaged in the business of farming and is not required to use the accrual method of accounting; or (c) it is eligible to use the cash method of accounting under Rev. Proc. 2002-28 (¶ 1515). Estates and nongrantor trusts cannot use this method.

Wage Expense Safe Harbor. A taxpayer using either the Section 861 method of cost allocation or the simplified deduction method may determine the amount of W-2 wages that is properly allocable to DPGR for a tax year by multiplying the amount of W-2 wages for the tax year by the ratio of the taxpayer's wage expense included in calculating qualified production activities income (QPAI) for the tax year to the taxpayer's total wage expense used in calculating the taxpayer's taxable income (or adjusted gross income, if applicable) for the tax year, without regard to any wage expense disallowed by Code Secs. 465, 469, 704(d), or 1366(d) (Reg. § 1.199-2(e)(2)).[241] A taxpayer that uses the Code Sec. 861 method of cost allocation or the simplified deduction method to determine QPAI must use the same expense allocation and apportionment methods that

---

References are to Standard Federal Tax Reports; Tax Research Consultant; and Practical Tax Explanations.

[236] ¶ 12,472C; BUSEXP: 6,108.05; § 6,015.20

[237] ¶ 12,472C, ¶ 12,472G; BUSEXP: 6,108.05; § 6,015.20

[238] ¶ 12,472C; BUSEXP: 6,108.10; § 6,015.20

[239] ¶ 12,472C; BUSEXP: 6,108.15; § 6,015.20

[240] ¶ 12,472C; BUSEXP: 6,108.20; § 6,015.20

[241] ¶ 12,472A; BUSEXP: 6,054.20; § 6,010

it uses to determine QPAI to allocate and apportion wage expense for purposes of this safe harbor. A taxpayer that uses the small business simplified overall method may use the small business simplified overall method safe harbor for determining the amount of W-2 wages that is properly allocable to DPGR. Under this safe harbor, the amount of W-2 wages that is properly allocable to DPGR is equal to the same proportion of W-2 wages that the amount of DPGR bears to the taxpayer's total gross receipts.

980H. Application to Pass-Through Entities. The deduction for domestic production activities (¶ 980A) is generally applied at the shareholder, partner, or similar level of a pass-through entity (Code Sec. 199(d)(1); Reg. § 1.199-5).[242] The entity allocates to each partner or shareholder its share of qualified production activities income (QPAI) and W-2 wages from the entity. Only an eligible entity may calculate QPAI and W-2 wages at the entity level. An eligible entity is:

    (1) an eligible Code Sec. 861 partnership,

    (2) an eligible widely-held pass-through entity, or

    (3) an eligible small pass-through entity (Rev. Proc. 2007-34).[243]

Entities that are ineligible to calculate QPAI and W-2 wages at the entity level include qualifying in-kind partnerships (under Reg. § 1.199-3(i)(7)) and EAG partnerships (as described in Reg. § 1.199-3(i)(8)).

If a taxpayer must combine QPAI and W-2 wages from a partnership, S corporation, trust, or estate with the taxpayer's total QPAI and W-2 wages from other sources, then for purposes of apportioning the taxpayer's interest expense, the taxpayer's interest in such partnership (and, where relevant in apportioning the taxpayer's interest expense, the partnership's assets), the taxpayer's shares in such S corporation, or the taxpayer's interest in such trust or estate shall be disregarded (Reg. § 1.199-4(d)).[244]

In addition, special rules permit patrons of agricultural or horticultural cooperatives to claim the deduction for their portion of any patronage dividend or per-unit allocation received that is allocable to the QPAI of the cooperative (Code Sec. 199(d)(3); Reg. § 1.199-6).[245] For a discussion of the application of the deduction to S corporations, see ¶ 312; for partnerships, see ¶ 431A; and for nongrantor trusts and estates, see ¶ 536.

Expenses of Professional Persons

981. Professional Persons. Expenses incurred for operating a car used in making professional calls, dues to professional organizations, rent paid for office space, and other ordinary and necessary business expenses are deductible by a professional person. Amounts for books and equipment may be deducted if the useful life of the item is not more than one year (Reg. § 1.162-6).[246]

No deduction is allowed for dues paid to any club organized for business, pleasure, recreation, or other social purposes (Code Sec. 274(a)(3); Reg. § 1.274-2(a)(2)(iii)).[247] However, this disallowance does not extend to dues paid to professional organizations (e.g., bar and accounting associations) or public service organizations (e.g., Kiwanis and Rotary clubs) (¶ 913A).

A professional who performs services as an employee and who incurs unreimbursed related expenses may deduct such expenses only as itemized deductions subject to the two-percent-of-adjusted-gross-income floor (¶ 941 and ¶ 1011).

Information Services. Amounts paid for subscriptions to professional journals and information services that have a useful life of one year or less, are deductible by a

---

References are to Standard Federal Tax Reports; Tax Research Consultant; and Practical Tax Explanations.

[242] ¶ 12,468, ¶ 12,472D; BUSEXP: 6,212; § 6,020.10
[243] ¶ 12,476.55; BUSEXP: 6,212.10, BUSEXP: 6,214; § 6,020.05
[244] ¶ 12,472C; BUSEXP: 6,108.10; § 6,015.20
[245] ¶ 12,468, ¶ 12,472E; BUSEXP: 6,204; § 6,020.05
[246] ¶ 8633; BUSEXP: 3,050; § 9,005.25
[247] ¶ 14,402, ¶ 14,405; BUSEXP: 24,658; § 9,625

lawyer, accountant or other taxpayer who buys a service in connection with the performance of his or her duties (*J.I. Peyser*, Dec. 13,076(M), 1 TCM 807 (1943); *G. Nehus*, Dec. 50,308(M), 68 TCM 1503 (1994)).[248] The cost of a professional library having a more permanent value should be capitalized.

Other Expenses. A deduction is allowed to members of the clergy, lawyers, merchants, professors, and physicians for expenses incurred in attending business conventions (¶ 959) (Reg. § 1.162-2).[249] For foreign conventions, see ¶ 960. A member of the medical profession is allowed a deduction for business entertainment, subject to the rules discussed at ¶ 910, so long as there is a direct relationship between the expense and the development or expansion of a medical practice (*R.A. Sutter*, Dec. 19,966, 21 TC 170 (1953) (Acq.)).[250] A doctor's staff privilege fee paid to a hospital is a capital expenditure (*G.L. Heigerick*, Dec. 27,846, 45 TC 475 (1966)).[251] For other deductions, see the Checklist at ¶ 57.

Farmer's Expenses

982. Farming Expenses. Deductions are permitted for expenses incurred in carrying on the business of farming, including those incurred in a horticultural nursery business (Reg. § 1.162-12).[252] Among allowable deductions are the following: cost of small tools expected to last one year or less; cost of feeding and raising livestock (excluding produce grown on the farm and labor of the taxpayer); and cost of gasoline, repairs, and upkeep of a car or truck used wholly in the business of farming, or a portion of the cost, if used for both farming and personal use. Special rules, however, apply to certain property produced in a farming business (¶ 999) and to farm tax shelters (¶ 1519). See ¶ 767 for income averaging rules. Expenses for the purchase of farm machinery or equipment, breeding, dairy or work animals, a car, and drilling water wells for irrigation purposes are capital items usually subject to depreciation.

Conservation Expenses. A farmer may generally deduct soil and water conservation expenditures that do not give rise to a deduction for depreciation, that are not otherwise deductible and that would increase the basis of the property absent the election to deduct them (Code Sec. 175; Reg. § 1.175-1—1.175-6).[253] However, current deductions for soil and water conservation expenses are limited to those that are consistent with a conservation plan approved by the Soil Conservation Service of the U.S.D.A. or, in the absence of a federally approved plan, a soil conservation plan of a comparable state agency. Expenses related to the draining or filling of wetlands or to land preparation for the installation or operation of center pivot irrigation systems may not be deducted under this provision. The deduction is limited annually to 25 percent of the taxpayer's gross income from farming. Excess expenses can be carried over to succeeding tax years, without time limitation, but in each year the total deduction is limited to 25 percent of that year's gross income from farming.

Deductible soil and water conservation expenses include such costs as: leveling; grading; construction, control, and protection of diversion channels, drainage ditches, outlets, and ponds; planting of windbreaks; and other treatment or moving of earth. Also deductible are endangered species recovery expenditures paid or incurred by a taxpayer engaged in the business of farming for the purpose of achieving site-specific management actions recommended in recovery plans approved pursuant to the Endangered Species Act of 1973 (P.L. 93-205). No current deduction is allowed for the purchase, construction, installation, or improvement of depreciable masonry, tile, metal, or wood structures, appliances, and facilities, such as tanks, reservoirs, pipes, canals, and pumps. Assessments levied by a soil or water conservation or drainage district in order to defray expenses made by the district may also be deductible.

Schedule F Loss Limitation. The amount of net farm losses that can be claimed for any tax year in which a taxpayer, other than a C corporation, has received applicable subsidies is limited to the greater of $300,000 ($150,000 for a married taxpayer filing

---

References are to Standard Federal Tax Reports; Tax Research Consultant; and Practical Tax Explanations.

[248] ¶ 8634.1206, ¶ 8634.1208; BUSEXP: 3,050; § 45,120.05

[249] ¶ 8527; BUSEXP: 24,160; § 9,515

[250] ¶ 8523.2717; BUSEXP: 24,160; § 9,610.05

[251] ¶ 8634.1154; BUSEXP: 9,100; § 10,201

[252] ¶ 8755; FARM: 9,050; § 36,101

[253] ¶ 12,060—¶ 12,066; FARM: 9,150; § 36,110.05

separately) or the taxpayer's aggregate net farm income for the five preceding tax years (Code Sec. 461(j)).[254] Any farm loss that exceeds this limitation is excess farm loss, which is not deductible in the tax year in which the taxpayer received the subsidies, but is carried forward to the next tax year and treated as a deduction.

983. Land Clearing Expenses. Land clearing expenditures must be capitalized and added to the farmer's basis in the land (*AMFAC, Inc.*, CA-9, 80-2 USTC ¶ 9630).[255] However, business expenses for ordinary maintenance activities related to property already used in farming (e.g., brush clearing) are currently deductible (*E.G. Barham*, DC Ga., 69-1 USTC ¶ 9356).[256]

984. Development Costs. Generally, farmers have the option of deducting or capitalizing certain developmental expenses that are ordinary and necessary business expenses (¶ 999). However, plants produced by farms that have a preproductive period of more than two years must be capitalized. For certain farms (corporations, partnerships, and tax shelters) that are required to use the accrual method, the expenses must be capitalized regardless of the length of the preproductive period. Special rules apply to farming syndicates (¶ 1521).

985. Expensing Fertilizer Costs. A farmer, other than a farm syndicate, may elect to deduct current expenses otherwise chargeable to capital account made for fertilizer, lime, ground limestone, marl, or other materials for enriching, neutralizing, or conditioning land used in farming. If no election is made, expenditures producing benefits extending over more than one year are capitalized and recovered by amortization (Code Sec. 180; Reg. § 1.180-1 and 1.180-2).[257] The election, which is effective only for the tax year claimed, is made by claiming the deduction on the return. For farm syndicates and prepayments by cash-basis farmers, see ¶ 1519, ¶ 1521, and ¶ 1539.

Landlord or Tenant Expenses

986. Landlord or Tenant. A tenant may deduct rent paid for business property, as well as any amounts such as property taxes and interest that the lease requires the tenant to pay on behalf of the landlord (Code Sec. 162(a)(3); Reg. § 1.162-11).[258] An amount paid by a *lessee* for cancellation of a lease on business property is generally deductible (*A.J. Cassatt*, CA-3, 43-2 USTC ¶ 9579).[259] However, payments by the *lessor* for the cancellation of a lease have generally been regarded as capital expenditures, amortizable over the unexpired term of the canceled lease (*Peerless Weighing & Vending Machine Corp*, Dec. 29,713, 52 TC 850 (1969)).[260]

Under the one-year rule, a cash-basis taxpayer can deduct otherwise allowable rent attributable to the current or a previous year in the year in which the taxpayer actually pays the rent (Reg. § 1.461-1(a)).[261] This is true even though most of the lease term is in the following year if the lease expires within a year of payment. Prepaid rent for a lease extending more than one year from the date of payment must be capitalized and amortized over the term of the lease. Some rental payments are subject to the uniform capitalization rules (¶ 990). For an improvement made by the lessee on leased premises, see ¶ 1234.

If an owner of property occupies part of the property as a personal residence and rents part of it, expenses and depreciation allocable to the rented space may be deductible (¶ 966).

Payments made under a conditional sales contract are not deductible as rent. A conditional sales contract generally exists when at least a portion of the rental payments is applied to the purchase of the property under advantageous terms (IRS Fact Sheet FS-2007-14).[262]

References are to Standard Federal Tax Reports; Tax Research Consultant; and Practical Tax Explanations.

[254] ¶ 21,802; FARM: 9,208; § 36,215

[255] ¶ 12,068.27; FARM: 9,102; § 36,101

[256] ¶ 8520.7455; FARM: 9,168; § 36,320.10

[257] ¶ 12,140; ¶ 12,141, ¶ 12,142; FARM: 9,064; § 36,115, § 36,320.20

[258] ¶ 8500; ¶ 8753; REAL: 12,050; § 18,605

[259] ¶ 8754.16; REAL: 12,252.10; § 18,605.15

[260] ¶ 13,709.417; REAL: 12,252.20; § 18,605.15

[261] ¶ 21,805; ACCTNG: 6,316; § 38,405

[262] ¶ 8754.5497; SALES: 42,056.15

Under certain conditions, taxpayers who are in the business of producing real property or tangible personal property for resale, or who purchase property for resale, may not claim rental or lease expenses as a current deduction. Instead, they must include some or all of these costs in the basis of the property they produce or acquire for resale under the uniform capitalization rules. These costs are recovered when the property is sold (IRS Fact Sheet FS-2007-14).

Mining Company's Expenses

987. Mine Exploration. Mining companies may elect to deduct domestic exploration expenses (except for oil or gas), provided that the amount deducted is recaptured once the mine reaches production stage or is sold (Code Sec. 617).[263] Recapture is accomplished by a company's electing either to (1) include in income for that year the previously deducted exploration expenditures chargeable to the mine, increase the basis of the property by the amount included in income, and subsequently recover this amount through depletion, or (2) forgo depletion from the property that includes or comprises the mine until deductions forgone equal exploration expenditures previously deducted.

Expenses not recaptured by one of these methods are recaptured on the sale or other disposition of the mining property with the amount recaptured treated as ordinary income. Certain transfers are not subject to these recapture rules (Code Sec. 617(b) and (d)(3)).[264]

Deductions allowed a corporation, other than an S corporation, for mineral exploration and development costs (¶ 988) must be reduced by 30 percent (Code Sec. 291(b)).[265] The 30 percent of expenses that cannot be deducted must be capitalized and amortized over a 60-month period on Form 4562. Taxpayers may also elect to capitalize mine exploration expenses and amortize them over a 10-year period (¶ 1450).

Geological and geophysical (G&G) expenditures paid or incurred in connection with oil and gas exploration or development in the United States must be amortized ratably over a 24-month period beginning on the mid-point of the tax year that the expenses were paid or incurred. If a property or project is abandoned or retired during the 24-month amortization period, any remaining basis must continue to be amortized (Code Sec. 167(h)).[266] Major integrated oil companies must ratably amortize any G&G costs over seven years.

988. Mine Development. Expenses paid or incurred with respect to a domestic mine or other natural deposit, other than oil or gas, after the existence of ores or minerals in commercially marketable quantities has been discovered can be deducted currently, unless the taxpayer elects to treat them as deferred expenses and deduct them ratably as the ore or mineral is sold (Code Sec. 616; Reg. § 1.616-1).[267] These expenses do not include those made for the acquisition or improvement of depreciable property. However, depreciation allowances are considered development costs.

The 30-percent reduction in the allowable deduction and the election to amortize over a 10-year period (discussed at ¶ 987 in the case of exploration expenses) applies also to mine development expenses (Code Sec. 291(b)).[268]

988A. Foreign Mine Exploration and Development. Foreign mining exploration and development expenses (other than oil, gas, or geothermal wells) are to be recovered over a 10-year, straight-line amortization schedule beginning with the tax year in which the costs were paid or incurred (Code Secs. 616(d) and 617(h)).[269] However, the taxpayer may elect to add such expenses to the adjusted basis of the property for purposes of computing cost depletion.

References are to Standard Federal Tax Reports; Tax Research Consultant; and Practical Tax Explanations.

[263] ¶ 24,110; FARM: 21,052; § 11,630
[264] ¶ 24,110; FARM: 21,058.20; § 11,630
[265] ¶ 15,190; FARM: 21,102; § 11,630
[266] ¶ 11,002; FARM: 21,176; § 11,501
[267] ¶ 24,090, ¶ 24,091; FARM: 21,110; § 11,630
[268] ¶ 15,190; FARM: 21,118; § 11,630
[269] ¶ 24,090, ¶ 24,110; FARM: 21,052; § 11,630

¶987

989. Oil, Gas, or Geothermal Well Drilling Expense. Operators of a domestic oil, gas, or geothermal well may elect to currently deduct intangible drilling and development costs (IDCs) rather than charge such costs to capital, recoverable through depletion or depreciation (Code Sec. 263(c); Reg. § 1.612-4).[270] The election is binding upon future years. IDCs generally include all expenses made by the operator incident to and necessary for the drilling of wells and the preparation of wells for the production of oil, gas, or geothermal energy that are neither for the purchase of tangible property nor part of the acquisition price of an interest in the property. IDCs include labor, fuel, materials and supplies, truck rent, repairs to drilling equipment, and depreciation for drilling equipment.

An integrated oil company (generally, a producer that is not an independent producer) must reduce the deduction for IDCs otherwise allowable by 30 percent (Code Sec. 291(b)).[271] The amount disallowed as a current expense deduction must be amortized over a 60-month period. Taxpayers may elect to capitalize, rather than currently deduct, IDCs and amortize these expenditures over a 60-month period (¶ 1450).

If the operator has elected to capitalize intangible drilling and development costs, and the well later proves to be nonproductive, i.e., a dry hole, the operator may elect to deduct those costs as an ordinary loss (Reg. § 1.612-4(b)(4)).[272] The election, once made, is binding for all years.

Foreign Wells. Operators may not opt to currently deduct IDCs for wells located outside the U.S. (Code Sec. 263(i)).[273] Such costs must be recovered over a 10-year straight-line amortization schedule or, at the operator's election, added to the adjusted basis of the property for cost depletion. Dry hole expenses incurred outside the U.S. are currently deductible.

989A. Advanced Mine Safety Equipment Expensing. A taxpayer may make an election to expense 50 percent of the cost of advanced mine safety equipment placed in service before January 1, 2014 (Code Sec. 179E).[274] The cost of any eligible equipment that is expensed under Code Sec. 179 cannot be taken into account in calculating this special deduction for mine safety equipment. The deduction is subject to recapture as ordinary income under the Code Sec. 1245 depreciation recapture rules.

> **Comment:** Absent further legislation, the expensing election for advanced mine safety equipment has expired for property placed in service after December 31, 2013. For the latest legislative updates, visit our website www.CCHGroup.com/TaxUpdates.

Uniform Capitalization Rules

990. Uniform Capitalization Rules. Taxpayers subject to the uniform capitalization rules are required to capitalize all direct costs and an allocable portion of most indirect costs that are associated with production or resale activities. The uniform capitalization rules apply to the following:

   (1) real or tangible personal property produced by the taxpayer for use in a trade or business or in an activity engaged in for profit;

   (2) real or tangible personal property produced by the taxpayer for sale to customers; or

   (3) real or personal property, both tangible and intangible, acquired by the taxpayer for resale. However, the uniform capitalization rules do not apply to intangible or intangible personal property acquired for resale if the taxpayer's annual gross receipts for the preceding three tax years do not exceed $10 million (Code Sec. 263A).[275]

References are to Standard Federal Tax Reports; Tax Research Consultant; and Practical Tax Explanations.

[270] ¶ 13,700, ¶ 23,949; FARM: 21,150; § 45,525.15

[271] ¶ 15,190; FARM: 21,154.10; § 45,525.15

[272] ¶ 23,949; FARM: 21,152.10; § 45,525.15

[273] ¶ 13,700; FARM: 21,152.20; § 45,525.15

[274] ¶ 12,139; BUSEXP: 19,000; § 10,255

[275] ¶ 13,800; BUSEXP: 9,050; § 10,301

Costs attributable to producing or acquiring property generally are capitalized by charging them to capital accounts or basis, and costs attributable to property that is inventory in the hands of the taxpayer generally are capitalized by including them in inventory.

Property Excepted from Rules. Among the classes of property excepted from the rules are:

(1) property produced by the taxpayer for its own use other than in a trade or business or in an activity conducted for profit;

(2) research and experimental expenditures (¶ 979);

(3) capital costs incurred in complying with EPA sulfur regulations (¶ 977A), intangible drilling and development costs (¶ 989), and mine development and exploration (¶ 987 and (¶ 988);

(4) any property produced by the taxpayer pursuant to a long-term contract;

(5) any costs incurred in raising, growing or harvesting trees (including the costs associated with the real property underlying such trees) other than trees bearing fruit, nuts, or other crops and ornamental trees (those which are six years old or less when severed from the roots); and

(6) costs, other than circulation expenditures, subject to amortization (¶ 1450).

990A. Writers, Photographers, and Artists. Expenses paid or incurred by a self-employed individual, including expenses of a corporation owned by a free-lancer and directly related to the activities of a qualified employee-owner, in the business of being a writer, photographer, or artist whose personal efforts create or may reasonably be expected to create the product are exempt from uniform capitalization rules (Code Sec. 263A(h)).[276] Generally, expenses for producing jewelry, silverware, pottery, furniture, and similar household items are not exempt.

991. Costs Required To Be Capitalized. Generally, direct material and labor costs and indirect costs must be capitalized with respect to property that is produced or acquired for resale (Code Sec. 263A(a)(2); Reg. § 1.263A-1(e)).[277] Direct material costs include the costs of those materials that become an integral part of the subject matter and of those materials that are consumed in the ordinary course of the activity. Direct labor costs include the cost of labor that can be identified or associated with a particular activity such as basic compensation, overtime pay, vacation pay, and payroll taxes.

Indirect costs include all costs other than direct material and labor costs. Indirect costs require a reasonable allocation to determine the portion of such costs that are attributable to each activity of the taxpayer. Indirect costs include: repair and maintenance of equipment or facilities; utilities; rental of equipment, facilities, or land; indirect labor and contract supervisory wages; indirect materials and supplies; depreciation, amortization and cost recovery allowance on equipment and facilities (to the extent allowable as deductions); certain administrative costs; insurance; contributions paid to or under a stock bonus, pension, profit-sharing, annuity, or other deferred compensation plan; rework labor, scrap and spoilage; and certain engineering and design expenses.

992. Costs Not Required To Be Capitalized. Costs that are not required to be capitalized with respect to property produced or acquired for resale include marketing, selling, advertising and distribution expenses (Reg. § 1.263A-1(e)(4)(iv)).[278] The IRS has established procedures that allow for the capitalization or amortization of package design costs (Rev. Proc. 98-39).[279] Other costs that need not be capitalized include bidding expenses incurred in the solicitation of contracts not awarded the taxpayer; certain general and administrative expenses; and compensation paid to officers attributa-

---

References are to Standard Federal Tax Reports; Tax Research Consultant; and Practical Tax Explanations.

[276] ¶ 13,800; BUSEXP: 9,062; § 10,305.10

[277] ¶ 13,800, ¶ 13,811; BUSEXP: 9,056; § 10,310.15

[278] ¶ 13,811; BUSEXP: 9,052; § 10,310.30

[279] ¶ 13,709.469; BUSEXP: 9,350; § 9,970

ble to the performance of services that do not directly benefit or are not incurred by reason of a particular production activity.

993. Interest Capitalization Rules. Interest costs paid or incurred during the production period and allocable to real property or tangible personal property produced by the taxpayer that has a class life of at least 20 years, an estimated production period exceeding two years, or an estimated production period exceeding one year and a cost exceeding $1 million must be capitalized (Code Sec. 263A(f)).[280]

994. Property Acquired for Resale. Unless an election is made to use the simplified resale method at ¶ 995, the rules applicable to the production of property apply to costs incurred with respect to property acquired for resale in a trade or business or in an activity conducted for profit (Code Sec. 263A(b)).[281] Property held for resale may include literary, musical, or artistic compositions; stocks; certificates, notes, bonds, debentures, or other evidence of indebtedness; or an interest in, right to subscribe to, or purchase of any of the foregoing, and other intangible properties. However, in the case of personal property acquired for resale, a taxpayer is not subject to the uniform capitalization rules if its average annual gross receipts for the three preceding tax years or, if less, the number of preceding tax years the taxpayer and any predecessor has been in existence, do not exceed $10 million. The uniform capitalization rules apply in the case of real property acquired for resale, regardless of the taxpayer's gross receipts.

995. Simplified Methods of Accounting for Resale Costs. Generally, taxpayers may elect to use one of the simplified resale methods for allocating costs to property acquired for resale (Reg. § 1.263A-3(d)).[282] However, in the case of a single trade or business that consists of both production and resale activities, only the simplified production method (¶ 996) is available. Under the simplified resale methods, preliminary inventory balances are calculated without the inclusion of the additional costs (listed later) required to be capitalized. The amount of additional costs attributable to prior periods and the amount of additional costs determined to be capitalized for the current period are then taken into account with the inventory balances as initially calculated in order to arrive at an ending inventory balance.

The following categories of costs are required to be capitalized with respect to property acquired for resale, regardless of whether a taxpayer elects one of the simplified resale methods: (1) off-site storage or warehousing; (2) purchasing; (3) handling, processing, assembly, and repackaging; and (4) certain general and administrative expenses (Reg. § 1.263A-3(c)).

996. Simplified Method of Accounting for Production Costs. An election to use the simplified production method may be made to account for the additional costs required to be capitalized with respect to property produced by the taxpayer that is: (1) stock in trade or other property properly includible in inventory, or (2) noninventory property held primarily for sale to customers in the ordinary course of business (Reg. § 1.263A-2(b)(2)(i)).[283] A modified simplified production method is provided for in proposed regulations that will be effective when published as final in the Federal Register (Prop. Reg. § 1.263A-2(c)).[284]

Categories of property eligible for the simplified production method also include properties constructed by a taxpayer for use in its trade or business if the taxpayer: (1) is also producing inventory property and the constructed property is substantially identical in nature and is produced in the same manner as the inventory property, or (2) produces such property on a routine and repetitive basis.

997. Simplified Service Cost Method. A simplified method is available for determining capitalizable mixed service costs for eligible property (Reg. § 1.263A-1).[285] The election to use the simplified method must be made independently from other allowable simplified methods.

References are to Standard Federal Tax Reports; Tax Research Consultant; and Practical Tax Explanations.

[280] ¶ 13,800; BUSEXP: 9,060; § 10,330.05

[281] ¶ 13,800; BUSEXP: 9,052.25; § 10,305.15

[282] ¶ 13,824; BUSEXP: 9,056.35; § 10,325.05

[283] ¶ 13,817; ACCTNG: 15,210.05; § 10,320.20

[284] ¶ 13,817C; ACCTNG: 15,210.05; § 10,320.20

[285] ¶ 13,811; ACCTNG: 15,212; § 10,315.15

999. Capitalization of Farming Business Expenses. The uniform capitalization rules apply to plants and animals produced by certain farming businesses (corporations, partnerships, and tax shelters) that are required to use the accrual method. For other farming businesses, the uniform capitalization rules apply only to plants produced in the farming business that have a preproductive period of more than two years (Code Sec. 263A(d)(1)).[286]

Generally, the rules do not apply to costs that are attributable to the replanting, cultivation, maintenance, and development of any plants (of the same type of crop) bearing an edible crop for human consumption (normally eaten or drunk by humans) that were lost or damaged as the result of freezing temperatures, disease, drought, pests, or casualty (Code Sec. 263A(d)(2)).[287] Replanting or maintenance costs may be incurred on property other than the damaged property if the acreage is not in excess of the acreage of the damaged property.

A farming business is a trade or business involving the cultivation of land or the raising or harvesting of any agricultural or horticultural commodity (Code Sec. 263A(e)(4)).[288] Examples include a nursery or sod farm; the raising of ornamental trees (including evergreen trees six years old or less when severed from their roots); the raising or harvesting of trees bearing fruit, nuts, or other crops; and the raising, shearing, feeding, caring for, training, and managing of animals.

Any farmer, other than a corporation, partnership, or tax shelter required to use the accrual method, may elect not to have the uniform capitalization rules made applicable to any plant produced in his or her business (Code Sec. 263A(d)(3) and (e); Reg. § 1.263A-1(b)(3)).[289] However, such election may not be made for any costs incurred within the first four years in which any almond or citrus trees were planted.

Unless IRS consent is obtained, farmers may only make the election not to have the uniform capitalization rules apply for the first tax year during which the farmer produces property to which the uniform capitalization rules apply (Code Sec. 263A(d)(3)).[290] Once the election is made, it is revocable only with the consent of the IRS.

Incentives for Economically Distressed Communities

999A. Tax Incentives for Distressed Communities. Special tax incentives have encouraged the development of economically distressed areas by businesses located in empowerment zones (¶ 999B), renewal communities (¶ 999C), and the District of Columbia Enterprise Community Zone (¶ 999D). The locations of qualifying empowerment zones and renewal communities are listed in the instructions to Form 8844.

999B. Empowerment Zones. The designation of certain geographic areas as an empowerment zone for purposes of enhanced tax benefits generally terminated on December 31, 2013 (Code Sec. 1391).[291]

> **Comment:** Absent further legislation, the work opportunity credit has expired for amounts paid to individuals in any targeted group who begin work for an employer after December 31, 2013. See ¶ 1365G. For the latest legislative updates, visit our website www.CCHGroup.com/TaxUpdates.

Work Opportunity Credit. The work opportunity credit may be claimed for certain first-year wages paid or incurred during the employer's tax year to "designated community residents" and "qualified summer youth employees" hired before January 1, 2014 and living within certain economically distressed areas (¶ 1365G) (Code Sec. 51(d)).[292]

Increased section 179 allowance for property placed in service in an empowerment zone. See ¶ 1208.

References are to Standard Federal Tax Reports; Tax Research Consultant; and Practical Tax Explanations.

[286] ¶ 13,800; FARM: 9,104; § 10,305.20

[287] ¶ 13,800; FARM: 9,104; § 36,320.15

[288] ¶ 13,800; FARM: 9,104; § 36,320.25

[289] ¶ 13,800, ¶ 13,811; FARM: 9,104; § 36,320.20

[290] ¶ 13,800; FARM: 9,104; § 36,320.20

[291] ¶ 32,385; BUSEXP: 57,000; § 10,001

[292] ¶ 4800; BUSEXP: 54,250; § 13,805.05

60-Percent Gain Exclusion for Small Business Stock. Taxpayers other than corporations may exclude 50 percent of the gain on the sale or exchange of qualified small business stock held for more than five years (¶ 1905) (Code Sec. 1202(a)(1)).[293] For gain attributable to periods before January 1, 2019, the amount that can be excluded is increased to 60 percent if the small business stock is stock in a corporation that qualifies as an empowerment zone business that was acquired after December 21, 2001 (Code Sec. 1202(a)(2)(C)). In general, the corporation must qualify as an enterprise zone during substantially all of the time the stock is held. In applying this rule, the end of the empowerment zone designation on December 31, 2013, is ignored in determining whether the corporation qualified as an enterprise zone during substantially all of the time the stock was held. Gain from the sale of small business stock of a qualified business entity in the District of Columbia enterprise zone is not eligible for the increased exclusion.

999C. Renewal Communities (Expired). Even though renewal community status terminates after December 31, 2009, the capital gain exclusion continues to be available.

Renewal Community Capital Gain Exclusion. Gross income does not include capital gain (or section 1231 gain) from the sale or exchange of a qualified community asset held for more than five years and acquired after December 31, 2001, and before January 1, 2010 (Code Sec. 1400F).[294] Gain attributable to periods before 2002 and after 2014 does not qualify for the exclusion.

If a qualified community asset is sold, or otherwise transferred, to a subsequent purchaser, it will qualify for the capital gain exclusion for the purchaser provided that the stock or partnership interest continues to represent an interest in a renewal community business or the tangible property continues to be used in a renewal community business (Code Secs. 1400B(b)(4)(B)(ii) and 1400F(b)(4)(B)).

Gain on tangible property that is substantially improved by a taxpayer before January 1, 2010, and any land on which such property is located qualifies for the exclusion if during any 24-month period beginning after December 31, 2001, additions to the basis of the property exceed the greater of the adjusted basis of the property at the start of the 24-month period or $5,000.

Special rules apply that limit the exclusion in the same way as with DC Zone assets (¶ 999D) (Code Secs. 1400B(e) and 1400F(c)(3)).[295]

999D. District of Columbia. Gross income does not include qualified capital gain from the sale or exchange of any DC Zone asset held for more than five years (Code Sec. 1400B).[296] In general, a DC Zone asset includes only (Code Sec. 1400B(b)):

(1) DC Zone business stock—stock originally issued after December 31, 1997, and acquired before January 1, 2012, for cash from a domestic corporation that is a DC Zone business;

(2) a DC Zone partnership interest—a capital or profits interest in a domestic partnership interest originally issued after December 31, 1997, and acquired before January 1, 2012, for cash from a partnership that is a DC Zone business; and

(3) DC Zone business property—tangible property acquired by purchase (as defined in Code Sec. 179(d)(2)) after December 31, 1997, and before January 1, 2012, the original use of which commences with the taxpayer in the taxpayer's DC Zone business. The property may not be acquired from a related person or another member of a controlled group.

A taxpayer who acquires stock, a partnership interest, or tangible property from another person in whose hands the asset was a DC Zone asset may also qualify for the exclusion.

References are to Standard Federal Tax Reports; Tax Research Consultant; and Practical Tax Explanations.

[293] ¶ 30,372; BUSEXP: 57,056.10; § 9,001

[294] ¶ 32,437; BUSEXP: 57,204.05; § 9,001

[295] ¶ 32,426, ¶ 32,437; SALES: 15,354.15; § 16,525.05

[296] ¶ 32,426; SALES: 15,352.15; § 16,525.05

Qualified capital gain is gain recognized on the sale or exchange of a DC Zone asset that is a capital asset or that is a Section 1231 asset (i.e., depreciable personal property and real property). It does not include gain attributable to periods before January 1, 1998, or after December 31, 2016, gain that would be recaptured as ordinary income under the Code Sec. 1245 depreciation recapture rules, gain that would be recaptured as ordinary income under the Code Sec. 1250 recapture rules if all depreciation on real property (rather than depreciation in excess of straight-line) was subject to recapture, and gain attributable to a transaction with a related person within the meaning of Code Sec. 267(b) or Code Sec. 707(b)(1).

District of Columbia Enterprise Zone. Prior to January 1, 2012, the District of Columbia Enterprise Zone (DC Zone) was treated as an empowerment zone, and qualifying taxpayers were generally entitled to the same special tax incentives (¶ 999B) applicable to other empowerment zones (Code Sec. 1400).[297] The $5,000 credit that was available to certain first-time homebuyers within the District of Columbia is no longer available after December 31, 2011 (¶ 1308). However, the termination of the DC Zone designation is disregarded for purposes of determining whether any property is a DC Zone asset eligible for the capital gain exclusion described above (Code Sec. 1400B(b)(5)).

References are to Standard Federal Tax Reports; Tax Research Consultant; and Practical Tax Explanations.

[297] ¶ 32,422; BUSEXP: 57,056.30; § 13,810

¶999D

Chapter 10

NONBUSINESS EXPENSES

Deductions, Generally

1001. Major Classifications. Deductions for individuals fall into two basic categories: those taken from gross income regardless of whether the taxpayer itemizes, and those taken from adjusted gross income if an eligible taxpayer elects to itemize deductions. Itemized deductions should be claimed only if they exceed the taxpayer's standard deduction (¶ 126). The standard deduction amount varies according to filing status. This amount, along with the taxpayer's personal and dependency exemptions, reduces adjusted gross income to arrive at taxable income.[1]

1003. Personal Expenses. A personal, living, or family expense is *not* deductible unless the Code specifically provides otherwise (Reg. §1.262-1).[2] Nondeductible expenses include, but are not limited to, rent and insurance premiums paid for the taxpayer's own dwelling, life insurance premiums paid by the insured, and payments for food, clothing, domestic help, and upkeep of an automobile.

Adjusted Gross Income

1005. Deductions Allowed. Adjusted gross income (AGI) is an intermediate figure between gross income and taxable income that is the starting point for computing certain deductions, credits, and other tax benefits that are based on or limited by income (Code Sec. 62; Temp. Reg. §1.62-1T).[3] See the chart at ¶ 4 for a listing of the 2014 AGI phaseout thresholds.

AGI is gross income minus deductions:

(1) on account of a trade or business carried on by the taxpayer, except for services as an employee (¶ 1006);

(2) for trade or business expenses paid or incurred by a qualified performing artist for services in the performing arts as an employee (¶ 941A);

(3) for allowed losses from the sale or exchange of property (¶ 1007);

(4) attributable to rental or royalty property (¶ 1089);

(5) for depreciation or depletion allowed to a life tenant of property, or to an income beneficiary of property held in trust, or to an heir, legatee, or devisee of an estate (¶ 1090);

References are to Standard Federal Tax Reports; Tax Research Consultant; and Practical Tax Explanations.

[1] ¶ 6020; FILEIND: 12,100; §1,010.15

[2] ¶ 13,601; INDIV: 39,052; §8,201, §8,205

[3] ¶ 6002, ¶ 6003; FILEIND: 9,000; §5,001

¶1005

(6) for contributions by self-employed persons to pension, profit-sharing, and annuity plans (¶ 2107);

(7) for cash payments to individual retirement accounts (IRAs), and to retirement savings plans of certain married individuals to cover a nonworking spouse (¶ 2157);

(8) for interest forfeited to a bank, savings association, etc., on premature withdrawals from time savings accounts or deposits (¶ 1111);

(9) for alimony payments (¶ 1008);

(10) for the amortization of reforestation expenses (¶ 1287);

(11) for certain repayments of supplemental unemployment compensation benefits to a trust described in Code Sec. 501(c)(9) or (c)(17) that are required because of receipt of trade readjustment allowances (¶ 1009);

(12) for jury duty pay remitted to employer (¶ 1010);

(13) for moving expenses (¶ 1073);

(14) for interest on education loans (¶ 1082);

(15) for contributions to an Archer medical savings account (MSA) (¶ 1020);

(16) for expenses paid or incurred by a fee-basis state or local government official for services performed (¶ 941D);

(17) for unreimbursed classroom expenses incurred by eligible educators (¶ 1084);

(18) for post-secondary tuition and related expenses (¶ 1082);

(19) for contributions to a health savings account (HSA) (¶ 1020A);

(20) for attorney fees and court costs paid in connection with an unlawful federal discrimination claim, or a whistleblower award for providing information on tax law violations (¶ 1010A);

(21) for travel expenses of National Guard and Armed Forces Reserve members while away from home to attend meetings and training sessions (¶ 941E); and

(22) for domestic production activities (also referred to as the manufacturer's deduction or DPAD) (¶ 980A).

Comment: Absent further legislation, the deduction for unreimbursed classroom expenses incurred by eligible educators and the deduction for post-secondary tuition and related expenses have expired for tax years beginning after December 31, 2013. For the latest legislative updates, visit our website www.CCHGroup.com/TaxUpdates.

The Code specifically allows a deduction from gross income for expenses paid or incurred in connection with the performance of services as an employee under a reimbursement or expense allowance arrangement with the employer or third party (Code Sec. 62(a)(2)(A)). In practice, employee expenses that are reimbursed under an accountable plan are *not* reported on the taxpayer's return. Generally, employee expenses that are not reimbursed or reimbursed under a nonaccountable plan are deductible, if adequately substantiated, only as miscellaneous itemized deductions subject to the two-percent-of-adjusted-gross-income floor and the 50-percent limit for meals and entertainment (¶ 942 and ¶ 943).

1006. Trade or Business Deductions. Expenses directly attributable to a trade or business carried on by a taxpayer are deducted from gross income. For this purpose, the performance of services as an employee is *not* considered to be a trade or business. However, the practice of a profession, not as an employee, is considered the conduct of a trade or business (Code Sec. 62(a)(1); Temp. Reg. § 1.62-1T(d)).[4] See ¶ 941 and following for business deductions that are available to employees.

References are to Standard Federal Tax Reports; Tax Research Consultant; and Practical Tax Explanations.

[4] ¶ 6002, ¶ 6003; FILEIND: 9,052; § 5,005, § 9,101

1007. Losses from Sales or Exchanges. Any allowable loss from the sale or exchange of property may be claimed as a deduction in arriving at adjusted gross income (AGI) (Code Sec. 62(a)(3); Temp. Reg. § 1.62-1T(c)(4)).[5] This includes allowable losses from sales or exchanges of capital assets; losses that are treated as losses from sales or exchanges of capital assets, i.e., losses on worthless stocks and bonds or nonbusiness bad debts; and any allowable losses from sales or exchanges of noncapital assets (¶ 1701). These deductions are allowed in addition to any losses attributable to a trade or business, or to losses incurred in connection with property held for the production of rents or royalties. An individual's capital loss deduction is generally limited to the individual's capital gains plus $3,000 of ordinary income (¶ 1752).

A loss on an involuntary conversion is deductible in computing AGI only if it is attributable to property used in a trade or business or to property held for the production of rents or royalties. A taxpayer may be entitled, however, to an itemized deduction for the involuntary conversion of property used for personal purposes if the loss arises from a casualty (¶ 1713) (Code Sec. 165(c)).[6]

1008. Deduction for Alimony Paid. Alimony (also referred to as maintenance or spousal maintenance) payments are deductible from gross income in the year paid, regardless of whether the taxpayer uses the cash or accrual method of accounting (Code Secs. 62(a)(10) and 215).[7] Back alimony is deductible in the year paid if it would have been deductible if paid on time.[8] See ¶ 771 and following for more details.

1009. Repayment of Supplemental Unemployment Compensation Benefits. Repayments of supplemental unemployment compensation benefits to trusts or voluntary employees' beneficiary associations (VEBAs) required because of subsequent receipt of trade readjustment allowances under the Trade Act of 1974 are deductible from gross income (Code Sec. 62(a)(12)).[9] Repayment of most other unemployment compensation benefits in a year following the year of receipt are deductible as an itemized deduction on Schedule A of Form 1040 (IRS Pub. 525). If the repayment of either type of unemployment compensation exceeds $3,000, the taxpayer may compute the tax for the tax year of the repayment by using the claim-of-right doctrine calculation as provided by Code Sec. 1341 (¶ 1543).[10]

1010. Jury Duty Pay. An employee can deduct jury duty pay surrendered to an employer who continued to pay the employee's normal salary while the employee was on jury duty (Code Sec. 62(a)(13)).[11] The deduction is claimed by entering the amount and "Jury Pay" on the dotted line next to line 36 of Form 1040 and including the amount in the total for that line.

1010A. Legal Fees and Costs. An individual can deduct from gross income attorney's fees and court costs incurred in connection with an action involving: (1) a claim of unlawful discrimination; (2) certain claims against the federal government; or (3) a private cause of action under the Medicare Secondary Payer statute (Code Sec. 62(a)(20)).[12] The deduction is limited to the amount includible in gross income on account of a judgment or settlement, whether as a lump sum or in periodic payments. The deduction is claimed by entering the amount and "UDC" on the dotted line next to line 36 of Form 1040 and including the amount in the total for that line.

An "above-the-line" deduction (formally referred to as an adjustment to gross income) is also allowed for court costs and attorney's fees paid by or on behalf of the taxpayer in connection with any whistleblower award under Code Sec. 7623(b) for providing information regarding tax law violations. The deduction cannot exceed the amount includible in gross income as a result of the award (Code Sec. 62(a)(21)).[13] The taxpayer claims this deduction by entering the amount and "WBF" on the dotted line next to line 36 of Form 1040 and including the amount in the total for that line.

For deductibility of legal fees associated with the production of income, see ¶ 1093.

References are to Standard Federal Tax Reports; Tax Research Consultant; and Practical Tax Explanations.

[5] ¶ 6002, ¶ 6003; FILEIND: 9,056; § 5,010

[6] ¶ 9802; SALES: 27,050; § 18,101

[7] ¶ 6002, ¶ 12,570; INDIV: 21,154; § 1,945

[8] ¶ 6094.80; INDIV: 21,154; § 1,945

[9] ¶ 6002; FILEIND: 9,074; § 5,035

[10] ¶ 31,880; FILEIND: 9,074; § 4,230.05

[11] ¶ 6002; FILEIND: 9,076; § 5,040

[12] ¶ 6002; FILEIND: 9,088; § 5,805

[13] ¶ 6002; FILEIND: 9,088

Floor on Miscellaneous Itemized Deductions

1011. Two-Percent Floor on Miscellaneous Itemized Deductions. Many expenses that are not deductible from gross income (¶ 1005) may be deductible from adjusted gross income (AGI) as itemized deductions, which are reported on Schedule A of Form 1040. A taxpayer should elect to itemize deductions, with certain exceptions, if they exceed the applicable standard deduction (¶ 126) (Code Sec. 63(d)).[14] Certain itemized deductions are treated as miscellaneous itemized deductions, which are allowed only to the extent that their total exceeds two percent of the individual's AGI (Code Sec. 67(a)).[15] See ¶ 1012 for a list of the itemized deductions *not* subject to the two-percent floor. Any limitation or restriction placed upon an itemized deduction, e.g., the 50-percent reduction for meals (¶ 916), generally applies prior to the two-percent-of-adjusted-gross-income floor (Reg. § 1.67-1T(a)(2)).[16]

Indirect deductions from pass-through entities are subject to the miscellaneous itemized limitation because they are treated as if they were incurred by the individual taxpayer. This rule applies to nonpublicly offered mutual funds, but does not apply to estates, certain trusts, cooperatives, certain publicly offered mutual funds (RICs), and real estate investment trusts (REITs) (Code Sec. 67(c); Temp. Reg. § 1.67-2T).[17] Estates and trusts are generally treated as individuals (¶ 528).

Statutory employees, e.g., full-time life insurance salespersons, are not treated as employees for purposes of deducting expenses incurred in their business. Thus, these expenses may be claimed as trade or business expenses on Schedule C of Form 1040, and are not treated as miscellaneous itemized deductions (¶ 941B).

1012. Itemized Deductions Not Subject to the Two-Percent Floor. The following itemized deductions, reported on Schedule A of Form 1040, are *not* subject to the two-percent-of-adjusted-gross-income (AGI) floor discussed at ¶ 1011 (Code Sec. 67(b)):[18]

    (1) interest (¶ 1043);

    (2) taxes (¶ 1021 and ¶ 1028);

    (3) personal casualty and theft losses (¶ 1121 and ¶ 1123);

    (4) charitable contributions (¶ 1058);

    (5) medical and dental expenses (¶ 1015);

    (6) impairment-related work expenses (¶ 1013);

    (7) estate tax in the case of income in respect of a decedent (¶ 191);

    (8) deductions allowable in connection with personal property used in a short sale (¶ 1944);

    (9) deductions relating to computation of tax when the taxpayer restores an amount in excess of $3,000 held under claim of right (¶ 1543);

    (10) deductions where annuity payments cease before an investment is recovered pursuant to Code Sec. 72(b)(3) (¶ 817);

    (11) amortizable bond premiums (¶ 1967);

    (12) deductions of taxes, interest, and business depreciation by a cooperative housing corporation tenant-stockholder (¶ 1040); and

    (13) gambling losses (¶ 785 and ¶ 1113).

1013. Impairment-Related Work Expenses. Ordinary and necessary business expenses incurred by a handicapped worker for attendant care services at the worker's place of employment, or for other expenses in connection with the worker's place of employment that are necessary for the individual to be able to work, are *not* subject to the two-percent-of-adjusted-gross-income floor (¶ 1011). Handicapped persons include individuals who have a physical or mental disability, including blindness or deafness that

---

References are to Standard Federal Tax Reports; Tax Research Consultant; and Practical Tax Explanations.

[14] ¶ 6020; FILEIND: 12,050; § 7,005

[15] ¶ 6060; FILEIND: 12,054; § 7,105.05

[16] ¶ 6061; INDIV: 39,100; § 7,105.05

[17] ¶ 6060, ¶ 6062; INDIV: 39,102; § 7,105.40

[18] ¶ 6060; FILEIND: 12,054; § 7,110.05

¶1011

limits employment, or a physical or mental impairment, including sight or hearing impairment, that substantially limits one or more major life activities (Code Sec. 67(d)).[19]

Phaseout of Itemized Deductions

1014. When AGI Exceeds Inflation-Adjusted Dollar Amount. For tax years beginning after December 31, 2012, taxpayers whose adjusted gross income (AGI) exceeds the applicable threshold amount must reduce the amount of allowable itemized deductions by the *lesser* of: (1) three percent of the excess of the taxpayer's adjusted gross income over the applicable threshold amount, or (2) 80 percent of allowable itemized deductions reduced by the deductions for medical expenses, investment interest, casualty and theft losses, and wagering losses (Code Sec. 68).[20]

The applicable threshold amount, as adjusted for inflation for 2014, is $305,050 for married individuals filing a joint return and surviving spouses; $279,650 for heads of households; $254,200 for single individuals; and $152,525 for married individuals filing separate returns (Code Sec. 68(b); Rev. Proc. 2013-35). The applicable threshold amount for 2015 is $309,900 for married individuals filing a joint return and surviving spouses; $284,050 for heads of households; $258,250 for single individuals; and $154,950 for married individuals filing separate returns (Rev. Proc. 2014-61).

The reduction is to be applied after application of the two-percent-of-adjusted-gross-income floor (¶ 1011) on itemized miscellaneous deductions has been taken into account (Code Sec. 68(d)). The reduced amount is reported on Schedule A of Form 1040.

No reduction of itemized deductions was required for tax years beginning before January 1, 2013, since the reduction of itemized deduction was phased out for these years.

Medical Expenses

1015. Medical and Dental Expenses. An itemized deduction is allowed for expenses paid during the tax year for the medical care of the taxpayer, the taxpayer's spouse, or a dependent to the extent that, for tax years beginning after December 31, 2012, the expenses exceed 10 percent of adjusted gross income (AGI) (7.5 percent for tax years beginning before January 1, 2013) (Code Sec. 213).[21] For taxpayers who attain age 65 before the close of the year, the threshold to claim an itemized deduction for unreimbursed medical expenses remains 7.5 percent of AGI for tax years beginning after December 31, 2012, but before January 1, 2017. On a joint return, the percentage limitation is based on the total AGI of both spouses. The expenses are reported on Schedule A of Form 1040.

The deduction may be taken for any person who was the taxpayer's dependent or spouse when the services were rendered or the expenses were paid (Reg. § 1.213-1(e)(3)).[22] For purposes of this deduction, dependent is defined at Code Sec. 152 (¶ 137), except that (1) dependent status is determined without regard to whether the dependent claims any dependency exemptions, files a joint return, or has gross income in excess of the exemption amount (Code Sec. 213(a); Reg. § 1.213-1(a)(3)) and (2) a child of divorced parents is treated as the dependent of both parents, even without a declaration by the custodial parent releasing the claim to the dependency exemption (¶ 139A) (Code Sec. 213(d)(5); Rev. Proc. 2008-48).

The deduction is limited to unreimbursed medical expenses (Code Sec. 213(a); Reg. § 1.213-1(g)). Reimbursement received for expenses deducted in a previous tax year is includible in gross income in the year received to the extent the expenses were previously deducted. Reimbursement for an earlier tax year in which no deduction was claimed is excludable from gross income.

Although medical expenses are generally deductible in the year paid, advance payments generally are *not* deductible until services are rendered (Reg. § 1.213-1(a)).[23]

References are to Standard Federal Tax Reports; Tax Research Consultant; and Practical Tax Explanations.

[19] ¶ 6060; INDIV: 36,400; § 7,110.35

[20] ¶ 6080; FILEIND: 12,056; § 7,015

[21] ¶ 12,540; INDIV: 42,000, INDIV: 42,300; § 7,201

[22] ¶ 12,541; INDIV: 42,356; § 7,205

[23] ¶ 12,541; INDIV: 42,250; § 7,215.05

Prepayments for lifetime care in a retirement home, nursing center, or similar institution are, however, deductible in the year paid if the obligation to pay was incurred at the time the payment was made and the promise to provide lifetime care was conditioned on the payment (Rev. Rul. 93-72). Charges to credit cards qualify as payment of medical expenses in the year the expenses are charged, regardless of when the credit card company is paid (Rev. Rul. 78-39).

See ¶ 1016 for the definition of medical expenses, ¶ 1017 for the treatment of drugs and supplies, ¶ 1018 for the treatment of medical expenses paid after death, ¶ 1019 for health insurance premiums, ¶ 1020 for deductible contributions to Archer medical savings accounts (MSAs), and ¶ 1020A for deductible contributions to health savings accounts (HSAs).

1016. Medical Expenses Defined. Medical expenses eligible to be deducted as itemized deductions (¶ 1015) include amounts paid for the diagnosis, cure, mitigation, treatment, or prevention of disease, or for the purpose of affecting any structure or function of the body. Medical expenses also include: transportation and lodging costs incurred on trips primarily for and essential to medical care; qualified long-term care services; and medical insurance, including premiums paid under the Social Security Act relating to supplementary medical insurance for the aged or for any qualified long-term care insurance contracts that do not exceed certain limits (Code Sec. 213).[24] The lodging deduction is limited to amounts that are not lavish or extravagant and cannot exceed $50 per night for each individual (Code Sec. 213(d)(2)). The lodging deduction may also be claimed for a person who must accompany the individual seeking medical care. Meals, however, are not deductible. Medical expenses do not include any amount allowable as a child or dependent care credit (¶ 1301) (Code Sec. 213(e)) or funeral expenses.[25]

The deduction is not limited to amounts paid for the least expensive form of medical care applicable. A physician's recommendation is unnecessary when the expenditures are for items that are wholly medical in nature and serve no other function. Thus, amounts paid by a healthy individual for self-initiated diagnostic tests and similar procedures, e.g., an annual physical, a full body scan or a self-administered pregnancy test kit, are deductible (Rev. Rul. 2007-72).

The costs of birth control pills prescribed by a physician, a legal abortion or a vasectomy are deductible (Rev. Ruls. 73-200, 73-201, and 73-603). Payments for psychiatric treatment of sexual inadequacy are medical expenditures, but marriage counseling fees are not (Rev. Rul. 75-319). The cost of fertility enhancement procedures are deductible if incurred in connection with *in vitro* fertilization or surgery (IRS Pub. 502). Costs incurred to obtain donated eggs, including donor, agency, testing and legal expenses, are also deductible (IRS Letter Ruling 200318017).

Expenses for elective cosmetic surgery are *not* deductible unless the surgery or procedure is necessary to ameliorate a deformity arising from, or directly related to, a congenital abnormality, a personal injury resulting from accident or trauma, or a disfiguring disease. Cosmetic surgery includes any procedure directed at improving the patient's appearance that does not meaningfully promote the proper function of the body or prevent or treat illness or disease (Code Sec. 213(d)(9)). Thus, costs to whiten teeth discolored by age are not deductible, but costs for breast reconstruction after a mastectomy and for vision correction by laser surgery are deductible (Rev. Rul. 2003-57). A weight-loss program is a medical expense if undertaken to relieve a disease or defect, such as obesity or hypertension (Rev. Rul. 2002-19). Smoking-cessation programs, whether or not prescribed, and prescription drugs to alleviate symptoms of nicotine withdrawal are also medical expenses, but over-the-counter gums or patches are not (Rev. Rul. 99-28).

When transportation expenses are deductible as a medical expense, the cost of operating a car for 2014 may be calculated at a standard rate of 23.5 cents per mile plus parking fees and tolls (Rev. Proc. 2010-51; Notice 2013-80).

References are to Standard Federal Tax Reports; Tax Research Consultant; and Practical Tax Explanations.

[24] ¶ 12,540; INDIV: 42,052; § 7,225

[25] ¶ 12,543.452; INDIV: 42,082.10; § 7,230

Special schooling for a physically or mentally handicapped child or one needing psychiatric treatment is deductible (Rev. Rul. 78-340). Amounts paid for inpatient treatment of alcoholism or drug addiction at a therapeutic center and for meals and lodging furnished as a necessary incident to the treatment are deductible (Rev. Rul. 73-325). Amounts paid to acquire, train, and maintain a dog or other service animal for assisting a blind, deaf, or physically disabled individual are deductible (Rev. Ruls. 55-261, 57-461, and 68-295).

The entire cost of maintenance in a nursing home or home for the aged, including meals and lodging, is a medical expense if an individual is there because of a physical condition and the availability of medical care is a principal reason for the individual's residence. If an individual is in such an institution primarily for personal or family reasons, then only that portion of the cost attributable to medical or nursing care, excluding meals and lodging, is deductible. Payments to perform both nursing care and housework may be deducted only to the extent of the nursing cost.[26]

Capital expenditures for home improvements and additions that are primarily for medical care qualify as a medical expense only to the extent that the cost of the improvement exceeds any increase in the value of the affected property (Reg. § 1.213-1(e)(1)).[27] The entire cost of any improvement that does not increase the value of the property is deductible. Deductions have been allowed for the installation of an elevator, a swimming pool, and a central air-conditioning system. Capital expenditures incurred to remove structural barriers to accommodate the condition of a physically handicapped person generally do not improve the value of the residence and, therefore, are fully deductible (Rev. Rul. 87-106). The entire cost of special equipment used to mitigate the effects of a physical impairment is also deductible.

See ¶ 59 for a checklist of medical expenses.

1017. Medicines and Drugs. In computing the deduction for medicine and drugs, only amounts paid for insulin and prescription medications may be taken into account (Code Sec. 213(b)).[28] Although amounts paid for over-the-counter (OTC) medicines or drugs are not taken into account in calculating the deduction, amounts paid for OTC equipment, supplies, or diagnostic devices may be deductible medical expenses (Rev. Rul. 2003-58).

> **Example:** In 2014, a taxpayer (who has not attained age 65 during the year) with an adjusted gross income of $48,000 paid $2,750 to a doctor for medical services, $3,325 to a hospital, $340 for prescription drugs, and $250 for OTC cold remedies and vitamins. His medical expense deduction is computed as follows:

Doctor	$2,750
Hospital	3,325
Medicine and drugs	340
OTC remedies and vitamins	0
2014 medical expenses	$6,415
Less: 10% of $48,000 (adjusted gross income)	4,800
Allowable deduction for 2014	$1,615

1018. Medical Expenses Paid After Death. A decedent's medical expenses that are paid by the decedent's estate within one year of the day after the decedent's death are treated as paid when incurred and may be deducted on the decedent's income tax return for the year incurred if the estate waives an estate tax deduction for the expenses (Reg. § 1.213-1(d)).[29] Alternatively, the estate may deduct the medical expenses as a claim against the estate for federal estate tax purposes (¶ 2925). Medical expenses disallowed for income tax purposes because of the 10-percent limitation (7.5 percent for tax years beginning after December 31, 2012, and before January 1, 2017, for taxpayers who have attained age 65 by the close of the year) (¶ 1015) may *not* be claimed on the

---

References are to Standard Federal Tax Reports; Tax Research Consultant; and Practical Tax Explanations.

[26] ¶ 12,543.726, ¶ 12,543.727; INDIV: 42,066; § 7,245, § 7,250

[27] ¶ 12,541; INDIV: 42,064; § 7,285.05

[28] ¶ 12,540; INDIV: 42,056; § 7,235

[29] ¶ 12,541; INDIV: 42,256; § 7,220

estate tax return when the estate allocates medical expenses between a decedent's final income tax and estate tax returns (Rev. Rul. 77-357).

1019. Health and Accident Insurance Premiums. A medical expense deduction is allowed for premiums paid for medical care insurance, including contact lens insurance, subject to the 10-percent limitation (7.5 percent for tax years after December 31, 2012, and before January 1, 2017, for taxpayers who have attained age 65 by the close of the year) (¶ 1015) (Code Sec. 213(d)(1)(D); Reg. § 1.213-1(e)(4)).[30] If the insurance contract provides payments for more than medical care, e.g., indemnity for loss of income or life, limb or sight, premiums are deductible only to the extent a reasonable charge for the medical care is stated separately in the contract or in a separate statement from the insurer. Premiums paid by a taxpayer under age 65 for insurance covering medical care expenses of the taxpayer, the taxpayer's spouse, or a dependent after the taxpayer turns 65 are considered to be medical expenses in the year paid if the premiums are payable on a level payment basis under the contract: (1) for a period of 10 years or more or (2) until the year the taxpayer reaches age 65, but in no case for a period of less than five years.

Premiums paid for a qualified long-term care insurance contract are a medical expense, but the deductible amount of the premium is limited by the age of the individual at the close of the tax year. The inflation-adjusted maximum deductible amount for 2014 is (Rev. Proc. 2013-35):

- age 40 or less, $370;
- more than age 40 but not more than 50, $700;
- more than age 50 but not more than 60, $1,400;
- more than age 60 but not more than 70, $3,720; and
- more than age 70, $4,660.

The maximum deductible amount for 2015 is (Rev. Proc. 2014-61):

- age 40 or less, $380;
- more than age 40 but not more than 50, $710;
- more than age 50 but not more than 60, $1,430;
- more than age 60 but not more than 70, $3,800; and
- more than age 70, $4,750.

Amounts paid as self-employment tax (¶ 2664) or as employment tax (¶ 2648) for hospital insurance under the Medicare program are *not* medical expenses. Similarly, the basic cost of Medicare insurance (Medicare A) is not deductible unless voluntarily paid by the taxpayer for coverage (Rev. Rul. 79-175). However, the cost of extra Medicare (Medicare B) is deductible (Rev. Rul. 66-216).

Self-employed persons can deduct from gross income 100 percent of amounts paid for health insurance coverage (¶ 908), including payments for both Medicare A and B (CCA 201228037).

1020. Archer Medical Savings Accounts. Eligible individuals may claim an above-the-line deduction (an adjustment to gross income) for contributions they make during the tax year to their Archer medical savings account (Archer MSA). Individuals who are self-employed or work for small employers may be able to maintain Archer MSAs to pay medical expenses, provided that the accounts are used in conjunction with a high deductible health insurance plan (HDHP) (Code Sec. 220; Notice 96-53).[31] The 2014 HDHP annual deductible amounts and limitations are:

References are to Standard Federal Tax Reports; Tax Research Consultant; and Practical Tax Explanations.

[30] ¶ 12,540, ¶ 12,541; INDIV: 42,100; § 7,240.05   [31] ¶ 12,670; INDIV: 42,500; § 42,601

¶1019

(1) a minimum deductible of $2,200, a maximum deductible of $3,250, and maximum out-of-pocket limitation of $4,350 for individual coverage; and

(2) a minimum deductible of $4,350, maximum deductible of $6,550, and maximum out-of-pocket limitation is $8,000 for family coverage (Rev. Proc. 2013-35).

The 2015 HDHP annual deductible amounts and limitations are (Rev. Proc. 2014-61):

(1) a minimum deductible of $2,200, a maximum deductible of $3,300, and maximum out-of-pocket limitation of $4,450 for individual coverage; and

(2) a minimum deductible of $4,450, maximum deductible of $6,650, and maximum out-of-pocket limitation is $8,150 for family coverage.

For a complete discussion of Archer MSAs, see ¶ 2037.

1020A. Health Savings Accounts. Eligible individuals with high-deductible health insurance plans (HDHP) may claim an adjustment to gross income (an above-the-line deduction) for contributions they make during the tax year to their health savings account (HSA). Individuals—and employees, through an employer's cafeteria plan—can establish HSAs to reimburse them for qualified medical expenses paid during the year (Code Sec. 223).[32] For a complete discussion on contributions, eligible individuals, the definition of high-deductible health plans, and taxation of distributions, see ¶ 2035.

Taxes, Generally

1021. Deductible Taxes. Taxes not directly connected with a trade or business or with property held for production of rents or royalties may be deducted only as an itemized deduction on Schedule A of Form 1040. These include the following (Code Sec. 164):[33]

(1) State, local, or foreign real property tax (¶ 1026 and ¶ 1028).

(2) State or local personal property tax (Reg. § 1.164-3(c)).

(3) State, local, or foreign income, war profits, or excess profits tax (¶ 1023 and ¶ 2475).

(4) Generation-skipping transfer tax imposed on income distributions (¶ 2942).

(5) State and local general sales tax (at the taxpayer's election and in lieu of state and local income taxes) (Code Sec. 164(b)(5)).

State and local taxes imposed on personal property are deductible if three conditions are met: the tax must be (1) *ad valorem*, i.e., substantially in proportion to the value of the property, (2) imposed on an annual basis, and (3) imposed with respect to personal property (Reg. § 1.164-3(c)).[34] Payment for car registration and licensing or a motor vehicle tax may be deductible as a personal property tax if it is imposed annually and assessed in proportion to the value of the car.

In tax years before January 1, 2014, taxpayers could elect to deduct *either* state and local income taxes or general state and local sales taxes (Code Sec. 164(b)(5)). If they elected to deduct the general state and local sales taxes paid, they could claim either the total amount paid by substantiation with receipts, or the amount from IRS tables plus the amounts of general state and local sales taxes paid on the purchase a motor vehicle, boat, or other items to be determined by the IRS (Notice 2005-31).

Comment: Absent further legislation, the election to claim state and local general sales tax in lieu of state and local income tax has expired for tax years beginning after December 31, 2013. For the latest legislative updates, visit our website www.CCHGroup.com/TaxUpdates.

If a foreign trust receives a gift or bequest from a covered expatriate (¶ 2412), a tax is imposed on the gift or bequest, and is payable by a U.S. citizen or resident beneficiary

---

References are to Standard Federal Tax Reports; Tax Research Consultant; and Practical Tax Explanations.

[32] ¶ 12,776; INDIV: 42,450; § 42,501

[33] ¶ 9500; INDIV: 45,000; § 7,301

[34] ¶ 9506; INDIV: 45,104; § 7,320

who receives from the trust a distribution attributable to the gift or bequest (¶ 516). The distribution recipient is allowed an income tax deduction under Code Sec. 164 for the amount of this tax paid or accrued, but only to the extent the tax is imposed on the portion of the distribution included in the recipient's gross income (¶ 2948) (Code Sec. 2801(a) and (e)(4)(B)).

See ¶ 1022 for when a tax is deductible, ¶ 1023 for the deductibility of foreign income and profits taxes, ¶ 1024 for the deductibility of advance payments of state income taxes, ¶ 1025 for nondeductible taxes, ¶ 1026 for the deductibility of taxes used to pay for local improvements, and ¶ 1027 for the deductibility of self-employment taxes. For discussion of real property taxes, see ¶ 1028.

1022. Taxes Deductible When Paid or Accrued. The deduction for taxes is allowed only for the year in which the taxes are paid or accrued (Code Sec. 164).[35] Cash-basis taxpayers deduct taxes in the year paid, including amounts withheld from wages, payments of estimated tax, and payments applicable to other tax years. Accrual-basis taxpayers may generally deduct taxes in the year they accrue (¶ 1515). A failure to deduct taxes in the proper year does not allow the taxpayer to deduct the taxes in a later year. Instead, the taxpayer must file an amended return for the year the taxes were paid or accrued.

The date when a tax becomes due and payable is not necessarily its accrual date. State income taxes accrue during the year in which the income is earned.[36] Uncontested additional assessments accrue at the same time they would have accrued upon a correct original assessment.[37] For accrual of real estate taxes, see ¶ 1031 and ¶ 1036.

A contested tax accrues when the taxpayer transfers cash or property to satisfy the tax, if the contest exists after the transfer and a deduction would have otherwise been allowed for the year of transfer. This rule does not apply to taxes imposed by a foreign country or U.S. possession (Code Sec. 461(f)).[38]

1023. Deduction of Foreign Income and Profits Taxes. Foreign income and profits taxes are deductible only if no credit under Code Sec. 901 is claimed for them on the taxpayer's U.S. income tax return (Code Sec. 275(a)(4)). The taxpayer must choose either the credit or the deduction; the taxes cannot be divided to support both a credit and a deduction. Foreign taxes accrue in the period for which they are imposed (¶ 2475 through ¶ 2485).

1024. Deduction of Advance Payments of State Income Taxes. Advance payments of estimated state income taxes made by a cash-basis taxpayer pursuant to state law are deductible in the year paid unless, on the date of payment, the taxpayer cannot reasonably determine that there is an additional amount owed (Rev. Rul. 82-208).

1025. Nondeductible Taxes. The taxes that cannot be deducted either as taxes or as business expenses are (Code Sec. 275):[39]

> (1) federal income taxes, including Social Security and railroad retirement taxes paid by employees and one-half of the self-employment taxes (¶ 2664);

> (2) federal war profits and excess profits taxes;

> (3) estate, inheritance, legacy, succession, and gift taxes (¶ 2901);

> (4) income, war profits, and excess profits taxes imposed by a foreign country or a U.S. possession, if the taxpayer chooses to take a foreign tax credit for these taxes (¶ 2475);

> (5) taxes on real property that must be treated as imposed on another taxpayer because of apportionment between buyer and seller (¶ 1032); and

---

References are to Standard Federal Tax Reports; Tax Research Consultant; and Practical Tax Explanations.

[35] ¶ 9500; INDIV: 45,200; § 7,310

[36] ¶ 9502.445, ¶ 21,817.115; INDIV: 45,202; § 7,310, § 7,325

[37] ¶ 9502.10; INDIV: 45,200; § 7,310

[38] ¶ 21,802; INDIV: 45,208; § 38,430.15

[39] ¶ 14,500; INDIV: 45,150; § 7,345

(6) certain additions to taxes imposed on public charities, private foundations, qualified pension plans, real estate investment trusts, stock compensation of insiders in expatriated corporations, golden parachute payments, and greenmail.

Drug Sale and Health Insurance Provider Fees. Nondeductible taxes also include the annual fee imposed on drug manufacturers and importers for U.S. branded prescription drug sales after December 31, 2010, and the annual fee imposed on certain health insurance providers after December 31, 2013 (Act Secs. 9008(f) and 9010(f) of the Patient Protection and Affordable Care Act (P.L. 111-148)).

1026. Deduction of Improvement Taxes. Any tax that is in reality an assessment for local benefits such as streets, sidewalks, and similar improvements is *not* deductible by a property owner, except where it is levied for the purpose of maintenance and repair or of meeting interest charges on local benefits. It is the taxpayer's burden to show the allocation of amounts assessed to the different purposes (Code Sec. 164(c)(1); Reg. § 1.164-4).[40]

1027. Deduction of Self-Employment Tax. A taxpayer can deduct one-half of the self-employment tax paid in the computation of the taxpayer's adjusted gross income for income tax purposes (¶ 1025). High-income taxpayers, however, are not able to deduct the additional 0.9-percent Medicare tax imposed on their self-employment income received after December 31, 2012 (Code Sec. 164(f)) (¶ 2664).

Real Property Taxes

1028. Deductibility of Real Property Taxes. Local, state, and foreign real property taxes are generally deductible only by the person upon whom they are imposed in the year in which they were paid or accrued (Code Sec. 164(a)(1); Reg. § 1.164-1(a)).[41] Real property taxes are taxes imposed on interests in real property and levied for the general public welfare. These taxes do not include taxes assessed for local benefits (¶ 1026) (Reg. § 1.164-3).[42] State or local tax includes only taxes imposed by a state, the District of Columbia, possessions of the U.S., or a political subdivision thereof. Foreign tax includes taxes imposed by the authority of a foreign country or its political subdivisions.

Stockholder-owners in a cooperative housing corporation may deduct their proportionate shares of the taxes paid by the corporation (¶ 1040). Condominium unit owners may also deduct real property taxes paid on their personal interests in the property (Rev. Rul. 64-31). Their homeowner association assessments, however, are not deductible as real property taxes because the assessments are not paid to the state or a political subdivision (Rev. Rul. 76-495).[43]

Ministers and military personnel are allowed to deduct taxes paid on their homes, even if they receive a parsonage or military allowance excludable from gross income (¶ 1050). Cash-basis mortgagors that pay taxes directly to the mortgagee are entitled to deduct the taxes in the year when the mortgagee pays the taxing authority.

1029. Real Property Construction Period Interest and Taxes. Interest and taxes on real property paid or incurred during the construction period generally must be capitalized (¶ 991 and ¶ 993) (Code Sec. 263A).[44]

1030. Carrying Charges on Real Property. If a taxpayer elects to capitalize taxes on unimproved and unproductive real property, no deduction is allowed for such taxes (¶ 1614) (Code Sec. 266).[45]

1031. Alternative Elections to Accrue Real Property Taxes for Accrual-Method Taxpayers. The economic performance rule generally delays an accrual-method taxpayer's deduction for real property taxes until they are paid (¶ 1540). An accrual basis seller or buyer, however, may elect to accrue real property taxes that are related to a definite period of time ratably over that period (Code Sec. 461(c); Reg. § 1.461-1(c)).[46]

References are to Standard Federal Tax Reports; Tax Research Consultant; and Practical Tax Explanations.

[40] ¶ 9500, ¶ 9508; INDIV: 45,156; § 7,315.05

[41] ¶ 9500, ¶ 9501; INDIV: 45,102; § 7,315.05

[42] ¶ 9506; INDIV: 45,100, IN-DIV: 45,156; § 7,315.05

[43] ¶ 9502.422, ¶ 9502.515; IN-DIV: 45,052; § 7,315.05

[44] ¶ 13,800; REAL: 3,054; § 10,320.05, § 10,330.05

[45] ¶ 14,100; REAL: 3,112; § 10,220

[46] ¶ 21,802, ¶ 21,805; INDIV: 45,206.10; § 7,315.15, § 38,440

Alternatively, if the real estate taxes are a "recurring item," a taxpayer may elect to accrue the taxes and claim the deduction on the date the tax is assessed or becomes a lien against the property (Code Sec. 461(h)(3); Reg. § 1.461-5).[47] Either election may be made without IRS consent for the first tax year in which a taxpayer accrues real property taxes. For later years, the IRS has provided automatic consent procedures for taxpayers to make the elections (Rev. Proc. 2011-14).

Making the Election. Whether a taxpayer should make the election to ratably accrue property taxes or adopt the recurring item exception to the economic performance rule depends on the taxpayer's tax year and lien date of the jurisdiction in which the real property is located. Except where taxes are prepaid, either option is more favorable than the payment rule.

> **Example 1:** X is a calendar-year, accrual-method taxpayer who owns Blackacre in Cook County, Illinois, where the real property tax year is the calendar year and 2014 real property taxes were assessed and became a lien on the property on January 1, 2014. One-half of the taxes are due on March 1, 2015, and the other half on August 1, 2015. Under its three options for accruing real property taxes, X would allocate its deduction between 2014 and 2015 as follows:
>
> - *Payment rule.* 2014: none. 2015: $^{12}/_{12}$.
> - *Ratable accrual.* 2014: $^{12}/_{12}$. 2015: none.
> - *Recurring item exception.* 2014: $^{12}/_{12}$ (provided that X adopted the recurring item exception on either a timely filed original return or on an amended return filed after paying the second installment but before September 15, 2015). 2015: none.

> **Example 2:** Assume X owns Greenacre in Alabama, where taxes for the fiscal year from October 1, 2014, to September 30, 2015, were assessed and became a lien on the property on October 1, 2014. Taxes are due on October 1, 2015. Under its three options for accruing real property taxes, X would allocate its deduction between 2014 and 2015 as follows:
>
> - *Payment rule.* 2014: none. 2015: $^{12}/_{12}$.
> - *Ratable accrual.* 2014: $^{3}/_{12}$. 2015: $^{9}/_{12}$.
> - *Recurring item exception.* 2014: none (because taxes are not due until more than 8½ months after end of 2014). 2015: $^{12}/_{12}$. However, X could advance its entire deduction into 2014 by prepaying its real property taxes on or before September 15, 2015.

1032. Apportionment of Real Property Tax Upon Sale. The real property tax deduction must be apportioned between the seller and the buyer according to the number of days in the real property tax year that each holds the property (¶ 1033). When property is sold during any real property tax year, the taxes are imposed upon the seller up to, but not including, the date of sale. The taxes are imposed on the buyer beginning with the date of sale. Proration is required whether or not the seller and purchaser actually apportion the tax (Reg. § 1.164-6(a) and (b)(1)).[48] When property is sold, however, before or after the real property tax year, see ¶ 1038.

> **Example 1:** A sells his farm to B on August 1, 2014. Both use the cash- and calendar-year basis of accounting. Taxes for the real property tax year, April 1, 2014, to March 31, 2015, become due and payable on May 15, 2015. B pays the real estate taxes when they fall due. Regardless of any agreement between the parties, for federal income tax purposes $^{122}/_{365}$ of the real estate taxes are treated as imposed upon A and are deductible by him.

> **Example 2:** Assume the same facts as in Example 1 above, except that A uses the accrual basis of accounting. If A has not elected to accrue the real property taxes ratably, he will be treated as having accrued $^{122}/_{365}$ of the taxes on the date of sale. The balance is deductible by B when she pays the taxes, if she is on the cash basis, unless the rule at ¶ 1035 applies because the seller (A) is personally liable for the taxes. If B is on the accrual basis, she follows the rules explained at ¶ 1031.

References are to Standard Federal Tax Reports; Tax Research Consultant; and Practical Tax Explanations.

[47] ¶ 21,802, ¶ 21,811; ACCTNG: 12,104.10; § 38,435.10

[48] ¶ 9603; INDIV: 45,300; § 7,315.10

1033. Real Property Tax Year Defined. The real property tax year is the period to which the tax relates under state law, local law, or the law imposing the tax. If a state and one or more local governmental units each imposes a tax, the real property tax year for each tax must be determined (Reg. § 1.164-6(c)).[49]

1034. Cash-Basis Sellers. The portion of the real estate tax imposed on a cash-basis seller under the rules described at ¶ 1032 may be deducted by the seller in the tax year of the sale, whether or not actually paid in that tax year, if: (1) the buyer is liable for the real estate tax for the real property tax year; or (2) the seller is liable for the real estate tax for the real property tax year and the tax is not payable until after the date of sale. When the tax is not a liability of any person, the person who holds the property at the time the tax becomes a lien on the property is considered liable for the tax (Reg. § 1.164-6(d)(1) and (3)).[50]

1035. Cash-Basis Buyers. The portion of the real estate tax imposed on a cash-basis buyer under the rules described at ¶ 1032 may be deducted by the buyer in the tax year of the sale, whether or not the tax is actually paid by the buyer in the tax year of the sale, if the seller is liable for the real estate tax. When the tax is not a liability of any person, the person who holds the property at the time the tax becomes a lien on the property is considered liable for the tax (Reg. § 1.164-6(d)(2) and (3)).[51]

1036. Accrual-Basis Buyers and Sellers. For accrual-basis buyers or sellers who do not elect ratable accrual for property taxes (¶ 1031), the portion of their tax liability (¶ 1032) that may not be deducted for any tax year by reason of their accounting method is treated as if accrued on the date of sale (Reg. § 1.164-6(d)(6)).[52]

1037. Excess Deduction. If a taxpayer deducted real estate taxes in excess of the portion of such tax treated as imposed upon the taxpayer under the rules discussed at ¶ 1032 in a tax year before the year of sale, the excess amount is included in the taxpayer's gross income in the year of sale, subject to the tax benefit rule (¶ 799) (Reg. § 1.164-6(d)(5)).[53]

> **Example:** A is a cash-basis taxpayer whose real property tax is due and payable on November 30 for the next calendar year, which is also the real property tax year. A paid the 2014 real property taxes on November 30, 2013, and deducted them on his 2013 income tax return. On June 30, 2014, A sold the real property. Only the taxes from January 1 through June 29, 2014, i.e., the $^{179}\!/_{365}$ portion, are treated as imposed on A. The excess amount deducted by A on his 2013 income tax return is includible in his gross income in 2014.

1038. Property Sold Before or After Real Property Tax Year. If property is sold after the real property tax becomes a personal liability or a lien but before the beginning of the related real property tax year (¶ 1033), the seller may not deduct any amount for real property taxes for the related real property tax year. To the extent that the buyer holds the property for that real property tax year, the buyer may deduct the amount of the taxes for the tax year in which they are paid or accrued. Conversely, where the property is sold before the tax becomes a personal liability or a lien but after the end of the related real property tax year, the buyer cannot deduct any amount for taxes for the related real property tax year. To the extent that the seller holds the property for that real property tax year, the seller may deduct the amount of the taxes for the tax year they are paid or accrued (Reg. § 1.164-6(b)(1)(ii) and (iii)).[54]

1040. Cooperative Housing Corporation. A tenant-stockholder may deduct amounts paid or accrued to the cooperative housing corporation (CHC) to the extent that they represent the tenant's proportionate share of: (1) real estate taxes on the apartment building or houses and the land on which they are situated; or (2) interest on debt contracted in the acquisition, construction, alteration, rehabilitation, or mainte-

---

References are to Standard Federal Tax Reports; Tax Research Consultant; and Practical Tax Explanations.

[49] ¶ 9603; INDIV: 45,312; § 7,315.10b
[50] ¶ 9603; INDIV: 45,316; § 7,315.10
[51] ¶ 9603; INDIV: 45,316; § 7,315.10
[52] ¶ 9603; INDIV: 45,318; § 7,315.10
[53] ¶ 9603; INDIV: 45,318; § 4,210, § 7,315.10
[54] ¶ 9603; INDIV: 45,308, INDIV: 45,310; § 7,315.10c

nance of such building, houses, or land (Code Sec. 216; Reg. § 1.216-1).[55] The limitations on deductible residential interest apply (¶ 1047).

For purposes of the deduction, a corporation is a CHC if:

- the corporation has only one class of outstanding stock;

- solely by reason of owning the stock, each stockholder is entitled to occupy a house or apartment in a building owned or leased by the corporation;

- no stockholder is entitled to receive any distribution which is not out of the corporation's earnings and profits, except on a partial or complete liquidation; and

- 80 percent or more of the corporation's gross income is derived from tenant-stockholders, 80 percent or more of the total square footage of its property is at all times used or available for use by the tenant-stockholders for residential purposes or purposes ancillary to residential use, or 90 percent or more of the corporation's expenses paid or incurred are for the acquisition, construction, management, maintenance, or care of the property for the tenant-stockholders' benefit.

Under the 80-percent-of-gross-income test, amounts received from tenant-stockholders to defray expenses for items like secretarial services, parking, utilities, recreation facilities, cleaning and related services are included in gross income derived from tenants, while amounts received from commercial leases and the operation of a business other than housing are excluded (Rev. Rul. 55-556). Income attributable to a unit that a governmental entity is entitled to occupy under a lease or stock ownership is also excluded (Code Sec. 216(b)(4); Reg. § 1.216-1(e)(4)).[56]

Interest

1043. Deduction of Interest Paid or Accrued. A taxpayer may generally deduct interest paid or accrued during the tax year on Schedule A of Form 1040 (Code Sec. 163).[57] Deductible interest must pertain to a debt of the taxpayer and result from a debtor-creditor relationship based upon a valid and enforceable obligation to pay a fixed or determinable sum of money. For example, interest paid by children on their parent's mortgage was *not* deductible.[58] There are numerous exceptions to and limitations on the deductibility of interest (¶ 937, ¶ 993, ¶ 1044—¶ 1056, ¶ 1948).

1044. Limitations on Interest Deduction. Interest deductions are limited or precluded for certain types of indebtedness.

Investment Indebtedness Interest. The deduction by noncorporate taxpayers is limited to net investment income (¶ 1094) (Code Sec. 163(d)).[59]

Life Insurance. Interest on loans incurred or continued to pay premiums on certain insurance contracts is nondeductible (¶ 909) (Code Sec. 264(a)).[60]

Mortgage Credit Certificates. The deduction for interest paid or accrued on indebtedness with respect to which a mortgage credit certificate has been issued is reduced by the amount of credit allowable (¶ 1306) (Code Sec. 163(g)).[61]

Personal Interest. Personal interest is *not* deductible (¶ 1045) (Code Sec. 163(h)).[62]

Prepaid Interest. Cash-basis taxpayers generally must capitalize prepaid interest and deduct it as if on the accrual basis (¶ 1055) (Code Sec. 461(g)).[63]

References are to Standard Federal Tax Reports; Tax Research Consultant; and Practical Tax Explanations.

[55] ¶ 12,600, ¶ 12,601; REAL: 9,200; § 7,445

[56] ¶ 12,600, ¶ 12,601; REAL: 9,108

[57] ¶ 9102; INDIV: 48,150; § 7,401

[58] ¶ 9104.264, ¶ 9104.344, ¶ 9104.728; INDIV: 48,200, IN-DIV: 48,200; § 7,405.10, § 7,405.15

[59] ¶ 9102; INDIV: 48,450; § 7,414.05

[60] ¶ 14,002; INDIV: 48,556; § 7,420.10

[61] ¶ 9102; INDIV: 48,050; § 13,020, § 18,515.05

[62] ¶ 9102; INDIV: 48,350; § 7,410

[63] ¶ 21,802; INDIV: 48,252; § 7,405.20d

Loan to Purchase and Carry Tax-Exempt Securities. A deduction for interest paid on a debt incurred or continued to purchase or carry tax-exempt bonds or other tax-exempt obligations is generally denied (¶ 970) (Code Sec. 265(a)).[64]

Related Taxpayers. Accrual-basis taxpayers are placed on the cash basis for interest owed to related cash-basis taxpayers (Code Sec. 267(a)).[65] A corporation is not allowed a deduction for excessive interest paid to a tax-exempt related person or on a loan guaranteed by certain tax-exempt or foreign related persons. For purposes of the disallowance, a corporate partner's distributive share of a partnership's interest income or expense is treated as the partner's interest income or expense, and its share of the partnership's liabilities is treated as the partner's liabilities (Code Sec. 163(j)).[66]

Judicial Exceptions. The courts have denied a deduction for the interest charged upon conversion of a life insurance policy to a higher-premium policy,[67] and for interest paid on loans to buy U.S. Treasury notes where there was nothing to be realized from the transaction beyond a tax deduction.[68]

1045. Nondeductible Personal Interest. Personal interest is *not* deductible (Code Sec. 163(h)).[69] Personal interest is any interest incurred by an individual other than:

   • interest paid or accrued on indebtedness properly allocable to a trade or business, other than services as an employee (¶ 937);

   • investment interest (¶ 1094);

   • interest taken into account in computing income or loss from a passive activity of the taxpayer (¶ 1165);

   • qualified residence interest (¶ 1047);

   • interest on the unpaid portion of the estate tax for the period during which there is an extension of time for payment of the tax on the value of a reversionary or remainder interest in property (¶ 1051); and

   • interest on qualified education loans (¶ 1082).

1047. Qualified Residence Interest (Home Mortgage Interest) Deduction. Although personal interest generally is not deductible (¶ 1045), interest payments attributable to purchase of a qualified residence (home mortgage interest) are deductible in the year paid or accrued. Qualified residence interest is interest that is paid or accrued during the tax year on acquisition and/or home equity indebtedness with respect to any qualified residence (¶ 1048) (Code Sec. 163(h)(3)).[70] Qualified residence interest also can include interest on a loan secured by a qualified residence in a state where the security instrument is otherwise restricted by a debtor protection law. Interest paid or accrued by a trust or estate is deductible if the debt is secured by a beneficiary's qualified residence. A qualified residence includes the taxpayer's principal residence, and one other residence, e.g., vacation home, that is not rented out at any time during the tax year, or that is used by the taxpayer for a number of days exceeding the greater of 14 days or 10 percent of the number of days that it is rented out at a fair rental value (Code Sec. 163(h)(4)).[71] Married taxpayers who file separate returns are treated as one taxpayer, with each entitled to take into account one residence unless both consent in writing to having only one taxpayer take into account both residences. For seller-provided financing, taxpayers deducting qualified residence interest must include on their Schedule A of Form 1040, the name, address and taxpayer identification number (TIN) of the person to whom interest is paid or accrued (Code Sec. 6109(h)).[72]

See ¶ 1048A for treatment of certain mortgage insurance premiums as qualified residence interest.

References are to Standard Federal Tax Reports; Tax Research Consultant; and Practical Tax Explanations.

[64] ¶ 14,050; INDIV: 48,552; § 7,420.05

[65] ¶ 14,150; INDIV: 48,254; § 7,405.10, § 9,140

[66] ¶ 9102; BUSEXP: 21,210; § 7,405.10

[67] ¶ 9104.45; INDIV: 48,556; § 7,405.10

[68] ¶ 9104.364; INDIV: 48,552; § 7,405.10

[69] ¶ 9102; INDIV: 48,350; § 7,410

[70] ¶ 9102; INDIV: 48,400; § 18,515.05

[71] ¶ 9102; INDIV: 48,400; § 18,515.10

[72] ¶ 36,960; REAL: 6,050; § 18,515.05

1048. Acquisition and Home Equity Indebtedness Defined. Acquisition indebtedness is debt incurred in acquiring, constructing, or substantially improving a qualified residence and is secured by the residence for purposes of the qualified residence mortgage interest deduction (¶ 1047). Refinanced debt remains acquisition debt to the extent that it does not exceed the principal amount of acquisition debt immediately before refinancing (Code Sec. 163(h)(3)(B)).[73] Home equity indebtedness is any nonacquisition debt that is secured by a qualified residence to the extent it does not exceed the fair market value of the residence reduced by any acquisition indebtedness (Code Sec. 163(h)(3)(C)). Interest on such debt is deductible even if the proceeds are used for personal expenditures (IRS Pub. 936).

Limitations. The amount of qualified mortgage interest (¶ 1047) that may be deducted is limited to interest on the aggregate amount of acquisition indebtedness that is not in excess of $1 million ($500,000 for married filing separately). The aggregate amount of home equity indebtedness may not exceed $100,000 ($50,000 for married filing separately). Interest attributable to debt over these limits is nondeductible personal interest (¶ 1045) (Code Sec. 163(h)(3)).[74]

The $1 million limit on acquisition indebtedness applies to the entire amount of acquisition debt incurred in acquiring the home, not to each co-owner's portion of the debt (CCA 200911007). The IRS has also ruled that home acquisition indebtedness may also constitute home equity indebtedness to the extent the debt *exceeds* $1 million, but subject to the $100,000 and fair market value limitations (Rev. Rul. 2010-25). The IRS will *not* follow Tax Court decisions which have disallowed such treatment for the portion of debt in excess of the $1 million.

> **Example 1:** A buys a home to be used as a principal residence for $375,000 that is secured by a mortgage in the amount of $350,000. The mortgage qualifies as home acquisition debt because the loan amount does not exceed the home's cost. Thus, since the acquisition indebtedness is less than $1 million, the entire amount of the interest payments is deductible.

> **Example 2:** The fair market value of B's home is $310,000, and the balance of the mortgage (home acquisition debt) is $295,000. B takes out a home equity loan in the amount of $42,500. B's home equity debt, on which interest payments will be deductible as qualified home equity indebtedness, is limited to $15,000: the smaller of (1) the $100,000 maximum limit or (2) the excess of the home's fair market value ($310,000) over the home acquisition debt ($295,000).

Pre-October 13, 1987, Indebtedness. Interest on acquisition indebtedness incurred on or before October 13, 1987, is fully deductible, and is not subject to the $1 million limitation. The amount of this grandfathered debt reduces the amount of the $1 million limitation available for new acquisition debt, e.g., for improvements.

Grandfathered debt is any debt incurred on or before October 13, 1987, that is secured by a qualified residence on that date and at all times thereafter before the interest is paid or accrued. It also includes debt secured by a qualified residence to refinance existing pre-October 13 debt, to the extent that the refinancing does not increase the principal amount or extend the term of the debt beyond the existing term of the acquisition debt immediately before the refinancing. If acquisition debt is not amortized over its term, as in the case of a balloon note, interest on any otherwise qualified refinancing is deductible for the term of the first refinancing for up to 30 years (Code Sec. 163(h)(3)(D)).[75]

1048A. Deduction of Mortgage Insurance Premiums. Certain premiums paid or accrued before January 1, 2014, for qualified mortgage insurance in connection with acquisition indebtedness (¶ 1048) are deductible as qualified residence interest (¶ 1047) (Code Sec. 163(h)(3)(E), and (4)(E)).[76] For every $1,000 by which the taxpayer's adjusted gross income (AGI) exceeds $100,000, however, the amount of premiums treated as interest is reduced by 10 percent. For married taxpayers filing separately, the

---

References are to Standard Federal Tax Reports; Tax Research Consultant; and Practical Tax Explanations.

[73] ¶ 9102; INDIV: 48,400; §18,515.15, §18,515.20

[74] ¶ 9102; REAL: 6,056.15; §18,515.15, §18,515.20

[75] ¶ 9102; REAL: 6,056

[76] ¶ 9102; REAL: 6,060; §18,520

amount of premiums treated as interest is reduced by 10 percent for every $500 that AGI exceeds $50,000. The deduction does not apply with respect to mortgage insurance contracts issued before January 1, 2007, or to premiums paid, accrued, or properly allocable to any period after December 31, 2013. Qualified mortgage insurance is that provided by the Department of Veterans Affairs (VA), the Federal Housing Administration (FHA), or the Rural Housing Administration (RHA), as well as private mortgage insurance.

For prepaid mortgage insurance, except VA or RHA contracts, amounts paid that are allocable to periods after the payment year are capitalized and treated as paid in the allocable periods. Prepaid premiums must be allocated ratably over the shorter of the stated term of the mortgage or 84 months, beginning with the month in which the insurance was obtained. If the mortgage is satisfied before the end of its term, no deduction is allowed for any premium allocable to periods after the mortgage is satisfied (Code Sec. 163(h)(4)(F); Reg. § 1.163-11).[77]

> **Comment:** Absent further legislation, the deduction for qualified mortgage insurance premiums has expired for amounts paid, accrued, or properly allocable to any period after December 31, 2013. For the latest legislative updates, visit our website www.CCHGroup.com/TaxUpdates.

1049. Deduction of Redeemable Ground Rents. Annual or periodic payments of redeemable ground rent, except amounts paid in redemption of this rent, are treated as interest paid on mortgage indebtedness (Code Sec. 163(c)).[78] Therefore, such ground rents are subject to the rules pertaining to qualified residences (¶ 1047). A redeemable ground rent is a ground rent payable under a freely assignable lease that, including possible renewal periods, is for a term in excess of 15 years, where the lessee has a right to terminate the lease and buy the lessor's interest in the land by paying a set amount, and the lessor's interest is primarily a security interest to protect the rental payments (Code Sec. 1055(c)(1); Reg. § 1.1055-1).[79]

1050. Deduction of Mortgage Interest of Ministers and Military Personnel. Ministers and military personnel are allowed to deduct mortgage interest on their qualified residences (¶ 1047) even though they receive a parsonage or military housing allowance that is excludable from gross income (Code Sec. 265(a)(6)).[80] Military personnel includes members of the Army, Navy, Air Force, Marine Corps, Coast Guard, National Oceanic and Atmospheric Administration, and Public Health Service (Rev. Rul. 87-32).

1051. Interest Paid on Delinquent or Deferred Taxes. Interest imposed on delinquent federal, state or local income taxes is generally nondeductible personal interest, regardless of the source of the income generating the tax liability (¶ 1045) (Temp. Reg. § 1.163-9T(b)(2)(i)(A)).[81] Interest on federal and state income tax deficiencies accruing after death is generally deductible by the estate as an administration expense (Rev. Rul. 69-402).

For estates of decedents dying after 1997, interest payable on any unpaid portion of federal estate tax during an extension period for payment of the tax where the estate consists largely of a closely-held business under Code Sec. 6166 (¶ 2939) is *not* deductible for federal income tax purposes (Code Sec. 163(k)).[82] However, any interest expense accrued for federal estate taxes during an extension for payment of tax under Code Sec. 6163 on the value of a reversionary or remainder interest in property, or under Code Sec. 6166 for estates of decedents who died before 1998, may be claimed as an administrative expense deduction from federal estate tax, or as an income tax deduction under Code Sec. 163(h)(2)(E)[83] if the right to an estate tax deduction for the interest has been waived (Code Sec. 642(g)).[84]

References are to Standard Federal Tax Reports; Tax Research Consultant; and Practical Tax Explanations.

[77] ¶ 9102, ¶ 9401D; REAL: 6,060; § 18,520

[78] ¶ 9102; REAL: 6,052.45; § 18,515.05

[79] ¶ 29,940, ¶ 29,941; REAL: 6,052.45; § 18,515.05

[80] ¶ 14,050; INDIV: 48,554; § 18,515.05

[81] ¶ 9400; INDIV: 48,352; § 28,440.30

[82] ¶ 9102; INDIV: 48,354; § 34,410.20

[83] ¶ 9102; INDIV: 48,350; § 7,410, § 32,310

[84] ¶ 24,280; ESTTRST: 9,200; § 32,310, § 32,320

Interest paid on sales and excise taxes incurred in connection with a trade or business or investment activity, and interest paid by a transferee for a C corporation's delinquent taxes, is not personal interest (Temp. Reg. § 1.163-9T(b)(2)(iii)).[85]

Prepaid Interest

1055. Deductibility of Prepaid Interest by Cash-Basis Taxpayers. A cash-basis taxpayer generally cannot take a current deduction for prepaid interest. Instead, the taxpayer must deduct prepaid interest over the period of the loan to the extent that the interest represents the cost of using the borrowed funds during each tax year in the period. Points paid on loans, other than certain home mortgage loans, are deducted ratably over the term of the loan (Code Sec. 461(g)).[86] Penalty payments made for the privilege of prepaying mortgage indebtedness are currently deductible as interest (Rev. Rul. 57-198).

The prepaid interest rule does not contemplate that interest will be treated as paid in equal payments over the term of the loan. Thus, interest paid on an amortizing loan as part of an equal constant payment, including principal and interest, is not subject to the prepaid interest rule merely because the payments consist of a larger interest portion in the earlier years of the loan than in later years.

Points on a home mortgage loan for the purchase or improvement of, and secured by, a principal residence are deductible in the year paid to the extent that the payment of points is an established practice in the area, and the amount paid does not exceed the points generally charged in the area for a home loan (Code Sec. 461(g)(2)).[87] Taxpayers may also choose to amortize points over the life of their loan if, for instance, the standard deduction in the year the points were paid exceeds the taxpayer's itemized deductions, including the points (IRS Letter Ruling 199905033).[88]

The IRS treats as deductible in the year paid any points paid by a cash-basis taxpayer that:

- are designated as points on the RESPA settlement statement (Form HUD-1), for example, as "loan origination fees," including amounts so designated on VA and FHA loans, "loan discount," "discount points," or "points;"

- are calculated as a percentage of the principal loan amount;

- are paid to acquire the taxpayer's principal residence in connection with a loan secured by that residence;

- are paid directly by the taxpayer, which may include earnest money, an escrow deposit, or down payment applied at closing, and not derived from loan proceeds; points paid by a seller, including points charged to the seller, are considered directly paid by the taxpayer from funds not derived from loan proceeds if they are subtracted by the taxpayer from the purchase price of the residence in computing its basis; and

- conform to an established business practice of charging points for loans for the acquisition of personal residences in the area.

No part of the points may be in lieu of appraisal, inspection, title, and attorney fees, property taxes, or other amounts that are ordinarily stated separately on the settlement statement (Rev. Proc. 94-27).

This safe harbor does not apply to points paid for a loan to acquire a principal residence to the extent the principal amount exceeds the limit on acquisition indebtedness (¶ 1048). Nor does it apply to points paid on home improvement loans, second or vacation home loans, refinancing or home equity loans, or lines of credit. The fact that a taxpayer cannot satisfy the requirements of the safe harbor does not necessarily mean that points are not currently deductible. It does mean that the IRS will not automatically consider them to be currently deductible.

References are to Standard Federal Tax Reports; Tax Research Consultant; and Practical Tax Explanations.

[85] ¶ 9400; INDIV: 48,350; § 7,410

[86] ¶ 21,802; INDIV: 48,256; § 7,405.20d, § 18,515.35, § 38,410.40

[87] ¶ 21,802; INDIV: 48,256; § 18,515.35

[88] ¶ 9402.55; INDIV: 48,256; § 38,410.40

Points paid to refinance a home mortgage are not deductible in full in the year paid, but must be deducted ratably over the period of the loan because they are incurred for the repayment of the taxpayer's existing indebtedness and are not paid in connection with the purchase or improvement of the home. The U.S. Court of Appeals for the Eighth Circuit, however, allowed a full deduction in the year paid for points on a long-term home mortgage loan refinancing a short-term balloon loan used to acquire the home (*J.R. Huntsman*, CA-8, 90-2 USTC ¶ 50,340, nonacq. except in the Eighth Circuit).[89] Also, the portion of the points allocable to the proceeds of a refinancing that are used for improvements may be deducted in the year paid. The portion allocable to the repayment of existing indebtedness or other purposes is deducted ratably over the period of the loan (Rev. Rul. 87-22).[90]

A loan discount, i.e., where a lender delivers to an individual borrower an amount smaller than the face amount of the loan and the difference is the agreed charge for the use of borrowed money, is interest (Rev. Rul. 75-12).

1056. Deductibility of Prepaid Interest by Accrual-Basis Taxpayers. Taxpayers who use the accrual method accrue and deduct interest ratably over the loan period, regardless of whether the interest is prepaid (Rev. Rul. 68-643).

Charitable Contributions

1058. Contributions by Individuals. Individuals who itemize their deductions are entitled to deduct contributions to a qualified charitable organization on Schedule A of Form 1040 (Code Sec. 170).[91] The charitable deduction for any one tax year is limited to a percentage of the individual taxpayer's contribution base determined by the type of organization receiving the donation and the type of property donated (¶ 1059). Any amount in excess of the percentage limitation for the tax year may be carried forward for a period of five years (¶ 1060). When spouses file a joint return, the percentage limitation depends on their aggregate contribution base. A limit also applies to the amount of a charitable deduction allowed for gifts of appreciated property (¶ 1062), and is imposed before applying the percentage limitation.

A charitable contribution is a contribution or gift to a qualifying organization (¶ 1061). Except in the case of a carryover of a deduction, a taxpayer may deduct the fair market value of property contributed to charity, subject to the percentage limitation, only in the year of payment (Reg. § 1.170A-1(a)).[92] Contributions charged to a bank credit card, however, are deductible in the year charged even though paid in a later year (Rev. Rul. 78-38).

Taxpayers who are recognized by the Alaska Eskimo Whaling Commission as whaling captains can claim a charitable contribution deduction of up to $10,000 per tax year for reasonable and necessary expenses paid in carrying out sanctioned Alaskan subsistence whale hunting activities (Code Sec. 170(n)).[93]

IRA Distributions. For tax years before January 1, 2014, individuals age 70½ or older may distribute up to $100,000 tax-free from their individual retirement accounts (IRAs) to certain charitable organizations without including the distribution in gross income (¶ 2165) (Code Sec. 408(d)(8)). The distribution must be made directly by the trustee to a 50-percent organization (¶ 1059), but *not* to a supporting organization or a donor advised fund (¶ 1061), and the entire distribution must otherwise be deductible as a charitable donation, disregarding the percentage limitations, even though the individual cannot claim a charitable deduction for the donation.

> **Comment:** Absent further legislation, this provision has expired for tax years beginning after December 31, 2013. For the latest legislative updates, visit our website www.CCHGroup.com/TaxUpdates.

References are to Standard Federal Tax Reports; Tax Research Consultant; and Practical Tax Explanations.

[89] ¶ 9402.62; INDIV: 48,256; § 18,515.35, § 38,410.40

[90] ¶ 9402.60; INDIV: 48,256; § 18,515.35

[91] ¶ 11,600; INDIV: 51,000; § 7,501

[92] ¶ 11,615; INDIV: 51,402; § 7,505.10

[93] ¶ 11,600; INDIV: 51,052.55

Special rules were enacted by the American Taxpayer Relief Act of 2012 (P.L. 112-240) to compensate for its late passage. Taxpayers may elect to treat any qualified charitable distribution made from an IRA after December 31, 2012, and before February 1, 2013, as being made on December 31, 2012. In addition, taxpayers may elect to treat any portion of distribution from an IRA made after November 30, 2012, and before January 1, 2013, as a qualified charitable distribution to the extent that such portion is transferred in cash following the distribution to a qualified charitable organization before February 1, 2013, and all other requirements for a qualified charitable distribution are otherwise satisfied.

1059. Percentage Limits on Individuals' Contributions. An individual's charitable deduction for any one tax year is limited to a percentage of the individual's contribution base determined by the type of organization receiving the donation and the type of property donated (Code Sec. 170(b)(1)).[94] The deduction limit also depends, in part, on whether the donation of property is made to the charitable organization or for its use (¶ 1063). A donation of an income interest in property is made for the use of the charity, whether or not it is transferred in trust. A donation of a remainder interest in property is made for the use of the organization if it is transferred in trust to be held and administered for the organization (Reg. § 1.170A-8(a)(2)).[95]

An individual's contribution base is the taxpayer's adjusted gross income (AGI), computed without regard to the charitable deduction and any net operating loss carryback (Code Sec. 170(b)(1)(G); Reg. § 1.170A-8(a)).[96] When a married couple files a joint return, the percentage limitations are applied against the couple's aggregate income.

Contributions of ordinary income property (¶ 1062) to tax-exempt organizations are limited to a maximum deduction of 50 percent of a taxpayer's contribution base (¶ 1058) for the tax year (Code Sec. 170(b)(1)(A); Reg. § 1.170A-9).[97] Contributions of capital gain property to tax-exempt organizations are limited to a maximum deduction of 30 percent of the taxpayer's contribution base for the tax year (¶ 1062) (Code Sec. 170(b)(1)(C)).[98] Tax-exempt organizations for this purpose include:

(1) churches or conventions or associations of churches (¶ 604);

(2) educational institutions;

(3) hospitals or medical research organizations, not including home health care organizations, convalescent homes, homes for children or the aged, or vocational institutions that train handicapped individuals;

(4) endowment foundations in connection with a state college or university;

(5) state, federal or local government units, if the contribution is made for exclusively public purposes;

(6) organizations referred to in Code Sec. 170(c)(2) (¶ 1061) normally receiving a substantial part of their support from the public or a governmental unit;

(7) private operating foundations (¶ 633);

(8) private nonoperating foundations (¶ 631 and ¶ 633) that distribute all contributions received to public charities and private operating foundations, or make certain other qualifying distributions, within 2½ months after the end of the tax year;

(9) private foundations (¶ 631) that pool all contributions into a common fund and allow a substantial contributor to designate a recipient charity, where income from the pool is distributed within 2½ months after the tax year in which it was realized and corpus attributable to any donor's contribution is distributed to a charity not later than one year after the death of the donor or surviving spouse with the right to designate the recipients of the corpus;

References are to Standard Federal Tax Reports; Tax Research Consultant; and Practical Tax Explanations.

[94] ¶ 11,600; INDIV: 51,250; § 7,565.05

[95] ¶ 11,661; INDIV: 51,250; § 7,505.05

[96] ¶ 11,600, ¶ 11,662; INDIV: 51,252; § 7,565.05

[97] ¶ 11,600; INDIV: 51,254; § 7,565.05, § 7,565.10

[98] ¶ 11,600; INDIV: 51,256; § 7,565.20

¶1059

(10) publicly supported organizations normally receiving

(a) more than ⅓ of their support in each tax year from the public and organizations listed at (1)—(6), above, in the form of grants, gifts, contributions, or membership fees, and gross receipts from an activity that is not an unrelated trade or business (less certain receipts), and

(b) not more than ⅓ of their support from gross investment income and unrelated business taxable income (less taxes); and

(11) certain supporting organizations (¶ 607).

The deduction limitation on contributions of ordinary income property to "other," non-50-percent, charitable organization donees—nonoperating foundations and organizations such as war veterans' and fraternal organizations, and public cemeteries—and on gifts *for the use of* 50-percent organization donees, is the lesser of: (1) 30 percent of the taxpayer's contribution base, or (2) the excess of 50 percent of the taxpayer's contribution base for the tax year over the amount of charitable contributions qualifying for the 50-percent deduction ceiling, including carryovers (Code Sec. 170(b)(1)(B)).[99] Contributions of capital gain property to these organizations are subject to a 20-percent contribution base limitation (Code Sec. 170(b)(1)(D)).[100]

Charitable contributions made by bona fide residents of U.S. possessions (¶ 2414) or Puerto Rico (¶ 2415) are deductible only to the extent allocable to income that is *not* excluded possession-source or Puerto Rico-source income (Reg. § 1.170A-1(j)(9)).[101]

For deduction limitations on charitable contributions by corporations, see ¶ 927.

Qualified Conservation Contributions. Individual donors who make a qualified conservation contribution (QCC) of real property (¶ 1063) in tax years beginning before January 1, 2014, are allowed to claim their QCC deduction against the 50-percent contribution base minus their deduction for all other charitable contributions, and any excess over this amount can be carried forward for 15 years. These rules are applied separately from the rules that apply to other donations (Code Sec. 170(b)(1)(E)).[102]

> **Comment:** Absent further legislation, this provision has expired for tax years beginning after December 31, 2013. For the latest legislative updates, visit our website www.CCHGroup.com/TaxUpdates.

Qualified Farmers and Ranchers. Qualified farmers and ranchers, i.e., individual taxpayers with more than 50 percent of gross income from farming or ranching, making a QCC of real property have their QCC deduction limited to 100 percent of the contribution base minus their deduction for all other charitable contributions, in tax years before January 1, 2014. The 100-percent limit only applies if the contribution includes a restriction that the property must remain generally available for agriculture or livestock production (Code Sec. 170(b)(1)(E)). The enhanced charitable deduction for QCC of real property by certain corporate farmers and ranchers for tax years beginning before January 1, 2014, is limited to the excess of the taxpayer's taxable income over the amount of other allowable charitable contributions, which is limited to 10 percent of taxable income (Code Sec. 170(b)(2)(B)).

> **Comment:** Absent further legislation, this provision has expired for tax years beginning after December 31, 2013. For the latest legislative updates, visit our website www.CCHGroup.com/TaxUpdates.

1060. Individuals' Five-Year Carryover. Individuals may carry forward for five years their charitable contributions that exceed the deductible ceiling for the year of the contribution (¶ 1059) (Code Sec. 170(b)(1)(D)(ii) and (d); Reg. § 1.170A-10).[103] The amount of the excess that may be deducted in any carryover year is limited to the lesser of: (1) the remaining portion of any excess contribution not already deducted or (2) an amount equal to 50 percent (or 30 percent for capital gain carryover) of the taxpayer's

---

References are to Standard Federal Tax Reports; Tax Research Consultant; and Practical Tax Explanations.

[99] ¶ 11,600; INDIV: 51,258; § 7,565.15

[100] ¶ 11,600; INDIV: 51,256; § 7,565.25

[101] ¶ 11,615; INDIV: 51,150; § 7,501

[102] ¶ 11,600; INDIV: 51,256, INDIV: 51,364; § 7,565.30

[103] ¶ 11,600, ¶ 11,663; INDIV: 51,262; § 7,570.05

contribution base (¶ 1058) after first deducting the sum of the charitable contributions (to which the 50-percent or 30-percent limitation applies) paid in the carryover year and any excess contributions that have precedence in order of time over the present carryover. The excess must be reduced to the extent that it reduces taxable income as computed for net operating loss (NOL) carrybacks and carryovers (¶ 1149) and increases the NOL deduction for a tax year succeeding the contribution year.

Qualified Conservation Contribution Carryover. If the value of a taxpayer's qualified conservation contribution (QCC) made in a tax year before 2014 (¶ 1059) exceeded the special higher limit for such a donation, the excess can be carried forward for 15 years (Code Sec. 170(b)(1)(E)(ii)).

1061. Contributions That Are Deductible. A charitable contribution is deductible only if it is a contribution or gift to, or for the use of, the following qualified organizations:

- the United States, a state, a local government, the District of Columbia, or a U.S. possession, for exclusively public purposes;

- a corporation, trust, or community chest, fund, or foundation, created or organized in the United States or a possession or under the law of the United States, a possession, a state, or the District of Columbia, organized and operated exclusively for religious, charitable, scientific, literary, or educational purposes, or to foster national or international amateur sports competition, or for the prevention of cruelty to children or animals; no part of the charity's net earnings may inure to the benefit of any private shareholder or individual. Also, the organization must not be disqualified for tax exemption under Code Sec. 501(c)(3) by attempting to influence legislation;

- a cemetery company owned and operated exclusively for the benefit of its members or any corporation chartered solely for burial purposes as a cemetery corporation and not operated for profit or for the benefit of any private shareholder or individual;

- a post or organization of war veterans, or its auxiliary society or unit, organized in the United States or its possessions, if no part of the net earnings inures to the benefit of any private shareholder or individual; or

- a domestic fraternal society, order, or association, operating under the lodge system, by only individual donors if the contributions are used exclusively for religious, charitable, scientific, literary or educational purposes, or for the prevention of cruelty to children or animals (Code Sec. 170(c)).[104]

Pew rents, building fund assessments, and periodic church dues are deductible (Rev. Rul. 70-47).

Clothing and Household Items. A deduction for a donation of clothing and household items is allowed only if the donated property is in good used condition or better. Household items do not include food, paintings, antiques, other objects of art, jewelry, gems, or collections. The IRS can deny a deduction for such donated property that is of minimal value. These restrictions do not apply if: (1) a deduction of more than $500 is claimed for the single clothing or household item, and (2) a qualified appraisal for that item is attached to the return (¶ 1071). For partnerships and S corporations, the restrictions are applied at the entity level, and denial of the deduction is at the partner or shareholder level (Code Sec. 170(f)(16)).[105]

Services. The value of service rendered to a charitable organization is *not* deductible as a contribution, e.g. the value of a blood donation (Reg. § 1.170A-1(g); Rev. Rul. 162).[106] An out-of-pocket, unreimbursed expense, e.g., uniforms, telephone, or equipment, incurred in rendering such service, however, is a deductible contribution (Rev. Rul. 84-61, modifying Rev. Rul. 58-279). No deduction is allowed for an out-of-pocket expenditure made by any person on behalf of a charitable organization other than an organization

---

References are to Standard Federal Tax Reports; Tax Research Consultant; and Practical Tax Explanations.

[104] ¶ 11,600; INDIV: 51,100; § 7,520.05, § 7,520.35

[105] ¶ 11,600; INDIV: 51,152; § 7,595

[106] ¶ 11,615, ¶ 11,620.65; INDIV: 51,056; § 7,540

described in Code Sec. 501(h)(5), i.e., churches, if the expenditure is made for the purpose of influencing legislation (Code Sec. 170(f)(6)). No charitable or business deduction is allowed for contributions made to organizations that conduct lobbying activities relating to matters of direct financial interest to the donor, unless the donor's direct conduct of the activities would have given rise to a business expense deduction (¶ 974) (Code Sec. 170(f)(9)).[107]

Certain payments made under leave-based donation programs, in which an employer makes charitable donations in exchange for an employee's election to forgo paid leave, have been deductible by the employer as compensation (¶ 906) but were neither includible in the employee's income nor deductible by the employee as a charitable contribution.[108]

Travel Expenses. Deductions are allowed for transportation or other travel expenses, including meals and lodging, incurred in the performance of services away from home on behalf of a charitable organization if there is no significant element of personal pleasure, recreation or vacation. If there is such an element, deductions are denied even though the expenses are paid directly by the individual, indirectly through a contribution to the organization, or by reimbursement by the organization. This rule does not apply to the extent that an individual pays for travel for third parties who are participants in the charitable activity. However, deductions are disallowed where two unrelated taxpayers pay each other's travel expenses or members of a group contribute to a fund that pays for all travel expenses (Code Sec. 170(j)).[109] Individuals who qualify for a deduction for the use of an automobile during the year may use the statutory standard mileage rate of 14 cents per mile, plus parking fees and tolls, in lieu of a deduction based on the actual expenses incurred. Depreciation and insurance are not includible in the deductible contribution (Code Sec. 170(i)).[110]

Fund-Raising Activities. An amount paid for a ticket to a charity event—e.g., a ball, bazaar, show, or athletic event—is presumed to represent the purchase price for an item of value. The burden is on the taxpayer to show either that the payment is not a purchase or that the payment exceeds the fair market value of the admission or other privileges associated with the event. The purchase price of a raffle ticket is not deductible (Rev. Rul. 83-130; Rev. Rul. 67-246, distinguished by Rev. Rul. 74-348, and amplified by Rev. Proc. 90-12).

> **Example:** A pays $20 to see a special showing of a motion picture, the net proceeds of which go to a qualified charitable organization. Printed on the ticket is "Contribution—$20." If the regular price for the movie is $9, A made a contribution of $11 to a qualified charitable organization.

A fund-raising organization that provides token benefits to contributors can advise them that their donations are fully deductible only if the token benefits have an insubstantial value. If items are mailed to potential donors, the organization can advise that a contribution is fully deductible only if the items are low cost, provided for free, and not distributed at the donor's request or consent (Rev. Procs. 90-12 and 92-49). A charity that receives a *quid pro quo contribution* in excess of $75 must provide a statement to the donor describing what portion of the donation represents consideration for goods or services (¶ 627) (Code Sec. 6115).[111]

Eighty percent of an otherwise deductible payment made to a college or university for the right to purchase tickets to an athletic event, including tickets to skyboxes, is treated as a charitable contribution regardless of whether the tickets would have been available if the payment had not been made (Code Sec. 170(l); IRS Letter Ruling 200004001).[112]

Transfers of property to a charitable organization that are directly related to the donor's business and made with a reasonable expectation of financial return equivalent

---

References are to Standard Federal Tax Reports; Tax Research Consultant; and Practical Tax Explanations.

[107] ¶ 11,600; INDIV: 51,118; § 7,540

[108] ¶ 11,620.522; INDIV: 51,056; § 4,110, § 7,540

[109] ¶ 11,600, ¶ 11,620.029; IN-DIV: 51,056; § 7,545

[110] ¶ 11,600; INDIV: 51,056; § 7,545

[111] ¶ 37,065; INDIV: 51,052; § 7,600.20

[112] ¶ 11,600, ¶ 11,680.10; IN-DIV: 51,052; § 7,510.75

to the value of the transfers do not qualify for a charitable deduction but may qualify as a trade or business expense (Reg. § 1.170A-1(c)(5)).[113]

Donor Advised Funds. The deduction for a contribution made to a donor advised fund (¶ 610) is allowed only if: (1) the fund's sponsoring organization is not a cemetery, a war veterans' organization, a lodge, or a "Type III supporting organization" that is not a "functionally integrated Type III supporting organization" (¶ 607 and ¶ 640), and (2) the donor obtains a contemporaneous written acknowledgment from the sponsoring organization that the organization has exclusive legal control over the assets contributed (Code Sec. 170(f)(18)).[114] Distributions from donor advised funds that are for noncharitable purposes are taxable, as are certain transactions between a donor advised fund and its donors, donor advisors, or related persons (Code Secs. 4966 and 4967).[115] The IRS has discretion to abate such taxes (¶ 647).

1062. Gifts of Appreciated Property. The amount of a noncash charitable contribution is generally the property's fair market value at the time of the contribution, reduced by limitations that apply to certain appreciated property (Code Sec. 170(e); Reg. §§ 1.170A-1(c) and 1.170A-4).[116] The deductible amount for appreciated property depends on whether it is ordinary income property, capital gain property, or a combination of both. The reduction rules described below do not apply if, due to the transfer of the contributed property, the donor recognizes income or gain in the same tax year in which the contribution is made.

Ordinary Income Property. Ordinary income property is property that, if sold at its fair market value on the date of contribution, would give rise to ordinary income or short-term capital gain. The deduction for such property is limited to the fair market value of the property less the amount that would be ordinary income. Such property includes inventory and stock in trade, artworks and manuscripts created by the donor, letters and memoranda, capital assets held for less than the required holding period for long-term capital gain treatment, and Code Sec. 306 stock (¶ 739 and ¶ 740) (Code Sec. 170(e)(1)(A); Reg. § 1.170A-4).[117]

Capital Gain Property. Capital gain property includes any asset on which a long-term capital gain would be realized if the taxpayer sold the asset for its fair market value on the date of contribution. As a general rule, gifts of capital gain property are deductible at their fair market value on the date of contribution. However, the individual's contribution must be reduced by the potential long-term gain (appreciation) if (Code Sec. 170(e)(1)(B)):

- the property is contributed to certain private nonoperating (grant-making) foundations (a deduction is, however, allowed for the fair market value of qualified appreciated stock, which is publicly traded stock that would produce long-term capital gain if sold (Code Sec. 170(e)(5)));

- the gift is tangible personal property put to a use that is unrelated to the purpose or function upon which the organization's exemption is based;

- the gift is tangible personal property which is "applicable property," but without regard to whether a deduction greater than the donor's basis has been allowed, that the organization sells, exchanges, or disposes of in the tax year when the contribution was made, and the organization has not made a certification regarding the property (see *"Recapture of Charitable Tax Benefits,"* following);

- the donation consists of patents, certain copyrights, trademarks, trade names, trade secrets, know-how, certain software, or similar intellectual property or applications or registrations of such property;

References are to Standard Federal Tax Reports; Tax Research Consultant; and Practical Tax Explanations.

[113] ¶ 11,615; INDIV: 51,150

[114] ¶ 11,600; INDIV: 51,100; § 7,520.40

[115] ¶ 34,317, ¶ 34,319; EX-EMPT: 24,000; § 33,720.05

[116] ¶ 11,600, ¶ 11,615, ¶ 11,632; INDIV: 51,200; § 7,525.05

[117] ¶ 11,600, ¶ 11,632; INDIV: 51,204; § 7,525.10

• the donation consists of taxidermy property contributed by the person who prepared, stuffed or mounted the property, or who paid or incurred the cost of preparation, stuffing or mounting; or

• the taxpayer elects to disregard the special 30-percent capital gains limitation in favor of the 50-percent limitation (Reg. § 1.170A-4(b)(2)).[118]

Combination Property. The charitable contribution deduction is specially computed if the donor's sale of the property at fair market value would have produced both ordinary income and capital gain (Code Sec. 170(e)). The fair market value is reduced by the ordinary income that would have resulted from the sale, and the remainder of the fair market value is treated as capital gain property, subject to the above rules. The types of property to which this special computation applies include property subject to depreciation recapture (¶ 1779 and ¶ 1788) and to recapture of farmland expenditures (¶ 1797), as well as interests in oil, gas, or geothermal property.

Recapture of Charitable Tax Benefits. If a donee organization disposes of applicable property within three years of the contribution and does not provide certification regarding the property, the donor taxpayer will be required to include as ordinary income for the year of the disposition the difference between the amount of the charitable deduction allowed for the donated capital gains property and the donor's basis. "Applicable property" is appreciated tangible personal property with a claimed value over $5,000, the use of which the donee certifies as related to its exempt function or purpose, and for which a deduction greater than the donor's basis is allowed. The certification is a written statement, signed under penalty of perjury by an officer of the donee, which either: (1) certifies that the property's use was *substantial and related* to the donee's exempt purpose, and describes how the property was used and how such use furthered the exempt purpose or (2) states the donee's intended use of the property at the time of the contribution and certifies that such use became impossible or infeasible to implement (Code Sec. 170(e)(7)).[119]

Food Inventories. Noncorporate and corporate taxpayers are allowed to claim an enhanced deduction for certain donations of food inventories for tax years beginning before January 1, 2014 (¶ 930A). For a taxpayer other than a C corporation, the total deduction for food inventory donations during the tax year is limited to a maximum of 10 percent of the taxpayer's net income from those trades or businesses making such donations (Code Sec. 170(e)(3)(C)).[120]

> **Comment:** Absent further legislation, the enhanced deduction for certain donations of food inventories has expired for tax years beginning after December 31, 2013. For the latest legislative updates, visit our website www.CCHGroup.com/TaxUpdates.

1062A. Donee Income from Intellectual Property. A donor is allowed an additional charitable deduction based on a sliding-scale percentage of net income received by, or accrued to, the donee that is allocable to donated qualified intellectual property over a 10-year period. Qualified intellectual property includes patents and other intellectual property (¶ 1062) but does not include property donated to certain private nonoperating (grant-making) foundations. This additional deduction is allowed only to the extent that the total amount calculated using the sliding scale exceeds the deduction amount claimed on the property contribution without regard to the additional amount. The donor must inform the donee at the time of the contribution of its intent to treat the donation as a qualified intellectual property contribution. A donee, other than certain private foundations, that receives or accrues net income during a tax year from any qualified intellectual property contribution must make an information return and provide a copy to the donor (Code Secs. 170(m) and 6050L(b); Notice 2005-41).[121]

References are to Standard Federal Tax Reports; Tax Research Consultant; and Practical Tax Explanations.

[118] ¶ 11,600, ¶ 11,632; INDIV: 51,200, INDIV: 51,206, INDIV: 51,254; § 7,525.15

[119] ¶ 11,600; INDIV: 51,200; § 7,525.15c

[120] ¶ 11,600; CCORP: 9,354; § 7,525.20

[121] ¶ 11,600, ¶ 36,260, ¶ 11,660.32; INDIV: 51,168; § 7,585

1063. Use of Property—Partial Interests. No charitable deduction is generally allowed for gifts to charity of the rent-free use of property and other nontrust gifts where less than the taxpayer's entire interest in the property is contributed, except in the following cases: (1) a contribution of an undivided portion of a taxpayer's entire interest in property, e.g., a one-fourth interest in property; (2) a contribution of a remainder interest in a personal residence or farm; (3) a qualified conservation contribution (QCC); or (4) where a charitable deduction would have been allowed had the interest been transferred in trust (¶ 538 and ¶ 1070) (Code Sec. 170(f)(3); Reg. § 1.170A-7).[122]

Additional Fractional Interest Charitable Contributions. The charitable deduction for additional contributions of tangible personal property in which the donor has previously contributed an undivided fractional interest is equal to the lesser of the fair market value of (1) the property used to determine the deduction for the initial fractional contribution, or (2) the property at the time of the additional contribution. The deduction will be recaptured if, on or before the earlier of the 10th anniversary of the initial fractional contribution or the donor's date of death, either (1) the donor fails to contribute the remaining interests to the donee, or (2) the donee fails to take substantial physical possession of the property and use it in a manner related to its exempt purpose. The recaptured amount will be subject to interest and an additional 10-percent tax (Code Sec. 170(o)).[123]

Qualified Conservation Contributions (QCC). A QCC is a contribution of a qualified real property interest to a qualified organization exclusively for conservation purposes that are protected in perpetuity. Qualified real property includes a donor's entire interest in real property other than an interest in subsurface oil, gas, or other minerals, and the right to access to such minerals, a remainder interest, and a restriction granted in perpetuity on the property's use (i.e., an easement). A qualified organization includes certain governmental units, public charities that meet certain public support tests, and certain supporting organizations. A qualified conservation purpose includes: (1) preserving land for public outdoor recreation or education; (2) protecting a relatively natural habitat of fish, wildlife, or plants; (3) preserving open space for the public's scenic enjoyment or under a governmental conservation policy that will yield significant public benefit; and (4) preserving an historically important land area or certified historic structure (Code Sec. 170(h)).[124]

For any QCC, the deduction is reduced by an amount equal to the contribution's fair market value multiplied by a fraction: the sum of the rehabilitation credits (¶ 1365B) allowed to the taxpayer for the five preceding tax years on any building that is part of the donation, over the building's fair market value on the contribution date (Code Sec. 170(f)(14)).

Facade Easements. A facade easement may qualify as a QCC. There are several requirements for contributions of facade easements regarding buildings located in registered historic districts and certified as being of historic significance. The easement must preserve the building's entire exterior and prohibit any change that is inconsistent with the exterior's historical character. Both the donor and donee must certify in writing that the donee: (1) is a qualified organization whose purpose is environmental protection, land conservation, or open space or historic preservation and (2) has the resources and a commitment to manage and enforce the restriction. The donor's return must include: (1) a qualified appraisal of the property interest (¶ 1071); (2) photographs of the building's entire exterior; and (3) a description of all restrictions on the building's development (Code Sec. 170(h)(4)(B)). Taxpayers who seek deductions over $10,000 for such contributions must submit a statutory $500 filing fee with their return (Code Sec. 170(f)(13)).

1064. Care of Unrelated Student in the Home. Charitable contributions include unreimbursed amounts spent to maintain a full-time elementary or high school student, who is *not* a dependent or relative, in the taxpayer's home under a written agreement with a program sponsored by a charitable organization providing educational opportunities for students. The deduction is limited to actual expenditures, up to $50 per month,

---

References are to Standard Federal Tax Reports; Tax Research Consultant; and Practical Tax Explanations.

[122] ¶ 11,600, ¶ 11,651; INDIV: 51,350; § 7,550.05—§ 7,550.20   [123] ¶ 11,600; INDIV: 51,354; § 7,550.15b   [124] ¶ 11,600; INDIV: 51,364; § 7,550.20

while the student is a member of the taxpayer's household. Dependent is defined at Code Sec. 152 (¶ 137), but without regard to whether the dependent claims dependency exemptions, files a joint return or has gross income in excess of the exemption amount (Code Sec. 170(g); Reg. § 1.170A-2).[125]

1065. Reduction for Interest. If a liability is assumed by the recipient or by any other person, or if the contributed property is subject to a liability, the contribution must be reduced by the interest paid by the taxpayer-donor, whether prepaid or to be paid in the future, attributable to any period after the contribution. If the gift is a bond, note, or other evidence of indebtedness, the amount of the contribution is further reduced by the interest that is paid or to be paid by the taxpayer-donor on indebtedness incurred or continued to purchase or carry such bond that is attributable to any period prior to the contribution (Code Sec. 170(f)(5); Reg. § 1.170A-3).[126]

1066. Contribution by Partnership. Although a partnership cannot claim a charitable deduction in figuring its taxable income, each partner is allowed a deduction for the partner's distributive share of the partnership's charitable contribution (¶ 417) (Code Secs. 702(a) and 703(a); Reg. § 1.702-1(a)).[127] See ¶ 1061 for special rules regarding partnership donations of clothing and household items.

1068. Denial of Deduction. A contribution is *not* deductible unless it is made to, or for the use of, an organization that qualifies as one of the types described at ¶ 1061. Contributions made directly to an individual or to groups of individuals are *not* deductible, including those made directly to individuals in the military.[128] Gifts to private schools and organizations, including churches, that practice racial discrimination in their admissions policies are not deductible (Rev. Rul. 75-231).

If a taxpayer makes a gift to a private foundation or a nonexempt trust, i.e., an annuity trust or unitrust, a deduction will be allowed only if the governing instrument specifically prohibits income accumulations and certain conflict-of-interest activities (¶ 635 and ¶ 644) (Code Sec. 508(d)).[129] The IRS has issued sample acceptable governing instrument clauses (Rev. Rul. 70-270). Many states have enacted statutes that accomplish the required governing instrument adjustments, and the IRS has published a list of those that satisfy the Code requirements (¶ 538 and ¶ 631) (Rev. Rul. 75-38).

An organization formed after October 9, 1969, and claiming exemption under Code Sec. 501(c)(3) (¶ 1061) must file notice of intent to be exempt (¶ 623), the exemption being retroactive to the date of organization only if the notice was timely. Contributions to such an organization are deductible only if the notice is filed. Contributions made to a late-filing organization are not deductible if made before the date of filing (Code Secs. 170(f)(1) and 508(d); Reg. § 1.508-1 and 1.508-2).[130] The IRS periodically updates and publishes a cumulative list of eligible organizations which may be searched on the IRS website, at http://www.irs.gov/Charities-&-Non-Profits/Exempt-Organizations-Select-Check (Rev. Proc. 2011-33).

Deductions are disallowed for contributions by a "substantial contributor" (¶ 635) to a foundation in a tax year in which there is an action resulting in a termination tax (¶ 649) (Code Secs. 170(f)(1) and 508(d); Reg. §§ 1.508-1 and 1.508-2).[131] Deductions are also denied for contributions made in connection with church-related tax avoidance schemes, i.e., the "donation" of assets to a personal "church" that effectively redistributes them to the donor. Deficiencies arising from the denial of deduction based on these schemes usually result in assessment of interest and penalties.[132]

1069. Gift of Future Interest in Tangible Personal Property. When a taxpayer transfers to a charitable organization a future interest in tangible personal property, such as a painting, manuscript, sculpture, or other art object, a charitable contribution deduction is *not* allowed until all intervening interests in, and rights to, the actual

---

References are to Standard Federal Tax Reports; Tax Research Consultant; and Practical Tax Explanations.

[125] ¶ 11,600, ¶ 11,621; INDIV: 51,120; § 7,535
[126] ¶ 11,600, ¶ 11,631; INDIV: 51,160
[127] ¶ 25,080, ¶ 25,081, ¶ 25,100; PART: 18,054; § 30,405

[128] ¶ 11,620.111; INDIV: 51,120; § 7,520.05
[129] ¶ 22,790; INDIV: 51,118
[130] ¶ 11,600, ¶ 22,790, ¶ 22,791, ¶ 22,792; INDIV: 51,100

[131] ¶ 11,600, ¶ 22,790, ¶ 22,791, ¶ 22,792; INDIV: 51,118
[132] ¶ 39,651G.225; INDIV: 51,118

possession or enjoyment of the property have expired or are held by persons other than the taxpayer, related taxpayers and controlled partnerships (Code Sec. 170(a)(3); Reg. § 1.170A-5).[133]

1070. Transfer in Trust. No deduction is allowed for the value of a contribution of a remainder interest that the donor transfers in trust unless the trust is a pooled income fund (¶ 593), a charitable remainder annuity trust, or a charitable remainder unitrust (¶ 590). If the donor gives *all* the interests in a trust to charity, however, a deduction is allowable (Code Sec. 170(f)(2); Reg. § 1.170A-6).[134]

1070A. Reporting, Recordkeeping and Substantiation. Taxpayers report their charitable contributions by entering the total amount contributed on Schedule A of Form 1040, but written records are required to substantiate the deductions.

Cash Donations. No deduction will be allowed for contributions of cash, checks or other monetary gifts, *regardless of the amount,* unless the donor maintains either: (1) a bank record, including a cancelled check, a bank or credit union statement, or a credit card statement; or (2) a receipt, letter, or other written communication from the donee, indicating the donee's name and the contribution date and amount (Code Sec. 170(f)(17); IRS Pub. 526).[135]

Payroll Deductions. For charitable contributions made by payroll deduction, the taxpayer must retain: (1) a pay stub, Form W-2 or other employer-furnished document indicating the amount withheld for payment to the donee organization; and (2) a pledge card or other document prepared by the donee organization, or at its direction, showing the donee's name. For contributions of $250 or more, the pledge card or other document must also include a statement that the donee does not provide goods or services in whole or partial consideration for any contributions made to it by payroll deduction; these requirements are in addition to those for contributions of $250 or more (see *Contributions of $250 or More,* following) (Notice 2006-110).

Lump-Sum Donations Through CFC. To substantiate a lump-sum charitable contribution made through the Combined Federal Campaign (CFC) or similar programs, e.g., the United Way campaigns, which distribute the amounts received to one or more qualified organizations (¶ 1061), the CFC organization must provide the donor with a written communication that includes the name of the donee organization that is the ultimate recipient of the contribution. This requirement is in addition to those for contributions of $250 or more (see *Contributions of $250 or More,* following) (Notice 2008-16).

Noncash Donations of Less than $250. For each noncash donation for which a deduction of less than $250 is claimed, the taxpayer generally must maintain a receipt from the donee, e.g., a letter or other written communication, indicating the donee's name, the date and location of the donation, and a detailed description, but not the value, of the donated property. If it would be impracticable to obtain a receipt, the donor must maintain reliable written records regarding each item contributed (Reg. § 1.170A-13(b)).[136]

Contributions of $250 or More. Charitable contributions of $250 or more must be substantiated by a contemporaneous written acknowledgment from the donee organization unless the donee files a return with the IRS reporting the information that would be included in the written acknowledgment. Generally, the acknowledgment must include: (1) the amount of cash contributed, and a description of any property contributed; (2) a description and good-faith estimate of the value of any goods or services with more than insubstantial value received in exchange for the contributions; and (3) if the donee provides any intangible religious benefits, a statement to that effect (Code Sec. 170(f)(8); Reg. § 1.170A-13(f)).[137]

References are to Standard Federal Tax Reports; Tax Research Consultant; and Practical Tax Explanations.

[133] ¶ 11,600, ¶ 11,634; INDIV: 51,350; § 7,560

[134] ¶ 11,600, ¶ 11,635; INDIV: 51,350; § 7,555.05, § 7,555.20

[135] ¶ 11,600; INDIV: 51,454; § 7,600.10a

[136] ¶ 11,685; INDIV: 51,454, INDIV: 51,456; § 7,600.05, § 7,600.10

[137] ¶ 11,600, ¶ 11,685; INDIV: 51,454; § 7,600.15

   Noncash Donations of More than $500. For property contributions for which a deduction of more than $500 is claimed, the taxpayer, other than a C corporation that is not a personal service corporation or closely-held C corporation, must include with its return for the tax year of the contribution a written description of the donated property and any other required information as the IRS may prescribe by regulation. If the documentation requirement is not met, the deduction will be denied unless the failure is due to reasonable cause and not to willful neglect. To determine the $500 threshold, all similar items of property donated to one or more donees are treated as a single item of property (Code Sec. 170(f)(11)).[138] Noncash contributions over $500 (over $5,000 for C corporations other than closely-held or personal service corporations) must be described in Section A of Form 8283, which is attached to the taxpayer's return. A noncash contribution that exceeds $5,000 must also be appraised and described in Section B of Form 8283 (¶ 1071) (Reg. § 1.170A-13(c)).[139]

   Donations of Clothing or Household Items. Donations of clothing or household items that are *not* in good used condition or better are allowed only if a deduction of more than $500 is claimed for a single item and a qualified appraisal (¶ 1071) for that item is attached to the return (¶ 1061).

   Vehicle Donations. Taxpayers donating to a charity a qualified vehicle, e.g., car, truck, boat, or aircraft, valued at over $500 must obtain from the charity and attach to his or her return either a Form 1098-C or a similar contemporaneous written acknowledgment of the contribution. The acknowledgment must identify the donor taxpayer, list the taxpayer's and the vehicle's identification numbers, and include a description and good faith estimate of the value of any goods or services provided by the charity in exchange for the vehicle. If the goods or services consist solely of intangible religious benefits, the acknowledgment must say so. If the charity sells the vehicle without significant intervening use or material improvement, the acknowledgment must also certify that the vehicle was sold in an arm's length transaction between unrelated parties, list the gross proceeds, and state that the deduction may not exceed the gross proceeds. If the charity retains the vehicle for its significant use or makes a material improvement, the acknowledgment must certify the use or improvement, the time frame the charity will use the vehicle, and that the vehicle will not be transferred before the use or improvement is completed. The taxpayer is then allowed to claim the fair market value of the vehicle as a charitable donation (Code Sec. 170(f)(12); Notice 2005-44; Notice 2006-1).[140]

   If the charity sells the vehicle to a needy individual at a price significantly below fair market value, or gratuitously transfers the vehicle, the taxpayer can claim the donated vehicle's fair market value only if the sale or transfer directly furthers the charity's purpose. However, if a charity sells the vehicle at auction, the IRS will not accept as substantiation an acknowledgment stating that the vehicle is to be transferred to a needy individual for significantly below fair market value. In that case, the donor taxpayer may claim a deduction greater than $500, but only to the extent that the gross sale proceeds exceed that amount and the donor substantiates the contribution with an acknowledgment listing the gross proceeds (Notice 2007-70, modifying Notice 2006-1).

   Qualified Conservation Contributions (QCCs). Documentation and certification requirements must be met for certain QCCs of facade easements (¶ 1063).

   Philippines Typhoon Relief. Individuals may elect to take a charitable deduction on their 2013 income tax return for contributions made after March 25, 2014, and before April 15, 2014, to qualified charities that provide relief to victims in areas affected by Typhoon Haiyan, which struck the Philippines on November 8, 2013 (Act Sec. 2 of the Philippines Charitable Giving Assistance Act (P.L. 113-92)). Taxpayers can deduct these contributions on either their 2013 or 2014 returns, but not both. Contributions may be made by cash, check, money order, credit card, charge card, debit card, or via text message. For donations by text message, the recordkeeping requirements can be met by a telephone bill showing the name of the donee organization, the date of the contribution and the contribution amount.

References are to Standard Federal Tax Reports; Tax Research Consultant; and Practical Tax Explanations.

[138] ¶ 11,600; INDIV: 51,456.15; § 7,600.10b

[139] ¶ 11,685; INDIV: 51,456.20; § 7,600.10b, § 7,600.25

[140] 11,600; INDIV: 51,152, INDIV: 51,460; § 7,590.05, § 7,590.15

1071. Appraisals for Noncash Contributions. A charitable deduction will be denied to any taxpayer for certain noncash contributions that fail to meet specific appraisal requirements. See ¶ 1070A for documentation requirements. An exception exists if the failure is due to reasonable cause and not to willful neglect. For purposes of determining the threshold dollar amounts for the reporting requirements (as described following), all similar items of noncash property, whether donated to a single donee or multiple donees, are aggregated and treated as a single property donation. For partnerships and S corporations, the requirements are applied at the entity level, but if the entities fail to meet the requirements, denial of the deduction will be made at the partner or shareholder level (Code Sec. 170(f)(11)).[141]

If a deduction of more than $5,000 is being claimed for a noncash donation, the taxpayer, including a C corporation, must:

- obtain a qualified appraisal of the property, and
- attach Form 8283 to its return for the tax year in which the donation is made; if a deduction of $500,000 or more is being claimed, the qualified appraisal itself must be attached to the return when filed.

These substantiation requirements do *not* apply to donations of:

- cash;
- patents and other intellectual property (¶ 1062);
- publicly-traded securities for which market quotations are readily available on an established securities market;
- inventory or property held by the taxpayer primarily for sale to customers in the ordinary course of his trade or business (¶ 1741); or
- a qualified vehicle sold by the donee organization without any significant intervening use or material improvement and for which an acknowledgment is provided (¶ 1070A).

A qualified appraisal is an appraisal prepared according to regulations or other IRS guidance, and conducted by a qualified appraiser under generally-accepted appraisal standards and other IRS guidance. A qualified appraiser must have either earned an appraisal designation from a recognized professional organization or otherwise meet minimum requirements, must regularly perform appraisals for pay, and must meet any other requirements prescribed by the IRS. A qualified appraiser must also demonstrate verifiable education and experience in valuing the type of property being appraised, and must not have been prohibited from practicing before the IRS during the three-year period ending on the appraisal date (Code Sec. 170(f)(11)(E); Reg. § 1.170A-13(c); Notice 2006-96).[142]

An appraisal summary, made on Section B of Form 8283, must be attached to the tax return on which the deduction of more than $5,000 is first claimed. Appraisals are also required if a taxpayer donates a number of similar items, whether or not to the same donee, such as stamps or coins, with a total value in excess of $5,000. For donations of publicly traded securities for which market quotations are *not* readily available on an established securities market, a partially completed appraisal summary is required if the claimed value exceeds $5,000. The appraisal summary only needs to be partially completed for nonpublicly traded stock with a claimed value between $5,000 and $10,000 (Reg. § 1.170A-13(c)).[143] The qualified appraisal requirement is waived for closely held and personal service corporations that contribute inventory, stock in trade, or other property normally held for sale in its business for the ill, needy, or infants (Notice 89-56).

Appraisal fees incurred by an individual in determining the fair market value of donated property are not treated as part of the charitable contribution, but they may be claimed as a miscellaneous deduction on Schedule A of Form 1040 (Rev. Rul. 67-461).

References are to Standard Federal Tax Reports; Tax Research Consultant; and Practical Tax Explanations.

[141] ¶ 11,600; INDIV: 51,456.20, INDIV: 51,458; § 7,600.25

[142] ¶ 11,600, ¶ 11,685; INDIV: 51,458.05, INDIV: 51,458.15; § 7,600.25

[143] ¶ 11,685; INDIV: 51,458.10; § 7,600.25b

Accuracy-Related Penalties. Appraisers are subject to civil penalties for certain appraisals that result in substantial or gross valuation misstatements (Code Sec. 6695A).[144]

Moving Expense

1073. Moving Expense Deduction. Employees and self-employed individuals may deduct as an adjustment to gross income (an above-the-line deduction) the reasonable expenses of moving themselves and their families if the move is related to starting work in a new location (Code Sec. 217).[145] The deduction is computed on Form 3903 and reported on Form 1040.

Deductible moving expenses are limited to the cost of (1) transportation of household goods and personal effects and (2) travel to the new residence, including lodging but not meals (Code Sec. 217(b)).[146] Where an automobile is used in making the move, a taxpayer may deduct either: (1) the actual out-of-pocket expenses incurred, i.e., gasoline and oil, but not repairs, depreciation, etc., or (2) a standard mileage allowance of 23.5 cents per mile plus parking fees and tolls for 2014 (Rev. Proc. 2010-51; Notice 2013-80).[147]

1075. Eligibility for Deduction. To deduct moving expenses (¶ 1073), a taxpayer must meet a distance test, a length-of-employment test and a commencement-of-work test. The new principal place of work must be at least 50 miles farther from the taxpayer's old residence than the old residence was from the taxpayer's old place of work. If there was no old place of work, the new place of work must be at least 50 miles from the old residence (Code Sec. 217(c)).[148]

During the 12-month period immediately following the move, the taxpayer must be employed full time for at least 39 weeks. A self-employed taxpayer must be employed or performing services full time for at least 78 weeks of the 24-month period immediately following the move and at least 39 weeks during the first 12 months. The full-time work requirement is waived, however, due to death, disability, involuntary separation from work, other than for willful misconduct, or transfer to another location for the benefit of the employer (Code Secs. 217(c) and (d)).

In general, the move must be in connection with the commencement of work at the new location and the moving expenses must be incurred within one year from the time the taxpayer first reports to the new job or business. If the move is not made within one year, the expenses ordinarily will not be deductible unless it can be shown that circumstances prevented the taxpayer from incurring the expenses within that period (Reg. § 1.217-2(a)(3)).[149]

An eligible taxpayer is permitted to deduct moving expenses even though the 39- or 78-week employment requirement has not been satisfied by the due date for the return including extensions for the tax year in which the moving expenses were incurred and paid. A taxpayer who fails to meet the requirements, however, must either file an amended return or include as gross income on the next year's return the amount previously claimed as expenses (Code Sec. 217(d); Reg. § 1.217-2(d)(3)).[150]

An individual who retires from an overseas job may deduct moving expenses incurred in returning to the United States. A surviving spouse or dependent who shared the residence of a decedent who worked outside the U.S. at the time of death may also deduct moving expenses incurred in returning to the U.S. within six months after the death (Code Sec. 217(i)).[151]

References are to Standard Federal Tax Reports; Tax Research Consultant; and Practical Tax Explanations.

[144] ¶ 39,971; PENALTY: 3,334; § 7,600.25

[145] ¶ 12,620; INDIV: 39,104; § 5,101

[146] ¶ 12,620; INDIV: 39,106.05; § 5,105.05

[147] ¶ 12,623.11; INDIV: 39,106.10; § 5,105.15

[148] ¶ 12,620; INDIV: 39,120; § 5,120.10

[149] ¶ 12,622; INDIV: 39,108; § 5,115

[150] ¶ 12,620, ¶ 12,622; INDIV: 39,120.20; § 5,120.15, § 5,125

[151] ¶ 12,620; INDIV: 39,124; § 5,101

1076. Reimbursement by Employer. Gross income does not include qualified moving expense reimbursements, which are amounts received directly or indirectly by an individual employee from an employer as a payment for or reimbursement of expenses that would be deductible as a moving expense if directly paid or incurred by the employee (¶ 2092) (Code Sec. 132(a)(6) and (g)).[152] Any amount, other than a qualified reimbursement, received or accrued, directly or indirectly, from the employer as a payment for or reimbursement of moving expenses must be included in the employee's gross income as compensation for services (Code Sec. 82)[153] and is considered wages subject to withholding (Code Sec. 3401(a)(15); Reg. § 31.3401(a)(15)-1).[154]

1077. Foreign Moves. The rules governing moving expenses incurred in connection with the commencement of work outside the U.S. and its possessions are similar to those discussed in ¶ 1073 and ¶ 1075. However, a deduction is also allowed for reasonable expenses of moving household goods and personal effects to and from storage, and of storing them while the new place of work abroad is the taxpayer's principal place of work (Code Sec. 217(h)).[155]

1078. Moves of Armed Forces Members. Gross income does not include moving and storage expenses that are furnished in kind by the military or cash reimbursements or allowances to the extent of expenses actually paid or incurred incident to a permanent change of station for a member of the U.S. Armed Forces on active duty. These expenses need not be reported and such moves are exempt from the time and mileage requirements (¶ 1075). An income exclusion is also provided for moving and storage expenses incurred by the spouse or dependents of such an Armed Forces member, even if they do not reside with the member either before or after the move (Code Sec. 217(g)). Reimbursements in excess of actual expenses are includible in the member's income as wages, while expenses in excess of reimbursements are deductible (Reg. § 1.217-2(g)(2)(ii)).[156]

Dues, Education, and Other Expenses

1080. Union Dues. Union dues, initiation fees and out-of-work-benefit assessments are deductible as an itemized deduction on Schedule A of Form 1040, subject to the two-percent-of-adjusted-gross-income (AGI) floor (¶ 1011) (Reg. § 1.162-15(c)).[157] The self-employed may deduct union dues as a business expense (¶ 1005).

1081. Job-Hunting Expenses. Individuals may deduct all expenses incurred in seeking employment in the *same* trade or business regardless of whether or not the search is successful. Such expenses include the typing, printing, and mailing of resumes, and travel and transportation expenses. Travel and transportation expenses to and from an area are deductible only if the trip relates primarily to seeking new employment. If the travel is primarily personal in nature, only the actual expenses of the search at the destination are deductible.[158]

Expenses are not deductible if an individual is seeking employment in a *new* trade or business even where employment is secured. Individuals cannot deduct job-hunting expenses if they are seeking their first job, entering a new trade or business, or if there is a substantial lack of continuity between the time of their past employment and the seeking of new employment.

Job-hunting expenses are deductible only as an itemized deduction on Schedule A of Form 1040, subject to the two-percent-of-adjusted-gross-income (AGI) floor (¶ 1011).

References are to Standard Federal Tax Reports; Tax Research Consultant; and Practical Tax Explanations.

[152] ¶ 7420; INDIV: 39,130; § 5,130

[153] ¶ 6374; INDIV: 39,130; § 5,130

[154] ¶ 33,502, ¶ 33,528; COMPEN: 33,116; § 5,130, § 22,110.10p

[155] ¶ 12,620; INDIV: 39,126; § 5,101

[156] ¶ 12,620, ¶ 12,622; INDIV: 39,122; § 5,135

[157] ¶ 8852, ¶ 8853.20; INDIV: 36,302; § 7,105.35

[158] ¶ 8524.25; INDIV: 36,250; § 7,105.15

1082. Education and Related Expenses. There are several types of deductions for education expenses. One of these tax benefits is that interest paid during the tax year on any qualified education loan is deductible as an adjustment to gross income, i.e., an above-the-line deduction, on Form 1040 or 1040A (Code Sec. 221).[159] The debt must be incurred by the taxpayer solely to pay qualified higher education expenses. The maximum deductible amount of interest is $2,500, but the amount of any deduction is reduced by an amount, but not below zero, that equals the otherwise allowable deduction times a fraction, the numerator being the excess of modified adjusted gross income (MAGI) over $50,000 ($100,000 for joint filers), which is annually adjusted for inflation, and the denominator being $15,000 ($30,000 for joint filers). For 2014, the maximum deduction is reduced when MAGI exceeds $65,000 ($130,000 for joint returns) and is completely eliminated when MAGI is $80,000 ($160,000 for joint returns) (Rev. Proc. 2013-35). For 2015, the maximum deduction is reduced when MAGI exceeds $65,000 ($130,000 for joint returns) and is completely eliminated when MAGI is $80,000 ($160,000 for joint returns) (Rev. Proc. 2014-61).

For tax years beginning before January 1, 2014, a taxpayer was able to take an adjustment to income (i.e., an above-the-line deduction) for qualifying tuition and related expenses for enrollment or attendance by the taxpayer, the taxpayer's spouse or dependent at any accredited post-secondary institution. The deductible amount was based on the taxpayer's adjusted gross income (AGI). The maximum deductible amount for tax years beginning after December 31, 2003, and before January 1, 2014, was $4,000 for taxpayers with AGI of $65,000 or less ($130,000 for joint filers) and $2,000 for taxpayers with AGI above $65,000 but less than or equal to $80,000 ($130,000 and $160,000, respectively, for joint filers). No deduction was available to taxpayers with AGI above $80,000 ($160,000 for joint filers) (Code Sec. 222).[160]

> **Comment:** Absent further legislation, the qualifying tuition and fees deduction has expired for tax years beginning after December 31, 2013. For the latest legislative updates, visit our website www.CCHGroup.com/TaxUpdates.

The taxpayer's own education expenses may qualify to be deducted as a business expense, even if they lead to a degree, if the education either: (1) maintains or improves skills *required* in the taxpayer's employment or other trade or business, including refresher courses, current developments courses, or academic or vocational courses, or (2) meets the express *requirements* of the taxpayer's employer, or of laws or regulations, *imposed* for a bona fide business purpose of the employer and as a condition to the taxpayer's retention of an established employment relationship, status, or rate of compensation (Reg. § 1.162-5).[161] Education in excess of the minimum requirement may qualify as education undertaken to maintain or improve the required skills.

Educational expenses that are personal or constitute an inseparable aggregate of personal and capital expenditures are not deductible, even though they may maintain or improve a skill or meet the express requirements of the employer or under law. Nondeductible capital or personal education expenses are those that: (1) are required of the taxpayer in order to meet the minimum educational requirements for qualification in the taxpayer's present employment, trade, or business or (2) qualify the taxpayer for a new trade or business.

The minimum education necessary to qualify for a position or other trade or business is determined from a consideration of such factors as requirements of the employer, laws or regulations, and the standards of the profession, trade, or business involved. The fact that an individual is already performing service in an employment status does not mean he or she has met the minimum educational requirements. However, once an individual has met the minimum requirements in effect when he or she enters the employment, profession, or trade or business, the individual is treated as continuing to meet those requirements even though they have changed. For these individuals, expenses for meeting the new requirements would be deductible.

References are to Standard Federal Tax Reports; Tax Research Consultant; and Practical Tax Explanations.

[159] ¶ 12,692; INDIV: 60,054; § 5,901

[160] ¶ 12,770; INDIV: 60,064; § 5,201, § 5,210

[161] ¶ 8631; INDIV: 60,102; § 7,901

¶1082

A change of duties is not a new trade or business if the new duties and the taxpayer's present employment involve the same general work. Thus, there is no new trade or business when a teacher moves from an elementary to a secondary school, from one subject to another, or from a teaching position to a principal's position (Reg. § 1.162-5(b)(3)).[162]

Unreimbursed expenditures for such items as tuition, books, laboratory fees, dues paid to professional societies, fees paid for professional journals, etc., are deducted by an employee as an itemized deduction, subject to the two-percent of AGI floor (¶ 1011) (Reg. § 1.162-6; IRS Pub. 970).[163] The cost of technical books of relatively permanent value used in connection with professional work is a capital expenditure and must be depreciated (IRS Pub. 946) (¶ 1240).[164]

Travel as a Form of Education. No deduction is allowed for travel as a form of education, such as when a French teacher spends summers in Paris to maintain familiarity with the language (Code Sec. 274(m)(2)).[165] Travel in pursuit of an education, however, may be deductible if the educational expense itself is deductible as a business expense; for example, a French teacher travels to Paris to take otherwise deductible classes that are offered only at the Sorbonne.[166]

1083. Uniforms and Special Clothing. The cost and upkeep of a uniform, including laundering and cleaning, are deductible only if the uniform is required as a condition of employment and is not adaptable to general wear. Uniform expense reimbursements paid under an accountable plan (¶ 943) are not reported on the employee's Form W-2 or included in the employee's income (Reg. § 1.62-2(c)(4)).[167] Costs that exceed the reimbursement are deductible as an itemized deduction, subject to the two-percent-of-adjusted-gross-income (AGI) floor (¶ 1011). Reimbursement made under a nonaccountable plan (¶ 943) must be included in income but may be deducted as an itemized deduction on Schedule A of Form 1040, subject to the two-percent of AGI floor and other limitations (Reg. § 1.62-2(c)(5)). Armed Forces reservists may deduct the unreimbursed cost, less nontaxable uniform allowance, of a uniform required at drills or other functions if they are prohibited from wearing it for regular use (Rev. Rul. 76-453, modifying Rev. Rul. 55-109).

A deduction is allowed for special items required in the employee's work that do not replace items of ordinary clothing, such as special work shoes and gloves, shop caps, and protective clothing.[168]

1084. Teachers' Classroom Expenses. Eligible educators were allowed an above-the-line deduction (an adjustment to gross income) of up to $250 for unreimbursed expenses incurred in connection with books, supplies (other than nonathletic supplies for courses in health or physical education), computer equipment and supplementary materials used in the classroom for tax years before January 1, 2014 (Code Sec. 62(a)(2)(D)).[169] An eligible educator is an individual who, for at least 900 hours during a school year, is a kindergarten through grade 12 teacher, instructor, counselor, principal, or aide in a school that provides elementary or secondary education as determined under state law (Code Sec. 62(d)(1)).

> **Comment:** Absent further legislation, the teacher's classroom expenses deduction has expired for tax years beginning after December 31, 2013. For the latest legislative updates, visit our website www.CCHGroup.com/TaxUpdates.

Production of Income

1085. Nontrade or Nonbusiness Expenses. An individual may deduct ordinary and necessary expenses paid or incurred for the production or collection of income, or for the management, conservation, or maintenance of property held for the production of

---

References are to Standard Federal Tax Reports; Tax Research Consultant; and Practical Tax Explanations.

[162] ¶ 8631; INDIV: 60,118.15; § 7,915.05

[163] ¶ 8633; INDIV: 60,100; § 7,105.10

[164] ¶ 8634.01; INDIV: 60,100; § 45,710.15

[165] ¶ 14,402; INDIV: 60,122; § 7,920.10

[166] ¶ 14,402.018; INDIV: 60,122; § 7,920.10

[167] ¶ 6004; INDIV: 36,200; § 5,310, § 7,105.10, § 7,105.20

[168] ¶ 8524.2658; INDIV: 36,202; § 7,105.20

[169] ¶ 6002; INDIV: 36,364; § 5,325

income, as long as the expenses are proximately related to these purposes and reasonable in amount (Code Sec. 212; Reg. § 1.212-1(d)).[170] The expenses are claimed as an itemized deduction on Schedule A of Form 1040, subject to the two-percent-of-adjusted-gross-income (AGI) floor (¶ 1011). Expenses attributable to property held for rents or royalties are deductible from gross income and are not subject to the two-percent of AGI floor (¶ 1089). No deduction is allowed for interest on indebtedness incurred or continued to purchase or carry obligations earning fully tax-exempt interest or other exempt income (¶ 1970) (Code Sec. 265(a)).[171]

1086. Investor's Expenses. Investment counsel fees, custodian fees, fees for clerical help, office rent, state and local transfer taxes, and similar expenses paid or incurred by individuals in connection with their investments are deductible as itemized deductions on Schedule A of Form 1040, subject to the two-percent-of-adjusted-gross-income (AGI) floor (¶ 1011) (Reg. § 1.212-1(g)),[172] except where they relate to rents and royalties (¶ 1089). A dealer or trader in securities is *not* an investor and may deduct these items as business expenses, subject to the uniform capitalization rules (¶ 990).[173]

1089. Expenses Attributable to Rental or Royalty Property. Ordinary and necessary expenses attributable to property held for the production of rents or royalties may be deducted in determining adjusted gross income (AGI) (Code Sec. 62(a)(4); Temp. Reg. § 1.62-1T(c))[174] even if the property is not actually producing income. These deductions include interest, taxes, depreciation, depletion, losses, etc. (Reg. § 1.212-1).[175]

Property held for the production of royalties includes intangible as well as tangible property. Therefore, depreciation on a patent or copyright may be deducted. Similarly, operating owners, lessees, sublessors, or sublessees, or purchasers of royalty interests can deduct their shares of a depletion allowance on natural resources (¶ 1201 and ¶ 1289).

Expenses must be pro rated if a property is devoted to rental purposes for part of a year and to personal use for the other part. See ¶ 966 for special rules governing the deduction of expenses of rental vacation homes. For the applicability of the at-risk and passive activity rules, see ¶ 1155 and ¶ 1165.

1090. Expenses of Life Tenant or Income Beneficiary. When property is held by one person for life, with the remainder to another person, the deduction for depreciation or depletion is allowed to the life tenant and is computed as if the life tenant were the absolute owner of the property (Reg. §§ 1.167(h)-1 and 1.611-1(c)).[176] After the life tenant's death, the deduction, if any, is allowed to the remainderman. For property held in trust or by an estate, the deduction is apportioned as explained at ¶ 530.

1091. Guardianship Expenses. A deduction is permitted for a reasonable amount paid or incurred for the services of a guardian or committee for a ward or minor and for other ordinary and necessary expenses incurred in connection with the production or collection of income inuring to the ward or minor, or in connection with the management, conservation, or maintenance of income-producing property belonging to the ward or minor (Reg. § 1.212-1(j)).[177] Expenses of a competency proceeding are deductible if the purpose of the proceeding is the management and conservation of income-producing property owned by the taxpayer.[178]

1092. Expenses Connected with the Determination of Tax. Any ordinary and necessary expense incurred in connection with the determination, collection, or refund of any tax is deductible as an itemized deduction on Schedule A of Form 1040, subject to

---

References are to Standard Federal Tax Reports; Tax Research Consultant; and Practical Tax Explanations.

[170] ¶ 12,520, ¶ 12,521; BUSEXP: 12,050; § 7,801, § 7,805, § 7,825

[171] ¶ 14,050; INDIV: 48,552; § 7,845.05

[172] ¶ 12,521; BUSEXP: 12,150; § 7,105.40, § 7,840.05, § 7,840.15

[173] ¶ 8521.1475, ¶ 8521.148; BUSEXP: 12,150; § 7,840.10

[174] ¶ 6002, ¶ 6003; FILEIND: 9,058; § 5,045, § 7,801, § 7,875.05

[175] ¶ 12,521; BUSEXP: 12,158.05; § 7,875.10

[176] ¶ 11,048, ¶ 23,922; DEPR: 15,258; § 5,015, § 11,015.30, § 11,605.15

[177] ¶ 12,521; BUSEXP: 12,210; § 7,801

[178] ¶ 12,523.13, ¶ 12,523.33; BUSEXP: 12,210; § 7,801

10

NONBUSINESS

the two-percent-of-adjusted-income (AGI) floor (¶ 1011) (Code Sec. 212(3)).[179] This includes tax return preparation fees allocable to an individual's Form 1040 and supporting schedules and forms. Form 1040 expenses attributable to a trade or business, including Schedules C, C-EZ, E, and F, however, are deductible from gross income and are *not* itemized deductions (Rev. Rul. 92-29, modifying Rev. Rul. 70-40).

This provision applies to income, estate, gift, property, and other taxes imposed at the federal, state, or local level (Reg. § 1.212-1(l)).[180] Legal expenses incurred in determining tax liability include legal fees paid for obtaining a ruling on a tax question (Rev. Rul. 89-68) and defending against a criminal indictment for tax evasion (Rev. Rul. 68-662). Expenses that pertain to both tax and nontax matters must be allocated and substantiated because only the tax element of the expense is deductible (Rev. Rul. 72-545).

Appraisal fees may be deductible as an expense paid in connection with the determination of income tax liability. Appraisal fees incurred in determining the fair market value of property donated to a charity or to establish the amount of loss are two examples of deductible expenses (Rev. Rul. 58-180; Rev. Rul. 67-461).

Credit or debit card convenience fees charged for electronic payment of federal individual income taxes, including estimated taxes, are deductible as miscellaneous itemized deductions (IRS News Release IR-2009-37).

1093. Legal Expenses. Legal expenses are deductible as miscellaneous itemized deductions on Schedule A of Form 1040, subject to the two-percent-of-adjusted-income (AGI) floor (¶ 1011), if they are paid or incurred for the production of income or for the management, conservation, or maintenance of income-producing property (Reg. § 1.212-1).[181] Legal expenses incurred in defending or perfecting title to property, in the acquisition or disposition of property, or in developing or improving property are *not* deductible and must be capitalized. Legal expenses paid or incurred in recovering investment property and amounts of income includible in gross income are generally deductible. The U.S. Court of Appeals for the Sixth Circuit has ruled, however, that legal expenses incurred in recovering stock are deductible only to the extent that they were allocable to the recovery of interest and dividends (*J.K. Nickell*, CA-6, 87-2 USTC ¶ 9585).

Divorce and Separation. Legal expenses paid by one spouse in resisting the other's monetary demands in connection with a divorce, separation or support decree are generally nondeductible personal expenses (¶ 1003). Legal expenses properly attributable to producing or collecting alimony under a divorce decree, separation agreement or support decree, however, may be deductible as a miscellaneous itemized deduction, subject to the two-percent of AGI floor (¶ 1011) (Reg. § 1.262-1(b)(7)).[182]

1094. Limitation on Investment Interest Deduction. A noncorporate taxpayer may deduct on Form 4952 interest paid on investment indebtedness to the extent of the taxpayer's net investment income (Code Sec. 163(d)).[183] Net investment income is the excess of investment income over investment expenses. The disallowed investment interest can be carried over to a succeeding tax year (Rev. Rul. 95-16).

Interest subject to the investment interest limitation is interest on debt properly allocable to property held for investment, which is generally defined as:

(1) property that produces interest, dividends (including qualified dividends), annuities, or royalties that are not derived in the ordinary course of a trade or business;

(2) property that produces gain or loss not derived in the ordinary course of a trade or business from the sale or exchange of property that either produces item (1) types of income or that is held for investment (but which is not an interest in a passive activity); and

---

References are to Standard Federal Tax Reports; Tax Research Consultant; and Practical Tax Explanations.

[179] ¶ 12,520; FILEIND: 12,050, BUSEXP: 12,064; § 7,835

[180] ¶ 12,521; INDIV: 45,112; § 7,835

[181] ¶ 12,521; BUSEXP: 18,050; § 7,105.45, § 7,855

[182] ¶ 12,523.3273, ¶ 13,601, ¶ 13,603.223; BUSEXP: 12,302; § 7,105.45

[183] ¶ 9102; INDIV: 48,450; § 7,414.05

(3) an interest in a trade or business activity that is not a passive activity and in which the taxpayer did not materially participate (Code Sec. 163(d)(5)(A); IRS Pub. 550).

It does not include qualified residence interest (¶ 1047), interest properly allocable to a rental real estate activity in which the taxpayer actively participates, within the meaning of the passive loss rule (¶ 1181), or interest that is taken into account in computing income or loss from a passive activity (¶ 1167).

Net capital gain from the disposition of investment property is not considered investment income. However, individuals may elect to treat all or any portion of such net capital gain as investment income by paying tax on the elected amounts at their ordinary income rates. The taxpayer may elect similar treatment for qualified dividend income (Code Sec. 163(d)(4)(B); Reg. § 1.163(d)-1).[184] Thus, the taxpayer loses the benefit of the otherwise applicable maximum capital gains tax rate with respect to the elected amount. The election must be made on Form 4952 on or before the due date of the return for the tax year in which the net capital gain or the qualified dividend income is recognized. The election is revocable with the consent of the IRS.

A noncorporate limited partner's distributive share of partnership interest expense incurred in the business of the partnership is subject to the limitation on the deduction of investment interest (Rev. Rul. 2008-12; Rev. Rul. 2008-38).

References are to Standard Federal Tax Reports; Tax Research Consultant; and Practical Tax Explanations.

[184] ¶ 9102; INDIV: 48,450; § 7,414.15

Chapter 11

LOSSES ☐ PASSIVE ACTIVITY LOSSES

Deduction of Losses

1101. Deductible Losses. A taxpayer may generally deduct losses which have not been compensated for by insurance or otherwise (Code Sec. 165(a); Reg. § 1.165-1).[1] In order to be deductible, a loss generally must be evidenced by a closed and completed transaction and fixed by identifiable events during the tax year, such as a sale, foreclosure, or condemnation. However, any loss arising from theft is treated as sustained during the tax year in which the taxpayer discovers the loss (¶ 1123). In addition, a special election exists for determining the year to deduct a loss attributable to a federally declared disaster (¶ 1133). Only a bona fide loss sustained by the taxpayer may be deducted, and the substance of a transaction, not its form, governs whether there is a deductible loss. Thus, a loss deduction may be disallowed for a transaction that lacks economic substance and is entered into solely for tax benefits.

No portion of a loss may be deducted if there is a reasonable prospect of recovery or reimbursement. Similarly, no deduction is generally allowed for a partial loss resulting from the decline in the value of property, except as reflected in inventory. An exception is provided for the deduction of an addition to a bad debt reserve and a charge-off of that part of a debt which is worthless (¶ 1137). A taxpayer may also claim a deduction for losses sustained from the abandonment of property (¶ 1109).

Losses realized by individuals may be deducted only if they are: (1) losses incurred in a trade or business; (2) losses incurred in a transaction entered into for profit; or (3) casualty and theft losses (Code Sec. 165(c); Reg. § 1.165-1(e)).[2] Individuals, as well as S corporations, partnerships, estates, and trusts, may deduct expenses attributable to activities not engaged in for profit only to the extent of the amount of gross income from the activity under the hobby loss rules (¶ 1195). Thus, an individual's personal losses that are not related to a business or profit-making activity may not be deducted unless they are the result of a casualty (¶ 1121) or theft (¶ 1123). In addition, there are a number of other special provisions that further limit an individual's ability to deduct losses, including the at-risk rules (¶ 1155), the passive activity loss rules (¶ 1165), and the related-party rules (¶ 1717).

Amount of Loss. The deduction for a loss cannot exceed the taxpayer's adjusted basis in the property (Code Sec. 165(b); Reg. § 1.165-1(c)).[3] Thus, the basis of the property must be adjusted for expenses, receipts, or losses properly chargeable to capital account, and for depreciation, obsolescence, amortization, and depletion to determine the amount of loss allowable as a deduction (¶ 1604). In addition, adjustments

---

References are to Standard Federal Tax Reports; Tax Research Consultant; and Practical Tax Explanations.

[1] ¶ 9802, ¶ 9803; BUSEXP: 30,100; § 16,905.05

[2] ¶ 9802, ¶ 9803; BUSEXP: 30,150; § 16,901

[3] ¶ 9802, ¶ 9803; BUSEXP: 30,202; § 16,905.15

must be made for any salvage value, as well as any insurance or other compensation received by the taxpayer.

The amount or character of a loss may be limited by a number of other rules. For example, capital losses are permitted to be deducted by a taxpayer but only to the extent allowed under the capital loss limitation rules (¶ 1752) (Code Sec. 165(f); Reg. § 1.165-1(c)(3)).[4] A worthless nonbusiness bad debt is only deductible as a short-term capital loss (¶ 1143). Special rules also apply for losses on small business stock (¶ 1911), losses on worthless securities (¶ 1916), losses on wash sales of securities (¶ 1935), and losses on debt obligations required to be in registered form (¶ 1963).

1103. Loss on Sale of Residence. A loss realized from a sale or exchange of residential property acquired and held as a personal residence is not deductible by an individual. A loss on the sale or exchange of residential property realized at the time it is being rented or otherwise used for income-producing purposes, however, is deductible (Reg. § 1.165-9).[5] If the property is used as the taxpayer's personal residence after having been acquired as income-producing property, then a loss realized on its sale or exchange at the time it is being used as a residence is not deductible. For the basis of residential or converted property, see ¶ 1626.

1105. Demolition Losses. A taxpayer may not deduct losses sustained in the demolition of buildings and their structural components, including certified historic structures. Any amount expended or loss sustained by an owner or lessee on account of the demolition of any structure must be capitalized as part of the basis of the land on which the structure was located (Code Sec. 280B).[6] The IRS has provided a safe harbor for certain structural modifications to a building that are not treated as a demolition and thus, not properly chargeable to the capital account with respect to the land on which the building is located (Rev. Proc. 95-27).[7] While demolition costs are nondeductible, a loss deduction may nonetheless be claimed by a taxpayer when depreciable business property is retired from use in a trade or business or from use in production of income (¶ 1109).

1107. Loss on Foreclosure or Tax Sale. The foreclosure of a mortgage by a judicial sale and disposition of the encumbered real estate is a sale of an asset. If the owner of an equity interest receives less than his or her basis in real estate when it is sold upon foreclosure, his or her investment may represent a deductible loss only if the property was used in a trade or business or a transaction entered into for profit.[8] The character of the loss—capital loss or ordinary loss—depends on the nature of the property foreclosed upon and whether or not it was a capital asset (¶ 1741) or section 1231 property (¶ 1747). The loss occurs when the redemption period expires or in the year the property becomes worthless. If there is no equity of redemption, however, the loss is fixed by the foreclosure sale and not by the decree of foreclosure that ordered the sale.[9] These principles also apply to a sale for delinquent taxes.[10]

If real property is disposed of by reason of foreclosure or similar proceedings, the amount of depreciation subject to recapture (¶ 1779) is determined as if the taxpayer ceased to hold the property on the date the proceedings began (Code Sec. 1250(d)(7)).[11]

1109. Abandonment and Obsolescence Losses. A taxpayer is allowed a deduction for a loss sustained in the abandonment of property used in a trade or business or a transaction entered into for profit. Depreciable property is abandoned when the taxpayer withdraws the property from use, or voluntarily and permanently gives up possession with the intention of ending ownership but without passing it on to someone else (Reg. § 1.167(a)-8(a)).[12] The abandonment loss equals the taxpayer's adjusted basis in the

---

References are to Standard Federal Tax Reports; Tax Research Consultant; and Practical Tax Explanations.

[4] ¶ 9802, ¶ 9803; BUSEXP: 30,102.05; § 16,901

[5] ¶ 10,102; BUSEXP: 30,158; § 16,930

[6] ¶ 14,900; BUSEXP: 39,150; § 16,915

[7] ¶ 14,901.60; BUSEXP: 39,156; § 16,915

[8] ¶ 9805.155, ¶ 10,103.54; BUSEXP: 30,268; § 18,205.20

[9] ¶ 21,817.45, ¶ 21,817.451; BUSEXP: 30,268; § 18,205.20

[10] ¶ 9808.453; BUSEXP: 30,268; § 18,205.20

[11] ¶ 31,000; DEPR: 18,260.15; § 11,710

[12] ¶ 11,020; BUSEXP: 39,104; § 16,910.05, § 16,910.10

abandoned property, less any salvage value, insurance, or other compensation that the taxpayer receives for the loss. An abandonment of property is not treated as a sale or exchange. Thus, an abandonment loss is an ordinary loss—regardless of whether or not the abandoned asset is a capital asset—and is reported on Form 4797 (IRS Pub. 544).

If a nondepreciable asset is abandoned following a sudden termination of its usefulness, an obsolescence loss is allowed in an amount equal to its adjusted basis. An obsolescence loss, in the case of nondepreciable property, is deductible in the tax year in which it is sustained, even though the overt act of abandonment or the loss of title to the property may not occur in that year (Reg. § 1.165-2).[13]

A taxpayer cannot deduct the costs of acquiring and developing creative property, i.e., screenplays, scripts, story outlines, and similar property for film development or production, as an abandonment loss unless the taxpayer establishes either: (1) an intent to abandon the property and an affirmative act of abandonment, or (2) identifiable events which show a closed and completed transaction establishing the property's worthlessness (Rev. Rul. 2004-58).[14] Mere nonuse of an asset does not constitute abandonment, and the treatment of abandonment losses for financial reporting purposes does not control their federal tax treatment. To minimize accounting disputes, the IRS has provided a safe harbor allowing taxpayers to amortize ratably over a 15-year period any creative property costs that have been properly written off by the taxpayer under the generally accepted accounting principles (GAAP) for financial reporting purposes (¶ 1229).

1111. Interest Forfeited on Premature Withdrawals. Interest that was previously earned on a time savings account or deposit with a savings institution and that is later forfeited because of premature withdrawals is deductible by an individual in computing adjusted gross income in the year when the interest is forfeited (Code Sec. 62(a)(9)).[15]

> **Example:** Tom Smith opened a four-year time savings account in January 2013. He was credited with $400 in interest earned for 2013 and reported this income on his 2013 return. He withdrew the funds in October 2014. This premature withdrawal triggered a penalty provision so that he received only $230 of interest for 2013, plus $195 in interest earned on the account for 2014. Thus, Tom has incurred a loss of $170 that should be claimed on his 2014 return. He should also report the $195 in interest earned for 2014 on his 2014 income tax return.

The necessary information is provided on Form 1099-INT. The deduction must be claimed on either Form 1040 or 1040A; no deduction is available on Form 1040EZ.

1113. Gambling Losses. A taxpayer can deduct gambling losses only to the extent of the amount of gambling winnings included in his or her gross income (Code Sec. 165(d); Reg. § 1.165-10).[16] For most taxpayers, deductible gambling losses are reported as miscellaneous itemized deductions not subject to the two-percent-of-adjusted-gross-income floor (¶ 1012). Professional gamblers, however, can deduct losses as an adjustment to gross income. Spouses who file a joint return can combine their gambling winnings and losses.

Casualty and Theft Losses

1121. Casualty Losses. An individual may deduct a loss from nonbusiness property only if it arises from fire, storm, shipwreck, or other casualty, or from theft (Code Sec. 165(c)(3)).[17] Each loss is subject to a $100 floor (¶ 1129), and net losses for the tax year are deductible only to the extent they exceed 10 percent of the taxpayer's adjusted gross income (AGI) (¶ 1131). However, an individual cannot claim a casualty loss deduction for damage to insured property unless a timely insurance claim is filed (Code Sec. 165(h)(5)(E)).[18] For a discussion of how to determine the amount of the deduction

---

References are to Standard Federal Tax Reports; Tax Research Consultant; and Practical Tax Explanations.

[13] ¶ 9901; BUSEXP: 39,102; § 16,910.15

[14] ¶ 9902.27; BUSEXP: 30,104.15; § 16,910.05

[15] ¶ 6002; FILEIND: 9,068; § 5,020

[16] ¶ 9802, ¶ 10,104; BUSEXP: 30,256; § 7,110.20, § 16,940.05

[17] ¶ 9802; INDIV: 54,050; § 7,701

[18] ¶ 9802; INDIV: 54,168; § 7,701

for a casualty loss, see ¶ 1127. Casualty and theft losses are reported on Form 4684. Theft losses are discussed at ¶ 1123.

A casualty loss is generally deductible only for the tax year in which the loss is sustained (¶ 1101) (Reg. § 1.165-7(a)(1)).[19] If the extent of the damage cannot reasonably be ascertained in the year of occurrence, however, the deduction can be taken in a later year when the extent of the damage is known. In addition, a special election exists for determining the year to deduct a loss attributable to a federally declared disaster (¶ 1133).

A casualty is the damage, destruction, or loss of property resulting from an identifiable event due to some sudden, unexpected, or unusual cause (IRS Pub. 547).[20] Examples of casualties include earthquakes, fires (not willfully set), floods, storms, hurricanes, tornados, volcanic eruptions, government-ordered demolition or relocation, mine cave-ins, shipwrecks, sonic booms, terrorist attacks, or vandalism. A casualty also includes damage that is a result of any ordinary automobile accident whether the taxpayer, or someone else driving his or her car, is at fault in a collision, or whether the other driver is at fault (Reg. § 1.165-7(a)(3)).[21] However, if a car accident was caused by the willful act or willful negligence of the taxpayer, or his or her agent, the casualty loss deduction is not allowed.

The damage or loss of property due to progressive deterioration is not considered a casualty and, therefore, is not deductible (IRS Pub. 547).[22] Examples include the weakening of property due to normal weather conditions, losses caused by drought to property not used in a trade or business or for the production of income unless the drought can be characterized as sudden or unusual, the deterioration and damage to a water heater, and damage to trees or other plants by normal infestations of fungi, disease, worms, or similar pests. The IRS takes the position that a casualty loss deduction for termite damage is not permitted because the "suddenness" test is not met, but some courts have allowed the deduction.[23]

A casualty loss is deductible only to the extent it is not compensated for by insurance or otherwise (¶ 1101). However, if there is no limitation on the manner in which money or property received as compensation for damaged property must be used, the amount received is a gift and does not reduce the amount of the taxpayer's casualty loss.[24] If, as the result of insurance or other reimbursement, a taxpayer realizes a gain from a casualty or theft loss, the taxpayer can defer recognition of the gain under the involuntary conversion rules by making an election and purchasing qualifying replacement property within the applicable replacement period (¶ 1713).

A casualty loss incurred with respect to either business or nonbusiness property can result in a net operating loss (NOL) (¶ 1147). The $100 floor and the 10-percent-of-AGI limitation are applied in the nonbusiness situation in determining an NOL.

Corrosive Drywall Damage. The IRS has issued safe harbor guidance for homeowners who have incurred property losses resulting from the effects of corrosive drywall installed in homes between 2001 and 2009 (Rev. Proc. 2010-36). Individuals who pay to repair the damages to their personal residences or household appliances resulting from the corrosive drywall may be able to treat certain unreimbursed amounts paid as a casualty loss in the year of payment.

1123. Theft Losses. A loss from the theft of property that is not compensated for by insurance or otherwise is generally deductible for the tax year in which the taxpayer discovers the loss (Code Sec. 165(e); Reg. § 1.165-8(a)).[25] No deduction may be claimed in the year of discovery, however, if a reimbursement claim exists with respect to which

---

References are to Standard Federal Tax Reports; Tax Research Consultant; and Practical Tax Explanations.

[19] ¶ 10,004; INDIV: 54,250; § 7,705.30

[20] ¶ 10,005.123—¶ 10,005.92; INDIV: 54,052, INDIV: 54,084; § 7,705.05

[21] ¶ 10,004; INDIV: 54,068; § 7,705.05

[22] ¶ 10,005.123—¶ 10,005.92; INDIV: 54,058; § 7,705.05

[23] ¶ 10,005.671; INDIV: 54,062; § 7,705.05

[24] ¶ 10,005.117; INDIV: 54,168; § 7,705.25

[25] ¶ 9802, ¶ 10,100; INDIV: 54,100; § 7,710.05, § 7,710.15

11 | LOSSES

there is a reasonable prospect of recovery (Reg. § 1.165-1(d)(3)).[26] As with casualty losses (¶ 1121), an individual cannot claim a deduction for theft of insured property unless a timely insurance claim is filed (Code Sec. 165(h)(5)(E)).[27] Theft includes the taking of money or property by robbery, larceny, burglary, blackmail, embezzlement, extortion, or kidnapping for ransom. Theft does not include property that was lost or misplaced. It also does not include the decline in value of stock acquired in the open market caused by the disclosure of accounting fraud by officers or directors of the corporation (IRS Pub. 547).[28] The deduction for theft losses is determined in the same way as for other casualty losses (¶ 1127). Casualty and theft losses are reported on Form 4684.

Losses from Ponzi-Type Schemes. Investors who incur losses from criminally fraudulent investment arrangements such as "Ponzi" schemes are entitled to claim a theft loss, rather than a capital loss (Rev. Rul. 2009-9).[29] The loss is deductible as a loss on a transaction entered into for profit, and it is not subject to the $100 floor (¶ 1129) or the 10-percent-of-adjusted-gross-income (AGI) limitation (¶ 1131) for personal theft losses, or the limitations on itemized deductions (¶ 1011 and ¶ 1014). The theft loss is deductible in the year it is discovered, and the amount of the deduction includes the amount invested in the scheme, less any amounts withdrawn, reimbursements, and claims as to which there is a reasonable prospect of recovery. If the theft loss deduction creates or increases a net operating loss (NOL) in the year the loss is deducted, the taxpayer may carry back up to three years and forward up to 20 years the portion of the NOL attributable to the theft loss (¶ 1149).

The IRS has also provided an optional safe harbor under which a qualified investor may deduct as a theft loss up to 95 percent of a qualified investment if the investor does not pursue any potential third-party recovery, or 75 percent of a qualified investment if the investor is pursuing or intends to pursue any potential third-party recovery. The deduction is reduced by the amount of any actual recovery and any recovery from insurance or the Securities Investor Protection Corporation (Rev. Proc. 2009-20, as modified by Rev. Proc. 2011-58).

1125. Loss on Bank Deposits. An individual may elect to treat the loss on a nonbusiness account in an insolvent or bankrupt financial institution as a personal casualty loss in the year in which the loss can reasonably be estimated (Code Sec. 165(l)).[30] If elected, the casualty loss deduction is subject to a $100 floor (¶ 1129) and the 10-percent-of-adjusted-gross-income (AGI) limitation (¶ 1131). The election is made on Form 4684.

Alternatively, an individual can elect to treat the loss as an ordinary loss arising from a transaction entered into for profit in the year the loss can be reasonably estimated, provided that no portion of the deposit is federally insured. The maximum amount that a taxpayer may claim as ordinary loss in any tax year is limited to $20,000 ($10,000 in the case of a married individual filing separately) for each financial institution, reduced by the amount of insurance proceeds that the taxpayer can reasonably expect to receive under state law (Code Sec. 165(l)(5)). The loss is deducted on Schedule A of Form 1040 as a miscellaneous itemized deduction subject to the two-percent-of-AGI limit (¶ 1011). The name of the financial institution and "Insolvent Financial Institution" should be written on the appropriate line of Schedule A. The calculation of the deducted loss should be included with the return (IRS Pub. 529).

Once made, either election applies to all losses on deposits in the financial institution during the tax year and it is revocable only with IRS consent. A taxpayer making either election is prohibited from deducting the loss as a bad debt deduction (Code Sec. 165(l)(6) and (7)). The elections cannot be made by an individual who is an owner of one percent or more of the value of the institution's stock, an officer of the institution, or

---

References are to Standard Federal Tax Reports; Tax Research Consultant; and Practical Tax Explanations.

[26] ¶ 9803; BUSEXP: 30,110; § 7,710.25

[27] ¶ 9802; INDIV: 54,168; § 7,701

[28] ¶ 10,101.237, ¶ 10,101.318; INDIV: 54,102; § 7,710.05, § 7,710.10

[29] ¶ 10,101.123; INDIV: 54,106.10; § 7,710.30

[30] ¶ 9802; INDIV: 54,082; § 7,105.55, § 7,705.10

a relative of an owner or officer (Code Sec. 165(l)(2)). If neither election is made, then the loss is treated as a nonbusiness bad debt in the year of final determination of the actual loss and is reported as a short-term capital loss on Form 8949 (¶ 1143 and ¶ 1752).

1127. Amount of Casualty or Theft Loss. The amount of a casualty loss (¶ 1121) which is deductible for business and income-producing property or nonbusiness property is the *lesser* of:

(1) the fair market value (FMV) of the property immediately before the casualty reduced by its FMV immediately after the casualty, or

(2) the adjusted basis of the property immediately before the casualty (Reg. § 1.165-7(b)).[31]

If business or income-producing property is totally destroyed, however, and the property's FMV immediately before the casualty is less than its adjusted basis, then the casualty loss is the adjusted basis of the property.

The amount of a theft loss (¶ 1123) which is deductible is the fair market value or the adjusted basis of the property stolen (Reg. § 1.165-8(c)).[32] When money is stolen, the theft loss is the amount stolen. The amount of a theft loss in the case of nonbusiness property other than money is the lesser of the value of the property or its adjusted basis. In the case of stolen business or income-producing property, the theft loss is the adjusted basis of the property stolen.

A personal casualty or theft loss is subject to a $100 floor (¶ 1129) and a 10-percent-of-adjusted-gross-income (AGI) limit (¶ 1131) in determining the allowable deduction. The $100 floor and AGI limit do not apply to a business or income-producing property casualty or theft loss.

A casualty or theft loss is reduced by any insurance or other compensation received by the taxpayer, and in the case of a casualty loss, it is also reduced by any salvage value (¶ 1101). An individual cannot claim a personal casualty or theft loss to the extent the loss is covered by insurance, unless a timely insurance claim is filed with respect to the loss (¶ 1121 and ¶ 1123).

When there is damage to different kinds of business property, losses must be computed separately for each single, identifiable property damaged or destroyed. This rule does not apply to nonbusiness property. Thus, if a tree is blown down in the front yard of a taxpayer's residence, the loss is the difference in the FMV of the taxpayer's whole property before and after damage to the tree (Reg. § 1.165-7(b)).[33]

The taxpayer's basis for property damaged or destroyed by casualty or theft is reduced by the amount allowable as a casualty or theft loss deduction, as well as by the amount of any insurance or other recovery for the loss (Rev. Rul. 71-161).[34]

1129. $100 Floor for Personal Casualty or Theft Losses. The deduction for a personal casualty (¶ 1121) or theft loss (¶ 1123) is limited to the amount that the loss from each casualty or theft exceeds $100 (Code Sec. 165(h)(1); Reg. § 1.165-7(b)(4)).[35] The $100 floor applies separately to the loss from each single casualty or theft, regardless of how many pieces of property are involved in the event. Thus, if several items of nonbusiness property are damaged or stolen in the course of a single casualty or theft, the $100 floor is applied only once against the sum of the allowable losses. In the case of married taxpayers filing a joint return, *only one* $100 floor applies to each casualty or theft loss; it does not matter if the property is owned jointly or separately. If married taxpayers file separate returns, each spouse is subject to the $100 limitation for

---

References are to Standard Federal Tax Reports; Tax Research Consultant; and Practical Tax Explanations.

[31] ¶ 10,004; BUSEXP: 30,212, INDIV: 54,152; § 7,705.10, § 7,705.15

[32] ¶ 10,100; BUSEXP: 30,212, INDIV: 54,152; § 7,705.10, § 7,710.20

[33] ¶ 10,004; BUSEXP: 30,212, INDIV: 54,152; § 7,705.10, § 7,705.15

[34] ¶ 10,005.16; SALES: 6,360.05; § 16,110.25

[35] ¶ 9802, ¶ 10,004; INDIV: 54,202, INDIV: 54,354; § 7,705.15

each casualty or theft loss. When property is used for both business and personal purposes, the $100 floor applies only to the net loss attributable to that portion of the property used for personal purposes.

1131. 10% of AGI Floor for Personal Casualty or Theft Losses. If a taxpayer's personal casualty (¶ 1121) or theft losses (¶ 1123) exceed his or her personal casualty or theft gains for the tax year, the excess generally is deductible only to the extent that it exceeds 10 percent of the taxpayer's adjusted gross income (AGI) for the year (Code Sec. 165(h)(2)).[36] For this purpose, gains and losses from personal casualties and thefts calculated on Form 4684 are netted without regard to holding periods for the initial determination of whether there was a gain or loss. The $100 floor (¶ 1129) is applied to each casualty or theft before this netting occurs. If the recognized gains exceed the recognized losses, the net gain is reported as a capital gain on Schedule D of Form 1040. If the recognized losses exceed the recognized gains after netting, the net loss is deductible as an itemized deduction on Schedule A of Form 1040 but only to the extent it exceeds 10 percent of the taxpayer's AGI.

> **Example 1:** A taxpayer who has AGI of $50,000 (without regard to casualty gains or losses), a $25,000 casualty gain, and a $15,000 casualty loss (after the $100 floor) will report a $10,000 capital gain on Schedule D.

> **Example 2:** A taxpayer who has AGI of $40,000, a $25,000 casualty loss (after the $100 floor), and a $15,000 casualty gain is allowed a $6,000 itemized deduction. The $10,000 loss resulting from netting the casualty gains against the casualty losses is deductible only to the extent that it exceeds 10 percent of AGI ($10,000 – $4,000 = $6,000).

Limitation for Estates and Trusts. The 10-percent-of-AGI limitation on personal casualty and theft losses applies to estates and trusts. AGI is computed in the same manner as it is for individuals, except that estates and trusts are allowed to deduct their administration expenses in arriving at AGI (Code Sec. 165(h)(5)(C)).[37] No deduction for a personal casualty or theft loss may be taken if, at the time of filing a decedent's return, the loss has been claimed for estate tax purposes (¶ 531).

1133. Disaster Loss. A taxpayer that sustains a loss occurring in a disaster area and attributable to a federally declared disaster can either (1) deduct the loss on the tax return for the year in which the loss occurred, or (2) elect to deduct the loss on the return for the preceding tax year (Code Sec. 165(i); Reg. § 1.165-11).[38] The disaster loss deduction is calculated using the same rules as those for any other personal casualty losses (¶ 1127). If, however, the taxpayer elects to claim a disaster loss on the return for the year immediately preceding the loss year, the 10-percent-of-adjusted-gross-income (AGI) limit (¶ 1131) is determined with respect to the preceding year's AGI. In addition, the IRS is authorized to issue guidance allowing the use of an appraisal used to secure a federal loan or loan guarantee as a result of federally declared disaster to establish the disaster loss amount.

The election to deduct a disaster loss in the tax year prior to the loss year is made by filing a return, an amended return, or a refund claim that clearly shows that the election is being made. The election applies to the entire loss sustained by the taxpayer in the disaster area during the disaster period. The election generally must be made by the due date of the tax return for the year of the loss without regard to extensions. For example, the election to deduct a 2014 disaster loss in 2013 must be made on or before April 15, 2015, for a calendar-year individual. A taxpayer may revoke the election within 90 days after it has been made; however, the Tax Court has held that revocation after the 90-day period is valid as long as the time for making the original election has not expired.[39]

References are to Standard Federal Tax Reports; Tax Research Consultant; and Practical Tax Explanations.

[36] ¶ 9802; INDIV: 54,204, IN-DIV: 54,206; § 7,705.15

[37] ¶ 9802; ESTTRST: 12,060.10; § 32,401

[38] ¶ 9802, ¶ 10,200; INDIV: 54,302; § 7,715.10

[39] ¶ 10,201.13; INDIV: 54,304; § 7,715.10

This special disaster loss treatment is also available for a personal residence rendered unsafe by a disaster in an area determined by the President of the United States to warrant federal government assistance if the taxpayer has been ordered by the state or local government within 120 days after the area is declared a disaster area to demolish or relocate the residence (Code Sec. 165(k)).[40] The amount of the deduction is reduced by any partial payments received from the state in the form of disaster aid.

Bad Debts

1135. Business Bad Debts. Business bad debts can generally be deducted from gross income as an ordinary loss when and to the extent that they become totally worthless (Code Sec. 166).[41] If a business bad debt is only partially worthless and is recoverable in part, then the worthless portion is deductible to the extent it is charged off during the tax year (¶ 1137). A business debt is a debt: (1) created or acquired in connection with the trade or business of the taxpayer who is claiming the deduction, or (2) the worthlessness of which has been incurred in the taxpayer's trade or business (Reg. § 1.166-5(b)).[42] If the taxpayer's primary motive for incurring the debt is not business related, then it is a nonbusiness debt and deductible only as a short-term capital loss (¶ 1143).

Only a bona fide debt qualifies for purposes of deducting a bad debt (Reg. § 1.166-1(c)).[43] A debt is considered bona fide if it arises from a true debtor-creditor relationship based on a valid and enforceable obligation to pay a fixed or determinable amount of money. For example, a business bad debt deduction is not available to shareholders who have advanced money to a corporation as a contribution to capital.[44] In addition, the bad debt deduction rules do not apply to a debt that is evidenced by a security (Code Sec. 166(e)).[45] If a security held by a taxpayer, other than a bank, becomes worthless during the tax year, it is treated as sold or exchanged at a loss on the last day of the tax year (¶ 1916). However, the bad debt rules do apply to any loss sustained by a bank resulting from the worthlessness of a security (¶ 2383).

Whether a debt is wholly or partially worthless is a question of fact, requiring consideration of all pertinent evidence, including the debtor's financial condition and the value of any security for the debt (Reg. § 1.166-2).[46] A debt becomes worthless when there is no longer any chance the amount owed will be paid. This can be evidenced (1) by the fact that legal action to enforce payment would result in an uncollectible judgment, or (2) upon a settlement in bankruptcy, although worthlessness may sometimes be determined after bankruptcy and before settlement. It is not necessary for the taxpayer to go to court to demonstrate worthlessness; the taxpayer only has to show that reasonable steps were taken to collect the debt, but he or she was unable to do so (IRS Pub. 535).

Guarantors. A taxpayer is eligible for a business bad debt deduction if in the course of a trade or business, the taxpayer pays an obligation as a guarantor, endorser, or indemnitor (Reg. § 1.166-9).[47] A noncorporate taxpayer is eligible for a nonbusiness bad debt deduction if the taxpayer pays an obligation as a guarantor, endorser, or indemnitor as part of a transaction entered into for profit. In the case of a business bad debt, no deduction is available if the agreement to act as guarantor, endorser, or indemnitor was not made in the course of the taxpayer's trade or business or a transaction for profit, if there is no legal obligation on the taxpayer to make the guaranty payment, or if the agreement was entered into after the debt became worthless.

Employee Loans. An employee's rendering of services for pay is a trade or business for purposes of the bad debt provisions. Therefore, a loan to an employer to protect a job

---

References are to Standard Federal Tax Reports; Tax Research Consultant; and Practical Tax Explanations.

[40] ¶ 9802, INDIV: 54,306; § 7,715.20

[41] ¶ 10,602; BUSEXP: 48,152; § 17,120.05

[42] ¶ 10,691; BUSEXP: 48,156; § 17,120.05

[43] ¶ 10,603; BUSEXP: 48,050; § 17,105

[44] ¶ 10,650.7301; BUSEXP: 48,108; § 17,120.10

[45] ¶ 10,602; BUSEXP: 48,154; § 16,555

[46] ¶ 10,604; BUSEXP: 48,250; § 17,110.05

[47] ¶ 10,753; BUSEXP: 48,400, BUSEXP: 48,402; § 17,125

11

LOSSES

can give rise to a business bad debt deduction if the employer defaults. If a loan by a shareholder-employee is intended to protect the shareholder's job rather than to protect the shareholder's investment in the company, then the failure to repay the loan results in a business bad debt deduction. The larger the shareholder's investment, the smaller his or her salary, and the larger his or her other sources of income, the more likely that a dominant nonbusiness motive exists for making the loan.[48]

1137. Accounting for Bad Debt Deduction. Bad debts are generally deductible in the tax year in which they become worthless (Code Sec. 166(a); Reg. § 1.166-3).[49] For nonbusiness debt (¶ 1143), the deduction is available when the debt becomes wholly worthless. A deduction is allowed for a business debt (¶ 1135) that becomes wholly or partially worthless, but only to the extent the debt is charged off of the taxpayer's books during the tax year. The bad debt deduction is not available for nonbusiness debts that are only partially worthless. A worthless debt arising from unpaid wages, rent, interest, or a similar item is not deductible unless the income that these items represent has been reported for income tax purposes by a taxpayer (Reg. § § 1.166-1(e) and 1.166-6(a)(2)).[50]

Generally, a taxpayer must use the specific charge-off method to claim a deduction for a business bad debt. If a business debt becomes totally worthless during the year, the taxpayer can deduct the entire amount in that year. If a business debt becomes partially worthless during the year, the taxpayer can deduct that amount of the debt charged off his or her books for the year (Reg. § 1.166-3). An exception to the charge-off rule exists for debt which has been significantly modified. Some accrual taxpayers may use the nonaccrual experience method of accounting for bad debts with respect to income to be received from the performance of services (¶ 1538). Small banks and thrift institutions can use the experience method of accounting to deduct bad debts (¶ 2383).

1139. Secured Bad Debt. When secured or mortgaged property is sold either to the secured party or to a third party for less than the amount of the debt, the creditor is entitled to a bad debt deduction (¶ 1135 and ¶ 1143) in an amount equal to the difference between the sale price and the amount of the debt, to the extent that the creditor can show that such difference is wholly or partially uncollectible (Reg. § 1.166-6).[51] No bad debt deduction is allowed if a mortgage is foreclosed and the creditor buys the mortgaged property at a price equal to the unpaid debt. However, loss or gain is realized on the transaction. It is measured by the difference between the amount of the obligations of the debtor that are applied to the purchase or bid price of the property and the fair market value of the property, to the extent that the obligations are capital or represent items the income from which has been returned by the creditor. See ¶ 1838 and ¶ 1841 for a discussion on repossession of property sold on the installment plan.

1141. Debts Owed by Political Parties. No deduction is generally allowable for a worthless debt owed by a political party. However, banks and accrual-basis taxpayers (¶ 1515) who are in the business of providing goods and services (e.g., polling, media, or organizational services) to political campaigns and candidates may deduct such bad debts (Code Sec. 271).[52]

1143. Nonbusiness Bad Debts. If a nonbusiness bad debt held by a taxpayer other than a corporation becomes *totally* worthless during the tax year, then the loss may be deducted as a short-term capital loss regardless of how long the taxpayer held the debt (Code Sec. 166(d); Reg. § 1.166-5).[53] Unlike business bad debts (¶ 1135), however, no deduction is permitted unless and until the debt becomes totally worthless. A nonbusiness bad debt is any debt *other than* one created or acquired in connection with the

---

References are to Standard Federal Tax Reports; Tax Research Consultant; and Practical Tax Explanations.

[48] ¶ 10,700.241; BUSEXP: 48,160.35, BUSEXP: 48,160.40; § 17,120.10

[49] ¶ 10,602, ¶ 10,605; BUSEXP: 48,250; § 17,101, § 17,112

[50] ¶ 10,603, ¶ 10,701; BUSEXP: 48,062, BUSEXP: 48,204; § 17,115

[51] ¶ 10,701; BUSEXP: 48,274, SALES: 6,064.10; § 17,110.10, § 17,115

[52] ¶ 14,306; BUSEXP: 48,068

[53] ¶ 10,602, ¶ 10,691; BUSEXP: 48,152, BUSEXP: 48,250; § 17,120.05

taxpayer's trade or business, or one that, when worthless, creates a loss that is incurred in the taxpayer's trade or business. For limitations on deduction of a capital loss, see ¶ 1752. For worthlessness of a debt evidenced by a bond or other security of a corporation or a government, see ¶ 1916.

Net Operating Losses (NOLs)

1145. Net Operating Loss (NOL). A net operating loss (NOL) from a trade or business may be claimed as a deduction in the current tax year equal to the aggregate amount of NOLs carried back or carried forward from other tax years (¶ 1149) (Code Sec. 172(a); Reg. § 1.172-1).[54] The NOL deduction, however, may not exceed the amount of taxable income for the year of the deduction. An NOL arises in any tax year when the taxpayer's deductible expenses for the year exceed its gross income, subject to certain adjustments (¶ 1147). The NOL deduction is available to most taxpayers, including corporations, individuals, estates and trusts, and participants in common trust funds. An NOL deduction is not claimed by a partnership or S corporation, but partners and S corporation shareholders use their distributive shares of partnership or S corporation income to calculate their individual NOLs (¶ 319 and ¶ 417). An NOL deduction also may not be claimed by regulated investment companies (¶ 2301) and life insurance companies (¶ 2370) (Code Secs. 805(b)(4) and 852(b)(2)(B)).[55]

Noncorporate Taxpayers. Individuals, estates, and trusts may use Form 1045 to claim a quick refund resulting from the *carryback* of an NOL (Code Sec. 6411; Reg. § 1.6411-1).[56] Form 1045 must be filed on or after the date for filing a tax return for the NOL year, but no later than one year after the end of the NOL year (¶ 2773). Form 1045 also contains schedules that can be used to determine the amount of NOL available for carryback or carryover, and the NOL deduction for each carryback year and the amount to be carried over.

As an alternative to Form 1045, an individual may file an amended return on Form 1040X for each carryback year to claim a refund from the *carryback* of an NOL. Form 1040X must generally be filed within three years after the due date of the return for the NOL year. Estates and trusts file an amended Form 1041 for each carryback year and check the "amended return" box. If an amended return is filed, the taxpayer must still attach the NOL computations using the Form 1045 computation schedules.

No special form is used to *carry over* an NOL deduction. If the taxpayer elects to waive the NOL deduction carryback (¶ 1149), however, a statement making the election must be attached to the return or amended return for the tax year. Individuals list an NOL carryover deduction as a negative figure on the "Other Income" line of Form 1040 or Form 1040NR. Estates and trusts include an NOL carryover deduction on Form 1041 with other deductions not subject to the two-percent-of-adjusted-gross-income limit.

Corporations. Corporations may file for a quick refund resulting from the *carryback* of an NOL using Form 1139. The form can be filed on or after the date on which the return for the NOL year is filed, but no later than one year after the end of the NOL year. Alternatively, a corporation may file an amended return on Form 1120X in place of Form 1139 for each carryback year. Form 1120X must be filed within three years of the due date including extensions for filing the return for the NOL year.

A corporation that expects an NOL in the current tax year may file Form 1138 to extend the time for payment of the tax for the immediately preceding tax year (Code Sec. 6164; Reg. § 1.6164-1).[57] The extension applies only to payments of tax that are required to be paid after Form 1138 is filed. The extension expires at the end of the month in which the return for the tax year of the expected NOL is required to be filed including extensions. However, if the corporation files Form 1139 before the extension period ends, the time for payments is further extended until the date that the IRS mails notice that it has allowed or disallowed the application (Reg. § 1.6164-5).[58]

References are to Standard Federal Tax Reports; Tax Research Consultant; and Practical Tax Explanations.

[54] ¶ 12,002, ¶ 12,003; BUSEXP: 45,000, BUSEXP: 45,050; § 17,001

[55] ¶ 25,770, ¶ 26,420; BUSEXP: 45,052

[56] ¶ 38,720, ¶ 38,722; BUSEXP: 45,256.05; § 17,025

[57] ¶ 37,240, ¶ 37,241; BUSEXP: 45,260; § 39,315.10

[58] ¶ 37,247; BUSEXP: 45,260.10; § 39,315.25

1147. Net Operating Loss (NOL) Defined. A net operating loss (NOL) for the tax year is the excess of allowable deductions over gross income, with certain modifications (Code Sec. 172(c); Reg. § 1.172-1).[59] For calculating the NOL, income and deductions from separate businesses are aggregated, and items that are excludable from gross income are generally excluded. The NOL for any tax year is determined under the law applicable to that tax year, without regard to the law applicable to the tax year to which the NOL is carried. A taxpayer with a short tax year cannot annualize an NOL.

Noncorporate Taxpayers. The following adjustments are made in computing the NOL of a noncorporate taxpayer (Code Sec. 172(d); Reg. § 1.172-3):[60]

(1) No deduction for NOL carryovers or carrybacks from other years is allowed.

(2) No deduction is allowed for personal or dependency exemptions.

(3) Nonbusiness capital losses are deductible only to the extent of nonbusiness capital gains determined without regard to the exclusion for gain from qualified small business stock (¶ 1905).

(4) Business capital losses are deductible only to the extent of the sum of (a) business capital gains determined without regard to the exclusion for gain from qualified small business stock, and (b) any nonbusiness capital gains that remain after deducting nonbusiness capital losses and excess nonbusiness deductions (item (5), below).

(5) Nonbusiness deductions are allowed only to the extent of nonbusiness income including net nonbusiness capital gains. Nonbusiness deductions generally include deductions not related to the taxpayer's trade or business, or employment—e.g., alimony, deductions for contributions to a retirement plan, health savings account (HSA) deductions, the standard deduction, and personal itemized deductions. Nonbusiness income generally includes income from passive investments, such as interest, dividends, annuities, as well at the taxpayer's share of nonbusiness income from a partnership or S corporation. The taxpayer's wages and salary are considered income that *is* attributable to the taxpayer's trade or business.

(6) The domestic production activities deduction (¶ 980A) is not allowed.

Corporations. The following adjustments are made in computing the NOL of a corporation (Code Sec. 172(d); Reg. § 1.172-2):[61]

(1) No deduction for NOL carryovers or carrybacks from other years is allowed.

(2) A corporation is entitled to deductions for dividends received from a domestic corporation, received on certain preferred stock of public utilities, received from certain foreign corporations, and paid on certain preferred stock of public utilities, without regard to the limitations, based on taxable income, imposed on such deductions in computing taxable income (¶ 223 and ¶ 231).

(3) The domestic production activities deduction is not allowed.

1149. Carryforward and Carryback of Net Operating Losses (NOLs). If a taxpayer has a net operating loss (NOL) for the current tax year (¶ 1147), then the loss may be carried back to prior tax years or carried forward to future years as a deduction against taxable income (¶ 1145). NOLs can generally be carried back to the two years preceding the loss year and then forward up to 20 years following the loss year (Code Sec. 172(b)(1)).[62] Special carryover periods, however, are available for NOLs attributable to casualties, disasters, farming losses, and certain other activities (¶ 1151). No deduction

---

References are to Standard Federal Tax Reports; Tax Research Consultant; and Practical Tax Explanations.

[59] ¶ 12,002, ¶ 12,003; BUSEXP: 45,100; § 17,005.05

[60] ¶ 12,002, ¶ 12,005; BUSEXP: 45,106; § 17,005.10

[61] ¶ 12,002, ¶ 12,004; BUSEXP: 45,104; § 17,005.15

[62] ¶ 12,002; BUSEXP: 45,150; § 17,010.05

is allowed in the year the loss is incurred. In determining the amount of an NOL carryback or carryover, the law in effect during the year to which the NOL is carried back or carried over is applied (Code Sec. 172(e)).

The NOL is first carried back to the second tax year preceding the loss year, then to the next earliest carryback year, and then forward to tax years after the loss year. If an NOL carryover is not fully absorbed in a carryback or carryover year, then the following adjustments must be made to taxable income in the carryback or carryover year (but not below zero) to determine the portion of the NOL still available to be carried to the next year in the carryback or carryover period (Code Sec. 172(b)(2); Reg. § 1.172-5).[63]

(1) The NOL deduction for the intervening year is computed by taking into account only carryback and carryovers from tax years *preceding* the loss year.

(2) For taxpayers other than corporations, capital losses are deductible only to the extent of capital gains.

(3) Personal and dependency exemptions are not allowed.

(4) The domestic production activities deduction (¶ 980A) is not allowed.

In a year in which an NOL is carried back, any income, deductions, or credits that are based on or limited to a percentage of adjusted gross income (AGI) must be recomputed based on AGI after applying the NOL deduction for the carryback year. The charitable contribution deduction, however, is not recomputed. Taxable income is recomputed taking into account the NOL and the preceding adjustments. Income tax, alternative minimum tax, and any credits that are based on or limited to the amount of tax are then recomputed.

Election to Forgo Carryback. A taxpayer may elect to waive the entire carryback period (Code Sec. 172(b)(3)).[64] If the election is made, the loss may be carried forward only. The election must be made by the return due date including extensions for the tax year of the NOL. The election may also be made on an amended return filed within six months of the due date of an original timely return excluding extensions. Refer to the instructions for Form 1045 or Form 1139 for specific statement requirements. Once made, the election is irrevocable.

Married Taxpayers. If a husband and wife were married and filed a joint return for each year considered in figuring NOL carrybacks and carryovers, their NOL is computed in the same manner as it is for one taxpayer (Reg. § 1.172-7).[65] If a husband and wife were married and filed separate returns for each year considered in figuring NOL carrybacks and carryovers, then each spouse is entitled to his or her own NOLs without regard to the income or deductions of the other spouse. Special rules apply for figuring the NOL carrybacks and carryovers of married people whose filing status changes for any tax year considered in figuring an NOL carryback or carryover.

1151. Special NOL Carryforward and Carryback Periods. A net operating loss (NOL) generally must be carried back to the two years preceding the loss year and then carried forward to the 20 years following the loss year (¶ 1149). Special carryover periods are available, however, for certain types of NOLs.

Casualties and Disasters. A three-year carryback period is available for: (1) an NOL of an individual arising from a fire, storm, shipwreck, other casualty, or theft, and (2) an NOL of a small business or taxpayer engaged in farming if the loss is attributable to a federally declared disaster (Code Sec. 172(b)(1)(F)).[66] A small business is one with an average annual gross receipts of $5 million or less. An eligible loss does not include a farming loss or qualified disaster loss described below.

References are to Standard Federal Tax Reports; Tax Research Consultant; and Practical Tax Explanations.

[63] ¶ 12,002, ¶ 12,007; BUSEXP: 45,200; § 17,015.15

[64] ¶ 12,002; BUSEXP: 45,152; § 17,010.15

[65] ¶ 12,009; BUSEXP: 45,208.05; § 17,020

[66] ¶ 12,002; BUSEXP: 45,154.35; § 17,010.20

Farming Loss. A farming loss may be carried back for five years (Code Sec. 172(b)(1)(G) and (i)).[67] A farming loss is the *smaller* of (1) the amount that would be the NOL for the tax year if only income and deductions attributable to farming businesses (¶ 999) were taken into account, or (2) the NOL for the tax year. A taxpayer may elect to waive the five-year carryback for a farming loss. In this case, the two-year carryback period generally applies. For ordering purposes, the farming loss is treated as a separate NOL to be taken into account *after* the remaining portion of the NOL for the tax year. A farming loss does not include a qualified disaster loss.

Federally Declared Disasters. A five-year NOL carryback period applies for qualified disaster losses (Code Sec. 172(b)(1)(J) and (j)).[68] A "qualified disaster loss" is the *lesser* of: (1) the sum of (a) losses occurring in a disaster area and attributable to a federally declared disaster occurring after 2007 and before 2010, plus (b) the qualified disaster expenses deduction allowable for the tax year (or which would be allowable if not otherwise treated as an expense); or (2) the NOL for the tax year. Remaining NOLs, if any, are subject to the general two-year carryback period. The qualified disaster loss is treated as a separate NOL to be taken into account *after* the remaining portion of the NOL for the tax year, and may not include losses attributable to property used in connection with golf courses, country clubs, massage parlors, hot tub or suntan facilities, liquor stores, or gambling or animal racing property. A taxpayer can elect to waive the five-year carryback period.

Other Disaster Area Losses. A five-year NOL carryback period was available for qualified losses incurred in 2005 in the Gulf Opportunity (GO) Zone and in 2008 in the Midwestern disaster area (Code Sec. 1400N(k); Division C, Act Sec. 702(a)(1)(A) and (d)(6) of the Emergency Economic Stabilization Act of 2008 (P.L. 110-343)).[69]

2008 and 2009 NOLs. A taxpayer can elect a three-, four- or five-year carryback period for an NOL for any tax year that ended after December 31, 2007, and began before January 1, 2010 (Code Sec. 172(b)(1)(H)).[70] The NOL amount that can be carried back to the fifth preceding tax year is limited to 50 percent of the taxpayer's taxable income for that preceding tax year. Most taxpayers can make the election for only one tax year (2008 or 2009); an eligible small business (one that met a $15 million or less gross receipts test for the year of the loss) may be able to elect an extended carryback period for 2008 and 2009 NOLs. If a taxpayer has elected this extended carryback period for 2008 or 2009 NOLs, then the three-year carryback period for casualty or theft losses of individuals, and NOLs of farmers or small businesses from federally declared disasters does not apply. A similar carryback election is allowed for operations losses of life insurance companies (¶ 2377).

Short Tax Years. If the IRS approves a request for a change in accounting period when the short period required to effect the change is a tax year in which the taxpayer has an NOL, the taxpayer can carry back the short-period NOL only if it is either (1) $50,000 or less, or (2) less than the full 12-month period NOL beginning with the first day of the short period as determined when the 12-month period has expired.[71]

Specified Liability Losses. A 10-year carryback period applies to specified liability losses (Code Sec. 172(b)(1)(C) and (f); Notice 2005-20).[72] A specified liability loss is the portion of an NOL that (1) is attributable to product liability or (2) arises out of satisfaction of a liability under federal or state law requiring land reclamation, nuclear power plant decommissioning, drilling platform dismantling, environmental remediation, or a payment under any workers' compensation act. For ordering purposes, the specified liability loss is treated as a separate NOL to be taken into account *after* the remaining portion of the NOL for the tax year.

References are to Standard Federal Tax Reports; Tax Research Consultant; and Practical Tax Explanations.

[67] ¶ 12,002; BUSEXP: 45,154.40; § 36,210

[68] ¶ 12,002; BUSEXP: 45,154.05; § 17,010.20

[69] ¶ 32,483, ¶ 32,487.056; BUSEXP: 57,304.45; § 10,001, § 17,010.05

[70] ¶ 12,002, ¶ 12,014.3202; BUSEXP: 45,154.55, BUSEXP: 45,154.60; § 17,010.17

[71] ¶ 12,014.30; NOL: 12,202; § 38,130.20

[72] ¶ 12,002; BUSEXP: 45,154.25; § 17,010.25

Real Estate Investment Trusts (REITs). An NOL from a REIT year—a tax year in which an entity operated as a real estate investment trust (¶ 2326)—cannot be carried back to any preceding tax year. An NOL from a non-REIT year cannot be carried back to a REIT year. A REIT NOL can be carried forward 20 years (Code Sec. 172(b)(1)(B); Reg. § 1.172-10).[73]

Corporate Equity Reduction Transactions (CERTs). A C corporation may not carry back a portion of its NOL if $1 million or more of interest expense is incurred in a "major stock acquisition" of another corporation or in an "excess distribution" by the corporation (Code Sec. 172(b)(1)(E) and (h)).[74] The amount subject to the limitation is the lesser of: (1) the corporation's deductible interest expense allocable to the CERT, or (2) the amount by which the corporation's interest expense for the current tax year exceeds the average interest expense for the three tax years preceding the tax year in which the CERT occurs.

Electric Utilities. For any tax year ending after 2005 and before 2009, an electric utility could elect a five-year carryback period for a portion of NOLs that arose in tax years 2003, 2004 and 2005. The carried-back NOL amount was limited to 20 percent of the sum of the taxpayer's electric transmission property capital expenditures and pollution control facility capital expenditures for the tax year preceding the tax year for which the election was made. Only one election could be made with respect to any NOL for a tax year, and an election could not be made for more than one tax year beginning in any calendar year (Code Sec. 172(b)(1)(I)).[75]

1153. NOL Carryovers Between Predecessors and Successors. A net operating loss (NOL) may generally be carried back or carried forward only by the taxpayer who sustained the loss (¶ 1145). A beneficiary of an estate or trust, however, is entitled to any carryover amount remaining unused after the last tax year of the estate or trust. Similarly, a bankruptcy estate succeeds to an individual debtor's NOLs (¶ 535). A successor corporation also is allowed to carry over the NOL and certain other items of its predecessor under specified conditions (¶ 2277).

At-Risk Limitations

1155. At-Risk Limitations on Losses. A taxpayer's deductible loss with respect to an activity is generally limited to the amount that the taxpayer has at risk with respect to the activity (Code Sec. 465).[76] The at-risk rules are designed to prevent taxpayers (¶ 1157) from offsetting trade, business, or professional income by losses from investments in activities (¶ 1159) that are largely financed by nonrecourse loans for which they are not personally liable. Even if it has been determined that the loss is deductible under the at-risk rules, the loss may still be limited by the passive activity loss rules (¶ 1165).

Under the at-risk rules, loss deductions are limited to the amount the taxpayer has at risk in the activity. This is the money and the adjusted basis of other property the taxpayer contributes to the activity. It also includes any amounts borrowed for use in the activity if the taxpayer has personal liability for repayment of the loan (recourse) or has pledged assets not used in the activity as security for the loan (Code Sec. 465(b)).[77]

Amounts are not at risk if they are borrowed from (1) a person who has an interest in the activity other than as a creditor, or (2) a person related to someone other than the taxpayer who has an interest in the activity. Exceptions are available for corporations that borrow from shareholders and qualified nonrecourse financing secured by real property used in an activity. Personal liability of the taxpayer for borrowed amounts generally hinges on whether the taxpayer is the ultimate obligor of the liability with no recourse against any other party.[78] The taxpayer is not considered at risk with respect to

---

References are to Standard Federal Tax Reports; Tax Research Consultant; and Practical Tax Explanations.

[73] ¶ 12,002, ¶ 12,012; BUSEXP: 45,154.15

[74] ¶ 12,002; NOL: 15,202

[75] ¶ 12,002; BUSEXP: 45,154.50

[76] ¶ 21,850; BUSEXP: 42,000; § 17,301

[77] ¶ 21,850; BUSEXP: 42,150; § 17,305.05

[78] ¶ 21,893.35; BUSEXP: 42,156.05; § 17,305.05

amounts protected against loss through nonrecourse financing, guarantees, stop-loss agreements, or similar arrangements.

Any loss not allowed because of the at-risk limitation is carried over to the following tax year, to be deducted subject to the same limitation (Code Sec. 465(a)(2)). The amount allowed as a loss for any year reduces the amount at risk for later years. Conversely, if a taxpayer's amount at risk at the end of any tax year is less than zero, the loss equal to the difference is recaptured (Code Sec. 465(e)).[79] Unused amounts generally are allowed when the activity is transferred or otherwise disposed (¶ 1161).

Form 6198 is used to compute the deductible loss, if any, under the at-risk rules. An activity subject to the passive loss rules must file Form 8582. If the activity is subject to both limitations, Form 6198 is completed first, and any allowable loss must be carried over to Form 8582.

For investment tax credit at-risk rules, see ¶ 1365A.

1157. Taxpayers Affected by At-Risk Rules. The at-risk rules (¶ 1155) apply to individuals, estates, and trusts (Code Sec. 465(a)(1)).[80] They apply to partners and S corporation shareholders at the partner or shareholder level, not at the entity level. Closely held corporations are generally subject to the at-risk rules if they meet the personal holding company stock ownership requirements (¶ 277). However, certain closely held corporations are not subject to the at-risk limits for any qualifying active business carried on; instead, each qualifying business of a corporation is treated as a separate activity (Code Sec. 465(c)(7)). In addition, if a closely held corporation is actively engaged in equipment leasing, the equipment leasing is treated as a separate activity not covered by the at-risk rules (Code Sec. 465(c)(4)).

1159. Activities Covered by At-Risk Rules. The at-risk limit on losses (¶ 1155) generally applies to all activities of a taxpayer engaged in as a trade or business, or for the production of income (Code Sec. 465(c)).[81] It also specifically applies to any taxpayer engaged in: the activity of holding, producing, or distributing motion picture films or video tapes; farming; leasing of section 1245 property; or exploring for or exploiting oil and gas resources or geothermal deposits. The at-risk rules do not apply to: (1) the holding of real property other than mineral property acquired before 1987 as an interest in a pass-through entity engaged in holding real property placed in service before 1987; (2) the leasing of equipment by closely held corporations (¶ 1157); or (3) a qualifying active business carried on by certain closely held corporations.

In the case of the specifically identified activities above, each film or tape, each piece of section 1245 property, each farm, and each oil, gas, or geothermal property is treated as a separate activity. However, for a partnership or an S corporation, all leased section 1245 properties that are placed in service in the same tax year are treated as a single activity (Code Sec. 465(c)(2)(B)).[82] Trade or business activities subject to the at-risk rules are to be aggregated and treated as a single activity if the taxpayer actively participates in the management of the trade or business or, where the trade or business is carried on by a partnership or S corporation, if 65 percent or more of the losses for the tax year are allocable to persons who actively participate in the management.

1161. Application of At-Risk Rules on Disposition of Activity. Under proposed regulations, when a taxpayer transfers or otherwise disposes of an activity, any gain realized on the transfer or disposition of the activity is treated as gain from the activity, which generally permits the taxpayer to recognize any losses suspended under the at-risk rules (¶ 1155) (Prop. Reg. § 1.465-66).[83] The same rules apply if a partnership liquidates a partner's interest or an S corporation completely redeems a shareholder's interest.

References are to Standard Federal Tax Reports; Tax Research Consultant; and Practical Tax Explanations.

[79] ¶ 21,850; BUSEXP: 42,200; § 17,315

[80] ¶ 21,850; BUSEXP: 42,050; § 17,301

[81] ¶ 21,850; BUSEXP: 42,100; § 17,310

[82] ¶ 21,850; BUSEXP: 42,106; § 17,310

[83] ¶ 21,883; BUSEXP: 42,210; § 17,320

Passive Activity Limits on Losses and Credits

1165. Passive Activity Defined. A passive activity is one that involves the conduct of any trade or business in which the taxpayer does not materially participate (Code Sec. 469(c); Temp. Reg. § 1.469-1T(e)).[84] Any rental activity is a passive activity whether or not the taxpayer materially participates (¶ 1181). However, there are special rules for real estate rental activities (¶ 1183) and real estate professionals (¶ 1185). Trading personal property that is actively traded, such as stocks and bonds, for the account of owners of interests in the activity is not a passive activity. For example, the activity of a partnership that trades stock using money contributed by the partners is not a passive activity.

Material participation in an activity requires that a taxpayer is involved in the operations of the activity on a regular, continuous, and substantial basis (Code Sec. 469(h); Temp. Reg. § 1.469-5T).[85] Generally, an individual is considered as materially participating in an activity during a tax year if he or she satisfies one of the following tests:

    (1) the individual participates more than 500 hours;

    (2) the individual's participation constitutes substantially all of the participation in the activity;

    (3) the individual participates for more than 100 hours and this participation is not less than the participation of any other individual;

    (4) the activity is a "significant participation activity" (see below) and the individual's participation in all significant participation activities exceeds 500 hours;

    (5) the individual materially participated in the activity for any five years of the 10 years that preceded the year in question;

    (6) the activity is a "personal service activity" (see below) and the individual materially participated in the activity for any three years preceding the tax year in question; or

    (7) the individual satisfies a facts and circumstances test that requires the individual to show participation on a regular, continuous, and substantial basis for more than 100 hours during the tax year.

With respect to test (7), an individual's participation in managing the activity does not count toward the 100-hour requirement if any other person received compensation for managing the activity or any other person spent more time managing the activity.

Special rules are provided for determining the material participation of certain retired or disabled farmers and participation in the activity of a personal service or closely held corporation (Temp. Reg. § 1.469-5T(h)).[86]

Limited Partners. A limited partner's share of income, losses, and credits from a partnership are treated as arising from a passive activity unless the limited partner participated in the activity for more than 500 hours, the limited partner materially participated in the activity five of the 10 preceding tax years, or the activity is a personal service activity in which the limited partner materially participated for any three preceding tax years. A general partner who also holds a limited partnership interest is not treated as a limited partner (Code Sec. 469(h)(2); Temp. Reg. § 1.469-5T(e)).[87]

Significant Participation Activity. A significant participation activity is one in which the taxpayer participates more than 100 hours during the tax year but does not materially participate under any of the other six tests set forth above (Temp. Reg. § 1.469-5T(c)).[88]

References are to Standard Federal Tax Reports; Tax Research Consultant; and Practical Tax Explanations.

[84] ¶ 21,960, ¶ 21,962; BUSEXP: 33,100; § 17,420.05

[85] ¶ 21,960, ¶ 21,965; BUSEXP: 33,150; § 17,435.05

[86] ¶ 21,965; BUSEXP: 33,158, BUSEXP: 33,164; § 17,435.25, § 17,435.35

[87] ¶ 21,960, ¶ 21,965; BUSEXP: 33,160; § 17,435.20

[88] ¶ 21,965; BUSEXP: 33,152; § 17,435.15

Personal Service Activity. A personal service activity involves the performance of personal service in the fields of health (including veterinary services), law, engineering, architecture, accounting, actuarial science, the performing arts, consulting, or any other trade or business in which capital is not a material income-producing factor (Temp. Reg. § 1.469-5T(d)).[89]

Definition of Participation. Any work done by an individual with respect to an activity in which the individual owns an interest is generally treated as participation (Reg. § 1.469-5(f)(1); Temp. Reg. § 1.469-5T(f)).[90] Participation does not include work that is not customarily done by an owner if one of the principal purposes for performing the work is to avoid the passive activity limitations. Furthermore, work done in an individual's capacity as an investor in an activity, such as studying and reviewing the activity's financial statements and operational reports, preparing summaries or analyses of the activity's finances or operations for personal use, and monitoring the finances or operations of the activity in a nonmanagerial capacity, is not counted as participation.

An individual's participation does include the participation of his or her spouse even if the spouse does not own an interest in the activity and separate returns are filed. Participation may be established by any reasonable means. It is not necessary to maintain contemporaneous daily records of participation. An approximate number of hours of participation may be based on appointment books, calendars, or narrative summaries.

1167. Passive Activity Income and Deductions. For purposes of the passive activity limit on losses (¶ 1169), passive income or loss generally is determined by aggregating gross income and deductions from all passive activities during the year (Temp. Reg. § 1.469-2T).[91] Certain types of income and deductions from a passive activity, however, are subject to special rules and must be excluded and reported separately as nonpassive income or deduction.

Portfolio income is excluded from passive activity income and expenses directly allocable to such income are not deductible in computing passive activity losses (Code Sec. 469(e)(1)).[92] Portfolio income includes interest, dividends, annuities, royalties, and gain or loss from the disposition of investment property not derived in the ordinary course of a trade or business. No exception is provided for the treatment of portfolio income arising from working capital, i.e., amounts set aside for the reasonable needs of the business.

Passive activity income also does not include: personal service income; income or gain from investments of working capital; income from intangible property if the taxpayer's personal efforts significantly contributed to its creation; refunds of state and local taxes; reimbursements of casualty and theft losses; and cancellation of debt income. Passive activity deductions do not include: qualified home mortgage interest expense, capitalization interest expense, and most other interest expenses properly allocable to a passive activity; state and local taxes; charitable contributions; disallowed miscellaneous itemized deductions; net operating losses (NOLs); and capital loss carrybacks and carryovers.

Certain self-charged interest income or deductions may be treated as passive activity gross income or deductions if the loan proceeds are used in a passive activity. Self-charged interest and expenses are items from a lending transaction between a taxpayer and a pass-through entity in which the taxpayer owns a direct or indirect interest (Reg. § 1.469-7).[93] These rules also apply to lending transactions between pass-through entities with identical ownership.

1169. Passive Activity Loss Limitations. Under the passive activity rules, losses and expenses attributable to passive activities may only be deducted from income

---

References are to Standard Federal Tax Reports; Tax Research Consultant; and Practical Tax Explanations.

[89] ¶ 21,965; BUSEXP: 33,152; § 17,435.15

[90] ¶ 21,964C, ¶ 21,965; BUSEXP: 33,154; § 17,435.10

[91] ¶ 21,963; BUSEXP: 33,350, BUSEXP: 33,400; § 17,450.05

[92] ¶ 21,960; BUSEXP: 33,354; § 17,450.10

[93] ¶ 21,965B; BUSEXP: 33,462.20; § 17,450.15

attributable to passive activities (Code Sec. 469).[94] Similarly, tax credits attributable to passive activities may only be used to offset taxes attributable to income from passive activities. A passive activity for this purpose is any activity that involves the conduct of a trade or business in which the taxpayer does not materially participate (¶ 1165). Any rental activity is a passive activity whether or not the taxpayer materially participates (¶ 1181). However, there are special rules for real estate rental activities (¶ 1183) and real estate professionals (¶ 1185). In determining a taxpayer's allowable loss, the at-risk rules (¶ 1155) are applied before the passive activity loss rules.

To the extent that the total deductions from passive activities exceed the total income from these activities for the tax year, the excess (the passive activity loss) is not allowed as a deduction for that year. Instead, the disallowed loss is suspended and carried forward as a deduction against income from the passive activity in the next succeeding tax year (Code Sec. 469(b)).[95] Any unused suspended losses are allowed in full when the taxpayer disposes of his or her entire interest in the activity in a fully taxable transaction (¶ 1177).

Tax credits arising with respect to passive activities are generally treated in the same manner as losses, except that suspended credits are not allowed on disposition of the activity (Code Sec. 469(a)(1)(B) and (d)).[96] Thus, credits may be used to offset the tax attributable to net passive income—the difference between the tax on all income, and the tax on taxable income other than net passive income. In both cases, the effect of credits is disregarded.

Unused credits can generally be carried forward indefinitely. However, the character of a credit relating to a passive activity changes, in effect, when the credit becomes allowable under the passive loss rules (either there is sufficient passive income to allow its use, or it is within the scope of the $25,000 benefit for real estate activities). At this time, the credit is aggregated with credits relating to nonpassive activities of the taxpayer to determine whether all such credits are allowable considering the other limitations that apply to the use of credits (¶ 1365).

Forms. Individuals, estates, and trusts use Form 8582 or Form 8582-CR to calculate their allowable passive losses and credits. Form 8582 generally must also be filed by a taxpayer that has an overall gain from business or rental passive activities for the year (even after including suspended passive losses from earlier tax years). However, Form 8582 does not need to be filed if the taxpayer actively participated in rental real estate activities. Form 8810 is used by personal service corporations and closely held C corporations to calculate passive activity losses and credits. Form 8825 is used by partnerships and S corporations to report income and deductible expenses from rental real estate activities.

1171. Passive Activity Losses of Publicly Traded Partnerships. Special rules apply to passive activity losses from publicly traded partnerships (PTPs) (Code Sec. 469(k)).[97] A PTP is a partnership whose interests are traded on an established securities market or are readily tradable on a secondary market or its substantial equivalent. A taxpayer's net income from a PTP may not be used to offset net losses from other PTPs or net losses from other passive activities. A disallowed loss from a PTP is carried forward and allowed as a deduction in a tax year when the PTP has net income or when the taxpayer disposes of his or her entire interest in the PTP. These rules apply to a regulated investment company or mutual fund (¶ 2301) holding an interest in a PTP, with respect to items attributable to the interest in the partnership.

1173. Taxpayers Covered by Passive Activity Rules. The passive activity rules (¶ 1169) apply to individuals, estates, trusts other than grantor trusts, and personal service corporations (Code Sec. 469(a)(2)).[98] Although the passive activity rules do not

[94] ¶ 21,960; BUSEXP: 33,000; § 17,401

[95] ¶ 21,960; BUSEXP: 33,200; § 17,470.05

[96] ¶ 21,960; BUSEXP: 33,250; § 17,495

[97] ¶ 21,960; BUSEXP: 33,458; § 17,415.15

[98] ¶ 21,960; BUSEXP: 33,050; § 17,405.05

11 LOSSES

apply to partnerships, S corporations, and grantor trusts directly, they are applied at the partner, shareholder, beneficiary, or grantor level. See ¶ 1171 for discussion of special rules applicable to publicly traded partnerships.

Closely Held C Corporations. C corporations are generally not subject to the passive activity rules. However, the passive activity rules do apply to a closely held C corporation (other than a personal service corporation) to the extent of its net active income. The corporation cannot use passive losses to offset portfolio income (¶ 1167). A closely held C corporation's net active income is equal to its taxable income, figured without any income or loss from a passive activity or any portfolio income or loss (Code Sec. 469(e)(2)).[99]

1175. Grouping Activities Under the Passive Activity Rules. In applying the passive activity rules (¶ 1165), one or more trade or business activities, or rental activities, may be treated as a single activity if the activities constitute an appropriate economic unit (Reg. § 1.469-4).[100] Whether activities constitute an appropriate economic unit depends upon all the relevant facts and circumstances. The following factors are given greatest weight in determining whether several activities can be combined:

- similarities or differences in types of business,
- extent of common control,
- extent of common ownership,
- geographical location, and
- business interdependencies among the activities.

Once activities are grouped together or kept separate, the taxpayer must be consistent in the treatment of these activities in subsequent tax years. A taxpayer generally may not regroup activities unless the original grouping was clearly inappropriate or became inappropriate due to a material change in facts and circumstances (Reg. § 1.469-4(e)).[101] A taxpayer is required to disclose their grouping and regrouping of activities in a written statement with the taxpayer's income tax return (Rev. Proc. 2010-13).[102] The statement must be filed for: (1) the first tax year in which two or more trade or business activities or rental activities are originally grouped as a single activity; (2) a tax year in which a taxpayer adds a new trade or business activity or a rental activity to an existing grouping; or (3) a tax year in which a taxpayer regroups activities. The IRS may disallow and regroup a taxpayer's grouping of activities if the grouping does not reflect an appropriate economic unit and has circumvention of the passive activity loss rules as a primary purpose (Reg. § 1.469-4(f)).[103]

A one-time regrouping of activities can be made by an individual, trust, or estate in the first tax year beginning after December 31, 2013, in which it satisfies the eligibility criteria for the net investment income (NII) tax (¶ 129) (Reg. § 1.469-11(b)(3)(iv)).[104] An individual, estate, or trust was also allowed to make the regrouping for any tax year beginning in 2013 if the eligibility criteria were met for that year. The term "eligibility criteria" means that (1) an individual, estate, or trust has net investment income, and (2) the individual's modified adjusted gross income (AGI) exceeds $250,000 for joint filers and surviving spouses, $125,000 for married filing separately, and $200,000 for all other individuals, or the estate's or trust's AGI exceeds the dollar amount for which the highest income tax bracket is imposed on an estate or trust ($12,150 for tax years beginning in 2014; $12,300 for tax years beginning in 2015). The determination of whether a taxpayer meets the eligibility criteria is made without regard to the effect of the regrouping and any regrouping applies to the tax year in which the regrouping is done and all subsequent tax years. The one-time regrouping generally must be made on an original return. It may be made on an amended return only if a change reported on

---

References are to Standard Federal Tax Reports; Tax Research Consultant; and Practical Tax Explanations.

[99] ¶ 21,960; BUSEXP: 33,054; § 17,405.15

[100] ¶ 21,964B; BUSEXP: 33,102; § 17,415.05

[101] ¶ 21,964B; BUSEXP: 33,102; § 17,415.10

[102] ¶ 21,966.579; BUSEXP: 33,102.35; § 17,415.25

[103] ¶ 21,964B; BUSEXP: 33,102.30; § 17,415.25

[104] ¶ 21,965F; BUSEXP: 33,102.33; § 17,415.20

the amended return causes the taxpayer to meet the eligibility criteria for the first time. If it is later determined that the taxpayer did not satisfy the eligibility criteria in a tax year in which a regrouping was made, the regrouping is void for the tax year it was made and all future years, unless the taxpayer's failure to satisfy the eligibility criteria is due to the carryback of a net operating loss.

Activities Conducted Through Entities. Activities conducted through a partnership, S corporation, personal service corporation, or closely-held corporation are first grouped at the entity level (Reg. § 1.469-4(d)(5)).[105] Once the entity groups its activities, a partner or shareholder may group those activities with each other, with activities conducted directly by the partner or shareholder, and with activities conducted through other entities. However, an activity that a taxpayer conducts through a C corporation may be grouped with another activity of the taxpayer only for purposes of determining whether the taxpayer materially or significantly participates in the other activity.

Rental Activities. A taxpayer generally may not treat an activity involving the rental of real property and an activity involving the rental of personal property as a single activity (Reg. § 1.469-4(d)(2)).[106] These two activities can be treated as a single activity only if the taxpayer provides the personal property in connection with the real property or the real property in connection with the personal property.

A rental activity may not be grouped with a trade or business activity unless either: (1) the rental activity is insubstantial in relation to the trade or business activity; or (2) the trade or business activity is insubstantial in relation to the rental activity (Reg. § 1.469-4(d)(1)).[107] There is a third alternative when each owner of the trade or business has the same proportionate ownership interest in the rental activity, in which case the portion of the rental activity that involves the rental of items of property to a trade or business activity may be grouped with the trade or business activity.

> **Example:** The Getaway Partnership owns a 10-story building in which it operates a travel agency on three floors and rents seven floors to tenants. The partnership is divided into two activities: a travel agency activity and a rental real estate activity. Deductions and credits attributable to the building are allocable to the travel agency activity only to the extent that they relate to the space occupied by the travel agency during the tax year.

Partial Disposition of Activity. If the taxpayer disposes of *substantially all* of an activity, he or she may treat the interest disposed of as a separate activity, provided that the taxpayer can establish the amount of gross income, deductions and credits allocable to that part of the activity for the tax year (Reg. § 1.469-4(g)).[108] Without this rule, taxpayers generally cannot claim suspended passive losses until they have disposed of their entire interest in an activity (¶ 1177).

1177. Disposition of Interest in Passive Activity. When a taxpayer disposes of his or her entire interest in a passive activity (¶ 1165) in a taxable transaction, the taxpayer's suspended passive activity losses (¶ 1169) may be applied against his or her nonpassive income (Code Sec. 469(g)).[109] Specifically, any net passive losses must first be applied against the taxpayer's net income or gain from passive activities. Any remaining loss from the activity is then classified as nonpassive and may be used to offset income from nonpassive activities, e.g., wages. Suspended credits are not allowed on the disposition of a passive activity.

Entire Interest. A disposition of a taxpayer's entire interest involves a disposition of the interest in all entities that are engaged in the activity. To the extent the activity is held in the form of a sole proprietorship, disposition of a taxpayer's entire interest includes disposition of all of the assets used or created in the activity. If a partnership or S corporation conducts two or more separate activities and the entity disposes of all the

---

References are to Standard Federal Tax Reports; Tax Research Consultant; and Practical Tax Explanations.

[105] ¶ 21,964B; BUSEXP: 33,102.20; § 17,415.15

[106] ¶ 21,964B; BUSEXP: 33,102.25; § 17,415.15

[107] ¶ 21,964B; BUSEXP: 33,102.25; § 17,415.15

[108] ¶ 21,964B; BUSEXP: 33,652; § 17,490.10

[109] ¶ 21,960; BUSEXP: 33,652; § 17,490.05

assets used or created in one activity, the disposition constitutes a disposition of the entire interest. The same rule applies to grantor trusts.[110] In some instances, a taxpayer may claim a deduction for suspended losses even though he or she disposes of less than his or her entire interest (¶ 1175).

Taxable Transactions. To qualify as a fully taxable disposition, the disposition generally must be a sale of the interest to a third party in an arm's-length transaction and must not be a sham, a wash sale, or a transfer of repurchase rights (Code Sec. 469(g)(1)).[111] If a taxpayer disposes of an interest in a passive activity in a taxable transaction with a related party as defined by Code Sec. 267(b) (¶ 1717) or with a controlled partnership as defined by Code Sec. 707(b)(1) (¶ 432) the suspended losses are not triggered. In these circumstances, the taxpayer is able to claim the loss only when the related person or controlled partnership disposes of the activity in a taxable transaction with an unrelated person. Abandonment is a fully taxable disposition.

Installment Sales. When a taxpayer sells his or her entire interest in a passive activity and reports the gain under the installment sale method (¶ 1801), only a portion of the suspended loss may be deducted in the year of the sale. Suspended losses are allowed in the year of sale and thereafter in the ratio that the gain recognized in a tax year bears to the total gross profit from the sale to be realized when payment is completed (Code Sec. 469(g)(3)).[112]

Death. A transfer of a taxpayer's entire interest by reason of the taxpayer's death causes suspended losses to be allowed in the year of death to the extent that they exceed the amount by which the basis of the interest is stepped up at death (¶ 1633) (Code Sec. 469(g)(2)).[113]

Gifts. Disposition of an interest in a passive activity by gift does *not* trigger suspended losses. Instead, the basis of the transferred interest is increased by the amount of such losses (Code Sec. 469(j)(6)).[114]

Nontaxable Exchanges. An exchange of a taxpayer's interest in a passive activity in a nonrecognition transaction, e.g., a like-kind exchange (¶ 1721), does not trigger suspended losses. However, to the extent that the taxpayer recognizes gain on the transaction, e.g., to the extent of boot received, the gain is treated as passive activity income against which passive losses may be deducted.[115]

Casualty or Theft. A casualty (¶ 1121) or theft (¶ 1123) loss involving property used in a passive activity does not constitute a complete disposition of the taxpayer's interest in the activity unless the casualty or theft results in a loss of all property used or created in the activity.[116]

Activity No Longer Passive. In the tax year that an activity ceases to be a passive activity, previously suspended losses from that activity are permitted to be claimed as deductions against the activity's net income (Code Sec. 469(f)(1)).[117] Similarly, prior year suspended passive activity credits may offset the current year's tax liability that is allocable to the current year's net income from the former passive activity. Tax liability for this purpose is figured on the net income as reduced by the prior year suspended losses.

Cessation of Closely Held C Corporation or PSC Status. If a closely held C corporation or a personal service corporation changes its status, suspended losses from prior years continue to be subject to the limitations that were imposed before the status changed (¶ 1173). Losses arising in years after the year in which the corporation's status changes are not subject to the passive activity rules (Code Sec. 469(f)(2)).

References are to Standard Federal Tax Reports; Tax Research Consultant; and Practical Tax Explanations.

[110] ¶ 21,966.0552; BUSEXP: 33,652.10; § 17,490.10

[111] ¶ 21,960; BUSEXP: 33,652.05, BUSEXP: 33,654; § 17,490.15, § 17,490.35

[112] ¶ 21,960; BUSEXP: 33,668; § 17,490.30

[113] ¶ 21,960; BUSEXP: 33,658; § 17,490.20

[114] ¶ 21,960; BUSEXP: 33,660; § 17,490.25

[115] ¶ 21,966.0553; BUSEXP: 33,662; § 17,490.15

[116] ¶ 21,966.0553; BUSEXP: 33,652.10; § 17,490.15

[117] ¶ 21,960; BUSEXP: 33,600; § 17,440

Rental Activities

1181. Rental Activities Subject to Passive Activity Rules. A rental activity is generally treated as a passive activity regardless of whether the taxpayer materially participates in the activity (¶ 1165) (Code Sec. 469(c)(2); Temp. Reg. § 1.469-1T(e)(3)).[118] An activity is a "rental activity" if (1) during the tax year, tangible property held in connection with the activity is used by customers or is held for use by customers, and (2) the gross income of the activity represents amounts paid mainly for the use of the tangible property. A taxpayer's rental real estate activity is not considered passive activity, however, if the taxpayer is a real estate professional (¶ 1185). In addition, if any one of the following tests is met, the activity is not considered to be a rental activity for purposes of the passive loss rules (¶ 1169):

- the average period of customer use of the property is seven days or less;

- the average period of customer use is 30 days or less and significant personal services are provided by or on behalf of the owner;

- without regard to the period of customer use, extraordinary personal services are provided by or on behalf of the owner;

- the rental of the property is incidental to a nonrental activity;

- the property is customarily made available during defined business hours for the nonexclusive use of customers; or

- the taxpayer provides property for use in an activity that is conducted by a partnership, S corporation, or joint venture in which the taxpayer owns an interest and the activity is not a rental activity.

If a taxpayer does not meet the requirements to be a real estate professional, but owns and actively participates in a rental real estate activity, then the taxpayer may deduct up to $25,000 of losses from a passive rental real estate activity from nonpassive income (¶ 1183).

1183. $25,000 Offset for Active Participation in Rental Real Estate Activity. Individuals who own and actively participate in a rental real estate activity may offset up to $25,000 of passive activity losses and credits ($12,500 for married filing separately) from the activity against nonpassive income (Code Sec. 469(i)).[119] To be eligible, the individual must own at least 10-percent by value of all interests in the activity throughout the year. The interest of an individual's spouse is taken into account in determining 10-percent ownership whether or not a joint return is filed. While the offset is available only to individual taxpayers who actively participate in rental real estate activities, a decedent's estate also qualifies for its tax years ending less than two years after the date of the decedent's death if it has an interest in a rental real estate activity in which the decedent actively participated in the year of death. A decedent's qualified revocable trust can also be treated as actively participating if both the trustee and the executor of the estate (if any) choose to treat the trust as part of the estate.

The active participation standard is less stringent than the material participation standard (¶ 1165). An individual may meet the active participation requirement if he or she participates in the making of management decisions (for example, approving new tenants, deciding on rental terms, approving expenditures) or arranges for others to provide services (for example, repairs) in a significant and bona fide sense. The requirement for active participation applies in the year in which the loss arose as well as the year in which the loss is allowed. However, real estate professionals may be able to treat rental property activities as nonpassive activities (¶ 1185).

The $25,000 maximum offset amount is reduced, but not below zero, by 50 percent of the amount by which the taxpayer's adjusted gross income (AGI) exceeds $100,000. It is completely phased out when AGI reaches $150,000 (Code Sec. 469(i)(3)). For this

---

References are to Standard Federal Tax Reports; Tax Research Consultant; and Practical Tax Explanations.

[118] ¶ 21,960; BUSEXP: 33,106; § 17,430.05

[119] ¶ 21,960; BUSEXP: 33,700; § 17,480.05

purpose, AGI is computed without regard to: taxable Social Security and railroad retirement benefits; the exclusion for qualified U.S. savings bonds used to pay higher education expenses; the exclusion for employer adoption assistance payments; passive activity income or loss included on Form 8582; any overall loss from a publicly traded partnership; rental real estate losses allowed to real estate professionals; the domestic production activities deduction; and deductions for contributions to IRAs and pension plans, for one-half of self-employment tax, interest on student loans, and higher education expenses.

Separate Returns. For married taxpayers who file separate returns and live apart, up to $12,500 of passive losses may be used to offset nonpassive income. This amount is reduced by 50 percent of the amount by which the taxpayer's modified AGI exceeds $50,000. The special allowance is completely phased out when modified AGI reaches $75,000. Married taxpayers who file separately and live together at any time during the tax year are not eligible for the special allowance (Code Sec. 469(i)(5)).

Offset of Credits. Passive activity credits attributable to rental real estate activities in which the taxpayer actively participates may be claimed under the $25,000 offset provision, but only after all eligible losses have been used. Special rules apply for the phaseout of the rehabilitation credit (¶ 1365B), low-income housing credit (¶ 1365K), and commercial revitalization deduction (Code Sec. 1400I).

1185. Real Estate Professionals. Real estate professionals may be able to treat rental real estate activities as nonpassive and thus not subject to the passive activity rules (¶ 1165) (Code Sec. 469(c)(7); Reg. § 1.469-9(g)).[120] To qualify:

- more than one-half of the personal services performed in trades or businesses by the taxpayer during the tax year must involve real property trades or businesses in which the taxpayer or the taxpayer's spouse materially participates; and

- the taxpayer must perform more than 750 hours of service during the tax year in real property trades or businesses in which the taxpayer or the taxpayer's spouse materially participates (¶ 1165).

These two requirements must be satisfied by one spouse if a joint return is filed. Personal services performed as an employee are not taken into account under either requirement unless the employee owns more than a five-percent interest in the employer. A real property trade or business is a business with respect to which real property is developed or redeveloped, constructed or reconstructed, acquired, converted, rented or leased, operated or managed, or brokered.

The exception for real estate professionals is applied as if each interest of the taxpayer in rental real estate is a separate activity. However, a taxpayer may elect to treat all interests in rental real estate as a single activity for purposes of satisfying the material participation requirements. To make the election, the taxpayer must file a statement with the taxpayer's original income tax return for the tax year declaring that he or she is a qualified taxpayer for the tax year and is making the election. Certain taxpayers may be permitted to make late elections (Rev. Proc. 2011-34).[121]

A closely held corporation qualifies as a real estate professional if more than 50 percent of its annual gross receipts for the tax year are from real property trades or businesses in which it materially participates.

Tax-Exempt Use Property

1191. Limits on Tax-Exempt Use Losses. A taxpayer leasing property to a government or other tax-exempt entity (i.e., sale-in, lease-out (SILO) arrangement) is not allowed to claim deductions that are related to the property (known as tax-exempt use property) to the extent that they exceed the taxpayer's income from the lease payments

---

References are to Standard Federal Tax Reports; Tax Research Consultant; and Practical Tax Explanations.

[120] ¶ 21,960, ¶ 21,965D;   [121] ¶ 21,966.568; BUSEXP:
BUSEXP: 33,106.40; § 17,430.15   33,106.40; § 17,430.15

(a tax-exempt use loss), subject to certain exceptions (Code Sec. 470).[122] Tax-exempt use property includes property owned by a partnership or other pass-through entity that has at least one tax-exempt partner and the allocations of partnership items attempt to inappropriately transfer the deductions from the tax-exempt partner to the taxable partners (Code Sec. 168(h)).[123]

Tax-exempt losses disallowed may be carried over to the next tax year and can be deducted to the extent of the taxpayer's net income from the property for that year. If property ceases to be tax-exempt use property during the lease term, the carried-over loss cannot be used to offset income from other property. If the property is disposed of, any disallowed loss is available under rules similar to passive activity losses (¶ 1177). However, the limitation on tax-exempt use property losses is applied before the passive activity rules (¶ 1169).

Hobby Losses

1195. Hobby Expenses and Losses. Expenses incurred by individuals, S corporations, partnerships, estates, and trusts that are attributable to an activity not engaged in for profit, i.e., a hobby, are generally deductible only to the extent of income produced by the activity (Code Sec. 183; Reg. § 1.183-1).[124] Specifically, if any activity is not engaged in for profit, deductions are allowed as follows:

(1) deductions a taxpayer can claim whether or not they are incurred with a hobby, e.g., taxes, interest, and casualty losses, are allowed even if they exceed hobby income;

(2) deductions that do not result in an adjustment to the basis of property, e.g., operating expenses, supplies, are allowed, but only to the extent that gross income from the hobby exceeds the deductions under category (1); and

(3) deductions that result in an adjustment to the basis of property, e.g., depreciation, amortization, are allowed, but only to the extent that gross income from the hobby that exceeds the deductions under category (1) and (2).

Individuals must claim the deductions in categories (2) and (3) above as miscellaneous itemized deductions on Schedule A of Form 1040, subject to the two-percent-of-adjusted-gross-income limitation (¶ 1011). If a partnership or S corporation carries on a hobby, the deduction limits apply at the entity level and are reflected in the individual shareholder's or partner's distributive shares.

Whether an activity is engaged in for profit is generally determined based on the facts and circumstances. However, an activity is presumed not to be a hobby if it produced a profit (gross income exceeded deductions) in any three of five consecutive tax years ending with the tax year in question, unless the IRS proves otherwise. An activity involving the breeding, training, showing, or racing of horses is presumed not to be a hobby if it produced a profit in two out of seven consecutive tax years. A special election on Form 5213 permits suspension of the presumption until after the fourth (or sixth, for horse breeding, training, showing, or racing) tax year after which the taxpayer first engages in the activity. Filing Form 5213 automatically extends the statute of limitations for the IRS to assess a deficiency for any deductions of the activity in any year in the five-year or seven-year period to two years after the due date of the return for the last year of the period.

References are to Standard Federal Tax Reports; Tax Research Consultant; and Practical Tax Explanations.

[122] ¶ 21,970; BUSEXP: 36,000   [123] ¶ 11,250; BUSEXP: 36,050   [124] ¶ 12,170, ¶ 12,171; BUSEXP:15,000; § 17,201

Chapter 12

DEPRECIATION, AMORTIZATION

AND DEPLETION

Allowance for Depreciation

1201. Property Subject to Depreciation. Taxpayers may deduct a reasonable allowance for the exhaustion, wear and tear of property used in a trade or business, or property held for the production of income (Reg. § 1.167(a)-1).[1] Depreciation is not allowable for property used solely for personal purposes, such as a residence.

Depreciation begins in the tax year that an asset is placed in service and ends in the tax year that it is retired from service or is fully depreciated (Reg. § 1.167(a)-10).[2] An asset is generally considered placed in service when it is in a condition or state of readiness and available for a specifically assigned function.

Methods of Depreciation. The Modified Accelerated Cost Recovery System (MACRS) (¶ 1236) applies to tangible property generally placed in service after 1986 and the Accelerated Cost Recovery System (ACRS) applies to property placed in service after 1980 and before 1987 (¶ 1252). Under MACRS and ACRS, the cost or other basis of an asset is generally recovered over a specific recovery period. Post-1980 depreciation on tangible assets first placed in service before 1981 is computed under the method elected for the years they were placed in service. For assets placed in service after 1970 and before 1981, the taxpayer had a choice of the Asset Depreciation Range (ADR) System (¶ 1282) or the general depreciation rules (¶ 1216). For tangible assets first placed in service before 1971, the taxpayer could have elected the Class Life System (CLS) for pre-1971 assets or the general depreciation rules. In no event may an asset

---

References are to Standard Federal Tax Reports; Tax Research Consultant; and Practical Tax Explanations.

[1] ¶ 11,003; DEPR: 15,050; § 11,005

[2] ¶ 11,024; DEPR: 15,652, DEPR: 3,054.104; § 11,020

¶1201

that is not subject to MACRS or ACRS be depreciated below a reasonable salvage value (Reg. § 1.167(a)-1(a)).[3]

Depreciation based on a useful life is calculated over the estimated useful life of the asset while actually used by the taxpayer and not over the longer period of the asset's physical life (Reg. § 1.167(a)-1(b)).[4] For rules governing the depreciation of self-constructed assets, see the uniform capitalization rules at ¶ 990–¶ 999.

Converted Residence. When an individual vacates a principal residence and offers it for sale, it may be depreciable for the period before the sale if the individual is seeking a profit based on the post-conversion appreciation in value. MACRS must be used to depreciate a residence converted to business use after 1986. For computation of depreciation when a home is used partly for business or rental purposes, see ¶ 961 and following. For depreciable basis, see ¶ 1203.

Estates and Trusts. For depreciation by an estate or trust, see ¶ 530.

Inventory. Depreciation is allowed for tangible property, but not for inventories, stock in trade, land apart from its improvements, or a depletable natural resource (Reg. § 1.167(a)-2).[5]

Farmers. Farm buildings and other physical farm property (except land) are depreciable. Livestock acquired for work, breeding, or dairy purposes may be depreciated unless included in inventory (Reg. § 1.167(a)-6(b)).[6]

Intangibles. An intangible business asset that is not amortizable over 15 years under Code Sec. 197 (¶ 1288) may be amortized under Code Sec. 167, generally using the straight-line method, provided that it has an ascertainable value and useful life that can be measured with reasonable accuracy.[7] Certain intangibles with no ascertainable useful life that are created by a taxpayer may be amortized over 15 years (Reg. § 1.167(a)-3(b)). See ¶ 1288A.

Software. Computer software that is not an amortizable Code Sec. 197 intangible (¶ 1288) may be depreciated using the straight-line method over 36 months beginning on the first day of the month the software is placed in service (Code Sec. 167(f)(1); Reg. § 1.167(a)-14(b)).[8] See ¶ 980. However, the cost of software developed for internal use or sale may be currently deducted as a research and development expense, amortized using the straight-line method over 60 months beginning on the date of completion of development, or amortized over 36 months from the date the software is placed in service (Rev. Proc. 2000-50). Off-the-shelf computer software may be expensed under Code Sec. 179 if placed in service in a tax year beginning after December 31, 2002, and before January 1, 2014 (Code Sec. 179(d)(1)). See ¶ 1208. Software included as part of the purchase price of a computer that has no separately stated cost is depreciated as part of the cost of the computer over a five-year recovery period (Reg. § 1.167(a)-14(b); Rev. Proc. 2000-50).

Web Site Development Costs. The IRS has not issued formal guidance on the treatment of web site development costs, but informal internal IRS guidance suggests that one appropriate approach is to treat these costs like an item of software and depreciate them over three years. It is clear, however, that taxpayers who pay large amounts to develop sophisticated sites have been allocating their costs to items such as software development (currently deductible like research and development costs under Code Sec. 174) and currently deductible advertising expense.[9]

Residential Mortgage-Servicing Rights. Depreciable residential mortgage-servicing rights that are not Code Sec. 197 intangibles may be depreciated under the straight-line method over 108 months (Code Sec. 167(f)(3)).[10]

References are to Standard Federal Tax Reports; Tax Research Consultant; and Practical Tax Explanations.

[3] ¶ 11,003; DEPR: 15,050; § 11,101

[4] ¶ 11,003; DEPR: 15,700; § 11,110

[5] ¶ 11,006; DEPR: 15,150; § 11,005

[6] ¶ 11,015; DEPR: 15,158, FARM: 9,078; § 36,320

[7] ¶ 11,008; DEPR: 15,162; § 11,005

[8] ¶ 11,002; DEPR: 15,162.85; § 11,535

[9] ¶ 13,720.01; BUSEXP: 18,852; § 11,005

[10] ¶ 11,002; DEPR: 15,162.90; § 11,540

Term Interests. The purchaser of a term interest in property held for business or investment is generally entitled to recover its cost over its expected life. However, no depreciation or amortization deduction is allowed for certain term interests in property for any period during which the remainder interest is held directly (or indirectly) by a related person (Code Sec. 167(e)).[11]

Form 4562. Form 4562 is generally used to claim the depreciation or amortization deduction and is attached to the taxpayer's tax return. Individuals and other noncorporate taxpayers (including S corporations) need not complete Form 4562 if their only depreciation (or amortization) deduction is for property (other than listed property (¶ 1211)) placed in service before the current tax year. Form 4562 must be filed if a section 179 deduction (including a carryover) is claimed in the current tax year.

Basis for Depreciation

1203. Cost or Other Basis Recoverable Through Depreciation Allowance. The cost of a depreciable asset, reduced by any amount claimed as an expense deduction under Code Sec. 179 (¶ 1208) or as first-year bonus depreciation (¶ 1237), may generally be recovered through depreciation. Other downward adjustments to cost may also be necessary to prevent a duplication of benefits received from credits and deductions claimed with respect to the property in the tax year of purchase. See ¶ 1365A for example for the effect of the investment credit on depreciable basis. When property held for personal use, such as a residence, is converted to business or income-producing use, the basis for depreciation is the lesser of the property's fair market value or adjusted basis on the date of conversion (Reg. § 1.167(g)-1; Reg. § 1.168(i)-4(b)).[12] In the case of a residence converted to business use after 1986, the Modified Accelerated Cost Recovery System (MACRS) must be used (¶ 1236).

When a building and land have been acquired for a lump sum, only the building is depreciated. The basis for depreciation cannot exceed the same proportion of the lump sum as the value of the building bore to the value of the entire property at the time of acquisition (Reg. § 1.167(a)-5). If property is subject to both depreciation and amortization, depreciation is allowable only for the portion that is not subject to amortization and may be taken concurrently with amortization.[13]

Section 179 Expense Election

1208. Election to Expense Certain Depreciable Business Assets. Taxpayers other than estates, trusts, and certain noncorporate lessors may elect an expense deduction for the cost of qualifying section 179 property placed in service during the tax year rather than treating the cost as a capital expenditure (Code Sec. 179).[14] The election is made on Form 4562 and is revocable only with IRS consent. The election is generally attached to the taxpayer's original return (including a late-filed original return). However, for property placed in service in tax years beginning before 2014, a taxpayer may make, revoke, or change an election without IRS consent on an amended return filed during the period prescribed for filing an amended return (Code Sec. 179(c)(2); Reg. § 1.179-5).[15]

> **Comment:** Absent further legislation, the ability to make, revoke, or change the election without IRS consent on an amended return has expired for property placed in service in tax years beginning after December 31, 2013. For the latest legislative updates, visit our website www.CCHGroup.com/TaxUpdates.

Dollar Limitation. The maximum Code Sec. 179 deduction is $25,000 for tax years beginning in 2014 and thereafter. The maximum deduction is $500,000 for tax years beginning in 2010 through 2013 (Code Sec. 179(b)(1)). Up to $250,000 of the $500,000 annual dollar limit for tax years beginning in 2010 through 2013 may be used to expense

---

References are to Standard Federal Tax Reports; Tax Research Consultant; and Practical Tax Explanations.

[11] ¶ 11,002; DEPR: 15,262; § 11,005

[12] ¶ 11,046; DEPR: 15,154; § 16,101

[13] ¶ 11,012, ¶ 11,014.021; SALES: 6,202; § 11,001

[14] ¶ 12,120, ¶ 12,126; DEPR: 12,000; § 9,801

[15] ¶ 12,120; DEPR: 12,050, DEPR: 12,150; § 9,830

qualified real property (discussed below). See also ¶ 1214 for a $25,000 deduction limit for any tax year on sport utility vehicles, short-bed trucks, and vans that are exempt from the luxury car depreciation caps.

> **Comment:** Absent further legislation, the maximum Code Sec. 179 deduction is only $25,000 for property placed in service in tax years beginning after 2013. At the time of publication, proposed legislation is pending before Congress to extend the increased deduction limit of $500,000 to property placed in service tax years beginning in 2014 and 2015. For the latest legislative updates, visit our website www.CCHGroup.com/TaxUpdates.

De Minimis Expensing Rule. Taxpayers may claim a current deduction for amounts paid or incurred to acquire or produce relatively low-cost units of property if specific requirements are met. See ¶ 903.

Investment Limitation. The maximum Code Sec. 179 dollar limitation is reduced dollar for dollar by the cost of qualified property placed in service during the tax year over an investment limitation. For tax years beginning in 2014 and thereafter the investment limitation is $200,000. The investment limitation is $2 million for tax years beginning in 2010 through 2013 (Code Sec. 179(b)(2)).

> **Comment:** Absent further legislation, the investment limitation is only $200,000 for property placed in service in tax years beginning after 2013. At the time of publication, proposed legislation is pending in Congress to extend the increased investment limitation to $2 million for property placed in service in tax years beginning in 2014 and 2015. For the latest legislative updates, visit our website www.CCHGroup.com/TaxUpdates.

Taxable Income Limitation. The total cost of property that may be expensed for any tax year cannot exceed the total amount of taxable income derived from the active conduct of any trade or business during the tax year, including employee salaries and wages (Code Sec. 179(b)(3)). An amount disallowed as the result of the taxable income limitation is carried forward. The deduction for carryforwards and the amounts expensed for qualifying property placed in service in a carryforward year, however, may not exceed the maximum annual dollar cost ceiling, investment limitation, or taxable income limitation for that year. Absent further legislation, no amount attributable to qualified real property (discussed below) may be carried over to a tax year beginning after 2013 (Code Sec. 179(f)(4)(A)).

Qualifying Section 179 Property. To qualify as section 179 property, the property must be tangible section 1245 property (new or used), depreciable under the Modified Accelerated Cost Recovery System (MACRS), and acquired by purchase for use in the active conduct of a trade or business (Code Sec. 179(d)).[16] Code Sec. 50(b) property and air conditioning and heating units do not qualify as section 179 property. Code Sec. 50(b) property includes property used predominantly outside of the United States, property used with respect to lodging, such as apartment buildings but not hotels and motels, and property used by tax-exempt organizations (unless the property is used predominantly in connection with an unrelated business income activity). A taxpayer may also make an election to treat qualified real property (discussed below) placed in service in certain tax years as section 179 property (Code Sec. 179(f)(1)).

Depreciable off-the-shelf computer software placed in service in tax years beginning in 2003 through 2013 may be expensed under Code Sec. 179 (Code Sec. 179(d)(1)(A)).[17] This is software described in Code Sec. 197(e)(3)(A)(i) that is readily available for purchase by the general public, is subject to a nonexclusive license, and has not been substantially modified, and which is depreciable over three years under Code Sec. 167(f)(1)(A).

> **Comment:** Absent further legislation, the election to expense off-the-shelf computer software has expired effective for property placed in service in tax years beginning after December 31, 2013. For the latest legislative updates, visit our website www.CCHGroup.com/TaxUpdates.

References are to Standard Federal Tax Reports; Tax Research Consultant; and Practical Tax Explanations.

[16] ¶ 12,120; DEPR: 12,200; §9,810　　[17] ¶ 12,120; DEPR: 12,200; §9,810

Qualified Real Property. A taxpayer may elect to treat the cost of qualified real property placed in service in a tax year that begins in 2010 through 2013 as section 179 property (Code Sec. 179(f); Notice 2013-59). The maximum amount of qualified real property that may be expensed is limited to $250,000. The expensed amount is counted toward the overall $500,000 annual expensing limit for those years, as discussed above.

> **Comment:** Absent further legislation, the election to expense qualified real property has expired effective for property placed in service in tax years beginning after December 31, 2013. For the latest legislative updates, visit our website www.CCHGroup.com/TaxUpdates.

> **Example 1:** A calendar-year taxpayer places $600,000 of qualified real property in service in 2013 and elects to treat the property as section 179 property. Assume that the taxpayer also places $400,000 of other section 179 property in service in 2013. The annual dollar limit for 2013 ($500,000) is not subject to reduction under the investment limitation because the taxpayer did not place more than $2 million of section 179 property in service in 2013 (only $1 million of section 179 property was placed in service). The taxpayer may elect to expense up to $250,000 of the cost of its qualified real property. If it elects to expense $250,000 of the qualified real property, then it may only elect to expense up to $250,000 of its other section 179 property in 2013.

Qualified real property is defined as:

> (1) qualified leasehold improvement property, described in Code Sec. 168(e)(6) (¶ 1234);

> (2) qualified restaurant property (i.e., a restaurant building or improvement described in Code Sec. 168(e)(7)) (¶ 1240); and

> (3) qualified retail improvement property, described in Code Sec. 168(e)(8) (¶ 1240).

The property must be depreciable and acquired by purchase for use in the active conduct of a trade or business. It does not include Code Sec. 50(b) property, and air conditioning or heating units, as discussed in *"Qualifying Section 179 Property,"* above.

No amount of a section 179 deduction attributable to qualified real property that is disallowed under the taxable income limitation may be carried over to a tax year beginning after 2013 (Code Sec. 179(f)(4)). To the extent that any amount attributable to qualified real property is not allowed to be carried over to a tax year beginning after 2013, the taxpayer is treated as if no section 179 election had been made. The amount of a disallowed carryover attributable to qualified real property placed in service in any tax year other than the taxpayer's last tax year beginning in 2013 is treated as property that was placed in service on the first day of the taxpayer's last tax year beginning in 2013. For the last tax year of the taxpayer beginning in 2013, the amount determined under the taxable business income limitation of Code Sec. 179(b)(3)(A) for the tax year is determined without regard to the carryover limitation rules for qualified real property.

> **Example 2:** A calendar year taxpayer pays for $150,000 of qualified real property in 2012 and elects to expense the entire amount. No other amount is expensed. The taxpayer's 2012 taxable income is $50,000. The taxpayer therefore has a $100,000 carryforward attributable to qualified real property for 2013. Assume that no portion of that carryforward is deductible in 2013 because the taxpayer expensed $500,000 of other property placed in service in 2013. The $100,000 carryforward may not be carried forward to 2014 and is treated as attributable to property placed in service on January 1, 2013, and may be depreciated. No depreciation claimed in 2013 on the $100,000 will reduce taxable income for purposes of determining the amount of the 2013 taxable income limitation.

If a taxpayer places both qualified real property that is treated as section 179 property and other types of section 179 property in service in a tax year in which there is a carryforward due to application of the taxable income limitation, the amount of the carryforward is allocated pro rata between the qualified real property and the other types of section 179 property that the taxpayer placed in service during the tax year and elected to expense (Code Sec. 179(f)(4)(D); Notice 2013-59).

The amount of qualified real property that is expensed under Code Sec. 179 is subject to the section 1245 ordinary income recapture rules (Code Sec. 1245(a)(3)(C)). Where only a portion of the cost of a qualified real property is expensed, a taxpayer may use any reasonable method to determine the amount of gain on the disposition of the qualified real property that is attributable to section 1245 property and section 1250 property, including the pro rata allocation methodology and gain allocation methodology described in Notice 2013-59. The section 1245 recapture amount is limited to the gain allocated to the section 1245 property.

Purchase Defined. Property is acquired by purchase unless it (1) is acquired from certain related persons, (2) is transferred between members of a controlled group, (3) has a substituted basis in whole or in part, or (4) is acquired from a decedent and has a basis determined under Code Sec. 1014(a) (i.e., a fair-market value basis) (Code Sec. 179(d)(2)).

Recapture. The Code Sec. 179 expense deduction is treated as depreciation for recapture purposes. Thus, gain on a disposition of section 179 property that is section 1245 property is treated as ordinary income to the extent of the Code Sec. 179 expense allowance claimed plus any depreciation claimed. Qualified real property is section 1250 property. However, as discussed above, the section 179 expense deduction claimed on qualified real property is subject to recapture as ordinary income under the rules that apply to section 1245 property (Code Sec. 1245(a)(3)(C)).

If business use of section 179 property fails to exceed 50 percent during any year of the property's depreciation period, a portion of the amount expensed is recaptured as ordinary income (Code Sec. 179(d)(10); Reg. § 1.179-1(e)). The recapture amount is the difference between the expense claimed and the depreciation that would have been allowed on the expensed amount for prior tax years and the tax year of recapture. Recapture is reported on Form 4797.

In the case of a listed property, such as a passenger automobile, the recapture rules described at ¶ 1211 for property used 50 percent or less for business apply in place of the preceding recapture rule.

Empowerment Zones. The section 179 dollar limit ($500,000 for tax years beginning in 2010 through 2013) is increased an additional $35,000 for section 179 property placed in service in designated empowerment zones by an enterprise zone business (Code Sec. 1397A).[18] The $35,000 increase is subject to recapture if the property is removed from the empowerment zone. In general, the qualifying property must be placed in service in the empowerment zone before January 1, 2014 (Code Secs. 1391(d)(1) and 1400).

Qualified Disaster Assistance Property. The section 179 dollar limit ($500,000 for tax years beginning in 2010 through 2013) was increased by the lesser of $100,000 or the cost of qualified disaster assistance property placed in service during the tax year that was also section 179 property. The investment limitation ($2 million for tax years beginning in 2010 through 2013) was increased by the lesser of $600,000 or the cost of qualified section 179 disaster assistance property placed in service during the tax year. Qualified disaster assistance property must rehabilitate property damaged, or replace property destroyed or condemned, as a result of a federally declared disaster. This provision applies to property placed in service after December 31, 2007, with respect to federally declared disasters declared after such date and occurring before January 1, 2010. The property generally had to be placed in service before the last day of the third calendar year following the date the disaster occurred (Code Sec. 179(e)).

References are to Standard Federal Tax Reports; Tax Research Consultant; and Practical Tax Explanations.

[18] ¶ 32,397; DEPR: 12,116;
§ 9,815.05

Limitations on Automobiles and Other Listed Property

1211. Business Usage Requirement for Listed Property. Depreciation deductions for "listed property" are subject to special rules (Code Sec. 280F).[19] Listed property includes: passenger automobiles (¶ 1214); other forms of transportation, if the property's nature lends itself to personal use (e.g., airplanes, boats, vehicles excluded from the definition of a passenger automobile); entertainment, recreational and amusement property; computers and peripheral equipment; and any other property specified by regulation. If an item of listed property is not used more than 50 percent for business, the deductions under the Modified Accelerated Cost Recovery System (MACRS) on the property must be determined under the alternative depreciation system (ADS) (Code Sec. 280F(b)(1)) (¶ 1247).

If the listed property satisfies the more-than-50-percent business use requirement in the tax year it is placed in service but fails to meet that test in a later tax year that occurs during any year of the property's ADS recovery period, depreciation deductions (including bonus depreciation) previously taken are subject to recapture (Code Sec. 280F(b)(2)). MACRS depreciation for years preceding the year in which the business use falls to 50 percent or less is recaptured to the extent that the MACRS depreciation (including any depreciation) for such years exceeds the depreciation that would have been allowed under ADS. Depreciation thereafter must be computed using ADS.

If the more-than-50-percent business use test is not satisfied in the tax year the property is placed in service, the property does not qualify for the Code Sec. 179 expensing election (¶ 1208). If the more-than-50-percent business use test is initially satisfied but is not met in a later tax year, the Code Sec. 179 expense deduction is treated as a depreciation deduction for purposes of the listed property depreciation recapture rule above. For example, if a taxpayer expenses the entire cost of a listed property, the difference between the amount expensed and the ADS deductions that would have been allowed on that amount prior to the recapture year is recaptured as ordinary income.

See ¶ 1214 for additional limits on passenger automobiles.

Reporting. Part IV of Form 4797 is used to calculate any recapture amount.

1214. Limitations on Passenger Automobiles, Including Trucks, SUVs, and Vans. The maximum depreciation deductions under the Modified Accelerated Cost Recovery System (MACRS) (including the Section 179 expensing deduction (¶ 1208) and first-year bonus depreciation allowance (¶ 1237)) that may be claimed for a passenger automobile other than a truck, including an SUV treated as a truck, or van placed in service in calendar year 2004 or later are shown in the chart below (Code Sec. 280F).[20] For earlier years, see IRS Publication 463.

For Cars Placed in Service		Depreciation Allowable in—				
After	Before	Year 1	Year 2	Year 3	Year 4, etc.	Authority
12/31/03	1/01/05	10,610 * 2,960	4,800	2,850	1,675	Rev. Proc. 2004-20
12/31/04	1/01/06	2,960	4,700	2,850	1,675	Rev. Proc. 2005-13
12/31/05	1/01/07	2,960	4,800	2,850	1,775	Rev. Proc. 2006-18
12/31/06	1/01/08	3,060	4,900	2,850	1,775	Rev. Proc. 2007-30
12/31/07	1/01/10	10,960 * 2,960	4,800	2,850	1,775	Rev. Proc. 2008-22, Rev. Proc. 2009-24
12/31/09	1/01/12	11,060 * 3,060	4,900	2,950	1,775	Rev. Proc. 2010-18, as modified by Rev. Proc. 2011-21

References are to Standard Federal Tax Reports; Tax Research Consultant; and Practical Tax Explanations.

[19] ¶ 15,100; DEPR: 3,500; § 11,301

[20] ¶ 15,100; DEPR: 3,504; § 11,330.05

12/31/11	1/01/14	11,160 * 3,160	5,100	3,050	1,875	Rev. Proc. 2012-23, Rev. Proc. 2013-21
12/31/13	1/01/15	3,160	5,100	3,050	1,875	Rev. Proc. 2014-21

* The higher first-year limit applies if the vehicle qualifies for bonus depreciation under the general provision of Code Sec. 168(k) and no election out is made. The higher limit does not apply if bonus depreciation is claimed under the authority of any other bonus depreciation provision, such as the provision for Gulf Opportunity Zone Property or Disaster Assistance Property. See ¶ 1237.

Assuming that the 200-percent declining balance method and half-year convention apply, a car placed in service in 2014 is subject to the first-year cap if the cost of the vehicle exceeds $15,800 ($15,800 × 20% = $3,160).

Trucks (including SUVs treated as trucks) and vans are subject to their own set of depreciation caps if placed in service after 2002. These caps (reproduced in the table below) reflect the higher costs associated with such vehicles. Keep in mind, however, that trucks and vans that have a loaded gross vehicle weight rating greater than 6,000 pounds are not subject to any caps (see below). *Also, certain trucks and vans placed in service after July 6, 2003, are not subject to the caps if, because of their design, they are not likely to be used for personal purposes (see below).* The following chart shows the depreciation caps for trucks and vans placed in service in calendar year 2003 and later.

For Trucks and Vans Placed in Service After	Before	Depreciation Allowable in—				
		Year 1	Year 2	Year 3	Year 4, etc.	Authority
12/31/02	5/06/03	7,960 * 3,360	5,400	3,250	1,975	Rev. Proc. 2003-75
5/05/03	1/01/04	11,010 * 3,360	5,400	3,250	1,975	Rev. Proc. 2003-75
12/31/03	1/01/05	10,910 * 3,260	5,300	3,150	1,875	Rev. Proc. 2004-20
12/31/04	1/01/06	3,260	5,200	3,150	1,875	Rev. Proc. 2005-13
12/31/05	1/01/07	3,260	5,200	3,150	1,875	Rev. Proc. 2006-18
12/31/06	1/01/08	3,260	5,200	3,050	1,875	Rev. Proc. 2007-30
12/31/07	1/01/09	11,160 * 3,160	5,100	3,050	1,875	Rev. Proc. 2008-22
12/31/08	1/01/10	11,060 * 3,060	4,900	2,950	1,775	Rev. Proc. 2009-24
12/31/09	1/01/11	11,160 * 3,160	5,100	3,050	1,875	Rev. Proc. 2010-18, as modified by Rev. Proc. 2011-21
12/31/10	1/01/12	11,260 * 3,260	5,200	3,150	1,875	Rev. Proc. 2011-21
12/31/11	1/01/13	11,360 * 3,360	5,300	3,150	1,875	Rev. Proc. 2012-23
12/31/12	1/01/14	11,360 * 3,360	5,400	3,250	1,975	Rev. Proc. 2013-21
12/31/13	1/01/15	3,460	5,500	3,350	1,975	Rev. Proc. 2014-21

* The higher first-year limit applies if the vehicle qualifies for bonus depreciation under the general provision of Code Sec. 168(k) and no election out is made. The higher limit does not apply if bonus depreciation is claimed under the authority of any other bonus depreciation provision, such as the provision for Gulf Opportunity Zone Property or Disaster Assistance Property. See ¶ 1237.

Assuming that the 200-percent declining balance method and half-year convention apply and that no bonus depreciation is claimed, a truck or van placed in service in 2014 is subject to the first-year cap if the cost of the vehicle exceeds $17,300 ($17,300 × 20% = $3,460).

The above maximum annual limits (often referred to as the luxury car limits) are based on 100-percent business use. If business use is less than 100 percent, the limits must be reduced to reflect the actual business use percentage.

For electric passenger automobiles built by an original equipment manufacturer and placed in service after August 5, 1997 and before 2007, the yearly statutory limits that apply to depreciation for luxury cars are tripled and then adjusted for inflation (Code Sec. 280F(a)(1)(C)(ii)).[21] The annual limits above apply to electric vehicles placed in service after 2006. The limits for electric vehicles placed in service before 2007 are located in the Revenue Procedures cited in the "Authority" column in the charts above.

For passenger vehicles that initially used nonclean-burning fuel, but were modified to allow them to be propelled by clean-burning fuel, the Code Sec. 280F limits do not apply to the cost of the installed device that equips the car to use clean-burning fuel. The balance of the car's cost remains subject to the Code Sec. 280F limits (Code Sec. 280F(a)(1)(C)).[22]

Passenger Automobile Defined. For purposes of the depreciation caps, a passenger automobile includes any four-wheeled vehicle manufactured primarily for use on public streets, roads, and highways that has an *unloaded* gross vehicle weight rating (GVWR) (i.e., curb weight fully equipped for service but without passengers or cargo) of 6,000 pounds or less (Code Sec. 280F(d)(5)(A)).[23] However, a truck or van is only treated as a passenger automobile subject to the caps if it has a *gross* vehicle weight rating (i.e., maximum total weight of a loaded vehicle as specified by the manufacturer) of 6,000 pounds or less (Code Sec. 280F(d)(5)(B)). A truck or van, therefore, is not subject to the depreciation caps if its GVWR exceeds 6,000 pounds. A sport utility vehicle is generally treated as a truck (even if built on a unibody (i.e., car chassis)) and, therefore, if its GVWR is in excess of 6,000 pounds it is also exempt from the caps. See footnoted material for further discussion of the definition of a "truck" as well as a list of SUVs, trucks, and vans with a GVWR in excess of 6,000 pounds.[24] Ambulances or hearses and vehicles used directly in the trade or business of transporting persons or property for hire (e.g., taxis and limousines) are not considered passenger automobiles subject to the caps regardless of their weight.

Luxury Car Depreciation Examples. The depreciation deduction that is claimed on the return for any tax year during a vehicle's recovery (depreciation) period is the lesser of the depreciation deduction for the tax year (computed as if there were no depreciation caps) or the cap that applies for the tax year.[25]

If, after the recovery period for a passenger automobile ends, the taxpayer continues to use the car in its trade or business, the unrecovered basis (referred to as "Sec. 280F unrecovered basis") may be deducted at the maximum annual rate provided in the chart above for the fourth and succeeding years. This rule permits depreciation deductions beyond the recovery period. Unrecovered basis is the difference between the cost of the vehicle and the amount of depreciation claimed on the return during the recovery period (or that would have been claimed on the return if business use had been 100 percent). The MACRS recovery period for a passenger automobile is five full years from the date the vehicle is deemed placed in service under the applicable half-year or mid-quarter convention (¶ 1245). Due to operation of the applicable convention, depreciation deductions are claimed over the six tax years that the five-year recovery period falls within.

The following example illustrates how depreciation is computed if the 50-percent bonus depreciation allowance is not claimed.

References are to Standard Federal Tax Reports; Tax Research Consultant; and Practical Tax Explanations.

[21] ¶ 15,100; DEPR: 3,504, BUSEXP: 18,704; § 11,330.05

[22] ¶ 15,100; DEPR: 3,504; § 11,330.05

[23] ¶ 15,100; BUSEXP: 24,852.05, DEPR: 12,150; § 840

[24] ¶ 15,108.022; DEPR: 3,502.052; § 840

[25] ¶ 15,108.40; DEPR: 3,600, DEPR: 3,504.15; § 11,330.10

¶1214

Example 1: On April 5, 2014, a calendar-year taxpayer purchased a car for $30,000. Business use of the car each year is 100 percent. Depreciation is computed under the general MACRS 200-percent declining-balance method over a five-year recovery period using a half-year convention subject to the luxury car limitations. Allowable depreciation during the regular recovery period (2014 through 2019) is computed as follows:

Year	100% Business-Use MACRS Depreciation	Luxury Car Limit	Deduction: Lesser of Col. 2 or 3	Sec. 280F Unrecovered Basis
2014.......	$6,000	$3,160	$3,160	$26,840
2015.......	9,600	5,100	5,100	21,740
2016.......	5,760	3,050	3,050	18,690
2017.......	3,456	1,875	1,875	16,815
2018.......	3,456	1,875	1,875	14,940
2019.......	1,728	1,875	1,728	13,212

Note that the unrecovered basis is computed by subtracting the depreciation that would have been allowed (taking the applicable cap into consideration) if business use was 100% (even if business use in less than 100%). Thus, for example, the unrecovered basis at the close of 2014 is $26,840 ($30,000 – $3,160). The $13,212 unrecovered basis at the close of the regular recovery period is deducted in the post recovery period years at the rate of $1,875 per year assuming 100-percent business use continues. The unrecovered basis is reduced by $1,875 each year regardless of the percentage of business use.

The following example shows how luxury car depreciation is computed if the 50-percent bonus deduction is claimed.

Example 2: On April 5, 2013, a calendar-year taxpayer purchased a new car for $30,000. Business use of the car each year is 100 percent. Depreciation is computed under the general MACRS 200-percent declining-balance method over a five-year recovery period using a half-year convention subject to the luxury car limitations. Allowable depreciation during the regular recovery period (2013 through 2018) is computed as follows:

Year	100% Business-Use MACRS Depreciation	Luxury Car Limit	Deduction: Lesser of Col. 2 or 3	Sec. 280F Unrecovered Basis
2013.......	$18,000	$11,160	$11,160	$18,840
2014.......	4,800	5,100	4,800	14,040
2015.......	2,880	3,050	2,880	11,160
2016.......	1,728	1,875	1,728	9,432
2017.......	1,728	1,875	1,728	7,704
2018.......	864	1,875	864	6,840

Beginning in 2019, the unrecovered basis is the $6,840 difference between the $30,000 cost and the sum of the return deductions claimed in 2013 through 2018. The unrecovered basis is deducted at the rate of $1,875 per year assuming that 100-percent business use continues. However, the unrecovered basis is reduced by $1,875 each year regardless of the percentage of business use.

Special Rules for Vehicles Subject to 100-Percent Bonus Depreciation in 2010 or 2011. If the 100-percent bonus deduction was claimed in 2010 or 2011 on a new car that is subject to the caps and a safe-harbor election was not made, a taxpayer claimed the amount of the first-year cap since this was less than the bonus depreciation allowance. No depreciation may be claimed in any succeeding years of the vehicle's recovery period because the depreciation deduction for each of those years computed as if there were no depreciation caps is $0 (the full cost is deemed deducted as a bonus depreciation allowance) and $0 is less than the cap amount for each of those years. To address this anomaly, a safe harbor election allowed a taxpayer to claim a 100-percent bonus depreciation deduction in the amount of the first-year cap in the year that the vehicle was placed in service and then determine its depreciation deductions for the remaining years in the recovery period by computing those deductions as if a 50-percent bonus depreciation allowance was claimed in the year the vehicle was placed in service. A taxpayer made this election by computing its depreciation deductions in accordance with the election (Rev. Proc. 2011-26).

12 DEPRECIATION

¶1214

$25,000 Section 179 Expensing Cap on Sport Utility Vehicles, Certain Trucks, and Certain Vans That Are Exempt from Luxury Car Depreciation Caps. The maximum amount of the cost of an SUV that may be expensed under Code Sec. 179 if the SUV is exempt from the luxury car caps (e.g., has a GVWR in excess of 6,000 pounds) is limited to $25,000, effective for SUVs placed in service after October 22, 2004. The $25,000 limitation also applies to exempt trucks with an interior cargo bed length of less than six feet and exempt passenger vans that seat fewer than ten persons behind the driver's seat. Exempt cargo vans are generally not subject to the $25,000 limitation (Code Sec. 179(b)(5)).

Exclusion from Depreciation Caps for Certain Trucks and Vans Not Likely To Be Used for Personal Purposes. Effective for trucks and vans placed in service after July 6, 2003, a truck or van that is a qualified nonpersonal use vehicle as defined in Reg. § 1.274-5(k) is excluded from the definition of a passenger automobile and is not subject to the annual depreciation limits (Reg. § 1.280F-6(c)(3)(iii)).[26] A qualified nonpersonal use vehicle generally is one that has been specially modified in such a way that it is not likely to be used more than a *de minimis* amount for personal purposes.

Reporting. The allowable depreciation deduction for any listed property, including automobiles, is reported on Form 4562 (Part V).

1215. Leased Listed Property Inclusion Amounts. The lessee of a passenger automobile (¶ 1214) used for business is required to include an additional amount in income to offset rental deductions for each tax year during which the vehicle is leased (Code Sec. 280F(c)(2); Reg. § 1.280F-7).[27] The inclusion amount is based on the cost of the vehicle and generally applies to a vehicle with a fair market value exceeding an inflation-adjusted dollar amount. The inclusion amount is not required on trucks, vans, and SUVs that would be exempt from the depreciation caps if owned by the lessee (e.g., an SUV treated as a truck with a GVWR in excess of 6,000 pounds).

Lease inclusion tables are issued annually by the IRS in the same revenue procedure in which the annual depreciation caps are issued (see list of these revenue procedures at ¶ 1214). The appropriate table is based on the calendar year that the vehicle was first leased. The same table is used for each year of the lease term.

Each revenue procedure includes a lease inclusion table for passenger automobiles and a lease inclusion table for trucks and vans (including SUVs treated as a truck). Prior to 2003, trucks and vans used the same table that applied to other passenger automobiles. Prior to 2007, electric vehicles had a separate lease inclusion table. Electric vehicles first leased in 2007 are now subject to the table that applies to passenger automobiles or trucks and vans, as appropriate. The inclusion tables for vehicles first leased in 2014 are reproduced below. For tables for vehicles first leased in earlier calendar years, see the STANDARD FEDERAL TAX REPORTER ¶ 15,108.048, Practical Tax Explanations § 850, or IRS Publication 463.

A lessee's inclusion amount for each tax year that the vehicle is leased is computed as follows: (1) use the fair market value of the vehicle on the first day of the lease term to find the appropriate dollar (inclusion) amounts on the IRS table (see below); (2) prorate the dollar amount from the table for the number of days of the lease term included in the tax year; and (3) multiply the prorated amount by the percentage of business and investment use for the tax year. For the last tax year during any lease that does not begin and end in the same tax year, the dollar amount for the preceding tax year should be used.

> **Example:** A car costing $25,500 is leased for four years by a calendar-year taxpayer beginning on April 1, 2014, and is used 100 percent for business. The annual dollar amounts from the table for leases beginning in 2014 are: $8 for the first tax year during the lease, $19 for the second tax year, $27 for the third tax year, $32 for the fourth tax year, and $38 for the fifth and following tax years. In

---

References are to Standard Federal Tax Reports; Tax Research Consultant; and Practical Tax Explanations.

[26] ¶ 15,107; DEPR: 3,502.05; § 11,305

[27] ¶ 15,100, ¶ 15,107; DEPR: 3,512; § 11,330.05

2014, the inclusion amount is $6.03 (275/365 × $8). The inclusion amounts for 2015, 2016, and 2017 are $19, $27, and $32, respectively, since the vehicle is leased for the entire year during these tax years. In 2018, the inclusion amount is $7.89 (90/365 × $32 (the dollar amount for 2017, the preceding tax year, is used in the last year of the lease)).

Listed Property Other Than Passenger Automobiles. Lessees of listed property other than passenger automobiles (¶ 1211) are required to include in income a usage-based inclusion amount in the first tax year that the business use percentage of such property is 50 percent or less (Code Sec. 280F(c); Reg. § 1.280F-7(b)).[28]

Reporting. The inclusion amount is reported on Form 2106 by employees, Schedule C (Form 1040) by the self-employed, and Schedule F by farmers.

Dollar Amounts for Passenger Automobiles
(That are not Trucks or Vans)
With a Lease Term Beginning in Calendar Year 2014
[Rev. Proc. 2014-21, I.R.B. 2014-11]

Fair Market Value of Passenger Automobile		*Tax Year During Lease*				
Over	*Not Over*	*1st*	*2nd*	*3rd*	*4th*	*5th and Later*
$18,500	$19,000	3	5	8	10	11
19,000	19,500	3	6	10	11	13
19,500	20,000	3	8	11	13	14
20,000	20,500	4	8	13	14	17
20,500	21,000	4	9	14	17	18
21,000	21,500	5	10	15	18	21
21,500	22,000	5	11	17	20	22
22,000	23,000	6	13	18	23	25
23,000	24,000	7	14	22	26	29
24,000	25,000	8	16	25	29	33
25,000	26,000	8	19	27	32	38
26,000	27,000	9	20	31	35	42
27,000	28,000	10	22	33	40	45
28,000	29,000	11	24	36	43	49
29,000	30,000	12	26	39	46	53
30,000	31,000	13	28	41	50	57
31,000	32,000	14	30	44	53	61
32,000	33,000	14	32	47	56	65
33,000	34,000	15	34	50	59	69
34,000	35,000	16	36	52	64	72
35,000	36,000	17	38	55	67	76
36,000	37,000	18	39	59	70	80
37,000	38,000	19	41	61	74	84
38,000	39,000	20	43	64	77	88
39,000	40,000	21	45	67	80	92
40,000	41,000	21	47	70	84	96
41,000	42,000	22	49	73	87	100
42,000	43,000	23	51	75	91	104
43,000	44,000	24	53	78	94	108
44,000	45,000	25	55	81	97	112
45,000	46,000	26	56	84	101	116

References are to Standard Federal Tax Reports; Tax Research Consultant; and Practical Tax Explanations.

[28] ¶ 15,100, ¶ 15,107; DEPR: 3,512.10; § 11,330.05

Dollar Amounts for Passenger Automobiles
(That are not Trucks or Vans)
With a Lease Term Beginning in Calendar Year 2014
[Rev. Proc. 2014-21, I.R.B. 2014-11]

Fair Market Value of Passenger Automobile		Tax Year During Lease				
Over	Not Over	1st	2nd	3rd	4th	5th and Later
46,000	47,000	27	58	87	104	120
47,000	48,000	28	60	90	107	124
48,000	49,000	28	62	93	111	127
49,000	50,000	29	64	96	114	131
50,000	51,000	30	66	98	118	135
51,000	52,000	31	68	101	121	139
52,000	53,000	32	70	104	124	143
53,000	54,000	33	72	106	128	147
54,000	55,000	34	74	109	131	151
55,000	56,000	34	76	112	135	155
56,000	57,000	35	78	115	138	159
57,000	58,000	36	80	118	141	163
58,000	59,000	37	81	121	145	167
59,000	60,000	38	83	124	148	171
60,000	62,000	39	86	128	153	177
62,000	64,000	41	90	134	159	185
64,000	66,000	43	94	139	167	192
66,000	68,000	44	98	145	173	201
68,000	70,000	46	102	150	180	209
70,000	72,000	48	105	156	188	216
72,000	74,000	50	109	162	194	224
74,000	76,000	51	113	168	200	232
76,000	78,000	53	117	173	208	239
78,000	80,000	55	120	179	215	247
80,000	85,000	58	127	189	226	261
85,000	90,000	62	137	203	243	281
90,000	95,000	67	146	217	260	301
95,000	100,000	71	156	231	277	320
100,000	110,000	77	170	253	303	349
110,000	120,000	86	189	281	337	389
120,000	130,000	95	208	310	370	428
130,000	140,000	103	228	337	405	467
140,000	150,000	112	247	366	438	507
150,000	160,000	121	266	394	473	545
160,000	170,000	130	284	423	507	585
170,000	180,000	138	304	451	541	624
180,000	190,000	147	323	479	575	663
190,000	200,000	156	342	507	609	703
200,000	210,000	164	361	536	643	742
210,000	220,000	173	380	565	676	781
220,000	230,000	182	399	593	710	821
230,000	240,000	190	418	622	744	860
240,000	and over	199	437	650	778	899

Dollar Amounts for Trucks and Vans
With a Lease Term Beginning in Calendar Year 2014
[Rev. Proc. 2014-21, I.R.B. 2014-11]

Fair Market Value of Truck or Van		*Tax Year During Lease*				
Over	*Not Over*	*1st*	*2nd*	*3rd*	*4th*	*5th and later*
$19,000	$19,500	2	4	5	7	8
19,500	20,000	2	5	7	8	10
20,000	20,500	3	6	8	10	12
20,500	21,000	3	7	10	11	14
21,000	21,500	3	8	11	14	15
21,500	22,000	4	9	12	15	18
22,000	23,000	5	10	15	17	21
23,000	24,000	5	12	18	21	24
24,000	25,000	6	14	20	25	28
25,000	26,000	7	16	23	28	32
26,000	27,000	8	18	26	31	36
27,000	28,000	9	20	28	35	40
28,000	29,000	10	21	32	38	44
29,000	30,000	11	23	35	41	48
30,000	31,000	11	26	37	45	52
31,000	32,000	12	27	41	48	56
32,000	33,000	13	29	43	52	60
33,000	34,000	14	31	46	55	64
34,000	35,000	15	33	49	58	68
35,000	36,000	16	35	51	62	72
36,000	37,000	17	37	54	65	76
37,000	38,000	18	38	58	69	79
38,000	39,000	18	41	60	72	83
39,000	40,000	19	43	63	75	87
40,000	41,000	20	44	66	79	91
41,000	42,000	21	46	69	82	95
42,000	43,000	22	48	72	85	99
43,000	44,000	23	50	74	89	103
44,000	45,000	24	52	77	93	106
45,000	46,000	24	54	80	96	111
46,000	47,000	25	56	83	99	115
47,000	48,000	26	58	86	102	119
48,000	49,000	27	60	88	106	123
49,000	50,000	28	62	91	109	127
50,000	51,000	29	63	95	113	130
51,000	52,000	30	65	97	117	134
52,000	53,000	31	67	100	120	138
53,000	54,000	31	69	103	123	142
54,000	55,000	32	71	106	126	146
55,000	56,000	33	73	108	130	150
56,000	57,000	34	75	111	133	154
57,000	58,000	35	77	114	137	157
58,000	59,000	36	79	116	141	161
59,000	60,000	37	80	120	144	165
60,000	62,000	38	84	123	149	172

12 | DEPRECIATION

¶1215

Dollar Amounts for Trucks and Vans
With a Lease Term Beginning in Calendar Year 2014
[Rev. Proc. 2014-21, I.R.B. 2014-11]

Fair Market Value of Truck or Van		Tax Year During Lease				
Over	Not Over	1st	2nd	3rd	4th	5th and later
62,000	64,000	40	87	130	155	180
64,000	66,000	41	91	136	162	187
66,000	68,000	43	95	141	169	195
68,000	70,000	45	99	146	176	203
70,000	72,000	47	102	153	182	211
72,000	74,000	48	107	158	189	219
74,000	76,000	50	110	164	196	227
76,000	78,000	52	114	169	203	235
78,000	80,000	54	118	175	209	243
80,000	85,000	57	124	185	222	256
85,000	90,000	61	134	199	239	276
90,000	95,000	65	144	213	256	295
95,000	100,000	70	153	227	273	315
100,000	110,000	76	168	248	298	345
110,000	120,000	85	187	277	332	383
120,000	130,000	93	206	305	366	423
130,000	140,000	102	225	334	400	462
140,000	150,000	111	244	362	434	501
150,000	160,000	120	263	390	468	541
160,000	170,000	128	282	419	502	580
170,000	180,000	137	301	447	536	619
180,000	190,000	146	320	475	571	658
190,000	200,000	154	339	504	604	698
200,000	210,000	163	358	532	639	736
210,000	220,000	172	377	561	672	776
220,000	230,000	180	397	589	706	815
230,000	240,000	189	416	617	740	854
240,000	and over	198	435	645	774	894

Depreciation Methods

1216. Methods of Computing Depreciation. Most tangible property placed in service after 1986 must be depreciated using the Modified Accelerated Cost Recovery System (MACRS) (¶ 1243). Depreciation for tangible property placed in service after 1980 and before 1987 is computed under ACRS (¶ 1252).

For tangible property placed in service before 1981, depreciation may be computed under the straight-line method (¶ 1224), the double declining-balance method (¶ 1226), the sum-of-the-years-digits method (¶ 1228), and other consistent methods (¶ 1231), depending on the taxpayer's election in the year the property was placed in service (Former Code Sec. 167(b)).[29] However, accelerated depreciation for pre-1981 realty is limited (Former Code Sec. 167(j)).

For an asset purchased before 1981, only a part of a full year's depreciation was allowed in the year it was placed in service. The allowable deduction was computed by

---

References are to Standard Federal Tax Reports; Tax Research Consultant; and Practical Tax Explanations.

[29] ¶ 11,037.021; DEPR: 15,306; § 10,301

multiplying the first full year's depreciation allowance by the months the property was owned and dividing by 12. The same rule applies in the year of sale.

1218. Methods for Depreciating Real Estate. Real property placed in service after 1986 is depreciated under the Modified Accelerated Cost Recovery System (MACRS) (¶ 1236). Real property placed in service after 1980 and before 1987 is depreciated under the Accelerated Cost Recovery System (ACRS) (¶ 1252). Additions and improvements to a building, including structural components of a building, placed in service after 1986 are depreciated under MACRS (see ¶ 1240). Post-1986 rehabilitation expenditures are also depreciated using MACRS (¶ 1236). Elements of a building that qualify as personal property may be separately depreciated under the cost segregation rules using shortened MACRS recovery periods (¶ 1240). Real property that is converted from personal use to residential rental property or nonresidential real property is depreciated as MACRS 27.5-year residential rental property or MACRS 39-year nonresidential real property even if the property was acquired for personal use prior to 1987.

1221. Change in Depreciation Method—Accounting Method Changes. A change in the method of computing depreciation is generally a change in accounting method that requires the consent of the IRS and the filing of Form 3115 (Reg. § 1.167(e)-1).[30] If the change from an impermissible accounting method to a permissible accounting method results in a negative (taxpayer favorable) Code Sec. 481(a) adjustment, the adjustment is taken into account in a single tax year. A positive adjustment is taken into account over four tax years—one-year if the positive adjustment is less than $25,000 and the taxpayer makes an election to include it in income in one year. No Code Sec. 481(a) adjustment is allowed when a taxpayer changes from one permissible method to another permissible method. These changes are applied on a "cut-off" basis.[31] Reg. § 1.446-1(e)(2)(ii)(d)(2) and (3) list changes in depreciation or amortization that are or are not considered a change in accounting method.

Although a taxpayer has not adopted an accounting method unless two or more returns have been filed, the IRS will allow a taxpayer who has only filed one return on which incorrect depreciation has been claimed to either file Form 3115 and claim a Code Sec. 481(a) adjustment on the current-year return or file an amended return. The asset must have been placed in service in the tax year immediately preceding the tax year of the change (Rev. Proc. 2007-16).

For changes that are not a change in accounting method, such as mathematical or posting errors, a taxpayer may only file amended returns for open years. Changes in accounting method are generally made by filing Form 3115. Procedures for changing from an impermissible method (e.g., where incorrect or no depreciation has been claimed) to a permissible method and from permissible to permissible methods with respect to pre-1986 property are generally governed by the automatic consent procedures of Rev. Proc. 2011-14 (Appendix Section 6). Otherwise, the advance consent procedures of Rev. Proc. 97-27 are followed.[32]

A taxpayer who has sold depreciable property without claiming any depreciation or all of the depreciation allowable may claim the depreciation by filing Form 3115 by the expiration of the period of limitations for filing an amended return for the year of the sale. The Form 3115 may be filed with the original federal tax return for the tax year in which the depreciable property is disposed (Rev. Proc. 2007-16).[33]

For depreciable property placed in service in a tax year ending before December 30, 2003, the IRS will not assert that a change in computing depreciation is a change in accounting method (IRS Chief Counsel Notice CC-2004-007, January 28, 2004, as clarified by Chief Counsel Notice 2004-24, July 14, 2004).[34]

References are to Standard Federal Tax Reports; Tax Research Consultant; and Practical Tax Explanations.

[30] ¶ 11,042; DEPR: 15,304; § 11,025

[31] ¶ 11,043.021; DEPR: 15,304.15; § 11,025

[32] ¶ 11,043.021; DEPR: 15,304; § 11,025

[33] ¶ 11,043.285; DEPR: 15,304; § 11,025

[34] ¶ 11,043.015; DEPR: 15,304.22

12 DEPRECIATION

1224. Straight-Line or Fixed-Percentage Method of Depreciation. The "straight-line" method of computing the depreciation deduction assumes that the depreciation sustained is uniform during the useful life of the property. The cost or other basis, less estimated salvage value, is deductible in equal annual amounts over the estimated useful life (Reg. § 1.167(b)-1).[35] An asset may not be depreciated below its salvage value. Straight-line depreciation under the Modified Accelerated Cost Recovery System (MACRS) and the Accelerated Cost Recovery System (ACRS) is generally computed in this manner, except that a recovery period is used instead of the useful life and salvage value is not considered (Code Sec. 168(b)(4))[36] (¶ 1243 and ¶ 1252).

1226. Declining-Balance Method of Depreciation. Under the declining-balance depreciation method, depreciation is greatest in the first year and smaller in each succeeding year (Reg. § 1.167(b)-2).[37] The depreciable basis (e.g., cost) is reduced each year by the amount of the depreciation deduction, and a uniform rate of 200 percent of the straight-line rate (double-declining balance or 200-percent declining balance method) or 150 percent of the straight-line rate (150-percent declining balance method) is applied to the resulting balances (Reg. § 1.167(b)-2).[38] Under the Modified Accelerated Cost Recovery System (MACRS) rules, the double-declining-balance method is used to depreciate 3-, 5-, 7-, and 10-year property and the 150-percent declining balance method is used to depreciate 15-and 20-year property (¶ 1243).

1228. Sum-of-the-Years-Digits Method of Depreciation. Under the sum-of-the-years-digits method of depreciation, changing fractions are applied each year to the original cost or other basis, less salvage value. The numerator of the fraction each year represents the remaining useful life of the asset and the denominator, which remains constant, is the sum of the numerals representing each of the years of the estimated useful life (the sum-of-the-years digits). This method, if elected, may be used for group, classified, or composite accounts (Reg. § 1.167(b)-3).[39]

1229. Income Forecast Method of Depreciation. The use of the income forecast method of depreciation only applies to film, videotape, sound recordings, copyrights, books, patents, and other property that may be specified by IRS regulations. The income forecast method may not be used to depreciate intangible property that is amortizable under Code Sec. 197 (¶ 1288) or consumer durables subject to rent-to-own contracts (¶ 1240) (Code Sec. 167(g)(6); Rev. Rul. 60-358).[40]

Under the income forecast method, the cost of an asset (less any salvage value) placed in service after September 13, 1995, is multiplied by a fraction, the numerator of which is the net income from the asset for the tax year and the denominator of which is the total net income forecast to be derived from the asset before the close of the 10th tax year following the tax year in which the asset is placed in service. The unrecovered adjusted basis of the property as of the beginning of the 10th tax year is claimed as a depreciation deduction in the 10th tax year following the tax year in which the asset was placed in service.

If the income forecast changes during the 10-year period, the formula is as follows: the unrecovered depreciable cost of the asset at the beginning of the tax year of revision is multiplied by a fraction. The numerator is the net income from the asset for the tax year of revision. The denominator is the revised forecasted total net income from the asset for the year of revision and the remaining years before the close of the 10th tax year following the tax year in which the asset was placed in service.

During the 3rd and 10th tax years after the asset is placed in service, a taxpayer is generally required to pay or may receive interest based on the recalculation of depreciation using actual income figures. This look-back rule does not apply to property that has a cost basis of $100,000 or less, or if the taxpayer's income projections were within 10 percent of the income actually earned.

References are to Standard Federal Tax Reports; Tax Research Consultant; and Practical Tax Explanations.

[35] ¶ 11,033; DEPR: 15,400; § 11,130

[36] ¶ 11,250; DEPR: 3,202; § 11,130

[37] ¶ 11,034; DEPR: 15,450; § 11,130

[38] ¶ 11,034; DEPR: 15,450; § 11,130

[39] ¶ 11,035; DEPR: 15,500; § 11,025

[40] ¶ 11,002; DEPR: 3,156.60, DEPR: 15,556; § 11,205

Effective for property placed in service after October 22, 2004, residuals and participations may be included in the adjusted basis of a property in the tax year that it is placed in service or excluded from adjusted basis and deducted in the year of payment (Code Sec. 167(g)(7)). Election guidance is provided in Notice 2006-47.

Reporting. Form 8866 is used to compute the look-back interest due or owed.

Creative Property Costs of Film Makers. A taxpayer may choose to amortize creative property costs ratably over 15 years beginning on the first day of the second half of the tax year in which the cost is written off for financial accounting purposes in accordance with Statement of Position 00-2 (SOP 00-2), as issued by the American Institute of Certified Public Accountants (AICPA) on June 12, 2000 (Rev. Proc. 2004-36).[41] Creative property costs are costs to acquire and develop for purposes of potential future film development, production, and exploitation: (1) screenplays; (2) scripts; (3) story out-lines; (4) motion picture production rights to books and plays; and (5) similar properties. If the election is not made, these costs are generally recovered under the income forecast method only if a film is actually produced. If a film is not made, deduction of the costs as a loss is usually denied (Rev. Rul. 2004-58).

Election to Expense First $15 Million of Film Costs. Effective for qualified film and television productions commencing after December 31, 2007, and before January 1, 2014, a taxpayer may elect to expense the first $15 million of production costs ($20 million for productions in low income communities or distressed areas) (Code Sec. 181). In the case of qualified film and television productions that commence after October 22, 2004, and before January 1, 2008, a taxpayer may only elect to expense productions with an aggregate cost that does not exceed $15 million ($20 million in low-income communi-ties or distressed areas). Election guidance is provided in Reg. § 1.181-2.

> **Comment:** Absent further legislation, the election to expense film costs has expired effective for productions commencing after December 31, 2013. For the latest legislative updates, visit our website www.CCHGroup.com/TaxUpdates.

1231. Other Consistent Depreciation Methods. In addition to the depreciation methods explained at ¶ 1224–¶ 1228, a taxpayer may use any other consistent method, such as the sinking fund method, if the total deductions during the first two-thirds of the useful life are not more than the total allowable under the declining-balance method (Reg. § 1.167(b)-4).[42]

Leased Property

1234. Lessee/Lessor Improvements, Lease Acquisition Costs. Unless a leasehold improvement placed in service before January 1, 2014, qualifies as 15-year leasehold improvement property or is a qualified improvement placed in service before January 1, 2014, to a retail building or a restaurant (see ¶ 1240), the cost of an addition or improvement made by the lessee or lessor to real property is depreciated under the Modified Accelerated Cost Recovery System (MACRS) in the same manner as the depreciation deduction for the real property would be calculated if the real property had been placed in service at the same time as the addition or improvement (Code Sec. 168(i)(6) and (8)(A); Reg. § 1.167(a)-4).[43] For example, permanent walls installed in a commercial building (structural components) are separately depreciated as 39-year real property beginning in the month that the walls are placed in service using the mid-month convention. If, upon termination of the lease, a lessee does not retain an improvement (made by the lessee), loss is computed by reference to the improvement's adjusted basis at the time of the lease termination. A lessor that disposes of or abandons a leasehold improvement (made by the lessor) upon termination of the lease may use the adjusted basis of the improvement at such time to determine gain or loss (Code Sec. 168(i)(8)(B); Reg. § 1.168(i)-8(c)(3)).

References are to Standard Federal Tax Reports; Tax Research Consultant; and Practical Tax Explanations.

[41] ¶ 20,620.6305; DEPR: 21,500; § 11,555

[42] ¶ 11,036; DEPR: 15,306; § 11,025

[43] ¶ 11,250, ¶ 11,010; DEPR: 3,052; § 11,105

12

DEPRECIATION

Leasehold additions and improvements that are section 1245 property (i.e., personal as opposed to real property) are generally depreciated over a shortened MACRS recovery period. See *Cost Segregation*, at ¶ 1240.

15-Year Qualified Leasehold Improvement Property. Qualified leasehold improvement property placed in service after October 22, 2004, and before January 1, 2014, is depreciated under MACRS over 15 years (39 years if the alternative depreciation system (ADS) applies) using the straight-line method and the half-year or mid-quarter convention, as applicable (Code Sec. 168(b)(3)(G), (e)(3)(E)(iv)), and (g)(3)(B)). Qualified leasehold improvement property is defined the same way as the term is defined in Code Sec. 168(k)(3) for purposes of the bonus depreciation deduction (¶ 1237) subject to an exception that generally prohibits an individual who acquires qualified leasehold improvement property from a lessor from treating the property as qualified leasehold improvement property (Code Sec. 168(e)(6)). Thus, the improvements must be made to the interior portion of nonresidential real property that is more than three years old by the lessor or lessee under or pursuant to the terms of a lease. Elevators and escalators, internal structural framework of the building, structural components that benefit a common area, and improvements relating to the enlargement of a building do not qualify (Code Sec. 168(k)(3)).

> **Comment:** Absent further legislation, leasehold improvement property placed in service after December 31, 2013 will be depreciated over 39 years as MACRS nonresidential real property. For the latest legislative updates, visit our website www.CCHGroup.com/TaxUpdates.

Lease Acquisition Costs. The cost of acquiring a lease is amortized over the lease term. A renewal period is counted as part of the lease term if less than 75 percent of the acquisition cost is attributable to the unexpired lease period (not counting the renewal period) (Code Sec. 178).[44]

Construction Allowances. A lessor must depreciate improvements made by the lessee with a qualified construction allowance as nonresidential real property. See ¶ 764.

1235. Sale v. Lease of Depreciable Property. Whether a transaction is treated as a lease or as a purchase for tax purposes is important in determining who is entitled to claim depreciation and other deductions for related business expenses.[45] In most situations, the rules for determining whether a transaction is a lease or a purchase evolved from a series of court decisions and IRS rulings. The rules generally look to the economic substance of a transaction, not its form, to determine who is the owner of the property for tax purposes when the parties characterize it as a lease (Rev. Proc. 2001-28, Rev. Proc. 2001-29).

Motor Vehicle Leases. A qualified motor vehicle lease agreement that contains a terminal rental adjustment clause (a provision permitting or requiring the rental price to be adjusted upward or downward by reference to the amount realized by the lessor upon the sale of the vehicle) is treated as a lease if, but for the clause, it would have been treated as a lease for tax purposes (Code Sec. 7701(h)).[46] This provision applies only to qualified agreements with respect to a motor vehicle (including a trailer).

Modified Accelerated Cost Recovery System (MACRS)

1236. MACRS in General. The Modified Accelerated Cost Recovery System (MACRS) is mandatory for most tangible depreciable property placed in service after December 31, 1986, unless transitional rules apply (Code Sec. 168).[47] Under MACRS, the cost of eligible property is recovered over a 3-, 5-, 7-, 10-, 15-, 20-, 27.5-, 31.5-, or

---

References are to Standard Federal Tax Reports; Tax Research Consultant; and Practical Tax Explanations.

[44] ¶ 12,100; SALES: 42,204; § 11,515

[45] ¶ 8754.022; SALES: 42,000; § 11,015

[46] ¶ 43,080; SALES: 42,104; § 11,015

[47] ¶ 11,250, ¶ 11,279; DEPR: 3,052; § 11,101

39-year period, depending upon the type of property (¶ 1240) by using statutory recovery methods (¶ 1243) and conventions (¶ 1245). Special transferee rules apply to property received in specified nonrecognition transactions (¶ 1248).

1237. MACRS Bonus Depreciation. Under the Modified Accelerated Cost Recovery System (MACRS), a bonus depreciation deduction is allowed for qualifying MACRS property acquired after December 31, 2007, and before January 1, 2014, if it is placed in service before January 1, 2014. The original use of the qualifying property must begin with the taxpayer after December 31, 2007. Property that is acquired pursuant to a written binding contract entered into after December 31, 2007, and before January 1, 2014, is deemed acquired before January 1, 2014 (Code Sec. 168(k)).[48]

> **Comment:** Absent further legislation, the bonus depreciation deduction has expired for property placed in service after December 31, 2013. At the time of publication, proposed legislation is pending in Congress to extend the deduction two years to property placed in service before January 1, 2016. For the latest legislative updates, visit our website www.CCHGroup.com/TaxUpdates.

The placed-in-service-deadline is extended one year (before January 1, 2015) for long production property that otherwise qualifies for bonus depreciation. Long production property is defined as property that (1) is subject to the Code Sec. 263A uniform capitalization rules, (2) has a production period greater than one year and a cost exceeding $1 million, and (3) has a MACRS recovery period of at least 10 years or is used in the trade or business of transporting persons or property for hire, such as commercial aircraft. However, only pre-January 1, 2014, progress expenditures are taken into account if the extended placed-in-service deadline applies (Code Sec. 168(k)(2)(B)). The extended placed-in-service deadline also applies to certain noncommercial aircraft acquired by purchase. Unlike commercial aircraft, 2014 progress expenditures on noncommercial aircraft placed in service before January 1, 2015, are eligible for bonus depreciation (Code Sec. 168(k)(2)(C)).

> **Comment:** Absent further legislation, the bonus depreciation deduction has expired for long-term production property and certain noncommercial aircraft placed in service after December 31, 2014. At the time of publication, proposed legislation is pending in Congress to extend the deduction for two years to long-term production property and certain noncommercial aircraft placed in service before January 1, 2017. For the latest legislative updates, visit our website www.CCHGroup.com/TaxUpdates.

The bonus depreciation rate is generally 50 percent. However, if qualifying MACRS property is acquired after September 8, 2010, and before January 1, 2012, and is placed in service before January 1, 2012, the rate is increased to 100 percent (Code Sec. 168(k)(5)). The original use of the property must begin with the taxpayer after September 8, 2010. In the case of long-production property and certain noncommercial aircraft, the 100-percent rate applies if the long-production property or noncommercial aircraft is acquired after September 8, 2010, and before January 1, 2013, and placed in service before January 1, 2013. The entire basis of the long-production property or noncommercial aircraft is eligible for the 100-percent rate if these deadlines are met. If long-production property or a noncommercial aircraft is acquired (or constructed, manufactured, or produced) pursuant to a written binding contract entered into after September 8, 2010, and before January 1, 2013, the 100-percent rate acquisition deadline is deemed satisfied (Rev. Proc. 2011-26, Section 3).

For purposes of the 50-percent bonus depreciation rate, property is generally deemed acquired when possession or control is taken (i.e., taxpayer has risk of loss) (Reg. §§ 1.48-2(b)(6) and 1.167(c)-1(a)(2)). For purposes of the 100-percent bonus depreciation rate, property is considered acquired when its cost is paid for by a cash-basis taxpayer or when its cost is incurred by an accrual-basis taxpayer (Rev. Proc. 2006-11, Section 3.02(1)(a)). Property constructed, manufactured, or produced by or for

---

References are to Standard Federal Tax Reports; Tax Research Consultant; and Practical Tax Explanations.

[48] ¶ 11,250; DEPR: 3,600; § 11,225

a taxpayer is deemed acquired for purposes of the 50-percent and 100-percent rates when work of a significant physical nature begins. Under an elective safe-harbor method, work of a significant physical nature begins when more than 10 percent of the total cost of a project has been paid for by a cash basis taxpayer or incurred by an accrual basis taxpayer (Reg. § 1.168(k)-1(b)(4)(iii); Rev. Proc. 2011-26, Section 3.02(1)(c)(2)).

If a larger self-constructed property does not qualify for bonus depreciation because its construction began before January 1, 2008, then individual components of the larger property, whether acquired or self-constructed, do not qualify for bonus depreciation (Reg. § 1.168(k)-1(b)(4)(iii)(C)(1) and (2)). However, if a larger constructed property does not qualify for the 100-percent rate solely because its construction began after December 31, 2007, and before September 9, 2010, a taxpayer may elect to claim the 100-percent rate on individual components of the property, whether acquired or self-constructed, that separately meet the requirements for the 100-percent rate (Rev. Proc. 2011-26, Section 3.02(1)(c)(2)).

Property purchased by a taxpayer in a sale-leaseback transaction within three months after the original purchaser placed the property in service may qualify for bonus depreciation if the original purchaser placed the property in service after December 31, 2007 (after September 8, 2010, for the 100-percent rate to apply). The last purchaser in a syndicated leasing transaction may also qualify if certain requirements are satisfied (Code Sec. 168(k)(2)(E)).

Property acquired pursuant to a written binding contract entered into before January 1, 2008, by the taxpayer or a related party does not qualify for bonus depreciation (Code Sec. 168(k)(2)(A)(iii) and (k)(2)(E)(iv)).

Bonus depreciation is treated as depreciation subject to recapture upon the sale of the property (Reg. § 1.168(k)-1(f)(3)). Unlike the section 179 expensing allowance (¶ 1208), there is no taxable income or investment limitation on the bonus depreciation allowance. There is no limit on the overall amount of bonus depreciation that may be claimed on qualifying property. The length of the tax year or date during the tax year that the qualifying property was placed in service does not affect the amount of the bonus depreciation deduction, except that a 100-percent rate applies to property acquired after September 8, 2010, and placed in service before January 1, 2012.

Qualifying Property. The bonus depreciation allowance is only available for: (1) new property ("original use" must begin with the taxpayer) that is depreciable under MACRS and has a recovery period of 20 years or less; (2) MACRS water utility property; (3) computer software depreciable over three years under Code Sec. 167(f) (¶ 980); or (4) qualified leasehold improvement property (defined below). Property that must be depreciated using the MACRS alternative depreciation system (ADS) (¶ 1247) does not qualify. If ADS is elected, however, the property may qualify. Listed property (¶ 1211), such as a passenger automobile (¶ 1214), that is used 50 percent or less for business, does not qualify. If business use of such a property falls to 50 percent or less, bonus depreciation and any amount expensed under Code Sec. 179 (¶ 1208) must be recaptured. Property amortized under Code Sec. 197 (¶ 1288) also does not qualify for bonus depreciation.

AMT. Bonus depreciation is allowed in full for alternative minimum tax purposes (AMT) (¶ 1430). If bonus depreciation is claimed, no AMT adjustment is required on the regular MACRS deductions (i.e., the deductions are allowed in full for AMT purposes) (Code Sec. 168(k)(2)(F); Reg. § 1.168(k)-1(d)(iii)).

Election Out. A taxpayer may elect out of bonus depreciation with respect to any class of property (Code Sec. 168(k)(2)(D)(iii)). The election out applies to all property in the class or classes of property for which the election is made. A taxpayer was allowed to elect a 50-percent bonus depreciation rate in place of the 100-percent bonus depreciation rate for any property class but only for a tax year that included September 8, 2010 (Rev. Proc. 2011-26, Section 4).

Qualified Leasehold Improvement Property. An improvement to an interior portion of nonresidential real property (whether or not depreciated under MACRS) by a lessor or

¶1237

lessee under or pursuant to a lease may qualify for bonus depreciation. The improvement must be placed in service more than three years after the building was first placed in service (i.e., the building must be more than three years old). The lessor and lessee may not be related persons. Expenditures for (1) the enlargement of a building, (2) any elevator or escalator, (3) any structural component that benefits a common area, or (4) the internal structural framework of the building do not qualify (Code Sec. 168(k)(3)). Retail improvement property (¶ 1240) and restaurant improvements (¶ 1240) that also meet the requirements of leasehold improvement property qualify for bonus depreciation (Rev. Proc. 2011-26, Section 3.03(1)(b)(3)).

Computation. The bonus depreciation deduction is claimed on the cost of the property after reduction by any Code Sec. 179 allowance (¶ 1208) claimed. Regular MACRS deductions are computed on the cost as reduced by any Code Sec. 179 allowance and bonus depreciation.

> **Example 1:** Taxpayer purchases qualifying five-year MACRS property subject to the half-year convention for $1,500 and claims a $600 Code Sec. 179 allowance. Using the 50-percent rate, bonus depreciation is $450 (($1,500 − $600) × 50%). Regular MACRS depreciation deductions are computed on a depreciable basis of $450 ($1,500 − $600 − $450). The regular first-year MACRS allowance is $90 ($450 × 20% (first-year table percentage)).

Election by Corporation to Forgo Bonus Depreciation and Claim Accelerated Research and/or AMT Credit Carryforward. A corporation may make an accelerated credit election in its first tax year ending after March 31, 2008, pursuant to which it will forgo the bonus depreciation deduction on eligible qualified property and in return claim a refundable credit (in each tax year that eligible qualified property is placed in service) for a portion of:

> (1) its unused general business credit carryforward that is attributable to research credits from tax years that began before January 1, 2006 (determined by using the ordering rules of Code Sec. 38(d)); and/or

> (2) its unused alternative minimum tax liability credit attributable to tax years that began before January 1, 2006 (Code Sec. 168(k)(4); Rev. Proc. 2009-33, modifying Rev. Proc. 2009-16 and Rev. Proc. 2008-65).[49]

The refundable AMT credit otherwise allowed to corporations making the accelerated credit election is subject to reduction under sequestration requirements of the Emergency Deficit Reduction Act of 1985 (P.L. 99-177, as amended by P.L. 112-25). Refund payments processed on or after October 1, 2013 and on or before September 30, 2014 will be reduced by the fiscal year 2014 sequestration rate of 7.2 percent irrespective of when the original or amended tax return is received by the IRS. The sequestration reduction rate will be applied unless and until a law is enacted that cancels or otherwise impacts the sequester. A sequestration rate of 38 percent applies for refunds processed on or after August 13, 2013, and on or before September 30, 2013. Corporations with refunds subject to the reduction will be notified by the IRS.

Foregone bonus depreciation not claimed on eligible qualified property that is "round 2 extension property" (generally, property placed in service in 2011 and 2012) or "round 3 extension property" (generally, property placed in service in 2013) may only be used to free up pre-January 1, 2006, AMT credits (Code Sec. 168(k)(4)(I) and (J)).

The computation of the refundable AMT credit is made on a worksheet provided with Form 8827. The computation of the refundable research credit was made on a worksheet found in Form 3800.

Effective for property placed in service after December 31, 2010, eligible qualified property is property that is acquired after March 31, 2008, and before January 1, 2014, and placed in service before January 1, 2014 (before January 1, 2015, for longer-period production property and certain noncommercial aircraft) and that is eligible for the

---

References are to Standard Federal Tax Reports; Tax Research Consultant; and Practical Tax Explanations.

[49] ¶ 11,279.0583; DEPR: 3,606;
§ 11,115.25c

bonus depreciation deduction. No binding written purchase contract may be in effect before April 1, 2008 (Code Sec. 168(k)(2)(A) and (k)(4)(D)).

Effective for property placed in service before January 1, 2011, eligible qualified property for purposes of the election to forgo bonus depreciation is property that is acquired after March 31, 2008, and before January 1, 2010, and placed in service before January 1, 2010 (before January 1, 2011, for longer-period production property and certain noncommercial aircraft) and that is eligible for the bonus depreciation deduction. No binding written purchase contract may be in effect before April 1, 2008 (Code Sec. 168(k)(2)(A) and (4)(D), prior to amendment by the Tax Relief, Unemployment Insurance Reauthorization, and Job Creation Act of 2010 (P.L. 111-312)).

The Small Business Jobs Act of 2010 (P.L. 111-240) extended bonus depreciation an additional year to include qualifying assets acquired after December 31, 2007, and before January 1, 2011, and placed in service after December 31, 2009, and before January 1, 2011 (before January 1, 2012, for property with a long production period and certain noncommercial aircraft). Property that qualifies for bonus depreciation only on account of this one-year extension is not treated as eligible qualified property (Former Code Sec. 168(k)(4)(D)(iv) and (v), effective for property placed in service after December 31, 2010).

A corporation that made the accelerated credit election in its first tax year ending after March 31, 2008, was allowed to make an election to exclude "extension property" (Code Sec. 168(k)(4)(H)(i)). If this election to exclude extension property was made, the corporation was allowed to claim bonus depreciation on the extension property and the extension property was not taken into account in determining the accelerated AMT and/or research credit.

Extension property is property that qualified for bonus depreciation solely by reason of the one-year extension that made bonus depreciation available to qualifying property placed in service in 2009 (in 2010 for property with a long production period and certain noncommercial aircraft) (Code Sec. 168(k)(4)(H)(iii)).

A corporation that did not make the accelerated credit election for its first tax year ending after March 31, 2008, was allowed to make an accelerated credit election that applied to eligible qualified property that is extension property (Code Sec. 168(k)(4)(H)(ii)).

If a corporation previously made an accelerated credit election for its first tax year ending after March 31, 2008, or made the above accelerated credit election for extension property for its first tax year ending after December 31, 2008, the election applies to "round 2 extension property," unless the corporation makes an election not to forgo bonus depreciation on round 2 extension property (Code Sec. 168(k)(4)(I)(ii)).

Round 2 extension property is property that is eligible qualified property (as defined above in Code Sec. 168(k)(4)(D)) solely by reason of the two-year extension of the bonus depreciation allowance for property acquired after December 31, 2007, and placed in service in 2011 or 2012, and in the case of longer-period production property and certain noncommercial aircraft, to property placed in service in 2013 (Code Sec. 168(k)(4)(I)(iv)).

If a corporation did not make the accelerated credit election in its first tax year ending after March 31, 2008, or the accelerated credit election for extension property for its first tax year ending after December 31, 2008, the corporation was allowed to make the accelerated credit election in its first tax year ending after December 31, 2010 for round 2 extension property (Code Sec. 168(k)(4)(I)(iii)).

Similar elections apply to "round 3 extension property." Thus, if a corporation has previously made an accelerated credit election for its first tax year ending after March 31, 2008, or with respect to extension property or round 2 extension property, the election applies to round 3 extension property unless an election not to forgo bonus depreciation on round 3 extension property is made. Alternatively, if a corporation made none of these accelerated credit elections, it may make an accelerated credit election and forgo bonus depreciation on round 3 extension property (Code Sec. 168(k)(4)(J)(ii) and (iii)).

Round 3 extension property is property that is eligible qualified property (as defined in Code Sec. 168(k)(4)(D)) solely by reason of the one-year extension of the bonus depreciation to property acquired after December 31, 2007, and placed in service in 2013, and in the case of longer-period production property and certain noncommercial aircraft, property placed in service in 2014 (Code Sec. 168(k)(4)(J)(iv)).

The total amount of the unused research and AMT credits that may be claimed for any tax year is generally equal to the bonus depreciation amount for that year. The bonus depreciation amount is 20 percent of the difference between: (1) the aggregate bonus depreciation and regular depreciation that would be allowed on eligible qualified property placed in service during the tax year if bonus depreciation was claimed; and (2) the aggregate depreciation that would be allowed on the eligible qualified property placed in service during the tax year if no bonus depreciation was claimed (Code Sec. 168(k)(4)(C)(i)).

The bonus depreciation amount for any tax year, however, may not exceed the "maximum increase amount" reduced (but not below zero) by the sum of the bonus depreciation amounts for all preceding tax years (Code Sec. 168(k)(4)(C)(ii)). The bonus depreciation amount, as limited by this rule, is referred to as the "maximum amount." The maximum increase amount is the lesser of $30 million or six percent of the sum of the "business credit increase amount" (i.e., unused research credits from tax years beginning before 2006) and the "AMT credit increase amount" (i.e., unused AMT credits from tax years beginning before 2006) (Code Sec. 168(k)(4)(C)(ii) and (iii); Rev. Proc. 2008-65, Section 5.03). When computing the maximum increase amount with respect to round 2 or 3 extension property, the business credit increase amount is disregarded (Code Secs. 168(k)(4)(I)(i)(II) and 168(k)(4)(J)(i)(II)) because the bonus depreciation amount may not be used to offset unused pre-2006 research credits.

A separate bonus depreciation amount, maximum amount, and maximum increase amount are computed and applied to eligible qualified property that is extension property, eligible qualified property that is round 2 extension property, eligible qualified property that is round 3 extension property, and other eligible qualified property (Code Sec. 168(k)(4)(H)(i)(II), (I)(ii), (I)(iii), (J)(ii), and (J)(iii); Rev. Proc. 2009-33, Section 5.02). This separate computation means that a corporation may claim a maximum $30 million of credits with respect to property that is not extension property or round 2 extension property, a maximum $30 million of credits with respect to property that is extension property, and a maximum $30 million of credits with respect to property that is round 2 extension property.

To claim a tax credit for an unused research credit from a tax year beginning before January 1, 2006, a corporation increases the Code Sec. 38(c) tax liability limitation for the tax year by the bonus depreciation amount for the tax year as computed above (Code Sec. 168(k)(4)(A)(iii) and (B)). The bonus depreciation amount allocated to the Code Sec. 38(c) tax liability limitation, however, may not exceed the corporation's pre-2006 research credit carryforwards reduced by any amount allocated to the Code Sec. 38(c) tax liability limitation under this provision in earlier tax years. The bonus depreciation amount may be allocated between the Code Sec. 38(c) tax liability limitation for the general business credit and the Code Sec. 53(c) tax liability limitation for the AMT tax credit. The amount allocated to the AMT tax liability limitation may not exceed the pre-2006 AMT credits reduced by any bonus depreciation amount allocated to the Code Sec. 53(c) tax liability limitation in previous tax years (Code Sec. 168(k)(4)(E)(ii)).

If an accelerated credit election is made, depreciation on the entire property is computed without claiming bonus depreciation and by using the MACRS straight-line method over the regular recovery period (Code Sec. 168(k)(4)(A)).

> **Example 2:** QPEX is a calendar-year corporation that places round 3 extension property that is 10-year MACRS property costing $100,000 in service in June 2013. QPEX made the accelerated credit election for its first tax year ending after March 31, 2008, and does not make the election to exclude round 3 extension property. It first computes the bonus depreciation and regular depreciation on the MACRS round 3 extension property. Bonus depreciation is $50,000 ($100,000 × 50%). Regular depreciation is $5,000 (($100,000 – $50,000 × 10% first- year percentage for

10-year property = $5,000). The $55,000 sum of the bonus depreciation and regular depreciation is reduced to $45,000 by the $10,000 depreciation that could be claimed in 2013 on the property if the bonus depreciation deduction was not claimed ($100,000 × 10% first- year percentage for 10-year property = $10,000). Assume that QPEX has $200,000 in unused pre-2006 AMT credits. The bonus depreciation amount is equal to the lesser of: (1) $9,000 ($45,000 × 20%); (2) $12,000 ($200,000 × 6% = $12,000)); or (3) $30 million. Since $9,000 is less than the amounts in items (2) and (3), the bonus depreciation amount is $9,000. In this situation QPEX could increase its AMT tax liability limitation by $9,000 and claim a refundable $9,000 AMT credit.

50-Percent Bonus Depreciation Allowance for Gulf Opportunity Zone Property (Expired). Taxpayers were allowed to claim a bonus depreciation allowance equal to 50 percent of the adjusted basis of qualified Gulf Opportunity Zone property acquired after August 27, 2005, and placed in service on or before December 31, 2007. (Code Sec. 1400N(d); Notice 2006-77).[50]

The placed-in-service deadline for nonresidential and residential property was extended to December 31, 2011, if the building was located in the Louisiana parishes of Calcasieu, Cameron, Orleans, Plaquemines, St. Bernard, St. Tammany, or Washington or the Mississippi counties of Hancock, Harrison, Jackson, Pearl River, or Stone. Bonus depreciation could have been claimed on portions of buildings (e.g., floors of multi-story buildings) that were placed in service by the December 31, 2011, deadline.

If the Gulf Zone bonus depreciation allowance was claimed, the bonus depreciation allowance and regular depreciation deductions on the property were allowed in full for AMT purposes. If business use drops to less than 80 percent, the deduction is subject to recapture under rules similar to those that apply to the Code Sec. 179 allowance (¶ 1208).

50-Percent Bonus Depreciation Allowance for Qualified Disaster Assistance Property. A taxpayer who suffered an economic loss attributable to a federally declared disaster declared after December 31, 2007, and that occurred before January 1, 2010, could have claimed an additional first-year depreciation deduction equal to 50 percent of the adjusted basis of qualified disaster assistance property (QDAP). The property must have been placed in service during the three calendar years that followed the date of the disaster (four calendar years for nonresidential and residential real property that was qualified disaster assistance property) and the property may not have been eligible for bonus depreciation under any other provision (Code Sec. 168(n)).[51]

50-Percent Bonus Depreciation Allowance for Mine Safety Equipment. A taxpayer may elect to deduct 50 percent of the cost of qualified advanced mine safety equipment paid or incurred, if the equipment is placed in service before January 1, 2014 (Code Sec. 179E).[52]

> **Comment:** Absent further legislation, the bonus depreciation deduction for mine safety equipment expires for property placed in service after December 31, 2013. For the latest legislative updates, visit our website www.CCHGroup.com/TaxUpdates.

50-Percent Bonus Depreciation Allowance for Qualified Reuse and Recycling Property. A 50-percent additional depreciation allowance may be claimed on the adjusted basis of qualified reuse and recycling property acquired and placed in service during the tax year. The property must be acquired by purchase, its original use must begin with the taxpayer, and it must have a useful life of a least five years, and no pre-September 1, 2008, binding acquisition contract may be in effect. Reuse and recycling property is machinery and equipment (not including buildings, real estate, rolling stock or equipment used to transport reuse and recyclable materials) that is used exclusively to collect, distribute, or recycle qualified reuse and recyclable materials. Machinery and equipment include appurtenances such as software necessary to operate the equipment. Qualified

---

References are to Standard Federal Tax Reports; Tax Research Consultant; and Practical Tax Explanations.

[50] ¶ 32,483, ¶ 12,126.54; DEPR: 3,650; § 11,225

[51] ¶ 11,250; SALES: 42,104; § 11,225.05

[52] ¶ 12,139; BUSEXP: 19,000; § 10,255

reuse and recyclable materials are scrap plastic, glass, textiles, rubber, packaging, and metal, as well as recovered fiber and electronic scrap. A taxpayer may elect out for any class of property (Code Sec. 168(m)).[53]

50-Percent Bonus Depreciation Allowance for Second Generation Biofuel Plant Property. A 50-percent additional depreciation allowance may be claimed on the adjusted basis of certain plant property acquired and placed in service after December 20, 2006, and before January 1, 2014, that is used to produce certain qualified biofuels (Code Sec. 168(l)).[54] For property placed in service after January 2, 2013, and before January 1, 2014, this bonus depreciation allowance may only be claimed on the adjusted basis of second generation biofuel plant property used to produce second generation biofuel. For purposes of the special allowance, second generation biofuel is defined under Code Sec. 40(b)(6)(E) and includes algae treated as qualified feedstock.

> **Comment:** Absent further legislation, the bonus depreciation deduction for plant property used to produce second generation biofuel expires for property placed in service after December 31, 2013. For the latest legislative updates, visit our website www.CCHGroup.com/TaxUpdates.

1238. Property Subject to MACRS. Most tangible depreciable property placed in service after 1986 is depreciated using the Modified Accelerated Cost Recovery System (MACRS). MACRS property is depreciable if it wears out, has a useful life that exceeds one year, and is used in a trade or business or for the production of income. This does not include: (1) property for which an election was made to use a depreciation method not expressed in terms of years, such as the unit of production or income forecast method; (2) public utility property (unless a normalization method of accounting is used); (3) motion picture films and videotapes; (4) sound recordings; (5) intangible property; and (6) property placed in service before 1987 that is excluded from MACRS under the anti-churning rules (Code Sec. 168(f)).[55] Public utility property that does not qualify under MACRS (Code Sec. 168(f)(2))[56] is depreciated under Code Sec. 167(a)[57] using the same depreciation method and useful life as is used to compute the rate-making depreciation allowance for the property.

1239. Accounting for MACRS Property in Item, Multiple Asset, and General Asset Accounts. Under the Modified Accelerated Cost Recovery System (MACRS), property may be accounted for individually in an item account or by placing a group of identically depreciated assets (i.e., assets with the same recovery period, depreciation method, convention, and placed-in-service tax year) in a multiple asset (pool) account (Reg. § 1.168(i)-7).[58] Alternatively, a taxpayer may elect to include a single asset or a group of identically depreciated assets in a general asset account (GAA) (Reg. § 1.168(i)-1).[59]

Depreciation (including bonus depreciation) on a GAA is computed on the combined bases of the assets in the multiple asset account or GAA (after reduction by any amounts expensed under Code Sec. 179) as if the multiple asset account or GAA is a single asset. Depreciation allowances determined for each GAA must be recorded in a depreciation reserve account for each account (Reg. § 1.168(i)-1(d)(1)). Similar rules apply to a multiple asset account (Reg. § 1.168(i)-7).

If a taxpayer disposes of an asset in a multiple asset account, then as of the first day of the tax year of disposition, the asset is placed into a single asset account and gain or loss is generally computed on the asset. In computing the adjusted depreciable basis of the asset disposed, the depreciation allowed or allowable for the asset is computed by using the depreciation method, recovery period, and convention applicable to the multiple asset account or pool in which the asset was included. The unadjusted depreciable basis of the multiple asset account is reduced by the unadjusted depreciable basis of

References are to Standard Federal Tax Reports; Tax Research Consultant; and Practical Tax Explanations.

[53] ¶ 11,250; DEPR: 3,800; § 11,235

[54] ¶ 11,250; DEPR: 3,850; § 11,220

[55] ¶ 11,250, ¶ 11,279.021; DEPR: 15,150; § 11,105

[56] ¶ 11,250; DEPR: 6,150; § 11,110

[57] ¶ 11,002; DEPR: 15,700; § 11,110

[58] ¶ 11,276P, ¶ 11,279.0372; DEPR: 15,210; § 11,105.07

[59] ¶ 11,275B, ¶ 11,279.038; DEPR: 3,559; § 11,140

12 DEPRECIATION

the asset disposed as of the first day of the tax year of disposition. The depreciation reserve of the multiple asset account is reduced by the depreciation allowed or allowable for the disposed asset in the tax years prior to the tax year of disposition (Reg. § 1.168(i)-8(h)(2)).

Generally, for a disposition that is not the disposition of all of the assets or the last asset in a GAA, the unadjusted depreciable basis of the GAA is not reduced. The asset is treated as having an adjusted depreciable basis of $0 immediately before the disposition and no loss is realized. The amount realized is recognized as ordinary income up to (1) the sum of the unadjusted depreciable basis of the account and the amount expensed under Code Sec. 179 for all assets in the account, and (2) reduced by amounts previously recognized as ordinary income (Reg. § 1.168(i)-1(e)(2)).

If all of the assets or the last asset in the account is disposed, a taxpayer may apply the preceding rule or elect to terminate the account and recognize gain or loss by reference to the adjusted basis of the GAA (i.e., unadjusted depreciable basis of the GAA less prior deprecation on assets in account) (Reg. § 1.168(i)-1(e)(3)(ii)).

In the case of a "qualifying disposition" a taxpayer may also elect to recognize gain or loss by reference to the adjusted basis of the disposed asset in the GAA. However, a qualifying disposition only includes a disposition that does not involve all of the assets or the last asset in the account and which is: (1) the direct result of a casualty or theft; (2) a deductible charitable contribution; (3) a direct result of a cessation, termination, or disposition of a business, manufacturing, or other income-producing process; and (4) certain nonrecognition transactions (Reg. § 1.168(i)-1(e)(3)(iii)).

Under temporary regulations that taxpayers were permitted to apply in a tax year beginning on or after January 1, 2012 and before January 1, 2014, the definition of a qualifying disposition included most sales or dispositions of an asset in a GAA (other than the last asset), including the retirement of a structural component of a building or component of other types of assets (Temp. Reg. § 1.168(i)-1T(e)(iii)(B)). The final regulations changed the definition of a qualifying disposition so as to prevent a taxpayer from electing to recognize gain or loss by reference to an asset's adjusted basis or the adjusted basis of a component of an asset upon its disposition from the GAA except in the limited circumstances described above that constitute a qualifying disposition (Reg. § 1.168(i)-1(e)(iii)(B)). As a result of this change, the IRS has issued guidance that allows taxpayers who made retroactive GAA elections for assets placed in service in tax years beginning before January 1, 2012, and timely GAA elections for assets placed in service in tax years beginning in 2012 or 2013 to revoke those elections by filing an accounting method change for any tax year beginning on or after January 1, 2012, and beginning before January 1, 2015 (Section 6.34 of the Appendix of Rev. Proc. 2011-14, as added by Rev. Proc. 2014-17 and modified by Rev. Proc. 2014-54). For taxpayers that applied the temporary GAA regulations and made qualifying disposition elections to claim losses on retired structural components of a building (or components of other types of property), in addition to revoking the GAA election, it is also necessary to preserve those losses by making the late partial disposition election described below by filing an accounting method change pursuant to Section 6.33 of the Appendix of Rev. Proc. 2011-14, as added by Rev. Proc. 2014-17 and modified by Rev. Proc. 2014-54.[60]

Structural Components of Buildings Not in a GAA. Under final regulations, a building, including its structural components, is treated as an asset and a taxpayer is permitted to claim a loss upon the retirement of a structural component of a building (or a component of any other asset, such as component of a machine) only by making a partial disposition election (Reg. § 1.168(i)-8(d)). If the partial disposition election is not made, depreciation continues on the retired structural component and no adjustment to the basis of the building is made. As noted above, the partial disposition election does not apply to assets, including buildings, that are placed in a GAA.

The final regulations apply to tax years beginning on or after January 1, 2014, but may also be applied to tax years beginning on or after January 1, 2012, and before

---

References are to Standard Federal Tax Reports; Tax Research Consultant; and Practical Tax Explanations.

[60] ¶ 11,279.038; DEPR: 3,559;
§ 11,140

¶1239

January 1, 2014. The final regulations are essentially identical to proposed regulations which a taxpayer may apply to tax years beginning on or after January 1, 2012, and before January 1, 2014 (Prop. Reg. § 1.168(i)-8). It is not necessary to apply either the final or proposed regulations to tax years beginning on or after January 1, 2012, and before January 1, 2014 (Reg. § 1.168(i)-8(j)).

Temporary regulations that were also optionally applicable to tax years beginning on or after January 1, 2012, and before January 1, 2014, treated a structural component of a building as a separate asset and the retirement of a structural component as a disposition that triggered recognition of a loss to the extent of the structural component's remaining adjusted basis unless the building was placed in a GAA (Temp. Reg. § 1.168(i)-8T). Taxpayers who applied the temporary regulations to tax years beginning on or after January 1, 2012, and before January 1, 2014, were also permitted to file an accounting method change to claim losses on retirements that occurred in pre-2012 tax years.

Taxpayers may make a late partial disposition election under the final regulations to claim retirement losses on retirements that occurred in tax years beginning before January 1, 2012, by filing a timely accounting method change for any tax year beginning on or after January 1, 2012, and beginning before January 1, 2015, pursuant to Section 6.33 of the Appendix of Rev. Proc. 2011-14, as added by Rev. Proc. 2014-17 and modified by Rev. Proc. 2014-54. The late election may also be made by filing an accounting method change under Section 6.33 for a retirement that occurred in a tax year that began on or after January 1, 2012, and ended on or before September 19, 2013, no later than the first or second tax year ending after the tax year in which the retirement occurred or by filing an amended return on or before 180 days from the due date including extensions of the taxpayer's return for the tax year of retirement, notwithstanding that the taxpayer may not have extended the due date (Reg. § 1.168(i)-8(d)(2)(iv); Proposed Reg. § 1.168(i)-8(d)(2)(iv)).[61]

Taxpayers who relied on the temporary regulations to claim retirement losses on structural components of buildings (or components of some other type of asset) must also make a late partial disposition election to preserve those losses by filing an accounting method change pursuant to Section 6.33 of the Appendix of Rev. Proc. 2011-14, as added by Rev. Proc. 2014-17 and modified by Rev. Proc. 2014-54, no later than their last tax year beginning before January 1, 2015. See Sec. 6.33(8)(b), Example 2.

1240. MACRS Depreciation Periods. The Modified Accelerated Cost Recovery System (MACRS) depreciation (recovery) period for an asset is based on its class life as of January 1, 1986, or is specifically prescribed by Code Sec. 168.[62] The recovery periods for MACRS assets can be found in a table that appears in IRS Pub. 946. This table is an updated version of the table that appears in Rev. Proc. 87-56. Under MACRS, assets are classified according to their class life as follows:

Three-Year Property. Three-year property includes property with a class life of four years or less. Any race horse placed in service after December 31, 2008, and before January 1, 2014, or any other horse over 12 years old at the time it is placed in service is classified as three-year property (Code Sec. 168(e)(1) and (3)). A race horse more than two years old at the time placed in service is three-year property (seven-year property if two years old or less when placed in service) if placed in service on or before December 31, 2008, or on or after January 1, 2014.[63] Certain "rent-to-own" consumer durable property (e.g., televisions and furniture) is three-year property (Code Sec. 168(e)(3)(iii)).[64] Breeding hogs (Rev. Proc. 87-56 Asset Class 01.236) and tractor units for use over the road (Rev. Proc. 87-56 Asset Class 00.26) are three-year property. A tractor unit is a highway truck designed to tow a trailer or semitrailer and that does not carry cargo on the same chassis as the engine (Reg. § 145.4051-1(e)(1)).

References are to Standard Federal Tax Reports; Tax Research Consultant; and Practical Tax Explanations.

[61] ¶ 11,279.0373; DEPR: 15,210; § 11,105.12

[62] ¶ 163.01, ¶ 11,279.021; DEPR: 15,150; § 11,110

[63] ¶ 11,250, ¶ 11,279.023; DEPR: 3,156.05; § 11,110

[64] ¶ 11,250; DEPR: 3,156.60; § 11,110

Five-Year Property. Five-year property generally includes property with a class life of more than four years and less than 10 years. This property includes: (1) cars, (2) light and heavy general-purpose trucks, (3) qualified technological equipment, (4) computer-based telephone central office switching equipment, (5) research and experimentation property that is Sec. 1245 property, (6) semi-conductor manufacturing equipment, (7) geothermal, solar and wind energy properties, (8) certain biomass properties that are small power production facilities, (9) computers and peripheral equipment, and (10) office machinery (typewriters, calculators, etc.) (Code Sec. 168(e)(1) and (3)).[65]

Furniture, appliances, window treatments, and carpeting used in residential rental property are five-year property (Announcement 99-82). Personal property used in wholesale or retail trade or in the provision of personal and professional services for which a specific recovery period is not otherwise provided is five-year property (Asset Class 57.0 of Rev. Proc. 87-56). For example, a professional library used by an accountant or attorney is five-year property. Examples of *personal* service businesses include hotels and motels, laundry and dry cleaning establishments, beauty and barber shops, photographic studios and mortuaries (Rev. Proc. 77-10). Examples of *professional* service businesses include services offered by doctors, dentists, lawyers, accountants, architects, engineers, and veterinarians (Rev. Proc. 77-10).

Five-year property also includes taxis (Rev. Proc. 87-56 Asset Class 00.22), buses (Rev. Proc. 87-56 Asset Class 00.23), airplanes not used in commercial or contract carrying of passengers or freight and all helicopters (Rev. Proc. 87-56 Asset Class 00.21), trailers and trailer-mounted containers (Rev. Proc. 87-56 Asset Class 00.27), breeding cattle and dairy cattle (Rev. Proc. 87-56 Asset Class 01.21), breeding sheep and breeding goats (Rev. Proc. 87-56 Asset Class 01.21), and assets used in construction by certain contractors, builders, and real estate subdividers and developers (Rev. Proc. 87-56 Asset Class 15.0).

Seven-Year Property. Seven-year property includes property with a class life of 10 years or more but less than 16 years (Code Sec. 168(e)(1)). This property includes office furniture, equipment and fixtures that are not structural components (Rev. Proc. 87-56 Asset Class 00.11). Desks, files, safes, overhead projectors, cell phones, fax machines and other communication equipment not included in any other class fall within this category. Seven-year property also includes: assets (except helicopters) used in commercial and contract carrying of passengers and freight by air (Rev. Proc. 87-56 Asset Class 45.0); certain livestock (Rev. Proc. 87-56 Asset Class 01.1); breeding or work horses 12 years old or less when placed in service (Rev. Proc. 87-56 Asset Class 01.221); other horses that are not three-year property (Rev. Proc. 87-56 Asset Class 01.225); assets used in recreation businesses (Rev. Proc. 87-56 Asset Class 80.0); and assets used in theme and amusement parks (Rev. Proc. 87-56 Asset Class 80.0). Railroad track and property (such as a fishing vessel) that does not have a class life and is not otherwise classified is seven-year property (Code Sec. 168(e)(3)(C)).[66]

10-Year Property. Ten-year property is property with a class life of 16 years or more and less than 20 years (Code Sec. 168(e)(1)).[67] This includes vessels, barges, tugs, and similar means of water transportation not used in marine construction or as a fishing vessel (Rev. Proc. 87-56 Asset Class 00.28). Effective for property placed in service after October 3, 2008, it also includes smart electric meters and qualified smart electric grid systems (Code Sec. 168(e)(3)(D)). MACRS deductions for trees or vines bearing fruit or nuts that are placed in service after 1988 are determined under the straight-line method over a 10-year recovery period (Code Sec. 168(b)(1)).[68] Single purpose agricultural or horticultural structures placed in service after 1988 are 10-year property (Code Sec. 168(e)(3)(D)(i)).

References are to Standard Federal Tax Reports; Tax Research Consultant; and Practical Tax Explanations.

[65] ¶ 11,250; DEPR: 3,156.10; § 11,110

[66] ¶ 11,250; DEPR: 3,156.15; § 11,110

[67] ¶ 11,250; DEPR: 3,156.20; § 11,110

[68] ¶ 11,250; DEPR: 3,156.20; § 11,110

¶1240

15-Year Property. Property with a class life of 20 years or more but less than 25 years is generally considered 15-year property (Code Sec. 168(e)(1)). It includes municipal wastewater treatment plants and telephone distribution plants and other comparable equipment used for the two-way exchange of voice, data communications, and retail motor fuels outlets (Code Sec. 168(e)(3)(E)).[69] A property qualifies as a retail motor fuels outlet (as opposed, for example, to a convenience store, which is 39-year real property) if: (1) 50 percent or more of gross revenues are derived from petroleum sales; (2) 50 percent or more of the floor space is devoted to petroleum marketing sales; or (3) the property is 1,400 square feet or less (Rev. Proc. 97-10).[70]

Fifteen-year property includes car wash buildings (and related land improvements), billboards, and section 1250 real property (including service station buildings) and depreciable land improvements used in marketing petroleum and petroleum products (Rev. Proc. 87-56 Asset Class 57.1). Water transportation assets (other than vessels) used in the commercial and contract carrying of freight and passengers by water are 15-year property (Rev. Proc. 87-56 Asset Class 44.0).

Land improvements not specifically included in any other asset class and otherwise depreciable are 15-year property (Rev. Proc. 87-56 Asset Class 00.3). Examples of land improvements include sidewalks, driveways, curbs, roads, parking lots, canals, waterways, drainage facilities, sewers (but not municipal sewers), wharves and docks, bridges, and nonagricultural fences. Landscaping and shrubbery is a depreciable land improvement if it is located near a building and would be destroyed if the building were replaced (Rev. Rul. 74-265; IRS Publication 946). Playground equipment is a land improvement (LTR 8848039).[71]

Depreciable gas utility clearing and grading costs incurred after October 22, 2004, to place pipelines into service are 15-year property (Code Sec. 168(e)(3)(E)(vi)).

15-Year Leasehold Improvement Property. See ¶ 1234.

15-Year Restaurant Improvements and Buildings. Qualified restaurant property placed in service after October 22, 2004, and before January 1, 2014, is 15-year MACRS property, depreciable using the straight-line method using the half-year or mid-quarter convention, as applicable (Code Sec. 168(e)(3)(E)(v)).[72] The ADS recovery period is 39 years. Qualified restaurant property is section 1250 property that is an improvement to a building. More than 50 percent of the building's square footage must be devoted to preparation of and seating for on-premises consumption of prepared meals. For restaurant improvements placed in service before 2009, the building must be more than three years old. For improvements placed in service after 2008, it is not necessary that the restaurant building be more than three years old (Code Sec. 168(e)(3)(E)(v) and (e)(7)).

> **Comment:** Absent further legislation, qualified restaurant property placed in service after December 31, 2013 will be depreciated as 39-year nonresidential real property. For the latest legislative updates, visit our website www.CCHGroup.com/TaxUpdates.

A restaurant building placed in service after December 31, 2008, and before January 1, 2014, is also included in the definition of qualified restaurant property and is depreciated as 15-year property using the straight-line method and half-year or mid-quarter convention if more than 50 percent of the building's square footage is devoted to preparation of and seating for the on-premises consumption of prepared meals. A 39-year ADS recovery period applies (Code Secs. 168(b)(3)(l) and (e)(7)(A)).

References are to Standard Federal Tax Reports; Tax Research Consultant; and Practical Tax Explanations.

[69] ¶ 11,250; DEPR: 3,156.25; § 11,110
[70] ¶ 11,279.34; DEPR: 3,156.25; § 11,110
[71] ¶ 11,279.0518; DEPR: 6,062.10; § 11,110
[72] ¶ 11,250; DEPR: 3,156.256; § 11,215

The Code Sec. 168(k) bonus depreciation deduction (¶ 1237) may not be claimed on qualified restaurant property placed in service after December 31, 2008, unless it meets the definition of qualified leasehold improvement property (¶ 1234) (Code Sec. 168(e)(7)(B); Rev. Proc. 2011-26).

15-Year Qualified Retail Improvement Property. Qualified retail improvement property placed in service after December 31, 2008, and before January 1, 2014, is depreciated under MACRS using a 15-year recovery period, the straight-line method, and the half-year or mid-quarter convention (Code Sec. 168(e)(3)(E)(ix)).[73] The ADS recovery period is 39 years. Qualified retail improvement property is an improvement to the interior portion of a building that is nonresidential real property. The improvement must be placed in service more than three years after the building was first placed in service. The improved interior portion must be open to the general public and used in the retail trade or business of selling tangible personal property to the general public. Elevators and escalators, internal structural framework of the building, structural components that benefit a common area, and improvements relating to the enlargement of a building do not qualify. Qualified retail improvement property is ineligible for bonus depreciation under Code Sec. 168(k) unless it also meets the definition of qualified leasehold improvement property (¶ 1234) (Code Sec. 168(e)(8); Rev. Proc. 2011-26).

> **Comment:** Absent further legislation, qualified retail improvement property placed in service after December 31, 2013 will be depreciated as 39-year nonresidential real property. For the latest legislative updates, visit our website www.CCHGroup.com/TaxUpdates.

20-Year Property. Twenty-year property includes property with a class life of 25 years and more, other than Code Sec. 1250 real property with a class life of 27.5 years or more. Water utility property and municipal sewers placed in service before June 13, 1996, and farm buildings (e.g., barns and machine sheds) are included within this class (Code Sec. 168(e)(1) and (3)).[74] Depreciable electric utility clearing and grading costs incurred after October 22, 2004, to place transmission and distribution lines into service are 20-year property (Code Sec. 168(e)(3)(F)).

25-Year Property. Water utility property and municipal sewers placed in service after June 12, 1996, is recovered over a 25 year recovery period (Code Sec. 168(c) and (e)(5)). The straight-line depreciation method is mandatory for 25-year property (Code Sec. 168(b)(3)(F)).

27.5-Year Residential Rental Property. Residential rental property has a recovery period of 27.5 years. Residential rental property includes buildings or structures with respect to which 80 percent or more of the gross rental income is from dwelling units (Code Sec. 168(e)(2)(A))[75] It also includes manufactured homes that are residential rental property and elevators and escalators.

Nonresidential Real Property. Nonresidential real property is Code Sec. 1250 real property (¶ 1786) that is not residential rental property or property with a class life (as provided in Rev. Proc. 87-56) of less than 27.5 years (Code Sec. 168(e)(2)(B)).[76] The cost of nonresidential real property generally placed in service after May 12, 1993, is recovered over 39 years. For property placed in service after 1986 and before May 13, 1993, cost is recovered over 31.5 years.

Farm Machinery and Equipment. Machinery and equipment, grain bins, and fences (but no other land improvements) used in specified agricultural activities are classified as MACRS 7-year property and have a 10-year ADS recovery period (Rev. Proc. 87-56 Asset Class 01.1). However, any machinery or equipment (other than any grain bin, cotton ginning asset, fence, or other land improvement) that is used in a farming business (as defined in Code Sec. 263A(e)(4)), the original use of which commences

---

References are to Standard Federal Tax Reports; Tax Research Consultant; and Practical Tax Explanations.

[73] ¶ 11,250; DEPR: 3,156.255; § 11,230
[74] ¶ 11,250; DEPR: 3,156.30; § 11,110
[75] ¶ 11,250; DEPR: 3,156.35; § 11,110
[76] ¶ 11,250; DEPR: 3,156.40; § 11,110

¶1240

with the taxpayer after December 31, 2008, and that is placed in service before January 1, 2010, is classified as MACRS 5-year property (Code Sec. 168(e)(3)(B)(vii)) and has a 10-year ADS recovery period (Code Sec. 168(g)(3)(B)). Property used in a farming business is depreciated using the 150-percent declining balance method as explained at ¶ 1243 (Code Sec. 168(b)(2)(B)).

Indian Reservation Property. For qualified Indian reservation property that is placed in service after 1993 and before January 1, 2014, special MACRS recovery periods are provided for both regular tax and alternative minimum tax purposes that permit faster write-offs (Code Sec. 168(j)).[77]

> **Comment:** Absent further legislation, Indian reservation property placed in service after December 31, 2013 will be depreciated using the generally applicable MACRS recovery periods. For the latest legislative updates, visit our website www.CCHGroup.com/TaxUpdates.

Additions and Improvements. Additions and improvements (including the cost of capitalized structural components) are depreciated under MACRS in the same way that the improved property would be depreciated if it were placed in service at the same time as the addition or improvement (Code Sec. 168(i)(6)).[78] For example, a new floor or roof added to a commercial building in 2014 is treated as 39-year MACRS nonresidential real property even if the building is depreciated under a pre-MACRS method. However, any elements of an addition or improvement to a building that qualify as personal property may be depreciated over a shorter recovery period as personal rather than real property by reason of the cost segregation rule described below. Special rules apply to leasehold improvement property (¶ 1234) and improvements to restaurants and buildings used in a retail business, as explained above.

Structural components. See ¶ 1239.

Roofs. The replacement of an entire roof (including the sheathing and rafters) or a significant portion of a roof that has deteriorated over time is a restoration that is capitalized as an improvement (Reg. § 1.263(a)-3(k)(7), Example 14; Temp. Reg. § 1.263(a)-3T(i)(5), Examples 12 and 13). The replacement of a worn and leaking waterproof membrane on a roof comprised of structural elements, insulation, and a waterproof membrane with a similar but new membrane is not required to be capitalized so long as the membrane was not leaking when the taxpayer placed the building in service (Reg. § 1.263(a)-3(j)(3), Example 13, and (k)(7), Example 15; Temp. Reg. § 1.263(a)-3T(i)(5), Example 14). Likewise the cost of replacing shingles that became leaky while the taxpayer owned the building with similar shingles is not capitalized (Reg. § 1.263(a)-3(g)(2)(ii), Example 3).

An otherwise deductible repair expense (e.g., the cost of replacing a portion of a roof) must be capitalized if the taxpayer claims a retirement loss deduction on the portion of the roof that is retired or a basis adjustment as a result of a casualty loss or casualty event, such as receipt of an insurance reimbursement (Reg. § 1.263(a)-3(k)(1)). However, a taxpayer may claim a repair expense deduction for otherwise deductible repair expenses in excess of the difference between (1) the basis reduction (e.g., to a building) required on account of a casualty loss or insurance payment, and (2) the cost of any expenditures that must be capitalized as a restoration expenditure without regard to the casualty loss rule (e.g., the cost of replacing an entire roof) (Reg. § 1.263(a)-3(k)(4); Reg. § 1.263(a)-3(k)(7), Examples 3, 4, and 5).

> **Example:** A taxpayer replaces an entire roof on account of a storm. The casualty loss basis reduction is $500,000 (the adjusted basis of the building) and the building's adjusted basis is reduced to $0. The taxpayer pays $350,000 to replace the entire roof and $400,000 for miscellaneous repair and cleaning expenses. The taxpayer must capitalize the cost of the replacement roof as a restoration expenditure because it is a major component and substantial structural

---

References are to Standard Federal Tax Reports; Tax Research Consultant; and Practical Tax Explanations.

[77] ¶ 11,250; DEPR: 3,156.55; § 11,120

[78] ¶ 11,250; DEPR: 6,052; § 11,110

part of the building structure. The taxpayer may deduct $250,000 ($400,000 – ($500,000 adjusted basis – $350,000)) of the repair and cleaning expenses as a repair expense and the remaining $150,000 is capitalized as a restoration expense (Reg. § 1.263(a)-3(k)(7), Example 5).

Cost Segregation. The Tax Court has ruled that elements of a building that are treated as personal property under the former investment tax credit rules (Reg. § 1.48-1(c)) may be separately depreciated under MACRS and ACRS as personal property (*Hospital Corp. of America*, 109 TC 21 (1997)).[79] The IRS has acquiesced to the court's holding that the former investment tax credit rules apply in determining whether an item is a structural component (i.e., real property) or personal property but nonacquiesced to its finding that various disputed items were in fact personal property under these rules (Notice of Acquiescence, 1999-35 I.R.B. 314). The separate depreciation of personal property elements of a building is referred to as cost segregation.

The determination of whether an item is personal property or a structural component will often depend upon the specific facts. However, the following items, if related to the operation and maintenance of a building, are examples of structural components: bathtubs, boilers, ceilings (including acoustical ceilings), central air conditioning and heating systems, chimneys, doors, electric wiring, fire escapes, floors, hot water heaters, HVAC units, lighting fixtures, paneling, partitions (if not readily removable), plumbing, roofs, sinks, sprinkler systems, stairs, tiling, walls, and windows (Reg. § 1.48-1(e)(2)).

1243. MACRS Recovery Methods. Under the Modified Accelerated Cost Recovery System (MACRS), the cost of depreciable property is recovered using (1) the applicable depreciation method, (2) the applicable recovery period, and (3) the applicable convention (Code Sec. 168(a)).[80]

The cost of property in the 3-, 5-, 7-, and 10-year classes is recovered using the 200-percent declining-balance method over three, five, seven, and ten years, respectively (i.e., the applicable recovery period), and the half-year convention (unless the mid-quarter convention applies), with a switch to the straight-line method in the year that maximizes the deduction (Code Sec. 168(b)(1)).[81] The cost of 15- and 20-year property is recovered using the 150-percent declining-balance method over 15 and 20 years, respectively, and the half-year convention (unless the mid-quarter convention applies), with a switch to the straight-line method to maximize the deduction (Code Sec. 168(b)(2)).[82] The cost of residential rental and nonresidential real property is recovered using the straight-line method and the mid-month convention over 27.5- and 39-year recovery periods, respectively (Code Sec. 168(b)(3)).[83]

Instead of the applicable depreciation method (200-percent declining balance method for 3-, 5-, 7-, and 10-year property and 150-percent declining balance method for 10- and 15-year property), taxpayers may irrevocably elect to claim straight-line MACRS deductions over the regular recovery period. The election applies to all property in the MACRS class for which the election is made that is placed in service during the tax year and is made on the return for the year the property is first placed in service (Code Sec. 168(b)(5)). For example, if the election is made for 3-year property, it applies to all 3-year property placed in service in the tax year of the election.

An election may be made to recover the cost of 3-, 5-, 7-, and 10-year property using the 150-percent declining-balance method over the regular recovery periods (the MACRS alternative depreciation system (ADS) recovery period for property placed in service before 1999) (¶ 1247) (Code Sec. 168(b)(2)(C)).[84] This election, like the straight-line election above, is made separately for each property class placed in service during the tax year of the election. A taxpayer may also elect the MACRS ADS with respect to any class of property (¶ 1247).

References are to Standard Federal Tax Reports; Tax Research Consultant; and Practical Tax Explanations.

[79] ¶ 11,279.25; DEPR: 6,058; § 11,110

[80] ¶ 11,250; DEPR: 3,200; § 11,115

[81] ¶ 11,250; DEPR: 3,202; § 11,115

[82] ¶ 11,250; DEPR: 3,202; § 11,115

[83] ¶ 11,250; DEPR: 3,202; § 11,115

[84] ¶ 11,250; DEPR: 3,202.05; § 11,115

¶1243

3-, 5-, 7-, and 10-year property used in the trade or business of farming must be depreciated under the 150-percent declining balance method unless an election was made to deduct preproductive period expenditures, in which case the ADS must be used (Code Sec. 168(b)(2)(B)). Consequently, Tables 1-8, below, may not be used for such property.

Computation of Deduction Without Tables. The MACRS deduction on personal property is computed by first determining the rate of depreciation (dividing the number one by the recovery period).[85] This basic rate is multiplied by 1.5 or 2 for the 150-percent or 200-percent declining-balance method, as applicable, to determine the declining balance rate. The adjusted basis of the property is multiplied by the declining-balance rate and the half-year or mid-quarter convention (whichever is applicable) is applied in computing depreciation for the first year. The depreciation claimed in the first year is subtracted from the adjusted basis before applying the declining-balance rate in determining the depreciation deduction for the second year.

Under the MACRS straight-line method (used, for example, on real property or if ADS applies), a new applicable depreciation rate is determined for each tax year in the applicable recovery period. For any tax year, the applicable depreciation rate (in percentage terms) is determined by dividing one by the length of the applicable recovery period remaining as of the beginning of such tax year. The rate is applied to the unrecovered basis of such property in conjunction with the appropriate convention. If as of the beginning of any tax year the remaining recovery period is less than one year, the applicable depreciation rate under the straight-line method for that year is 100 percent.

Example 1: An item of five-year property is purchased by a calendar-year taxpayer in January ("Year 1") at a cost of $10,000. No Code Sec. 179 expense allowance or bonus depreciation is claimed. The 200-percent declining-balance method and half-year convention apply. Depreciation computed without the use of the IRS tables is determined as follows: the declining-balance depreciation rate is determined and compared with the straight-line rate. A switch is made to the straight-line rate in the year depreciation equals or exceeds that determined under the declining-balance method. The applicable rate is applied to the unrecovered basis. The 200-percent declining-balance depreciation rate is 40 percent (1 divided by 5 (recovery period) times 2). The straight-line rate (which changes each year) is 1 divided by the length of the applicable recovery period remaining as of the beginning of each tax year (after considering the applicable convention for purposes of determining how much of the applicable recovery period remains as of the beginning of the year). For year four, the straight-line rate is .40 (1 divided by 2.5), which is the same as the declining balance rate. For year five, the straight-line rate is .6667 (1 divided by 1.5). For year six, the straight-line rate is 100 percent because the remaining recovery period is less than one year.

Year	Method	Rate	Unrecovered Basis		Depreciation
1	DB	.40	× $ 10,000 × .5 (half-yr. conv.)		= $ 2,000
2	DB	.40	× (10,000 – 2,000)	= $8,000 ..	= 3,200
3	DB	.40	× (8,000 – 3,200)	= 4,800 ..	= 1,920
4	DB	.40	× (4,800 – 1,920)	= 2,880 ..	= 1,152
5	SL	.6667	× (2,880 – 1,152)	= 1,728 ..	= 1,152
6	SL	1.000	× (1,728 – 1,152)	= 576 ..	= 576
				0	
				Total ..	$10,000

The computation of MACRS without tables is discussed in detail by the IRS in Rev. Proc. 87-57.

Computation of Deduction Using Tables. MACRS depreciation tables, which contain the annual percentage depreciation rates to be applied to the unadjusted basis of property in each tax year, may be used to compute depreciation instead of the above rules.[86] The tables incorporate the appropriate convention and a switch from the

---

References are to Standard Federal Tax Reports; Tax Research Consultant; and Practical Tax Explanations.

[85] ¶ 11,279.027; DEPR: 3,204.05; § 11,130

[86] ¶ 164.01; DEPR: 3,204; § 11,130

declining-balance method to the straight-line method in the year that the latter provides a depreciation allowance equal to, or larger than, the former. The tables may be used for any item of property (that otherwise qualifies for MACRS) placed in service in a tax year.

Selected MACRS depreciation tables are reproduced below. A complete set of tables is at ¶ 164 of the STANDARD FEDERAL TAX REPORTER and at § 820 of the Practical Tax Explanations. Tables for the TAX RESEARCH CONSULTANT are located in the "Tax Rates and Tables" publication.

If a table is used to compute the annual depreciation allowance for any item of property, it must be used throughout the entire recovery period of such property. However, a taxpayer may not continue to use a table if there are any adjustments to the basis of the property for reasons other than (1) depreciation allowances or (2) an addition or improvement to such property that is subject to depreciation as a separate item of property. The IRS MACRS depreciation tables may not be used in situations involving short tax years (¶ 1244).

Example 2: Depreciation on five-year property purchased by a calendar-year taxpayer in January of the current tax year at a cost of $10,000 is computed under the general MACRS 200-percent declining-balance method over a five-year recovery period using the half-year convention. No amount is expensed under Code Sec. 179 or claimed as a bonus depreciation deduction.

If the depreciation tables provided by the IRS are used, depreciation is computed as follows: the applicable depreciation rate in Table 1 under the column for a five-year recovery period for the applicable recovery year is applied to the cost of the property.

Year	Rate	Unadj. Basis	Depreciation		Basis		
1	.20 ×	$ 10,000 =	$ 2,000	($10,000 –	$2,000)	=	$8,000
2	.32 ×	10,000 =	3,200	(8,000 –	3,200)	=	4,800
3	.192 ×	10,000 =	1,920	(4,800 –	1,920)	=	2,880
4	.1152 ×	10,000 =	1,152	(2,880 –	1,152)	=	1,728
5	.1152 ×	10,000 =	1,152	(1,728 –	1,152)	=	576
6	.0576 ×	10,000 =	576	(576 –	576)	=	0
		Total	$10,000				

Table 1. General Depreciation System
Applicable Depreciation Method: 200 or 150 Percent
Declining Balance Switching to Straight Line
Applicable Recovery Periods: 3, 5, 7, 10, 15, 20 years
Applicable Convention: Half-year

If the Recovery Year is:	and the Recovery Period is:					
	3-year	5-year	7-year	10-year	15-year	20-year
	the Depreciation Rate is:					
1	33.33	20.00	14.29	10.00	5.00	3.750
2	44.45	32.00	24.49	18.00	9.50	7.219
3	14.81	19.20	17.49	14.40	8.55	6.677
4	7.41	11.52	12.49	11.52	7.70	6.177
5		11.52	8.93	9.22	6.93	5.713
6		5.76	8.92	7.37	6.23	5.285
7			8.93	6.55	5.90	4.888
8			4.46	6.55	5.90	4.522
9				6.56	5.91	4.462
10				6.55	5.90	4.461
11				3.28	5.91	4.462
12					5.90	4.461
13					5.91	4.462
14					5.90	4.461
15					5.91	4.462
16					2.95	4.461
17						4.462
18						4.461
19						4.462
20						4.461
21						2.231

Table 2. General Depreciation System
Applicable Depreciation Method: 200 or 150 Percent
Declining Balance Switching to Straight Line
Applicable Recovery Periods: 3, 5, 7, 10, 15, 20 years
Applicable Convention: Mid-quarter (property placed in
service in first quarter)

If the Recovery Year is:	and the Recovery Period is:					
	3-year	5-year	7-year	10-year	15-year	20-year
	the Depreciation Rate is:					
1	58.33	35.00	25.00	17.50	8.75	6.563
2	27.78	26.00	21.43	16.50	9.13	7.000
3	12.35	15.60	15.31	13.20	8.21	6.482
4	1.54	11.01	10.93	10.56	7.39	5.996
5		11.01	8.75	8.45	6.65	5.546
6		1.38	8.74	6.76	5.99	5.130
7			8.75	6.55	5.90	4.746
8			1.09	6.55	5.91	4.459
9				6.56	5.90	4.459
10				6.55	5.91	4.459
11				0.82	5.90	4.459
12					5.91	4.460
13					5.90	4.459
14					5.91	4.460
15					5.90	4.459
16					0.74	4.460
17						4.459
18						4.460
19						4.459
20						4.460
21						0.565

12 DEPRECIATION

Table 3. General Depreciation System
Applicable Depreciation Method: 200 or 150 Percent
Declining Balance Switching to Straight Line
Applicable Recovery Periods: 3, 5, 7, 10, 15, 20 years
Applicable Convention: Mid-quarter (property placed in
service in second quarter)

If the Recovery Year is:	and the Recovery Period is:					
	3-year	5-year	7-year	10-year	15-year	20-year
	the Depreciation Rate is:					
1	41.67	25.00	17.85	12.50	6.25	4.688
2	38.89	30.00	23.47	17.50	9.38	7.148
3	14.14	18.00	16.76	14.00	8.44	6.612
4	5.30	11.37	11.97	11.20	7.59	6.116
5		11.37	8.87	8.96	6.83	5.658
6		4.26	8.87	7.17	6.15	5.233
7			8.87	6.55	5.91	4.841
8			3.33	6.55	5.90	4.478
9				6.56	5.91	4.463
10				6.55	5.90	4.463
11				2.46	5.91	4.463
12					5.90	4.463
13					5.91	4.463
14					5.90	4.463
15					5.91	4.462
16					2.21	4.463
17						4.462
18						4.463
19						4.462
20						4.463
21						1.673

Table 4. General Depreciation System
Applicable Depreciation Method: 200 or 150 Percent
Declining Balance Switching to Straight Line
Applicable Recovery Periods: 3, 5, 7, 10, 15, 20 years
Applicable Convention: Mid-quarter (property placed in
service in third quarter)

If the Recovery Year is:	and the Recovery Period is:					
	3-year	5-year	7-year	10-year	15-year	20-year
	the Depreciation Rate is:					
1	25.00	15.00	10.71	7.50	3.75	2.813
2	50.00	34.00	25.51	18.50	9.63	7.289
3	16.67	20.40	18.22	14.80	8.66	6.742
4	8.33	12.24	13.02	11.84	7.80	6.237
5		11.30	9.30	9.47	7.02	5.769
6		7.06	8.85	7.58	6.31	5.336
7			8.86	6.55	5.90	4.936
8			5.53	6.55	5.90	4.566
9				6.56	5.91	4.460
10				6.55	5.90	4.460
11				4.10	5.91	4.460
12					5.90	4.460
13					5.91	4.461
14					5.90	4.460
15					5.91	4.461
16					3.69	4.460
17						4.461
18						4.460
19						4.461
20						4.460
21						2.788

Table 5. General Depreciation System
Applicable Depreciation Method: 200 or 150 Percent
Declining Balance Switching to Straight Line
Applicable Recovery Periods: 3, 5, 7, 10, 15, 20 years
Applicable Convention: Mid-quarter (property placed in
service in fourth quarter)

If the Recovery Year is:	and the Recovery Period is:					
	3-year	5-year	7-year	10-year	15-year	20-year
	the Depreciation Rate is:					
1	8.33	5.00	3.57	2.50	1.25	0.938
2	61.11	38.00	27.55	19.50	9.88	7.430
3	20.37	22.80	19.68	15.60	8.89	6.872
4	10.19	13.68	14.06	12.48	8.00	6.357
5		10.94	10.04	9.98	7.20	5.880
6		9.58	8.73	7.99	6.48	5.439
7			8.73	6.55	5.90	5.031
8			7.64	6.55	5.90	4.654
9				6.56	5.90	4.458
10				6.55	5.91	4.458
11				5.74	5.90	4.458
12					5.91	4.458
13					5.90	4.458
14					5.91	4.458
15					5.90	4.458
16					5.17	4.458
17						4.458
18						4.459
19						4.458
20						4.459
21						3.901

Table 6. General Depreciation System
Applicable Depreciation Method: Straight Line
Applicable Recovery Period: 27.5 years
Applicable Convention: Mid-month

If the Recovery Year is:	And the Month in the First Recovery Year the Property is Placed in Service is:											
	1	2	3	4	5	6	7	8	9	10	11	12
	the Depreciation Rate is:											
1	3.485	3.182	2.879	2.576	2.273	1.970	1.667	1.364	1.061	0.758	0.455	0.152
2	3.636	3.636	3.636	3.636	3.636	3.636	3.636	3.636	3.636	3.636	3.636	3.636
3	3.636	3.636	3.636	3.636	3.636	3.636	3.636	3.636	3.636	3.636	3.636	3.636
4	3.636	3.636	3.636	3.636	3.636	3.636	3.636	3.636	3.636	3.636	3.636	3.636
5	3.636	3.636	3.636	3.636	3.636	3.636	3.636	3.636	3.636	3.636	3.636	3.636
6	3.636	3.636	3.636	3.636	3.636	3.636	3.636	3.636	3.636	3.636	3.636	3.636
7	3.636	3.636	3.636	3.636	3.636	3.636	3.636	3.636	3.636	3.636	3.636	3.636
8	3.636	3.636	3.636	3.636	3.636	3.636	3.636	3.636	3.636	3.636	3.636	3.636
9	3.636	3.636	3.636	3.636	3.636	3.636	3.636	3.636	3.636	3.636	3.636	3.636
10	3.637	3.637	3.637	3.637	3.637	3.637	3.636	3.636	3.636	3.636	3.636	3.636
11	3.636	3.636	3.636	3.636	3.636	3.636	3.637	3.637	3.637	3.637	3.637	3.637
12	3.637	3.637	3.637	3.637	3.637	3.637	3.636	3.636	3.636	3.636	3.636	3.636
13	3.636	3.636	3.636	3.636	3.636	3.636	3.637	3.637	3.637	3.637	3.637	3.637
14	3.637	3.637	3.637	3.637	3.637	3.637	3.636	3.636	3.636	3.636	3.636	3.636
15	3.636	3.636	3.636	3.636	3.636	3.636	3.637	3.637	3.637	3.637	3.637	3.637
16	3.637	3.637	3.637	3.637	3.637	3.637	3.636	3.636	3.636	3.636	3.636	3.636
17	3.636	3.636	3.636	3.636	3.636	3.636	3.637	3.637	3.637	3.637	3.637	3.637
18	3.637	3.637	3.637	3.637	3.637	3.637	3.636	3.636	3.636	3.636	3.636	3.636
19	3.636	3.636	3.636	3.636	3.636	3.636	3.637	3.637	3.637	3.637	3.637	3.637
20	3.637	3.637	3.637	3.637	3.637	3.637	3.636	3.636	3.636	3.636	3.636	3.636
21	3.636	3.636	3.636	3.636	3.636	3.636	3.637	3.637	3.637	3.637	3.637	3.637
22	3.637	3.637	3.637	3.637	3.637	3.637	3.636	3.636	3.636	3.636	3.636	3.636
23	3.636	3.636	3.636	3.636	3.636	3.636	3.637	3.637	3.637	3.637	3.637	3.637
24	3.637	3.637	3.637	3.637	3.637	3.637	3.636	3.636	3.636	3.636	3.636	3.636
25	3.636	3.636	3.636	3.636	3.636	3.636	3.637	3.637	3.637	3.637	3.637	3.637
26	3.637	3.637	3.637	3.637	3.637	3.637	3.636	3.636	3.636	3.636	3.636	3.636
27	3.636	3.636	3.636	3.636	3.636	3.636	3.637	3.637	3.637	3.637	3.637	3.637
28	1.970	2.273	2.576	2.879	3.182	3.485	3.636	3.636	3.636	3.636	3.636	3.636
29	0.000	0.000	0.000	0.000	0.000	0.000	0.152	0.455	0.758	1.061	1.364	1.667

12 DEPRECIATION

¶1243

Table 7. General Depreciation System
Applicable Depreciation Method: Straight Line
Applicable Recovery Period: 31.5 years
Applicable Convention: Mid-month

If the Recovery Year is:	And the Month in the First Recovery Year the Property is Placed in Service is:											
	1	2	3	4	5	6	7	8	9	10	11	12
	the Depreciation Rate is:											
1	3.042	2.778	2.513	2.249	1.984	1.720	1.455	1.190	0.926	0.661	0.397	0.132
2	3.175	3.175	3.175	3.175	3.175	3.175	3.175	3.175	3.175	3.175	3.175	3.175
3	3.175	3.175	3.175	3.175	3.175	3.175	3.175	3.175	3.175	3.175	3.175	3.175
4	3.175	3.175	3.175	3.175	3.175	3.175	3.175	3.175	3.175	3.175	3.175	3.175
5	3.175	3.175	3.175	3.175	3.175	3.175	3.175	3.175	3.175	3.175	3.175	3.175
6	3.175	3.175	3.175	3.175	3.175	3.175	3.175	3.175	3.175	3.175	3.175	3.175
7	3.175	3.175	3.175	3.175	3.175	3.175	3.175	3.175	3.175	3.175	3.175	3.175
8	3.175	3.174	3.175	3.174	3.175	3.174	3.175	3.175	3.175	3.175	3.175	3.175
9	3.174	3.175	3.174	3.175	3.174	3.175	3.174	3.175	3.174	3.175	3.174	3.175
10	3.175	3.174	3.175	3.174	3.175	3.174	3.175	3.174	3.175	3.174	3.175	3.174
11	3.174	3.175	3.174	3.175	3.174	3.175	3.174	3.175	3.174	3.175	3.174	3.174
12	3.175	3.174	3.175	3.174	3.175	3.174	3.175	3.174	3.175	3.174	3.175	3.174
13	3.174	3.175	3.174	3.175	3.174	3.175	3.174	3.175	3.174	3.175	3.174	3.175
14	3.175	3.174	3.175	3.174	3.175	3.174	3.175	3.174	3.175	3.174	3.175	3.175
15	3.174	3.175	3.174	3.175	3.174	3.175	3.174	3.175	3.174	3.175	3.174	3.175
16	3.175	3.174	3.175	3.174	3.175	3.174	3.175	3.174	3.175	3.174	3.175	3.174
17	3.174	3.175	3.174	3.175	3.174	3.175	3.174	3.175	3.174	3.175	3.174	3.174
18	3.175	3.174	3.175	3.174	3.175	3.174	3.175	3.174	3.175	3.174	3.175	3.174
19	3.174	3.175	3.174	3.175	3.174	3.175	3.174	3.175	3.174	3.175	3.174	3.175
20	3.175	3.174	3.175	3.174	3.175	3.174	3.175	3.174	3.175	3.174	3.175	3.175
21	3.174	3.175	3.174	3.175	3.174	3.175	3.174	3.175	3.174	3.175	3.174	3.175
22	3.175	3.174	3.175	3.174	3.175	3.174	3.175	3.174	3.175	3.174	3.175	3.174
23	3.174	3.175	3.174	3.175	3.174	3.175	3.174	3.175	3.174	3.175	3.174	3.174
24	3.175	3.174	3.175	3.174	3.175	3.174	3.175	3.174	3.175	3.174	3.175	3.174
25	3.174	3.175	3.174	3.175	3.174	3.175	3.174	3.175	3.174	3.175	3.174	3.175
26	3.175	3.174	3.175	3.174	3.175	3.174	3.175	3.174	3.175	3.174	3.175	3.175
27	3.174	3.175	3.174	3.175	3.174	3.175	3.174	3.175	3.174	3.175	3.174	3.175
28	3.175	3.174	3.175	3.174	3.175	3.174	3.175	3.174	3.175	3.174	3.175	3.174
29	3.174	3.175	3.174	3.175	3.174	3.175	3.174	3.175	3.174	3.175	3.174	3.175
30	3.175	3.174	3.175	3.174	3.175	3.174	3.175	3.174	3.175	3.174	3.175	3.174
31	3.174	3.175	3.174	3.175	3.174	3.175	3.174	3.175	3.174	3.175	3.174	3.175
32	1.720	1.984	2.249	2.513	2.778	3.042	3.175	3.174	3.175	3.174	3.175	3.174
33	0.000	0.000	0.000	0.000	0.000	0.000	0.132	0.397	0.661	0.926	1.190	1.455

Table 7A. General Depreciation System
Applicable Depreciation Method: Straight-Line
Applicable Recovery Period: 39 years
Applicable Convention: Mid-month—taken from the IRS Pub. 946

If the Recovery Year is:	And the Month in the First Recovery Year the Property is Placed in Service is:											
	1	2	3	4	5	6	7	8	9	10	11	12
	the Depreciation Rate is:											
1	2.461	2.247	2.033	1.819	1.605	1.391	1.177	0.963	0.749	0.535	0.321	0.107
2—39	2.564	2.564	2.564	2.564	2.564	2.564	2.564	2.564	2.564	2.564	2.564	2.564
40	0.107	0.321	0.535	0.749	0.963	1.177	1.391	1.605	1.819	2.033	2.247	2.461

Table 7B. Alternative Depreciation System
Applicable Depreciation Method: Straight-Line
Applicable Recovery Period: 40 years
Applicable Convention: Mid-month

If the Recovery Year is:	and the Month in the First Recovery Year the Property is Placed in Service is:											
	1	2	3	4	5	6	7	8	9	10	11	12
	the Depreciation Rate is:											
1	2.396	2.188	1.979	1.771	1.563	1.354	1.146	0.938	0.729	0.521	0.313	0.104
2—40	2.500	2.500	2.500	2.500	2.500	2.500	2.500	2.500	2.500	2.500	2.500	2.500
41	0.104	0.312	0.521	0.729	0.937	1.146	1.354	1.562	1.771	1.979	2.187	2.396

¶1243

Table 8. General and Alternative Depreciation Systems
Applicable Depreciation Method: Straight Line
Applicable Recovery Periods: 2.5 — 50 years
Applicable Convention: Half-year

If the Recovery Year is:	and the Recovery Period is:														
	2.5	3.0	3.5	4.0	4.5	5.0	5.5	6.0	6.5	7.0	7.5	8.0	8.5	9.0	9.5
	the Depreciation Rate is:														
1	20.00	16.67	14.29	12.50	11.11	10.00	9.09	8.33	7.69	7.14	6.67	6.25	5.88	5.56	5.26
2	40.00	33.33	28.57	25.00	22.22	20.00	18.18	16.67	15.39	14.29	13.33	12.50	11.77	11.11	10.53
3	40.00	33.33	28.57	25.00	22.22	20.00	18.18	16.67	15.38	14.29	13.33	12.50	11.76	11.11	10.53
4		16.67	28.57	25.00	22.23	20.00	18.18	16.67	15.39	14.28	13.33	12.50	11.77	11.11	10.53
5				12.50	22.22	20.00	18.19	16.66	15.38	14.29	13.34	12.50	11.76	11.11	10.52
6						10.00	18.18	16.67	15.39	14.28	13.33	12.50	11.77	11.11	10.53
7								8.33	15.38	14.29	13.34	12.50	11.76	11.11	10.52
8									7.14	13.33	12.50	11.77	11.11	10.53	
9												6.25	11.76	11.11	10.52
10														5.56	10.53

If the Recovery Year is:	and the Recovery Period is:														
	10.0	10.5	11.0	11.5	12.0	12.5	13.0	13.5	14.0	14.5	15.0	15.5	16.0	16.5	17.0
	the Depreciation Rate is:														
1	5.00	4.76	4.55	4.35	4.17	4.00	3.85	3.70	3.57	3.45	3.33	3.23	3.13	3.03	2.94
2	10.00	9.52	9.09	8.70	8.33	8.00	7.69	7.41	7.14	6.90	6.67	6.45	6.25	6.06	5.88
3	10.00	9.52	9.09	8.70	8.33	8.00	7.69	7.41	7.14	6.90	6.67	6.45	6.25	6.06	5.88
4	10.00	9.53	9.09	8.69	8.33	8.00	7.69	7.41	7.14	6.90	6.67	6.45	6.25	6.06	5.88
5	10.00	9.52	9.09	8.70	8.33	8.00	7.69	7.41	7.14	6.90	6.67	6.45	6.25	6.06	5.88
6	10.00	9.53	9.09	8.69	8.33	8.00	7.69	7.41	7.14	6.90	6.67	6.45	6.25	6.06	5.88
7	10.00	9.52	9.09	8.70	8.34	8.00	7.69	7.41	7.14	6.90	6.67	6.45	6.25	6.06	5.88
8	10.00	9.53	9.09	8.69	8.33	8.00	7.69	7.41	7.15	6.89	6.66	6.45	6.25	6.06	5.88
9	10.00	9.52	9.09	8.70	8.34	8.00	7.69	7.41	7.14	6.90	6.67	6.45	6.25	6.06	5.88
10	10.00	9.53	9.09	8.69	8.33	8.00	7.70	7.40	7.15	6.89	6.66	6.45	6.25	6.06	5.88
11	5.00	9.52	9.09	8.70	8.34	8.00	7.69	7.41	7.14	6.90	6.67	6.45	6.25	6.06	5.89
12			4.55	8.69	8.33	8.00	7.70	7.40	7.15	6.89	6.66	6.45	6.25	6.06	5.88
13					4.17	8.00	7.69	7.41	7.14	6.90	6.67	6.45	6.25	6.06	5.89
14							3.85	7.40	7.15	6.89	6.66	6.46	6.25	6.06	5.88
15									3.57	6.90	6.67	6.45	6.25	6.06	5.89
16											3.33	6.46	6.25	6.06	5.88
17													3.12	6.07	5.89
18															2.94

If the Recovery Year is:	and the Recovery Period is:														
	17.5	18.0	18.5	19.0	19.5	20.0	20.5	21.0	21.5	22.0	22.5	23.0	23.5	24.0	24.5
	the Depreciation Rate is:														
1	2.86	2.78	2.70	2.63	2.56	2.500	2.439	2.381	2.326	2.273	2.222	2.174	2.128	2.083	2.041
2	5.71	5.56	5.41	5.26	5.13	5.000	4.878	4.762	4.651	4.545	4.444	4.348	4.255	4.167	4.082
3	5.71	5.56	5.41	5.26	5.13	5.000	4.878	4.762	4.651	4.545	4.444	4.348	4.255	4.167	4.082
4	5.71	5.55	5.41	5.26	5.13	5.000	4.878	4.762	4.651	4.545	4.444	4.348	4.255	4.167	4.082
5	5.72	5.56	5.40	5.26	5.13	5.000	4.878	4.762	4.651	4.546	4.444	4.348	4.255	4.167	4.082
6	5.71	5.55	5.41	5.26	5.13	5.000	4.878	4.762	4.651	4.545	4.445	4.348	4.255	4.167	4.082
7	5.72	5.56	5.40	5.26	5.13	5.000	4.878	4.762	4.651	4.546	4.444	4.348	4.255	4.167	4.082
8	5.71	5.55	5.41	5.26	5.13	5.000	4.878	4.762	4.651	4.545	4.445	4.318	4.255	4.167	4.082
9	5.72	5.56	5.40	5.27	5.13	5.000	4.878	4.762	4.651	4.546	4.444	4.348	4.255	4.167	4.081
10	5.71	5.55	5.41	5.26	5.13	5.000	4.878	4.762	4.651	4.545	4.445	4.348	4.255	4.167	4.082
11	5.72	5.56	5.40	5.27	5.13	5.000	4.878	4.762	4.651	4.546	4.444	4.348	4.256	4.166	4.081
12	5.71	5.55	5.41	5.26	5.13	5.000	4.878	4.762	4.651	4.545	4.445	4.348	4.255	4.167	4.082
13	5.72	5.56	5.40	5.27	5.13	5.000	4.878	4.762	4.651	4.546	4.444	4.348	4.256	4.166	4.081
14	5.71	5.55	5.41	5.26	5.13	5.000	4.878	4.762	4.651	4.545	4.445	4.348	4.255	4.167	4.082
15	5.72	5.56	5.40	5.27	5.13	5.000	4.878	4.762	4.651	4.546	4.444	4.348	4.256	4.166	4.081
16	5.71	5.55	5.41	5.26	5.12	5.000	4.878	4.762	4.651	4.545	4.445	4.348	4.255	4.167	4.082
17	5.72	5.56	5.40	5.27	5.13	5.000	4.878	4.762	4.652	4.546	4.444	4.347	4.256	4.166	4.081
18	5.71	5.55	5.41	5.26	5.12	5.000	4.878	4.762	4.651	4.545	4.445	4.348	4.255	4.167	4.082
19		2.78	5.40	5.27	5.13	5.000	4.878	4.761	4.652	4.546	4.444	4.347	4.256	4.166	4.081
20				2.63	5.12	5.000	4.879	4.762	4.651	4.545	4.445	4.348	4.255	4.167	4.082
21						2.500	4.878	4.761	4.652	4.546	4.444	4.347	4.256	4.166	4.081
22								2.381	4.651	4.545	4.445	4.348	4.255	4.167	4.082
23										2.273	4.444	4.347	4.256	4.166	4.081
24												2.174	4.255	4.167	4.082
25														2.083	4.081

If the Recovery Year is:	and the Recovery Period is:														
	25.0	25.5	26.0	26.5	27.0	27.5	28.0	28.5	29.0	29.5	30.0	30.5	31.0	31.5	32.0
	the Depreciation Rate is:														
1	2.000	1.961	1.923	1.887	1.852	1.818	1.786	1.754	1.724	1.695	1.667	1.639	1.613	1.587	1.563
2	4.000	3.922	3.846	3.774	3.704	3.636	3.571	3.509	3.448	3.390	3.333	3.279	3.226	3.175	3.125
3	4.000	3.922	3.846	3.774	3.704	3.636	3.571	3.509	3.448	3.390	3.333	3.279	3.226	3.175	3.125
4	4.000	3.922	3.846	3.774	3.704	3.636	3.571	3.509	3.448	3.390	3.333	3.279	3.226	3.175	3.125
5	4.000	3.922	3.846	3.774	3.704	3.636	3.571	3.509	3.448	3.390	3.333	3.279	3.226	3.175	3.125
6	4.000	3.921	3.846	3.774	3.704	3.636	3.571	3.509	3.448	3.390	3.333	3.279	3.226	3.175	3.125
7	4.000	3.922	3.846	3.774	3.704	3.636	3.571	3.509	3.448	3.390	3.333	3.279	3.226	3.175	3.125
8	4.000	3.921	3.846	3.774	3.704	3.636	3.571	3.509	3.448	3.390	3.333	3.279	3.226	3.175	3.125
9	4.000	3.922	3.846	3.773	3.704	3.637	3.572	3.509	3.448	3.390	3.333	3.279	3.226	3.175	3.125
10	4.000	3.921	3.846	3.774	3.704	3.636	3.571	3.509	3.448	3.390	3.333	3.279	3.226	3.174	3.125
11	4.000	3.922	3.846	3.773	3.704	3.637	3.572	3.509	3.448	3.390	3.333	3.279	3.226	3.175	3.125
12	4.000	3.921	3.846	3.774	3.704	3.636	3.571	3.509	3.448	3.390	3.333	3.279	3.226	3.174	3.125
13	4.000	3.922	3.846	3.773	3.703	3.637	3.572	3.509	3.448	3.390	3.334	3.279	3.226	3.175	3.125
14	4.000	3.921	3.846	3.773	3.704	3.636	3.571	3.509	3.448	3.390	3.333	3.279	3.226	3.174	3.125
15	4.000	3.922	3.846	3.774	3.703	3.637	3.572	3.509	3.449	3.390	3.334	3.278	3.226	3.175	3.125
16	4.000	3.921	3.846	3.773	3.704	3.636	3.571	3.509	3.448	3.390	3.333	3.279	3.226	3.174	3.125
17	4.000	3.922	3.846	3.774	3.703	3.637	3.572	3.509	3.449	3.390	3.334	3.278	3.226	3.175	3.125
18	4.000	3.921	3.846	3.773	3.704	3.636	3.571	3.508	3.448	3.390	3.333	3.279	3.226	3.174	3.125
19	4.000	3.922	3.846	3.774	3.703	3.637	3.572	3.509	3.449	3.390	3.334	3.279	3.226	3.175	3.125
20	4.000	3.921	3.847	3.773	3.704	3.636	3.571	3.508	3.448	3.390	3.333	3.279	3.226	3.174	3.125
21	4.000	3.922	3.846	3.774	3.703	3.637	3.572	3.509	3.449	3.389	3.334	3.278	3.225	3.175	3.125
22	4.000	3.921	3.847	3.773	3.704	3.636	3.571	3.508	3.448	3.390	3.333	3.279	3.226	3.174	3.125
23	4.000	3.922	3.846	3.774	3.703	3.637	3.572	3.509	3.449	3.389	3.334	3.278	3.225	3.175	3.125
24	4.000	3.921	3.847	3.773	3.704	3.636	3.571	3.508	3.448	3.390	3.333	3.279	3.226	3.174	3.125
25	4.000	3.922	3.846	3.774	3.703	3.637	3.572	3.509	3.449	3.389	3.334	3.278	3.225	3.175	3.125
26	2.000	3.921	3.847	3.773	3.704	3.636	3.571	3.508	3.448	3.390	3.333	3.279	3.226	3.174	3.125
27			1.923	3.774	3.703	3.637	3.572	3.509	3.449	3.389	3.334	3.278	3.225	3.175	3.125
28					1.852	3.636	3.571	3.508	3.448	3.390	3.333	3.279	3.226	3.174	3.125
29							1.786	3.509	3.449	3.389	3.334	3.278	3.225	3.175	3.125
30									1.724	3.390	3.333	3.279	3.226	3.174	3.125
31											1.667	3.278	3.225	3.175	3.125
32													1.613	3.174	3.125
33															1.562

If the Recovery Year is:	and the Recovery Period is:														
	32.5	33.0	33.5	34.0	34.5	35.0	35.5	36.0	36.5	37.0	37.5	38.0	38.5	39.0	39.5
	the Depreciation Rate is:														
1	1.538	1.515	1.493	1.471	1.449	1.429	1.408	1.389	1.370	1.351	1.333	1.316	1.299	1.282	1.266
2	3.077	3.030	2.985	2.941	2.899	2.857	2.817	2.778	2.740	2.703	2.667	2.632	2.597	2.564	2.532
3	3.077	3.030	2.985	2.941	2.899	2.857	2.817	2.778	2.740	2.703	2.667	2.632	2.597	2.564	2.532
4	3.077	3.030	2.985	2.941	2.899	2.857	2.817	2.778	2.740	2.703	2.667	2.632	2.597	2.564	2.532
5	3.077	3.030	2.985	2.941	2.899	2.857	2.817	2.778	2.740	2.703	2.667	2.632	2.597	2.564	2.532
6	3.077	3.030	2.985	2.941	2.899	2.857	2.817	2.778	2.740	2.703	2.667	2.632	2.597	2.564	2.532
7	3.077	3.030	2.985	2.941	2.898	2.857	2.817	2.778	2.740	2.703	2.667	2.632	2.597	2.564	2.532
8	3.077	3.030	2.985	2.941	2.899	2.857	2.817	2.778	2.740	2.703	2.667	2.631	2.597	2.564	2.532
9	3.077	3.030	2.985	2.941	2.898	2.857	2.817	2.778	2.740	2.703	2.667	2.632	2.597	2.564	2.532
10	3.077	3.030	2.985	2.941	2.899	2.857	2.817	2.778	2.740	2.703	2.667	2.631	2.598	2.564	2.532
11	3.077	3.030	2.985	2.941	2.898	2.857	2.817	2.778	2.740	2.703	2.667	2.632	2.597	2.564	2.532
12	3.077	3.030	2.985	2.941	2.899	2.857	2.817	2.778	2.740	2.703	2.667	2.631	2.598	2.564	2.532
13	3.077	3.030	2.985	2.941	2.898	2.857	2.817	2.778	2.740	2.703	2.667	2.632	2.597	2.564	2.532
14	3.077	3.030	2.985	2.941	2.899	2.857	2.817	2.778	2.740	2.703	2.667	2.631	2.598	2.564	2.531
15	3.077	3.031	2.985	2.941	2.898	2.857	2.817	2.778	2.740	2.703	2.666	2.632	2.597	2.564	2.532
16	3.077	3.030	2.985	2.941	2.899	2.857	2.817	2.778	2.740	2.703	2.667	2.631	2.598	2.564	2.531
17	3.077	3.031	2.985	2.941	2.898	2.857	2.817	2.778	2.740	2.703	2.666	2.632	2.597	2.564	2.532
18	3.077	3.030	2.985	2.841	2.899	2.857	2.817	2.778	2.740	2.702	2.667	2.631	2.598	2.564	2.531
19	3.077	3.031	2.985	2.941	2.898	2.857	2.817	2.778	2.739	2.703	2.666	2.632	2.597	2.564	2.532
20	3.077	3.030	2.985	2.941	2.898	2.857	2.817	2.778	2.740	2.702	2.667	2.631	2.598	2.564	2.531
21	3.077	3.031	2.985	2.941	2.899	2.857	2.817	2.778	2.739	2.703	2.666	2.632	2.597	2.564	2.532
22	3.077	3.030	2.985	2.941	2.898	2.857	2.817	2.777	2.740	2.702	2.667	2.631	2.598	2.564	2.531
23	3.077	3.031	2.985	2.941	2.899	2.857	2.817	2.778	2.739	2.703	2.666	2.632	2.597	2.564	2.532
24	3.077	3.030	2.985	2.941	2.898	2.857	2.817	2.777	2.740	2.702	2.667	2.631	2.598	2.564	2.531
25	3.077	3.031	2.985	2.942	2.899	2.857	2.817	2.778	2.739	2.703	2.666	2.632	2.597	2.564	2.532
26	3.077	3.030	2.985	2.941	2.898	2.857	2.817	2.777	2.740	2.702	2.667	2.631	2.598	2.564	2.531
27	3.077	3.031	2.985	2.942	2.899	2.857	2.817	2.778	2.739	2.703	2.666	2.632	2.597	2.564	2.532
28	3.077	3.030	2.985	2.941	2.898	2.858	2.817	2.777	2.740	2.702	2.667	2.631	2.598	2.564	2.531
29	3.077	3.031	2.985	2.942	2.899	2.857	2.817	2.778	2.739	2.703	2.666	2.632	2.597	2.564	2.532
30	3.077	3.030	2.985	2.941	2.898	2.858	2.817	2.777	2.740	2.702	2.667	2.631	2.598	2.564	2.531
31	3.076	3.031	2.986	2.942	2.899	2.857	2.817	2.778	2.739	2.703	2.666	2.632	2.597	2.564	2.532
32	3.077	3.030	2.985	2.941	2.898	2.858	2.816	2.777	2.740	2.702	2.667	2.631	2.598	2.564	2.531
33	3.076	3.031	2.986	2.942	2.899	2.857	2.817	2.778	2.739	2.703	2.666	2.632	2.597	2.565	2.532
34		1.515	2.985	2.941	2.898	2.858	2.816	2.777	2.740	2.702	2.667	2.631	2.598	2.564	2.531
35				1.471	2.899	2.857	2.817	2.778	2.739	2.703	2.666	2.632	2.597	2.565	2.532
36						1.429	2.816	2.777	2.740	2.702	2.667	2.631	2.598	2.564	2.531
37								1.389	2.739	2.703	2.666	2.632	2.597	2.565	2.532
38										1.351	2.667	2.631	2.598	2.564	2.531
39												1.316	2.597	2.565	2.532
40														1.282	2.531

12 DEPRECIATION

If the Recovery Year is: — and the Recovery Period is: — the Depreciation Rate is:

Year	40.0	40.5	41.0	41.5	42.0	42.5	43.0	43.5	44.0	44.5	45.0	45.5	46.0	46.5	47.0
1	1.250	1.235	1.220	1.205	1.190	1.176	1.163	1.149	1.136	1.124	1.111	1.099	1.087	1.075	1.064
2	2.500	2.469	2.439	2.410	2.381	2.353	2.326	2.299	2.273	2.247	2.222	2.198	2.174	2.151	2.128
3	2.500	2.469	2.439	2.410	2.381	2.353	2.326	2.299	2.273	2.247	2.222	2.198	2.174	2.151	2.128
4	2.500	2.469	2.439	2.410	2.381	2.353	2.326	2.299	2.273	2.247	2.222	2.198	2.174	2.151	2.128
5	2.500	2.469	2.439	2.410	2.381	2.353	2.326	2.299	2.273	2.247	2.222	2.198	2.174	2.151	2.128
6	2.500	2.469	2.439	2.410	2.381	2.353	2.326	2.299	2.273	2.247	2.222	2.198	2.174	2.151	2.128
7	2.500	2.469	2.439	2.410	2.381	2.353	2.326	2.299	2.273	2.247	2.222	2.198	2.174	2.150	2.128
8	2.500	2.469	2.439	2.410	2.381	2.353	2.326	2.299	2.273	2.247	2.222	2.198	2.174	2.150	2.128
9	2.500	2.469	2.439	2.410	2.381	2.353	2.325	2.299	2.273	2.247	2.222	2.198	2.174	2.151	2.128
10	2.500	2.469	2.439	2.410	2.381	2.353	2.326	2.299	2.273	2.247	2.222	2.198	2.174	2.151	2.128
11	2.500	2.469	2.439	2.410	2.381	2.353	2.325	2.299	2.273	2.247	2.222	2.198	2.174	2.150	2.128
12	2.500	2.469	2.439	2.410	2.381	2.353	2.326	2.299	2.273	2.247	2.222	2.198	2.174	2.151	2.128
13	2.500	2.469	2.439	2.410	2.381	2.353	2.325	2.299	2.273	2.247	2.222	2.198	2.174	2.150	2.128
14	2.500	2.469	2.439	2.409	2.381	2.353	2.326	2.299	2.273	2.247	2.222	2.198	2.174	2.151	2.128
15	2.500	2.469	2.439	2.410	2.381	2.353	2.325	2.299	2.273	2.247	2.222	2.198	2.174	2.151	2.128
16	2.500	2.469	2.439	2.409	2.381	2.353	2.326	2.299	2.273	2.247	2.222	2.198	2.174	2.151	2.128
17	2.500	2.469	2.439	2.410	2.381	2.353	2.325	2.299	2.273	2.247	2.222	2.198	2.174	2.150	2.127
18	2.500	2.469	2.439	2.409	2.381	2.353	2.326	2.299	2.273	2.247	2.222	2.198	2.174	2.151	2.128
19	2.500	2.469	2.439	2.410	2.381	2.353	2.325	2.299	2.273	2.247	2.222	2.198	2.174	2.150	2.127
20	2.500	2.469	2.439	2.409	2.381	2.353	2.326	2.299	2.273	2.247	2.222	2.198	2.174	2.151	2.128
21	2.500	2.469	2.439	2.410	2.381	2.353	2.325	2.299	2.273	2.247	2.222	2.198	2.174	2.150	2.127
22	2.500	2.469	2.439	2.409	2.381	2.353	2.326	2.299	2.273	2.247	2.222	2.198	2.174	2.150	2.128
23	2.500	2.469	2.439	2.410	2.381	2.353	2.325	2.299	2.272	2.247	2.222	2.198	2.174	2.151	2.128
24	2.500	2.469	2.439	2.409	2.381	2.353	2.326	2.299	2.273	2.247	2.222	2.198	2.174	2.150	2.127
25	2.500	2.469	2.439	2.410	2.381	2.353	2.325	2.299	2.272	2.247	2.222	2.198	2.174	2.151	2.128
26	2.500	2.469	2.439	2.409	2.381	2.353	2.326	2.299	2.273	2.247	2.222	2.198	2.174	2.151	2.128
27	2.500	2.469	2.439	2.410	2.381	2.353	2.325	2.299	2.272	2.247	2.223	2.198	2.174	2.151	2.127
28	2.500	2.469	2.439	2.409	2.381	2.353	2.326	2.299	2.272	2.247	2.222	2.198	2.174	2.151	2.128
29	2.500	2.469	2.439	2.410	2.381	2.353	2.325	2.299	2.272	2.247	2.223	2.198	2.174	2.150	2.127
30	2.500	2.469	2.439	2.409	2.381	2.353	2.326	2.299	2.273	2.248	2.222	2.197	2.174	2.151	2.128
31	2.500	2.469	2.439	2.410	2.381	2.353	2.325	2.299	2.272	2.247	2.223	2.198	2.174	2.150	2.127
32	2.500	2.470	2.439	2.409	2.381	2.353	2.326	2.299	2.272	2.248	2.222	2.197	2.174	2.151	2.128
33	2.500	2.469	2.439	2.410	2.381	2.353	2.325	2.298	2.272	2.247	2.223	2.198	2.174	2.151	2.128
34	2.500	2.470	2.439	2.409	2.381	2.353	2.326	2.299	2.273	2.248	2.222	2.197	2.174	2.150	2.127
35	2.500	2.469	2.439	2.410	2.381	2.353	2.325	2.298	2.272	2.247	2.223	2.198	2.174	2.151	2.128
36	2.500	2.470	2.139	2.409	2.381	2.353	2.326	2.299	2.273	2.247	2.222	2.198	2.174	2.150	2.127
37	2.500	2.469	2.439	2.410	2.381	2.353	2.325	2.298	2.272	2.247	2.223	2.198	2.174	2.150	2.127
38	2.500	2.470	2.439	2.409	2.381	2.353	2.326	2.299	2.273	2.248	2.222	2.197	2.174	2.151	2.128
39	2.500	2.469	2.439	2.410	2.381	2.353	2.325	2.298	2.272	2.247	2.223	2.198	2.174	2.150	2.127
40	2.500	2.470	2.439	2.409	2.381	2.353	2.326	2.299	2.273	2.248	2.222	2.197	2.173	2.151	2.128
41	1.250	2.469	2.439	2.410	2.380	2.352	2.325	2.298	2.272	2.247	2.223	2.198	2.174	2.150	2.127
42			1.220	2.409	2.381	2.353	2.326	2.299	2.273	2.248	2.222	2.197	2.173	2.151	2.128
43					1.190	2.352	2.325	2.298	2.272	2.247	2.223	2.198	2.174	2.150	2.127
44							1.163	2.299	2.273	2.248	2.222	2.197	2.173	2.151	2.128
45									1.136	2.247	2.223	2.198	2.174	2.150	2.127
46											1.111	2.197	2.173	2.151	2.128
47													1.087	2.150	2.127
48															1.064

If the Recovery Year is:		47.5	48.0	and the Recovery Period is: 48.5	49.0	49.5	50.0
				the Depreciation Rate is:			
1	. . . . . .	1.053	1.042	1.031	1.020	1.010	1.000
2	. . . . . .	2.105	2.083	2.062	2.041	2.020	2.000
3	. . . . . .	2.105	2.083*	2.062	2.041	2.020	2.000
4	. . . . . .	2.105	2.083	2.062	2.041	2.020	2.000
5	. . . . . .	2.105	2.083	2.062	2.041	2.020	2.000
6	. . . . . .	2.105	2.083	2.062	2.041	2.020	2.000
7	. . . . . .	2.105	2.083	2.062	2.041	2.020	2.000
8	. . . . . .	2.105	2.083	2.062	2.041	2.020	2.000
9	. . . . . .	2.105	2.083	2.062	2.041	2.020	2.000
10	. . . . . .	2.105	2.083	2.062	2.041	2.020	2.000
11	. . . . . .	2.105	2.083	2.062	2.041	2.020	2.000
12	. . . . . .	2.105	2.083	2.062	2.041	2.020	2.000
13	. . . . . .	2.105	2.083	2.062	2.041	2.020	2.000
14	. . . . . .	2.105	2.083	2.062	2.041	2.020	2.000
15	. . . . . .	2.105	2.083	2.062	2.041	2.020	2.000
16	. . . . . .	2.105	2.083	2.062	2.041	2.020	2.000
17	. . . . . .	2.105	2.083	2.062	2.041	2.020	2.000
18	. . . . . .	2.105	2.083	2.062	2.041	2.020	2.000
19	. . . . . .	2.105	2.084	2.062	2.041	2.020	2.000
20	. . . . . .	2.105	2.083	2.062	2.041	2.020	2.000
21	. . . . . .	2.105	2.084	2.062	2.041	2.020	2.000
22	. . . . . .	2.105	2.083	2.062	2.041	2.020	2.000
23	. . . . . .	2.105	2.084	2.062	2.041	2.020	2.000
24	. . . . . .	2.105	2.083	2.062	2.041	2.020	2.000
25	. . . . . .	2.105	2.084	2.062	2.041	2.020	2.000
26	. . . . . .	2.106	2.083	2.062	2.041	2.020	2.000
27	. . . . . .	2.105	2.084	2.062	2.041	2.020	2.000
28	. . . . . .	2.106	2.083	2.062	2.041	2.020	2.000
29	. . . . . .	2.105	2.084	2.062	2.041	2.020	2.000
30	. . . . . .	2.106	2.083	2.062	2.041	2.020	2.000
31	. . . . . .	2.105	2.084	2.062	2.041	2.021	2.000
32	. . . . . .	2.106	2.083	2.062	2.041	2.020	2.000
33	. . . . . .	2.105	2.084	2.062	2.041	2.021	2.000
34	. . . . . .	2.106	2.083	2.062	2.040	2.020	2.000
35	. . . . . .	2.105	2.084	2.062	2.041	2.021	2.000
36	. . . . . .	2.106	2.083	2.062	2.040	2.020	2.000
37	. . . . . .	2.105	2.084	2.061	2.041	2.021	2.000
38	. . . . . .	2.106	2.083	2.062	2.040	2.020	2.000
39	. . . . . .	2.105	2.084	2.061	2.041	2.021	2.000
40	. . . . . .	2.106	2.083	2.062	2.040	2.020	2.000
41	. . . . . .	2.105	2.084	2.061	2.041	2.021	2.000
42	. . . . . .	2.106	2.083	2.062	2.040	2.020	2.000
43	. . . . . .	2.105	2.084	2.061	2.041	2.021	2.000
44	. . . . . .	2.106	2.083	2.062	2.040	2.020	2.000
45	. . . . . .	2.105	2.084	2.061	2.041	2.021	2.000
46	. . . . . .	2.106	2.083	2.062	2.040	2.020	2.000
47	. . . . . .	2.105	2.084	2.061	2.041	2.021	2.000
48	. . . . . .	2.106	2.083	2.062	2.040	2.020	2.000
49	. . . .		1.042	2.061	2.041	2.021	2.000
50	. . . .				1.020	2.020	2.000
51	. . . .						1.000

12 DEPRECIATION

1244. MACRS Short Tax Years. Special rules are provided for determining deductions under the Modified Accelerated Cost Recovery System (MACRS) when: (1) property is placed in service in a short tax year (any tax year with less than 12 months); (2) a short tax year occurs during the recovery period of property; or (3) a disposition of property occurs before the end of the recovery period (Rev. Proc. 89-15). If any of the above situations exist, refinements are made to the use of the applicable conventions and the MACRS depreciation tables at ¶ 1243 may *not* be used.[87]

The mid-month convention is applied without regard to the length of the tax year. For example if residential rental property is placed in service in the first month of a six-month tax year, 5 ½ months depreciation is claimed.

Under the half-year convention, property placed in service or disposed of in a short tax year is deemed placed in service or disposed on the midpoint of the short tax year, which always falls on either the first day or the midpoint of the month.

Under the mid-quarter convention, property is deemed placed in service or disposed on the midpoint of the quarter, which always falls on either the first day or the midpoint of a month, in the short tax year that it is placed in service or disposed.

Depreciation for the first recovery year in the recovery period is computed by multiplying the basis in the property by the applicable depreciation rate. The depreciation allowance allocable to the first tax year that includes a portion of the first recovery year is derived by multiplying the depreciation for the first recovery year by a fraction. The numerator is the number of months (including fractions of months) the property is deemed to be in service during the tax year under the applicable convention and the denominator is 12.

The correlation of a depreciation allowance between recovery years and tax years after the first tax year in the recovery period may be made under either an allocation or a simplified method.

1245. Applicable MACRS Conventions. Specified averaging conventions apply to depreciation computations made under the Modified Accelerated Cost Recovery System (MACRS) (Code Sec. 168(d)).[88] The recovery period begins on the date on which the property is placed in service under the applicable convention. The depreciation table percentages take into account the applicable convention in the first and last year of the regular recovery period. However, if property is disposed of prior to the end of the regular recovery period, the result obtained by using the table percentage for the year of disposition must be adjusted to take into account the applicable convention.

Half-Year Convention. Under the half-year convention, which can apply to any property other than residential rental and nonresidential real property, an asset is treated as placed in service or disposed of in the middle of the tax year. Thus, one-half of a full year's depreciation is allowed in the tax year in which the asset is placed in service regardless of the date that the asset is placed in service during the tax year.

A half-year of depreciation is allowed in the tax year of disposition if there is a disposition of property before the end of the recovery period.[89] The table percentage for the year of disposition does not take this into account; therefore, only one-half of the depreciation as computed using the applicable table percentage is allowed.

> **Example 1:** Five-year property with a depreciable basis of $1,000 and subject to the half-year convention is placed in service in 2012 and sold in 2014. Using Table 1 at ¶ 1243, 2012 depreciation is $200 ($1,000 × 20%); 2013 depreciation is $320 ($1,000 × 32%); and 2014 depreciation is $96 ($1,000 × 19.20% × 50% to reflect half-year convention in year of disposition).

Mid-Month Convention. A mid-month convention applies to residential rental property, including low-income housing, and nonresidential real property. Property is deemed placed in service or disposed of during the middle of the month. The deduction

---

References are to Standard Federal Tax Reports; Tax Research Consultant; and Practical Tax Explanations.

[87] ¶ 11,279.053; DEPR: 3,202; DEPR: 3,350, DEPR: 3,252; § 11,130

[88] ¶ 11,250; DEPR: 3,252; § 11,125

[89] ¶ 11,279.037; DEPR: 3,252; § 11,125

is based on the number of months the property was in service. Thus, one-half month's depreciation is allowed for the month the property is placed in service and for the month of disposition if there is a disposition of property before the end of the recovery period.

> **Example 2:** A commercial building costing $100,000 is purchased by a calendar-year taxpayer in February 2013 and sold in August 2014. Using Table 7A at ¶ 1243, 2013 depreciation is $2,247 ($100,000 × 2.247% (first-year percentage for property placed in service in second month of tax year)) and 2014 depreciation is $1,603 ($100,000 × 2.564% (second-year percentage for property placed in service in second month) × 7.5/12 to reflect 7.5 months in service in 2014 (January through mid-August) under the mid-month convention).

Mid-Quarter Convention. Under the mid-quarter convention, all property placed in service or disposed of during any quarter of a tax year is treated as placed in service at the midpoint of the quarter (Code Sec. 168(d)(3); Reg. § 1.168(d)-1).[90] Depreciation under the mid-quarter convention may be determined using Tables 2-5.

The mid-quarter convention applies to all property, other than nonresidential real property and residential rental property, if more than 40 percent of the aggregate bases of such property is placed in service during the last three months of the tax year. Property placed in service and disposed of within the same tax year is disregarded for purposes of the 40-percent test.

In determining whether the mid-quarter convention is applicable, the aggregate basis of property placed in service in the last three months of the tax year must be computed regardless of the length of the tax year. Thus, if a short tax year consists of three months or less, the mid-quarter convention applies regardless of when the depreciable property is placed in service during the tax year.

The bonus depreciation deduction (¶ 1237) does not reduce the aggregate basis of property taken into account for purposes of determining whether the mid-quarter convention applies. However, any amount properly expensed under Code Sec. 179 (¶ 1208) does reduce aggregate basis. Thus, a taxpayer may be able to avoid the mid-quarter convention (if desired) by allocating the Code Sec. 179 deduction to property placed in service in the last quarter. No similar reduction is made for the amount of bonus depreciation. Also, the mid-quarter convention does not operate to reduce the deduction otherwise allowable under Code Sec. 179 or for bonus depreciation.

> **Example 3:** A calendar-year taxpayer places $100 of used five-year property in service in the first quarter of 2013 and $100 of new 10-year property in service in the fourth quarter. The taxpayer claims a 50% bonus depreciation allowance on the 10-year property. The mid-quarter convention applies to the five-year property and to the 10-year property because 50% of the aggregate adjusted basis of the property placed in service in 2013 (without regard to the bonus depreciation allowance) was placed in service in the fourth quarter. If the bonus depreciation allowance was not claimed on the 10-year property and the entire basis of the 10-year property was expensed under section 179, the half-year convention would apply to the five-year property placed in service in the first quarter.

For purposes of the 40-percent test, depreciable basis does not include adjustments resulting from transfers of property between members of the same affiliated group filing a consolidated return.

If the MACRS deduction for property subject to the mid-quarter convention is computed without tables, depreciation for the first year is determined by computing the depreciation for the full tax year and then multiplying it by the following percentages for the quarter of the tax year the property is placed in service: first quarter, 87.5%; second quarter, 62.5%; third quarter, 37.5%; and fourth quarter, 12.5%. In the year of disposition (whether or not the table percentages are used) the deduction for a full year is multiplied by the following percentages for the quarter in which the asset is disposed of: first quarter, 12.5%; second quarter, 37.5%; third quarter, 62.5%, and fourth quarter 87.5%.

References are to Standard Federal Tax Reports; Tax Research Consultant; and Practical Tax Explanations.

[90] ¶ 11,260; DEPR: 3,252.15;
§ 11,125

1247. MACRS Alternative Depreciation System (ADS). The Modified Accelerated Cost Recovery System (MACRS) alternative depreciation system (ADS) must be used for (1) tangible property used outside the United States, (2) tax-exempt use property, (3) tax-exempt bond-financed property, (4) property imported from a foreign country for which an Executive Order is in effect because the country maintains trade restrictions or engages in other discriminatory acts, and (5) property for which an ADS election has been made (Code Sec. 168(g)).[91] Mandatory ADS property does not qualify for bonus depreciation (¶ 1237).

Under ADS, the deduction is computed by applying the straight-line method, the applicable convention and the applicable longer recovery period (12 years for personal property with no class life, 40 years for real property, 50 years for railroad grading and tunnel bores, and the class life for all other property) for the respective class of property (Code Sec. 168(g)(2)(C)).[92] ADS is also used to compute the earnings and profits of a foreign or domestic corporation. The allowable depreciation deductions for luxury cars and other types of listed property used 50 percent or less in business are also determined under this method (¶ 1211 and ¶ 1214).

Electing ADS. In lieu of the regular MACRS deduction, taxpayers may irrevocably elect to apply the MACRS alternative depreciation system to any class of property for any tax year (Code Sec. 168(g)(7)).[93] If elected, ADS applies to all property in the MACRS class placed in service during the tax year. For example, if the election is made for five-year property, it applies to all five-year property placed in service in the tax year of the election. For residential rental property and nonresidential real property, the election is made on a property-by-property basis. Property for which ADS is elected may qualify for bonus depreciation (¶ 1237).

1248. Special Transferee Rules for Depreciation. A transferee in certain corporate and partnership transactions is treated as the transferor and must use the latter's recovery period and method in computing the deduction under the Modified Accelerated Cost Recovery System (MACRS) for the portion of the transferee's basis that does not exceed the transferor's adjusted basis in the property (Code Sec. 168(i)(7)).[94] This rule applies to nonrecognition transfers under Code Sec. 332 (subsidiary liquidations) (¶ 2261); transfers to a controlled corporation (¶ 1731); transfers related to certain reorganizations (¶ 2209); contributions to a partnership (¶ 443); certain partnership distributions (¶ 453); and transactions between members of the same affiliated group during any tax year for which a consolidated return is made by such group. It does not apply to transactions relating to the sale or exchange of 50 percent or more of the total interest in a partnership's capital and profits within a 12-month period (Code Sec. 708(b)(1)(B)).

1249. Recapture Upon Disposition of Depreciable Property. See ¶ 1779.

1250. Depreciable Property in Like-Kind Exchanges and Involuntary Conversions. The exchanged basis (i.e., carryover basis) of property under the Modified Accelerated Cost Recovery System (MACRS) acquired in a like-kind exchange or involuntary conversion for other MACRS property is depreciated by applying the following rules (Reg. § 1.168(i)-6).[95]

(1) If the replacement MACRS property has the same or a shorter recovery period and the same or a more accelerated depreciation method than the relinquished MACRS property, the exchanged (carryover) basis is depreciated over the remaining recovery period of, and using the depreciation method and convention of, the relinquished MACRS property.

(2) If the recovery period of the replacement MACRS property is longer than that of the relinquished MACRS property, the exchanged basis is depreciated over

---

References are to Standard Federal Tax Reports; Tax Research Consultant; and Practical Tax Explanations.

[91] ¶ 11,250; DEPR: 3,456; § 11,135

[92] ¶ 11,250; DEPR: 3,450, DEPR: 3,458; § 11,135

[93] ¶ 11,250; DEPR: 3,460; § 11,135

[94] ¶ 11,250; DEPR: 3,306.05; § 11,150

[95] ¶ 11,276K; DEPR: 3,306.30; § 18,055

the remainder of the recovery period that would have applied to the replacement MACRS property if the replacement MACRS property had originally been placed in service when the relinquished MACRS property was placed in service by the acquiring taxpayer.

(3) If the depreciation method of the replacement MACRS property is less accelerated than that of the relinquished MACRS property, the exchanged basis is depreciated beginning in the year of replacement using the less accelerated depreciation method of the replacement MACRS property that would have applied to the replacement MACRS property if the replacement MACRS property had originally been placed in service when the relinquished MACRS property was placed in service by the acquiring taxpayer.

The excess basis of the replacement property (i.e., the noncarryover basis usually attributable to additional cash paid for the replacement property) is separately depreciated as if originally acquired in the year of replacement.

These rules are effective for like-kind exchanges and involuntary conversions in which the time of disposition and replacement both occur after February 27, 2004. A taxpayer, however, may apply the regulations retroactively (Reg. § 1.168(i)-6(k)). A taxpayer may also elect not to apply the regulations to a post-effective date exchange or conversion and depreciate the entire basis of the acquired property as a single depreciable asset beginning in the tax year of replacement (Reg. § 1.168(i)-6(i) and (j)).

Bonus depreciation may be claimed on the entire basis of qualifying acquired property (¶ 1237) (Reg. § 1.168(k)-1(f)(5)). However, only the excess basis (noncarryover basis) may qualify for expensing under Code Sec. 179 even if an election not to apply the regulations is made (Reg. § 1.168(i)-6(g) and (i)).

Accelerated Cost Recovery System (ACRS)

1252. Pre-1987 ACRS in General. The Accelerated Cost Recovery System (ACRS) must be used to compute the depreciation deduction for most tangible depreciable property placed in service after 1980 and before 1987 (Code Sec. 168, prior to 1987).[96] Cost recovery methods and periods are the same for both new and used property, and salvage value is disregarded in computing ACRS allowances. Post-1980 depreciation on tangible assets first placed in service before 1981 is computed using the method elected by the taxpayer when the property was placed in service (including the Class Life ADR depreciation system (¶ 1284) and other methods of depreciation discussed at ¶ 1216).

Under ACRS, the cost of eligible property is recovered over a 3-year, 5-year, 10-year, 15-year, 18-year, or 19-year period, depending on the type of property. ACRS applies to recovery property, as defined at ¶ 1255. The deduction is determined by applying the statutory table percentage for the appropriate class of property to its unadjusted basis. The unadjusted basis of property under ACRS is the basis of the property as determined for purposes of computing gain or loss), unadjusted for depreciation, amortization or depletion. It does not include that portion of the basis for which there is an election to amortize (¶ 1287) or to expense the cost of Code Sec. 179 property (¶ 1208) (Code Sec. 168(d)(1), prior to 1987).[97]

For personal ACRS recovery property placed in service after 1980 and before 1987, one-half year's depreciation is allowed, regardless of how long it is held in the year that it is placed in service. No deduction is allowed in the year of disposition of personal recovery property. Special prorations by month (using a mid-month convention) are provided for real recovery property (¶ 1261).

Straight-Line Election. An election to recover costs by using a straight-line method over the regular recovery period or a longer recovery period was also available under ACRS and was made on the taxpayer's return for the year in which the property was placed in service (Code Sec. 168(f)(4), prior to 1987).[98]

References are to Standard Federal Tax Reports; Tax Research Consultant; and Practical Tax Explanations.

[96] ¶ 11,258.01; DEPR: 3,054; § 11,001   [97] ¶ 11,258.041; DEPR: 3,104; § 11,001   [98] ¶ 11,258.031; DEPR: 3,404.15; § 11,001

12

DEPRECIATION

1255. ACRS Recovery Property. For purposes of the Accelerated Cost Recovery System (ACRS), recovery property is tangible depreciable property that is placed in service after 1980 and before 1987. It does not include property for which an election is made to compute depreciation on a method not based on a depreciation period (unit-of-production method, income forecast method, etc.), public utility property for which the normalization method of accounting is not used, intangible assets such as patents and copyrights (¶ 1201), property for which an election to amortize was made, or motion picture films and videotapes (Code Sec. 168(c) and (e), prior to 1987).[99] For purposes of determining the class of recovery property into which an asset falls, recovery property is defined as either Code Sec. 1245 class property or Code Sec. 1250 class property.

Code Sec. 1245 class property includes tangible section 1245 property, as defined at ¶ 1785, other than elevators and escalators, and certain rapidly amortized realty. Code Sec. 1250 class property includes tangible section 1250 property, as defined at ¶ 1786, and elevators and escalators.

1258. ACRS Personal Property. Under the Accelerated Cost Recovery System (ACRS), the statutory percentage for personal property placed in service after 1980 and before 1987 is determined using prescribed percentage tables based on the type of property (3-year, 5-year, 10-year or 15-year). These table percentages are not reproduced because such property should generally be fully depreciated at this time. The tables, however, are contained in ACRS (Prop. Reg. § 1.168-2). No recovery deduction is generally allowed in the year of disposition of ACRS personal property.

1261. ACRS Real Property. Under the Accelerated Cost Recovery System (ACRS), the unadjusted basis of real property is recovered over a period of 19 years for real property placed in service after May 8, 1985, and before 1987. For real property placed in service after March 15, 1984, and before May 9, 1985, unadjusted basis is recovered over a period of 18 years. A 15-year recovery period applies to real property placed in service after 1980 and before March 16, 1984, and to low-income housing.[100]

In computing the ACRS deduction, a full-month convention is used for real recovery property placed in service before March 16, 1984, and for low-income housing, and a mid-month convention is used for real recovery property (other than low-income housing) placed in service after March 15, 1984. Under the full-month convention, real property placed in service at any time during a particular month is treated as placed in service on the first day of such month, thereby permitting a full month's cost recovery for the month the property is placed in service. For a disposition at any time during a particular month before the end of a recovery period, no cost recovery is permitted for such month of disposition. Under the mid-month convention, real property placed in service at any time during a particular month is treated as placed in service in the middle of such month, thereby permitting one-half month's cost recovery for the month the property is placed in service. For a disposition of real property during a month before the end of a recovery period, one-half month's cost recovery is allowed for the month of disposition.

In using the following tables, there are separate rate schedules depending upon the month in the first tax year that the property is placed in service. Further, where real property is sold before the end of the recovery period, the ACRS deduction for the year of disposition is to reflect only the months of the year during which the property was in service. For a short tax year, appropriate adjustments must also be made to the table amounts (¶ 1270). A complete set of ACRS depreciation tables is provided in IRS Publication 534.

References are to Standard Federal Tax Reports; Tax Research Consultant; and Practical Tax Explanations.

[99] ¶ 11,258.01, ¶ 11,258.045; DEPR: 3,058.20; § 11,001

[100] ¶ 11,258.025; DEPR: 3,158; § 11,001

Table I *18-Year Real Property*
(placed in service after June 22, 1984) for Which Alternate ACRS Method
Over a 35-Year Period Is Elected

Year	Month Placed in Service				
	1-2	3-6	7-10	11	12
1st	3%	2%	1%	0.4%	0.1%
2-30th	3%	3%	3%	3%	3%
31st	2%	2%	2%	2.6%	2.9%
32-35th	2%	2%	2%	2%	2%
36th		1%	2%	2%	2%

Table II *18-Year Real Property*
(placed in service after March 15 and before June 23, 1984)
15-Year Real Property and Low-Income Housing
(placed in service before May 9, 1985) for Which Alternate
ACRS Method Over a 35-Year Period Is Elected

Year	Month Placed in Service		
	1-2	3-6	7-12
1st	3%	2%	1%
2-30th	3%	3%	3%
31-35th	2%	2%	2%
36th		1%	2%

Table III *Low-Income Housing (placed in service after May 8, 1985)*
for Which Alternate ACRS Method Over a 35-Year Period Is Elected

Year	Month Placed in Service											
	1	2	3	4	5	6	7	8	9	10	11	12
1st	2.9%	2.6%	2.4%	2.1%	1.9%	1.7%	1.4%	1.2%	1.0%	0.7%	0.5%	0.2%
2-20th	2.9%	2.9%	2.9%	2.9%	2.9%	2.9%	2.9%	2.9%	2.9%	2.9%	2.9%	2.9%
21-35th	2.8%	2.8%	2.8%	2.8%	2.8%	2.8%	2.8%	2.8%	2.8%	2.8%	2.8%	2.8%
36th		0.3%	0.5%	0.8%	1.0%	1.2%	1.5%	1.7%	1.9%	2.2%	2.4%	2.7%

Table IV *19-Year Real Property*
for Which Alternate ACRS Method Over a 35-Year Period Is Elected

Year	Month Placed in Service											
	1	2	3	4	5	6	7	8	9	10	11	12
1st	2.7%	2.5%	2.3%	2.0%	1.8%	1.5%	1.3%	1.1%	0.8%	0.6%	0.4%	0.1%
2-20th	2.9%	2.9%	2.9%	2.9%	2.9%	2.9%	2.9%	2.9%	2.9%	2.9%	2.9%	2.9%
21-35th	2.8%	2.8%	2.8%	2.8%	2.8%	2.8%	2.8%	2.8%	2.8%	2.8%	2.8%	2.8%
36th	0.2%	0.4%	0.6%	0.9%	1.1%	1.4%	1.6%	1.8%	2.1%	2.3%	2.5%	2.8%

Table V *18-Year Real Property*
(placed in service after June 22, 1984) 19-Year Real Property for Which
Alternate ACRS Method Over a 45-Year Period Is Elected

Year	Month Placed in Service											
	1	2	3	4	5	6	7	8	9	10	11	12
1st	2.1%	1.9%	1.8%	1.6%	1.4%	1.2%	1%	0.8%	0.6%	0.5%	0.3%	0.1%
2-11th	2.3%	2.3%	2.3%	2.3%	2.3%	2.3%	2.3%	2.3%	2.3%	2.3%	2.3%	2.3%
12-45th	2.2%	2.2%	2.2%	2.2%	2.2%	2.2%	2.2%	2.2%	2.2%	2.2%	2.2%	2.2%
46th	0.1%	0.3%	0.4%	0.6%	0.8%	1%	1.2%	1.4%	1.6%	1.7%	1.9%	2.1%

12 DEPRECIATION

Table VI *18-Year Real Property*
(placed in service after March 15 and before June 23, 1984) 15-Year Real Property
and Low-Income Housing (placed in service after December 31, 1980) for Which
Alternate ACRS Method Over a 45-Year Period Is Elected

Year	Month Placed in Service											
	1	2	3	4	5	6	7	8	9	10	11	12
1st	2.3%	2%	1.9%	1.7%	1.5%	1.3%	1.2%	0.9%	0.7%	0.6%	0.4%	0.2%
2-10th	2.3%	2.3%	2.3%	2.3%	2.3%	2.3%	2.3%	2.3%	2.3%	2.3%	2.3%	2.3%
11-45th	2.2%	2.2%	2.2%	2.2%	2.2%	2.2%	2.2%	2.2%	2.2%	2.2%	2.2%	2.2%
46th		0.3%	0.4%	0.6%	0.8%	1%	1.1%	1.4%	1.6%	1.7%	1.9%	2.1%

1264. ACRS: Predominant Use Outside the United States. Under the Accelerated Cost Recovery System (ACRS), the unadjusted basis of personal property used outside the United States is recovered over a period equal to the ADR class life for that property as of January 1, 1981.[101] No recovery deduction is generally allowed in the year of disposition of personal recovery property used predominantly outside the United States. The unadjusted basis of real property and low income housing used predominantly outside the United States is to be recovered over a period of 35 years. For real recovery property (other than low-income housing) placed in service after March 15, 1984, a mid-month convention is used. There are separate rate schedules depending on the month in the first tax year that the property is placed in service.

1267. ACRS: Components of Sec. 1250 Class Property. Under the Accelerated Cost Recovery System (ACRS), structural components of section 1250 class property may not be depreciated separately. Composite depreciation is required on the entire building, unless the components qualify for amortization elections (Code Sec. 168(f)(1), prior to 1987).[102] Components that are considered personal property can be separately depreciated under the cost segregation rules. See ¶ 1240.

Substantial Improvements. If a taxpayer made a substantial improvement to a building, it was treated as a separate building rather than as one or more components. The taxpayer could use the regular ACRS deduction or elect the straight-line ACRS deduction for the improvement over the regular or a longer recovery period regardless of the ACRS method that is used for the rest of the building.

Components and improvements placed in service after 1986 are depreciated using the Modified Accelerated Cost Recovery System (MACRS) even if the building is not MACRS property (¶ 1240).

1270. ACRS: Short Tax Years. For a tax year of less than 12 months, the amount of the deduction under the Accelerated Cost Recovery System (ACRS) is the amount that bears the same relationship to the amount of the deduction as the number of months and partial months in the short year bears to 12 (Code Sec. 168(f)(5), prior to 1987).[103] For real property and low-income housing placed in service or disposed of in a short tax year, the above rule generally does not apply and the deduction is based on the number of months the property is in service during the year, regardless of the length of the tax year and regardless of the recovery period and method used.

Any unrecovered allowance (the difference between the recovery allowance properly allowable for the short tax year and the recovery allowance that would have been allowable if such year were not a short tax year) is claimed in the tax year following the last year in the recovery period (Prop. Reg. §1.168-2(f)(3)).[104] However, there is a maximum limitation on the amount of an unrecovered allowance that may be claimed as a recovery allowance in a tax year. The unrecovered allowance claimed as a recovery allowance in the tax year following the last year of the recovery period may not exceed the amount of the recovery allowance permitted for the last year of the recovery period, assuming that such year consists of 12 months. Any remainder is carried forward until exhausted.

References are to Standard Federal Tax Reports; Tax Research Consultant; and Practical Tax Explanations.

101 ¶ 162.01; DEPR: 6,106; §11,001

102 ¶ 11,258.05; DEPR: 3,206.45; §11,001

103 ¶ 11,258.055; DEPR: 3,354; §11,001

104 ¶ 11,252; DEPR: 3,354; §11,001

Class Life ADR System

1282. Post-1980 Depreciation Under ADR. If the Asset Depreciation Range (ADR) System was elected for tangible assets first placed in service after 1970 and before 1981, post-1980 depreciation on such assets must be computed under the ADR System.[105]

1284. ADR in General. Under the Asset Depreciation Range (ADR) System, all tangible assets were placed in specific classes. A class life or "asset guideline period" was given for each class of assets in Reg. § 1.167(a)-11.[106] In addition, each class of assets other than land improvements and buildings was given a range of years or "asset depreciation range" that was about 20 percent above and below the class life. For details on the ADR system, see ¶ 11,029.01 and following of the STANDARD FEDERAL TAX REPORTER, DEPR: 15,800 of the Tax Research Consultant and § 11,025.10 and § 11,025.15 of Practical Tax Explanations.

Deductions for Refiners

1285. Deduction for EPA Sulfur Regulation Compliance Costs of Small Refiners. Small business refiners may elect to immediately deduct as an expense up to 75 percent of the qualified capital costs paid or incurred during the tax year for the purpose of complying with the Highway Diesel Fuel Sulfur Control Requirements of the Environmental Protection Agency (EPA) (Code Sec. 179B). Costs paid or incurred with respect to any facility of a small business refiner during the period beginning on January 1, 2003, and ending on the earlier of the date that is one year after the date on which the taxpayer must comply with the applicable EPA regulations or December 31, 2009, qualify for the deduction. Election guidance is provided in Temp. Reg. § 1.179B-1T(d).

1285A. Expensing Election for New or Expanded Refineries. A taxpayer may elect to expense 50 percent of the cost of qualified refinery property placed in service after August 8, 2005, and before January 1, 2014 (Code Sec. 179C; Reg. § 1.179C-1).[107] The property must be placed in service before January 1, 2010, if its construction is not subject to a written binding contract entered into after June 14, 2005, and before January 1, 2010, or, in the case of self-constructed property, construction did not begin after June 14, 2005, and before January 1, 2010. The original use of the refinery property must commence with the taxpayer. An improvement to an existing refinery can qualify if the improvement increases production capacity by specified levels.

> **Comment:** Absent further legislation, the expensing election for qualified refinery property expires for property placed in service after December 31, 2013. For the latest legislative updates, visit our website www.CCHGroup.com/TaxUpdates.

Deduction for Energy Efficiency Improvements

1286. Deduction for Energy Efficiency Improvements to Depreciable Buildings. A taxpayer may deduct the cost of certain energy efficiency improvements installed on or in a depreciable building located in the United States, effective for improvements placed in service after December 31, 2005, and before January 1, 2014 (Code Sec. 179D; Notice 2006-52, as clarified by Notice 2008-40; Notice 2012-26, modifying Notice 2008-40).[108] The deduction applies to energy efficient commercial building property, which is depreciable property installed as part of a building's (1) interior lighting systems, (2) heating, cooling, ventilation, and hot water systems, or (3) envelope as part of a certified plan to reduce the total annual energy and power costs of these systems by at least 50 percent in comparison to a reference building that meets specified minimum standards. The deduction is limited to the lesser of the cost of the qualifying property reduced by the aggregate amount deducted in any prior tax year or the product of $1.80 and the total square footage of the building reduced by the aggregate amount deducted in any prior tax year.

References are to Standard Federal Tax Reports; Tax Research Consultant; and Practical Tax Explanations.

[105] ¶ 11,029.01; DEPR: 15,800; § 11,001

[106] ¶ 11,026; DEPR: 15,812; § 11,001

[107] ¶ 12,137, ¶ 12,137A; BUSEXP: 18,900; § 10,245

[108] ¶ 12,138, ¶ 12,138D.20; BUSEXP: 18,950; § 10,250

Comment: Absent further legislation, the deduction for energy efficiency improvements expires for property placed in service after December 31, 2013. For the latest legislative updates, visit our website www.CCHGroup.com/TaxUpdates.

A taxpayer may also claim a partial deduction for the costs of property that meet energy savings targets set by the IRS in Notice 2006-52, as modified by Notice 2012-26. The deduction is determined by substituting $.60 for $1.80.

For property placed in service on or after March 12, 2012, the taxpayer may use the following energy savings percentages to determine if a partial deduction is available: (1) building envelope—10 percent; heating, cooling, ventilation, and hot water systems—15 percent; and interior lighting systems—25 percent; or (2) building envelope—10 percent; heating, cooling, ventilation, and hot water systems—20 percent; and interior lighting systems—20 percent.

The deduction is generally claimed by the building's owner. However, in the case of a public building, the person primarily responsible for designing the property may claim the deduction. The deduction reduces the depreciable basis of the building and is treated as a depreciation deduction for section 1245 recapture purposes (Code Sec. 1245(a)(3)(C)).

The Department of Energy maintains a list of the software that must be used to calculate power consumption and energy costs for purposes of certifying the required energy savings necessary to claim the deduction (Notice 2008-40). The certification is not attached to the taxpayer's return but must be retained as part of the taxpayer's books and records. The deduction is claimed on the "Other deductions" line of the taxpayer's return. There is no special form for computing the deduction.

Taxpayers who failed to claim a Code Sec. 179D deduction may file an automatic accounting method change to do so (Rev. Proc. 2011-14, Appendix Section 8.04, as amended by Rev. Proc. 2012-39).

Allowance for Amortization

1287. Property Subject to Amortization. Amortization is the recovery of certain capital expenditures, that are not ordinarily deductible, in a manner that is similar to straight-line depreciation. That portion of the basis of property that is recovered through amortization deductions may not also be depreciated.

Pollution Control Facilities. Taxpayers may elect to amortize over a 60-month period the cost of certified pollution control facilities added to or used in connection with a plant in operation before 1976. The amortization deduction is available only for the portion of the facility's basis attributable to the first 15 years of its recovery period if it has a recovery period under the Modified Accelerated Cost Recovery System (MACRS) in excess of 15 years. The remaining basis is depreciable. An air pollution control facility placed in service after April 11, 2005, in connection with a coal-fired plant placed in operation after 1975 qualifies for an 84-month amortization period (Code Sec. 169). The 60-month amortization period continues to apply to an air pollution facility placed in service after April 11, 2005, in connection with a coal-fired plant placed in operation before 1976 (Code Sec. 169).[109]

Architectural and Transportation Barriers. Business taxpayers can elect to deduct up to $15,000 of the costs of removing certain architectural and transportation barriers for handicapped or elderly persons in the year paid or incurred instead of capitalizing and depreciating such costs (Code Sec. 190).[110]

References are to Standard Federal Tax Reports; Tax Research Consultant; and Practical Tax Explanations.

[109] ¶ 11,502; DEPR: 21,150; § 11,501

[110] ¶ 12,260; BUSEXP: 9,102.35; § 10,220

Reforestation Expenditures. A taxpayer (other than a trust) may elect to expense up to $10,000 of qualified reforestation expenditures each tax year for each qualified timber property. A taxpayer may also elect (including a trust or estate) to amortize over 84 months amounts for which a current deduction is not elected (Code Sec. 194).[111] Election guidance is provided in Notice 2006-47.

Start-Up and Organizational Costs. See ¶ 904.

Oil and Gas Geological and Geophysical Expenditures. Geological and geophysical (G&G) expenditures paid or incurred in connection with oil and gas exploration or development in the United States must be amortized ratably over a 24-month period beginning on the mid-point of the tax year that the expenses were paid or incurred. If a property or project is abandoned or retired during the 24-month amortization period, any remaining basis must continue to be amortized (Code Sec. 167(h)).[112] Major integrated oil companies, however, must ratably amortize any G&G costs over five years (Code Sec. 167(h)(5)).

Musical Compositions and Copyrights (Expired). For tax years beginning before January 1, 2011, a taxpayer could elect five-year ratable amortization of capitalized expenses paid or incurred in creating or acquiring a musical composition (including the accompanying words) or a copyright to a musical composition if the expenses were not exempt from capitalization as the qualified creative expenses of an individual (¶ 990A), the expenses were not amortizable under Code Sec. 197 because acquired as part of the acquisition of a trade or business, or the taxpayer uses a simplified UNICAP method for property acquired for resale (¶ 995) (Code Sec. 167(g)(8)). The provision is effective for expenses paid or incurred with respect to property placed in service in tax years beginning after December 31, 2005.

1288. Amortization of Section 197 Intangibles. The capitalized cost of goodwill and most other intangibles used in a trade or business or for the production of income are ratably amortized over a 15-year period generally beginning in the month of acquisition (Code Sec. 197).[113] Intangibles amortizable under this provision are referred to as section 197 intangibles.

The following intangibles are section 197 intangibles: (1) goodwill, going concern value, and covenants not to compete entered into in connection with the acquisition of a trade or business (¶ 1743); (2) workforce in place; (3) information base; (4) a patent, copyright, formula, design, or similar item; (5) any customer-based intangible; (6) any supplier-based intangible; (7) any license, permit, or other right granted by a governmental unit or agency; and (8) any franchise, trademark, or trade name (Code Sec. 197(d)).[114]

Self-created intangibles are generally not amortized under Code Sec. 197 unless created in connection with the acquisition of a trade or business. Exceptions are provided for government-granted licenses, permits, and rights, covenants not to compete entered into in connection with the purchase of a business, and franchises, trademarks, and trade names (Code Sec. 197(c)(2)).[115] However, certain self-created intangibles without an ascertainable useful life may be amortized over 15 years under Reg. § 1.167(a)-3(b) (¶ 1288A).

The following intangibles are specifically excluded from the definition of a section 197 intangible: (1) interests in a corporation, partnership, trust, or estate; (2) interests under certain financial contracts; (3) interests in land; (4) computer software not acquired in connection with the purchase of a business, or that is readily available for purchase by the general public, is subject to a nonexclusive license, and has not been substantially modified (¶ 980); (5) certain separately acquired rights and interests, including an interest in a patent or copyright or an interest in a film, sound recording,

References are to Standard Federal Tax Reports; Tax Research Consultant; and Practical Tax Explanations.

[111] ¶ 12,330; FARM: 24,100; § 11,505

[112] ¶ 11,002; FARM: 21,176; § 11,550

[113] ¶ 12,450; DEPR: 21,050; § 11,401

[114] ¶ 12,450; DEPR: 21,052; § 11,405

[115] ¶ 12,450; DEPR: 21,052.60; § 11,415

videotape, book, or similar property; (6) interests under existing leases of tangible property; (7) interests under existing indebtedness; (8) sports franchises acquired on or before October 22, 2004; (9) residential mortgage servicing rights not acquired in connection with the acquisition of a business; and (10) professional fees and transaction costs incurred in a corporate organization or reorganization (Code Sec. 197(e)).[116]

No loss may be claimed when an amortizable section 197 intangible is disposed of if any other section 197 intangibles acquired in the same transaction are retained. The bases of the retained section 197 intangibles are increased by the amount of the unrecognized loss (Code Sec. 197(f)).[117]

1288A. 15-Year Safe-Harbor Amortization for Certain Self-Created Intangibles. A taxpayer is permitted to amortize certain created intangibles that do not have readily ascertainable useful lives over a 15-year period using the straight-line method and no salvage value (Reg. § 1.167(a)-3(b); Rev. Proc. 2006-12, as modified by Rev. Proc. 2006-37).[118] For example, amounts paid to acquire memberships or privileges of indefinite duration, such as a trade association membership, are covered by this safe harbor.

A taxpayer may use the 15-year amortization period on any intangible other than: (1) any intangible acquired from another person; (2) created financial interests; (3) any intangible that has a useful life that can be estimated with reasonable accuracy; or (4) an intangible asset for which an amortization period or useful life is specifically prescribed or proscribed by the Code, regulations, or other published IRS guidance. In addition, amounts paid to facilitate an acquisition of a trade or business, a change in the capital structure of a business entity, and certain other similar transactions described in Reg. § 1.263(a)-5 do not qualify. The 15-year amortization period is extended to 25 years for an intangible benefit described in Reg. § 1.263(a)-4(d)(8). These are intangibles created by transferring ownership of real property to another person or by making a monetary contribution for the acquisition or improvement of real property owned by another person. However, for the treatment of impact fees, see Rev. Rul. 2002-9, which requires developers to allocate the cost of impact fees to the basis of the buildings constructed.

What Is Depletion?

1289. Deduction for Depletion. A deduction for depletion is allowed in determining the taxable income from natural resources. The deduction is similar to depreciation in that it allows the taxpayer to recover the cost of an asset over the resources' productive life. Depletion is the exhaustion of natural resources, such as mines, wells, and timberlands, as a result of production. The right to a depletion allowance is based upon the taxpayer's economic interest in the property (Reg. § 1.611-1(b)(i)).[119] An economic interest exists if the taxpayer (1) has acquired by investment any interest in minerals in place or in standing timber, and (2) looks to the income from the extraction of the minerals or severance of the timber for a return on investment.

The basic method of computing depletion is cost depletion (Code Sec. 612).[120] The basis upon which the deduction is allowed is the adjusted basis of the property (Reg. § 1.612-1).[121] Determination of cost depletion first requires an estimate of the number of units (tons, barrels, etc.) that make up the deposit. Then that part of the cost or other adjusted basis of the property that is allocable to the depletable reserves is divided by the number of units. The quotient is the cost depletion per unit. This amount, multiplied by the number of units extracted and sold during the year, determines the cost depletion deductible for the year. Each year the cost basis of the property is reduced, but not below zero, by the amount of depletion deducted for that year, whether cost or percentage depletion was used. The remaining basis is used in computing cost depletion for the next year.

References are to Standard Federal Tax Reports; Tax Research Consultant; and Practical Tax Explanations.

[116] ¶ 12,450; DEPR: 21,054; § 11,410

[117] ¶ 12,450; DEPR: 21,056.05; § 11,425

[118] ¶ 11,008, ¶ 11,009.135; BUSEXP: 9,104.20; § 11,415

[119] ¶ 23,922; FARM: 15,052; § 11,610

[120] ¶ 23,940, ¶ 23,942; FARM: 15,100; § 11,615

[121] ¶ 23,941; FARM: 15,106; § 11,615

An alternative method of computing depletion, known as percentage depletion, may be used for almost all depletable property, other than timber (Reg. § 1.611-1(a)(1)).[122] Under this method, a flat percentage of *gross income* from the property is taken as the depletion deduction. The percentage depletion deduction may not exceed 50 percent (100 percent in the case of oil or gas properties) of the *taxable income* from the property computed without regard to the depletion allowance or the qualified domestic production activities deduction under Code Sec. 199. See ¶ 1294 for special rules concerning independent producers and royalty owners. In computing taxable income, the deductible mining expenses must be decreased by the amount of section 1245 gains allocable to the property (Code Sec. 613(a)).[123] If cost depletion results in a greater deduction, cost depletion must be used (Reg. § 1.613-1).[124]

Ordinarily, the lease of a mineral property requires the lessee to make an advance payment, known as a bonus or advance royalty. In such a case, the lessor's cost depletion allowance must be allocated between the advance lump-sum payment and the royalties received during the period of extraction (Reg. § 1.612-3).[125] Unlike bonuses or advance royalties, "shut-in" oil payments and delay rentals are not depletable (*F.I. Johnson*, CA-5, 61-1 USTC ¶ 9307).[126]

Coal and iron ore royalties retained upon the disposition of coal and iron ore generally held for more than one year before mining are eligible for percentage depletion for any tax year in which the maximum rate of tax imposed on net capital gain equals or exceeds the maximum rate for ordinary income (Code Sec. 631(c)).[127]

Depletion is subject to recapture as ordinary income upon the sale or other disposition of an oil, gas, geothermal, or other mineral property at a gain (Code Sec. 1254).[128] Recapture is limited to the amount by which the depletion deduction reduced the adjusted basis of the disposed property.

Mineral Production Payments

1291. Mineral Production Payments. A mineral production payment is treated as a loan by the owner of the production payment to the owner of the mineral property (Code Sec. 636).[129] Thus, a carved-out mineral production payment—created when the owner of a mineral property sells or carves out a portion of the future production with payment secured by an interest in the minerals—is treated as a mortgage loan on the mineral property rather than as an economic interest in the property. All the income from the property is taxed to the seller (owner of the working interest) and is subject to depletion by him. The owner of the production payment does not get depletion.

When the owner of a mineral interest sells the working interest, a retained production payment is treated as a purchase money mortgage loan and not as an economic interest in the mineral property. Accordingly, all the income from the property is taxed to the purchaser and is subject to depletion by him. The seller who retains the production payment is not entitled to depletion.

Percentage Depletion

1294. Oil and Gas Production. A 22-percent depletion rate is allowed for oil and gas production in the case of regulated natural gas and natural gas sold under a fixed contract (but not certain casinghead gas contracts); a 10-percent rate applies to geopressurized methane gas wells (Code Sec. 613A(b)).[130]

References are to Standard Federal Tax Reports; Tax Research Consultant; and Practical Tax Explanations.

[122] ¶ 23,922; FARM: 24,054; § 11,620

[123] ¶ 23,960; FARM: 15,308; § 11,620

[124] ¶ 23,961; FARM: 15,100; § 11,620

[125] ¶ 23,946; FARM: 15,116; § 11,615

[126] ¶ 23,963.60; FARM: 18,260; § 11,615

[127] ¶ 24,150; FARM: 18,350; § 11,625

[128] ¶ 31,060; FARM: 21,200; § 16,710.05

[129] ¶ 24,170; FARM: 18,208; § 11,610

[130] ¶ 23,980; FARM: 15,202; § 11,625

A 15-percent depletion rate applies to independent producers and royalty owners with limitations based on average daily production (Code Sec. 613A(c)).[131] The rate applies to an average daily production of 1,000 barrels of oil and six million cubic feet of gas. The percentage depletion deduction is generally limited to the lesser of 65 percent of the *taxable income* before the depletion allowance (Code Sec. 613A(d)(1))[132] or 100 percent of the *taxable income from the property* before the depletion allowance (see ¶ 1289). For purposes of the 65-percent limit, taxable income is computed without regard to any net operating loss carryback, capital loss carryback, or qualified domestic production activities deduction under Code Sec. 199. Any portion of a depletion allowance disallowed under the 65-percent limit may be carried over. Percentage depletion is also denied for lease bonuses, advance royalty payments, or other amounts payable without regard to actual production from an oil, gas or geothermal property (¶ 1296) (Code Secs. 613(e)(3) and 613A(d)(5)).[133]

The 100-percent taxable income limit on percentage depletion deductions for oil and gas properties is suspended for marginal properties for tax years (1) beginning after December 31, 1997, and before January 1, 2008, or (2) beginning after December 31, 2008, and before January 1, 2012 (Code Sec. 613A(c)(6)(H)).[134] Thus, the limitation is not suspended for tax years beginning after 2011, but is suspended for tax years beginning in 2009, 2010, and 2011.

The 15-percent depletion rate for marginal oil or gas production properties held by independent producers or royalty owners increases by one percent (up to a maximum 25-percent rate) for each whole dollar that the reference price for crude oil for the preceding calendar year is less than $20 per barrel (Code Sec. 613A(c)(6)).[135] The allowance for depletion is computed using the increased rate with respect to the portion of the taxpayer's average daily marginal production of domestic crude oil and natural gas that does not exceed the taxpayer's depletable quantities of those products. An election may be made to have this rule apply to the pro rata portion of marginal production. The applicable percentage for marginal production for tax years beginning in 2001 through 2014 is 15 percent (Notice 2014-63).

1296. Geothermal Deposits. Geothermal deposits (geothermal reservoirs consisting of natural heat that is stored in rocks or in an aqueous liquid or vapor (whether or not under pressure)) are eligible for a 15-percent depletion allowance (Code Sec. 613(e)).[136]

1298. Coal or Other Minerals. Percentage depletion is allowed, under Code Sec. 613(b)[137] at the following percentages of gross income from the property:

(a) 22%—sulphur and uranium; and, if from deposits in the United States, anorthosite, clay, laterite, and nephelite syenite (to the extent that alumina and aluminum compounds are extracted therefrom), asbestos, bauxite, celestite, chromite, corundum, fluorspar, graphite, ilmenite, kyanite, mica, olivine, quartz crystals (radio grade), rutile, block steatite talc, and zircon, and ores of the following metals: antimony, beryllium, bismuth, cadmium, cobalt, columbium, lead lithium, manganese, mercury, molybdenum, nickel, platinum and platinum group metals, tantalum, thorium, tin, titanium, tungsten, vanadium and zinc.

(b) 15%—if from deposits in the United States, gold, silver, copper, iron ore, and oil shale (except shale described in (e) below).

(c) 14%—metal mines (other than metals from deposits in the United States to which the 22-percent rate in (a) applies), rock asphalt, and vermiculite; if (a) above and (e) and (f) below do not apply, ball clay, bentonite, china clay, sagger

---

References are to Standard Federal Tax Reports; Tax Research Consultant; and Practical Tax Explanations.

[131] ¶ 23,980; FARM: 15,206; § 11,625

[132] ¶ 23,980; FARM: 15,218; § 11,625

[133] ¶ 23,960, ¶ 23,980; FARM: 15,206; § 11,625

[134] ¶ 23,980; FARM: 15,150; § 11,625

[135] ¶ 23,980; FARM: 15,216; § 11,625

[136] ¶ 23,960; FARM: 15,158; § 11,625

[137] ¶ 23,960; FARM: 15,154; § 11,625

clay, and clay used or sold for use for purposes dependent on its refractory properties.

(d) 10%—asbestos from deposits outside the United States, brucite, coal, lignite, perlite, sodium chloride, and wollastonite.

(e) 7½%—clay and shale used or sold for use in the manufacture of sewer pipe or brick, and clay, shale, and slate used or sold for use as sintered or burned lightweight aggregates.

(f) 5%—gravel, peat, pumice, sand, scoria, shale (except shale described in (b) and (e) above) and stone (except stone falling within the general 14-percent group described in (g)); clay used, or sold for use, in the manufacture of drainage and roofing tile, flower pots, and kindred products; also, if from brine wells, bromite, calcium chloride, and magnesium chloride.

(g) 14%—all other minerals not included in any of the categories listed above. For purposes of this paragraph, the term "all other minerals" does not include (A) soil, sod, dirt, turf, water, or mosses; (B) minerals from sea water, the air, or similar inexhaustible sources; or (C) oil and gas wells.

Gross income from the property, on which percentage depletion is based, is the amount of income that comes from the extraction of the ores or minerals from the ground and the application of mining processes, including mining transportation (Code Sec. 613(c)).[138] Mining processes include certain specified treatment processes. The percentage depletion allowance is generally based on the mined product after application of those treatment processes applied by "ordinary" miners. Hence, an integrated miner-manufacturer computes gross income from mining at the point when the nonintegrated miner disposes of the product. Gross income is computed by use of the representative market or field price. However, when it is impossible to determine such a field price, and where the IRS does not determine that a more appropriate method should be used, the proportionate profits method must be used (Reg. § 1.613-4(d)).[139]

References are to Standard Federal Tax Reports; Tax Research Consultant; and Practical Tax Explanations.

[138] ¶ 23,960; FARM: 15,258; § 11,620

[139] ¶ 23,967; FARM: 15,264; § 11,620

12 DEPRECIATION

Chapter 13

TAX CREDITS

Nonrefundable Credits

1301. Child and Dependent Care Credit. A nonrefundable credit is allowed for a portion of qualifying child or dependent care expenses paid for the purpose of allowing the taxpayer, and the taxpayer's spouse if filing a joint return to be gainfully employed (Code Sec. 21).[1] The credit is computed on Form 2441 for filers of Form 1040 and Form 1040A. The credit cannot be claimed on Form 1040EZ. To be eligible for the credit, the taxpayer must incur employment-related expenses in providing care for one of the following qualified individuals:

- a dependent of the taxpayer who is a qualifying child of the taxpayer and has not attained the age of 13 (¶ 137A);

- a dependent of the taxpayer who is a qualifying child or qualifying relative of the taxpayer (¶ 137B) (determined without regards to whether the individual may be claimed as a dependent by another taxpayer, has income in excess of the dependency exemption amount, or files a joint return with his or her spouse) and is physically or mentally incapable of caring for himself or herself and who has the same principal place of abode as the taxpayer for more than half of the year; or

- the taxpayer's spouse, if the spouse is physically or mentally incapable of caring for himself or herself and has the same principal place of abode as the taxpayer for more than half of the year.

Amount of Credit. The maximum amount of employment-related expenses to which the credit may be applied is $3,000, if one qualifying individual is involved, or $6,000, if two or more qualifying individuals are involved, less excludable employer dependent care assistance program payments (¶ 2065) (Code Sec. 21(c)). The credit amount is equal to the amount of qualified expenses multiplied by an applicable percentage determined by the taxpayer's adjusted gross income (AGI). Taxpayers with an AGI of $15,000 or less use the highest applicable percentage of 35 percent. For taxpayers with an AGI over $15,000, the credit is reduced by one percentage point for each $2,000 of AGI, or fraction thereof, over $15,000 (Code Sec. 21(a)(2)). The minimum applicable percentage of 20 percent is used by taxpayers with an AGI greater than $43,000. Thus, the maximum dependent care credit amount is $1,050 for one qualifying dependent and $2,100 for two or more qualifying dependents.

Example: A widower paid a housekeeper $5,000 during the year to take care of his home and 10-year-old daughter while he is working. His AGI was $25,000.

References are to Standard Federal Tax Reports; Tax Research Consultant; and Practical Tax Explanations.

[1] ¶ 3502; INDIV: 57,050; § 12,201

Since there is only one qualifying child, the maximum credit he can claim is $900 (30 percent of $3,000).

Qualifying Expenses. Qualifying expenses include expenses paid for household services and for the care of a qualifying individual that allow the taxpayer, and the taxpayer's spouse if filing a joint return, to work or look for work. Services outside the home qualify if they involve the care of a qualified individual who regularly spends at least eight hours a day in the taxpayer's home. Payments to a relative may be qualifying expenses unless the taxpayer claims a dependency exemption for the relative or if the relative is the taxpayer's child and under age 19. No expenses incurred to send a child or other dependent to an overnight camp are considered qualifying expenses for credit purposes.

Qualifying employment-related expenses are considered in determining the credit only to the extent of earned income—wages, salary, remuneration for personal services, net self-employment income, etc. For married taxpayers, expenses are limited to the earned income of the lower-earning spouse. Thus, if one spouse is generally not working, no credit is allowed. However, if the nonworking spouse is physically or mentally incapable of caring for himself or herself or is a full-time student at an educational institution for at least five calendar months during the year, the earned income amount is assumed to be—for each month of disability or school attendance—$250 if there is one qualifying individual or $500 if there are two or more qualifying individuals (Code Sec. 21(d)(2)).

Claiming the Credit. A married taxpayer *must* file a joint return to claim the credit. For this purpose, a married person living apart from his or her spouse under the circumstances described at ¶ 173 is considered unmarried. Also, a divorced or legally separated taxpayer having custody of a child who is disabled or under the age 13 is entitled to the credit even though he or she has released the right to a dependency exemption for the child (¶ 139A) (Code Sec. 21(e)(5)). Taxpayers must provide each qualifying individual's taxpayer identification number in order to claim the credit (generally a Social Security number), as well as an identifying number of the dependent care service provider (either their Social Security number or employer identification number (EIN)) (Code Sec. 21(e)(9) and (10)).

1302. Credit for the Elderly or the Permanently and Totally Disabled. A tax credit is available to individuals who are (1) 65 years of age before the close of the tax year or (2) under age 65 but are retired and were permanently and totally disabled when they retired (Code Sec. 22).[2] Married taxpayers must file a joint return to claim the credit unless the spouses live apart throughout the tax year. The credit is computed on Schedule R of Form 1040 and 1040A.

The credit is 15 percent of an applicable initial amount based on an individual's filing status and reduced by certain income. For individuals age 65 or older, the applicable initial amount is as follows:

Single individual	$5,000
Married individuals, joint return, one spouse is a qualified individual . .	5,000
Married individuals, joint return, both spouses are qualified individuals	7,500
Married individual, separate return	3,750

This initial amount is then reduced by amounts received as pension, annuity, or disability benefits that are excludable from gross income and are payable under the Social Security Act (Title II), the Railroad Retirement Act of 1974, a Veterans Affairs program, or that are otherwise excludable under a non-Code provision. No reduction is made for pension, annuity or disability benefits for personal injuries or sickness payable from a Veterans Affairs program.

The maximum amount determined above is further reduced by one-half of the excess of the taxpayer's adjusted gross income (AGI) over the following levels, based on filing status (Code Sec. 22(d)):

References are to Standard Federal Tax Reports; Tax Research Consultant; and Practical Tax Explanations.

[2] ¶ 3550; INDIV: 57,100;
§ 12,501

13

TAX CREDITS

Single taxpayer	$7,500
Married taxpayers, combined AGI on joint return	10,000
Married individual filing separately	5,000

For permanently and totally disabled individuals under age 65, the applicable initial amount noted may not exceed the amount of disability income for the tax year. In determining their initial amounts, special rules apply to a married couple filing a joint return where both spouses qualify for the credit and at least one of them is under age 65. Disability income means the total amount that is included in an individual's gross income for the tax year under Code Secs. 72 (¶ 817) or 105(a) (¶ 2015) to the extent the amount constitutes wages, or payments in lieu of wages, for periods during which the individual is absent from work due to permanent and total disability (Code Sec. 22(c)(2)(B)).

An individual is considered permanently and totally disabled for this purpose if he or she is unable to engage in any substantial gainful activity by reason of any medically determinable physical or mental impairment that can be expected to result in death or to last for a continuous period of not less than 12 months. The impairment should be substantiated by a letter from a certified physician kept in the taxpayer's records (Code Sec. 22(e)(3)).

Example: Alex, age 66 and single, has AGI of $9,000 for the year and receives $4,000 of nontaxable Social Security benefits for the year. To determine his credit, he would make the following computation:

Initial amount	$5,000
Less: nontaxable Social Security benefits	4,000
Reduced initial amount	$1,000
Less: one-half of AGI above $7,500	750
Amount eligible for credit	$250
Credit: $250 × 15%	$38

1303. Credits for Higher Education Tuition. There are two education-related tax credits: the American Opportunity (modified Hope) tax credit (AOTC) and the lifetime learning credit. The AOTC replaces the Hope scholarship credit for tax years beginning after December 31, 2008, and before January 1, 2018. The credits may be claimed on Form 8863 by individuals for qualified tuition expenses incurred by students pursuing college or graduate degrees, or vocational training (Code Sec. 25A).[3] The credits are elective, generally nonrefundable (except for the AOTC which is 40-percent refundable), and cannot be claimed using the same expenses for which another tax benefit is also received. The credits are also not permitted to be claimed by more than one taxpayer in the same year—for example, they may be claimed either by the parents or by the dependent child, but not by both (¶ 137). Higher income parents whose adjusted gross income (AGI) would result in the phaseout of the dependency exemption may waive claiming the dependency exemption to allow their student dependent to claim an educational credit (Reg. § 1.25A-1(f)(1)). This does not entitle the student dependent to claim a personal exemption on his or her tax return (¶ 135).

American Opportunity Tax Credit. The AOTC is a modification of the Hope scholarship credit for tax years beginning after December 31, 2008, and before January 1, 2018 (Code Sec. 25A(i)).[4] The credit amount is the sum of 100 percent of the first $2,000 of qualified tuition and related expenses, plus 25 percent of the next $2,000 of qualified tuition and related expenses for a total maximum credit of $2,500 per eligible student per year. The credit is available for the first four years of a student's post-secondary education. Up to 40 percent of the credit amount is refundable should the taxpayer's tax liability be insufficient to offset the nonrefundable credit amount. The credit amount phases out ratably for taxpayers with modified AGI (MAGI) between $80,000 and

---

References are to Standard Federal Tax Reports; Tax Research Consultant; and Practical Tax Explanations.

[3] ¶ 3820; INDIV: 60,150; § 12,401

[4] ¶ 3820; INDIV: 60,152; § 12,417

¶1303

$90,000 ($160,000 and $180,000 for joint filers) (Code Sec. 25A(i)(4)). MAGI is defined as AGI determined without regard to the exclusions for foreign earned income, foreign housing expenses (¶ 2402), and U.S. possession income (¶ 2414 and ¶ 2415). The AOTC may not be taken by married taxpayers who file separate returns (Code Sec. 25A(g)).

Lifetime Learning Credit. The lifetime learning credit is equal to 20 percent of the amount of qualified tuition expenses paid on the first $10,000 of tuition, an amount which is not inflation adjusted. In contrast to the AOTC, the maximum lifetime learning credit is calculated per taxpayer and does not vary based on the number of eligible students in the taxpayer's family. A student is eligible for the lifetime learning credit if the student is enrolled in one or more courses at a qualified educational institution. The allowable amount of the lifetime learning credit is reduced for taxpayers who have MAGI above certain amounts. The phaseout of the credits begins for single taxpayers in 2014 when MAGI reaches $54,000 ($55,000 in 2015) and completely phases out when MAGI reaches $64,000 ($65,000 in 2015). For joint filers, the phaseout range is $108,000 ($110,000 in 2015) to $128,000 ($130,000 in 2015) in 2014 (Code Sec. 25A(d); Rev. Proc. 2013-35; Rev. Proc. 2014-61). The lifetime learning credit may not be taken by married taxpayers who file separate returns (Code Sec. 25A(g)).

Hope Scholarship Credit. For tax years beginning after December 31, 2017, the Hope scholarship credit amount per eligible student is equal to 100 percent of the first $1,000 of qualified tuition expenses and 50 percent of the second $1,000 of qualified tuition paid during the year, indexed for inflation. An eligible student for the Hope credit is any individual who:

- has not elected to claim the Hope credit in any two earlier years;
- has not completed the first two years of post-secondary education before the beginning of the current tax year;
- is enrolled at least half-time in a program that leads to a degree, certificate, or other recognized educational credentials; and
- has not been convicted of any Federal or State felony class drug offense for possession or distribution.

Qualified Expenses. The education credits are available for qualified tuition and related expenses incurred for the taxpayer, the taxpayer's spouse, or the taxpayer's dependent who is an eligible student at a qualified educational institution (Code Sec. 25A(f) and (i)(3)). Qualified expenses generally do not include room and board, books, unless required for enrollment, as well as student health fees, or transportation. However, for purposes of claiming the AOTC, qualifying expenses include course materials. The amount of qualified tuition and related expenses paid with any tax-free funds such as scholarships or Pell grants reduces the amount available for claiming the credits. A qualified educational institution is any post-secondary educational institution eligible to participate in a student aid program administered by the Department of Education (Code Sec. 25A(f)(2)).

Coordination with Other Provisions. To coordinate the education credits with other provisions of the Code, educational expenses eligible for the credits must first be reduced by tax-free educational assistance such as scholarships or fellowships (¶ 865), veterans' educational assistance allowances, employer-provided educational assistance (¶ 2067), or any other educational assistance excluded from gross income, other than gifts, bequests, devises, or inheritances (Reg. § 1.25A-5(c)). Taxpayers are then permitted to elect to claim either the AOTC or the lifetime learning credit for a student in any tax year.

The expenses used to claim an educational credit also reduce the amount of eligible expenses available for purposes of determining the exclusion amount of distributions from Coverdell educational savings accounts (¶ 867) or qualified tuition programs (QTPs) (¶ 869). Since any excess distributions from Coverdell account or QTP over the eligible educational expenses are includible in gross income and subject to a 10-percent additional tax, not claiming an educational credit may result in a lower tax liability. However, taxpayers should be aware that the 10-percent additional tax for excess distributions from Coverdell accounts or QTPs is waived if the excess is caused by

¶1303

claiming an educational credit. Taxpayers who receive distributions in excess of eligible expense from both an Coverdell account and QTP in the same year must allocate the expenses between the two distributions. Finally, only after eligible expenses are reduced by an educational credit and distributions from Coverdell accounts or QTPs, the remaining expenses may be used to determine the exclusion amount for Series EE United States Savings Bonds (¶ 730) (Code Secs. 25A(g)(2), 135(d)(2), 529(c)(3)(B), and 530(d)(2)(C)).[5]

1304. Retirement Savings Contributions Credit. Eligible low-income taxpayers may claim a nonrefundable credit for contributions to elective deferral plans or individual retirement accounts (IRAs) (Code Sec. 25B).[6] The credit is referred to as the retirement savings contributions credit or the savers credit. The credit amount equals the eligible taxpayer's applicable percentage, determined by filing status and adjusted gross income (AGI), multiplied by the total qualified retirement savings contributions, not to exceed $2,000 for the tax year. The maximum credit amount is $1,000. The credit is in addition to the exclusion or deduction from gross income for making elective deferrals and IRA contributions that are otherwise allowed.

Eligibility. To be eligible for the credit, a taxpayer making a contribution to a qualified retirement savings plan must be at least 18 years of age at the close of the tax year, must not be claimed as a dependent by someone else (¶ 137), and must not be a full-time student (¶ 137A). A qualified retirement savings plan contribution is the sum of:

- contributions to a traditional or Roth IRA, other than rollover contributions (Code Sec. 219(e));

- any elective deferrals of compensation to a 401(k), 403(b) tax-sheltered annuity, or SIMPLE or SEP plan (Code Sec. 402(g)(3));

- any elective deferrals of compensation to a Code Sec. 457(b) plan of a state or local government or tax-exempt organization; and

- any voluntary employee contributions to any qualified retirement plan (Code Sec. 4974(c)).

The amount of contributions to be taken into account in determining the credit must be reduced by any distributions from such qualified retirement plans over a test period (Code Sec. 25B(d)(2)). The test period is period including the current tax year, the two preceding tax years, and the following tax year up to the due date of the return including extensions. Distribution amounts that qualify as a trustee-to-trustee transfer or as a rollover distribution to another qualified retirement account are not included in the reduction calculation.

Claiming the Credit. Form 8880 is used to calculate the amount of the credit. For 2014, the credit is phased out when AGI exceeds $60,000 for joint return filers, $45,000 for heads of households, and $30,000 for single and married filing separately (Notice 2013-73). For 2015, the credit is phased out when AGI exceeds $61,000 for joint return filers, $45,750 for heads of households, and $30,500 for single and married filing separately (IRS News Release IR-2014-99). The applicable percentage is the percentage as determined by the inflation adjusted income ranges for 2014 in the following table:

Adjusted Gross Income						Applicable percentage
Joint return		Head of a household		All other cases		
Over	Not over	Over	Not over	Over	Not over	
$0	$36,000	$0	$27,000	$0	$18,000	50
36,000	39,000	27,000	29,250	18,000	19,500	20
39,000	60,000	29,250	45,000	19,500	30,000	10
60,000	—	45,000	—	30,000	—	0

References are to Standard Federal Tax Reports; Tax Research Consultant; and Practical Tax Explanations.

[5] ¶ 3820, ¶ 7550, ¶ 22,940, ¶ 22,950; INDIV: 60,150; § 1,810, § 12,420

[6] ¶ 3835; INDIV: 57,550; § 12,701

The applicable percentage is the percentage as determined by the inflation adjusted income ranges for 2015 in the following table:

Adjusted Gross Income						Applicable percentage
Joint return		Head of a household		All other cases		
Over	Not over	Over	Not over	Over	Not over	
$0	$36,500	$0	$27,375	$0	$18,250	50
36,500	39,500	27,375	29,625	18,250	19,750	20
39,500	61,000	29,625	45,750	19,750	30,500	10
61,000	—	45,750	—	30,500	—	0

1305. Child Tax Credit. Taxpayers who have one or more qualifying children that they may claim as dependents (¶ 137) may be entitled to a child tax credit of $1,000 per child (Code Sec. 24).[7] The credit is allowed only for tax years consisting of 12 months. The credit is calculated using a worksheet in the Instructions to Form 1040.

Qualifying Child. The definition of qualifying child for purposes of the child tax credit is the same as that for claiming a dependency exemption (¶ 137A) except that the child must not have attained the age of 17 by the end of the year. In addition, the qualifying child must be either a U.S. citizen, national, or resident of the United States (Code Sec. 24(c)).

Limitation on Child Tax Credit. The child tax credit begins to phase out when the taxpayer's modified adjusted gross income (MAGI) reaches $110,000 for joint filers, $55,000 for married taxpayers filing separately, and $75,000 for single taxpayers. The credit is reduced by $50 for each $1,000, or fraction thereof, of MAGI above the threshold amount (Code Sec. 24(b)). MAGI is defined as AGI determined without regard to the exclusions for foreign earned income, foreign housing expenses (¶ 2402), and U.S. possession income (¶ 2414 and ¶ 2415).

Nonrefundable Portion of Child Tax Credit. The child tax credit is generally a nonrefundable personal credit. For tax years beginning after December 31, 2011, all nonrefundable personal tax credits are allowed to the full extent of the taxpayer's regular tax liability, reduced by the foreign tax credit, and alternative minimum tax (AMT) liability (Code Sec. 26(a)).[8]

Refundable Amount of Child Tax Credit. For tax years beginning before January 1, 2018, a portion of the child tax credit is refundable for all taxpayers (referred to as the additional child tax credit), regardless of the amount of the taxpayer's regular tax or AMT liabilities. The credit is refundable in an amount equal to the lesser of the unclaimed portion of the nonrefundable credit amount or 15 percent of the taxpayer's earned income in excess of $3,000 (Code Sec. 24(d)(4)).[9] Military families may elect to include otherwise excludable combat zone pay in their earned income when calculating the refundable portion of the credit. Taxpayers with three or more children may use an alternative method to calculate their refundable child tax credit. Under this method, the refundable credit is the excess of the taxpayer's share of Social Security taxes, including one-half of any self-employment taxes, over his or her earned income credit for the tax year (¶ 1322). The additional child tax credit is claimed on Schedule 8812.

1306. Mortgage Interest Credit. Low-income homeowners who obtain qualified mortgage credit certificates (MCCs) from state or local governments may claim a tax credit on Form 8396 during any tax year for which the certificate is in effect for a portion of the interest paid or incurred (Code Sec. 25; IRS Pub. 530).[10] An MCC is in effect for interest attributable to the period beginning on the date the certificate is issued and ending when either (1) it is revoked by the issuing authority, or (2) the taxpayer sells

---

References are to Standard Federal Tax Reports; Tax Research Consultant; and Practical Tax Explanations.

[7] ¶ 3760; INDIV: 57,450; § 12,101

[8] ¶ 3850; INDIV: 57,200; § 12,005

[9] ¶ 3760; INDIV: 57,454.10; § 12,120.15

[10] ¶ 3800; INDIV: 57,150; § 13,020.05

the residence or ceases to use it as a personal residence. Any mortgage interest claimed as an itemized deduction must be reduced by any credit claimed (Code Sec. 163(g)).

Amount of Credit. The credit is equal to the product of: (1) the certificate credit rate, which may not be less than 10 percent or more than 50 percent, and (2) the interest paid or accrued by the taxpayer for the year on the remaining principal of the certified indebtedness, plus a limited carryforward, if any. If the credit rate exceeds 20 percent, the tax credit for any year may not exceed $2,000 (Code Sec. 25(a)(2)(A)).

Tax Liability Limitation. The amount of the mortgage interest credit cannot exceed the limit on nonrefundable personal credits under Code Sec. 26(a) (¶ 1315), reduced by all nonrefundable credits other than the mortgage interest credit, the adoption credit (¶ 1307), the credit for residential energy efficient property (¶ 1342), and the credit for first-time homebuyers in the District of Columbia (¶ 1308) (Code Sec. 25(e)(1)).[11] Any unclaimed credit amount may be carried over to each of three succeeding tax years. The carryover amount is added to the current year credit amount and subject to the same tax liability limitation.

Recapture of Tax Benefit. A recapture of the tax benefit received from MCCs is triggered if the home is disposed of by the taxpayer, or ceases to be the taxpayer's principal place of residence during the first nine years after the testing date (Code Secs. 25(i) and Code Sec. 143(m)). The testing date is the date the taxpayer becomes liable either in whole or in part of the federal-subsidized debt on the principal residence. The recapture amount equals the product of the federally-subsidized amount of indebtedness times the holding period percentage times the income percentage. This recapture amount is treated as an addition to tax for the disposition tax year and calculated using Form 8828.

1307. Adoption Credit. For tax years beginning after December 31, 2011, an individual may claim a nonrefundable credit for qualified adoption expenses for each eligible child (Code Sec. 23).[12] The maximum credit amount for the 2014 tax year is $13,190 ($13,400 for 2015). The credit is phased out ratably in 2014 for taxpayers with a modified adjusted gross income (MAGI) over $197,880 ($201,010 in 2015). No credit is allowed to taxpayers with a MAGI over $237,880 ($241,010 in 2015) (Rev. Proc. 2013-35; Rev. Proc. 2014-61). MAGI is defined as AGI determined without regard to the exclusions for foreign earned income, foreign housing expenses (¶ 2402), and U.S. possession income (¶ 2414 and ¶ 2415). The credit amount and the phase out range are adjusted annually for inflation.

The nonrefundable adoption credit replaced the refundable credit under Code Sec. 36C, which was in effect for tax years beginning after December 31, 2009, and before January 1, 2012 (¶ 1327A).

Qualified Adoption Expenses. Qualified adoption expenses include reasonable and necessary adoption fees, court costs, attorney fees, and other expenses which are directly related to the legal adoption of an eligible child. Expenses incurred in violation of state or federal law or in connection with the adoption of a child of the taxpayer's spouse are not eligible for the credit. Costs associated with a surrogate parenting arrangement are also ineligible for use in claiming the credit (Code Sec. 23(d)(1)).

Expenses used to claim any other deduction or credit may not be used to claim the adoption credit (Code Sec. 23(b)(3)). This includes amounts excluded from gross income that are paid or incurred by an employer for the employee's qualified adoption expenses pursuant to an adoption assistance program (¶ 2063). The dollar limitation for the exclusion is identical to the dollar limitation for the credit ($13,190 for 2014). However, any qualified adoption expenses incurred in excess of the amount provided under an employer's adoption assistance program may be used to claim the adoption credit.

References are to Standard Federal Tax Reports; Tax Research Consultant; and Practical Tax Explanations.

[11] ¶ 3800; INDIV: 57,158; § 13,020.10

[12] ¶ 3700; INDIV: 57,350; § 12,301

Eligible Child and Special Needs Child. For purposes of the adoption credit, an eligible child is an individual who has not attained the age of 18 as of the time of the adoption or who is physically or mentally incapable of caring for himself or herself. This definition also includes a child with special needs. A special needs child is any child who, as determined by the state, should not or cannot be returned to the home of his or her parents, is a citizen or resident of the United States, and a specific factor or condition makes it reasonable to conclude that the child cannot be placed with adoptive parents unless assistance is provided (Code Sec. 23(d)(2) and (d)(3)).

Claiming the Credit. Adoption expenses incurred or paid during a tax year prior to the year in which the adoption is finalized may be claimed as a credit in the tax year following the year the expense were incurred. Adoption expenses incurred during the year the adoption becomes final or in the year following the finalization of the adoption are claimed in the year they were incurred (Code Sec. 23(a)(2)). Adoption expenses for any qualified child who is not a U.S. citizen or resident cannot be claimed as a credit until the adoption is finalized (Code Sec. 23(e)). Taxpayers who adopt a child with special needs are allowed to claim the full amount of the credit regardless of actual expenses paid or incurred in the year the adoption becomes final (Code Sec. 23(a)(3)). Married couples must file a joint return in order to claim the credit unless the special rules for married individuals who are separated or living apart apply (¶ 173). The credit must be claimed on Form 8839 with proper documentation attached.

Carryovers. As noted above, for tax years beginning after December 31, 2011, the adoption credit is nonrefundable. In addition, all nonrefundable personal tax credits are allowed to the full extent of the sum of the taxpayer's regular tax and minimum tax liabilities (¶ 1315). Thus, the adoption credit may be claimed against both regular tax liability, reduced by any foreign tax credit claimed, and the minimum tax liability. The adoption credit can be carried forward for up to five years if the credit exceeds the sum of the taxpayer's regular tax and minimum tax liability reduced by the sum of the other nonrefundable credits, except the adoption credit, residential energy efficient property credit, and the first-time homebuyer credit for the District of Columbia (Code Sec. 23(c)).[13]

1308. Credit for First-Time Homebuyer in the District of Columbia (Expired). First-time homebuyers who purchased a principal residence in the District of Columbia from an unrelated person before January 1, 2012, could claim a nonrefundable credit of up to $5,000 of the purchase price ($2,500 in the case of a married person filing separately) (Code Sec. 1400C).[14] The credit was nonrefundable, however, any unused credit can be carried over to the next succeeding year (or years) (Code Sec. 1400C(d)). Form 8859 is used to claim a carryforward of any unused credit.

1309. Alternative Minimum Tax Credit. Taxpayers are permitted a tax credit against their regular income tax liability for some or all of alternative minimum tax (AMT) paid in previous years (¶ 1401). The minimum tax credit is allowed for the amount of adjusted net minimum tax for all tax years reduced by the minimum tax credit for all prior tax years (Code Sec. 53).[15] Any unused credit may be carried forward indefinitely as a credit against regular tax liability. It is limited, however, to the extent that the regular tax liability reduced by other nonrefundable credits exceeds the tentative minimum tax for the tax year. The credit may not be used to offset any future AMT liability. Special rules allowed individuals with long-term unused minimum tax credit to claim an additional refundable credit amount in 2007 through 2012 (¶ 1327). The credit is claimed by individuals, trusts, and estates on Form 8801 and by corporations on Form 8827.

References are to Standard Federal Tax Reports; Tax Research Consultant; and Practical Tax Explanations.

[13] ¶ 3700; INDIV: 57,366; § 12,301

[14] ¶ 32,428; INDIV: 57,500; § 13,005

[15] ¶ 4870; FILEIND: 30,452; § 15,510.05

For noncorporate taxpayers, the adjusted net minimum tax is the taxpayer's AMT liability reduced by the amount that would have been the taxpayer's AMT liability if only certain specified adjustments and preferences had been taken into account (Code Sec. 53(d)(1)).[16] The adjustments include those related to standard deduction, personal exemptions, medical and dental expenses, miscellaneous itemized deductions, taxes, and interest expenses (¶ 1435). The preference items include certain depletion deductions exceeding adjusted basis, tax-exempt interest on specified private activity bonds, and the exclusion of gain on the sale of qualified small business stock (¶ 1425). In determining corporate credits for prior year minimum tax liability, adjusted net minimum tax is the taxpayer's AMT for the year.

Limitation on Nonrefundable Credits

1315. Limitation on Nonrefundable Credits. The use of nonrefundable personal tax credits against an individual's regular tax and alternative minimum tax (AMT) or minimum tax liability has been made permanent (Code Sec. 26(a)).[17] For tax years beginning after December 31, 2011, all nonrefundable personal tax credits are allowed to the full extent of the sum of the taxpayer's regular tax liability, reduced by any applicable foreign tax credit, and minimum tax liability.

Refundable Credits

1321. Credit for Taxes Withheld on Wages. A taxpayer is allowed a credit against his or her income tax liability for income taxes withheld from his or her salary or wages (Code Sec. 31).[18] A taxpayer is also allowed a special refund of any Social Security taxes which were over-withheld from his or her wages. Excess Social Security taxes may be withheld where an individual works for more than one employer during the year and earns more than the Social Security wage base of $117,000 in 2014 in total. The maximum amount of Social Security taxes that may be withheld is 6.2 percent of the wage base (¶ 2648). The same rule applies to excess withheld railroad retirement taxes. Since there is no wage base for calculating Medicare taxes, there can be no over-withholding of such taxes. The special refund for over-withheld Social Security taxes may be claimed as a credit on Form 1040. However, if the individual is not required to file an income tax return, he or she may file a special refund claim (Reg. § 31.6413(c)-1).[19] A nonresident alien (or foreign corporation) is allowed a credit against income tax liability for taxes withheld on U.S. source income that is not effectively connected with a U.S. trade or business (Code Sec. 33).[20] For a discussion on the withholding of tax on payments other than wages to nonresident aliens, see ¶ 2455.

1322. Earned Income Credit. A refundable earned income credit (EIC) is available to certain low-income individuals (Code Sec. 32).[21] To be eligible to claim the credit, a taxpayer must have earned income with an adjusted gross income (AGI) below a certain level, have a valid Social Security number, use a filing status other than married filing separately, be a U.S. citizen or resident alien, have no foreign income, and not have investment income above a certain amount. The amount of credit varies depending on the number of the taxpayer's qualifying children and their AGI level.

Amount of Credit. The credit amount is determined by multiplying an applicable credit percentage by the individual's earned income that does not exceed a maximum earned income amount. In 2014, the maximum earned income amount for taxpayers with one qualifying child is $9,720, with two or more qualifying children is $13,650, and with no qualifying child is $6,480 (Rev. Proc. 2013-35). For 2015, the amounts are $9,880, $13,870, and $6,580, respectively (Rev. Proc. 2014-61). The credit amount is then reduced by a limitation amount determined by multiplying the applicable phaseout percentage by the excess of the amount of the individual's AGI (or earned income, if greater) over a phaseout amount. The earned income amount and the phaseout amount

---

References are to Standard Federal Tax Reports; Tax Research Consultant; and Practical Tax Explanations.

[16] ¶ 4870; FILEIND: 30,452; § 15,510.05

[17] ¶ 3850; INDIV: 57,200; § 12,005

[18] ¶ 4060; INDIV: 57,302, IN-DIV: 57,308; § 12,801, § 12,805

[19] ¶ 38,754; IRS: 33,108; § 12,801, § 12,805

[20] ¶ 4100; INTL: 3,554.05, IN-DIV: 57,308; § 12,801, § 12,805

[21] ¶ 4080; INDIV: 57,250; § 12,601

are adjusted yearly for inflation. The amount of allowable credit is determined through the use of the tables that appear at ¶ 87.

The credit and phaseout percentages limit the maximum amount of credit that may be claimed (Code Sec. 32(b)(1)). For 2014, the maximum earned income credit for taxpayers with one qualifying child is $3,305, with two qualifying children is $5,460, with three or more qualifying children is $6,143, and with no qualifying children is $496 (Rev. Proc. 2013-35). For 2015, the amounts are $3,359, $5,548, $6,242, and $503, respectively (Rev. Proc. 2014-61).

Credit Limitations. For 2014, the credit begins to phase out when taxpayers with a filing status of single, surviving spouse, or head of household and with one or more qualifying children have an AGI of $17,830, and with no qualifying children have an AGI of $8,110. Phaseout of the credit is complete when taxpayers with a filing status of single, surviving spouse, or head of household with one qualifying child have an AGI of $38,511; with two qualifying children have an AGI of $43,756; with three or more qualifying children have an AGI of $46,997; and with no qualifying children have an AGI of $14,590. The credit amount begins to phase out when taxpayers with a filing status of married filing jointly and with one or more qualifying children have an AGI of $23,260, and with no qualifying children have an AGI of $13,540. Phaseout of the credit is complete when taxpayers with a filing status of married filing jointly with one qualifying child have an AGI of $43,941; with two qualifying children have an AGI of $49,186; with three or more qualifying children have an AGI of $52,427; and with no qualifying children have an AGI of $20,020 (Rev. Proc. 2013-35).

For 2015, the credit begins to phase out when taxpayers with a filing status of single, surviving spouse, or head of household and with one or more qualifying children have an AGI of $18,110, and with no qualifying children have an AGI of $8,240. Phaseout of the credit is complete when taxpayers with a filing status of single, surviving spouse, or head of household with one qualifying child have an AGI of $39,131; with two qualifying children have an AGI of $44,454; with three or more qualifying children have an AGI of $47,747; and with no qualifying children have an AGI of $14,820. The credit amount begins to phase out when taxpayers with a filing status of married filing jointly and with one or more qualifying children have an AGI of $23,630, and with no qualifying children have an AGI of $13,750. Phaseout of the credit is complete when taxpayers with a filing status of married filing jointly with one qualifying child have an AGI of $44,651; with two qualifying children have an AGI of $49,974; with three or more qualifying children have an AGI of $53,267; and with no qualifying children have an AGI of $20,330 (Rev. Proc. 2014-61).

Earned Income. The credit is based on earned income, which includes all wages, salaries, tips, and other employee compensation including union strike benefits, plus the amount of the taxpayer's net earnings from self-employment determined with regard to the deduction for one-half of self-employment taxes (¶ 923). Earned income is determined without regard to community property laws (Code Sec. 32(c)(2)). It also does not include: (1) interest and dividends; (2) welfare benefits, including AFDC payments; (3) veterans' benefits; (4) pensions or annuities; (5) alimony; (6) Social Security benefits; (7) workers' compensation; (8) unemployment compensation; (9) taxable scholarships or fellowships that are not reported on Form W-2; (10) fixed or determinable periodic income of a nonresident alien not connected with a U.S. business (¶ 2431); (11) amounts received for services performed by prison inmates while in prison; or (12) payments received from work activities, including work associated with the refurbishing of public housing if sufficient private sector employment is not available and from community service programs (Sections 407(d)(4) and (7) of the Social Security Act). The earned income credit calculation is based on the taxpayer's AGI (Code Sec. 2(a)(2)(B) and (c)(2)).

Members of the Armed Forces. Taxpayers that are members of the Armed Forces are allowed to elect to treat combat pay that is otherwise excludable from gross income (¶ 895) as earned income for purposes of claiming the earned income credit (Code Sec. 32(c)(2)(B)(vi)). The election applies to all excludable combat pay received by the taxpayer.

13

TAX CREDITS

¶1322

Qualifying Child. A qualifying child for purposes of claiming the earned income credit is generally the same as for claiming the dependency exemption without regard to the support test (¶ 137A) (Code Sec. 32(c)(3)). In addition, the relationship, residency, and age tests must be met with the following modifications. For the residency test, the child must have the same principal place of abode as the taxpayer for more than half of the tax year and the abode must be located within the United States. A qualifying child for the earned income credit does not include a child who is married unless the taxpayer is entitled to claim him or her as a dependent. The taxpayer claiming the qualifying child must include the name, age and taxpayer identification number (¶ 2579) of the qualifying child on the return. Finally, the rules for determining among several taxpayers who may claim a child as a qualifying child for purposes of the earned income credit are the same as for determining who may claim a qualifying child for the dependency exemption (¶ 139).

No Qualifying Child. An individual who does not have a qualifying child may be eligible for the credit if: (1) the principal residence of the individual is in the United States for more than half of the tax year; (2) the individual, or the spouse of the individual, is at least age 25 and under age 65 before the close of the tax year; and (3) the individual is not claimed as a dependent by another (Code Sec. 32(c)(1)(A)(ii)).

Disqualifying Income. The earned income credit may not be claimed by taxpayers whose investment income exceeds $3,350 for 2014 ($3,400 for 2015) (Code Sec. 32(i); Rev. Proc. 2013-35; Rev. Proc. 2014-61). Disqualified income includes an individual's capital gain net income and net passive income in addition to interest, dividends, tax-exempt interest, and nonbusiness rents or royalties. The credit may also not be claimed by taxpayers who are not eligible to work in the United States. For example, a nonresident alien usually cannot claim an earned income credit (Code Sec. 32(c)(1)). Also, a person who claims a foreign earned income exclusion cannot claim an earned income credit (¶ 2402).

Claiming the Credit. Taxpayers claiming the credit must provide their Social Security or taxpayer identification) number, as well as the Social Security or taxpayer identification numbers of their spouse and dependents, if any. Failure to provide all required Social Security or taxpayer identification numbers is treated as a mathematical error (Code Sec. 6213(g)(2)).[22] Married persons must file a joint return in order to claim the credit. However, a married person living apart from a spouse under circumstances described at ¶ 173 need not file a joint return to claim the credit. Taxpayers with one or more qualifying children complete Schedule EIC of Form 1040 or Form 1040A. Taxpayers with no qualifying children may use Form 1040EZ to determine whether they are eligible to claim the earned income credit. Credit amounts are determined by using the tables at ¶ 87. The credit may be claimed only for a full 12-month tax year, except in the case of death.

1324. First-Time Homebuyer Credit (Expired). A refundable first-time homebuyer credit was available to qualified individuals and certain long-term homebuyers who purchased, or were under contract to purchase, a home before May 1, 2010, to be used as their principal residence (Code Sec. 36).[23] Special rules were enacted for military and government personal. The credit, however, must be recaptured in years after the purchase under certain circumstances. The credit and any recapture of the credit are reported on Form 5405.

Recapture Rules for Pre-2009 purchases. For residences purchased after April 8, 2008, and before January 1, 2009, the amount of the credit that could be claimed was equal to the lesser of 10 percent of the purchase price or $7,500 ($3,750, if married, filing separate). The $7,500 credit amount must be recaptured over a 15-year period beginning in the second year after the year in which the residence is purchased—the 2010 income tax return. The recapture amount is treated as an addition to tax for each year of the recapture period and is equal to 6.67 percent of the credit amount claimed (or 1/15 of the credit amount). If the taxpayer disposes of or ceases to use the home as a principal

---

References are to Standard Federal Tax Reports; Tax Research Consultant; and Practical Tax Explanations.

[22] ¶ 37,545; IRS: 27,206.50;   [23] ¶ 4186; INDIV: 57,950;
§ 39,515.10   § 13,010

¶1324

residence within the 15-year recapture period, any remaining amount of the credit must be recaptured in the year of disposition.

Recapture Rules for Post-2008 purchases. The amount of the first-time homebuyer credit claimed must be recaptured if the home, purchased after December 31, 2008, ceases to be the principal residence of the taxpayer at any time within the 36-month period from the date of purchase. The recapture amount is claimed as an addition to tax in the year the property is disposed of by the taxpayer or ceases to be the taxpayer's principal residence. The recapture amount cannot exceed the amount of gain from the sale of the home to an unrelated third party. Exceptions are provided to the required recapture due to:

- death of the taxpayer;

- involuntary conversion of the property (¶ 1713) if the taxpayer acquires a new principal residence within two years; however, the accelerated recapture rule will apply to the new principal residence during the remainder of the recapture period;

- transfer between spouses or incident to a divorce; However, the transferee steps into the shoes of the transferor in respect to the recapture and accelerated recapture rules.

Special Rules for Certain Governmental and Military Personnel. Certain government officials and Armed Forces personnel serving on qualified official extended duty for at least 90 days during the period beginning after December 31, 2008, and before May 1, 2010, could claim the first-time homebuyer credit on any purchase made before May 1, 2011. The same one-year time extension also applied to purchases that were under written binding contract before May 1, 2011, and the purchase was completed before July 1, 2011.

Recapture of the credit amount is waived in the case of disposition or cessation of the use of the home as a principal residence in the event the individual (if married, their spouse) receives orders for qualified official extended duty service. Qualified official extended duty service is defined as service on qualified official extended duty as a member of the Armed Forces, the Foreign Service, or an employee of the intelligence community (Code Sec. 36(f) and (h)).

1326A. Refundable Adoption Credit (Expired). For tax years beginning after December 31, 2009, and before January 1, 2012, taxpayers could claim a refundable credit based on the amount of qualified adoption expenses incurred for adopting an eligible child (Code Sec. 36C).[24] The credit was phased out ratably for taxpayers with a modified adjusted gross income (AGI) over a threshold amount. The adoption credit is a nonrefundable personal credit for tax years beginning after December 31, 2011 (¶ 1307).

1327. Refundable Long-Term Unused Minimum Tax Credit (Expired). For individuals with a long-term unused minimum tax credit for tax years before January 1, 2013, the minimum tax credit allowable for that year (¶ 1309) was not less than the AMT refundable credit amount, regardless of the minimum tax credit otherwise allowed to the taxpayer (Code Sec. 53(e)).[25] The credit was calculated on Form 8801.

A long-term unused minimum tax credit for a tax year was the portion of the minimum tax credit attributable to the adjusted net minimum tax (¶ 1309) for tax years before the third tax year immediately preceding such tax year. For this purpose, the credits were treated as allowed on a first-in, first-out (FIFO) basis.

The AMT refundable credit amount was, with respect to any tax year, the amount (not in excess of the long-term unused minimum tax credit for such tax year) equal to the greater of: (1) 50 percent of the long-term unused minimum tax credit for such tax year or (2) the amount (if any) of the AMT refundable credit amount determined for the taxpayer's preceding tax year.

References are to Standard Federal Tax Reports; Tax Research Consultant; and Practical Tax Explanations.

[24] ¶ 4198; INDIV: 57,350;   [25] ¶ 4870; FILEIND: 30,452;
§ 12,301   § 15,510.15

1329. Credit for Federal Tax on Gasoline, Special Fuels. A credit for federal excise taxes on gasoline and special fuels may be taken where the fuel item is used for: (1) farming purposes, (2) nonhighway purposes of a trade or business, (3) operation of intercity, local, or school buses, or (4) certain nontaxable purposes (Code Sec. 34).[26] The credit is computed on Form 4136 or the taxpayer can file a claim for refund on Form 8849 or a credit against fuel tax liability on Form 720.

1330. Credit for Capital Gain Tax. Undistributed capital gain of a regulated invest-ment company (RIC) must be included proportionately in the gross income of its shareholders (Code Sec. 852(b)(3)). The capital gain tax that the company pays on this gain is treated as having been paid by the shareholders and is allowed as a credit against the tax (Code Sec. 852(b)(3)(D)(ii)).[27] In order to claim the credit, Copy B of Form 2439 must be attached to the taxpayer's return (¶ 2305).

Health Care Credits

1331. Health Insurance Premium Assistance Refundable Credit. Effective for tax years ending after December 31, 2013, certain individuals who purchase qualified health care coverage through an American Health Benefit Exchange are entitled to a refund-able income tax credit equal to the premium assistance credit amount (Code Sec. 36B(a)).[28]

Eligibility for Premium Credit. A qualified individual is defined as a person who:

- is seeking to enroll in a qualified health plan in the individual market offered through an Exchange and residing in the state in which the Exchange is established,

- has a household income of at least 100 percent, but no more than 400 percent, of the federal poverty line (FPL) for a family of that size,

- if married, must file a joint return, and

- cannot be claimed as a dependent on another taxpayer's return (¶ 137) (Code Sec. 36B(c)(1)).

Lawful resident aliens who are ineligible for Medicaid and have household income below 100 percent of the FPL for a family of that size are imputed to have a household income equal to 100 percent of the FPL and eligible for the credit (Reg. § 1.36B-2(b)(5)). An individual who is not a U.S. citizen, national, or alien lawfully present in the United States is not eligible (Code Sec. 36B(e)). Qualified individuals do not include individuals who are incarcerated unless the incarceration is pending the disposition of charges (Code Sec. 5000A). The individual may, however, be allowed a tax credit if a family member is enrolled in a qualified plan (Reg. § 1.36B-2(b)(4)).

Family size is equal to the number of individuals the taxpayer is allowed as personal and dependency exemptions for the tax year. This may include individuals who are not subject to or are exempt from the Code Sec. 5000A penalty (Reg. § 1.36B-1(d)). House-hold income equals the taxpayer's modified adjusted gross income (MAGI) and includes all income of individuals who are the taxpayer's dependents if a tax return is required to be filed. Household income does not include the MAGI of a family member who files a tax return solely to report tax under a different Code section (i.e. other than Code Sec. 5000A), such as a Code Sec. 72(t) early distribution penalty (Reg. § 1.36B-1(e)(1)(ii)). MAGI is AGI increased by any amount of excluded foreign income, foreign housing allowance expenses, tax-exempt interest, and Social Security and tier 1 Railroad Retire-ment benefits (Code Sec. 36B(d)(2)(B)).

Credit Amount. The premium assistance credit amount for any tax year is the sum of the premium assistance amounts for all of the taxpayer's coverage months during the tax year (Code Sec. 36B(b)). The premium assistance amount for any coverage month is the lesser of:

References are to Standard Federal Tax Reports; Tax Research Consultant; and Practical Tax Explanations.

[26] ¶ 4150; BUSEXP: 54,800; § 13,501

[27] ¶ 26,420; RIC: 3,260; § 19,205.05

[28] ¶ 4196; HEALTH: 3,300; § 42,015.05

- the monthly premium for one or more qualified health plans offered in the individual market Exchange within a state covering the taxpayer, the taxpayer's spouse, or any dependent of the taxpayer who is enrolled through the Exchange, or

- the excess, if any, of the adjusted monthly premium for the applicable second lowest cost silver plan with respect to the taxpayer over an amount equal to $\frac{1}{12}$th of the product of the applicable percentage and the taxpayer's household income for the tax year.

Under proposed regulations, to apply to tax years ending after December 31, 2013, but which may be relied on for tax years ending before January 1, 2015, if a qualified health plan is terminated before the last day of a month and, as a result, the issuer reduces or refunds a portion of the monthly premium, the premium assistance amount for the coverage month is prorated (Prop. Reg. § 1.36B-3(d)(2)).

Coverage Month. A coverage month is any month in which the taxpayer, the taxpayer's spouse, or any dependent is covered by a qualified health plan enrolled in through an Exchange and the premium is paid by the taxpayer or through advance payment of the premium assistance credit (Code Sec. 36B(c)(2)). A coverage month does *not* include any month that the individual is eligible for minimum essential coverage outside the individual market. A month also is *not* a coverage month if the taxpayer's share of premiums is not paid in full by the unextended due date for filing the taxpayer's income tax return for the tax year (Reg. § 1.36B-3(c)(1)). An employee is *not* considered to be eligible for minimum essential coverage outside of the market if the coverage is an employer-sponsored plan, including a grandfathered health plan, and either of these exceptions apply:

- the employee's required contribution is unaffordable for the employee or a related individual—it would exceed 9.5 percent of the employee's household income for 2014 (9.56 percent for 2015 (Rev. Proc. 2014-37)); and

- the plan provides less than 60 percent coverage for total allowed costs.

An employee uses the employee's cost for self-only coverage to determine whether the coverage is affordable—if the required contribution would exceed 9.5 percent of the employee's household income for 2014 (Reg. § 1.36B-2(c)(3)(v)(A)). The affordability of coverage for any related individuals of an employee is also determined by using the employee's cost of self-only coverage.

The applicable second lowest cost silver plan is the second lowest cost silver plan of the individual market Exchange in the rating area where the taxpayer resides. It must be offered through the same Exchange offering the qualified health plan and provide (1) self-only coverage for single taxpayers with no dependents or those who purchase self-only coverage, and (2) family coverage for all other taxpayers (Code Sec. 36B(b)(3)). The adjusted monthly premium for an applicable second lowest cost silver plan is the monthly premium that would be charged for the plan if each individual covered under a qualified health plan were covered by that silver plan, and the premium was adjusted only for the age of each individual pursuant to section 2701 of the Public Health Service Act. The applicable percentage is between 2.0 percent and 9.5 percent of a taxpayer's household income for any tax year with respect to a taxpayer whose household income is between 100 and 400 percent of the FPL for that tax year; for the 2015 tax year, the applicable percentage is between 2.01 percent and 9.56 percent (Rev. Proc. 2014-37). If there is at least one silver level plan offered on an Exchange that does not cover all members of a taxpayer's coverage family under one policy and premium, the premium for the applicable plan is the single premium or the combination of premiums that is the second lowest cost silver option for covering the entire family (Reg. § 1.36B-3(f)(3)).

The IRS has provided the following rules for determining, for purposes of the premium tax credit, whether, or when, certain individuals are eligible for minimum essential coverage (1) under the Medicaid, Medicare, Children's Health Insurance Program (CHIP), or TRICARE programs, or (2) through self-funded student health plans and state high risk pools (Notice 2013-41):

- An individual who may not re-enroll in CHIP for a period of time called the lockout period due to a failure to pay premiums is treated as eligible for CHIP and not eligible for qualified health plan coverage subsidized by the premium tax credit during the lockout period.

- An individual who is terminated from Medicaid or CHIP for failure to pay premiums is treated as eligible for Medicaid or CHIP during any period for which the individual would be eligible for Medicaid or CHIP except for the failure to pay premiums.

- An individual who may not enroll in CHIP during a pre-enrollment waiting period may be eligible for qualified health plan coverage subsidized by the premium tax credit during this period.

- An individual is eligible for minimum essential coverage under Medicaid or Medicare in the following circumstances only upon a favorable determination of eligibility by the responsible agency: (1) Medicaid coverage requiring a finding of disability or blindness; and (2) Medicare coverage based solely on a finding of disability or illness.

- An individual is eligible for minimum essential coverage under the following programs only if the individual is enrolled in the coverage: (1) Medicare Part A coverage requiring payment of premiums; (2) state high risk pools; (3) student health plans; and (4) TRICARE programs.

Advance Payment of Credit. The premium assistance credit must be reduced, but not below zero, by the amount of any advance payment of the credit (Code Sec. 36B(f)). If the advance payments for a tax year exceed the premium assistance credit allowed, the excess is an increase to the tax imposed for the tax year. For taxpayers with household incomes less than 400 percent of the FPL for the tax year, the increase is limited to between $600 and $2,500 ($300 and $1,250 for unmarried taxpayers other than surviving spouses and heads of household).

1332. Health Insurance Costs Credit. Eligible individuals may claim a refundable tax credit for the cost of qualified health insurance for themselves and qualified family members during each eligible coverage month. The credit is 72.5 percent of the costs during coverage months beginning after February 12, 2011, and ending before January 1, 2014. The credit is 80 percent during coverage months beginning after April 30, 2009, and ending on or before February 12, 2011 (Code Sec. 35).[29] An eligible coverage month occurs when, on the first day of the month during the taxpayer's tax year, the taxpayer: (1) is an eligible individual; (2) is covered by a qualified health insurance plan on which the taxpayer paid the premiums; (3) has no other specified coverage, including under Medicare or COBRA; and (4) is not imprisoned by any federal, state, or local authority. Taxpayers determine their eligibility and claim the credit on Form 8885 and attaching to their return along with copies of the required documentation. See also IRS Pub. 502.

> **Comment:** Absent further legislation, the health insurance costs credit has expired for tax years beginning after December 31, 2013. For the latest legislative updates, visit our website www.CCHGroup.com/TaxUpdates.

Eligible Individuals. The credit is available only to individuals receiving or who are eligible to receive trade adjustment assistance (TAA) (or TAA-alternative payments) and retirees age 55 or older receiving benefits from the Pension Benefit Guaranty Corporation (PBGC) (Code Sec. 35(c)). A qualifying family member of an eligible individual includes the taxpayer's spouse and any dependents to which the taxpayer is entitled to an exemption (¶ 137) (Code Sec. 35(d)). A spouse is not considered a qualifying family member if the taxpayer is married at the end of the year, both are considered eligible individuals, and each files a separate income tax return (Code Sec. 35(g)(5)). However, the rules for head of household status relating to separated parents and individuals living apart for six months apply (¶ 173). In the case of separated or divorced parents, dependents are considered qualifying family members only for the custodial parent (¶ 139A) (Code Sec. 35(d)(2)).

References are to Standard Federal Tax Reports; Tax Research Consultant; and Practical Tax Explanations.

[29] ¶ 4170; HEALTH: 15,152; § 42,315

Qualifying Premiums. Premiums paid by taxpayers for coverage in a qualified health insurance plan as defined in Code Sec. 35(e)(1) are to be taken into account in determining the health insurance costs credit. Qualified health insurance does *not* include either a flexible spending or similar arrangement (¶ 2041) or any insurance whose coverage is substantially for "excepted benefits" under Code Sec. 9832(c) (Code Sec. 35(e)(3)).

Insurance coverage that qualifies as other specified coverage under Code Sec. 35(f) includes: (1) any insurance which is considered to be for medical care under a health plan maintained by the employer of the taxpayer or the taxpayer's spouse where at least 50 percent of the cost is paid or incurred by the employer; (2) any insurance coverage under a cafeteria plan (¶ 2045) in which the premiums are paid or incurred by the employer in lieu of a right to receive cash benefits or other qualified benefits under a cafeteria plan; (3) participation in Medicare, Medicaid, or State Child Health Insurance Program (SCHIP); and (4) participation in a health benefits plan for federal employees and military personnel. The credit is also coordinated with the COBRA premium assistance provision (¶ 1391) to prevent double benefits.

Coordination with Other Provisions. Amounts taken into account for the determination of the health insurance costs credit may not be used in computing either the health insurance costs for the self-employed deduction (¶ 908) or the itemized deduction for medical/dental costs (¶ 1015). Amounts received from health savings account (HSAs) (¶ 2035) or Archer medical saving accounts (¶ 2037) may not be used to compute the health insurance costs credit. Payment made for the benefit of a third party who is not a qualifying family member cannot be included in the amount of premiums paid for qualified health insurance in determining the credit (Code Sec. 35(g)(1), (2) and (3)).

Advance Payment. The advance payment program makes monthly payments on behalf of eligible individuals directly to providers of qualified health insurance. The advance payments cannot equal more than the credit percentage (72.5, 80, or 65 percent) of the anticipated health insurance costs of the eligible taxpayer. The aggregate amount of all advance payments during the tax year reduces the health insurance costs credit amount dollar for dollar but not below zero (Code Secs. 35(g)(8)(A) and 7527). The Secretary of the Treasury is allowed to refund to the taxpayer amounts paid prior to the advance payment program making premiums payments.

Additional Requirements for State Plans. State health plans must make an election to be considered a qualified health insurance plan for the health insurance costs credit. In addition to the election, several additional requirements must be satisfied (Code Sec. 35(e)(2)). The IRS maintains a list of available qualified state plans on the internet at http://www.irs.gov/Individuals/HCTC:-List-of-State-Qualified-Health-Plans.

1333. Small Employer Health Insurance Credit. An eligible small employer may claim a tax credit if it makes nonelective contributions that pay for at least one-half of the cost of health insurance premiums for the coverage of its participating employees (Code Sec. 45R).[30] The credit is computed on Form 8941 and is claimed as a component of the general business credit (¶ 1365).

Credit Amount. The credit amount for tax years beginning after 2013 is equal to 50 percent of the lesser of:

(1) the total amount of nonelective contributions the employer makes on behalf of its employees during the tax year under a contribution arrangement for premiums for qualified health plans offered to its employees through a state-sponsored market exchange (i.e., through a Small Business Health Options Program (SHOP)), or

(2) the total amount of nonelective contributions that would have been made during the tax year if each employee taken into account in item (1) had enrolled in

---

References are to Standard Federal Tax Reports; Tax Research Consultant; and Practical Tax Explanations.

[30] ¶ 4500ZN; HEALTH: 9,200; § 42,115.05

a qualified health plan that had a premium equal to the average premium for the small group market in the rating area in which the employee enrolls for coverage (Code Sec. 45R(b)).

The credit amount for tax years beginning before 2014 is equal to 35 percent of the lesser of:

(1) the total amount of nonelective contributions the employer makes on behalf of its employees during the tax year under a contribution arrangement for the payment of premiums for qualified health insurance coverage (as defined in Code Sec. 9832(b)(1)) of its employees, or

(2) the total amount of nonelective contributions that would have been made during the tax year if each employee taken into account in item (1) had enrolled in a qualified health plan that had a premium equal to the average premium for the small group market in the state in which the employer is offering health insurance coverage or the area within the state specified by the Secretary of Health and Human Services (HHS) (Code Sec. 45R(a), (b) and (g)).

The contribution arrangement must require an employer to make a nonelective contribution on behalf of each employee who enrolls in a qualified health plan offered by the employer in an amount equal to a uniform percentage, but not less than 50 percent, of the premium cost of the plan (Code Sec. 45R(d)(4) and (g)(3)). An employer contribution is considered a nonelective contribution so long as it is not made through a salary reduction arrangement (Code Sec. 45R(e)(3)). For tax years beginning after 2013, the contribution arrangement must offer the insurance through an Exchange. For tax years beginning before 2014, the arrangement is not required to offer the insurance through an Exchange.

Credit Phaseout. The credit amount is reduced, but not below zero, by the sum of:

- the credit amount multiplied by the number of the employer's full-time equivalent employees for the tax year in excess of 10, divided by 15; and

- the credit amount multiplied by the employer's average annual wages in excess of the applicable dollar amount for the tax year ($25,800 in 2015, $25,400 in 2014), divided by the applicable dollar amount (Code Sec. 45R(c); Rev. Proc. 2014-61; Rev. Proc. 2013-35).

Eligible Small Employer Defined. An employer determines its status as an eligible small employer each tax year. An employer is an eligible small employer if, during the tax year:

- the employer has 25 or fewer full-time equivalent employees;

- the average annual wages of these employees is not greater than twice the applicable dollar amount for the tax year ($25,800 in 2015, $25,400 in 2014); and

- the employer has a qualified health care arrangement in effect (Code Sec. 45R(d)(1); Rev. Proc. 2014-61;Rev. Proc. 2013-35).

Full-Time Equivalent Employee Defined. The number of full-time equivalent employees during a tax year is equal to the total number of hours for which employees were paid wages by the employer divided by 2,080. The result, if not a whole number, is rounded to the next lowest whole number. In making this computation, only the first 2,080 hours of each employee's wages are taken into account. Hours in excess of this amount are not counted (Code Sec. 45R(d)(2)). For purposes of determining average annual wages and the number of full-time equivalent employees, hours of service worked by, and wages paid to, a seasonal worker are not taken into account unless the worker works for the employer on more than 120 days during the tax year (Code Sec. 45R(d)(5)(A)).

Employee Defined. For purposes of the credit, the following individuals are not considered employees (Code Sec. 45R(e)(1)):

(1) any self-employed individual (as defined in Code Sec. 401(c)(1));

(2) any two-percent shareholder (as defined in Code Sec. 1372(b)) of an eligible small business which is an S corporation;

(3) any five-percent owner (as defined in Code Sec. 416(i)(1)(B)(i)) of an eligible small business; or

(4) any individual who bears any of the familial relationships of a qualifying relative (¶ 137B) to an individual described in items (1), (2), or (3), above, or is a qualifying relative dependent with the same principal abode as the individual and is a member of the individual's household.

Leased employees as defined in Code Sec. 414(a) are considered employees (Code Sec. 45R(e)(1)).

Wages Defined. Wages for purposes of the credit are defined by reference to Code Sec. 3121(a), relating to the definition of wages for purposes of the Federal Insurance Contributions Act (FICA) but without regard to any dollar limitation (Code Sec. 45R(e)(4)) (¶ 2648).

Additional Rules. The following special rules described in Code Sec. 52 relating to the work opportunity credit (Code Sec. 51) apply to the small employer health insurance credit (Code Sec. 45R(e)(5)(B)):

• an estate or trust must apportion the credit between itself and its beneficiaries based on income allocable to each (Code Sec. 52(d));

• in computing the credit, a regulated investment company (RIC), real estate investment trust (REIT), and cooperative organization (Code Sec. 1381(a)) must apply rules similar to the rules provided in Code Sec. 46(e) and (h), as in effect prior to the date of enactment of the Revenue Reconciliation Act of 1990 (P.L. 101-508) (Code Sec. 52(e)).

A third special rule seems to suggest that the small employer health insurance credit is not available to a tax-exempt organization, other than a tax-exempt cooperative described in Code Sec. 521 (Code Secs. 45R(e)(5)(B) and Code Sec. 52(c)). This reference appears to be erroneous. In fact, Code Sec. 45R provides special computation rules applicable to certain tax-exempt organizations. See following, under *Special Computation Rules for Tax-Exempt Eligible Small Employers.*

Certain Persons Treated as Single Employer. All controlled groups, partnerships, and affiliated service groups treated as a single employer under Code Sec. 414(b), (c), (m), or (o) are treated as one employer (Code Sec. 45R(e)(5)(A)).

General Business Credit. The small employer health insurance credit is a component of the general business credit (Code Sec. 38(b)(36)) (¶ 1365). Any portion of the credit that is not claimed by the expiration of the 20-year carryforward period may be claimed as a deduction in the first tax year after expiration of the carryforward period (Code Sec. 196(c)(14)).

Deduction for Premiums Is Reduced by Credit Amount. The deduction for employer-paid premiums for qualified health plans or, in the case of tax years beginning before 2014 for health insurance coverage, is reduced by the amount of the small employer health insurance credit determined with respect to those premiums (Code Sec. 280C(h)).

Credit Period After 2013. The small employer health insurance credit may only be claimed for two consecutive tax years beginning after 2013 (Code Sec. 45R(g)). The credit period is the two-consecutive-tax-year period beginning with the first tax year in which the employer offers one or more qualified health plans to its employees through an SHOP Exchange (Code Sec. 45R(e)(2)). The credit period does not begin until the first year the employer files a return claiming the credit (Reg. § 1.45R-1(a)(3)).

No credit period is treated as beginning with a tax year beginning before 2014 (Code Sec. 45R(g)(1)). A transitional rule applies to an employer's first tax year beginning in 2014, if:

¶1333

(1) the employer's health plan year does not begin on the first day of the tax year;

(2) the employer has a health plan in effect as of August 26, 2013;

(3) the employer offers one or more qualified health plans to its employees through a SHOP Exchange as of the first day of its 2014 plan year.

Such an employer is treated as if coverage was offered through a SHOP Exchange for the entire 2014 tax year if the health coverage that was provided from the first day of the tax year through the day prior to the first day of the 2014 plan year would have qualified for a credit under the rules applicable in the 2013 tax year discussed previously. The 2014 tax year begins the start of the two-year credit period if the employer uses this transitional rule (Reg. § 1.45R-3(i)(1)).

Special Computation Rules for Tax-Exempt Eligible Small Employers. The credit percentage for a tax-exempt eligible small employer is 35 percent for tax years beginning after 2013, and 25 percent for tax years beginning before 2014 (Code Sec. 45R(b) and (g)(2)(A)). A tax-exempt eligible small employer is an eligible small employer that is a Code Sec. 501(c) organization that is exempt from tax (Code Sec. 45R(f)(2)). Other tax-exempt organizations generally are not eligible to claim the credit. However, a farmers' cooperative is eligible to claim the credit as a taxable employer if it otherwise meets the requirements (Notice 2010-82). If the credit exceeds the amount of payroll taxes of the organization during the calendar year in which the tax year begins, then the credit amount is limited to the amount of the payroll taxes (Code Sec. 45R(f)(1)).

Payroll taxes are defined as amounts required to be withheld from the tax-exempt organization's employees for Medicare under Code Sec. 3101(b) and income tax withholding under Code Sec. 3401(a), and amounts of the taxes imposed on the tax-exempt organization for Medicare under Code Sec. 3111(b) (Code Sec. 45R(f)(3)(A)). The special rule contained in Code Sec. 24(d)(2)(C), which treats amounts paid pursuant to an agreement entered into by American employers with respect to foreign affiliates that are the equivalent of social security taxes imposed by Code Sec. 3101 or railroad retirement taxes (Code Sec. 3201(a)), applies (Code Sec. 45R(f)(3)(B)).

Energy Credits

1341. Nonbusiness Energy Property Credit. A nonrefundable tax credit is available to individuals for the installation of nonbusiness energy property, such as residential exterior doors and windows, insulation, heat pumps, furnaces, central air conditioners, and water heaters (Code Sec. 25C).[31] The credit applies to qualified energy efficiency improvements and qualified energy property placed in service before January 1, 2014. The property must be installed in, or on, a dwelling unit in the United States that is owned and used by the taxpayer as the taxpayer's principal residence. Original use of the property must commence with the taxpayer. The credit is claimed on Form 5695.

> **Comment:** Absent further legislation, the nonbusiness energy property credit has expired effective for property placed in service after December 31, 2013. For the latest legislative updates, visit our website www.CCHGroup.com/TaxUpdates.

The credit may be claimed against regular tax liability and alternative minimum tax liability. An unused credit may not be carried forward (Notice 2013-70). The basis of the residence is reduced by the allowed credit (Code Sec. 25C(f); Instructions to Form 5695).

Credit Amount. For property placed in service in 2011, 2012, or 2013, the credit amount is equal to 10 percent of the amount paid or incurred for qualified energy efficiency improvements during the tax year, and 100 percent of the amount paid or incurred for qualified energy property during the tax year, up to a set amount depending on the type of property (Code Sec. 25C(b)). The maximum credit amount for qualified energy property is $200 for exterior windows and skylights, reduced by the aggregate

---

References are to Standard Federal Tax Reports; Tax Research Consultant; and Practical Tax Explanations.

[31] ¶ 3839; INDIV: 57,800;
§ 13,201

credit allowed for exterior windows and skylights in prior years; $50 for any advanced main air circulating fan; $150 for any qualified furnace or boiler; and $300 for any other item. For all nonbusiness energy property, there is a $500 maximum lifetime credit.

Qualified Energy Efficiency Improvements. Qualified energy improvements include any energy efficient building envelope component that meets certain energy conservation criteria (Code Sec. 25C(c)). A building envelope component is defined as any insulation material or system which is designed to prevent heat loss or gain, exterior windows (including skylights), exterior doors, and any metal roof with either pigmented coating or cooling granules designed to reduce heat gain.

Qualified Energy Property. Qualified energy property is defined as energy-efficient building property, qualified natural gas, propane, or oil furnace or hot water boiler, or an advance main air circulating fan that meet specific performance and quality standards (Code Sec. 25C(d)). Qualified energy-efficient building property includes electric heat pump water heaters, qualified electric heat pumps, qualified central air conditioners, and qualified stoves that use biomass fuels.

1342. Residential Energy Efficient Property Credit. A nonrefundable tax credit is available to help individual taxpayers pay for residential alternative energy equipment installed on or in connection with a dwelling unit located in the United States and used as a residence by the taxpayer (Code Sec. 25D).[32] The credit is available for the cost of eligible solar water heaters, solar electricity equipment, fuel cell plants, qualified small wind energy property, and qualified geothermal heat pump property placed in service before January 1, 2017 (Code Sec. 25D(g)). Cooperative and condominium dwellers can claim the credit by splitting the cost of installing equipment with other unit owners. The credit is claimed on Form 5695.

Credit Amount. The credit amount is equal to 30 percent of the cost of eligible property, but the maximum amount of credit for the installation of qualified fuel cell property for any tax year is $500 per half kilowatt hour (Code Sec. 25D(b)(1)). The credit cannot exceed the excess of the sum of the taxpayer's regular tax and alternative minimum tax minus the sum of the taxpayer's other personal nonrefundable credits (plus the foreign tax credit) (Code Sec. 25D(c)(1)). Any excess amount is carried over and added to the credit amount for the next tax year. The credit allowed reduces the basis of the residence (Code Sec. 25D(f); Instructions to Form 5696).

Qualifying Property. Qualifying solar heating property is any property used to heat water for use in a dwelling unit that receives at least half of its energy from the sun. None of the cost allocated to heat a swimming pool or hot tub may be considered a qualified expenditure. Qualifying solar electric property is any property that generates electricity from solar energy to be used in a dwelling unit. Qualified fuel cell property is any fuel cell property with a nameplate capacity of least 0.5 kilowatt hours of electricity generated by using an electrochemical process with an electricity-generating efficiency greater than 30 percent. Qualified small wind energy property is any wind turbine that generates electricity for use in the residence of the taxpayer. It does not include any wind facility for which a credit can be claimed for electricity produced from renewable resources (¶ 1365N). Qualified geothermal heat pump property is any property that uses the ground or ground water as a thermal source to heat a dwelling unit (Code Sec. 25D(d)).

Alternative Motor Vehicle Credit

1345. Alternative Motor Vehicle Credit. Taxpayers who buy a motor vehicle may be eligible for the alternative motor vehicle credit (Code Sec. 30B).[33] The credit amount is equal to the sum of the following component credits: (1) a qualified fuel cell motor vehicle credit (¶ 1346); (2) an advanced lean burn technology motor vehicle credit (¶ 1347); (3) a qualified hybrid motor vehicle credit (¶ 1348); (4) a qualified alternative motor vehicle credit (¶ 1349); and (5) a plug-in conversion credit (¶ 1350). Of these five

---

References are to Standard Federal Tax Reports; Tax Research Consultant; and Practical Tax Explanations.

[32] ¶ 3844; INDIV: 57,850; § 13,301

[33] ¶ 4059A; INDIV: 57,702; § 12,905.05

component credits, only the qualified fuel cell motor vehicle credit is available to be claimed currently. The individual components comprising the alternative motor vehicle credit are calculated based on various factors such as vehicle weight, vehicle fuel efficiency, lifetime fuel savings, etc. Each has a different phaseout or termination rule. The credit amount claimed is the sum of the components applicable to a particular vehicle, whether used for personal or business purposes. The credit is claimed on Form 8910.

Common Requirements. There are distinct requirements for each of the five components of the credit. However, three requirements are common to each of the components: (1) the original use of the vehicle must commence with the taxpayer; (2) the vehicle must be acquired for use or lease by the taxpayer and not for resale; (3) the vehicle must be made by a manufacturer; and (4) the vehicle must be primarily used in the United States.

Any credit amount claimed under the alternative motor vehicle credit for personal use is treated as a nonrefundable personal credit (¶ 1315) (Code Sec. 30B(g)(2)). Taxpayers with qualified motor vehicles that are used in a trade or business and subject to depreciation claim the alternative motor vehicle credit as a part of, and subject to, the rules of the general business credit (¶ 1365). Thus, any unused credit in a tax year is eligible to be carried back three years and forward 20 years. A seller claiming the alternative motor vehicle credit for a vehicle sold to a tax-exempt entity can only claim the credit as a part of the general business credit (Code Sec. 30B(h)(6)).

1346. Fuel Cell Motor Vehicle Credit. The first component of the alternative motor vehicle credit is a qualified fuel cell motor vehicle credit for qualifying vehicles placed in service after December 31, 2005, and purchased before January 1, 2015 (Code Sec. 30B(b)).[34] In addition to the common requirements for qualifying vehicles (¶ 1345), there are specific requirements for a vehicle to be classified as a qualified fuel cell motor vehicle. The vehicle must be propelled by power derived from one or more cells which convert chemical energy directly into electricity by combining oxygen with hydrogen fuel. In addition, if the vehicle is a passenger vehicle or light truck, it must be certified to meet specific environmental emission standards.

The amount of the credit is calculated based on the gross vehicle weight rating (GVWR) of the vehicle, supplemented by the fuel efficiency of the vehicle relative to the 2002 model-year city fuel economy. The credit can range from $8,000 for vehicles under 8,500 pounds GVWR and up to $40,000 for vehicles over 26,000 pounds GVWR. Qualified fuel cell vehicles that meet the definition of either a passenger automobile or light truck and meet certain standards for increased fuel efficiency may increase their credit amount based on the increase in fuel efficiency over the 2002 city fuel economy standards. The increase in the credit amount ranges from $1,000 up to $4,000. A list of qualified fuel cell vehicles eligible for the credit, and their credit amount is available on the IRS website at http://www.irs.gov/Businesses/Corporations/Qualified-Fuel-Cell-Vehicles.

1347. Advanced Lean Burn Technology Vehicle Credit (Expired). The second component of the alternative motor vehicle credit is the advanced lean burn technology motor vehicle credit for qualifying vehicles placed in service after December 31, 2005, and purchased before January 1, 2011 (Code Sec. 30B(c)).[35] In addition to the common requirements for qualifying vehicles (¶ 1345), there were specific requirements for classification as an advanced lean burn technology motor vehicle. An advanced lean burn technology motor vehicle was a passenger vehicle or light truck with an internal combustion engine that: (1) was designed to operate primarily using more air than is necessary for complete combustion of the fuel, (2) incorporated direct injection, and (3) achieved at least 125 percent of the 2002 model year city fuel economy. Additionally, 2004-and-later model vehicles had to meet specified environmental emission standards based on gross vehicle weight rating (GVWR).

References are to Standard Federal Tax Reports; Tax Research Consultant; and Practical Tax Explanations.

[34] ¶ 4059A; INDIV: 57,704; § 12,905.10

[35] ¶ 4059A; INDIV: 57,706; § 12,905.15

The credit amount was calculated based on the fuel efficiency of the vehicle relative to the 2002 model year city fuel economy supplemented by a conservation credit based on the vehicle's lifetime fuel savings. The range of the credit amount was from $400 to $2,400. The credit amount could have been increased by a conservation credit, which ranges from $250 to $1,000. The advanced lean burn technology motor vehicle credit began to phase out after a manufacturer sold a specific quantity of qualifying vehicles. A list of advanced lean-burn technology vehicles eligible for the credit, and their credit amount is still available on the IRS website at http://www.irs.gov/Businesses/Corporations/Qualified-Advanced-Lean-Burn-Technology-Vehicles.

1348. Hybrid Motor Vehicle Credit (Expired). The third component of the alternative motor vehicle credit was the qualified hybrid motor vehicle credit for qualifying vehicles placed in service after December 31, 2005, and purchased before either January 1, 2010, or January 1, 2011, depending on the size of the vehicle (Code Sec. 30B(d)).[36] The qualified hybrid motor vehicle credit for passenger automobiles or light trucks with a gross vehicle weight rating (GVWR) of no more than 8,500 pounds terminated for vehicles purchased after December 31, 2010. The credit for heavy vehicles terminated for vehicles purchased after December 31, 2009. In addition to the common requirements for qualifying vehicles (¶ 1345), there were requirements specific to the qualified hybrid motor vehicle credit. The vehicle had to draw propulsion energy from both an internal combustion or heat engine and a rechargeable energy storage system. In addition, the vehicle must have had received a certificate of conformity that it meets or exceeds specific environmental emission standards. The vehicle must have also met the maximum available power standards required for the vehicle's GVWR.

The amount of the credit allowed for a qualified vehicle with a GVWR of 8,500 pounds or less was the sum of the amounts determined for fuel economy and the conservation credit. The credit amount ranged from $400 up to $2,400. The credit amount for qualified hybrid motor vehicles that are passenger automobiles or light trucks with a GVWR of no more than 8,500 pounds could be increased by a conservation credit, which ranges from $250 up to $1,000. Thus, the credit ranged from $400 to $3,400. The hybrid motor vehicle credit began to phase out after a manufacturer sold a specific quantity of qualifying vehicles. A list of qualified hybrid vehicle eligible for the credit, and their credit amount is still available on the IRS website at http://www.irs.gov/uac/Summary-of-the-Credit-for-Qualified-Hybrid-Vehicles.

1349. Alternative Fuel Motor Vehicle Credit (Expired). The fourth component of the alternative motor vehicle credit was the qualified alternative fuel motor vehicle credit for qualifying vehicles placed in service after December 31, 2005, and purchased before January 1, 2011 (Code Sec. 30B(e)).[37] In addition to the common requirements of qualifying vehicles (¶ 1345), the vehicle must have been capable of operating on an alternative fuel (e.g., compressed natural gas, liquefied natural gas, liquefied petroleum gas, hydrogen or any liquid consisting of at least 85-percent methanol).

The amount of the credit allowed for a qualifying vehicle was calculated as the applicable percentage of the incremental cost of any new vehicle placed into service during the tax year. The applicable percentage was 50 percent, plus 30 percent if the vehicle had received a certificate of conformity that it met or exceeded specific environmental emission standards. The incremental cost of a new qualified alternative motor vehicle was the amount by which the manufacturer's suggested retail price (MSRP) of the vehicle exceeded the MSRP of a gasoline-or diesel-powered version of the same model. However, the incremental cost was limited with respect to the vehicle's gross vehicle weight rating (GVWR) (Code Sec. 30B(E)(3)).

Credit for Mixed-Fuel Vehicles. The credit for qualified alternative fuel motor vehicles also applied to vehicles that qualified as mixed-fuel vehicles, but at a fraction of the credit amount. In addition to the common requirements of qualifying vehicles (¶ 1345), there were two additional requirements for qualification as a mixed-fuel vehicle. The

---

References are to Standard Federal Tax Reports; Tax Research Consultant; and Practical Tax Explanations.

[36] ¶ 4059A; INDIV: 57,708; § 12,905.20

[37] ¶ 4059A; INDIV: 57,710; § 12,905.25

vehicle must have been certified by the manufacturer as being able to efficiently operate on a mixture of an alternative fuel and a petroleum-based fuel. The vehicle must also have received either a certificate of conformity that it met or exceeded specific environmental emission standards.

The credit amount allowed for a mixed fuel vehicle was 70 percent of the credit that would be allowed as if the vehicle qualified for the alternative fuel motor vehicle credit and was a 75/25 mixed-fuel vehicle or 90 percent of the credit allowed as if the vehicle qualified for the alternative fuel motor vehicle credit and was a 90/10 mixed-fuel vehicle. A 75/25 mixed-fuel vehicle operated using at least 75-percent alternative fuel and no more than 25-percent petroleum-based fuel, while a 90/10 mixed-fuel vehicle operated using at least 90-percent alternative fuel and no more than 10-percent petroleum-based fuel.

1350. Plug-In Electric Drive Motor Vehicle Conversion Credit (Expired). The fifth component of the alternative motor vehicle credit was the plug-in electric drive motor vehicle conversion credit for qualifying vehicles placed in service after February 17, 2009, and converted before January 1, 2012 (Code Sec. 30B(i)).[38] The credit was available for converting an existing vehicle into a vehicle that, in addition to the common requirements of qualifying vehicles (¶ 1345), was a qualified plug-in electric drive motor vehicle under Code Sec. 30D (¶ 1351).

The plug-in conversion credit was equal to 10 percent of the cost of converting the vehicle, up to $40,000, for a maximum credit of $4,000. The credit was treated as part of the alternative motor vehicle credit and could have been claimed even if another alternative motor vehicle credit under Code Sec. 30B was claimed for the same motor vehicle in any preceding tax year.

1351. Qualified Plug-In Electric Drive Motor Vehicle Credit. A tax credit is allowed for the purchase price of a qualified plug-in electric drive motor vehicle acquired after December 31, 2009, and placed in service during the tax year (Code Sec. 30D).[39] The credit amount is $2,500 plus, $417 in the case of a vehicle which draws propulsion energy from a battery with not less than five kilowatt hours of capacity, and an additional $417 for each kilowatt hour of battery capacity in excess of five kilowatt hours. The additional amount cannot exceed $5,000. Thus, the maximum credit amount per vehicle is $7,500 (Code Sec. 30D(b)). For qualified vehicles used in a trade or business, the credit is claimed as a portion of the general business credit (¶ 1365). For qualified vehicles used for personal use, the credit is treated as a nonrefundable personal credit (¶ 1315). The credit is claimed using Form 8936.

Qualified Vehicles. To qualify as a plug-in electric drive vehicle, the vehicle must: (1) be made by a manufacturer, (2) be acquired for use or lease but not resale, (3) have its original use commencing with the taxpayer, (4) be treated as a motor vehicle for purposes of Title II of the Clean Air Act, (5) have a gross vehicle weight rating of not more than 14,000 pounds, and (6) be propelled to a significant degree by an electric motor that draws electricity from a battery with a capacity of not less than four kilowatt hours and that is capable of being recharged from an external source of electricity (Code Sec. 30D(d)(1)). The term "motor vehicle" means any vehicle that has at least four wheels and is manufactured primarily for use on public streets, roads, and highways (Code Sec. 30D(d)(2)). The plug-in electric drive motor vehicle credit has been expanded to cover 2- and 3-wheeled plug-in electric vehicles acquired during 2012 or 2013 (see below).

Phaseout. The credit begins to phaseout after 200,000 vehicles have been sold for use in the United States. The phaseout period begins with the second calendar quarter following the calendar quarter in which the 200,000th unit is sold. For the first two quarters of the phaseout period, the credit is cut to 50 percent of the full credit amount. The credit is cut to 25 percent for the third and fourth quarters of the phaseout period. Thereafter, no credit is allowed (Code Sec. 30D(e)).

References are to Standard Federal Tax Reports; Tax Research Consultant; and Practical Tax Explanations.

[38] ¶ 4059A; INDIV: 57,712;   [39] ¶ 4059L; INDIV: 58,000;
§ 12,905.30   § 12,915.15

Special Rules. No qualified plug-in electric drive motor vehicle credit is allowed for property used predominantly outside of the United States. The amount of any other deduction or credit claimed with respect to the vehicle is reduced by the amount of the qualified plug-in electric drive vehicle credit. The individual's basis in the vehicle is reduced by the amount of credit claimed. The IRS is required to issue regulations providing for the recapture of the credit in the event the vehicle no longer qualifies for the credit. Taxpayers have the option to elect out of claiming this credit for a qualified vehicle. Finally, a vehicle is not eligible to be a qualified vehicle unless it is in compliance with the Clean Air Act for applicable makes and models of the vehicle and satisfies the motor vehicle standards under Title 49 of the United States Code (Code Sec. 30D(f)).

2- and 3-Wheeled Plug-in Electric Vehicles. The plug-in electric drive motor vehicle credit has been extended to cover 2- and 3-wheeled plug-in electric vehicles acquired during 2012 or 2013 (Code Sec. 30D(g)). The credit is equal to the applicable amount with respect to each new qualified 2- or 3-wheeled plug-in electric drive vehicle. The applicable amount is equal to the lesser of 10 percent of the cost of the vehicle or $2,500.

In order for a vehicle to qualify as a 2- or 3-wheeled plug-in electric drive vehicle, the vehicle must have 2 or 3 wheels, be made by a manufacturer, and be acquired for use or lease by the taxpayer and not resale. The original use of the vehicle must begin with the taxpayer. In addition, the vehicle must:

(1) have a gross vehicle weight rating of less than 14,000 pounds;

(2) be primarily manufactured for use on public streets, roads, and highways;

(3) be able to achieve a speed of at least 45 miles an hour;

(4) be propelled to a significant extent by an electric motor drawing electricity from a battery having a capacity of at least 2.5 kilowatt hours that can be recharged from an external source; and

(5) be acquired after December 31, 2011, and before January 1, 2014.

The IRS has issued guidance regarding certification of vehicles eligible for this credit (Notice 2013-67).

> **Comment:** Absent further legislation, the credit for 2- and 3-wheeled plug-in electric drive vehicles has expired for vehicles acquired after December 31, 2013. For the latest legislative updates, visit our website www.CCHGroup.com/TaxUpdates.

1354. Certain Plug-In Electric Vehicle Credit (Expired). A credit was allowed for the cost of acquiring certain electrically powered two-wheeled, three-wheeled, and low-speed vehicles acquired after February 17, 2009, and before January 1, 2012 (Code Sec. 30).[40] The credit was equal to 10 percent of the cost of each qualified plug-in electric vehicle the taxpayer placed in service during the tax year with a maximum credit of $2,500 per vehicle. A vehicle qualifies for the credit if it was a qualified plug-in electric vehicle (¶ 1351), except that the battery for a 2- or 3-wheel vehicle must have had a capacity of not less than 2.5 kilowatt hours and the vehicle must have been low-speed as defined under section 571.3 of title 49 of the Code of Federal Regulations. The credit was claimed using Form 8834.

Any credit amount claimed reduced the taxpayer's basis in the vehicle. The amount of any other deduction or credit claimed with respect to the vehicle is reduced by the credit amount. The seller of a qualified vehicle to a tax-exempt entity could claim the credit after full disclosure of the available credit amount to the tax-exempt buyer. The vehicle could not be used outside the United States. The credit amount is subject to recapture if the vehicle ceases to be a qualifying vehicle. Taxpayers also had the option to elect not to claim this credit for a qualifying vehicle.

References are to Standard Federal Tax Reports; Tax Research Consultant; and Practical Tax Explanations.

[40] ¶ 4053; INDIV: 58,010; § 12,920

1355. Alternative Fuel Vehicle Refueling Property Credit. Taxpayers are permitted a credit for the installation of qualified alternative fuel refueling property placed in service before 2014 (before 2015 for refueling property related to hydrogen) (Code Sec. 30C).[41] The credit is claimed on Form 8911 regardless of whether the property is personal or used in a trade or business. Taxpayers may elect not to have the credit apply to otherwise qualifying property.

> **Comment:** Absent further legislation, the alternative fuel vehicle refueling property credit for refueling property unrelated to hydrogen has expired for property placed in service after December 31, 2013. For the latest legislative updates, visit our website www.CCHGroup.com/TaxUpdates.

Credit Amount. The credit amount is 30 percent of the cost of alternative fuel vehicle refueling property placed in service by the taxpayer during the tax year, with a per-location limit of $30,000 for property subject to depreciation (such as a commercial or retail refueling stations) and $1,000 for personal use property (such as residential property). In 2009 and 2010, the credit amount is 50 percent of the cost of non-hydrogen-related property and 30 percent of the cost of hydrogen-related property, with a per-location limit of $50,000 for non-hydrogen-related property subject to depreciation, $2,000 for non-hydrogen-related personal use property, $200,000 for hydrogen-related property subject to depreciation, and $1,000 for hydrogen-related personal use property.

If the credit is attributable to property that is subject to the rules of depreciation, then it is considered to be part of the general business credit (¶ 1365). The amount of the credit that is not attributable to depreciable property cannot exceed the excess of the taxpayer's regular income tax liability (as defined in Code Sec. 26(b)) reduced by the sum of nonrefundable personal credits and the foreign tax credit over the taxpayer's tentative minimum tax (Code Sec. 30C(d)).

Credits for property sold to a tax-exempt entity may be claimed by the seller but only if the seller discloses in a written document the amount of credit allowable. For purposes of claiming this credit for property sold to a tax-exempt entity, the property is treated as if it is depreciable property, and thus is subject to the business tax credit limitation rule. Qualifying property used outside the United States cannot be used to claim the credit. The qualifying property's basis must be reduced by the amount of the credit claimed. However, should the property cease to be qualifying property, the credit may be recaptured. Taxpayers also have the option to elect not to claim this credit (Code Sec. 30(e)).

Qualifying Property. Qualifying alternative fuel vehicle refueling property is property used for storing a clean-burning fuel or for dispensing clean-burning fuel into the fuel tank of a motor vehicle, but only if the property is located at the point where the fuel is delivered into the tank of the vehicle. It also includes any equipment that is used to recharge a motor vehicle that is propelled by electricity, but only if the property is located at the point where the vehicles are recharged. Only the following fuels shall be considered clean burning:

- any fuel that is at least 85 percent by volume consisting of ethanol, natural gas, compressed natural gas, liquefied natural gas, liquefied petroleum gas, or hydrogen;

- any fuel mixture that consists of a combination of at least two fuels which include biodiesel, diesel fuel, or kerosene with at least 20 percent of the volume being biodiesel without regard to any kerosene in the mixture; and

- electricity (Code Sec. 30C(c)).

References are to Standard Federal Tax Reports; Tax Research Consultant; and Practical Tax Explanations.

[41] ¶ 4059F; INDIV: 57,750; § 12,910

Foreign Tax Credit

1361. Foreign Tax Credit. An individual taxpayer may either deduct foreign income taxes paid or accrued as an itemized deduction on Schedule A of Form 1040 or claim them as a tax credit against his or her U.S. income tax liability (¶ 2475) (Code Sec. 27).[42] The credit is claimed by individuals on Form 1116 unless the total foreign taxes paid are less than $300 for single filers ($600 for joint filers). For these taxpayers, the credit may be claimed directly on Form 1040 if all filing requirements are satisfied (¶ 2476). A corporate taxpayer may also either deduct foreign income taxes paid or accrued or elect to claim such payments as a credit against its U.S. income tax liability. Form 1118 is used to calculate the amount of credit in a single tax year.

1362. U.S. Possessions Credit. A U.S. domestic corporation with a substantial portion of business in a U.S. possession may elect to claim a tax credit for taxes paid on business income derived from the possession and qualified investment income earned in the possession (Code Secs. 30A and 936).[43] The credit is generally unavailable to new claimants for tax years beginning after 1995 and is phased out for existing credit claimants for tax years beginning before 2006. A U.S. corporation that is an existing credit claimant with respect to American Samoa may still claim a version of the credit for tax years beginning before January 1, 2014 (Act Sec. 119(d) of the Tax Relief and Health Care Act of 2006 (P.L. 109-432), as amended by Act Sec. 330 of the American Taxpayer Relief Act of 2012 (P.L. 112-240)). In addition, other domestic corporations that have qualified production activities income (¶ 980B) from American Samoa can claim the credit for the first two tax years beginning after December 31, 2011, and before January 1, 2014. Form 5735 is used to figure the credit for economic activity in American Samoa.

General Business Credits

1365. General Business Credit. The general business credit is a limited, nonrefundable credit that is claimed after all other nonrefundable credits (¶ 1315) are claimed, other than the minimum tax credit. The general business credit for a tax year is the sum of: (1) the business credit carried forward to the current year, (2) the amount of the current year business credit, and (3) the business credit carried back to the year (Code Sec. 38).[44]

The current year general business credit is the sum of:

- the investment credit (¶ 1365A);
- the work opportunity credit (¶ 1365G);
- the alcohol fuels credit (¶ 1365I);
- the research activities credit (¶ 1365J);
- the low-income housing credit (¶ 1365K);
- the disabled access credit (¶ 1365M);
- the renewable electricity production credit (¶ 1365N);
- the empowerment zone employment credit (¶ 1365O);
- the Indian employment credit (¶ 1365Q);
- the employer Social Security credit (FICA tip credit) (¶ 1365R);
- the orphan drug credit (¶ 1365S);
- the new markets credit (¶ 1365T);
- the small employer pension plan start-up costs credit (¶ 1365U);
- the employer-provided child care facilities and services credit (¶ 1365V);
- the qualified railroad track maintenance credit (¶ 1365W);
- the biodiesel fuels credit (¶ 1365X);
- the low sulfur diesel fuel production credit (¶ 1365Y);

References are to Standard Federal Tax Reports; Tax Research Consultant; and Practical Tax Explanations.

[42] ¶ 4002; INTLOUT: 3,000; § 13,401   [43] ¶ 4058, ¶ 28,380; INTL: 27,000; § 13,435   [44] ¶ 4250; BUSEXP: 54,000; § 13,601

- the distilled spirits credit (¶ 1365Z);
- the advanced nuclear power facility production credit (¶ 1365AA);
- the nonconventional source fuels credit (¶ 1365BB);
- the energy efficient home credit (¶ 1365CC);
- the energy efficient appliance credit (¶ 1365DD);
- the alternative motor vehicle credit (portion allocable to a trade or business) (¶ 1345);
- the alternative fuel vehicle refueling property credit (portion allocable to a trade or business) (¶ 1355);
- the mine rescue team training credit (¶ 1365GG);
- the agricultural chemical security credit (¶ 1365HH);
- the differential wage payment credit (¶ 1365II);
- the carbon dioxide sequestration credit (¶ 1365JJ);
- the qualified plug-in electric drive motor vehicle credit (portion allocable to a trade or business) (¶ 1351);
- the credit for certain plug-in electric vehicles (expired) (¶ 1354);
- the small employer health insurance credit (¶ 1333);
- the new hire retention credit (expired) (¶ 1365FF);
- the credit for contributions to selected community development corporations (CDCs); and
- general credits from an electing large partnership (¶ 482–¶ 488).

Each of these credits is computed separately on its applicable IRS form. The credit computation form is attached to Form 3800, and the credit amount is reported on Form 3800. It is not necessary to attach a credit computation form if the taxpayer is not a partnership or S corporation and the taxpayer's only source for the credit is from a partnership, S corporation, estate, trust, or cooperative. However, an exception may apply if the taxpayer is claiming an investment credit (Form 3468) or a biodiesel credit (Form 8864), the taxpayer is an estate or trust and a credit is allocated to beneficiaries, or the taxpayer is a cooperative and the credit is allocated to patrons. See Form 3800 instructions for details.

Ordering rules. For any tax year, carryforwards of the general business credit to the tax year are deemed used first (starting with the earliest carryforwards), followed by the general business credit earned in the tax year, and then by any carryback to the tax year. If the tax liability limit discussed below is exceeded for the tax year, the components of the general business credit are generally deemed used in the order given above (Code Sec. 38(d); Form 3800 instructions).

Tax Liability Limitations. The general business credit may not exceed a limitation based on the amount of tax liability (Code Sec. 38(c)(1)). Generally, the general business credit may not exceed net income tax less the greater of the taxpayer's tentative minimum tax liability or 25 percent of net regular tax liability above $25,000. However, the limitation is determined separately for the portion of the credit attributable to the alcohol fuels credit, the low-income housing credit attributable to buildings placed in service after 2007, the renewable electricity production credit for electricity or refined coal produced at a facility placed in service after October 22, 2004, and during the 4-year period beginning on the date the facility was originally placed in service, the FICA tip credit, railroad track maintenance credit, the credit for small employer health insurance premiums, the energy credit component of the investment credit, the rehabilitation credit component of the investment credit attributable to expenditures for periods after 2007, and the work opportunity credit (Code Sec. 38(c)(4)). When calculating the limitation as it applies to these specified credits, the tentative minimum tax is to be treated as zero, which results in these credits being fully allowable against both the regular and alternative minimum tax (AMT) liabilities of the taxpayer.

For the empowerment zone employment credit (¶ 1365O), the credit amount may not exceed the excess of the net income tax over the greater of 75 percent of the taxpayer's tentative minimum tax liability or 25 percent of net regular tax liability above $25,000. This result is then reduced by the general business credit allowed for the tax year other than the empowerment zone employment credit and the specified credits listed above (Code Sec. 38(c)(2)).

For purposes of calculating these limitations, net income tax is the sum of the taxpayer's regular tax liability as defined in (Code Sec. 26(b)) and AMT liability as defined in Code Sec. 55 (¶ 1401), less all other nonrefundable credits (Code Secs. 21—30D). Net regular tax liability is the regular tax liability reduced by these credits (Code Sec. 38(c)(1)).

For a married couple filing separate returns, the $25,000 figure is limited to $12,500 for each spouse. If, however, one spouse has no current credit or unused credit, the spouse having current credit or unused credit may use the full $25,000 figure in determining his or her credit for the year. For a controlled group of corporations, the group may divide the $25,000 figure among its members in any way the members choose. For an estate or trust, the $25,000 figure is reduced to an amount that bears the same ratio to $25,000 as the portion of the estate's or trust's income that is not allocated to the beneficiaries bears to the total income of the estate or trust (Code Sec. 38(c)(6)).

Carrybacks and Carryforwards of Unused Credits. When the credit exceeds the tax liability limitation in any year, the excess or unused amount may be carried back one year and forward 20 years (15-year carryforward for credits that arise in tax years beginning before 1998) (Code Sec. 39).[45] The order in which these credits are claimed in any carryback or carryforward year is as follows: (1) carryforwards to that year on a first-in, first-out (FIFO) basis, (2) the business credit earned in that year, and (3) the carrybacks to that year on a FIFO basis.

A special carryback period of five years applies for the 2010 tax year of small businesses (Code Sec. 39(a)(4)). Eligible small business credits of an eligible small business determined for its first tax year beginning in 2010 may be carried back five years and forward 20 years. Eligible small business credits are the credits described in Code Sec. 38(b), which comprise the current year business credit component of the general business credit. An eligible small business is a sole proprietorship, partnership, or non-publicly traded corporation with $50 million or less in average annual gross receipts during the three tax years preceding the first tax year beginning in 2010. The eligible small business credits determined for 2010 may be claimed against the eligible small business's regular and AMT liabilities.

Separate carryback and carryforward records must be maintained for the amount of the general business credit attributable to the empowerment zone employment credit, and to each of the other components of the general business credit. Separate record-keeping is necessary because the empowerment zone employment credit may offset up to 25 percent of the taxpayer's AMT (Code Sec. 38(c)(2)(A)). Several of the credits that remain unused at the end of the carryforward period, or when the taxpayer ceases to exist, may be claimed as a deduction in the following year (Code Sec. 196).[46]

1365A. Investment Credit–Generally. Taxpayers may claim an investment credit which is the sum of the rehabilitation credit (¶ 1365B), the energy credit (¶ 1365C), the qualifying advanced coal project credit (¶ 1365D), the qualifying gasification project credit (¶ 1365E), the qualifying advanced energy project credit (¶ 1365F), and the qualifying therapeutic discovery project credit (¶ 1365LL) (Code Sec. 46).[47] The investment credit is claimed on Form 3468 and is one of the components of the general business credit, subject to the tax liability limitation and the carryover rules (¶ 1365).

The amount of investment credit allowed on investment credit property of a partnership for a tax year is generally apportioned among partners according to the ratio in which the partners divide the general profits of the partnership. The investment credit amount on an S corporation's investment credit property for a tax year is apportioned among the shareholders on a daily basis according to each shareholder's proportion of

13 **TAX CREDITS**

References are to Standard Federal Tax Reports; Tax Research Consultant; and Practical Tax Explanations.

[45] ¶ 4300; BUSEXP: 54,058; § 13,605.15

[46] ¶ 12,400; BUSEXP: 54,058.10; § 13,605.20

[47] ¶ 4502; BUSEXP: 51,050; § 13,701

¶1365A

ownership. The investment credit amount allowed on investment credit property of an estate or trust is apportioned between the estate or trust and the beneficiaries on the basis of the income allocable to each.

At-Risk Limitation. No investment credit is allowed for investment credit property to the extent that the property is financed with nonqualified nonrecourse borrowing (Code Sec. 49).[48] Thus, the credit base of investment credit property is reduced by the amount of nonqualified nonrecourse financing regarding the property, as determined at the close of the tax year in which the property is placed in service.

Nonqualified nonrecourse financing is any nonrecourse financing which is not qualified commercial financing. Qualified commercial financing is any financing of property if: (1) the property is acquired from an unrelated person; (2) the amount of the nonrecourse financing does not exceed 80 percent of the property's credit base; and (3) the financing is borrowed from a qualified person, or represents a loan from any Federal, state or local government or instrumentality, or which is guaranteed by any Federal, state or local government or instrumentality. The credit base is equal to the sum of the portion of the basis of a qualified rehabilitation building attributable to qualified rehabilitation expenditures, the basis of energy property, and the basis of any property that is part of a qualifying advanced coal project, a qualifying gasification project or a qualified advanced energy project. A qualified person is any person who actively and regularly engages in the business of lending money and is not the person from whom the property was acquired, a person who receives a fee with respect to the taxpayer's investment in the property, or a person who is related to the taxpayer (Code Sec. 49(a)(1)(D)).

Decreases in nonqualified recourse financing on the property in tax years following the year in which the property was placed in service increase the credit base of the property. This rule does not apply if the decrease occurs through the surrender or other use of property financed by nonqualified nonrecourse financing. Similarly, increases in nonqualified nonrecourse financing on the property in tax years following the year in which the property was placed in service decrease the credit base of the property and trigger recapture (Code Sec. 49(a)(2) and (b)).

The limitation applies to investment credit property placed in service by individuals and by certain closely held corporations engaged in business activities that are subject to the loss limitation rules of the at-risk rules (¶ 1155). For a partnership or S corporation, the investment credit at-risk limitation applies at the partner or shareholder level (Code Sec. 49(a)(1)(E)).

The investment credit at-risk limitation does not apply to certain energy property. To come within this exception, nonqualified nonrecourse financing may not exceed 75 percent of the basis of energy property at the close of the tax year in which the property is placed in service. In addition, any nonqualified nonrecourse financing for such property must be a level payment loan (a loan repaid in substantially equal installments, including both principal and interest).

An increase in the amount at risk is treated as if it occurred in the year that the property was first placed in service for purposes of computing the investment credit and for computing any recapture of such credit. However, the investment credit attributable to the increase in the amount at risk is claimed by the taxpayer during the tax year in which the decrease in the amount of nonqualified nonrecourse financing occurs.

If at the close of a tax year there is a net increase in the amount of nonqualified nonrecourse financing regarding such property, thereby causing a decrease in the taxpayer's amount at risk, the investment credit must be recomputed and the decrease in investment credits for previous tax years is recaptured as additional tax in the year that the net increase in nonqualified nonrecourse financing occurs.

Ineligible Property. No investment credit is allowed for the following types of property: (1) property used predominantly outside the United States except in limited circumstances; (2) property used predominantly to furnish lodging (or in connection

---

References are to Standard Federal Tax Reports; Tax Research Consultant; and Practical Tax Explanations.

[48] ¶ 4750; BUSEXP: 51,400;
§ 13,730.05

¶1365A

with the furnishing of lodging), except in the case of nonlodging commercial facilities, a hotel or motel furnishing accommodations predominantly to transients, certified historic structures to the extent of that portion of the basis attributable to qualified rehabilitation expenditures, and energy property; and (3) property used by a tax-exempt organization (other than a farmers' cooperative) unless it is used predominantly in an unrelated trade or business (Code Sec. 50(b)).[49] Generally, property used by, or leased to, a governmental unit, foreign person, or foreign entity is not eligible for the investment credit. However, the portion of the property attributable to qualified rehabilitation expenditures or held under a short-term lease (generally under six months) does qualify for the investment credit.

Basis Reduction. The basis of property for which an investment credit is claimed is reduced by the full amount of the credit except for the energy credit property whose basis is reduced by 50 percent of the credit amount (¶ 1365B) (Code Sec. 50(c)).[50] The reduced basis is used to compute depreciation and any gain or loss on the disposition of property.

If the investment credit is recaptured on property for which an investment credit downward basis adjustment was made, the basis of the property immediately before the event resulting in recapture must be increased by the recapture amount and by 50 percent of the recapture amount for an energy credit. In determining the amount of gain that is recaptured as ordinary income on a sale or disposition of depreciable personal property (Code Sec. 1245) or depreciable real property (Code Sec. 1250), the amount of the investment credit downward basis adjustment is treated as a deduction allowed for depreciation. Thus, the basis adjustment is treated as depreciation subject to ordinary income recapture. For section 1250 property, the recapture applies only to the excess of depreciation claimed over depreciation computed under the straight-line method, with the latter computed on the basis without reduction for the applicable investment credit downward basis adjustment.

If an investment credit for which a downward basis adjustment was made does not result in a tax benefit because it remains unused at the end of the 20-year credit carryover period for tax years after December 31, 1997 (15-year general business credit carryforward period for tax years prior to January 1, 1998), a deduction is allowed under Code Sec. 196 to the taxpayer for 50 percent of the unused energy and 100 percent of any other unused investment credit attributable to the basis reduction.

Special Investment Credit Rules. Special limitations apply to the amount of investment credit that may be claimed by regulated invesment companies, real estate investment trusts, noncorporate lessors, and certain other regulated companies (Code Sec. 50(d)).[51]

Early Disposition. When investment credit property is disposed of by the taxpayer (including dispositions due to casualties or thefts), or ceases to be investment credit property before the end of its recapture period, the tax for the year of disposal or cessation is increased by the amount of the credit that is recaptured (Code Sec. 50(a)).[52] A taxpayer subject to recapture must file Form 4255.

The amount of the recapture is a percentage of the original credit claimed, depending on how long the property is held before recapture is required. The recapture percentages are 100 percent within the first full year after placement in service, 80 percent within the second full year, 60 percent within the third full year, 40 percent within the fourth full year, 20 percent within the fifth full year, and zero thereafter. Advance rehabilitation or energy credits on progress expenditures are also subject to recapture. Special recapture rules apply to certain energy property.

References are to Standard Federal Tax Reports; Tax Research Consultant; and Practical Tax Explanations.

[49] ¶ 4752; BUSEXP: 51,250; § 13,701

[50] ¶ 4752; BUSEXP: 51,056; § 13,740

[51] ¶ 4752; BUSEXP: 51,650, BUSEXP: 51,606; § 13,701

[52] ¶ 4752; BUSEXP: 51,450, BUSEXP: 51,500; § 13,735

¶**1365A**

13 TAX CREDITS

The recapture rules do not apply to the following transfers: (1) a transfer between spouses or incident to divorce (¶ 778) (but a later disposition by the transferee will result in recapture to the same extent as if the disposition had been made by the transferor at that later date), (2) a transfer because of death, and (3) a transfer to which Code Sec. 381(a) (concerning carryovers after corporate acquisitions) applies. Similarly, the recapture rules do not apply where there is a mere change in the form of operating a business, provided that the property is retained in the business and the taxpayer retains a substantial interest in the business.

1365B. Rehabilitation Credit. A part of the investment credit (¶ 1365A), the rehabilitation investment credit is 20 percent of qualified rehabilitation expenses (QREs) for certified historic structures and 10 percent of QREs for qualified rehabilitated buildings (QRBs) first placed in service before 1936 (other than certified historic structures) (Code Sec. 47).[53] An election may also be made to claim an advance rehabilitation investment credit. No energy credit (¶ 1365C) is allowed on that portion of the basis of property that is attributable to QREs (Code Sec. 48(a)(2)(B)). Certain restrictions also apply to property which is used as lodging (Code Sec. 50(b)).

Eligibility. A building and its structural components constitute a QRB if they are substantially rehabilitated for the tax year and placed in service by any person before the beginning of the rehabilitation. Property other than a certified historic structure must also satisfy: (1) the applicable wall retention test, (2) an age requirement, and (3) a location-of-rehabilitation requirement (Code Sec. 47(c)(1); Reg. § 1.48-12(b)).[54] Property is considered substantially rehabilitated only if the expenditures during an elected 24-month measurement period (60-month period for phased rehabilitations) ending with or within the tax year are greater then the adjusted basis of the property or $5,000.

QREs do not include: (1) an enlargement or new construction; (2) the cost of acquisition; (3) noncertified rehabilitation of a certified historic structure; (4) rehabilitation of tax-exempt use property; (5) expenditures, generally, that are not depreciated under the MACRS straight-line method over specified recovery periods; or (6) a lessee-incurred expenditure if, on the date the rehabilitation of the building is completed, the remaining term of the lease (determined without regard to renewal periods) is less than the applicable recovery period (Reg. § 1.48-12(c)).

The rehabilitation investment credit for QREs generally must be claimed in the tax year in which the property attributable to the expenditures is placed in service, provided that the building is a QRB for such tax year (Code Sec. 47(b)). The credit may be claimed before the date the property is placed in service under the rules for qualified progress expenditures (Code Sec. 47(d)).

Buildings in Disaster Areas. The rehabilitation tax credit percentage is increased for certified historic structures or QRBs in the Gulf Opportunity (GO) Zone and the Midwest disaster area. The tax credit percentage is increased from 20 to 26 percent for any certified historic structure and from 10 to 13 percent for QRBs provided the structure or building is located in either disaster area. For the GO Zone, the increase applies to QRE that are paid or incurred on or after August 28, 2005, and before January 1, 2012 (Code Sec. 1400N(h)). For the Midwest disaster area, the increase applies to QREs made on building or structures damaged or destroyed by the Midwestern storms and that are paid or incurred on or after the applicable disaster date, and before January 1, 2012 (Division C, Act Sec. 702(a)(1)(A) and (d)(5) of the Emergency Economic Act of 2008 (P.L. 110-343).

Advance Credits for Progress Expenditures. An election may be made to claim an advance rehabilitation investment credit for progress expenditures on certain rehabilitated buildings before such property is placed in service (Code Sec. 47(d)).[55] Property qualifying for an advance rehabilitation investment credit on progress expenditures includes a building that is being rehabilitated by, or for, the taxpayer, if the normal

---

References are to Standard Federal Tax Reports; Tax Research Consultant; and Practical Tax Explanations.

[53] ¶ 4600; BUSEXP: 51,152; § 13,705

[54] ¶ 4600, ¶ 4609; BUSEXP: 51,154; § 13,705

[55] ¶ 4600; BUSEXP: 51,160; § 13,705

rehabilitation period for the building is two or more years and it is reasonable to expect that the building will be a QRB when it is placed in service.

The amount of QREs that are considered progress expenditures for which an advance rehabilitation investment credit may be claimed is the amount of QREs properly chargeable to the capital account for self-rehabilitated buildings. For non-self-rehabilitated buildings, the amount is the lesser of: (a) the QRE paid to another person for the rehabilitation of the building during the tax year, or (b) the portion of the overall cost of the rehabilitation completed during the tax year.

1365C. Energy Credit. A part of the investment credit (¶ 1365A), the business energy investment credit is generally equal to 10 percent of the taxpayer's basis in qualified energy property placed in service during the tax year. Effective for property placed in service before 2017, the credit percentage is increased to 30 percent for (1) qualified fuel cell property, (2) equipment that uses solar energy to generate electricity, to heat or cool a structure, or provide solar process heat (except used to heat a swimming pool), (3) equipment that uses solar energy to illuminate the inside of a structure using fiber-optic distributed sunlight, and (4) qualified small wind energy property (Code Sec. 48).[56] The credit for qualified fuel cell property may not exceed $1,500 for each 0.5 kilowatt of capacity. Qualified energy property eligible for the 10-percent credit generally includes microturbine property and other energy property, including combined heat and power system property, geothermal heat pump systems, and public utility property.

To qualify for the credit, the energy property must be depreciable (or amortizable) and must meet performance and quality standards prescribed by IRS regulations. In addition, the taxpayer must complete the construction, reconstruction, or erection of the property or, if the property is acquired, the taxpayer must be the first person to use it. The basis of all energy property prior to the credit determination is reduced by any tax-exempt or subsidized financing. No energy credit is allowed for that portion of the basis of property for which a rehabilitation investment credit (¶ 1365B) is claimed. An advance energy investment credit may be claimed under special rules for progress expenditures. The energy credit may be claimed against the alternative minimum tax.

Investment Credit Election. A taxpayer may make an irrevocable election to treat certain qualified property that is part of a qualified investment credit facility as energy property eligible for a 30-percent investment credit (Code Sec. 48(a)(5)). If the election is made, no renewable electricity production credit is allowed under Code Sec. 45 (¶ 1365N) for any tax year with respect to the qualified investment credit facility. For purposes of the election, qualified investment credit facilities are facilities otherwise eligible for the renewable electricity production credit that produce electricity using wind or solar power, closed-loop biomass, open-loop biomass, geothermal energy, landfill gas, municipal solid waste (trash), hydropower, or marine and hydrokinetic renewable energy. In order to qualify for the election, the qualified investment credit facility must be placed in service after 2008, and the construction of the facility must begin before January 1, 2014. Qualified property which is eligible for the 30-percent investment credit if the election is made is tangible personal property, or other tangible property (not including a building or its structural components), but only if such property is used as an integral part of the qualified investment credit facility. In addition, the property must be depreciable or amortizable, constructed, reconstructed, erected, or acquired by the taxpayer, and the original use of the property must commence with the taxpayer.

Coordination With Section 1603 Grants Authorized. The Secretary of Treasury is authorized to provide a grant to each person who places into service specified energy property that is either: (1) an electricity production facility otherwise eligible for the renewable electricity production credit under Code Sec. 45 or (2) qualifying property otherwise eligible for the energy investment credit under Code Sec. 48 (Act Sec. 1603(a)

References are to Standard Federal Tax Reports; Tax Research Consultant; and Practical Tax Explanations.

[56] ¶ 4651; BUSEXP: 51,102; § 13,710

of the American Recovery and Reinvestment Act of 2009 (P.L. 111-5), as amended by the Tax Relief, Unemployment Insurance Reauthorization, and Job Creation Act of 2010 (P.L. 111-312)). In order to be eligible for the grant, the specified energy property must be:

- placed in service during 2009, 2010, or 2011, or
- placed in service after 2011 and before the credit termination date for such property, if construction of the property began during 2009, 2010, or 2011.

No energy credit (Code Sec. 48) or electricity production credit (Code Sec. 45) is allowed for the year of the grant or any subsequent year (Code Sec. 48(d)). In the event that a credit amount was claimed for the facility prior to the grant being made, the credit amount is recaptured by adding the prior claimed credit amounts to the tax liability of the grant year. The taxpayer must adjust any carryovers of general business credits to reflect the amount of the recaptured credit. The energy credit and electricity production credit may not be claimed on account of the reduction of a section 1603 grant by reason of the sequestration rules (Notice 2014-39).

1365D. Qualified Advanced Coal Project Credit. A qualifying advanced coal project credit may be claimed as a component of the investment credit (¶ 1365A) (Code Sec. 48A).[57] The credit is available only to taxpayers who have applied for and received certification that their project satisfies the relevant requirements outlined by the IRS, in consultation with the Secretary of Energy. The credit is equal to 20 percent of qualified investments in integrated combined cycle projects, 15 percent of qualified investments in other advanced coal-based projects, and 30 percent of qualified investments in advanced coal-based generation technology projects. The IRS is required to recapture any tax benefits should the project fail to maintain carbon dioxide separation and sequestration.

1365E. Qualified Gasification Project Credit. A qualifying gasification project credit may be claimed as a component of the investment credit (¶ 1365A) (Code Sec. 48B).[58] The credit is available only to taxpayers who have applied for and received certification that their project satisfies the relevant requirements outlined by the IRS, in consultation with the Secretary of Energy. The credit is equal to 20 percent of qualified investments in qualifying gasification projects, increased to 30 percent for qualifying gasification projects that include equipment that separates and sequesters at least 75 percent of the project's total carbon dioxide emissions. A qualifying gasification facility is one that combines coal, petroleum residue, biomass, or other materials with steam under high pressure to create a synthetic gas, or "syngas." The IRS is authorized to recapture any tax benefits if the project fails to attain or maintain the 75-percent separation and sequestration requirement.

1365F. Advanced Energy Project Credit. A tax credit is allowed equal to 30 percent of a taxpayer's qualified investment for the tax year with respect to any qualifying advanced energy project (Code Sec. 48C).[59] The credit is part of the investment credit (¶ 1365A) and the basis of any property that is part of a qualifying advanced energy project is included in the credit base for purposes of applying the investment credit at-risk limitation rules under Code Sec. 49. The credit is not allowed for any qualified investment for which a credit is also allowed for the energy credit, the qualifying advanced coal project credit, or the qualifying gasification project credit.

A qualifying advanced energy project is a project that re-equips, expands, or establishes a manufacturing facility for the production of: (1) property designed to be used to produce energy from the sun, wind, or geothermal deposits (within the meaning of Code Sec. 613(e)(2)) or other renewable resources; (2) fuel cells, microturbines, or an energy storage system for use with electric or hybrid-electric motor vehicles; (3) electric grids to support the transmission of intermittent sources of renewable energy, including storage of such energy; (4) property designed to capture and sequester carbon dioxide emissions; (5) property designed to refine or blend renewable fuels or to

---

References are to Standard Federal Tax Reports; Tax Research Consultant; and Practical Tax Explanations.

[57] ¶ 4672; BUSEXP: 51,700; § 13,715

[58] ¶ 4676; BUSEXP: 51,750; § 13,720

[59] ¶ 4685; BUSEXP: 51,800; § 13,725

produce energy conservation technologies (including energy-conserving lighting technologies and smart grid technologies); (6) new qualified plug-in electric drive motor vehicles, qualified plug-in electric vehicles, or components which are designed specifically for use with such vehicles, including electric motors, generators, and power control units; or (7) other advanced energy · property designed to reduce greenhouse gas emissions as may be determined by the Secretary of Treasury (Code Sec. 48C(c)(1)). Any portion of the qualified investment in the qualifying project must be certified by the Secretary of Treasury as eligible for the credit. A qualifying project does not include any portion of a project for the production of any property used in the refining or blending of any transportation fuel (other than renewable fuels).

1365G. Work Opportunity Tax Credit. The work opportunity credit is available for wages paid by employers who hire individuals from certain targeted groups of hard-to-employ individuals (Code Sec. 51).[60] The credit is generally 40 percent of the first $6,000 of qualified wages ($3,000 for qualified summer youth employees) paid to each member of a targeted group during the first year of employment and 25 percent in the case of wages attributable to individuals meeting only minimum employment levels described below. The credit is taken for first-year wages paid to eligible individuals who begin work before January 1, 2014, unless an election is made not to claim the credit. Any business deduction for such wages must be reduced by the amount of the credit, as computed on Form 5884.

> **Comment:** Absent further legislation, the work opportunity credit is not available for targeted group members that begin work after December 31, 2013. For the latest legislative updates, visit our website www.CCHGroup.com/TaxUpdates.

Tax Liability Limitations. Although the work opportunity credit is a component of the general business credit (¶ 1365), credit amounts are not subject to the general business credit tax liability limitation rule but are to be calculated separately. The credit limitation formula is changed to treat the tentative minimum tax as zero, allowing taxpayers to fully utilize the credit against both the regular tax and the minimum tax liabilities (Code Sec. 38(c)(4)). The credit limitation calculation applies to any carrybacks of such credit amounts to any previous year. No credit is allowed for wages paid to an individual for services rendered at the employer's plant or facility that are substantially similar to services performed by employees who are participants in a strike or who are affected by a lockout.

Minimum Employment Period. An employee must have completed a minimum of 120 hours of service for the wages to be taken into account for calculation of the work opportunity credit. The hours-of-service test is the only way the minimum employment period is measured for purposes of the credit. If the 120-hour test is met but the employee fails to perform at least 400 hours of service, the employer is entitled to a credit of 25 percent. For 400 or more hours of service, the percentage is 40 percent of the employee's wages (Code Sec. 51(i)(3)).

Target Groups. Wages paid to individuals who are certified members of one of the following groups qualify for the work opportunity credit (Code Sec. 51(d)):

- a qualified IV-A recipient (the individual must be a member of a family that received Temporary Assistance for Needy Families (TANF) assistance for any 9 of the 18 months before the hire date);

- a qualified veteran;

- a qualified ex-felon (the individual must have a hire date within one year of being released from prison);

- a vocational rehabilitation referral (the individual must have a physical or mental handicap resulting in a substantial handicap to employment and be referred to the employer upon completion of rehabilitative services);

References are to Standard Federal Tax Reports; Tax Research Consultant; and Practical Tax Explanations.

[60] ¶ 4800; BUSEXP: 54,250; § 13,805.05

- a qualified summer youth employee (the individual must be a new hire who performs services between May 1 and September 15, be 16 or 17 years of age on the later of the hire date or May 1, and must live in an empowerment zone while such designation is in effect) (the maximum qualified wages is $3,000 with the maximum credit amount being $1,200);

- a designated community resident (the individual must be at least 18 years of age but less than 40 years of age on the hiring date and live in an empowerment zone or rural renewal county while such designation is in effect);

- a qualified food stamps recipient (the individual must be at least 18 of age but younger than 40 years of age and be a member of a family that either received food stamp benefits for the six months before the hire date or received food stamp benefits for three of the five months before the hire date but lost the benefits for failure to comply with the program's work requirements);

- a qualified supplemental security income (SSI) recipient (the individual must have received SSI within 60 days before the hire date); or

- a long-term family assistance recipient (the individual must be a member of a family that received the maximum amount of IV-A (TANF) assistance over an 18-month period ending within two years of the hire date) (up to $10,000 are considered qualified first year wages, up to $10,000 are considered qualified second year wages, and the credit percentage equals 50 percent for the second year (maximum credit amount of $5,000)).

Comment: Absent further legislation, empowerment zone designations terminate December 31, 2013 (Code Sec. 1391(d)(1)(A)(i)). Thus, wages paid or incurred for services performed after December 31, 2013, by a designated community resident or qualified summer youth employee who lives in an empowerment zone does not qualify for the work opportunity credit. For the latest legislative updates, visit our website www.CCHGroup.com/TaxUpdates.

Certifications. An employer of an individual who is a member of a targeted group must either have the individual certified by an authorized local agency prior to the individual's first day of work or file an application for certification of the individual within 28 days of the first day of work (Code Sec. 51(d)(12)). Employers use Form 8850 to pre-screen employees and to make a written request that the local agency certify an employee as being a member of a targeted group. Employers are permitted to submit Form 8850 electronically. Two alternative methods of certification using electronic signatures are also permitted (Notice 2012-13).

The 28-day deadline was extended in the case of an employer who hired a targeted group member other than a qualified veteran on or after January 1, 2012, and before April 1, 2013 or hired a qualified veteran on or after January 1, 2013 and before April 1, 2013. In such case, certification requests on Form 8850 needed to be filed no later than April 29, 2013 (Notice 2013-14).

Special rules apply to qualified veterans. A veteran is a qualified veteran if the veteran is certified as falling within one of the following categories (Code Sec. 51(d)(3), (d)(13)(D)):

- a member of a family receiving assistance under a supplemental nutrition assistance program under the Food and Nutrition Act of 2008 for at least a 3-month period ending during the 12-month period ending on the hiring date;

- a veteran entitled to compensation for a service-connected disability and either has a hiring date which is not more than 1 year after discharge or release from active duty or has aggregate periods of unemployment during the 1-year period ending on the hiring date which equal or exceed 6 months;

- a veteran with aggregate periods of unemployment during the 1-year period ending on the hiring date which equal or exceed 4 weeks (but less than 6 months); or

- a veteran with aggregate periods of unemployment during the 1-year period ending on the hiring date which equal or exceed 6 months

Although the qualified wage limit is generally $6,000 for a targeted group member, the limit is increased to: (a) $12,000 for an individual who is a qualified veteran by reason of being entitled to compensation for a service-connected disability and having a hiring date which is not more than 1 year after discharge; (b) $24,000 for an individual who is a qualified veteran by reason of being entitled to compensation for a service-connected disability and having aggregate periods of unemployment during the 1-year period ending on the hiring date which equal or exceed 6 months; and (c) $14,000 for an individual who is a qualified veteran by reason of having aggregate periods of unemployment during the 1-year period ending on the hiring date which equal or exceed 6 months (Code Sec. 51(b)(3)).

Tax-Exempt Organizations and Qualified Veterans. Tax-exempt organizations, other than exempt farmers' cooperatives (¶ 698) generally cannot claim the work opportunity credit (Code Sec. 52(c)). However, Code Sec. 501(c) exempt organizations (¶ 602 and ¶ 692) that employ qualified veterans may take advantage of the credit. The credit rate in such circumstances is reduced from 40 percent to 26 percent of qualified wages. These exempt organizations must use Form 5884-C to claim the credit. The form is filed separately and is not attached to any other return filed by the exempt organization. The credit is allowed against the tax-exempt employer's Federal Insurance Contribution Act (FICA) tax obligation on wages paid to the veteran within one year of hiring (Code Sec. 3111(e)). The liability on the organization's employment tax return is not reduced by the credit; rather, the credit is processed separately and the amount properly claimed is refunded to the exempt organization. This is likely to occur after the filing of the return, so organizations are cautioned not to reduce their FICA obligation on their returns in anticipation of the refund (Notice 2012-13).

1365I. Alcohol Fuels Credit. Producers of alcohol fuels or mixtures are entitled to a tax credit for any sale or use occurring before January 1, 2012, with the exception of the second generation biofuel producer credit (discussed below) (Code Sec. 40).[61] The alcohol fuels credit is the sum of the alcohol mixture credit, the alcohol credit, the small ethanol producer credit, and the second generation biofuel producer credit (formerly, the cellulosic biofuel producer credit) The credit is computed on Form 6478 and is a component of the general business credit (¶ 1365), but the credit limitation is calculated separately from the general business credit limitation. The alcohol fuels credit amount may be claimed against both the regular and the alternative minimum tax liability (Code Sec. 38(c)(4)).

Alcohol Mixture Credit. The alcohol mixture credit was equal to 60 cents per gallon of nonethanol alcohol of at least 190 proof (45 cents per gallon of nonethanol alcohol of at least 150 proof but less than 190 proof) utilized in the production of a qualified mixture fuel (alcohol mixed with gasoline or a special fuel) that was used by the producer or that was sold in the producer's trade or business in the United States prior to January 1, 2012. The alcohol mixture credit was 45 cents per gallon of ethanol alcohol of at least 190 proof (33.33 cents per gallon of ethanol alcohol of at least 150 proof but less than 190 proof) (Code Sec. 40(b)(1), (d)(7), and (h)(1)).

Alcohol Credit. The alcohol credit was equal to 60 cents per gallon of nonethanol alcohol of at least 190 proof (45 cents per gallon of nonethanol alcohol of at least 150 proof but less than 190 proof) not mixed with gasoline or a special fuel (other than any denaturant) that was used by a person as a fuel in a trade or business or that was sold at retail and placed in the fuel tank of the purchaser's vehicle in the United States prior to January 1, 2012. The alcohol credit was 45 cents per gallon of ethanol alcohol of at least 190 proof (33.33 cents per gallon of ethanol alcohol of at least 150 proof but less than 190 proof) not mixed with gasoline or a special fuel (other than any denaturant) (Code Sec. 40(b)(2), (d)(7), and (h)(1)).

Small Ethanol Producer Credit. An eligible small ethanol producer (a producer with a production capacity of up to 60 million gallons of alcohol per year) could have claimed

---

References are to Standard Federal Tax Reports; Tax Research Consultant; and Practical Tax Explanations.

[61] ¶ 4302; BUSEXP: 54,100; § 14,205

the small ethanol producer credit of 10 cents per gallon on production of up to 15 million gallons per year of ethanol sold or used for purposes of fuel or added to a fuel mixture in the user's trade or business in the United States prior to January 1, 2012. The 15 million annual limitation of the production of ethanol was determined without regard to any qualified cellulosic biofuel production (discussed below) (Code Sec. 40(b)(4)(C)). The ethanol must have been used by the producer for specific purposes or sold to another person who used the ethanol for those purposes. The specific purposes were: (1) to be used in a trade or business to produce an alcohol mixture (other than casual off-farm production), (2) to be used as a fuel in a trade or business, or (3) for selling to another person at retail and putting the ethanol in the buyer's fuel tank.

Second Generation Biofuel Producer Credit (formerly, Cellulosic Biofuel Production Credit). The second generation biofuel producer credit is equal to $1.01 per gallon of qualified second generation biofuel produced by a qualified second generation biofuel producer before January 1, 2014 (Code Sec. 40(b)(6)). Second generation biofuel is defined as any liquid fuel produced from lignocellulosic or hemicellulosic matter or, with respect to fuels sold or used after January 2, 2013, from any cultivated algae, cyanobacteria, or lemna, that is available on a renewable or recurring basis and that meets the Environmental Protection Agency registration requirements for fuel and fuel additives established under section 211 of the Clear Air Act. The fuel called "black liquor," as well as crude tall oil (made by reacting acid with black liquor soap), does not qualify for the credit. Renewable sources of lignocellulosic and hemicellulosic matter include energy crops and trees, wood and wood residues, plants, grasses, agricultural residues, fibers, animal wastes, and other waste material, including municipal solid waste.

The second generation biofuel must be used by the producer for specific purposes or sold to another person who will use the second generation biofuel for those purposes. The specified purposes are: (1) to use in a trade or business to produce an alcohol mixture (other than casual off-farm production), (2) to use as a fuel in a trade or business, or (3) to sell to another person at retail and putting the ethanol in the buyer's fuel tank. A qualified second generation biofuel producer is one that is registered with the IRS as a second generation biofuel producer whose production is produced and used in its entirety within the United States. The second generation biofuel claimed under Code Sec. 40 cannot also be claimed under Code Sec. 40A as renewable diesel or biodiesel.

Special Rules. Special rules apply for partnerships, S corporations, and other pass-through entities which include allocation to patrons of farm cooperatives. All taxpayers have the option of electing to not claim the alcohol fuels credit. Any excise tax exemption claimed with respect to alcohol produced for alcohol fuels reduces the amount of the income tax credit. The carryforward period for the alcohol fuels credit is limited to three tax years after the relevant fuel's termination year. An alcohol fuels credit carryforward that is unused at the end of the carryforward period is deductible in the following tax year (Code Sec. 196).

Recapture of Credit. If the alcohol fuels credit is claimed, the producer must pay a tax on each gallon at the original credit rate if the producer separates alcohol from the mixture, uses the alcohol mixture other than as fuel, mixes alcohol on which the credit was allowed for retail sale, uses the alcohol other than as fuel, or for ethanol fuel or second generation biofuel, does not use the fuel for the required purpose (Code Sec. 40(d)(3)). The tax must be reported on Form 720.

1365J. Credit for Increased Research Expenditures. A credit for incremental research expenses (computed on Form 6765) is claimed as one of the components of the general business credit (¶ 1365) (Code Sec. 41).[62] The credit is available for amounts paid or incurred through December 31, 2013 (Code Sec. 41(h)(1)(B)).

References are to Standard Federal Tax Reports; Tax Research Consultant; and Practical Tax Explanations.

[62] ¶ 4350; BUSEXP: 54,150; § 13,901

Comment: Absent further legislation, the research credit has expired for amounts paid or incurred after December 31, 2013. For the latest legislative updates, visit our website www.CCHGroup.com/TaxUpdates.

The credit is subject to the general business credit's tax liability limitation and carryover rules (¶ 1365). The research credit that remains unused at the end of the carryforward period is allowed as a deduction in the year following the expiration of such period (Code Sec. 196). The credit does not apply to unused amounts claimed under the reduced research credit election.

Amount of Credit. Unless an election is made to use the alternative simplified credit computation (discussed below), the research credit is the sum of: (1) 20 percent of the excess of qualified research expenses for the current tax year over a base period amount, (2) 20 percent of the basic research payments made to a qualified organization, and (3) 20 percent of the amounts paid or incurred by a taxpayer in carrying on any trade or business to an energy research consortium for qualified energy research (Code Sec. 41(a)). Special base period adjustments are required where there is an acquisition or disposition of the major portion of a business that paid or incurred research expenses.

Base Amount. For purposes of calculating the credit, the base period amount is the product of the taxpayer's fixed-base percentage and average annual gross receipts for the four tax years preceding the credit period (Code Sec. 41(c)). The base amount may not be less than 50 percent of the qualified research expenses for the credit year. The fixed-base percentage (aggregate qualified research expenses compared to aggregate gross receipts for 1984 through 1988 tax years) may not exceed 16 percent.

Start-Up Company. A start-up company's fixed-base percentage is three percent for each of the first five tax years for which it has qualified research expenses. The fixed-base percentage for the sixth through tenth tax years in which qualified research expenses were incurred is a portion of the percentage which qualified research expenses bear to gross receipts for specified preceding years. For subsequent tax years, the fixed-base percentage is the whole percentage that qualified research expenses bear to gross receipts for any five years selected by the taxpayer from the fifth through tenth tax years. The definition of a start-up company includes a taxpayer who has both gross receipts and qualified research expenses for the first time in a tax year that begins after 1983 (Code Sec. 41(c)(3)(B)).

Alternative Simplified Credit. Taxpayers may elect an alternative method to calculate the increased research activities credit amount using an alternative simplified credit (Code Sec. 41(c)(5)). Under the alternative simplified credit method, a taxpayer can claim an amount equal to 14 percent of the amount by which the qualified research expenses exceed 50 percent of the average qualified research expenses for the three preceding tax years (Code Sec. 41(c)(5)). If the taxpayer has no qualified research expenses for any of the preceding three years, then the credit is equal to six percent of the qualified research expenses for the current tax year. If the taxpayer makes the election to use the alternative simplified credit method, the election is effective for succeeding tax years unless revoked with the consent of the IRS.

Deduction for Research and Experimental Expenditures. A taxpayer claiming the credit must reduce the business deduction for research and experimental expenditures (¶ 979) by the amount of the research credit (Code Sec. 280C(c)). Capitalized expenses must also be reduced by the amount of the research credit that exceeds the amount otherwise allowable as a deduction for such expenses. An annual irrevocable election is available to claim a reduced research credit and thereby avoid reducing the research expense deduction (or capital expenditures). Under the election, the research credit must be reduced by the product of the research credit computed in the regular manner and the maximum corporate tax rate.

Qualified Research Expenses. Qualified research expenses for purposes of calculating the credit are the same as those for the business deduction (¶ 979) other than expenses for foreign research, research in the social sciences, arts or humanities, or subsidized research. However, research eligible for the credit is limited to research undertaken to discover information that is technological in nature and intended to be useful in the development of a new or improved business component. Further, the

¶1365J

research must relate to elements of a process of experimentation for a functional purpose (i.e., it must relate to a new or improved function, performance, reliability, or quality).

Qualified research expenses cover in-house expenses for the taxpayer's own research (i.e., wages, including income from employees' exercise of stock options, for substantially engaging in or directly supervising or supporting research activities, supplies, and computer use charges) and 65 percent of amounts paid or incurred for qualified research done by a person other than an employee of the taxpayer. The percentage is increased to 75 percent of amounts paid or incurred for qualified research performed by a qualified research consortium. A qualified research consortium is a tax-exempt organization under either Code Sec. 501(c)(3) or (c)(6). The consortium must be operating primarily to conduct energy research and it must have at least five unrelated customers, with no single person accounting for more than 50 percent of the revenues of the organization.

Qualified Energy Research Expenditures. The 20-percent credit amount applies to expenditures to an energy research consortium for qualified energy research only. The percent limitation placed on outside research does not apply energy research. Amounts paid or incurred for any energy research conducted outside of the United States, Puerto Rico, or U.S. possession cannot be taken into account in determining the 20 percent of amounts paid or incurred by a taxpayer in carrying on any trade or business during the tax year to an energy research consortium under Code Sec. 41(a)(3) (Code Sec. 41(f)(6)(C)).

Special Rule for Pass-Through Entities. For individuals with interests in unincorporated businesses, partners, trust or estate beneficiaries, or S corporation shareholders, any allowable pass-through of the credit cannot exceed the amount of tax attributable to the individual's taxable income allocable to that individual's interest in the entity (Code Sec. 41(g)).

1365K. Low-Income Housing Credit. A nonrefundable income tax credit is available on a per-unit basis for low-income units in qualified low-income buildings in qualified low-income housing projects (Code Sec. 42).[63] The owner of a qualified low-income housing project that is constructed, rehabilitated, or acquired may claim the credit over a 10-year period in an amount equal to the applicable credit percentage appropriate to the type of project, multiplied by the qualified basis allocable to the low-income units in each qualified low-income building.

The taxpayer begins to claim the credit with the tax year in which the project is placed in service or, at the taxpayer's election, the next tax year (but only if the building is a qualified low-income building as of the close of the first year of such period). The first-year credit is reduced to reflect the time during the year that any low-income units are unoccupied. If the reduction is made, a credit is allowed in the eleventh year in an amount equal to the reduction. The credit is calculated on Form 8586 and is a component of the general business credit. Thus, it is subject to the general business credit's tax liability limitation and carryover rules (¶ 1365).[64] The credit cannot be claimed for otherwise qualified buildings unless the owner of the building is subject to an enforceable 30-year low-income use agreement with the housing agency (Code Sec. 42(h)(6)). However, the credit is not limited or disallowed by the rules applicable to activities not entered into for profit (¶ 1195) (Reg. § 1.42-4).[65]

The applicable credit rates are the appropriate percentages issued by the IRS for the month in which the building is placed in service. Different percentages are provided for new construction or rehabilitation, subsidized construction or rehabilitation, and the acquisition of existing housing (¶ 86). An irrevocable election is available to determine the credit percentage applicable to a building in advance of the date that it is placed in service.

References are to Standard Federal Tax Reports; Tax Research Consultant; and Practical Tax Explanations.

[63] ¶ 4380; BUSEXP: 54,200; § 14,420

[64] ¶ 4380; BUSEXP: 54,224; § 14,420

[65] ¶ 4384A; BUSEXP: 54,218; § 14,420

Rehabilitation expenditures are generally treated as expenditures for a separate new building provided that the expenditures are allocable to, or substantially benefit, low-income units and that they are incurred during any 24-month period and are at least equal to the greater of 20 percent of the adjusted basis of the building or $6,000 per low-income unit, adjusted annually for inflation ($6,600 in 2015, $6,500 in 2014, and $6,400 in 2013) (Code Sec. 42(e); Rev. Proc. 2014-61; Rev. Proc. 2013-35 and Rev. Proc. 2012-41). The limits are 10 percent of adjusted basis and $3,000 for buildings that are allocated a credit dollar amount on or before July 30, 2008. A qualified low-income housing project is any project for residential rental property that meets requirements for low-income tenant occupancy, gross rent restrictions, state credit authority, and IRS certification. The project must continue to meet these requirements for 15 years or recapture of a portion of the credit may be required using Form 8611. A qualified low-income building must be subject to MACRS depreciation.

State Allocations. The low-income housing credit can be claimed for any tax year, but generally only to the extent that the owner of a qualified low-income building receives a housing credit allocation from a state or local housing credit agency (Code Sec. 42(h)).

1365M. Disabled Access Credit. An eligible small business is entitled to a nonrefundable tax credit for expenditures incurred to make a business accessible to disabled individuals (Code Sec. 44).[66] The credit is 50 percent of the amount of eligible access expenditures for a year that exceed $250 but that do not exceed $10,250. The credit is computed on Form 8826 and is a component of the general business credit. Thus, it is subject to the tax liability limitation and the carryover rules of the general business credit (¶ 1365). Any unused credit remaining at the end of the carryforward period is lost. No other deduction or credit is permitted for any amount for which a disabled access credit is allowed.

Eligibility. An eligible small business is any person that elects to claim the disabled access credit that had gross receipts (less returns and allowances) for the preceding tax year that did not exceed $1 million or that employed no more than 30 full-time employees during the preceding tax year. Eligible access expenditures include reasonable and necessary amounts paid or incurred by an eligible small business for the purpose of enabling the business to comply with the requirements of the Americans with Disabilities Act of 1990.

Eligible expenditures also include expenditures: (1) for the purpose of removing architectural, communication, physical, or transportation barriers that prevent a business from being accessible to, or usable by, disabled individuals (other than amounts for new construction); (2) to provide qualified interpreters or other effective methods of making aurally delivered materials available to hearing-impaired individuals; (3) to provide qualified readers, taped texts, and other effective methods of making visually delivered materials available to visually impaired individuals; (4) to acquire or modify equipment or devices for disabled individuals; or (5) to provide other similar services, modifications, materials, or equipment.

1365N. Credit for Electricity Produced from Renewable Sources. A credit is available for the domestic production of electricity from qualified energy resources at a qualified facility, if the electricity is sold to an unrelated third party (Code Sec. 45).[67] The credit is also allowed for the sale of certain refined coal produced within the United States at a qualified refined coal production facility, but only if sold to an unrelated person. The credit for refined coal production may not be claimed if production from the facility was eligible for the nonconventional fuel source credit for any tax year (¶ 1365BB).

Credit Amounts and Limitations. The credit amount for electricity produced in a qualified wind, closed-loop biomass, geothermal energy, or solar facility is 2.3 cents per kilowatt hour in 2014. Electricity produced in qualified open-loop biomass, small irriga-

---

References are to Standard Federal Tax Reports; Tax Research Consultant; and Practical Tax Explanations.

[66] ¶ 4400; BUSEXP: 54,350; § 14,101

[67] ¶ 4410; BUSEXP: 54,550; § 14,215

tion power, landfill gas, trash combustion, qualified hydroelectric, and marine and hydrokinetic energy facilities generate a credit amount of 1.1 cents per kilowatt-hour in 2014. The credit amount for production of refined coal in 2014 is $6.601 per ton and for Indian coal it is $2.317 per ton (Notice 2014-36).

The credit is reduced in the same ratio as the excess of the reference price for the calendar year in which the sale occurs over eight cents bears to three cents. The reference price and the eight-cent threshold amount are each adjusted annually by multiplying them by an inflation adjustment factor for the calendar year in which the sale occurs.

For 2014, the inflation adjustment factor for qualified energy resources and refined coal is 1.5088 and for Indian coal is 1.1587. The reference price for electricity produced from wind is 4.85 cents per kilowatt-hour; for refined coal production the reference price for 2002 is 31.90 and for 2014 is $56.88 per ton; the reference prices for electricity produced from closed-loop biomass, open-looped biomass, geothermal energy, solar energy, small irrigation power, municipal solid waste, and qualified hydropower production facilities has not been determined for calendar year 2014. The phaseout of the credit for electricity produced by wind does not apply for calendar year 2014, nor does it apply to refined coal sold in calendar year 2014. The phaseout of the credit for production of electricity from closed-loop biomass, open-looped biomass, geothermal energy, solar energy, small irrigation power, municipal solid waste, qualified hydroelectric production, and marine and hydrokinetic energy does not apply during calendar year 2014 (Notice 2014-36).

The credit is claimed on Form 8835 and is one of the components of the general business credit (¶ 1365). The credit limitation for the renewable energy source credit is determined separately from the other general business credits. In the calculation of the tax liability limitation, the tentative minimum tax is to be treated as zero. The result is that the renewable energy source credit amounts are available to be used against both the regular and the alternative minimum tax liabilities for the current year (Code Sec. 38(c)(4)).

Qualified Energy Facilities. The credit for electricity from renewable energy sources can be claimed over a 5-or 10-year period depending on the facility. The following facilities qualify for the 5-year period: (1) open-loop biomass facilities that use agricultural livestock waste nutrients originally placed in service after October 22, 2004, and on or before August 8, 2005; (2) open-loop biomass facilities that do not use agricultural livestock waste nutrients originally placed in service before January 1, 2005; (3) geothermal facilities originally placed in service after October 22, 2004, and on or before August 8, 2005; (4) solar facilities originally placed in service after October 22, 2004, and on or before August 8, 2005; (5) small irrigation power facilities originally placed in service after October 22, 2004, and on or before August 8, 2005; (6) landfill gas facilities originally placed in service after October 22, 2004, and on or before August 8, 2005; and (7) trash combustion facilities (or certain new units placed in service in connection with an existing trash combustion facility) originally placed in service after October 22, 2004, and on or before August 8, 2005.

The following facilities qualify to claim the credit for the 10-year period for electricity from a renewable energy source: (1) wind facilities originally placed in service after December 31, 1993, and the construction of which begins before January 1, 2014; (2) open-loop biomass facilities originally placed in service after August 8, 2005, and the construction of which begins before January 1, 2014; (3) closed-loop biomass facilities modified to use closed-loop biomass to co-fire with coal, other biomass, or both originally placed in service after December 31, 1992, and the construction of which begins before January 1, 2014; (4) any other closed-loop biomass facilities originally placed in service after December 31, 1992, and the construction of which begins before January 1, 2014; (5) geothermal facilities originally placed in service after August 8, 2005, and the construction of which begins before January 1, 2014; (6) solar facilities originally placed in service after August 8, 2005, and before January 1, 2006; (7) small irrigation power facilities originally placed in service after August 8, 2005, and before October 3, 2008; (8) landfill gas facilities originally placed in service after August 8, 2005, and the construc-

¶1365N

tion of which begins before January 1, 2014; (9) trash facilities (or new units placed in service in connection with an existing trash facility) originally placed in service after August 8, 2005, and the construction of which begins before January 1, 2014; (10) refined coal production facilities placed in service after October 22, 2004, and before January 1, 2010; (11) qualified hydropower facilities placed in service after August 8, 2005, and the construction of which begins before January 1, 2014 (and 10-year period begins on date such improvements are placed in service); and (12) marine and hydrokinetic renewable energy facility, originally placed in service on or after October 3, 2008, and the construction of which begins before January 1, 2014 (Code Sec. 45(d)). In the case of Indian coal, the credit may be claimed over an eight-year period from an Indian coal production facility placed in service after January 1, 2006, and before January 1, 2014.

Construction Starting Date. Construction on a facility is deemed to begin prior to January 1, 2014, if a taxpayer either begins physical work of a significant nature prior to January 1, 2014 or pays or incurs at least five percent of the total cost of the facility prior to January 1, 2014. A special rule that applies to a single project consisting of multiple facilities allows a taxpayer that pays or incurs at least three percent but less than five percent of the total cost of the project before January 1, 2014, to treat the number of individuals facilities with a total aggregate cost not greater than twenty times the amount paid or incurred before January 1, 2014, as eligible for the credit (Notice 2014-46, clarifying and modifying Notice 2013-29, and Notice 2013-60).

13650. Empowerment Zone Credit. Employers located in empowerment zones are entitled to a 20-percent wage credit on the first $15,000 of annual wages paid or incurred for services performed within an empowerment zone by residents of the empowerment zone (¶ 999) (Code Sec. 1396). The empowerment zone designation terminates December 31, 2013. The credit is computed on wages paid during the calendar year that ends within the employer's tax year (Code Sec. 1391(d)(1)(A)(i)).[68] The credit is claimed on Form 8844 and, although part of the general business credit (¶ 1365), is not a part of the general business credit tax liability limitation computation.

> **Comment:** Absent further legislation, empowerment zone designations terminate December 31, 2013 (Code Sec. 1391(d)(1)(A)(i)). Thus, the empowerment zone credit may not be claimed for wages paid or incurred after December 31, 2013. For the latest legislative updates, visit our website www.CCHGroup.com/TaxUpdates.

1365Q. Indian Employment Credit. A nonrefundable credit is available to employers for certain wages and health insurance costs paid or incurred in a tax year that begins on or before December 31, 2013, for qualified full- or part-time employees who are enrolled members of an Indian tribe or their spouses (Code Sec. 45A).[69] The credit is equal to 20 percent of the excess of eligible employee qualified wages and health insurance costs paid or incurred during a tax year over the amount of the costs paid or incurred during 1993. However, the credit is available only for the first $20,000 of qualified wages and health insurance costs paid for each qualified employee. Also, no deduction is allowed for the portion of wages equal to the amount of the credit. Qualified wages are wages paid or incurred by an employer for services performed by a qualified employee excluding wages for which a work opportunity credit (¶ 1365G) is allowed. Qualified health insurance costs are costs paid or incurred by an employer for a qualified employee, except for costs paid under a salary reduction agreement.

> **Comment:** Absent further legislation, the Indian employment credit has expired for tax years beginning after December 31, 2013. For the latest legislative updates, visit our website www.CCHGroup.com/TaxUpdates.

Eligibility. An individual who receives more than 50 percent of wages from services performed in the trade or business of the employer is a qualified employee for any period *only* if: (1) the individual was an enrolled member of an Indian tribe or the spouse

---

References are to Standard Federal Tax Reports; Tax Research Consultant; and Practical Tax Explanations.

[68] ¶ 32,393; BUSEXP: 54,650; § 13,810

[69] ¶ 4430; BUSEXP: 54,700; § 13,815

thereof; (2) substantially all of the services performed during the period by the employee for the employer were performed within an Indian reservation; and (3) the principal place of abode of the employee while performing the services was on or near the reservation on which the services are performed. Ineligible employees include employees who receive wages exceeding an dollar amount, adjusted annually for inflation ($45,000 in 2013) (Code Sec. 45A(c)(3)).

The credit is calculated on Form 8845 and is claimed as one of the components of the general business credit (¶ 1365). Thus, it is subject to the tax liability limitation and carryover rules. Any unused credit at the end of the carryforward period is allowed as a deduction in the year following the expiration of the period (Code Sec. 196).

1365R. Credit for Employer-Paid Social Security Taxes on Employee Cash Tips (FICA Tip Credit). An employer in the food and beverage industry may claim a nonrefundable income tax credit for a portion of the employer's Social Security and Medicare taxes (FICA taxes) paid or incurred on employee tips (Code Sec. 45B).[70] Employee tip income is treated as employer-provided wages for purposes of FICA taxes (Code Sec. 3121(q)). The credit is equal to the employer's FICA obligation to an employee attributable to excess tips treated as wages for purposes of satisfying the minimum wage provisions of the Fair Labor Standards Act. No credit may be claimed for the employer's portion of FICA taxes on the tips used to meet the Federal minimum wage rate. For purposes of calculating the credit only, the minimum wage rate has been permanently established at the amount in effect on January 1, 2007, or $5.15 per hour.

The credit is allowed for tips received from customers in connection with the providing, delivering, or serving of food or beverages for consumption if the tipping of employees delivering or serving food or beverages by customers is customary. The credit is available whether or not the employee reported the tips and regardless of where the services were performed. The employer may not deduct any amount considered in determining this credit to claim any other tax benefit. An election may be made to have this credit not apply.

The FICA tip credit is claimed on Form 8846 and is a component of the general business credit (¶ 1365). For purposes of determining the amount of the FICA tip credit that may be claimed in the current tax year and any credit carrybacks from the current tax year, the tentative minimum tax is considered zero and the credit amount is not subject to the general business credit tax liability limitation rule but is calculated separately (Code Sec. 38(c)(4)(A)). The result of setting the minimum tax at zero and reducing the net tax liability allows taxpayers to claim the maximum amount of the FICA tip credit against both their regular and the alternative minimum tax liabilities. Any credit that remains unused at the end of the carryover period is lost.

1365S. Credit for Clinical Testing Expenses for Certain Drugs for Rare Diseases and Conditions (Orphan Drug Credit). A credit, commonly known as the orphan drug credit, is allowed for an amount equal to 50 percent, subject to limitations, of the clinical testing expenses to develop drugs to treat rare diseases and conditions (Code Sec. 45C).[71] The credit is claimed on Form 8820 and is a component of the general business credit. Thus, it is subject to the general business credit's tax liability limitation and carryover rules (¶ 1365).

1365T. New Markets Tax Credit. The new markets tax credit is available for equity investments made in low-income community through a qualified community development entity (CDE) (Code Sec. 45D).[72] The credit is equal to five percent of the equity investment for the first three allowance dates and six percent of the equity investment for the next four allowance dates. The total credit available is equal to 39 percent of the investment over seven years. Active involvement of the low-income communities is required with strict penalties if the investment is terminated before seven years.

References are to Standard Federal Tax Reports; Tax Research Consultant; and Practical Tax Explanations.

[70] ¶ 4450; BUSEXP: 54,400; § 14,005

[71] ¶ 4470; BUSEXP: 54,450; § 14,405

[72] ¶ 4480; BUSEXP: 54,900; § 14,430

The equity investment must be made within five years after the date that the CDE receives an allocation of the new markets tax credit limitation amount specified for the calendar year (Code Sec. 45D(b)(1)). The limitation amount for calendar year 2013 is $3.5 billion (Code Sec. 45D(f)).

> **Comment:** Absent further legislation, there is no allocation of the new markets tax credit limitation for calendar years beginning after 2013. For the latest legislative updates, visit our website www.CCHGroup.com/TaxUpdates.

The new markets tax credit is a component of the general business credit, subject to its tax liability limitation and carryover rules (¶ 1365). The credit is calculated on Form 8874. Any unused credit at the end of the carryforward period is allowed as a deduction in the following tax year under Code Sec. 196. Any termination event requires recapture of the credit amount claimed, treated as an addition to tax in the termination year. Any amount carried forward or carried back will need to be adjusted accordingly. Finally, claiming the new markets tax credit necessitates an adjustment in the basis of the investment in the CDE.

1365U. Small Employer Pension Plan Startup Costs Credit. Eligible small businesses may claim a credit for qualified startup costs incurred in establishing and administering an eligible employer benefit plan for their employees (Code Sec. 45E).[73] The credit equals 50 percent of the qualified startup costs incurred to create or maintain a new employee retirement plan. The credit is limited to $500 in any tax year and it may be claimed for qualified costs incurred in each of the three years beginning with the tax year in which the plan becomes effective. The credit is part of the general business credit and subject to the tax liability limitation and carryover rules of the general business credit (¶ 1365). Form 8881 is used to calculate and claim the credit.

Eligibility. An eligible small business is one that has not employed more than 100 employees who received at least $5,000 of compensation from that employer in the preceding year. A business is not eligible if during the preceding three tax years it established or maintained a qualified employer plan with respect to which contributions were made, or benefits were accrued, for substantially the same employees as are in the new qualified employer plan. An eligible plan includes a new qualified defined contribution or defined benefit plan (¶ 2101), savings incentive match plans for employees (SIMPLEs) (¶ 2187), or simplified employee pension plans (SEP) (¶ 2189).

Qualified startup costs are any ordinary and necessary expenses incurred to establish or administer an eligible plan or to educate employees about retirement planning. Qualified costs are not deductible to the extent that they are effectively offset by the tax credit. The credit is applied to the first $1,000 of qualified costs incurred in the first year the new plan is effective and in each of the following two years. The employer may elect to take the credit in the year immediately preceding the first year the new plan is effective or elect not to claim the credit for a tax year.

1365V. Employer-Provided Child Care Credit. Businesses may claim a tax credit for qualified expenses related to either an employer-provided child care center or a service related to locating qualified child care (Code Sec. 45F).[74] The credit for a given tax year is the sum of 25 percent of the qualified child care expenditures and 10 percent of the qualified resource and referral expenditures. The maximum amount of credit allowed in any given year is $150,000. Form 8882 is used to calculate and claim the credit. The credit is part of the general business credit and is subject to its tax liability limitation and carryover rules (¶ 1365).

No double benefit is allowed for expenditures used to claim the employer-provided child care credit and the basis of the qualified child care facility must be reduced by the amount of the credit taken. In addition, there is no deduction allowed in the year following the final year of any carryforward of unused employer-provided child care credit. If a qualified child care facility ceases to operate as a qualified child care facility (or there is a change in ownership), the business may have to recapture part or all of the

13 TAX CREDITS

References are to Standard Federal Tax Reports; Tax Research Consultant; and Practical Tax Explanations.

[73] ¶ 4491; BUSEXP: 54,950; § 14,010

[74] ¶ 4493; BUSEXP: 55,000; § 14,015

credit claimed. In the event of recapture, the tax liability of that tax year must be increased by an amount equal to the applicable percentage times the aggregate decrease in the general business credit as if all previously allowed employer-provided child care credits with respect to the employer's child care facility had been zero (Code Sec. 45F(d)(2)(A)). Any carryforward or carryback amounts of the employer-provided child care credit must also be adjusted.

Qualifying Facility. A qualified child care facility is a facility whose principal use is to provide child care assistance and that meets the requirements of all applicable laws and regulations of the state and local government in which it is located, including the licensing requirements applicable to a child care facility. The principal use requirement is waived for facilities located in the principal residence of the operator of the facility. Additional requirements include that: (1) enrollment must be open to the employees of the taxpayer during the tax year; (2) at least 30 percent of the enrollees at the facility are the dependents of the taxpayer's employees (¶ 133), in the event the facility is the principal trade or business of the taxpayer; and (3) the use of the child care facility cannot discriminate in favor of highly compensated employees (¶ 2017).

Qualifying Expenditures. Qualified child care expenditures are amounts paid or incurred: (1) to acquire, construct, rehabilitate, or expand property which is to used as a qualified child care facility of the taxpayer; (2) for the operating costs of a qualified child care facility, including the costs related to the training of employees, scholarship programs, and providing increased compensation for employees with high levels of child care training; or (3) under a contract with a qualified child care facility to provide child care services to the taxpayer's employees. Costs associated with item (1) must qualify for depreciation or amortization and must not be the principal residence of the taxpayer. Expenses for items (2) and (3) cannot exceed the fair market value of such care. Further, qualified child care resources and referral expenditures are expenses paid or incurred by the taxpayer under a contract to provide child care services to the taxpayer's employees. These expenditures cannot discriminate in favor of highly compensated employees.

1365W. Railroad Track Maintenance Credit. An income tax credit is available to small-and mid-sized railroad companies for qualified railroad track maintenance expenses (Code Sec. 45G).[75] The credit is equal to 50 percent of the qualified expenses paid or incurred by an eligible taxpayer in tax years beginning before January 1, 2014. The credit cannot exceed $3,500 multiplied by the number of miles of railroad track owned or leased by the eligible taxpayer as of the close of the tax year. Eligible taxpayers are Class II and Class III railroad companies and persons who operate over their rail lines or provide related rail services. The credit is a part of the general business credit but is not subject to the tax liability limitation rule. Instead, the credit is allowed against the sum of the regular income tax and alternative minimum tax liabilities (Code Sec. 38(c)). The credit is subject to the general business credit's carryover rules (¶ 1365). No provision is made for deduction of unused credits at the end of the carryforward period or if the taxpayer ceases to exist. The credit is claimed on Form 8900.

> **Comment:** Absent further legislation, the railroad track maintenance credit has expired for expenses paid or incurred in tax years beginning after December 31, 2013. For the latest legislative updates, visit our website www.CCHGroup.com/TaxUpdates.

1365X. Biodiesel Fuels Credit. A producer of biodiesel fuels may claim a credit equal to the sum of the biodiesel mixture credit, the biodiesel credit, and the small agri-biodiesel producer credit (Code Sec. 40A).[76] The credit is computed on Form 8864 and may be claimed for fuels sold or used before January 1, 2014. The credit is part of the general business credit and is subject to its tax liability limitation and carryover rules (¶ 1365). Any unused credit at the end of the carryforward period, or if the taxpayer ceases to exist, may be claimed as a deduction (Code Sec. 196). No credit is allowed for

---

References are to Standard Federal Tax Reports; Tax Research Consultant; and Practical Tax Explanations.

[75] ¶ 4495; BUSEXP: 55,050; §14,415

[76] ¶ 4310; BUSEXP: 55,100; §14,220

any biodiesel which is produced outside the United States for use as a fuel outside the United States.

> **Comment:** Absent further legislation, the biodiesel fuels credit has expired for sales or uses after December 31, 2013. For the latest legislative updates, visit our website www.CCHGroup.com/TaxUpdates.

The biodiesel mixture credit is $1.00 for each gallon of biodiesel used by the taxpayer in the production of a qualified biodiesel mixture. A qualified biodiesel mixture is a mixture of biodiesel and diesel fuel, determined without regard to any use of kerosene, which is sold by the taxpayer producing the mixture to any person for use as a fuel or is used as a fuel by the taxpayer producing the mixture. The sale or use by the taxpayer must be in the taxpayer's trade or business. Casual off-farm production is not eligible for the credit (Code Sec. 40A(b)(1)).

The biodiesel credit is $1.00 for each gallon of biodiesel which is not in a mixture with diesel fuel and which is used by the taxpayer as a fuel in a trade or business or is sold by the taxpayer at retail to a person and placed in the fuel tank of the person's vehicle (Code Sec. 40A(b)(2)). Biodiesel fuels are defined as monoalkyl esters of long chain fatty acids derived from plant or animal matter that meet the requirements for fuels or fuel additives imposed by the Environmental Protection Agency and which meet the requirements of the American Society of Testing and Materials D6751 (Code Sec. 40A(d)(1)).

The small agri-biodiesel producer credit of any eligible small agri-biodiesel producer is 10 cents for each gallon of qualified agri-biodiesel production. Qualified agri-biodiesel production means any agri-biodiesel which is produced by an eligible small agri-biodiesel producer and: (1) is sold by the producer to another person (a) for use by the other person in the production of a qualified biodiesel mixture in the other person's trade or business (other than casual off-farm production), (b) for use by the other person as a fuel in a trade or business, or (c) who sells the agri-biodiesel at retail to another person and places the agri-biodiesel in the fuel tank of such other person; or (2) is used or sold by the producer for any of these purposes.

An eligible agri-biodiesel fuel producer's production of qualified agri-biodiesel cannot exceed 15 million gallons per tax year (Code Sec. 40A(b)(4)). An eligible small agri-biodiesel producer is a person with a productive capacity for agri-biodiesel not in excess of 60 million gallons per tax year (Code Sec. 40A(e)(1)). Agri-biodiesel is biodiesel derived solely from virgin oils, including esters derived from virgin vegetable oils from corn, soybeans, sunflower seeds, cottonseeds, canola, crambe, rapeseeds, safflowers, flaxseeds, rice bran, and mustard seeds, camelina, and animal fats (Code Sec. 40A(d)(2)).

If a credit was claimed on biodiesel used in the production of a qualified biodiesel fuel mixture, a tax equal to the $1 per gallon credit rate is imposed on any person who separates the biodiesel from the mixture or does not use the mixture as a fuel. A $1 per gallon tax is imposed on any person who mixes biodiesel or uses it other than as a fuel if the biodiesel credit was claimed with respect to the retail sale of the biodiesel. A 10 cent per gallon tax is imposed on a person who does not use agri-biodiesel production for which a credit was claimed for one of the qualifying purposes described above (Code Sec. 40A(d)(3)).

1365Y. Low Sulfur Diesel Fuel Production Credit (Expired). A credit of five cents per gallon was available to small business refiners for the production of low sulfur diesel fuel unless an election out from claiming the credit was made (Code Sec. 45H).[77] The credit was intended to subsidize the costs incurred by small refiners to comply with Environmental Protection Agency (EPA) regulations requiring refiners to produce diesel fuel with a low sulfur content (15 parts per million or less). The maximum credit available was 25 percent of the qualified costs incurred by the refiner in bringing the refining facility into compliance with the EPA's Highway Diesel Fuel Sulfur Control

---

References are to Standard Federal Tax Reports; Tax Research Consultant; and Practical Tax Explanations.

[77] ¶ 4497; BUSEXP: 55,150; § 14,225

Requirements. The credit applied only to costs incurred between January 1, 2003, and December 31, 2009, or if earlier, one year after the date on which the taxpayer had to comply with the EPA requirements. The credit was claimed on Form 8896.

1365Z. Distilled Spirits Excise Tax Carrying Credit. An income tax credit is available for wholesalers, qualified distillers, and importers that carry distilled spirits subject to excise taxes in inventory (Code Sec. 5011).[78] The credit is generally calculated to equal the approximate interest charges that the eligible taxpayer would incur while holding the distilled spirits in inventory. The credit is a component of the general business credit and is subject to its tax liability limitation and carryover rules (¶ 1365). The credit is claimed on Form 8906.

1365AA. Advanced Nuclear Power Facilities Production Credit. A tax credit is available to taxpayers that produce electricity from an advanced nuclear power facility (Code Sec. 45J).[79] The credit is equal to 1.8 cents times the number of kilowatt hours of electricity produced at a qualifying advanced nuclear power facility and sold to an unrelated person during the tax year. It may only be claimed during the eight-year period beginning on the date the facility was originally placed in service. A qualifying advanced nuclear power facility is any advanced nuclear facility owned by the taxpayer that uses nuclear energy to produce electricity and was placed in service after August 8, 2005, and before January 1, 2021. Any nuclear facility with a reactor design (or a substantially similar design of comparable capacity) approved before 1994 by the Nuclear Regulatory Commission is not a qualifying advanced nuclear power facility. Certain limitations restrict the amount of credit that may be claimed in any tax year, including that the credit is part of the general business credit and as such is subject to the tax liability limitation and carryover rules (¶ 1365).

1365BB. Nonconventional Source Fuel Production Credit. A tax credit is allowed for the domestic production of qualified fuels derived from nonconventional sources produced by the taxpayer within the United States or U.S. possession and sold to unrelated persons (Code Sec. 45K).[80] The credit is available for coke or coke gas produced in facilities placed in service before January 1, 1993, or after June 30, 1998, and before January 1, 2010, that is sold during the period beginning after the later of January 1, 2006, or the year the facility is placed in service but no later than four years after the start of such period. The credit is no longer available for fuel produced from biomass and liquid, gaseous, or solid synthetic fuels.

The credit is a component of the general business credit and is subject to the ordering, tax liability limitation, and carryover rules of the general business credit (¶ 1365). The credit amount is reduced pro rata by any grants, tax-exempt bonds, and subsidized energy financing the project receives. No double benefits are allowed as the credit amount is reduced by any credit amount claimed as an energy credit and/or enhanced oil recovery credit. The credit is claimed on Form 8907.

Credit Amount. The credit is equal to $3 multiplied by the barrel-of-oil equivalent of qualified fuels produced and sold by the taxpayer to an unrelated third party. The $3 amount is annually adjusted for inflation (Code Sec. 45K(a) and (b)(2)). The inflation adjustment factor for calendar year 2013 is 1.1975. Thus, the inflation-adjusted credit amount per barrel-of-oil equivalent sold in calendar year 2013 is $3.59 (Notice 2014-25). The inflation factor is determined and published no later than April 1st for the preceding calendar year.

1365CC. Energy Efficient Home Credit. Eligible contractors who build an energy-efficient home acquired by a person for use as a residence before January 1, 2014, can claim an income tax credit of up to $2,000 (Code Sec. 45L).[81] Eligible contractors also include manufacturers of energy-efficient manufactured homes. A residence qualifies as an energy-efficient home if it is located in the United States and is certified to have an annual heating and/or cooling consumption at least 50 percent less than a comparable

---

References are to Standard Federal Tax Reports; Tax Research Consultant; and Practical Tax Explanations.

[78] ¶ 34,965; BUSEXP: 55,250   [80] ¶ 4050; BUSEXP: 54,500;   [81] ¶ 4500I; BUSEXP: 55,350;
[79] ¶ 4500A; BUSEXP: 55,300;   § 14,240   § 14,315
§ 14,235

house with at least 10 percent of the 50 percent saving coming from the building envelope. A reduced credit of $1,000 is available for homes with a heating or cooling consumption at least 30 percent less than a comparable house and for homes with the Energy Star label. The credit is a component of the general business credit and is subject to the tax liability limitation and carryover rules of the general business credit (¶ 1365). The credit is claimed on Form 8908.

> **Comment:** Absent further legislation, the energy efficient home credit has expired for residences acquired after December 31, 2013. For the latest legislative updates, visit our website www.CCHGroup.com/TaxUpdates.

1365DD. Energy Efficient Appliance Credit. An income tax credit is available to taxpayers that manufacture energy-efficient home appliances in calendar years after 2005 and before 2014 (Code Sec. 45M).[82] The total credit available for a tax year is equal to the sum of the credit separately calculated for each type of qualified energy-efficient appliance (dishwashers, clothes washers, and refrigerators) produced by the taxpayer during the calendar year ending with or within that tax year. The credit for each type of qualified appliance is determined by multiplying the eligible production for that type of appliance by the type's applicable amount. The maximum credit is reduced each subsequent year by the amount of credit, if any, claimed in the prior year. In addition, there are sub-limits for each type of home appliance. This credit is a component of the general business credit and is subject to its tax liability limitations and carryover rules (¶ 1365). The credit is claimed on Form 8909.

> **Comment:** Absent further legislation, the energy efficient appliance credit has expired for appliances manufactured after December 31, 2013. For the latest legislative updates, visit our website www.CCHGroup.com/TaxUpdates.

1365FF. Employee Retention Credit (Expired). An employee retention credit is available for qualified individuals hired after February 3, 2010, and before January 1, 2011 (Act Sec. 102 of the Hiring Incentives to Restore Employment Act (P.L. 111-147)).[83] Qualified employers who retain qualified individuals as employees for 52 consecutive weeks can increase any current year general business credit (¶ 1365) by up to $1,000 per retained worker. Thus, the additional general business credit amount cannot be claimed until after the retained worker remains employed for 52 consecutive weeks. Qualified employees are individuals who:

- certified that he or she has not been employed for more than 40 hours during the 60-day period ending on the date that he or she was hired,

- was not hired to replace another employee unless that employee separated from the employer voluntarily or for cause, and

- is not a related individual as defined in Code Sec. 51(i)(1).

1365GG. Mine Rescue Team Training Credit. Eligible employers are entitled to a tax credit for mine rescue team training expenses paid or incurred in tax years beginning after December 21, 2005, and before January 1, 2014 (Code Sec. 45N).[84] The credit is equal to the lesser of: (1) 20 percent of the training program costs paid or incurred during the tax year for each qualified mine rescue team employee, including wages paid while attending the training program, or (2) $10,000. An eligible employer is any taxpayer that employs individuals as miners in underground mines located in the United States. A qualified mine rescue team employee is a full-time miner employee who is eligible for more than six months of the tax year to serve as a mine rescue team member because he or she has met certain training requirements. To prevent any double benefits that may arise from the claiming of this credit, eligible mine employers cannot claim as a wage the amount of any mine rescue team training credit determined

---

References are to Standard Federal Tax Reports; Tax Research Consultant; and Practical Tax Explanations.

[82] ¶ 4500N; BUSEXP: 55,400; § 14,320

[83] ¶ 4250; BUSEXP: 54,070; § 13,835

[84] ¶ 4500S; BUSEXP: 55,450; § 14,435

for the tax year (Code Sec. 280C). The mine rescue team training credit is claimed on Form 8923 and is a component of the general business credit subject to its tax liability limitation and carryover rules (¶ 1365).

> **Comment:** Absent further legislation, the mine rescue team training credit has expired for amounts paid or incurred in tax years beginning after December 31, 2013. For the latest legislative updates, visit our website www.CCHGroup.com/TaxUpdates.

1365HH. Agricultural Chemicals Security Credit (Expired). For qualified chemical security expenditures paid or incurred after May 22, 2008, and before January 1, 2013, eligible agricultural businesses may claim the agricultural chemical security credit (Code Sec. 45O).[85] The credit is equal to 30 percent of the qualified chemical security expenditures. The credit limit is $100,000 per facility reduced by the aggregate amount of this credit claimed in the previous five years. In addition, each taxpayer has an annual limit of $2 million. The taxpayer is defined to include controlled groups under rules set out in Code Sec. 41(f). The taxpayer's deductible expenses are reduced by the amount of credit claimed. In addition, the credit is a component of the general business credit subject to its tax liability limitation and carryover rules (¶ 1365). The credit is claimed on Form 8931.

Eligibility. Eligible agricultural businesses are businesses that: (1) sell agricultural products, including certain specified agricultural chemicals, at retail predominantly to farmers and ranchers, or (2) manufacture, formulate, distribute, or aerially apply specified agricultural chemicals. Qualified chemical expenditures are amounts paid or incurred for: (1) employee security training and background checks, (2) limitations and prevention of access to controls of specified agricultural chemicals stored at a facility, (3) tagging, locking tax valves, and chemical additives to prevent the theft of specified agricultural chemicals or to render such chemicals unfit for illegal use, (4) protection of the perimeter of specified agricultural chemicals, (5) installation of security lighting, cameras, recording equipment and intrusion detection sensors, (6) implementation of measures to increase computer or computer network securities, (7) conducting security vulnerability assessments, (8) implementing a site security plan, and (9) other measures provided for by regulation.

1365II. Employer Credit for Differential Wage Payments to Military Personnel. Eligible employers making differential wage payments after June 17, 2008, and before January 1, 2014, can claim a tax credit equal to 20 percent of eligible payments for each employee (Code Sec. 45P).[86] An eligible differential wage payment is a payment that: (1) must be made by an employer to an individual with respect to any period during which the individual is performing services in the uniformed armed forces on active duty for a period of more than 30 days, and (2) must represent all or a portion of the wages that the individual would have received from the employer if the individual were performing services for the employer (Code Sec. 3401) (¶ 895 and ¶ 2609). The differential wage payment is limited to $20,000 per employee paid during the tax year.

A qualified employee is an individual who has been employed by the employer for a period of 91 days immediately preceding the period for which any differential wage payments were made. A qualified employer is a small business employer that: (1) employs an average of fewer than 50 individuals on any day during the tax year, and (2) provides differential wage payments to every qualified employee under a written plan. The deduction for wages is reduced by the amount of differential wage payment credit claimed as well as reducing any other credit related to compensation paid to eligible employees. The credit is a component of the general business credit subject to its tax liability limitation and carryover rules (¶ 1365). The credit is claimed on Form 8932.

> **Comment:** Absent further legislation, the differential wage payment credit has expired for payments made after December 31, 2013. For the latest legislative updates, visit our website www.CCHGroup.com/TaxUpdates.

References are to Standard Federal Tax Reports; Tax Research Consultant; and Practical Tax Explanations.

[85] ¶ 4500W; BUSEXP: 55,550; § 14,445

[86] ¶ 4500Z; BUSEXP: 55,500; § 14,020

1365JJ. Carbon Dioxide Capture Credit. Taxpayers may claim a tax credit for the capture and transport of carbon dioxide from an industrial source after October 3, 2008, for use in enhanced oil recovery or for permanent storage in a geologic formation (Code Sec. 45Q).[87] The credit is $20 per metric ton of qualified carbon dioxide that is captured by the taxpayer at a qualified facility and disposed of in secure geological storage. The credit is $10 per metric ton of qualified carbon dioxide that is captured by the taxpayer at a qualified facility, used as a tertiary injectant in a qualified enhanced oil or natural gas recovery project, and disposed of in secure geologic storage. The $20 and $10 credit amounts are adjusted for inflation. The inflation adjusted amounts for calendar year 2014 are $21.51 per metric ton of qualified CO2 under Code Sec. 45Q(a)(1) and $10.75 per metric ton of qualified CO2 under Code Sec. 45Q(a)(2) (Notice 2014-40).

The credit is recaptured with respect to any qualified carbon dioxide that ceases to be captured, disposed of, or used as a tertiary injectant in accordance with the credit requirements (Code Sec. 45Q(d)(6)). The credit is attributable to the person that captures and physically or contractually ensures the disposal, or the use as a tertiary injectant, of the qualified carbon dioxide, except to the extent provided by regulations (Code Sec. 45Q(d)(5)). The credit applies with respect to qualified carbon dioxide before the end of the calendar year in which the IRS, in consultation with the Environmental Protection Agency, certifies that 75-million metric tons of qualified carbon dioxide have been captured or disposed of or used as a tertiary injectant (Code Sec. 45Q(e)). The credit is a component of the general business credit subject to its tax liability limitation and carryover rules (¶ 1365). The credit is claimed on Form 8933.

Eligibility. Qualified carbon dioxide is carbon dioxide captured from an industrial source that would otherwise be released into the atmosphere as an industrial emission of greenhouse gas and that is measured at the source of capture and verified at the point of disposal or injection. Qualified carbon dioxide includes the initial deposit of captured carbon dioxide used as a tertiary injectant, but does not include carbon dioxide that is recaptured, recycled, and reinjected as part of the enhanced oil and natural gas recovery process (Code Sec. 45Q(b)). Only carbon dioxide captured and disposed of or used within the United States or its possessions (including the continental shelf areas as defined in Code Sec. 638) is taken into account in computing the credit (Code Sec. 45Q(d)(1)).

1365LL. Therapeutic Discovery Project Credit (Expired). A tax credit was allowed for 50 percent of an eligible taxpayer's qualified investment for tax years beginning in 2009 and 2010 with respect to any qualifying therapeutic discovery project (Code Sec. 48D).[88] The credit was part of the investment credit (¶ 1365A), and the basis of any property that was part of a qualifying therapeutic discovery project was included in the credit base for purposes of applying the investment credit at-risk limitation rules under Code Sec. 49 (Code Secs. 46(6) and 49(a)(1)(C)(vi)).

Tax Credit Bonds

1371. Tax Credit Bonds. As an alternative to traditional tax-exempt bonds, states and local governments may issue tax credit bonds for certain purposes. Unlike tax-exempt bonds, tax credit bonds are not interest-bearing obligations. Rather, the taxpayer holding a tax credit bond on a credit-allowance date is entitled to a tax credit. The credit can be claimed against both the regular income tax and alternative minimum tax liabilities. To standardize the tax treatment of these bonds, they must meet certain requirements regarding the determination of the amount of the credit bond holders are entitled to receive. In addition, in order for a bondholder to qualify for the tax credit, the bond must meet certain requirements with respect to proceeds, expenditures, arbitrage, maturity limitations, and conflicts of interest (Code Sec. 54A)).[89]

Credit Amount. A taxpayer holding a tax credit bond on a credit-allowance date is entitled to a tax credit calculated on Form 8912. If the bond is held by a partnership or S

References are to Standard Federal Tax Reports; Tax Research Consultant; and Practical Tax Explanations.

[87] ¶ 4500ZH; BUSEXP: 55,600; § 14,450

[88] ¶ 4700; BUSEXP: 51,850; § 13,728

[89] ¶ 4882; BUSEXP: 55,800; § 14,501

13 | TAX CREDITS

corporation, the allocation of the credit to the shareholders or partners is treated as a distribution (Code Sec. 54A(g)). If the bond is held by a regulated investment company (RIC) or real estate investment trust (REIT), the credit is allocated and any interest treated as gross income is distributed to the shareholders or beneficiaries under procedures to be prescribed by the Secretary of the Treasury (Code Sec. 54A(h)).

The amount of the credit with respect to any allowance date is 25 percent of the annual credit amount determined on that allowance date (Code Sec. 54A(b)). The allowance dates are: March 15, June 15, September 15, and December 15. The annual credit amount is determined by multiplying the bond's applicable credit rate by the face amount on the holder's bond. The applicable credit rate is set by the Secretary of the Treasury at a rate that would permit issuance of a tax credit bond without discount and interest cost to the issuer. The taxpayer holding a tax credit bond on a quarterly credit-allowance date is entitled to a tax credit (Code Sec. 54A(a) and (e)(1)). The credit accrues quarterly and is includible in gross income as if it were an interest payment on the bond (Code Sec. 54A(f)).

The credit in a tax year cannot be larger than the sum of the taxpayer's regular tax liability plus minimum tax liability, minus the total of the taxpayer's credits against tax. The subtracted credits do not include refundable credits or the qualified tax bond credit itself (Code Sec. 54A(c)). Unused qualified tax credit bond amounts may be carried over to succeeding tax years. Special rules apply to S corporation, partnership, regulated investment companies, and real estate investment trust bond holders.

Reporting Requirements. The qualified issuer must submit reports similar to reports required under Code Sec. 149(e) for tax-exempt bonds (Code Sec. 54A(d)(3)). For other return purposes, the credit is reported as an interest payment (Code Sec. 6049(d)(9)). Holders of tax credit bonds receiving a credit amount of $10 or more are issued a Form 1099-INT.

Refundable Credit Election. To stimulate the rebuilding and improvement of local and state infrastructure, issuers of certain tax credit bonds may elect to claim a refundable credit generally equal to the amount of interest that would be payable to the holders of the bonds (Code Sec. 6431(f)). The election may be made only for bonds issued after March 18, 2010. The election can be made by issuers of new clean renewable energy bonds (¶ 1374), qualified energy conservation bonds (¶ 1375), qualified zone academy bonds other than those issued under the 2011 bond limitation or any carryforward of such allocation (¶ 1376), and qualified school construction bonds (¶ 1377). The election is similar to the alternative election available to issuers of Build America bonds (¶ 1378).

1373. Qualified Forestry Conservation Bonds. State and local governments, or qualified nonprofit organizations, may generally issue up to $500 million in qualified forestry conservation credit bonds (QFCB) after May 22, 2008, for the acquisition of forest and forest lands that are subject to conservation restrictions (Code Sec. 54B).[90] The purpose of the bonds is the acquisition of forest and forest lands from an unrelated third person that meets the following requirements: (1) some portion of the land acquired must be adjacent to United States Forest Service Land; (2) at least half of the land acquired must be transferred to the United States Forest Service at no net cost, and not more than half of the land acquired may either remain with or be donated to a state; (3) all of the land must be subject to a habitat conservation plan for native fish approved by the United States Fish and Wildlife Service; and (4) the amount of acreage acquired must be at least 40,000 acres. QFCB are tax credit bonds subject to rules similar to those that apply to qualified tax credit bonds (¶ 1371).

1374. New Clean Renewable Energy Bonds (NCREBs). New clean renewable energy bonds (NCREBs) provide a federal subsidy to allow nonprofit electricity produc-ers, including cooperatives and government-owned utilities, to compete more evenly

---

References are to Standard Federal Tax Reports; Tax Research Consultant; and Practical Tax Explanations.

[90] ¶ 4890; BUSEXP: 55,804; § 14,510.10

with for-profit companies that can take advantage of the production tax credit under Code Sec. 45 (Code Sec. 54C).[91] NCREBs are tax credit bonds subject to rules similar to those that apply to qualified tax credit bonds (¶ 1371).

An NCREB is a bond issued as part of an issue if: (1) 100 percent of the available project proceeds of the issue are to be used for capital expenditures incurred by governmental bodies, public power providers, or cooperative electric companies for one or more qualified renewable energy facilities; (2) the bond is issued by a qualified issuer; and (3) the issuer designates the bond as an NCREB (Code Sec. 54C(a)). Qualified renewable energy facilities are facilities that produce electrical power and are owned by a public power provider, a governmental body or a cooperative electric company and that qualify under the renewable electricity production credit (Code Sec. 45). Qualified facilities include wind facilities, closed-loop biomass facilities, open-loop biomass facilities, geothermal or solar energy facilities, small irrigation power facilities, landfill gas facilities, trash combustion facilities, and qualified hydropower facilities (Code Sec. 54C(d)(1)).

1375. Qualified Energy Conservation Bonds. State and local governments, or qualified nonprofit organizations, are authorized to issue qualified energy conservation bonds (QECBs) to finance energy conservation projects, including capital expenditures, research expenditures, expenses for mass commuting facilities, demonstration projects, and public education campaigns (Code Sec. 54D).[92] The bonds are subject to the requirements for tax credit bonds (¶ 1371) with the annual tax credit limited to 70 percent of the face amount times the applicable credit rate.

1376. Qualified Zone Academy Bond Credit. State and local governments were authorized to issue qualified zone academy bonds (QZAB) through 2013 to be used to improve certain eligible public schools (54E and Code Secs. 1397E).[93] QZABs issued after October 3, 2008, are subject to the requirements for qualified tax credit bonds (¶ 1371). QZABs issued prior to October 3, 2008, are subject to the provisions under Code Sec. 1397E.

1377. Qualified School Construction Tax Credit Bonds. Tax credit bonds known as qualified school construction bonds could be issued through December 31, 2010 (Code Sec. 54F).[94] The bonds must satisfy the requirements for qualified tax credit bonds (¶ 1371) (Code Sec. 54A(d)(1)(E)). A bond is a qualified school construction bond if: (1) 100 percent of the available project proceeds of the issue of which it is a part are to be used for the construction, rehabilitation, or repair of a public school facility or to acquire land on which a facility funded by the same issue is to be built; (2) the bond is issued by a state or local government within the jurisdiction of which the school is located; and (3) the issuer designates the bond as a qualified school construction bond (Code Sec. 54F(a)).

1378. Build America Bonds. State and local governments could issue taxable build America bonds through January 1, 2011, which provide the bondholder with both taxable interest and a tax credit (Code Sec. 54AA).[95] A build America bond is any obligation, other than a private activity bond, that meets these three requirements: (1) the bond must be issued before January 1, 2011; (2) the issuer must make an irrevocable election to have Code Sec. 54AA apply to the bond; and (3) but for that election, the interest on the bond would have been excludable under Code Sec. 103 (Code Sec. 54AA(d)(1)).

For purposes of the rules under Code Sec. 149(b) that exclude federally guaranteed bonds from the category of tax-exempt bonds, build America bonds are not treated as federally guaranteed by virtue of their cash payment or credit features. Also, for purposes of the rules under Code Sec. 148 that exclude arbitrage bonds from the

References are to Standard Federal Tax Reports; Tax Research Consultant; and Practical Tax Explanations.

[91] ¶ 4897; BUSEXP: 55,806; § 14,510.15

[92] ¶ 4902; BUSEXP: 55,808; § 14,510.20

[93] ¶ 32,405, ¶ 4910; BUSEXP: 57,150; § 14,510.25

[94] ¶ 4918; BUSEXP: 55,812; § 14,510.30

[95] ¶ 4932; BUSEXP: 55,814; § 14,515

¶1378

category of tax-exempt bonds, the yield on build America bonds must be determined without regard to the credit. Finally, build America bonds cannot have an issue price that has more than a *de minimis* amount of premium over the stated principal amount of the bond (a *de minimis* amount is generally ¼ of one percent of the stated redemption price at maturity, multiplied by the number of years to maturity) (Code Sec. 54AA(d)(2)).

Unlike tax credit bonds, which provide a tax credit in lieu of interest payments, build America bonds pay interest to the bondholders and also provide a tax credit. The bondholder must include the interest in gross income but is allowed a credit against federal income tax liability for a portion of the interest payments received (Code Sec. 54AA(a) and (f)(1)). The credit is itself treated as interest that is includible in gross income (Code Sec. 54AA(f)(2)). The tax credit is equal to 35 percent of the interest payable on the interest payment date of the bond (Code Sec. 54AA(b)). The interest payment date is any date on which the bondholder of record is entitled to a payment of interest under the bond (Code Sec. 54AA(e)).

Tax Liability Limitations. The credit cannot exceed the excess of the sum of the bondholder's regular tax liability and alternative minimum tax liability over the sum of the credits allowed under Code Secs. 21 through 54E, not including Code Secs. 31 through 37 and the build America bond credit itself. Any unused credit may be carried forward to succeeding tax years (Code Sec. 54AA(c)).

Rules similar to Code Sec. 54(g), (h) and (i) apply for purposes of the credit (Code Sec. 54AA(f)(2)). Thus, in the case of a build America bond held by a partnership or S corporation, the allocation of the credit to the partners or shareholders is treated as a distribution. For build America bonds held by a real estate investment trust (REIT), the credit is allowed to the respective beneficiaries (and any gross income included in income with respect to the credit is treated as distributed to them) under procedures to be prescribed by the Treasury Secretary.

Qualified Bonds Issued Before 2011. State and local governments may elect to issue certain build America bonds as qualified bonds before January 1, 2011. Qualified bonds are issued in exchange for a payment credit , determined in accordance with Code Sec. 6431. The payment credit to the issuer is in lieu of the credit that would otherwise be allowed to the bondholder and is generally equal to 35 percent of the interest paid on the bond (Code Sec. 54AA(g)(1)).

1380. Midwestern Tax Credit Bonds (Expired). States located in the Midwestern disaster area were authorized to issue Midwestern tax credit bonds during 2009 which could be used, in effect, to extend the maturity of existing obligations by two years at lower interest costs (Code Sec. 1400N(l)).[96] These bonds were subject to the requirements of tax credit bonds as discussed in ¶ 1371.

1385. Mutual Fund Election to Pass-Through Tax Credit Bond Credits. Regulated investment companies (RICs) may elect to pass through to their shareholders credits attributable to tax credit bonds held by the entity, replacing the required pass-through of the credits (Code Sec. 853A).[97] If the election is made, the RIC is not allowed any credits attributable to the tax credit bonds and includes in gross income, as interest, the amount of income that the entity would have included if the election did not apply, increasing the amount of the dividends paid by the same amount.

In order to qualify for the election, a RIC must hold directly or indirectly, one or more tax credit bonds on one or more applicable dates during the tax year and must also meet the 90 percent distribution requirements of a RIC under Code Sec. 852(a)(1). The RIC must also have been taxed as a RIC under Code Sec. 852 for all tax years ending on or after November 8, 1983, or have no accumulated earnings and profits from a tax year to which the RIC provisions did not apply.

References are to Standard Federal Tax Reports; Tax Research Consultant; and Practical Tax Explanations.

[96] ¶ 32,483; BUSEXP: 57,302.15; § 10,001

[97] ¶ 26,448; RIC: 3,366; § 14,505

Where the election is made, shareholders of the RIC are to include in income the shareholder's proportionate share of the interest income attributable to the credits and are simultaneously allowed the proportionate share of credits (Code Sec. 853A(b)(3)). A RIC must report to shareholders in a written notice the shareholder's proportionate share of credits and gross income in respect of the credits. The shareholder's proportionate share of credits and gross income in respect of the credits cannot exceed the amounts so designated by the RIC in the notice.

Miscellaneous Credits

1391. COBRA Premium Credit (Expired). A temporary reduction in premiums for COBRA coverage was provided to assistance eligible individuals who were involuntarily terminated from their employment (Code Sec. 6432).[98] An assistance eligible individual was treated for purposes of COBRA continuation coverage as having paid the premium required for coverage if the individual pays 35 percent of the premium. In effect, the individual was provided with a 65-percent reduction in premiums. An assistance eligible individual is any qualified beneficiary if: (1) at any time during the period beginning on September 1, 2008, and ending on May 31, 2010, the qualified beneficiary is eligible for COBRA continuation coverage; (2) the beneficiary elects such coverage; and (3) the qualifying event for which the beneficiary would otherwise lose health plan coverage is the involuntary termination of the covered employee's employment during such period (Act Sec. 3001(a)(3) and (a)(17) of the American Recovery and Reinvestment Act of 2009 (P.L. 111-5), as amended by the Department of Defense Appropriations Act, 2010 (P.L. 111-118), the Temporary Extension Act of 2010 (P.L. 111-144), and the Continuing Extension Act of 2010 (P.L. 111-157)).

The 65-percent premium reduction or subsidy terminated with the first month beginning on or after the earlier of: (1) the date that is 15 months after the first day of the first month for which the subsidy applies, (2) the end of the maximum required period of continuation coverage for the beneficiary under the Code's COBRA rules or the applicable state or federal law, or (3) the date the assistance eligible individual is eligible for coverage under Medicare or any other employer-sponsored health plan.

A person to whom premiums for COBRA continuation coverage were payable was reimbursed for the amount of premiums not paid by plan beneficiaries because of the temporary subsidy. The reimbursement was made in the form of a credit against the person's liability for payroll taxes.

References are to Standard Federal Tax Reports; Tax Research Consultant; and Practical Tax Explanations.

[98] ¶ 38,935; HEALTH: 24,118; § 42,845.05

Chapter 14

ALTERNATIVE MINIMUM TAX

	Par.
AMT Liability	1401
AMT Preferences and Adjustments	1425
Credits Against Minimum Tax	1470

AMT Liability

1401. Alternative Minimum Tax (AMT) Liability. The alternative minimum tax (AMT) is a separate method of determining tax liability designed to ensure that taxpayers do not completely avoid income tax through the use of deductions, exemptions, losses, and credits. All taxpayers subject to regular income tax are generally subject to the AMT, including individuals, estates, trusts, and corporations (Code Secs. 55(a) and 59(c)).[1] Partnerships and S corporations are not subject to the AMT. Instead, partners and shareholders compute their AMT liability separately by taking into account their share of partnership or S corporation items. Special rules apply, however, to partners of an electing large partnership using a simplified pass-through system (¶ 1455).

A taxpayer's AMT for a tax year is the excess of the taxpayer's tentative minimum tax over regular tax liability. AMT must be paid in addition to the regular tax liability and other federal taxes owed (¶ 1420). For example, if a taxpayer's tentative minimum tax for a tax year is $75,000 while regular tax liability is $50,000, the taxpayer must pay an AMT liability of $25,000 in addition to the $50,000 regular tax liability for a total tax liability of $75,000.

Tentative Minimum Tax. For an individual, estate, or trust, tentative minimum tax is equal to 26 percent of the taxpayer's alternative minimum taxable income (AMTI) up to a certain threshold amount, plus 28 percent of any AMTI in excess of the threshold amount (Code Sec. 55(b) and (d)(4); Rev. Proc. 2013-35; Rev. Proc. 2014-61).[2] For tax years beginning in 2014, the threshold amount is $182,500 ($91,250 if married filing separately). For tax years beginning in 2015, the threshold amount is $185,400 ($92,700 if married filing separately). For corporations, tentative minimum tax is 20 percent of AMTI, but certain small corporations and corporations in their first year of existence are exempt from the AMT (¶ 1415). A taxpayer's AMTI for this purpose is the taxpayer's regular taxable income increased by AMT tax preference items and modified by AMT adjustments (¶ 1405). A certain amount of AMTI is exempt from tax (¶ 1410).

Both corporate and noncorporate taxpayers may claim the AMT foreign tax credit in computing their tentative minimum tax (¶ 1470). Subject to limits, any AMT liability of a taxpayer may also be reduced by nonrefundable personal credits and general business credits (¶ 1475). Form 6251 is used by individuals to compute AMT. Estates and trusts use Schedule I of Form 1041. Corporations use Form 4626.

Net Capital Gain and Qualified Dividends. The taxation of net capital gains and qualified dividends for AMT purposes is the same as for regular income tax purposes (¶ 1736 and ¶ 1738), including the netting of capital gains and losses by noncorporate taxpayers into separate tax-rate groups (¶ 1739) (Code Sec. 55(b)(3)). The capital gain or loss amounts, however, may differ from the regular tax amounts because of AMT tax preferences and adjustments affecting the basis of capital assets in computing AMTI.

References are to Standard Federal Tax Reports; Tax Research Consultant; and Practical Tax Explanations.

[1] ¶ 5100, ¶ 5400; FILEIND: 30,000; § 15,005

[2] ¶ 5100; FILEIND: 30,400; § 15,005, § 15,110.05

¶1401

Minimum Tax on a Minor Child. A child who is subject to the kiddie tax (¶ 103) is subject to the AMT. The child computes tentative minimum tax in the same manner as any individual taxpayer. Thus, all adjustments and preferences apply, and AMT liability on the child's net unearned income is computed under the rules that apply to other taxpayers except that the child's exemption amount is limited (¶ 1410). The child's exemption amount and his or her ultimate AMT liability are not dependent on the computation of the parent's AMTI or AMT exemption amount.

1405. Alternative Minimum Taxable Income (AMTI). A taxpayer's alternative minimum taxable income (AMTI) for purposes of determining alternative minimum tax (AMT) liability (¶ 1401) is the taxpayer's regular taxable income modified by AMT tax preference items and various AMT adjustments (Code Sec. 55(b)(2); Reg. § 1.55-1).[3] All provisions of the Code and regulations that apply in determining regular taxable income also generally apply in determining AMTI. If, however, the taxpayer's regular income tax is determined by reference to an amount other than regular taxable income, then that amount is treated as taxable income for AMT purposes (e.g., unrelated business taxable income (¶ 655), real estate investment trust (REIT) taxable income (¶ 2329), and life insurance company taxable income (¶ 2370)). Nonresident aliens and foreign corporations only include income effectively connected with a U.S. trade or business in their AMTI (¶ 2429). AMTI does not include fixed or determinable annual or periodic (FDAP) income (¶ 2431).

AMT tax preference items and adjustments involve alterations to various deductions or exclusions allowed in computing regular taxable income. Tax preference items are deductions or exclusions that are allowed in computing regular taxable income but that are not allowed in computing AMTI. This includes the exclusion of gain from qualified small business stock, depletion deductions for natural resources, and interest earned on tax-exempt private activity bonds (¶ 1425). Thus, tax preferences items can only increase a taxpayer's AMTI. Taxpayers may avoid having some of these deductions classified as tax preference items if they elect to capitalize the expenses and deduct them ratably over specified periods for regular tax purposes (¶ 1450).

AMT adjustments are items of income or deductions that are computed differently in determining AMTI than they are for regular taxable income. The result is that adjustments may increase or decrease AMTI. For example, all taxpayers must recompute depreciation, the expensing of mining exploration and development costs, income from long-term contracts, and net operating losses (NOLs) in computing AMTI (¶ 1430).

Individuals, estates, and trusts must also make specific adjustments for itemized deductions, personal exemptions, the standard deduction, and incentive stock options (¶ 1435). In determining the AMTI of an individual, estate, or trust, however, any reference to the taxpayer's adjusted gross income (AGI) or modified AGI is treated as a reference to the taxpayer's AGI or modified AGI as determined for regular tax purposes (Reg. § 1.55-1(b)). Corporations must make specific adjustments to various items in calculating AMTI that only pertain to them, including adjusted current earnings (¶ 1440). In addition, the reduction or cutback of certain corporate preference items for regular tax purposes must generally be applied before a corporation applies the AMT rules (¶ 1445).

In computing the AMTI of a noncorporate taxpayer, the passive activity loss limitations generally apply with certain modifications (¶ 1460). However, a taxpayer cannot deduct any losses from tax-shelter farming activities. The limitations on the deductibility of other losses, including losses subject to the at-risk rules (¶ 1155), partnership losses by partners (¶ 425), and S corporation losses by shareholders (¶ 321) do apply in determining a taxpayer's AMTI (Code Sec. 59(h)).[4] These limitations are applied separately, taking into account all AMT tax preferences and adjustments. Thus, the amount of losses suspended and carried over may differ for AMT and regular tax purposes.

References are to Standard Federal Tax Reports; Tax Research Consultant; and Practical Tax Explanations.

[3] ¶ 5100; ¶ 5100B; FILEIND: 30,050; § 15,005, § 15,110.05

[4] ¶ 5400; FILEIND: 30,150; § 15,401

¶1405

1410. AMT Exemption Amounts. A certain amount of alternative minimum taxable income (AMTI) (¶ 1405) of a taxpayer is exempt from the alternative minimum tax (AMT) (Code Sec. 55(d); Rev. Proc. 2013-35; Rev. Proc. 2014-61).[5] The exemption amounts for an individual, estate, or trust are adjusted annually for inflation for tax years beginning after 2012.

For an individual, the AMT exemption amount for tax years beginning in 2014 is $82,100 if married filing jointly or surviving spouse, $52,800 if unmarried, and $41,050 if married filing separately. The exemption amount for tax years beginning in 2015 is $83,400 if married filing jointly or surviving spouse, $53,600 if unmarried, and $41,700 if married filing separately.

For an estate or trust (other than an electing small business trust (¶ 304)), the AMT exemption amount is $23,500 for tax years beginning in 2014 and is $23,800 for tax years beginning in 2015. The AMT exemption is zero in the case of the portion of an electing small business trust that is treated as a separate trust (Code Sec. 641(c)(2)(B)).[6]

For a corporation, the AMT exemption amount is $40,000 for any tax year; it is not adjusted annually for inflation. In the case of a controlled group of corporations (¶ 291), the single $40,000 exemption is shared by all members of the group (Code Sec. 1561(a)(3)).[7]

Phaseout of AMT Exemption Amount. For all taxpayers (individuals, estates, trusts, and corporations), the AMT exemption amount is phased out or reduced 25 percent for each $1 of the excess of the taxpayer's AMTI over certain threshold amounts (Code Sec. 55(d)(3) and (d)(4); Rev. Proc. 2013-35; Rev. Proc. 2014-61).[8] The thresholds for an individual, estate, and trust are adjusted annually for tax years beginning after 2012.

For an individual, the threshold amount for tax years beginning in 2014 is $156,500 if married filing jointly or surviving spouse, $117,300 if unmarried, and $78,250 if married filing separately. Thus, the AMT exemption amount for an individual is completely phased out in 2014 when AMTI reaches $484,900 if married filing jointly or surviving spouse, $328,500 if unmarried, and $242,450 if married filing separately. For tax years beginning in 2015, the threshold amount is $158,900 if married filing jointly or surviving spouse, $119,200 if unmarried, and $79,450 if married filing separately. The AMT exemption amount is completely phased out in 2015 when AMTI reaches $492,500 if married filing jointly or surviving spouse, $333,600 if unmarried, and $246,250 if married filing separately.

For an estate or trust, the threshold amount for tax years beginning in 2014 is $78,250. Thus, the AMT exemption amount of an estate or trust is completely phased out in 2014 when its AMTI reaches $172,250. For tax years beginning in 2015, the threshold amount for an estate or trust is $79,450, and the AMT exemption amount is completely phased out when AMTI reaches $174,650.

For a corporation, the threshold amount is $150,000 for any tax year and is not adjusted annually for inflation. Thus, the $40,000 AMT exemption amount of a corporation is completely phased out when its AMTI reaches $310,000 for any tax year.

AMT Exemption Amount for a Child. A child who is subject to the kiddie tax (¶ 103) is subject to AMT and computes his or her tentative minimum tax in the same manner as any individual taxpayer. The AMTI exemption amount of a child subject to the kiddie tax, however, is limited to the sum of the child's earned income for the year, plus $7,250 for 2014 ($7,400 for 2015) (Code Sec. 59(j); Rev. Proc. 2013-35; Rev. Proc. 2014-61).[9]

References are to Standard Federal Tax Reports; Tax Research Consultant; and Practical Tax Explanations.

[5] ¶ 5100; FILEIND: 30,402; § 15,015, § 15,115

[6] ¶ 24,260; SCORP: 166.35; § 32,605.25

[7] ¶ 33,340; CCORP: 42,058

[8] ¶ 5100; FILEIND: 30,402; § 15,015, § 15,115

[9] ¶ 5400; FILEIND: 30,404.15; § 1,515

1415. AMT Exemption for Small Corporations. A corporation is generally subject to the alternative minimum tax (AMT) at a flat rate of 20 percent (¶ 1401) on alternative minimum taxable income (AMTI) (¶ 1405). However, a small corporation that meets a gross receipts test will not be liable for the AMT so long as it remains a small corporation—its tentative minimum tax will be treated as zero (Code Sec. 55(e)).[10]

For a corporation to qualify as an exempt small corporation, its average gross receipts must not exceed $7.5 million for all three-tax-year periods prior to the year for which qualification is sought. The threshold is reduced to $5 million for the corporation's first three-year-period (or portion thereof). If the tax year is the first year of the corporation's existence, then the corporation is generally treated as an exempt small corporation regardless of its gross receipts for the year. In applying the small corporation exemption, any reference to the corporation includes its predecessor and any related corporation. An exempt small corporation may also be exempt from using the accrual method of accounting (¶ 1515).

Once a corporation qualifies as a small corporation, it will continue to be exempt from AMT for so long as its average annual gross receipts for all three prior tax-year periods does not exceed $7.5 million. If a corporation ceases to be a small corporation, it cannot qualify as such for any subsequent tax year. The AMT in such circumstances will only apply prospectively.

> **Example:** XYZ is a calendar-year corporation that is first incorporated in 2013. It is neither aggregated with an existing related corporation, nor treated as having a predecessor. It will qualify as a small corporation for 2013, regardless of its gross receipts for the year. In order to qualify as a small corporation for 2014, XYZ's gross receipts for 2013 must be $5 million or less. If XYZ qualifies for 2014, it will also qualify for 2015 if its average gross receipts for the two-tax-year period including 2013 and 2014 is $7.5 million or less. If XYZ does not qualify for 2014, it cannot qualify for 2015 or any subsequent year. If XYZ qualifies for 2014, it will qualify for 2015 if its average gross receipts for the three-tax-year period including 2012, 2013, and 2014 is $7.5 million or less.

AMT Credit for Small Corporations. Taxpayers may be eligible to claim a tax credit based upon their AMT liability for the prior tax year (¶ 1309). However, the credit allowed against the regular tax of an exempt small corporation is limited to the amount by which the corporation's regular tax liability (reduced by other credits) exceeds 25 percent of the excess (if any) of the corporation's regular tax (reduced by other credits) over $25,000 (Code Sec. 55(e)(5)).[11]

1420. Regular Tax Compared with Tentative Minimum Tax. A taxpayer is subject to the alternative minimum tax (AMT) to the extent that tentative minimum tax exceeds regular tax liability (¶ 1401). A taxpayer's regular tax liability for this purpose is regular income tax liability under the Code reduced by the foreign tax credit used for regular income tax purposes (¶ 1361), and by the U.S. possession or Puerto Rico economic activity credit (¶ 1362) (Code Sec. 55(c)).[12] It does not include any increase in tax due to the recapture of the investment tax credit (¶ 1365A) or the low-income housing credit (¶ 1365K). The income averaging rules for farmers and fishermen also do not apply when determining the taxpayer's regular tax liability (¶ 767). Taxes excluded from regular tax liability are (Code Sec. 26(b)):

- alternative minimum tax (AMT);

- tax imposed on a corporation for environmental purposes (Code Sec. 59A);

- additional tax on early distributions from retirement plans (Code Sec. 72(m)(5)(B), (q), (t), and (v));

- tax that arises out of the recapture of mortgage bond federal subsidies (Code Sec. 143(m));

References are to Standard Federal Tax Reports; Tax Research Consultant; and Practical Tax Explanations.

[10] ¶ 5100; STAGES: 9,120.15; § 15,105.15   [11] ¶ 5100; SCORP: 356.30; § 15,105.25   [12] ¶ 5100; FILEIND: 30,400, INDIV: 57,200; § 15,005, § 15,110.05

- the additional tax on certain distributions from Coverdell education savings accounts (Code Sec. 530(d)(4));

- accumulated earnings tax (Code Sec. 531);

- tax on personal holding companies (Code Sec. 541);

- tax on foreign expropriation loss recoveries (Code Sec. 1351(d));

- tax on the built-in gains of an S corporation (Code Sec. 1374);

- tax on an S corporation's passive investment income (Code Sec. 1375);

- tax on nonqualified withdrawals from certain Merchant Marine capital construction funds (Code Sec. 7518(g)(6));

- 30-percent withholding tax on the fixed or determinable annual or periodical (FDAP) income of nonresident aliens and foreign corporations (Code Secs. 871(a) and 881);

- excise tax on the transfer of a residual interest in a real estate mortgage investment company (REMIC) to a "disqualified organization" (Code Sec. 860E(e));

- foreign corporations' branch profits taxes (Code Sec. 884);

- interest on tax liabilities deferred under the installment method (Code Secs. 453(l)(3) and 453A(c));

- the "tax" on certain transfers of high-yield interests to disqualified holders (Code Sec. 860K);

- the additional tax on Archer medical savings account (MSA) distributions not used for qualified medical expenses (Code Sec. 220(f)(4));

- the penalty imposed for distributions from Medicare Advantage medical savings accounts that were not used for qualified medical expenses (Code Sec. 138(c)(2));

- taxes relating to certain failures to maintain high deductible health plan coverage (Code Secs. 106(e)(3)(A)(ii), 223(b)(8)(B)(i)(II), and 408(d)(9)(D)(i)(II));

- tax relating to recapture of certain deductions for fractional gifts (Code Sec. 170(o)(3)(B));

- the additional tax on health savings account (HSA) distributions not used for qualified medical expenses (Code Sec. 223(f)(4));

- the additional tax under Code Sec. 409A(a)(1)(B) and (b)(4)(A) on income from nonqualified deferred compensation plans;

- the recapture of the first-time homebuyer credit under Code Sec. 36(f); and

- the tax (including interest and an additional tax) imposed on certain compensation that is deferred under a nonqualified deferred compensation plan (Code Sec. 457A(c)(1)(B)).

AMT Preferences and Adjustments

1425. AMT Tax Preference Items. In determining a taxpayer's alternative minimum taxable income (AMTI) (¶ 1405), a taxpayer's regular taxable income for the tax year is increased by certain tax preference items (Code Sec. 57).[13] A corporation generally must reduce or cut back certain tax preference items before calculation of its AMTI (¶ 1445). Tax preference items include the following:

- Seven percent of any gain realized on the sale of qualified small business stock and excluded from gross income under Code Sec. 1202 is generally treated as a tax preference item (¶ 1905). Since the exclusion generally equals 50 percent

---

References are to Standard Federal Tax Reports; Tax Research Consultant; and Practical Tax Explanations.

[13] ¶ 5300; FILEIND: 30,100, FILEIND: 30,250; § 15,301

of the realized gain, 3.5 percent of the gain recognized is treated as a tax preference item. For qualified stock acquired after February 17, 2009, and before September 28, 2010, the exclusion amount is 75 percent, 5.25 percent of the recognized gain is treated as a tax preference item. For qualified stock acquired after September 27, 2010, and before January 1, 2014, none of the excluded gain is treated as a tax preference item since the exclusion is 100 percent (Code Sec. 1202(a)(4)).[14]

• Tax-exempt interest (less any related expenses) on certain tax-exempt private activity bonds issued after August 7, 1986, is a tax preference item (except for bonds issued in 2009 and 2010).

• The amount by which the depletion deduction (¶ 1289) claimed by a taxpayer (other than an independent oil and gas producer) for an interest in a property exceeds the adjusted basis of the interest at the end of a tax year is a tax preference item.

• If a taxpayer deducts intangible drilling costs (IDCs) (¶ 989), the difference between the amount allowed as a deduction and the amount that would have been deductible if the costs had been capitalized and ratably amortized over a 120-month period is a tax preference item to the extent it exceeds 65 percent of the taxpayer's net income from oil, gas, and geothermal properties. An independent producer is not subject to this rule, but its AMTI may not be reduced by more than 40 percent of the AMTI that would otherwise be determined if the taxpayer took the IDC tax preference into account and did not compute an alternative tax net operating loss deduction (¶ 1430). A taxpayer may avoid having deductions for IDCs classified as a tax preference item by electing to capitalize the expenses and deduct them over a 60-month period for regular income tax purposes (¶ 1450).

• The accelerated depreciation of real property, leased personal property, leased recovery property, and pollution control facilities placed in service before 1987 is treated as a tax preference item to the extent that it was a preference item under prior law, unless the taxpayer elected to apply MACRS to the property for regular tax purposes.

1430. AMT Adjustments for All Taxpayers. In determining a taxpayer's alternative minimum taxable income (AMTI) (¶ 1405), certain deductions must be recomputed in a less favorable manner than is allowed when determining the taxpayer's regular taxable income. The adjustments are usually required in order to eliminate time value tax savings that result from the acceleration of deductions or the deferral of income. Some adjustments are made solely by noncorporate taxpayers (¶ 1435), while others are made solely by corporate taxpayers (¶ 1440). Both noncorporate and corporate taxpayers must make the following adjustments when determining AMTI.

Depreciation. For MACRS property placed in service after 1998, if the 200-percent declining balance method is used for regular tax purposes for 3-, 5-, 7-, or 10-year property, then the 150-percent declining balance method and regular tax depreciation period must be used in calculating AMTI (Code Sec. 56(a)(1)).[15] For all other MACRS property placed in service after 1998, no AMT adjustment is required as AMT and regular tax depreciation are computed in the same way.

For MACRS property placed in service after 1986 and before 1999, if the 200-percent declining balance method is used for regular income tax purposes for 3-, 5-, 7-, or 10-year property, then the 150-percent declining balance method and the alternative depreciation system (ADS) recovery period must be used in calculating AMTI. If the 150-percent declining balance method is used for 15-or 20-year property, then the 150-percent declining balance method and the ADS recovery period are used in calculating AMTI. If the 150-percent declining balance method election is in effect for regular tax purposes

References are to Standard Federal Tax Reports; Tax Research Consultant; and Practical Tax Explanations.

[14] ¶ 30,372; FILEIND: 30,256; § 15,305

[15] ¶ 5200; FILEIND: 30,102; § 15,230

¶1430

for 3-, 5-, 7-, 10-, 15-, or 20-year property, then no adjustment is required for AMT purposes as the AMT and regular tax depreciation are computed the same way.

In the case of 27.5-year residential real property or 31.5-or 39-year real property placed in service after 1986 and before 1999, AMT depreciation is computed using the straight-line method and ADS recovery period (40 years). If the straight-line election is in effect for regular tax purposes for 3-, 5-, 7-, 10-, 15-, or 20-year property, then for AMT purposes the straight-line method and ADS recovery period must be used. If the ADS method (elective or nonelective) is used for regular tax purposes, then no adjustment is required in calculating AMTI, as AMT and regular tax depreciation are computed the same way on real and personal property subject to the ADS method.

> **Comment:** A benefit of the AMT depreciation adjustment is that depreciation for all property is combined in calculating AMTI. This allows the netting of excess MACRS deductions with excess AMT deductions. A taxpayer with excess MACRS deductions on new property may offset them against AMT deductions on old property and, thus, may be able to avoid paying AMT on these deductions.

No AMT adjustment of depreciation is required for the following property:

• any qualified property for which bonus depreciation or special depreciation allowance was claimed (¶ 1237) if the basis for AMT purposes is the same as for regular income tax purposes (Code Sec. 168(k)(2)(G)), including qualified disaster assistance property (Code Sec. 168(n)(2)(D)), qualified reuse and recycling property (Code Sec. 168(m)(2)(D)), cellulosic biofuel plant property (Code Sec. 168(l)(5)), qualified New York Liberty Zone property (Code Sec. 1400L(b)(2)(E)), qualified Gulf Opportunity Zone property (Code Sec. 1400N(d)(4)), and Kansas disaster area qualified recovery assistance property (Act Sec. 15345(a)(1) and (d)(1) of P.L. 110-246);

• any portion of property the taxpayer elected to expense under Code Sec. 179 (¶ 1208), as well as any other property depreciated under a method not expressed in a term of years such as the unit-of-production method (but not the retirement-replacement-betterment or similar method) (Code Sec. 56(a)(1)(B));

• motion picture films, videotapes, or sound recordings;

• public utility property if a normalization method of accounting is not used;

• certain natural gas gathering lines placed in service after April 11, 2005, which are treated as MACRS 7-year property regardless of whether owned by a producer or a nonproducer; and

• any qualified Indian reservation property (Code Sec. 168(j)(3)).

Disposition of Property. The AMT adjustments for depreciation, pollution control facilities, incentive stock options, and circulation, research, and experimental expenses (¶ 1435) are taken into account in determining the related property's basis for AMT purposes. Thus, the AMT gain or loss from the disposition of the property may be different from the gain or loss for regular tax liability. The difference between regular tax gain or loss and AMT gain or loss is an adjustment in computing the taxpayer's AMTI (Code Sec. 56(a)(6) and (b)(3)).[16] The difference is taken into account as a negative adjustment in calculating AMTI if the AMT gain is less than the regular tax gain, the AMT loss is more than the regular tax loss, or there is an AMT loss and a regular tax gain.

> **Example:** A taxpayer purchased a piece of property for $100,000 and claimed a total of $25,000 of depreciation deductions resulting in an adjusted basis of $75,000 for regular tax purposes. In AMTI calculations made during the same tax years, the taxpayer claimed adjusted depreciation deductions totaling $10,000 resulting in an adjusted basis of $90,000 for AMT purposes. If the taxpayer sells the property in the current tax year for $150,000, his regular tax gain is $75,000 ($150,000 –

References are to Standard Federal Tax Reports; Tax Research Consultant; and Practical Tax Explanations.

[16] ¶ 5200; FILEIND: 30,054; § 15,245, § 15,425

$75,000) and his AMT gain is $60,000 ($150,000 – $90,000). The $15,000 difference is a negative adjustment in calculating the taxpayer's AMTI.

Mining Exploration and Development Costs. A taxpayer who has expensed mining exploration and development expenses (or amortized the costs in computing regular tax liability (¶ 987 and ¶ 988)) must capitalize and amortize the expenses over a 10-year period in calculating AMTI, beginning with the tax year in which the expenses were incurred (Code Sec. 56(a)(2)).[17] If a tax loss is incurred from a mine, the deduction from AMTI is the lesser of the loss allowed for the costs had they remained capitalized or all expenses which have been capitalized but not yet amortized. When property that generated mining exploration and development deductions is sold, its adjusted basis must be computed under the AMT rules in order to determine the gain or loss from the sale for AMT purposes. The AMT adjustment for mining exploration and development costs does not have to be made if the taxpayer elects an optional 10-year amortization period for regular tax purposes (¶ 1450).

Long-Term Contracts. A taxpayer must use the percentage-of-completion method of accounting (¶ 1551) to determine AMTI from long-term contracts (other than home construction contracts) (Code Sec. 56(a)(3)).[18] This method replaces all other accounting methods, such as the completed contract or cash basis method. The percentage-of-completion is determined using simplified cost allocation procedures in the case of construction contracts of certain small contractors if the contract has an estimated duration of less than two years.

Alternative Tax Net Operating Losses. Net operating loss (NOL) deductions must be recomputed in calculating AMTI (Code Sec. 56(a)(4) and (d)).[19] The alternative tax NOL (ATNOL) is generally computed in the same manner as an ordinary NOL (¶ 1145) except that all AMT adjustments are taken into account first, and tax preference items reduce ATNOL (¶ 1425) to the extent they increased the amount of the NOL for the tax year. The ATNOL may not offset more than 90 percent of AMTI, determined without regard to the ATNOL deduction and the domestic production activities deduction. However, the 90 percent limit does not apply to certain qualified disaster losses. Unused ATNOLs are carried forward or back to the earliest year in which they can be used, according to the same rules as NOLs including the election to forgo the carryback period (¶ 1149). The amount of ATNOLs carried forward or back is reduced by 90 percent of the AMTI for any year to which they are carried, whether or not the taxpayer is liable for the AMT in that year.

> **Example:** A taxpayer's income for a tax year is $75,000, while her losses total $100,000, of which $20,000 is from tax preference items. Her NOL for regular taxation is $25,000. In computing AMTI, tax preference items cannot be used. Consequently, only $80,000 of the losses may offset income, leaving the taxpayer with an ATNOL of $5,000.

Pollution Control Facilities. For property placed in service after 1986 and before 1999, the five-year amortization method for depreciating pollution control facilities (¶ 1287) must be replaced by the alternative depreciation system (ADS) (¶ 1247) (Code Sec. 56(a)(5)).[20] The pollution control facility adjustment is computed under MACRS using the straight-line method for property placed in service after 1998. When the pollution control facility is sold, its adjusted basis must be computed under the AMT rules in order to determine the gain or loss from the sale for AMT purposes.

Domestic Production Activities Deduction. The domestic production activities deduction is allowed for both individuals and corporations against the AMT (¶ 980A). The deduction is equal to nine percent of the lesser of (1) the taxpayer's qualified production activities income determined without regard to available AMT adjustments, or (2) the taxpayer's taxable income (or in the case of a corporation its AMTI), determined without regard to the deduction (Code Sec. 199(a) and (d)(6)).

References are to Standard Federal Tax Reports; Tax Research Consultant; and Practical Tax Explanations.

[17] ¶ 5200; FILEIND: 30,106; § 15,255

[18] ¶ 5200; FILEIND: 30,202; § 15,240

[19] ¶ 5200; FILEIND: 30,156; § 15,415

[20] ¶ 5200; FILEIND: 30,110

¶1430

1435. AMT Adjustments for Noncorporate Taxpayers. In addition to alternative minimum tax (AMT) adjustments that affect all taxpayers (¶ 1430), individuals and other noncorporate taxpayers must make a number of adjustments to various tax items in calculating alternative minimum taxable income (AMTI) that only pertain to them (¶ 1405).

Itemized Deductions. Individuals are entitled to claim itemized deductions in calculating AMTI with certain adjustments (Code Sec. 56(b)).[21] The limit on itemized deductions that applies for regular tax purposes does not apply for AMT purposes (¶ 1014).

An individual may not claim state, local, or foreign income or property taxes paid during the tax year (including state and local sales taxes paid in lieu of income taxes, if applicable) (¶ 1021) in calculating AMTI. If the taxes are refunded to the taxpayer, they are not included in AMTI even though the recovered taxes are included in gross income for regular tax purposes. The only taxes that reduce a noncorporate taxpayer's AMTI are business taxes that reduce adjusted gross income (AGI) and generation-skipping transfer taxes paid on income distributions.

Itemized deductions may be claimed for medical expenses in computing AMTI to the extent they exceed 10 percent of the taxpayer's AGI (¶ 1015). The adjustment is applicable to all individuals, including taxpayers who otherwise may claim medical expenses to the extent they exceed 7.5 percent of AGI for regular tax purposes. This includes (i) individuals who have attained age 65 in any tax year after December 31, 2012, and before January 1, 2017, and (ii) all individuals for tax years beginning before January 1, 2013.

An itemized deduction may also be claimed in computing AMTI for qualified housing interest, which is similar to the qualified residence interest deduction that may be claimed for regular tax purposes (¶ 1047) (Code Sec. 56(e)).[22] However, qualified housing interest only encompasses interest paid on acquisition indebtedness; it does not include interest paid on home equity indebtedness. In addition, the interest deduction for AMT purposes is limited to only the acquisition of a house, apartment, condominium, or mobile home.

Investment interest expenses are generally deductible in computing AMTI to the same extent as regular tax liability—that is limited to the taxpayer's net investment income (¶ 1094) (Code Sec. 56(b)(1)(C)). However, investment interest does not include qualified housing interest for AMT purposes even if it is otherwise allocable to property held for investment. In addition, tax-exempt interest on private activity bonds is included in investment income for AMT purposes, and interest expended to carry the bonds is included in investment interest expenses.

A noncorporate taxpayer cannot claim any miscellaneous itemized deductions subject to the two-percent AGI floor in calculating AMTI (¶ 1011). For example, legal expenses are generally deductible as a miscellaneous itemized deduction and therefore cannot be deducted for AMTI. Attorney fees and court costs paid in connection with an unlawful federal discrimination claim or whistleblower award for providing information on tax law violations, however, are deductions taken into account as an above-the-line deduction in computing the individual's AGI and can therefore be claimed as a deduction to AMTI (¶ 1010A).

Personal Exemptions and the Standard Deduction. Personal exemption deductions may not be claimed against AMTI, including the personal exemption deduction allowed to a decedent's estate or a trust (¶ 133 and ¶ 534). In addition, the standard deduction is not allowed in computing AMTI, including the additional standard deduction for each elderly and blind taxpayer (¶ 126) (Code Sec. 56(b)(1)(E)).[23]

Incentive Stock Options. An individual does not recognize gain or loss when an incentive stock option (ISO) is granted or exercised for regular tax purposes (¶ 1925).

References are to Standard Federal Tax Reports; Tax Research Consultant; and Practical Tax Explanations.

[21] ¶ 5200; FILEIND: 30,300; § 15,205

[22] ¶ 5200; FILEIND: 30,310.05; § 15,220.05

[23] ¶ 5200; FILEIND: 30,302; § 15,205

Instead, gain or loss is recognized when the stock is sold. The individual, however, must make an adjustment for AMT purposes by increasing AMTI by the amount the stock's fair market value exceeds the option price at the time the individual's rights to the stock are freely transferable or not subject to a substantial risk of forfeiture (Code Sec. 56(b)(3)).[24] This generally occurs when the option is exercised. The basis of stock acquired through the exercise of the ISO is increased for AMT purposes by the amount of the AMT adjustment. There is no AMT adjustment of basis if the stock is nontransferable and subject to a substantial risk of forfeiture. The individual in such circumstances may make a Code Sec. 83(b) election to take the AMT adjustment into account in the tax year (¶ 713). There is no AMT adjustment if the option is exercised and the stock is disposed of in the same tax year. Although the exercise of an ISO can trigger an AMT liability, a taxpayer may be able to recover the liability through the AMT credit in future years (¶ 1309).

> **Comment:** The price of stock acquired through an ISO may substantially decrease in value after the option is exercised. As a result, the taxpayer may not realize any actual income or a loss when the stock is sold. If the stock is sold at a loss, the taxpayer would be subject to $3,000 limit on deducting capital losses for regular tax purposes. Thus, even though the individual could have a significant AMT liability from exercising the ISO, he or she could have a loss for regular tax purposes from selling the stock which cannot be used against the AMT liability. To alleviate this problem, if a taxpayer has any long-term unused AMT credit, then a portion of the credit may be used to offset regular tax liability as a result of any excess losses (¶ 1327).

Circulation, Research, and Experiment Expenses. Circulation expenses which are expensed for regular tax purposes (¶ 971) must be capitalized for AMTI calculations and ratably amortized over a three-year period starting with the tax year in which the expenses are incurred. Similarly, research and experiment expenses which are expensed for regular tax purposes (¶ 979) must be capitalized for AMT purposes and ratably amortized over a 10-year period (Code Sec. 56(b)(2)).[25] The adjustment for circulation expenses applies to any individual or personal holding company (¶ 277). The adjustment for research and experiment expenses applies only to an individual, unless the individual has materially participated (¶ 1165) in the activity that generated the expenses. Neither adjustment has to be made if the taxpayer elects to amortize the circulation, research, or experiment expenses for regular income tax purposes (¶ 1450).

If a loss is sustained on property that generated the circulation, research, or experiment expenses, a deduction is allowed equal to the lesser of the unamortized expenses or the amount that would be allowed as a loss had the expenses remained capitalized. The adjusted basis of such property must be computed under the AMT rules in order to determine the gain or loss from the sale for AMT purposes (¶ 1430). The difference between the regular tax gain or loss and the recomputed AMT gain or loss is a tax preference adjustment in the year of sale.

1440. AMT Adjustments for Corporate Taxpayers. In addition to alternative minimum tax (AMT) adjustments that affect all taxpayers (¶ 1430), a corporation must make a number of adjustments to various tax items in calculating alternative minimum taxable income (AMTI) (¶ 1405) that pertain only to corporations.

Adjusted Current Earnings. A portion of the difference between the AMTI and the adjusted current earnings (ACE) of a corporation—other than an S corporation, regulated investment company (RIC) (¶ 2301), real estate investment trust (REIT) (¶ 2326), or real estate mortgage investment conduit (REMIC) (¶ 2343)—is treated as an adjustment to AMTI (Code Secs. 56(c)(1) and (g)).[26] This adjustment does not attempt to recapture the tax benefit derived by a corporation from the use of a particular tax deduction or exclusion. Instead, it is aimed at recapturing some of the overall tax savings enjoyed by a corporation that reports large earnings to its shareholders and

---

References are to Standard Federal Tax Reports; Tax Research Consultant; and Practical Tax Explanations.

[24] ¶ 5200; FILEIND: 30,204; § 15,245   [25] ¶ 5200; FILEIND: 30,112; § 15,250, § 15,252   [26] ¶ 5200; STAGES: 9,120.05; § 15,125.05

creditors, but pays little or no tax. To achieve recapture, a corporation's AMTI must be increased by 75 percent of the amount by which its ACE exceeds its AMTI, computed without the adjustments for ACE or alternative tax net operating losses (ATNOLs) (¶ 1430).

> **Example:** A corporation has AMTI of $100,000 before it makes adjustments for ACE or ATNOLs. The current tax year's ACE amounts to $200,000, leaving the corporation with an ACE adjustment of $75,000 (.75 × ($200,000 − $100,000)), which increases AMTI to $175,000 ($100,000 + $75,000).

Similarly, a corporation's AMTI is reduced by 75 percent of the excess of the corporation's pre-adjustment AMTI over its ACE. The reduction cannot exceed the excess of the total positive adjustments for all prior years over the total negative adjustments for all prior years. In a given tax year, this ceiling is determined by limiting the amount of AMTI available for reduction to the excess of prior year increases in AMTI caused by the ACE adjustment over prior year reductions caused by an ACE shortfall.

> **Example:** In a corporation's current tax year it calculates ACE of $50,000 and AMTI of $70,000. Multiplying the difference between AMTI and ACE by 0.75 leaves the corporation with a possible $15,000 that may possibly be used to reduce AMTI. In its prior tax years, the corporation calculated an overall positive ACE adjustment of $10,000. This amount serves as a limit on the amount by which AMTI may be reduced in the current year, leaving the corporation with only a $10,000 reduction of AMTI rather than a $15,000 reduction. The possible reduction of $5,000 that remains may not be carried over to later tax years.

The computation of a corporation's ACE begins with its AMTI as a base, but determined without regard to the ACE adjustment and the ATNOL deduction. This AMTI is then adjusted to determine ACE. Many of the adjustments are similar to the adjustments made by a corporation in determining its earnings and profits for purposes of the taxation of dividend distributions to shareholders (¶ 748). The adjustments include (but are not limited to) the following.

- A corporation that has pre-1994 depreciable assets remaining in service must adjust the depreciation in calculating ACE. For most depreciable property placed in service before 1994, ACE depreciation is computed using the alternative depreciation system (ADS) (straight-line method) (¶ 1247).

- Income that is exempt from regular tax and AMT liability but that is included in the computation of earnings and profits must be included in the computation of ACE. For example, ACE includes tax-exempt interest from investments in state or local bonds (except bonds issued in 2009 and 2010 and certain housing bonds). Income from the discharge of indebtedness, however, does not have to be included in this adjustment. Expenses incurred in earning tax-exempt income, while not deductible in determining regular tax or AMT, are deductible in determining ACE.

- If a corporation does not claim a deduction against earnings and profits, it may generally not claim the deduction in the computation of ACE (except for certain 100-percent dividends and dividends from 20-percent-owned corporations).

- Intangible drilling costs (IDC) (¶ 989), the costs of organizing a corporation (¶ 237), and the costs of circulating periodicals (¶ 971) which may be expensed or amortized for regular tax purposes must be capitalized in computing ACE.

- ACE must be increased or decreased by an increase or decrease in a corporation's LIFO recapture amount, which is the amount by which the value of the corporation's inventory under the FIFO method of inventory valuation exceeds the value under the LIFO method.

- The installment method of accounting (¶ 1801) may not be used in the computation of ACE except to the extent that it is used to calculate preadjustment AMTI. Rather, income from installment sales must be included in ACE in the year in which property is sold.

¶1440

- Income that has built up on a life insurance contract must be included in a corporation's ACE.

- The cost depletion method (¶ 1289) must be used to determine depletion deductions of corporations other than independent oil and gas producers and royalty owners.

- A corporation that has undergone an ownership change in which new shareholders have acquired more than half of the value of the corporation's stock must undertake a wholesale recomputation of the basis of its assets so that the adjusted basis of each asset immediately after an ownership change becomes its proportionate share of the fair market value of the assets immediately before the change.

- ACE may not include a loss from the exchange of one pool of debt obligations for another pool that consists of obligations with the same effective interest rates and maturities as obligations in the first pool.

- The adjusted basis of assets for purposes of making ACE adjustments is determined under these ACE adjustment rules.

- No adjustment related to the earnings and profits effect of charitable contributions is made to ACE.

- A property and casualty insurance company that elects to be taxed only on taxable investment income for regular tax purposes determines its ACE without regard to underwriting income or underwriting expense.

Merchant Marine Capital Construction Funds. Contributions made by shipping companies to capital construction funds (established under § 607 of the Merchant Marine Act of 1936, 46 U.S.C. 1177) may not be deducted and a fund's earnings (including gains or losses) may not be excluded from AMTI (Code Sec. 56(c)(2)).[27] No reduction in the basis of a vessel, barge, or container is made to reflect amounts withdrawn from a fund if the amounts have been included in AMTI.

Blue Cross and Blue Shield Organizations. The special deduction from regular tax allowed to Blue Cross and Blue Shield organizations under Code Sec. 833 for 25 percent of their annual claims and administrative expenses (less the prior tax year's adjusted surplus) may not be claimed against AMTI (Code Sec. 56(c)(3)).[28]

1445. AMT Interaction with Corporate Preference Cutbacks. The tax benefit a corporation derives from certain tax preferences generally must be reduced or cut back 20 or 30 percent (Code Secs. 59(f) and 291).[29] The cutback rules of Code Sec. 291 are applied before the calculation of a corporation's alternative minimum taxable income (AMTI) (¶ 1405). The cutbacks are made to the following tax preferences.

- If a corporation sells or otherwise disposes of section 1250 property (¶ 1786), the 20 percent of any excess of the amount that would have been treated as recapture income had the property been section 1245 property (¶ 1785), over the amount recaptured as ordinary income under Code Sec. 1250, must be recaptured as ordinary income. The cutback does not apply to any disposition of property to the extent Code Sec. 1250 does not apply or that was part of a certified pollution control facility that elected to amortize expenses (¶ 1287). Also, if a real estate investment trust (REIT) (¶ 2326) disposes of section 1250 property, gain which is treated as not coming from ordinary income and is distributed to shareholders as a capital gain dividend is excluded from ordinary income treatment. Corporate shareholders of a REIT must treat capital gain dividends as subject to the 20-percent ordinary income treatment.

References are to Standard Federal Tax Reports; Tax Research Consultant; and Practical Tax Explanations.

[27] ¶ 5200; INDIV: 33,558
[28] ¶ 5200; EXEMPT: 15,160.10
[29] ¶ 5,400, ¶ 15,190; DEPR: 18,266, FARM: 15,154.35, FARM: 21,154.10; § 26,020.05

14

MINIMUM TAX

- The percentage depletion deduction (¶ 1298) of a corporation for iron ore and coal (including lignite) must be reduced by 20 percent of the excess of the percentage depletion deduction (determined before the 20-percent reduction is made), over the adjusted basis (determined without including the depletion deduction) of the minerals at the close of the tax year.

- There must be a 20-percent reduction in the amount of deductions claimed by a financial institution (defined under Code Sec. 585) for certain interest expenses on debts incurred to purchase tax-exempt obligations acquired after December 31, 1982, and before August 8, 1986.

- The basis of certified pollution control facilities that are used for computing rapid amortization deductions must be reduced by 20 percent. ACRS depreciation must be used to depreciate the reduced basis.

- A corporation's (including an integrated oil company's) deductions for intangible drilling costs and mineral exploration and development costs (¶ 987, ¶ 988, and ¶ 989) must be reduced by 30 percent. Reduced deductions may be deducted ratably over a 60-month period that starts with the month in which costs are paid or incurred. If the related property is disposed, the deductions may be recaptured.

1450. Election to Avoid Tax Preference Status. A taxpayer can avoid having an alternative minimum tax (AMT) preference or adjustment for certain expenses if the taxpayer elects to capitalize the expenses and deduct them ratably over specified periods for regular tax purposes beginning with the tax year (or month) in which the expenses were made (Code Sec. 59(e)).[30] Taxpayers may limit their elections to only a portion of their deductions, leaving the remaining deductions subject to AMT. A three-year period may be claimed for circulation expenses (¶ 971), a 60-month period may be claimed for intangible drilling costs (IDC) that begins with the month in which they are paid or incurred (¶ 989), and a 10-year period may be claimed for research and experiment expenses (¶ 979) and mineral exploration and development expenses (¶ 987 and ¶ 988). The election for deductions allowed to partnerships and S corporations is made by the partners or shareholders, rather than by the partnership or the corporation.

1455. Net AMT Adjustment of Electing Large Partnerships. A partnership is not subject to the alternative minimum tax (AMT) and its partners generally compute their AMT liability separately by taking into account their share of partnership items (¶ 1401). However, in the case of an electing large partnership using a simplified reporting system of partnership items (¶ 482), AMT tax preference items and adjustments are computed at the partnership level with the partnership reporting to its partners a net AMT adjustment for passive loss limitation activities and other activities (Code Sec. 772).[31] The net AMT adjustment is determined by using the adjustments applicable to individuals in the case of noncorporate partners (¶ 1435) and the adjustments applicable to corporations in the case of corporate partners (¶ 1440). Except as provided in regulations, the applicable net AMT adjustment is treated as a deferral tax preference for purposes of computing the minimum tax credit (¶ 1309).

1460. Losses Not Allowed for AMT. In computing alternative minimum taxable income (AMTI) (¶ 1405), a taxpayer subject to the passive activity loss rules (¶ 1169) may claim passive activity losses when computing AMTI only to the extent they exceed income from passive activities unless the taxpayer is insolvent, in which case the insolvent taxpayer may claim the otherwise disallowed losses. Losses from a tax shelter farm activity are also not allowed in computing AMTI unless the taxpayer is insolvent.

Passive Activity Losses. The passive activity rules of Code Sec. 469 apply in computing the AMTI of an individual, estate, trust, closely-held C corporation, or personal

---

References are to Standard Federal Tax Reports; Tax Research Consultant; and Practical Tax Explanations.

[30] ¶ 5400; FILEIND: 30,114; § 15,250, § 15,252, § 15,255, § 15,320

[31] ¶ 25,608; PART: 18,452.25; § 15,025

¶1450

service corporation (Code Sec. 58(b)).[32] Thus, deductions for passive losses may be claimed only against passive income. The taxpayer must take into account AMT adjustments and tax preference items before computing income, deductions, and credits from a passive activity for AMT purposes. AMT passive activity gain or loss is computed without regard to qualified housing interest, as opposed to qualified residence interest for regular tax purposes (¶ 1435). The amount of a disallowed AMT passive activity loss is reduced by the amount of a taxpayer's insolvency at the close of the tax year (Code Sec. 58(c)).

> **Example:** In calculating his regular tax, a taxpayer has a passive loss deduction of $15,000 for net losses from real estate rentals. The losses are partially based on MACRS deductions. His AMT liability must be determined by computing depreciation deductions under the alternative depreciation system (ADS). This leaves him with a passive loss deduction of only $5,000 against AMTI. Since he already has adjusted his depreciation deductions in determining whether there is a passive loss, he does not have to include them as part of any adjustment for depreciation in calculating AMTI.

Passive Farm Tax Shelter Losses. Noncorporate taxpayers, as well as personal service corporations, may not deduct losses from a tax shelter farm activity in computing AMTI (Code Sec. 58(a)).[33] A tax shelter farm activity is a farm syndicate (¶ 1521) or passive farm activity in which the taxpayer (or the taxpayer's spouse) is not a material participant (¶ 1165). The taxpayer must take into account AMT adjustments and tax preference items in determining the amount of gain or loss from a tax shelter farm activity. The amount of a disallowed loss is reduced by the amount of a taxpayer's insolvency at the close of the tax year (Code Sec. 58(c)). Taxpayers may not net income and losses from various farming tax shelters to determine an overall loss or gain. Each tax shelter must be regarded separately. Farm losses that have been disallowed as deductions from AMTI in one tax year may be claimed as deductions from farm income from the same farm activity in the succeeding tax year. Taxpayers who dispose of their interest in a tax shelter farm activity are allowed to claim their losses against AMTI.

1465. AMT Liability of REITs, RICs, and Common Trust Funds. Tax preference items and adjustments which are treated differently for alternative minimum tax (AMT) purposes (¶ 1405) than for regular tax purposes must be apportioned between regulated investment companies (RICs) (¶ 2301) or real estate investment trusts (REITs) (¶ 2326), and their shareholders and holders of beneficial interests. Participants in common trust funds must apportion these items among themselves on a pro rata basis (Code Sec. 59(d)).[34]

Credits Against Minimum Tax

1470. Alternative Minimum Tax Foreign Tax Credit. The alternative minimum tax (AMT) foreign tax credit may be claimed by taxpayers in computing their tentative minimum tax (¶ 1401). The AMT foreign tax credit is similar to the foreign tax credit for regular income tax purposes (¶ 2475), except that it is limited to the foreign tax on foreign source alternative minimum taxable income (AMTI) instead of foreign tax on regular taxable income (Code Sec. 59(a)).[35] Thus, the AMT foreign tax credit cannot exceed the taxpayer's tentative minimum tax multiplied by the ratio of the taxpayer's foreign source AMTI to worldwide AMTI. Alternatively, the taxpayer may elect to compute the AMT foreign tax credit limit by multiplying the tentative minimum tax by the ratio of the taxpayer's foreign source regular taxable income to worldwide AMTI. Amounts disallowed by the foreign tax credit limitation may be carried back one year and forward 10 years, subject to the same limitation in those years for both regular tax and AMT purposes.

References are to Standard Federal Tax Reports; Tax Research Consultant; and Practical Tax Explanations.

[32] ¶ 5350; FILEIND: 30,152; § 15,405

[33] ¶ 5350; FILEIND: 30,154; § 15,410

[34] ¶ 5400; FILEIND: 30,404.25; § 15,025

[35] ¶ 5400; FILEIND: 30,352; § 15,505

1475. Other Tax Credits Under AMT. Nonrefundable personal credits that may be claimed by an individual are allowed in full against the taxpayer's combined regular tax liability and alternative minimum tax (AMT) liability (Code Sec. 26(a)).[36] A taxpayer's regular tax liability for this purpose is regular income tax liability under the Code reduced by the foreign tax credit used for regular income tax purposes and the U.S. possession credit (¶ 1420).

The general business credit (¶ 1365) that a taxpayer can claim during a tax year may not exceed the excess of net income tax over the greater of the taxpayer's tentative minimum tax or 25 percent of the taxpayer's net regular tax liability over $25,000 (Code Sec. 38(c)).[37] For this purpose, net income tax is the sum of the taxpayer's regular tax liability and AMT liability, reduced by all other nonrefundable and other credits. The tax liability limitation is determined separately for the general business credit attributable to the alcohol fuels credit (¶ 1365I), the low-income housing credit (¶ 1365K), the renewable electricity production credit (¶ 1365N), the FICA employer tip credit (¶ 1365R), the railroad track maintenance credit (¶ 1365W), the small employer health insurance credit (¶ 1333), the rehabilitation credit (¶ 1365B), the business energy credit (¶ 1365C), and the work opportunity credit (¶ 1365G). The limitation is also made separately for the empowerment zone employment credit, substituting 75 percent of tentative AMT for 100 percent of AMT.

1480. AMT and Possessions Tax Credit. Corporate income for which the Puerto Rico economic activity credit or the possessions tax credit may be claimed (¶ 1362) is not includible in alternative minimum taxable income (AMTI) (¶ 1405) and therefore is not subject to the minimum tax (Code Sec. 59(b)).[38]

References are to Standard Federal Tax Reports; Tax Research Consultant; and Practical Tax Explanations.

[36] ¶ 3850; INDIV: 57,200; § 12,005

[37] ¶ 4250; BUSEXP: 54,056; § 15,515.15

[38] ¶ 5400; INTL: 27,066

Chapter 15

TAX ACCOUNTING

	Par.

Accounting Period

1501. Tax Year. Taxable income is computed on the basis of a taxpayer's tax year (Code Sec. 441).[1] A tax year is the annual accounting period regularly used by a taxpayer in keeping books and records to compute income. This period is usually a calendar year of 12 months ending on December 31 or a fiscal year of 12 months ending on the last day of any month other than December. A taxpayer may elect to use a 52-53 week fiscal year that always ends on the same day of the week, rather than the last day of the month (¶ 1503). Special rules exist when a taxpayer must file a return for a period that is less than 12 months (short-period return) (¶ 1505).

> **Example 1:** A corporation began doing business on August 15, 2014. The end of its first tax year cannot be later than July 31, 2015, because a tax year may not cover more than a 12-month period and must end on the last day of a month, unless it is a 52-53 week tax year.

A new taxpayer may adopt either a calendar or a fiscal year on their first tax return, but certain taxpayers are required to adopt a specific tax year (Reg. § 1.441-1).[2] An existing taxpayer must follow IRS procedures to change his or her tax year (¶ 1513). If a taxpayer adopts an improper tax year, such as a fiscal year (other than a 52-53 week tax year) that does not end on the last day of a calendar month, the IRS may require the taxpayer to adopt a proper tax year or to request IRS approval to change tax years (Rev. Rul. 85-22).[3]

> **Example 2:** Assume that the new corporation in Example 1 determines there is no advantage in keeping its books on the basis of any year other than the calendar year. Therefore, it adopts the calendar-year basis. It should close its books as of December 31, 2014, and file its first return for the short period from August 15, 2014, through December 31, 2014. This is its first tax year. All its later tax years will be full calendar years until its dissolution or until it changes to a fiscal year.

A fiscal year will be recognized only if it is established as the taxpayer's annual accounting period and only if the taxpayer keeps his or her books accordingly. A taxpayer who has no annual accounting period, does not keep adequate records, or whose present tax year does not qualify as a fiscal year must compute taxable income on a calendar-year basis (Reg. § 1.441-1).[4]

Partnerships. A partnership generally must use the same tax year as that of its owners, unless the partnership can establish a business purpose for having a different tax year (Code Sec. 706(b); Reg. § 1.706-1).[5] The tax year of the owners for this purpose is the tax year of the partner(s) owning the majority interest in the partnership—the tax

---

References are to Standard Federal Tax Reports; Tax Research Consultant; and Practical Tax Explanations.

[1] ¶ 20,302; ACCTNG: 24,050; § 38,101

[2] ¶ 20,303; ACCTNG: 24,052; § 38,105

[3] ¶ 20,307.70; ACCTNG: 24,058; § 38,135.20

[4] ¶ 20,303; ACCTNG: 24,052; § 38,110

[5] ¶ 25,160, ¶ 25,161; ACCTNG: 24,352; § 30,120.05

year of the partner(s) owning in total more than a 50-percent interest in partnership profits and capital (¶ 416). If there is no majority interest tax year, the partnership must adopt the same tax year as that of its principal partners, each of whom must have at least a 5-percent interest in partnership profits or capital. When neither condition is met, the partnership must use the tax year that produces the least aggregate deferral of income to the partners.

Corporations. An S corporation or a personal service corporation (PSC) (¶ 273) must generally use the calendar year unless the entity can establish a business purpose for having a different tax year (Code Secs. 441(i) and 1378(b)).[6] The ownership tax year of an S corporation generally satisfies the business purpose requirement. A corporation is not considered a PSC unless more than 10 percent of its stock, by value, is held by employee-owners. If a corporation is a member of an affiliated group filing a consolidated return, all members of that group must be considered in determining whether the corporation is a PSC.

Section 444 Election of Nonrequired Year. A partnership, S corporation, or PSC may make a section 444 election on Form 8716 to use a tax year other than a required tax year if the deferral period of the elected year is generally not longer than three months (Code Sec. 444).[7] To neutralize the tax benefits resulting from such a tax year, an electing partnership or S corporation must compute and make any required payments, i.e., the amount of tax that would otherwise be due from partners and stockholders had the entity used the required tax year, exceeding $500 (Code Sec. 7519; Temp. Reg. § 1.7519-2T).[8] The required payment is due on or before May 15 of the calendar year following the calendar year in which the election year begins. An electing PSC must make minimum distributions to its employee-owners by the end of a calendar year falling within a tax year to avoid certain deduction deferrals for amounts paid to employee-owners (Code Sec. 280H).[9]

The section 444 election must be made by the earlier of: (1) the 15th day of the fifth month following the month that includes the first day of the tax year for which the election is first effective, or (2) the due date, without extensions, of the return that results from the election (Code Sec. 444(d); Temp. Reg. § 1.444-3T).[10] The election remains in effect until an entity changes its tax year or otherwise terminates such an election. The election may not be made by an entity that is a member of a tiered structure unless the tiered structure consists only of partnerships or S corporations or both, all of which have the same tax year.

Common Trust Funds. Common trust funds, certain investment funds maintained by a bank (¶ 2389), are required to adopt the calendar year as their tax year (Code Sec. 584(i)).[11]

DISCs. The tax year of a domestic international sales corporation (DISC) (¶ 2498) must be the same as that of the shareholder or group of shareholders with the same tax year who have the highest percentage of voting power. Voting power is determined on the basis of total combined voting power of all classes of stock of the corporation entitled to vote. If two or more shareholders or groups are tied for the highest percentage, the tax year used is that of any such shareholder or group (Code Sec. 441(h)).[12]

1503. 52- or 53-Week Accounting Period. A taxpayer may elect to use a fiscal tax year that varies from 52 to 53 weeks if that period always ends on the same day of the week (Monday, Tuesday, etc.) and that day is either the last such day in a calendar month or the closest such day to the last day of a calendar month (Code Sec. 441(f); Reg. § 1.441-2).[13]

References are to Standard Federal Tax Reports; Tax Research Consultant; and Practical Tax Explanations.

[6] ¶ 20,302, ¶ 32,260; ACCTNG: 24,354, ACCTNG: 24,356; § 27,120, § 28,410.15

[7] ¶ 20,600; ACCTNG: 24,450; § 38,115.05

[8] ¶ 42,770, ¶ 42,773; ACCTNG: 24,500; § 38,115.10

[9] ¶ 15,160; ACCTNG: 24,550; § 38,115.15

[10] ¶ 20,600, ¶ 20,604; ACCTNG: 24,450; § 38,115.05

[11] ¶ 23,630; RIC: 12,304.15

[12] ¶ 20,302; ACCTNG: 24,110.10

[13] ¶ 20,302, ¶ 20,304; ACCTNG: 24,302; § 38,105

Example: A new taxpayer wishes to have its accounting period end on the last Monday in August. In 2014, its tax year ends on August 25, completing a 52-week year (August 27, 2013, through August 25, 2014). In 2015, its tax year ends on August 31, completing a 53-week year (August 26, 2014, through August 31, 2015). With this type of tax year, most of the taxpayer's tax years are 52 weeks long. As an alternative, the taxpayer could select a tax year that ends on the Monday that is nearest to the end of August. In 2014, therefore, the tax year ends on September 1 (the Monday nearest the end of August). In 2015, the tax year ends on August 31.

If a pass-through entity or an owner of a pass-through entity, or both, use a 52-53-week tax year and the tax year of the entity and owner end with reference to the same calendar month, then for purposes of determining the tax year in which items of income, gain, loss, deductions, or credits from the entity are taken into account by the owner, the owner's tax year will be deemed to end on the last day of the entity's tax year. Under this rule, a pass-through entity is a partnership, S corporation, trust, estate, closely held real estate investment trust (¶ 2326), common trust fund (¶ 2389), controlled foreign corporation (¶ 2487), or passive foreign investment company (¶ 2490) (Reg. § 1.441-2(e)).[14]

1505. Short-Period Return. A return for a period of less than 12 months may need to be filed by a taxpayer who changes its annual accounting period (¶ 1513) or is in existence during only part of what would otherwise be the tax year (Code Sec. 443; Reg. § 1.443-1).[15]

Taxpayers who are not in existence for a full 12-month period include:

(1) a corporation that begins business or goes out of business at any time other than the beginning or end of its accounting period,

(2) an individual taxpayer who dies prior to the end of the accounting period, and

(3) a decedent's estate that comes into existence on the date of the decedent's death and adopts an accounting period ending less than 12 months from that date.

If the taxpayer is not in existence for a full tax year, the tax is computed as if the return had actually covered a full tax year. When a short period occurs as a result of a change in accounting period, the tax is computed on an annualized basis (¶ 1507). An alternative relief method is also available for taxpayers that change their accounting period (¶ 1509). Short-period returns of decedents and dissolving corporations, and the first return of a new corporation, however, are not required to be annualized.

If a change to or from a 52-53 week tax year results in a short period of 359 days or more, the tax is computed as if the return had actually covered a full tax year. If the short period is less than seven days, the short period becomes a part of the following tax year. If the short period is more than six days but less than 359 days, the tax is computed under the annualized method (Code Sec. 441(f)(2)).[16] Special annualization rules apply to taxpayers that make such a change (¶ 1507).

1507. General Method for Annualizing Income for Short Periods. When there has been a change in an accounting period that necessitates the filing of a short-period return (¶ 1505), income for the period must be converted to an annual basis. This conversion is generally accomplished by: (1) multiplying the taxpayer's modified taxable income for the short period by 12 and (2) dividing the result by the number of months in the short period. The tax is computed on the resulting taxable income except that individuals must use the tax rate schedules to compute the tax and not the tax tables. The tax so computed is divided by 12 and multiplied by the number of months in the

References are to Standard Federal Tax Reports; Tax Research Consultant; and Practical Tax Explanations.

[14] ¶ 20,304; ACCTNG: 24,308; § 38,105

[15] ¶ 20,500, ¶ 20,501; ACCTNG: 24,250; § 38,140.05

[16] ¶ 20,302; ACCTNG: 24,306; § 38,140.15

short period (Code Sec. 443).[17] See ¶ 1509 for an alternative method for annualizing income for short periods.

The modified taxable income for the short period is the gross income for the period less any allowable deductions. However, in the case of an individual, no standard deduction is allowed, only itemized deductions (Code Sec. 63(c)(6)(C)). In addition, the deduction for personal exemptions is only allowed in proportion to the ratio that the number of months in the short period bears to 12.

Example: Tom has been making his returns on the basis of a fiscal year ending April 30. He changes to a year ending June 30 in 2014. He must file his return for the year ending April 30, 2014, on or before August 15, 2014. On or before October 15, 2014, he must file his return for the short period of two months beginning May 1, 2014, and ending June 30, 2014. His gross income for the short period is $9,600, and his itemized deductions total $600. He is married, age 60, and has no dependents. His wife has no income or deductions. The tax before credits on their joint return is computed as follows:

Gross income	$9,600
Itemized deductions[*]	600
Net income	9,000
Less 2/12 of $7,900 (2 × $3,950) exemptions	1,317
Modified taxable income for short period	7,683
Annualized taxable income—$7,683 × 12/2	46,098
Tax on $46,098	6,007
Tax for short period, 2/12 of $6,007	1,001

---

* Assume that the itemized deductions are not miscellaneous itemized deductions and that amounts are rounded up to the nearest dollar.

When a short-period return is filed, the taxpayer's self-employment tax (¶ 2664) should be computed on the actual self-employment income for the short period and not prorated for a portion of a 12-month period.[18] A net operating loss deduction (¶ 1145) should be applied against actual income for the short period before annualizing (Rev. Proc. 2002-39, modified by Rev. Proc. 2003-34 and Rev. Proc. 2003-79).[19]

A taxpayer that is changing to or from a 52-53-week fiscal tax year and that must annualize income will apply the same rules as other taxpayers in determining the income of the short period, but will calculate income on an annual basis by multiplying the income of the short period by 365 and dividing the result by the number of days in the short period (Code Sec. 441(f)(2)(B)(iii)). Tax is computed on that annualized income and, as computed, is multiplied by the ratio of the number of days in the short period to 365; the resulting figure is the tax for the short year.

1509. Alternative Method for Annualizing Income for Short Periods. An alternative method is provided for annualizing income when computing tax for a short-period return (¶ 1505) (Code Sec. 443(b)(2); Reg. § 1.443-1(b)(2)).[20] Under this method, the tax for the short period is the greater of:

(1) a tax on the actual taxable income for the 12-month period beginning with the start of the short period (using the law in effect for that 12-month period) multiplied by the modified taxable income (¶ 1507) for the short period and divided by the modified taxable income for the 12-month period, or

(2) a tax on the modified taxable income for the short period.

References are to Standard Federal Tax Reports; Tax Research Consultant; and Practical Tax Explanations.

[17] ¶ 20,500; ACCTNG: 24,260; § 38,140.10, § 38,140.15

[18] ¶ 35,203.30; INDIV: 63,058; § 38,140.15

[19] ¶ 20,406.27; ACCTNG: 24,260; § 38,140.15

[20] ¶ 20,500, ¶ 20,501; ACCTNG: 24,260.15; § 38,140.25

If a taxpayer does not exist at the end of the 12-month period described in (1), above, or if a corporate taxpayer has distributed substantially all its assets before the end of that period, the tax is computed by using a 12-month period ending with the last day of the short period. In such cases, in order to claim the benefits of the alternative method, the taxpayer must attach a return covering the 12-month period ending on the last day of the short year to the return initially computed for the short period.

If there was a change in accounting period resulting in a short period (¶ 1513), the taxpayer must first compute the tax using the general annualization method and file the return. If the alternate method would result in lower taxes, a claim for credit or refund must be filed no later than the due date by which a return would have been required to be filed if the 12-month period beginning with the short period were considered a tax year. The application of the taxpayer for use of the alternate method is considered as a claim for credit or refund.

1513. Change of Accounting Period. The change from one accounting period (¶ 1501) to another generally requires prior permission of the IRS and requires the filing of a return for the short period (¶ 1505). To request IRS approval to change, Form 1128 generally must be filed by the due date of the taxpayer's return, not including extensions, for the first effective year. A change in the accounting period will be approved where it is established that a substantial business purpose exists for making the change but generally will not be approved where the sole purpose of the change is to maintain or obtain a preferential tax status (Reg. § 1.442-1(b)).[21] The IRS will consider all the facts and circumstances relating to the change, including the tax consequences. Among the non-tax factors is the effect of the change on the taxpayer's annual cycle of business activity. The agreement between the taxpayer and the IRS under which the change is carried out will, in appropriate cases, provide terms, conditions, and adjustments necessary to prevent a substantial distortion of income that would otherwise result from the change. For example, effects that would constitute substantial distortions of income include:

(1) deferring a substantial portion of the taxpayer's income or shifting a substantial portion of deductions from one year to another so as to reduce substantially the taxpayer's tax liability;

(2) causing a similar deferral or shift in the case of any other person, such as a partner, a beneficiary, or an S corporation shareholder; or

(3) creating a short period in which there is either: (a) a substantial net operating loss, capital loss or credit, including a general business credit; or (b) a substantial amount of income to offset an expiring net operating loss, capital loss, or credit (Reg. § 1.442-1(b)(3)).[22]

Non-Individual Taxpayers. Automatic approval procedures are provided for certain corporations that have not requested a tax year change within the most recent 48-month period ending with the last month of the requested tax year (Rev. Proc. 2006-45, modified by Rev. Proc. 2007-64). Automatic approval procedures are also provided for trusts and certain partnerships, S corporations, electing S corporations, and personal service corporations that have not requested a tax year change within the most recent 48-month period ending with the last month of the requested tax year, that meet certain conditions (Rev. Proc. 2006-46). If the automatic approval procedures do not apply, the IRS has provided other procedures for taxpayers to follow in order to obtain the IRS's prior approval of an adoption, change, or retention in an annual accounting period through application to the IRS national office (Reg. § 1.442-1(b)(3); Rev. Proc. 2002-39, modified by Rev. Procs. 2003-34 and 2003-79).[23]

Individuals. Certain individuals may also follow automatic approval procedures (Reg. § 1.442-1(b)(3); Rev. Proc. 2003-62). The only individual who may change his or

---

References are to Standard Federal Tax Reports; Tax Research Consultant; and Practical Tax Explanations.

[21] ¶ 20,401, ¶ 20,406.41; ACCTNG: 24,200; § 38,101

[22] ¶ 20,401; ACCTNG: 24,200; § 38,120.20, § 38,125.10, § 38,130.25

[23] ¶ 20,401; ACCTNG: 24,200; § 38,120.05, § 38,125.05, § 38,130.05

her tax year without IRS consent is a newly married individual who is adopting the annual accounting period of his or her spouse to file a joint return (Reg. § 1.442-1(d)).[24]

Improper Tax Year. As an alternative to the above procedures, any taxpayer may correct a prior adoption of an improper tax year by filing Form 1128 with an amended return on a calendar year basis (Rev. Proc. 85-15).[25]

Accounting Method

1515. Cash v. Accrual Basis. Taxable income must be computed not only on the basis of a fixed accounting period (¶ 1501) but also in accordance with a method of accounting regularly employed in keeping the taxpayer's books (Code Sec. 446; Reg. § 1.446-1(a)).[26] A "method of accounting" includes the overall method of accounting for income and expenses, as well as the method of accounting for special items such as depreciation. There are two common overall methods of accounting for income: the cash basis and the accrual basis.

The cash basis (cash receipts and disbursements) is the method of accounting used by most individuals. Income is generally reported in the year that it is actually or constructively received in the form of cash or its equivalent or other property. The constructive receipt of income is income not actually received but within the taxpayer's control (¶ 1533). There is no constructive receipt, however, if there are substantial limits or restrictions on the right to receive it. Deductions or credits are generally taken for the year in which the related expenditures were actually paid, unless they should be taken in a different period to more clearly reflect income, such as depreciation allowances and prepaid expenses (Reg. § 1.446-1(c)(1)(i)).[27]

Under the accrual method, income is accounted for when the taxpayer has the right to receive it—when all events that determine that right have occurred. It is not the actual receipt but the *right to receive* that governs. Expenses are deductible on the accrual basis in the year incurred—when all the events have occurred that fix the amount of the item and determine the liability of the taxpayer to pay it (Reg. § 1.446-1(c)(1)(ii)).[28] See ¶ 1540 for a discussion of this "all-events test" as it relates to economic performance.

The accounting method used must clearly reflect income (¶ 1525). An approved standard method of accounting, i.e., the cash basis or the accrual basis, ordinarily is regarded as clearly reflecting income. A taxpayer may use one accounting method to keep his or her personal books and another for the books of his or her trade or business. A taxpayer may use different accounting methods if the taxpayer has two or more separate businesses as long as separate and distinct sets of records are maintained. However, the use of multiple accounting methods is not permitted if there is a creation or shifting of profits or losses between the taxpayer's various trades or businesses (Reg. § 1.446-1).[29] Generally, and except as otherwise required, a hybrid method of accounting combining two or more methods of accounting—such as a combination of the cash method as the taxpayer's overall method of accounting and the accrual method for inventories—may be used so long as the combination clearly reflects income and is consistently used (Reg. § 1.446-1(c)(1)(iv)).[30]

Taxpayers that are required to use inventories (¶ 1553) must use the accrual method to account for purchases and sales (Reg. § 1.446-1(c)(2)).[31] Furthermore, the following taxpayers must generally use the accrual method of accounting as their overall method of accounting for tax purposes:

    (1) C corporations,

    (2) partnerships that have a C corporation as a partner,

References are to Standard Federal Tax Reports; Tax Research Consultant; and Practical Tax Explanations.

[24] ¶ 20,401; ACCTNG: 24,152; § 38,110

[25] ¶ 20,406.15; ACCTNG: 24,166; § 38,110

[26] ¶ 20,606, ¶ 20,607; ACCTNG: 200; § 38,201

[27] ¶ 20,607; ACCTNG: 208; § 38,210, § 38,215.05

[28] ¶ 20,607; ACCTNG: 210; § 38,220.05

[29] ¶ 20,607; ACCTNG: 208.05; § 38,205.05

[30] ¶ 20,607; ACCTNG: 6,400; § 38,225

[31] ¶ 20,607; ACCTNG: 15,060; § 38,215.05

¶1515

(3)　charitable trusts that are subject to the tax on unrelated trade or business income (¶ 655), but only for that income, and

(4)　tax shelters (Code Sec. 448(a) and (d) (6)).[32]

Qualified personal service corporations (¶ 273) are treated as individuals rather than as corporations for purposes of category (2), above.

Notwithstanding the general requirement that these taxpayers use the accrual method, the cash method of accounting may be used instead if the entity is not a tax shelter and:

(1)　is engaged in a farming or tree-raising business, unless the taxpayer is a corporation or has a corporation as a partner (¶ 1519),

(2)　is a qualified personal service corporation, or

(3)　is an eligible small business (Code Sec. 448(b)).

A small business is exempt from using the accrual method if it has met the $5-million-or-less gross receipts test for all prior tax years beginning after 1985. An entity meets the $5-million gross receipts test if the average annual gross receipts for the three tax years ending with the prior tax year does not exceed $5 million (Temp. Reg. § 1.448-1T(f)).[33] Furthermore, most businesses that are required to account for inventories may use the cash method if average annual gross receipts do not exceed $1 million (Rev. Proc. 2001-10). Certain other small businesses required to account for inventories may also use the cash method if average annual gross receipts do not exceed $10 million (Rev. Proc. 2002-28).[34]

1516. Prorating Income of Accrual-Method Taxpayers. When the effective date of a tax rate change occurs within a tax year, an accrual-method taxpayer (¶ 1515) must compute the tax for the entire tax year by using both the old and the new rates (Code Sec. 15).[35] The final tax is the sum of (1) the tax calculated at the old rates that is proportionate to the portion of the tax year before the effective date of the new tax, and (2) the tax calculated at the new rates that is proportionate to the portion of the tax year beginning with the effective date. When the tax rate change involves the highest rate of income tax, the taxpayer must compute the tax for the year by using a weighted average of the highest rates before and after the change determined on the basis of the respective portions of the tax year before the date of change and on or after the date of change.

1519. Accrual Accounting for Farm Corporations. Corporations, and partnerships having a corporation as a partner, that are engaged in the business of farming are required to use the accrual method of accounting (¶ 1515) (Code Sec. 447).[36] In addition, these taxpayers are required to capitalize their preproductive period expenses (¶ 999). All farming corporations are subject to the accrual accounting rule except:

• S corporations,

• corporations or partnerships engaged in the trade or business of operating a nursery or sod farm, or raising or harvesting trees, other than fruit and nut trees, and

• corporations having annual gross receipts of $1 million or less for each prior tax year beginning after 1975, including the receipts of predecessor corporations and members of a controlled group.

A family corporation meets the gross-receipts test if its gross receipts do not exceed $25 million for each prior tax year beginning after 1985. A family corporation is defined as:

References are to Standard Federal Tax Reports; Tax Research Consultant; and Practical Tax Explanations.

[32] ¶ 20,800; ACCTNG: 6,050; § 38,215.05

[33] ¶ 20,801B; ACCTNG: 208.15; § 38,215.10

[34] ¶ 20,803.75; ACCTNG: 6,050, ACCTNG: 15,058; § 38,215.10

[35] ¶ 3385; ACCTNG: 24,310.10, FILEIND: 15,054.25; § 38,140.10

[36] ¶ 20,700; FARM: 3,060; § 36,315.10

- any corporation in which at least 50 percent of the total combined voting power of all classes of voting stock and at least 50 percent of all other classes of the corporation's stock are owned by members of the same family, or
  - any of the closely held corporations described in Code Sec. 447(h).

If a corporation or qualified partnership (each of the partners of which is a corporation) has, for a 10-year period ending with its first tax year after 1975, and for all subsequent years, used an annual accrual method of accounting with respect to its trade or business of farming, and the entity raises crops that are harvested a year or more after planting, it may continue to use this method.

1521. Expenses of Farming Syndicates. A farming syndicate is a tax shelter and must use the accrual method of accounting (¶ 1515) (Code Secs. 448(d) and 461(i)(4)).[37] A farming syndicate is any farming partnership or enterprise, other than a corporation that is not an S corporation, if at any time: (1) interests in the enterprise or partnership have been offered for sale in an offering required to be registered with any federal or state agency having authority to regulate such offering, or (2) more than 35 percent of the losses during any period are allocable to limited partners or limited entrepreneurs (Code Sec. 464(c)).[38] An individual is not treated as a limited partner or limited entrepreneur if the individual:

(1) has his or her principal residence on the farm on which the farming enterprise is being carried on;

(2) has an interest attributable to active participation in management of the farming enterprise for a period of not less than five years;

(3) actively participates in the management of a farming enterprise as his or her principal business activity, regardless of whether he or she actively participates in the management of the enterprise in question; or

(4) actively participates in the management of another farming enterprise involving the raising of livestock (or is so treated under either (1) or (2)) and owns an interest in an enterprise involving the further processing of the livestock raised in the enterprise.

If an individual meets any of these conditions, any member of his or her family who owns an interest in a farming enterprise that is attributable to the individual's active participation is not treated as a limited partner or limited entrepreneur.

1525. Accounting Method Prescribed by IRS. The IRS can prescribe a method of accounting (¶ 1515) that will clearly reflect income if, in the IRS's opinion, the method used by the taxpayer fails to do so (Code Sec. 446(b)).[39] If the IRS requires a change in accounting methods, the taxpayer must compute an income adjustment due to the change, referred to as a section 481(a) adjustment (¶ 1531).

1529. Change of Accounting Method. A taxpayer generally may not change his or her method of accounting (¶ 1515) without obtaining advance permission from the IRS (Code Sec. 446(e); Reg. § 1.446-1(e)).[40] A change of accounting method includes a change in the overall plan of accounting as well as a change in the treatment of any material item. In most cases, a method of accounting is not established for an item unless there is a pattern of consistent treatment. A change in the treatment of a material item is one involving the timing of its inclusion in income or deduction; not the traditional accounting meaning dealing with the relationship of amounts.

IRS consent is required whether the change is made from an acceptable or an unacceptable method. If the taxpayer fails to file a request to change his or her method of accounting, the absence of IRS consent to the change will not prevent the imposition of or diminish the penalties, i.e., additions to tax (Code Sec. 446(f)).[41] A taxpayer that

References are to Standard Federal Tax Reports; Tax Research Consultant; and Practical Tax Explanations.

[37] ¶ 20,800, ¶ 21,802; ACCTNG: 12,352
[38] ¶ 21,840; PART: 18,302
[39] ¶ 20,606; ACCTNG: 21,110; § 38,620
[40] ¶ 20,606, ¶ 20,607; ACCTNG: 21,102; § 38,610.05
[41] ¶ 20,606; ACCTNG: 21,050; § 38,610.05

changes its method of accounting for a tax year generally must make certain adjustments to its income, referred to as section 481(a) adjustments (¶ 1531).

Changes in accounting method include, but are not limited to:

(1) a change from the cash to the accrual basis;

(2) any change in the method of valuing inventories (¶ 1571);

(3) a change in depreciation or amortization method (¶ 1221);

(4) a change from the cash or accrual basis to one of the long-term contract methods (¶ 1551), from one of the long-term contract methods to the cash or accrual basis, or from one long-term contract method to another;

(5) a change involving the adoption, use, or discontinuance of any other specialized basis, i.e., the crop method (¶ 1569); and

(6) a change where the Code and regulations specifically require that IRS consent be obtained.

The IRS will automatically approve certain taxpayers' changes of accounting method. This approval is granted for the tax year for which the taxpayer requests the change if the taxpayer complies with the automatic change procedures included in Rev. Proc. 2011-14.[42] The IRS frequently modifies Rev. Proc. 2011-14 to add other accounting method changes to the list of changes that are eligible for the automatic consent procedures. For changes of accounting method which are *not* granted automatic approval by the IRS, taxpayers must comply with a separate set of request procedures included in Rev. Proc. 97-27, modified by Rev. Procs. 2002-19, 2007-67, 2009-39, 2011-14, and 2012-39.[43]

Application for permission to change the taxpayer's method of accounting must generally be filed on Form 3115 during the tax year in which the taxpayer desires to make the proposed change (Reg. § 1.446-1(e)(3)(i)).[44]

1531. Adjustments Required by Changes in Method of Accounting. Taxpayers who voluntarily change their method of accounting with the IRS's permission (¶ 1529), or who are compelled by the IRS to make a change because the method used does not clearly reflect income (¶ 1525), must make certain adjustments to income in the year of the change (Code Sec. 481(a); Reg. § 1.481-1).[45] The adjustments are those determined to be necessary to prevent duplication or omission of items. Since the adjustments for the year of change might result in the bunching of income, two statutory methods of limiting the tax in the changeover year may be applied if the adjustments for the changeover year increase taxable income by more than $3,000 (Reg. § 1.481-2).[46] If both limitations apply, the one resulting in the lower tax should be used.

Under the first method, the old method of accounting must have been used in the two preceding years; if so, the tax increase in the changeover year is limited to the tax increases that would result if the adjustments were spread ratably over that year and the two preceding years. Under the second method, the taxpayer must be able to reconstruct his or her income under the new method of accounting for one or more consecutive years immediately preceding the changeover year. The increase in the changeover year's tax because of the adjustments may not be more than the net tax increases that would result if the adjustments were allocated back to those preceding years under the new method. Any amounts that cannot be allocated back must be included in the changeover year's income for purposes of computing the limitation.

In addition to the statutorily prescribed methods of allocation limiting the tax in the changeover year, IRS guidance provides that the adjustment period for a voluntary accounting method change is one tax year (the year of change) for a net negative section 481(a) adjustment and four tax years (the year of change and next three tax

---

References are to Standard Federal Tax Reports; Tax Research Consultant; and Practical Tax Explanations

[42] ¶ 20,620.285; ACCTNG: 21,102.05; § 38,610.10

[43] ¶ 20,620.284; ACCTNG: 21,102; § 38,610.20

[44] ¶ 20,607; ACCTNG: 21,104; § 38,615

[45] ¶ 22,270, ¶ 22,271; ACCTNG: 21,150; § 38,625.05

[46] ¶ 22,272; ACCTNG: 21,152; § 38,625.10

years) for a net positive section 481(a) adjustment. A net positive section 481(a) adjustment is taken into account ratably over the adjustment period for taxpayers that agree to the IRS conditions. A taxpayer may elect to use a one-year adjustment period (the year of change) in lieu of the four-year adjustment period otherwise provided for a positive adjustment if the net adjustment is less than $25,000 (Rev. Procs. 97-27 and 2011-14).[47] Moreover, a taxpayer may request approval of an alternative method of allocating the amount of the adjustments (Reg. § 1.481-4).[48]

A change in accounting method resulting from limitations placed on the use of the cash method of accounting (¶ 1515) is treated as a change initiated by the taxpayer with the consent of the IRS. The related section 481(a) adjustment is includible in income over a period generally not exceeding four years (Code Sec. 448(d)(7)).[49]

Timing of Income and Expenses

1533. Constructive Receipt of Income for Cash-Basis Taxpayers. It is not always necessary that a taxpayer take possession of money or property representing income before it is considered received. Income that is constructively received is taxed to a cash-basis taxpayer (¶ 1515) as though it had been actually received (Reg. § 1.451-2(a)).[50] There is constructive receipt when income is credited without restriction and made available to the taxpayer. There must be no substantial limitation or condition on the taxpayer's right to bring the funds within his or her control. An insubstantial forfeiture provision, a notice requirement, or the loss of bonus interest for deposits or accounts in certain financial institutions is not a substantial limitation.

Common examples of constructive receipt include matured and payable interest coupons, interest credited on savings bank deposits, and dividends unqualifiedly made subject to a stockholder's demand. However, if a dividend is declared payable on December 31 and the corporation follows a practice of paying the dividend by checks mailed so that the shareholders will not receive them until January of the following year, the dividend is not considered to be constructively received by the stockholders in December (Reg. § 1.451-2(b)).[51] For the time of receipt by shareholders of certain mutual fund dividends, see ¶ 2309. Accrued interest on an unwithdrawn insurance policy dividend is gross income to the taxpayer for the first tax year during which the interest may be withdrawn.

Salaries credited on corporate books are taxable to an officer in the year when the officer may withdraw the compensation at will if the corporation has funds available to pay the salaries without causing financial difficulties. Bonuses that are based on yearly sales and that are otherwise not available to an officer are taxable in the year of receipt.[52]

Accrued interest on a deposit that may not be withdrawn at the close of an individual's tax year because of an institution's actual or threatened bankruptcy or insolvency is not includible in the depositor's income until the year in which that interest is withdrawable (Code Sec. 451(g)).[53]

Constructive receipt does not give rise to constructive payment. Thus, for example, the fact that the negotiable note of a responsible and solvent maker, received in payment of salary, interest, rent, etc., must be reported by a recipient on the cash basis as income to the extent of its fair market value when received does not mean that the maker (on a cash basis) may also deduct the same amount at that time. Delivery of a note is not a payment on the cash basis, and the deduction may be taken only in the year when the note is paid. Giving collateral to secure the note does not change the promise to pay into an actual payment.[54]

References are to Standard Federal Tax Reports; Tax Research Consultant; and Practical Tax Explanations.

[47] ¶ 22,277.40; ACCTNG: 21,158, ACCTNG: 21,162; § 38,625.05

[48] ¶ 22,275; ACCTNG: 21,156; § 38,625.05

[49] ¶ 20,800; ACCTNG: 21,164.15; § 38,625.05

[50] ¶ 21,007; ACCTNG: 6,150; § 38,315.05

[51] ¶ 21,007, ¶ 21,009.1235; ACCTNG: 6,210, ACCTNG: 6,218; § 3,101, § 38,315.15

[52] ¶ 21,009.17; ACCTNG: 6,152.10; § 38,315.05

[53] ¶ 21,002; ACCTNG: 6,218; § 38,315.15

[54] ¶ 21,817.185; ACCTNG: 6,262; § 38,315.05

1537. Prepaid Income. Payments received in advance are usually income to an accrual-basis or cash-basis taxpayer (¶ 1515) in the year of receipt, provided that there is no restriction on the use of those payments. This is true even though the payments are returnable on the happening of some specified event. A distinction must be made, however, between prepayments that may be refunded for services or goods and deposits over which the taxpayer does not have complete dominion and control on receipt.[55] For example, a utility company was not required to include deposits from uncreditworthy customers in income on receipt because it was required to return the deposit on request by a customer who established creditworthiness.

Prepaid Merchandise. Inclusion in the year of receipt is also required for advance payments received on the sale of merchandise. However, under certain circumstances the IRS permits accrual-basis sellers to include certain advance payments in income in the tax year in which those payments are properly accruable under the method of accounting used for tax purposes if they are reported at that time or later for financial reporting purposes (Reg. § 1.451-5).[56] If the method used for financial reporting results in an earlier accrual, then the advance payments are taxed according to the financial reporting method. When a long-term contract method of accounting (¶ 1551) is used, advances are included in income under that method without regard to how the income from these payments is accounted for in the seller's financial reports.

An advance payment for this purpose is any amount received by an accrual-basis taxpayer under an agreement (1) for the sale or other disposition in a future tax year of goods held by the taxpayer primarily for sale to customers in the ordinary course of his or her trade or business, or (2) for the building, installation, construction, or manufacture of items by the taxpayer where the agreement is not completed within that tax year. An exception exists where substantial advance payments for inventoriable goods have been received and goods are on hand or available to satisfy the agreement in the year of receipt. Payments for gift certificates are substantial when received, but in other cases, advance payments are not substantial until they exceed the cost of goods to be sold. In such cases, all advance payments received by the last day of the second tax year following the year in which the substantial advance payments are received and not previously included in income under the taxpayer's method of accounting must be included in income in the second tax year (Reg. § 1.451-5(c)).[57]

Certain manufacturers, wholesalers and retailers that receive advance payments for multi-year service warranty contracts may elect to recognize income from advance payments as a series of equal payments over the life of the contracts. This election is permitted only if an eligible taxpayer purchases insurance to cover its obligations under a service warranty contract within 60 days after the sale of the contract (Rev. Proc. 97-38).[58]

Prepaid Services and Mixed Prepayments. Taxpayers who receive advance payments for services and advance payments for the transfer of both goods and services are allowed a limited deferral beyond the tax year of receipt for certain advance payments (Rev. Proc. 2004-34, modified by Rev. Proc. 2011-18, modified by Rev. Proc. 2013-29).[59] Excludable payments generally include the payment for services; the sale of goods other than those for which the taxpayer uses a method of deferral allowed for advance payments of goods discussed previously; the use of intellectual property, including license or lease; the use of property ancillary to the provision of services, e.g., hotel rooms, booths at trade shows, campsites, and banquet facilities; the sale, lease, or license of computer software; guaranty or warranty contracts ancillary to any of the above; subscriptions; memberships in an organization; an eligible gift card sale; or any combination of the above. An eligible gift card sale is a sale in which the taxpayer is primarily liable to the customer and the gift card is redeemable by the taxpayer or an entity legally obligated to the taxpayer.

References are to Standard Federal Tax Reports; Tax Research Consultant; and Practical Tax Explanations.

[55] ¶ 21,005.7039; ACCTNG: 6,152, ACCTNG: 9,104; § 38,310.05

[56] ¶ 21,016; ACCTNG: 9,200; § 38,310.10

[57] ¶ 21,016; ACCTNG: 9,206; § 38,310.10

[58] ¶ 20,620.20; ACCTNG: 9,484.25

[59] ¶ 21,005.7043; ACCTNG: 27,154; § 38,310.10

The term "advance payment" does not include: rent, other than that paid for the use of intellectual property, computer software, and property ancillary to the provision of services; insurance premiums to the extent governed by the taxation of insurance companies; payments with respect to financial instruments, such as debt instruments, deposits, letters of credit, notional principal contracts, options, forward contracts, futures contracts, foreign currency contracts, credit card agreements, and financial derivatives; payments with respect to service warranty contracts; payments with respect to warranty and guaranty contracts under which a third party is the primary obligor; certain payments with respect to nonresident aliens and foreign corporations; and payments in property transferred in connection with the performance of services to which the restricted property rules of Code Sec. 83 apply (¶ 713).

Qualifying taxpayers generally may defer to the next succeeding tax year the inclusion in gross income for federal income tax purposes of advance payments to the extent the advance payments are not recognized in revenues for financial statement purposes or, in certain cases, are not earned in the tax year of receipt. Except in the case of certain short tax years, the IRS does not permit deferral to a tax year later than the next succeeding tax year. These rules neither restrict a taxpayer's ability to use the methods of deferral for the advance payment of merchandise (see "*Prepaid Merchandise,*" previously), nor limit the period of deferral available under that regulation.

> **Example 1:** Advance payment for 48 dancing lessons under a one-year contract is received on November 1, 2014, by a calendar-year taxpayer. Eight lessons are given in 2014. The remaining lessons are provided in 2015. In its applicable financial statement, the dance studio recognizes $\frac{1}{6}$ of the payment in revenues for 2014 and $\frac{5}{6}$ of the payment in revenues for 2015. If the dance studio, an accrual-basis taxpayer, elects the deferral method, $\frac{1}{6}$ of the payment is includible in 2014 income and $\frac{5}{6}$ of it is taxable as 2015 income, even if not all of the remaining 40 lessons are given in 2015.

> **Example 2:** Assume the same facts as in Example 1, except that the advance payment is received for a 2-year contract under which up to 96 lessons are provided. The dance studio provides eight lessons in 2014, 48 lessons in 2015, and 40 lessons in 2016. In its applicable financial statement, the studio recognizes $\frac{1}{12}$ of the payment in revenues for 2014, $\frac{6}{12}$ of the payment in revenues for 2015, and $\frac{5}{12}$ of the payment in gross revenues for 2016. For federal income tax purposes, the studio must include $\frac{1}{12}$ of the payment in gross income for 2014 and the remaining $\frac{11}{12}$ of the payment in gross income for 2015.

Certain accrual-basis membership organizations and publishers can defer prepaid dues and subscription income (Code Secs. 455 and 456).[60]

Accrued Income. In certain situations, cash-basis taxpayers may be required to report income that has not yet been received, and accrual-basis taxpayers may compute income in a manner that differs from general accrual principles. For example, both accrual-basis and cash-basis taxpayers may be required to use present value concepts to compute and report income arising out of a section 467 rental agreement (¶ 1541), original issue discount (OID) from any debt obligation held by the taxpayer (¶ 1952), and amounts arising from debt instruments issued for property (¶ 1868, ¶ 1954). In addition, an accrual-method publisher of magazines, paperbacks, or records may elect to exclude from gross income the income attributable to the qualified sale of magazines, paperbacks, or records that are returned before the close of the merchandise return period (Code Sec. 458).[61]

1538. Accruing Income Doubtful of Collection. On the accrual basis of accounting (¶ 1515), income such as interest is taxable as it accrues even though it is received at a later date. However, if there is a real doubt that the interest is collectible when it becomes due, it need not be accrued.[62] On the other hand, where the uncollectible item

---

[60] ¶ 21,510, ¶ 21,520; ACCTNG: 9,250, ACCTNG: 9,300; § 38,320.45

[61] ¶ 21,540; ACCTNG: 12,206; § 38,320.20

[62] ¶ 5704.32; ACCTNG: 9,058; § 38,220.10

arises from a sale of property, the proper procedure is to report the sale and then take a bad debt deduction as appropriate (¶ 1135 and ¶ 1143).

An accrual-basis taxpayer is generally not required to accrue as income any amount to be received for the performance of services that, based on experience, will not be collected (Code Sec. 448(d)(5); Reg. § 1.448-2(a)).[63] This treatment is an accounting method that must be elected by the taxpayer. The nonaccrual experience method of accounting is limited to amounts to be received for the performance of qualified services (health, law, engineering, architecture, accounting, actuarial science, performing arts, or consulting) and for services provided by certain small businesses.

1539. Prepaid Expenses of Cash-Basis Taxpayers. Cash-basis taxpayers (¶ 1515) may deduct certain prepaid *expenses* in the year paid under certain conditions (Code Sec. 461; Reg. § 1.461-1).[64] A distinction is made between expenditures that are more in the nature of expenses and those that are capital in nature. If the payment creates an asset having a useful life extending substantially beyond the end of the tax year in which the payment is made, the expenditure may not be deductible, or may be deductible only in part, in that year. If payment is made for a capital asset or is capital in nature, a deferment and charge-off for depreciation, amortization, or other comparable allowance are proper (¶ 1201). Taxpayers are generally not required to capitalize amounts paid for a right or benefit, such as rent or insurance, that does not extend beyond the earlier of: (1) 12 months after the first date on which the taxpayer realizes the right or benefit, or (2) the end of the tax year following the tax year in which the payment is made (Reg. § 1.263(a)-4(f)(1)).[65] Special rules apply to certain rental agreements (¶ 1541).

> **Example:** Jonathan Mathis, a calendar-year taxpayer who uses the cash basis of accounting, signs a three-year business property lease on December 1 of the tax year and agrees to pay $18,000 upfront plus a monthly rental of $1,000 for 36 months. He can deduct only $1,500 for the tax year ($1,000 rent plus ⅟₃₆ of $18,000). The $18,000 is an amount paid for securing the lease and must be amortized over the lease term.

Cash-basis farmers and ranchers can deduct prepaid feed costs in the year of payment if:

(1) the advance feed expenditure is a payment and not a deposit;

(2) the payment is for a business purpose; and

(3) the deduction does not cause a material distortion of income.[66]

No deduction is generally allowed, however, to a cash-basis farmer, other than farming syndicates, in the year of prepayment for advance payments for feed, seed, fertilizer, or other supplies to the extent those prepayments exceed 50 percent of total deductible farming expenses, excluding prepaid supplies) (Code Sec. 464(f)).[67] For rules applicable to farming syndicates, see ¶ 1521. The limitation does not apply to a "farm-related taxpayer" if:

(1) the aggregate prepaid farm supplies for the preceding three tax years are less than 50 percent of the aggregate deductible farming expenses, other than prepaid farm supplies, for that period, or

(2) the taxpayer has excess prepaid farm supplies for the tax year by reason of any change in business operation directly attributable to extraordinary circumstances.

A farm-related taxpayer is one whose principal residence is on a farm, who has a principal occupation of farming, or who is a family member of such a taxpayer. The family of an individual includes brothers and sisters, whether by whole or half blood, spouse, ancestors, and lineal descendants (Code Sec. 464(c)(2)(E)). It may also include a corporation that is engaged full-time in farming activities.

References are to Standard Federal Tax Reports; Tax Research Consultant; and Practical Tax Explanations.

[63] ¶ 20,800, ¶ 20,802; ACCTNG: 9,058.10; § 38,320.25

[64] ¶ 21,802, ¶ 21,805; ACCTNG: 6,266; § 38,410.05

[65] ¶ 13,704C; BUSEXP: 9,104.20; § 10,210.40

[66] ¶ 21,817.205; FARM: 9,054; § 38,410.20

[67] ¶ 21,840; FARM: 9,054; § 38,410.20

Estimated state income taxes paid in advance are deductible by a cash-basis taxpayer in the year paid (Rev. Rul. 56-124).[68]

See ¶ 1055 for a discussion of the allowance of deductions for prepaid interest payments.

1540. Expenses of Accrual-Basis Taxpayers. Under the "all-events" test, an accrual-basis taxpayer (¶ 1515) is generally entitled to deduct the face amount of an accrued expense in the tax year in which (1) all of the events have occurred that determine the fact of liability, and (2) the amount of the liability can be determined with reasonable accuracy (Code Sec. 461(h)).[69] The all-events test is not treated as met before economic performance occurs with respect to the particular item of expense or obligation that underlies the taxpayer's liability. For a liability of a taxpayer that requires a payment for property or services, economic performance is deemed to occur as the property or services are provided to the taxpayer. If the liability arises out of the taxpayer's use of property, economic performance occurs as the taxpayer uses the property (Reg. § 1.461-4(d)).[70]

> **Example 1:** A partner on the accrual basis contractually obligates itself in October 2014 to pay Techno Inc. $10,000 for research and development to be performed in 2015. No amount is deductible before performance is rendered in 2015.

Taxpayers are permitted to accrue payments before services are rendered or property is received if the taxpayer can reasonably expect the services or property to be provided within 3½ months after payment.

> **Example 2:** An accrual-method, calendar-year taxpayer makes payment on December 1, 2014, for goods it expects to receive by March 12, 2015. It may deduct the payment or otherwise take it into account for its 2014 tax year.

If the liability of the taxpayer requires him or her to provide services or property, then economic performance occurs as the taxpayer incurs costs. However, economic performance with respect to the drilling of an oil or gas well is considered to have occurred within a tax year if drilling commences within 90 days after the close of the tax year.

> **Example 3:** Zop Corp., a calendar-year, accrual-method taxpayer, sells lawn mowers under a three-year warranty that obligates it to make reasonable repairs to each mower it sells. In 2014, Zop repairs 12 mowers sold in 2013 at a cost of $2,500. Economic performance with respect to Zop's liability to perform services under the warranty occurs as Zop incurs costs in connection with the liability. Consequently, the $2,500 expense incurred by Zop is a deduction for the 2014 tax year.

Certain manufacturers, wholesalers and retailers that make advance payments to purchase insurance policies that cover their obligations under multi-year service warranty contracts must capitalize the cost of the policies and deduct that cost ratably over the life of the policies. This rule applies regardless of whether the taxpayer uses the cash or accrual method (Rev. Proc. 97-38).[71]

Economic performance generally occurs only when payment is made to the person to whom the liability is owed. Payment is considered to be economic performance for the following:

> (1) liabilities to another person arising out of any workers' compensation, tort, or breach of contract claims against the taxpayer or any violation of law by the taxpayer;

> (2) rebates and refunds;

> (3) awards, prizes, and jackpots;

References are to Standard Federal Tax Reports; Tax Research Consultant; and Practical Tax Explanations.

[68] ¶ 21,817.1875; ACCTNG: 6,318; § 38,410.25

[69] ¶ 21,802; ACCTNG: 12,050; ACCTNG: 12,100; § 38,430.05

[70] ¶ 21,810; ACCTNG: 12,102; § 38,435.05

[71] ¶ 20,620.20; ACCTNG: 9,484.25

(4) insurance, warranty and service contracts; and

(5) taxes other than creditable foreign taxes (Reg. § 1.461-4(g)).[72]

Under certain limited circumstances, an irrevocable payment to a court-ordered settlement fund that completely extinguishes specified tort liabilities will also constitute economic performance (Code Sec. 468B).[73]

Recurring Items. Certain recurring items are treated as incurred in advance of economic performance by taxpayers other than tax shelters. Under this exception, an item is treated as incurred during a tax year if:

(1) the all-events test, without regard to economic performance, is satisfied during that year;

(2) the economic performance test is met within the shorter of 8½ months or a reasonable time after the close of the year;

(3) the item is recurring in nature and the taxpayer consistently treats similar items as incurred in the tax year in which the all-events test is met; and

(4) either the item is not material or accrual of the item in the year that the all-events test is met results in a better matching against the income to which it relates than accrual of the item in the tax year of economic performance (Code Sec. 461(h)(3); Reg. § 1.461-5).[74]

In determining whether an item is material or whether a more proper matching against income results from deduction of an expense prior to economic performance, the treatment of the expense on financial statements is to be taken into account but will not necessarily govern the tax treatment of the expense.

An item is recurring if it can generally be expected to be incurred from one tax year to the next (Reg. § 1.461-5(b)(3)). However, a taxpayer may treat a liability as recurring even if it is not incurred in each tax year. Also, a liability that has never previously been incurred may be treated as recurring if it is reasonable to expect that it will be incurred on a recurring basis in the future.

A taxpayer may adopt the recurring item exception as part of its method of accounting for any type of expense for the first tax year in which that type of expense is incurred. Any change to or from the recurring item exception is generally treated as a change in the taxpayer's method of accounting (¶ 1529) (Reg. § 1.461-5(d)). Tax shelters are generally prohibited from using the recurring item exception (Code Sec. 461(i)).[75]

1540A. Accruing Uncertain and Contingent Liabilities. On the accrual-basis of accounting (¶ 1515), expenses are deductible in the tax year when all events have occurred that fix the amount of the item and determine the liability of the taxpayer to pay it (¶ 1540). Thus, there can be no accrual of an expense until any contingency disappears and the liability becomes fixed and certain (Reg. § 1.461-1).[76] Similarly, an accrual-method taxpayer generally cannot accrue a liability that the taxpayer is contesting, as the liability is not fixed and certain. However, if the taxpayer is contesting an asserted liability and transfers money or property to provide for the satisfaction of the liability, the taxpayer can take a deduction in the year of the transfer if the contest continues to exist after the transfer and the liability would otherwise be allowed as a deduction in the year of transfer or an earlier tax year (Code Sec. 461(f)).[77]

See ¶ 1547 for a discussion of reserves for contingent or estimated expenses.

1540B. Accruing Interest and Expenses Owed to Related Taxpayers. When different methods of accounting (¶ 1515) are used by related taxpayers, accrued interest and expenses owed to a related taxpayer may not be deducted until the time that the interest or expense payment is includible in the gross income of the cash-basis payee (Code Sec. 267(a)(2)).[78] Thus, an accrual-basis payor is placed on the cash basis for the purpose of

---

References are to Standard Federal Tax Reports; Tax Research Consultant; and Practical Tax Explanations.

[72] ¶ 21,810; ACCTNG: 12,102.20; § 38,435.05

[73] ¶ 21,950; ACCTNG: 12,214; § 38,435.20

[74] ¶ 21,802, ¶ 21,811; ACCTNG: 12,104.10; § 38,435.10

[75] ¶ 21,802; ACCTNG: 12,354; § 38,435.10

[76] ¶ 21,805; ACCTNG: 12,056; § 38,430.10

[77] ¶ 21,802; ACCTNG: 12,058; § 38,430.15

[78] ¶ 14,150; ACCTNG: 12,150, ACCTNG: 12,152.10; § 9,140, § 27,125.25

deducting business expenses and interest owed to a related cash-basis taxpayer. The deduction is deferred until the cash-basis payee takes the item into income.

A related person for this purpose includes persons described in Code Sec. 267(b) (¶ 1717), as well as a personal service corporation (PSC) and any of its employee-owners (¶ 273). Thus, a PSC may not deduct payments made to owner-employees before the tax year in which such persons must include the payment in gross income. A special pass-through entity rule treats a partnership or an S corporation as related to a taxpayer who owns any capital or profits interest in the partnership or stock of the S corporation and persons related to that taxpayer (Code Sec. 267(e)).

1541. Deferred Payments Under Certain Rental Agreements. Lessors and lessees of certain leaseback and long-term rental agreements that involve the use of property must report income and expenses arising out of those agreements by applying statutory accrual-basis and present-value principles (Code Sec. 467; Reg. § 1.467-1).[79] This treatment, in effect, is an extension of the principles embodied in the rules on taxation of original issue discount (¶ 1952). Although the rules under Code Sec. 467 apply to the use of property, the IRS is given authority to extend similar rules to agreements for services.

Section 467 rental agreements cover tangible property with respect to which either (1) at least one amount, allocable to the use of property in the calendar year, is to be paid after the close of the following calendar year (deferred payments), or (2) there are increases in the amount to be paid as rent under the agreement (stepped rents). A section 467 rental agreement does not encompass a rental agreement in which the sum of the amounts to be paid is $250,000 or less.

Regardless of the accounting method used (¶ 1515), the lessor or lessee of any such agreement must report for any tax year the sum of: (1) the accrued rental payments, and (2) any interest for the year (calculated at the rate of 110 percent of the applicable federal rate compounded semiannually (¶ 83)) on unpaid rents (amounts that were attributed to a prior tax year but are still unpaid as of the current tax year).

The accrued rental payments—except in tax-avoidance transactions and agreements that do not allocate rents—are calculated by (1) allocating rents in accordance with the agreement, and (2) including the present value of rents allocable to the period but paid after the close of the period. In tax-avoidance transactions and agreements that do not allocate rents, the rent that accrues during the tax year is equal to the allocable portion of the "constant rental amount." The constant rental amount is equal to the amount which, if paid as of the close of each lease period, would result in an aggregate present value equal to the present value of the aggregate payments required under the lease.

1543. Claim-of-Right Doctrine. Under the claim-of-right doctrine, payments must be included in gross income if the taxpayer receives them without restriction under a claim of right.[80] This is true even though the taxpayer may discover in a later year that he or she had no right to the payments in the earlier year and is required to repay the same amount. The taxpayer may deduct the repayments in the year in which they are made.

When the repayments exceed income for the year of repayment, or when the income (after subtraction of those repayments) is taxed at a rate lower than that at which the income in the year of inclusion was taxed, the deduction does not compensate the taxpayer adequately for the tax paid in the earlier year. The law eliminates this inequity if the amount repaid exceeds $3,000. In that case, the taxpayer is required to reduce his or her tax for the year of repayment by the amount of tax for the previous year which was attributable to inclusion of this amount; any excess is to be claimed as a refund. If a smaller tax liability results from simply deducting the repaid amount in the year of repayment, the taxpayer is to claim the deduction instead (Code Sec. 1341; Reg. § 1.1341-1).[81]

References are to Standard Federal Tax Reports; Tax Research Consultant; and Practical Tax Explanations.

[79] ¶ 21,910, ¶ 21,910D; REAL: 12,356; § 38,410.35
[80] ¶ 21,005.1251; ACCTNG: 27,000; § 38,310.05
[81] ¶ 31,880, ¶ 31,881; ACCTNG: 27,500; § 4,230.05

In either case, the adjustment is made for the year of repayment. The return for the prior year—the year in which the item was received—is not reopened; in no case will there be an allowance for interest on the tax paid for the earlier year.

Example: In 2013, a single taxpayer reported taxable income of $55,000 (adjusted gross income of $65,000 minus $3,900 personal exemption, minus $6,100 standard deduction), consisting entirely of sales commissions, on which he paid a tax of $9,679. In 2014, it is determined that the commissions were erroneously computed for 2013. Accordingly, the taxpayer pays back $6,000 of the commissions. His taxable income for 2014, without regard to the $6,000 repayment, is $13,200.

The tax for 2014 will be computed as follows:

(a) Tax on $7,200 ($13,200 less $6,000)		$720
(b) Tax on $13,200		1,526
Less: Difference between—		
Tax paid for 2013 on $55,000	9,679	
Tax payable in 2013 on $49,000		
($55,000 – $6,000)	8,179	1,500
		26

The tax for 2014 is the lesser of the amount computed under (a) or (b). In this case, the amount computed under (b) is less than the amount computed under (a). Thus, the tax for 2014 is $26, the amount computed under (b).

When the tax for the year of restoration under a claim of right is reduced by the amount of the tax already paid on the item in a previous year, the amount restored is not considered for any purpose. For example, taxpayers cannot use that amount in computing a net operating loss for the year of restoration (Reg. §1.1341-1(b)(2)).[82] The reduction of tax in the year of repayment does not apply where the taxpayer did, in fact, have an unrestricted right to receive the amount in the prior year and the obligation to repay arose as the result of subsequent events.

1545. Dealer's Reserve for Income. Dealers who discount customers' installment paper with financial institutions that withhold a small percentage of the price and credit it to a reserve account as security for the dealer's guaranty of payment of the installment paper must accrue those credits as income in the year when the installment paper is transferred to the financial institution.[83] This has been applied to accrual-basis home sellers who guarantee buyers' loans by requiring them to accrue as income in the year of sale the proceeds pledged as loan security to the lender. As to a cash-basis taxpayer, however, the pledged amounts are taxable to him only as they become available for withdrawal (the pledged amount was in a restricted savings account and could be withdrawn in specified amounts only as the buyer reduced the loan principal by certain amounts).

1547. Reserve for Estimated Expense. Although reserves for contingent liabilities are often set up in business practice, amounts credited to them are generally not deductible for income tax purposes because the fact of liability is not fixed.[84] For example, advance deductions have been denied for additions to a reserve for expected cash discounts on outstanding receivables, amounts credited by a manufacturer to a reserve for possible future warranty service, and additions to a reserve covering estimated liability of a carrier for tort claims. However, to the extent that the Code specifically provides for a deduction for a reserve for estimated expenses, the economic performance rules (¶1540) do not apply (Code Sec. 461(h)(5)).[85]

References are to Standard Federal Tax Reports; Tax Research Consultant; and Practical Tax Explanations.

[82] ¶31,881; ACCTNG: 27,558; §38,310.05

[83] ¶31,882.25; ACCTNG: 9,406; §38,320.05

[84] ¶21,817.688; ACCTNG: 12,200; §38,430.10

[85] ¶21,802; ACCTNG: 12,104; §38,430.10

1549. Accrual of Vacation and Sick Leave Pay. The deduction for vacation and sick leave pay is generally limited to the amount of pay earned during the year to the extent (1) the amount is paid to employees during the year, or (2) the amount is vested as of the last day of the tax year and is paid to employees within 2.5 months after the end of the year. If the vacation or sick leave pay is not paid until after the expiration of that period, the employer may deduct vacation pay when paid and sick leave pay in its tax year that includes the last day of the employee's tax year for which the payment is reported as income by the employee (Code Sec. 404(a)(5); Temp. Reg. §1.404(b)-1T).[86] However, vacation and sick leave pay incurred with respect to the production of real and tangible personal property or with respect to property acquired for resale is considered a direct labor cost that must be capitalized by taxpayers subject to the uniform capitalization rules (¶991) (Reg. §1.263A-1(e)(2)(i)(B)).[87]

Regardless of whether or not vested vacation pay is considered deferred compensation, FICA and FUTA taxes may be deducted by an accrual basis taxpayer prior to the tax year that the FICA and FUTA taxes are actually paid if: (1) all events have occurred to establish the fact of the taxpayer's liability for the FICA and FUTA taxes, (2) the amount of the payroll tax liability can be determined with reasonable accuracy, and (3) the taxpayer properly adopts the recurring item exception (¶1540) as a method of accounting with respect to the payroll taxes (Rev. Rul. 2007-12).[88]

Long-Term Contracts

1551. Long-Term Contract Method of Accounting. Taxable income from a long-term contract generally must be accounted for under the percentage-of-completion method of accounting (Code Sec. 460).[89] A taxpayer who has entered into a small construction contract or home construction contract, however, may use an exempt contract method of accounting (¶1552).

A long-term contract is a building, installation, construction, or manufacturing contract that is not completed within the tax year in which it is entered into. A manufacturing contract is not to be considered long term unless the contract involves the manufacture of (1) unique items not normally carried in the finished goods inventory or (2) items normally requiring more than 12 calendar months to complete, regardless of the duration of the actual contract.

Percentage-of-Completion Method. Under the percentage-of-completion method, gross income is reported annually according to the percentage of the contract completed in that year. The completion percentage must be determined by comparing costs allocated and incurred before the end of the tax year with the estimated total contract costs (cost-to-cost method or simplified cost-to-cost method). Thus, for a particular tax year, the taxpayer includes a portion of the total contract price in gross income as the taxpayer incurs allocable contract costs for the year. Any contract income that has not been included in the taxpayer's gross income by the end of the tax year in which the contract is completed is included in gross income for the following tax year (Code Sec. 460(b); Reg. §1.460-4(b)).[90]

Modified Percentage-of-Completion Method (10-Percent Method). A taxpayer may elect to defer the recognition of income and accounting for costs until the first tax year in which at least 10 percent of the estimated total costs of the contract have been incurred (Code Sec. 460(b)(5)).

Look-Back Rule. To the extent that the percentage-of-completion method applies to a long-term contract, a taxpayer who errs in his or her estimate of the contract price or costs must look back and recompute his or her tax liability on the basis of the actual contract price and costs for the years for which that method was used. A taxpayer will either pay or receive interest at the rate for overpayment of tax (¶2765), compounded daily and figured on Form 8697, on the amount by which the recomputed tax liability for

---

References are to Standard Federal Tax Reports; Tax Research Consultant; and Practical Tax Explanations.

[86] ¶18,330, ¶18,354; ACCTNG: 12,300; §38,435.15

[87] ¶13,811; ACCTNG: 15,208.10; §10,310.10

[88] ¶21,817.128; ACCTNG: 12,052.15; §9,365

[89] ¶21,550; ACCTNG: 33,000; §38,230.05

[90] ¶21,550, ¶21,555; ACCTNG: 33,100; §38,230.20

a year exceeds or is less than the previously reported tax liability (Code Sec. 460(b); Reg. § 1.460-6).[91] Only one rate of interest will apply for each "accrual period," the period which begins on the date after the original return due date for the tax year and which ends on the original return due date for the following tax year. The applicable overpayment rate of interest is the overpayment rate in effect for the calendar quarter in which the accrual period begins. The look-back method does not have to be applied in computing taxable income with respect to home construction contracts, long-term construction contracts of small businesses, and small long-term contracts. Taxpayers can also elect not to apply the look-back method when the differences between estimated and actual amounts are *de minimis*.

Pass-through entities, i.e., partnerships, S corporations, and trusts, that are not closely held must use a simplified look-back method if substantially all of the income under a long-term contract is from sources in the United States (Code Sec. 460(b)(4)). A closely held entity is an entity where 50 percent or more of the value of the beneficial interests are owned by five or fewer persons. The amount of taxes deemed overpaid or underpaid under a contract in any year is determined at the entity level and is the product of the amount of contract income overreported or underreported for the year times the top marginal tax rate applicable for the year, i.e., the top corporate tax rate, or the top individual tax rate if more than 50 percent of the beneficial interests in the entity are held by individuals.

Allocation and Capitalization of Costs. A taxpayer generally must allocate costs to long-term contracts accounted for under the percentage-of-completion method in the same manner as direct and indirect costs are capitalized to property produced by a taxpayer under the uniform capitalization rules (Code Sec. 460(c); Reg. § 1.460-5).[92] Thus, the taxpayer must allocate to each long-term contract all direct costs and certain indirect costs properly allocable to the long-term contract. While bonus depreciation (¶ 1237) is generally taken into account when allocating contract costs, solely for purposes of determining the percentage of completion, the cost of qualified property is taken into account as if the bonus depreciation rules had not been enacted.

Under the general cost allocation method, research and experimental expenses, other than independent research and development expenses, must be allocated to the contract. However, independent research and development expenses, expenses incurred in making unsuccessful bids and proposals, and marketing, selling, and advertising costs may be expensed. Production period interest generally must be allocated to the contract (¶ 1561). Contributions to a pension or annuity plan, whether related to current or past services, are subject to the long-term contract rules and are treated as costs allocable to a long-term contract.

A taxpayer can elect to use a simplified cost-to-cost method of allocation if all the taxpayer's contracts are accounted for under the percentage-of-completion method and the 10-percent method is not used (Reg. § 1.460-5(c)). Small construction and home construction contracts accounted for under an exempt contract method are not subject to the general cost allocation rules (¶ 1552). Special rules are also provided for allocating costs to cost-plus long-term contracts and to federal long-term contracts.

1552. Exempt Contract Methods of Accounting. Although taxable income from a long-term contract generally must be accounted for under the percentage-of-completion method of accounting (¶ 1551), income from a small construction contract or a home construction contract may be taken into account using the exempt-contract-percentage-of-completion method or the completed contract method. The look-back rule and the cost allocation rules, except for the allocation of production period interest, are not required for these contracts (Code Sec. 460(e); Reg. § 1.460-4).[93] A taxpayer may change his or her method of accounting to conform with either of these special methods only after securing permission from the IRS (¶ 1529). Eligible taxpayers are not required to use these methods of accounting and may instead elect any other permissible method, such as a cash, accrual, or hybrid method (¶ 1515).

References are to Standard Federal Tax Reports; Tax Research Consultant; and Practical Tax Explanations.

[91] ¶ 21,550, ¶ 21,557; ACCTNG: 33,200; § 38,230.55

[92] ¶ 21,550, ¶ 21,556; ACCTNG: 33,300; § 38,230.55

[93] ¶ 21,550, ¶ 21,555; ACCTNG: 33,066, ACCTNG: 33,152; § 38,230.15, § 38,230.30

Small Construction Contracts. A small construction contract is a construction contract expected to be completed within two years that is performed by a taxpayer whose average annual gross receipts for the three prior tax years does not exceed $10 million.

Home and Residential Construction Contracts. A home construction contract is any construction contract where 80 percent or more of the estimated total contract costs are reasonably expected to be attributable to dwelling units contained in buildings with four or fewer dwelling units, and to improvements to real property related to such dwelling units. A home construction contract related to buildings with more than four dwelling units is a residential construction contract, for which the availability of the exempt contract methods is limited (see *Percentage-of-Completion/Capitalized Cost Method* later).

Exempt-Contract-Percentage-of-Completion Method. Under the exempt-contract-percentage-of-completion method, the taxpayer includes in income the portion of the total contract price that corresponds to the percentage of the entire contract that the taxpayer has completed during the tax year. The percentage is determined by using any method of cost comparison that clearly reflects income and is used consistently (Reg. § 1.460-4(c)).

Completed Contract Method. Under the completed contract method, the taxpayer does not report income until the tax year in which the contract is completed and accepted (Reg. § 1.460-4(d)). Expenses allocable to the contract are deductible in the year in which the contract is completed. Expenses not allocated to the contract, i.e., period costs, are deductible in the year in which they are paid or incurred, depending on the method of accounting employed.

Percentage-of-Completion/Capitalized-Cost Method. For residential construction contracts, the taxpayer may report 70 percent of the income using the percentage-of-completion method and the remaining 30 percent using an exempt contract method (Reg. § 1.460-4(e)).

Inventories

1553. Requirement to Use Inventories. A taxpayer generally must use inventories to clearly reflect income where the production, purchase, or sale of merchandise is an income-producing factor (Code Sec. 471(a); Reg. § 1.471-1).[94] To figure taxable income, a taxpayer must value inventory at the beginning and end of each tax year. This valuation depends on the items included in inventory (¶ 1557) and the method of valuation (¶ 1559). Inventory practices must be consistent from year to year. A taxpayer whose average annual gross receipts do not exceed $1 million or a taxpayer engaged in an eligible trade or business whose average annual gross receipts do not exceed $10 million is generally not required to use inventories or the accrual method of accounting (Rev. Procs. 2002-28 and 2001-10). However, a taxpayer who does not otherwise use inventories must treat merchandise inventory in the same manner as a material or supply that is not incidental (¶ 903). A farmer may also use the cash method of accounting for purchases and sales. See the accrual method requirement for certain farming corporations at ¶ 1519. However, any taxpayer, including a farmer, who uses inventories must use the accrual method of accounting for purchases and sales.

1557. Items Included in Inventory. An inventory is an itemized list, with valuations, of goods held for sale or consumption in a manufacturing or merchandising business. Taxpayers must usually verify the amount of items in inventory by a physical count of the items as of the last day of the tax year. Taxpayers may use estimates of inventory shrinkage that are confirmed by a physical count after year-end if the taxpayer normally does a physical inventory count at each location on a regular and consistent basis and the taxpayer makes proper adjustments to those inventories and to its estimating methods to the extent the estimates are greater than or less than the actual shrinkage (Code Sec. 471(b)).[95]

References are to Standard Federal Tax Reports; Tax Research Consultant; and Practical Tax Explanations.

[94] ¶ 22,202, ¶ 22,203; ACCTNG: 15,052; § 38,501

[95] ¶ 22,202; ACCTNG: 15,252.20; § 38,515.10

Inventory should include all finished or partly finished goods and only those raw materials and supplies which have been acquired for sale or which will physically become a part of merchandise intended for sale (Reg. § 1.471-1).[96] Merchandise should be included in inventory only if title to it is vested in the taxpayer. A seller should include in inventory goods under contract for sale but not yet segregated and applied to the contract and goods out on consignment. The seller should not include goods sold, including containers, where title has passed to the buyer. A buyer should include in inventory merchandise purchased, including containers, where title has passed to him or her, even where the merchandise is in transit or has not been physically received.

It is necessary to identify the particular goods in inventory so that proper costs can be applied to the quantities. Identification of inventories is ordinarily accomplished by the first-in, first-out (FIFO) rule (¶ 1564), unless the items are specifically identified. A taxpayer can also elect to identify inventory items by use of the last-in, first-out (LIFO) rule (¶ 1565).

Real property held for sale by a dealer may not be inventoried because each parcel of real estate is unique.[97] Likewise, capital assets, equipment, accounts, notes, investments, cash, or similar assets may not be included in inventories. For inventories of farmers and dealers in securities, see ¶ 1569 and ¶ 1903.

1559. Valuation of Inventory. An inventory must conform to the best accounting practice in the particular trade or business and must clearly reflect income (Reg. § 1.471-2(a) and (b)).[98] An inventory that, under the best accounting practice, can be used in a balance sheet showing the financial position of the taxpayer will generally be regarded as clearly reflecting income. In determining whether income is clearly reflected, great weight is given to consistency in inventory practice, but a legitimate accounting system will be disallowed where it distorts income.

Two methods commonly used to value inventories are the cost method (¶ 1561) and the lower of cost or market method (¶ 1563) (Reg. § 1.471-2(c) and (d)).[99] Opening and closing inventories must be valued by the same method. If the lower of cost or market method is used, it must be consistently applied to each item in the inventory. Cost and market value are determined as to each item, and the lower amount is included in the inventory valuation. A taxpayer is not permitted to inventory the entire stock at cost and also at market and use the lower of the two results (Reg. § 1.471-4).[100] Deviations are permitted, however, as to goods inventoried under the last-in, first-out (LIFO) identification method (¶ 1565) and as to animals inventoried under the "unit-livestock-price" method (¶ 1569).

The IRS will also generally accept the rolling-average inventory valuation method used to value inventories for financial accounting purposes as clearly reflecting income for federal income tax purposes (Rev. Proc. 2008-43, modified by Rev. Proc. 2008-52). However, if inventory is held for several years or costs fluctuate substantially, the rolling-average cost method may not clearly reflect income, depending on the particular facts and circumstances. Moreover, if the taxpayer does not use the rolling-average method for financial accounting purposes, then that method may not accurately determine costs or clearly reflect income for tax purposes. Special rules apply to dealers in securities (¶ 1903).

Whether the cost or the lower of cost or market method is used, inventoried goods that are unsalable, or unusable in normal transactions because of wear and tear, obsolescence, or broken lots, should be valued at bona fide selling price, less cost of selling (Reg. § 1.471-2(c)).[101] A bona fide selling price is the actual offering of goods during a period ending not later than 30 days after inventory date. Adjustment of the

---

References are to Standard Federal Tax Reports; Tax Research Consultant; and Practical Tax Explanations.

[96] ¶ 22,203; ACCTNG: 15,056; § 38,505.05
[97] ¶ 22,204.36; ACCTNG: 15,058; § 38,505.05
[98] ¶ 22,205; ACCTNG: 15,152; § 38,501
[99] ¶ 22,205; ACCTNG: 15,250; § 38,535.05
[100] ¶ 22,209; ACCTNG: 15,254; § 38,535.15
[101] ¶ 22,205; ACCTNG: 15,256; § 38,515.20

valuation on a reasonable basis, not less than scrap value, is permitted in the case of unsalable or unusable raw material or partly finished goods.

1561. Inventory at Cost: Uniform Capitalization Rules. Uniform capitalization rules govern the inclusion in inventory or capital accounts of all allocable costs that are incurred with respect to real and tangible personal property that is produced by the taxpayer or acquired for resale and would otherwise be considered in computing taxable income (Code Sec. 263A(a) and (b); Reg. § 1.263A-2).[102] For this purpose, tangible personal property includes a film, sound recording, videotape, book, or similar property. Except for the interest capitalization rules, the uniform capitalization rules also apply to costs incurred with respect to real or personal, whether tangible or intangible, property that is acquired for resale. Certain small businesses with average annual gross receipts not exceeding $10 million for the three previous years that acquire personal property for resale are exempt from these rules.

Costs attributable to inventory must be added to costs of producing or acquiring the inventory, and costs attributable to producing other property must be capitalized. Direct material and labor costs, as well as the portion of indirect costs allocable to that property, are subject to these rules (Reg. § 1.263A-1(a)(3)).

The uniform capitalization rules replace the inventory cost rules of Code Sec. 471 (¶ 1553) in the case of property to which they apply. The rules do not apply to inventories valued at market under either the market method or the lower of cost or market method (¶ 1563) if the market valuation used by the taxpayer generally equals the property's fair market value, i.e., price of sale to customers less direct disposition costs. However, the uniform capitalization rules do apply in determining the market value of any inventory for which market is determined with reference to replacement cost or reproduction cost.

The uniform capitalization rules do not apply to property produced for personal use or pursuant to a long-term contract (¶ 1551); timber, including certain ornamental trees; costs deductible as Code Sec. 174 research and experimental expenditures (¶ 979); costs associated with certain oil, gas, and other mineral property, foreign drilling, and amortizable or developmental expenditures; and costs, other than circulation expenditures, subject to the 10-year amortization rule for certain alternative minimum tax preference items. Certain costs incurred by an individual or personal service corporation (¶ 273) engaged in the business of being a writer, photographer, or artist (¶ 990A) that are otherwise deductible are also exempt from those rules. In addition, the following costs may be currently deducted: marketing and selling expenses and general and administration expenses that do not directly benefit production or the acquisition of inventory (¶ 1450) (Code Sec. 263A(c) and ((h)); Reg. § 1.263A-1(e)(4)).[103]

Interest Capitalization Rules. Interest costs paid or incurred during the production period to finance the construction, building, installation, manufacture, development, or improvement of real or tangible personal property that is produced by the taxpayer must be capitalized in certain cases (Code Sec. 263A(f); Reg. § 1.263A-8).[104] Property subject to the interest capitalization requirement includes property that is produced by the taxpayer for use in its trade or business or in an activity for profit and that has (1) a long useful life (real property or any other property with a class life of 20 years or more), (2) an estimated production period exceeding two years, or (3) an estimated production period exceeding one year and a cost exceeding $1 million. The production period begins on the date on which production of the property starts and ends on the date on which the property is ready to be placed in service or is ready to be held for sale. Capitalization of interest is not required for property acquired for resale, e.g., inventory held by a dealer, and interest that constitutes qualified residence interest (¶ 1047).

References are to Standard Federal Tax Reports; Tax Research Consultant; and Practical Tax Explanations.

[102] ¶ 13,800, ¶ 13,817; ACCTNG: 15,200; § 38,535.10

[103] ¶ 13,800, ¶ 13,811; BUSEXP: 9,050; § 10,305.05

[104] ¶ 13,800, ¶ 13,852; BUSEXP: 9,060; § 10,330.05

¶1561

In applying the interest capitalization rules, a taxpayer is treated as producing any property that is produced for the taxpayer under a contract (Code Sec. 263A(g)(2)).[105] Thus, the portion of the taxpayer-customer's interest expense allocable to costs required to be capitalized, including progress payments, advances to the contractor, and an allocable portion of the general and administrative expenses of the taxpayer, must be capitalized.

In determining whether interest expense is allocable to the production of property, interest on a debt that financed production or construction costs of a particular asset is first allocated and capitalized as part of the cost of the item (Reg. §§ 1.263A-9 and 1.263A-11).[106] If the production or construction costs for an asset exceed the amount of this direct debt, interest on other loans is also subject to capitalization under an avoided-cost rule to the extent of the excess. An assumed interest rate based on the average interest rates on the taxpayer's outstanding debt, excluding debt specifically traceable to production or construction, may be used for this purpose. For this purpose, production or construction expenditures include cumulative production costs (including previously capitalized interest) required to be capitalized.

Interest relating to property used to produce property subject to the interest capitalization rules is also subject to capitalization to the extent that interest is allocable to the produced property as determined under the above rules (Code Sec. 263A(f)(3)).[107]

For flow-through entities, i.e., partnerships, S corporations, estates, and trusts, the interest capitalization rules are applied first at the entity level and then at the beneficiary level (Code Sec. 263A(f)(2)(C)).

Farming Businesses. For the uniform capitalization rules pertaining to farm businesses, see ¶ 999.

Inventory at Cost: Code Sec. 471 Rules. The following rules are to be used to value inventory at cost where the uniform capitalization rules do not apply. For merchandise on hand at the beginning of the year, cost is the amount at which it was included in the closing inventory of the preceding period. For merchandise *bought* after the beginning of the year, cost means the invoice price less trade or other discounts, except cash discounts approximating a fair interest rate, which may be deducted from cost, or reported as income, at the option of the taxpayer. Cost also includes transportation or other acquisition charges. For merchandise *produced* by the taxpayer, the costs attributed to inventoried goods must be determined under the uniform capitalization rules (see previously).

1563. Inventory at "Cost or Market". If a cost or market inventory is used, the market value of each item is compared with the cost of the item (¶ 1559), and the lower of the two values must be used for that item (Reg. § 1.471-4).[108]

> **Example:** A lumber dealer has three grades of lumber at the end of his tax year. They are valued as follows:

Grade	Cost	Market	Lower of Two
A	$45,000	$60,000	$45,000
B	20,000	15,000	15,000
C	5,000	5,000	5,000
	$70,000	$80,000	$65,000

If the lumber dealer is using the cost method, his ending inventory is valued at $70,000. If the dealer is using the lower of cost or market method, the ending inventory is valued at $65,000.

References are to Standard Federal Tax Reports; Tax Research Consultant; and Practical Tax Explanations.

[105] ¶ 13,800; BUSEXP: 9,060; § 10,330.10

[106] ¶ 13,856, ¶ 13,864; ACCTNG: 15,208; § 10,330.15

[107] ¶ 13,800; BUSEXP: 9,060; § 10,330.15

[108] ¶ 22,209; ACCTNG: 15,254; § 38,535.15

Under normal conditions, market value is the prevailing current bid price at the inventory date in the volume in which the items are usually purchased by the taxpayer. If a current bid price is unobtainable, the best available evidence of fair market value must be used. Specific purchases or sales by the taxpayer or others, or compensation paid for cancellation of contracts for purchase commitments, may be used.

The market value of goods in process and finished goods, for a manufacturer or processor, is reproduction cost. This is the total that materials, labor and factory burden or overhead would cost at current prices to bring the article to a comparable state of completion. The market price basis does not apply to goods on hand or in the process of manufacture for delivery under firm sale contracts at fixed prices entered into before the inventory date where the taxpayer is protected against actual loss. Such goods must be inventoried at cost.

A merchant may also use the "retail method" to approximate the lower of cost or market of goods in inventory (Reg. § 1.471-8).[109] The retail selling prices of goods on hand at the end of the year are multiplied by a ratio or cost complement to arrive the value of ending inventory. Minor changes in the way the ratio is computed apply for tax years beginning after December 31, 2014.

If inventories are valued at cost under the lower of cost or market method, that valuation is subject to the uniform capitalization rules at ¶ 1561.

1564. "First-In, First-Out" (FIFO) Rule. The "first-in, first-out" (FIFO) method of identifying inventory assumes that items purchased or produced first are the first items sold, consumed or otherwise disposed (Code Sec. 471; Reg. § 1.471-2).[110] Accordingly, items in inventory at the end of the year are matched with the costs of similar items that were most recently purchased or produced. The FIFO method of valuation is utilized for items taken in inventory that have been so commingled that they cannot be identified with specific invoices; thus, they are considered to be the items most recently purchased or produced. The cost is the actual cost of the items purchased and produced during the period in which the quantity of items in inventory was acquired. In the absence of an election to use the last-in, first-out (LIFO) method (¶ 1565), inventory is identified under the FIFO method.

1565. "Last-In, First-Out" (LIFO) Rule. The "last-in, first-out" (LIFO) method of identifying inventory is based on cost values (Code Sec. 472).[111] Under the LIFO method, inventory is taken at cost, but the items contained in the inventory are treated as being, first, those contained in opening inventory, to the extent of the opening inventory (whether or not they are physically on hand), and, second, those acquired during the tax year. The items treated as still in the opening inventory are taken in order of acquisition, except for the first year in which the method is used. For that year, the items in the opening inventory are taken at the average cost of those items. The closing inventory of the preceding year must also be adjusted and an amended return filed to reflect the changes. In the case of a retailer or certain manufacturers, items deemed to have been purchased during the year, that is, inventory increases, may be taken, at the taxpayer's election, on the basis of the most recent purchases, or at average cost for the year, or in order of acquisition.

A taxpayer need not obtain advance permission from the IRS to elect to use the LIFO method but must adopt it on the return for the year in which the method is first used. In addition, the taxpayer must file a Form 970 with the return and accept any modifications or adjustments required by the IRS. The election applies only to the class or classes of goods specified in the application. Although the election to adopt LIFO must generally cover the entire inventory of a business, manufacturers or processors may elect to have the method apply to raw materials only, including those in finished goods and work-in-process (Reg. § 1.472-1(h)).[112] Furthermore, if LIFO is used for tax

---

References are to Standard Federal Tax Reports; Tax Research Consultant; and Practical Tax Explanations.

[109] ¶ 22,217, ¶ 22,217B; ACCTNG: 15,256.35; § 38,535.20

[110] ¶ 22,202, ¶ 22,205; ACCTNG: 15,154; § 38,520

[111] ¶ 22,230; ACCTNG: 18,050; § 38,525.05

[112] ¶ 22,231; ACCTNG: 18,100; § 38,525.07

purposes, it generally must also be used in preparing annual financial statements for credit purposes or for the purpose of reports to stockholders, partners, or proprietors. For purposes of this "report rule," all members of the same group of financially related corporations are treated as one taxpayer.

As an alternative to the regular LIFO method, a taxpayer with numerous items in an inventory may use the dollar-value LIFO method (¶ 1567).

1567. Dollar-Value LIFO Method. Instead of determining quantity increases of each item in the inventory and then pricing them, as is required under the regular last-in, last (LIFO) method (¶ 1565), the "dollar-value" LIFO method may be used (Reg. § 1.472-8).[113] The increase in LIFO value is determined by comparing the total dollar value of the beginning and ending inventories at base year (the first LIFO year) prices and then converting any dollar-value increase to current prices by means of an index. Taxpayers are allowed, under the dollar-value LIFO method, to determine base year dollars through the use of government indexes (Code Sec. 472(f)).[114]

Simplified Dollar-Value LIFO Method. Small businesses, those with average gross receipts for the three preceding years of $5 million or less, may elect to use a simplified dollar-value LIFO method to account for their inventories (Code Sec. 474).[115] The method requires separate inventory pools for each major category in the applicable government price index. The election applies to all succeeding years unless the taxpayer obtains IRS permission to change to another method or becomes ineligible to use that method. If elected, it must be used to value all LIFO inventories.

1569. Special Methods for Farmers. In addition to the standard cost (¶ 1561) and the lower of cost or market (¶ 1563) methods for valuing inventory, a farmer on the accrual basis has a choice of two other systems. The "farm-price" method provides for the valuation of inventories at market price less the direct cost of disposition. If this method is used, it must be applied to the entire inventory except livestock which the taxpayer has elected to inventory under the "unit-livestock-price" method (Reg. § 1.471-6(d)).[116]

The "unit-livestock-price" method—adoptable when the farmer raises his or her own livestock or purchases young animals and raises them to maturity—provides for the valuation *of different classes* of animals at a standard unit price for each animal within a class. This method, once elected, must be applied to all livestock raised to maturity or purchased before maturity and raised to maturity, whether held for sale or for breeding, draft or dairy purposes. This includes unweaned calves. Unit prices assigned to classes must account for normal cost of production. For purchased livestock, the cost should be increased in accordance with unit prices only for animals acquired in the first six months of the tax year (Reg. § 1.471-6(g)).[117]

The "crop" basis of accounting may be used with IRS consent for crops which have not been gathered and disposed of during the tax year in which they are planted (Reg. § 1.61-4(c)).[118] The entire cost of producing the crop must be deducted no earlier than in the year in which the crop income is realized.

1571. Change in Inventory Accounting. A change in the method used to account for an inventory can be made only when authorized by the IRS. A change from a cash method to an inventory method is, in effect, a change to the accrual method of accounting for purchases and sales (Reg. § 1.446-1(c)(2); Rev. Proc. 2011-14).[119] Permission to make such a change must generally be requested within the tax year that the change is to be effective (¶ 1529), with the exception of an election to change to the last-in, first-out (LIFO method). An election to use this method may be made by a statement

---

References are to Standard Federal Tax Reports; Tax Research Consultant; and Practical Tax Explanations.

[113] ¶ 22,239; ACCTNG: 18,200; § 38,525.10

[114] ¶ 22,230; ACCTNG: 18,204; § 38,525.10

[115] ¶ 22,260; ACCTNG: 18,250; § 38,525.15

[116] ¶ 22,213; FARM: 3,110; § 36,325

[117] ¶ 22,213; FARM: 3,112; § 36,325

[118] ¶ 5601; FARM: 3,064; § 36,315.15

[119] ¶ 20,607, ¶ 20,620.243; ACCTNG: 15,300; § 38,601

on Form 970 attached to the first tax return in which it is used; however, adjustments will be required to prevent duplications and omissions of income and expenses (Reg. §§ 1.472-3 and 1.472-4).[120]

Allocation and Reconstruction of Income

1573. Allocation by IRS. When two or more organizations, trades, or businesses are owned or controlled by the same interests, the IRS may allocate gross income, deductions, or credits between them if it determines that this action is necessary to prevent evasion of taxes or to clearly reflect income (Code Sec. 482).[121] Moreover, the IRS is specifically authorized by statute to allocate any income, deduction, credit, exclusion, or other allowance between certain personal service corporations (¶ 273) and their employee-owners when the principal purpose of forming or using such a corporation is to avoid or evade income tax (¶ 1575).

1575. Acquisitions to Avoid Tax. If a taxpayer acquires control of a corporation, directly or indirectly, to evade or avoid income tax by securing the benefit of a deduction, credit, or other allowance that would not otherwise be enjoyed, then that deduction, credit or other allowance will not be permitted. The same rules of disallowance apply to a corporation that acquires property of another corporation that was not controlled by the acquiring corporation or its stockholders and that acquires a basis determined by reference to the basis in the hands of the transferor corporation (Code Sec. 269).[122] The IRS is authorized to deny an acquiring corporation the carryover and other tax benefits of a subsidiary corporation, acquired in a qualified stock purchase for which an election of asset acquisition treatment is not made, if the subsidiary corporation is liquidated under a plan adopted within two years of the acquisition date and the principal purpose of the liquidation is tax avoidance or evasion. For a discussion of the use or formation of a personal service corporation (PSC) by another entity to avoid or evade income tax and the IRS's authority to allocate amounts between the PSC and its employee-owners in order to clearly reflect income, see ¶ 273.

1577. Income Reconstruction. When a taxpayer has kept either inadequate or no books or records, the IRS has authority to compute income in order to clearly reflect the taxpayer's income (Code Sec. 446(b)).[123] The methods for reconstructing income vary depending on the facts and circumstances, and the records that are available. The IRS has developed several methods for reconstructing a taxpayer's income. The methods used most often are:

(1) *Bank deposits and expenditures method.* All bank deposits are assumed to represent income unless the taxpayer can establish otherwise. Although the taxpayer is given an opportunity to show that the deposits do not represent income, the IRS is not required to link the bank deposits with an identified income-producing activity.[124]

(2) *Net worth method.* An opening net worth or total value of assets at the beginning of a given year is established. The IRS then shows increases in the taxpayer's net worth for each subsequent year and calculates the difference between the adjusted net values of the assets at the beginning and end of each year under examination. Nondeductible expenses are added to the increases. If the resulting amount is greater than reported taxable income for that year, then the excess is treated as unreported taxable income.[125]

(3) *Percentage or unit mark-up method.* This method is used where inventories are a necessary income-producing factor but have not been kept or were incorrectly taken. Net income is determined by applying certain percentages, such as gross profits to sales, net income to gross income, or net income to sales, derived from other taxpayers in similar types of businesses.[126]

References are to Standard Federal Tax Reports; Tax Research Consultant; and Practical Tax Explanations.

[120] ¶ 22,234, ¶ 22,235; ACCTNG: 18,102; § 38,601

[121] ¶ 22,280; ACCTNG: 30,050; § 38,010.10

[122] ¶ 14,250; CONSOL: 71,050; § 9,135

[123] ¶ 20,606; ACCTNG: 3,152; § 39,730.05

[124] ¶ 20,620.416; ACCTNG: 3,156; § 39,730.15

[125] ¶ 20,620.52; ACCTNG: 3,154; § 39,730.15

[126] ¶ 20,620.548; ACCTNG: 3,162; § 39,730.15

Chapter 16

BASIS FOR GAIN OR LOSS

Computing Gain or Loss

1601. Basis. The rules on determining the basis for computing gain or loss or depreciation on property acquired in most common transactions are outlined below, with references to the paragraphs where additional details appear. This basis, after adjustments described at ¶ 1611—¶ 1617, is subtracted from the amount realized to determine the amount of gain or loss from a sale or other disposition (Code Sec. 1001).[1] Except where other rules are prescribed, the basis for gain or loss is determined under the law in effect when the property is sold or disposed.

Type of acquisition	Basis for gain or loss
Bargain purchases	
arm's-length	Cost (¶ 789)
corporation's, from nonstockholder	Cost (¶ 1660)
corporation's, from stockholder	Cost, unless saving is paid-in surplus (¶ 1660)
employee's	Cost plus amount taxable as compensation for services (¶ 789)
relative or friend	Cost, unless saving is a gift (¶ 1630)
stockholder's	Cost plus amount taxable as a dividend (¶ 789)
Bequests	For property acquired from a decedent, basis generally is fair market value at the date of the decedent's death (¶ 1633—¶ 1639)
Cash purchases	Cost (¶ 1604)
mortgage also assumed, or property taken subject to the mortgage	Full price, including mortgage amount (¶ 1725)
purchase money mortgage also given	Full purchase price (¶ 1725)
purchase notes also given	Full purchase price (¶ 1725)
redeemable ground rent assumed, or property taken subject to ground rent	Full purchase price (¶ 1725)
Community property	
survivor (death of spouse)	See "Bequests," above
Corporate property	
acquired for stock by controlled corporation	Transferor's basis (¶ 1660)
acquired for stock in taxable exchange	Fair market value of stock at time of exchange (¶ 1648)
contributions by nonstockholders	Zero (¶ 1660)
paid-in surplus	Transferor's basis (¶ 1660)
Dividend property	
corporate, stockholder of domestic corporation	Fair market value (¶ 735)
corporate, stockholder of foreign corporation	Fair market value (¶ 735)
noncorporate, stockholder	Fair market value (¶ 735)
Divorce or separation agreement	Transferors' basis (¶ 1734)

References are to Standard Federal Tax Reports; Tax Research Consultant; and Practical Tax Explanations.

[1] ¶ 29,220; SALES: 9,050; § 16,015

Type of acquisition	Basis for gain or loss
Gift property	Donor's basis, increased by gift tax in some cases; basis for loss *limited* to lesser of donor's basis or fair market value at time of gift (¶ 1630)
Inventory	Last inventory value (¶ 1561)
Joint tenancy	
after death of one tenant	Basis depends on amount contributed by each joint tenant toward the original purchase price (¶ 1634, ¶ 1636)
Lessor's acquisitions of lessee's improvements	Zero, if excluded from income (¶ 764)
Life estate	Zero, if disposed of after October 9, 1969 (¶ 1633)
Livestock	
inventory	Last inventory value (¶ 767)
purchased	Cost (¶ 767)
raised by accrual-basis farmer	Cost of raising (¶ 767)
raised by cash-basis farmer	Zero, if costs were charged to expense (¶ 767)
Mortgaged property (or property subject to redeemable ground rent)	Basis includes mortgage (or ground rent) (¶ 1725)
Partners' property	
partnership interest in exchange for contribution	Partners' adjusted basis of property contributed (¶ 443)
partnership interest purchased	Cost (¶ 434)
received in distribution other than liquidation	Partnership's adjusted basis at time of distribution (limited to partner's basis of his interest) (¶ 456)
received in partnership liquidation	Adjusted basis of partnership interest less cash received (¶ 456)
Partnership property	
after transfer of partnership interest or distributions to partners	Unaffected, unless election is made to adjust values (¶ 459, ¶ 467)
capital contribution	Partner's adjusted basis (¶ 443)
Purchase for more than value	Cost (¶ 1604), but excess may be a gift
Rehabilitated buildings, other than certified historic structures, for which investment credit on qualified expenditures available	Basis is reduced by allowable investment credit and the recaptured credit is added to basis (¶ 1365A)
Repossessed property after installment sale	
personal property	Fair market value (¶ 1838)
real property reacquired in satisfaction of purchaser's indebtedness secured by property	Adjusted basis of indebtedness plus gain resulting from reacquisition and reacquisition costs (¶ 1843)
Spousal transfers	Transferor's basis (¶ 1734)
Stock	
acquired in wash sale	Basis of stock sold, adjusted for difference between selling price of sold stock and purchase price of acquired stock (¶ 1935)
bonus stock	Allocable portion of basis of old stock (¶ 1620, ¶ 1682)
nontaxable stock dividend	Allocable share of basis of stock on which declared (¶ 1620, ¶ 1682)
qualified small business stock rollover	Cost, reduced by gain rolled over (¶ 1907)
purchased	Cost, if adequately identified (¶ 1975)
received for services	Amount reported as income, plus cash paid (¶ 1681)
S corporation	See ¶ 315, ¶ 317
specialized small business investment company stock rollover	Cost, reduced by gain rolled over (¶ 1907)
taxable stock dividend	Fair market value when issued (¶ 733A)
Stock rights	
nontaxable	Allocable share of basis of stock unless rights value is less than 15% of stock value (¶ 733A, ¶ 1682)
taxable	Fair market value when issued (¶ 733A)
Transfer in trust	Grantor's basis, plus gain or minus loss, upon transfer (¶ 1678)

1604. Adjusted Basis of Property. To determine the gain or loss from a sale or other disposition of property, the amount realized must be compared with the basis of the property to the taxpayer—generally measured by the original capital investment, adjusted to the date of sale (¶ 1611—¶ 1617) (Code Sec. 1011; Reg. § 1.1011-1).[2] In most situations, the basis of property is its cost to the taxpayer (Code Sec. 1012).[3] When property is acquired in a fully taxable exchange, the cost of the property acquired is the fair market value of the property given up.[4] Since, in an arm's-length transaction, both are presumed to be equal in value, the basis of the acquired property can be expressed as its fair market value.

1607. "Substituted" or Carryover Basis. A "substituted" basis is one that is continued or carried over from one taxpayer to another, or from one piece of property to another. The taxpayer has a substituted or carryover basis in property received as a gift (¶ 1630), in a transfer in trust (¶ 1678), in a tax-free exchange (¶ 1651), or acquired from a decedent dying in 2010 whose estate elects not to have federal estate tax apply (¶ 1633). The taxpayer also has a substituted basis in a personal residence purchased before May 7, 1997, if the recognition of gain realized on the sale of a prior residence was deferred under former Code Sec. 1034.[5]

Property Acquired by Purchase

1611. Additions to Basis of Property. In computing gain or loss on the sale of business or investment property, or gain on the sale of personal property, the cost or other basis must be *adjusted* for any expenditure, receipt, loss, or other item that is a capital expenditure (Code Sec. 1016(a)(1); Reg. § 1.1016-2).[6] This necessitates an addition for improvements made to the property since its acquisition.[7] For example, the cost of capital improvements such as an addition, new roof, newly installed central air conditioning, or electrical rewiring is added to the owner's basis. Other components that add to the cost basis of property include: brokers' commissions and lawyers' fees incurred in buying real estate; expenditures incurred in defending or perfecting the title to property;[8] zoning costs;[9] the capitalized value of a redeemable ground rent (Code Sec. 1055); and sales tax, freight, installation and testing costs, excise taxes, and revenue stamps.[10]

Settlement Fees and Other Costs. The basis of real property includes settlement fees and closing costs such as abstract fees, charges for installing utility services, legal fees (including title search and preparation of the sales contract and deed), recording fees, surveys, transfer taxes, owner's title insurance, and amounts owed by the seller but paid by the buyer, such as back taxes or interest, recording or mortgage fees, charges for improvements or repairs, and sales commissions (Code Sec. 1012; Reg. § 1.1012-1(b); Rev. Rul. 68-528).[11] Amounts placed in escrow for future payments of items such as insurance and taxes do not increase basis. The creation of a mortgage does not diminish the owner's basis in a property. When a buyer assumes an existing mortgage and pays cash or other consideration, the buyer's basis in the property includes the outstanding portion of the mortgage and the value of the other consideration, and the seller realizes a benefit in the amount of the mortgage and the additional consideration (*B.B. Crane*, SCt, 47-1 USTC ¶ 9217).[12] Fees and costs related to getting a loan to purchase the property are not included in the basis of the property.

Assessments. Assessments for improvements or other items that increase the value of property are added to the basis of the property and not deducted as a tax. Such

---

References are to Standard Federal Tax Reports; Tax Research Consultant; and Practical Tax Explanations.

[2] ¶ 29,310, ¶ 29,311; SALES: 9,050, SALES: 6,350; § 16,005

[3] ¶ 29,330; SALES: 6,050; § 16,105.05

[4] ¶ 29,335.33; SALES: 6,060; § 16,105.15

[5] ¶ 29,426.01; SALES: 6,250; § 16,101

[6] ¶ 29,410, ¶ 29,413; SALES: 6,352; § 16,110.10

[7] ¶ 29,412.84; SALES: 6,352.05; § 16,110.10

[8] ¶ 29,412.844; SALES: 6,352.20; § 16,105.30

[9] ¶ 13,709.659; SALES: 6,352.05; § 16,110.10

[10] ¶ 29,335.967, ¶ 29,335.577; SALES: 6,056.05; § 16,110.10

[11] ¶ 29,330, ¶ 29,331, ¶ 29,313.40; BUSEXP: 9,402.05; § 16,110.10

[12] ¶ 29,313.60; SALES: 6,054; § 18,505.05

improvements may include streets, sidewalks, water mains, sewers, and public parking facilities. The amount of such an assessment may be a depreciable asset. For example, the cost of a mall enclosure paid for by a business taxpayer through an assessment is depreciable. Assessments for maintenance or repairs, or for meeting interest charges on the improvements, are currently deductible as a real property tax, although the burden is on the taxpayer to show the allocation of the amounts assessed to the different purposes (Code Sec. 164(c)(1); Reg. § 1.164-4; Rev. Rul. 70-62).[13] Legal fees for obtaining a decrease in an assessment levied against property to pay for local improvements are added to the basis of the property and are not a deductible business expense.

Taxes. Any tax paid in connection with the acquisition of a property is treated as part of the cost of the property. A tax paid in connection with the disposition of a property reduces the amount realized on the disposition (Code Sec. 164(a)).[14]

In computing the cost of real property, the buyer cannot take into account any amount paid to the seller as reimbursement for real property taxes which are treated as imposed upon the purchaser (¶ 1032). This rule applies whether or not the sales contract calls for the buyer to reimburse the seller for real estate taxes paid or to be paid by the seller. However, where the buyer pays or assumes liability for real estate taxes imposed upon the seller, the taxes are considered part of the cost of the property. It is immaterial whether or not the sales contract specifies that the sale price has been reduced by, or is in any way intended to reflect, real estate taxes allocable to the seller (Reg. § 1.1012-1(b)).[15]

Checklist. Common expenses and the corresponding deduction rules may be found at ¶ 57.

1614. Additions to Basis for Carrying Charges. A taxpayer may elect to treat taxes or other carrying charges (such as interest) on some property as capital charges rather than as an expense of the tax year (Code Sec. 266; Reg. § 1.266-1).[16] The items chargeable to the capital account are:

(1) in the case of unimproved and unproductive real property: annual taxes, interest on a mortgage, and other carrying charges;

(2) in the case of real property, whether improved or unimproved and whether productive or unproductive: interest on a loan, taxes of the owner of such property measured by compensation paid to the owner's employees, taxes of the owner on the purchase of materials or on the storage, use or other consumption of materials, and other necessary expenditures, paid or incurred for the development or improvement of the property up to the time the development or construction work has been completed;

(3) in the case of personal property, taxes of an employer measured by compensation for services rendered in transporting machinery or other fixed assets to the plant or installing them, interest on a loan to buy such property or to pay for transporting or installing it, and taxes of the owner imposed on the purchase of such property or on the storage, use or other consumption, paid or incurred up to the date of installation or the date when the property is first put to use by the taxpayer, whichever is later; and

(4) any other taxes and carrying charges, otherwise deductible, which are chargeable to the capital account under sound accounting principles.

The election must be made by filing a statement with the taxpayer's original return indicating which items the taxpayer elects to treat as chargeable to the capital account (Reg. § 1.266-1(c)).[17] The election in (1) above is effective only for the year in which it is made. The election in (2) is effective until the development or construction work has

---

References are to Standard Federal Tax Reports; Tax Research Consultant; and Practical Tax Explanations.

[13] ¶ 8526.453, ¶ 9500, ¶ 9508; REAL: 3,104; § 7,315.05

[14] ¶ 9500; SALES: 6,354; § 16,110.25, § 16,430

[15] ¶ 29,331; REAL: 15,302; § 16,105.25

[16] ¶ 14,100, ¶ 14,101; SALES: 6,354, BUSEXP: 9,304; § 10,220

[17] ¶ 14,101; SALES: 6,354.05; § 10,220

been completed. The election in (3) is effective until the property is installed or first put to use, whichever date is later. The IRS determines whether the election in (4) is effective.

1617. Reductions in Basis. In order to determine the amount of gain or loss realized on the sale, exchange, or other disposition of property (or for figuring allowable depreciation, depletion, or amortization), the unadjusted basis of property (¶ 1601) must be decreased by any items that represent a return of capital for the period during which the property has been held by the taxpayer (Code Sec. 1016(a)).[18] These include:

- deductions previously allowed or allowable for depreciation, depletion, or amortization (¶ 1201 and following);

- the Code Sec. 179 expense deduction for certain depreciable business assets (¶ 1208), as well as the expense deduction for energy efficient commercial business property (¶ 1286), small business refiner capital costs incurred to comply with Environmental Protection Agency sulfur regulations (¶ 1285), and clean-fuel vehicles placed in service before 2006;

- any loss recognized from an involuntary conversion, as well as any money received that was not invested in replacement property (¶ 1687);

- gain from the sale of qualified small business stock or publicly traded securities excluded from gross income and rolled over to the basis of qualified replacement stock (¶ 1907 and ¶ 1909);

- casualty or theft loss deductions, as well as the amount of any insurance or other recovery for the loss (¶ 1127);

- tax-free dividends by corporations (¶ 733A) and nonliquidating distributions by a partnership to a partner (¶ 447); and

- the investment credit (except for 50 percent of the energy credits) (¶ 1365A).

Depreciation. The basis of property is reduced by the amount of depreciation claimed, or if greater, the depreciation which should have been claimed under the method chosen (Code Sec. 1016(a)(2); Reg. § 1.1016-3).[19] If no depreciation or insufficient depreciation was claimed, the basis is nonetheless reduced by the full amount of depreciation that should have been claimed. In order to mitigate the effect of this rule, the IRS has issued procedures that allow the taxpayer to change to a proper method of accounting for depreciation and claim a downward adjustment to income that reflects the additional amount of depreciation that should have been claimed (¶ 1221). If excess depreciation was claimed on an asset, the basis of the asset is reduced by the amount of depreciation that should have been claimed plus the part of the excess depreciation deducted that actually reduced the taxpayer's tax liability.

Percentage Depletion. Even though a percentage depletion allowance is in excess of cost or other basis, it is not necessary to use a negative basis (less than zero) in computing gain on the sale of mineral property (¶ 1294–¶ 1298).[20]

Motor Vehicles. The basis of a motor vehicle is reduced by any deduction or tax credit the taxpayer claimed with respect to the purchase including the credit for alternative motor vehicles (¶ 1345), the credit for certain qualified plug-in electric vehicles purchased after February 17, 2009, and before 2012 (¶ 1354), the credit for new qualified plug-in electric drive motor vehicles purchased after 2009 (¶ 1351), and the credit for alternative fuel vehicle refueling property, whether commercial or residential (¶ 1355). The basis of an automobile must also be reduced by the amount of any gas guzzler tax imposed by Code Sec. 4064 when use of the vehicle begins not more than one year after the first retail sale (Code Sec. 1016(d)).[21]

References are to Standard Federal Tax Reports; Tax Research Consultant; and Practical Tax Explanations.

[18] ¶ 29,410; SALES: 6,350; § 16,110.25

[19] ¶ 29,410, ¶ 29,414; SALES: 6,364; § 16,110.20

[20] ¶ 29,412.675; FARM: 18,068; § 11,610

[21] ¶ 29,410; SALES: 6,372.50

Easements. Generally, the amount received for granting an easement for a limited use or for a limited period reduces the basis of the affected part of the property (Rev. Rul. 68-291).[22] Gain is recognized to the extent that the amount received exceeds the basis of the affected part. The granting of a perpetual easement that denies the grantor any beneficial use of the property may be considered a sale of property even though the grantor retains legal title.

Residential Property. The basis of a personal residence or dwelling unit is reduced by certain tax credits the taxpayer claimed with respect to the property. This includes the nonbusiness energy credit allowed for qualified energy efficiency improvements and residential energy property (¶ 1341), and the residential energy efficient property credit allowed for amounts spent on alternative energy equipment such as solar or fuel cell equipment (¶ 1342). An eligible contractor who has constructed and claimed a credit a for qualified new energy-efficient home must also reduce his or her basis in the property to the extent that the credit is claimed (¶ 1365CC). In addition, the basis of a dwelling unit for which an excludable energy conservation subsidy was provided by a public utility must be reduced by the amount of the subsidy (¶ 889).

Homes Purchased Before May 7, 1997. The basis of a home purchased before May 7, 1997, must be reduced to reflect any gain realized on the sale of the prior home but deferred under former Code Sec. 1034.

Adoption Credit. The basis of a residence must be reduced by the amount of the adoption tax credit that was claimed with respect to improvements that increased that basis of the home (¶ 1307).

Child Care Credit. The basis of facilities acquired, constructed, rehabilitated, or expanded, and with respect to which an employer-provided child care credit (¶ 1365V) is allowed, must be reduced by the amount of the credit. If there is a recapture of the credit on the disposition of such property, the basis of the property is increased by the amount recaptured (Code Sec. 1016(a)(28)).

Canceled Debt. A taxpayer must reduce certain tax attributes by an amount excluded from gross income as the result of a discharge of indebtedness in a Title 11 bankruptcy case, a discharge of indebtedness during insolvency, or a discharge of qualified farm indebtedness (¶ 855).

Railroad Track. For tax years before January 1, 2014, eligible small and mid-sized railroad companies must reduce the basis of track on which they have been allowed a railroad track maintenance credit (¶ 1365W).

Substituted Basis. Where the basis of the property is a substituted basis (¶ 1607), the same adjustments must be made for the period the property was held by the transferor, donor, or grantor, or during the period the property was held by the person for whom the basis is to be determined (Code Sec. 1016(b)).[23]

1620. Apportionment of Cost or Other Basis. When a sale is made of parts of property purchased as a unit, as in a subdivision of real estate, allocation of the total basis is required (Reg. § 1.61-6).[24] Other instances where allocation of the cost or other basis is necessary include stock of different classes received as a dividend or pursuant to a reorganization, a split-up, split-off, or spin-off (¶ 2205); stock received as a bonus with the purchase of stock of a different character; stock purchase warrants attached to debenture bonds; and depreciable and nondepreciable property purchased for a lump sum.

Trade or Business Purchased. Applicable asset acquisition rules require the allocation of the purchase price of a trade or business among the assets in proportion to their

---

References are to Standard Federal Tax Reports; Tax Research Consultant; and Practical Tax Explanations.

[22] ¶ 29,412.813; SALES: 6,356.05; § 16,110.25

[23] ¶ 29,410; SALES: 6,374; § 16,101

[24] ¶ 5605; SALES: 6,200, SALES: 6,216; § 16,115

fair market values in the following classes and the following order (Code Sec. 1060; Reg. § § 1.338-6 and 1.1060-1):[25]

> • Class I asset: Cash and general deposit accounts (including savings and checking accounts), other than certificates of deposits held in banks, savings and loan associations, and other depository institutions.

> • Class II asset: Actively traded personal property, as well as certificates of deposit and foreign currency, even if they are not actively traded personal property.

> • Class III asset: Assets that the taxpayer marks to market at least annually for federal income tax purposes.

> • Class IV asset: Stock in trade of the taxpayer or other property of a kind that would properly be included in the inventory of the taxpayer if on hand at the close of the tax year, or property held by the taxpayer primarily for sale to customers in the ordinary course of its trade or business.

> • Class V asset: All assets other than Class I, II, III, IV, VI, and VII assets.

> • Class VI asset: Code Sec. 197 intangibles, except goodwill and going concern value.

> • Class VII asset: Goodwill and going concern value whether or not they qualify as section 197 intangibles.

Before making the above allocation, the purchase price is first reduced by any cash and general deposit accounts (savings and checking) which the acquired business holds as assets. The buyer and seller of the assets of a trade or business are bound by any written agreements allocating consideration to the transferred assets. However, any allocation that is not found to be fair market value will be disregarded. The buyer and seller must attach Form 8594 to their income tax returns for the year of sale to report the allocation.

Land and Buildings. When a building and land are purchased for a lump sum, the purchase price must be allocated between the land and building on the basis of their fair market values. If the fair market values are uncertain, the allocation may be based on their assessed values for real estate tax purposes (Reg. § § 1.61-6(a) and 1.167(a)-5).[26]

Subdivided Lots. The basis of each lot of a subdivided property is equal to the purchase price of the entire property multiplied by a fraction, the numerator of which is the fair market value of the lot and the denominator of which is the fair market value of the entire property. The cost of common improvements is also allocated among the individual lots. A developer who sells subdivided lots before development work is completed may include, with IRS consent, an allocation of the estimated future cost for common improvements in the basis of the lots sold (Rev. Proc. 92-29).[27] There is a special rule relating to the recognition of capital gain on the sale of subdivided lots (¶ 1762).

1623. Allocation of Basis—Bargain Sale to Charity. If a charitable deduction is available (¶ 1062), the basis of property sold to charity for less than its fair market must be allocated between the portion of the property "sold" and the portion "given" to charity, based on the fair market value of each portion. Thus, the seller-donor realizes some taxable gain even if the selling price did not exceed the seller-donor's cost or other basis for the entire property (Code Sec. 1011(b); Reg. § 1.1011-2).[28] The adjusted basis of the portion of property sold to a charity is computed as:

References are to Standard Federal Tax Reports; Tax Research Consultant; and Practical Tax Explanations.

[25] ¶ 16,281, ¶ 30,060, ¶ 30,061; SALES: 33,052; § 18,401

[26] ¶ 5605, ¶ 11,012; SALES: 6,202.05; § 16,115

[27] ¶ 29,313.576; SALES: 6,216; § 38,430.10

[28] ¶ 29,310, ¶ 29,312; INDIV: 51,300, INDIV: 51,302; § 7,530

$$\frac{\text{Amount realized (fair market value of part sold)}}{\text{Fair market value of entire property}} \times \frac{\text{Adjusted basis of entire property}}{}$$

1626. Basis of Residential or Converted Property. Where property has been continually occupied by the taxpayer as a residence since its acquisition, no adjustment of the basis is made for depreciation because none is allowable. The cost of permanent improvements to the property is added to the basis, as are special assessments paid for local benefits that improve the property (¶ 1611). Recoveries against a builder for defective construction reduce the basis.[29]

If residential property is converted to rental property, an adjustment should be made for depreciation from the date of the conversion. Thus, the basis for gain in the case of rented residential property is the taxpayer's cost or other statutory basis, less depreciation allowable while the property was rented or held for rental.

The basis for loss may not exceed the value at the time the residence was converted to rental use, taking into account subsequent basis adjustments, including reduction for allowable depreciation. This is only a limitation; if a smaller loss results from the use of the adjusted cost basis, it must be used (Reg. § 1.165-9(b)).[30] The value of the property upon conversion to rental use has no effect on the basis for gain. If converted property is sold for a price that is greater than the basis for loss but less than the basis for gain, there is no gain or loss.

If rental property is converted to a personal residence, adjustments to basis for depreciation end on the date of the conversion. Any gain on the sale of the property will be recognized (subject to the exclusion rules at ¶ 1705) and may be subject to depreciation recapture (¶ 1779). Loss will not be recognized.

Property Acquired by Gift or Bequest

1630. Basis of Property Acquired by Gift. For property acquired by gift, the basis to the donee is generally the same as it would be in the hands of the donor or the last preceding owner by whom it was not acquired by gift (Code Sec. 1015(a); Reg. § 1.1015-1).[31] However, the basis for loss is the adjusted basis of the property prior to the date of the gift (¶ 1611—¶ 1617) or the fair market value of the property at the time of the gift, whichever is lower. In some cases, there is neither gain nor loss on the sale of property received by gift because the selling price is less than the basis for gain and more than the basis for loss.

If a gift was made on or after September 1, 1958, and before 1977, the basis of the property is increased by the amount of the gift tax paid (¶ 2903), but not above the fair market value of the property at the time of the gift. As to gifts made before September 2, 1958, and held by the donee on that date, the basis is also increased by the amount of the gift tax, but not by more than any excess of the fair market value of the property at the time of the gift over the basis of the property in the hands of the donor at the time of the gift (Code Sec. 1015(d); Reg. § 1.1015-1).[32]

In the case of a gift made after 1976 on which the gift tax is paid, the basis of the property is increased by the amount of gift tax attributable to the net appreciation in value of the gift. The net appreciation for this purpose is the amount by which the fair market value of the gift exceeds the donor's adjusted basis immediately before the gift (Code Sec. 1015(d)(6)).[33]

Zero basis generally applies to a life estate acquired by gift (¶ 1633).

References are to Standard Federal Tax Reports; Tax Research Consultant; and Practical Tax Explanations.

[29] ¶ 29,412.9968; SALES: 6,356.10; § 16,110.10

[30] ¶ 10,102; REAL: 15,054; § 16,930

[31] ¶ 29,390, ¶ 29,391; SALES: 6,102; § 16,205

[32] ¶ 29,390, ¶ 29,391; SALES: 6,104.10; § 16,210.05, § 28,605.25

[33] ¶ 29,390; SALES: 6,104.05; § 16,210.15

1633. Basis of Property Acquired from a Decedent. The basis of any real or personal property acquired from a decedent is generally its fair market value on the date of the decedent's death or on the alternate valuation or special use valuation date (¶ 2922) (Code Sec. 1014).[34] If there is no federal estate tax liability, the basis of the property is its fair market value as of the date of the decedent's death for the purpose of state inheritance or transmission taxes (Reg. § 1.1014-3(a); Rev. Rul. 54-97).[35] Fair market value is presumptive, and may be rebutted by clear and convincing evidence. There are certain exceptions to the basis of property acquired from a decedent equaling fair market value (¶ 1636 and ¶ 1639), including property subject to a qualified conservation easement and income in respect of the decedent (¶ 182) (Code Sec. 1014(a)(4) and (c)).[36]

Decedents Dying in 2010. Effective for decedents dying in 2010, the executor of the decedent's estate had the option to elect out of the federal estate tax. If the election was made, a modified carryover basis rule applied to property acquired from the decedent. Specifically, the property recipient received a basis equal to the lesser of the property's adjusted basis in the hands of the decedent or its fair market value on the date of the decedent's death. Executors had the option to elect to increase the basis of estate property by up to $1.3 million (plus an increase for certain carryovers and unrealized losses of the decedent), with an additional basis increase of up to $3 million in the case of property passing to a surviving spouse. However, the basis of any property could not be increased above its fair market value in the decedent's hands on the date of the decedent's death (former Code Sec. 1022).[37] The IRS provided optional safe harbor procedures for determining modified carryover basis (Rev. Proc. 2011-41).[38]

Term Interests. In most instances, a zero basis is assigned to a life estate that was acquired by gift or bequest and sold or disposed of after October 9, 1969. Interests covered by this exception to the usual rules are: (1) life interests in property; (2) interests for a term of years in property; and (3) income interests in trusts. The zero basis requirement does not apply where the life tenant and remainderman sell their interests simultaneously so that the entire ownership of the property is transferred to another person or group of persons (Code Sec. 1001(e); Reg. §§ 1.1001-1 and 1.1014-5(b)).[39]

1634. Basis in Property Held in Joint Tenancy. A decedent's interest in property held in a joint tenancy (with a right of survivorship) or as tenants by the entirety that passes to the other owner by operation of law is considered property acquired from a decedent (Code Sec. 1014(b)(9); Reg. §§ 1.1014-2(b) and 1.1014-6(a)(1)).[40] Thus, the basis of the property in the hands of the survivor will generally depend upon the amount contributed by each joint tenant toward the original purchase price and, in the case of depreciable property, the manner in which income is divided under local (state) law.

> **Example 1:** Tom Smith and Susan Jones (unmarried) purchased a townhouse for $100,000, which they held as joint tenants with right of survivorship. Tom contributed $30,000 and Susan $70,000. Susan died when the property was worth $200,000; 70 percent of the fair market value ($140,000) is included in her estate. Tom's basis in the property is $170,000 ($30,000 + $140,000).

> **Example 2:** Assume that Tom and Susan held the townhouse as a rental property and that $25,000 of depreciation was allowed prior to Susan's death. If Tom and Susan are entitled to one-half of the income from the property under local law, Tom's basis would be reduced by $12,500 to $157,500 ($170,000 – $12,500).

For purposes of the federal estate tax, the entire value of jointly held property with the right of survivorship is included in a decedent's gross estate except for the portion of the property for which the surviving joint tenant furnished consideration (¶ 2919). If the

---

References are to Standard Federal Tax Reports; Tax Research Consultant; and Practical Tax Explanations.

[34] ¶ 29,370; ESTGIFT: 54,000; § 16,305.05

[35] ¶ 29,373, ¶ 29,380.38; ESTGIFT: 54,058.05; § 16,305.15

[36] ¶ 29,370; ESTGIFT: 54,102, ESTGIFT: 15,758; § 16,305.40, § 32,930

[37] ¶ 29,496; ESTGIFT: 51,060.10; § 16,310

[38] ¶ 29,498.10; ESTGIFT: 51,060.10; § 16,310

[39] ¶ 29,220, ¶ 29,221, ¶ 29,375; ESTGIFT: 54,056; § 2,115.30

[40] ¶ 29,370, ¶ 29,372, ¶ 29,376; ESTGIFT: 54,206; § 16,305.20

joint tenants are spouses, then it is a qualified joint interest and it does not matter who furnished the consideration for the property—one-half of the value is included in the gross estate of the first spouse to die. The surviving spouse's basis in the remaining portion of the qualified joint interest is one-half of the original cost (regardless of the amount that the survivor actually contributed) reduced by any depreciation deductions allocable to the surviving spouse (IRS Pub. 559).

> **Example 3:** Assume the same facts as in Example 1, except that Tom and Susan are married. Tom's basis in the property is $150,000 ($50,000 (one-half of original cost) + $100,000 (one-half of fair market value included in Susan's estate).

1636. Carryover Basis Elections. Executors and administrators of estates of decedents dying after 1976 and before November 7, 1978, could elect to determine the basis under the otherwise repealed carryover basis rules.[41] The time for elections expired July 31, 1980, but valid elections will continue to affect computation of gain on dispositions of property to which such elections apply.

1639. Appreciated Property Reacquired by Donor from Decedent. For property acquired from a decedent who dies after December 31, 1981, the basis of the property when reacquired by the donor following the decedent's death is equal to the decedent's adjusted basis in the property immediately before the decedent's death if: (1) appreciated property was acquired by the decedent after August 13, 1981, as a gift; (2) the decedent received the gift within one year before his death; and (3) following the decedent's death, the donor of the gift, or the donor's spouse, reacquires the property (Code Sec. 1014(e)).[42]

Property Acquired by Exchange

1648. Basis of Property Transferred to Corporation in a Taxable Exchange. When a corporation acquires property for its stock in an exchange taxable to the transferor, its basis for the property is the fair market value of the stock on the date of the exchange. If the stock has no established market value at that time, it may be considered to be the equivalent of the fair market value of the property received.[43]

1651. Basis of Property Acquired in a Tax-Free Exchange. If property is acquired in an exchange on which no gain or loss is recognized, the basis of the property is the same as that for the property exchanged (Code Sec. 1031(d); Reg. § 1.1031(d)-1).[44] Substitute basis (¶ 1607) applies to:

- like-kind exchange of property held for productive use or investment (¶ 1721);

- exchange of stock for stock of the same corporation (¶ 1728);

- exchange of property solely for stock or securities of a "controlled" corporation (¶ 1731); and

- exchange of stock or securities solely for stock or securities in a reorganization (¶ 2229).

Trade-in arrangements under which a taxpayer sells old equipment used in a trade or business to a dealer and purchases new equipment of like kind from the dealer are like-kind exchanges qualifying for nonrecognition treatment if the sale of the old equipment and the purchase of the new equipment are mutually dependent transactions, even if they are not simultaneous. The basis of the new equipment, for gain or loss or depreciation, is ordinarily the total of the adjusted basis of the trade-in plus whatever additional cash is needed. In effect, the basis of the new property is its purchase price, increased or decreased according to whether the trade-in value of the old equipment is greater or less than its depreciated cost. Special depreciation rules may apply to like-kind exchanges (¶ 1250).

References are to Standard Federal Tax Reports; Tax Research Consultant; and Practical Tax Explanations.

[41] ¶ 44,438.70; ESTGIFT: 54,060; § 16,101

[42] ¶ 29,370; ESTGIFT: 54,104; § 16,305.35

[43] ¶ 29,225.272; SALES: 6,060, SALES: 6,068; § 16,105.15

[44] ¶ 29,602, ¶ 29,612; SALES: 6,250; § 18,040

1657. Basis of Boot Acquired in an Otherwise Tax-Free Exchange. In a like-kind exchange, a taxpayer may receive money or other property (commonly referred to as boot) that is not of a like-kind (¶ 1723). The taxpayer recognizes gain from the transaction to the extent of the boot's fair market value. In such exchanges, the cost or other applicable basis of the property acquired is the same as that of the property exchanged, decreased by the amount of any money received by the taxpayer in the transaction and increased by the amount of gain or decreased by the amount of loss recognized in the exchange. If boot is received in an exchange that is tax free in part, the cost or other basis of the property disposed of must be allocated between the property received tax free and such "other property," assigning to the "other property" an amount equivalent to its fair market value (Code Sec. 1031(d)).[45]

1660. Basis of Property Transferred to a Corporation. The basis of property acquired by a corporation from a shareholder in exchange for stock in a Code Sec. 351 transaction in which the shareholder controls the corporation immediately after the exchange (¶ 203), as well as the basis of property from a shareholder as paid-in surplus or as a contribution to capital, is the same to the corporation as it was in the hands of the shareholder, increased by the amount of gain recognized by the shareholder on the transfer (Code Sec. 362(a); Reg. § 1.362-1).[46] If property is acquired by a corporation in a reorganization, the basis of the transferor (increased by any recognized gain) generally also follows through to the transferee corporation. However, carryover basis will not apply if the property acquired by the corporation consists of stock or securities in another corporation that is a party to the reorganization unless the stock or securities were acquired as consideration for the transfer (Code Sec. 362(b)). Rules for property acquired subject to a built-in loss (¶ 1667) and for property acquired upon liquidation of a subsidiary may apply (¶ 2261).

Property contributed to a corporation by nonstockholders on or after June 22, 1954, has a zero basis. Money contributed by an outsider on or after that date reduces the basis of corporate property acquired with it within 12 months after the contribution is received. To the extent that the contribution is not used to acquire property within this 12-month period, it reduces, as of the last day of the period, the basis of any other property held by the company (Code Sec. 362(c)).

1667. Limitations on Built-In Losses. If a corporation receives property in an exchange with an owner who is *not* subject to U.S. tax, and the property's fair market value is less than the transferee's adjusted basis of all property received in the exchange (i.e., there is a built-in loss), the corporate transferee's basis in the property received is its fair market value immediately after the transfer (Code Sec. 362(e)).[47] Thus, the foreign loss is not recognized for U.S. tax purposes. This treatment applies to property acquired by the corporation from a shareholder in exchange for stock in a Code Sec. 351 transaction in which the shareholder controls the corporation immediately after the exchange (¶ 203), as well as the basis of property from a shareholder as paid-in surplus or as a contribution to capital (¶ 1660).

Similarly, if a corporation acquires property in a section 351 exchange with an owner who *is* subject to U.S. tax, and the transferred property's adjusted basis exceeds its fair market value, the corporate transferee's basis in the property is generally limited to its fair market value immediately after the transaction. Any required basis reduction is allocated among the transferred properties in proportion to their built-in losses immediately before the transaction. For this type of exchange, the transferor owner and transferee controlled corporation can make an irrevocable election to limit the owner's basis in the stock received—rather than the corporation's basis in the property—to the aggregate fair market value of the transferred property (Reg. § 1.362-4(d)).[48]

References are to Standard Federal Tax Reports; Tax Research Consultant; and Practical Tax Explanations.

[45] ¶ 29,602; SALES: 6,252; § 18,040

[46] ¶ 16,610, ¶ 16,611; CCORP: 3,204, CCORP: 39,302; § 26,135

[47] ¶ 16,610; CCORP: 39,304.10; § 26,135

[48] ¶ 16,611CE; CCORP: 39,304.10; § 26,135

1669. Assumption of Liabilities. The assumption of liabilities by a shareholder in a Code Sec. 351 exchange with a controlled corporation (¶ 203) or in a reorganization (¶ 2229) is not treated as the equivalent of cash (¶ 2233). In a determination of basis after such transfers, the corporation whose liabilities were assumed (or whose property was taken subject to the liabilities) will treat the assumption or acquisition as money received, to the extent of the liabilities (Code Secs. 358(d) and 1031(d)).[49] This rule applies only to the corporation whose liabilities are assumed. It has no effect on the corporation that assumes the debts.

1672. Discharge of Debt. Under some conditions, a taxpayer realizes no income from a discharge of debt (¶ 855). Any amount of debt discharged and excluded from gross income reduces the basis of the property securing the debt (Code Sec. 1017).[50] Regulations prescribe the sequence of allocation where the debt is, or must be treated as, a general liability (Reg. § § 1.108-4 and 1.1017-1).[51]

Other Acquired Property

1678. Basis of Property Transferred in Trust. If property is acquired by a transfer in trust, other than by a transfer in trust by gift, bequest, or devise—for example, sale to the trust by the grantor—after December 31, 1920, its basis is the same as it would be in the hands of the trust's grantor, increased by the gain, or decreased by the loss, recognized to the grantor under the law in effect as of the date of such transfer (Code Sec. 1015(b)).[52] When an existing charitable remainder trust is split pro rata into separate trusts, one for each beneficiary, the original trust's basis in the assets is split pro rata among the new trusts (Rev. Rul. 2008-41).

1681. Basis of Stock or Other Property Received for Services. If stock or other property is given to an employee as compensation for personal services instead of cash, the fair market value of the property is income to the employee unless the property is subject to a substantial risk of forfeiture (¶ 713). The fair market value of the property included in income becomes its basis to the employee (Code Sec. 83; Reg. § 1.83-4(b)).[53] If the property is sold to the employee for less than its market value, the difference between the amount paid and the value of the property is also income. In this case, the employee's basis for the property is the cash cost, plus the amount reported as income.

A taxpayer who receives property subject to a substantial risk of forfeiture may make a Code Sec. 83(b) election to include the fair market value of the property (less any amount paid for the property) in income in the year that the property is received (¶ 713). The basis for determining gain or loss when the property is sold is the amount included in income in the election year, plus the amount paid for the property (Reg. § 1.83-2(a)).[54]

Corporations may grant their employees the option to purchase stock in the corporation (¶ 1923—¶ 1931). For purposes of determining an individual's basis in property transferred in connection with the performance of services, rules similar to the annuity basis rules under Code Sec. 72(w) apply (Code Sec. 83(c)(4)) (¶ 821).

1682. Basis of Stock Received in Nontaxable Distributions. If a shareholder in a corporation receives stock or stock rights in a nontaxable distribution (¶ 733A), the basis of the old stock is allocated between the old stock and new stock in proportion to the fair market value of each on the date of the distribution (not the record date) (Code Sec. 307; Reg. § 1.307-1).[55] If only part of the stock dividend is nontaxable, the basis of the old stock is allocated between the old stock and the part of the new stock that is not taxable.

References are to Standard Federal Tax Reports; Tax Research Consultant; and Practical Tax Explanations.

[49] ¶ 16,550, ¶ 29,602; SALES: 27,300, CCORP: 39,256.05; § 26,130

[50] ¶ 29,430; SALES: 6,368; § 3,420.15

[51] ¶ 7003E, ¶ 29,431; SALES: 6,368.10; § 3,420.10

[52] ¶ 29,390; SALES: 6,110; § 16,205

[53] ¶ 6380, ¶ 6384; SALES: 6,062; § 21,430.05

[54] ¶ 6382; COMPEN: 18,302; § 21,475.05

[55] ¶ 15,500, ¶ 15,501; SALES: 6,302.10; § 26,235.10

This rule applies with respect to stock rights only if such rights are exercised or sold. If exercised, the basis of the stock rights is added to the cost of the stock acquired. If sold, the basis allocable to the stock rights is used to determine the taxpayer's gain or loss. If the stock rights are allowed to expire, the basis of the shares with respect to which the rights were distributed remains intact.

If the fair market value of the stock rights on the date of distribution is less than 15 percent of the fair market value of the stock with respect to which the distribution is made, the basis of the stock rights is deemed to be zero unless the taxpayer elects to make a basis allocation (Code Sec. 307(b); Reg. § 1.307-2).[56] The election must be made in a statement attached to the shareholder's return for the year in which the rights are received. It is irrevocable with respect to the rights for which it is made. The election must be made for all the rights received in a particular distribution by the shareholder on stock of the same class received by the shareholder at the time of the distribution.

> **Example:** Bob bought 100 shares of Yeta Company common stock at $125 per share and later received 100 rights entitling him to purchase 20 shares of new common stock in Yeta Company at $100 per share. When the rights were distributed, the old shares had a fair market value of $120 per share, and the rights had a fair market value of $3 each. Three weeks later, Bob sold his rights for $4 each. He elects to apportion basis.

Cost of old stock on which rights were distributed	$12,500.00
Market value of old stock at date of distribution of rights .	12,000.00
Market value of rights at date of distribution	300.00
Cost apportioned to old stock after distribution of rights (12,000/12,300 of $12,500)	12,195.12
Cost apportioned to rights (300/12,300 of $12,500)	304.88
Selling price of rights	400.00
Gain ($400 – $304.88)	$95.12

In determining gain or loss from any later sale of the stock on which the rights were distributed, the adjusted cost of the old stock is $12,195.12, or $121.95 a share.

The holding period of nontaxable stock rights includes the holding period of the stock on which the rights are distributed. The holding period of the stock acquired by the exercise of the rights begins on the date that the rights are exercised (Code Sec. 1223(4) and (5); Reg. § 1.1223-1(e) and (f)).[57]

1684. Basis of Equipment for Which Medical Deduction Claimed. The basis of equipment whose cost qualifies as a medical expense (¶ 1016) does not include that portion of its cost that has been claimed as an itemized deduction because such amounts are not properly capitalized. However, the equipment's basis includes that portion of the cost that is nondeductible because of the 10-percent of adjusted gross income (AGI) floor (7.5-percent of AGI floor if the taxpayer or his or her spouse has attained age 65 in tax years after 2012 and before 2017; 7.5-percent of AGI floor for all taxpayers in tax years before 2013) (¶ 1015).

To determine this portion, the total amount of the AGI limitation is multiplied by a fraction whose numerator is the cost of the equipment and whose denominator is the total amount of the taxpayer's medical expenses. Similarly, if a taxpayer's total allowable itemized deductions exceed the taxpayer's AGI, or are limited by the overall limitation on itemized deductions of high-income taxpayers (¶ 1014), that portion of the equipment's cost attributable to the nondeductible expenses may also be included in the equipment's basis (Reg. § 1.1016-2).[58]

References are to Standard Federal Tax Reports; Tax Research Consultant; and Practical Tax Explanations.

[56] ¶ 15,500, ¶ 15,501B; SALES: 6,302.15; § 26,235.10

[57] ¶ 30,460, ¶ 30,461; SALES: 15,162.30; § 16,540.05

[58] ¶ 29,413; SALES: 6,360.10; § 7,285.10

¶1684

1687. Basis of Property Acquired Through Involuntary Conversion. The basis of property purchased as the result of an involuntary conversion (¶ 1713) on which gain is not recognized is the cost of the replacement property less the amount of gain not recognized on the conversion. If qualifying replacement property is received as the result of an involuntary conversion, the replacement property's basis is the same as the basis of the involuntarily converted property decreased by any loss recognized on the conversion and any money received and not spent on qualifying replacement property. The basis is increased by any gain recognized on the conversion and any cost of acquiring the replacement property (Code Sec. 1033(b); Reg. § 1.1033(b)-1).[59] Special depreciation rules may apply (¶ 1250).

1693. Basis of Property Transferred Between Spouses. No gain or loss is recognized on a transfer of property from an individual to, or in trust for the benefit of, a spouse or a former spouse if the transfer to the former spouse is incident to the divorce of the parties (¶ 1734). In such case, the basis of the transferred property in the hands of the transferee is the transferor's adjusted basis in the property. The carryover basis rule does not apply to a spouse (or former spouse) who is a nonresident alien (Code Sec. 1041(d)). Nonrecognition of gain is not permitted with respect to the transfer of property in trust to the extent that the sum of the amount of any liabilities assumed, plus the amount of any liabilities to which the property is subject, exceeds the total of the adjusted basis of the property transferred (Code Sec. 1041(e)).[60] The transferee's basis is adjusted to take into account any gain recognized.

Valuation Rules

1695. Indeterminate Fair Market Value. Only in rare and extraordinary cases does property have no determinable fair market value (Reg. § 1.1001-1).[61] If the fair market value of an asset received in an exchange (such as a contract to receive royalties) cannot be determined with fair certainty, gain is not realized on the exchange until after the total payments received under the contract exceed the cost (or other basis) of the property surrendered in exchange.[62] The Tax Court has applied the *Cohan* rule (estimated or approximate value) to estimate the value of patents, patent applications, and stock rights, where the taxpayer could not prove their exact value.[63]

1697. Valuation of Securities and Real Estate. The fair market value of securities traded on the open market, or on a recognized exchange, is ordinarily the average of the high and low quoted prices on the valuation date. If only a minimal number of shares are traded on the valuation date, or if other abnormal market conditions exist, an alternative valuation method may be necessary.[64]

When corporate stock is not sold on the open market, its fair market value depends upon many factors, including the nature and history of the business, economic outlook and condition of the industry, book value of stock and financial condition of the business, earning capacity of the company, dividend-paying capacity, goodwill, prior sales, size of the block to be valued, and market price of similar but listed stock.[65] Isolated sales of small portions of the stock or forced sales are not considered evidence of fair market value.[66]

Restrictive sales agreements must be considered in the valuation of stock. If the stock is subject to a repurchase option, its value may not exceed the amount for which it may be repurchased. If there are restrictions making sale of stock impossible, and its value is highly speculative, it does not have a fair market value.[67]

References are to Standard Federal Tax Reports; Tax Research Consultant; and Practical Tax Explanations.

[59] ¶ 29,640, ¶ 29,644; SALES: 6,254; § 18,145.05

[60] ¶ 29,800; SALES: 6,262; § 18,230

[61] ¶ 29,221; VALUE: 1,000; § 16,405

[62] ¶ 29,225.153; ACCTNG: 6,114; § 16,405

[63] ¶ 8520.586, ¶ 16,612.175; SALES: 6052; § 26,410.15

[64] ¶ 29,225.187, ¶ 29,225.242; VALUE: 3,100; § 34,110.20

[65] ¶ 29,225.228; VALUE: 9,050; § 34,110.20

[66] ¶ 29,225.234; VALUE: 9,062.05; § 34,110.20

[67] ¶ 29,225.2563; VALUE: 9,200; § 34,110.20

There are three principal methods used in determining the fair market value of real property:[68]

(1) the comparable sales method, which involves gathering information on sales of property similar to the subject property and then making adjustments (both positive and negative) for various differences between the *comparables* and the property being appraised;

(2) the capitalization of income method, which estimates a property's fair market value based upon future benefits (cash-flow) to be derived from the ownership of the property; and

(3) the replacement cost method, which is based on the principle of substitution and estimates the fair market value of real property based on the assumption that a prudent person (in other words, a willing buyer) would not pay more for a property than it would cost to acquire a similar site and erect a comparable structure (less accrued depreciation).

Other factors that may be appropriate to consider with regard to a fair market value determination of real property include:

(1) the development potential of the property with regard to its highest and best potential and realistic use;

(2) the possibility of zoning changes that may either enhance or diminish the marketability of the property;

(3) the taxpayer's ability to acquire adjacent parcels of property allowing for expanded and, in many cases, enhanced uses;

(4) leases, debt, and other encumbrances on the property; and

(5) environmental concerns, restrictions, and hazards.

Appraisal affidavits of a retrospective nature, standing alone, are generally not accorded great weight.[69]

References are to Standard Federal Tax Reports; Tax Research Consultant; and Practical Tax Explanations.

[68] ¶ 11,660.555; VALUE: 15,100

[69] ¶ 29,225.1055; VALUE: 1,104; § 7,600.25

16 | BASIS

Chapter 17

SALES AND EXCHANGES

CAPITAL GAINS

Sales and Exchanges of Property

1701. Gain or Loss from Sale or Exchange of Property. Gain or loss from the sale or exchange of property generally must be recognized for income tax purposes (Code Sec. 1001(c)).[1] A taxpayer has gain if the amount realized from the sale or exchange is more than the taxpayer's adjusted basis in the property. A taxpayer has a loss when the adjusted basis of the property is more than the amount realized from the sale or exchange (Code Sec. 1001(a)).[2] However, not all gains and losses have to be recognized for income tax purposes.

In order to determine the tax consequences of a sale or exchange, the following questions must be answered:

(1) What is the amount realized in the transaction (¶ 1703)?

(2) What is the taxpayer's adjusted basis in the property (¶ 1601—¶ 1697)?

(3) Is the gain or loss on the transaction recognized (¶ 1719—¶ 1734)?

(4) Do the capital gain and loss provisions apply (¶ 1735—¶ 1744)?

(5) Is any part of the gain attributable to depreciation recapture (¶ 1779)?

Installment Payments. When real or personal property is sold by a nondealer and part or all of the selling price is to be paid after the year of sale, the recognized gain from the sale must be reported on the installment method, unless the taxpayer elects otherwise (¶ 1801).

Rollover into SSBIC Stock. Individuals and C corporations may elect to defer the recognition of capital gain from the sale of publicly traded securities if the sale proceeds are invested in the stock of or a partnership interest in a specialized small business investment company (SSBIC). These rollovers are subject to cumulative limits (¶ 1909).

Gain from Small Business Stock. Noncorporate taxpayers may generally exclude from gross income a percentage of any gain from the sale or exchange of qualified small

---

References are to Standard Federal Tax Reports; Tax Research Consultant; and Practical Tax Explanations.

[1] ¶ 29,220; SALES: 9,050; § 16,005, § 16,010

[2] ¶ 29,220; SALES: 9,052; § 16,015

¶1701

business stock held for more than five years and issued after August 10, 1993 (¶ 1905). The excluded gain is given special treatment for alternative minimum tax (AMT) preference purposes (¶ 1425). A noncorporate taxpayer may also elect to roll over the realized gain from the sale of qualified small business stock held for more than six months if other small business stock is purchased during the 60-day period beginning on the date of sale (¶ 1907).

Virtual Currency. Convertible virtual currency (e.g., Bitcoin) that has an equivalent value in or acts as a substitute for real currency is treated as property for federal tax purposes (¶ 785) (Notice 2014-21).[3] Thus, the sale or exchange of virtual currency results in gain or loss. The character of the gain or loss generally depends on whether the virtual currency is a capital asset in the hands of the taxpayer. The basis of virtual currency that a taxpayer "mines" or receives as payment for goods or services is the fair market value of the virtual currency in U.S. dollars as of the date of receipt.

Insurance Company Demutualization. A mutual insurance company is demutualized when it converts into a stock company and issues cash and/or shares to its policyholders in exchange for their equity interests. The IRS has held that a policyholder has zero basis in the surrendered equity interest (Rev. Rul. 71-233), but some courts have disagreed, and instead treated sales proceeds of demutualized stock as a return of capital.[4]

1703. Amount Realized. The amount realized on a sale or exchange of property is the total of monies received plus the fair market value of all other property or services received (Code Sec. 1001(b); *International Freighting Corp., Inc.,* CA-2, 43-1 USTC ¶ 9334).[5] Property with no readily determinable fair market value is generally treated as equal in value to the property for which it was exchanged (*Philadelphia Park Amusement Co.,* CtCls, 54-2 USTC ¶ 9697).[6] Part of the basis in a larger property generally must be allocated to any portion of that property that is disposed of. However, if basis or fair market value cannot be ascertained or apportioned, the open-transaction doctrine may defer recognition of any gain until the taxpayer's basis in the larger property has been recovered (*E.A. Fisher,* FedCl, 2008-2 USTC ¶ 50,481, aff'd, per curiam, CA-FC, 2010-1 USTC ¶ 50,289).[7] Generally, the amount realized includes any liabilities from which the seller is relieved as a result of the sale or exchange (Reg. § 1.1001-2).[8]

The amount realized on the receipt of an annuity in exchange for property is the fair market value of the annuity contract at the time of the exchange. The entire gain or loss is recognized at the time of the exchange, regardless of the taxpayer's method of accounting (Prop. Reg. § 1.1001-1(j)).[9]

A taxpayer who makes a gift of property on condition that the donee pay the resulting gift taxes realizes gain to the extent that the gift taxes paid by the donee exceed the donor's basis in the property (*V.P. Diedrich,* SCt, 82-1 USTC ¶ 9419).[10]

Gain or Loss from Sale of Residence

1705. Exclusion of Gain from Sale of Principal Residence. An individual may exclude from gross income up to $250,000 of gain ($500,000 if married filing a joint return or surviving spouse) realized on the sale or exchange of a principal residence (Code Sec. 121).[11] The individual must meet an ownership test and a use test for at least two years during the five years preceding the sale or exchange (¶ 1707). An individual cannot use the exclusion more frequently than once every two years. A partial or reduced exclusion may be available even if a taxpayer does not meet the ownership and use requirements, or has used the exclusion within the previous two years (¶ 1709).

References are to Standard Federal Tax Reports; Tax Research Consultant; and Practical Tax Explanations.

[3] ¶ 29,225.1038; SALES: 45,600; § 19,601

[4] ¶ 29,225.1726, ¶ 31,829.13; SALES: 9,104.10, VALUE: 1,108; INDIV: 30,100, CCORP: 6,054; § 16,105.15

[5] ¶ 29,220, ¶ 29,225.1013; SALES: 9,100; § 16,401

[6] ¶ 29,225.1523; SALES: 9,104.10; § 16,405

[7] ¶ 5700.225; SALES: 36,404; § 16,105.15

[8] ¶ 29,223; SALES: 9,108; § 16,410

[9] ¶ 29,221D; SALES: 9,106; § 3,245.10

[10] ¶ 29,226.3062; SALES: 3,056.10; § 32,830.30

[11] ¶ 7260; REAL: 15,152; § 1,601

Married Individuals. The maximum amount of gain that may be excluded is $500,000 for married individuals filing jointly in the tax year of the sale or exchange if:

(1) either spouse meets the ownership test with respect to the property,

(2) both spouses meet the use test with respect to the property, and

(3) neither spouse is ineligible for exclusion by virtue of a sale or exchange of a residence within the prior two years (Code Sec. 121(b)(2); Reg. § 1.121-2).[12]

A married couple's exclusion is determined on an individual basis. For instance, if Spouse A is eligible for the exclusion, but Spouse B used the exclusion within the previous two years, Spouse A is entitled to a maximum exclusion of $250,000. Once both spouses satisfy the eligibility rules and two years have passed since either of them used the exclusion, they may exclude up to $500,000 of gain on their joint return.

Surviving Spouse. A surviving spouse may use the full $500,000 exclusion if the sale occurs within two years after the other spouse's death and requirements (1)–(3) listed above are met immediately before the date of death (Code Sec. 121(b)(4); Reg. § 1.121-4(a)).[13] For this purpose, a surviving spouse is considered as owning and living in the home for the same period as the deceased spouse, so long as the surviving spouse does not remarry before the sale (Code Sec. 121(d)(2)).

> **Example 1:** Erik purchases and begins living in his home in 2000. On July 10, 2013, he marries Helen and they both live in Erik's home. Erik dies on March 3, 2014, and Helen inherits the home. On June 1, 2014, Helen, who has not remarried, sells the home. Helen satisfies the ownership and use tests because she can include the time that Erik owned and used the home.

Gain Allocable to Nonqualified Use. Gain that is allocable to periods of nonqualified use may not be excluded from gross income (Code Sec. 121(b)(4)[(5)]).[14] Nonqualified use is generally any use other than as a principal residence; thus, this rule significantly limits the exclusion for second homes and vacation homes. However, a period of nonqualified use does not include: (1) any period before January 1, 2009; (2) any portion of the five-year period ending on the date the property is sold that is after the last date the property is used as the principal residence; (3) any period of 10 years or less when the taxpayer or the taxpayer's spouse is serving on qualified official extended duty as a member of the U.S. uniformed services or U.S. Foreign Service, or an employee of the intelligence community; or (4) any period of two years or less for temporary absence due to a change of employment, health conditions, or other unforeseen circumstances.

> **Example 2:** On January 1, 2014, Eleanor buys a residence for $400,000 and uses it as rental property for two years, claiming $20,000 of depreciation deductions. On January 1, 2016, she converts the property to her principal residence. She moves out on January 13, 2018, and sells the property for $700,000 on January 1, 2019. The portion of the gain attributable to the depreciation deductions ($20,000) is included in income (see "*Gain Recognized to Extent of Depreciation*," below). Of the remaining $300,000 gain, 40 percent (two years divided by five years), or $120,000, is allocated to the nonqualified use and is not eligible for the exclusion. The period from January 14, 2018, to January 1, 2019, is after she last used it as her primary residence, so it is not a period of nonqualified use. Thus, the remaining gain of $180,000 is excluded from Eleanor's gross income.

Like-Kind Exchanges. A taxpayer may qualify for both the exclusion of gain from the sale or exchange of a principal residence and nonrecognition of gain from a like-kind exchange (¶ 1721). If the residence was acquired in a like-kind exchange, the exclusion does not apply if the individual (or any person whose basis in the property is derived from the individual's basis) sells or exchanges the residence during the five-year period that begins on the date the residence was acquired (Code Sec. 121(d)(10)).[15]

References are to Standard Federal Tax Reports; Tax Research Consultant; and Practical Tax Explanations.

[12] ¶ 7260, ¶ 7262; REAL: 15,152.10; § 1,615.10

[13] ¶ 7260, ¶ 7264; REAL: 15,152.10; § 1,615.15

[14] ¶ 7260; REAL: 15,152.05; § 1,615.20

[15] ¶ 7260; REAL: 15,160; § 1,640

¶1705

Example 3: Wallace obtains a single family home in a like-kind exchange on September 1, 2009. After renting it out for 18 months, he moves in and uses it as his principal residence, beginning March 1, 2011. If Wallace sells the home before September 1, 2014, the exclusion is not available.

Gain Recognized to Extent of Depreciation. The exclusion of gain on the sale or exchange of a principal residence does not apply to the extent of any depreciation allowable with respect to the rental or business use of the residence after May 6, 1997 (Code Sec. 121(d)(6); Reg. § 1.121-1(d)(1)).[16] This rule applies to the amount of depreciation allowed if the taxpayer can establish that it was less than the amount allowable (Code Sec. 1250(b)(3)).[17]

Remainder Interests. The exclusion applies to gain on the sale or exchange of a remainder interest in a principal residence, provided the buyer is not a member of the taxpayer's family or other related entity as defined by Code Sec. 267(b) or 707(b) (Code Sec. 121(d)(8)).[18] See ¶ 432 and ¶ 1717 for discussion of related persons.

Expatriates. The exclusion is not available to nonresident aliens who relinquish U.S. citizenship or long-term resident status and are subject to the mark-to-market rules for higher-income expatriates (¶ 2412) (Code Sec. 121(e)).[19]

Involuntary Conversions. For purposes of determining excludable gain from the sale of a principal residence, the destruction, theft, seizure, requisition, or condemnation of the property is treated as a sale or exchange (Code Sec. 121(d)(5); Reg. § 1.121-4(d)).[20] In addition, the ownership and use of property acquired in an involuntary conversion generally includes the ownership and use of the property treated as sold or exchanged. For purposes of the involuntary conversions rules (¶ 1713), the amount realized on the conversion is reduced by the excluded gain.

Property Acquired from Decedents. Estates, heirs and revocable trusts established by a decedent generally cannot exclude any gain on the sale of the decedent's principal residence. However, the exclusion can be used if the decedent died in 2010 and the estate elects to have the modified carryover basis rules apply (¶ 1633) (Code Sec. 121(d)(11), prior to repeal by the Tax Relief, Unemployment Insurance Reauthorization, and Job Creation Act of 2010 (P.L. 111-312); Act Sec. 301 of P.L. 111-312).[21]

Reporting Requirements. If all of the gain from the sale of a home is excludable, the sale does not have to be reported on the seller's tax return. If, however, the individual can exclude only some of the gain or receives a Form 1099-S, then the sale or exchange is reported on Form 8949. If the home was sold under the installment method and gain is recognized (¶ 1801), the sale is reported on Form 6252. Sale of the business or rental portion of the property (¶ 1707) may have to be reported on Form 4797.

1707. Ownership and Use Requirements. An individual's gain on the sale or exchange of a principal residence may be excluded from gross income (¶ 1705) if, during the five-year period that ends on the date of the sale or exchange, the individual owned and used the property as a principal residence for periods aggregating two years or more (i.e., a total of 730 days (365 × 2)) (Code Sec. 121(a); Reg. § 1.121-1(c)).[22] The ownership and use tests may be met during nonconcurrent periods, provided that both tests are met during the five-year period that ends on the date of sale. If a taxpayer does not meet the ownership and use requirements, or used the exclusion within the two-year period ending on the sale date, a reduced exclusion may be available (¶ 1709).

The home or dwelling unit does not have to be the taxpayer's principal residence at the time it was purchased or sold. Although a principal residence may include the surrounding land, the exclusion applies only if the house or dwelling unit was actually used as the taxpayer's principal residence for at least two years during the five years preceding the sale (*D.A Gates*, 135 TC 1, Dec. 58,259).[23] Short temporary absences for

---

References are to Standard Federal Tax Reports; Tax Research Consultant; and Practical Tax Explanations.

[16] ¶ 7260, ¶ 7261; DEPR: 18,112; § 1,615.25

[17] ¶ 31,000; DEPR: 18,262.10; § 11,710

[18] ¶ 7260; REAL: 15,152.05; § 1,625.10

[19] ¶ 7260; REAL: 15,152.05; § 1,610.25

[20] ¶ 7260, ¶ 7264; REAL: 15,158; § 1,625.15

[21] ¶ 7260; REAL: 15,150; § 1,610.30

[22] ¶ 7260, ¶ 7261; REAL: 15,156; § 1,610.05

[23] ¶ 7266.72; REAL: 15,156.10; § 1,610.05

¶1707

17
SALES

vacations or seasonal absences are counted as periods of use, even if the taxpayer rents out the property during these periods. However, absence for an entire year is not considered a short temporary absence.

Divorced Individuals. If a residence is transferred to an individual incident to a divorce, the time the individual's spouse or former spouse owned the residence is added to the individual's period of ownership (Code Sec. 121(d)(3); Reg. §1.121-4(b)).[24] An individual who owns a residence is deemed to use it as a principal residence during the time the individual's spouse or former spouse has use of the home under a divorce or separation agreement.

Incapacity. An individual who becomes physically or mentally incapable of self-care is deemed to use a home as a principal residence while the individual owns the residence and resides in a licensed care facility (e.g., a nursing home), as long as the individual owned and used the home as a principal residence for periods totalling at least one year during the five years preceding the sale or exchange (Code Sec. 121(d)(7)).[25]

Relief for Military, Foreign Service, Peace Corps, and Intelligence Personnel. A special exception to the two-out-of-five-year rule applies if the taxpayer or the taxpayer's spouse serves on qualified official extended duty as a member of the U.S. uniformed services or U.S. Foreign Service, or an employee of the intelligence community; or serves outside the United States as a Peace Corps employee on qualified official extended duty or as a Peace Corps enrolled volunteer or volunteer leader (Code Sec. 121(d)(9) and (12); Reg. §1.121-5).[26] In this case, the taxpayer may elect to suspend the five-year test period by not including the gain in gross income on the tax return filed for the year of the sale. The suspension period cannot last more than 10 years, and the election may be made with respect to only one property. The taxpayer may revoke the election at any time.

Qualified official extended duty is any extended duty while serving at a duty station that is at least 50 miles from the individual's principal residence or while residing in government quarters under government orders (Code Sec. 121(d)(9)(C)). Extended duty is any period of active duty due to a call or order for a period in excess of 90 days or for an indefinite time.

Allocation for Partial Use. An individual cannot claim the exclusion for any portion of the gain that is allocable to the portion of the property that is separate from the actual residence (the dwelling unit) and not used as a residence (Reg. §1.121-1(e)).[27] The basis of mixed-use property and the amount realized must be allocated under the same method used to determine the depreciation adjustments. The IRS has provided a number of examples to illustrate the allocation rules in various situations.

If part of the home was used for a business (e.g., home office) or to produce rental income, the individual does not need to allocate the basis of the property and the amount realized from the sale or exchange between the business portion of the home and the residential portion. However, gain must be recognized to the extent of claimed depreciation (¶1705). The rule is different when a separate part of the property was used for business purposes or rental income (e.g., the individual owned an apartment building and lived in one unit and rented out the other units). Generally, if the separate part of the property is used for business or rental purposes in the year of sale, the individual must treat the sale of the property as the sale of two properties: the dwelling unit and the business or rental property.

> **Example:** Bob sold his main home in 2014 at a $30,000 gain. He meets the ownership and use tests to exclude the gain. However, he used part of the home as a business office in 2011 and claimed $500 depreciation. Because the business office was part of his home (not separate from it), he does not have to allocate the basis and amount realized between the business and residential portions of the property. In addition, he does not have to report any part of the gain on Form 4797. Bob reports his gain, exclusion, and taxable gain of $500 on Form 8949.

References are to Standard Federal Tax Reports; Tax Research Consultant; and Practical Tax Explanations.

[24] ¶7260, ¶7264; REAL: 15,152.10; §1,610.10

[25] ¶7260; REAL: 15,156.10; §1,610.15

[26] ¶7260, ¶7265; REAL: 15,156.15; §1,610.20

[27] ¶7261; REAL: 15,156.20; §1,610.35

¶1707

Trusts and Single-Owner Entities. An individual is treated as owning a residence while (i) it is owned by a grantor trust (¶ 571) and the individual is treated as the owner of the trust or the portion of the trust that includes the residence, or (ii) it is owned by the individual's single-member disregarded entity (¶ 402A) (Reg. § 1.121-1(c)(3)).[28]

Co-ops. A taxpayer who owns stock in a cooperative housing corporation as a tenant-stockholder (¶ 1040) may be able to exclude gain on the sale or exchange of the stock if, during the five-year period ending on the date of sale or exchange, the taxpayer owned the stock for at least two years and lived in the house or apartment as a principal residence for at least two years (Code Sec. 121(d)(4); Reg. § 1.121-4(c)).[29]

1709. Reduced Exclusion of Gain from Sale of Principal Residence. A partial or reduced exclusion of gain from the sale or exchange of a principal residence (¶ 1705) may be possible when an individual fails to meet the ownership and use requirements (¶ 1707) or has used the exclusion within two years of the sale. The reduced exclusion is available if, based on the facts and circumstances, the primary reason for the sale of the home is a qualified individual's change in place of employment, health reasons, or unforeseen circumstances (Code Sec. 121(c); Reg. § 1.121-3).[30] A qualified individual for this purpose is the taxpayer, the taxpayer's spouse, a co-owner of the residence, or a person whose principal place of abode is in the same household as the taxpayer.

Change in Place of Employment. The primary reason test is satisfied if the sale or exchange is due to a change in the location of a qualified individual's employment (Reg. § 1.121-3(c)). A safe harbor exists if the qualified individual's new place of employment is at least 50 miles farther from the residence sold or exchanged than was the former place of employment; if there was no former place of employment, the distance between the qualified individual's new place of employment and the residence sold or exchanged must be at least 50 miles. Employment includes beginning a job with a new employer, continuing a job with an existing employer, or beginning or continuing self-employment.

Health Reasons. The primary reason test is satisfied if the reason for the sale or exchange is to obtain, provide, or facilitate the diagnosis, cure, mitigation, or treatment of disease, illness, or injury of a qualified individual; or to obtain or provide medical or personal care for a qualified individual suffering from a disease, illness, or injury (Reg. § 1.121-3(d)). A qualified individual includes a qualified individual's child, sibling, parent, niece, nephew, or in-law, as well as a descendant of the taxpayer's grandparent. A sale or exchange that is merely beneficial to the individual's general health does not qualify. A safe harbor exists if a physician recommends a change of homes for health reasons (Reg. § 1.121-3(f)).

Unforeseen Circumstances. The primary reason test is satisfied if the sale or exchange is due to an event that the taxpayer could not reasonably have anticipated before buying and occupying the residence (Reg. § 1.121-3(e)). A sale or exchange due to the individual's preference for a different residence or improvement in financial position does not qualify. A safe harbor exists for the following situations:

- involuntary conversion of the home (¶ 1713);

- damage to the home from natural or man-made disasters or acts of war or terrorism;

- a qualified individual's:

    — death,

    — loss of employment entitling the individual to unemployment compensation,

    — change in employment status resulting in the taxpayer's inability to pay housing costs and reasonable basic living expenses,

---

References are to Standard Federal Tax Reports; Tax Research Consultant; and Practical Tax Explanations.

[28] ¶ 7261; REAL: 15,156.05; § 1,610.25

[29] ¶ 7260, ¶ 7264; REAL: 9,304, REAL: 15,156.05; § 1,610.25

[30] ¶ 7260, ¶ 7263; REAL: 15,166; § 1,620.05

— divorce or legal separation, or

— multiple births resulting from a single pregnancy; or

• other events that the IRS designates as safe harbors.

Other Factors. If the disposition of the residence does not satisfy one of the safe harbor tests described above, the IRS considers all the facts and circumstances when determining whether the primary reason for the sale or exchange is due to a change in place of employment, health, or unforeseen circumstances. Relevant factors include: (1) the circumstances giving rise to the sale; (2) the taxpayer's financial ability to maintain the property; (3) material changes that impact the suitability of the property as the taxpayer's residence; and (4) the taxpayer's use of the property as a residence during the ownership period (Reg. § 1.121-3(b)).

Computing the Reduced Exclusion. The reduced exclusion is computed by multiplying the maximum allowable exclusion ($250,000 or $500,000) by a fraction (Reg. § 1.121-3(g)). The numerator is the shortest of (a) the period that the taxpayer owned the property during the five-year period ending on the sale or exchange date; (b) the period that the taxpayer used the property as a principal residence during the five-year period ending on the sale or exchange date; or (c) the period between the date of the most recent prior sale or exchange to which the exclusion applied and the current sale or exchange date. The denominator of the fraction is either 730 days or 24 months, depending on the whether the numerator is expressed in days or months.

> **Example 1:** Al Jackson is an unmarried taxpayer who owned and used a principal residence for 12 months. He then sold the home because he was unable to care for himself after sustaining injuries in an accident. Jackson had not excluded gain from the sale of a residence within the prior two years. He may exclude up to $125,000 of any gain that he realizes from the sale ($250,000 maximum exclusion × 12/24 = $125,000).

> **Example 2:** On September 1, 2013, Bill and Ruth Green purchased a townhouse in Boston for $450,000. A few months later, Ruth received an offer of employment in Atlanta, and on July 1, 2014, the Greens sold their townhouse and moved to Atlanta. Because they owned and resided in the townhouse for 10 months, they may exclude up to $208,333 of their realized gain ($500,000 maximum exclusion × 10/24 = $208,333).

Involuntary Conversion

1713. Gain or Loss from Involuntary Conversion. An involuntary conversion occurs when property is destroyed, stolen, seized, condemned, or disposed of under the threat of condemnation and the taxpayer receives other property or money (usually insurance proceeds or a condemnation award) as compensation. To the extent the compensation exceeds the basis of the converted property, the taxpayer realizes gain (¶ 1701).

There are two specific sets of circumstances, however, under which gain from compulsory or involuntary conversion of property is not recognized for tax purposes (Code Sec. 1033; Reg. § § 1.1033(a)-1, 1.1033(a)-2):[31]

• When property is converted involuntarily or by compulsion into other property that is similar or related in service or use, no gain is currently recognized. The basis of the old property is transferred to the new property (¶ 1687). This nonrecognition rule is mandatory.

• When property is involuntarily converted into money (e.g., insurance proceeds after fire destroys a building), or into property that is not similar or related in service or use, the owner may elect to postpone the recognition of gain that is invested in replacement property within a specified replacement period (¶ 1715). Thus, an electing taxpayer recognizes gain on the conversion only to the extent that the amount realized exceeds the cost of the replacement property. A taxpayer

---

References are to Standard Federal Tax Reports; Tax Research Consultant; and Practical Tax Explanations.

[31] ¶ 29,640, ¶ 29,641, ¶ 29,642; SALES: 27,050; § 18,101

¶1713

elects to defer the reinvested gain simply by excluding it from gross income on the tax return for the tax year in which it is realized, and providing details of the involuntary conversion in a statement attached to the return (see *Reporting Requirements* below).

Loss. Loss from an involuntary conversion is deductible only if the converted property was used in a business or for the production of income (¶ 1101). However, casualty or theft losses on personal property may be deductible (¶ 1121 and ¶ 1123). For a discussion of the treatment of certain gains and losses from involuntary conversions as capital gains and losses, see ¶ 1748.

Residence. An individual whose principal residence is involuntarily converted may exclude up to $250,000 of the realized gain ($500,000 in the case of a joint return or the return of a surviving spouse) as if the home had been sold (¶ 1705) (Code Sec. 121(d)(5)).[32] Gain that exceeds the exclusion may be deferred if it is used to purchase replacement property. The sale of the underlying land within a reasonable period of time following the destruction of a principal residence can qualify as part of the involuntary conversion of the residence (Rev. Rul. 96-32).[33]

Livestock. Livestock that is destroyed, sold or exchanged because of disease is treated as involuntarily converted (Code Sec. 1033(d); Reg. §1.1033(d)-1).[34] Sales or exchanges of livestock (except poultry) in excess of the number that would normally be sold, made solely on account of drought, flood, or other weather-related conditions, may also be entitled to involuntary conversion treatment (Code Sec. 1033(e); Reg. §1.1033(e)-1).[35] The generally applicable two-year period for purchasing replacement property is extended to four years when the weather-related condition results in the area being eligible for assistance from the federal government. The IRS can further extend the replacement period if the weather-related condition continues for more than three years. For instance, the replacement period for livestock that is involuntarily converted due to persistent drought in the taxpayer's region is extended until the end of the taxpayer's first tax year ending after the region's first drought-free year (Notice 2006-82). Each year, the IRS publishes a list of the counties that suffered droughts sufficient to extend the replacement period (Notice 2014-60).[36]

If, due to drought, flood, other weather-related conditions, or soil or other environmental contamination, it is not feasible for a farmer to reinvest the proceeds from involuntarily converted livestock in property similar or related in service or use, the proceeds may be invested in other property used for farming (Code Sec. 1033(f)).[37] If the conversion was due to soil or other environmental contamination, even real property can qualify as replacement property.

Reporting Requirements. Form 4797 is used to report the gain or loss from an involuntary conversion (other than from casualty or theft) of business property, capital assets used in a business, or capital assets used in connection with a transaction entered into for profit. Form 4684 is used to report involuntary conversions from casualties and thefts. Gains from involuntary conversions (other than from casualty or theft) of capital assets not held for business or profit are reported by individuals, estates, and trusts on Form 8949 (for tax years before 2013, estates and trusts reported such gains on Schedule D of Form 1041).

A separate statement that reports all details connected to the involuntary conversion must be attached to the tax return for the year in which gain is realized (Reg. §1.1033(a)-2(c)(2)).[38] These details include a description of the property, the date and type of conversion, computation of the gain, the decision to replace the converted property, and expiration of the replacement period. If the taxpayer elects to defer gain, but then decides not to replace the converted property, or fails to expend all of the deferred gain on replacement property within the replacement period, the taxpayer must

---

References are to Standard Federal Tax Reports; Tax Research Consultant; and Practical Tax Explanations.

[32] ¶ 7260; REAL: 15,158, SALES: 27,104; § 1,625.15

[33] ¶ 29,650.508; SALES: 27,104; § 18,140.10

[34] ¶ 29,640, ¶ 29,646; FARM: 3,206; § 18,115

[35] ¶ 29,640, ¶ 29,647; FARM: 3,206; § 36,015.10

[36] ¶ 29,650.127; FARM: 3,206; § 36,015.10

[37] ¶ 29,640; SALES: 27,160; § 18,130

[38] ¶ 29,642; SALES: 27,200; § 18,160

recompute the tax liability in an amended return for the year(s) for which the election was made. If the taxpayer elects nonrecognition after filing the return and paying tax for the tax year(s) in which gain is realized but before the replacement period expires, the taxpayer should file a credit or refund claim for each year that gain was reported. The taxpayer must report all of the details of the replacement of converted property in the return for the year of replacement, even if no gain is realized in that year.

The IRS may assess a deficiency attributable to realized gain on an involuntary conversion within three years from the date the taxpayer notifies the IRS of the replacement of the converted property, an intention not to replace, or a failure to replace within the required period (Code Sec. 1033(a)(2)(C); Reg. § 1.1033(a)-2(c)(5)).

1715. Replacement Property. A taxpayer does not recognize gain on an involuntary conversion (¶ 1713) to the extent that the converted property is replaced with property that is similar or related in service or use (Code Sec. 1033(a)).[39] When money or dissimilar property is received, gain is generally recognized. However, if the taxpayer buys qualifying replacement property within the replacement period, the taxpayer can elect to postpone the recognition of gain. Even under this rule, gain must still be recognized to the extent that the net proceeds from the involuntary conversion are not invested in replacement property.

Replacement Property. Replacement property can be (1) other property similar or related in service or use to the property converted, or (2) stock with a controlling interest (at least 80-percent control) in a corporation owning such other property. An actual purchase must take place (e.g., title must pass); an enforceable contract to purchase is not sufficient.[40] If real property used in the taxpayer's trade or business (other than inventory or property held primarily for sale) or held for investment has been condemned or is under threat of condemnation, however, replacement property that is of a "like-kind" (¶ 1721) is treated as similar or related in service or use if it is held either for productive use in trade or business or for investment (Code Sec. 1033(g); Reg. § 1.1033(g)-1).[41] The like-kind test does not apply to acquisitions of 80-percent control of a corporation owning such property or to involuntary conversions by fire, storm, or other casualty. A taxpayer may elect to treat an outdoor advertising display as real property except when the Code Sec. 179 expense election has been made (¶ 1208).

Basis of Replacement Property. If property is compulsorily or involuntarily converted directly into property that is similar or related in service or use, the basis of the acquired property is the same as the basis of the property converted (¶ 1687).

Property Acquired from Related Persons. Certain taxpayers cannot defer the recognition of gain on an involuntary conversion if the replacement property is acquired from a related person, unless the related person obtained the property from an unrelated person during the replacement period (Code Sec. 1033(i)).[42] See ¶ 432 and ¶ 1717 for discussion of related persons. The prohibition applies to a C corporation, a partnership if more than a 50 percent of its interest is owned by C corporations, and any other taxpayer who realizes gain of more than $100,000 during the year from involuntary conversions. If the property is owned by a partnership or S corporation, the $100,000 limitation applies to both the entity and each partner or shareholder.

Replacement Period. Purchase of the replacement property, or of 80-percent control of a corporation that owns such property, must be completed within a period that begins on the actual date of the destruction, condemnation, etc., or the date on which the threat or imminence of condemnation or requisition begins, whichever is earlier (Code Sec. 1033(a)(2)(B)).[43] The replacement period generally ends two years after the close of the first tax year in which any gain on the conversion is realized. The replacement period for condemned real property used in a trade or business or held for investment is three years. The replacement period is four years for a principal residence (¶ 1705) in a

---

References are to Standard Federal Tax Reports; Tax Research Consultant; and Practical Tax Explanations.

[39] ¶ 29,640; SALES: 27,150; § 18,125, § 18,135.05

[40] ¶ 29,650.204; SALES: 27,152; § 18,125

[41] ¶ 29,640, ¶ 29,648; SALES: 27,158; § 18,135.20

[42] ¶ 29,640; SALES: 27,152.05; § 18,135.15

[43] ¶ 29,640; SALES: 27,164; § 18,135.05

¶1715

federally declared disaster area, and for certain involuntarily converted livestock (¶ 1713). The replacement period is five years for property located in the Kansas disaster area that is converted on or after May 4, 2007, due to tornadoes and storms occurring on that date, and in the Midwestern disaster area that is converted on or after May 20, 2008, and before August 1, 2008, due to severe storms, tornados or flooding occurring during that period.[44] Taxpayers may also apply for an extension of the applicable time period (see "*Application for Extension,*" below).

> **Example:** Laura has a $100,000 basis in a commercial building. The building is destroyed by fire, and Laura receives a $120,000 settlement from her insurance company, thus realizing a gain of $20,000. If she acquires a new building for the same use for $120,000 (or more) within the prescribed replacement period, she may elect not to recognize any gain on the involuntary conversion. If the replacement building costs only $110,000, Laura must recognize $10,000 of gain if she elects nonrecognition treatment. Without her election, she must recognize the entire $20,000 gain.

Real Property. If business or investment real property (other than inventory) is condemned (other than through casualty or theft), the replacement period ends three years, rather than two years, after the close of the first tax year in which any of the gain is realized (Code Sec. 1033(g)(4)).[45]

Principal Residence in Federal Disaster Area. Special rules apply to a principal residence, including its contents, that is located in a disaster area and is involuntarily converted as the result of a federally declared disaster (Code Sec. 1033(h)(1)).[46] Generally, insurance proceeds (i.e., insurance reimbursement for scheduled items) for the residence or its contents are treated as a common pool of funds received for the conversion of a single item of property. The taxpayer must use insurance funds received for scheduled property to purchase property that is similar or related in service or use to the converted residence (or its contents) in order to avoid gain recognition (Rev. Rul. 95-22).[47] Gain is recognized only to the extent that the pool of funds exceeds the cost of any replacement property acquired. For unscheduled items, the taxpayer recognizes no gain upon receiving insurance funds, regardless of how those funds are used.

The replacement period for a principal residence involuntarily converted as the result of a federally declared disaster is four years after the close of the first tax year in which any gain upon the conversion is realized (Code Sec. 1033(h)(1)(B)). For this purpose, a principal residence can include a home that the taxpayer does not own (Code Sec. 1033(h)(4)).

Business or Investment Property in Federal Disaster Area. Business or investment property that is located in a disaster area and is compulsorily or involuntarily converted as a result of a federally declared disaster need not be replaced with similar or related property (Code Sec. 1033(h)(2)).[48] Replacement property is deemed to be similar or related in service or use if it is tangible property held for productive use in a trade or business. The replacement period is generally two years.

Application for Extension. The IRS may extend the replacement period upon a written application submitted to the Internal Revenue Center where the taxpayer's return is filed (Code Sec. 1033(a)(2)(B); Reg. § 1.1033(a)-2(c)(3)).[49] The IRS does *not* provide a form for extension requests. The application should explain in detail why the taxpayer is unable to replace the converted property within the replacement period. It should be filed before the statutory replacement period expires, but the IRS may accept a late request if it is made within a reasonable period of time after the replacement period expires and there is reasonable cause for the untimely filing. The IRS may grant an extension if the replacement property is being built during the replacement period, but it will not grant an extension based on the scarcity or high price of replacement property (Rev. Rul. 60-69).[50]

References are to Standard Federal Tax Reports; Tax Research Consultant; and Practical Tax Explanations.

[44] ¶ 29,650.048; SALES: 27,164; § 18,135.05

[45] ¶ 29,640; SALES: 27,164; § 18,135.20

[46] ¶ 29,640; SALES: 27,066; § 18,140.10

[47] ¶ 29,650.317; SALES: 27,066; § 18,140.10

[48] ¶ 29,640; SALES: 27,066; § 18,140.15

[49] ¶ 29,640, ¶ 29,642; SALES: 27,164; § 18,135.05

[50] ¶ 29,650.202; SALES: 27,164; § 18,135.05

1716. Condemnation Award. If only a portion of a tract of land is appropriated by a government authority, the condemnation award may have two components: (1) compensation for the converted portion; and (2) severance damages for the retained portion. Severance damages may be paid, for example, when access to the owner's land has been impaired, or because the owner must replace fences and plant trees to restore the retained property to its former use. The entire award is considered compensation for the condemned property unless both parties stipulate that a specific amount was paid for severance damages (Rev. Rul. 59-173).[51] The owner's net severance damages (i.e., gross severance damages minus legal expenses and other costs) reduce the basis of the retained property. Any excess of the severance damages over the owner's basis is gain (Rev. Rul. 68-37). However, the owner may elect not to recognize the gain that is reinvested in replacement property (¶ 1715) (Rev. Rul. 83-49).

Transactions Between Related Persons

1717. Losses Not Allowed in Transactions Between Related Persons. A loss from a sale or exchange is generally not recognized when the parties to the transaction are related persons (Code Sec. 267(a); Reg. § 1.267(a)-1).[52] However, a loss might be recognized when the buyer subsequently sells or exchanges the property at a gain.

Related Persons. The term "related persons" includes:

(1) Members of a family (brother, sister, spouse, ancestor, or lineal descendant);

(2) An individual and a corporation if the individual owns (directly or indirectly) more than 50 percent in value of the outstanding stock;

(3) Corporations that are members of the same controlled group of corporations;

(4) A grantor and a fiduciary of any trust;

(5) A fiduciary of one trust and a fiduciary of another trust, if the same person is grantor of both trusts;

(6) A fiduciary and a beneficiary of the same trust;

(7) A fiduciary of a trust and a beneficiary of another trust, if the same person is a grantor of both trusts;

(8) A fiduciary of a trust and a corporation, if more than 50 percent in value of the outstanding stock is directly or indirectly owned by or for the trust or a grantor of the trust;

(9) An exempt charitable or educational organization and a person who controls it (including an individual's family members);

(10) A corporation and a partnership if the same persons own (a) more than 50 percent in value of the outstanding stock of the corporation, and (b) more than 50 percent of the capital interest or profits interest in the partnership;

(11) S corporations if the same persons own more than 50 percent in value of the outstanding stock of each corporation;

(12) An S corporation and a C corporation if the same persons own more than 50 percent in value of the outstanding stock of each corporation; or

(13) An executor and a beneficiary of an estate, unless the sale or exchange satisfies a pecuniary bequest (Code Sec. 267(b); Reg. § 1.267(b)-1).[53]

Stock Ownership. In determining stock ownership: (1) stock held by a corporation, partnership, estate, or trust is considered owned proportionately by its shareholders, partners, or beneficiaries; (2) individuals are considered to own stock owned by their families, as defined above; and (3) an individual's stock in a corporation includes stock owned by the individual's partner (Code Sec. 267(c)).[54]

References are to Standard Federal Tax Reports; Tax Research Consultant; and Practical Tax Explanations.

[51] ¶ 29,650.504; SALES: 27,106, § 18,105

[52] ¶ 14,150, ¶ 14,151; SALES: 39,100; § 17,601

[53] ¶ 14,150, ¶ 14,153; SALES: 39,150; § 17,605.10

[54] ¶ 14,150; SALES: 39,154.25; § 17,605.15

Previously Disallowed Loss. The related transferee's gain on a subsequent disposal of the property is reduced (but not below zero) by the amount of any loss that was denied to the original transferor because of the related-person rules (Code Sec. 267(d); Reg. § 1.267(d)-1).[55]

> **Example:** Asa sells business property with a $15,000 basis to his son, Ben, for $5,000. Asa's $10,000 realized loss is not deductible because he sold the property to a related person. Later, Ben sells the property for $18,000 to an unrelated person. Ben's realized gain is $13,000 ($18,000 minus $5,000). However, only $3,000 of this gain is recognized ($13,000 realized gain minus Asa's $10,000 unrecognized loss).

Tax-Free Exchanges

1719. Gain or Loss from Exchange of Property. Gains from exchanges of property are generally recognized for tax purposes (Code Sec. 1001(c)).[56] Some types of exchanges, however, do not result in recognized gain or deductible loss. These include like-kind exchanges (¶ 1721—¶ 1723), exchanges of insurance or annuity contracts (¶ 1724), mortgaged real estate (¶ 1725), government obligations (¶ 1726), stock exchanged for stock in the same corporation (¶ 1728) or for property (¶ 1729), transfers of property to a corporation controlled by the transferor (¶ 1731), exchanges by certain government employees to avoid conflicts of interest (¶ 1732), sales of stock to an employee stock ownership plan (¶ 1733), and transfers between spouses or former spouses (¶ 1734).

1721. Like-Kind Exchanges. No gain or loss is recognized upon the exchange of property held for productive use in a trade or business or for investment if the property received is of a like kind and is held either for productive use in a business or for investment (Code Sec. 1031(a)(1); Reg. § 1.1031(a)-1).[57] The nonrecognition rule generally does *not* apply to stock in trade or other property held primarily for sale, stocks, bonds, notes, certificates of trust, beneficial interests, partnership interests, securities, evidences of indebtedness or interest, or choses in action (Code Sec. 1031(a)(2)).[58] However, stock in certain mutual ditch, reservoir, or irrigation companies is not excluded from like-kind exchange treatment if the stock is treated as real property or an interest in real property under applicable state law (Code Sec. 1031(i)).

The like-kind exchange rules also do not apply to exchanges of property the taxpayer uses for personal purposes (e.g., home or family car) (IRS Pub. 544). A dwelling unit such as a vacation home, however, is generally treated as held for business purposes if (i) the taxpayer rented out the unit for at least two weeks in each of the two years before the exchange, and similarly rents out the property received for at least two weeks in the first two years after the exchange, and (ii) the taxpayer's personal use of the units in those years is minimal (Rev. Proc. 2008-16).[59] The disposition of a property used as a home and then converted to use as business property may be both a like-kind exchange and a sale of a principal residence qualifying for an exclusion of gain (¶ 1705) (Rev. Proc. 2005-14).

Trade-in Arrangements. A like-kind exchange occurs when a taxpayer sells old trade or business equipment to a dealer and purchases new equipment of like kind from the same dealer in reciprocal and mutually dependent transactions, even though the parties execute separate contracts and treat the sale and purchase as unrelated transactions for recordkeeping purposes (Rev. Rul. 61-119).[60]

Related Persons. If property received in a like-kind exchange between certain controlled partnerships (¶ 432) or related persons (¶ 1717) is disposed of within two years after the last transfer involved in the exchange, the original exchange does not

---

References are to Standard Federal Tax Reports; Tax Research Consultant; and Practical Tax Explanations.

[55] ¶ 14,150; ¶ 14,155; SALES: 39,110; § 17,605.20

[56] ¶ 29,220; SALES: 3,050; § 16,010

[57] ¶ 29,602, ¶ 29,603; SALES: 30,000; § 18,001, § 18,005.05

[58] ¶ 29,602; SALES: 30,150; § 18,010.05

[59] ¶ 29,608.2495; SALES: 30,200, § 18,005.10, § 18,060

[60] ¶ 29,608.1178; SALES: 30,312; § 18,015.20

17

SALES

qualify for nonrecognition treatment (Code Sec. 1031(f)).[61] The taxpayer takes the previously unrecognized gain or loss into account on the date of the subsequent disposition of the exchanged property by the taxpayer or the related party. The use of a qualified intermediary does not prevent a like-kind exchange from being treated as a related party transaction. The running of the two-year period may be suspended when the holder of the exchanged property has substantially diminished the risk of loss by the use of a put option (¶ 1921), short sale (¶ 1944), the holding by another person of a right to acquire such property, or any other transaction (Code Sec. 1031(g)).[62] These related-person rules do not apply if: (1) neither the original exchange nor the disposition had the avoidance of federal income tax as one of its principal purposes; (2) the disposition was due to the death of either related party; or (3) the disposition was due to the compulsory or involuntary conversion of the property (¶ 1713) (Code Sec. 1031(f)(2)).

Like-Kind Property Defined. Property is of like kind if it is of the same nature or character (Reg. § 1.1031(a)-1(b) and (c)).[63] All facts and circumstances are considered in determining whether properties are of like kind, including state law and federal tax law classifications. Federal income tax law determines whether the properties are of the same nature or character (CCA 201238027).[64]

Most exchanges of real property qualify as like-kind exchanges. However, real property located in the United States and real property located outside the United States are not like-kind (Code Sec. 1031(h)(1)).[65] Leaseholds with at least 30 years to run are generally like-kind to fee simple interests (Reg. § 1.1031(a)-1(c)).[66]

Personal properties are of like kind if they are of a like kind or class. Depreciable tangible personal properties are of a like class if they fall within the same general asset class or the same product class (Reg. § 1.1031(a)-2(b)).[67] Asset classes for depreciable tangible personal property are those used for depreciation purposes, as set forth in Rev. Proc. 87-56. Product classes are determined by reference to the six-digit product codes of the North American Industrial Classification System (NAICS). Personal property predominantly used in the United States and personal property predominantly used outside of the United States are not like-kind property (Code Sec. 1031(h)(2)).[68]

Exchanges involving intangible personal property or nondepreciable tangible personal property may qualify for like-kind exchange treatment only if the properties are of like kind (Reg. § 1.1031(a)-2(c)).[69] For example, an exchange of a copyright on a novel for a copyright on another novel would generally be a like-kind exchange. However, an exchange of a copyright on a novel for a copyright on a song would not be a like-kind exchange. The goodwill or going concern value of one business and the goodwill or going concern value of another business are *not* like-kind. Intangibles such as trademarks, trade names, mastheads and other customer-based intangibles that can be separately described and valued apart from goodwill can qualify as like-kind property.[70]

Substituted Basis. For the basis of property received in a like-kind exchange, see ¶ 1651.

Reporting. Form 8824 is used to report a like-kind exchange. If there is any gain recognized because the taxpayer transferred and received more than one group of like-properties or boot (¶ 1723), then Schedule D of the taxpayer's return is used to report gains of capital assets not held for business or profit, Form 4797 is used to report gains of assets held for business or profit, or Form 6252 is used to report gain from an installment sale.

References are to Standard Federal Tax Reports; Tax Research Consultant; and Practical Tax Explanations.

[61] ¶ 29,602, ¶ 29,608.2493; SALES: 30,206.10; § 18,020

[62] ¶ 29,602; SALES: 30,206.10; § 18,020

[63] ¶ 29,603; SALES: 30,100; § 18,005.15

[64] ¶ 29,608.1103; SALES: 30,100; § 18,005.15

[65] ¶ 29,602; SALES: 30,100, SALES: 30,160; § 18,010.20

[66] ¶ 29,603; SALES: 30,110, § 18,005.15

[67] ¶ 29,606; SALES: 30,102; § 18,005.15

[68] ¶ 29,602; SALES: 30,162; § 18,010.20

[69] ¶ 29,606; SALES: 30,118; § 18,010.05

[70] ¶ 29,608.2654; SALES: 30,150; § 18,010.05

¶1721

1722. Deferred Like-Kind Exchanges. An exchange of property may qualify for like-kind treatment (¶ 1721) even if the replacement property is received after the relinquished property has been transferred, provided that identification and receipt requirements are satisfied (Code Sec. 1031(a)(3); Reg. § 1.1031(k)-1).[71] This type of transaction is known as a "Starker exchange." The replacement property must be (i) identified within 45 days after the relinquished property is transferred, and (ii) received within 180 days or, if earlier, by the due date (including extensions) of the income tax return for the tax year in which the relinquished property was transferred. The deadlines may be extended if the parties are affected by a federally declared disaster (Rev. Proc. 2007-56).[72] Property not in existence or still under construction may qualify as replacement property in a deferred exchange (Reg. § 1.1031(k)-1(e)).[73]

Identifying Replacement Property. The period for identifying replacement property begins on the date that the relinquished property is transferred and ends at midnight on the 45th day thereafter (Code Sec. 1031(a)(3)(A); Reg. § 1.1031(k)-1(b)(2)).[74] The replacement property must be unambiguously described and designated as replacement property in either: (1) a written agreement covering the exchange that is signed by all parties before the end of the identification period; or (2) a written document signed by the taxpayer and hand delivered, mailed, telecopied, or otherwise sent before the end of the identification period to a person involved in the exchange (such as an intermediary, escrow agent, or title company) other than the taxpayer, the taxpayer's agent, or a related party (Reg. § 1.1031(k)-1(c)).[75] A street address or legal description is generally an adequate identification of real property. A taxpayer may identify up to three replacement properties regardless of their fair market values, or any number of replacement properties whose aggregate value does not exceed 200 percent of the aggregate value of all relinquished properties.

Safe Harbors. The taxpayer may not actually or constructively receive cash or other property and then use the proceeds to buy the replacement property (Reg. § 1.1031(k)-1(f)). However, a party to a deferred like-kind exchange is not considered to be in actual or constructive receipt of money or other property if the transaction involves: (1) qualifying security or guarantee arrangements; (2) qualified escrow accounts or trusts; (3) a qualified intermediary; or (4) the transferor's entitlement to receive interest or a growth factor (Reg. § 1.1031(k)-1(g)).[76]

Parking Transactions. An additional safe harbor may apply to a "reverse-Starker exchange" or "parking transaction"—an exchange in which replacement property is acquired before the relinquished property is transferred (Rev. Proc. 2000-37, modified by Rev. Proc. 2004-51).[77] The replacement property is "parked" with a third party (the accommodation party) until it is transferred to the ultimate transferee in a simultaneous or deferred exchange. The parties use a Qualified Exchange Accommodation Arrangement (QEAA) in which a person other than the taxpayer or a disqualified person holds title to the property. The combined time period that the relinquished and replacement properties are held in the QEAA cannot exceed 180 days. Under the safe harbor, the IRS will not challenge the qualification of property as either replacement property or relinquished property or the treatment of the exchange accommodation titleholder as the beneficial owner of the property. The safe harbor is not available, however, if the replacement property was owned by the taxpayer within the 180-day period ending on the date that title or other qualified indicia of ownership of the property is transferred to the exchange accommodation titleholder.

References are to Standard Federal Tax Reports; Tax Research Consultant; and Practical Tax Explanations.

[71] ¶ 29,602, ¶ 29,619; SALES: 30,600; § 18,015.05

[72] ¶ 29,620.80; SALES: 36,102.30; § 18,015.30

[73] ¶ 29,619; SALES: 30,606; § 18,015.15

[74] ¶ 29,602, ¶ 29,619; SALES: 30,602.05; § 18,015.10

[75] ¶ 29,619; SALES: 30,602.10; § 18,015.10

[76] ¶ 29,619; SALES: 30,608, SALES: 30,610; § 18,035.05

[77] ¶ 29,620.10; SALES: 30,614; § 18,015.25

Interest on Funds Held by Intermediaries. Escrow accounts, trusts, and funds used to facilitate deferred exchanges (exchange funds) are generally treated as loaned by the taxpayer to an exchange facilitator (Reg. §1.468B-6).[78] Interest is imputed to the taxpayer under Code Sec. 7872 (¶ 795), unless the exchange facilitator pays sufficient interest. The exchange facilitator is deemed to receive the same amount as compensation for its services, and has an offsetting deduction for its interest "payment" to the taxpayer. The exchange facilitator must take into account all items of income, deduction, and credit attributable to the exchange fund. Exchange funds include relinquished property, cash, or cash equivalents held in an escrow account, trust, or fund to secure the transferee's obligation to transfer replacement property or the proceeds from a transfer of the relinquished property. An exchange facilitator is a qualified intermediary (QI), transferee, escrow holder, trustee or other party that holds exchange funds for a taxpayer in a deferred exchange under an escrow, trust or exchange agreement. Exchange funds are not treated as loans if the escrow agreement, trust agreement, or exchange agreement specifies that the earnings attributable to the exchange funds are payable to the taxpayer. In this situation, the taxpayer must take into account all items of income, deduction, and credit attributable to the exchange funds.

Safe Harbor for Bankrupt Qualified Intermediaries. The IRS has provided a safe harbor method for reporting gain or loss for a taxpayer undertaking a deferred like-kind exchange if the qualified intermediary defaults on its obligations (Rev. Proc. 2010-14).[79] Taxpayers are generally allowed to avoid recognition of gain until payment is received.

Direct Deeding of Property. In an exchange of real property involving three parties—the taxpayer, a qualified intermediary, and a third party that supplies the replacement property—the exchange may qualify as like kind even if the third party deeds the replacement property directly to the taxpayer (Rev. Rul. 90-34).[80] Therefore, it is not necessary for the transferee to take title to the replacement property and then transfer title to the taxpayer.

1723. Cash or Other Property Received in a Like-Kind Exchange. If money or property not of a like-kind (commonly referred as to "boot") is received by a taxpayer as part of a like-kind exchange (¶ 1721), the taxpayer recognizes gain from the transaction to the extent of the boot's fair market value (Code Sec. 1031(b); Reg. §1.1031(b)-1).[81] A taxpayer who receives boot cannot deduct any loss on the exchange (Code Sec. 1031(c); Reg. §1.1031(c)-1).[82] Boot may consist of cash, relief from indebtedness (¶ 1725), property that is not like kind to the property being exchanged, or property excluded from like-kind treatment. Boot is often given to equalize the value of the like-kind properties being exchanged.

> **Example:** Bill exchanges real estate, with a basis of $10,000, for real estate with a fair market value of $12,000 and $4,000 in cash. His *realized* gain of $6,000 ($16,000 value received minus $10,000 basis) is *recognized* only to the extent of the $4,000 cash he received. His basis for the replacement real estate is $10,000 ($10,000 basis in old property, minus $4,000 cash received, plus $4,000 *recognized* gain).

See ¶ 1728 for situations involving stock exchanged for stock in the same corporation, and ¶ 1731 for discussion of the tax-free transfer of property to a controlled corporation.

1724. Exchange of Insurance or Annuity Contracts. A life insurance, endowment, annuity, or qualified long-term care insurance policy is considered property for federal tax purposes, so any gain or loss realized on a sale or exchange of the policy is ordinarily taxable. However, no gain or loss results from an exchange of:

- a life insurance contract for another life insurance contract, or an endowment, annuity, or qualified long-term care insurance contract;

References are to Standard Federal Tax Reports; Tax Research Consultant; and Practical Tax Explanations.

[78] ¶ 21,950H; ACCTNG: 12,222; § 18,035.15

[79] ¶ 29,621.75; SALES: 30,610.15; § 18,035.20

[80] ¶ 29,621.30; SALES: 30,510

[81] ¶ 29,602, ¶ 29,609; SALES: 30,250; § 18,030

[82] ¶ 29,602, ¶ 29,611; SALES: 30,250; § 18,030

- an endowment contract for another endowment contract that provides for regular payment beginning at a date no later than the date payments would have begun under the contract exchanged, or for an annuity or long-term care insurance contract;

  - an annuity contract for another annuity contract if both are payable over the life of the same annuitant, or for a qualified long-term care insurance contract; or

    - a qualified long-term care insurance contract for another qualified long-term care insurance contract (Code Sec. 1035; Reg. § 1.1035-1).[83]

Gain or loss may be recognized if the exchange has the effect of transferring property to any person other than a United States person. Policyholders who surrender life insurance or annuity contracts of a financially troubled insurance company may qualify for nonrecognition treatment if, within 60 days, all cash received is reinvested in another policy or contract issued by another insurance company or in a single custodial account (Rev. Proc. 92-44; Rev. Proc. 92-44A).[84]

A partial exchange of the cash surrender value of an existing annuity contract for a second annuity contract is a tax-free exchange only if no amount, other than an amount received as an annuity for a period of 10 years or more or during one or more lives, is received during the 180 days beginning on the date of the transfer (Rev. Proc. 2011-38).[85] A subsequent direct transfer is not taken into account. These rules do not apply to partial annuitizations (¶ 817). Different rules applied to transfers completed before October 24, 2011 (Rev. Proc. 2008-24).

1725. Like-Kind Exchange of Mortgaged Real Estate. A taxpayer who relinquishes mortgaged real estate in a like-kind exchange (¶ 1721) receives boot (¶ 1723) equal to the amount of the mortgage from which the taxpayer is relieved (Code Sec. 1031(d); Reg. §§ 1.1031(b)-1(c), 1.1031(d)-2).[86] If mortgaged property is exchanged for mortgaged property, the net reduction of the mortgage indebtedness is treated as boot. It is immaterial whether a mortgage is assumed by the purchaser or whether the property is acquired subject to a mortgage.

> **Example:** Kathy's relinquished property has a fair market value of $100,000 and an adjusted basis of $75,000, and is subject to a $70,000 mortgage. Her replacement property has a fair market value of $60,000 and is subject to a $30,000 mortgage. Her entire realized gain must be recognized:

Fair market value of property received	$60,000
Less mortgage on that property	30,000
	$30,000
Mortgage on property transferred by Kathy	70,000
Total consideration received	$100,000
Less basis of property transferred	75,000
Gain realized	$25,000

The total realized gain is recognized because it is less than the $40,000 net mortgage reduction.

1726. Exchange of Government Obligations. Obligations issued by the United States may be exchanged tax-free for other such obligations (except to the extent that money is received in the exchange) (Code Sec. 1037; Reg. § 1.1037-1).[87] Municipal or state bonds may be exchanged under a refunding agreement with no recognized gain or loss, provided that there are no material differences in the terms of the exchanged bonds (Rev. Rul. 81-169).[88]

References are to Standard Federal Tax Reports; Tax Research Consultant; and Practical Tax Explanations.

[83] ¶ 29,680, ¶ 29,681; INDIV: 30,502; § 3,250.10

[84] ¶ 29,682.30; INDIV: 30,502; § 3,250.10

[85] ¶ 29,682.108; INDIV: 30,502.10; § 3,250.10

[86] ¶ 29,602, ¶ 29,609, ¶ 29,614; SALES: 30,256, SALES: 30,258; § 18,030

[87] ¶ 29,720, ¶ 29,721; SALES: 27,252; § 18,220

[88] ¶ 29,226.1117; SALES: 24,510

1728. Stock Exchanged for Stock of the Same Corporation. An exchange of common stock for common stock of the same corporation, or preferred stock for preferred stock of the same corporation, does not result in recognized gain or deductible loss (Code Sec. 1036; Reg. § 1.1036-1).[89] However, gain (but not loss) may be recognized if cash or other property (boot) is received (¶ 1723). Nonqualified preferred stock is not treated as stock for these purposes.

1729. Stock Exchanged for Property. A corporation does not recognize gain or loss upon the receipt of money or other property in exchange for its own stock, including treasury stock, regardless of the nature of the transaction or the facts and circumstances involved (Code Sec. 1032; Reg. § 1.1032-1).[90] This treatment does not apply if a corporation acquires shares of its own stock unless it acquires those shares in exchange for shares of its own stock, including treasury stock. Also, no gain or loss is recognized by a corporation upon the lapse or acquisition of an option, or with respect to a securities futures contract, to buy or sell its own stock, including treasury stock. See ¶ 736 for discussion of the nonrecognition of gain or loss when a corporation distributes its stock to shareholders.

1731. Tax-Free Transfer of Property to Controlled Corporation. No gain or loss is recognized if one or more persons (individuals, trusts or estates, partnerships, or corporations) transfer property to a corporation solely in exchange for its stock and, immediately after the transfer, are in control of the transferee corporation (Code Sec. 351; Reg. § 1.351-1).[91] See ¶ 203 for further discussion of tax-free contributions of property to a corporation in exchange for stock. See ¶ 1660 for discussion of the basis of the property transferred to the controlled corporation.

1732. Dispositions of Property to Avoid Conflicts of Interest. An officer or employee of the executive branch or a judicial officer of the federal government who sells property in order to comply with conflict-of-interest requirements may elect to recognize gain only to the extent that the amount realized is more than the adjusted basis of any permitted property that the taxpayer purchases during the 60-day period beginning on the sale date (Code Sec. 1043).[92] Permitted property includes any U.S. obligation or diversified investment fund approved by the Office of Government Ethics. The nonrecognized gain reduces basis in the permitted property. The deferral option is also available to any spouse, minor, or dependent child whose ownership of property is attributable to the federal officer or employee under any applicable conflict-of-interest law. These deferral rules also apply to sales by a trustee if any person subject to the rules has a beneficial interest in the principal or income of the trust. Form 8824 is used to report conflict-of-interest sales.

1733. Tax-Free Sale of Stock to ESOP. Taxpayers (other than C corporations) may elect to sell qualified securities to an employee stock ownership plan (ESOP) (¶ 2103) or worker-owned cooperative and replace the securities with other securities without recognition of gain (Code Sec. 1042; Temp. Reg. § 1.1042-1T).[93] The taxpayer makes the election by attaching a statement to its original or amended return for the tax year in which the sale occurs.

1734. Transfers of Property Between Spouses or Former Spouses. No gain or loss is recognized on transfers of property from an individual to a spouse or to a former spouse incident to a divorce (Code Sec. 1041; Temp. Reg. § 1.1041-1T).[94] The transferor's basis for the transferred property is carried over to the transferee. A transfer to a former spouse must occur within one year after the date on which the marriage ceased, or must be related to the cessation of the marriage. This nonrecognition treatment is not available for transfers to spouses or former spouses who are nonresident aliens.

References are to Standard Federal Tax Reports; Tax Research Consultant; and Practical Tax Explanations.

[89] ¶ 29,700, ¶ 29,701; SALES: 27,300; § 18,215

[90] ¶ 29,622, ¶ 29,623; CCORP: 3,152; § 26,801

[91] ¶ 16,402, ¶ 16,403; CCORP: 3,050; § 26,110.05

[92] ¶ 29,840; SALES: 27,350; § 18,240

[93] ¶ 29,820, ¶ 29,821; RETIRE: 75,354.05; § 24,825.15

[94] ¶ 29,800, ¶ 29,801; INDIV: 21,050; § 18,230

Treatment of Capital Gain or Loss

1735. Characterization of Gain or Loss. Gain or loss realized on the disposition of property generally is recognized for federal income tax purposes (¶ 1701). The tax treatment of gain or loss is determined by its character. Gain or loss on the sale or exchange of property that is not a capital asset is ordinary income or ordinary loss, respectively (Code Secs. 64 and 65).[95] Individuals, estates, and trusts may be eligible for lower tax rates on their net long-term gain from the sale of a capital asset (¶ 1736). Whether a capital gain or loss is long-term or short-term depends on whether the taxpayer held the capital asset for at least one year (¶ 1737). Corporate taxpayers must include both net long-term and short-term capital gains in gross income (¶ 1738). Deductions for capital losses that exceed capital gains may be limited for all taxpayers (¶ 1752).

Capital gain or loss can arise only from a sale or exchange of a capital asset (¶ 1741 and ¶ 1742). Taxpayers must follow specific procedures in calculating their recognized capital gain or loss (¶ 1739). Special rules prevent taxpayers from converting all or a part of what would otherwise be capital gain into ordinary income (¶ 1740).

Reporting Requirements. Taxpayers report the details of their sales and other dispositions of capital assets on Form 8949, and then carry the relevant dollar amount totals to Schedule D of their tax returns. Prior to the 2011 tax year for individuals, the 2012 tax year for corporations and partnerships, and the 2013 tax year for trusts and estates, the details of sales and exchanges of capital assets were reported directly on Schedule D in most situations.

1736. Tax on Capital Gains—Individual, Estate, Trust. For individuals, estates, and trusts, a number of different tax rates can apply to net capital gains for regular income tax and alternative minimum tax (AMT) purposes. The capital gains rate on net capital gains and qualified dividend income (¶ 733) for individuals is 20 percent if the taxpayer is in the 39.6-percent income tax bracket, 15 percent if in the 25-, 28-, 33-, or 35-percent income tax bracket, and 0 percent if in the 10- or 15-percent income tax bracket. For estates and trusts, the rate is 20 percent if the taxpayer is in the 39.6-percent income tax bracket, 15 percent if in the 25-, 28-, or 33-percent income tax bracket, and 0 percent if in the 15-percent income tax bracket (Code Sec. 1(h)(1)).[96] (In 2012, the capital gains tax rate was generally 15 percent, or 0 percent for individuals in the 10-percent or 15-percent income tax bracket, and estates and trusts in the 15 percent income tax bracket.) For all tax years, the capital gains tax rate is 25 percent for unrecaptured Code Sec. 1250 gain (¶ 1779), and 28 percent for collectibles and gain on qualified small business stock (¶ 1905).

To calculate net capital gain (or loss) for the tax year, a noncorporate taxpayer must first net short and long-term capital gains and losses for each of the rate groups separately (¶ 1739). Capital gain or loss is short or long term depending on how long the taxpayer held the property prior to its sale or other disposition (¶ 1737). Net capital gain that the taxpayer elects to treat as investment interest (¶ 1094) is subtracted from the total net capital gain in order to determine the amount subject to the maximum capital gains rate (Code Sec. 1(h)(2)).

Depreciable Real Estate. A 25-percent tax rate is imposed on long-term capital gain attributable to certain prior depreciation that was claimed on real property (Code Sec. 1(h)(1)(E) and (6)(A)).[97] This depreciation is referred to as "unrecaptured Section 1250 gain" and is the excess of:

> (1) the amount of long-term capital gain (not otherwise treated as ordinary income) that would be treated as ordinary income if Code Sec. 1250(b)(1) included all depreciation and the applicable percentage that applied under Code Sec. 1250(a) was 100, over

> (2) the excess of 28-percent rate loss over 28-percent rate gain.

Even under these capital gains rules, Code Sec. 1250 continues to treat some prior claimed depreciation as ordinary income (¶ 1779) (usually the amount claimed in excess of the amount allowable under the straight-line method).

References are to Standard Federal Tax Reports; Tax Research Consultant; and Practical Tax Explanations.

[95] ¶ 6030, ¶ 6040; SALES: 15,050; § 16,020

[96] ¶ 3260; SALES: 15,200; § 16,525.10

[97] ¶ 3260; SALES: 15,202.70; § 16,525.10

Example: William Drake sold a building for $1 million, realizing a $600,000 gain. The building had originally cost $700,000. Over the years, Drake had claimed $300,000 in depreciation, including $100,000 that was in excess of that allowed under the straight-line method. Thus, $200,000 of the total claimed depreciation is classified as unrecaptured Section 1250 gain, because if Code Sec. 1250 had applied to all depreciation, and not only additional depreciation, $300,000 of Drake's long-term capital gain would have been treated as ordinary income. The $100,000 in excess depreciation is taxed as ordinary income, the $200,000 in unrecaptured Section 1250 gain is subject to a capital gains rate of 25 percent, and the remaining $300,000 of gain is subject to regular capital gains rates.

Under MACRS, all depreciation on real property must be computed under the straight-line method (¶ 1780). As a result, any gain on the sale of MACRS real property that was held more than 12 months and that is due to claimed deprecation is unrecaptured Section 1250 gain and subject to a maximum capital gains rate of 25 percent.

Collectibles. Generally, collectibles (e.g., stamps, antiques, gems, and most coins) are taxed at the tax rate of 28 percent even if held more than 12 months (Code Sec. 1(h)(4)(A)(i) and (5)).[98]

Small Business Stock. Noncorporate taxpayers may exclude from gross income a certain percentage of capital gain from the sale or exchange of qualified small business stock held for more than five years and issued after August 10, 1993 (¶ 1905). This excluded capital gain (section 1202 gain) is not used in computing the taxpayer's long-term capital gain or loss, and it is not investment income for purposes of the investment interest limitation. However, the capital gain that is *not* excluded is taxed at the maximum 28 percent capital gains rate (Code Sec. 1(h)(4)(A)(ii) and (7)).[99]

Pass-Through Entities. A pass-through entity—including an S corporation, partnership, estate, trust, regulated investment company (mutual fund), and real estate investment trust (REIT)—allocates capital gains to its shareholders or beneficiaries (Code Sec. 1(h)(10)).[100] Capital gain distributions from a mutual fund are taxed as long-term capital gains regardless of how long the shareholder owned the fund shares (¶ 2311). If capital gain distributions are automatically reinvested in the fund, the reinvested amount is the basis of the additional shares (IRS Pub. 550).

1737. Holding Period for Capital Assets. The holding period for a capital asset (¶ 1741) is the length of time that the taxpayer owns the property before disposing of it. The classification of the taxpayer's holding period as short-term or long-term determines the tax treatment of any recognized gain or loss (¶ 1736 and ¶ 1739, respectively). Long-term gain or loss arises from assets held for more than one year, while short-term gain or loss arises from assets held for one year or less (Code Secs. 1222 and 1223; Reg. § 1.1223-1).[101]

Calculating the Holding Period. When determining how long an asset was held, the taxpayer generally begins counting on the date after the day the property was acquired. The same date of each following month is the beginning of a new month regardless of the number of days in the preceding month (Rev. Rul. 66-7).[102] The date the asset is disposed of is part of the holding period. If an asset is acquired on the last day of a month, the first day on which it may be considered to have been held for more than one year is the first day of the *13th* calendar month following the calendar month of acquisition. However, there are special rules for assets acquired in a tax-free exchange, by gift or inheritance, or in an involuntary conversion.

Example: An asset acquired on March 31, 2013, must be held until April 1, 2014, in order to be considered held for more than one year.

References are to Standard Federal Tax Reports; Tax Research Consultant; and Practical Tax Explanations.

[98] ¶ 3260; SALES: 15,202.65; § 16,525.10

[99] ¶ 3260; SALES: 15,300; § 16,525.10

[100] ¶ 3260; SALES: 15,202.90; § 16,525.10

[101] ¶ 30,440, ¶ 30,460, ¶ 30,461; SALES: 15,150; § 16,540.05

[102] ¶ 30,463.3997, ¶ 30,463.4099; SALES: 15,152; § 16,540.05

Tax-Free Exchange. When property is received in a tax-free exchange (¶ 1719), the holding period of the property given up by the taxpayer is added ("tacked on") to the holding period of the property that the taxpayer receives (Code Sec. 1223).[103]

Gift. The holding period of property acquired by gift or transfer in trust includes the time the property was held by both the donor and the donee if, as is usually the case, the donee takes the donor's basis (Code Sec. 1223(2)).[104] However, when the fair market value at the time of the gift is used as the donee's basis (¶ 1630), the holding period starts the day after the gift was made (IRS Pub. 544).

Inherited. When property is acquired from a decedent, its basis in the hands of the heir or beneficiary is stepped up to its fair market value, and it is automatically deemed to have been held for more than one year (Code Sec. 1223(9)).[105] However, if the decedent died in 2010 and the executor elected to have the carryover basis rule (¶ 1633) rather than the estate tax apply, the taxpayer's holding period of the property is the same as the decedent's, whether or not the executor allocates any basis increase to the property (Rev. Proc. 2011-41).[106]

Involuntary Conversion. The holding period of property acquired in an involuntary conversion (¶ 1713) includes the holding period of the property converted if the basis of the new property is determined by reference to the basis of the old property (Code Sec. 1223(1)(A)).[107]

Stock. The holding period for stock and securities purchased on an exchange begins on the day following the day of purchase (the trade date), and ends on, and includes, the date of sale (rather than the day when payment is received and delivery is made (the settlement date)) (Rev. Rul. 66-97; Rev. Rul. 93-84).[108] The holding period for stock received in a nontaxable stock distribution or in a "spin-off" includes the holding period of the related stock on which the distribution is made (Code Sec. 1223(1) and (4)).[109]

Options. When assets are acquired by the exercise of a purchase option, the holding period starts the day after the option is exercised.[110]

Partnership Property. A partner's holding period for property received as a distribution from the partnership includes the period for which the partnership held the property (Code Sec. 735(b)).[111]

Treasury Obligations. In determining the holding period of U.S. Treasury notes and bonds sold at auction on the basis of yield, the acquisition date is the date the Secretary of Treasury, through news releases, gives notification of the successful bidders (Rev. Rul. 78-5).[112] The acquisition date of U.S. Treasury notes sold through an offering on a subscription basis at a specified yield is the date the subscription is submitted.

1738. Corporate Capital Gains. A corporation must include both long-term and short-term capital gains in gross income to the extent the gains exceed capital losses for the year. As a result, capital gains of a corporation are generally taxed at ordinary corporate income tax rates (¶ 219). A corporation may pay an alternative tax of 35 percent on net capital gain instead of the regular income tax in any year in which the top corporate income tax rate exceeds 35 percent (determined without regard to the additional taxes on corporations with taxable incomes over $100,000 or over $15 million) (Code Sec. 1201(a)).[113] The net capital gain on which the alternative tax is imposed cannot exceed the corporation's taxable income. Net capital gain equals the excess of the net long-term capital gain for the tax year minus the net short-term capital loss for

---

References are to Standard Federal Tax Reports; Tax Research Consultant; and Practical Tax Explanations.

[103] ¶ 30,460; SALES: 15,178; § 16,540.15

[104] ¶ 30,460; SALES: 15,178.05; § 16,540.25

[105] ¶ 30,460; SALES: 15,164; § 16,540.30

[106] ¶ 29,380.762; ESTGIFT: 51,060.10; § 16,310

[107] ¶ 30,460; SALES: 15,178.30; § 18,145.05

[108] ¶ 30,463.3746; ¶ 30,463.4383; SALES: 15,162; § 16,540.10

[109] ¶ 30,460; SALES: 15,178.25; § 16,540.10

[110] ¶ 30,463.4013; SALES: 15,154.05; § 16,540.10

[111] ¶ 25,400; SALES: 15,178.15; § 30,535.10

[112] ¶ 30,463.67; SALES: 15,162.45

[113] ¶ 30,352; SALES: 15,210; § 16,527.10

the tax year (Code Sec. 1222(11)).[114] As the maximum rate currently is 35 percent, the alternative tax has no immediate impact on corporations.

Timber Gains. Qualified timber gains of C corporations for the first and second tax years ending after May 22, 2008, are subject to a reduced capital gains rate of 15 percent if the timber was held for more than 15 years (Code Sec. 1201(b)). Only the portion of the corporation's total timber gains properly allocable to the period after May 22, 2008, is eligible for the lower rate in the first tax year; only the portion allocable to the period of the year on or before May 22, 2009, is eligible for the lower rate in the second tax year. See ¶ 1772 for discussion of the election to treat timber cutting as a sale or exchange.

See ¶ 1752 and ¶ 1756 for treatment of corporate capital losses.

1739. Netting of Gains and Losses. Noncorporate taxpayers have to use specific netting procedures to calculate their recognized capital gain or loss for the tax year (Code Sec. 1(h)(1); Notice 97-59).[115] The gains and losses within each tax rate group are netted in order to arrive at a net gain or loss for the group. Generally, there are three tax rate groups—15 percent (20 percent for individuals, estates, and trusts in the 39.6-percent income tax bracket), 25 percent, and 28-percent (¶ 1736). After the basic netting process within each group has been completed, the following ordering rules must be applied.

- *Short-term capital gains and losses.* Short-term capital losses (including short-term capital loss carryovers (¶ 1754)) are applied first to reduce short-term capital gains, if any, that would otherwise be taxable at ordinary income tax rates. A net short-term loss is then used to reduce any net long-term capital gain from the 28-percent group. Any remaining short-term loss is then used to reduce gain from the 25-percent group, and then to reduce net gain from the 15-percent group (20-percent group for taxpayers in the 39.6-percent income tax bracket).

- *Long-term capital gains and losses.* A net loss from the 28-percent group (including long-term capital loss carryovers) is used first to reduce gain from the 25-percent group, then to reduce net gain from the 15-percent group (20-percent group for taxpayers in the 39.6-percent income tax bracket). A net loss from the 15-percent group (20-percent group) is used first to reduce net gain from the 28-percent group, and then to reduce gain from the 25-percent group.

1740. Gain from Conversion Transactions. Capital gain from the disposition or termination of a position that is part of a financial "conversion transaction" is subject to recharacterization as ordinary income (Code Sec. 1258).[116] The amount of capital gain treated as ordinary income is generally equal to the interest that would have accrued on the taxpayer's net investment at a yield equal to 120 percent of the applicable federal rate (AFR) compounded semiannually (¶ 83), or 120 percent of the federal short-term rates compounded daily if the term of the conversion transaction is indefinite.

A conversion transaction is generally a transaction in which a taxpayer's return on an investment is attributable to the time value of money, but an attempt is made to make the return appear to be attributable to market risk, thus making it seem to be capital gain rather than ordinary income. In addition, the transaction must be:

- a transaction in which the taxpayer acquires property and on a substantially contemporaneous basis enters into a contract to sell the property (or substantially identical property) at a predetermined price;

- a tax straddle (¶ 1948);

- marketed or sold as producing capital gains from a transaction in which the taxpayer's expected return is substantially from the time value of the net investment; or

- specified by the IRS in regulations.

References are to Standard Federal Tax Reports; Tax Research Consultant; and Practical Tax Explanations.

[114] ¶ 30,440; SALES: 15,202.55; § 16,527.05

[115] ¶ 3260, ¶ 3285.55; SALES: 15,206.15; § 16,525.05

[116] ¶ 31,125; SALES: 15,250

Example: Sam Jones purchases stock on January 2, 2012, for $100 and agrees on the same day to sell it to Wendell Johnson on January 2, 2014, for $115. A portion of the $15 gain from the sale of the stock equal to 120 percent of the AFR compounded semiannually for two years and applied to the $100 investment is recharacterized as ordinary income.

Transactions of options dealers and commodities traders in the normal course of their trade or business of dealing in options or trading section 1256 contracts (¶ 1947) are *not* conversion transactions (Code Sec. 1258(d)(5)).[117] This exception does not apply to certain gains allocated to limited partners and limited entrepreneurs as defined in Code Sec. 464(e)(2).

Constructive Ownership Transactions. The amount of long-term capital gains that a taxpayer may recognize from certain constructive ownership transactions that arise from specified financial assets may be limited (Code Sec. 1260).[118] These financial assets include any equity interest in a pass-through entity (a partnership, S corporation, regulated investment company (mutual fund), or real estate investment trust). The long-term gain is limited to the amount of gain that the taxpayer would have recognized if the financial asset had been held directly by the taxpayer during the term of the derivative contract. Any additional gain is recognized as ordinary income. Tax liability is increased by the amount of interest that would have accrued on the underpayment that would have arisen if the recharacterized ordinary income had been included in gross income.

1741. Capital Asset. A capital gain or loss arises from the sale or exchange of a capital asset. A capital asset is any property held by a taxpayer, whether or not connected with a trade or business (Code Sec. 1221; Reg. § 1.1221-1).[119] The following items, however, are *not* capital assets:

- stock in trade, inventory, and property held primarily for sale to customers in the ordinary course of the taxpayer's trade or business;
- a note or account receivable acquired in the ordinary course of trade or business for services rendered or from the sale of stock in trade or property held primarily for sale in the ordinary course of business;
- depreciable business property;
- real property used in the taxpayer's trade or business;
- a copyright, a literary, musical or artistic composition, a letter or memorandum, or similar property (but not a patent or invention) held by the taxpayer who created it, or by a taxpayer whose basis in the property is determined by reference to the basis of the person who created it, or in the case of a letter, memorandum or similar property, a taxpayer for whom such property was prepared or produced;
- a U.S. government publication (including the *Congressional Record*) held by a taxpayer who received it (or by another taxpayer whose basis in the publication is determined in whole or in part by reference to the original recipient's basis) other than by purchase at the price at which the publication is offered to the public;
- commodities derivative financial instruments held by commodities derivatives dealers;
- hedging transactions (¶ 1949) entered into in the normal course of the taxpayer's business; and
- supplies of a type regularly used or consumed by the taxpayer in the ordinary course of business.

Although creative works are generally not capital assets in the hands of their creators, a taxpayer may elect to treat the sale or exchange of a musical composition or a copyright in a musical work created by the taxpayer's personal efforts (or having a basis determined by the reference to the creator's basis) as the sale or exchange of a capital asset (Code Sec. 1221(b)(3); Reg. § 1.1221-3).[120] The election is made separately for each composition or copyright sold by reporting the transaction as a sale of a capital asset on Form 8949. (Prior to the 2011 tax year for individuals, the 2012 tax year for corporations and partnerships, and the 2013 tax year for trusts and estates, the election was made on Schedule D of the relevant tax return.)

References are to Standard Federal Tax Reports; Tax Research Consultant; and Practical Tax Explanations.

[117] ¶ 31,125; SALES: 15,252.25
[118] ¶ 31,140; SALES: 45,500

[119] ¶ 30,420, ¶ 30,421; SALES: 15,100; § 16,505.05

[120] ¶ 30,420, ¶ 30,425; SALES: 15,108.15; § 16,505.20

Personal Property. Gain from the sale of an individual's household furnishings, personal residence, or automobile is generally taxed under the capital gains rates. However, loss from the sale is not recognized unless the property was held for the production of income (¶ 1003 and ¶ 1101) (Reg. § 1.262-1(b)(4)).[121] For example, an individual who sells a residence that was partially used as rental property must allocate the original cost of the building, the selling price, depreciation (applicable to the rental portion only), and selling expenses between the personal and rental portions of the building as if there were two separate transactions (¶ 1707). Only the loss allocable to the rental portion of the home may be a capital loss. The gain or loss associated with the sale of a personal residence is discussed at ¶ 1103, ¶ 1626, and ¶ 1705.

Securities. Stock and securities generally are considered to be held for production of income so that a loss on their sale is a capital loss, except in the hands of a dealer who holds them for sale to customers (¶ 1903).[122] Gain or loss from the sale, exchange or termination of a securities futures contract may be eligible for capital gain treatment (Code Sec. 1234B).[123]

Noncapital Assets. The sale or exchange of property results in ordinary income or loss if the property is classified as a noncapital asset. The definition of "capital asset" must be broadly interpreted, so a noncapital asset must come within one of the statutory categories of noncapital assets listed above (*Arkansas Best Corp.*, SCt, 88-1 USTC ¶ 9210).[124] The U.S. Supreme Court rejected the contention that ordinary income and loss treatment should apply to an asset that is otherwise capital simply because it is acquired for business purposes. Therefore, bank stock that was acquired by a holding company in order to prevent damage to the holding company's business reputation was a capital asset even though it was acquired for a business purpose, because the stock did not fall within any of the exclusion categories. In an earlier decision, the Supreme Court ruled that assets held as part of hedging transactions that were an integral part of a business's inventory-purchase system were noncapital assets because they were inventory (*Corn Products Refining*, SCt, 55-2 USTC ¶ 9746).[125]

Special Rules. Special rules apply when the sale involves section 1231 property (¶ 1747), patents (¶ 1767), depreciable property (¶ 1779), farm property (¶ 1797), and partnership interests (¶ 434).

1742. Sale or Exchange Requirement. The capital gain and loss provisions (¶ 1735) apply to the sale or exchange of a capital asset (¶ 1741) (Code Sec. 1222; Reg. § 1.1222-1).[126] In the case of real estate, a sale or exchange occurs on the earlier of the date of conveyance or the date when the burden and benefits of ownership pass to the purchaser.[127] A sale or exchange occurs when there is a corporate liquidation (¶ 2253), when securities become worthless (¶ 1916), and upon any failure to exercise a privilege or option on property that would have been a capital asset if acquired (¶ 1919).

When bonds with past-due interest are purchased "flat" (i.e., the bonds were in default of interest payments), aggregate interest payments that are for the prepurchase period and are in excess of the purchase price but less than the face value of the bonds are properly characterized as capital gains, because they are considered to be amounts received on retirement of the bonds (Rev. Rul. 60-284).[128] The sale of an endowment insurance policy before its maturity or of a paid-up annuity contract before the annuity starting date results in ordinary income (*E.J. Arnfeld*, CtCls, 58-2 USTC ¶ 9692).[129]

1743. Sale of a Trade or Business. When a trade or business is sold, generally each asset of the business is treated as being sold separately in determining the seller's income, gain or loss and the buyer's basis in each of the assets (Rev. Rul. 55-79).[130] The

---

References are to Standard Federal Tax Reports; Tax Research Consultant; and Practical Tax Explanations.

[121] ¶ 13,601; SALES: 15,206.05; § 8,201

[122] ¶ 30,422.684; SALES: 15,104.30; § 16,505.05

[123] ¶ 30,640; SALES: 45,550; § 18,845.10

[124] ¶ 30,422.6865; SALES: 15,118.05

[125] ¶ 30,426.15; SALES: 15,118.10

[126] ¶ 30,440, ¶ 30,441; SALES: 15,050; § 16,520.05

[127] ¶ 21,005.8838; SALES: 3,110; § 16,540.10

[128] ¶ 5704.3075; SALES: 24,508; § 45,415.15

[129] ¶ 30,422.58; INDIV: 30,212, INDIV: 30,356; § 45,450.10

[130] ¶ 30,422.125; SALES: 33,050; § 18,401

seller must allocate the purchase price among the assets in order to determine the amount and character of any recognized gain or loss. The buyer must allocate the purchase price among the assets to determine any allowable depreciation or amortization (Code Sec. 1060(a); Reg. § 1.1060-1(a)).[131] The buyer and seller may agree in writing to allocations of part or all of the consideration involved in the transaction and the fair market value of any assets transferred. The allocation generally is binding on both parties, unless the IRS determines that it is inappropriate (¶ 1620).

Reporting. Generally, the purchaser and the seller each must file Form 8594 to report the sale of assets used in a trade or business when the purchaser's basis in the assets is determined wholly by the amount paid. The form is attached to the tax return for the year in which the sale took place.

1744. Sale of Depreciable Assets Between Related Taxpayers. Capital gain treatment (¶ 1735) is denied when depreciable property (including patent applications) is sold or exchanged between related taxpayers (Code Sec. 1239; Reg. § 1.1239-1).[132] This rule applies to sales or exchanges between:

* a person and all entities that the person controls;

* a taxpayer and any trust in which the taxpayer or the taxpayer's spouse has a beneficiary interest that is not a remote contingent interest; and

* an executor and the beneficiary of the same estate, unless the sale or exchange is in satisfaction of a pecuniary bequest.

For purposes of this rule, entities that are controlled by a taxpayer include:

* a corporation if the taxpayer owns (directly or indirectly) more than 50 percent of the value of its stock;

* a partnership if the taxpayer owns (directly or indirectly) more than 50 percent of the capital or profits interest; and

* certain entities that are related persons with respect to the taxpayer, including two corporations that are members of the same controlled group, a corporation and a partnership if the same persons own more than 50 percent of each, and two S corporations, or an S corporation and a C corporation, if the same persons own more than 50 percent of the stock of each.

Section 1231

1747. Section 1231 Property Used in Trade or Business. Business real estate and depreciable business property is generally excluded from the definition of capital assets (¶ 1741). However, if the business property qualifies as "section 1231 property," gain or loss realized from the sale, exchange, or involuntary conversion of the property may nonetheless qualify as capital gain or loss. Specifically, if a taxpayer's section 1231 gains exceed its section 1231 losses, then all of the taxpayer's section 1231 gains and losses are generally treated as long-term capital gains and losses (¶ 1736) (Code Sec. 1231(a)).[133] On the other hand, if the taxpayer's section 1231 losses exceed its section 1231 gains, then all of the taxpayer's section 1231 gains and losses are treated as ordinary income and losses. Taxpayers use Form 4797 to report the sale or exchange of section 1231 property.

Section 1231 Property. Section 1231 property includes:

* property used in the trade or business subject to depreciation and held more than one year, but not including: property includible in inventory; property held primarily for sale to customers; a copyright, a literary, musical or artistic composition, or a letter, memorandum, or similar property; and certain federal government publications;

References are to Standard Federal Tax Reports; Tax Research Consultant; and Practical Tax Explanations.

[131] ¶ 30,060, ¶ 30,061; SALES: 33,052; § 18,401   [132] ¶ 30,730, ¶ 30,731; SALES: 39,200; § 17,615   [133] ¶ 30,572; SALES: 21,100; § 16,805

- real property used in the trade or business and held for more than one year, but not including property includible in inventory or held primarily for sale to customers;

- trade or business property held for more than one year and compulsory or involuntarily converted (¶ 1748);

- capital assets held for more than one year in connection with a trade or business or a transaction entered into for profit, and compulsory or involuntarily converted;

- an unharvested crop on land used in the trade or business and held for more than one year, if the crop and land are sold, exchanged, or involuntarily converted at the same time to the same person;

- certain livestock, but not poultry (¶ 1750); and

- timber, domestic iron ore, and coal (¶ 1772) (Code Sec. 1231(b); Reg. §§ 1.1231-1 and 1.1231-2).[134]

When section 1231 property is subject to depreciation recapture, the section 1231 gain is the amount by which the total gain exceeds the amounts recaptured and taxed at ordinary income rates (¶ 1779). Also, the recapture of certain farmland expenses may cause a reduction in section 1231 gain (¶ 1797). A gain or loss that is disallowed by other provisions of the law (e.g., a loss on a sale between family members) is not taken into account in determining section 1231 gains and losses (Code Sec. 1231(a)(4); Reg. § 1.1231-1(d)).

Recapture of Net Section 1231 Losses. A taxpayer with a net section 1231 gain for the tax year (section 1231 gains that exceed section 1231 losses) must recapture past net section 1231 losses by treating the current year's net section 1231 gain as ordinary income to the extent of the unrecaptured net section 1231 losses for the five previous tax years (Code Sec. 1231(c)).[135] The losses are recaptured on a first-in, first-out (FIFO) basis (IRS Pub. 544).

> **Example:** Mary has a net section 1231 gain of $23,000 for 2014. She had a net section 1231 loss of $12,000 in 2012 and a net section 1231 loss of $15,000 in 2013. For 2014, under the recapture rules, Mary must include her $23,000 net section 1231 gain as ordinary income (i.e., she recaptures the $12,000 loss from 2012 and $11,000 of the $15,000 loss from 2013). The $4,000 balance of the loss from 2013 remains outstanding, and available for recapture if Mary realizes any net section 1231 gain during 2015-2018.

1748. Compulsory or Involuntary Conversion of Section 1231 Property. The capital gain and ordinary loss rules of Code Sec. 1231 apply to gains and losses realized from the compulsory or involuntary conversion of section 1231 property (¶ 1747), unless the nonrecognition rules for involuntary conversions (¶ 1713) apply (Code Sec. 1231(a)(3)(A)(ii); Reg. § 1.1231-1(d)(4) and (e)).[136] For this purpose, recognized gains and losses resulting from theft or seizure or an exercise of power of requisition or condemnation are treated as section 1231 gains or losses. When casualty or theft gains and losses result in a net loss, the transactions are not grouped with other section 1231 transactions. Instead, the net loss is treated as an ordinary loss.

Personal Assets—Casualty and Theft Losses. Casualty and theft losses on personal assets (those not used in a trade or business or for investment) are excluded from Code Sec. 1231. Instead, gains and losses that exceed the $100 floor per loss (¶ 1129) from personal casualties and thefts are grouped separately. Any resulting net loss may be claimed as an itemized deduction to the extent it exceeds 10 percent of the taxpayer's adjusted gross income (AGI) (¶ 1131). A net gain is classified as a capital gain. The period of time that the taxpayer owned the property determines whether the gain is long term or short term. Generally, taxpayers use Form 4684 to initially report a casualty loss and then report it as an itemized deduction on Schedule A of Form 1040.

References are to Standard Federal Tax Reports; Tax Research Consultant; and Practical Tax Explanations.

[134] ¶ 30,572, ¶ 30,573, ¶ 30,574; SALES: 21,100; § 16,805

[135] ¶ 30,572; SALES: 21,250; § 16,830

[136] ¶ 30,572, ¶ 30,573; SALES: 21,052; § 16,820

¶1748

1750. Livestock as Section 1231 Property. Capital gain and ordinary loss treatment under Code Sec. 1231 applies to the sale, exchange, or involuntary conversion of livestock (not including poultry) held for draft, breeding, dairy or sporting purposes (¶ 1747) (Code Sec. 1231(b)(3); Reg. § 1.1231-2).[137] To qualify for this treatment, horses and cattle must be held for at least 24 months and all other livestock must be held for at least 12 months. The holding period begins on the date of acquisition rather than on the date the animal is actually placed in one of the above uses. Livestock includes fur-bearing animals such as chinchillas, mink, and foxes.[138] For treatment of involuntary conversions of livestock due to disease or weather conditions, see ¶ 1713. For treatment of forced sales due to weather conditions (e.g., flood or drought), see ¶ 767.

1751. Canceled Leases and Distributor's Agreements. An amount received by a lessee for cancellation of a lease is treated as received in exchange for the lease. This rule applies also to amounts received by a distributor of goods for the cancellation of a distributor's agreement if the taxpayer has a substantial capital investment in the distributorship (Code Sec. 1241; Reg. § 1.1241-1).[139] If the lease or agreement is section 1231 property (¶ 1747), the taxpayer has a section 1231 gain or loss (Rev. Rul. 2007-37).[140]

Capital Loss Limitation, Carryover, Carryback

1752. Limitation on Capital Losses. To determine the deductibility of capital losses (¶ 1735), the taxpayer totals all capital gains and losses, both long term and short term, incurred during the year. Capital losses are deductible only to the extent of the capital gains plus, in the case of noncorporate taxpayers, up to $3,000 in ordinary income (Code Sec. 1211(b); Reg. § 1.1211-1(b)).[141] Thus, both net long-term capital losses and net short-term capital losses may be used to offset up to $3,000 of an individual's ordinary income ($1,500 for married individuals filing separate returns). There are special rules for married persons, whether filing joint or separate returns (¶ 1757). Unused losses are carried forward (¶ 1754).

> **Example:** Janet Green is a single individual with $30,000 of ordinary income, a net short-term capital loss of $3,500 and a net long-term capital loss of $300. Her capital loss deduction is limited to $3,000 for the current tax year. The remaining $800 is carried forward.

Corporations. A corporation may use capital losses to offset only capital gains and not ordinary income (Code Sec. 1211(a); Reg. § 1.1211-1(a)).[142] However, its capital losses may be carried back or carried forward (¶ 1756).

1754. Capital Loss Carryover of Noncorporate Taxpayers. Individuals and other noncorporate taxpayers may carry over a net capital loss (¶ 1739) to future tax years until the loss is used (Code Sec. 1212(b)).[143] A capital loss that is carried over to a later tax year retains its long-term or short-term character. In determining the amount of the capital loss that can be carried over, short-term capital gain is increased by the lesser of:

- the ordinary income offset (whether $3,000 or the amount of the overall net loss), or

- taxable income increased by the sum of that offset and the deduction for personal exemptions (¶ 133). Any excess of allowable deductions over gross income for the loss year is treated as negative taxable income for this purpose.

A short-term capital loss carryover first offsets short-term gain in the carryover year. Any remaining net short-term capital loss first offsets net long-term capital gain, and then up to $3,000 of ordinary income ($1,500 for married individuals filing separate returns) (¶ 1752). A long-term capital loss carryover first reduces long-term capital gain in the carryover year, then net short-term capital gain, and finally up to $3,000 of ordinary income.

References are to Standard Federal Tax Reports; Tax Research Consultant; and Practical Tax Explanations.

[137] ¶ 30,572, ¶ 30,574; FARM: 3,252; § 16,805
[138] ¶ 30,575.154; FARM: 3,252; § 16,805
[139] ¶ 30,750, ¶ 30,751; SALES: 24,354.05; § 16,520.30

[140] ¶ 30,752.24; SALES: 24,354.05; § 16,520.30
[141] ¶ 30,390, ¶ 30,391; SALES: 15,206.05; § 16,530
[142] ¶ 30,390, ¶ 30,391; SALES: 15,210, SALES: 15,212; § 16,535

[143] ¶ 30,400; SALES: 15,208; § 16,530

Example: Jack Crowe has taxable income of $30,000 and files a joint return. In computing taxable income, he reports a net short-term capital loss of $1,000 and a net long-term capital loss of $6,000. He uses his $1,000 net short-term loss to offset $1,000 of ordinary income; he then uses $2,000 of his net long-term capital loss to offset $2,000 of ordinary income. The remaining $4,000 of his net long-term capital loss is carried over to the following tax year ($4,000 is carried over because it is less than his taxable income of $30,000 increased by the ordinary income offset of $3,000 and the deduction for personal exemptions).

Code Sec. 1256 Contract Loss. An individual (but not an estate, trust, or corporation) may elect to carry back a net section 1256 contract loss (¶ 1947) to the three prior tax years (Code Sec. 1212(c)).[144]

1756. Corporate Capital Loss Carryover and Carryback. A corporation may carry back a net capital loss (¶ 1738) to each of the three tax years preceding the loss year (Code Sec. 1212(a); Reg. § 1.1212-1(a)).[145] Any excess may be carried forward for five years following the loss year. However, the carryback cannot cause or increase a net operating loss (¶ 1145) in the carryback year. Any carryback or carryover is treated as short-term capital loss for the carryover year. As such, it is grouped with any other capital losses for the carryover year and is used to offset any capital gains. Any undeducted loss remaining after the three-year carryback and the five-year carryover is not deductible.

Foreign expropriation losses can be carried over for 10 years but are ineligible for the three-year carryback. A foreign expropriation capital loss is the sum of the capital losses sustained (either directly or on securities that become worthless) by reason of the expropriation, intervention, seizure, or similar taking of property by the government of any foreign country, or any political subdivision, agency, or instrumentality thereof.

For tax years beginning after December 22, 2010, a regulated investment company or mutual fund (¶ 2301) can carry forward net capital losses indefinitely, and the treatment of the components of those losses as long-term or short-term is preserved (Code Sec. 1212(a)(3)). For tax years beginning before December 23, 2010, however, a mutual fund can carry net capital losses forward only for eight years, and any losses carried forward are treated as short-term capital losses in the carryover year (Code Sec. 1212(a)(1)(C)(i), prior to amendment by the Regulated Investment Company Modernization Act of 2010 (P.L. 111-325)).

A quick refund procedure is available for corporate net operating loss carrybacks or capital loss carrybacks (¶ 2773).

1757. Capital Gain or Loss of Spouses. Spouses who file a joint return compute all of their aggregate capital gains and losses (¶ 1735) as if they were the gains and losses of one person (Reg. § 1.1201-1(d)).[146] If the spouses file separate returns, the capital loss deduction (¶ 1752) for each is limited to $1,500 (one-half of the limit for a joint return) (Code Sec. 1211(b)(1)).[147] If they file separate returns for a year after a net capital loss was reported on a joint return, any carryover is allocated on the basis of the individual net capital loss of the spouses for the prior year (Reg. § 1.1212-1(c)).[148]

1758. Capital Gain or Loss of Partnerships and S Corporations. The capital gains and losses of a partnership or S corporation are generally segregated from its ordinary net income and carried separately into the income of the individual partners or shareholders. Partners (¶ 431) and shareholders (¶ 309) treat their distributive share of the capital gain or loss as if it were their own capital gain or loss. The same rule applies for Code Sec. 1231 transactions (¶ 1747) (Code Secs. 702(a) and 1366(a)).[149] S corporations may be taxed on capital gains in very limited situations (¶ 337).

References are to Standard Federal Tax Reports; Tax Research Consultant; and Practical Tax Explanations.

[144] ¶ 30,400; SALES: 48,108; § 45,420.10

[145] ¶ 30,400, ¶ 30,401; SALES: 15,214; § 16,535

[146] ¶ 30,353; SALES: 15,206.10; § 16,530

[147] ¶ 30,390; SALES: 15,206.10; § 16,530

[148] ¶ 30,401; SALES: 15,208; § 16,530

[149] ¶ 25,080, ¶ 32,080; PART: 18,104, SCORP: 402; § 28,405, § 30,410

Reporting. Generally, partnerships and S corporations use Form 8949 to report capital gains and losses not required to be reported on any other form. Partnerships then use Schedule D of Form 1065 to determine the overall gain or loss from the transactions reported on Form 8949. The net gains and losses from Schedule D are entered on Schedule K, and each partner's share is entered on Schedule K-1 of Form 1065. S corporations similarly use Schedule D of Form 1120S to determine the overall gain or loss from the transactions reported on Form 8949. The net gains and losses from Schedule D are entered on Schedule K, and each shareholder's share is entered on Schedule K-1 of Form 1120S. (Prior to 2012, partnerships and S corporations reported capital gains and losses only on Schedule D of their respective returns).

1760. Gains or Losses of Investors, Dealers, and Traders. In order to determine whether a taxpayer's gains or losses on securities are ordinary or capital in nature (¶ 1735), it must be determined if the taxpayer entered into the transaction as an investor, dealer, or trader.

Investors. An investor is a taxpayer whose activities are limited to occasional transactions for his or her own account. The level of activity is less than that associated with a trade or business.[150] Gains and losses of an investor are subject to the capital gains and loss rules (¶ 1736).

Dealers. A dealer regularly purchases securities from, and sells securities to, customers in the ordinary course of a trade or business. Because they are in the business of buying and selling, the gains and losses of dealers are classified as ordinary gain or loss unless the securities are held primarily for personal investment (Code Sec. 1236).[151] Securities that are held by a dealer for personal investment purposes must be clearly identified in the dealer's records before the close of the day on which they were acquired and must never be held primarily for sale to the dealer's customers. Similarly, capital gain and loss treatment does not apply to real estate sales by a dealer in realty unless the property was held as an investment (¶ 1762). See ¶ 1903 for further discussion of the mark-to-market requirement for dealers in securities.

Traders. A securities trader (including a "day trader") buys and sells securities for the trader's own account. A trader is one who seeks to profit from short-term changes in value rather than long-term investments. The taxpayer's trading activity must be substantial, frequent, regular, and continuous.[152] Because a trader's securities are not held primarily for sale to customers (¶ 1741), the gains and losses are generally treated as capital in nature, and are reported on Form 8949. However, traders that make a mark-to-market election report their gains and losses on Form 4797. Traders claim their business expenses on Schedule C of Form 1040 because they are in the business of trading. For the rules concerning the commissions paid by traders when buying and selling securities, see ¶ 1983.

Subdivision of Real Estate

1762. Subdivision and Sale of Real Estate. Noncorporate taxpayers and S corporations are not treated as real estate dealers solely because they subdivide a tract of land for sale (Code Sec. 1237(a)).[153] At least part of the gain on the sale of a lot or parcel is treated as capital gain when:

- the taxpayer has not previously held the tract or any lot or parcel thereof for sale in the ordinary course of business and, in the same tax year as the sale occurs, does not hold any other real estate for sale in the ordinary course of business (this rule automatically disqualifies a real estate dealer);

- no substantial improvements are made while the tract is held by the taxpayer or under a sale contract between the taxpayer and the buyer; and

---

References are to Standard Federal Tax Reports; Tax Research Consultant; and Practical Tax Explanations.

[150] ¶ 8521.1475; SALES: 45,052; §7,840.10
[151] ¶ 30,670; SALES: 45,054; § 18,805.05
[152] ¶ 30,422.6811; SALES: 45,058; § 18,805.15
[153] ¶ 30,690; REAL: 15,500; § 16,560.05

¶1762

- the taxpayer held the lot for at least five years (but there is no minimum holding period requirement if the taxpayer acquired the lot by inheritance or devise).

There is an exception to the substantial improvement rule above. Certain improvements, such as water, sewage, drainage, or road installations, are not considered substantial improvements if the property (including inherited property) is held for at least 10 years and would not have been marketable at the prevailing local price for similar building sites without such improvements (Code Sec. 1237(b)(3); Reg. § 1.1237-1(c)).[154] The taxpayer must also elect *not* to adjust the basis of the property (or other property) for the improvement costs or deduct them as expenses. The election is reported with the tax return for the year in which the lots covered by the election are sold. The election must include certain information, including a plat of the subdivision and a list of all the improvements.

The profits realized on the sales of the first five lots or parcels from the same tract are classified as capital gains (Code Sec. 1237(b)(1); Reg. § 1.1237-1(e)(2)).[155] However, beginning in the year in which the sixth sale or exchange is made, gain on each sale is taxed as ordinary income to the extent of five percent of the selling price. Selling expenses are deducted first from the five percent that would otherwise be considered ordinary income and then are used to reduce the capital gain on the sale or exchange (Code Sec. 1237(b)(2)). The selling expenses cannot be deducted from other income as ordinary business expenses.

Example 1: Mark subdivides a tract of land that he bought approximately 10 years ago and sells three lots for $50,000 each. The adjusted basis for each lot is $30,000. Selling expenses for each lot total $600. Mark has a long-term capital gain of $19,400 from the sale of each lot ($50,000 - $30,000 - $600).

Example 2: Same facts as in Example 1, except that Mark sells three additional lots under the same terms. Because he sold more than five lots, five percent of the selling price, or $2,500, could be characterized as ordinary income. However, this amount is reduced by his $600 in selling expenses. Thus, the sale of each lot produces $1,900 in ordinary income ($2,500 -$600), and $17,500 in long-term capital gain ($50,000 - $30,000 -$2,500).

If a taxpayer sells or exchanges any lots or parcels from a tract, and then does not sell or exchange any others for a period of five years from the last sale or exchange, the taxpayer can sell another five lots without having a portion of the gain taxed as ordinary income (Reg. § 1.1237-1(g)(2)).[156]

A taxpayer that buys a tract of land with the intent to subdivide and sell it as separate lots or parcels must measure gain or loss on every lot or parcel sold on the basis of an equitable (not ratable) apportionment (such as their relative assessed valuations for real estate tax purposes) of the cost of the subdivision (Reg. § 1.61-6(a)).[157]

Patents, Royalties, and Franchises

1767. Sale or Exchange of Patents. The transfer of all substantial rights to a patent, or an undivided interest in such rights, is treated as the sale of a capital asset (¶ 1741) held for more than 12 months (Code Sec. 1235(a); Reg. §§ 1.1235-1 and 1.1235-2).[158] The payment for the patent may be a lump-sum, a periodic payment, or contingent upon the productivity or use of the property transferred. These rules do not apply to transfers by gift or inheritance. The rules do apply to a transfer by the original inventor or another individual who acquired the patent from the original inventor before the invention was tested successfully under operating conditions. The inventor's employer and certain related persons are not eligible for long-term capital gain treatment if they acquire the patent from the inventor.

[154] ¶ 30,690, ¶ 30,691; REAL: 15,510; § 16,560.20

[155] ¶ 30,690, ¶ 30,691; REAL: 15,504; § 16,560.10

[156] ¶ 30,691; REAL: 15,506; § 16,560.10

[157] ¶ 5605; REAL: 15,504; § 3,015, § 16,560.10

[158] ¶ 30,650, ¶ 30,651, ¶ 30,652; SALES: 24,050; § 18,705.05

1772. Timber, Coal or Iron Ore. A taxpayer may elect to treat the cutting of timber (for sale or for use in a trade or business) as a sale or exchange of the timber during the year. The taxpayer must have owned the timber or held the contract right to cut the timber for more than one year (Code Sec. 631; Reg. § 1.631-1).[159] Under Code Sec. 1231, this timber is considered to be property used in the trade or business, so that gain may be treated as long-term capital gain under certain conditions (¶ 1747). In order to make the election, a taxpayer must generally file Form T with the tax return for the year in which the election is to be effective.

Timber, coal, or domestic iron ore royalties are generally subject to Code Sec. 1231 treatment when the owner or a holder (including a lessee) disposes of the timber, coal or ore while retaining an economic interest in it (Code Sec. 631(b) and (c); Reg. § § 1.631-2 and 1.631-3).[160] An outright sale of timber also qualifies. This treatment is not available for iron ore mined outside the United States, or for coal or iron ore dispositions between related parties or persons owned and controlled by the same interests.

1774. Transfers of Franchises, Trademarks, or Trade Names. Amounts received from the transfer of a franchise, trademark, or trade name are generally treated as ordinary income if the transferor retains any significant power, right, or continuing interest over the transferred asset (Code Sec. 1253).[161] Ordinary income treatment also applies to amounts received from the transfer, sale, or other disposition of a franchise, trademark, or trade name that are contingent on the transferred asset's productivity, use, or disposition. Amounts paid or incurred on account of the transfer of a franchise, trademark, or trade name are amortized over 15 years under Code Sec. 197 (¶ 1288). Amortization is claimed on Form 4562.

Contingent serial payments paid or incurred on account of a transfer, sale, or other disposition of a trademark, trade name, or franchise may be treated as a deductible business expense (¶ 901) if the payments are contingent on the asset's productivity, use, or disposition; and the contingent amounts are paid as part of a series of payments that are: (1) payable at least annually throughout the term of the transfer agreement; and (2) substantially equal in amount or payable under a fixed formula (Code Sec. 1253(d)(1)).

Disposition of Depreciable Property

1779. Depreciation Recapture Rules. A taxpayer that sells or disposes of depreciable or amortizable property must treat realized gain as ordinary income (rather than capital gain) to the extent of depreciation or amortization deductions previously allowed or allowable for the property. The recapture of depreciation or amortization applies to section 1245 property (¶ 1785) and section 1250 property (¶ 1786). The recapture rules apply notwithstanding any other Code provision (Reg. § § 1.1245-6 and 1.1250-1(c)).[162]

Section 1245 Property. Gain realized from the disposition of section 1245 property is treated as ordinary income to the extent the adjusted basis of the property is exceeded by the lower of: (1) the recomputed basis of the property; (2) the amount realized upon a sale, exchange, or involuntary conversion of the property; or (3) the fair market value of the property in the case of any other disposition (Code Sec. 1245(a)).[163] For this purpose, recomputed basis is the property's adjusted basis plus previously allowed or allowable depreciation or amortization. Amortization deductions include amounts expensed for the following: Code Sec. 179 property (¶ 1208); clean-fuel vehicles and refueling property under Code Sec. 179A; capital costs of compliance with EPA sulfur regulations (¶ 1285); refinery property (¶ 1285A); energy efficient commercial buildings (¶ 1286); mine safety equipment (¶ 989A); film and television production costs (¶ 977B); and expenditures for removal of architectural and transportation barriers to the handicapped and elderly, reforestation, or tertiary injectants (¶ 1287).

References are to Standard Federal Tax Reports; Tax Research Consultant; and Practical Tax Explanations.

[159] ¶ 24,150, ¶ 24,151; FARM: 24,150; § 11,615.20, § 16,805
[160] ¶ 24,150, ¶ 24,153, ¶ 24,155; FARM: 18,250, FARM:

24,200; § 11,615.20, § 11,625.25, § 16,805
[161] ¶ 31,040; SALES: 24,300; § 18,745

[162] ¶ 30,908, ¶ 31,001; DEPR: 18,054; § 16,815
[163] ¶ 30,902; DEPR: 18,200; § 11,705.05

Section 1250 Property. Gain on the sale or other disposition of section 1250 property is treated as ordinary income to the extent of the excess of post-1969 depreciation allowances over the depreciation that would have been available under the straight-line method (¶ 1780) (Code Sec. 1250).[164] However, if section 1250 property is held for one year or less, all depreciation (and not just the excess over straight-line depreciation) is recaptured (Code Sec. 1250(b)(1)). See ¶ 1736 for capital gains treatment of unrecaptured Section 1250 gain. In the case of a sale to a related party (¶ 1717), gain that is not recaptured may still be treated as ordinary income (¶ 1744). Different holding periods and recapture percentages may apply to substantial improvements made to section 1250 property that are considered separate property for recapture purposes, and also to property that consists of more than one element (Code Sec. 1250(f)).[165]

For residential rental property, certain types of government assisted housing, subsidized housing, section 1250 property for which rapid depreciation of rehabilitation expenditures was claimed, and property mortgaged under the Housing Act of 1949, depreciation recapture is reduced by one percent for each full month the property is held over a specified period (Code Sec. 1250(a)(1)(B) and (2)(B)).

Dispositions. Depreciation recapture is triggered by the disposition of depreciable property, including sales, exchanges, and involuntary conversions. Special rules apply for transfers by gift or at death (¶ 1788), certain tax-free corporate or partnership transactions (¶ 1789), disposal in a like-kind exchange or involuntary conversion where gain is not recognized (¶ 1790), and property distributed by a partnership (¶ 1792). A disposition of section 1245 property includes a sale in a sale-and-leaseback transaction and a transfer upon the foreclosure of a security interest, but does not include a mere transfer of title to a creditor upon creation of a security interest or to a debtor upon termination of a security interest (Reg. § 1.1245-1).[166]

Installment Sale. In the case of disposal of section 1245 or section 1250 property in an installment sale, any income recaptured as ordinary income is recognized in the year of the disposition, and any gain in excess of the recapture income is reported under the installment method (¶ 1823).

Investment Credit Basis Reductions. For recapture purposes, the amount of an investment credit downward basis adjustment is treated as a deduction allowed for depreciation (¶ 1365A).

Additional Recapture for Corporations. For C corporations, the amount treated as ordinary income on the sale or other disposition of section 1250 property is increased by 20 percent of the additional amount that would be treated as ordinary income if the property were subject to recapture under the rules for section 1245 property (Code Sec. 291(a)(1)).[167]

Reporting Recapture. Form 4797 is used to calculate and report the amount of recaptured depreciation. A taxpayer subject to recapture of an investment credit downward basis adjustment must file Form 4255.

1780. Depreciation Subject to Recapture. In general, depreciation on tangible property placed in service after 1986 is determined under the Modified Accelerated Cost Recovery System (MACRS). Property placed in service after 1980 and before 1987 is covered under the Accelerated Cost Recovery System (ACRS). See ¶ 1216 and following for the methods of computing allowable depreciation deductions.

MACRS. Gain on the disposition of tangible personal property is treated as ordinary income to the extent of previously-allowed MACRS deductions (¶ 1779). If property from a general asset account is disposed of, the full amount of proceeds realized on the disposition is treated as ordinary income to the extent the unadjusted depreciable basis of the account (increased by amounts allowed as deductions under Code Secs. 179 and 190 for assets in the account) exceeds previously recognized ordinary income from prior dispositions (Code Sec. 168(i)(4); Reg. § 1.168(i)-1(e)).[168]

References are to Standard Federal Tax Reports; Tax Research Consultant; and Practical Tax Explanations.

[164] ¶ 31,000; DEPR: 18,250; § 11,710
[165] ¶ 31,000; DEPR: 18,264

[166] ¶ 30,903; DEPR: 18,052; § 11,705.05
[167] ¶ 15,190; DEPR: 18,266; § 26,020.10

[168] ¶ 11,250, ¶ 11,275B; DEPR: 3,554; § 11,145

Residential rental property and nonresidential real property that is placed in service after 1986 and is subject to the MACRS rules must be depreciated under the straight-line MACRS method (¶ 1243). Thus, there is no recapture of depreciation upon disposition of such property because no depreciation in excess of straight-line depreciation could have been taken.

ACRS. Gain on the disposition of personal recovery property and nonresidential real recovery property is treated as ordinary income to the extent of previously-allowed ACRS deductions (¶ 1779).[169] Gain on the disposition of residential rental real recovery property is treated as ordinary income to the extent that ACRS deductions exceed straight-line ACRS depreciation over the recovery period applicable to such property. Consequently, there is no recapture if the straight-line ACRS method was elected for real property.

On the disposition of assets from mass asset accounts, taxpayers recognize the amount of the proceeds realized as ordinary income to the extent of the unadjusted basis in the account less any amounts previously included in income. Any excess proceeds realized are treated as capital gain, unless a nonrecognition provision applies. Regarding the recovery of depreciation, the mass asset account is treated as though there was no disposition of the asset, and the unadjusted basis of the property is left in the capital account until fully recovered in future years (Prop. Reg. § 1.168-2(h)).[170]

Amounts Excluded from Depreciation Adjustments. In determining the amount of additional depreciation taken before the disposition of section 1250 property, a taxpayer's depreciation adjustments do *not* include amortization of emergency facilities, pollution control facilities, railroad grading and tunnel bores, child care facilities, expenditures to remove architectural and transportation barriers to the handicapped and elderly, or tertiary injectant expenses (Code Sec. 1250(b)(3)).[171]

1785. Code Sec. 1245 Property. Code Sec. 1245 property is property that is or has been depreciable (or subject to amortization under Code Sec. 197) and is either:

- personal property (tangible and intangible); or

- other tangible property (not including a building or its structural components) used as an integral part of:

  — manufacturing, production, or extraction; or

  — the furnishing of transportation, communications, electrical energy, gas, water, or sewage disposal services (Code Sec. 1245(a)(3); Reg. § 1.1245-3).[172]

The term "other tangible property" includes research facilities or facilities for the bulk storage of fungible commodities used in connection with the activities listed above. A leasehold of section 1245 property is also treated as section 1245 property. Livestock is considered section 1245 property, and depreciation on purchased draft, breeding, dairy and sporting livestock is recaptured as ordinary income when sold. Raised livestock generally has no basis for depreciation, but to the extent that it does have a basis and is depreciated, it is subject to recapture (IRS Pub. 225).

Section 1245 property also includes any real property that has an adjusted basis reflecting adjustments for special amortization for the following: Code Sec. 179 property (¶ 1208); clean-fuel vehicles and refueling property under Code Sec. 179A; capital costs of compliance with EPA sulfur regulations (¶ 1285); refinery property (¶ 1285A); energy efficient commercial buildings (¶ 1286); mine safety equipment (¶ 989A); railroad grading and tunnel bores; child care facilities; and expenditures for removal of architectural and transportation barriers to the handicapped and elderly, reforestation, or tertiary injectants (¶ 1287). Section 1245 property also includes single purpose agricultural and horticultural structures, and storage facilities used in connection with the distribution of petroleum products.

References are to Standard Federal Tax Reports; Tax Research Consultant; and Practical Tax Explanations.

[169] ¶ 30,909.023; DEPR: 18,166; § 11,001

[170] ¶ 11,252; DEPR: 3,560

[171] ¶ 31,000; DEPR: 18,262; § 11,710

[172] ¶ 30,902, ¶ 30,905; DEPR: 18,150; § 11,705.10

1786. Code Sec. 1250 Property. Code Sec. 1250 property is any real property that is or has been depreciable under Code Sec. 167 but is not subject to recapture under Code Sec. 1245. This includes all intangible real property (such as leases of land or section 1250 property), buildings and their structural components, and all other tangible real property except section 1245 property (Code Sec. 1250(c); Reg. § 1.1250-1(e)).[173] For real property that is section 1245 property rather than section 1250 property, see ¶ 1785.

1788. Disposition of Depreciable Property by Gift or Death. The recapture of depreciation as ordinary income when section 1245 or section 1250 property is sold or otherwise disposed (¶ 1779) does not apply to dispositions by gift or transfers at death (except a taxable transfer of section 1245 or section 1250 property in satisfaction of a specific bequest of money) (Code Secs. 1245(b) and 1250(d); Reg. § § 1.1245-4 and 1.1250-3).[174] Upon a later sale, however, the donee realizes the same amount of ordinary income that the donor would have realized had the donor retained the property and sold it (except in the case of a tax-exempt donee). Also, if the taxpayer contributes section 1245 or section 1250 property to a charitable organization, the allowable charitable contribution deduction is reduced by the amount that would have been treated as ordinary income had the taxpayer sold the asset at its fair market value (¶ 1062).

1789. Disposition of Depreciable Property in Tax-Free Corporate or Partnership Transaction. When section 1245 or section 1250 property is disposed of in certain tax-free transactions (i.e., Code Secs. 332, 351, 361, 721, or 731), the transferor takes into account the deprecation recapture treated as ordinary income (¶ 1779) only to the extent that gain is recognized under those sections (Code Secs. 1245(b)(3) and 1250(d)(3); Reg. § § 1.1245-4(c) and 1.1250-3(c)).[175] However, when there is an otherwise tax-free transfer to a tax-exempt organization (other than a cooperative described in Code Sec. 521), the gain is recognized in full to the transferor. On a later sale of section 1245 or section 1250 property received in one of these tax-free transactions, the transferee realizes depreciation recapture to the extent of the transferor's unrecognized unrecaptured section 1245 or section 1250 gain plus depreciation deducted by the transferee (not to exceed the actual gain).

1790. Disposition of Depreciable Property in Like-Kind Exchange or Involuntary Conversion. If section 1245 or section 1250 property is exchanged for like-kind property (¶ 1721) or is involuntarily converted (¶ 1713), depreciation recapture (¶ 1779) is recognized to the extent of any gain recognized on the exchange (if money or other property is received) or on the conversion (when the conversion proceeds are not all spent on replacement property), plus the fair market value of any property received in the exchange or acquired as replacement property that is not section 1245 or section 1250 property (Code Secs. 1245(b)(4) and 1250(d)(4); Reg. § § 1.1245-4(d) and 1.1250-3(d)).[176] When this occurs, the basis of the acquired property is determined under the like-kind exchange or involuntary conversion rules (Reg. § § 1.1245-5 and 1.1250-3(d)).[177]

> **Example:** Greg exchanges section 1245 property with an adjusted basis of $10,000 for like-kind property with a fair market value of $9,000 and unlike property with a fair market value of $3,500. He must recognize gain of $2,500 because he received unlike property. His basis in the acquired property is $12,500 ($10,000 adjusted basis of the transferred property plus $2,500 recognized gain), of which $3,500 (fair market value) is allocated to the unlike property and the remaining $9,000 is allocated to the like-kind property.

References are to Standard Federal Tax Reports; Tax Research Consultant; and Practical Tax Explanations.

[173] ¶ 31,000, ¶ 31,001; DEPR: 18,252; § 11,710

[174] ¶ 30,902, ¶ 30,906, ¶ 31,000, ¶ 31,003; DEPR:

18,102, DEPR: 18,104; § 11,705.15, § 11,710

[175] ¶ 30,902, ¶ 30,906, ¶ 31,000, ¶ 31,003; DEPR: 18,106; § 11,705.15, § 11,710

[176] ¶ 30,902, ¶ 30,906, ¶ 31,000, ¶ 31,003; DEPR: 18,108; § 18,145.05

[177] ¶ 30,907, ¶ 31,003; SALES: 30,452; § 11,705.20, § 11,710

1792. Partnership Distribution of Depreciable Property. For purposes of the depreciation recapture rules (¶ 1779), the basis of section 1245 or section 1250 property distributed by a partnership to a partner is determined by reference to the partnership's adjusted basis in the property (Code Secs. 1245(b)(5) and 1250(d)(5); Reg. §§ 1.1245-4(f) and 1.1250-3(f)).[178]

For recomputing the basis of the property in the hands of the partner, the amount of the depreciation or amortization adjustments for section 1245 property, or the additional depreciation for distributed section 1250 property, attributable to pre-distribution periods is equal to: (1) the amount of gain that would have been treated as ordinary income under the recapture rules had the partnership sold the property at fair market value immediately before the distribution; minus (2) any gain treated as ordinary income under the partnership rules for distributions of receivables or inventory items (¶ 436).

1793. Corporate Distribution of Depreciable Property. A corporation that distributes a dividend consisting of section 1245 or section 1250 property might be required to recognize ordinary income under the depreciation recapture rules (¶ 1779), even though it would not normally recognize gain under the corporate distribution rules (¶ 736) (Reg. §§ 1.1245-1(a), 1.1245-6(b), and 1.1250-1(c)).[179]

A corporation's transfer of section 1245 property or section 1250 property to a shareholder for less than fair market value is not treated as a sale, exchange, or involuntary conversion for depreciation recapture purposes (Reg. §§ 1.1245-1(c) and 1.1250-1(a)). Accordingly, the corporation's gain for recapture purposes is the amount by which the property's adjusted basis is exceeded by the lower of the property's fair market value on the disposition date or the property's recomputed basis.

If a corporation transfers section 1245 property or section 1250 property to a shareholder in a sale or exchange for less than fair market value, the disposition will not be treated as a sale, exchange, or involuntary conversion for depreciation recapture purposes (Reg. §§ 1.1245-1(c) and 1.1250-1(a)). Accordingly, the corporation's gain for recapture purposes will be the amount by which the property's adjusted basis is exceeded by the lower of the property's fair market value on the disposition date or the property's recomputed basis.

If the transferee's basis in the property is determined solely by the corporate distribution rules (¶ 735), no depreciation adjustments are reflected in the adjusted basis of section 1245 property, and no additional depreciation is reflected in the adjusted basis of section 1250 property, on the date that the transferee acquires the property (Reg. §§ 1.1245-2(c) and 1.1250-2(e)).[180]

Farmers' Recapture

1797. Recapture on Land Sale. If farm land held for less than 10 years is disposed of, the lesser of the gain realized or a percentage of the total post-1969 deductions for soil and water conservation and land clearing expenses must be recaptured as ordinary income on Form 4797 (Code Sec. 1252).[181] The recapture percentage is 100 percent if the land is held for five years or less, and declines 20 percent for each additional year (to 80 percent in the sixth year, 60 percent in the seventh year, 40 percent in the eighth year, and 20 percent in the ninth year). There is no recapture after the ninth year. See ¶ 982 concerning deductions for conservation expenses. Exceptions to this recapture rule exist for transfers by gift, transfers at death, and transfers in certain tax-free transactions (Reg. § 1.1252-2).[182]

References are to Standard Federal Tax Reports; Tax Research Consultant; and Practical Tax Explanations.

[178] ¶ 30,902, ¶ 30,906, ¶ 31,000, ¶ 31,003; DEPR: 18,106.05; § 30,535.20, § 30,555

[179] ¶ 30,903, ¶ 30,908, ¶ 31,001; DEPR: 18,054

[180] ¶ 30,904, ¶ 31,002; DEPR: 18,204.05, DEPR: 18,262

[181] ¶ 31,020; FARM: 9,168; § 36,030.10

[182] ¶ 31,022; FARM: 9,168.20; § 36,030.10

17

CAPITAL GAINS

Chapter 18

INSTALLMENT SALES

DEFERRED PAYMENTS

Installment Method

1801. Use of Installment Method. The installment method is a special way of reporting gains (not losses) from sales of property when at least one payment is received in a tax year after the year of sale (deferred payments). Under the installment method, gain from the sale is prorated and recognized over the years in which payments are received (Code Sec. 453).[1] As a result, each payment received usually consists of interest, return of basis, and gain on the sale.

The installment method must be used for installment sales unless the taxpayer elects not to use the installment method (¶ 1803) or it is otherwise prohibited. This rule applies to both cash and accrual basis taxpayers (¶ 1515). The installment method generally is not available for most sales by dealers (¶ 1808), sales of property of a type that would be included in inventory (¶ 1553), sales of personal property under a revolving credit plan (¶ 1805), sales of publicly traded property (¶ 1805), or sales of depreciable property between related taxpayers (¶ 1835). Thus, payments for such sales are treated as if they are received in the year of disposition, even if the taxpayer expects to receive some payments in future years.

Gain Calculation. The amount of gain from an installment sale that is taxable in a given year is calculated by multiplying the payments received in that year by the gross profit ratio for the sale (Code Sec. 453(c)).[2] The gross profit ratio is equal to the anticipated gross profit divided by the total contract price (¶ 1813). However, gain from installment sales of depreciable property subject to recapture under Code Sec. 1245 or Code Sec. 1250 is determined under a special rule (¶ 1823).

> **Example:** On December 1, 2014, Bob Smith sells vacant land that he has held for investment purposes for a number of years. His basis in the land is $12,000. The total contract price is $15,000. Bob receives a $5,000 down payment, with the $10,000 balance due in monthly installments of $500 each, plus interest at the applicable federal rate, beginning on January 1, 2015. His anticipated gross profit from the sale is $3,000. His gross profit percentage is 20% ($3,000 gross profit ÷ $15,000 contract price). Under the installment method, Bob must report $1,000

References are to Standard Federal Tax Reports; Tax Research Consultant; and Practical Tax Explanations.

[1] ¶ 21,402; SALES: 36,050; § 18,301   [2] ¶ 21,402; SALES: 36,100; § 18,320

¶1801

($5,000 × 20%) as long-term capital gain in 2014, $1,200 ($6,000 × 20%) in 2015, and $800 ($4,000 × 20%) in 2016. The interest is reported as ordinary income.

Although use of the installment method determines when gain from an installment sale is reported, it does not affect the characterization of the gain as capital gain or ordinary income. The proper characterization depends on the nature of the asset sold (¶ 1735 and ¶ 1741).

Reporting Requirements for Gain. Gain from an installment sale is reported on Form 6252, which must be filed with the tax return in the year of sale and in each year payments are received. The gain calculated on Form 6252 is carried over and entered on Schedule D of the taxpayer's return or Form 4797, or both, as appropriate.

1803. Election Not to Use Installment Method. If a taxpayer elects not to use the installment method (¶ 1801), the entire gain is reported in the year of the sale, even though not all of the sale proceeds are received in that year (Code Sec. 453(d); Temp. Reg. § 15A.453-1(d)).[3] The election is made by individuals, corporations, partnerships, estates, and trusts by simply reporting the gain on Form 8949 or Form 4797, whichever applies. (Prior to the 2011 tax year for individuals, the 2012 tax year for corporations and partnerships, and the 2013 tax year for estates and trusts, these taxpayers made the election by reporting the gain on either Form 4797 or Schedule D of their respective tax return, whichever applied.) The election must be made by the due date, including extensions, of the tax return for the year in which the installment sale occurs. If a taxpayer files a timely return without an election out, the taxpayer can elect out by filing an amended return within six months of the due date, excluding extensions (Reg. § 301.9100-2). The IRS will otherwise permit late elections only in rare circumstances if the taxpayer can show good cause for not making the election by the due date. An election out can be revoked only with IRS approval, but revocation is not allowed if one of its purposes is to avoid federal income tax, or if the tax year in which any payment was received has closed.

1805. Publicly Traded Property and Revolving Credit Plans. The installment method (¶ 1801) may *not* be used for: (1) sales of personal property under a revolving credit plan; (2) sales of stock or securities that are traded on an established securities market; or (3) to the extent provided by regulations, sales of other kinds of property that are regularly traded on an established market. All payments to be received from such sales are treated as received in the year of disposition (Code Sec. 453(k)).[4]

1808. Dealer Dispositions by Installment Sale. Dealers in real or personal property may not use the installment method to report the gain from dealer dispositions (Code Sec. 453(b)(2)(A) and (l)(1)).[5] A dealer disposition includes:

- any disposition of personal property by a person who regularly sells or otherwise disposes of such property on an installment plan; and

- any disposition of real property that is held by the taxpayer for sale to customers in the ordinary course of the taxpayer's trade or business.

Certain types of installment transactions by a dealer, however, are not considered dealer dispositions and as a result the installment method of reporting may be used (Code Sec. 453(l)(2)).[6] These include:

- the disposition of any property used or produced in the trade or business of farming;

- the disposition in the ordinary course of the taxpayer's trade or business of:

    — any residential lot, provided that the dealer or any related person is not obligated to make any improvements to the lot; or

---

References are to Standard Federal Tax Reports; Tax Research Consultant; and Practical Tax Explanations.

[3] ¶ 21,402, ¶ 21,404; SALES: 36,056; § 18,315

[4] ¶ 21,402; SALES: 36,052.05; § 18,310.20, § 18,310.25

[5] ¶ 21,402; SALES: 36,250; § 18,310.10

[6] ¶ 21,402; SALES: 36,054; § 18,310.10

18

INSTALLMENT SALE

— a timeshare right to use or own residential real property for not more than six weeks per year, or a right to use specified campgrounds for recreational purposes.

A timeshare right to use or own property held by an individual's spouse, children, grandchildren, or parents is treated as held by the individual.

Payment of Interest. To use the installment method for the sale of residential lots and timeshares, the taxpayer must pay interest on the amount of tax attributable to the installment payments received during the year. The interest is calculated for the period beginning on the date of sale and ending on the date the payment is received (Code Sec. 453(l)(3)).[7] The amount of interest is based upon the applicable federal rate in effect at the time of sale, compounded semiannually (¶ 1875).

Computation of Income

1813. Amount of Income for Installment Sales. For nondealer dispositions of property (¶ 1808) that are not subject to the depreciation recapture provisions of Code Sec. 1245 or Code Sec. 1250, the amount of income reported from an installment sale in any tax year (including the year of sale) is equal to the payments received during the year multiplied by the gross profit ratio for the sale (Code Sec. 453(c); Temp. Reg. § 15A.453-1(b)(2)).[8] Payments include all amounts actually or constructively received in the tax year under the installment obligation (¶ 1819).

The gross profit ratio is the gross profit on the installment sale divided by the total contract price. The gross profit is the selling price of the property minus its adjusted basis. The selling price of the property is not reduced by any existing mortgage or encumbrance, or by any selling expenses, but is reduced by any imputed interest (¶ 1859).

The total contract price (denominator of gross profit ratio) is the selling price minus that portion of qualifying indebtedness (¶ 1815) which the buyer assumes or takes the property subject to that does not exceed the seller's basis in the property (adjusted to reflect commissions and other selling expenses). In the case of an installment sale that is a partially nontaxable like-kind exchange (¶ 1723), the gross profit is reduced by that portion of the gain that is not recognized, and the total contract price is reduced by the value of the like-kind property received (Code Sec. 453(f)(6)).[9]

For certain nondealer sales of property over $150,000, a special interest charge may apply (¶ 1825).

1815. Qualifying Indebtedness for Installment Sales. For the purpose of determining the total contract price of an installment sale of property (¶ 1813), qualifying indebtedness includes:

(1) any mortgage or other indebtedness encumbering the property; and

(2) any indebtedness not secured by the property but incurred or assumed by the purchaser incident to the acquisition, holding or operation of the property in the ordinary course of business or investment (Temp. Reg. § 15A.453-1(b)(2)(iv)).[10]

Qualifying indebtedness does not include an obligation of the seller incurred incident to the *disposition* of the property, or an obligation functionally unrelated to the acquisition, holding or operation of the property. Any obligation incurred or assumed in contemplation of disposition of the property is not qualifying indebtedness if recovery of the seller's basis is accelerated.

Wrap-Around Mortgage. When property encumbered by an outstanding mortgage is sold in exchange for an installment obligation equal to the mortgage, the installment

---

References are to Standard Federal Tax Reports; Tax Research Consultant; and Practical Tax Explanations.

[7] ¶ 21,402; SALES: 36,054.10; § 18,310.10

[8] ¶ 21,402, ¶ 21,404; SALES: 36,100; § 18,320

[9] ¶ 21,402; SALES: 36,114.05; § 18,350

[10] ¶ 21,404; SALES: 36,106; § 18,320

¶1813

obligation is said to "wrap around" the mortgage. The seller generally uses the payments received from the installment obligation to pay the "wrapped" mortgage. In this situation, the IRS will follow the Tax Court's position and will not treat the buyer as having taken the property subject to, or as having assumed, the seller's mortgage (*Professional Equities, Inc.,* 89 TC 165, Dec. 44,064 (1987) (Acq.)).[11] As a result, the seller does not have to reduce the total contract price by the amount of the wrapped mortgage.

1819. Installment Payments. When determining the amount of reportable income under the installment method (¶ 1813), a payment includes all amounts actually or constructively received in the tax year under an installment obligation, as well as:

(1) evidence of indebtedness of a person other than the buyer;

(2) evidence of indebtedness of the buyer that is payable on demand or readily tradable, including a bond issued with coupons or in registered form;

(3) a bank certificate or treasury note;

(4) qualifying indebtedness (¶ 1815) assumed or taken subject to by the buyer, to the extent it exceeds the seller's basis for the sold property as adjusted for selling expenses;

(5) seller's indebtedness to the buyer that is canceled; and

(6) indebtedness on the sold property (for which the seller is not personally liable) when the buyer is the obligee of the indebtedness (Code Sec. 453(f)(3), (f)(4), and (f)(5); Temp. Reg. § 15A.453-1(b)(3)).[12]

Debt instruments in registered form that the seller can establish are not readily tradable are not considered payments. In addition, like-kind property received in a partially tax-free exchange (¶ 1723) that is part of an installment sale transaction is not treated as a payment for purposes of determining the amount of income to be reported under the installment method (Code Sec. 453(f)(6)).[13]

1821. Contingent Payment Sales. A contingent payment sale must be reported on the installment method (¶ 1801) unless the seller elects not to use the installment method (Temp. Reg. § 15A.453-1(c)).[14] A contingent payment sale is a sale or other disposition of property in which the total selling price is not determinable by the close of the tax year in which the sale or disposition occurs. It does not include transactions with respect to which the installment obligation represents, under applicable principles of tax law: (1) a retained interest in the property which is the subject of the transaction; (2) an interest in a joint venture or partnership; (3) an equity interest in a corporation; (4) or similar transaction, regardless of the existence of a stated maximum selling price or a fixed payment term.

In a contingent payment sale, the basis of the property sold (including selling expenses, but not those of real estate dealers) is allocated to payments received in each tax year and recovered as follows:

- for sales with a stated maximum selling price, basis is recovered according to a profit ratio based on the stated maximum selling price;

- for sales with a fixed payment period, basis is recovered ratably over the fixed period; and

- for sales with neither a maximum selling price nor a fixed payment period, basis is recovered ratably over a 15-year period.

Alternate methods of basis recovery may be required when the normal method would substantially and inappropriately accelerate or defer the recovery of basis.

References are to Standard Federal Tax Reports; Tax Research Consultant; and Practical Tax Explanations.

[11] ¶ 21,412.80; SALES: 36,106; § 18,320

[12] ¶ 21,402, ¶ 21,404; SALES: 36,102; § 18,325

[13] ¶ 21,402; SALES: 36,114.05; § 18,350

[14] ¶ 21,404; SALES: 36,112; § 18,330.05

1823. Installment Sale of Property Subject to Depreciation Recapture. For install-ment sales of real or personal property to which the depreciation recapture provisions of Code Sec. 1245 or Code Sec. 1250 apply (¶ 1779), any recapture income must be reported in the year of disposition, whether or not an installment payment is received in that year (Code Sec. 453(i)).[15] The amount of ordinary income reported in the year of sale is added to the property's basis, and this adjusted basis is used in determining the remaining profit on the disposition. The remaining profit amount is used to compute the gross profit percentage to be applied to each installment payment.

> **Example:** On December 1, 2014, Bob sells a rental building for a total contract price of $100,000, plus interest at the applicable federal rate. He receives a note due in yearly installments of $20,000, plus interest, beginning January 1, 2015. Bob's adjusted basis in the building is $20,000. Assume that $10,000 of the total $80,000 gain is attributable to depreciation that must be recaptured as ordinary income under Code Sec. 1250 (¶ 1780). The $10,000 must be included in Bob's ordinary income for 2014 (the year of sale). The $10,000 is added to his $20,000 adjusted basis for purposes of determining the gross profit on the remaining gain. There-fore, gross profit is, $70,000 ($100,000 − $30,000). Of each $20,000 payment received in the following years, $14,000 is includible in income ($20,000 × ($70,000 ÷ $100,000)).

If a portion of the capital gain from an installment sale of depreciable real property consists of unrecaptured section 1250 gain, and another portion consists of other capital gains (¶ 1736), the taxpayer is required to take the unrecaptured section 1250 gain into account before the other capital gains are received (Reg. § 1.453-12).[16]

1825. Special Interest Rule for Nondealers of Property. A special interest charge may apply to an installment obligation that arises from a nondealer disposition of real or personal property (¶ 1813) under the installment method if the sales price is over $150,000 (Code Sec. 453A).[17] The interest charge does not apply to nondealer disposi-tions of property used in the business of farming or personal use property. For this purpose, personal use property is property that is not substantially used in connection with the taxpayer's trade or business or in an investment activity. The interest charge also does not apply to dispositions of timeshares and residential lots (but the interest payment rule described in ¶ 1808 does apply).

Generally, the interest charge is imposed on the tax deferred under the installment method with respect to outstanding installment obligations. However, the interest charge will not apply unless the face amount of all obligations held by the taxpayer that arose during and remain outstanding at the close of the tax year exceeds $5 million.

If any indebtedness is secured by a nondealer installment obligation that arises from the disposition of any real or personal property having a sales price over $150,000, the net proceeds of the secured indebtedness will be treated as a payment received on the installment obligation on the later of the date that the indebtedness is secured or the date that the net proceeds are received.

The interest is not reported on Form 6252, but rather is entered as an additional tax on the taxpayer's return. For individuals, it is included on the line for "Other taxes" on Form 1040. For estates and trusts, it is included on the line for "Total tax" on Schedule G of Form 1041. For corporations, it is entered on Schedule J of Form 1120.

Related-Party Sales

1833. Installment Sale to Related Persons. When a person makes an installment sale of property (¶ 1801) to a related person who sells the property before the install-ment payments are made in full, the amount realized by the related person from the second sale is treated as being received by the initial seller at the time of the second sale (Code Sec. 453(e)).[18] However, the resale rule does not generally apply if the second sale takes place more than two years after the first sale. A related person for this purpose includes the seller's spouse, child, grandchild and other lineal descendants,

---

References are to Standard Federal Tax Reports; Tax Research Consultant; and Practical Tax Explanations.

[15] ¶ 21,402; SALES: 36,108; § 18,355.05

[16] ¶ 21,425; SALES: 36,100; § 18,355.05

[17] ¶ 21,450; SALES: 36,150; § 18,375.05

[18] ¶ 21,402; SALES: 36,200; § 18,360

parent, grandparent and other ancestors, brother, sister, controlled corporation, partnership, certain trusts, estate, or executor (Code Sec. 453(f)(1)).

In applying the resale rule, the amount treated as received by the initial seller is limited to:

> (1) the *lesser* of—
>
>> (a) the total amount realized from the second disposition before the close of the tax year of disposition; or
>>
>> (b) the total contract price for the first disposition;
>
> (2) *minus* the sum of—
>
>> (a) the total amount received from the first disposition before the close of the year of the second disposition; and
>>
>> (b) the total amount treated as received for prior years under the resale rule.

There are a number of exceptions to the resale rule. Any sale or exchange of stock to the issuing corporation is not treated as a first disposition. An involuntary conversion (¶ 1713), and any transfer thereafter, is not treated as a second disposition if the first disposition occurred before the threat or imminence of the conversion. Any transfer after the earlier of the death of the person making the first disposition or the death of the person acquiring the property in the first disposition, and any transfer thereafter, is not treated as a second disposition. Further, the resale rule does not apply if it is established to the IRS's satisfaction that neither disposition had federal income tax avoidance as one of its principal purposes.

1835. Installment Sale of Depreciable Property Between Related Persons. The installment method (¶ 1801) generally cannot be used for installment sales of depreciable property between related persons. As a result, all payments are deemed received in the year of sale. However, the installment method may be used if the IRS is satisfied that tax avoidance was not one of the principal purposes of the sale (Code Sec. 453(g)).[19] For this purpose, the term "related person" is defined in Code Sec. 1239(b) (¶ 1744) and includes corporations and partnerships that are more than 50-percent owned, either directly or indirectly, by the same person.

Repossessions of Property

1838. Repossession of Personal Property. When personal property that was sold in an installment sale (¶ 1801) is repossessed, the repossession is treated as a disposition of the installment obligation (¶ 1846) (IRS Pub. 537).[20] Gain or loss is measured by subtracting the seller's basis in the obligation from the fair market value of the property on the date of repossession (and the value of any other property received from the buyer). If the seller did not use the installment method to report the gain on the original sale, the seller's basis in the obligation is equal to the face value of the obligation minus all principal payments that the seller received on the obligation. If the seller used the installment method to report the gain on the original sale, the seller's basis in the obligation is determined by multiplying the unpaid balance of the obligation by the seller's gross profit percentage, and then subtracting that amount from the unpaid balance. The character of the gain or loss, if any, on the repossession is the same as on the original sale.

If the installment obligation is not completely satisfied by repossession of the property, and the seller is unable to collect the balance of the debt, the seller may be able to claim a bad debt deduction for the portion of the obligation that is not satisfied through repossession (¶ 1135 and ¶ 1143).

References are to Standard Federal Tax Reports; Tax Research Consultant; and Practical Tax Explanations.

[19] ¶ 21,402; SALES: 36,204; § 18,310.30

[20] ¶ 21,406.048; SALES: 36,452; § 18,365.10

1841. Repossession of Real Property. When real property is sold on the installment method (¶ 1801) and the seller accepts an installment debt secured by the property, the seller will recognize only a limited amount of gain and no loss upon repossession of the property (Code Sec. 1038; Reg. § 1.1038-1).[21] Gain on the repossession is limited to the lesser of:

(1) the amount by which the amount of money and the fair market value of other property (other than obligations of the purchaser) received, prior to the reacquisition, with respect to the sale of such property, exceeds the amount of the gain on the sale of such property returned as income for periods prior to the reacquisition; or

(2) the amount by which the price at which the real property was sold exceeded its adjusted basis, reduced by the sum of (a) the amount of the gain on the sale of such property returned as income for periods prior to the reacquisition of such property, and (b) the amount of money and the fair market value of other property (other than obligations of the purchaser received with respect to the sale of such property) paid or transferred by the seller in connection with the reacquisition of such property.

The same rules apply when an estate or beneficiary repossesses real property that had been sold by a decedent on the installment method (Code Sec. 1038(g)).[22]

Repossession of Principal Residence. Special rules apply if a seller repossesses a principal residence that was sold under the installment method and gain realized from the sale was excluded from gross income (¶ 1705). If the seller resells the residence within one year of repossession, the original sale and the resale are treated as one transaction and realized gain is determined on the combined sale and resale (Code Sec. 1038(e); Reg. § 1.1038-2).[23] If the resale does not take place within one year, the general rules for repossessions of real property apply.

1843. Basis After Repossession of Real Property. The seller's basis in repossessed real property (¶ 1841) is generally the adjusted basis of the debt secured by the property (determined at the time of the repossession), increased by any gain recognized at the time of the repossession and by the seller's repossession costs (Code Sec. 1038(c)).[24] If the debt to the seller is not discharged as a result of the repossession, the basis of the debt is zero. If, before repossession, the seller has treated the secured debt as having become worthless or partially worthless, then, upon repossession, the seller is considered to have received an amount equal to the amount that was treated as worthless. However, the seller's adjusted basis in the debt is increased by the same amount (Code Sec. 1038(d)).

Dispositions of Installment Obligations

1846. Dispositions or Transfers of Installment Obligations. Gain or loss is generally recognized when an installment obligation is sold, disposed of, or satisfied other than at face value (Code Sec. 453B).[25] The character of any resulting gain or loss on the disposition of an installment obligation is determined by the character of the original asset that was sold (¶ 1741). The amount of gain or loss is the difference between the basis of the obligation and either:

(1) the amount realized, if the obligation is satisfied other than at face value or is sold or exchanged; or

(2) the fair market value of the obligation, if the obligation is distributed or disposed of other than by sale or exchange.

References are to Standard Federal Tax Reports; Tax Research Consultant; and Practical Tax Explanations.

[21] ¶ 29,740, ¶ 29,741; SALES: 36,454; § 18,365.15

[22] ¶ 29,740, ¶ 29,742; EST-TRST: 9,166; § 18,365.15

[23] ¶ 29,740, ¶ 29,742; REAL: 6,156.35; § 18,365.20

[24] ¶ 29,740; REAL: 6,156.25; § 18,365.15

[25] ¶ 21,470; SALES: 36,350; § 18,370

For this purpose, the basis of the obligation to the transferor is the excess of the face value of the obligation over the income that would have been returnable had the obligation been satisfied in full. To determine the basis, the unpaid balance of the installment obligation is multiplied by the gross profit percentage, and the result is subtracted from the unpaid balance. The result is the basis in the installment obligation (IRS Pub. 537).

The cancellation or lapse of an installment obligation is treated as a disposition other than a sale or exchange. This includes a self-canceling installment note that is extinguished at the death of the holder (*R.E. Frane Est.*, CA-8, 93-2 USTC ¶ 50,386).[26] Therefore, gain or loss is computed based on the fair market value of the obligation.

Transfers Between Spouses. The transfer of an installment obligation between spouses or incident to divorce (other than a transfer in trust) will not trigger recognition of gain (Code Sec. 453B(g)).[27] Thus, the same tax treatment applies to the transferee spouse that would have applied to the transferor spouse.

Transfers at Death. The transfer of an installment obligation at the death of the obligee (other than to the buyer) is not a taxable disposition requiring the recognition of any gain or loss (Code Sec. 453B(c)).[28] Instead, the gain portion of any installment obligation acquired from a decedent is considered income in respect of a decedent (¶ 182). The taxpayer who receives such installment payments (estate, beneficiary, etc.) must report as income the same portion of the payments that would have been taxable income to the decedent. The amount considered to be an item of gross income in respect of the decedent is the excess of the face value of the obligation over its basis in the hands of the decedent.

While the transfer of an installment obligation upon a seller's death is generally not a taxable disposition, the seller's estate is deemed to have made a taxable disposition if the obligation is transferred by bequest, devise, or inheritance to the obligor or if the estate allows the obligation to become unenforceable. If the decedent and obligor-recipient of the obligation were related persons (¶ 1833), the fair market value of the obligation may not be determined at less than its face amount (Code Sec. 691(a)(5)).[29]

Corporate Liquidations

1856. Installment Obligations Received from Liquidating Corporations. Liquidating corporations, other than certain liquidating S corporations (¶ 1858), that distribute installment obligations to shareholders in exchange for their stock must currently recognize gain or loss from the distribution (¶ 1846). However, a shareholder that receives a qualifying installment obligation may treat the exchange as though it were an ordinary sale of stock for an installment obligation. Thus, the shareholder may be able to use the installment method to report the gain from the exchange (Code Sec. 453(h)(1)(A); Reg. § 1.453-11(a)(1)).[30]

If the liquidating corporation is traded on an established securities market, installment sale treatment is generally not available (¶ 1805). However, a shareholder *may* use the installment method if the stock of the liquidating corporation is not traded on an established market, even if the obligation arose from the sale by the liquidating corporation of securities that are traded on an established market (so that the liquidating corporation could not have used the installment method). For this rule to apply, the liquidating corporation must not have been formed or used to avoid the prohibition against using the installment method for publicly traded stock (Reg. § 1.453-11(c)(5)).

References are to Standard Federal Tax Reports; Tax Research Consultant; and Practical Tax Explanations.

[26] ¶ 21,471.15; SALES: 36,352.15

[27] ¶ 21,470; SALES: 36,354.40; § 18,370

[28] ¶ 21,470; SALES: 36,354.35; § 18,370

[29] ¶ 24,900; SALES: 36,352.15; § 18,370

[30] ¶ 21,402, ¶ 21,419; SALES: 36,354.20; § 26,710

18

INSTALLMENT SALE

Gain on the transfer of a qualifying installment obligation to a shareholder during a liquidation is not immediately taxed to the shareholder. Instead, the payments received under the installment obligation are treated as payments for the stock, and any gain is included in the shareholder's income as payments are received. This rule applies when:

(1) stockholders exchange their stock in the corporation in a Code Sec. 331 liquidation (¶ 2253);

(2) the corporation, during the 12-month period beginning with the adoption of the plan of liquidation, had sold some or all of its assets in exchange for an installment note;

(3) the corporation, within that 12-month period, distributes the installment notes acquired in connection with those sales to the shareholders in exchange for their stock; and

(4) the liquidation is completed within that 12-month period.

This rule does not apply to obligations arising from a sale of inventory, stock in trade, or assets held for sale to customers in the ordinary course of business, unless those assets are sold in a bulk sale (Code Sec. 453(h)(1)(B)).

Subsidiary Liquidations. In a complete liquidation of a subsidiary, in which gain or loss on distributions of property is generally not recognized by the parent or the subsidiary (¶ 2261), the distribution of installment obligations will not cause recognition of gain or loss (Code Sec. 453B(d)).[31]

1858. Installment Obligation Received in S Corporation Liquidations. If an installment obligation is distributed by an S corporation in a complete liquidation (¶ 2253), and the receipt of the obligation is not treated as payment for stock in a complete 12-month liquidation (¶ 1856), then the corporation generally does not recognize gain or loss on the distribution. This is true even for accrual-basis S corporations (Code Sec. 453B(h)).[32]

Imputed Interest

1859. Inadequate or Unpaid Interest on Deferred Payments. When a sale or exchange of property involves the issuance of a debt instrument with deferred payments, such as with an installment sale (¶ 1801), the instrument generally should provide for the payment of adequate interest. If the instrument does not provide for the payment of adequate stated interest, interest income must be imputed to the seller or holder of the debt under the original issue discount (OID) rules of Code Sec. 1274 (¶ 1954) or the unstated interest rules of Code Sec. 483 (¶ 1868). The unstated interest rules will apply only if the transaction does not come within the scope of the OID rules (Code Sec. 483(d)(1)).[33]

If neither the unstated interest rules nor OID rules apply, interest may be imputed under other Code sections (Reg. §§ 1.483-1(a) and (c)(3); Reg. § 1.1274-1(b)).[34] For example, interest is imputed to certain obligations given in exchange for services or for the use of property under Code Secs. 404 and 467 (¶ 906 and ¶ 1541). Further, the interest imputation rules of Code Sec. 7872 apply to certain below-market demand loans (¶ 795).

In addition, the unstated interest rules and OID rules do not apply to transfers of property between spouses or incident to divorce (¶ 778), to cash method debt instruments (¶ 1954), or to a purchaser who gives debt when buying personal use property.

The following steps should be taken with respect to deferred contracts:

(1) determine whether the transaction is covered by either the unstated interest rules or the OID rules (¶ 1868 and ¶ 1954);

---

[31] ¶ 21,470; SALES: 36,354.20; § 18,370

[32] ¶ 21,470; SCORP: 352.45; § 28,905.10

[33] ¶ 22,290; ACCTNG: 36,304; § 18,355.10

[34] ¶ 22,291, ¶ 31,301; ACCTNG: 36,154.05

(2) test for unstated interest or OID;

(3) compute the total unstated interest or OID under the contract; and

(4) apportion the unstated interest or OID over the payments.

1868. Scope of Code Sec. 483. The unstated interest rules of Code Sec. 483 impute interest income (¶ 1872) on any payments on the sale or exchange of property that are due more than six months after the sale or exchange if any payments are due more than one year after the sale or exchange (Code Sec. 483).[35] The rules under Code Sec. 483 do not apply in the following situations:

(1) debt instruments for which an issue price is determined under Code Sec. 1273(b)(1), (2) or (3), or Code Sec. 1274;

(2) sales for $3,000 or less;

(3) with respect to the buyer, any purchase of personal property or educational services (under Code Sec. 163(b)) on an installment basis if the interest charge cannot be ascertained and is treated as six percent; and

(4) sales or exchanges of patents (¶ 1767) to the extent of any payments that are contingent on the productivity, use or disposition of the property transferred.

1872. Testing for and Imputing Unstated Interest. The imputed interest rules of Code Sec. 483 apply (¶ 1868) when there is "unstated interest," which is the excess of the total payments (excluding any interest payments) due more than ·six months after the date of sale over the total of their present values (including the present values of any interest payments). Generally, present value is determined by using a discount rate equal to the applicable federal rate (AFR) determined under Code Sec. 1274(d) (¶ 1875) (Code Sec. 483(b); Reg. §§ 1.483-2 and 1.483-3).[36] However, the discount rate will not exceed six percent, compounded semiannually, in the case of transfers of land between family members. This rule only applies if the aggregate sales price of all land sales between the family members does not exceed $500,000, and if no party to the sale is a nonresident alien (Code Sec. 483(e); Reg. § 1.483-3(b)).[37] In addition, a discount rate not in excess of nine percent (if less than the AFR), compounded semiannually, applies to most debt instruments given in consideration for the sale or exchange of property if the stated principal amount does not exceed a certain amount adjusted for inflation (¶ 1954).

1875. Adequate Stated Interest. A debt instrument with deferred payments is considered to have adequate stated interest for purposes of the unstated interest rules of Code Sec. 483 (¶ 1859) if the stated principal amount is less than or equal to its imputed principal amount (Code Secs. 483(b) and 1274(b) and (c); Reg. §§ 1.483-2(b) and 1.1274-2(c)).[38] The imputed principal amount is determined by totaling the present values of all principal and interest payments due on the instrument discounted at the applicable federal rate (AFR) (¶ 83). Payments within six months after the sale are taken into account.

The AFR is the lowest rate in effect for any month in the three-calendar-month period ending with the first calendar month in which there is a binding written contract. It is determined by reference to the term of the debt instrument, including renewal and extension options, as shown in the following table (Code Sec. 1274(d); Reg. §§ 1.483-3(a) and 1.1274-4(a)).[39]

Term of Debt Instrument:	Applicable Federal Rate:
Not over 3 years	Federal short-term rate
Over 3 years but not over 9 years .	Federal mid-term rate
Over 9 years	Federal long-term rate

References are to Standard Federal Tax Reports; Tax Research Consultant; and Practical Tax Explanations.

[35] ¶ 22,290; ACCTNG: 36,300; § 19,505.05

[36] ¶ 22,290, ¶ 22,292, ¶ 22,294; ACCTNG: 36,308; § 19,510.10

[37] ¶ 22,290, ¶ 22,294; ACCTNG: 36,308.25; § 19,510.15

[38] ¶ 22,290, ¶ 22,292, ¶ 31,300, ¶ 31,302; ACCTNG: 36,310; § 19,510.05

[39] ¶ 22,294, ¶ 31,300, ¶ 31,304; ACCTNG: 36,162; § 19,410.10

¶1875

For sale and leaseback transactions, the discount rate is 110 percent of the AFR, compounded semiannually (Code Sec. 1274(e); Reg. § 1.1274-4(a)(2)).[40] For transactions in which a debt instrument is given in consideration for the sale or exchange of property (other than new Code Sec. 38 property) and the stated principal amount of the instrument does not exceed an inflation-adjusted amount ($5,557,200 for 2014, and $5,468,200 for 2013), a nine-percent rate may be substituted for the AFR (Code Sec. 1274A; Rev. Rul. 2013-23; Rev. Rul. 2012-33).[41] The discount rate will not exceed six percent, compounded semiannually, in the case of transfers of land between family members, but this rule only applies if the aggregate sales price of all land sales between the family members during the calendar year does not exceed $500,000, and no party to the transaction is a nonresident alien (Code Sec. 483(e); Reg. § 1.483-3(b)).[42]

1881. Assumptions of Debt. If any person in connection with the sale or exchange of property assumes any debt instrument or acquires any property subject to any debt instrument, in determining whether the unstated interest rules apply, the assumption or acquisition is not generally taken into account. However, when the instrument's terms and conditions are modified in a manner that would constitute an exchange, the unstated interest rules may be applied (Reg. § 1.483-1(d)).[43]

Treatment of Interest

1883. Treatment of Imputed Interest. The amount of unstated interest determined under Code Sec. 483 is classified as interest for tax purposes (Reg. § 1.483-1(a)(2)).[44] As a result, it may be deductible by the buyer. Unstated interest is not deductible, however, by the issuer of a debt instrument given in consideration for the sale or exchange or personal use property (Reg. § 1.483-1(c)(3)).[45] Instead, the unstated interest must be accrued by the holder. Personal use property means any property substantially all the use of which by the taxpayer is not in connection with the taxpayer's trade or business or activities engage in for profit (Code Sec. 1275(b)(3)).[46]

Reporting Requirements. The reporting of unstated interest depends upon whether the seller is on the cash or accrual basis. Cash basis sellers include unstated interest as interest income in the year payments are received. Sellers on the accrual basis include unstated interest in income in the year payments are due (Reg. § 1.446-2(a)).[47]

References are to Standard Federal Tax Reports; Tax Research Consultant; and Practical Tax Explanations.

[40] ¶ 31,300, ¶ 31,304; ACCTNG: 36,308.20

[41] ¶ 31,320, ¶ 31,322.30; ACCTNG: 36,308; § 19,315.10

[42] ¶ 22,290, ¶ 22,294; ACCTNG: 36,308.25; § 19,510.15

[43] ¶ 22,291; ACCTNG: 36,264; § 19,505.10

[44] ¶ 22,291; ACCTNG: 36,302; § 19,515

[45] ¶ 22,291; ACCTNG: 36,306.30; § 19,505.10

[46] ¶ 31,340; ACCTNG: 36,224; § 19,315.10, § 19,505.10

[47] ¶ 20,610; ACCTNG: 36,200; § 19,310.05

Chapter 19

SECURITIES TRANSACTIONS

Taxation of Securities Transactions

1901. Securities Transactions. Securities such as stocks and bonds held for investment are generally capital assets. Calculating gain or loss from the sale of securities follows the same rules that apply to other capital assets (¶ 1701). There are, however, a number of special rules that apply to the sale or exchange of certain securities, including securities held by dealers (¶ 1903), worthless securities (¶ 1916), options to buy securities (¶ 1919), wash sales (¶ 1935), short sales (¶ 1944), tax straddles (¶ 1948), and a corporation dealing in its own stocks or bonds (¶ 1729). In addition, gain on the sale of qualified small business stock may be either excluded from gross income (¶ 1905) or rolled over to other small business stock (¶ 1907). A taxpayer may also rollover gain from the sale of publicly traded securities to an interest in a specialized small business investment company (¶ 1909). Losses from the sale of stock in certain small businesses may be treated as ordinary losses (¶ 1911 and ¶ 1913).

1903. Dealer in Securities. Securities held for sale by dealers to their customers in the ordinary course of a trade or business are not capital assets (¶ 1741). Thus, gain or loss realized from the sale or disposition is treated as ordinary gain or loss unless the securities are held primarily for personal investment (Code Sec. 1236; Reg. § 1.1236-1).[1] Securities that are held by a dealer for personal investment purposes must be clearly identified in the dealer's records before the close of the day on which they are acquired and must never be held primarily for sale to the dealer's customers. See ¶ 1760 for a discussion of the distinction between a dealer, trader, and investor.

Mark-to-Market Requirements. Dealers in securities must use the mark-to-market method of accounting for reporting gains and losses from the disposition of securities (Code Sec. 475(a)).[2] Under the mark-to-market rules, any security that is inventory in the hands of a dealer must be included in inventory at its fair market value. A securities dealer may use the fair market value as reported on the dealer's financial statements for this purpose (Reg. § 1.475(a)-4).[3]

Any security that is not classified as inventory in the dealer's hands and that is held at the close of the tax year is treated as if it were sold at its fair market value on the last business day of the year. The dealer must recognize any gain or loss that results from the deemed sale. Any gain or loss recognized is taken into account when calculating the dealer's gain or loss when the security is actually sold or exchanged.

References are to Standard Federal Tax Reports; Tax Research Consultant; and Practical Tax Explanations.

[1] ¶ 30,670, ¶ 30,671; SALES: 45,054; § 18,805.05

[2] ¶ 22,265; SALES: 45,350; § 38,235.05

[3] ¶ 22,265E; SALES: 45,362; § 38,235.05

The mark-to-market rules generally apply to all securities held by a dealer, other than those they hold as investments or not for sale to customers in the ordinary course of the taxpayer's trade or business (Code Sec. 475(b)).[4] The rules also do not apply to debt instruments acquired in the ordinary course of a trade or business or securities that are hedges of certain positions (¶ 1949). In order for a security to be exempt from the mark-to-market requirements, it must be clearly identified in the dealer's records before the close of the day on which it is acquired, originated, or entered into.

Commodity dealers, as well as traders in securities or commodities, may elect to have the mark-to-market requirements apply to their noninvestment positions (Code Sec. 475(e) and (f)).[5] For a commodities dealer, the election applies to commodities held by the dealer in the same manner as securities held by a dealer. A trader in securities or commodities that elects mark-to-market treatment must recognize gain or loss on any security or commodity held in connection with the trading business as if the security or commodity were sold at fair market value on the last business day of the tax year.

The mark-to-market election must be made by the due date (not including extensions) of the tax return for the year prior to the year for which the election becomes effective. For example, the election must have been made by April 15, 2014, to be effective for 2014. The election is made by attaching a statement to the taxpayer's timely-filed return or request for extension to file his or her return (Rev. Proc. 99-17; Rev. Proc. 2011-14).[6] If a taxpayer is not required to file a tax return, the election is made by placing a statement in the taxpayer's books and records no later than March 15 of the election year. The election may be made without the consent of the IRS, and in the case of trader of securities or commodities, may be made separately for each trade or business of the taxpayer. Once made, the election continues to apply to every tax year of the taxpayer until it is revoked with the IRS's consent.

Gains and Losses on Small Business Stock

1905. Exclusion of Gain from Small Business Stock. A noncorporate taxpayer can exclude from gross income 50 percent of any gain from the sale or exchange of qualified small business stock held for more than five years (Code Sec. 1202).[7] The exclusion is increased to 75 percent for qualified small business stock acquired after February 17, 2009, and before September 28, 2010, and to 100 percent for qualified stock acquired after September 27, 2010, and before January 1, 2014. The exclusion is 60 percent if the stock is issued by a corporation in an empowerment zone (¶ 999B).

Eligible gain from any single issuer is subject to a cumulative limit for any given tax year to the greater of: (1) $10 million reduced by the aggregate amount of eligible gain taken in prior years ($5 million for married individuals filing separately); or (2) 10 times the taxpayer's adjusted basis of all qualified stock of the issuer disposed of during the tax year. For alternative minimum tax (AMT) purposes, seven percent of the excluded gain is a tax preference item (¶ 1425). However, none of the excluded gain is a preference item for the disposition of stock acquired after September 27, 2010, and before January 1, 2014 (Code Sec. 1202(a)(4)). The sale or exchange of qualified small business stock is reported on Form 8949 (except individuals use Schedule D of Form 1040 for tax years before 2011, and estates and trusts use Schedule D of Form 1041 for tax years before 2013).

Qualified Small Business Stock. To be eligible as qualified small business stock, the stock must be issued after August 10, 1993, and acquired by the taxpayer at its original issue (directly or through an underwriter) in exchange for money, property, or as compensation for services provided to the corporation (Code Sec. 1202(c) and (d); Reg. § 1.1202-2).[8] Qualified stock that is converted to other stock of the corporation (such as preferred stock) is treated as qualified stock. Qualified stock acquired by exercising

---

References are to Standard Federal Tax Reports; Tax Research Consultant; and Practical Tax Explanations.

[4] ¶ 22,265; SALES: 45,354; § 38,235.15

[5] ¶ 22,265; SALES: 45,360; § 38,235.20

[6] ¶ 22,268.20; SALES: 45,360.15; § 38,235.20

[7] ¶ 30,372; SALES: 15,300; § 16,605.05

[8] ¶ 30,372, ¶ 30,374; SALES: 15,304.05; § 16,605.10

options or warrants, or converting debt, is deemed acquired at original issue. Small business stock is not qualified if it has been the subject of certain redemptions that are more than *de minimis*. A taxpayer who acquires qualified stock by gift or inheritance is treated as having acquired such stock in the same manner as the transferor and adds the transferor's holding period to his or her own. Gain on qualified stock held by a partnership, S corporation, regulated investment company, or common trust fund is excludable if the entity held it for more than five years and if the partner, shareholder, or participant to whom the gain passes held his or her interest in the entity when the stock was acquired, and only to the extent his or her share of the entity has not increased (Code Sec. 1202(g)).

The issuing corporation must be a domestic C corporation (other than a regulated investment company (¶ 2301), cooperative, or other similar pass-through corporation). Both before and immediately after the qualified stock's issuance, the corporation must have aggregate gross assets that do not exceed $50 million. All corporations that are members of the same parent-subsidiary controlled group are treated as one corporation in applying this test. In addition, during substantially all of the taxpayer's holding period, at least 80 percent of the value of the corporation's assets must be used in the active conduct of one or more qualified trades or businesses. For this purpose, the performance of services in the fields of health, law, engineering, architecture, etc., will not be a qualified trade or business, nor are the hospitality, farming, insurance, finance or mineral extraction industries. However, a specialized small business investment company (SSBIC), licensed under section 301(d) of the Small Business Investment Act of 1958, will meet the active business test (¶ 1909).

1907. Rollover of Gain from Small Business Stock. A noncorporate taxpayer may elect to roll over capital gain from the sale of qualified small business stock (¶ 1905) held for more than six months if other qualified small business stock is purchased during the 60-day period beginning on the date of sale (Code Sec. 1045; Reg. § 1.1045-1).[9] The replacement stock must meet the active business requirement for the six-month period following its purchase. Except for purposes of determining the six-month active business test, the holding period of the stock purchased includes the holding period of the stock sold. Gain will only be recognized to the extent that the amount realized on the sale exceeds the cost of the replacement stock. The basis of the newly purchased stock must be reduced by the amount of gain rolled over. Special rules apply for partnerships that want to roll over gain from a business that is held in the form of qualified small business stock. The sale of the stock is reported on Form 8949 (except individuals use Schedule D of Form 1040 for tax years before 2011, partnerships use Schedule D of Form 1065 for tax years before 2012, and estates and trusts use Schedule D of Form 1041 for tax years before 2013; a partnership must also attach a statement to Form 1065 that identifies the stock and adjustments to each partner's basis in the replacement stock).

1909. Rollover of Gain from Publicly Traded Securities. Individual and C corporations may elect to defer recognition of capital gain realized upon the sale of publicly traded securities if the sale proceeds are used within 60 days to purchase common stock or a partnership interest in a specialized small business investment company (SSBIC) (Code Sec. 1044; Reg. § 1.1044(a)-1).[10] To the extent that the sale proceeds exceed the cost of the SSBIC common stock or partnership interest, gain must be recognized. For this purpose, an SSBIC is a corporation or partnership licensed under section 301(d) of the Small Business Investment Act of 1958 to finance small business concerns owned by disadvantaged persons.

An individual taxpayer (as well as married individuals filing a joint return) can roll over no more than $50,000 of gain in any given tax year or $500,000 during his or her lifetime ($25,000 and $250,000, respectively, for a married individual filing separately). In the case of a joint return, the amount of gain excluded for any tax year must be allocated

---

References are to Standard Federal Tax Reports; Tax Research Consultant; and Practical Tax Explanations.

[9] ¶ 29,850, ¶ 29,852; SALES: 15,308; § 16,610.05

[10] ¶ 29,845, ¶ 29,845B; SALES: 27,400; § 16,615, § 18,245

equally between the spouses for purposes of applying the limit in a subsequent tax year. For a C corporation, the annual and cumulative limits are $250,000 and $1 million, respectively. All corporations that are members of the same controlled group are treated as one taxpayer for this purpose, and any gain excluded by the predecessor of a C corporation is treated as gain excluded by the successor corporation. The deferred gain is reflected as a basis reduction. Basis is not reduced, however, when calculating gain eligible for the exclusion for qualified small business stock (¶ 1905).

The election to roll over gain into an SSBIC must be made by the due date (including extensions) for the taxpayer's return for the year in which the publicly traded securities are sold. The election is made by reporting the entire gain from the sale on Form 8949 (except individuals use Schedule D of Form 1040 for tax years before 2011, and C corporations use Schedule D of Form 1120 for tax years before 2012). A separate statement must also be attached to taxpayer's return showing how the nonrecognized gain was calculated, the SSBIC in which the sale proceeds were invested, the date the SSBIC stock or partnership interest was purchased, and the basis of the SSBIC interest. Once made, the election is revocable only with the IRS's consent.

1911. Losses on Small Business Stock (Section 1244 Stock). A loss sustained by an individual on the sale, exchange, or worthlessness of small business stock (referred to as section 1244 stock) may be treated as an ordinary loss, even if the stock is a capital asset in the taxpayer's hands (Code Sec. 1244).[11] The maximum amount deductible as an ordinary loss in any tax year is $50,000 ($100,000 for married individuals filing a joint return).

Any loss claimed as an ordinary loss is treated as a loss from a trade or business of the taxpayer in computing a net operating loss (NOL) for the tax year (¶ 1145) and reported on Form 4797. Any loss in excess of the dollar limits is treated as a capital loss and reported on Form 8949 (except Schedule D of Form 1040 is used for tax years before 2011). Any gain on the disposition of section 1244 stock is capital gain if the stock was a capital asset in the taxpayer's hands (¶ 1741). Gains and losses that are within the ordinary loss limit are not offset, even if the transactions are in stock of the same company.

For stock to qualify as section 1244 stock, it must be stock of a domestic corporation (including preferred stock) issued after November 6, 1978, and meet the following requirements (additional requirements must be met for stock issued after June 30, 1958, and before November 7, 1978):

- the stock must have been issued to the taxpayer or a partnership in which the taxpayer was a partner at the time in exchange for money or property other than stock or securities;

- the issuing corporation must be a small business corporation, meaning that at the time the stock was issued the aggregate amount of money and other property (taken into account at its adjusted basis) received by the corporation as a contributions to capital and as a paid-in surplus (not only for the stock in question but any previously issued stock) did not exceed $1 million (qualification as a small business corporation under the S corporation rules does not automatically qualify its stock as section 1244 stock); and

- during the corporation's five most recent tax years ending before the date the stock is sold by the taxpayer, more than 50 percent of its gross receipts must have been derived from sources other than royalties, rents, dividends, interest, annuities, and gains from the sales of securities (the corporation must be largely an operating company, meaning that ordinary loss treatment is not available to corporations with little or no gross receipts) (Reg. §§ 1.1244(c)-1 and 1.1244(c)-2).[12]

References are to Standard Federal Tax Reports; Tax Research Consultant; and Practical Tax Explanations.

[11] ¶ 30,790; SALES: 18,200; § 16,620.05

[12] ¶ 30,793, ¶ 30,794; SALES: 18,100; § 16,620.15

1913. Losses on Small Business Investment Company Stock (SBIC). A loss sustained on the sale, exchange, or worthlessness of stock in a small business investment company (SBIC) (¶ 2392) may be treated by a taxpayer as an ordinary loss on Form 4797, even if the stock is a capital asset in the taxpayer's hands (Code Sec. 1242; Reg. § 1.1242-1(b)).[13] The SBIC must be licensed to operate as an SBIC at the time the loss is sustained by the taxpayer. In addition, the loss is not subject to the limitations on the allowance of nonbusiness deductions in computing net operating losses (NOLs) (¶ 1145). When a taxpayer has several transactions involving the stock of the SBIC, each transaction is considered separately to determine if the taxpayer's loss is an ordinary loss; transactions are not netted. A loss sustained on the closing of a short sale of SBIC stock (¶ 1944) with other SBIC stock acquired only for the purpose of closing the short sale will not be treated as an ordinary loss, but instead as a capital loss under the short sale rules (Rev. Rul. 63-65).

Worthless Securities

1916. Worthless Securities. A security that becomes completely worthless during the tax year is treated as sold or exchanged on the last day of the tax year (Code Sec. 165(g); Reg. § 1.165-5).[14] If the security is a capital asset (¶ 1741), the resulting loss is generally a capital loss subject to the limits on capital losses (¶ 1752). If the security is not a capital asset, the loss is an ordinary loss subject to the limits on ordinary losses (¶ 1101). The amount of the loss is the taxpayer's adjusted basis in the security, less any amount compensated for by insurance.

> **Example:** On December 10, 2014, Judy Green purchased shares of Xetco Corporation for $5,000. On May 1, 2015, she received formal notification that the shares of Xetco were worthless. In claiming a capital loss for the worthless shares on her 2015 tax return, Judy must treat the shares as becoming worthless on December 31, 2015. As a result, her $5,000 capital loss is recognized as long term even though she did not own the shares for more than 12 months before they became worthless.

A security becomes totally worthless when it has no value or potential value as the result of an identifiable event. The abandonment of a security establishes the worthlessness of the security to the taxpayer. To abandon a security, the taxpayer must permanently surrender and relinquish all rights in a security and receive no consideration for the exchange. Deductions for partial worthlessness are generally not allowed.

For this purpose, a security includes stock, the right to subscribe for or receive stock, and bonds, debentures, notes, certificates, or other evidence of indebtedness issued with interest coupons or in registered form by a corporation or government to pay a fixed or determinable sum of money. A worthless debt that does not meet the definition of a security (e.g., because it was not issued by a corporation or government) is treated as a bad debt (¶ 1135 and ¶ 1143).

Securities held by a securities dealer as inventory are not considered capital assets, and a loss from worthlessness is an ordinary loss (¶ 1903). An ordinary loss may also be claimed for losses from worthless securities that are section 1244 stock (¶ 1911), issued by a small business investment company (SBIC) (¶ 1913), held by a small business investment company (¶ 2392), securities in an affiliated corporation, or securities held by a bank or other financial institution (¶ 2383).

Options

1919. Options to Buy or Sell Property. Gain or loss from the sale or exchange of an option to buy or sell property, including a cash settlement option and an option on a section 1256 contract (¶ 1947), is considered gain or loss from the sale or exchange of the underlying property (Code Sec. 1234; Reg. § 1.1234-1).[15] Thus, a capital gain or loss results only if the option covers property that would be a capital asset in the hands of the

19 | SECURITIES

References are to Standard Federal Tax Reports; Tax Research Consultant; and Practical Tax Explanations.

[13] ¶ 30,753, ¶ 30,754; SALES: 18,304; § 45,410.15

[14] ¶ 9802, ¶ 10,000; BUSEXP: 30,262; § 16,935

[15] ¶ 30,610, ¶ 30,611; SALES: 45,202; § 19,110, § 19,115

taxpayer (¶ 1741). The length of time the taxpayer held the option determines whether the capital gain or loss is short term or long term unless the sale or exchange is part of a hedging transaction (¶ 1949). If the underlying property is section 1231 property, then any gain or loss from the sale or exchange of the option may be section 1231 gain or loss (¶ 1747).

If the holder of an option incurs a loss from the failure to exercise the option, then the option is deemed to have been sold or exchanged on the date it expired. In the case of the grantor of an option for stock, securities, commodities, or commodity futures (including an option granted as part of a straddle (¶ 1948)), gain or loss from any closing transaction and gain on the lapse of the option is treated as a short-term capital gain or loss. See ¶ 1921 for a discussion of holders and writers of options on securities (puts and calls).

The characterization rules above do not apply to gain or loss realized on the sale or exchange of an option by a dealer who holds options primarily for sale to customers (¶ 1903). They also do not apply to gain realized from the sale or exchange of an employee stock option (¶ 1925 and ¶ 1927), an option to lease property, an option to buy or sell inventory, an option equivalent to a dividend, an option involving section 306 stock (¶ 739), and an option included as part of a short sale (¶ 1944).

1921. Puts and Calls. Puts are options to sell, and calls are options to buy, stock, securities, or commodities at a set price on or before a specified date. Puts and calls are issued by writers (grantors) to holders for premiums. They end when the option is exercised by the holder, the option lapses, or due to a closing transaction (Rev. Rul. 78-182; IRS Pub. 550).[16]

Holders of Puts and Calls. The purchase of a put option or call option is not a taxable event. The cost of purchasing the put or call, however, is a nondeductible capital expenditure (Rev. Rul. 71-521).[17] If the holder sells a put or call without exercising it, the difference between its cost and the amount received is either a long-term or short-term capital gain or loss, depending on how long it was held (¶ 1919). If the option expires, its cost is either a long-term or short-term capital loss, depending on the taxpayer's holding period, which ends on the expiration date. If the holder exercises a call, its cost is added to the basis of the security purchased. If the holder exercises a put, the amount realized on the sale of the underlying security is reduced by the cost of the put when computing gain or loss on the sale of the stock. That gain or loss is long term or short term depending on the taxpayer's holding period for the underlying security (Rev. Rul. 78-182; IRS Pub. 550).[18] The acquisition of a put is considered a short sale, and the exercise, sale, or lapse of the put is a closing of the short sale (¶ 1944).

Writers of Puts and Calls. If a taxpayer writes or grants a call or put option, the premium received is not included in income at the time of receipt. Instead it is deferred until the option expires, the taxpayer buys or sells the underlying security when the option is exercised, or the taxpayer engages in a closed transaction.

When the option expires, the premium can then be treated as a short-term capital gain. If a call is exercised and the taxpayer sells the underlying security, then the premium is added to the amount realized on the sale and any gain or loss is long-term or short-term depending on the taxpayer's holding period of the security. If a put is exercised and the taxpayer buys the underlying security, then the premium reduces its basis in the security. The taxpayer's holding period on the security begins on the date of the purchase, not on the date the put was written.

The taxpayer can also terminate a put or call through a closing transaction—such as repurchasing the option or substituting the original option by purchasing another option with identical terms. If the taxpayer closes the transaction, the difference between the premium originally received and the amount paid in the closing transaction is short-term capital gain or loss.

References are to Standard Federal Tax Reports; Tax Research Consultant; and Practical Tax Explanations.

[16] ¶ 30,614.14; SALES: 45,200; § 19,105　　[17] ¶ 30,592.70; SALES: 45,202; § 19,120　　[18] ¶ 30,614.14; SALES: 45,200; § 19,105

Example 1: Ten call options were issued on April 8 for $4,000. The options expired in December without being exercised. The holder (buyer) of the options recognizes a short-term capital loss of $4,000. The writer of the options recognizes a short-term capital gain of $4,000.

Example 2: Assume the same facts as in Example 1, except that, on May 10, the options were sold for $6,000. The holder (buyer) of the options who sold them recognizes a short-term capital gain of $2,000. If the writer of the options bought them back, he or she would recognize a short-term capital loss of $2,000.

Example 3: Assume the facts as in Example 1, except that the options were exercised on May 27. The holder (buyer) adds the cost of the options to the basis of the stock bought through the exercise of the options. The writer adds the amount received from writing the options to the amount realized from selling the stock. The gain or loss is short term or long term, depending on the holding period of the stock.

1923. Nonstatutory Stock Options. An employee or independent contractor granted a stock option as compensation for the performance of services is generally subject to the rules regarding restricted property transfers (¶ 713) when the option is granted or exercised, unless it is an incentive stock option (ISO) (¶ 1925) or an option granted under an employee stock purchase plan (ESPP) (¶ 1929) (Code Sec. 83(e)(1); Reg. § 1.83-7).[19]

A nonstatutory stock option with a readily ascertainable fair market value when granted is subject to the restricted property rules on the grant date. The taxpayer has ordinary income equal to the stock's fair market value on the grant date, less any amount paid. A nonstatutory stock option without a readily ascertainable fair market value when granted is subject to the restricted property rules when it is exercised or disposed of by the taxpayer, even if the fair market value becomes ascertainable before the option is exercised or disposed. If the option is exercised, the taxpayer has ordinary income equal to the stock's fair market value at the exercise date or when substantially vested, less the exercise price.

If a nonstatutory stock option is sold or disposed in an arm's-length transaction, the taxpayer is considered to have exercised the option and has income equal to the amount of money or property received, less the exercise price. If the sale or disposition is not an arm's-length transaction, the taxpayer is not considered to have exercised the option. The taxpayer must, nonetheless, include in income as compensation the amount of money or property received. In addition, when the transferee exercises the option, the taxpayer (transferor) has additional income equal to the fair market value of stock acquired by the transferee, less the exercise price and any amount the taxpayer received from the sale of the option. A sale or disposition of a nonstatutory stock option to a related person is not treated as an arm's-length transaction for this purpose. If the holder of an option incurs a loss on failure to exercise the option, then it is deemed to have been sold or exchanged on the date it expired (¶ 1919).

Readily Ascertainable Market Value. A stock option generally has a readily ascertainable fair market value if it is actively traded on an established securities market (Reg. § 1.83-7(b)).[20] Even if the option is not actively traded on an established securities market, it will be considered to have a readily ascertainable value if taxpayer can demonstrate that the option is transferable, immediately exercisable, there is no condition or restriction on the underlying property that would have a significant effect on its fair market value, and the fair market value of the option privilege is readily ascertainable.

Sale of Stock. Stock acquired through the exercise of a nonstatutory stock option is treated as any other investment property when sold or exchanged (IRS Pub. 525). The taxpayer's basis in the stock is the amount paid for the stock, plus any amount included in income upon grant or exercise of the option. The taxpayer's holding period begins

---

References are to Standard Federal Tax Reports; Tax Research Consultant; and Practical Tax Explanations.

[19] ¶ 6380, ¶ 6388; COMPEN: 18,500; § 21,701

[20] ¶ 6388; COMPEN: 18,502, COMPEN: 18,504; § 21,710.05

when the option was acquired if it had a readily ascertainable value, or the date the option was exercised if it did not.

Employer's Deduction. An employer may deduct the value of a nonqualified stock option as a business expense for the tax year in which the option is included in the gross income of the employee (Code Sec. 83(h); Reg. § 1.83-6(a)).[21] When the employer and the employee have different tax years, the employer generally claims the deduction in the tax year in which, or with which, the employee's tax year ends. If the option's market value, however, is not readily ascertainable at the time of grant, and the employee's rights in the stock are substantially vested upon exercise, the employer may take the deduction in accordance with its usual method of accounting.

Reporting Requirements. In most situations, when an employee exercises a nonqualified stock option, the employer is required to report the excess of the fair market value of the stock received over the amount that the employee paid for that stock (i.e., "the spread") on the employee's Form W-2.

1925. Incentive Stock Options. An incentive stock option (ISO) is an option granted by a corporation (or related corporation) to an employee giving him or her the right to purchase stock of the employer, often at a discount. Unlike a nonstatutory stock option (¶ 1923), if certain requirements are met, no gain or loss is generally realized by the employee when an ISO is granted or exercised (Code Sec. 421(a)).[22] Instead, the employee is not subject to income tax until shares acquired by the exercise of the option are sold. See ¶ 1927 for a discussion of ISO plan requirements.

Gain or loss from the sale of the stock received in an ISO is a capital gain or loss if: (1) the taxpayer does not dispose of the stock for at least two years from the date on which the option is granted; and (2) the stock is held for at least one year after the option is exercised (Code Sec. 422(a); Reg. § 1.422-1(a)).[23] The amount of gain or loss is the difference between the amount the taxpayer paid for the stock (the option price) and the amount the taxpayer received when he or she sold the stock. The taxpayer must remain an employee of the corporation from the time the option is granted until three months before the option is exercised (one year if the taxpayer ceased employment because of permanent and total disability). In the event the holder of an ISO dies, the deceased's executor, administrator, or representative may exercise the option but he or she does not have to exercise the option within three months after the death of the employee (Reg. § 1.421-2(c)).[24]

If the employee sells the stock before the required holding period ends (a disqualifying disposition), gain on the sale is ordinary income equal to the fair market value of the stock when the option was exercised, less the exercise price (Code Sec. 421(b); Reg. § 1.421-2(b)).[25] Any excess gain is capital gain, and any loss is a capital loss. The gain is recognized for the tax year in which the sale occurs. In addition, any gain from a disqualifying disposition is excluded from wages for FICA and FUTA tax purposes and is not subject to income tax withholding (Code Secs. 3121(a)(22) and 3306(b)(19)).

Basis of ISO. An employee's basis in an ISO is the amount that the employee paid for the option. If the employee did not pay for the option and the option lapses, the employee does not have a deductible loss because he or she does not have a basis. An employee's basis in stock purchased through an ISO is the amount he or she paid for the stock when the option was exercised (plus any amount he or she paid for the option).

Annual Dollar Limit. The maximum value of stock with respect to which ISOs may first become exercisable in any one year is $100,000. Stock is valued when the option is granted. Options are taken into account in the order in which they are granted, and options issued under ISO plans of any parent, subsidiary, or predecessor corporation are taken into account (Code Sec. 422(d)).[26]

References are to Standard Federal Tax Reports; Tax Research Consultant; and Practical Tax Explanations.

[21] ¶ 6380, ¶ 6386; COMPEN: 18,508; § 21,720

[22] ¶ 19,602; COMPEN: 24,050; § 21,510

[23] ¶ 19,800, ¶ 19,801A; COMPEN: 24,150; § 21,525.05

[24] ¶ 19,609; COMPEN: 24,152; § 21,520.15

[25] ¶ 19,602, ¶ 19,609; COMPEN: 24,056, COMPEN: 24,154; § 21,530.10

[26] ¶ 19,800; COMPEN: 24,116; § 21,515.40

¶1925

Minimum Tax. The favorable tax treatment of ISOs does not apply for purposes of the alternative minimum tax (AMT). Instead, the *excess* of the (1) fair market value of the stock received upon the exercise of the option, over (2) the amount paid for the stock, plus any amount paid for the ISO, must generally be recognized as an AMT adjustment (¶ 1435). As a result, individuals who have exercised ISOs to purchase stock with a high fair market value which declined before they could sell it maybe left with large AMT liabilities and no cash to pay them.

1927. Incentive Stock Options Plan Requirements. A stock option granted by an employer to an employee must satisfy several requirements to qualify for favorable tax treatment as an incentive stock option (ISO) (¶ 1925) (Code Sec. 422(b); Reg. § 1.422-2).[27] ISOs must be granted under a plan adopted by the granting corporation and approved by its shareholders that sets out the total number of shares that may be issued under options and the employees who may receive the options. The plan must be approved by the stockholders within 12 months before or after the date such plan is adopted.

The options must be granted within 10 years from the date the plan is adopted or approved, whichever is earlier. Further, the options must be exercisable within 10 years from the date of the grant. The option price may not be less than the fair market value of the stock at the time the option is granted, and the option may not be transferable other than at the grantee's death. The option may be exercised only by the employee. Finally, the employee, *at the time the option is granted*, may not own stock with more than 10 percent of the total combined voting power of all classes of stock of the employer corporation or its parent or any subsidiary.

1929. Employee Stock Purchase Plans. An employee stock purchase plan (ESPP) may grant employees the option to purchase stock in their employer or the employer's parent or subsidiary. Unlike a nonstatutory stock option (¶ 1923), if certain requirements are met, no gain or loss is generally realized by the employee when an option is granted or exercised under an ESPP (Code Sec. 421(a)).[28] Instead, the employee is not subject to income tax until shares acquired by the exercise of the option are sold. See ¶ 1931 for a discussion of ESPP plan requirements.

Gain or loss from the sale of the stock received in an ESPP is a capital gain or loss if: (1) the taxpayer does not dispose of the stock for at least two years from the date on which the option is granted; and (2) the stock is held for at least one year after the option is exercised (Code Sec. 423(a)).[29] The amount of gain or loss is the difference between the amount the taxpayer paid for the stock (the option price) and the amount the taxpayer received when he or she sold the stock. The taxpayer must remain an employee of the corporation from the time the option is granted until three months before the option is exercised (one year if the taxpayer ceased employment because of permanent and total disability). In the event the employee dies, his or her executor, administrator, or representative may exercise the option but he or she does not have to exercise the option within three months after the death of the employee (Reg. § 1.421-2(c)).[30]

If the option price is less than 100 percent (but not less than 85 percent) of the fair market value of the stock, then the favorable tax treatment does not apply when the taxpayer disposes of the stock (Code Sec. 423(c)).[31] Instead, the employee recognizes ordinary income in the amount of the *lesser* of:

- the excess of the fair market value of the shares when sold or on the employee' death, over the option price, or

- the excess of the fair market value of the shares when the option was granted, over the option price.

References are to Standard Federal Tax Reports; Tax Research Consultant; and Practical Tax Explanations.

[27] ¶ 19,800, ¶ 19,801C; COMPEN: 24,100; § 21,515.05

[28] ¶ 19,602; COMPEN: 21,050; § 21,601

[29] ¶ 19,900; COMPEN: 21,054; § 21,625.10

[30] ¶ 19,609; COMPEN: 21,054.15; § 21,625.10

[31] ¶ 19,900; COMPEN: 21,054.10; § 21,625.10

The balance of any gain is treated as capital gain. If the taxpayer realizes any loss from the sale, then it is a capital loss.

If the employee sells the stock before the required holding period ends (a disqualifying disposition), gain on the sale is ordinary income equal to the fair market value of the stock when the option was exercised, less the exercise price (Code Sec. 421(b); Reg. § 1.421-2(b)).[32] Any excess gain is capital gain, and any loss is a capital loss. The gain is recognized for the tax year in which the sale occurs. In addition, any gain from a disqualifying disposition is excluded from wages for FICA and FUTA tax purposes and is not subject to income tax withholding (Code Secs. 3121(a)(22) and 3306(b)(19)).

An ESPP is different from an employee stock ownership plan (ESOP) (¶ 2103). While both plans involve employee ownership of company stock, an ESOP is a retirement plan that holds employer stock for the benefit of participating employees.

1931. Employee Stock Purchase Plan Requirements. An employee stock purchase plan (ESPP) must satisfy several requirements in order for options acquired under the plan to qualify for favorable tax treatment (¶ 1929) (Code Sec. 423(b)).[33] ESPPs are written, shareholder-approved plans under which employees are granted options to purchase shares of their employer's stock or the stock of a parent or subsidiary corporation.

An ESPP cannot grant options to any employee who has more than five percent of the voting power or value of the employer's stock, or that of any parent or subsidiary of the employer. All full-time employees must be included in the plan, except those with less than two years of employment, highly compensated employees (¶ 2114), part-time employees, and seasonal workers. The plan must be nondiscriminatory, though it may limit the amount of stock any employee can buy, and the amount of stock that each employee may become entitled to buy may be tied to compensation.

The option price may not be less than the *lesser* of 85 percent of: (1) the fair market value of the stock at the time the option is granted, or (2) the fair market value of the stock at the time the option is exercised. The option cannot be exercised later than 27 months from the date the option is granted (or five years from the date the option is granted, if the option price is based on the fair market value of the stock at the time the option is exercised). No employee can acquire the right to buy more than $25,000 of stock per year (valued at the time the option is granted).

Wash Sales

1935. Wash Sales of Stock or Securities. Under the wash sale rule, a taxpayer who realizes a loss upon a sale or other disposition of stock or securities may not claim a deduction for the loss unless the loss is incurred in the ordinary course of a trade or business as a securities dealer (¶ 1903) (Code Sec. 1091; Reg. § 1.1091-1).[34] A wash sale occurs if the taxpayer sells or disposes of the stock or securities, and within 30 days before or after that date (the 61-day period) the taxpayer acquires, or enters into a contract or option to acquire, substantially identical stock or securities (¶ 1937). The acquisition of substantially identical stock or securities through a traditional IRA or Roth IRA cannot be used to avoid the wash sale rule (Rev. Rul. 2008-5).

If the wash sale rule applies, only a portion of the total loss is disallowed if a taxpayer acquires less stock or securities during the 61-day period than he or she sold. The nondeductible loss is allocated to the stock or securities disposed of in the order of their time of acquisition. When the amount of stock and securities acquired during the 61-day period is more than the amount sold, the shares acquired that resulted in the nondeductibility of the loss are determined by the order of their acquisition.

References are to Standard Federal Tax Reports; Tax Research Consultant; and Practical Tax Explanations.

[32] ¶ 19,602, ¶ 19,609; COM-PEN: 21,054; § 21,625.10

[33] ¶ 19,900; COMPEN: 21,052; § 21,610.05

[34] ¶ 30,180, ¶ 30,181; SALES: 45,150; § 18,905

A loss realized on the closing of a short sale of stock or securities (¶ 1944) is disallowed under the wash sale rule if within 30 days before or after the closing of the sale substantially identical stock or securities are sold or another short sale of substantially identical stock or securities is entered. The wash sale rule also applies to a loss realized on the sale, exchange, or termination of a securities futures contract to sell stock or securities. It does not apply to losses from sales or trades of commodity futures contracts and foreign currencies.

The disallowance of a loss under the wash sale rule does not apply to stock or securities acquired in a nontaxable exchange. This includes stock or securities acquired by gift, bequest, or devise, or through a nonrecognition transaction such as a like-kind exchange, exchange of property for stock, exchange of stock for stock, and spousal transfer incident to divorce. The wash sale rule also does not apply to any loss attributable to a section 1256 contract (¶ 1947) (Code Sec. 1256(f)(5)).[35] The wash sale rule will also not apply to a redemption of shares in a money market fund (MMF) after October 13, 2014, that results in a loss if the MMF has a share price that has a floating net asset value (NAV) but is subject to the same investment limits as other MMFs (Rev. Proc. 2014-45; Prop. Reg. § 1.446-7).[36] Under proposed regulations taxpayers may rely on for tax years ending on or after July 28, 2014, aggregate gain or loss is determined for each computation period for this purpose. In addition, no gain or loss is determined for any particular redemption of a taxpayer's shares in a floating NAV fund.

When a loss is disallowed because of the wash sale rule, the disallowed loss is added to the cost basis of the new stock or securities (unless the new stock or securities are acquired through an IRA). The adjustment postpones the loss deduction until the disposition of the new stock or securities (Code Sec. 1091(d); Reg. § 1.1091-2).[37] The taxpayer's holding period of the new stock or securities includes the holding period of the stock or securities sold (Code Sec. 1223(3)).[38]

> **Example:** Betty buys 100 shares of Rapid Corporation stock for $1,000 on January 1, 2014. She sells these shares on January 2, 2015, for $750 and within 30 days from the sale Betty buys another 100 shares of Rapid Corporation for $800. Because Betty purchased substantially identical stock, she cannot deduct the $250 loss that she realized on the sale. Betty, however, adds the disallowed loss of $250 to the cost of her new shares. As a result, her basis in the new shares is $1,050 ($800 cost, plus the $250 loss she could not claim under the wash sale rule). If she sells the new shares on March 31, 2015, any gain is long-term capital gain.

The wash sale rule applies without regard to the gain or loss realized on the sale of separate lots of the same stock or security. Thus, where the wash sale rule applies to deny deductions for losses for one lot, any gain realized on a separate lot is not reduced by the losses (Rev. Rul. 70-231).[39] In addition, the wash sale rule does not specifically apply when stock is sold at a loss and a party related to the seller, such as his or her spouse, reacquires the stock within the prohibited 61-day period. The loss, however, may be disallowed under the related party rules of Code Sec. 267 (¶ 1717) on the ground that there is an indirect sale to the spouse (*J. P. McWilliams*, SCt, 47-1 USTC ¶ 9289).[40]

1937. Substantially Identical Stock or Securities. In determining whether stock or securities are substantially identical subject to the wash sale rule (¶ 1935), all facts and circumstances must be considered. Ordinarily, stocks or securities of one corporation are not considered substantially identical to stocks or securities of another corporation. They may, however, be substantially identical in some cases such as in a reorganization—the stocks and securities of the predecessor and successor corporations may be substantially identical (IRS Pub. 550).

Bonds or preferred stock of a corporation are not ordinarily considered substantially identical to the common stock of the same corporation. When the bonds or

References are to Standard Federal Tax Reports; Tax Research Consultant; and Practical Tax Explanations.

[35] ¶ 31,100; SALES: 45,150; § 18,910

[36] ¶ 20,618, ¶ 30,183.1115; SALES: 45,150; § 18,905

[37] ¶ 30,180, ¶ 30,182; SALES: 45,164; § 18,920

[38] ¶ 30,460; SALES: 45,164; § 18,925

[39] ¶ 30,183.11; SALES: 45,160; § 18,930

[40] ¶ 30,183.109; SALES: 45,166.10

preferred stock are convertible into common stock of the same corporation, however, the relative values, price changes, and other circumstances may make these bonds or preferred stock and the common stock substantially identical (Rev. Rul. 77-201).[41]

1942. Share Lending Agreements. No gain or loss is recognized by a taxpayer on an exchange of securities if the exchange is made as part of a qualifying securities lending arrangement in which the taxpayer transfers the securities and later receives identical securities in return (Code Sec. 1058).[42] In effect, the taxpayer is merely lending securities to the other party to the transaction. This provision is designed to mitigate delays that a broker may face in obtaining securities by allowing the broker to borrow securities without creating tax consequences for the lender. However, the provision is available to any taxpayer that lends securities, not just those that lend to brokers. This treatment applies only if the securities lending agreement requires the borrower to return securities to the taxpayer that are identical to those which were lent. The taxpayer's basis in the securities received is the same as the taxpayer's basis in the securities that were loaned to the borrower.

Short Sales

1944. Short Sales. A short sale is a transaction in which a taxpayer sells shares of stock or property that he or she does not own or wish to transfer at the time of the time of sale. The taxpayer sells short by: (1) borrowing property (usually from a broker) and delivering it to the buyer; and (2) closing or covering the transaction at a later date by purchasing substantially identical property and delivering it to the lender, or making delivery out of property the taxpayer held at the time of the sale (Code Sec. 1233(a); Reg. § 1.1233-1(a)).[43]

Generally, the seller does not recognize gain or loss on the transaction until he or she delivers the property to the lender and the short sale is closed. However, if the property that has been sold short becomes substantially worthless, the seller must recognize gain as if the short sale were closed when the property became substantially worthless (Code Sec. 1233(h)).[44] In addition, entering a short sale of an appreciated financial position may cause the taxpayer to be treated as making a constructive sale at the time that the taxpayer entered into the transaction (¶ 1945).

The gain or loss on a closed short sale is the difference between the amount realized on the sale of the borrowed property and the taxpayer's adjusted basis in the property used to close the transaction. Generally, the character of that gain or loss is determined by reference to the character of the property used to close the sale in the hands of the taxpayer. Thus, a taxpayer will have capital gain or loss if the property used to close the short sale is a capital asset (¶ 1741). Hedging transactions, however, generally result in ordinary income or loss (¶ 1949). If a short seller has a gain on the transaction when the replacement property is purchased, the gain is recognized at that time. A loss is not recognized until the replacement property is delivered to the lender (Rev. Rul. 2002-44).[45]

Holding Period. Generally, short sellers determine whether they have a short-term or long-term capital gain or loss by determining the amount of time they held the property that they deliver to the lender to close out the short sale.

> **Example:** On January 2, Mary Edwards enters into an agreement to sell 100 shares of Niftexo Corp. for $10 a share to Susan Croft. Mary does not own any Niftexo shares, so she borrows the 100 shares from her broker and delivers these shares to Susan. On May 1, Mary purchases 100 shares of Niftexo at a price of $15 a share. The same day she delivers these shares to her broker in order to replace the shares she had borrowed. Her recognized loss of $500 is short term because her holding period of the Niftexo shares is determined by the amount of time she held the shares (i.e., less than one day).

References are to Standard Federal Tax Reports; Tax Research Consultant; and Practical Tax Explanations.

[41] ¶ 30,183.14; SALES: 45,154; § 18,915

[42] ¶ 30,000; SALES: 3,302.35; § 18,855

[43] ¶ 30,590, ¶ 30,591; SALES: 45,100; § 19,001

[44] ¶ 30,590; SALES: 45,120; § 19,005

[45] ¶ 30,463.4383; SALES: 45,102

Gain from the short sale of a capital asset is short-term capital gain, however, if the taxpayer owned substantially identical property for one year or less on the date of the short sale, or if the taxpayer acquired substantially identical property after the short sale and by the date the sale is closed (Code Sec. 1233(b); Reg. § 1.1233-1(c)).[46] The holding period of the substantially identical property begins on the closing of the short sale or on the date the property is sold, whichever happens first. In addition, any loss realized on the short sale of a capital asset is a long-term capital loss if the taxpayer owned substantially identical property for more than one year (Code Sec. 1233(d)). The loss is long term even when the property used to close the short sale is held by the seller for one year or less. A taxpayer can avoid the prohibition of losses from short sale if the position is part of a mixed straddle (¶ 1948).

Special holding period rules apply to brokers' arbitrage transactions (Code Sec. 1233(f); Reg. § 1.1233-1(f)).[47] Losses on short sales of stock or securities are also subject to the wash sales rule (¶ 1935).

1945. Constructive Sale Treatment of Short Sales. Under certain circumstances, appreciated financial positions must be treated as being constructively sold at the time that the taxpayer entered into the transaction (Code Sec. 1259(a)).[48] The taxpayer must recognize gain as if the position were sold, assigned, or otherwise terminated at its fair market value *as of the date of the constructive sale* and immediately repurchased. Any gain or loss subsequently realized on the position is adjusted to reflect the gain recognized. The taxpayer's holding period begins as if the taxpayer had first acquired the position on the date of the constructive sale.

An appreciated financial position is generally any position with respect to any stock, debt instrument, or partnership interest if there would be gain if the position were sold, assigned, or otherwise terminated at its fair market value (Code Sec. 1259(b)). It does not include any position that is subject to mark-to-market requirements (¶ 1903), including section 1256 contracts (¶ 1947). It also does not include any position or hedge of a position with regard to straight debt if:

- the debt unconditionally entitles the holder to receive a specified principal amount;

- interest payments are payable based on a fixed rate or, to the extent provided in regulations, at a variable rate; and

- the debt is not convertible into stock of the issuer or any related person as defined by Code Sec. 267(b) or Code Sec. 707(b) (¶ 432 and ¶ 1717).

A constructive sale generally is one of four specified types of transactions offsetting an appreciated financial position that has the effect of substantially eliminating both the taxpayer's risk of loss and chance for further gain on the position. They include: short sales (¶ 1944); notional principal contracts; forward or futures contracts; or the purchase of property to cover the position if the appreciated position is itself a short position (Code Sec. 1259(c)). Contracts for the sale of appreciated financial assets that are not publicly traded are excluded from the definition of a constructive sale if the contract settles within one year after the date it was entered. A safe harbor is also provided for certain short-term hedges that would otherwise be treated as constructive sales if three conditions are satisfied:

- the transaction is closed on or before the end of the 30th day after the end of the tax year in which the transaction was entered;

- the taxpayer holds the appreciated financial position throughout the 60-day period beginning on the date the transaction is closed; and

References are to Standard Federal Tax Reports; Tax Research Consultant; and Practical Tax Explanations.

[46] ¶ 30,590, ¶ 30,591; SALES: 45,104; § 19,010.10   [47] ¶ 30,590, ¶ 30,591; SALES: 45,112   [48] ¶ 31,130; SALES: 45,450

¶1945

19

SECURITIES

• at no time during that 60-day period is the taxpayer's risk of loss with respect to the position reduced by a circumstance that would be described in Code Sec. 246(c)(4) if references to stock included references to such position.

The "closed transaction" exception also applies to certain reestablished positions.

1946. Payments in Lieu of Dividends on Short Sales. A taxpayer who borrows stock to make a short sale (¶ 1944) may have to make payments to the lender in lieu of dividends distributed during the short position. The payments may be deductible as investment interest expense as an itemized deduction (¶ 1094) if the short sale is held open for at least 46 days (more than one year if extraordinary dividends are involved). If the short sale is closed by the 45th day after the date of the short sale (one year or less in the case of an extraordinary dividend), the short seller cannot claim the deduction and must instead increase the basis of the stock used to close the short sale by the amount of the payment (Code Sec. 263(h)).[49] The 45-day and one-year periods are suspended for any period in which the borrower holds options to buy substantially identical property or holds one or more positions in such property.

Commodities and Related Instruments

1947. Section 1256 Contracts. Each section 1256 contract held by a taxpayer at the end of the tax year is generally subject to mark-to-market requirements and treated as sold at its fair market value on the last business day of the year (Code Sec. 1256).[50] The mark-to-market rule also applies if the taxpayer's obligation (or rights) under a section 1256 contract is terminated or transferred during the tax year.

Any capital gains or losses arising from a section 1256 contract as a result of the mark-to-market requirement are treated as if they are 60 percent long-term and 40 percent short-term without regard to the taxpayer's actual holding period. Form 6781 is used by a taxpayer to report gains and losses from all section 1256 contracts that are open at the end of the year or that were closed during the year. An individual who has a net section 1256 contract loss for the tax year may elect to carry the loss back three years instead of carrying it over to the next year (¶ 1754).

A section 1256 contract includes regulated futures contracts, foreign currency contracts, nonequity options, dealer equity options, and dealer securities futures contracts. However, the mark-to-market rules do not apply to hedging transactions (¶ 1949), equity options, and section 1256 contracts that are part of a mixed straddle if an election is made to exclude them from mark-to-market treatment (¶ 1948).

1948. Tax Straddles. A tax straddle is any set of offsetting positions such as a futures contract, a forward contract, or an option on actively traded personal property (including stock) that seeks to diminish an investor's risk of loss (Code Sec. 1092).[51] Any loss realized with respect to a straddle position may be deducted only to the extent that the loss exceeds the taxpayer's unrealized gain in the offsetting position. Unused losses are carried forward to the taxpayer's next tax year. A taxpayer must report on Form 6781 each position in actively traded personal property (whether or not it is part of a straddle) on which the taxpayer has unrecognized gain at the end of the tax year.

The loss deferral rule does not apply if a straddle is identified on the taxpayer's books before the close of the day on which it is acquired. If there is a loss from any position in an identified straddle, the taxpayer must increase the basis of each of the positions that offset the loss position by the same ratio to the loss as the unrecognized gain for the offsetting position bears to the total unrecognized gain for all the offsetting positions. The loss deferral rule also does not apply to hedging transactions (¶ 1949), straddles consisting entirely of qualified covered call options, and straddles consisting entirely of section 1256 contracts (¶ 1947).

Wash Sale and Short Sales. A modified wash sale rule (¶ 1935) applies to any disposition of a position in a straddle and denies a deduction of a loss if there is

---

References are to Standard Federal Tax Reports; Tax Research Consultant; and Practical Tax Explanations.

[49] ¶ 13,700; SALES: 45,118.05; § 19,015

[50] ¶ 31,100; SALES: 48,100; § 18,830.05

[51] ¶ 30,200; SALES: 48,150; § 45,425.30

unrecognized gain in a successor position (Temp. Reg. § 1.1092(b)-1T).[52] In addition, a modified short sale rule (¶ 1944) applies to a straddle suspending the taxpayer's holding during the time he or she holds offsetting and successor positions (Temp. Reg. § 1.1092(b)-2T).[53]

Mixed Straddles. A mixed straddle is a straddle in which at least one, but not all, of the positions is a section 1256 contract (¶ 1947), with each position being properly identified as part of the straddle. A taxpayer may elect not to have mark-to-market rules apply to the section 1256 contracts that are a part of the mixed straddle (Code Sec. 1256(d)).[54] If the taxpayer elects out of the mark-to-market rules, the straddle is subject to the loss deferral rule, the modified wash sale, and the modified short sale rules. Alternatively, a taxpayer may elect to offset gains and losses from positions that are part of a mixed straddle by (1) separately identifying each mixed straddle to which such treatment applies, or (2) establishing a mixed straddle account with respect to a class of activities for which gains and losses will be recognized and offset on a periodic basis (Code Sec. 1092(b); Temp. Reg. § 1.1092(b)-3T; Temp. Reg. § 1.1092(b)-4T).[55]

Interest and Carrying Charges. Interest and carrying charges incurred with respect to a straddle position are not permitted, except to the extent the interest and carrying charges are offset by current income generated by the position. Any excess must be capitalized (Code Sec. 263(g)).[56]

1949. Hedging Transactions. A hedging transaction is one a taxpayer enters into in the normal course of business primarily to reduce the risk of changes in interest rates, price changes, or currency fluctuations (Code Sec. 1221(a)(7); Reg. § 1.1221-2).[57] The property involved in a hedging transaction is generally not classified as a capital asset (¶ 1741). As a result, gain or loss on most hedging transactions is classified as ordinary income or loss. This rule also applies when a short sale or option is part of a hedging transaction (¶ 1944). In order to be classified as a hedging transaction, the transaction must be entered into in the normal course of the taxpayer's business in order to manage risk. The determination of whether a transaction was entered into in order to manage the taxpayer's business risk is based upon all the facts and circumstances. A transaction that is not a hedging transaction may be a straddle (¶ 1948).

Identification. The hedging transaction must be identified before the close of the day on which the taxpayer entered into the transaction (Reg. § 1.1221-2(f)). The taxpayer must identify the property that is being hedged within 35 days after the transaction is entered into. The taxpayer's identification of the hedged property must be unambiguous and become part of the taxpayer's books and records.

Corporate Bonds and Other Debt Instruments

1950. Discounts, Premiums, and Issue Expenses of Corporate Bonds. The tax effects to a corporation from the issuance of bonds and from the reacquisition of such bonds depends upon whether the bonds are issued at face value, at a discount, or at a premium. A corporation generally does not realize gain or loss upon the issuance of a bond or other debt instrument (Reg. § 1.61-12(c)).[58] If, however, a corporation repurchases a bond for less than its adjusted issue price, then it will realize income from the discharge of indebtedness (¶ 855). In the case of a bond repurchased at a discount during 2009 or 2010, the corporation can elect to defer the discharge of indebtedness income and recognize it ratably over a five-year period beginning in 2014 and through 2018 (Code Sec. 108(i)).[59]

[52] ¶ 30,201; SALES: 48,156; § 45,425.30

[53] ¶ 30,202; SALES: 48,158; § 45,425.30

[54] ¶ 31,100; SALES: 48,200; § 45,425.30

[55] ¶ 30,200, ¶ 30,203, ¶ 30,204; SALES: 48,200; § 45,425.30

[56] ¶ 13,700; SALES: 48,160, BUSEXP: 9,502.05; § 45,425.30

[57] ¶ 30,420, ¶ 30,424; SALES: 15,114, SALES: 48,250; § 16,505.40

[58] ¶ 5,801; CCORP: 3,158; § 3,401

[59] ¶ 7002; SALES: 12,252; § 3,420.40

In the case of bonds issued at a discount, the discount is amortized and deductible by the corporation over the life of the bond. If bonds are issued at a premium on or after March 2, 1998, the amount of the premium is amortized as an offset to the corporation's otherwise allowable interest deduction with the portion of bond premium allocable to the accrual period based on constant yield (Reg. § 1.163-13(a)).[60] Any amount allocable to a bond's conversion feature is not part of the bond premium (Code Sec. 171(b)(1)).[61] See ¶ 1967 for the tax treatment of a premium paid by the buyer of a bond. Any expenses related to issuing the bond (i.e., printing, advertising, legal fees) are amortized over the life of the bond and deducted as business expenses.[62]

1952. Original Issue Discount. Any holder of any debt instrument that has an original issue discount (OID) must include in gross income an amount equal to the sum of the daily portions of the OID for each day during the tax year on which the holder held the debt instrument (Code Sec. 1272).[63] The basis of the debt instrument in the hands of the holder is increased by the amount required to be included in gross income. The OID requirement does not apply to short-term obligations with a fixed maturity of less than one year, tax-exempt obligations, U.S. savings bonds, and certain loans between natural persons. It also does not apply to any holder who has purchased the debt instrument at a premium or to any holder that is a life insurance company.

OID on a debt instrument is the excess of the stated redemption price at maturity over the issue price (Code Sec. 1273).[64] Under a special *de minimis* rule, if the difference is less than 0.25 percent of the redemption price multiplied by the number of full years from the date of issue to the date of maturity, then the OID is zero.

The stated redemption price at maturity includes all payments provided by the obligation other than qualified interest payments. These are amounts actually and unconditionally payable at fixed, periodic intervals of one year or less, based on a fixed interest rate and outstanding principal amount. Debt instruments that are publicly offered or that are issued for money or publicly traded property have their issue price determined based on those objective features. Special rules determine issue price when publicly offered debt instruments are part of investment units. For debt instruments that are issued for property, services, or the right to use property, but none of which is publicly traded, the issue price may be the stated principal amount, or the imputed principal amount (¶ 1954).

Interest Deduction. In the case of any debt instrument issued after July 1, 1982, the portion of OID allowable as a deduction to the issuer for any tax year is equal to the aggregate daily portions of the OID for days during that tax year (Code Sec. 163(e)).[65] The daily portions of OID for any day is determined by allocating to each day in any accrual period a ratable portion of the increase during the accrual period in the adjusted issue price of the debt instrument (Code Sec. 1272(a)(3)).[66]

Information Statement for Recipients. Any issuer with any bond outstanding or any other evidence of indebtedness in registered form issued at a discount must generally furnish the holder and the IRS with an information statement (Form 1099-OID) for the calendar year if there is OID of at least $10 (Code Sec. 6049).[67]

Stripped Bonds and Stripped Coupons. Special OID rules govern stripped bonds and stripped coupons purchased or sold after July 1, 1982 (Code Sec. 1286(a)).[68] Under this type of arrangement, one taxpayer strips an interest coupon from a bond and sells either the bond or the coupon. The bond and the coupon are treated as separate debt instruments issued with OID. The buyer of a stripped bond treats as OID the bond's

---

References are to Standard Federal Tax Reports; Tax Research Consultant; and Practical Tax Explanations.

[60] ¶ 9,302D; BUSEXP: 21,214
[61] ¶ 11,850; CCORP: 3,154; § 11,530
[62] ¶ 5804.22; CCORP: 3,156; § 19,350
[63] ¶ 31,260; ACCTNG: 36,200; § 19,310.05
[64] ¶ 31,280; ACCTNG: 36,100; § 19,315.05
[65] ¶ 9102; BUSEXP: 21,102; § 7,405.20
[66] ¶ 31,260; ACCTNG: 36,214; § 19,310.10
[67] ¶ 36,020; ACCTNG: 36,550; § 19,320.10
[68] ¶ 31,480; ACCTNG: 36,350; § 19,335

value at maturity minus the price paid. The buyer of a stripped coupon treats as OID the interest to be paid on the due date of the coupon minus the price paid.

The seller of stripped bonds or stripped coupons must include in income the interest that accrued before the date of sale that was not previously included in income. Market discount must also be included in the seller's income. Both of these included items increase the seller's basis in the bonds and coupons. The seller then allocates the adjusted basis between the item kept (e.g., the bond) and the item sold (e.g., the coupon) based on the fair market value of the items. The difference between the sales price of the item and its adjusted basis is the seller's gain or loss.

Stripped Stock. Preferred stock purchased after April 30, 1993, that has been stripped of some or all of its dividend rights is treated in the same manner as stripped bonds. OID is equal to the stated redemption price minus the amount paid for the stock (Code Sec. 305(e)).[69]

Tax-Exempt and Stripped Tax-Exempt Bonds. OID on a tax-exempt bond is generally treated as tax-exempt interest (¶ 1956). However, when a tax-exempt bond is stripped, only a portion of the OID is treated as coming from a tax-exempt obligation (Code Sec. 1286(d)).[70] The balance is treated as OID on a taxable obligation. The Code contains the rules for determining the tax-exempt portion of the OID.

1954. Original Issue Discount for Debt Instruments Issued for Property. In determining the original issue discount (OID) of certain debt instruments issued for property (¶ 1952), the issue price may be determined by the stated principal amount of the instrument when there is adequate stated interest, or the imputed principal amount if there is not adequate stated interest (Code Sec. 1274).[71] This rule applies to debt instruments given in consideration for the sale or exchange of property if: (1) the stated redemption price at maturity exceeds either the stated principal amount (when there is adequate stated interest) or the imputed principal amount; and (2) some or all of the payments due under the instrument are due more than six months after the date of the sale or exchange. The rule does not apply to:

- sales for $250,000 or less;
- sales of principal residences by individuals (¶ 1707);
- sales of farms by individuals, estates, testamentary trusts, or small business corporations or partnerships for $1 million or less;
- land transfers between related parties that are covered by Code Sec. 483(e);
- sales of patents for amounts that are contingent on the productivity, use, or disposition of the property transferred (¶ 1767); or
- in the case of the borrower, sales or exchanges of personal use property (Code Sec. 1275(b)).[72]

If a debt-for-property transaction is not covered by these rules, the transaction may be subject to the imputed interest rules of Code Sec. 483 (¶ 1868). In addition, certain annuity contracts governed by Code Sec. 72 are excluded from the definition of "debt instrument" (Code Sec. 1275(a)(1)(B)).[73]

Adequate Stated Interest. A debt instrument generally provides for adequate stated interest if its stated principal amount is less than or equal to the imputed principal amount—the sum of the present value of all principal and interest payments due on the instrument (Code Sec. 1274(c)(2)).[74] Except in the case of a potentially abusive situation, present value of all payments due on the instrument is generally determined based on the lowest applicable federal rate in effect (¶ 83) in the three-month period (1) ending with the first month in which there is a binding written contract, or (2) ending with the

[69] ¶ 15,400; ACCTNG: 36,356
[70] ¶ 31,480; ACCTNG: 36,500; § 19,335

[71] ¶ 31,300; ACCTNG: 36,150; § 19,315.10
[72] ¶ 31,340; ACCTNG: 36,154.45; § 19,315.10

[73] ¶ 31,340; ACCTNG: 36,054.05
[74] ¶ 31,300; ACCTNG: 36,158, ACCTNG: 36,160; § 19,315.10

19

SECURITIES

month in which the sale or exchange occurred (Code Sec. 1274(b)). The AFR is determined by reference to the term of the debt instrument, including renewal and extension options. In situations where the imputed interest rules of Code Sec. 483 apply to a debt instrument (¶ 1868), payments due within six months after the sale are taken into account at face value.

For a sale-leaseback transaction, a rate equal to 110 percent of the AFR applies in determining the present value of payments (Code Sec. 1274(e)). The AFR may not exceed nine percent, compounded semiannually, if the debt instrument is given in consideration for the sale or exchange of property (other than new Code Sec. 38 property) and the stated principal amount of the instrument does not exceed an inflation-adjusted amount ($5,557,200 for 2014) (Code Sec. 1274A; Rev. Rul. 2013-23).[75] The AFR may not exceed six percent, compounded semiannually, in the case of transfers of land between family members if the aggregate sales price of all prior land sales between the family members during the calendar year does not exceed $500,000. However, this limit does not apply if any party to the sale is a nonresident alien (Code Sec. 483(e); Reg. § 1.483-3(b)).[76]

Joint Election. For sales or exchanges of property (other than new Code Sec. 38 property), the lender and borrower may jointly elect out of the rules for OID on debt issued for property, and take the interest on the debt instrument into account under the cash method of accounting (Code Sec. 1274A(c); Rev. Rul. 2013-23).[77] The election can be made only if:

- the stated principal amount of the instrument does not exceed an inflation-adjusted amount ($3,969,500 for 2014);

- the lender is on the cash-basis method of accounting and is not a dealer with respect to the property sold or exchanged; and

- these rules would otherwise have applied to the transaction.

1956. Original Issue Discount on Tax-Exempt Bonds. For tax-exempt obligations issued after September 3, 1982, and acquired after March 1, 1984, original issue discount (OID) is accrued in the same manner as that provided for OID on obligations issued by corporations and others under the constant yield method (¶ 1952) for purposes of determining interest expense deduction and the adjusted basis of the holder (Code Sec. 1288).[78] For purposes of determining the interest expense deduction, the reduction normally required where a subsequent holder pays an acquisition premium is disregarded. For tax-exempt obligations with a maturity of less than one year, interest is computed in the same manner as for short-term taxable obligations. The tables at ¶ 84 present applicable federal interest rates that have been adjusted to account for tax-exempt interest.

1958. Market Discount Bonds. Gain from the sale of a market discount bond is treated as ordinary interest income to the extent of accrued market discount (Code Sec. 1276).[79] A market discount bond is a bond that was purchased at a discount, other than obligations that mature within one year of issuance, U.S. savings bonds, certain installment obligations, and tax-exempt bonds purchased before May 1, 1993.

The accrued market discount on a bond is generally determined under a ratable accrual method where the accrued market discount equals the amount bearing the same ratio to the market discount on the bond as the number of days that the taxpayer held the bond bears to the number of days after the date of acquisition to the maturity date. Alternatively, the taxpayer can make an affirmative election to determine the accrued market discount under a constant interest method where the accrued market discount is equal to the total amount that would have been includible in a taxpayer's gross income

---

References are to Standard Federal Tax Reports; Tax Research Consultant; and Practical Tax Explanations.

[75] ¶ 31,320, ¶ 31,322.30; ACCTNG: 36,162.20; § 19,315.10

[76] ¶ 22,290, ¶ 22,294; ACCTNG: 36,308.25; § 19,510.15

[77] ¶ 31,320, ¶ 31,322.30; ACCTNG: 36,154.65; § 19,315.10

[78] ¶ 31,520; ACCTNG: 36,502.10, ACCTNG: 36,502.15; § 3,105.05

[79] ¶ 31,360; ACCTNG: 36,400; § 19,325.05

using the constant yield method for debt instruments with original issue discount (OID) for all periods during which the bond was held. The election is revocable only with the consent of the IRS and applies to all market discount bonds acquired during and after the tax year of the election. The election is made by filing a statement with the taxpayer's timely filed tax return that states that the market discount has been included in income. The statement should also indicate how the amount included in income was calculated (Rev. Proc. 92-67; Rev. Proc. 2011-14).[80]

Any partial payment of principal on a market discount bond is ordinary income to the extent of accrued market discount on the bond for obligations acquired after October 22, 1986 (Code Sec. 1276(a)(3)).[81] The payment that is included in gross income reduces the amount of accrued market discount.

Net direct interest expenses on debt incurred to purchase or continue a market discount bond acquired after July 18, 1984, may be deducted only to the extent that the expenses exceed the market discount allocable to the number of days the bond is held by the taxpayer (Code Sec. 1277).[82] The taxpayer may elect to take any deferred interest deduction in a subsequent year to the extent of net interest income from the market discount bond. Any deferred interest expense that remains (whether or not the election is made) is deducted in the year of disposition.

1961. Discount on Short-Term Obligations. Certain holders of short-term obligations must include in gross income: (1) an amount equal to the sum of the daily portions of the acquisition discount for each day during the tax year that the holder held the bond; and (2) any other interest payable on the obligation (Code Sec. 1281).[83] The holder of any short-term obligation is required to increase the obligation's basis by amounts required to be included. An obligation for this purpose includes a bond, debenture, note, certificate, or other evidence of debt, but not a tax-exempt obligation, which has a fixed maturity date not more than one year from the date of issue (Code Sec. 1283(a)(1)).[84] For short-term, nongovernmental obligations, the accrual requirement applies to original issue discount (OID), as opposed to acquisition discount.

Accrual of acquisition discount on short-term obligations is required for: (1) accrual method taxpayers; (2) banks; (3) brokers and dealers who hold short-term obligations for sale to customers in the ordinary course of trade or business; (4) regulated investment companies (¶ 2301) and common trust funds (¶ 2389); (5) persons who identify short-term obligations as part of a hedging transaction (¶ 1949); and (6) persons who strip a short-term bond of its interest coupons (¶ 1952) (or any person whose basis in such instruments is determined by reference to the basis in the hands of such persons). Obligations held by pass-through entities (partnerships, S corporations and trusts) are subject to mandatory accrual of acquisition discount and interest if the pass-through entity acquires the obligation during the required accrual period (or if it acquires the obligation to avoid mandatory accrual).

Net direct interest expense incurred with respect to a short-term obligation is deductible only to the extent that it exceeds the sum of: (1) the acquisition discount (excess of stated redemption price over basis) for each day during the year that the bond is held by the taxpayer, and (2) the amount of any interest payable on the obligation that accrues during the year but is not included in gross income for that year because of the taxpayer's accounting method. The daily portion of the acquisition discount is equal to the total discount divided by the number of days from the acquisition date to the maturity date (Code Secs. 1282(a) and 1283(b)(1)).[85] The interest deduction is deferred in a manner similar to that applicable to market discount bonds (¶ 1958).

References are to Standard Federal Tax Reports; Tax Research Consultant; and Practical Tax Explanations.

[80] ¶ 31,361.40; ACCTNG: 36,404; § 19,325.05

[81] ¶ 31,360; ACCTNG: 36,408.15; § 19,325.05

[82] ¶ 31,380; ACCTNG: 36,410; § 19,325.10

[83] ¶ 31,420; ACCTNG: 36,452; § 19,330.05

[84] ¶ 31,460; ACCTNG: 36,452; § 19,330.05

[85] ¶ 31,440, ¶ 31,460; ACCTNG: 36,458; § 19,330.10

1963. Unregistered Obligations. Most corporate and government debt obligations are required to be in registered form for the payor to deduct interest (Code Sec. 163(f)(1)).[86] An excise tax is imposed on issues of registration-required obligations (other than tax-exempt bonds) that are not in registered form (Code Sec. 4701).[87] The excise tax is equal to one percent of the principal amount of the obligation multiplied by the number of calendar years (or portions thereof) during the period beginning on the date of issuance of the obligation and ending on the date of maturity.

If a registration-required obligation is not in registered form, any gain realized on its sale or other disposition is taxed as ordinary income (Code Sec. 1287)[88] and loss deductions are denied (Code Sec. 165(j))[89] unless the issuance of the obligation was subject to the excise tax or certain other specified exceptions apply. Issuers of registration-required obligations face the loss of deductions for interest (including original issue discount (¶ 1952)) on the bonds and cannot reduce earnings and profits by the amount of any interest on the obligation (Code Sec. 312(m)).[90]

1965. Exchanges of U.S. Obligations. Some types of U.S. savings bonds may be exchanged tax free for other types of U.S. savings bonds (¶ 730) (Code Sec. 1037).[91] If the original bond was issued at a discount, an amount equal to what would have been ordinary income from original issue discount (¶ 1952) if the exchange had been taxable is treated ordinary income when the bond received in exchange is disposed of or redeemed at a gain.

1967. Bond Premium Amortization by Bondholder. When a bond owner has paid a premium over the face amount of a taxable bond, he or she has the option of (1) amortizing the premium by deducting it over the life of the bond, or (2) not amortizing and treating the premium as part of basis (Code Sec. 171(a); Reg. § 1.171-4).[92] The amortization method is elected by reporting the amortization on the tax return for the first year the election is to apply and attaching a statement to the tax return that the amortization election is being made. No amortization is allowed for tax-exempt bonds. However, a reduction in the basis of the bond by the amount of the bond premium is required (Code Sec. 1016(a)(5)).[93] For a dealer in municipal bonds, see ¶ 1970.

The amount of bond premium that can be amortized for the tax year (and deducted currently) is calculated under a constant yield method (Code Sec. 171(b); Reg. § 1.171-2).[94] Under this method, the amount of the amortizable bond premium and the amount attributable to a particular tax year must be determined on the basis of the taxpayer's yield to maturity, using the taxpayer's basis in the obligation and compounding at the close of each accrual period. If a bond is received in an exchange and the basis of the bond is determined at least in part from the basis of the property given up in the exchange, the basis of the bond cannot exceed its fair market value immediately after the exchange for purposes of determining bond premium. This rule generally does not apply to an exchange of securities in a reorganization.

Premium on Convertible Bond. Amortization is not allowed for any part of a premium that is paid for the conversion feature in a convertible bond. A corporation's deduction for the premium it is called upon to pay to repurchase its own convertible indebtedness is generally limited to the amount of the normal call premium (Code Sec. 249(a)).[95]

1970. Dealer in Tax-Exempt Bonds. A dealer in tax-exempt obligations must amortize any premiums just as if the interest on the bonds had been taxable. A dealer who does not inventory securities or who inventories them at cost must reduce the adjusted basis of any municipal bonds sold during the year by the total amortization for the period they were held. A dealer who values inventories other than at cost (for

---

References are to Standard Federal Tax Reports; Tax Research Consultant; and Practical Tax Explanations.

[86] ¶ 9102; BUSEXP: 30,252; § 19,340

[87] ¶ 33,941; BUSEXP: 30,252; § 19,340

[88] ¶ 31,500; SALES: 24,404.05; § 19,340

[89] ¶ 9802; SALES: 24,404.05

[90] ¶ 15,600; CCORP: 12,104.30

[91] ¶ 29,720; SALES: 27,250; § 18,220

[92] ¶ 11,850, ¶ 11,854; DEPR: 21,200; § 45,415.20

[93] ¶ 29,410; DEPR: 21,210; § 45,415.20

[94] ¶ 11,850, ¶ 11,852; DEPR: 21,200; § 45,415.20

[95] ¶ 13,400; BUSEXP: 9,454.05

example, market value) must annually reduce his or her cost of securities sold by amortization on municipal bonds held during the year (Code Sec. 75; Reg. § 1.75-1).[96]

When a tax-exempt obligation is purchased and is sold or otherwise disposed of within 30 days after acquisition, matures, or is callable more than five years after it is acquired, an amortization adjustment must be made unless the bond is sold or disposed of at a gain. Thus, a dealer who inventories at other than cost and holds at the end of the year a bond maturing or callable more than five years after acquisition does not have to reflect amortization on it in the cost of securities sold. If it is sold at a gain, no amortization adjustment is to be made. If it is not sold at a gain, the cost of securities sold is then reduced by the amortization for the entire period it was held.

Accounting Issues

1973. Reporting and Time of Sale for Publicly Traded Securities. A cash or accrual method taxpayer other than a dealer (¶ 1903) who sells stock or securities traded on an established securities market generally must recognize gains and losses on the trade date, rather than the settlement date (Rev. Rul. 93-84).[97] The holding period for such stock or securities is also measured by using the trade date as the date sold and not the settlement date (¶ 1737). Gain or loss on a short sale of securities, however, is recognized on the settlement date as set by exchange rules (¶ 1944). The installment method of reporting is not available for sales of stock or securities traded on an established securities market (¶ 1805).

1975. Identification of Securities Sold. If a taxpayer can adequately identify the shares of securities sold or exchanged, his or her basis is the cost or other basis of the particular shares of stock or bond. An adequate identification is made if the taxpayer can show the certificates representing shares of stock from a lot which the taxpayer acquired on a certain date, or for a certain price, and which were delivered to the taxpayer's broker or other transferee. If a taxpayer buys and sells securities at various times in varying quantities and cannot adequately identify the shares that are sold, then the basis and holding period of the shares sold are generally determined on a first-in, first-out (FIFO) basis (Reg. § 1.1012-1(c)).[98] Most courts hold, however, that after a nontaxable reorganization in which the taxpayer receives shares of stock in another corporation in exchange for the original shares, the FIFO rule is not applicable.[99] In the case of the sale, exchange, or other disposition of a specified security on or after an applicable date (¶ 1980), the basis reported by the broker on Form 1099-B must be calculated on an account by account basis (Code Sec. 1012(c)).[100] Thus, the broker may be required to use different basis computation methods for different accounts.

A shareholder in a regulated investment company (RIC) or mutual fund (¶ 2301) may elect to figure gain or loss of identical shares using an average basis if the shareholder (1) acquired the shares at various times and prices, and (2) left the shares on deposit in an account handled by a custodian or agent who acquires or redeems shares of the RIC or mutual fund (Code Sec. 1012(d); Reg. § 1.1012-1(e)).[101] Shares are identical for this purpose if they have the same Committee on Uniform Security Identification Procedure (CUSIP) number or other security identifier number permitted by the IRS. The option to use an average basis is available only with respect to mutual fund shares and, beginning after 2010, dividend reinvestment plans. For periods on or after October 18, 2010, the average basis is determined by averaging the basis of all shares of identical stock in an account regardless of the taxpayer's holding period. For periods before October 18, 2010, a shareholder figures average basis using either the single-category method or a double-category method in which all shares in the mutual fund account at the time of each disposition are categorized as either short-term or long-term shares.

References are to Standard Federal Tax Reports; Tax Research Consultant; and Practical Tax Explanations.

[96] ¶ 6250, ¶ 6251; ACCTNG: 15,256.15

[97] ¶ 21,005.892; SALES: 45,300; § 18,310.25

[98] ¶ 29,331; SALES: 6,212; § 16,115

[99] ¶ 29,336.451; SALES: 6,212.25; § 16,115

[100] ¶ 29,330; SALES: 6,068; § 39,120.12

[101] ¶ 29,330, ¶ 29,331; SALES: 6,212.35, SALES: 6,212.45; § 19,220.05, § 19,220.20

¶1975

1980. Basis and Holding Period Reporting for Securities. If a broker is required to file a return on Form 1099-B with respect to the gross proceeds of the sale of a covered security (¶ 2565), the broker must also report the customer's adjusted basis in the security and whether any gain or loss with respect to the security is long-term or short-term (Code Sec. 6045(g); Reg. § 1.6045-1).[102] A "covered security" is any specified security acquired through a transaction in the account in which the security was held, or was transferred to that account from an account in which the security was a covered security if the broker receiving custody of the security receives a statutory statement with respect to the transfer.

A "specified security" includes: (1) any share of stock in a corporation; (2) a note, bond, debenture or other evidence of indebtedness (other than certain interests in a real estate mortgage investment conduit (REMIC) (¶ 2343), a debt instrument where payments may be accelerated, and pools of debt instruments affected by prepayments); (3) a commodity, or a contract or a derivative with respect to a commodity; (4) any securities futures contract; (5) on option on one or more specified securities, or a warrant or stock right; and (6) other financial instruments as determined by the IRS. Special rules apply to broker reporting on sales by S corporations, short sales (¶ 1944), and options transactions. The applicable date of the basis reporting requirements depends on the type of specified security that is sold. The applicable date is:

- January 1, 2011, for corporate stock, generally;

- January 1, 2012, for stock in a regulated investment company or mutual fund (¶ 2301) and stock acquired in connection with a dividend reinvestment plan (DRP);

- January 1, 2014, for an option granted or acquired on or after that date;

- January 1, 2014, for a debt instrument for which a yield and maturity can be determined (e.g., a debt instrument that provides a single fixed payment schedule or alternative payment schedule), however, short-term debt instruments with a fixed maturity of less than one year are exempted from basis reporting; and

- January 1, 2016, for a debt instrument with more complex features (e.g., variable rate, inflation-indexed, or contingent payment), convertible debt, stripped bond or coupon, tax credit bond, and a debt instrument issued by a non-U.S. issuer or that requires payment in a foreign currency.

The broker must generally determine adjusted basis of a covered security under the first-in, first-out (FIFO) method (¶ 1975) unless the taxpayer adequately identifies the stock sold. For any stock for which an average basis method is allowed, such as stock in a mutual fund acquired in connection with a dividend reinvestment plan, the customer's adjusted basis is determined according to the broker's default method, unless the customer notifies the broker that he or she elects another acceptable method regarding the account in which the stock is held. Basis is determined without regard to the wash sale rule (¶ 1935) unless the acquisition and sale transactions resulting in a wash sale occur in the same account and are in identical securities.

Securities Transfers Between Accounts. Every broker (and any other person specified in regulations) that transfers a covered security to another broker must furnish to the transferee broker a written statement that permits the transferee broker to satisfy the basis and holding-period reporting requirements (Code Sec. 6045A; Reg. § 1.6045A-1).[103] The written statement must be furnished no later than 15 days after the date of the transfer, except as provided otherwise by the IRS, or the transferor could be subject to a penalty (¶ 2823).

References are to Standard Federal Tax Reports; Tax Research Consultant; and Practical Tax Explanations.

[102] ¶ 35,920, ¶ 35,923; FILEBUS: 9,252, FILEBUS: 9,256; § 39,120.12

[103] ¶ 35,931, ¶ 35,932; FILEBUS: 9,252, FILEBUS: 9,256; § 39,120.12

¶1980

Organizational Actions Affecting Basis. Issuers of specified securities must file Form 8937 describing any organizational action (e.g., stock split, merger, acquisition) that affects the basis of the security, the quantitative effect on the basis from such action, and any other information required by the IRS (Code Sec. 6045B; Reg. § 1.6045B-1).[104] A copy of Form 8937 must also be given to each security holder of record or the holder's nominee as of the date of the organizational action. Form 8937 must be filed by the earlier of 45 days after the organizational action or January 15 of the year following the calendar year during which the organizational action took place. However, no return is required for organizational actions which occur before the applicable date with respect to that security.

An issuer is not required to file Form 8937 if, by the filing due date, the issuer posts a completed and signed Form 8937 in a readily accessible format in a dedicated area of its primary public website, and keeps that form accessible on its website (or its successor's primary public website) for 10 years. If the issuer satisfies these public reporting requirements, then it is treated as having furnished a copy of Form 8937 to all holders and nominees. Form 8937 also is not required to be filed if the issuer reasonably determines that all recipients of the securities are exempt recipients. In addition, Form 8937 is not required if the issuer is an S corporation and the corporation reports the information on a timely-filed Schedule K-1 of Form 1120S. Penalties may be imposed for failure to file correct information returns in connection with organizational actions, failure to furnish correct statements to holders or nominees, or failure to provide required publicly-available information (¶ 2823).

1983. Commissions Paid on Securities. Commissions and other transaction costs paid to facilitate the sale of securities generally must be capitalized (Reg. § 1.263(a)-1(e); Temp. Reg. § 1.263(a)-1T(d)).[105] In the case of dealers in securities, however, commissions and other amounts paid to facilitate the sale of a security are treated as ordinary and necessary business expenses. Traders and investors treat the amounts capitalized as a reduction in the amount realized from the sale. They are taken into account either in the tax year in which the sale occurs or in the tax year in which the sale is abandoned if a loss deduction is permitted. The capitalized amount is not added to the basis of the property. See ¶ 1760 for information concerning the proper classification of a taxpayer as a trader, dealer, or investor. Ordinary and necessary expenses for investment advice, including a "wrap fee" on a brokerage account, paid by an investor in lieu of commissions on individual trades, are deductible investment expenses and are claimed as miscellaneous itemized deductions on the individual's Schedule A of Form 1040 in the year paid (Reg. § 1.212-1(g)).[106]

References are to Standard Federal Tax Reports; Tax Research Consultant; and Practical Tax Explanations.

[104] ¶ 35,934, ¶ 35,935; FILEBUS: 9,380; § 39,120.12

[105] ¶ 13,701, ¶ 13,702BC; SALES: 9,152; § 7,105.40

[106] ¶ 12,521; BUSEXP: 12,154.05; § 7,840.05

Chapter 20

HEALTH AND EMPLOYEE BENEFITS

Employer Health Insurance Mandate

2001. Employer Health Insurance Mandate. For any month beginning on or after January 1, 2015 (for employers with 100 or more full-time employees), and January 1, 2016 (for employers with 50 or more full-time employees), an applicable large employer may be assessed a nondeductible penalty known as a shared responsibility payment if either:

- the employer fails to offer at least 95 percent (70 percent for 2015) of its full-time employees (and after 2015, their dependents) the opportunity to enroll in minimum essential coverage under an eligible employer-sponsored plan (¶ 2003), or

- the employer offers its full-time employees (and after 2015, their dependents) the opportunity to enroll in minimum essential coverage under an eligible employer-sponsored plan but the coverage is unaffordable to the employee or does not provide minimum value (¶ 2005) (Code Sec. 4980H; Notice 2013-45; T.D. 9655, Preamble).[1]

An applicable large employer may be liable for either type of assessable payment in any calendar month, but not both. Minimum essential coverage for this purpose means coverage under an employer-sponsored plan offered in the small or large group market within a state and which meets the requirements for group health plans or group health insurance coverage under section 2791 of the Public Health Service Act (Code Sec. 5000A(f); Reg. § 54.4980H-1(a)(27)).[2]

Applicable Large Employer. An applicable large employer is any employer that employed on average at least 50 full-time employees, full-time equivalents (FTEs), or some combination on business days during the preceding calendar year (Code Sec. 4980H(c)(2); Reg. §§ 54.4980H-1(a)(4) and 54.4980H-2).[3] FTEs are determined by adding all hours of service for the month for employees who were not full-time employees (but no more than 120 hours per employee), and dividing by 120. An employer not in existence during an entire preceding calendar year is an applicable large employer for the current year if it is reasonably expected to employ an average of 50 or more full-time employees (including FTEs) on business days during the current calendar year.

An exemption to the 50-employee threshold applies if the employer has more than 50 employees for 120 days or less during the preceding calendar year, but the employees in excess of 50 are seasonal workers. A seasonal worker is an employee who performs labor or services on a seasonal basis including, but not limited to, certain agricultural workers and retail workers employed during holiday season.

In applying the 50-employee threshold, an employer includes all common law employers, including for-profit businesses, tax-exempt organizations, and government

---

References are to Standard Federal Tax Reports; Tax Research Consultant; and Practical Tax Explanations.

[1] ¶ 34,619ZA, ¶ 34,619ZD.35; HEALTH: 6,050; § 42,101

[2] ¶ 34,619ZBF, ¶ 34,962; HEALTH: 6,050; § 42,101

[3] ¶ 34,619ZA, ¶ 34,619ZBF, ¶ 34,619ZBI; HEALTH: 6,052; § 42,105

entities (Federal, State, local, and Indian tribes). Employers with common ownership such as controlled groups under Code Sec. 414(b) or (c), or related employers such as an affiliated service group under Code Sec. 414(m), are combined for the 50 employee threshold. Moreover, any references to an employer include references to the employer's predecessors and successors.

Full-Time Employee. A full-time employee for purposes of determining applicable large employer status is an employee who was employed on average at least 30 hours of service per week or 130 hours of service in a calendar month (Code Sec. 4980H(c)(4); Reg. §§54.4980H-1(a)(21) and 54.4980H-3).[4] Employee is defined under the common law standard, i.e., right to control, direct, etc. It does not include a leased employee, sole proprietor, partner in partnership, or two-percent or more S corporation shareholder, unless services are provided as both an employee and nonemployee.

An hour of service includes each hour for which the employee is paid or entitled to be paid for services performed in the United States for the employer, including periods of paid leave. For hourly employees, the employer calculates hours of service using records of hours worked and for which payment is made or due. For non-hourly employees, an employer can count actual hours worked and for which payment is due, or apply a days-worked equivalency (8 hours of service) or weeks-worked equivalency (40 hours of service). An employer may use different methods for different classifications of non-hourly employees as long as the categories are reasonable and consistently applied.

Safe harbors are provided allowing an employer the option of using either a look-back method or monthly measurement method to determine full-time employee status (Reg. §54.4980H-3).[5] Look-back measurements are provided for ongoing employees, new employees, and employees with a change in employment status.

Offer of Coverage. An employer is treated as offering coverage for a calendar month if it offers the coverage for that month to at least 95 percent (70 percent for 2015) of its full-time employees and (after 2015) their dependents (Reg. §§54.4980H-4(b) and 54.4980H-5(b)).[6] An offer occurs if the employee has the opportunity to elect to enroll in or decline coverage at least once during the plan year. Failure to offer coverage for any day of a calendar month is treated as failure to offer coverage for the entire month.

A full-time employee is treated as having been offered coverage only if the employer also offers coverage to the employee's dependents. A dependent is the employee's child who is under the age of 26. It does not include anyone other than children, such as the employee's spouse. If an employee or dependent enrolls in coverage but fails to pay his or her share of premiums on a timely basis, the employer is nonetheless treated as offering coverage for that coverage period.

Reporting Requirements. For tax years beginning on or after January 1, 2015, employers and insurance are required to file an annual information return with the IRS reporting health care coverage provided to employees and other individuals (¶ 2567) (Code Secs. 6055 and 6056; Notice 2013-45).

2003. Penalty for Employers Not Offering Health Care Coverage. For any month beginning on or after January 1, 2015, an applicable large employer (¶ 2001) is liable for a shared responsibility payment (assessable payment) if:

- the employer fails to offer to its full-time employees (and after 2015, their dependents) the opportunity to enroll in minimum essential coverage under an eligible employer-sponsored group health plan for any month, and

- at least one full-time employee is certified as having enrolled in a qualified health plan through a Health Insurance Exchange and eligible to receive a premium tax credit (¶ 1331) or cost-sharing reduction payment (Code Sec. 4980H(a); Reg. § 54.4980H-4; Notice 2013-45).[7]

References are to Standard Federal Tax Reports; Tax Research Consultant; and Practical Tax Explanations.

[4] ¶ 34,619ZA, ¶ 34,619ZBF, ¶ 34,619ZBL; HEALTH: 6,052; § 42,110

[5] ¶ 34,619ZBL; HEALTH: 6,056; § 42,110

[6] ¶ 34,619ZBO, ¶ 34,619ZBR; HEALTH: 6,054; § 42,125

[7] ¶ 34,619ZA, ¶ 34,619ZBO, ¶ 34,619ZD.35; HEALTH: 6,054; § 42,130.10

The assessable payment for an employer not offering coverage with respect to any calendar month equals the number of the employer's full-time employees reduced by 30 (by 80 in 2015 (T.D. 9655, Preamble)), multiplied by 1/12 of $2,000 (i.e., $166.67 per month). The $2,000 amount is adjusted for inflation after 2014 (Code Sec. 4980H(a), (c)(1) and (c)(5)).

The 30-employee reduction applies only for purposes of calculating the assessable payment (Code Sec. 4980H(c)(2)(D)). It does not apply for determining if the employer is an applicable large employer (i.e., 50 employee threshold). Also, a full-time employee does not include a full-time equivalent (FTE) employee for purposes of the payment calculation (Code Sec. 4980H(c)(2)(E)). Employers with common ownership or otherwise related are allowed only one 30-employee reduction which is allocated ratably among all the related employers.

An employer must pay the assessable payment upon notice and demand by IRS; it is not required to be included with the employer's tax return (Code Sec. 4980H(d)). The payment is assessed and collected in the same manner as an assessable penalty. However, it is not deductible as a business expense (Code Sec. 4980H(c)(7)).

2005. Penalty for Employers Offering Health Care Coverage. For any month beginning on or after January 1, 2015, an applicable large employer (¶ 2001) is liable for a shared responsibility payment (assessable payment) if:

- the employer offers minimum essential coverage under an eligible employer-sponsored group health plan to its full-time employees (and after 2015, their dependents) for any month, but

- at least one full-time employee is certified as having enrolled in a qualified health plan through a Health Insurance Exchange and eligible to receive an applicable premium tax credit (¶ 1331) or cost-sharing reduction payment because the coverage is not affordable to the employee or does not provide minimum value (Code Sec. 4980H(b); Reg. § 54.4980H-5; Notice 2013-45).[8]

Affordability. Coverage for an employee is affordable if the employee's share of the premium for self-only coverage, not family coverage, does not exceed 9.5 percent of the employee's annual household income (adjusted to 9.56 percent in 2015 (Rev. Proc. 2014-37)). The affordability test applies to the lowest-cost option available to the employee that also meets the minimum value requirement.

Safe harbors are provided for an employer to determine if coverage is affordable to an employee based on the employee's Form W-2 wages, the employee's rate of pay, or the federal poverty line. An employer may choose one or more safe harbors for all of its employees or any reasonable category of employees, so long as it is done on a uniform and consistent basis. The safe harbors only apply for purposes of the assessable payment; they do not affect an employee's eligibility for a premium tax credit.

Minimum Value. An employer-sponsored group health plan fails to provide minimum value if the plan's share of the total allowed costs of benefits provided under the plan is less than 60 percent of the costs (Prop. Reg. § 1.36B-6).[9] An eligible employer-sponsored plan may determine whether it provides minimum value by: (1) a minimum value calculator provided by the IRS and the Department of Health and Human Services (HHS); (2) actuarial certification; (3) certain safe harbor plan designs that will be specified in future guidance; or (4) for plans in the small group market, meeting the requirements for metal level coverage (bronze, silver, gold, or platinum).

Calculation of Assessable Payment. The assessable payment for an employer offering health care coverage with respect to any calendar month equals the number of the employer's full-time employees who receive a premium tax credit or cost-sharing reduction, multiplied by 1/12 of $3,000 (i.e., $250 per month). The $3,000 amount is adjusted for inflation after 2014 (Code Sec. 4980H(b) and (c)(5); Reg. § 54.4980H-5).[10]

References are to Standard Federal Tax Reports; Tax Research Consultant; and Practical Tax Explanations.

[8] ¶ 34,619ZA, ¶ 34,619ZBR, ¶ 34,619ZD.35; HEALTH: 6,054; § 42,130.15

[9] ¶ 4196U; HEALTH: 3,310; § 42,120

[10] ¶ 34,619ZA, ¶ 34,619ZBR; HEALTH: 6,054; § 42,130.15

The assessable payment for any calendar month is capped at the number of the employer's full-time employees for the month (minus up to 30; up to 80 in 2015 (T.D. 9655, Preamble)), multiplied by 1/12 of $2,000. The cap ensures that the payment for an employer that offers coverage can never exceed the assessable payment the employer would owe if it did not offer coverage (¶ 2003).

An employer must pay the assessable payment upon notice and demand by IRS; it is not required to be included with the employer's tax return (Code Sec. 4980H(d)). The payment is assessed and collected in the same manner as an assessable penalty. However, it is not deductible as a business expense (Code Sec. 4980H(c)(7)).

Health and Welfare Benefits

2011. Welfare Benefit Plans. A welfare benefit plan or welfare benefit fund is any fund through which an employer provides welfare benefits to employees, independent contractors, or their beneficiaries (Code Sec. 419).[11] Welfare benefits are benefits other than deferred compensation or transfers of restricted property, such as accident or health benefits, disability or death benefits, unemployment benefits, severance benefits, vacation, or similar benefits.

An employer may deduct contributions paid or accrued to a welfare benefit fund to the extent that the contributions do not exceed the qualified cost of the fund for the tax year, reduced by the after-tax income of the fund. If the employer's contributions to the fund are more than its qualified cost, the excess is carried over to the next tax year. Welfare benefits provided directly by an employer are deductible only in the tax year the employee includes the benefits in gross income or would include such benefits in gross income if they were taxable to the employee (¶ 906) (Code Sec. 404(b)(2)(A)).[12] An employer may not accrue and deduct unpaid welfare benefits.

A welfare benefit fund's qualified cost is the direct cost the employer would have been able to deduct using the cash method of accounting if it paid for the benefits directly (Code Sec. 419(c)). The qualified cost also includes any addition to a qualified asset account. A qualified asset account is a reserve set aside for the payment of disability benefits, medical benefits, supplemental unemployment benefits (SUB) or severance pay benefits, and life insurance or death benefits (Code Sec. 419A).[13]

The allowable addition to a qualified asset account for a tax year is the amount that will bring the account to a level (the "account limit") that is reasonably and actuarially necessary to fund the payment of incurred but unpaid benefits. In the case of post-retirement medical and life insurance benefits, the allowable addition is the amount required to fund the payment of such benefits on a level basis over the working lives of the covered employees based on current medical costs. For employers who do not support higher additions to a qualified asset account by actuarial certifications, there are safe harbor additions for the various benefits. Limits are placed on the level of disability and SUB or severance pay benefits that may be considered in establishing the account limit for such benefits.

VEBAs. Collectively bargained voluntary employees' beneficiary associations (VEBAs) are exempt from the account limits applicable to welfare benefit funds (Code Sec. 419A(f)(5)). Thus, employer contributions to VEBAs are deductible and earnings on assets of such VEBAs are tax exempt. In addition, VEBAs that are funded solely with employee contributions are also exempt from the account limits if: (1) the VEBA covers at least 50 employees; and (2) no employee is entitled to a refund with respect to amounts in the fund, other than a refund based on the experience of the entire fund. VEBAs are tax-exempt trusts that provide life, sickness, accident and other benefits to members or their dependents or beneficiaries and meet certain nondiscrimination requirements (Code Secs. 501(c)(9) and 505).[14]

References are to Standard Federal Tax Reports; Tax Research Consultant; and Practical Tax Explanations.

[11] ¶ 19,295; COMPEN: 42,100; § 9,345

[12] ¶ 18,330; COMPEN: 42,050; § 9,345

[13] ¶ 19,298; COMPEN: 42,150; § 9,345

[14] ¶ 22,602, ¶ 22,711; COMPEN: 54,100; § 33,005

2013. Employer Contributions to Accident and Health Plans. Contributions by an employer to an accident or health plan that provides coverage for personal injuries or sickness incurred by the employee and his or her spouse, dependent, and child under the age of 27, are excluded from the employee's gross income (Code Sec. 106; Reg. § 1.106-1).[15] If a plan provides other benefits in addition to accident and health benefits, the exclusion applies only to the part of the employer's contributions that is allocable to accident and health benefits. See ¶ 2015 for a further discussion of accident and health plans. See ¶ 322 and ¶ 421 for treatment of an S corporation shareholder or partner in a partnership whose accident or health insurance premiums are paid by the S corporation or partnership.

An employer generally contributes to an accident or health plan by paying a portion of the premium for accident and health insurance, or by contributing to a separate trust or fund that provides benefits directly or through insurance. A qualified long-term care insurance contract is generally treated as an accident and health insurance contract for this purpose (¶ 2019). However, employer contributions for the cost of long-term care insurance provided through a flexible spending account or similar arrangement (¶ 2041) are included in the employee's wages for income tax purposes (they are excluded from wages for FICA and FUTA purposes) (Code Sec. 106(c)).

Employer contributions to an employee's health savings account (HSA) (¶ 2035) or Archer medical savings account (MSA) (¶ 2037) may be excluded from an employee's gross income as employer-provided coverage for medical expenses under an accident or health plan to the extent they do not exceed the HSA or MSA limits (Code Sec. 106(b) and (d)). If an employer makes such contributions, it must make comparable contributions on behalf of all employees with comparable coverage during the same period (Code Secs. 4980E and 4980G).[16] Employer contributions paid for COBRA continuation coverage of a former employee (¶ 2021) may also be excluded as coverage under an accident or health plan (IRS Pub. 15-B).

2015. Accident and Health Benefits. Amounts received by an employee under an employer-financed accident and health plan are generally excluded from gross income if received as:

- reimbursements for medical care of the employee, his or her spouse, dependent, and child under the age of 27 to the extent the medical expenses were not deducted by the employee in a prior tax year (Code Sec. 105(b); Reg. § 1.105-2);[17] or

- payments for permanent injury or loss of bodily function (i.e., disability) of the employee, spouse, or dependent, so long as the payments are based on the nature of the injury rather than length of time the employee is absent from work (Code Sec. 105(c); Reg. § 1.105-3).[18]

Amounts received by an employee through an accident and health insurance that are not reimbursements of medical expenses, but are instead payments for personal injuries or sickness, generally are included in gross income if they are attributable to contributions by the employer that were not included in the employee's gross income or paid directly by the employer (Code Sec. 105(a); Reg. § 1.105-1).[19] Amounts the employee receives that are not attributable to employer contributions, such as benefits attributable to the employee's own contributions, are not included in gross income.

Employee. An employee for this purpose includes any current, retired, and former employee, as well as a widow or widower of a retired employee and any individual who dies while an employee. It also includes a leased employee who provides services on substantially full-time basis (IRS Pub. 15-B). Self-employed individuals are not considered employees and the cost of their employer-provided accident and health insurance is included in their gross income (Code Sec. 105(g); Reg. § 1.105-5(b)),[20] although a

---

References are to Standard Federal Tax Reports; Tax Research Consultant; and Practical Tax Explanations.

[15] ¶ 6800, ¶ 6801; HEALTH: 12,102; § 42,220

[16] ¶ 34,615, ¶ 34,619B; HEALTH: 9,306; § 42,515.35, § 42,615.10

[17] ¶ 6700, ¶ 6703; HEALTH: 12,104; § 42,215

[18] ¶ 6700, ¶ 6705; HEALTH: 12,200; § 42,215

[19] ¶ 6700, ¶ 6701; HEALTH: 12,104; § 42,215

[20] ¶ 6700, ¶ 6708; HEALTH: 12,100; § 42,215

deduction from gross income is available (¶ 908) (Code Sec. 162(l)). Partners in a partnership and two-percent or greater shareholders of an S corporation who are employees are considered to be self-employed.

Dependents. The definition of a dependent for this purpose is the same as for claiming the dependency exemption, but without regard to whether the dependent claims dependency exemptions (¶ 137), files a joint return (¶ 138), or has gross income in excess of the exemption amount (¶ 137A). If certain conditions are met, the IRS will treat the child of divorced or separated parents as a dependent of both parents under an employer accident and health plan (Code Sec. 105(b) and (c)).

Same-Sex Spouses. Same-sex couples who were legally married in a jurisdiction that recognizes same-sex marriages treated as married for all federal tax purposes, even if the couple lives in a jurisdiction that does not recognize the validity of same-sex marriages (¶ 152) (Rev. Rul. 2013-17; *E. Windsor*, SCt, 2013-2 USTC ¶ 50,400).[21]

Accident and Health Plan. An accident and health plan is any arrangement of an employer that provides benefits to employees and their spouses, dependents, and children under age 27 in the event of personal injury or sickness (Code Sec. 105(e); Reg. § 1.105-5(a)).[22] The plan may be insured or not insured, and does not need to be in writing. A qualified long-term care insurance contract is generally treated as an accident and health insurance contract for this purpose (¶ 2019). A sickness and disability fund for employees maintained by a state, the District of Columbia, or an Indian tribal government are also treated the same as an employer accident and health plan (Code Sec. 7871(a)(6)(A)). Qualified health care benefits provided by an Indian tribal government may also be excluded from gross income (¶ 2027). An employer's accident and health plan must not discriminate in favor of highly compensated individuals (¶ 2017).

COBRA Coverage. A group health plan provided by an employer must offer each qualified beneficiary who would otherwise lose coverage as a result of a qualifying event, an opportunity to elect continuation coverage referred to as COBRA continuation coverage (¶ 2021).

Railroad Unemployment Insurance. Benefits paid to an employee under the Railroad Unemployment Insurance Act for sick days are included in the employee's gross income unless an illness is due to an on-the-job injury (Code Sec. 105(i)).[23]

Annuity Rules. Amounts received as accident or health benefits are generally not taxable under the annuity rules of Code Sec. 72 (Reg. § 1.72-15).[24] However, some employer-established plans pay participants both amounts taxable under the annuity rules (¶ 817) and amounts excludable from gross income as payments under an accident or health plan. Specific rules are provided for determining which amounts are excludable in these cases. Benefits attributable to the employee's contributions are excludable from gross income under the rules at ¶ 851.

2017. Nondiscrimination Requirements for Employer Health Plans. An employer's self-insured medical reimbursement plan must not discriminate in favor of highly compensated individuals in terms of eligibility for coverage or benefits offered under the plan (Code Sec. 105(h); Reg. § 1.105-11).[25] The Code requires that for plan years beginning on or after September 23, 2010, similar nondiscrimination requirements apply to group health plans other than self-insured plans (Code Sec. 9815). However, compliance for group health plans will not be required until additional guidance is issued (Notice 2011-1). For a discussion of employer health reimbursement arrangements (HRAs), see ¶ 2039.

Excess reimbursements paid to a highly compensated individual that fails to meet the nondiscrimination requirements are includible in the individual's gross income. A highly compensated employee is an employee who is one of the five highest paid

---

References are to Standard Federal Tax Reports; Tax Research Consultant; and Practical Tax Explanations.

[21] ¶ 3320.15; FILEIND: 3,200; § 1,210.10

[22] ¶ 6700, ¶ 6708; HEALTH: 12,104; § 42,225

[23] ¶ 6700; HEALTH: 12,104

[24] ¶ 6124; INDIV: 30,152.05; § 42,225

[25] ¶ 6700, ¶ 6711; HEALTH: 9,050; § 42,155.10

officers, among the highest paid 25 percent of all employees, or a shareholder owning more than 10 percent of the company's stock.

The entire amount of a reimbursement with respect to a benefit that is available only to highly compensated individuals is treated as an excess reimbursement includible in income. In the case of a plan that discriminates in terms of eligibility, the includible excess reimbursement is equal to all the medical expenses for which the highly compensated individual was reimbursed times a fraction—the numerator of which is the total amount reimbursed to all participants who are highly compensated individuals and the denominator is the total amount reimbursed to all employees under the plan for such plan year. If the plan discriminates in terms of eligibility *and* benefits, any amount which is included in income by reason of the benefits not being available to all other participants is not to be taken into account in determining the excess reimbursements that result from the plan being discriminatory in terms of eligibility.

There is no eligibility discrimination if the plan benefits (1) at least 70 percent of all employees or 80 percent of all eligible employees if at least 70 percent of all employees are eligible, or (2) a class of employees found by the IRS not to be discriminatory in favor of highly compensated individuals. Certain employees, such as part-time workers, employees with less than three years of service, employees under age 25, and employees excluded as a result of a collective bargaining agreement, may be excluded from coverage. There is no benefits discrimination if the self-insured medical expense plan provides the same benefits for non-highly compensated employees as it does for highly compensated employees.

2019. Long-Term Care Insurance. A qualified long-term care insurance contract is treated as an accident and health insurance contract, and any employer plan providing coverage under a qualified long-term care insurance contract is treated as an accident and health plan (Code Sec. 7702B).[26] Amounts received under the contract other than dividends and refunds are excluded from the recipient's gross income as amounts received for personal injuries and sickness (¶ 2015). The exclusion does not apply to long-term care insurance coverage provided under a cafeteria plan (¶ 2045) or flexible spending arrangement (¶ 2041) (Code Secs. 106(c) and 125(f)).[27] Premiums paid by an individual for a qualified long-term care insurance contract may be deducted as a medical expense (¶ 1019).

A qualified long-term care insurance contract is an insurance contract that provides only coverage of qualified long-term care services including necessary diagnostic, preventive, and treatment services or personal care services required by a chronically ill individual and prescribed by a licensed health care practitioner (Code Sec. 7702B(b) and (c)).[28] In addition, the contract must be guaranteed renewable, must not provide a cash surrender value, and meets certain consumer protection provisions.

2021. COBRA Continuation Coverage. A group health plan provided by an employer with 20 or more employees must offer each covered employee, as well as his or her spouse and dependent, who would lose coverage as a result of a qualifying event, an opportunity to elect to continue coverage referred to as COBRA coverage (Code Sec. 4980B).[29] A qualifying event with respect to a covered employee includes death, termination of employment or reduction of hours, divorce or legal separation, eligibility for Medicare, a dependent child ceasing to be a dependent, or bankruptcy of the employer. Group health plans that fail to provide COBRA coverage to qualified beneficiaries are subject to an excise tax.

The option to elect COBRA coverage must allow the qualified beneficiary to purchase medical coverage under the company plan at group, rather than individual, rates for at least 18 months for most qualified beneficiaries (36 months in limited circumstances). The plan may require the beneficiary to pay premiums for the continuation coverage not to exceed 102 percent of the applicable premium for the coverage

---

References are to Standard Federal Tax Reports; Tax Research Consultant; and Practical Tax Explanations.

[26] ¶ 43,166; COMPEN: 45,066; § 7,240.15

[27] ¶ 6800, ¶ 7320; COMPEN: 45,066

[28] ¶ 43,166; COMPEN: 45,066; § 7,240.15

[29] ¶ 34,600; HEALTH: 24,100; § 42,801

period. The continuation coverage must be identical to the coverage provided to similarly situated beneficiaries under the plan for whom no qualifying event has occurred.

2023. Wellness Programs; Employee Assistance Programs. Wellness programs or employee assistance programs (EAPs) are generally part of an employer's overall health promotion for employees and may be one of several methods used to reduce health care costs. Although many EAPs are initiated to deal with drug and alcohol abuse, EAPs may also address family problems, stress, job termination, finances, and retirement. Because EAPs commonly provide treatment for drug and alcohol abuse and other similar health and medical problems, they often qualify as employee welfare benefit plans (¶ 2011). However, if an EAP merely provides referrals and does not pay for any services or benefits, the EAP will not be deemed to be an employee welfare benefit plan (Pension Welfare Benefits Administration (PWBA) Opinion Letter 91-26A).

2025. Disability Benefits. Disability income plans are employer plans, some mandated by state law, that provide full or partial income replacement for employees who become disabled. To the extent an employer offers such coverage under an accident and health plan, whether benefits received by employees are taxable depends on who pays for the premiums and whether they are paid on an after-tax basis (¶ 2015) (Code Sec. 105(a)).

2027. Indian Health Care Benefits. Qualified health care benefits provided by Indian tribal governments to a member of an Indian tribe or to a member's spouse or dependents are excluded from the beneficiary's gross income (Code Sec. 139D).[30] A qualified health care benefit includes:

- any health service provided or purchased by the Indian Health Service through a grant, contract or compact with an Indian tribe or tribal organization, or through a program funded by the Indian Health Service;

- medical care provided or purchased, or reimbursements for such medical care, by an Indian tribe or tribal organization for a member of an Indian tribe, member's spouse or dependent;

- coverage under an accident or health insurance plan provided by an Indian tribe or tribal organization for medical care to a member of an Indian tribe, member's spouse or dependent; and

- any other medical care provided by an Indian tribe or tribal organization that supplements, replaces or substitutes for medical care programs and services provided by the federal government to Indian tribes or their members.

The exclusion does not apply to Indian health care benefits that are not includible in the beneficiary's gross income under another provision in the Code or to any benefit for which the beneficiary may claim a deduction.

2028. Indian General Welfare Benefits. Indian general welfare benefits provided to, or on behalf of, a member of an Indian tribe, the member's spouse, or dependents are excluded from the recipient's gross income (Code Sec. 139E, as added by the Tribal General Welfare Exclusion Act of 2014 (P.L. 113-168)).[31] An Indian general welfare benefit is any payment made, or services provided, under an Indian tribal government program administered under specific guidelines and which does not discriminate in favor of members of the governing body of the Indian tribe. A program will not fail to be treated as an Indian tribal government program solely by reason of it being established by tribal custom or government practice. Benefits under the program must be available to any tribal member and must be for the promotion of general welfare. In addition, benefits must not be lavish or extravagant, and not provided as compensation for services. Any items of cultural significance, reimbursement of costs, or cash honorarium for participation in cultural or ceremonial activities for the transmission of tribal culture will not be treated as compensation.

References are to Standard Federal Tax Reports; Tax Research Consultant; and Practical Tax Explanations.

[30] ¶ 7649N; INDIV: 33,512; § 3,715

[31] ¶ 7649V; INDIV: 33,364; § 4,050

2029. Subsidies for Retiree Prescription Drug Plans. An employer that provides a qualified retiree prescription drug plan to its retired employees is eligible for a special subsidy payment each year from the federal government based on the cost of providing the coverage to qualified retirees (Social Security Act, § 1860D-22). The subsidy payment is excludable from the employer's gross income for both regular tax and alternative minimum tax (AMT) purposes (Code Sec. 139A).[32] For tax years beginning after 2012, the amount otherwise allowable as a deduction to the employer for retiree prescription drug costs is reduced by the amount of the excludable subsidy received by the employer. For tax years beginning before 2013, the value of any subsidy received by the employer is disregarded in calculating the employer's business deduction for prescription drug costs. Therefore, an employer can claim a deduction for prescription drug expenses incurred during such tax years even though the employer also received an excludable subsidy related to the same expenses.

2031. Medical Loss Ratio Rebates. Health insurance issuers may be required to pay medical loss ratio (MLR) rebates to policyholders in the form of either cash payments or premium reductions. For policies purchased on the individual market, MLR rebates are taxable or nontaxable depending on whether the individual deducted the premium payments (www.irs.gov, IRS FAQs, Medical Loss Ratio (MLR)). If the individual did not deduct the premiums for the year, an MLR rebate received in the following year is excluded from income whether received as cash or premium reduction. If the individual deducted the premiums, then an MLR rebate received in the following year is treated as the recovery of an itemized deduction under the tax benefit rule (¶ 799).

For policies purchased by an employee through an employer-sponsored group health plan, MLR rebates are taxable or nontaxable depending on whether the employee used pre-tax or after-tax dollars to pay the health insurance premiums. If the employee used pre-tax dollars, then any MLR rebate received is subject to income and employment taxes. If the employee used after-tax dollars and MLR rebates are paid only to employees who participated in the plan both in the year the premiums were paid and in the year the rebates are received, then a rebate is not included in income if the employee did not deduct the premiums. If, however, MLR rebates are provided to all employees participating in the group health plan in the year the rebates are paid, regardless of whether the employee participated in the plan in the year the premiums were paid, then the rebates are not included in income if the employee used after-tax dollars.

HSAs, HRAs, and FSAs

2035. Health Savings Accounts (HSAs). A health savings account (HSA) is a trust or custodial account established for the exclusive purpose of paying for qualified medical expenses of the account beneficiary (Code Sec. 223).[33] HSAs can be established by employees through an employer's cafeteria plan (¶ 2045).

Eligibility. To be eligible to establish an HSA in any month, an individual:

- must be covered by a high-deductible health plan (HDHP) on the first day of the month,

- must not be covered by any other plan that is not a HDHP,

- must not be enrolled in Medicare, and

- cannot be claimed as a dependent on another person's tax return (Code Sec. 223(c)(1)).[34]

Exceptions exist for permitted coverage under certain non-HDHPs. Permitted coverage includes coverage for accidents, disability, dental care, vision care, long term care or prescription drugs. Also allowed is permitted insurance for a specified disease or illness, insurance paying a fixed amount per day (or other period) for hospitalization, and insurance if substantially all the coverage relates to liabilities for workers' compensation, ownership or use of property (for example, auto insurance), or torts.

References are to Standard Federal Tax Reports; Tax Research Consultant; and Practical Tax Explanations.

[32] ¶ 7649; HEALTH: 9,250   [33] ¶ 12,776; INDIV: 42,450; § 42,501   [34] ¶ 12,776; INDIV: 42,460.05; § 42,510.05

While covered by an HSA, an individual generally may not be covered by a health flexible spending arrangement (FSA) (¶ 2041) or health reimbursement account (HRA) (¶ 2039) sponsored by the individual's employer or spouse's employer unless it is a limited purpose FSA or HRA, a suspended HRA, a post-deductible health FSA or HRA, or a retirement HRA. However, coverage under a general purpose health FSA during a grace period is disregarded in determining if tax deductible contributions can be made to an HSA for that period if the balance in the health FSA at the end of the plan year is zero or the entire remaining balance in the health FSA at the end of the plan year is contributed to an HSA in a qualified HSA distribution.

A taxpayer who is an eligible individual for an HSA on the first day of the last month of a tax year is treated as eligible during every month of that tax year. If the taxpayer ceases to be eligible during the period beginning with the last month of the tax year and ending on the last day of the 12th month following that month, he or she must include in gross income an amount equal to the amount actually contributed minus the sum of the monthly contribution limits to which the individual would otherwise have been entitled. An additional 10-percent tax is imposed on this amount. Recapture does not apply if the taxpayer is ineligible due to death or disability (Code Sec. 223(b)(8); Notice 2008-52).[35]

Dependent. The definition of a dependent for purposes of an HSA is the same as for claiming a dependency exemption, but determined without regard to whether the dependent claims dependency exemptions (¶ 137), files a joint return (¶ 138), or has gross income in excess of the exemption amount (¶ 137A) (Code Sec. 223(d)(2)(A)). If certain conditions are met, the IRS will treat the child of divorced or separated parents as a dependent of both parents, without a declaration by the custodial parent releasing the claim to the dependency exemption (¶ 139A) (Rev. Proc. 2008-48).[36]

Contributions. Contributions made to an HSA by an eligible individual outside the employment context are deductible by the individual in determining adjusted gross income. The maximum an individual can deduct for 2014 is $3,300 for self-only coverage or $6,550 for family coverage (Rev. Proc. 2013-25). The maximum amount an individual can deduct for 2015 is $3,350 for self-only coverage or $6,650 for family coverage (Rev. Proc. 2014-30). Excess contributions are includible in gross income and subject to a six-percent excise tax. Individuals who reach age 55 by the end of the tax year can increase their annual contributions by $1,000. Contributions cannot be made after the participant attains age 65 or the participant is enrolled in Medicare, but in either circumstance withdrawals for qualified medical expenses continue to be excluded from gross income (Notice 2008-59, amplifying Notice 2004-2; Notice 2004-50).[37]

Married Taxpayers. For married taxpayers, if either spouse has family coverage under any health plan, then both will be treated as having only family coverage under the plan. If each spouse has family coverage under different plans, then both spouses are treated as having coverage under the plan with the lowest deductible (Code Sec. 223(b)(5)). If only one spouse is an eligible individual, only that spouse may contribute to an HSA (Notice 2004-50). If one or both spouses have family coverage, the contribution limit is the lowest deductible amount, divided equally between the spouses unless they agree on a different division, and further reduced by any contribution to an Archer MSA. Both spouses may make the catch-up contributions for individuals age 55 or over without exceeding the family coverage limit (Notice 2008-59, amplifying Notice 2004-2).

If a husband and wife are each eligible to make catch-up contributions, each spouse can make such contributions only to his or her own HSA. The maximum annual contribution limit for a married couple is the statutory maximum for family coverage where: (1) one spouse has family coverage and the other spouse has self-only coverage, regardless of whether the family coverage includes the spouse with self-only coverage; or (2) both spouses have family coverage, regardless of whether each spouse's family coverage covers the other spouse. A married taxpayer covered under an HDHP can contribute to an HSA for use with qualifying out-of-pocket medical expenses even if his

References are to Standard Federal Tax Reports; Tax Research Consultant; and Practical Tax Explanations.

[35] ¶ 12,776, ¶ 12,785.25; HEALTH: 18,050; § 42,515.10

[36] ¶ 6702.27; PLANIND: 3,254.05, INDIV: 42,460.05; § 1,215.40

[37] ¶ 12,785.25; INDIV: 42,454.05; § 42,540

¶2035

or her spouse's coverage is nonqualifying family coverage, as long as the taxpayer is not covered by the spouse's policy (Rev. Rul. 2005-25).

HDHP Defined. An HDHP is a plan with (1) an annual deductible of at least $1,250 for 2014 ($1,300 for 2015) for self-only coverage or $2,500 for 2014 ($2,600 for 2015) for family coverage; and (2) an annual out-of-pocket expenses limit of $6,350 for 2014 ($6,450 for 2015) for self-only coverage or $12,700 for 2014 ($12,900 for 2015) for family coverage (Rev. Proc. 2013-25; Rev. Proc. 2014-30). Out-of-pocket expenses include deductibles, co-payments and other amounts (other than premiums) that must be paid for plan benefits (Code Sec. 223(c)(2); Notice 2008-59, amplifying Notice 2004-2).[38]

Distributions. Distributions from an HSA are excluded from the account beneficiary's gross income only if used to pay or be reimbursed for qualified medical expenses incurred during the coverage period (Code Sec. 223(f)).[39] Qualified medical expenses are those specified in the plan that would generally qualify as an itemized deduction and incurred by the account beneficiary, his or her spouse, or dependents (¶ 1016). Nonprescription medicines (other than insulin) are not considered qualified medical expenses under an HSA (Code Sec. 223(d)(2)). In addition, health insurance premiums are not qualified medical expenses under an HSA unless for long-term care insurance, COBRA continuation coverage, health care coverage while receiving unemployment compensation, or Medicare. Distributions from an HSA not used for qualified medical expenses are included in the account beneficiary's gross income and subject to a 20 percent additional tax, unless made after the beneficiary reaches age 65, dies, or becomes disabled. The additional tax is not treated as a tax liability for purposes of the alternative minimum tax (¶ 1420).

Contributions by Partnership or S Corporation. Contributions made by a partnership or S corporation to a partner's or shareholder's HSA are generally treated as payments to the partner or shareholder and includible in gross income. The individual partner or shareholder may treat the contribution as an above-the-line deduction (an adjustment to gross income). However, a contribution to the partner's HSA by the partnership for services rendered is treated as a guaranteed payment, and the partnership may deduct the contribution as a business expense. Similarly, a contribution by the S corporation to a two-percent shareholder's HSA for services rendered is deductible by the S corporation and included in the shareholders income (Notice 2005-8).[40]

Distributions to Fund HSAs. An eligible individual can make a one-time qualified HSA distribution directly from his or her IRA to his or her HSA (¶ 2165). The amount that can otherwise be contributed to the HSA for the tax year of the distribution is reduced by the amount contributed from the IRA, and the individual cannot deduct the distribution amount as an HSA contribution (Code Sec. 223(b)(4)(C); Notice 2008-51).[41] An eligible individual can also roll over distributions from another HSA or Archer MSA into an HSA. The taxpayer does not have to be an eligible individual to make a rollover contribution from an existing HSA to a new HSA. An employer could also make a one-time distribution from an employee's health FSA or health HRA to the employee's HSA before January 1, 2012 (Code Sec. 106(e)).

2037. Archer Medical Savings Accounts (MSAs). An Archer medical savings account (MSA) is a trust or custodial account established for the exclusive purpose of paying for qualified medical expenses of the account beneficiary, his or her spouse, or dependents (Code Sec. 220).[42] Archer MSAs operate almost exactly the same as health savings accounts (HSAs) (¶ 2035). New Archer MSAs may *not* be established after 2007. However, an individual can still utilize an Archer MSA if he or she was an active participant in the MSA before January 1, 2008, or he or she became an active participant for a tax year ending after December 31, 2007, by reason of coverage under a high deductible health plan (HDHP) of an Archer MSA participating employer.

References are to Standard Federal Tax Reports; Tax Research Consultant; and Practical Tax Explanations.

[38] ¶ 12,776, ¶ 12,785.25; INDIV: 42,450; § 42,510.10

[39] ¶ 12,776; INDIV: 42,460; § 42,520.10, § 42,525

[40] ¶ 12,785.25; INDIV: 42,454.10; § 42,515.05

[41] ¶ 12,776; HEALTH: 9,306; § 42,515.40

[42] ¶ 12,670; INDIV: 42,500, INDIV: 42,510; § 42,601

To qualify for an Archer MSA, an individual or spouse must be either an employee of a small employer or self-employed person that maintains high-deductible health plan (HDHP). A small employer for this purpose is generally an employer who had an average of 50 or fewer employees during either of the last two calendar years. Like HSAs, the individual can have no other health care coverage, including under Medicare. An HDHP under an Archer MSA has higher annual deductibles and lower out-of-pocket limits than under an HSA: (1) for individual coverage, the minimum deductible is $2,200 for 2014 ($2,200 for 2015), the maximum deductible is $3,250 for 2014 ($3,300 for 2015), and the maximum out-of-pocket limitation is $4,350 for 2014 ($4,450 for 2015); and (2) for family coverage, the minimum deductible is $4,350 for 2014 ($4,450 for 2015), the maximum deductible is $6,550 for 2014 ($6,650 for 2015), and the maximum out-of-pocket limitation is $8,000 for 2014 ($8,150 for 2015) (Rev. Proc. 2013-35; Rev. Proc. 2014-61).

Contributions. Within the limits, contributions to an Archer MSA are deductible if made by an eligible individual and excludable from income if made by an employer on behalf of an eligible individual (employer contributions must be reported on the employee's W-2). Annual contributions to an Archer MSA are limited to 75 percent of the deductible of the required health insurance plan (65 percent if a self-only plan). Contributions are also limited by an employee's compensation or the income earned from a self-employed individual's business (Code Sec. 220(b)). Excess contributions are subject to an excise tax. Eligible individuals may claim an above-the-line deduction (an adjustment to gross income) for contributions they make during the tax year to their Archer MSA.

Distributions. Distributions from an Archer MSA are excluded from the account beneficiary's gross income only if used to pay or be reimbursed for qualified medical expenses incurred during the coverage period (Code Sec. 220(f)). Qualified medical expenses are those specified in the plan that would generally qualify as an itemized deduction and incurred by the account beneficiary, his or her spouse, or dependents (¶ 1016). Nonprescription medicines (other than insulin) are not considered qualified medical expenses under an HSA. In addition, health insurance premiums are not qualified medical expenses under an HSA unless for long-term care insurance, COBRA continuation coverage, and health care coverage while receiving unemployment compensation. Distributions from an HSA not used for qualified medical expenses are included in the account beneficiary's gross income and subject to a 20 percent additional tax, unless made after the beneficiary reaches age 65, dies, or becomes disabled. The additional tax is not treated as a tax liability for purposes of the alternative minimum tax (¶ 1420).

Medicare Advantage MSAs. Medicare Advantage MSAs are medical savings accounts that must be used in conjunction with a high deductible Medicare Advantage MSA health plan (Code Sec. 138).[43] Individuals eligible for Medicare are permitted to have their Medicare benefits deposited directly into a Medicare Advantage MSA and can make trustee-to-trustee transfers from Archer MSAs to these MSAs. Income earned on the account and withdrawals used to pay health care expenses are not included in the individual's income.

2039. Health Reimbursement Arrangements (HRAs). A health reimbursement arrangement (HRA) is an employer-funded plan that reimburses employees for qualified medical care expenses (Notice 2002-45, amplified by Rev. Rul. 2006-36).[44] An HRA is funded solely by employer contributions and may not be funded through employee salary deferrals under a cafeteria plan (¶ 2045). The plan must provide reimbursements up a maximum dollar amount for a coverage period. Any unused amounts in the HRA can be carried forward for reimbursements in later years.

To the extent an HRA constitutes an employer-provided accident or health plan (¶ 2015), coverage and reimbursements of qualified medical care expenses are generally excludable from the employee's gross income. An HRA may be offered in conjunction

---

References are to Standard Federal Tax Reports; Tax Research Consultant; and Practical Tax Explanations.

[43] ¶ 7630; INDIV: 42,466; § 42,615

[44] ¶ 6702.73; HEALTH: 18,100; § 42,401

with other provided health benefits, such as a group health plan or health FSA (¶ 2041). HRAs must be integrated with an employer's minimum essential coverage, and reimbursements cannot be used to obtain individual coverage on a health exchange (except for stand-alone retiree plans and plans with fewer than two participants).[45]

Distributions from an HRA can only be used to reimburse the employee for his or her qualified medical expenses incurred during the coverage period. Qualified medical expenses are those specified in the plan that would generally qualify as an itemized deduction and incurred for the employee, spouse, dependent, or child under the age of 27 (¶ 1016). Nonprescription medicines (other than insulin) are not considered qualified medical expenses under an HRA (Code Sec. 106(f)).[46]

2041. Flexible Spending Arrangements (FSAs). A flexible spending arrangement (FSA) is an employer-established benefit program under which amounts credited to an employee's account may be used to reimburse the employee for health care, dependent care, or adoption expenses that would otherwise be excludable from the employee's gross income if paid by the employer (Prop. Reg. § 1.125-5).[47] An FSA may be funded by employer contributions or by a salary reduction agreement with pre-tax dollars as part of a cafeteria plan (¶ 2045).

Generally, the plan must provide either a maximum dollar limit or maximum percentage of compensation that can be contributed through a cafeteria plan. In the case of a health FSA, however, the maximum contribution is limited to $2,500 for 2014 ($2,550 for 2015) (Code Sec. 125(i); Rev. Proc. 2013-35; Rev. Proc. 2014-61).[48] If the plan allows salary reduction contributions to a health FSA in excess of the annual dollar amount, then the employee will be subject to tax on distributions from the health FSA. In the case of a dependent or adoption FSAs, the maximum contribution is limited to the amount the employee could exclude under a adoption assistance program (¶ 2063) or dependent care assistance program (¶ 2065).

An FSA generally may not be used to defer compensation; any balance remaining in the account at the end of the plan year is forfeited (use-it-or-lose-it rule) (Prop. Reg. § 1.125-5(c); Notice 2005-42).[49] A plan may permit, however, a grace period of up to 2½ months after the end of the plan year (March 15 for calendar year plans) during which qualified expenses incurred during the period can be paid from any amounts left in the account at the end of the previous year. The employer is not permitted to refund any balance in an FSA account to an employee.

Beginning in the 2013 plan year, a cafeteria plan may allow up to $500 of any balance remaining in a health FSA at the end of the year to be carried over to pay or reimburse qualified medical expenses incurred in the next year (Notice 2013-71). The carried over amount does not count against the maximum contribution an employee can make to the health FSA ($2,500 for 2014; $2,550 for 2015). Any unused amount in a health FSA at the end of the year in excess of $500 (or lower amount specified in the plan) is forfeited. A plan that adopts the carryover option may not also provide the 2½ month grace period.

Special Rules for Health FSAs. Health FSA plans must comply with the rules applicable to other accident and health plans, including the nondiscrimination requirements for highly compensated employees (¶ 2017). Distributions from a health FSA can only be used to reimburse the employee for qualified medical expenses incurred during the coverage period. Qualified medical expenses are those specified in the plan that would generally qualify as an itemized deduction and incurred for the employee, spouse, dependent, or child under the age of 27 (¶ 1016). Nonprescription medicines (other than insulin) are not considered qualified medical expenses under an FSA (Code Sec. 106(f)).[50]

Qualified Reservist Distribution. A cafeteria plan may allow for distribution of any remaining balance of a health FSA for any reason to a participant who is called to active

---

References are to Standard Federal Tax Reports; Tax Research Consultant; and Practical Tax Explanations.

[45] ¶ 34,963.054; HEALTH: 18,108; § 42,405
[46] ¶ 6800; HEALTH: 18,100; § 42,401
[47] ¶ 7323F; COMPEN: 51,200; § 42,701
[48] ¶ 7320, ¶ 7324.35; COMPEN: 51,200; § 42,701
[49] ¶ 7323F; COMPEN: 51,212; § 42,710
[50] ¶ 6800; HEALTH: 18,150; § 42,710

duty for a period of at least 180 days due to his or her membership in a reserve unit of the military (Code Sec. 125(h)). The distribution must be made between the date of the order and the last day for which reimbursements can be made during the plan year.

Family and Medical Leave Act. The Family and Medical Leave Act (P.L. 103-3) (FMLA) imposes certain requirements on employers regarding coverage, including family coverage, under group health plans for employees taking FMLA leave and regarding the restoration of benefits to employees who return from FMLA leave. Reg. § 1.125-3 provides guidance on the effect of the FMLA on the operation of cafeteria plans.

Cafeteria Plans

2045. Cafeteria Plans. Cafeteria plans are employer-sponsored benefit packages that offer employees a choice between taking cash and receiving qualified benefits which may be excluded from gross income (Code Sec. 125; Prop. Reg. § 1.125-1).[51] If a participant chooses cash, it is includible in gross income as compensation. If qualified benefits are chosen, they are excludable to the extent allowed under the Code. A cafeteria plan cannot offer anything other than cash or qualified benefits. Cafeteria plan elections must be made before the start of the plan year and are generally irrevocable unless the employee experiences a change in status (i.e., marital status, number of dependents, etc.). Special transition relief is available for an employee who wishes to modify or revoke a salary reduction election for accident and health coverage offered through a fiscal year cafeteria plan and purchase health care coverage through an American Health Benefit Exchange (see later) beginning with the 2014 calendar year (Notice 2013-71). In addition, as of September 18, 2014, employers may permit revoked elections for employees expected to average less than 30 hours of service per week who nevertheless are still eligible for coverage under the employer plan, and for employees who would like to cease employer coverage and buy coverage through an exchange without a period of duplicate or no coverage (Notice 2014-55).

A cafeteria plan may include any of the following qualified benefits: accident and health benefits (¶ 2015) including benefits under a flexible spending arrangement (¶ 2041), adoption assistance benefits (¶ 2063), dependent care assistance benefits (¶ 2065), disability coverage (¶ 2025), group-term life insurance (¶ 2055), health savings accounts (HSAs) (¶ 2035), and 401(k) plans (¶ 2104). A qualified benefit does *not* include benefits under an Archer MSA (¶ 2037), scholarships and fellowship grants (¶ 865), educational assistance benefits (¶ 2067), long-term care insurance (¶ 2019), or statutory fringe benefits under Code Sec. 132 (¶ 2085).

Highly compensated employees are not entitled to exclude any benefit under a cafeteria plan attributable to a plan year in which the plan discriminates in favor of the highly compensated employees with respect to participation, contributions, and benefits. Key employees are not entitled to exclude any benefit attributable to a plan year in which the statutory qualified benefits provided to all key employees exceed 25 percent of the total of such benefits provided to all employees under the plan. In such cases, the benefits must be included in the gross income of the highly compensated employee or key employee for the tax year in which the plan year ends (Code Sec. 125(b)). An employer who maintains a cafeteria plan is generally required to file an information return (Code Sec. 6039D).[52] However, the reporting requirement for cafeteria plans has been suspended indefinitely (Notice 2002-24).

Generally, a plan that provides deferred compensation is *not* included in the definition of a cafeteria plan. However, elective contributions under a qualified cash or deferred arrangement, profit-sharing plan, stock bonus plan, such as a 401(k) plan, or contributions by an educational institution for post-retirement group life insurance are permitted.

American Health Benefit Exchange Plans. An American Health Benefit Exchange and Small Business Health Options Program (SHOP) Exchange, run either by a state or

[51] ¶ 7320, ¶ 7321; COMPEN: 51,000; § 20,801   [52] ¶ 35,660; COMPEN: 51,058; § 39,155.25

the federal government, are available in every state beginning January 1, 2014. These exchanges, or marketplaces, provide qualified individuals and small businesses with access to health plans, possibly at subsidized prices. Qualified health plans offered through such an exchange cannot be provided by employers through a cafeteria plan unless the employer is exchange-eligible (Code Sec. 125(f)(3)). An exchange-eligible employer is a small employer electing to make all of its full-time employees eligible for one or more qualified health plans offered in the small group market through an exchange (Act Sec. 1312(f)(2)(A) of the Patient Protection and Affordable Care Act (P.L. 111-148)). A small employer is an employer who employed an average of at least one, but not more that 100, employees on business days during the preceding plan year and employs at least one employee on the first day of the current plan year (Act Sec. 1304(b)(2) of P.L. 111-148). The small group market is the health insurance market under which employees obtain health insurance coverage through a group health plan maintained by a small employer (Act Sec. 1304(a)(3) of P.L. 111-148). Beginning in 2017, the definition of an exchange-eligible employer is expanded to include large employers in addition to small employers (Act Sec. 1312(f)(2)(B) of P.L. 111-148).

2047. Simple Cafeteria Plans. Certain small employers can establish simple cafeteria plans under which the nondiscrimination requirements applicable to regular cafeteria plans (¶ 2045), as well as the nondiscrimination rules applicable to group-term life insurance (¶ 2055), accident and health plans (¶ 2015), and dependent care assistance programs (¶ 2065), are considered satisfied (Code Sec. 125(j)).[53] A simple cafeteria plan is a cafeteria plan established and maintained by an eligible employer that meets certain contribution, eligibility, and participation requirements.

Eligible Employers. To be eligible to establish a simple cafeteria plan, an employer must have employed an average 100 or fewer employers on business days during either of the two preceding years. An employer that was not in existence throughout the preceding year may be considered as an eligible employer if it reasonably expects to average 100 or fewer employees on business days during the current year. If an employer has 100 or fewer employees for the year and establishes a simple cafeteria plan, then it is treated as an eligible employer for any subsequent year even if the employer employs more than 100 employees in the subsequent year, unless the employer employs an average of 200 or more employees during the subsequent year.

For purposes of determining the qualification of a business that has recently changed ownership, the fact that the previous owner had 100 or fewer employees in a preceding year is used to determine eligibility of the current ownership to establish a simple cafeteria plan. Also, any person treated as a single employer for purposes of the work opportunity credit (¶ 1365G) or for purposes of deferred compensation rules for leased employees under Code Sec. 414(n) or Code Sec. 414(o) are treated as one person for purposes of simple cafeteria plans.

Contribution Requirements. The contribution requirements of a simple cafeteria plan are met if the employer is required by the plan to make a contribution to provide qualified benefits on behalf of each qualified employee in an amount equal to: (1) a uniform percentage of at least two percent of the employee's compensation for the year; or (2) at least six percent of the employee's compensation for the plan year or twice the amount of the salary reduction contributions of each qualified employee, whichever is less (Code Sec. 125(j)(3)). If the employer bases the satisfaction of the contribution requirements on the second option, it will not be treated as met if the rate of contributions with respect to any salary reduction contribution of a highly compensated or key employee is greater than that with respect to any other employee.

Employee Eligibility and Participation Requirements. The minimum eligibility and participation requirements of a simple cafeteria plan are met if all employees who had at least 1,000 hours of service for the preceding plan year are eligible to participate. In addition, each employee eligible to participate may elect any benefit under the plan, subject to terms and conditions applicable to all participants (Code Sec. 125(j)(4)). An

---

References are to Standard Federal Tax Reports; Tax Research Consultant; and Practical Tax Explanations.

[53] ¶ 7320; COMPEN: 51,250;
§ 20,840.05

¶2047

employer may elect to exclude from the plan, regardless of the satisfaction of the 1,000 hour requirement, employees: (1) who have not attained the age of 21 before the close of the plan year; (2) who have less than one year of service with the employer; (3) who are covered under a collective bargaining agreement; or (4) who are nonresident aliens working outside the United States whose income did not come from a U.S. source.

Other Employee Benefits

2055. Group-Term Life Insurance. An employee may exclude from gross income the cost of the first $50,000 of group-term life insurance on the employee's life provided under a policy carried directly or indirectly by the employer (Code Sec. 79(a) and (c); Reg. §§ 1.79-1 and 1.79-3).[54] The cost of coverage in excess of $50,000 is included in the employee's gross income and subject to employment taxes, reduced by any amount the employee paid toward the insurance. The cost in excess of $50,000 is not the employer's actual cost in providing coverage. Instead, the cost is determined under a Uniform Premium Table (see below) which provides a per-month premium cost for $1,000 of insurance based on the employee's age as of the end of the employee's tax year. The $50,000 limit relates to the group-term life insurance coverage which the employee receives during any part of the tax year.

In the case of certain disabled or retired employees, the full cost of employer-provided group-term life insurance coverage is excluded from the employee's income (Code Sec. 79(b) and (d); Reg. § 1.79-2; Temp. Reg. § 1.79-4T).[55] A full exclusion is also available if the employer or a charity is the beneficiary of the insurance benefits. On the other hand, key employees must include the cost of all benefits they receive under plans that do not satisfy nondiscrimination requirements. In addition, coverage on the life of the employee's spouse or dependents is not excluded unless it qualifies as a de minimis fringe benefit (¶ 2089).

Group-term life insurance is insurance that provides for a general death benefit that is excluded from gross income (¶ 803) and provided to a group of at least 10 full-time employees at some time during the year (Reg. § 1.79-1; IRS Pub. 15-B). An employee includes any current common-law employee, former employee, or leased employee, as well as a statutory employee who is a full-time salesperson. An employee does not include a self-employed person, partner, or 2-percent S corporation shareholders. The amount of insurance provided to each employee must be computed under a formula that precludes individual selection. In addition, the policy must not provide any permanent benefits.

Table 1

Cost Per $1,000 of Protection for One-Month Period

Age	Cost
Under 25	5 cents
25 through 29	6 cents
30 through 34	8 cents
35 through 39	9 cents
40 through 44	10 cents
45 through 49	15 cents
50 through 54	23 cents
55 through 59	43 cents
60 through 64	66 cents
65 through 69	$1.27
70 and above	$2.06

Example: X Corp. pays the premiums on a $70,000 group-term insurance policy on the life of its president, Fox, who is 51 years old at the end of 2014. The IRS-established uniform cost for $1,000 of group-term coverage for twelve months is $2.76 ($0.23 × 12) (Reg. § 1.79-3(d)(2)). The cost of the policy includible in Fox's gross income is computed as follows:

References are to Standard Federal Tax Reports; Tax Research Consultant; and Practical Tax Explanations.

[54] ¶ 6360, ¶ 6362, ¶ 6364; COMPEN: 48,100; § 21,005.05

[55] ¶ 6360, ¶ 6363, ¶ 6366; COMPEN: 48,100; § 21,005.05

Total insurance coverage	$70,000.00
Tax-free insurance	50,000.00
Insurance coverage subject to tax	$20,000.00
Taxable cost of policy includible in Fox's gross income ($2.76 × 20)	$55.20

2057. Split-Dollar Life Insurance. A split-dollar life insurance arrangement is an arrangement where the premiums, cash-surrender value, or death benefits are split between an owner and non-owner of a life insurance policy (Reg. § 1.61-22).[56] Ownership and benefits are most often split between an employer and an employee, but they may also be split between a corporation and shareholder, or between family members. A split-dollar arrangement entered into, or materially modified after September 17, 2003, is taxed under either the economic benefit rule or the loan rule depending upon which party owns the contract, and the relationship of the owner to the non-owner.

Owner of the Contract. The owner of a contract is generally the person named as the policy owner (Reg. § 1.61-22(c)). If two or more persons are named as policy owners and each has an undivided interest in every right and benefit, those persons are treated as owners of separate contracts. However, an employer is treated as the owner of the policy if the only benefit available under the arrangement is the value of the current life insurance protection (i.e., in non-equity arrangement).

Economic Benefit Rule. Under the economic benefit rule, the owner of the life insurance contract is treated as transferring economic benefits to the non-owner (Reg. § 1.61-22(d)). Depending on the relationship between the parties, the economic benefits may constitute compensation, a distribution under Code Sec. 301, a gift, or another type of income. Both the owner and non-owner must account for the economic benefits fully and consistently, reduced by any consideration paid by the non-owner for the economic benefits. The economic benefit rule generally applies to compensatory arrangements in which the employer is the owner of the contract—for example, endorsement split-dollar arrangements, in which the employer is formally designated as the owner of the insurance contract and endorses the contract to specify the portion of the insurance proceeds payable to the employee's beneficiary (Reg. § 1.61-22(b)(3)(ii)). The value of the benefit provided under such an arrangement is the cost of any current life insurance protection provided to the employee (Reg. § 1.61-22(d)).

Loan Rule. Under the loan rule, the non-owner is treated as lending premium payments to the owner (Reg. § 1.7872-15). The rule generally applies to collateral assignments in which the employee is designated as the owner of the contract and the employer pays all or a portion of the premiums, the payment is a loan under general principals of federal tax law, and repayment is secured by the insurance policy's death benefits or cash surrender value. If a split-dollar loan does not provide for sufficient interest, the loan is a below-market split-dollar loan and is subject to the below market interest rules (¶ 795).

Deferred Compensation. Because certain types of split-dollar life insurance arrangements provide for deferred compensation, the requirements of Code Sec. 409A may apply (¶ 2197).

Pre-September 18, 2003, Arrangements. For a split-dollar arrangement entered into on or before September 17, 2003, or not materially modified thereafter, an employee is taxed on the value of economic benefits received. The economic benefit primarily consists of the value of the protection the employee receives over the premiums the employee pays. Certain other benefits might also be taxed, such as policy dividends received by the employee. The value of the economic benefit is determined using the P.S. 58 rate table contained in Rev. Rul. 55-747,[57] the insurance company's lower published term rates, or the Table 2001 group-term rates (¶ 2055) (Notice 2002-8, revoking Notice 2001-10).

References are to Standard Federal Tax Reports; Tax Research Consultant; and Practical Tax Explanations.

[56] ¶ 5906E; COMPEN: 48,150; § 21,010.05

[57] ¶ 5508.24; COMPEN: 48,150; § 21,005.20

¶2057

2059. Employer-Provided Vehicle. An employee who uses an employer-provided vehicle for more than *de minimis* personal use receives a taxable fringe benefit from his or her employer (Reg. § 1.61-21(a)).[58] The fair market value of the fringe benefit is included in the employee's wages for income and employment tax purposes, and may be deducted by the employer as compensation. The fair market value is generally the cost to the employee of leasing a comparable car at a comparable price for a similar period in an arms-length transaction (Reg. § 1.61-21(b)(4)). Under certain conditions, however, the employer may elect to use one of the following special valuation rules described below: automobile lease valuation rule, cents-per-mile, or commuting value (Reg. § 1.61-21(c)). Separate rules are used for valuing flights by an employee on employer-provided noncommercial aircraft.

Automobile Lease Valuation. The value of the personal use of an employer-provided car may be computed under annual lease value tables (Reg. § 1.61-21(d)).[59] The annual lease value of an automobile is computed by first determining the FMV of the automobile on the first date it was made available to any employee for personal use. Under a safe-harbor, the employer's cost can be substituted for FMV, provided certain conditions are met. FMV is reduced when an employee contributes an amount toward the purchase or lease of the automobile. In addition, if the automobile is part of a fleet of at least 20, then the FMV of each automobile can be treated as equal to the fleet-average value.

Once the FMV is established, the annual lease value table prepared by the IRS and reproduced below, is used to determine the annual lease value that corresponds to the FMV. The annual lease values include the FMV of maintenance and insurance for the automobile but do not include the cost of gasoline provided by the employer. The fuel provided can be valued either at its FMV or at 5.5 cents per mile for all miles driven within the United States, Canada, or Mexico by the employee. If continuous personal use of a company car is for less than a year, but at least 30 days, the employee may prorate the car's annual lease value. The values in the table are based on an assumed four-year lease term.

Automobile fair market value (1)	Annual Lease Value (2)
$ 0 to 999	$600
1,000 to 1,999	850
2,000 to 2,999	1,100
3,000 to 3,999	1,350
4,000 to 4,999	1,600
5,000 to 5,999	1,850
6,000 to 6,999	2,100
7,000 to 7,999	2,350
8,000 to 8,999	2,600
9,000 to 9,999	2,850
10,000 to 10,999	3,100
11,000 to 11,999	3,350
12,000 to 12,999	3,600
13,000 to 13,999	3,850
14,000 to 14,999	4,100
15,000 to 15,999	4,350
16,000 to 16,999	4,600
17,000 to 17,999	4,850
18,000 to 18,999	5,100
19,000 to 19,999	5,350
20,000 to 20,999	5,600
21,000 to 21,999	5,850
22,000 to 22,999	6,100
23,000 to 23,999	6,350
24,000 to 24,999	6,600
25,000 to 25,999	6,850
26,000 to 27,999	7,250
28,000 to 29,999	7,750

References are to Standard Federal Tax Reports; Tax Research Consultant; and Practical Tax Explanations.

[58] ¶ 5906; COMPEN: 33,150; § 8,035

[59] ¶ 5906; COMPEN: 33,152; § 8,055.10

Automobile fair market value (1)	Annual Lease Value (2)
30,000 to 31,999	8,250
32,000 to 33,999	8,750
34,000 to 35,999	9,250
36,000 to 37,999	9,750
38,000 to 39,999	10,250
40,000 to 41,999	10,750
42,000 to 43,999	11,250
44,000 to 45,999	11,750
48,000 to 49,999	12,750
50,000 to 51,999	13,250
52,000 to 53,999	13,750
54,000 to 55,999	14,250
56,000 to 57,999	14,750
58,000 to 59,999	15,250

For vehicles having a fair market value in excess of $59,999, the Annual Lease Value is equal to: (0.25 × the fair market value of the automobile) + $500.

Cents-Per-Mile Valuation. The value of the personal use of an employer-provided vehicle may be determined by multiplying personal use mileage, provided it is at least 10,000 miles, by the standard mileage rate (56 cents per mile in 2014) if certain requirements are satisfied (Reg. § 1.61-21(e); Rev. Proc. 2010-51; Notice 2013-80).[60] For a passenger automobile first made available to an employee in calendar year 2014, the FMV of the vehicle cannot exceed $16,000, and for a truck or van, the fair market value cannot exceed $17,300 (Reg. § 1.61-21(e); Notice 2014-11). Fuel provided by the employer must be valued separately, at either its FMV or at 5.5 cents per mile for miles driven in North America (Reg. § 1.61-21(d)(3)(ii)(B)).

Commuting Valuation. If certain requirements are met, the use of an employer-provided commuting vehicle is valued at $1.50 each way, i.e., to and from work, per employee (Reg. § 1.61-21(f)).[61] Even if two or more employees commute in the vehicle, e.g., a car pool, each employee includes $1.50 each way in income. To qualify, personal use of the vehicle must be *de minimis* and the employer must require the employee or employees to commute to and/or from work in the vehicle for bona-fide noncompensatory business reasons.

Employer-Provided Transportation Due to Unsafe Conditions. If it is unsafe for an employee, who would normally do so, to walk or use public transportation to get to work and certain other requirements are met, the employee includes only $1.50 per one-way commute ($3.00 per round trip commute) in income with respect to cab fare or an employer-provided vehicle (Reg. § 1.61-21(k)).[62]

Chauffeur Services. The fair market value of chauffeur services is determined separately from the value of the availability of an employer-provided automobile (Reg. § 1.61-21(b)(5)). The services of a chauffeur may generally be valued by reference to either (1) the fair market value of these services as determined in an arm's-length transaction, or (2) the compensation of the chauffeur.

Noncommercial Aircraft Flights. The value of personal flights, domestic or international, on employer-provided noncommercial aircraft is determined under an IRS formula that is based on Standard Industry Fare Level (SIFL) flight mileage rates, a terminal charge and the weight of the aircraft (Reg. § 1.61-21(g)).[63] If a trip made primarily for business purposes includes business and personal flights, the excess of the value of all the actual flights over the value of the flights that would have been taken if there had been no personal flights is includible in gross income. If the trip is primarily personal, the value of the personal flights that would have been taken if there had been no business flights is includible in gross income. No amount is included in income if the

---

References are to Standard Federal Tax Reports; Tax Research Consultant; and Practical Tax Explanations.

[60] ¶ 5906, ; COMPEN: 33,154; § 8,055.15

[61] ¶ 5906; COMPEN: 33,156; § 8,055.20

[62] ¶ 5906; COMPEN: 33,152.20, COMPEN: 33,156, COMPEN: 33,160; § 21,130.10, § 21,130.15

[63] ¶ 5906; COMPEN: 33,202; § 21,105.10

¶2059

employee takes a personal trip on a noncommercial aircraft and at least one-half of the aircraft's seating capacity is occupied by employees whose flights are primarily business related and excludable from income.

Frequent Flyer Miles. The IRS will not try to tax the personal use of airline frequent flyer miles or other in-kind promotional benefits attributable to the taxpayer's business or official travel. Any future guidance on the taxability of these benefits will be applied prospectively. This relief does not apply to travel or other promotional benefits that are converted to cash, to compensation that is paid in the form of travel or other promotional benefits, or to other circumstances where these benefits are used for tax-avoidance purposes (Announcement 2002-18).[64]

2063. Adoption Assistance Programs. Qualified adoption expenses incurred by a taxpayer for the adoption of an eligible child and paid to a third party or reimbursed to an employee by an employer under a written adoption assistance program are excludable from the employee's gross income (Code Sec. 137).[65] An adoption assistance program is a written plan that (1) benefits employees who qualify under rules set up by the employer which do not favor highly compensated employees or their dependents; (2) does not pay more than five percent of its payments each year to shareholders or owners of more than five percent of the stock; (3) provides for adequate notice to employees of their eligibility; and (4) requires employees to provide reasonable substantiation of qualified expenses that are to be paid or reimbursed.

The rules for the exclusion generally parallel the rules for the adoption expense credit. Thus, an eligible child and qualified adoption expenses are defined as they are for purposes of the credit (¶ 1307). The aggregate amount of payments that may be excluded from income (for both special needs adoptions and other adoptions) is $13,190 for 2014 ($13,400 for 2015) (Rev. Proc. 2013-35; Rev. Proc. 2014-61). The exclusion is phased out for higher income taxpayers the same as for the adoption credit when modified adjusted gross income is between $197,880 and $237,880 for 2014 (between $201,010 and $241,010 for 2015).

2065. Dependent Care Assistance Benefits. An employee may exclude from gross income amounts paid or incurred by an employer for dependent care assistance services provided to the employee under a written plan (Code Sec. 129).[66] The maximum amount excluded cannot exceed $5,000 for the tax year ($2,500 if married filing separately). Any amount exceeding the limit is includible in the employee's gross income for the year in which the services are provided, even if the payment for the services is received in a subsequent year. The exclusion also cannot exceed the employee's earned income if unmarried, or earned income of the lower-earning spouse if married.

Dependent care assistance means the payment for services (or providing services) which if paid by the employee would entitle him or her to claim the child and dependent care credit (¶ 1301). In other words the expenses must be incurred for household services for care of a child or other dependent to enable the employee to work. A dependent care assistance plan generally must not discriminate in favor of employees who are highly compensated. If a plan would qualify as a dependent care assistance program except for the fact that it fails to meet discrimination, eligibility, or other requirements, then despite the failure the plan may still be treated as a dependent care assistance program in the case of employees who are not highly compensated.

The exclusion of dependent care assistance benefits does not apply unless the name, address, and taxpayer identification number of the person performing the child or dependent care services are included on the return of the employee benefiting from the exclusion. The exclusion may be claimed even though the information is not provided if it can be shown that the taxpayer exercised due diligence in attempting to provide this information.

References are to Standard Federal Tax Reports; Tax Research Consultant; and Practical Tax Explanations.

[64] ¶ 5907.35; BUSEXP: 24,906.15; § 3,085

[65] ¶ 7600; COMPEN: 36,650; § 4,025

[66] ¶ 7380; COMPEN: 36,600; § 20,001

2067. Educational Assistance Programs. Up to $5,250 of payments received by an employee for tuition, fees, books, supplies, etc., under an employer's educational assistance program may be excluded from gross income (Code Sec. 127; Reg. §§ 1.127-1 and 1.127-2).[67] This benefit is available for both undergraduate and graduate-level courses. Excludable assistance payments may not cover tools or supplies that the employee retains after completion of the course or the cost of meals, lodging, or transportation. Although the courses covered by the plan need not be job related, an exception applies to courses involving sports, games, or hobbies. These courses may only be covered if they involve the employer's business or are required as part of a degree program.

An educational assistance program is a separate written plan that provides educational assistance only to employees, subject to various limitations. An employee for this purpose includes a current employee, as well as a former employee who retired, left on disability, or was laid off. It also includes a partner who performs services for a partnership and a leased employee who has provided services on a substantially full-time basis for at least a year (Rev. Rul. 96-41). A program that provides benefits to spouses or dependents of employees is not a qualified program.

Reports and Records. An employer who maintains an educational assistance plan must maintain records and file an information return (Form 5500) for the plan (Code Sec. 6039D).[68] However, the reporting requirement for educational assistance plans has been suspended indefinitely (Notice 2002-24).

2069. Employee Achievement Award. An employee achievement award is excludable from an employee's gross income to the extent the cost of the award is deductible by the employer ($400 for nonqualified awards or $1,600 for qualified awards) (Code Sec. 74(c); Prop. Reg. § 1.74-2).[69] See ¶ 919 for a discussion of the employer's deduction and the definition of an employee achievement award. If the cost of an award exceeds the dollar limitations, then the employee must include in gross income the greater of excess of the fair market value or the cost to the employer of the award over the dollar limitation, but not in excess of the fair market value of the award. The exclusion is not available for any award made by a sole proprietorship to the sole proprietor.

2071. Vacation Pay. A vacation pay plan is an employer plan that provides compensation to employees for specified periods of vacation, including vacation time that has been earned but not actually taken. Such a plan also generally includes compensation for specified holidays, whether or not those days are actually taken.[70]

Vacation pay plans, like other employee benefit plans, can take a wide variety of forms: the benefits may be vested or unvested; the plan may be funded or unfunded; and the plan may be a single-employer plan or a multiemployer plan. Vacation pay is taxable and is subject to income tax withholding (Code Sec. 61; Reg. § 31.3401(a)-1(b)(3)). Vacation pay is also subject to FICA and FUTA taxes (Code Secs. 3121(a) and 3306(b)).

Vacation pay is generally deductible by a an employer as reasonable compensation for prior services rendered (Code Sec. 162; Reg. § 1.162-7). An additional discussion of vacation pay deductions can be found at ¶ 1549.

2073. Leave Sharing. An employee who deposits accrued leave in an employer-sponsored leave bank for use by other employees adversely affected by a major disaster under a major disaster leave sharing plan does not realize income or wages with respect to the deposited leave, provided the plan treats the amounts paid to the leave recipient as wages subject to income tax withholding and payroll taxes (Notice 2006-59).[71]

If an employee participates in a leave donation program under which employees may elect to forgo vacation, sick, or personal leave in exchange for employer making cash contributions to charitable organizations, the contributing employee may not claim an expense, charitable contribution, or loss deduction for the contributed leave. However, the IRS will not assert that such cash payments constitute income or wages of the employee with respect to donations made to a charitable organization before January 1, 2014, for the relief of victims of Hurricane Sandy, as well as donations made before

References are to Standard Federal Tax Reports; Tax Research Consultant; and Practical Tax Explanations.

[67] ¶ 7350, ¶ 7351, ¶ 7352; COMPEN: 36,554; § 20,101
[68] ¶ 35,660; PENALTY: 3,208.20; § 39,155.25
[69] ¶ 6200, ¶ 6203; INDIV: 33,154; § 3,060.15
[70] ¶ 5507.47; COMPEN: 12,212; § 22,110.10
[71] ¶ 11,620.522; COMPEN: 6054; § 3,005.25, § 22,110.10

January 1, 2016, for the relief of victims of the Ebola virus disease outbreak in Guinea, Liberia, and Sierra Leone (Notice 2012-69; Notice 2014-68).[72]

Amounts deposited in a leave bank to be used by employees experiencing medical emergencies are not taxable to contributing employees but they are included in the gross income of the recipients subject to income tax withholding and payroll taxes (Rev. Rul. 90-29). The IRS has not granted favorable tax treatment to other leave-sharing plans.

2075. Severance Pay. A severance pay plan is a plan that provides payments to employees upon termination of employment. Depending upon the facts and circumstances, severance pay arrangements can qualify as a welfare plan or a retirement plan or may be exempt from certain federal requirements. Generally, the payments are proportionate to length of employment.[73] The plan may be a permanent program or a limited program—e.g., an "open-window" program that offers a group of employees cash payments, increased pension benefits, or both as inducements to voluntarily retire or to separate from employment within a certain time period. The plan may cover voluntary separations, involuntary separations, or both, and may place conditions on payment of benefits—e.g., no benefits are provided if the employee goes to work for a competitor or for a successor employer. In addition, the plan may deny benefits if the employee is terminated for cause.

Golden Parachutes. In a golden parachute agreement, a corporate employer states that it will pay a key employee or a number of key employees an amount over and above other compensation in the event of a change in ownership or control of the corporation or a substantial portion of the corporation's assets (¶ 907). The tax consequences applicable to golden parachute payments are triggered merely by the payment of the requisite amount of compensation, and a termination of employment is not literally required. As a practical matter, however, golden parachute payment provisions in an employment agreement or employer's benefits plan usually are designed to be triggered upon loss of employment within a designated period of time following the acquisition of the employer.

2077. Same-Sex Marriage and Domestic Partner Benefits. Employers may offer benefits to an employee's domestic partner, including health care insurance (medical, dental, vision), access to an employee assistance plan, and dependent life insurance. Employers often require a written affidavit affirming the relationship and may require various documentation, e.g., joint mortgage or lease, proof of registration under a local ordinance, drivers' license, tax returns, bank statements, or joint credit statements.

Registered domestic partnerships, civil unions, and other similar formal relationships recognized under state law are not considered a "marriage" for federal income tax purposes (Rev. Rul. 2013-17). Thus, while employer-provided health benefits are tax free for spouses (including same-sex spouses) and dependents of an employee (¶ 2015), the cost of providing the benefit to a domestic partner who is not legally married to the employee or cannot be claimed as the employee's dependent (¶ 137) is included in the employee's gross income. Additionally, if a domestic partner is a not the employee's spouse or dependent, contributions for a partner's coverage must be on an after-tax basis, and the domestic partner is not eligible for reimbursement from health care FSAs.

Same-Sex Spouses. The IRS has ruled same-sex couples who were legally married in a jurisdiction that recognizes same-sex marriages will be treated as married for all federal tax purposes, even if the couple lives in a jurisdiction that does not recognize the validity of same-sex marriages (¶ 152). The ruling is generally effective as of September 16, 2013, but taxpayers may rely on it retroactively for any open tax year to make claims for refunds or adjustments of taxes with respect to employer-provided benefits. Specific guidance has been provided for employers and employees to make claims for refunds or adjustments of overpayments of employment taxes and income tax withholding for benefits provided to same-sex spouses (Notice 2013-61).[74]

References are to Standard Federal Tax Reports; Tax Research Consultant; and Practical Tax Explanations.

[72] ¶ 11,620.1005; INDIV: 27,208; § 22,110.10

[73] ¶ 5507.297; COMPEN: 27,202; § 9,345

[74] ¶ 38,519.395, ¶ 38,770.13; PAYROLL: 9,352; § 22,235.25

20 | HEALTH/BENEFITS

Fringe Benefits Under Code Sec. 132

2085. Fringe Benefits Under Code Sec. 132. Certain fringe benefits provided by an employer to an employee are excluded from an employee's gross income for income tax purposes, and from wages for purposes of income tax withholding and FICA and FUTA taxes (Code Sec. 132).[75] These include: no-additional-cost services (¶ 2087), qualified employee discounts (¶ 2088), *de minimis* fringe benefits (¶ 2089), working condition fringe benefits (¶ 2090), qualified transportation fringe benefits (¶ 2091), qualified moving expense reimbursements (¶ 2092), qualified retirement planning services (¶ 2093), on-premises athletic facilities (¶ 2094), and qualified military base realignment and closure fringe benefits (¶ 2095). Employers providing fringe benefits must meet certain nondiscrimination requirements in order for such benefits to apply to favored groups.

Any fringe benefit that does not qualify for exclusion under Code Sec. 132, or any other Code provision, is includible in the recipient's gross income and wages at the excess of its fair market value over any amount paid by the employee for the benefit (unless excluded under another specific statutory provision) (¶ 713). Employers are generally allowed a trade or business expense deduction for the value or a portion of the value of the fringe benefit provided to employees (¶ 906).

For purposes of no-additional-cost services, qualified employee discounts, and on-premise athletic facilities, the exclusion under Code Sec. 132 applies to benefits provided to: (1) employees, their spouses, and dependent children; (2) former employees who separated from service because of retirement or disability, as well as their spouses and dependent children; (3) the widow or widower of a deceased employee; and (4) the dependent children of deceased employees (Code Sec. 132(h); Reg. § 1.132-1(b)).[76] For purposes of working condition fringes, the exclusion applies to benefits provided to employees, independent contractors, directors, and partners who perform services for a partnership.

2087. No-Additional-Cost-Services. No-additional-cost-services provided by an employer to employees are excluded from gross income and wages as a fringe benefit (¶ 2085) (Code Sec. 132(b); Reg. § 1.132-2).[77] No-additional-cost-services are free services provided to all employees by an employer where the employer incurs no substantial additional cost in providing the service, and the service is normally offered to the employer's customers in the line of business, such as free travel on a standby basis for airline employees. The exclusion is available only if the service is available to employees on a nondiscriminatory basis.

2088. Qualified Employee Discounts. Discounts provided to employees on their purchase of qualified property or services of their employer are excluded from gross income and wages as a fringe benefit (¶ 2085) (Code Sec. 132(c); Reg. § 1.132-3).[78] Qualified employee discounts are discounts provided to all employees on the selling price of certain property or services in the ordinary line of business. In the case of merchandise, the discount cannot exceed the gross profit percentage of the price at which the property is offered to customers. For services, the discount cannot exceed 20 percent of the price at which the service is offered to customers. In order to be excluded, the discounts must be available to employees on a nondiscriminatory basis. Moreover, employees do not receive income if they pay at least fair market value for damaged, distressed, or returned property.

2089. *De Minimis* Fringe Benefits. If the value of any property or service provided to an employee is so minimal that accounting for the property or service would be unreasonable or administratively impracticable for an employer, it is a *de minimis* fringe benefit that is excluded from the employee's gross income and wages (¶ 2085) (Code Sec. 132(e); Reg. § 1.132-6).[79] Examples include limited use of copy machines, occasional parties or picnics, meal money or transit fare due to overtime work, holiday gifts with a

References are to Standard Federal Tax Reports; Tax Research Consultant; and Practical Tax Explanations.

[75] ¶ 7420; COMPEN: 36,000; § 21,101

[76] ¶ 7420, ¶ 7422; COMPEN: 33,050; § 21,101

[77] ¶ 7420, ¶ 7423; COMPEN: 36,050; § 21,105.05

[78] ¶ 7420, ¶ 7424; COMPEN: 36,100; § 21,110.05

[79] ¶ 7420, ¶ 7427; COMPEN: 36,300; § 21,120.05

small market value, tickets occasionally provided for entertainment events, and employer-furnished coffee and doughnuts. In determining whether the *de minimis* exclusion applies, the frequency with which similar fringe benefits are provided by an employer to its employees is taken into account. A subsidized eating facility operated by an employer for the benefit of employees is treated as a *de minimis* fringe benefit if the eating facility is located on or near the employer's business premises, and the revenue derived from such facility normally equals or exceeds the direct operating costs of such facility (Reg. § 1.132-7).

Meals and Lodging. Meals are excluded from an employee's gross income and wages as a *de minimis* fringe benefit if furnished on the business premises of the employer for the convenience of the employer (Code Sec. 119; Reg. § 1.119-1).[80] Lodging is also excluded from an employee's gross income and wages if furnished for the convenience of the employer on the business premises of the employer, and as a condition of employment.

Meals are regarded as furnished for the convenience of the employer if they are furnished for a substantial noncompensatory business reason of the employer (even if the meals also serve a compensatory purpose). If more than one-half of the employees who are furnished meals by the employer are furnished meals for the convenience of the employer, then all meals furnished on the premises of the employer are considered to be for the convenience of the employer. Therefore, the meals are fully deductible by the employer, instead of possibly being subject to the 50-percent limit on business meal deductions, and excludable by the employees. The business premises of the employer for this purpose generally means the place of employment of the employee. It can include a camp located in a foreign country if an employee is furnished lodging (¶ 2406).

Faculty Housing. The value of campus lodging furnished to employees by educational or medical research institutions is excludable from the employee's gross income and wages if an adequate rental is charged. A rental is considered inadequate and thus the exclusion will not apply to the extent of the excess of: (1) the lesser of (a) five percent of the appraised value of the lodging or (b) an amount equal to the average of the rentals paid by nonemployees or nonstudents during the year for comparable lodging provided by the institution; over (2) the rent paid by the employee for the calendar year (Code Sec. 119(d)).[81] The appraised value of lodging will be determined as of the close of the calendar year in which the tax year begins or, in the case of a rental period not greater than one year, at any time during the calendar year in which such period begins.

2090. Working Condition Fringe Benefits. Working condition fringe benefits provided to an employee may be excluded from gross income and wages as a fringe benefit (¶ 2085) provided the cost the property or service would have been deductible by the employee as a business expense had the employee bought the item on his or her own (Code Sec. 132(d); Reg. § 1.132-5).[82] The general nondiscrimination rules applicable to fringe benefits do not apply to working condition fringes; therefore, they can be provided exclusively or on more favorable terms to executives. Examples of working condition fringes include use of a company vehicle, airplane transportation, travel expenses including meals and lodging, allowances for business use of cell phones, computers, and internet service, entertainment, and club dues. Denial of a deduction to an employer for its payment of travel expenses of a spouse, dependent, or other individual accompanying an employee on business travel does not preclude those items from qualifying as working condition fringe benefits.

Employer-Provided Cell Phones. An employer-provided cell phone and similar equipment provided to the employee for noncompensatory business purposes is excluded from an employee's gross income and wages as a working condition fringe benefit (Notice 2011-72).[83] A noncompensatory business purpose is any substantial reason relating to the employer's business, other than providing compensation, such as the

References are to Standard Federal Tax Reports; Tax Research Consultant; and Practical Tax Explanations.

[80] ¶ 7220, ¶ 7221; COMPEN: 36,500; § 21,205, § 21,210

[81] ¶ 7220; COMPEN: 36,508; § 21,230

[82] ¶ 7420, ¶ 7426; COMPEN: 36,250; § 21,115.05

[83] ¶ 7438.80; COMPEN: 36,258; § 21,115.22

20 HEALTH/BENEFITS

¶2090

employer's need to contact employees during work-related emergencies, or the employer's requirement that the employee be available to speak with clients away from the office or outside normal workday hours. The business substantiation requirements for the working condition fringe exclusion are automatically satisfied. Personal use of an employer-provided cell-phone, provided primarily for noncompensatory business purposes, is excluded from an employee's gross income and wages as a *de minimis* fringe benefit (¶ 2089). Employers that require employees to use their personal cell phones primarily for noncompensatory business reasons may treat reimbursements of the employees' reasonable expenses as nontaxable. This does not mean, however, that cell phones used for primarily personal reasons are exempt from tax or from the substantiation requirements.

Employer-Provided Vehicles. The value of an employee's *business-use* of an employer-provided automobile is excludable from the employee's gross income and wages as a working condition fringe benefit. The value of employee's *personal use* of an employer-provided automobile is generally included in the employee's income and wages. The employer, however, may elect not to withhold income tax on the value of the employee's personal use (Code Sec. 3402(s)).[84] The employer must notify the employee of the election, and must include the value of the benefit on a timely filed Form W-2. An employer who elects not to withhold income tax for an employer-provided automobile is still required to withhold FICA taxes.

2091. Qualified Transportation Fringe Benefits. Commuting expenses to and from a place of business and home are generally not deductible. However, qualified transportation fringe benefits provided by an employer to an employee may be excluded from the employee's gross income and wages as a fringe benefit (¶ 2085) (Code Sec. 132(f); Reg. § 1.132-9).[85] A qualified transportation fringe benefit includes employer-provided transit passes, qualified parking, van pooling, and qualified bicycle commuting reimbursement.

For 2014 and 2015, the maximum that may be excluded for qualified parking is $250 per month, but only $130 for employer-provided transit passes and van pooling (Rev. Proc. 2013-35; Rev. Proc. 2014-61). The exclusion for qualified bicycle commuting reimbursement is limited to a per employee limitation of $20 per month multiplied by the number of qualified bicycle commuting months during the calendar year.

> **Comment:** Absent further legislation, the monthly exclusion amount for employer-provided transit passes and van pool benefits will no longer equal the monthly exclusion amount for qualified parking for tax years beginning after December 31, 2013. For the latest legislative updates, visit our website www.CCHGroup.com/TaxUpdates.

An employer may simultaneously provide an employee with a transit pass, qualified parking, and van pooling. However, an employee may not receive a bicycle commuting expense reimbursement for any month in which the employee receives any other qualified transportation fringe benefit. Employers who provide any qualified transportation fringe benefits for their employees may offer employees a choice between cash and one or more qualified transportation benefits without causing the employees to lose the exclusion from income for noncash transportation fringe benefits. The amount of cash offered is includible in the employee's income only to the extent that the employee chooses the cash option.

Qualified parking for this purpose is parking provided on or near the business premises of the employer, or on or near a location from which the employee commutes to work by mass transit, in a commuter highway vehicle, or by car pool. It does not include parking on or near property used by the employee for residential purposes. Van pooling is transportation in a qualifying commuter highway vehicle if that transportation is in connection with travel between the employee's residence and the place of employment. A qualifying commuter vehicle must seat at least six adults (excluding the driver) and at least 80 percent of its mileage use must be reasonably expected to be for

---

References are to Standard Federal Tax Reports; Tax Research Consultant; and Practical Tax Explanations.

[84] ¶ 33,542; COMPEN: 33,350;   [85] ¶ 7420, ¶ 7429B; COMPEN:
§ 22,110.10   36,350; § 21,125.05

employees' commuting purposes and for trips when the vehicle is at least one-half full (excluding the driver).

2092. Qualified Moving Expenses Reimbursements. An employee may exclude any qualified moving expenses reimbursement from gross income and wages as a fringe benefit (¶ 2085) (Code Sec. 132(g)).[86] A qualified moving expenses reimbursement includes any amount received, directly or indirectly, by the employee from the employer as payment or reimbursement of expenses that would be deductible as moving expenses if directly paid or incurred by the employee (¶ 1073). It does not include a payment for, or a reimbursement of, an expense actually deducted by the employee in a prior tax year. Expenses that would be deductible if paid directly or incurred by the employee include the reasonable expenses of moving household goods and personal effects from a former residence to a new residence, as well as the expense of traveling to the new residence, including lodging during the period of travel.

2093. Qualified Retirement Planning Services. Qualified retirement planning services provided to an employee and his or her spouse by an employer that maintains a qualified plan are excludable from the employee's gross income and wages as fringe benefits (¶ 2085) (Code Sec. 132(m)).[87] Qualified retirement planning services consist of retirement planning advice and information. The exclusion applies to a highly compensated employee only if retirement planning services are available on substantially the same terms to each member of the group of employees that is normally provided with education and information about the employer's qualified plan. In determining the exclusion's application to highly compensated employees, the IRS may allow employers to take into account employee circumstances other than compensation and position in providing advice to classifications of employees.

2094. Athletic Facilities. The value of an on-premises athletic facility provided by an employer is a fringe benefit (¶ 2085) that is excluded from an employee's gross income (Code Sec. 132(j)(4); Reg. § 1.132-1(e)(3)).[88] The athletic facility must be located on the employer's premises, operated by the employer, and be used on a substantially exclusive basis by employees, their spouses, and dependent children. The athletic facility need not be located on the employer's business premises, only on premises owned or leased by the employer. However, the exclusion does not apply to any athletic facility that is a facility for residential use. In addition, employer-paid country club or health club memberships are not qualifying athletic facilities unless owned (or leased) and operated by the employer and substantially all the use of the facility is by employees, their spouses, and dependent children.

2095. Military Base Realignment and Closure Benefits. Qualified military base realignment and closure payments are excluded from an individual's gross income and wages as a fringe benefit (¶ 2085) (Code Sec. 132(n)).[89] The exclusion applies to payments made under the Department of Defense Homeowners Assistance Program (HAP) as in effect February 17, 2009, where: (1) there was a base closure or realignment; (2) the property was purchased before July 1, 2006, and sold between July 1, 2006, and September 30, 2012; (3) the property is the owner's primary residence; and (4) the owner has not previously received benefits under HAP. The payments are intended to compensate military personnel and certain civilian employees for a reduction in the fair market value (FMV) of their homes resulting from military or Coast Guard base closure or realignment.

References are to Standard Federal Tax Reports; Tax Research Consultant; and Practical Tax Explanations.

[86] ¶ 7420; COMPEN: 33,116; § 21,135

[87] ¶ 7420; COMPEN: 36,700; § 21,145

[88] ¶ 7420, ¶ 7422; COMPEN: 36,450; § 21,140

[89] ¶ 7420; COMPEN: 6,610; § 4,065.25

Chapter 21

RETIREMENT PLANS

Types of Retirement Plans

2101. Retirement Plans—Introduction. An employer may establish a pension, profit-sharing, or stock bonus plan that qualifies for certain tax benefits (Code Sec. 401).[1] These are called "qualified plans" and they are entitled to certain tax benefits, including: (1) a tax exemption for the trust established to provide benefits (Code Sec. 501(a); Reg. § 1.401(f)-1(c)(1));[2] (2) a current deduction by the employer for contributions made to the trust (Code Sec. 404);[3] and (3) tax deferral for the employee on the employer's contributions and earnings (Code Secs. 402(a) and 403(a)(1)).[4] To receive these benefits, employer-provided retirement plan must meet the qualification requirements of Code Sec. 401 (¶ 2111).

There are two broad categories of qualified retirement plans: defined contribution plans and defined benefit plans. Defined contribution plans include profit-sharing, stock bonus, and money purchase plans in which a separate account is provided for each employee covered by the plan and the employee's retirement benefit is based on the contributions to the account, as well as any income, expenses, gains, losses, and forfeitures of other accounts that may be allocated to the account (Code Sec. 414(i)).[5] Defined benefit plans include pension and annuity plans that offer a specific retirement benefit to employees, usually in the form of a monthly retirement pension based on the employee's wages and years of service with the employer (Code Sec. 414(j)).[6] An employer's annual contributions to the plan are based on actuarial assumptions and are not allocated to individual accounts maintained for the employees (Reg. § 1.401-1(b)(1)(i)).[7]

As an alternative to a qualified plan, an employer may establish and contribute to an IRA-based plan such as a savings incentive match plan for employees (SIMPLE IRA) (¶ 2181) or simplified employee pension (SEPs) (¶ 2189), or an employer may merely enable employees to choose to make direct contributions via payroll deductions to an individual retirement account (IRA) they have established. An eligible small business with 100 or fewer employees may claim a credit for the start-up costs incurred in establishing certain benefit plans (¶ 1365U). Outside the employment relationship, individuals who have compensation during a year may establish and make contributions to a traditional IRA (¶ 2155) or Roth IRA (¶ 2171) to save for their retirement. Educational employers (¶ 2191) and tax exempt and government employers (¶ 2193) may establish specialized plans. All of these plans and accounts mirror the tax treatment

---

References are to Standard Federal Tax Reports; Tax Research Consultant; and Practical Tax Explanations.

[1] ¶ 17,502; RETIRE: 100; § 24,101

[2] ¶ 18,100, ¶ 22,602; RETIRE: 100; § 24,101

[3] ¶ 18,330; RETIRE: 100; § 24,101

[4] ¶ 18,202, ¶ 18,270; RETIRE: 100; § 24,101

[5] ¶ 19,150; RETIRE: 3,000; § 24,115

[6] ¶ 19,150; RETIRE: 6,000; § 24,120.05

[7] ¶ 17,504; RETIRE: 100; § 24,120.10

accorded to qualified plans: current deduction for the employers, tax-free accumulation of earnings, and possible deferral of tax for the participant until the benefits are received. Rules vary, but they tend to favor nondiscriminatory benefits that reach rank and file employees.

Nonqualified deferred compensation plans are different. In general, the employer's deduction is matched to the tax year of the service provider's inclusion in income. These plans are typically aimed narrowly at executives or directors rather than rank and file employees, and may be conditioned on performance (¶ 2197).

2102. Profit-Sharing and Money Purchase Plans. A profit-sharing retirement plan is a type of defined contribution plan (¶ 2101) to which the employer makes discretionary contributions, so long as the plan provides a definite formula for allocating the contributions among participants and distributing accumulated funds (Code Sec. 401(a)(27); Reg. § 1.401-1(b)(1)(ii)).[8] The term "profit-sharing plan" is a misnomer because the employer does not have to make a profit for the year in order to make a contribution (other than a self-employed individual), and the plan may be maintained by a tax-exempt organization. In fact, the employer is not required to contribute every year or any particular percentage of profits or other particular amount, but contributions must be substantial and recurring. A profit-sharing plan can also be coordinated with the employer's paid time off plan so that the cash value of each employee's unused time off, either at the end of each year or at the termination of the employee's employment, is contributed to the employee's account under the plan as a nonelective employer contribution or as an elective deferral by the employee such as with a 401(k) plan (¶ 2104). In either case, the contributions are subject to the generally applicable nondiscrimination rules (¶ 2114) and limits on contributions (¶ 2115). A money purchase plan is a type of defined contribution plan that operates like a profit-sharing plan except that the employer's annual contributions are fixed under the terms of the plan (Reg. § 1.401-1(b)(1)(i)).[9] For example, under a money purchase plan, the employer may be required to contribute five percent of each participating employee's wages, regardless of whether the employer shows a profit for the year.

2103. Stock Bonus Plans and ESOPs. A stock bonus plan is a defined contribution plan (¶ 2101) that must generally follow the same rules as a profit-sharing plan (¶ 2102) except that distributed benefits usually are in the form of employer stock (Reg. § 1.401-1(b)(1)(iii)).[10] An employee stock ownership plan (ESOP) is a special type of stock bonus plan that, if certain requirements are met, provides special tax advantages including the following (Code Secs. 409 and 4975(e)(7)):[11]

- An ESOP will qualify for an exemption from certain of the prohibited transaction rules that apply in the case of loans made by disqualified persons to qualified plans (¶ 2136) (Code Sec. 4975(d)(3)).[12]

- Under some circumstances, a shareholder, other than a C corporation, may elect not to recognize gain on the sale of qualified securities to an ESOP (Code Sec. 1042).[13] Nonrecognition depends upon the shareholder purchasing qualified replacement property within a specific period of time.

- A C corporation is entitled to a deduction for dividends on its stock held by an ESOP that are: (1) paid in cash directly to participants in the ESOP, (2) paid to the ESOP and subsequently distributed to the participants in cash no later than 90 days after the end of the plan year in which the dividends are paid to the ESOP, or (3) used to repay an ESOP loan (Code Sec. 404(k)).[14] In addition, C corporations may deduct dividends that are, at the election of plan participants or their beneficiaries, paid to an ESOP and reinvested in qualified employer securities.

References are to Standard Federal Tax Reports; Tax Research Consultant; and Practical Tax Explanations.

[8] ¶ 17,502, ¶ 17,504; RETIRE: 3,100; § 24,115.10

[9] ¶ 17,504; RETIRE: 33,206; § 24,115.20

[10] ¶ 17,504; RETIRE: 3,450; § 24,115.15

[11] ¶ 18,950, ¶ 34,400; RETIRE: 75,000; § 24,801

[12] ¶ 34,400; RETIRE: 75,302; § 24,825.10

[13] ¶ 29,820; RETIRE: 75,350; § 24,825.15

[14] ¶ 18,330; RETIRE: 75,204; § 24,815.15

• Contributions to an ESOP that are used to pay the principal on loans that were incurred to purchase employer securities may be deducted to the extent that they do not exceed 25 percent of the compensation paid to participants (Code Sec. 404(a)(9)).[15] This contribution rule does not apply to S corporations.

2104. 401(k) Plans (Cash or Deferred Arrangements). A profit-sharing (¶ 2102) or stock-bonus (¶ 2103) retirement plan can include a cash or deferred arrangement (CODA) under which each participating employee has the option of receiving an amount of their compensation in cash or having it contributed pre-tax to the plan (Code Secs. 401(k) and 402(e)(3); Reg. §§ 1.401(k)-1 and 1.402(a)-1(d)).[16] The contribution is referred to as an elective contribution or elective deferral. A profit-sharing or stock-bonus plan with this type of arrangement is known as a 401(k) plan. If the plan meets certain requirements, the normal constructive receipt rules are preempted and the employees do not have to recognize the deferred amounts immediately in gross income. Certain eligible employers (¶ 2183) may also adopt a savings incentive match plan for employees (SIMPLE) option as part of a 401(k) plan. Generally, a SIMPLE 401(k) must meet the same requirements that apply to other 401(k) plans except for the nondiscrimination and top-heavy rules. It is also subject to special rules on contributions, deductions, and vesting (¶ 2185).

A partnership may maintain a 401(k) plan and individual partners may make elective deferrals to the plan based on their compensation for the services they provide to the partnership (Reg. § 1.401(k)-1(a)(6)(i)).[17] A sole proprietor is also permitted to maintain a 401(k) plan with elective deferrals based on net earnings from the business. In fact, most self-employed individuals will find that their tax deductible contributions to a 401(k) plan will be greater than those allowed to other types of self-employed retirement plans (¶ 2107). The Federal Thrift Savings Plan provides federal employees with the same savings and tax benefits that private employers offer their employees with 401(k) plans (¶ 2110).

A 401(k) plan must meet the following specific requirements, in addition to the general requirements for all qualified plans (¶ 2111):

• the plan must not require as a condition of participation that an employee complete more than one year of service with the employer;

• the plan must not condition any other employee benefit (apart from matching contributions) upon an employee's election to make contributions to the 401(k) plan;

• the plan must provide that the participant's right to the value of his or her account that is attributable to elective contributions be fully vested at all times;

• the plan must not provide for distributions merely by reason of a stated period of participation or the lapse of a fixed number of years; and

• the plan must be prohibited from distributing amounts attributable to elective contributions *earlier* than one of the following events:

— severance from employment, death or disability;

— termination of the plan without establishment or maintenance of another defined contribution plan (¶ 2101) (Code Sec. 401(k)(10));

— attainment of age 59½; or

— employee hardship (¶ 2129) (however, distributions at age 59½ or for hardship are not permitted in the case of a money purchase pension plan).

A 401(k) plan that includes a qualified Roth contribution program (¶ 2121) may permit a qualified rollover contribution from a participant's non-Roth account to the participant's designated Roth account within the same plan (¶ 2147) (Code Sec. 402A(c)(4)(B)).

References are to Standard Federal Tax Reports; Tax Research Consultant; and Practical Tax Explanations.

[15] ¶ 18,330; RETIRE: 75,202.15; § 24,815.10

[16] ¶ 17,502, ¶ 18,202, ¶ 18,110B, ¶ 18,203; RETIRE: 3,200; § 24,701

[17] ¶ 18,110B; RETIRE: 3,206; § 24,705.10

2105. Pension and Annuity Plans. A pension or annuity plan is a employer-provided defined benefit plan (¶ 2101) providing specific benefits to an employee or beneficiaries generally in the form of an annuity based on a formula reflecting the compensation and years of service of the employee. For example, under a flat benefit plan the benefit for each participant is a fixed dollar amount, as long as a minimum number of years of service is reached. A formula for this type of plan could base a monthly retirement benefit upon a percentage of compensation multiplied by monthly compensation. On the other hand, under a unit benefit plan, greater benefits are generally provided for a long-service employee than for a short-term employee with the same average compensation. A formula for this type of plan could be a monthly retirement benefit based on a percentage of monthly compensation multiplied by years of service.

In either case, the employer (or other sponsor) must make required minimum contributions to the plan based on actuarial assumptions and calculations of the amount necessary to fund the promised benefits (¶ 2133). Employee contributions are sometimes required or voluntary. Instead of funding the plan directly, an employer may buy an insurance policy or annuity contract to fund the plan (Code Secs. 403(a)(1) and 404(a)(2)).[18] Employers with 500 or fewer employees may establish a plan that combines a defined benefit plan with a 401(k) plan (¶ 2109).

2106. IRA-Based Retirement Plans. In addition to individuals being able to set up a individual retirement account (IRA) (¶ 2155 and ¶ 2171), an employer may also establish and contribute to an IRA-based plan for providing retirement benefits to employees. In these arrangements, a separate IRA account is established and maintained on behalf of each participating employee. The employer's contributions to the accounts are deductible as compensation but generally are not recognized as income by the employee until distributed. There are three types of IRA-based plans. Under a simplified employee pension (SEP) plan, the employer makes contributions directly to a traditional IRA (called a SEP-IRA) set up by or for each eligible employee (¶ 2189). Certain eligible employers may also establish a savings incentive match plan for employees (SIMPLE) in which employees are allowed salary reduction contributions to an IRA and the employer makes matching or nonelective contributions to the account (¶ 2181). Finally, under a payroll deduction IRA, an employer may establish a traditional or Roth IRA to which an employee authorizes a payroll deduction to be contributed to the account.

2107. Retirement Plans Covering Self-Employed Participants. No distinction is generally made between pension, profit-sharing, and other retirement plans (¶ 2101) established by corporations and those established by individual proprietors and partnerships. Retirement plans maintained by self-employed individuals are generally referred to by the name used for that particular plan type—SEP-IRA (¶ 2189), self-employed 401(k) plan (¶ 2104), or SIMPLE IRA (¶ 2181).

Even though there is general parity between retirement plans established by a self-employed individual and plans established by other business entities, special rules have to be considered. For example, the term "employee" generally includes a participant in a plan of an unincorporated enterprise who is a partner or a sole proprietor (Code Sec. 401(c)).[19] When references are made to the employer, a sole proprietor is treated as his or her own employer. However, a partnership is considered to be the employer of each partner. As a result, sole proprietors may establish their own retirement plans. Only a partnership may establish a retirement plan for its partners.

Contributions and deductions for a self-employed participant covered by a qualified plan are subject to the same basic rules that apply to participants who are common law employees. However, a special computation must be made to figure the maximum deduction for contributions made by a self-employed taxpayer as an employer for

---

References are to Standard Federal Tax Reports; Tax Research Consultant; and Practical Tax Explanations.

[18] ¶ 18,270, ¶ 18,330; RETIRE: [19] ¶ 17,502; RETIRE: 60,052;
6,150, RETIRE: 33,254;   § 24,135.10
§ 24,120.15

himself or herself. Generally, the deduction limits are based, in part, on the compensation paid to eligible employees participating in the plan. For this purpose, a self-employed individual's compensation is his or her earned income, defined as the net earnings from self-employment (¶ 2670) reduced by: (1) the deduction allowed for contributions made on behalf of the self-employed participant and (2) the deduction from gross income that is allowed for 50 percent of the self-employment tax paid by the self-employed participant (¶ 923) (Code Sec. 401(c)(2)(A)).[20]

Since a self-employed taxpayer's deductions for contributions on his or her own behalf and his or her net earnings are dependent on each other, the deduction for the taxpayer's own contributions must be determined indirectly by reducing the contribution rate provided in the plan (referred to as the percentage equivalent adjustment). In IRS Pub. 560, the IRS provides a rate table or rate worksheet to determine the reduced contribution rate for this purpose, depending on whether the plan's contribution rate is a whole percentage or not. For example, under the rate table, if the maximum plan contribution rate is 15 percent, the maximum deduction percentage for contributions to the self-employed individual's own plan is 13.0435 percent, while the 15 percent rate applies to other employees. Similarly, if the plan's maximum contribution rate is 25 percent, a 20 percent rate applies to the self-employed individual, and the 25 percent rate applies to other employees.[21]

401(k) Plan for the Self Employed. In general, the same rules that apply to 401(k) plans established by other types of entities apply to the 401(k) plans of self-employed taxpayers (¶ 2104) (Reg. § 1.401(k)-1(a)(6)(i)). This makes a 401(k) plan more advantageous than other types of self-employment plans because the taxpayer may make both employer contributions and elective employee contributions subject to the general limit for additions to defined contributions plans (¶ 2115). Self-employed 401(k) plans may also offer the possibility of being able to make loans to participating employees (¶ 2152).

Retirement Contribution for Partner. A partnership's deduction for retirement contributions on behalf of a partner must be allocated solely to that partner (Reg. § 1.404(e)-1A(f)).[22] It cannot be allocated among all of the partners pursuant to the partnership agreement (¶ 428).

Contribution Is Not a Business Expense. A contribution to a qualified plan for the benefit of a self-employed individual is not a business expense of that individual (*D.L. Gale,* DC-IL, 91-2 USTC ¶ 50,356).[23] Thus, it is not deductible on Schedule C of Form 1040 or on Form 1065 and is not deductible in calculating self-employment tax. For a sole proprietorship, the contribution is claimed as an adjustment to gross income on Form 1040. For a partnership, the contribution is shown on Schedule K-1 of Form 1065 and deducted from gross income on the partner's Form 1040 (¶ 431).

2108. Hybrid Benefit Plans. There are several types of hybrid plans that combine elements of defined contribution plans and defined benefit plans (¶ 2101).

Cash Balance Plans. Cash balance plans are hybrid defined benefit plans that provide guaranteed benefits for employees that are insured by the Pension Benefit Guaranty Corporation (PBGC). These plans establish a separate hypothetical account for each employee. The employer credits a specified percentage of compensation to each account and credits each account with interest earned to mimic the allocations of actual contributions under a defined contribution plan such as a money purchase plan. The amounts to be contributed are actuarially determined to ensure sufficient funds to provide the promised benefit. If at retirement the balance in a participant's individual account is less than the amount promised by the employer, the participant will receive the promised amount. Participants may elect to receive their benefit in a lump-sum or as an annuity. Since benefits are not based solely on actual contributions and forfeitures allocated to an employee's account and the actual investment experience and expenses

---

References are to Standard Federal Tax Reports; Tax Research Consultant; and Practical Tax Explanations.

[20] ¶ 17,502; RETIRE: 60,100; § 24,330.05

[21] ¶ 17,933.036; RETIRE: 60,202; § 24,330.05

[22] ¶ 18,359; PART: 21,260; § 24,305.30

[23] ¶ 18,347.17; RETIRE: 60,214; § 24,330.05

of the plan allocated to the account, the arrangement is treated as a defined benefit plan rather than as a defined contribution plan. Accordingly, the plan is required to provide definitely determinable benefits, use a fixed interest rate, and adhere to the minimum funding standards.[24]

Floor Offset Plans. A floor offset plan is a defined contribution plan with a defined benefit floor. Under such a plan, an employee who leaves employment before retirement age receives the amount in his or her individual account. However, an employee who continues to work until retirement receives the greater of the defined contribution accumulation or the promised defined benefit pension. The defined contribution and defined benefit portions of the combined floor-offset plan must comply with statutory requirements applicable to both plans (i.e., the actuarial equivalence rule governing lump-sum distributions of accrued benefits).[25]

Pension Equity Plans. Under a pension equity plan (PEP plan), benefits accrue on a level basis. Employee earn credits for each year they have worked. Upon termination, employees receive a lump-sum payment or an annuity that is based on accumulated credits and final average pay.[26]

Target Benefit Plan. A target benefit plan is a plan under which an employer establishes a target benefit for its employees but where each employee's actual benefit is based on the amount in his or her individual account. The IRS defines a target benefit plan as a money purchase pension plan (¶ 2102) in which:

(1) the plan indicates a stated benefit commencing at the plan's normal retirement date;

(2) contributions necessary to fund the stated benefit with respect to a participant are determined under the individual level premium funding method using actuarial assumptions or factors stated in the plan;

(3) the contributions, and any forfeitures reducing those contributions, are allocated and separately accounted for with respect to each such participant; and

(4) the benefits provided under the plan are provided solely from the contribution amounts allocated in paragraph (3), employee contributions and any income, expenses and gains, reduced by any losses.

Because it is a money purchase pension plan, it is considered a defined contribution plan. However, the employer contributions are determined actuarially, as though the plan were a defined benefit plan. The employer does not guarantee the targeted amount; its only obligation is to pay whatever benefit can be provided by the amount in the participant's account.[27]

Small Employer Combined Plans. Small employers may establish a combined qualified retirement plan that consists of a defined benefit plan and a defined contribution plan incorporating a cash or deferred arrangement (401(k) plan) (¶ 2109).

2109. Defined Benefit and 401(k) Plans (DB/K Plans). Small employers may establish a combined defined benefit/401(k) plan (a "DB/K" plan) under which the relevant Code provisions are applied separately to the defined benefit (¶ 2101) portion of the plan and the 401(k) portion (¶ 2104) (Code Sec. 414(x)).[28] A small employer for this purpose is an employer who employed an average of at least two but not more than 500 employees on business days during the preceding calendar year and who employs at least two employees on the first day of the plan year.

The assets of the DB/K plan must be held in a single trust and must be clearly identified and allocated to the defined benefit plan and the applicable defined contribution plan to the extent necessary for the separate application of the Code and ERISA. Thus, for example, the Code Sec. 415 limitations apply separately to contributions under the 401(k) plan and to benefits under the defined benefit plan, both of which are part of

---

References are to Standard Federal Tax Reports; Tax Research Consultant; and Practical Tax Explanations.

[24] ¶ 19,076.0345; RETIRE: 39,058; § 24,270.05

[25] ¶ 17,710; RETIRE: 39,206; § 24,120.17

[26] ¶ 19,050; RETIRE: 39,058; § 24,001

[27] ¶ 19,200; RETIRE: 36,304; § 24,115.20

[28] ¶ 19,150; RETIRE: 3,500; § 24,901

¶2109

the DB/K plan (¶ 2115). Similarly, the spousal protection rules apply to the defined benefit plan but not to the 401(k) plan. In addition, the DB/K plan must also meet certain benefit, contribution, vesting, and nondiscrimination requirements.

Defined Benefit Plan Requirements. A defined benefit plan that is part of a DB/K plan must provide each participant with a benefit of not less than the applicable percentage of the participant's final average pay. For this purpose, final average pay is determined using the consecutive-year period (not exceeding five years) during which the participant has the greatest aggregate compensation. The applicable percentage is the lesser of (1) one percent multiplied by the participant's years of service or (2) 20 percent (Code Sec. 414(x)(2)(B)(i) and (ii)). Any benefits provided under a defined benefit plan that is part of a DB/K plan (including any benefits provided in addition to required benefits) must be fully vested after three years of service (Code Secs. 414(x)(2)(D)(i) and 404(a)(1)(D)(i)).[29]

Cash Balance Plans. A special rule applies to a Code Sec. 411(a)(13)(B) applicable defined benefit plan, under which the accrued benefit is calculated as the balance of a hypothetical account or as an accumulated percentage of the participant's final average compensation, and which meets the interest credit requirements of Code Sec. 411(b)(5)(B)(i). Such a plan is treated as meeting the benefit requirement if each participant receives a pay credit for each plan year of not less than a certain percentage of compensation that is determined based on the participant's age. If the participant is age 30 or less, then the percentage is two percent; if the participant is over age 30 but less than age 40, then the percentage is four percent; if the participant is age 40 or over but less than age 50, then the percentage is six percent; and if the participant is age 50 or over, the percentage is eight percent. A defined benefit plan that is part of a DB/K plan must provide the required benefit to each participant, regardless of whether the participant makes elective deferrals to the applicable defined contribution plan that is part of the DB/K plan (Code Sec. 414(x)(2)(B)(iii) and (iv)).

Defined Contribution Plan Requirements. Certain automatic enrollment and matching contribution requirements must be met with respect to a 401(k) plan that is part of a DB/K plan. First, the qualified cash or deferred arrangement under the plan must constitute an automatic contribution arrangement (Code Sec. 414(x)(2)(C)(i)(I)). An automatic contribution arrangement must generally provide that each employee eligible to participate in the arrangement is treated as having elected to make elective contributions in an amount of four percent of the employee's compensation. The employee, however, may elect not to make such contributions or to make contributions at a different rate. The automatic contribution arrangement must also meet certain notice requirements (Code Sec. 414(x)(5)(B)).[30]

Second, the employer must make matching contributions on behalf of each employee eligible to participate in the arrangement in an amount equal to 50 percent of the employee's elective deferrals, but no more than four percent of the compensation. The rate of matching contributions with respect to any elective deferrals for highly compensated employees (¶ 2114) must not be greater than the matching contribution rate for non-highly compensated employees. Matching contributions in addition to the required matching contributions can also be made (Code Sec. 414(x)(2)(C)(i)(II)).

The employer can also make nonelective contributions under the 401(k) plan. These contributions, however, are not taken into account in determining whether the matching contribution requirement is met (Code Sec. 414(x)(2)(C)(ii)).

Matching contributions under the 401(k) plan (including contributions in excess of the required matching contributions) are fully vested when made, while nonelective contributions are fully vested after three years of service.

Other Requirements. All contributions, benefits, and other rights and features that are provided under a defined benefit plan or an applicable defined contribution plan that is part of a DB/K plan must be provided uniformly to all participants (Code Sec. 414(x)(2)(E)). This requirement applies regardless of whether nonuniform contribu-

---

References are to Standard Federal Tax Reports; Tax Research Consultant; and Practical Tax Explanations.

[29] ¶ 19,150, ¶ 18,330; RETIRE: [30] ¶ 19,150; RETIRE: 3,504;
3,502; § 24,910   § 24,915

tions, benefits, or other rights or features could be provided without violating the nondiscrimination rules. However, it is intended that a plan will not violate the uniformity requirement merely because benefits accrued for periods before a defined benefit or defined contribution plan became part of a DB/K plan are protected.

Reporting. A DB/K plan is treated as a single plan for purposes of the annual reporting rules (Code Sec. 414(x)(6)(B)). All the information required with respect to the defined benefit plan and the 401(k) plan that are part of the DB/K plan must be provided in a single Form 5500. In addition, only a single summary annual report must be provided to the participants.

Termination of the Plan. In the case of a termination of an eligible DB/K plan, the defined benefit and 401(k) components of the DB/K plan must be terminated separately (Code Sec. 414(x)(1)).

2110. Federal Thrift Savings Plan. The Federal Thrift Savings Plan (TSP) provides employees of the federal government with the same savings and tax benefits that private employers offer their employees with 401(k) plans (¶ 2104) (Code Sec. 7701(j)).[31] However, nondiscrimination rules that apply to cash or deferred arrangements do not apply to the TSP.

Qualified Plan Requirements

2111. Qualified Retirement Plan Requirements—Introduction. A "qualified plan" is a pension plan that features a tax-exempt trust to which employers contribute. These contributions are currently deductible, earnings accumulate tax-free, and participants are taxed on the payment of benefits. To be a qualified plan, the plan must satisfy the requirements of Code Sec. 401. A plan that is out of compliance risks losing its qualified status in which case (among other things) participants are taxed immediately for current and past employer contributions, the trust income is taxable, and rollovers are prohibited (¶ 2101).[32]

A qualified plan must be written, permanent, and for the exclusive benefit of employees or their beneficiaries. In addition, the plan must meet requirements regarding:

- participation and coverage (¶ 2112);
- minimum vesting standards (¶ 2113);
- nondiscrimination requirements for contributions and benefits (¶ 2114);
- limitations on contributions and benefits (¶ 2115);
- deduction of employer contributions (¶ 2117);
- elective deferrals to 401(k) and other plans (¶ 2121);
- distributions of benefits (¶ 2125);
- minimum distributions requirements (¶ 2127);
- payment of joint and survivor annuities (¶ 2130);
- anti-assignment of benefits (¶ 2131);
- top-heavy plans (¶ 2132);
- minimum funding standards (¶ 2133); and
- prohibited transactions of retirement plans (¶ 2136).

The annual accounting period adopted by the plan is called the plan year and it may or may not coincide with the employer's tax year. If there is a trust associated with plan, then it must be a valid written domestic trust established by the employer.

Not all employer-sponsored pension plans are Code Sec. 401 qualified plans. Such plans include Code Sec. 403(b) plans for educational employers (¶ 2191), Code Sec. 457 plans for government and tax-exempt employers (¶ 2193), and IRA-based plans for small employers (¶ 2181 and ¶ 2189). These plans are taxed similarly to qualified plans, and

---

References are to Standard Federal Tax Reports; Tax Research Consultant; and Practical Tax Explanations.

[31] ¶ 43,080; RETIRE: 3,400; § 24,701

[32] ¶ 17,507; RETIRE: 100; § 24,201

they are subject to similar though simplified participation, coverage and nondiscrimination requirements.

2112. Participation and Coverage Requirements for Retirement Plans. A qualified retirement plan (¶ 2111) must satisfy minimum participation and coverage requirements (Code Sec. 410).[33]

Participation. The minimum participation requirement provides that a plan is limited in the age and service tests that can be imposed on employees before allowing them to participate in the plan. A qualified plan may generally not condition an employee's participation in the plan on the completion of more than one year of service or the attainment of more than 21 years of age, whichever occurs later (Code Sec. 410(a)).[34] Once these conditions are met, an employee must be eligible to participate within six months or, if earlier, by the first day of the plan's next accounting year. However, participation may be conditioned on completion of two years of service if, after no more than two years of service, each participant has a vested right to their entire accrued benefit under the plan

Coverage. The minimum coverage requirement limits the ability of a plan to adopt employee classification standards that disproportionately favor highly compensated employees (¶ 2114) for coverage in comparison to non-highly compensated employees. The requirement may be met by a plan in one of two ways:

- "Ratio percentage test"—the percentage of rank-and-file employees who benefit from the plan divided by the percentage of highly compensated employees who benefit must equal at least 70 percent (Code Sec. 410(b)(1); Reg. § 1.410(b)-2(b)(2));[35]

- "Average benefit test"—(a) the plan must benefit employees under a classification set up by the employer and found by the IRS not to discriminate in favor of highly compensated employees, and (b) the average benefit percentage for non-highly compensated employees must be at least 70 percent of the average benefit percentage for highly compensated employees; an employee's "benefit percentage" comprises the employer-provided contributions (including forfeitures) or benefits under all qualified plans of the employer, expressed as a percentage of the employee's compensation (Code Sec. 410(b)(2); Reg. §§ 1.410(b)-2, 1.410(b)-4 and 1.410(b)-5).[36]

A defined benefit plan (¶ 2101) must also benefit at least the lesser of: (1) 50 employees or (2) the greater of 40 percent of all employees or two employees (one employee if there is only one employee) (Code Sec. 401(a)(26)).[37]

2113. Vesting Requirements for Retirement Plans. A qualified retirement plan (¶ 2111) must satisfy minimum vesting requirements (Code Sec. 411(a)).[38] Employee contributions must be vested (i.e., nonforfeitable) at all times, including those made through elective deferral of compensation (¶ 2121).

For defined contribution plans (¶ 2101), employer contributions (including matching contributions) must be vested at least as quickly as they would be under one of the following methods:

- *Graded Vesting*—20 percent of an employee's accrued benefit derived from employer contributions must vest after two years of service and an additional 20 percent must vest after each additional year of service;[39] after six years of service, the employee must be 100 percent vested;

References are to Standard Federal Tax Reports; Tax Research Consultant; and Practical Tax Explanations.

[33] ¶ 18,970; RETIRE: 12,000; § 24,250.05, § 24,255.05

[34] ¶ 18,970; RETIRE: 12,150, RETIRE: 12,200; § 24,250.05

[35] ¶ 18,970, ¶ 18,988; RETIRE: 12,056; § 24,255.10

[36] ¶ 18,970, ¶ 18,988, ¶ 18,990, ¶ 18,991; RETIRE: 12,058; § 24,255.15

[37] ¶ 17,502; RETIRE: 12,100; § 24,120.25

[38] ¶ 19,050; RETIRE: 18,050; § 24,260

[39] ¶ 19,050; RETIRE: 18,102; § 24,260

- *Cliff Vesting*—an employee has no vested interest in the accrued benefit derived from employer contributions until the employee has completed three years of service but then must be 100 percent vested.[40]

For defined benefit plans (¶ 2101), all employees' interests in their accrued benefits derived from employer contributions must vest at least as quickly as they would under either a three-to-seven-years graded vesting schedule or a five-year cliff vesting schedule (Code Sec. 411(a)(2); Notice 2007-7).[41]

2114. Nondiscrimination Requirements for Retirement Plans. A qualified retirement plan (¶ 2111) must provide either contributions or benefits that do not discriminate in favor of highly compensated employees (Code Sec. 401(a)(4)).[42] This is satisfied if: (a) either the contributions or benefits provided are nondiscriminatory in amount; (b) the benefits, rights and features under the plan are available in a nondiscriminatory manner; and (c) the plan is nondiscriminatory in effect, including plan amendments, terminations, and grants of past service credit.

Highly Compensated Employees. An employee is generally considered highly compensated for this purpose if he or she: (1) was a five-percent owner at any time during the current or preceding year, or (2) had compensation from the employer for the preceding year in excess of $115,000 for 2014, $120,000 for 2015 (Code Sec. 414(q)(1); Notice 2013-73; IRS News Release IR-2014-99).[43] The employer may elect to limit employees treated as highly compensated employees under (2) to those who are in the top 20 percent of employees when ranked on the basis of compensation paid during the year. Part-time employees, minors, union members, and any employee who works less than six months during the year may be excluded from the top-paid group.

Actual Contribution Percentage (ACP) Test. A special nondiscrimination test applies to employee contributions and matching contributions by employers to a qualified plan (Code Sec. 401(m); Reg. § 1.401(m)-1).[44] Matching contributions are those made by the employer on account of a contribution by a participant or because of an elective contribution by a participant under a 401(k) plan. The test is satisfied if the actual contribution percentage (ACP) for the group of eligible highly compensated employees for the plan year does not exceed the greater of (1) 125 percent of such percentage for all other eligible employees for the preceding plan year, or (2) the lesser of 200 percent of such percentage for all other eligible employees for the preceding plan year or such percentage for all other eligible employees for the preceding plan year plus two percentage points. The ACP test can be satisfied by the plan adopting one of the alternative safe harbors for meeting the actual deferral percentage (ADP) test for 401(k) plans (¶ 2123).

Failure to satisfy the ACP test will not result in disqualification of the plan if the excess contributions (and the income allocable to them) are distributed within 12 months following the plan year in which they arose (Code Sec. 401(m)(6)(A)).[45] However, the employer is subject to a 10-percent tax based on the amount of the excess contributions unless the contributions (and the income allocable to them) are distributed to the highly compensated employees within 2½ months after the plan year in which they arose (Code Sec. 4979(f)(1)).[46] The amount of a corrective distribution (other than the portion representing the employee's contributions) is included in the employee's gross income. The 10-percent additional tax on early distributions (¶ 2151) does not apply (Code Sec. 401(m)(7)).[47]

2115. Contribution and Benefit Limits for Retirement Plans. A qualified retirement plan (¶ 2111) must limit the contributions and benefits that may be provided to

---

References are to Standard Federal Tax Reports; Tax Research Consultant; and Practical Tax Explanations.

[40] ¶ 19,050; RETIRE: 18,102; § 24,265

[41] ¶ 19,050; RETIRE: 18,102; § 24,260

[42] ¶ 17,502; RETIRE: 39,000; § 24,245.05

[43] ¶ 19,150; RETIRE: 3,210.30; § 24,140

[44] ¶ 17,502, ¶ 18,121; RETIRE: 27,150; § 24,705.30

[45] ¶ 17,502; RETIRE: 27,154; § 24,705.35

[46] ¶ 34,520; RETIRE: 27,154; § 24,705.35

[47] ¶ 17,502; RETIRE: 27,154; § 24,705.35

each individual plan participant (Code Sec. 415).[48] See ¶ 2117 and ¶ 2119 for the limits imposed on the deduction of employer contributions.

Defined Contribution Plan. The maximum annual addition that may be made to a participant's account in a defined contribution plan (¶ 2101) may not exceed the *lesser* of 100 percent of the participant's compensation (see below) or $52,000 for 2014, $53,000 for 2015 (Notice 2013-73; IRS News Release IR-2014-99).[49] The term "annual addition" includes employer and employee contributions, as well as forfeitures allocated to the account under the plan.

Defined Benefit Plan. The maximum annual retirement benefit for any participant of a defined benefit plan (¶ 2101) may not exceed the *lesser* of 100 percent of the participant's average compensation for the participant's three consecutive calendar years of highest compensation (see below) or $210,000 for 2014, $210,000 for 2015 (Code Sec. 415(b); Notice 2013-73; IRS News Release IR-2014-99).[50] The maximum annual benefit is actuarially reduced when retirement benefits are paid before age 62 and increased when benefits are not paid until after age 65. If certain requirements are met, an annual benefit of up to $10,000 may be provided by the plan even if that exceeds the 100 percent of compensation limit. The benefit limit and the compensation limit are reduced in the case of individuals with less than 10 years of service with the employer.

Compensation Limit. The maximum compensation that may be taken into account when determining the limit on contributions and benefits of an employee, and when applying the nondiscrimination rules (¶ 2114), is $260,000 for 2014, $265,000 for 2015 (Code Sec. 401(a)(17); Reg. § 1.401(a)(17)-1(a); Notice 2013-73; IRS News Release IR-2014-99).[51] For purposes of the limitation on contributions to a defined contribution plan, an employee's compensation includes any compensation received from the employer maintaining the plan included in gross income or net earnings from self-employment, as well as any elective deferrals (¶ 2121) or other amounts contributed by the employer at the employee's election that may be excluded from an employee's gross income (e.g., cafeteria plan benefits (¶ 2045)) (Code Sec. 415(c)(3)).[52]

2117. Deduction of Employer Contributions to Retirement Plans. Subject to annual limits (¶ 2119), employers are allowed to deduct their contributions to a qualified retirement plan (¶ 2111) to the extent they are otherwise deductible under the Code as an ordinary and necessary expense or paid for the production of income (Code Sec. 404(a)).[53] The deductions are allowed whether or not the rights of the employees to the contributions are forfeitable. However, contributions are generally deductible only for the tax year when paid regardless of whether the taxpayer uses the cash or accrual method of accounting, unless contributions in excess of the annual limits must be carried over to later years.

A deductible contribution is generally deemed made on the last day of the tax year if it is paid no later than the due date (including extensions) of the taxpayer's return. However, in the case of most defined benefit plans, the minimum required contribution for a plan year must be paid (¶ 2133) within 8½ months after the close of the plan year (Code Sec. 430(j)). As a result, the required funding date may actually come before the last day for making deductible contributions. Payments made on a date other than the valuation date for the plan year of a defined benefit plan must be adjusted for interest accruing for the period from the valuation date to the payment date. Elective and matching contributions under a 401(k) plan (¶ 2121) and other types of defined contribution plans are not deductible by the employer for a tax year if they are attributable to compensation earned by participants after the end of that tax year (Rev. Rul. 90-105; Rev. Rul. 2002-46).[54]

References are to Standard Federal Tax Reports; Tax Research Consultant; and Practical Tax Explanations.

[48] ¶ 19,200; RETIRE: 36,050; § 24,275.05

[49] ¶ 19,200; RETIRE: 36,200; § 24,275.15

[50] ¶ 19,200; RETIRE: 36,150; § 24,275.10

[51] ¶ 17,502, ¶ 17,902; RETIRE: 36,350; § 24,145

[52] ¶ 19,200; RETIRE: 75,104.05; § 24,145

[53] ¶ 18,330; RETIRE: 33,354; § 24,305.05

[54] ¶ 18,347.27; RETIRE: 33,356; § 24,305.30

¶2117

S Corporations. A retirement plan established by an S corporation is generally governed by the same rules that apply to plans established by other corporations. As a result, S corporation shareholders are not entitled to claim retirement plan deductions based on their pro rata share of pass-through income from the S corporation. A court has ruled that this income could not be treated as earnings from self-employment for retirement plan purposes (*A.R. Durando*, CA-9, 95-2 USTC ¶ 50,615).

2119. Limits on Deduction of Employer Contributions to Retirement Plans. There are limits on the annual deductions that may be claimed for an employer's contributions to a qualified retirement plan (¶ 2117).

Defined Contribution Plans. The maximum deduction allowed for contributions to a defined contribution plan (¶ 2101), including profit-sharing, stock-bonus, and money purchase plans (except as provided otherwise in regulations), is 25 percent of the compensation of all the participants in the plan (Code Sec. 404(a)(3)).[55] However, contributions that are in excess of the maximum amount allowed to be made to the plan (¶ 2115) may not be deducted (Code Sec. 404(j)).[56] See ¶ 2181 and ¶ 2185 for the deduction limits that apply to SIMPLE IRAs and SIMPLE 401(k) plans, respectively.

Defined Benefit Plans. The maximum deduction allowed for contributions to a defined benefit plan (¶ 2101) generally is determined actuarially based on the expected costs of the plan (Code Sec. 404(a)(1)(A)). The deduction is subject to both a floor of the annual contributions necessary to satisfy the minimum funding standard (¶ 2133) and a ceiling of the full funding limitation for the plan. The amount that can be deducted for any year cannot exceed the greater of the following:

- *Level Funding Method*—The limit is an amount necessary to provide, for all participants under the plan, the remaining unfunded cost of their past and current service credits distributed as a level amount or level percentage of compensation over the remaining service of each participant. Under this method, the past service liability for each participant is deducted ratably over the employee's projected years of service until retirement.

- *Normal Cost Method*—The limit is an amount equal to the normal ("current") cost of the plan plus, if past service or other supplementary credits are provided, an amount not in excess of that necessary to amortize these credits in equal payments over 10 years. However, all defined benefit plans may deduct 100 percent of their unfunded current liability (Code Sec. 404(a)(1)(D)(i)).[57]

Employer Maintaining More Than One Type of Plan. If an employer makes contributions to a defined contribution plan and also to a defined benefit plan, there is an overall limit on the deduction of these contributions. The deduction is limited to the *greater* of: (1) 25 percent of the compensation paid or accrued for that year to the participants in all such plans, or (2) the amount necessary to satisfy the minimum funding standards of Code Sec. 412. The overall limitation does not apply when no individual is a participant in more than one plan maintained by the employer (Code Sec. 404(a)(7)).[58] Also, the overall deduction limit does not apply when only elective deferrals are made to any of the employer's defined contribution plans during the tax year.

Elective Deferrals. Elective deferrals (¶ 2121) made by employees are not taken into account when determining deduction limits for stock bonus and profit-sharing plans, combination defined benefit and defined contribution plans, and ESOPs (Code Sec. 404(n)).

Compensation. In applying the annual deduction limits, the amount of an employee's compensation that may be taken into account is limited in the same manner as for determining contributions and benefits (¶ 2115) (Code Sec. 404(l)).[59] However, compensation for purposes of the deduction limits includes certain amounts that are generally

---

References are to Standard Federal Tax Reports; Tax Research Consultant; and Practical Tax Explanations.

[55] ¶ 18,330; RETIRE: 33,202, RETIRE: 60,202; § 24,305.15

[56] ¶ 18,330; RETIRE: 33,200; § 24,310

[57] ¶ 18,330; RETIRE: 33,252; § 24,305.10

[58] ¶ 18,330; RETIRE: 33,306; § 24,305.20

[59] ¶ 18,330; RETIRE: 36,350; § 25,305.15

excluded from gross income (e.g., elective deferrals and certain disability benefits and elective deferrals) (Code Sec. 404(a)(12)).

Carryovers. When an employer's contribution exceeds the maximum deductible amount for the year, the excess amount may be carried over and deducted in later tax years. However, the total of the carryovers and the regular contributions in the carryover year may not exceed the deductible limit for that year (Code Sec. 404(a)(1)(E) and (3)(A)(ii)).[60] Similarly, if the 25 percent overall limit for contributions to different types of plans is exceeded, the excess may be carried over. The combination of carryovers and regular deductions for any succeeding year may not exceed 25 percent of the compensation paid to participants in that year (Code Sec. 404(a)(7)(B)).[61]

2121. Elective Deferrals to 401(k) Plans. A qualified retirement plan (¶ 2111) may include a cash or deferred arrangement (i.e., 401(k) plan) under which a participating employee has the option of receiving compensation in cash or having it contributed pre-tax to the plan (¶ 2104). The contribution is referred to as an elective contribution or elective deferral. An employee's elective deferral is subject to an annual limit (Code Sec. 402(g)).[62] The limit is $17,500 for 2014, $18,000 for 2015 (Notice 2013-73; IRS News Release IR-2014-99). The limit does not just apply to each 401(k) plan to which the employee makes elective deferrals, but instead applies to the aggregate amount of all the elective deferrals made by the employee for the year to all plans which permit such contributions, including other 401(k) plans, SEP-IRAs (¶ 2181) and 403(b) annuity plans (¶ 2191) (but not 457 plans (¶ 2193)). Special nondiscrimination rules for 401(k) plans may further limit the amount of elective deferrals (but not catch-up contributions) that can be made by highly compensated employees (¶ 2123).

> **Example:** Tony, age 45, works for two employers. Each of the employers offers a 401(k) plan and Tony participates in both plans. During 2014, Tony deferred $11,500 of his wages into the 401(k) plan of Employer A and $6,500 of his wages into the 401(k) plan of Employer B. For 2014, Tony has made an excess deferral of $500 ($18,000 in aggregate deferrals – $17,500 maximum deferral allowable).

Catch-Up Contributions. An individual who will be at least 50 years of age by the end of the tax year may make additional "catch-up" contributions to a qualified plan allowing elective deferrals including 401(k) plan, 403(b) annuity plan, 457 plan, SIMPLE 401(k), SIMPLE IRA, and certain SEPs. The maximum amount of the catch-up contribution depends upon the type of plan involved. The maximum catch-up contribution to a 401(k), 403(b) annuity plan, 457 plan, and certain SEPs is $5,500 for 2014, $6,000 for 2015. The maximum catch-up contribution to a SIMPLE 401(k) or SIMPLE IRA is $2,500 for 2014, $3,000 for 2015 (Code Sec. 414(v); Notice 2013-73; IRS News Release IR-2014-99).[63] Catch-up contributions may only be made if the plan permits this type of contribution.

Excess Deferrals. Elective deferrals that exceed the annual limit are included in the employee's income and subject to a 10-percent penalty (Code Secs. 402(g) and 4979).[64] The employee may generally withdraw the excess contribution from the plan before April 15 of the following tax year along with any attributable income. If the employee has made elective deferrals to more than one plan, then the employee can designate the amount of the excess that is to be withdrawn from each plan. If the excess contribution remains in the plan past the April 15 distribution date, it will be taxed a second time when distributed (Reg. § 1.402(g)-1(e)(8)(iii)).[65] The 10-percent penalty will not apply if the excess is distributed within 2½ months following the plan year in which the excess contribution was made.

Matching Contributions. Matching contributions made to a 401(k) plan by the employer are not treated as an employee's elective contributions and therefore, not

---

References are to Standard Federal Tax Reports; Tax Research Consultant; and Practical Tax Explanations.

[60] ¶ 18,330; RETIRE: 33,300; § 25,305.15

[61] ¶ 18,330; RETIRE: 33,306; § 24,305.20

[62] ¶ 18,202; RETIRE: 3,254; § 24,710.10

[63] ¶ 19,150, ¶ 19,198.25; RETIRE: 27,102.35; § 24,710.15

[64] ¶ 18,202, ¶ 34,520; RETIRE: 3,254.05; § 24,710.10

[65] ¶ 18,220, ¶ 34,520; RETIRE: 3,254; § 24,710.10

¶2121

subject to the annual limit on deferrals. In addition, matching contributions made by a self-employed person to a 401(k) plan are not treated as part of the individual's elective contributions (Code Sec. 402(g)(8)).[66]

After-Tax Roth Contributions. Plans that allow employees to make pre-tax elective deferrals may also allow participating employees to designate all or part of their elective deferrals to the plan to be treated as after-tax Roth contributions (Code Sec. 402A).[67] The designated Roth contributions are generally treated the same as pre-tax elective deferrals under the plan for purposes of limits on deferrals and nondiscrimination requirements, except that the plan must account for them separately. While the employee must include the Roth contributions in gross income, distributions are subject to rules similar to the rules applicable to distributions from a Roth IRA (¶ 2173). However, unlike a Roth IRA, amounts held in a Roth 401(k) account are subject to the required minimum distribution (RMD) rules (¶ 2127).

2123. Nondiscrimination Requirements for 401(k) Plans. A special nondiscrimination requirement applies to elective deferrals made to a 401(k) plan (but not catch-up contributions) (¶ 2121) (Code Sec. 401(k)(3); Reg. § 1.401(k)-2).[68] The plan will not be treated as qualified unless the actual deferral percentage (ADP) for eligible highly compensated employees (¶ 2114) for the plan year bears a relationship to the ADP for all other eligible employees for the preceding plan year that meets either of the following tests:

- the ADP for the group of eligible highly compensated employees is not more than the actual ADP of all other eligible employees multiplied by 1.25, or

- the excess of the ADP for the group of eligible highly compensated employees over that of all other eligible employees is not more than 2 percentage points, and the ADP for the group of eligible highly compensated employees is not more than the ADP of all other eligible employees multiplied by 2.

The employer may elect to calculate the ADP test for rank-and-file employees with reference to the current year rather than the preceding year. However, the election once made may not be revoked without IRS permission. In the case of a test year which is the first year of the plan (other than a successor plan), the ADP of rank-and-file employees for the preceding plan year will be deemed to be three percent or, if the employer elects, the ADP calculated on the basis of rank-and-file employees for the first plan year. If the 401(k) plan provides for matching employer contributions or allows employees contributions to be made on an after-tax basis, then a separate nondiscrimination test generally applies to those contributions.

A plan can avoid failing to satisfy the ADP test by having the employer make qualified nonelective contributions or qualified matching contributions that are treated as elective contributions under the plan and that, in combination with the elective deferrals, satisfy the nondiscrimination requirements. The plan can also limit the elective deferrals by highly compensated employees to prevent any excess contributions or allow the highly compensated employees the option to have any excess contributions distributed back to them or recharacterized (Code Sec. 401(k)(8); Reg. § 1.401(k)-2(b)(1)). An employer may also adopt one of three designed-based safe harbors to satisfy the ADP test for its 401(k) plan. The ADP test will be deemed satisfied if:

- a prescribed level of matching or nonelective contributions are made under the plan on behalf of all eligible non-highly compensated employees and if employees are provided a timely notice describing their rights and obligations under the plan (Code Sec. 401(k)(12) and (m)(11); Reg. § 1.401(k)-3);[69]

References are to Standard Federal Tax Reports; Tax Research Consultant; and Practical Tax Explanations.

[66] ¶ 18,202; RETIRE: 3,210.20, RETIRE: 3,254.05; § 24,710.25

[67] 18,230; RETIRE: 3,258; § 24,725.05

[68] ¶ 17,502, ¶ 18,110; RETIRE: 3,210; § 24,705.35

[69] ¶ 17,502, ¶ 18,111C; RETIRE: 3,210.60; § 24,705.35

- the plan meets the requirements for a qualified automatic contribution arrangement where eligible employees are uniformly treated as having elected to have the employer make elective contributions equal to a qualified percentage of compensation (no more than 10 percent, but at least three percent in the first year, four percent for the second year, five percent for the third year, and six percent for the fourth year) (Code Sec. 401(k)(13) and (m)(12)); or

- the plans meets the contribution and vesting requirements applicable to SIMPLE 401(k) plans (¶ 2185).

2125. Distribution Requirements for Retirement Plans. An qualified retirement plan (¶ 2111) must provide that the payment of benefits under the plan will begin (unless the participant elects otherwise) no later than the 60th day after the *latest* of the close of the plan year in which:

- the participant attains the earlier of age 65 or the normal retirement age specified in the plan;

- the participant marks the 10th anniversary of enrollment in the plan; or

- the participant terminates service with the employer (Code Sec. 401(a)(14)).[70]

See ¶ 2141 for a discussion of the taxation of distributions from retirements plans.

Mandatory Cash-Outs. Generally, a qualified plan is restricted from distributing any portion of a participant's accrued benefits in any form without the participant's (or surviving spouse's) consent. However, the plan may pay out the balance of a participant's account without the participant's consent if the present value of the benefit does not exceed $5,000 (Code Sec. 411(a)(11)(A)).[71] If the present value of the benefit exceeds $1,000, and the participant does not elect otherwise, a mandatory distribution must be transferred directly to an traditional IRA (¶ 2155) established by the plan for the benefit of the participant (Code Sec. 401(a)(31)(B); Notice 2005-5).

Phased Retirement Arrangements. A qualified plan is allowed to provide that a distribution may be made to an employee who has attained age 62 and who is not separated from employment at the time of the distribution but instead is in a phased retirement program (i.e., working retirement) (Code Sec. 401(a)(36)).

Death Benefits for Participants Serving in the Military. Survivors of a participant who has died while performing qualified military service are entitled to any benefits that would have been provided under the plan (other than benefit accruals relating to the period of military service) had the participant returned and then terminated employment on account of death (Code Sec. 401(a)(37)). Thus, survivor benefits such as accelerated vesting or ancillary life insurance benefits that are contingent upon a participant's termination of employment on account of death must be provided to the beneficiaries of a participant who has died during qualified military service. This requirement applies to qualified plans, 403(b) annuity plans (¶ 2191), and 457 plans (¶ 2193).

2127 Required Minimum Distributions (RMDs). All types of qualified retirement plans (¶ 2101), as well as traditional IRAs (¶ 2155), 403(b) annuity plans (¶ 2191), and 457 plans (¶ 2193) must satisfy a minimum distribution requirement in which distribution of an employee's or IRA owner's interest must begin by the "required beginning date" (Code Sec. 401(a)(9); Reg. § 1.401(a)(9)-1).[72] For most individuals, this is April 1 of the calendar year following *the later of:* (1) the calendar year in which the participant attains age 70½ or (2) the calendar year in which the employee retires. In the case of a five-percent owner (¶ 2132) or IRA owner, the required beginning date is April 1 of the year following the year in which the individual reaches age 70½.

If the employee's entire interest is not distributed by the required beginning date, then the employee's interest must generally be paid out over a period that does not exceed the life or life expectancy of the participant or the combined lives or life

---

References are to Standard Federal Tax Reports; Tax Research Consultant; and Practical Tax Explanations.

[70] ¶ 17,502; RETIRE: 42,106; § 24,425

[71] ¶ 19,050; RETIRE: 42,104; § 24,430

[72] ¶ 17,502, ¶ 17,723C; RETIRE: 42,150; § 24,440.10

expectancies of the participant and his or her designated beneficiary (Code Sec. 401(a)(9)(A)).[73] The required minimum distribution (RMD) rules vary depending upon whether distributions begin before or after the employee's death. However, distributions made to a participant or the beneficiary of a participant must satisfy the RMD rules in each calendar year. The RMD for a particular year is generally equal to the participant's accrued benefit or account balance as of the end of the prior year, divided by the appropriate distribution period (Reg. §§ 1.401(a)(9)-5 and 1.401(a)(9)-6).

A plan participant may exclude the value of a Qualifying Longevity Annuity Contract (QLAC) from the account balance used to determine RMDs prior to annuitization (Reg. § 1.401(a)(9)-6, Q&A 3(d)). QLACs are permissible for qualified plans, as well as for Code Sec. 403(b) plans (Reg. § 1.403(b)-6(e)(9)) and IRAs (Reg. § 1.408-8, Q&A 12). The QLAC rules apply to contracts purchased on or after July 2, 2014.[74]

Required Distributions Before Participant's Death. If RMDs begin while the participant is alive, the distribution period is derived from one of two tables (Reg. § 1.401(a)(9)-9). The *Uniform Lifetime Table* (reproduced below) is used to determine the distribution period for lifetime distributions to an unmarried individual or to a married individual if the individual's spouse is either: (1) not the sole designated beneficiary or (2) the sole designated beneficiary and not more than 10 years younger than the individual. The *Joint and Last Survivor Table* is used to determine the distribution period for lifetime distributions to a married individual whose spouse is the sole beneficiary and is more than 10 years younger than the individual.

Required Distributions After Participant's Death. If required distributions have been made to the participant before his or her death, then any remaining benefit payable to a beneficiary may be payable over the longer of the life expectancy of the beneficiary or of the participant (Code Sec. 401(a)(9)(B)(i); Reg. § 1.401(a)(9)-5, Q&A-5(a)).[75]

If required distributions have not been made to the participant before his or her death, then the participant's entire interest is to be distributed to the beneficiary within five years after the death (Code Sec. 401(a)(9)(B)(ii)).[76] The 2009 calendar year is ignored in counting the five-year period (Code Sec. 401(a)(9)(H)). However, most beneficiaries will be able to take advantage of one of two exceptions to the five-year distribution rule (Reg. § 1.401(a)(9)-5, Q&A-5(b)). First, the five-year rule does not apply when:

- any portion of the participant's interest is payable to (or for the benefit of) a designated beneficiary;

- the portion of the participant's interest to which the beneficiary is entitled will be distributed over the life of the beneficiary or over a period not extending beyond the life expectancy of the beneficiary (for this purpose, the *Single Life Table* provided in the regulations and reproduced below is used to determine an individual beneficiary's life expectancy) (Reg. § 1.401(a)(9)-9); and

- the distributions commence no later than one year after the date of the participant's death (Code Sec. 401(a)(9)(B)(iii)).[77]

Second, the five-year rule does not apply if:

- the designated beneficiary is the participant's surviving spouse;

- the portion of the participant's interest to which the surviving spouse is entitled will be distributed over the life of that spouse (or over a period not exceeding his or her life expectancy); and

- the distributions commence no later than the date on which the participant would have attained age 70½ (Code Sec. 401(a)(9)(B)(iv)).[78]

References are to Standard Federal Tax Reports; Tax Research Consultant; and Practical Tax Explanations.

[73] ¶ 17,502; RETIRE: 42,158.10; § 24,440.15

[74] ¶ 17,725I, ¶ 18,278H, ¶ 18,917A; RETIRE: 42,174.45; § 24,440.15

[75] ¶ 17,502, ¶ 17,725G; RETIRE: 42,160; § 24,440.20

[76] ¶ 17,502; RETIRE: 42,162; § 24,440

[77] ¶ 17,502; RETIRE: 42,162.10; § 24,440.20

[78] ¶ 17,502; RETIRE: 42,162.15; § 24,440.20

If the surviving spouse dies before payments are required to begin, the five-year rule is to be applied as if the surviving spouse were the participant. Payments to a surviving spouse under a qualified joint and survivor annuity (¶ 2130) will satisfy this second exception.

Estate planners use these rules strategically to maximize the distribution period for an inherited IRA by pegging the distribution period to an individual's (preferably, a young individual's) life expectancy to preserve IRA assets as long as possible (Reg. § 1.401(a)(9)-5, Q&A-5(b), (c)).[79]

Final Determination of Beneficiary. A beneficiary must be designated as of the date of the employee's death. However, the final determination of who is a beneficiary is not made until September 30 of the year following the calendar year of death (Reg. § 1.401(a)(9)-4, Q&A-4(a)). As a result, if an individual does not remain a beneficiary on the September 30 deadline, the individual is not taken into consideration when determining the RMDs that must be made from the retirement account. For example, individuals who are named beneficiaries as of the time of the participant's death may not be beneficiaries by the September 30 deadline because they have disclaimed their right to any portion of the retirement account.

Penalty for Failure to Receive RMDs. An excise tax is imposed on an employee or beneficiary who does not take an RMD. The tax is 50 percent of the amount by which the RMD exceeds the distribution actually made (Code Sec. 4974).[80] Part or all of the tax may be waived if any of the RMD shortfall is due to reasonable error and if steps are taken to correct it. The penalty is reported on Form 5329. If the individual believes that part or all of the tax should be waived due to reasonable error, a statement of explanation should be attached along with Form 5329. Any tax due must be paid at the time Form 5329, along with the statement of explanation, is filed.

Uniform Lifetime Table

Age of employee	Distribution period	Age of employee	Distribution period
70	27.4	92	10.2
71	26.5	93	9.6
72	25.6	94	9.1
73	24.7	95	8.6
74	23.8	96	8.1
75	22.9	97	7.6
76	22.0	98	7.1
77	21.2	99	6.7
78	20.3	100	6.3
79	19.5	101	5.9
80	18.7	102	5.5
81	17.9	103	5.2
82	17.1	104	4.9
83	16.3	105	4.5
84	15.5	106	4.2
85	14.8	107	3.9
86	14.1	108	3.7
87	13.4	109	3.4
88	12.7	110	3.1
89	12.0	111	2.9
90	11.4	112	2.6
91	10.8	113	2.4
		114	2.1
		115+	1.9

References are to Standard Federal Tax Reports; Tax Research Consultant; and Practical Tax Explanations.

[79] ¶ 17,725G; RETIRE: 66,456.20

[80] ¶ 34,380; RETIRE: 42,652; § 24,450.15

¶2127

Single Life Table (for use by beneficiaries)

Age	Life Expectancy	Age	Life Expectancy	Age	Life Expectancy	Age	Life Expectancy
0 ...	82.4	27 ...	56.2	55 ...	29.6	83 ...	8.6
1 ...	81.6	28 ...	55.3	56 ...	28.7	84 ...	8.1
2 ...	80.6	29 ...	54.3	57 ...	27.9	85 ...	7.6
3 ...	79.7	30 ...	53.3	58 ...	27.0	86 ...	7.1
4 ...	78.7	31 ...	52.4	59 ...	26.1	87 ...	6.7
5 ...	77.7	32 ...	51.4	60 ...	25.2	88 ...	6.3
6 ...	76.7	33 ...	50.4	61 ...	24.4	89 ...	5.9
7 ...	75.8	34 ...	49.4	62 ...	23.5	90 ...	5.5
8 ...	74.8	35 ...	48.5	63 ...	22.7	91 ...	5.2
9 ...	73.8	36 ...	47.5	64 ...	21.8	92 ...	4.9
10 ...	72.8	37 ...	46.5	65 ...	21.0	93 ...	4.6
11 ...	71.8	38 ...	45.6	66 ...	20.2	94 ...	4.3
12 ...	70.8	39 ...	44.6	67 ...	19.4	95 ...	4.1
13 ...	69.9	40 ...	43.6	68 ...	18.6	96 ...	3.8
14 ...	68.9	41 ...	42.7	69 ...	17.8	97 ...	3.6
15 ...	67.9	42 ...	41.7	70 ...	17.0	98 ...	3.4
16 ...	66.9	43 ...	40.7	71 ...	16.3	99 ...	3.1
17 ...	66.0	44 ...	39.8	72 ...	15.5	100 ...	2.9
18 ...	65.0	45 ...	38.8	73 ...	14.8	101 ...	2.7
19 ...	64.0	46 ...	37.9	74 ...	14.1	102 ...	2.5
20 ...	63.0	47 ...	37.0	75 ...	13.4	103 ...	2.3
21 ...	62.1	48 ...	36.0	76 ...	12.7	104 ...	2.1
22 ...	61.1	49 ...	35.1	77 ...	12.1	105 ...	1.9
23 ...	60.1	50 ...	34.2	78 ...	11.4	106 ...	1.7
24 ...	59.1	51 ...	33.3	79 ...	10.8	107 ...	1.5
25 ...	58.2	52 ...	32.3	80 ...	10.2	108 ...	1.4
26 ...	57.2	53 ...	31.4	81 ...	9.7	109 ...	1.2
		54 ...	30.5	82 ...	9.1	110 ...	1.1
						111+...	1.0

2129. Hardship Distributions from 401(k) Plans. A 401(k) plan may allow hardship distributions up to the amount of the participant's elective deferrals (¶2121). A hardship distribution is one that (1) is made because of the employee's immediate and heavy financial need and (2) does not exceed the amount necessary to satisfy that need (Reg. § 1.401(k)-1(d)(3)).[81] Types of expenses that satisfy the requirement of immediate and heavy financial need include:

- medical expenses of the employee, spouse, and dependents;

- expenditures (excluding mortgage payments) to purchase a principal residence for the employee;

- post-secondary tuition for the employee, spouse, or dependents;

- expenditures to stave off eviction or foreclosure with respect to the employee's principal residence;

- burial or funeral expenses for the employee's deceased parent, spouse, or dependents; and

- expenses for the repair of casualty damage to the employee's principal residence.

An immediate and heavy financial need also includes any amounts necessary to pay any income taxes or penalties reasonably anticipated to result from the distribution. To the extent allowed under the plan, if medical, tuition, or funeral expenses incurred on behalf of the employee's spouse or dependent are deemed to be an immediate and heavy financial need, the incurring of the same expenses with regard to the employee's beneficiary under the plan can also be considered an immediate and heavy financial need (Notice 2007-7).

References are to Standard Federal Tax Reports; Tax Research Consultant; and Practical Tax Explanations.

[81] ¶ 18,110; RETIRE: 3,302; § 24,715.15

A distribution will be treated as necessary to satisfy the employee's immediate and heavy financial need if the following requirements are met:

- the distribution is not in excess of the amount needed to satisfy the financial need;
- the employee has obtained all distributions and nontaxable loans available under all plans of the employer; and
- the distribution triggers the suspension of elective contributions on behalf of the employee and other employee contributions to any deferred compensation plan of the employer for at least six months.

Example: Bill takes a hardship distribution from his 401(k) plan on April 1, 2015. In order to satisfy one of the safe harbor requirements, Bill will not be able to make any elective deferrals or after-tax contributions to the plan until October 1, 2015 (i.e., six-month suspension of contributions).

A hardship distribution is included in the employee's income and subject to the 10-percent additional tax on early distributions unless an exception applies (¶ 2151). A hardship distribution generally may *not* be rolled over into an IRA or other type of retirement plan (Code Sec. 402(c)(4)(C)).[82]

2130. Joint and Survivor and Pre-Retirement Annuities. A qualified retirement plan (¶ 2111) that pays benefits in the form of an annuity must generally provide for the payment in the form of a joint and survivor annuity for the participant and the surviving spouse (Code Secs. 401(a)(11)(A)(i) and 417).[83] The annuity must be the actuarial equivalent of an annuity for the single life of the employee, and the survivor portion may not be less than 50 percent of the annuity paid during the joint lives of the employee and spouse. A pre-retirement survivor annuity must be provided for the surviving spouse of a vested participant who dies prior to the earliest retirement age. An employee may "elect out" of either the joint and survivor or pre-retirement survivor annuity. However, the election may only be made with the written consent of the spouse and the consent must be witnessed by a notary public or plan representative. The spouse's consent cannot be given in a prenuptial agreement (Reg. § 1.401(a)-20).[84]

2131. Anti-Assignment of Retirement Plan Benefits. A qualified retirement plan (¶ 2111) must provide that benefits under the plan may not be assigned or otherwise transferred (Code Secs. 401(a)(13) and 414(p)).[85] An exception is made for assignments ordered by a qualified domestic relations order (QDRO) issued under a state's domestic relations law (¶ 2144). In addition, a participant's benefits may be reduced when the individual has committed a breach of fiduciary duty or committed a criminal act against the plan.

2132. Top-Heavy Retirement Plans. More stringent qualification requirements must be met by qualified retirement plans (¶ 2111) and 403(b) annuity plans (¶ 2191) that primarily benefit an employer's key employees. These plans are referred to as "top-heavy plans" (Code Sec. 416(a)).[86] Most qualified plans must include language stating that they will comply with the top-heavy rules if they become top heavy. However, the top-heavy requirements do not apply to SIMPLE IRAs plans (¶ 2181) or SIMPLE 401(k) (¶ 2185). A plan is top heavy if the accrued benefits or account balances of key employees are more than 60 percent of the total benefits or balances under the plan.

Accelerated Vesting. For any plan year in which a plan is top heavy, the benefits of each employee for that year must *either* be: (1) 100 percent vested if the employee has at least three years of service or (2) 20 percent vested after two years of service with a 20 percent increase for each later year of service (Code Sec. 416(b)).[87] See ¶ 2113 for the general vesting requirements.

Minimum Benefits and Contributions. In any plan year in which a defined benefit plan is top heavy, each participating non-key employee must be provided with a retirement benefit that is not less than two percent of average annual compensation

---

References are to Standard Federal Tax Reports; Tax Research Consultant; and Practical Tax Explanations.

[82] ¶ 18,202; RETIRE: 3,302; § 24,455.10

[83] ¶ 17,502, ¶ 19,260; RETIRE: 42,200; § 24,435.10

[84] ¶ 17,729; RETIRE: 42,212; § 24,435.25

[85] ¶ 17,502, ¶ 19,150; RETIRE: 9,300; § 24,230.20

[86] ¶ 19,250; RETIRE: 21,050; § 24,280

[87] ¶ 19,250; RETIRE: 21,302; § 24,280.10

(¶ 2115) for the employee's five consecutive years of highest compensation, multiplied by years of service (up to a maximum of ten years of service) (Code Sec. 416(c)(1)).[88] In any plan year in which a defined contribution plan is top heavy, each participating non-key employee must be provided with a contribution that is not less than three percent of such employee's compensation for that year. Employer matching contributions are taken into account when determining if this contribution requirement has been met. If the contribution rate for the key employee receiving the largest contribution is less than three percent, then the contribution rate for such key employee is used to determine the minimum contribution for non-key employees (Code Sec. 416(c)(2)).[89]

Key Employee Defined. A key employee is defined as an employee who, at any time during the plan year, is:

- an officer with compensation in excess of $170,000 for 2014, $170,000 for 2015 (Code Sec. 416(i)(1); Notice 2013-73; IRS News Release IR-2014-99);[90]

- a more-than-five-percent owner, or

- a more-than-one-percent owner who received more than $150,000 (not subject to an inflation adjustment) in compensation.

In the case of a corporate employer, an employee is a five-percent owner when the employee owns more than five percent of the employer's outstanding stock or stock possessing more than five percent of the total combined voting power of all of the employer's stock. When the employer is not a corporation, a five-percent owner is any employee who owns more than five percent of the capital or profits interest in the employer. An employee is also treated as owning stock owned by certain members of the employee's family or, in the case of any employer that is not a corporation, by partnerships, estates, trusts or corporations in which the employee has an interest (Code Sec. 416(i)(1)(B)). The same rules apply to determine whether an individual owner is a one-percent owner.

2133. Minimum Funding Standards of Defined Benefits Plans. Employers maintaining single-employer defined benefit plans (¶ 2101) are required to make minimum contributions to the plan each year based on the plan's assets (reduced by credit balances), funding target, and target normal cost (Code Secs. 412, 430, and 436, as amended by the Cooperative and Small Employer Charity Pension Flexibility Act (P.L. 113-97)).[91] Full funding of plans is required, with existing shortfalls generally required to be eliminated over seven years, unless a special funding schedule has been elected. Multiemployer collectively bargained plans and Cooperative and Small Employer Charity (CSEC) plans operate under different sets of rules (substantially the same rules under which all plans operated prior to 2008) that require a funding standard account (Code Secs. 431 and 433, as amended by P.L. 113-97).[92] Failure to meet minimum funding requirements or correct shortfalls will generally subject the employer to an excise tax (Code Sec. 4971).[93] However, a temporary waiver of the minimum funding requirements may be provided to an employer that is unable to satisfy the minimum funding standard for a plan year without "substantial business hardship." The employer may be required to provide security to the plan as a condition for the waiver. In addition, no plan amendment that has the effect of increasing plan liabilities may generally be adopted during the waiver period.

2136. Prohibited Transactions of Retirement Plans. Certain transactions between a qualified employees' trust and a plan fiduciary or other "disqualified person" are prohibited (Code Sec. 4975(c)).[94] The disqualified person who engages in the prohibited transaction is liable for excise taxes based upon the amount of the prohibited transaction. The basic excise tax rate is 15 percent. If the prohibited transaction is not corrected before the IRS assesses the tax or mails a notice of deficiency regarding it, the excise tax rate increases to 100 percent (Code Sec. 4975(b)).[95]

References are to Standard Federal Tax Reports; Tax Research Consultant; and Practical Tax Explanations.

[88] ¶ 19,250; RETIRE: 21,354.05; § 24,280.15

[89] ¶ 19,250; RETIRE: 21,356; § 24,280.15

[90] ¶ 19,250; RETIRE: 21,102; § 24,280.20

[91] ¶ 19,100, ¶ 20,151, ¶ 20,211; RETIRE: 30,000; RETIRE: 57,200; § 24,120.30

[92] ¶ 20,171, ¶ 20,202; RETIRE: 30,500; RETIRE: 30,650; RE-TIRE: 57,200; § 24,120.30

[93] ¶ 34,320; RETIRE: 30,502; § 24,120.30

[94] ¶ 34,400; RETIRE: 48,250; § 24,020.20

[95] ¶ 34,400; RETIRE: 48,250; § 51,201.25

Plan Loans. Loans of plan assets to owners of the employer, including owner-employees, are generally prohibited transactions. Loans of IRA assets to the account owner are always prohibited, but a loan from an employer plan may qualify for an exception to the rule (Code Sec. 4975(f)(6)(B)(iii)). Loans from employer plans to disqualified persons are not prohibited if (Code Sec. 4975(d)(1)):

- loans are available to all participants on a reasonably equivalent basis;
- the plan must explicitly provide for such loans;
- the loan must have a reasonable rate of interest; and
- the loan must be adequately secured.

For this purpose, the term "owner-employee" is defined as: (1) a self-employed person who owns the entire interest in an unincorporated trade or business (i.e., a sole proprietor) or (2) an individual who owns more than a 10-percent capital or profits interest in a partnership (Code Sec. 401(c)(3)).[96]

2137. Retirement Plan Returns (Form 5500). A qualified retirement plan (¶ 2111) generally must file Form 5500 (and accompanying schedules) each tax year to report detailed information concerning various aspects of employee benefit plans (e.g., accountant's report, information concerning the fiduciary and financial information) (Code Sec. 6058).[97] Small plans meeting certain eligibility requirements (generally plans with less than 100 participants) must file Form 5500-SF. However, some plans (one-participant plans) generally may file a simpler Form 5500-EZ if a plan's only participants are an individual and spouse who together own the business (whether or not incorporated) for which the plan is established. Form 5500-EZ may also be used by the plan of a partnership if the only participants are partners and their spouses. Form 5500-SF or 5500-EZ need not be filed if certain conditions are met (e.g., the plan, and any other plan of the employer, had total assets of $250,000 at the end of the plan year, unless it is the plan's final year).

If a Form 5500, Form 5500-SF, or Form 5500-EZ has to be filed, as a general rule, the form and its required schedules have to be filed no later than the last day of the seventh month after the plan year ends (e.g., July 31 for calendar year plans). A one-time extension of up to 2½ months may be obtained by filing Form 5558. An automatic extension for filing Form 5500, Form 5500-SF, or Form 5500-EZ will be granted if certain conditions are met (e.g., the plan year and the employer's tax year are the same and the employer has been granted an extension to file its tax return). Form 5500 and Form 5500-SF must be filed electronically with the Department of Labor. Form 5500-EZ must be filed on paper with the IRS. A one-participant plan that is eligible to file may elect to file Form 5500-SF electronically through the Department of Labor's system rather than filing a Form 5500-EZ on paper with the IRS.[98]

A plan may also be required to file the stand-alone Form 8955-SSA to report certain information regarding separated participants with deferred vested benefits under the plan. Form 8955-SSA must be filed with the IRS by the last day of the seventh month following the last day of that plan year (plus extensions). It should not be filed with Form 5500 or Form 5500-SF. A one-time extension to file Form 8955-SSA (up to 2½ months) may be obtained by filing Form 5558 on or before the normal due date (not including any extensions).

Various penalties may be imposed for the failure to timely file the required Form 5500 series form, schedules, reports, or Form 8955-SSA (Code Secs. 6652 and 6692).[99]

> **Comment:** The IRS is instituting a one-year pilot program for late filers of Form 5500-EZ, under which penalties are waived if a qualifying taxpayer's filings are brought up to date (Rev. Proc. 2014-32).[100] The program runs from June 2, 2014, to June 2, 2015, and might be made permanent after that.

References are to Standard Federal Tax Reports; Tax Research Consultant; and Practical Tax Explanations.

[96] ¶ 17,502; RETIRE: 48,322; § 24,020.25

[97] ¶ 36,500; RETIRE: 51,356; § 24,530.05

[98] ¶ 39,480; RETIRE: 51,356; § 24,530.05

[99] ¶ 39,480, ¶ 39,935; RETIRE: 51,356; § 24,530.05

[100] ¶ 39,490.1295; RETIRE: 78,052.10; § 24,530.05

2138. Retirement Plans Terminations. An employer that establishes a qualified retirement plan (¶ 2111) can terminate the plan when it has sufficient assets to satisfy benefit liabilities or in a distress situation. On termination, partial termination, or complete discontinuance of contributions to plan, all affected employees have certain nonforfeitable rights. Depending on type of plan being terminated and whether termination is standard termination or distress termination, the plan administrator must comply with specific requirements. For this purpose, whether a partial termination has occurred is determined on a case-by-case basis (Reg. § 1.411(d)-2(b)). A special rule applies where a defined benefit plan ceases or reduces future benefit accruals. In this case, a partial termination occurs if a potential reversion to the employer or employees who maintain the plan is created or increased. Multiemployer plans are subject to the vesting, participation, and benefit accrual rules that generally apply to all qualified plans. However, there are special funding and termination rules for multiemployer plans regarding special amortization periods (Code Sec. 412(b)(2)).

A defined contribution plan (¶ 2101) is considered terminated on the date when it is voluntarily terminated by the employer or employers who maintain it. A defined benefit plan is terminated when it is voluntarily terminated by the plan administrator or when it is terminated by the Pension Benefit Guaranty Corporation (PBGC) (Reg. § 1.411(d)-2(c)). The PBGC is a corporation operated under the Department of Labor whose primary purpose is to administer a pension plan termination insurance program for beneficiaries provided in ERISA.

Voluntary Termination. A qualified defined benefit plan may be voluntarily terminated through either a standard termination or a distress termination. The type of termination that the plan administrator uses depends on whether there are, or appear to be, assets sufficient to satisfy PBGC guaranteed benefits. In determining if there are sufficient plan assets to pay benefits in a standard termination, claims are divided into six categories: (1) voluntary employee contributions that are nonforfeitable; (2) mandatory employee contributions, plus interest; (3) annuities provided with employer contributions that have been, or could have been, in pay status at least three years prior to plan termination; (4) the participant's basic-type benefits that do not exceed the guarantee limits; (5) all other nonforfeitable benefits; and (6) all plan benefits not allocated to the above five categories (29 CFR § 4044, Secs. 11-16).

On the other hand, a distress termination of a defined benefit plan may be initiated by the plan administrator or the PBGC. Initiating a distress termination requires several steps: (1) notice of intent to terminate given to participants, (2) filing forms with PBGC, (3) PBGC review, (4) determination of whether requirements are met, (5) notice of benefit distribution, (6) issuances of notices, (7) distribution of benefits, and (8) filing of post-distribution certificate (ERISA § 4041).

Involuntary Terminations. A defined benefit may be involuntarily terminated by the PBGC if it makes a determination that: (1) the plan has not met the minimum funding standard; (2) the plan will be unable to pay benefits when due; (3) there has been a distribution under the plan to a participant who is a substantial owner, the distribution has a value of $10,000 or more, the distribution is not made by reason of the death of the participant, and, immediately after the distribution, the plan has nonforfeitable benefits that are not funded; or (4) the possible long-run loss to the PBGC may be expected to increase unreasonably if the plan is not terminated (ERISA § 4042(a)). When a termination occurs, (1) the termination must not have the effect of discriminating in favor of highly compensated employees (¶ 2114), (2) the plan administrator must notify the IRS, (3) all benefits or contributions that are not allocated to employees must be so allocated, (4) benefits must become nonforfeitable, and (5) the plan's assets must be distributed as soon as administratively feasible.

2139. Employee Plan Compliance Resolution System (EPCRS). The Employee Plan Compliance Resolution System (EPCRS) is a comprehensive system of correction programs for sponsors of plans intended to be qualified retirement plans (¶ 2111), 403(b) annuity plans (¶ 2191), SIMPLE IRAs (¶ 2181), and SEPs (¶ 2189) that have not met the qualification requirements for a period of time. Plan sponsors should generally follow the correction procedures found in Rev. Proc. 2013-12. The IRS may extend EPCRS to cover other arrangements as well. EPCRS includes the following correction programs.

Self-Correction Program (SCP). The SCP is available to correct operational failures for qualified plans and 403(b) annuity plans, as well as SEPs and SIMPLE IRAs provided the SEP or SIMPLE IRA is established and maintained on a document approved by the IRS. In addition, in the case of a qualified plan that is the subject of a favorable determination letter from the IRS or in the case of a 403(b) annuity plan, the plan sponsor generally may correct significant and insignificant operational failures without payment of any fee or sanction. SEPs and SIMPLE IRAs are eligible for SCP only to correct insignificant operational failures. SCP may also be used to correct significant operational failures for qualified plans or 403(b) plans (Rev. Proc. 2013-12). A plan can self correct an operational failure if given all the facts and circumstances the failure is insignificant. Self correction is available even if the plan or sponsor is under examination and even if the operational failure is discovered on examination.

Voluntary Correction Program (VCP). The VCP provides general procedures for correction of operational, plan document, demographic, and employer eligibility qualification failures for qualified plans, 403(b) annuity plans, SEPs, and SIMPLE IRAs. A plan sponsor may, at any time prior to audit, pay a limited fee and receive the IRS's approval for a correction. Under VCP, there are special procedures for anonymous submissions and group submissions. If the plan or plan sponsor is under examination, VCP is not available. However, while the plan or plan sponsor is under examination, insignificant operational failures can be corrected under the SCP and, if correction has been substantially completed before the plan or plan sponsor is under examination, significant operational failures can be corrected under SCP (Rev. Proc. 2013-12). VCP is for correction of failures raised by the plan sponsor or failures identified by the IRS in processing the application. Consideration under VCP does not preclude a subsequent examination of the plan or plan sponsor by the IRS with respect to the tax year(s) involved with respect to matters outside the compliance statement. Absent unusual circumstances, a plan that has been properly submitted under VCP will not be examined while the submission is pending. This does not, however, preclude concurrent examination of the plan sponsor's other plan.

Closing Agreements Programs (Audit CAP). If a failure is identified on audit and has not been corrected through the SCP or the VCP, the plan sponsor may correct the failure and pay a sanction. The sanction imposed will take into account the nature, extent and severity of the failure as well as the extent to which correction occurred before audit. The Audit Closing Agreement Program (Audit CAP) is available for qualified plans for correction of all failures found on examination that have not been corrected in accordance with SCP or VCP (Rev. Proc. 2013-12 modifying and superseding Rev. Proc. 2008-50). If the IRS and the plan sponsor cannot reach an agreement regarding the correction or the failure(s) or the amount of the sanction, the plan will be disqualified or, in the case of a 403(b) annuity plan, SEP, or SIMPLE IRA, the plan cannot rely on the effect of EPCRS. The sanction under Audit CAP is a negotiated percentage of the maximum payment amount. For 403(b) annuity plans, SEPs and SIMPLE IRAs, the sanction is a negotiated percentage of the total sanction amount.

Taxation of Distributions and Rollovers

2141. Taxation of Distributions from Retirement Plans. Generally, distributions from a qualified retirement plan (¶ 2111) are taxed to the recipient unless the distribution is an eligible rollover distribution (¶ 2145) or attributable to designated Roth contributions (¶ 2121). The tax treatment of a distribution depends on the form of the distribution. If the plan distribution takes the form of an annuity, it is taxable under the annuity rules (¶ 817 and ¶ 839) (Code Secs. 402(a) and 403(a)(1)). For this purpose, the benefits derived from the employee's contributions to a defined contribution plan and the earnings on them may be treated as a separate contract from benefits derived from the employer's contributions (Code Sec. 72(d)(2)).[101] A participant's separate account in a defined benefit plan is treated as a defined contribution plan if the plan provides a benefit derived from employer contributions that is based partly on the balance of the separate account (Code Sec. 414(k)(2)).[102]

References are to Standard Federal Tax Reports; Tax Research Consultant; and Practical Tax Explanations.

[101] ¶ 6102; RETIRE: 42,302; § 24,405.10

[102] ¶ 19,150; RETIRE: 42,302; § 24,405.10

If a plan distribution is not in the form of an annuity, the following rules apply (Code Sec. 72(e); Reg. § 1.72-11):[103]

- If a distribution is made *before* the annuity starting date, it is treated in much the same way as an annuity distribution; that is, there is excluded from gross income that portion of the distribution that bears the same ratio to the distribution as the investment in the contract bears to the value of the contract (Code Sec. 72(e)(2)(B)). The total amount excluded cannot exceed the employee's investment in the contract.

- A non-annuity distribution made *on or after* the annuity starting date is generally included in full in gross income unless it reduces the dollar amount of subsequent annuity payments (Code Sec. 72(e)(2)(A)).

U.S. Civil Service Retirement Benefits. Retired federal employees generally receive annuity payments under the Civil Service Retirement System (CSRS) or the Federal Employee Retirement System (FERS). The portion of the payment that represents the employee's after-tax contributions to the retirement plan is not taxed. Form 1099-R will generally show the nontaxable portion of the CSRS or FERS payment as calculated under the simplified method (¶ 839) (IRS Pub. 721).

Death In Line of Duty. The amount paid as a survivor annuity to the spouse, former spouse, or child of a "public safety officer" killed in the line of duty is generally excludable from the recipient's gross income when the annuity is provided under a governmental retirement plan (Code Sec. 101(h)). The term "public safety officer" includes law enforcement officers, firefighters, and members of an ambulance crew, or public rescue squad (Act Sec. 1204 of the Omnibus Crime Control and Safe Streets Act of 1968 (P.L. 90-351)). A chaplain killed in the line of duty may also be classified as a public safety officer for purposes of this exclusion.

Victims of Terrorism. If certain requirements are met, death benefits paid by an employer due to the death of an employee who was a victim of a terrorist act may be excluded from income (Code Sec. 101(i)). For this purpose, a self-employed individual may be considered an employee.

Hurricane Sandy Relief. The IRS provided relief to taxpayers who were adversely affected by Hurricane Sandy by relaxing procedural and administrative rules that normally apply to plan loans and hardship distributions (Announcement 2012-44). The six-month ban on 401(k) and 403(b) contributions that normally affects employees who take hardship distributions does not apply for these distributions. To qualify, hardship withdrawals must be made by February 1, 2013.

Employer Securities. Distributions of an employer's securities under circumstances not involving a lump-sum distribution (¶ 2143) are subject to the above rules except for unrealized appreciation attributable to shares that were purchased with the employee's own contributions (Code Sec. 402(e)(4)(A)).[104] That appreciation is not taxed until the securities are sold.

Loss. An employee may claim a loss on his or her return if the employee receives, entirely in cash or worthless securities, a distribution of his or her entire benefit from a qualified plan and the distribution is less than the employee's remaining basis in the plan (Rev. Rul. 72-305). The deductible loss is claimed on Schedule A (Form 1040) as a miscellaneous itemized deduction that is subject to the two-percent of adjusted gross income floor.

References are to Standard Federal Tax Reports; Tax Research Consultant; and Practical Tax Explanations.

[103] ¶ 6102, ¶ 6113; RETIRE: 42,550, INDIV: 30,100; § 24,405.10

[104] ¶ 18,202; RETIRE: 42,402; § 24,301

2143. Lump-Sum Distributions from Retirement Plans. Special rules apply in determining the taxable portion of a lump-sum distribution from a qualified retirement plan (¶ 2111). A lump-sum distribution is a distribution of a participant's entire interest in a qualified plan within a single tax year of the recipient due to one of the following circumstances:

- the death of the employee,
- the employee has attained age 59½,
- on account of the employee's separation from service from the employer (as common-law employee), or
- after a participant who is a self-employed individual becomes totally and permanently disabled (Code Sec. 402(e)(4)(D)).[105]

The rules applicable to lump-sum distributions are applied without regard to community property laws. As a result, a lump-sum distribution is considered to belong entirely to the participant, rather than half to the participant and half to his or her spouse (*R.L. Karem*, 100 TC 521, Dec. 49,091).[106] However, a spouse may acquire an interest in retirement plan assets by means of a qualified domestic relations order (QDRO) (¶ 2144).

Determining Taxable Amount. The entire amount of the lump-sum distribution is not always subject to taxation. To determine the taxable portion of the lump-sum distribution, the following items must be subtracted from the total amount of the distribution:

- nondeductible amounts contributed to the plan by the participant (less any previous distributions the participant received that were not includible in gross income),
- any premiums paid by the plan to furnish a participant with life insurance protection that were included in gross income,
- any repayments of loans from the plan that were included in gross income (¶ 2152),
- the current actuarial value of any annuity contract that was included in the lump-sum distribution, and
- net unrealized appreciation in any employer securities that were distributed as part of the lump-sum distribution (unless the taxpayer elects to be taxed on this appreciation).

If the net unrealized appreciation is excluded from gross income upon distribution of the securities, tax is deferred until the securities are sold or exchanged. The cost or other basis of the employer securities is included in the taxable portion of the distribution (Code Sec. 402(e)(4)(B)).[107]

Born Before January 2, 1936. Employees born before January 2, 1936 (or their beneficiaries), may elect to have their lump-sum distributions from a qualified plan taxed under favorable rates. The election is also available to the employee's beneficiaries, including a spouse or former spouse who was named as an alternate payee under a QDRO. The recipient (employee, beneficiary, or alternate payee) must elect to use this special tax treatment for all such amounts received during the tax year (Code Sec. 402(d)(4)(B), prior to amendment by the Small Business Job Protection Act of 1996 (P.L. 104-188)). Also, this special treatment is *not* available if any portion of the lump-sum distribution is rolled over into another plan (Code Sec. 402(d)(4)(K), prior to amendment by P.L. 104-188).[108]

References are to Standard Federal Tax Reports; Tax Research Consultant; and Practical Tax Explanations.

[105] ¶ 18,202; RETIRE: 42,350; § 24,405.20

[106] ¶ 18,207.11; RETIRE: 42,058.10; § 24,405.20

[107] ¶ 18,202; RETIRE: 42,356; § 24,410

[108] ¶ 18,202; RETIRE: 42,360.15; § 24,405.20; § 46,640.15

2144. Retirement Plans Distributions Incident to Divorce or Separation. A distribution made by a qualified retirement plan (¶ 2111) to an alternate payee (e.g., spouse, ex-spouse, child or other dependent of the participant) under the terms of a qualified domestic relations order (QDRO) is taxable to the alternate payee and not to the participant (Code Secs. 402(e)(1)(A) and 414(p)).[109] A QDRO is a judgment, decree, or order (including approval of a property settlement agreement) made under a state's domestic relations or community property law. The QDRO must relate to the provision of child support, alimony, or marital property rights to a spouse, former spouse, child, or other dependent of a plan participant. In order to be "qualified," the order must meet specified requirements as to content and generally may not require the plan to pay benefits that are not otherwise payable under the terms of the plan.

Payment of the entire amount due the spouse or ex-spouse under a QDRO is eligible for special tax averaging treatment for lump-sum distributions if it would be eligible had it been paid to the participant (¶ 2143). All qualified plans must permit a participant (or a spouse or ex-spouse of a participant who is an alternate payee under a QDRO) to elect to have any distribution that is eligible for rollover treatment transferred directly to an eligible transferee plan specified by the participant (Code Sec. 401(a)(31)). The participant's "investment in the contract" is allocated between the participant and the spouse or ex-spouse, pro rata, on the basis of the present value of all benefits awarded to the spouse or ex-spouse and the present value of all benefits reserved to the participant (Code Sec. 72(m)(10)).[110]

Rollover Distributions. When a participant's spouse or former spouse is awarded all or part of the participant's interest in a qualified retirement plan by a QDRO, the distribution of any part of that interest to the spouse or former spouse may be rolled over on the same terms that would apply if the distribution were made to the participant (¶ 2145) (Code Sec. 414(p)(10)).[111]

Transfers of IRAs. The transfer of all or a portion of an IRA to a spouse or former spouse under a divorce or separation instrument that meets the definition established by Code Sec. 71(b)(2) is a nontaxable transaction as to both parties, and the IRA is thereafter treated as that of the spouse or former spouse (Code Sec. 408(d)(6)).[112] Accordingly, the spouse or former spouse may roll over to another IRA or IRAs all or any part of the interest transferred to him or her (¶ 2167).

2145. Rollovers Distributions from Retirement Plans. A distribution from an qualified retirement plan (¶ 2111) may be excluded from gross income if the recipient rolls over the distribution to another qualified plan or IRA (Code Sec. 402(c)).[113] All distributions from a qualified plan are eligible for rollover treatment except:

- a distribution that is one of a series of substantially equal periodic payments, made over the life (or life expectancy) of the participant or the joint lives (or joint life expectancies) of the participant and his or her beneficiary;
- a distribution that is one of a series of substantially equal periodic payments made over a specified period of 10 years or more;
- distributions required under the minimum distribution rules (¶ 2127); and
- hardship distributions from 401(k) plans (¶ 2129) (Code Sec. 402(c)(4)).[114]

Eligible rollover distributions from qualified plans, 403(b) annuity plans, and 457 plans may be rolled over to any type of plan. Similarly, distributions from a traditional IRA generally are permitted to be rolled over into any type plan (¶ 2167). A distribution from a designated Roth account in a qualified plan may be rolled over only to another designated Roth account or to a Roth IRA (¶ 2175). Special rules apply for rollover distributions by successor after death of participant (¶ 2148) and incident to divorce or separation (¶ 2144).

References are to Standard Federal Tax Reports; Tax Research Consultant; and Practical Tax Explanations.

[109] ¶ 18,202, ¶ 19,150; RETIRE: 42,250; § 24,460.05

[110] ¶ 6102; RETIRE: 42,304; § 24,460.15

[111] ¶ 19,150; RETIRE: 9,308.05; § 24,460.15

[112] ¶ 18,902; RETIRE: 66,708; § 25,460

[113] ¶ 18,202; RETIRE: 42,450; § 25,445.05

[114] ¶ 18,202; RETIRE: 42,450; § 24,455.10

A rollover distribution generally must be made within 60 days of receipt of the distribution. The IRS has the authority to grant a waiver of the 60-day rule in situations involving equity, good conscience, or situations beyond the control of the individual. Acceptable excuses might include: (1) military service in a combat zone or during a Presidentially declared disaster; (2) errors committed by a financial institution; or (3) inability to complete a rollover due to death, disability, hospitalization, incarceration, restrictions imposed by a foreign country, or postal error (Code Sec. 402(c)(3)).

Direct Transfers. A qualified plan must allow an employee to elect to have any distribution that is eligible to be rolled over transferred directly to a qualified plan or traditional IRA unless the plan reasonably believes that the employee will receive distributions eligible to be rolled over of less than $200 (Code Secs. 401(a)(31)(C) and 402(c)(2), Reg. §1.401(a)(31)-1).[115] Plans that are eligible to receive direct rollovers generally are the same plans that can receive rollovers, except qualified plans are required to allow direct transfers to qualified plans only if they are defined contribution plans (Code Sec. 401(a)(31)(E)). The defined contribution plan that accepts the transfer must agree to separately account for the pre-tax and after-tax portions of the amount that is transferred (Code Sec. 401(a)(31)(C)(i)). After-tax contributions from qualified retirement plans can also be rolled over in a direct trustee-to-trustee transfer to a defined benefit plan or a 403(b) annuity plan (Code Sec. 402(c)(2)(A)). The transferee plan must separately account for after-tax contributions and earnings. A traditional IRA to which the pre-tax and post-tax amounts are rolled over does not have to separately account for these amounts. A rollover that includes both pre-tax and post-tax amounts is considered as coming first from pre-tax amounts (Code Sec. 402(c)(2)).

Mandatory Rollovers. A qualified plan must provide for a direct rollover (i.e., a trustee to trustee transfer) from the plan into an IRA when the plan makes a mandatory distribution of the participant's benefit (an involuntary cash-out) (Code Sec. 401(a)(31)). The rule applies when a mandatory distribution from a qualified plan exceeds $1,000 and the plan specifies that nonforfeitable benefits that do not exceed $5,000 must be distributed immediately. However, the employee must have the right to elect to receive the distribution or have it rolled over into another IRA or qualified plan (Notice 2005-5).

Withholding. If a distributee does not elect a direct transfer, and receives the distribution and then transfers the funds to an eligible plan within 60 days, the payor of the distribution must withhold 20 percent of the distribution (Code Sec. 3405(c)).[116] If the distributee does elect a direct transfer, there is no withholding.

Written Explanation. The plan administrator must provide a written explanation to a recipient of the distribution options (including the direct trustee-to-trustee transfer option) within a reasonable period of time before making an eligible rollover distribution (Code Sec. 402(f)).[117]

2147. Rollover Distributions of After-Tax Roth Contributions. A qualified retirement plan (¶ 2111) that allows participating employees to designate part of their elective deferrals as after-tax Roth contributions (¶ 2121) may permit a rollover of a distribution from a participant's non-Roth account to the participant's designated Roth account within the same plan (Code Sec. 402A(c)(4)). The intra-plan non-Roth to Roth rollover rules mirror the eligible retirement plan to Roth IRA rollover rules (¶ 2175). Both kinds of rollovers adopt the traditional IRA to Roth IRA conversion rules. The distribution to be rolled over must be otherwise allowed under the plan; thus, an employer may have to amend its non-Roth plan to allow in-service distributions or distributions prior to normal retirement age.

The converted amount is includible in gross income as a distribution for the tax year in which the amount is distributed or transferred. This amount is reduced by any after-tax contributions included in the amount rolled over. A special rule applies if the rollover was done in 2010. In that case, the amount the taxpayer would have included in gross income in 2010 is instead included in equal installments in 2011 and 2012, unless

---

References are to Standard Federal Tax Reports; Tax Research Consultant; and Practical Tax Explanations.

[115] ¶ 17,502, ¶ 18,202,   [116] ¶ 33,620; RETIRE: 42,700;   [117] ¶ 18,202; RETIRE: 42,466;
¶ 17,925A; RETIRE: 42,500;   § 24,445.20   § 24,455.40
§ 24,455.40

¶2147

the taxpayer elected to include it all in 2010. Any election for any distribution during a tax year may not be changed after the due date for such tax year.

2148. Rollover Distributions After Death of Participant. When a distribution from a qualified retirement plan (¶ 2111) that would be eligible for rollover treatment if made to the employee is received by the participant's surviving spouse, the spouse may roll that distribution into an account maintained in the survivor's name under the same terms and conditions that would have applied to the employee (¶ 2145) (Code Sec. 402(c)(9)).[118] Successors other than a surviving spouse who receive a distribution from a qualified plan are not entitled to roll over that distribution to an IRA or to another qualified plan account in their own name. Instead, a nonspouse beneficiary can roll a qualified plan distribution into an IRA established in the name of the decedent. The IRA is treated as an inherited IRA. This allows the beneficiary to take distributions from the IRA in accordance with the required minimum distribution rules (¶ 2127) instead of taking the entire distribution into income in the year of the plan distribution (Code Sec. 402(c)(11)). The surviving spouse of the owner of an IRA is also eligible to roll over any amount received from that IRA to another IRA or qualified plan (¶ 2167). However, this cannot be done by any other successor to the IRA.

2151. Penalty for Early Distribution from Retirement Plans. Taxable distributions from a qualified retirement plan (¶ 2141) or traditional IRA (¶ 2165) are generally subject to an 10-percent additional tax if they are made before the participant reaches age 59½ (Code Sec. 72(t)).[119] However, the 10-percent additional tax will *not* apply to:

- eligible distributions that are timely and properly rolled over into an IRA or other qualified plan (¶ 2145);

- distributions upon death or disability of the participant;

- distributions after separation from service that are part of a series of substantially equal periodic payments (not less frequently than annually) over the life (or life expectancy) of the participant or the joint lives (or life expectancies) of the participant and the beneficiary;

- distributions other than from a SEP (¶ 2189) or traditional IRA (¶ 2163) after the participant's separation from service, provided the separation from service occurred during or after the calendar year in which the participant reached age 55 (Notice 87-13) (age 50, in the case of distributions from a government plan to a retired police officer, firefighter, or emergency medical services provider);

- distributions to a nonparticipant under a qualified domestic relations order (QDRO) (¶ 2144);

- distributions not exceeding deductible medical expenses (determined without regard to whether deductions are itemized);

- certain distributions by employee stock ownership plans (ESOPs) of dividends on employer securities;

- distributions made on account of the IRS's levy against the participant's account;

- qualified reservist distributions (¶ 2160); and

- distributions from federal retirement plans that are made under a phased retirement program.

Additional Tax on IRA Distributions. The exceptions to the 10-percent additional tax described above generally apply to IRA distributions except for distributions to a participant who has reached age 55 and has separated from service. Also, though the transfer of an IRA interest under a divorce or separation agreement is not a taxable event, subsequent distributions from a transferred IRA are not excluded from the additional tax. Some additional exceptions to the tax apply for IRA distributions only (¶ 2169).

References are to Standard Federal Tax Reports; Tax Research Consultant; and Practical Tax Explanations.

[118] ¶ 18,202; RETIRE: 42,460.05; § 24,455.30

[119] ¶ 6102; RETIRE: 66,454; § 25,450.25

SIMPLE Plan Penalty. For employees who withdraw any amount from a SIMPLE IRA (¶ 2181) during the first two years of participation, the 10-percent additional tax is increased to 25 percent (Code Sec. 72(t)(6)).

Reporting Requirements. The 10-percent additional tax on early distributions is generally reported on Form 5329. If an exception to the tax exists, the individual should provide this information on Form 5329. However, if no exception exists and distribution "Code 1" (i.e., early distribution) is correctly shown in the Form 1099-R received by the individual, then Form 5329 does not need to be filed. Instead, the amount of the additional tax should be reported directly on the individual's Form 1040.

2152. Retirement Plan Loans. Unless certain requirements are met, a loan to a participant from a qualified retirement plan is treated as a distribution and included in the participant's gross income. A pledge or assignment of any part of a participant's interest in a plan is treated as a loan for this purpose (Code Sec. 72(p)(1); Reg. § 1.72(p)-1). The exceptions do not apply unless loan limitations and level amortization of the loan is required, with payments that occur not less frequently than quarterly (Code Sec. 72(p)(2)(C); Reg. § 1.72(p)-1, Q&A-4, -9, and -10). The loan must also be subject to an enforceable agreement.[120]

Allowable Loans. Subject to specific dollar limits, a loan will not be treated as a distribution if the loan must be repaid within five years or the loan proceeds must be used (within a reasonable time after the date of the loan) to acquire a dwelling unit that is to be used as the principal residence of the participant. When determining if a plan loan is allowable, all plans of the employer are treated as a single plan (Code Sec 72(p)(2)(D)(ii)). As a general rule, the *refinancing* of a home loan does not qualify under this exception (Reg. § 1.72(p)-1, Q&A-8(a)). However, the repayment of a loan from a third party that was used to acquire the principal residence may qualify under the exception.

> **Example 1:** On July 1, 2014, Betty purchased a home that she used as a principal residence. She paid a portion of the purchase price with a $50,000 loan from Global Bank. On August 1, 2014, Betty borrowed $50,000 from her 401(k) plan. A few days later, Betty used the money from the plan loan to pay the $50,000 she owed Global Bank. Based on these facts, the plan loan would be treated as having been used to acquire Betty's principal residence. As a result, Betty's plan loan would *not* be treated as a taxable distribution.

Loan Limits. A loan from a qualified plan will be treated as a distribution only to the extent that, when added to the balances of all other loans to the participant (whenever made), the proceeds exceed the *lesser* of $50,000 or half the present value (but not less than $10,000) of the plan participant's vested benefits under the plan. The $50,000 amount must be reduced by the excess (if any) of: (1) the highest outstanding balance of loans from the plan during the one-year period ending on the day preceding the date of the loan over (2) the outstanding balance of those loans on the date of the loan (Code Sec. 72(p)(2)).[121]

> **Example 2:** Jane Smith is a participant in her employer's qualified profit-sharing plan. She wishes to borrow the maximum amount subject to the five-year repayment rule on July 1, 2014. On that date, the value of her vested interest in the plan is $120,000. Her highest loan balance during the period July 1, 2013, through June 30, 2014, was $40,000, and her balance on July 1, 2014, is $35,000. The maximum amount that Jane may borrow on July 1, 2014, is $10,000. This is the amount that, when added to her $35,000 loan balance, does not exceed $45,000. The $45,000 amount is determined by reducing the $50,000 loan limit by the excess of her highest loan balance for the past year ($40,000) over the loan balance at the time of the new loan ($35,000).

References are to Standard Federal Tax Reports; Tax Research Consultant; and Practical Tax Explanations.

[120] ¶ 6102, ¶ 6133; RETIRE: 42,154, RETIRE: 42,802.05; § 24,465.15

[121] ¶ 6102; RETIRE: 42,804.05; § 24,465.15

¶2152

Traditional IRAs

2155. Traditional Individual Retirement Accounts (IRAs). Individuals who receive compensation, including alimony, that is includible in gross income and who are under age 70½ throughout the tax year are entitled to make contributions to traditional individual retirement accounts (IRAs) (Code Sec. 219). Amounts earned in a traditional IRA are not taxed until distributions are made (Code Sec. 408(e)(1)).[122] Contributions to a traditional IRA generally may be deducted. However, when the individual, or the individual's spouse, is an active participant in an employer-maintained retirement plan, the deduction may be reduced or eliminated (¶ 2157) (Code Sec. 219(g)).[123] Nondeductible contributions may be made to a traditional IRA (¶ 2160) (Code Sec. 408(o)).[124] Roth IRAs are discussed at ¶ 2171.

IRA Contributions. The maximum combined contribution that can be made to all of an individual's traditional and Roth IRAs is $5,500 for 2014, $5,500 for 2015 (Notice 2013-73; IRS News Release IR-2014-99). An individual who will be at least age 50 by the end of the tax year is allowed to make additional contributions to a traditional or Roth IRA. Under this catch-up rule, the maximum contribution amount for an individual who has attained age 50 before the end of the taxable year is generally $1,000 (Code Sec. 219(b)(5)(B)).

Individuals have until the due date of their tax returns to make contributions to their IRAs for the return year (generally April 15). Filing extensions are *not* taken into account. If the contribution is made by the due date, it will be treated as having been made on the last day of the tax year for which the return is filed (Code Sec. 219(f)(3)).[125] A deduction may be claimed for a contribution even though the contribution had not yet been made when the return is filed. However, the contribution must be made by the due date of the tax return (Rev. Rul. 84-18).[126]

If a contribution to a traditional IRA is *less* than the allowable maximum for that year, the individual cannot contribute more in a later year to make up the difference. If a contribution is *more* than the allowable maximum, the excess contribution may be withdrawn on or before April 15 or carried over and deducted in later years to the extent that the actual contributions in those later years are less than the allowable maximum (Code Sec. 219(f)(6)).[127] However, the excess contribution is subject to a six percent tax each year until it is corrected (Code Sec. 4973(a)).[128] The individual reports the six percent tax on Form 5329. Individuals with low to moderate incomes may be able to claim a nonrefundable credit based upon their contributions to IRAs (traditional and/or Roth) as well as other types of qualified retirement plans (¶ 1304).

Compensation. For purposes of determining an individual's eligibility to make contributions to an IRA, the term "compensation" includes earned income and alimony. It also includes differential wage payments received by a reservist from his or her civilian employer (Code Sec. 219(f)(1)). Compensation does *not* include pensions, annuities, or other forms of deferred compensation. However, under a safe-harbor rule, the IRS will accept as compensation the amount properly shown on the individual's Form W-2 as wages, tips, and other compensation, less any amount properly shown for nonqualified plans (Rev. Proc. 91-18).[129] The compensation of a self-employed person is the individual's earned income (¶ 2107). Combat pay earned by a member of the Armed Forces and excluded from gross income (¶ 895) may be treated as compensation for purposes of the limit on IRA contributions.

References are to Standard Federal Tax Reports; Tax Research Consultant; and Practical Tax Explanations.

[122] ¶ 18,902; RETIRE: 66,500; § 25,401

[123] ¶ 12,650; RETIRE: 66,200; § 25,415.15

[124] ¶ 18,902; RETIRE: 66,250; § 25,420

[125] ¶ 12,650; RETIRE: 66,208; § 25,425.05, § 46,525.10

[126] ¶ 18,922.87; RETIRE: 66,208; § 25,425.05, § 46,525.10

[127] ¶ 12,650; RETIRE: 66,356.15; § 25,430.05

[128] ¶ 34,360; RETIRE: 66,354; § 25,430.05

[129] ¶ 18,922.1063; RETIRE: 66,206; § 25,415.10

Tax Refunds. A taxpayer may choose to have a refund of federal income taxes directly deposited into up to three separate accounts, including an IRA. The IRA must be established before the request for the direct deposit is made. The deposit counts against the taxpayer's annual contribution limit. Thus, the taxpayer should inform the IRA trustee which year the direct deposit contribution is for. The taxpayer must also verify that the direct deposit is made to the IRA by the due date of his or her return for that year without regard to extensions. A direct deposit request of an entire refund into an IRA should be made on a taxpayer's Form 1040. However, if a taxpayer chooses to have a refund split and deposited in up to three different accounts, then Form 8888 is used.

Allowable Investments. Although IRAs may hold almost any investment, they are generally prohibited from investing in "collectibles" (e.g., antiques and stamps). However, certain U.S. gold and silver bullion coins minted since October 1986 may be held by an IRA. An IRA may also hold certain platinum and state-issued coins, as well as gold, silver, platinum, and palladium bullion (Code Sec. 408(m)(3)).[130]

Deemed IRAs. Qualified plans may allow employees to make voluntary contributions to a separate account that will be deemed to be a traditional IRA or Roth IRA if the account meets all the requirements of the particular type of IRA (Code Sec. 408(q)). The employee must designate the contribution as a deemed IRA contribution. An employee's contributions to this account count against the annual limit on IRA contributions (Reg. § 1.408(q)-1(a)).

Modified Adjusted Gross Income. When determining the taxpayer's AGI for deduction limitation rules, the taxpayer's AGI is modified by taking into account Code Sec. 86 (the inclusion in income of Social Security and Railroad Retirement benefits) and Code Sec. 469 (the disallowance of passive activity losses) but not Code Sec. 135 (exclusion of interest on educational U.S. Savings Bonds), Code Sec. 137 (exclusion of employer-paid adoption assistance), Code Sec. 221 (deduction for student loan interest), Code Sec. 222 (deduction for tuition and related expenses), Code Sec. 199 (deduction for domestic production activities), Code Sec. 911 (foreign earned income and housing exclusion), and the deduction for contributions to IRAs (Code Sec. 219(g)(3)(A)).[131]

2157. Deductible Contributions to IRAs—In General. Contributions to a traditional IRA generally may be deducted subject to the contribution limits (¶ 2155). The maximum deduction may be reduced when the individual or spouse is an active participant in a qualified retirement plan (¶ 2111), SIMPLE IRA (¶ 2181), SEP (¶ 2189), or a Code Sec. 501(c)(18) trust created before June 25, 1959 (Code Sec. 219(g)).[132] An eligible 457 deferred compensation plan is not treated as a plan for this purpose. When an individual is an active participant in an employer's plan, the amount of the deductible IRA contribution depends upon the individual's adjusted gross income and filing status. See ¶ 2158 for phaseout for married individuals filing jointly. See ¶ 2159 for phaseout for married individuals filing separately and single filers. See ¶ 2160 for discussion of nondeductible contributions.

Active Participant Defined. The determination on active participant status is made without regard to whether an individual's rights under an employer-sponsored plan are nonforfeitable (Code Sec. 219(g)). In the case of a defined benefit plan, an individual who is not excluded under the eligibility provisions of the plan is considered to be an active participant if he or she is eligible to participate for any part of the plan year ending with or within the tax year, even though the individual has elected not to do so, has failed to make a mandatory contribution, or has failed to meet the minimum service requirements (Reg. § 1.219-2). In the case of a defined contribution plan, an individual is considered an active participant if contributions or forfeitures are allocated to the individual's account for the plan year that ends with or within that tax year. Finally, an individual is an active participant for any tax year in which the individual makes a

---

References are to Standard Federal Tax Reports; Tax Research Consultant; and Practical Tax Explanations.

[130] ¶ 18,902; RETIRE: 66,458.10; § 25,470   [131] ¶ 12,650; RETIRE: 66,202; § 25,415.15   [132] ¶ 12,650; RETIRE: 66,202; § 25,415.15

voluntary or mandatory employee contribution (Notice 87-16).[133] Social Security and Railroad Retirement (Tier I or Tier II) are not retirement arrangements for purposes of determining active participation. If an individual receives benefits from a previous employer's plan, the individual is not covered by the plan. An individual is also *not* considered an active participant in an employer-sponsored plan merely because the individual's spouse is an active participant (Code Sec. 219(g)(7)).[134] An employer should have marked the box labeled "Retirement Plan" on the employee's Form W-2 if the employee participated in an employer plan for the year.

Social Security Recipients. An employed individual, either the taxpayer or the spouse, who is covered by a retirement plan, currently receiving Social Security benefits, and wants to determine the allowable deduction for contributions to a traditional IRA must compute taxable Social Security benefits twice. The first computation is for the purpose of determining the tentative amount of Social Security benefits that must be included in gross income if the individual did not make any IRA contribution. This computation determines the amount of hypothetical adjusted gross income for purposes of the IRA phaseout provision. The second computation determines the actual amount of taxable Social Security benefits by taking into account the deductible IRA contribution that was determined under the first computation. The worksheets necessary for these computations are found in IRS Pub. 590 (¶ 716).

2158. Deductible IRA Contribution Limits—Married Filing Jointly. When a married couple files a joint return, each spouse may make deductible contributions to his or her IRA. For 2014, the IRAs of the spouse with the greater amount of compensation ("higher-paid spouse") may receive deductible contributions of up to the *lesser* of: (1) $5,500, or $6,500 if catch-up contributions are allowable ($5,500 and $6,500, respectively, for 2015), as reduced for active participation, or (2) his or her compensation (Code Sec. 219(c); Notice 2013-73; IRS News Release IR-2014-99).[135] The IRAs of the spouse with the lesser amount of compensation ("lower-paid spouse") may receive deductible contributions for 2014 equal to the *lesser* of:

- $5,500, or $6,500 if catch-up contributions are allowable ($5,500 and $6,500, respectively, for 2015), as reduced for active participation, or

- the sum of:

  - the compensation of the lower-paid spouse, and

  - the compensation of the higher-paid spouse, reduced by: (i) the deduction allowed to the higher-paid spouse for IRA contributions, (ii) the amount of any designated nondeductible IRA contribution on behalf of the higher-paid spouse, and (iii) the amount of any contribution on behalf of the higher-paid spouse to a Roth IRA (¶ 2171).

AGI Limits for Joint Filers. If both individuals on a joint return are active participants in an employer's qualified retirement plan, their ability to claim a deduction for contributions made to traditional IRAs depends upon the amount of their modified adjusted gross income (AGI) (¶ 2155). The allowable IRA deduction for joint filers will be reduced when modified AGI is between $96,000 and $116,000 for 2014, and between $98,000 and $118,000 for 2015 (Notice 2013-73; IRS News Release IR-2014-99). For information regarding the IRA deduction limits for married persons filing separately and single filers, see ¶ 2159.

> **Example 1:** Ralph and Alice file a joint return for 2014. They are both employed and both are covered by their employers' qualified plans. Their modified AGI for 2014 is $120,000. Since they are both active participants in qualified plans sponsored by their employers and their modified AGI exceeds the high end of the phaseout range for 2014 (i.e., $116,000), they are not allowed to make deductible IRA contributions for 2014. They may make nondeductible contributions to traditional IRAs. As an alternative, they should consider the tax advantages of making their contributions to Roth IRAs.

References are to Standard Federal Tax Reports; Tax Research Consultant; and Practical Tax Explanations.

[133] ¶ 18,922.865; RETIRE: 66,202; § 25,415.15   [134] ¶ 12,650; RETIRE: 66,202; § 25,415.15   [135] ¶ 12,650; RETIRE: 66,302; § 25,415.15

An individual will *not* be considered an active participant in an employer-sponsored plan merely because the individual's spouse is treated as an active participant (Code Sec. 219(g)(7)).[136] However, if an individual is not an active participant and is married to someone who is covered, the deductible contribution is phased out if the couple's modified AGI (jointly computed) is between $181,000 to $191,000 for 2014, and between $183,000 and $193,000 for 2015.

> **Example 2:** Bob is covered by a 401(k) plan sponsored by his employer. His wife, Betty, is not employed. The couple files a joint income tax return for 2014, with a modified AGI of $120,000. Betty may make a deductible contribution to a traditional IRA for the year because she is not an active participant in an employer-sponsored retirement plan and their combined modified AGI is below $181,000. However, Bob may not make a deductible IRA contribution because their combined modified AGI is above the phaseout range for active participants who are married and filing jointly ($96,000 to $116,000 for 2014).

> **Example 3:** Assume the same facts as in Example 2, except that the couple's modified AGI was $200,000 for 2014. Neither Bob nor Betty would be able to make a deductible contribution to a traditional IRA.

2159. Deductible IRA Contribution Limits—Single or Married Filing Separately. For a single individual, head of household, or a married individual who files separately, contributions to traditional IRAs are generally deductible to the extent that they do not exceed the *lesser* of: (1) the individual's compensation for that year that is includible in gross income; or (2) for 2014, $5,500, or $6,500 if catch-up contributions are allowable ($5,500 and $6,500, respectively, for 2015) (Code Sec. 219(b)(1); Notice 2013-73; IRS News Release IR-2014-99).[137] However, the maximum allowable deduction may be reduced when the individual is an active participant in an employer-maintained retirement plan (¶ 2157). For information regarding the IRA deduction limits for married individuals filing jointly, see ¶ 2158.

Single Individuals or Head of Household. When a single individual or head of household is an active participant in an employer's retirement plan, the IRA deduction begins to phase out when modified adjusted gross income (AGI) (¶ 2155) is between $60,000 and $70,000 for 2014, and between $61,000 and $71,000 for 2015 (Code Sec. 219(g); Notice 2013-73; IRS News Release IR-2014-99).

Married Filing Separately. When an individual files as "married filing separately" and the individual, or the spouse, is an active participant in an employer's retirement plan, the IRA deduction begins to phase out when the individual's modified AGI exceeds $0. The deduction is completely phased out when modified AGI is $10,000 or more. This phaseout range is not adjusted for inflation. When determining if an individual is married or single for the purpose of determining which IRA deduction limit applies, spouses who file separate returns and live apart at all times during a tax year are *not* considered to be married during that tax year (Code Sec. 219(g)(4)).

2160. Nondeductible Contributions to Traditional IRAs. An individual may make nondeductible contributions to a traditional IRA (¶ 2155). These contributions may not exceed the *excess* of: (1) the maximum allowable contribution for the year over (2) the amount actually allowed as a deduction for the year (¶ 2157) (Code Sec. 408(o)(2)(B)).[138] In applying this rule, an individual may elect to treat otherwise deductible contributions as nondeductible contributions. However, the tax advantages of funding a Roth IRA should be considered before making nondeductible contributions to a traditional IRA (¶ 2171).

> **Example:** In 2014, Bill Webb, age 48 and single, had earned income of $53,000 and a modified adjusted gross income (AGI) of $61,000. He is an active participant in his employer's 401(k) plan. Since his modified AGI exceeds $60,000, a maximum contribution to a traditional IRA would not be fully deductible. Bill determines that

---

References are to Standard Federal Tax Reports; Tax Research Consultant; and Practical Tax Explanations.

[136] ¶ 12,650; RETIRE: 66,202; § 25,415.15

[137] ¶ 12,650; RETIRE: 66,200, RETIRE: 66,202; § 25,415.15

[138] ¶ 18,902; RETIRE: 66,250; § 25,420

his maximum deductible contribution would be $4,950. As a result, he could make an additional $550 nondeductible IRA contribution.

Nondeductible contributions may be made up to and including the due date of the return for the tax year. A filing extension does *not* extend the due date for making the contribution (Code Sec. 219(f)(3)). The same deadline applies to deductible IRA contributions and Roth IRA contributions. Nondeductible contributions to a traditional IRA must be reported on Form 8606, which is attached to Form 1040 or Form 1040A.

Reservist Contributions. Certain "qualified reservist distributions" are not subject to the tax on early distributions and may be recontributed to an IRA as a nondeductible contribution without counting against the dollar limits applicable to IRA contributions (Code Sec. 72(t)(2)(G)). A qualified reservist distribution is a distribution that is made:

- from an IRA or from an individual's elective deferrals under an employer plan (for example, a 401(k) or 403(b) annuity plan);

- to an individual who is a reservist who was called to active duty for a period of more than 179 days or for an indefinite period; and

- during the period beginning on the date the reservist was called to active duty and ending on the date the active duty ended.

The distribution may be recontributed at any time within the two years after the end of the active duty period. A reservist who took a distribution after being called up and paid the early distribution penalty may file a claim for refund of the penalty.

2161. Excess Contributions to IRAs. Annual contributions to a traditional IRA (¶ 2155) and/or Roth IRA (¶ 2171) in excess of the allowable amount are subject to a cumulative six percent tax, which is reported on Form 5329 (Code Sec. 4973).[139] See ¶ 2165 for a discussion on the taxation of distributions from a traditional IRA.

2163. Distribution Requirements of Traditional IRAs. Traditional IRAs (¶ 2155) are subject to the same required minimum distribution (RMD) rules that apply to qualified employer-provided retirement plans (¶ 2127) (Code Sec. 408(a)(6) and (b)(3)).[140] This means that distributions to the owner or beneficiary of a traditional IRA must begin no later than April 1 following the calendar year in which the owner reaches age 70½ (Reg. § 1.408-8, Q&A-3). A few special rules affecting RMDs from IRAs are discussed below.

Inherited Traditional IRA: Spouse. A surviving spouse may elect to treat an inherited traditional IRA as his or her own by having the account redesignated as an account belonging to the surviving spouse as owner rather than beneficiary. Alternatively, the surviving spouse will be treated as having made this election if: (1) any amounts in the IRA are not distributed within the time period that applied to the decedent or (2) the surviving spouse makes contributions (including rollover contributions) to the inherited IRA that are subject, or are deemed subject, to the lifetime distribution requirements. In order to make the election, the surviving spouse must be the sole beneficiary of the IRA and have an unlimited right to withdraw amounts from it (Reg. § 1.408-8, Q&A-5).[141] When a trust is named as the beneficiary of the IRA, this requirement has not been satisfied even if the spouse is the sole beneficiary of the trust. When the surviving spouse makes the election, he or she is treated as the owner of the IRA for all purposes. If the election is not made, then the RMDs are determined as though the spouse was the beneficiary of the IRA.

Inherited Traditional IRA: Nonspouse. A nonspouse beneficiary who inherits an IRA cannot treat it as his or her own account but must take RMDs determined under the rules applicable to beneficiaries receiving distributions from a qualified plan. When an individual other than the decedent's spouse receives a lump sum distribution from an IRA, in general, the individual may not roll over that distribution into another IRA; it must be distributed within a certain period (Code Sec. 408(d)(3)(C)). The distribution,

---

References are to Standard Federal Tax Reports; Tax Research Consultant; and Practical Tax Explanations.

[139] ¶ 34,360; RETIRE: 66,350; § 25,430.05

[140] ¶ 18,902; RETIRE: 66,400, RETIRE: 66,450; § 25,475.05

[141] ¶ 18,917A; RETIRE: 42,160.20; § 25,445.15

minus the aggregate amount of the owner's nondeductible IRA contributions, is taxed as ordinary income in the year the distribution is received (Rev. Rul. 92-47).[142]

Trust Named as Beneficiary. When a trust is named as the beneficiary of the IRA, the beneficiaries of the trust will be treated as the deceased individual's beneficiaries if certain requirements are met (Reg. §1.401(a)(9)-4, Q&A-5). The requirements include: (1) validity of the trust, (2) identification of the trust's beneficiaries, and (3) the delivery of proper documentation to the plan administrator (Reg. §1.401(a)(9)-4, Q&A-6).

More Than One IRA. If an individual is required to receive an RMD from more than one traditional IRA in a calendar year, the amount of the minimum distribution from each IRA must be calculated separately and the separate amounts totalled. However, the total may be withdrawn from one or more of the IRAs in whatever amounts the individual chooses (Reg. §1.408-8, Q&A-9).[143]

Planning and Due Diligence Considerations. For families that are not in immediate need of inherited IRA funds, it can make sense to stretch out the RMD period as long as possible in order to protect the IRA assets from tax. Careful designation of beneficiaries can help to peg the RMD period to the life expectancy of an individual beneficiary. Inherited IRAs are subject to a number of special rules and deadlines in the year following the owner's death, including rules for identifying designated beneficiaries, disclaiming interests, providing the IRS with trust information, and slicing an inherited IRA into multiple IRAs.[144]

2165. Taxation of Distributions from Traditional IRAs. If an individual never made nondeductible contributions to a traditional IRA (¶ 2160), then any distributions from the IRA are fully taxable to the owner or beneficiary as ordinary income (Code Sec. 408(d)(1); Reg. §1.408-4(a)). However, if nondeductible contributions were made, the owner has a *cost basis* in the IRA. An individual's cost basis in distributions made from a traditional IRA is the sum of the nondeductible contributions made to the IRA minus any prior withdrawals or distributions of nondeductible contributions (Notice 87-16). The recovery of this basis is not recognized as taxable income. As a result, the individual must determine how much of the IRA distribution is nontaxable. The taxable and nontaxable portions of the distribution are generally determined under the same rules that apply to annuity payments (¶ 817) (Code Secs. 72 and 408(d)(1) and (2)).[145] When applying these rules:

- all traditional IRAs of an individual, including SIMPLE IRAs (¶ 2181) and SEPs (¶ 2189), are treated as a single contract;

- all distributions during the individual's tax year are treated as one distribution;

- the value of the contract, the income on the contract, and the investment in the contract are calculated (after adding back distributions made during the year) as of the close of the calendar year in which the tax year of the distribution begins; and

- total withdrawals excludable from income in all tax years cannot exceed the taxpayer's investment in the contract in all tax years.

Charitable Distributions. For tax years beginning before January 1, 2014, individuals age 70 ½ or older may distribute up to $100,000 tax-free from their IRAs to certain charitable organizations without including the distribution in gross income (Code Sec. 408(d)(8)). The entire distribution must otherwise be deductible as a charitable contribution, disregarding the percentage limitations, even though the individual cannot claim a charitable deduction for the donation (¶ 1058).

References are to Standard Federal Tax Reports; Tax Research Consultant; and Practical Tax Explanations.

[142] ¶ 18,922.26; RETIRE: 66,502.05, RETIRE: 66,804, § 25,445.30

[143] ¶ 18,917A; RETIRE: 66,456; § 25,475.05

[144] ¶ 18,917A; RETIRE: 66,456.20; RETIRE: 66,812; RETIRE: 66,814; § 25,475.10

[145] ¶ 18,902, ¶ 6102; RETIRE: 66,500; § 25,450.15

> **Comment:** Absent further legislation, the exclusion from gross income for qualified charitable distributions from a taxpayer's IRAs has expired for tax years beginning after December 31, 2013. For the latest legislative updates, visit our website www.CCHGroup.com/TaxUpdates.

HSA Funding Distributions. An individual may make a one-time transfer of funds from his or her IRA distribution directly to the IRA owner's health savings account (HSA) without recognizing income on the distribution (Code Sec. 408(d)(9); Notice 2008-51).[146] The transfer can only be made, however, if it would otherwise be a taxable distribution. The dollar amount excluded cannot exceed the annual limitation on the individual's HSA contribution for the year (¶ 2035). The exclusion is lost if the individual ceases to be eligible to contribute to an HSA during the twelve months after the contribution. In such a case, the distribution is subject to tax and a 10-percent penalty is imposed.

Reporting Requirements. Form 8606 is used to report the taxable portion of an IRA distribution if the individual ever made nondeductible contributions to an IRA.

Estate Tax. If the distributee is the beneficiary of the IRA owner and the value of the IRA is included in the owner's estate for federal estate tax purposes, the distributee is entitled to deduct the estate tax allocable to the IRA (¶ 191) (Rev. Rul. 92-47).[147]

Return of Contributions. A distribution from a traditional IRA that represents the return of a contribution made for a particular tax year will not be included in the individual's income if (Code Sec. 408(d)(4)):[148]

- the distribution is made before the due date, including extensions, of the individual's tax return for that year;
- no deduction is allowed with respect to the contribution; and
- the distribution includes any net income earned by the contribution.

The net income earned by the contribution is included in income for the tax year in which the contribution was made even if the distribution is received in the following year.

Recognizing Loss on an IRA. An IRA owner can recognize a loss on traditional IRA investments, but only when all amounts from all of the owner's traditional IRA accounts have been distributed and the total distributions are less than any unrecovered basis in the accounts. The recognized loss is claimed on Schedule A as a miscellaneous itemized deduction, subject to the two-percent floor (IRS Pub. 590). If the individual never made nondeductible contributions to any of the traditional IRAs, the realized loss cannot be deducted because the individual has no tax basis in the IRAs.

2167. Rollover Distributions from IRAs. A distribution from a traditional IRA (¶ 2163) may be excluded from gross income if the recipient rolls over the distribution to another traditional IRA or returns it to the same IRA (Code Sec. 408(d)(3); Rev. Proc. 2003-16).[149] A distribution from a traditional IRA may also be rolled over into a qualified plan (¶ 2111), 403(b) annuity plan (¶ 2191), or 457 plan (¶ 2193) provided that the plan accepts rollover contributions. All distributions from a qualified plan are eligible for rollover treatment except for required minimum distributions (RMDs) (¶ 2127). A rollover of after-tax Roth contributions can be made from one IRA to another IRA. However, after-tax Roth contributions in an IRA cannot be rolled over into an employer's qualified plan. See ¶ 2175 regarding a rollover from a traditional IRA into a Roth IRA. See ¶ 2181 regarding rollovers from a SIMPLE IRA.

The rollover or return of an IRA distribution must generally be accomplished within 60 days after the withdrawal. It is not necessary that the entire amount withdrawn be transferred, but only the amount that is transferred during the 60-day period will not be taxed. Any portion of the withdrawal that is not rolled over within the 60-day period will

---

References are to Standard Federal Tax Reports; Tax Research Consultant; and Practical Tax Explanations.

[146] ¶ 18,902; HEALTH: 18,050; § 25,450

[147] ¶ 18,922.26; RETIRE: 66,806.05; § 7,110.10

[148] ¶ 18,902; RETIRE: 66,356.05; § 25,430.10

[149] ¶ 18,902; RETIRE: 42,450, RETIRE: 66,700; § 25,445.10

be taxed as ordinary income and may be subject to the 10-percent additional tax for early distributions (¶ 2169). The IRS has the authority to grant a waiver of the 60-day rule in situations involving equity, good conscience, or situations beyond the control of the individual.

Once-Per-12-Month Rule. Once an individual has made a tax-free rollover, he or she must wait at least one year from the date of receipt of the amount withdrawn before becoming eligible to engage in another rollover. Historically, the IRS applied this generously for taxpayers by applying it on an IRA-by-IRA basis, rather than on a taxpayer-by-taxpayer basis. Accordingly, a taxpayer with multiple IRAs could roll over amounts from each IRA during the course of a 12-month period, as long as the taxpayer only did it once per IRA. Starting in 2015, the once-per-12-month rule applies on a taxpayer-by-taxpayer basis. Accordingly, if a taxpayer has multiple IRAs, a rollover from one prevents the taxpayer from rolling over again within 12-months from any of the taxpayer's IRAs (Code Sec. 408(d)(3)(B)). Note that this waiting period rule does not apply to trustee-to-trustee direct transfers.[150]

2169. Penalty for Early Distributions from IRAs. Generally, if the individual is under age 59½, a distribution from a traditional IRA (¶ 2165) or nonqualified distribution from a Roth IRA (¶ 2173) is subject to the 10-percent additional tax on taxable early distributions. Many of the exceptions to the tax on early distributions that apply to distributions from qualified employer-provided retirement plans (¶ 2151) also apply to early distributions from an IRA with the exception for early retirements (Code Sec. 72(t)(3)(A)).[151] In addition, the following exceptions apply to early distributions from an IRA but not to distributions from a qualified retirement plan. If an exception applies, it may be necessary to file Form 5329.

Medical Insurance Premiums of Unemployed Individuals. To the extent that they do not exceed qualifying medical insurance premiums, distributions from an IRA, SIMPLE IRA (¶ 2181), or SEP (¶ 2189) to certain unemployed individuals are *not* subject to the 10-percent additional tax (Code Sec. 72(t)(2)(D)).[152] Eligible unemployed individuals are those who have received federal or state unemployment compensation for 12 consecutive weeks. A self-employed individual will be treated as having received unemployment compensation if, under federal or state law, the individual would have received unemployment compensation but for being self-employed.

Qualifying premiums are deductible premiums for the medical care of the unemployed individual, spouse and dependents. The distributions must be received in the tax year during which unemployment compensation is received or in the following year. In determining whether the premiums are deductible, the 10-percent-of-adjusted-gross-income floor (7.5 percent for all individuals before 2013 and, for tax years beginning after December 31, 2012, and before January 1, 2017, for individuals who have attained age 65 by the close of such tax year) for medical expenses (¶ 1015) is ignored. This exception to the 10-percent additional tax ceases to apply after the individual has been reemployed for 60 days (not necessarily consecutive) after initial unemployment.

Education Expenses. The 10-percent additional tax does not apply if the individual uses the IRA distribution to pay for "qualified higher education expenses" for the individual, the individual's spouse or child, or a grandchild of the individual or the individual's spouse. Qualified expenses include tuition at a post-secondary educational institution, books, fees, supplies and equipment (Code Sec. 72(t)(2)(E)).[153]

First-Time Homebuyer Expenses. The 10-percent additional tax does not apply if the individual uses the IRA distribution for certain expenses of a first-time homebuyer. Only $10,000 during the individual's lifetime may be withdrawn without a penalty for this purpose. Qualified expenses include acquisition costs, settlement charges and closing costs. The principal residence may be for the individual or the individual's spouse, child

---

References are to Standard Federal Tax Reports; Tax Research Consultant; and Practical Tax Explanations.

[150] ¶ 18,922.75; RETIRE: 66,704; § 25,445.10

[151] ¶ 6102; RETIRE: 66,506; 25,450.25

[152] ¶ 6102; RETIRE: 42,554.216; 25,450.25

[153] ¶ 6102; INDIV: 60,056; 25,450.25

¶2169

or grandchild, or an ancestor of the individual or the individual's spouse. In order to be considered a "first-time homebuyer," the person buying the residence (and spouse, if married) must not have had an ownership interest in a principal residence during the two-year period ending on the date that the new home is acquired (Code Sec. 72(t)(2)(F)).[154]

Return of Nondeductible Contributions. The 10-percent additional tax does not apply to the portion of the distribution that represents a return of nondeductible IRA contributions (i.e., the individual's cost basis in the IRA) (¶ 2165).

Roth IRAs

2171. Roth IRAs. A Roth IRA is a type of IRA consisting of after-tax contributions (Code Sec. 408A).[155] A Roth IRA generally is treated like a traditional IRA (¶ 2155) except that contributions to a Roth IRA cannot be deducted from income and qualified distributions from the Roth IRA are excludable from gross income (¶ 2173).

Roth IRA Contributions. The maximum contribution that can be made to individual's Roth and traditional IRAs is $5,500 for 2014, $5,500 for 2015 (Code Sec. 408A(c); Reg. § 1.408A-3; Notice 2013-73; IRS News Release IR-2014-99).[156] The limit is the amount that may be contributed to *both* types of IRAs combined, not the amount that may be contributed to each type. An individual who will be at least age 50 by the end of the tax year is allowed to make additional "catch-up" contributions to a Roth or traditional IRA. The maximum amount of the annual catch-up contribution is $1,000 (Code Sec. 219(b)(5)). Rollover contributions into a Roth IRA are not counted against the annual contribution limit. In addition, unlike traditional IRAs, individuals may make contributions to a Roth IRA after reaching age 70½.

Income Limits. The ability of an individual to make a contribution to a Roth IRA depends upon the amount of the individual's modified adjusted gross income (AGI) (Code Sec. 408A(c)(3); Notice 2013-73; IRS News Release IR-2014-99). For 2014, the allowable Roth IRA contribution is phased out when modified AGI is between $114,000 and $129,000 for single filers, and between $181,000 and $191,000 for joint filers. For 2015, the modified AGI phase-out range is between $116,000 and $131,000 for single filers, and between $183,000 and $193,000 for joint filers. The phase-out range remains between $0 and $10,000 for individuals who are married filing separately. Modified AGI is generally calculated as it is for traditional IRAs. However, for Roth IRA purposes, modified AGI does not include the income reported from the conversion of a traditional IRA into a Roth IRA.

Deemed Roth IRAs. Qualified plans may allow employees to make voluntary contributions to an account that will be deemed to be a Roth IRA if the account meets all the requirements of a Roth IRA (Code Sec. 408(q)).[157] An employee's contribution to this account counts towards the maximum annual contribution that may be made to a Roth IRA.

Losses in Roth IRA. Like a traditional IRA, the owner of a Roth IRA can recognize a loss on investments in the account only when all the amounts in all the owner's Roth IRA accounts have been distributed and the total distributions are less than the individual's unrecovered basis in the accounts. The basis is the total amount of the nondeductible contributions in the Roth IRAs. The recognized loss is claimed on Schedule A as a miscellaneous itemized deduction, subject to the two-percent-of-adjusted-gross-income floor (IRS Pub. 590). The loss rule applies separately to each kind of IRA. Thus, to report a loss on a Roth IRA, all the Roth IRAs owned by the individual have to be liquidated, and to report a loss on a traditional IRA, all the traditional IRAs owned by the individual have to be liquidated.

References are to Standard Federal Tax Reports; Tax Research Consultant; and Practical Tax Explanations.

[154] ¶ 6102; RETIRE: 42,554.224; § 25,450.25

[155] ¶ 18,925; RETIRE: 66,750; § 25,501

[156] ¶ 18,925, ¶ 18,927; RETIRE: 66,752; § 25,510

[157] ¶ 18,902; RETIRE: 66,058.10; § 25,405.25

Military Death Gratuity. An individual who receives a military death gratuity or payment under the Servicemembers' Group Life Insurance (SGLI) program may contribute an amount up to the sum of the gratuity and SGLI payments received to a Roth IRA, notwithstanding the annual contribution limit and the income phase-out of the contribution limit that otherwise apply to contributions to Roth IRAs. The contribution must be made within one year of the receipt of the payment (Code Sec. 408A(e)). These contributions are generally treated as though they were a rollover from another Roth IRA. This option is available for amounts paid in connection with deaths from injuries occurring on or after June 17, 2008.

2173. Taxation of Distributions from Roth IRAs. Qualified distributions from a Roth IRA (¶ 2171) are not included in the recipient's gross income nor are they subject to the 10-percent additional tax for early withdrawals (¶ 2169) (Code Sec. 408A(d); Reg. § 1.408A-6).[158] To be treated as a qualified distribution, the Roth IRA distribution, including distributions allocable to rollover contributions, may not be made before the end of the five-year period beginning with the first tax year for which the individual made a contribution to the Roth IRA. The five-year holding period ends on the last day of the individual's fifth consecutive tax year after the holding period started. Generally, each Roth IRA owner has only one five-year period for all of the Roth IRAs that the individual owns.

> **Example:** Jack Martin made his first contribution to a Roth IRA on September 15, 2010, for the 2010 tax year. On December 27, 2011, Jack made another contribution to a Roth IRA, for the 2011 tax year. On December 30, 2012, he made another contribution to a Roth IRA for the 2012 tax year. The five-year holding period for all of Jack's Roth IRAs is considered to have started on January 1, 2010. Distributions made after December 31, 2014, will have satisfied the five-year holding period.

In addition to satisfying the five-year holding period, a distribution will constitute a qualified distribution only if it is (Code Sec. 408A(d)(2)):[159]

- made on or after the date on which the individual attains age 59½,
- made to a beneficiary (or the individual's estate) on or after the individual's death,
- attributable to the individual being disabled, or
- a distribution to pay for qualified first-time homebuyer expenses (¶ 2169).

Pre-Death Requirements. The *pre-death* required minimum distribution (RMD) requirements (¶ 2127) that apply to qualified plans and traditional IRAs do *not* apply to Roth IRAs (Code Sec. 408A(c)(5)).[160] Thus, owners of Roth IRAs are not required to take distributions by April 1 of the year following the calendar year in which they attain age 70½. As a general rule, the *post-death* RMD rules do apply to Roth IRAs (Reg. § 1.408A-6, Q&A-14). If the sole beneficiary is the decedent's spouse, the spouse may delay distributions until the decedent would have attained age 70½ or may treat the Roth IRA as his or her own.

Nonqualified Distributions. When an individual receives a nonqualified distribution from a Roth IRA, a portion of the distribution may be includible in gross income. In order to determine the amount that is includible in gross income, specific ordering rules are applied under which regular Roth contributions are deemed to be withdrawn first, then amounts transferred from traditional IRAs starting with amounts first transferred (Code Sec. 408A(d)(4)). Withdrawals of transferred amounts are then treated as coming first from amounts that were included in income. Earnings are treated as withdrawn after contributions (Reg. § 1.408A-6, Q&A-8). Thus, no amount is includible in gross income until all the after-tax contributions have been distributed. If an individual receives a nonqualified distribution from a Roth IRA that is includible in gross income, then the 10-percent additional tax for early distributions will generally apply. However, the same exceptions that apply to early distributions from traditional IRAs (¶ 2169) will also apply to the nonqualified Roth IRA distributions.

References are to Standard Federal Tax Reports; Tax Research Consultant; and Practical Tax Explanations.

[158] ¶ 18,925, ¶ 18,928; RE-   [159] ¶ 18,925; RETIRE: 66,758;   [160] ¶ 18,925; RETIRE: 66,758;
TIRE: 66,758; § 25,525.10   § 25,525.10   § 25,525.10

Reporting Roth IRA Distributions. Distributions from Roth IRAs are reported on Form 8606. If the 10-percent additional tax on early distributions applies, it is reported on Form 5329.

2175. Rollovers and Conversions of Roth IRAs. Taxpayers can make qualified rollover contributions to a Roth IRA (¶ 2171) from another Roth IRA, a traditional IRA (¶ 2155), and from certain qualified plans (Code Sec. 408A(c)(6) and (e)).[161] However, unlike rollovers to traditional IRAs (¶ 2145), qualified rollovers to Roth IRAs may result in the inclusion in income of an amount equal to the amount that would be includible if it were not part of a qualified rollover distribution.

Rollovers from Roth IRAs. In the case of a qualified rollover from another Roth IRA, amounts distributed from the Roth IRA must be contributed either to the same or to another Roth IRA within 60 days of receiving the distribution. However, once a qualified rollover has been made, any other distributions received within the twelve months after the distribution rolled over was received cannot be rolled over. In the case of an individual with more than one Roth IRA, the once-per-12-month restriction applies separately to each Roth IRA.

Conversions of Traditional IRAs. A taxpayer can convert an eligible retirement plan to a Roth IRA as long as the amount contributed to the Roth IRA satisfies the definition of a qualified rollover contribution (Code Sec. 408A(e)). Generally, amounts transferred or converted from a traditional IRA into a Roth IRA must be included in gross income for the tax year in which the amount is distributed or transferred to the extent it does not represent a return of basis. Taxpayers who made a conversion in 2010 must recognize the conversion amount ratably in gross income in 2011 and 2012, unless the taxpayer elected to recognize it all in 2010. If a taxpayer opted to include a 2010 conversion in income ratably in 2011 and 2012, a distribution of conversion amounts before 2012 results in the acceleration of income.[162]

The 10-percent additional tax on early distributions does not apply to the taxable conversion amount. However, if within the five-year period starting with the year in which an individual made a conversion contribution of an amount from a traditional IRA to a Roth IRA, the individual takes a distribution from a Roth IRA of an amount that is attributable to the portion of the conversion contribution that was included in income, then the individual will be liable for the 10-percent additional tax unless one of the exceptions to the tax applies (¶ 2169) (Reg. § 1.408A-6, Q&A-5(c)). The five-year period is separately determined for each conversion contribution made to a Roth IRA. Individuals can correct a failed Roth conversion by making a proper recharacterization election (¶ 2177).

Rollovers from Qualified Plans. Distributions from qualified retirement plans (¶ 2145), 403(b) annuity plans (¶ 2191), or 457 plans (¶ 2193) can be rolled over directly into a Roth IRA. Such rollovers are treated the same as under the conversion rules for traditional IRAs, though rollovers from designated Roth accounts are treated as rollovers from another Roth IRA (Notice 2009-75). In addition, the rollover contribution must meet the rollover requirements applicable to the specific type of retirement plan.

2177. Recharacterization of IRA Contributions. An individual who has made contributions to a traditional IRA (¶ 2155) or Roth IRA (¶ 2171) may later decide that a contribution to an IRA of the other type is more advantageous. If certain requirements are met, the contribution can be recharacterized and treated as having been originally made to the desired type of IRA (Code Sec. 408A(d)(6)).[163] Recharacterizing an IRA contribution requires transferring amounts previously contributed to a traditional or Roth IRA (plus any resulting net income or minus any resulting net loss) to a new IRA of the opposite type and electing to have the amounts treated as having been transferred to the second IRA at the time they actually were contributed to the first IRA (Reg. § 1.408A-5, Q&A-1). The transfer must be from trustee to trustee. Generally, taxpayers have until the due date (including extensions) of the tax return for the year in which the

---

References are to Standard Federal Tax Reports; Tax Research Consultant; and Practical Tax Explanations.

[161] ¶ 18,925; RETIRE: 66,760; § 25,530

[162] ¶ 18,925; RETIRE: 66,706; § 25,515.20

[163] ¶ 18,925; RETIRE: 66,762; § 25,520.05

contribution was made to make the recharacterization. A recharacterization must be reported on the taxpayer's tax return. In certain situations, Form 8606 must be filed, along with a statement explaining the nature of the recharacterization (IRS Pub. 590). Once a Roth IRA has been recharacterized back to a (new) traditional IRA, the (new) traditional IRA can be (re)converted back to a Roth IRA, provided the taxpayer meets the eligibility requirements in the reconversion year (¶ 2179).

2179. Roth IRA Reconversions. A "reconversion" is a conversion from a traditional IRA (¶ 2155) to a Roth IRA (¶ 2171) of an amount that had previously been recharacterized as a contribution to the traditional IRA after having been earlier converted to a Roth IRA (¶ 2177). An IRA owner who converts an amount from a traditional IRA to a Roth IRA during any tax year and then transfers that amount back to a traditional IRA by means of a recharacterization may not reconvert that amount from the traditional IRA to a Roth IRA before the *later* of: (1) the beginning of the tax year following the tax year in which the amount was converted to a Roth IRA or (2) the end of the 30-day period beginning on the day on which the IRA owner transfers the amount from the Roth IRA back to a traditional IRA by means of a recharacterization (regardless of whether the recharacterization occurs during the tax year in which the amount was converted to a Roth IRA or the following tax year) (Reg. § 1.408A-5, Q&A-9(a)(1)).[164]

SIMPLE Plans and SEPs

2181. SIMPLE IRA Plans. An eligible small employer (¶ 2187) may adopt a "Savings Incentive Match Plan for Employees" (SIMPLE) IRA retirement plan for its employees (Code Sec. 408(p)).[165] A SIMPLE IRA plan is a written salary reduction agreement that lets eligible employees elect to have the employer make payments as elective contributions to a SIMPLE IRA of the employee or to the employee directly in cash. The plan may be designed so that elective contributions are made only if the employee affirmatively elects to have them made or as an automatic contribution unless the employee affirmatively opts out (Notice 2009-66). The employer is required to make contributions to its employees' SIMPLE IRAs as either matching contributions of up to three percent of compensation or as nonelective contributions. No contributions other than the employee's salary reduction contributions and employer contributions may be made to a SIMPLE IRA. However, a rollover from another SIMPLE IRA may be received (Code Sec. 408(d)(3)(G)).[166] See ¶ 2183 for a discussion of employee and employer contributions to a SIMPLE IRA.

All contributions under a SIMPLE IRA plan must be made to SIMPLE IRA set up by the employer for each eligible employee. A SIMPLE IRA must meet the same requirements that apply to traditional IRAs (¶ 2155). It may not be designated as a Roth IRA (¶ 2171), but contributions to a SIMPLE IRA are not taken into account in determining the Roth IRA contribution limit (Code Sec. 408A(f)). Each eligible employee must have the right to elect during the 60-day period preceding the beginning of any calendar year (and the 60-day period preceding the employee's first day of eligibility) to participate in the plan for that calendar year or to modify the amount of his or her elective contributions for that calendar year (Code Sec. 408(p)(5)).[167] In addition, an employee may terminate participation in the SIMPLE plan at any time during a calendar year. However, the plan may prohibit reentry until the beginning of the following calendar year.

Distributions from a SIMPLE IRA are taxable to the employee (or the beneficiary or estate of the employee) under the same rules that govern distributions from traditional IRAs (¶ 2163) (Code Sec. 408(p)(1)(A)).[168] This includes the 10-percent additional tax that applies to early distributions from an IRA (¶ 2169) except that the tax is increased to 25 percent when the employee takes an early distribution within two years after the employee's first participation in a SIMPLE IRA plan (Code Sec. 72(t)(6)).[169] The two-year period begins on the first day on which contributions made by the individual's

---

References are to Standard Federal Tax Reports; Tax Research Consultant; and Practical Tax Explanations.

[164] ¶ 18,927D; RETIRE: 66,764; § 25,520.15

[165] ¶ 18,902; RETIRE: 63,550; § 25,101

[166] ¶ 18,902; RETIRE: 63,756; § 25,145.15

[167] ¶ 18,902; RETIRE: 63,606; § 25,125.05

[168] ¶ 18,902; RETIRE: 63,756; § 25,145.10

[169] ¶ 6102; RETIRE: 63,756; § 25,145.10

employer are deposited in the individual's SIMPLE IRA (Notice 98-4). If the employee has participated in the SIMPLE IRA for at least two years, a distribution may be rolled over into other types of retirement plans including qualified plans (¶ 2111), 403(b) annuity plans (¶ 2191), and 457 plans (¶ 2193) (Code Sec. 408(d)(3)(A)). If the employee has not participated in the SIMPLE plan for two years, the distribution may only be rolled over into another SIMPLE plan (Code Sec. 408(d)(3)(G)).

Establishing SIMPLE IRAs. The IRS has issued two model forms that may be used by employers that want to establish a SIMPLE IRA for their employees. Form 5304-SIMPLE is used when the employer permits each employee to choose the financial institution that will receive the SIMPLE IRA contributions. Form 5305-SIMPLE is used when the employer designates the financial institution that will receive the contributions. In that case, an employee must be given a reasonable period of time each year in which to transfer his or her SIMPLE IRA balance without cost or penalty from the designated financial institution to a SIMPLE IRA at another financial institution. Both forms also contain information that can be used to notify employees of the existence of the plan. Although the completed forms do not have to be filed with the IRS, they must be kept in order to show that the plan was adopted by the employer.

2183. SIMPLE IRAs—Employee and Employer Contributions. Contributions to an employee's SIMPLE IRA (¶ 2181) are limited to: (1) employee contributions made under a salary reduction agreement, and (2) employer contributions that are made as either matching contributions or nonelective contributions (Code Sec. 408(p)(2)).[170] However, a rollover from another SIMPLE IRA may be received (Code Sec. 408(d)(3)(G)).[171]

Employee Contributions. An employee's elective contributions to a SIMPLE IRA under a salary reduction agreement are limited to $12,000 for 2014, $12,500 for 2015 (Code Sec. 408(p)(2); Notice 2013-73; IRS News Release IR-2014-99).[172] In addition, employees who will be at least age 50 by the end of the year are allowed to make additional catch-up contributions of $2,500 for 2014, $3,000 for 2015 (Code Sec. 414(v)(2)(B)(ii)). The maximum dollar limit is the only limit on employee contributions. An employer may not place a limit on the percentage of salary an employee may elect to defer in the plan (except in order to comply with the annual dollar limit). The employer must deposit the employee's elective contributions into the SIMPLE IRA within 30 days after the end of the month in which the amounts would have been paid to the employee. Elective contributions by an employee are fully vested when made (Code Sec. 408(p)(3)).[173]

Matching Contributions. If an employee makes an elective contribution to a SIMPLE IRA, then the employer generally must make a matching contribution in an amount not exceeding three percent of the employee's compensation for the calendar year (¶ 2185). An employer may elect to limit its matching contribution to a smaller percentage of compensation but not less than one percent. The election may *not* be made by an employer in more than two out of every five years. If the SIMPLE account did not exist during the full five-year period, the election may still be made in up to two of the years in which it did exist. Employees must be notified of the employer's election to contribute less than three percent a reasonable time before the beginning of the 60-day period at the end of each calendar year during which employees designate the amount of their election contributions for the following calendar year. Matching contributions to SIMPLE IRAs that are made on behalf of self-employed individuals are not treated as elective contributions made by the individuals (Code Sec. 408(p)(9)).

References are to Standard Federal Tax Reports; Tax Research Consultant; and Practical Tax Explanations.

[170] ¶ 18,902; RETIRE: 63,606; § 25,120.10

[171] ¶ 18,902; RETIRE: 63,756; § 25,145.15

[172] ¶ 18,902; RETIRE: 63,650; § 25,120.10

[173] ¶ 18,902; RETIRE: 63,612, RETIRE: 63,614; § 25,130.05

¶2183

Example 1: Ralph, age 52, participates in his employer's SIMPLE IRA plan and for 2014 his salary will be $50,000. He elects to defer the maximum amount into the plan ($14,500). Under the plan, the employer makes a maximum matching contribution for each participating employee, up to the three percent limit. Therefore, the employer will make a $1,500 ($50,000 × three percent) matching contribution to Ralph's SIMPLE IRA.

Nonelective Contributions. Instead of making matching contributions, an employer may elect to make nonelective contributions of two percent of the compensation for each employee who is eligible to participate in the plan and who has at least $5,000 of compensation from the employer for the calendar year (Code Sec. 408(p)(2)(B)(ii)).[174]

Example 2: Assume the same facts as in Example 1, above, except that Ralph's employer decided to base its contributions on the nonelective contributions option. In this situation, Ralph would still be allowed to contribute $14,500 to his SIMPLE IRA. However, the employer's contribution would be $1,000 ($50,000 × two percent).

Vesting. The employee's right to both matching contributions and nonelective contributions of the employer (and the earnings on these contributions) in a SIMPLE IRA must be fully vested at all times (Code Sec. 408(p)(3)).[175]

Employer's Deduction. An employer can deduct SIMPLE IRA contributions in the tax year with or within which the calendar year for which the contributions were made ends. Contributions for a particular tax year may be deducted if they are made for that tax year and are made by the due date, including extensions, of the employer's tax return for that year (Code Sec. 404(m)).[176]

2185. SIMPLE 401(k) Plans. An eligible small employer (¶ 2187) may adopt a "Savings Incentive Match Plan for Employees" (SIMPLE) retirement plan as part of a 401(k) plan (¶ 2104). A SIMPLE 401(k) is a simplified plan which generally must meet the same requirements that apply to other 401(k) plans except that in lieu of satisfying the nondiscrimination test for elective deferrals and matching contributions (¶ 2123), a SIMPLE 401(k) plan must satisfy the following requirements (and also will not be subject to the rules for "top-heavy plans" (¶ 2132)).

Employee Contributions. Each employee eligible to participate in the SIMPLE 401(k) plan must have the right to make annual elective contributions, expressed as a percentage of compensation but not exceeding $12,000 for 2014, $12,500 for 2015. An employee age 50 or over may make an additional catch-up contribution of $2,500 for 2014, $3,000 for 2015 (Code Sec. 414(v)(2)(B)(ii); Notice 2013-73; IRS News Release IR-2014-99).[177] Nondeductible employee contributions and rollover contributions may not be made to a SIMPLE 401(k).

Employer Contributions. The employer generally must make matching contributions for each participant in a SIMPLE 401(k) in an amount not exceeding three percent of the employee's compensation (Code Sec. 401(k)(11)(B)).[178] Instead of making matching contributions, an employer may elect to make nonelective contributions of two percent of compensation for each employee who is eligible to participate in the arrangement and who has at least $5,000 of compensation. Employees must be notified that the employer has chosen to make the two-percent contribution within a reasonable period of time before the 60th day before the beginning of the calendar year.

Compensation. SIMPLE compensation means the sum of wages, tips, and other compensation from the eligible employer subject to federal income tax withholding. It also includes the employee's elective contributions made under any other qualified plan, including a SIMPLE IRA plan, a salary reduction simplified employee pension (SAR-SEP), a 403(b) annuity plan, and compensation deferred under a section 457 plan required to be reported by the employer on Form W-2. For self-employed individuals, SIMPLE compensation means net earnings from self-employment determined prior to

---

References are to Standard Federal Tax Reports; Tax Research Consultant; and Practical Tax Explanations.

[174] ¶ 18,902; RETIRE: 63,654.10; § 25,120.20

[175] ¶ 18,902; RETIRE: 63,612, RETIRE: 63,614; § 25,130.05

[176] ¶ 18,330; RETIRE: 63,700; § 25,145.15

[177] ¶ 19,150; RETIRE: 27,102.20; § 24,720.15

[178] ¶ 17,502; RETIRE: 3,350; § 24,720.15

subtracting any contributions made under the SIMPLE 401(k) plan on behalf of the individual (Reg. § 1.401(k)-4(e)(5)).

Employer's Deduction. An employer's deduction for contributions to a defined contribution plan is generally limited to the *greater* of: (1) 25 percent of the compensation paid or accrued during the tax year to beneficiaries under a stock bonus or profit-sharing plan, or (2) the amount that the employer is required to contribute to a SIMPLE 401(k) plan for the year (Code Sec. 404(a)(3)(A)(i)(I) and (II)).[179] Thus, an employer's deduction for its contributions to a SIMPLE 401(k) may be greater than the general limit of 25 percent of compensation paid (¶ 2119).

Vesting. All contributions to a SIMPLE 401(k) must be fully vested when made, and the plan cannot impose any restrictions on withdrawals (Code Sec. 401(k)(11)).[180]

Establishing a SIMPLE 401(k). The IRS has issued a model amendment that may be used by employers that want to adopt a plan that contains a SIMPLE 401(k) plan (Rev. Proc. 97-9).[181] The model amendment includes provisions for employee contributions, employer options concerning its contributions, and notification to employees.

2187. SIMPLE Plans—Eligible Employers and Employees. A SIMPLE IRA plan (¶ 2181) or SIMPLE 401(k) (¶ 2185) may only be established by an employer that has 100 or fewer eligible employees who received at least $5,000 in compensation during the preceding tax year (Code Sec. 408(p)(2)(C)(i)).[182] Any type of employer can establish a SIMPLE plan, including tax-exempt entities, governmental entities, and employers of domestic workers even though the compensation of domestic workers may not be subject to income tax withholding. The employer may generally not make contributions to any other qualified plan starting with the year the SIMPLE plan goes into effect. However, employers may adopt a SIMPLE plan for noncollectively bargained employees and at the same time maintain a qualified plan for collectively bargained employees (Code Sec. 408(p)(2)(D)).[183]

If the employer has established a SIMPLE plan, an employee must be eligible to participate in any calendar year if he or she received at least $5,000 of compensation from the employer during *any* of the *two* preceding calendar years and is reasonably expected to receive at least $5,000 in compensation during the current calendar year (Code Sec. 408(p)(4)).[184] Nonresident alien employees and employees covered by a collective bargaining agreement may be excluded from participation.

If an individual is not self-employed, compensation means the amount described in Code Sec. 6051(a)(3) (wages, tips, and other compensation from the employer subject to income tax withholding under Code Sec. 3401(a)), and amounts described in Code Sec. 6051(a)(8), including elective contributions made under a SIMPLE IRA plan, and compensation deferred under a section 457 plan. Compensation does not include amounts deferred under a cafeteria plan. For purposes of applying the 100-employee limitation, and in determining whether an employee is eligible to participate (i.e., whether the employee had $5,000 in compensation for any two preceding years), an employee's compensation also includes the employee's elective deferrals under a 401(k) plan, a salary reduction SEP (SARSEP) and a section 403(b) annuity contract.

A self-employed individual is treated as an employee and may participate in a SIMPLE plan if the minimum compensation requirement is met (Code Sec. 408(p)(6)).[185] For this purpose, compensation means net earnings from self-employment (Schedule SE of Form 1040) before subtracting any contributions made to a SIMPLE IRA. Self-employed persons who have elected out of the self-employment tax on religious grounds under Code Sec. 1402(g) may base their retirement plan contributions, including contributions to SIMPLE IRAs, on their self-employment income that is exempt from self-employment tax.

References are to Standard Federal Tax Reports; Tax Research Consultant; and Practical Tax Explanations.

[179] ¶ 18,330; RETIRE: 63,700; § 24,305.15

[180] ¶ 17,502; RETIRE: 3,350; § 24,720.25

[181] ¶ 18,112.80; RETIRE: 3,352; § 24,720.35

[182] ¶ 18,902; RETIRE: 63,552; § 25,110.05

[183] ¶ 18,902; RETIRE: 63,552; § 25,110.15

[184] ¶ 18,902; RETIRE: 63,602; § 25,115.05

[185] ¶ 18,902; RETIRE: 63,602; § 25,115.05

¶2187

2189. Simplified Employee Pensions (SEPs). A simplified employee pension (SEP) is an arrangement under which an employer makes contributions to the IRAs of each of its employees (Code Sec. 408(k)).[186] Annual contributions by an employer to a SEP are excluded from the employee's gross income to the extent that the contributions do not exceed the *lesser* of 25 percent of the participant's compensation or $52,000 for 2014, $53,000 for 2015 (Code Sec. 402(h); Notice 2013-73; IRS News Release IR-2014-99).[187] The maximum amount of compensation that may be considered is $260,000 for 2014, $265,000 for 2015. If the employer exceeds the annual limit on contributions, the employee is generally taxed on the amount of the excess contribution and subject to a six-percent excise tax if not withdrawn (¶ 2161). In the case of a SEP established by an unincorporated employer, the compensation of a self-employed partici-pant (partner or proprietor) is earned income.

The employer must decide each year whether and how much to contribute to a SEP plan. If any contribution is made to a plan, nondiscriminatory employer contributions must be made for each employee who has reached age 21, performed services for the employer during at least three of the immediately preceding five years, and received at least $550 of compensation for 2014, $600 for 2015 (Code Sec. 408(k)(2); Notice 2013-73; IRS News Release IR-2014-99). Unlike traditional IRAs, the account owner of a SEP-IRA can make contributions after reaching age 70½ (Code Sec. 219(b)(2)).[188]

In order to deduct its SEP contributions for a particular year, the employer must make the contributions by the due date (including extensions) of its tax return for that tax year (Code Sec. 404(h)).[189] The contributions are made to the SEP-IRAs that have been established by, or for, each eligible employee. Although the employer's deduction cannot exceed 25 percent of the employee's compensation (¶ 2119), any excess can be carried over and deducted in later years subject to the percentage limitation. In addition, when an employer maintains another type of defined contribution plan, the contributions to a SEP must be taken into account when determining compliance with the annual limit imposed on deductible contributions to the plans (Code Sec. 404(h)(2)).[190]

Employee Contributions. In plan years beginning before 1997, an employer could include a salary reduction agreement (cash or deferred arrangement) as part of its SEP—commonly know as SARSEP. New SARSEPs cannot be established after 1996 (Sec. 1421(c) of Small Business Job Protection Act of 1996 (P.L. 104-188)).[191] SARSEPs established before 1997 are allowed to continue but subject to the rules for traditional IRAs regarding contribution and deduction limits (¶ 2155).

Establishing a SEP-IRA. Most employers are able to establish a SEP plan by completing a Form 5305-SEP. The form is *not* filed with the IRS. Instead, it is retained by the employer as evidence that a SEP plan has been established. All eligible employees must be given a copy of the Form 5305-SEP. Certain employers should not use Form 5305-SEP, e.g., employers that are currently maintaining another qualified plan or use the services of leased employees. An employer may establish a SEP-IRA for a particular year as late as the due date, including extensions, for its income tax return for that year.

Distributions. Distributions from a SEP are taxed under the rules that apply to distributions from a traditional IRA (¶ 2163) (Code Secs. 402(h)(3) and 408(d)).[192]

Top-Heavy SEP. If a SEP is top heavy (¶ 2132), each participant who is not a key employee must be provided with a contribution that is not less than three percent of his or her compensation. If the rate for the key employee receiving the largest contribution is less than three percent, the contribution rate for that employee is used to determine the minimum contribution for non-key employees (Code Sec. 408(k)(1)(B)).[193]

References are to Standard Federal Tax Reports; Tax Research Consultant; and Practical Tax Explanations.

[186] ¶ 18,902; RETIRE: 63,050; § 25,005

[187] ¶ 18,202; RETIRE: 63,050; § 45,040.20

[188] ¶ 18,902; RETIRE: 63,102; § 25,010.10

[189] ¶ 18,330; RETIRE: 63,204; § 25,015

[190] ¶ 18,330; RETIRE: 63,202; § 25,015

[191] ¶ 18,902; RETIRE: 63,150; § 25,020

[192] ¶ 18,202, ¶ 18,902; RETIRE: 63,256; § 25,010.20

[193] ¶ 18,902; RETIRE: 63,114; § 25,010.30

Sec. 403(b), Sec. 457, and Nonqualified Plans

2191. Sec. 403(b) Plans (Tax Sheltered Annuities). A public school system or tax-exempt educational, charitable, or religious organization may provide retirement benefits for its employees through the purchase of annuities or by contributing to a custodial account invested in mutual funds (Code Sec. 403(b)(1) and (7)).[194] This type of retirement plan is commonly referred to as a "403(b) annuity plan" or "tax-sheltered annuity" (TSA). Generally, the employee's rights in the annuity or account must be nonforfeitable.

Limit on Annual Addition. There is a limit imposed on the total amount of the annual addition that may be made to an employee's 403(b) account. This annual limit is sometimes called the maximum amount contributable (MAC). The annual addition or MAC is made up of the following three types of contributions:

- elective contributions made by the employee,

- nonelective contributions made by the employer, and

- after-tax contributions made by the employee (Code Sec. 403(b)(1)).[195]

Generally, the annual addition cannot be more than the *lesser* of 100 percent of the employee's compensation or $52,000 for 2014, $53,000 for 2015 (¶ 2115) (Code Sec. 415(c)(1); Notice 2013-73; IRS News Release IR-2014-99). There are also limits on the amount of elective deferrals that generally apply to all of an employee's deferrals (¶ 2121) under any 403(b) annuity plan, 401(k) plan, SIMPLE 401(k) (¶ 2185), and SEP (¶ 2189) (Code Sec. 402(g)(3)). However, employees are not required to coordinate their maximum deferral under a 457 plan (¶ 2193) with their contributions made to 403(b) plans (Code Sec. 457(c), prior to amendment by the Economic Growth and Tax Relief Reconciliation Act of 2001 (P.L. 107-16)). Employees who will be at least age 50 by the end of the year may make "catch-up contributions" to a 403(b) plan. The maximum catch-up contribution to a 403(b) plan is $5,500 for 2014, $6,000 for 2015 (Code Sec. 414(v); Notice 2013-73; IRS News Release IR-2014-99). Qualified employees of certain organizations, e.g., schools, hospitals, churches, and home health service organizations, who are covered by an annuity contract under a 403(b) plan may defer additional amounts of their compensation (Code Sec. 402(g)(7)). For this purpose, a qualified employee is one who has completed 15 years of service with the organization.

Distributions. Payments to an employee from a 403(b) plan are taxed under the annuity rules explained at ¶ 817. However, any employee contributions that were excluded from wages are not treated as part of the employee's investment in the contract. Distributions may generally be made because of the employee's death, disability, severance from employment, attainment of age 59½, or financial hardship (Code Sec. 403(b)(7)(A)(ii) and (b)(11)). Distributions that do not meet these requirements are subject to the 10-percent additional tax on early distributions (¶ 2151). The required minimum distribution (RMD) rules also apply (¶ 2127) (Reg. § 1.403(b)-3).

Rollovers. Distributions from a 403(b) annuity plan may be rolled over into an IRA or another 403(b) plan, as well as to other types of employer plans, for example a 401(k) plan or 457 plan (Code Sec. 403(b)(8)(A)). Although the employee has the right to make the rollover, the other plans are not required to accept the rollover. The spousal rollover rules that apply to other types of employer sponsored plans and the written explanation requirements also apply to a beneficiary under a qualified annuity plan (Code Sec. 403(a)(4)(B)). A 403(b) plan that includes a qualified Roth contribution program may now permit a qualified rollover contribution from a participant's non-Roth account to the participant's designated Roth account within the same plan (Code Sec. 402A(c)(4)(B)).

References are to Standard Federal Tax Reports; Tax Research Consultant; and Practical Tax Explanations.

[194] ¶ 18,270; RETIRE: 69,056.10, RETIRE: 69,054.15; § 25,205.10, § 25,210.05

[195] ¶ 18,270; RETIRE: 69,058; § 25,215.10

2193. Sec. 457 Plans (Deferred Compensation Plans of Exempt Employers). Special rules apply to certain deferred compensation plans sponsored by state and local governments and private tax-exempt organizations, commonly referred to as 457 plans (Code Sec. 457(a)).[196] Under a state or local government plan, compensation deferred under the plan is only included in income when it is paid to the employee. However, for plans of tax-exempt organizations, deferred compensation is includible when paid or made available. As with other types of qualified retirement plans, special requirements have to be met by 457 plans.

Availability of Benefits. Compensation is deferred for any calendar month under a 457 plan only if an agreement providing for deferral is entered into before the beginning of that month (Code Sec. 457(b)(4)). Benefits are not considered to be made available under the plan if the participant or beneficiary may elect, before any benefits become payable, to defer payment of some or all of them to a fixed or determinable future time. In addition, amounts deferred under an eligible plan are not considered to be made available to the participant solely because the individual may choose among various investment options under the plan, whether before or after benefit payments have commenced (Reg. § 1.457-8(b)(2)).[197] After benefits have become payable but before payments have commenced, the participant or beneficiary may elect to defer them to a date later than that originally elected. Only one such election may be made (Code Sec. 457(e)(9)(B)).[198]

Limitation on Deferral. The maximum amount that can be deferred is the *lesser* of 100 percent of the participant's includible compensation or $17,500 for 2014, $18,000 for 2015 (Code Sec. 457(e)(15); Notice 2013-73; IRS News Release IR-2014-99).[199] Participants in a 457 plan are permitted to make additional deferrals of income for one or more of the last three tax years that end before normal retirement age (Code Sec. 457(b)(3)). The allowable deferral for such participants is increased, up to a limit of twice the standard dollar amount for the year, by the amount of allowable deferrals not made in previous plan years. Alternatively, employees covered by a 457 plan who will be at least 50 years of age by the end of the year are able to make special catch-up contributions to the plan (Code Sec. 414(v)). The maximum catch-up contribution is $5,500 for 2014, $6,000 for 2015 (Notice 2013-73; IRS News Release IR-2014-99). However, during the last three years of employment that end before attaining normal retirement age, a special formula is used to determine the maximum contribution (Code Sec. 457(e)(18)).

Other Requirements. A 457 plan must satisfy the required minimum distribution (RMD) rules that are generally imposed on qualified plans (¶ 2127) (Code Sec. 457(d)(2)). Distributions of deferred amounts must not be made available before the calendar year in which the participant attains age 70½, is severed from employment, or is faced with an unforeseen emergency (Code Sec. 457(d)(1)).[200] An unforeseeable emergency must be defined in the plan as: (1) a severe financial hardship to the participant that results from a sudden unexpected illness or accident of the participant or his or her spouse or dependent, or (2) a loss of the participant's property due to casualty or other similar extraordinary and unforeseeable circumstances beyond the control of the participant.

Hardship withdrawals may not be made to the extent that the financial hardship can be relieved by insurance, liquidation of the participant's assets (if liquidation would not cause financial hardship), or by stopping deferrals under the plan. In addition, withdrawal of amounts for unforeseeable emergencies is permitted only to the extent reasonably needed to satisfy the emergency. The need for funds to purchase a new home or to meet the college expenses of the participant's children is *not* an unforeseeable emergency (Reg. § 1.457-6(c)(2)(i)). To the extent allowed under the plan, if the occurrence of an event with regard to the employee's spouse or dependent would be a

---

References are to Standard Federal Tax Reports; Tax Research Consultant; and Practical Tax Explanations.

[196] ¶ 21,531; COMPEN: 15,150; § 25,301

[197] ¶ 21,532; COMPEN: 15,156; § 25,310.10

[198] ¶ 21,531; COMPEN: 15,156; § 25,310.10

[199] ¶ 21,531; COMPEN: 15,152.25; § 25,305.20

[200] ¶ 21,531; COMPEN: 15,152.40; § 25,305.30

hardship, the occurrence of the same event with regard to the employee's beneficiary under the plan would also be a hardship (Notice 2007-7, Q&A-5).

Rollovers. An employee participating in a 457 plan may roll over distributions into a IRAs, 401(k) plans, and 403(b) annuity plans (Code Sec. 457(e)(16)). Similarly, in some circumstances, assets from these plans may be rolled over into another 457 plan. A 457 plan that includes a qualified Roth contribution program may permit a qualified rollover contribution from a participant's non-Roth account to the participant's designated Roth account within the same plan (Code Sec. 402A(c)(4)(B)).

Roth 401(k) Plans. A 457 plan may allow participants to designate elective deferrals as Roth contributions. An applicable retirement plan for purposes of offering a qualified Roth contribution program includes eligible deferred compensation plans offered by state and local governments (Code Sec. 402A(e)(1)(C)). Elective deferrals for these purposes include any elective deferral of compensation by an individual under an eligible deferred compensation plan of an eligible employer that is a state or local government (Code Sec. 402A(e)(2)(B)).

Ineligible Plans. Compensation deferred under a nonqualified deferred compensation plan (¶ 2197) of a state or local government or other tax-exempt organization that is not an eligible 457 plan is includible in the income of a participant or beneficiary for the first tax year in which there is no substantial risk of forfeiture (Code Sec. 457(f)(1)(A) and (2)(E)).[201]

2195. Sec. 457A Plans (Tax-Indifferent Parties). In general, any compensation which is deferred under a nonqualified deferred compensation plan (¶ 2197) of a nonqualified entity, e.g., a foreign entity not subject to a comprehensive income tax, is includible in the service provider's gross income when there is no substantial risk of forfeiture of the rights to the compensation (Code Sec. 457A(a)). If the amount of any compensation is not determinable at the time that it is otherwise includible in gross income, then, in addition to income inclusion when the amount is determinable, the tax imposed for the year in which the compensation is includible in income must be increased by 20 percent of the amount of the compensation, plus an interest charge.

Effective Date. This rule generally applies to amounts deferred which are attributable to services performed after December 31, 2008. In the case of any amount deferred to which the rule does not apply solely by reason of the fact that the amount is attributable to services performed before January 1, 2009, to the extent that amount is not includible in gross income in a tax year beginning before 2018, the amount will be includible in gross income in the later of the last tax year beginning before 2018 or the tax year in which there is no substantial risk of forfeiture of the rights to such compensation.

With respect to a deferred amount attributable to services performed before January 1, 2009, a change in the time and form of payment to conform the date of distribution to the date the amount may be required to be included in income under the Code Sec. 457A special timing rule will not be treated as an impermissible acceleration under the nonqualified deferred compensation rules of Code Sec. 409A, provided that the change was established in writing and was effective on or before December 31, 2011 (Notice 2009-8).

2197. Nonqualified Deferred Compensation Plans. An employer may maintain a retirement or other deferred compensation plan for a group of selected employees that is not a qualified retirement plan (¶ 2111). Unless certain plan design and funding requirements are met, all compensation deferred under a nonqualified plan for the current year and all preceding tax years is includible in income of plan participants to the extent they are not subject to a substantial risk of forfeiture (¶ 713) and not previously included in gross income (Code Sec. 409A(a)(1)).[202] Any amount included in gross income will also be subject to a penalty of 20 percent of the deferred compensation, plus interest. See ¶ 2199 for a discussion of funding rules for nonqualified plans.

References are to Standard Federal Tax Reports; Tax Research Consultant; and Practical Tax Explanations.

[201] ¶ 21,531; COMPEN: 15,158; § 22,110.20

[202] ¶ 18,952; COMPEN: 15,066; § 25,601

Distributions. To avoid immediate inclusion of deferrals and the penalty, a nonqualified plan must allow distributions only if they are "permissible payments" triggered by the employee's separation from service from the employer, the employee's death or disability, a time specified under the plan, upon a change in the effective ownership or control of the employer, or in the event of an unforeseeable emergency (Code Sec. 409A(a)(2)).[203] Distributions to key employees resulting from a separation from service must also not be allowed until six months after the separation, unless the former employee dies in the interim.

Actual distributions from a nonqualified plan are included in the income of the employee in the year in which the distributions are made in accordance with the rules applicable to annuities (¶ 817) (Code Secs. 402(b) and 403(c)).[204] If the distributions do not take the form of an annuity, they are considered to be derived first from plan earnings and asset appreciation (taxable gain), rather than from the employee's investment (basis) in the plan. The participant's basis in a nonqualified plan is increased by any amounts included in his or her income for contributions, if any, made by the plan sponsor.

Acceleration of Benefits. A nonqualified plan generally cannot permit the acceleration of the time or schedule of any payment under the plan (Code Sec. 409A(a)(3)).[205] Exceptions are permitted for: domestic relations orders; *de minimis* cash-out provisions; payment of employment taxes; cancellations of deferrals due to disability, hardships, or unforeseen circumstances; and as an offset of debts.

Election Rules. A nonqualified plan must meet certain requirements regarding the participants' elections to defer compensation and to receive distributions (Code Sec. 409A(a)(4)).[206] Compensation for services performed during a tax year generally can be deferred only if the participant's election to defer is made before the close of the preceding tax year. In the case of any performance-based compensation that is based on services performed over a period of at least 12 months, the election may be made no later than six months before the end of the period. For new employees, a deferral election may be made within 30 days after the date the participant becomes eligible to participate. A participant is "new" for this purpose if at least 24 months have passed since the employee was an active participant in the plan or the plan aggregated with the plan.

Reporting. The total amount of deferrals under a nonqualified deferred compensation plan are required to be shown on an individual's Form W-2 or Form 1099-MISC even if the amount of deferred compensation is not currently taxable (Code Secs. 6041(g) and 6051(a)(13)).

2199. Nonqualified Deferred Compensation Plans—Funding Rules. The income tax treatment of contributions to a nonqualified deferred compensation plan (¶ 2197) depends on whether the plan is funded or unfunded. If an employer funds a nonqualified plan with contributions or the payment of premiums for an annuity, it is transferring restricted property to the plan participant under Code Sec. 83 in connection with the performance of services (¶ 713). The plan participant generally must include the contributions or amount of the premiums in gross income in the first year that the rights to the contributions or premium amounts are transferable or are not subject to a substantial risk of forfeiture (Code Secs. 402(b)(1) and 403(c)). If, however, one of the reasons the deferred compensation plan fails to be a qualified deferred compensation plan is the failure to satisfy the minimum participation or coverage requirements (¶ 2112), then highly compensated employees (¶ 2114) must include their vested accrued benefits, reduced by their own investment, in income for the tax year with or within which the tax year of the trust ends (Code Sec. 402(b)(4)).[207] Contributions to unfunded deferred compensation plans are discussed at ¶ 723 and ¶ 906.

Employer's Deduction. The employer is entitled to a deduction for contributions to, or premiums paid under, a nonqualified deferred compensation plan on behalf of an

---

References are to Standard Federal Tax Reports; Tax Research Consultant; and Practical Tax Explanations.

[203] ¶ 18,952; COMPEN: 15,056.10; § 25,601

[204] ¶ 18,202, ¶ 18,270; COMPEN: 15,200; § 25,610.10

[205] ¶ 18,952; COMPEN: 15,056.10; § 25,601

[206] ¶ 18,952; COMPEN: 15,056.10; § 22,110.20

[207] ¶ 18,202; RETIRE: 39,700; § 24,105.10

¶2199

employee in the tax year of the employer in which an amount attributable to the contribution is includible in the gross income of the employee (Code Sec. 404(a)(5)).[208] If more than one employee participates, this rule applies only if separate accounts are maintained for each employee.

Plan Income. In the case of a nonqualified plan funded through a trust, the trust is not tax-exempt and the plan's earnings are generally taxable to the trust (Code Sec. 641).[209] The grantor trust rules (¶ 571) ordinarily do not apply to a nonqualified plan. Therefore, the participant is not usually treated as the owner of his or her share of the trust's assets and is not subject to tax on the trust's income. However, if a participant's contributions as of any date exceed the employer's contributions on behalf of the participant, the participant is treated as the owner of the portion of the trust attributable to his or her contributions and is subject to tax on the income from that portion (Reg. § 1.402(b)-1(b)(6)).[210]

Other Funding Rules. If a nonqualified deferred compensation plan uses an offshore trust, or places assets outside the United States, the plan will generally *not* defer the compensation (Code Sec. 409A(b)).[211] Also, if the plan provides that its assets will become restricted to the payment of benefits under the plan if there is a change in the employer's financial health, or if the assets actually become so restricted, the plan will not defer compensation. These rules apply to all deferred compensation, regardless of when it was deferred.

A nonqualified plan will also not defer compensation to the extent of contributions made on behalf of or restricted to benefits for certain employees at a time when the employer or its defined benefit plan are experiencing financial difficulties. This provision applies if the plan is in at-risk status under Code Sec. 430(i), if the plan sponsor is in bankruptcy, and if, during the 12-month period beginning six months before the plan terminates, the plan is underfunded.

References are to Standard Federal Tax Reports; Tax Research Consultant; and Practical Tax Explanations.

[208] ¶ 18,330; COMPEN: 15,250; § 25,605

[209] ¶ 24,260; PLANIND: 15,064; § 25,610.10

[210] ¶ 18,208; COMPEN: 15,106; § 25,610.10

[211] ¶ 18,952; PLANRET: 3,206.40; § 25,610.20, § 45,040.10

Chapter 22

CORPORATE ACQUISITIONS

REORGANIZATIONS

LIQUIDATIONS

Corporate Division

2201. "Spin-Off," "Split-Off," "Split-Up," and "Splint-Off" Exchanges. The benefits of nonrecognition of gain apply to receipt of stock in connection with corporate distributions known as "spin-offs," "split-offs," "split-ups," or "splint-offs."

Spin-Off. A "spin-off" occurs when a corporation distributes pro rata stock or securities in a controlled corporation (at least 80-percent stock ownership). Shareholders do not typically surrender any of their stock in the controlling corporation (Code Sec. 355; Reg. § 1.355-1).[1] A new or existing corporation may be used for the spin-off.

Split-Off. In a "split-off," a parent corporation distributes to some or all of its shareholders stock in a newly formed or pre-existing controlled corporation, under the same conditions as in a "spin-off," except that the shareholders surrender a part of their stock in the parent corporation for the stock in the controlled corporation. The distribution may be pro rata but usually is not.

Split-Up. In a "split-up," the distributing corporation's shareholders surrender all shares held in the distributing corporation and in return receive new shares in two or more subsidiaries the distributing corporation controlled immediately before the distribution. The subsidiaries may be pre-existing or newly formed.

Splint-Off. In a "splint-off," some of the distributing corporation's shareholders surrender their shares in exchange for stock of the controlled corporation (as in a split-off). Other shareholders receive stock of the controlled corporation pro rata without surrendering any of their stock of the distributing corporation (as in a spin-off).

To attain nonrecognition treatment in a spin-off, split-off, split-up, or splint-off, the distributing and controlled corporations must immediately after the transaction be engaged in the active conduct of a trade or business (Code Sec. 355(b); Reg. § 1.355-3).[2] This requirement does not apply to the distributing corporation if immediately before the distribution, it had no assets other than stock in the controlled corporation. The trade or business must have been actively conducted throughout the five-year period immediately preceding the date of the distribution.

In addition to the active business requirement, the transaction must have a valid corporate business purpose, and it cannot be primarily a tax-avoidance device (Reg. § 1.355-2(b)).[3] If, however, a corporate business purpose can be achieved through a nontaxable transaction that does not involve the distribution of stock of a controlled corporation and which is neither impractical nor unduly expensive, then the separation

---

References are to Standard Federal Tax Reports; Tax Research Consultant; and Practical Tax Explanations.

[1] ¶ 16,460, ¶ 16,462; REORG: 30,050, REORG: 30,052

[2] ¶ 16,460, ¶ 16,464; REORG: 30,106

[3] ¶ 16,463; REORG: 30,114

¶2201

is not carried out for that corporate business purpose. Other limitations relate to continuity of interest on the part of the owners (Reg. § 1.355-2(c)),[4] the amount of securities distributed, taxable acquisitions within five years, and receipt of other property or "boot" (Code Sec. 355(a)(3)).[5]

Basis Rules. With an exchange of stock or securities, the basis of the old stock or securities becomes the basis of the new stock or securities ("substituted basis") (Code Sec. 358).[6] If the exchange is partially taxable, the basis of the old stock or securities is decreased by the sum of the money and fair market value of "other property" received and increased by the amount of gain recognized and the amount treated as a dividend. If any loss is recognized, the basis of the property received is decreased by that amount. If some old stock is retained, the basis is allocated as though the stock were first surrendered and then received in the exchange.

Morris Trust Rules. Restrictions have been imposed on certain spin-offs that follow the fact pattern of *Morris Trust*, SCt, 66-2 USTC ¶ 9718 (Code Sec. 355(e)).[7] If either the controlled or distributing corporation is acquired pursuant to a plan or arrangement in existence on the date of distribution, gain is generally recognized by the distributing corporation as of the date of the distribution. Recognition can be avoided if more than 50 percent of the historical shareholders retain ownership in the distributing and acquiring corporations. Acquisitions occurring within the four-year period beginning two years before the date of distribution are presumed to have occurred pursuant to a plan or arrangement.

Reporting Requirements. The distributing corporation in a divisive Code Sec. 355 transaction is required to file a statement with its tax return for the year of the distribution (Reg. § 1.355-5).[8] A shareholder or security holder of the distributing corporation that is a significant distributee must also file an information statement with his or her return for the tax year in which the distribution is received. A significant distributee is any shareholder of the distributing corporation who received stock in the distribution and owned, immediately before the distribution, at least five percent (by vote or value) of the stock of the distributing corporation if the stock owned by the shareholder is publicly traded, or at least one percent (by vote or value) of the distributing corporation's stock if the stock owned by the shareholder is not publicly traded.

The distributing corporation and its shareholders and security holders who are required to file information statements in connection with the Code Sec. 355 transaction must keep records that contain information regarding the amount, basis and fair market value of all property distributed or exchanged in the transaction, and any liabilities assumed or extinguished as part of the transaction.

Corporate Reorganization

2205. Tax-Free Exchange in Reorganization. A corporation that is a party to a reorganization (¶ 2221) and its shareholders and security holders are eligible for nonrecognition of gain or loss on the reorganization exchange. To achieve the favorable tax treatment, reorganization transactions must satisfy strict statutory and nonstatutory requirements (¶ 2209).

A corporation generally recognizes no gain or loss on the exchange of property solely for stock or securities of another corporation if the corporation is a party to the reorganization and the exchange is made pursuant to a plan of reorganization (Code Sec. 361).[9] If the corporation receives other property or money ("boot") in addition to the stock or securities, it does not recognize gain on the exchange if the boot is distributed pursuant to the plan of reorganization. The transferee corporation does not recognize gain or loss on the receipt of property in exchange for its own stock (Code Sec. 1032).[10]

References are to Standard Federal Tax Reports; Tax Research Consultant; and Practical Tax Explanations.

[4] ¶ 16,463; REORG: 30,116	[7] ¶ 16,460, ¶ 16,466.10;	[9] ¶ 16,580; CCORP: 39,302
[5] ¶ 16,460; REORG: 30,104.05	REORG: 30,112	[10] ¶ 29,622; CCORP: 39,304.05
[6] ¶ 16,550; REORG: 30,152.15	[8] ¶ 16,465C; REORG: 30,158	

No gain or loss is generally recognized by shareholders or security holders who exchange, pursuant to a plan of reorganization, stock or securities of a corporation that is a party to the reorganization solely for stock or securities of that corporation or another corporation that is a party to the reorganization (Code Sec. 354).[11] However, gain (but not loss) may be recognized on the receipt of boot (Code Sec. 356).[12] The recognized gain equals the lesser of the amount of gain realized on the exchange or the amount of boot received. Gain on the boot is typically capital gain, unless the exchange has the effect of the distribution of a dividend, in which case the boot is taxed as ordinary income (¶ 2237).

Basis Rules. The basis of stock and securities received by a corporate transferor in a reorganization is generally the same as the basis of the property transferred to the acquiring corporation, adjusted for any gain or loss recognized on the exchange and the value of any boot received (Code Sec. 358(a)).[13] The basis of boot received by the transferor corporation from the acquiring corporation is its fair market value at the time of the exchange. Property received by the transferee corporation has the same basis in the hands of the transferee as it had in the hands of the transferor ("carryover basis"), increased by the amount of gain recognized by the transferor on the transfer (Code Sec. 362(b)).[14] The property acquired by the transferee corporation does not take a carryover basis, however, if it consists of stock or securities in a corporation that is a party to the corporate reorganization.

The basis of stock or securities received by shareholders in the reorganization exchange is the same as the basis of stock or securities they surrendered in the exchange (Code Sec. 358(a)).[15] If boot is received, the basis of the nonrecognition property received by a shareholder is equal to the basis of the stock or securities exchanged in the reorganization, adjusted for any amount of gain or loss recognized and the fair market value of the boot. The shareholder's basis in any boot received is its fair market value.

2209. "Reorganization" Defined. A qualified reorganization must fall within one of seven categories—each referred to by a letter corresponding to the statutory provisions of Code Sec. 368; Reg. § 1.368-2.[16] In each category, there cannot be a tax-free reorganization unless there is an exchange of properties as distinguished from a sale.

Type A reorganization: a statutory merger or consolidation (that is, a merger or consolidation accomplished pursuant to state law or the laws of a foreign jurisdiction, including certain mergers involving disregarded entities) (Reg. § 1.368-2(b));[17]

Type B reorganization: the acquisition by one corporation of the stock of another corporation, in exchange solely for all or a part of its own or its parent's voting stock (¶ 2211), if the acquiring corporation has control of the other corporation immediately after the acquisition, whether or not it had control before the acquisition;

Type C reorganization: the acquisition by one corporation of substantially all of the properties of another corporation (¶ 2217) in exchange solely for all or a part of its own voting stock or its controlling parent's voting stock (¶ 2211), followed by the acquired corporation's distribution of all its property pursuant to the plan of reorganization (unless this requirement is waived by the IRS);

Type D reorganization: a transfer by a corporation of all or a part of its assets to another corporation if, immediately after the transfer, the transferor or one or more of its shareholders is in control of the corporation to which the assets are transferred; the term "shareholders" includes those who were shareholders immediately before the transfer, but only if the stock or securities of the corporation to which the assets are transferred are distributed under the plan of reorganization in a transaction described at ¶ 2201 or ¶ 2205;

Type E reorganization: a recapitalization (¶ 2225);

References are to Standard Federal Tax Reports; Tax Research Consultant; and Practical Tax Explanations.

[11] ¶ 16,431; CCORP: 39,252
[12] ¶ 16,490; CCORP: 39,254
[13] ¶ 16,550; CCORP: 39,302.15
[14] ¶ 16,610; CCORP: 39,304.10
[15] ¶ 16,550; CCORP: 39,256
[16] ¶ 16,750, ¶ 16,752; CCORP: 39,052
[17] ¶ 16,752; REORG: 6,050

Type F reorganization: a mere change in the identity, form, or place of organization of one corporation; or

Type G reorganization: a transfer by a corporation in bankruptcy of all or part of its assets to another corporation, but only if stock or securities of the transferee corporation are distributed to the shareholders tax free or partially tax free (¶ 2247).

80-Percent Control Test. For purposes of the corporate reorganization rules, the term "control" means the ownership of stock possessing at least 80 percent of the combined voting power of all classes of stock entitled to vote and at least 80 percent of the total number of shares of all other classes of stock of the corporation (Code Sec. 368(c)).[18] The 80-percent control requirement is changed to 50 percent in the case of nondivisive D reorganizations (Code Secs. 304(c) and 368(a)(2)(H)(i)).[19]

In order for the control requirement to be satisfied, it is not necessary that the acquiror acquire 80 percent (or 50 percent) of the target's stock in the reorganization, nor that control be attained in the transactions that constitute the reorganization. Rather, it is sufficient that the acquiring corporation is in control of the target corporation immediately after the transaction (Code Sec. 368(a)(1)(B)).[20] Thus, a corporation can acquire stock in one of its subsidiaries in a tax-free reorganization.

S Corporation Reorganization Using QSubs. When an S corporation merges into a newly formed corporation in a transaction qualifying as a Type F reorganization, the newly formed surviving corporation meets the requirements of an S corporation, and the acquiring corporation elects to treat the transferor S corporation as a qualified sub-chapter S subsidiary (QSub), the reorganization does not terminate the S election (Rev. Ruls. 64-250 and 2008-18).[21] The QSub must retain and use its employer identification number (EIN) when it is treated as a separate corporation for federal tax purposes.

Triangular Reorganizations. Tax-free reorganizations are often structured as triangular reorganizations, which involve use of a subsidiary to acquire the target corporation. There are five types of triangular reorganizations (Reg. § 1.358-6(b)(2)):[22]

 (1) triangular B reorganizations;

 (2) triangular C reorganizations;

 (3) triangular G reorganizations;

 (4) forward triangular mergers (the acquiring corporation uses the stock of its parent to acquire substantially all the properties of the target corporation); and

 (5) reverse triangular mergers (parent stock is used to acquire the target corporation, but an acquisition subsidiary of the parent merges into the target, and the target becomes an 80-percent-owned subsidiary of the parent).

2211. Exchange of Stock or Property Solely for Voting Stock. In a B reorganization (¶ 2209), the exchange of stock "solely for voting stock" means that the acquiring corporation cannot use cash or nonvoting stock in the exchange, or the reorganization becomes taxable (Reg. § 1.368-2(c)).[23]

The "solely" requirement is relaxed for a C reorganization (¶ 2209) in that "substantially all the assets" (¶ 2217) must be acquired solely for voting stock. If at least 80 percent of the value of all the property of the transferor corporation is acquired solely for voting stock, the remaining properties may be acquired for money or other property (Code Sec. 368(a)(2)(B)).[24] If the acquiring corporation does transfer money or property in addition to voting stock, then for the purpose of determining whether at least 80 percent of the assets are acquired for voting stock, the amount of any liability assumed by the acquiring corporation or the amount of any liability to which the property acquired is subject is also treated as money paid for the property.

References are to Standard Federal Tax Reports; Tax Research Consultant; and Practical Tax Explanations.

[18] ¶ 16,750; CCORP: 39,052, REORG: 12,054, REORG: 15,058

[19] ¶ 15,375, ¶ 16,750; REORG: 18,052.10

[20] ¶ 16,750; CCORP: 39,052, REORG: 12,054

[21] ¶ 32,053.69; SCORP: 304.10; § 28,920

[22] ¶ 16,552F; REORG: 9,050, REORG: 9,100, REORG: 27,400

[23] ¶ 16,752; REORG: 12,052

[24] ¶ 16,750; REORG: 15,100

2217. Substantially All Requirement in C Reorganizations. What constitutes "substantially all" of the properties of a corporation for purposes of a C reorganization (¶ 2209) is not precisely defined in the Code or regulations. However, a special rule provides that a reorganization may still qualify as a C corporation if the acquiring corporation acquires at least 80 percent of all of the target corporation's property solely for voting stock of the acquiring corporation or its parent (Code Sec. 368(a)(1)(C) and (a)(2)(B)).[25] Some courts have held that a transfer of approximately two-thirds in value of the assets, or 68 percent or even 75 percent of all the corporate property, is not "substantially all." Other courts have held that 85.2 percent or even 90 percent, which included all property except cash, was substantially all. The IRS interprets the substantially all requirement, for the purpose of issuing ruling letters, as requiring a transfer of assets representing at least 90 percent of the fair market value of the net assets and at least 70 percent of the fair market value of the corporation's gross assets held immediately before the transfer (Rev. Proc. 77-37).[26]

2221. Party to a Reorganization—Plan of Reorganization. The reorganization provisions provide for the nonrecognition solely of the gains and losses of the parties to reorganizations and their shareholders and security holders (¶ 2205 and ¶ 2229). A party to a organization includes a corporation resulting from a reorganization and both corporations in a reorganization resulting from the acquisition by one corporation of stock or properties of another (Code Sec. 368(b); Reg. § 1.368-2(f)).[27] In an A, B, C, or G reorganization (¶ 2209), a party to a reorganization includes a controlling corporation if its stock is exchanged and likewise includes a controlled subsidiary that receives any of the assets or stock exchanged.

A plan of reorganization is required in connection with a tax-free exchange (Reg. § 1.368-2(g)).[28] The plan does not need to be a formal written document. However, the safest practice would be to incorporate the plan into the corporate records. The plan may be amended as circumstances change so long as the reorganization remains in compliance with the reorganization requirements (¶ 2209).

2225. Recapitalization. For a transaction to qualify as a recapitalization or E reorganization (¶ 2209), there must be a reshuffling of the capital structure of a corporation (*Southwest Consolidated Corp.*, SCt, 42-1 USTC ¶ 9248).[29] For example, an E reorganization occurs when a corporation discharges outstanding bond indebtedness by issuing preferred stock to the shareholders in exchange for the bonds instead of paying them off in cash, when 25 percent of a corporation's preferred stock is surrendered for cancellation and no-par-value common stock is issued, or when previously authorized but unissued preferred stock is issued in exchange for outstanding common stock (Reg. § 1.368-2(e)).[30]

2229. Receipt of Stock, Securities or Other Property. No gain or loss is generally recognized by a shareholder or securities holder if stock or securities in a corporation that is party to a reorganization (¶ 2221) are exchanged solely for stock or securities of another corporation, and the exchange is made pursuant to a plan of reorganization (¶ 2209) or a corporate division (¶ 2201) (Code Sec. 354).[31] An exchange of securities in a reorganization is tax free only to the extent that the principal amount received does not exceed the principal amount surrendered. Nonrecognition treatment also does not apply if securities are received and no securities are surrendered. The term "securities" is not defined by the Code or regulations for this purpose. Under case law, however, an instrument with a term of less than five years generally is not a security.[32]

If a shareholder or security holder receives money or other property ("boot") in the exchange, it can result in gain recognition, dividend treatment (¶ 2237), or in the case of a corporate division, treatment as a corporate distribution (Code Sec. 356).[33] Securities

---

References are to Standard Federal Tax Reports; Tax Research Consultant; and Practical Tax Explanations.

[25] ¶ 16,750; REORG: 15,056

[26] ¶ 16,753.53; REORG: 15,056

[27] ¶ 16,750, ¶ 16,752; CCORP: 39,054

[28] ¶ 16,752; CCORP: 39,056, REORG: 3,200

[29] ¶ 16,753.476; REORG: 24,050

[30] ¶ 16,752; REORG: 24,052

[31] ¶ 16,431; CCORP: 39,250

[32] ¶ 16,433.61; CCORP: 39,252.05

[33] ¶ 16,490; CCORP: 39,254

received in a Code Sec. 351 exchange are treated as boot for this purpose (¶ 1731). In addition, nonqualified preferred stock is treated as boot (Code Sec. 351(g)).[34] Any liabilities of the shareholder or security holder assumed by a party to the organization are not considered boot (¶ 2233).

If no boot is received in a corporate reorganization or division, the shareholders or security holders retain for the stock or securities they receive the same basis that they had in the stock or securities they surrendered in the exchange (Code Sec. 358).[35] If boot is received, the basis of the nonrecognition property received by a shareholder or security holder is equal to the basis of the stock or securities exchanged in the reorganization, adjusted for the amount of gain or loss recognized, any amount treated as a dividend (¶ 2237), and the amount of the boot received. The basis determined for nonrecognition stock and securities must be allocated among all classes of stock or securities involved in the transaction. The basis of any boot is its fair market value.

2233. Assumption of Liabilities in Reorganizations. A release from liabilities assumed by a transferee or a disposition of property subject to liabilities in a reorganization (¶ 2209), a transfer of property to a controlled corporation (¶ 1731), or certain bankruptcy reorganizations or foreclosures (¶ 2247) is not money or other property ("boot") received by the taxpayer and does not prevent the transaction from being tax free (Code Sec. 357).[36] However, if the principal purpose of the assumption of liabilities is to avoid income tax, or the purpose is not a bona fide business purpose, the liability assumed is treated as boot (unless the taxpayer can prove to the contrary).

If the liabilities assumed, or to which the property is subject, exceed the total basis of all the properties transferred in a Code Sec. 351 exchange or divisive D reorganization involving a corporate division, the excess is treated as gain from a sale or exchange of a capital asset or a noncapital asset, depending on the nature of the encumbered asset transferred (Code Sec. 357(c)). See ¶ 1669 for a discussion of the basis of property after an assumption of liabilities. A liability is excluded from this exception if it is assumed in a Code Sec. 351 transfer and the payment of the liability by the transferor would give rise to a deduction or would be basically the equivalent of a payment made in liquidation of the interest of a retiring or deceased partner, unless such liability resulted in the creation of, or the increase in, the basis of any property. The liability is excluded, however, to the extent incurring the liability results in the creation of, or an increase in, the basis of any property.

2237. Dividend Distribution in Reorganization. A distribution of money or other property ("boot") to a stockholder as part of a plan of reorganization (¶ 2229) may be taxed as a dividend if it has the effect of a taxable dividend, even if the money or other property is received in an exchange which is, in part, tax free (Code Sec. 356; Reg. § 1.356-1).[37] The constructive ownership rules discussed at ¶ 743 are applied in determining dividend equivalency. For this purpose, a distribution is taxable as a dividend, not to exceed the recognized gain, to the extent the distributing company has earnings and profits sufficient to cover the distribution.

2241. Liquidation as Part of Reorganization. Under a plan of reorganization (¶ 2209), a corporation often acquires, for all or part of its stock, all of the stock in another corporation from the stockholders of the latter. As the final step in the reorganization, the acquiring corporation may liquidate the latter company, acquiring those assets by surrendering its own stock. This last step in the reorganization may be accomplished tax free under Code Sec. 332 (¶ 2261).

2247. Reorganizations of Bankrupt or Insolvent Corporations. Corporate restructurings ordered pursuant to certain bankruptcy, foreclosure, or similar proceedings may qualify as corporate reorganizations (¶ 2209) (Code Sec. 368(a)(1)(G)).[38] To qualify for nonrecognition treatment, a G reorganization must meet six requirements:

References are to Standard Federal Tax Reports; Tax Research Consultant; and Practical Tax Explanations.

[34] ¶ 16,402; CCORP: 3,102.05
[35] ¶ 16,550; CCORP: 39,256

[36] ¶ 16,520; CCORP: 39,252.15, CCORP: 39,302.20; § 26,125.05

[37] ¶ 16,490, ¶ 16,491; CCORP: 39,254.15
[38] ¶ 16,750; REORG: 27,050

- the debtor/target corporation must transfer all or part of its assets to an acquiring corporation;

  - the transfer must take place in a Title 11 or similar case;

  - the stock or securities of the acquiring corporation must be distributed as part of a plan of reorganization;

  - there must be continuity of interest;

  - there must be continuity of business enterprise; and

  - There must be a business purpose for the transaction.

2249. Reporting Requirements. Each corporation that is a party to a reorganization (¶ 2221) must file a statement with its tax return for the tax year of the reorganization exchange (Reg. § 1.368-3(a)).[39]

Certain shareholders and security holders of the target corporation ("significant holders") must also file an information statement with their return for the tax year of the reorganization exchange (Reg. § 1.368-3(b) and (c)).[40] A target shareholder is a significant holder if the shareholder receives stock in the reorganization exchange and owns, before the exchange, at least five percent (by vote or value) of the target's total outstanding stock if the stock owned by the shareholder is publicly traded or at least one percent (by vote or value) of the target's total outstanding stock if the stock owned by the shareholder is not publicly traded. A security holder in the target corporation who receives stock or securities in the exchange is a significant holder and is required to file a statement if, immediately before the exchange, the security holder owned securities in the target with a basis of $1 million or more.

Corporate parties and shareholders and security holders who are required to file information statements in connection with a reorganization must keep records that contain information regarding the amount, basis, and fair market value of all property transferred or exchanged in the transaction, and any liabilities assumed or extinguished as part of the transaction (Reg. § 1.368-3(d)).[41]

Corporate Liquidation

2253. Gain or Loss to Shareholders in Corporate Liquidations. Amounts distributed in a complete liquidation of a corporation are usually treated as full payment in exchange for the stock (Code Sec. 331; Reg. § 1.331-1).[42] The shareholder's gain or loss from a distribution is determined by comparing the amount distributed to the cost or other basis of the stock. Assuming that the stock is a capital asset, the gain or loss to the shareholder is capital.

If property is received in a distribution in a complete liquidation and gain or loss is recognized on receipt of the property, the basis of the property in the hands of the person receiving it is the fair market value of the property at the time of the distribution (Code Sec. 334(a)).[43] When a parent corporation liquidates an 80-percent controlled subsidiary, the parent corporation's basis in the property received is generally the same as the liquidating subsidiary's basis in the property unless the subsidiary recognizes gain from the transfer (¶ 2261). If property received in a complete liquidation is subject to a liability, the recipient's recognition of gain or loss is adjusted accordingly (¶ 1672).

A distribution that is one of a series of distributions in redemption of all of a corporation's stock pursuant to a plan is treated as a complete liquidation (Code Sec. 346(a)).[44] If a distribution is made as one of a series of distributions intended eventually to result in a complete liquidation of the corporation, no gain is realized by the shareholder until the entire cost of the stock is recovered. If a complete liquidation covers two or more consecutive tax years, the distribution first offsets the shareholder's

References are to Standard Federal Tax Reports; Tax Research Consultant; and Practical Tax Explanations.

[39] ¶ 16,754; REORG: 3,252
[40] ¶ 16,754; REORG: 3,254

[41] ¶ 16,754; REORG: 3,252, REORG: 3,254
[42] ¶ 16,002, ¶ 16,003; CCORP: 27,100; § 26,710

[43] ¶ 16,150; CCORP: 27,122; § 26,710
[44] ¶ 16,351; CCORP: 27,050

basis for the stock and the excess is gain in the year received. The gain is not allocable to all of the years in which distributions were received (Rev. Rul. 85-48).[45]

Partial Liquidation. A distribution of corporate assets to a *noncorporate* shareholder is treated as made in exchange for stock (whether or not stock is actually surrendered) if the distribution is in a partial liquidation of the corporation. The distribution must not be essentially equivalent to a dividend (determined by reference to the effect on the corporation rather than the effect on the shareholders), but rather must be made pursuant to a plan and must occur within the tax year in which the plan is adopted or within the succeeding tax year. A distribution qualifies as a partial liquidation if it is attributable to the corporation's ceasing to conduct a trade or business that it actively conducted for at least five years ending with the date of the distribution and if the corporation continues to conduct at least one other trade or business immediately after the distribution (Code Sec. 302(b)(4) and (e)).[46] A corporation may also rely on the common law doctrine of "corporate contraction" to establish a partial liquidation—contraction of the business of the corporation.

2257. Recognition of Gain or Loss by Corporation in Complete Liquidation. Property distributed in a complete liquidation of a corporation is generally deemed to have been sold by the corporation at its fair market value and any gain or loss is recognized by the liquidating corporation (Code Sec. 336).[47] If the distributed property is subject to a liability or if the distributee assumes a liability upon the distribution, the fair market value of the property is deemed to be no less than the amount of the liability. The following exceptions to this general recognition rule apply:

(1) No gain or loss is recognized upon any distribution of property to shareholders in a tax-free reorganization (¶ 2205 and ¶ 2209), except that gain may be recognized on the distribution of appreciated property that is not a qualified property (Code Secs. 336(c) and 361(c)(4)).[48]

(2) No gain or loss is generally recognized in connection with the complete liquidation of a controlled subsidiary into its parent corporation, except that gain (but not loss) is recognized with respect to any property distributed to minority shareholders (¶ 2261).

(3) No loss is recognized with respect to a distribution of property to a related person within the meaning of Code Sec. 267 (¶ 1717), unless the property (a) is distributed to all shareholders on a pro rata basis and (b) was not acquired by the liquidating corporation in a Code Sec. 351 transaction or as a contribution to capital during the five years preceding the distribution (Code Sec. 336(d)(1)).[49]

(4) Recognition of loss may be limited if the distributed property was initially acquired by the liquidating corporation, either by tax-free transfer to a controlled corporation or as a contribution to capital, as part of a plan a principal purpose of which was the recognition of loss on the property in connection with the liquidation. In these circumstances, the basis of the property for purposes of determining loss is reduced, but not below zero, by the excess of the adjusted basis of the property on the date of contribution over its fair market value. There is a presumption of a tax-avoidance purpose with respect to any such transfer within the two-year period prior to the adoption of the plan of liquidation (Code Sec. 336(d)(2)).[50]

(5) No gain or loss is recognized if a corporation owning 80 percent or more of the voting power and value of another corporation elects to treat any disposition (sale, exchange, or distribution) of the subsidiary's stock as a disposition of all of the subsidiary's assets (Code Sec. 336(e); Reg. § § 1.336-0—1.336-5).[51]

References are to Standard Federal Tax Reports; Tax Research Consultant; and Practical Tax Explanations.

[45] ¶ 16,004.163; CCORP: 27,108

[46] ¶ 15,325; CCORP: 21,700; § 26,330.05

[47] ¶ 16,200; CCORP: 27,150; § 26,715

[48] ¶ 16,200, ¶ 16,580; CCORP: 27,156

[49] ¶ 16,200; CCORP: 27,160.05; § 26,720.10

[50] ¶ 16,200; CCORP: 27,160.15; § 26,720.15

[51] ¶ 16,200, ¶ 16,201— ¶ 16,211; CCORP: 27,218

2259. Reporting Requirements for Complete Liquidations. Certain shareholders of a liquidating corporation who transfer stock to the liquidating corporation in exchange for property must file a statement with their return for the tax year of the liquidating exchange (Reg. § 1.331-1(d)).[52] The statement must include the fair market value and basis of the transferred stock and a description of the property received in the exchange.

The reporting requirement applies to a "significant shareholder"—a shareholder who owns at least five percent (by vote or value) of the liquidating corporation's total outstanding stock if the stock owned by the shareholder is publicly traded or at least one percent (by vote or value) of the liquidating corporation's total outstanding stock if the stock owned by the shareholder is not publicly traded. A shareholder need not file a statement if the property is part of a distribution made pursuant to a resolution providing that the distribution is made in a complete liquidation, and the liquidating corporation is completely liquidated and dissolved within one year after the distribution.

The liquidating corporation must file Form 966 within 30 days after it adopts a plan of liquidation (Code Sec. 6043(a); Reg. §§ 1.6043-1 and 1.6043-2).[53] The liquidating corporation must also file a separate Form 1099-DIV for each shareholder to whom a liquidating distribution of $600 or more is made and furnish a copy to the shareholder.

2261. Liquidation of Subsidiary. If distributions in a complete liquidation are made by a subsidiary to a parent corporation (owning at least 80 percent by value and voting power of the subsidiary), then no gain or loss on the distributions is recognized by either the parent corporation or the liquidating subsidiary (Code Secs. 332 and 337).[54] For this purpose, the 80-percent control requirement must be met by direct ownership and not by reason of the aggregation rules. In addition, property distributed to a controlling domestic corporation in satisfaction of a debt owed by the liquidating subsidiary is treated as a distribution in liquidation for these purposes (Code Sec. 337(b)(1)). However, the distribution of earnings by a U.S. holding company to a foreign corporation in a complete liquidation is treated as a taxable dividend if the U.S. holding company was in existence for less than five years (Code Sec. 332(d)).

If a minority shareholder receives property in such a liquidation, the minority shareholder may recognize gain or loss on the distribution (¶ 2253), while the liquidating corporation may recognize gain, but not loss (¶ 2257). Gain or loss also is recognized on distributions to 80-percent distributees that are foreign corporations (¶ 2492) and tax-exempt organizations, unless the property is used by that organization in a trade or business unrelated to its tax-exempt purpose (Code Sec. 337(b)(2)).

Basis. After a complete liquidation of a subsidiary, the parent corporation usually holds the distributed assets with the same basis that the assets formerly had in the hands of the subsidiary. However, the basis of the property in the hands of the parent corporation is the fair market value at the time of the distribution if: (1) the subsidiary recognizes gain or loss with respect to the property; or (2) the parent's aggregate adjusted basis in the property exceeds its fair market value immediately after the liquidation in the case of a loss importation transaction where the built-in loss property was not subject to tax in the hands of the subsidiary but is subject to tax in the hands of the parent (Code Sec. 334(b)).[55]

Reporting Requirements. The parent corporation must include a statement with its tax return for the year in which it receives a distribution from the liquidating subsidiary (Reg. § 1.332-6(a)).[56] The liquidating subsidiary must timely file Form 966 and its final income tax return (Code Sec. 6043(a); Reg. §§ 1.332-6(b) and 1.6043-1).[57] Both the liquidating subsidiary and the parent corporation must also retain permanent records

---

References are to Standard Federal Tax Reports; Tax Research Consultant; and Practical Tax Explanations.

[52] ¶ 16,003; CCORP: 27,054

[53] ¶ 35,880, ¶ 35,881, ¶ 35,883; FILEBUS: 9,352, CCORP: 27,054; § 26,740

[54] ¶ 16,050, ¶ 16,225; CCORP: 27,202, CCORP: 27,210; § 26,730.10, § 26,730.20

[55] ¶ 16,150; CCORP: 27,214.05; § 26,730.10

[56] ¶ 16,051E; CCORP: 27,202.30

[57] ¶ 35,880, ¶ 16,051E, ¶ 35,881; FILEBUS: 9,352, CCORP: 27,202.30; § 26,740

regarding the liquidation (Reg. § 1.332-6(d)).[58] These records must specifically include information regarding the amount, basis, and fair market value of the distributed property, and any liability assumed or extinguished as part of the liquidation.

2263. Code Sec. 336(e) Elections. A corporation that owns at least 80 percent of the total voting power and 80 percent of the total value of the stock of another corporation (target) and sells, exchanges, or distributes 80 percent or more of the total voting power and 80 percent or more of the total value of the stock in a qualified stock disposition may make an election to treat the sale, exchange, or distribution as a disposition of all the assets of the target corporation (Code Sec. 336(e) election). In such circumstance, no gain or loss is recognized on the sale, exchange, or distribution of the stock (Code Sec. 336(e); Reg. § 1.336-2).[59] The Code Sec. 336(e) election is available for qualified stock dispositions occurring on or after May 15, 2013.

A qualified stock disposition is any disposition or series of dispositions in which the seller sells, exchanges, or distributes—or any combination thereof—stock equal to 80 percent or more of the voting power and 80 percent or more of the total value of a domestic target corporation during the 12-month disposition period. Thus, the seller may retain a portion of the target stock. The 12-month disposition period is the 12-month period beginning with the date of the first sale, exchange, or distribution of stock included in a qualified stock disposition (Reg. § 1.336-1(b)).[60]

A disposition is any sale, exchange, or distribution of stock, but only if: (1) the basis of the stock in the hands of the purchaser is not determined by reference to the adjusted basis of the stock in the hands of the person from whom the stock is acquired or from a decedent; (2) the stock is not sold, exchanged, or distributed in a transaction to which Code Sec. 351, 354, 355, or 356 applies and is not sold, exchanged, or distributed in any transaction described in regulations in which the transferor does not recognize the entire amount of the gain or loss realized in the transaction (an exception applies to a distribution of stock to an unrelated person in which the full amount of stock gain would be recognized in certain Code Sec. 355 transactions); and (3) the stock is not sold, exchanged, or distributed to a related person.

Stock disposed of by the seller to another person that is reacquired by the seller during the 12-month disposition period is not considered as disposed of by the seller. If a seller retains any target stock after the 12-month disposition period, the seller is treated as purchasing the retained stock from an unrelated person on the day after the disposition date for its fair market value. The holding period for the retained stock starts on the day after the disposition date. For this purpose, the fair market value of all the target stock equals the grossed-up amount realized on the sale, exchange, or distribution of recently disposed stock of the target.

A seller for this purpose is any domestic corporation that makes a qualified stock disposition of stock of another corporation. A seller includes both a transferor and a distributor of target stock. A purchaser is one or more persons that receive the stock of another corporation in a qualified stock disposition. A target corporation is any domestic corporation the stock of which is sold, exchanged, or distributed by another domestic corporation in a qualified stock disposition.

2265. Acquisition of Stock Treated as Acquisition of Assets. If a parent corporation purchases 80-percent control of a second corporation (the target) within a 12-month period, the parent may irrevocably elect to have the target treated as if it had sold and purchased its own assets (Code Sec. 338; Reg. § 1.338-3).[61] If the election is made, the target corporation is treated as a new corporation after the date of acquisition of 80-percent control. The hypothetical sale is deemed to have occurred on the date of acquisition of control. The target's tax year as the "selling corporation" ends on that date, its carryovers and other tax attributes disappear, and as the "purchasing corporation," it becomes a member of the affiliated group including the parent on the day

---

References are to Standard Federal Tax Reports; Tax Research Consultant; and Practical Tax Explanations.

[58] ¶ 16,051E; CCORP: 27,202.30

[59] ¶ 16,200, ¶ 16,205; CCORP: 27,162

[60] ¶ 16,203; CCORP: 27,162.

[61] ¶ 16,275, ¶ 16,278; CCORP: 30,000

following that date. Gain or loss is recognized by the target as though it had sold all of its assets at fair market value in a single transaction on the acquisition date. Recapture items are typically taken into account on the final return of the "selling corporation." The election is to be made no later than the 15th day of the 9th month beginning after the month in which 80-percent control is acquired. The parent is not required to liquidate the target corporation, but if it does, it succeeds to the basis of the target's assets, as increased by the hypothetical purchase.

There are detailed rules to ensure consistency of treatment for acquisitions of stock or assets by and from members of an affiliated group of corporations (Reg. § 1.338-4(h)).[62] A consolidated group may treat a sale of its 80-percent-controlled target as a sale of the target corporation's underlying assets. The assets receive a stepped-up basis to fair market value, and the selling consolidated group recognizes gain or loss attributable to the assets, but there is no separate tax on the seller's gain attributable to the stock. This treatment also applies in situations when the selling affiliated group owns 80 percent of the target's stock by value and voting power but does not file a consolidated return (Code Sec. 338(h)(10)).[63]

Carryforwards

2277. Carryovers in Certain Corporate Acquisitions. In a tax-free asset acquisition, certain tax attributes may be transferred or are carried over to the acquiring corporation (Code Sec. 381; Reg. § 1.381(a)-1).[64] This applies to a parent after complete liquidation of a subsidiary (¶ 2261), as well as a tax-free A, C, D, F, or G reorganization (¶ 2209). In the case of D and G reorganizations, however, the carryover of certain tax attributes only applies to acquisitive reorganizations, where substantially all of the assets are acquired and distributed, not to divisive reorganizations.

The carryover provisions are mandatory, even though in some cases they work to the disadvantage of the successor. They do not apply after a split-up, split-off, spin-off, or splint-off type of divisive reorganization (¶ 2201), or a partial liquidation. The tax-attribute items covered are listed in Code Sec. 381(c) and include, but are not limited to, net operating losses (NOLs), unused general business credits, capital loss carryovers, method of computing depreciation, and method of accounting. Even if a tax attribute properly carries over to an acquiring corporation, the acquiring corporation's ability to use the attribute may be limited (¶ 2281). If an acquiring corporation makes an election to treat the target corporation as having purchased its own assets (¶ 2265), there is no carryforward of attributes of the subsidiary for the periods prior to the parent's acquisition.

Carrybacks. Carrybacks of net operating losses (¶ 1149) and net capital losses (¶ 1756) are permitted from one corporate entity to another only in the case of an F reorganization—a mere change in identity, form, or place of organization (¶ 2209).

2281. Limitations on Use of Carryforwards in Corporate Acquisitions. After a reorganization or other change in corporate ownership, the use of certain carryforwards may be limited or prohibited (¶ 2277). The carryforwards involved concern:

  (1) net operating losses (NOLs);

  (2) unused general business credit;

  (3) corporate minimum tax credit;

  (4) foreign tax credit; and

  (5) capital loss carryovers (Code Secs. 382 and 383).[65]

After an ownership change, the amount of *income* that a corporation may offset each year by preacquisition NOL carryforwards (¶ 2285) is generally limited to an amount determined by multiplying the value of the equity of the corporation just prior to the ownership change by the federal long-term tax-exempt rate (¶ 85) in effect on the date

---

References are to Standard Federal Tax Reports; Tax Research Consultant; and Practical Tax Explanations.

[62] ¶ 16,279; CCORP: 30,300   [64] ¶ 17,002, ¶ 17,003; REORG: [65] ¶ 17,101, ¶ 17,200; REORG:
[63] ¶ 16,275; CCORP: 30,150   33,150   33,200, REORG: 33,250

of the change (Code Sec. 382).[66] Any unused limitation may be carried forward and added to the next year's limitation. In addition, NOL carryforwards are eliminated completely unless the business continuity requirements for reorganizations are satisfied for the two-year period following the ownership change. The annual income limitation is reduced by the recognition of any built-in losses and increased by the recognition of built-in gains. An exception to the limitations on NOL carryforwards is provided in bankruptcy situations, with certain restrictions.

Two kinds of ownership changes can trigger the income limitation: a change involving a five-percent shareholder, and any tax-free reorganization other than divisive and F reorganizations (¶ 2209). In either case, one or more of the five-percent shareholders must have increased their percentage of ownership in the corporation by more than 50 percent over their lowest pre-change ownership percentage (generally within three years of the ownership change). Similar rules apply to the other carryforwards, including those for net capital losses, unused general business credit, and foreign taxes (Code Sec. 383; Reg. § 1.383-1).[67]

Pre- and Post-change Allocation. A loss corporation must allocate NOLs or taxable income and net capital loss or gain for the change year between the pre-change period and the post-change period either by: (1) ratably allocating an equal portion to each day in the change year; or (2) electing to treat its books as closed on the date of the change (Reg. § 1.382-6).[68] If a "closing of the books" election is made, the amounts allocated to either period may not exceed the NOL or taxable income and net capital loss or gain for the change year.

Worthless Stock. In order to prevent a double tax benefit, the NOLs of a corporation may not be carried forward after an ownership change if a shareholder with 50-percent-or-more control (prior to the ownership change) claims, within three years, a worthless stock deduction with respect to the stock (Code Sec. 382(g)(4)(D)).[69]

Tax Avoidance Purpose. NOLs and other carryforwards may be disallowed if an acquisition is made with a tax avoidance purpose (¶ 1575).

2285. Limitation on Preacquisition Losses. A corporation (or any member of its affiliated group) may not use its preacquisition losses (net operating losses (NOLs), net built-in losses, net capital losses, and credit carryforwards, ¶ 2281) against the built-in gains of a company:

    (1) whose assets are acquired in an A, C, or D reorganization (¶ 2209); or

    (2) that becomes directly or indirectly controlled (80-percent ownership of its stock by vote and value) by the acquiring corporation.

The restriction generally applies to built-in gains recognized within five years of the acquisition date, unless 50 percent or more of the gain company has been owned by the loss corporation (or a member of its group) for five years prior to the acquisition (Code Sec. 384).[70]

The unrealized built-in gains of either the acquired or acquiring corporation are subject to the restriction. It applies to any successor corporation to the same extent as to its predecessor, and all members of the same affiliated group before the acquisition are treated as one corporation.

References are to Standard Federal Tax Reports; Tax Research Consultant; and Practical Tax Explanations.

[66] ¶ 17,101; REORG: 33,200
[67] ¶ 17,200, ¶ 17,204; REORG: 33,250
[68] ¶ 17,111; REORG: 33,208
[69] ¶ 17,101; REORG: 33,200
[70] ¶ 17,300; REORG: 33,300

Chapter 23

SPECIAL CORPORATE STATUS

Mutual Funds

2301. Qualification as a Mutual Fund. Mutual funds (regulated investment companies) are domestic corporations that act as investment agents for their shareholders, typically investing in corporate and government securities and distributing income earned from the investments as dividends. Mutual funds may escape corporate taxation because, unlike ordinary corporations, they are entitled to claim a deduction for dividends paid (¶ 259) to shareholders against their ordinary income and net capital gain. A corporation qualifies as a mutual fund if it makes an irrevocable election to be treated as such by filing Form 1120-RIC, and it meets all of the following requirements (Code Sec. 851).[1]

- The corporation must be registered under the Investment Company Act of 1940 as a management company, unit investment trust, business development company, or as a type of common trust fund.

- At least 90 percent of its gross income must be derived from dividends, interest, payments with respect to certain securities loans, gains from the sale or disposition of stock, securities, or foreign currencies, or other income derived from the business of investing, including the net investment income of qualified publicly traded partnerships.

- At the close of each quarter of the tax year, at least 50 percent of its total assets must be invested in cash, government securities, securities of other mutual funds, or the securities of other issuers (so long as the securities of any given issuer do not exceed five percent of the value of the mutual fund's assets or 10 percent of the issuer's outstanding voting securities).

- At the close of each quarter of the tax year, no more than 25 percent of the total value of its assets may be invested in the securities of any one issuer (other than government securities or securities of other mutual funds), the securities of two or more issuers controlled by the mutual fund and engaged in a related trade or business, or the securities of one or more qualified publicly traded partnerships.

- The corporation must distribute at least 90 percent of its annual investment company taxable income (¶ 2303) and its net tax-exempt interest income (¶ 2307) to its shareholders (there is no threshold for net capital gains) (Code Sec. 852(a)).[2]

2303. Taxation of Mutual Funds. A mutual fund (regulated investment company) (¶ 2301) is subject to taxation at regular corporate income tax rates on its investment company taxable income (Code Sec. 852(b); Reg. § 1.852-3).[3] Investment company taxable income is computed on Form 1120-RIC in the same manner as the taxable income of an ordinary corporation (¶ 221) with the following adjustments:

- gross income is the fund's ordinary income (net capital gains are not included);

References are to Standard Federal Tax Reports; Tax Research Consultant; and Practical Tax Explanations.

[1] ¶ 26,400; RIC: 3,000, RIC: 3,050; § 19,201, § 45,430.05

[2] ¶ 26,420; RIC: 3,060; § 19,201, § 45,430.05

[3] ¶ 26,420, ¶ 26,424; RIC: 3,200; § 19,201, § 45,430.05

- a deduction is allowed for any ordinary dividends paid (¶ 259), but no deduction is allowed for dividends of capital gains or tax-exempt interest;
- no deduction is allowed for dividends received;
- no deduction is allowed for net operating losses (NOLs);
- taxable income of a short tax year is not annualized;
- if the fund so elects, taxable income is computed by disregarding the short-term discount obligation rules of Code Sec. 454(b); and
- a deduction is allowed for the tax imposed on the fund if it fails to meet the asset test or gross income test (¶ 2301).

For purposes of the dividends-paid deduction, dividends declared and payable by a mutual fund in October, November, or December of a calendar year are treated as paid on December 31 of that year if they are actually paid in January of the following calendar year (Code Sec. 852(b)(7)).[4] See ¶ 2323 for discussion of the treatment of certain dividends declared after the close of the mutual fund's tax year.

A mutual fund, other than a publicly traded mutual fund, generally may not claim a deduction for dividend distributions if it singles out one class of shareholders or one or more members of a class of shareholders for special dividend treatment, unless such treatment was originally intended when the dividend rights were created (Code Sec. 562(c); Rev. Rul. 89-81).[5] However, the IRS has issued guidance describing the conditions under which distributions to mutual fund shareholders may vary and nevertheless be deductible, including the treatment of distributions to shareholders that differ as a result of the allocation and payment of fees and expenses (Rev. Proc. 99-40).[6]

Excise Taxes. A nondeductible excise tax is generally imposed on a mutual fund that does not satisfy minimum distribution requirements (Code Sec. 4982).[7] The tax is four percent of the excess of any required distribution for the calendar year over the amount actually distributed for the calendar year. For this purpose, the required distribution is the sum of 98 percent of the fund's ordinary income for the year, plus 98.2 percent of its net capital gain income for the one-year period ending October 31 of the calendar year. Special rules apply to how a mutual fund treats post-October 31 capital gains and foreign currency losses. For excise tax purposes, amendments made in 2010 to the capital loss carryover rules (¶ 2305) apply beginning with any net capital loss recognized in the period that determines a mutual fund's required distribution for calendar year 2011 (Rev. Rul. 2012-29).[8]

Built-in Gains Tax. A mutual fund may be subject to a modified version of the built-in gains tax imposed on S corporations (¶ 337) if property owned by a C corporation becomes property of the mutual fund when the corporation qualifies as a mutual fund, or if property of a C corporation is transferred to the mutual fund (Reg. § 1.337(d)-7).[9] The tax does not apply, however, if the corporation makes a deemed sale election to recognize gain and loss as if it sold the converted property to an unrelated person at fair market value. The tax also does not apply if the corporation otherwise recognizes gain or loss on the conversion transaction, or if the corporation's gain is not recognized in a like-kind exchange or an involuntary conversion.

2305. Capital Gains and Losses of Mutual Funds. A mutual fund (regulated investment company) (¶ 2301) may avoid corporate level tax on its net capital gains by distributing such gains to shareholders. If the mutual fund elects to retain some of its net capital gains, then it is subject to tax at regular capital gains rates (¶ 1738) on the excess of its net capital gains for the tax year over the amount of any capital gains dividends paid during the year (Code Sec. 852(b)(3)).[10] Form 2438 is used to figure and report the fund's capital gains. Although the fund is taxed on its undistributed net capital

---

References are to Standard Federal Tax Reports; Tax Research Consultant; and Practical Tax Explanations.

[4] ¶ 26,420; RIC: 3,460; § 19,205.50

[5] ¶ 23,470, ¶ 26,433.50; RIC: 3,204.10

[6] ¶ 26,433.28; RIC: 3,204.10

[7] ¶ 34,640; RIC: 3,212; § 19,201, § 45,430.05

[8] ¶ 34,642.10; RIC: 3,212; § 19,201, § 45,430.05

[9] ¶ 16,241H; RIC: 3,550

[10] ¶ 26,420; RIC: 3,250; § 19,205.05, § 45,430.10

gains, it may elect to designate to its shareholders some or all of its undistributed gains and the tax paid on those gains. Form 2439 is used to notify each shareholder of his or her portion of the undistributed capital gains and tax paid for the year (¶ 2309 and ¶ 2311). The mutual fund must also report any undistributed long-term capital gains not designated to shareholders and any net short-term capital gain on Form 8949 and Schedule D (Form 1120).

Capital Loss Carryovers. If a mutual fund has a net capital loss for a tax year, any excess of the net short-term capital loss over the net long-term capital gain is treated as a short-term capital loss arising on the first day of the next tax year, and any excess of the net long-term capital loss over the net short-term capital gain is treated as a long-term capital loss arising on the first day of the next tax year (Code Sec. 1212(a)(3)(A)).[11] There is no limit to the number of tax years that a net capital loss of a mutual fund may be carried over.

If a net capital loss under the general corporate capital loss carryback and carryover rules (¶ 1756) is carried over to a tax year of a mutual fund, amounts treated as a long-term or short-term capital loss arising on the first day of the next tax year under the capital loss carryover rules for mutual funds (discussed above) are determined without regard to amounts treated as a short-term capital loss under the general corporate capital loss carryover rule. Further, in determining the reduction of a carryover by capital gain net income for a prior tax year under the general corporate capital loss carryover rule, any capital loss treated as arising on the first day of the prior tax year under the capital loss carryover rules for mutual funds is taken into account in determining capital gain net income for the prior year (Code Sec. 1212(a)(3)(B)). Capital gain net income is the excess of gains from the sale or exchange of capital assets over losses from such sales or exchanges (Code Sec. 1222(9)).[12]

2307. Tax-Exempt Interest of Mutual Funds. A mutual fund (regulated investment company) (¶ 2301) may pay tax-exempt interest earned on state or local bonds to its shareholders in the form of exempt-interest dividends, but only if the bonds represent at least 50 percent of the value of the fund's assets at the close of each quarter of its tax year (Code Sec. 852(b)(5)).[13] Form 1099-INT is used to inform shareholders of dividends identified as tax-exempt interest dividends (¶ 2309 and ¶ 2311).

An upper-tier mutual fund that is a qualified fund of funds may pass through exempt-interest dividends to its shareholders without having to meet the 50-percent asset requirement (Code Sec. 852(g)).[14] A qualified fund of funds is a mutual fund if, at the close of each quarter of the tax year, at least 50 percent of the value of its total assets is represented by interests in other mutual funds.

If a mutual fund shareholder receives an exempt-interest dividend with respect to any share held for six months or less, then any loss on the sale or exchange of such share is generally disallowed to the extent of the exempt-interest dividend (Code Sec. 852(b)(4)).[15] However, the disallowance of a loss on the sale or exchange of mutual fund shares on which exempt-interest dividends have been paid does not apply, except as otherwise provided by regulations, to a regular dividend paid by a mutual fund that declares exempt-interest dividends on a daily basis in an amount not less than 90 percent of its net tax-exempt interest and distributes such dividends on a monthly or more frequent basis.

2309. Designation of Mutual Fund Distributions. A mutual fund (regulated investment company) (¶ 2301) must report in written statements furnished to its shareholders the portions of distributions made during the tax year that are capital gains dividends (¶ 2305) and exempt-interest dividends (¶ 2307), as well as any foreign tax credits (¶ 2320), tax credit bond credits (¶ 2320), dividends that qualify for the dividends-received deduction (¶ 223), and passed-through ordinary dividends eligible for the

---

References are to Standard Federal Tax Reports; Tax Research Consultant; and Practical Tax Explanations.

[11] ¶ 30,400; RIC: 3,252; § 16,535

[12] ¶ 30,440; SALES: 15,202.45; § 16,535

[13] ¶ 26,420; RIC: 3,300; § 19,205.05, § 45,430.10

[14] ¶ 26,420; RIC: 3,302; § 19,205.35

[15] ¶ 26,420; RIC: 3,304, SALES: 45,406.20; § 19,230.10

reduced tax rate for qualified dividends (¶ 2311) (Code Secs. 852(b)(3)(C) and (5), 853(c), 853A(c), and 854(b)).[16] Capital gain dividends, dividends received from a tax-exempt corporation, and dividends received from a qualified real estate investment trust (REIT) (¶ 2326) are not eligible for the dividends-received deduction (Code Sec. 854(a) and (b)(2)). The aggregate amount that the mutual fund can report as dividends eligible for the dividends-received deduction is limited to its aggregate dividends received from domestic corporations for the tax year. The aggregate amount that the mutual fund can report as qualified dividend income is limited to its qualified dividend income for the tax year (Code Sec. 854(b)(1)(C)).

Additionally, within 60 days after the close of its tax year, a mutual fund must report and notify its shareholders of the portion of distributions made during the tax year that is designated as undistributed capital gain (Code Sec. 852(b)(3)(D)).

2311. Taxation of Mutual Fund Distributions. The tax treatment of a distribution received from a mutual fund (regulated investment company) (¶ 2301) depends on how the distribution is designated (¶ 2309). Distributions not designated as capital gain dividends are generally treated by shareholders as ordinary income to the extent of the fund's earnings and profits. However, all or a portion of the distribution of an ordinary dividend may be a qualified dividend eligible to be taxed at capital gains rates (¶ 733) if the aggregate amount of qualified dividends received by the fund during the year is less than 95 percent of its gross income (Code Sec. 854(b)(1)(B)).[17] Distributions reported as tax-exempt interest dividends may generally be excluded from the shareholder's gross income (Code Sec. 852(b)(5)(B)).[18] However, exempt-interest dividends derived from private activity bonds constitute tax preference items for alternative minimum tax (AMT) purposes (¶ 1425).

Distributions received from a mutual fund reported as capital gain dividends may be treated as long-term capital gains by the shareholder for income and AMT purposes, regardless of how long the shareholder held the shares (Code Sec. 852(b)(3)(B)).[19] Similarly, capital gains that the fund elects to pass through to the shareholder are treated as long-term capital gains (¶ 2305). The shareholder is entitled to a credit or refund for its portion of any capital gain taxes paid by the mutual fund on the undistributed capital gains (Code Sec. 852(b)(3)(D)). In addition, the shareholder may increase the basis of its mutual fund shares by the difference between the undistributed capital gains and its deemed portion of taxes paid. The mutual fund must designate distributions as undistributed capital gain dividends, reporting the designation and providing shareholders a written notice within 60 days of the end of its tax year (¶ 2309).

If a shareholder receives a capital gain dividend or has capital gain passed through by the fund with respect to any share or beneficial interest, and holds the share for six months or less, then any loss on the sale of that share is treated as a long-term capital loss to the extent of any long-term capital gain (Code Sec. 852(b)(4)).[20] In addition, the amount of loss that may be claimed must also be reduced by the amount of any exempt-interest dividend received on the shares. These rules do not apply to losses incurred on the disposition of mutual fund shares or beneficial interests pursuant to a plan that provides for the periodic liquidation of such shares or interests. For purposes of determining whether a taxpayer has held mutual fund shares for six months or less, rules similar to those for the dividends-received deduction are applied (¶ 223). A mutual fund shareholder may also not claim a loss from the sale or exchange of mutual fund shares if the wash sale rules apply (¶ 1935).

A distribution that is not out of a mutual fund's earnings and profits is a return of the shareholder's investment. Return-of-capital distributions are generally not subject to tax, and they reduce the shareholder's basis in the mutual fund shares. On the other hand, mutual fund distributions that are automatically reinvested by the shareholder into more

---

References are to Standard Federal Tax Reports; Tax Research Consultant; and Practical Tax Explanations.

[16] ¶ 26,420, ¶ 26,440, ¶ 26,448, ¶ 26,460; RIC: 3,400; § 19,205.05

[17] ¶ 26,460; RIC: 3,400; § 19,205.10, § 19,205.15

[18] ¶ 26,420; RIC: 3,304; § 19,205.35

[19] ¶ 26,420; RIC: 3,250; § 19,205.20, § 19,205.25

[20] ¶ 26,420; RIC: 3,258; § 19,230.15

shares of the fund are taxed as if they had actually been received by shareholder in cash. Thus, reinvested ordinary dividends and reinvested capital gain distributions are generally taxed as income, reinvested exempt-interest dividends are not reported as income, and reinvested return-of-capital distributions are reported as a return of capital (IRS Pub. 550).

2313. Earnings and Profits of Mutual Funds. Dividends from a mutual fund (regulated investment company), just like dividends from most other corporations, must be paid out of earnings and profits (¶ 747—¶ 757) (Code Secs. 301, 312, 316, 561, 562(a), and 852(a)(1)).[21] Thus, a mutual fund must maintain sufficient current or accumulated earnings and profits to satisfy annual dividend distribution requirements. There should also be enough earnings and profits to avoid the excise tax on the undistributed income (¶ 2303).

A mutual fund's earnings and profits are generally computed under the rules that apply to ordinary corporations. However, mutual funds do not reduce their current earnings and profits by any amount they are unable to claim as a deduction from taxable income in that year (Code Sec. 852(c)(1)).[22] Net capital loss for a tax year is not taken into account in determining earnings and profits; but any capital loss treated as arising on the first day of the following tax year is taken into account in determining earnings and profits for that year (subject to the application of the net capital loss rule for that year). Also, deductions disallowed in computing mutual fund taxable income with respect to tax-exempt interest are allowed in calculating a mutual fund's current earnings and profits (but not accumulated earnings and profits).

If a mutual fund that is not a calendar-year taxpayer makes distributions to its shareholders with respect to any class of stock of the company in excess of the sum of its current and accumulated earnings and profits (i.e., a portion of the distribution constitutes return of capital or capital gain), its current earnings and profits must be allocated first to distributions during the mutual fund's tax year that are made before January 1 (Code Sec. 316(b)(4)).[23] If a mutual fund has more than one class of stock, this rule applies separately to each class of stock, so that distributions made during the corporation's tax year are considered to be made to the shares with higher priority before they are made to shares with lower priority (Rev. Rul. 69-440).[24]

A company that has failed to qualify as a mutual fund because it has not purged itself of non-mutual fund earnings and profits may still qualify if it distributes those earnings and profits with interest to its shareholders (Code Sec. 852(e)).[25] In order to qualify, distributions must be specifically designated as non-mutual fund distributions and take place within the 90-day period that begins on the date the corporation is determined not to be a mutual fund (¶ 2317). This option is not available if the corporation was determined not to be a mutual fund because it engaged in fraudulent tax evasion.

2315. Redemption of Mutual Fund Shares. A redemption of stock by a corporation, including a mutual fund (regulated investment company) (¶ 2301), is generally treated as an exchange of stock if the redemption falls within one of four categories of transactions (Code Sec. 302):[26] (1) a redemption that is not essentially equivalent to a dividend; (2) a substantially disproportionate redemption; (3) a redemption that terminates the shareholder's interest in the corporation; or (4) a partial liquidation, in the case of a noncorporate shareholder. Redemptions of corporate stock are discussed in ¶ 742—¶ 745. Because transactions that fall within one of these four categories are treated as exchanges of stock, they normally result in capital gain treatment to the shareholder. If the redemption does not fall within any of these categories, it is treated as a Code Sec. 301 distribution of property that generally results in dividend treatment.

References are to Standard Federal Tax Reports; Tax Research Consultant; and Practical Tax Explanations.

[21] ¶ 15,302, ¶ 15,600, ¶ 15,702, ¶ 23,450, ¶ 23,470, ¶ 26,420; RIC: 3,204.15; § 26,601

[22] ¶ 26,420; RIC: 3,204.15; § 19,201

[23] ¶ 15,702; RIC: 3,204.15

[24] ¶ 15,704.755; CCORP: 12,166, RIC: 3,204.15

[25] ¶ 26,420; RIC: 3,202

[26] ¶ 15,325; CCORP: 21,104; § 26,301

Special rules apply to redemptions of mutual fund shares. A distribution in redemption of stock of a publicly offered mutual fund is treated as an exchange for stock if the redemption is upon the demand by the stockholder and the mutual fund issues only stock that is redeemable upon the demand of the stockholder. A publicly offered mutual fund is a fund whose shares are: (1) continuously offered pursuant to a public offering; (2) regularly traded on an established securities market; or (3) held by or for no fewer than 500 persons at all times during the tax year (Code Sec. 67(c)(2)(B)).[27] Additionally, the loss disallowance and deferral rules for transactions between related persons (¶ 1717) do not apply to any redemption of stock of a fund-of-funds mutual fund if the mutual fund issues only stock that is redeemable upon the demand of the stockholder and the redemption is upon the demand of another mutual fund (Code Sec. 267(f)(3)(D)).[28]

2317. Deficiency Dividends of Mutual Funds. If there is a determination that adjustments are needed to certain amounts that a mutual fund (regulated investment company) (¶ 2301) reports for a tax year, and if the adjustments could cause the entity to lose its mutual fund status, the mutual fund may avoid disqualification by making deficiency dividend distributions, and may claim a deduction for such dividends paid (Code Sec. 860; Reg. §§ 1.860-1—1.860-5).[29] A deficiency dividend is a distribution of property (including money) that would have been includible in calculating the entity's dividends-paid deduction had the property been distributed during the tax year. The distribution must be made within 90 days after the determination date, and before the entity files a deficiency dividend deduction claim, which must be filed on Form 976 within 120 days after the determination date.

For a mutual fund, an adjustment can be: (1) an increase in its investment company taxable income, determined without regard to the dividends-paid deduction; (2) an increase in the amount of the excess of its net capital gain over its deduction for capital gain dividends paid; or (3) a decrease in its dividends-paid deduction (determined without regard to capital gains dividends). A determination is a final decision by a court, a closing agreement, an agreement between the IRS and the entity relating to its tax liability, or a statement by the entity attached to its amendment or supplement to a tax return for the relevant tax year. Filing Form 8927 is treated as a "self-determination" by the entity for these purposes (Rev. Proc. 2009-28).[30]

The deficiency dividend deduction is not available if part of the adjustment is due to fraud with intent to evade tax or willful failure to file a timely income tax return.

2318. Basis in Mutual Fund Shares. A shareholder's basis in the shares of a mutual fund (regulated investment company) (¶ 2301) is usually the cost to purchase the shares, including any fees or load charges incurred to acquire or redeem them (¶ 1975). Fees or load charges are not added to the shareholder's original basis if the shareholder acquires a reinvestment right, disposes of the shares within 90 days of being purchased, and acquires new shares in the same (or another) mutual fund for which the fee or load charge is reduced or waived because of the reinvestment right (Code Sec. 852(f)).[31] In such cases, the omission of the load charge from basis applies to the extent the charge does not exceed the reduction in the load charge for the new investment. To the extent that a load charge is not taken into account in determining the purchaser's gain or loss, it is treated as incurred in connection with the acquisition of the second-acquired shares.

The treatment of load charges applies only if the original mutual fund stock is disposed of within 90 days after the date it was originally acquired and the taxpayer acquires stock in the same or another mutual fund during the period beginning on the date of the disposition of the original stock, and ending on January 31 of the calendar year following the calendar year that includes the date of such disposition for this rule to apply.

References are to Standard Federal Tax Reports; Tax Research Consultant; and Practical Tax Explanations.

[27] ¶ 6060; RIC: 3,204.10; § 19,210.07

[28] ¶ 14,150; SALES: 39,100; § 19,210.07

[29] ¶ 26,580, ¶ 26,581— ¶ 26,585; RIC: 3,500

[30] ¶ 42,625.435; RIC: 3,500

[31] ¶ 26,420; SALES: 6,068, SALES: 45,404.05; § 19,215.05

The original basis of mutual fund shares acquired by reinvesting distributions (even exempt-interest dividends) is the amount of the distributions used to buy each full or fractional share (¶ 1975). A shareholder's original basis in shares acquired by gift is generally the donor's adjusted basis (¶ 1630). However, if the fair market value of the shares was more than the donor's adjusted basis, then the shareholder's basis is the donor's adjusted basis at the time of the gift, plus all or part of any gift tax paid. A shareholder's basis in mutual fund shares that are inherited is generally the fair market value of the shares at the decedent's death (or the alternate valuation date if the estate chooses) (¶ 1633). No matter how a shareholder's original basis is determined, it must be adjusted for post-acquisition occurrences such as reinvestment of distributions and return of capital distributions (¶ 2311).

2320. Tax Credit Elections. A mutual fund (regulated investment company) (¶ 2301) may elect to have its foreign tax credit (¶ 2475) claimed by its shareholders on their tax returns instead of its own. The election can only be made if more than 50 percent of the value of the fund's total assets at the close of the tax year consists of stock or securities in foreign corporations and it has distributed at least 90 percent of its investment company taxable income (¶ 2303) and net tax-exempt interest (¶ 2307) for the year (Code Sec. 853).[32]

An upper-tier mutual fund that is a qualified fund of funds may pass through foreign tax credits to its shareholders without having to meet the 50-percent asset requirement (Code Sec. 852(g)).[33] A qualified fund of funds is a mutual fund at least 50 percent of the total value of whose assets (as measured at the close of each quarter of its tax year) is represented by interests in other mutual funds.

A mutual fund may also elect to pass through to its shareholders credits attributable to tax credit bonds (¶ 1371) held by the mutual fund (Code Sec. 853A).[34]

2323. Mutual Fund Distributions After Tax Year Ends. A mutual fund (regulated investment company) may declare and pay spillover dividends after the close of a tax year that are considered made out of a mutual fund's earnings and profits for that year (Code Sec. 855(a); Reg. § 1.855-1).[35] Spillover dividends are included in the calculation of mutual fund taxable income for that year and are considered in determining whether the mutual fund met its distribution requirements for the year. Spillover dividends must be declared no later than the fifteenth day of the ninth month following the close of the tax year to which the dividend relates, or the extended due date for the mutual fund's return for the tax year, whichever comes later. The dividend must be paid to shareholders in the 12-month period after the close of the tax year to which the dividend relates, but no later than the date of the first dividend payment *of the same type of dividend* (e.g., capital gains or ordinary) after the declaration.

The shareholder generally must treat such a dividend as received in the tax year in which the distribution is made. This does not apply, however, to dividends declared in October, November, or December that are treated as paid on December 31 of a calendar year even though they are actually paid in January of the following calendar year (¶ 2303) (Code Sec. 855(b)).

Real Estate Investment Trusts

2326. Qualification as a REIT. A corporation, trust, or association that acts as an investment agent specializing in real estate and real estate mortgages may elect to be a real estate investment trust (REIT) (Code Sec. 856).[36] REITs may escape corporation taxation because, unlike ordinary corporations, they are entitled to claim a deduction for dividends paid to shareholders against their ordinary income and net capital gains (¶ 259). An entity qualifies as a REIT if it makes an election to be treated as such by filing Form 1120-REIT, and it meets certain requirements as to ownership and organization, source of income, investment of assets, and distribution of income to shareholders.

References are to Standard Federal Tax Reports; Tax Research Consultant; and Practical Tax Explanations.

[32] ¶ 26,440; RIC: 3,350; § 19,240.10

[33] ¶ 26,420; RIC: 3,352; § 19,240.10

[34] ¶ 26,448; RIC: 3,364; § 14,505

[35] ¶ 26,480, ¶ 26,481; RIC: 3,450

[36] ¶ 26,500; RIC: 6,050; § 19,201, § 45,440.05

¶ 2320

The REIT election may be revoked voluntarily, but the organization will be prohibited from making a new REIT election for the four tax years after revocation. An organization may elect REIT status even if it fails the ownership test in the first year.

Ownership and Organization Requirements. To be eligible for REIT status, an entity must be taxable as a domestic corporation (Code Sec. 856(a)). Foreign corporations, trusts, and associations, as well as financial institutions such as banks and insurance companies, are not eligible. An eligible entity must be managed by one or more trustees or directors during the entire tax year. It must also adopt a calendar-year accounting period (Code Sec. 859).[37] An entity making a REIT election may change its accounting period to a calendar year without seeking IRS approval.

Beneficial ownership in a REIT must be evidenced by transferable shares or certificates of interest. The REIT must have at least 100 beneficial owners for at least 335 days of a 12-month tax year (Code Sec. 856(a) and (b)). Ownership cannot be closely held as determined under the personal holding company rules (¶ 285) (Code Sec. 856(h)).[38] However, attribution to another partner in a partnership is ignored. In addition, a pension trust generally is not treated as a single owner, but any REIT shares or certificates of interest held by the trust are treated as directly held by its beneficiaries. The look-through rule does not apply if persons disqualified from dealings with the pension trust own five percent or more of the value of the REIT and the REIT has accumulated earnings and profits attributable to a year it did not qualify as a REIT.

Income Requirements. An entity must satisfy the following income tests each tax year in order to qualify as a REIT (Code Sec. 856(c)(2) and (3)):[39]

- at least 95 percent of the entity's gross income must be from rents from real property, gain from the disposition of real property, dividends, interest, gains from dispositions of stock and securities, abatements and refunds of real property taxes, income and gain from foreclosure property, consideration received or accrued for agreeing to make loans secured by real property mortgages or interests or to purchase or lease real property, and certain mineral royalty income earned from real property owned by a timber REIT; and

- at least 75 percent of the entity's gross income must be from real property sources, which include rents from real property, interest on real property mortgages, gain from the disposition of real property or mortgage interests, dividends and gain from the disposition of shares in other qualifying REITs, abatements and refunds of real property taxes, income and gain from foreclosure property, consideration received or accrued for agreeing to make loans secured by real property mortgages or interests or to purchase or lease real property, and qualified temporary investment income.

For both tests, an entity's gross income does not include the gross income from prohibited transactions (¶ 2329), foreign currency gains in the form of passive foreign exchange gains, or real estate foreign exchange gains (Code Sec. 856(n)),[40] as well as gains from hedging transactions entered into by the entity to reduce the risk of debt incurred to acquire or hold real estate or to manage the risk of currency fluctuations (Code Sec. 856(c)(5)(G)).[41] The IRS has the authority to designate income as not constituting gross income for purposes of the REIT income tests. Alternatively, the IRS may designate nonqualified income as qualified income (Code Sec. 856(c)(5)(J)).[42]

Rents from real property generally include: rents from interests in real property; amounts received for customary services (utilities, maintenance), even if separate charges are made for such services; and rent attributable to personal property incidental to rental of real property if the amount allocable to personal property is 15 percent or less of the total rent (Code Sec. 856(d)).[43] Rents from real property do *not* include amounts received from: (1) any noncorporate person in which the REIT owns 10 percent

References are to Standard Federal Tax Reports; Tax Research Consultant; and Practical Tax Explanations.

[37] ¶ 26,560; RIC: 6,050, RIC: 6,052; § 38,135.10
[38] ¶ 26,500; RIC: 6,052.30
[39] ¶ 26,500; RIC: 6,054; § 45,440.05
[40] ¶ 26,500; RIC: 6,054.05
[41] ¶ 26,500; RIC: 6,054.05, RIC: 6,054.15
[42] ¶ 26,500; RIC: 6,054
[43] ¶ 26,500; RIC: 6,056

¶2326

or more in that person's assets or profits; (2) a corporation, if the REIT owns 10 percent or more of either the voting stock or the value of all shares issued by the corporation; or (3) amounts received based on income or profits of a tenant or debtor (unless certain conditions are met). Rents from real property also do not include rents that depend on income or profits derived by any person from the property; exceptions exist to this general prohibition.

Amounts paid to a REIT by a taxable REIT subsidiary (¶ 2340) are not excluded from the definition of if rents from real property at least 90 percent of the property at issue is rented to unrelated parties at rents comparable to those paid by other tenants for comparable space (Code Sec. 856(d)(8)). In addition, a taxable REIT subsidiary may lease a qualified lodging facility or a qualified health care property, and the rents paid are treated as rents from real property so long as the facility is operated by an eligible independent contractor for a fee.

An entity that fails to meet either of the income tests for any tax year may still qualify as a REIT if it identifies the failure on a separate schedule prescribed by the IRS and the failure is due to reasonable cause and not willful neglect (Code Sec. 856(c)(6)).[44] The REIT also must pay a tax equal to the greater of the amount by which the entity fails to meet either the 95-percent or 75-percent income test, multiplied by the fraction of the REIT's taxable income over its gross income for the tax year (Code Sec. 857(b)(5)).[45]

Asset Requirements. A REIT must meet the following requirements regarding its assets at the close of each quarter of the tax year:

- at least 75 percent of the value of its total assets must consist of real estate assets (including interests in a REMIC (¶ 2343)), cash items (including receivables), and government securities;

- no more than 25 percent of the value of its total assets can be invested in securities other than those representing real estate assets or government securities;

- no more than 25 percent of the value of total assets can be invested in securities of taxable REIT subsidiaries (¶ 2340); and

- except for government securities and securities of taxable REIT subsidiaries, no more than five percent of the value of its total assets can be invested in the securities of any one issuer, and investment in the securities of any one issuer cannot exceed 10 percent of the total value or voting power of that issuer's outstanding securities (Code Sec. 856(c)(4)).[46]

For purposes of the limitation that a REIT may not hold more than 10 percent of the value of the outstanding securities of a single issuer, certain obligations are not treated as securities of an issuer, including straight debt securities, loans to an individual or estate, section 467 rental agreements (¶ 1541), or any obligation to pay rents from real property (Code Sec. 856(m)).[47] A straight debt security is debt payable on demand or on a specified date where the interest rate and interest payments are not contingent on profits, the borrower's discretion, or similar factors, and there is no convertibility (directly or indirectly) into stock (Code Sec. 1361(c)(5)(B)).[48] However, special rules permit certain contingencies of straight debt.

An entity that fails to meet any of the asset requirements for a particular tax quarter (other than the 5-percent and 10-percent asset tests) may still qualify as a REIT if:

(1) it identifies the failure on a separate schedule prescribed by the IRS;

(2) failure is due to reasonable cause and not willful neglect;

(3) the assets causing the failure are disposed of within six months of the last day of the quarter in which the failure occurred; and

(4) the REIT pays an excise tax (Code Sec. 856(c)(7)).[49]

References are to Standard Federal Tax Reports; Tax Research Consultant; and Practical Tax Explanations.

[44] ¶ 26,500; RIC: 6,054.20   [46] ¶ 26,500; RIC: 6,072   [48] ¶ 32,021; RIC: 6,072.10
[45] ¶ 26,520; RIC: 6,054.20   [47] ¶ 26,500; RIC: 6,072.10   [49] ¶ 26,500; RIC: 6,072.25

¶2326

The tax is the greater of $50,000 or the tax on the net income generated by the assets during the period of failure at the highest corporate rate (¶ 219). A REIT will not lose its exempt status for a *de minimis* failure to meet the 5- or 10-percent asset requirements if the failure is due to ownership of assets the total value of which does not exceed the lesser of one percent of the total value of the REIT's assets at the end of a tax quarter or $10 million. The REIT must dispose of the assets causing the failure within six months of the last day of the quarter in which the failure occurred.

Distribution of Income. To qualify as a REIT, an entity generally must distribute to its shareholders during the tax year the sum of 90 percent of its ordinary taxable income (determined without the deduction for dividends paid and excluding net capital gain) (¶ 2329) and 90 percent of its net income from foreclosure property (less the tax imposed on that income), minus its excess noncash income (Code Sec. 857(a)).[50] The IRS has the authority to waiver this requirement if failure is due to distributions necessary to avoid imposition of the excise tax on undistributed REIT income.

Other Failures. If an entity fails to satisfy one or more requirements of REIT qualification other than the income tests or asset requirements, then the entity may still retain REIT qualification if the failure is due to reasonable cause and not willful neglect. However, the REIT must pay a penalty of $50,000 for each failure (Code Sec. 856(g)(5)).[51]

2329. Taxation of REITs. An entity that qualifies as a real estate investment trust (REIT) (¶ 2326) is subject to regular corporate income tax rates on its taxable income (Code Sec. 857(b)).[52] A REIT's taxable income is computed on Form 1120-REIT in the same manner as an ordinary corporation with the following adjustments.

• A deduction is allowed for dividends paid (¶ 259), but without regard to dividends attributable to the net income from foreclosure property.

• Net income from foreclosure property or a prohibited transaction is disregarded.

• The special deductions available to corporations (¶ 223—¶ 231), including the dividends-received deduction, are not allowed, but the deduction for organizational expenditures (¶ 237) is allowed.

• Any tax imposed on redetermined rents, redetermined deductions, and excess interest under Code Sec. 857(b)(7), and any tax imposed for failures to meet the income, asset, or other REIT qualification requirements (¶ 2326), are deducted.

• Taxable income is not annualized in the case of a change in accounting periods.

For purposes of the dividends-paid deduction, dividends declared and payable in October, November, or December of a calendar year are treated as paid on December 31 of that year if they are actually paid in January of the following calendar year (Code Sec. 857(b)(9)).[53] See ¶ 2339 for discussion of the treatment of dividends declared after the close of the REIT's tax year.

Capital Gains. If a REIT has any net capital gains in the tax year, the tax imposed on REIT taxable income is the lesser of: (1) the regular corporate tax on REIT taxable income; or (2) the regular corporate tax on REIT taxable income, determined by excluding net capital gains and by computing the deduction for dividends paid without capital gain dividends, plus 35 percent on the excess of the net capital gain minus any capital gain dividends paid (Code Sec. 857(b)(3)).[54]

A REIT may avoid the tax on its net capital gains by distributing the gains to its shareholders (¶ 2331). The REIT must designate any distributions as capital gain dividends in a written notice to the shareholders or beneficiaries with its annual report or within 30 days of the end of the tax year. For purposes of determining the maximum

---

References are to Standard Federal Tax Reports; Tax Research Consultant; and Practical Tax Explanations.

[50] ¶ 26,520; RIC: 6,074
[51] ¶ 26,500; RIC: 6,078.05
[52] ¶ 26,520; RIC: 6,100
[53] ¶ 26,520; RIC: 6,104; § 19,205.50
[54] ¶ 26,520; RIC: 6,108

amount of capital gain dividends that a REIT may pay for a tax year, the REIT may not offset its net capital gains with the amount of any net operating losses (NOLs) (¶ 1145). In addition, the REIT must increase the amount of any NOL carryover to the extent it pays capital gains dividends in excess of its net income.

If the REIT does retain any net capital gains, it may elect to designate to its shareholders some or all of those undistributed amounts and the tax it paid on those gains. The REIT must make the designation in a written notice to its shareholders at any time before the end of the 60-day period after the close of its tax year, or that is mailed with its annual report for the tax year. The REIT uses Form 2438 to report and determine its tax on undistributed capital gains, and Form 2439 to inform each shareholder of his or her portion of the undistributed gains and any tax paid. Form 2439 must be provided within 60 days of the close of the REIT's tax year. The REIT must also report any undistributed long-term capital gains not designated to shareholders and any net short-term capital gain on Form 8949 and Schedule D (Form 1120).

Net Operating Losses. NOLs in a tax year that an entity is a REIT may only be carried forward, while NOLs in a tax year an entity is not a REIT may not be carried back to any year the entity was a REIT (¶ 1151) (Code Sec. 172(b)(1)(B)).[55]

Built-in Gains Tax. A REIT may be subject to a modified version of the built-in gains tax imposed on S corporations (¶ 337) if property owned by a C corporation becomes property of the REIT when the corporation qualifies as a REIT (¶ 2326), or if property of a C corporation is transferred to the REIT (Reg. § 1.337(d)-7).[56] The tax does not apply, however, if the corporation makes a deemed sale election to recognize gain and loss as if it sold the converted property to an unrelated person at fair market value. The tax also does not apply if the corporation otherwise recognizes gain or loss on the conversion transaction, or if the corporation's gain is not recognized in a like-kind exchange or an involuntary conversion.

Other Taxes. In addition to the tax on its taxable income, a REIT may be subject to the following additional taxes:

- a tax for failure to meet the REIT asset or income requirements for the tax year (¶ 2326);

- a tax at the highest corporate rate on net income from foreclosure property (Code Sec. 857(b)(4));[57]

- a 100-percent tax on the net income derived from a prohibited transaction (e.g., disposition of property, other than foreclosure property, that is held for sale to customers in the ordinary course of business) (Code Sec. 857(b)(6));[58]

- a four-percent excise tax on the amount of any taxable income that is undistributed at the end of the tax year, and calculated and paid on Form 8612 (Code Sec. 4981);[59] and

- a 100-percent tax on the excess portion of rents, deductions, and interest that must be reduced to clearly reflect income when a REIT and taxable REIT subsidiary (¶ 2340) engage in transactions other than those at arm's length (Code Sec. 857(b)(7)).[60]

2331. Taxation of REIT Distributions. Distributions received from a real estate investment trust (REIT) (¶ 2326) not designated as capital gain dividends are generally treated by shareholders as ordinary income to the extent of the REIT's earnings and profits. However, all or a portion of the distribution of a ordinary dividend may be a qualified dividend eligible to be taxed at capital gains rates (¶ 733). The amount a REIT can designate as qualified dividend income is limited to the sum of: (1) the REIT's qualified dividend income for the tax year; (2) the excess of the sum of REIT taxable income for the preceding tax year and the income subject to tax under the Code Sec. 337(d) regulations for that preceding tax year, over the taxes payable by the REIT under the REIT rules (¶ 2329) and the Code Sec. 337(d) regulations for that preceding tax

---

References are to Standard Federal Tax Reports; Tax Research Consultant; and Practical Tax Explanations.

[55] ¶ 12,002; RIC: 6,110   [57] ¶ 26,520; RIC: 6,114   [59] ¶ 34,620; RIC: 6,120
[56] ¶ 16,241H; RIC: 6,124   [58] ¶ 26,520; RIC: 6,116   [60] ¶ 26,520; RIC: 6,122

year; and (3) the amount of earnings and profits that were distributed by the REIT for the tax year and accumulated in tax years in which the entity was not a REIT. The amount of qualified dividends must be specified by the REIT in a written notice to shareholders no later than 60 days after the close of the tax year (Code Sec. 857(c)(2)).[61]

Distributions in excess of the REIT's earnings and profits (other than deficiency dividends (¶ 2337)) constitute a return of the shareholder's basis (¶ 754). Dividends received from a REIT do not qualify for the dividends-received deduction for corporations (¶ 223).

Distributions designated as capital gain dividends are treated as long-term capital gains by the shareholders, regardless of how long they held their interests in the REIT (Code Sec. 857(b)(3)).[62] This includes any undistributed capital gains designated by the REIT (¶ 2329). Shareholders are entitled to a credit or refund for their portion of any capital gain taxes paid by the REIT on the undistributed capital gains. In addition, a shareholder must increase the basis of his or her REIT shares by the difference between his or her portions of the undistributed capital gains and the deemed taxes paid. Certain capital gain distributions from REITs to foreign investors are treated as REIT dividends that are not capital gains (Code Sec. 857(b)(3)(F)).

If a shareholder receives a capital gain dividend or the REIT has designated undistributed capital gains with respect to any share or beneficial interest, and the shareholder holds the share for six months or less, then any loss on the sale of that share is treated as a long-term capital loss to the extent of the long-term capital gain dividend (Code Sec. 857(b)(8)).[63] This rule does not apply to losses incurred on the disposition of REIT stock or a beneficial interest under a plan that provides for the periodic liquidation of such shares or interests. For purposes of determining whether a taxpayer has held REIT stock or beneficial interest for six months or less, rules similar to those for the dividends-received deduction are applied (¶ 223).

2337. Deficiency Dividends of REITs. If there is a determination that adjustments are needed to certain amounts that a real estate investment trust (REIT) (¶ 2326) reports for a tax year, and if the adjustments could cause the entity to lose its REIT status, the REIT may avoid disqualification by making deficiency dividend distributions, and may claim a deduction for the dividends paid (Code Sec. 860; Reg. §§1.860-1—1.860-5).[64] For a REIT, an adjustment can be: (1) an increase in the sum of its taxable income (determined without regard to its dividends-paid deduction and excluding any net capital gain), plus the excess of its net income from foreclosure property minus the tax on the foreclosure property net income; (2) an increase in the amount of the excess of its net capital gain over its deduction for capital gain dividends paid; or (3) a decrease in its dividends-paid deduction (determined without regard to capital gains dividends). See ¶ 2317 for further discussion of the deficiency dividend procedure, which is the same as that for mutual funds (regulated investment companies).

2339. REIT Distributions After Tax Year Ends. A real estate investment trust (REIT) (¶ 2326) that declares a dividend (including a capital gain dividend) before the due date for filing its return for a tax year (including extensions), but distributes the dividend after the close of the tax year, can treat the dividend as having been paid during the tax year if the entire declared dividend is paid within the 12-month period following the close of the tax year and no later than the date of the first regular dividend payment after the declaration (Code Sec. 858; Reg. § 1.858-1).[65] The shareholder must generally treat the dividend as received in the tax year in which the distribution is made. This rule does not apply, however, to dividends declared in October, November, or December that are treated as paid on December 31 of a calendar year even though they are actually paid in January of the following calendar year (¶ 2329).

References are to Standard Federal Tax Reports; Tax Research Consultant; and Practical Tax Explanations.

[61] ¶ 26,520; RIC: 6,150, RIC: 6,200; § 19,205.05, § 45,440.10

[62] ¶ 26,520; RIC: 6,108, RIC: 6,200; § 19,205.20, § 45,440.10

[63] ¶ 26,520; RIC: 6,150; § 19,230.15, § 45,440.10

[64] ¶ 26,580, ¶ 26,581—¶ 26,585; RIC: 6,106

[65] ¶ 26,540, ¶ 26,541; RIC: 6,104.05

2340. REIT Subsidiaries. A real estate investment trust (REIT) (¶ 2326) may own a qualified REIT subsidiary and treat all of the subsidiary's assets, liabilities, and items of income, deduction, and credit as its own (Code Sec. 856(i)).[66] A qualified subsidiary is any corporation other than a taxable REIT subsidiary, all of the stock of which is held by the REIT. A taxable REIT subsidiary is any corporation that is owned, in whole or in part, by the REIT and that both entities jointly elect (using Form 8875) to treat as a taxable REIT subsidiary (Code Sec. 856(l)). A taxable REIT subsidiary can be used by the REIT to provide noncustomary services to its tenants or to manage and operate properties without causing the amounts received or accrued to be disqualified as rents from real property. The election to be treated as a taxable REIT subsidiary can only be revoked with the consent of both the REIT and the subsidiary.

Real Estate Mortgage Investment Conduits

2343. Qualification as a REMIC. A real estate mortgage investment conduit (REMIC) is an entity that holds a fixed pool of mortgages and issues multiple classes of interests to investors (Code Sec. 860D; Reg. § 1.860D-1).[67] A REMIC is treated like a partnership for federal tax purposes with its income passed through to its interest holders (¶ 2344). Thus, a REMIC is not subject to taxation on its income, although it is subject to taxes on prohibited transactions (¶ 2355), income from foreclosure property (¶ 2356), and on certain contributions received after its start-up day (¶ 2357). It also may be required to withhold taxes on amounts paid to foreign holders of regular or residual interests (¶ 2367).

An entity qualifies as REMIC if it makes an irrevocable election to be treated as such by filing Form 1066 during its first tax year of existence, and if it meets certain requirements as to its investors (¶ 2344) and assets (¶ 2345). If an entity ceases to qualify as a REMIC at any time during the tax year, it will not be treated as a REMIC for that or any later tax year. A REMIC is required to file an information return with the IRS on Form 8811 within 30 days of its start-up day (and 30 days from any change of information provided in a previously-filed Form 8811) identifying its representative for reporting tax information (Reg. § 1.6049-7).[68]

2344. Investors' Interests. In order to qualify as a real estate mortgage investment conduit (REMIC) (¶ 2343), all of the interests in the entity must be either regular interests or residual interests, and there must be only one class of residual interests (Code Sec. 860D; Reg. § 1.860D-1).[69] However, a *de minimis* interest that is neither a regular nor a residual interest can be created to facilitate the REMIC creation.

A regular interest is any interest that is issued on the start-up day of the REMIC with fixed terms and that is designated as a regular interest (Code Sec. 860G(a)(1); Reg. § 1.860G-1).[70] A regular interest may be issued in the form of debt, stock, interest in a partnership or trust, or any other form permitted by state law, as long as it unconditionally entitles the holder to receive a specific principal amount and interest based on a fixed rate (or permitted variable rate). An interest-only regular interest may also be issued that entitles the holder to receive interest payments determined by reference to the interest payable on qualified mortgages, rather than a specified principal amount.

An interest does not fail to qualify as a regular interest merely because the timing of principal payments may be contingent on the prepayments on qualified mortgages or the amount of income from permitted investments (¶ 2345). In addition, an interest does not fail to be a regular interest solely because the specified principal amount may be reduced as a result of a nonoccurrence of a contingent payment with respect to a reverse mortgage loan held by the REMIC if the REMIC's sponsor reasonably believes on the start-up day that all principal and interest due under the regular interest will be paid at or prior to the REMIC's liquidation. The REMIC must file Form 1099-INT for each regular interest holder (and provide a copy to the interest holder) that has been paid or to which

---

References are to Standard Federal Tax Reports; Tax Research Consultant; and Practical Tax Explanations.

[66] ¶ 26,500; RIC: 6,072.20, RIC: 6,072.30

[67] ¶ 26,660, ¶ 26,661; RIC: 9,050; § 45,445.05

[68] ¶ 36,036; RIC: 9,052

[69] ¶ 26,660, ¶ 26,661; RIC: 9,050; § 45,445.05

[70] ¶ 26,720, ¶ 26,720A; RIC: 9,056; § 45,445.10

has accrued $10 or more of interest during the calendar year (Reg. § 1.6049-7).[71] If the REMIC is also reporting original issue discount (OID) (¶ 1952), it can report both the interest and OID on Form 1099-OID.

A residual interest is an interest issued on the REMIC's start-up day that is not a regular interest and that is designated as a residual interest (Code Sec. 860G(a)(2)).[72] There may be only one class of residual interests, and any distribution with respect to such interests must be pro rata. Furthermore, a REMIC must have reasonable arrangements to ensure that residual interests are not held by certain disqualified organizations (governments, exempt organizations, cooperatives) (Code Sec. 860D(a)(3) and (6)).[73] For each quarter of its tax year, a REMIC must send a Schedule Q of Form 1066 to residual interest holders reporting their share of the REMIC's income or loss (Reg. § 1.860F-4(e)).[74]

REMIC Interests as Assets in Other Contexts. Regular and residual interests in a REMIC are treated as real estate assets for purposes of determining whether an organization qualifies as a real estate investment trust (REIT) (¶ 2326). However, if for any calendar quarter less than 95 percent of the REMIC's assets are real estate assets, the REIT is treated as holding directly its proportionate share of the assets and income of the REMIC (Code Sec. 856(c)(5)(E); Reg. § 1.856-3(b)).[75] If one REMIC owns interests in another REMIC, then the character of the second REMIC's assets flow through for purposes of making this determination. Any regular or residual interest in a REMIC can also qualify as an asset for purposes of determining whether an organization is a domestic building and loan association (Code Sec. 7701(a)(19); Reg. § 301.7701-13A).[76] If 95 percent or more of REMIC assets qualify as an asset for this purpose, then the entire interest in the REMIC can qualify as an asset.

2345. Qualified Mortgages and Permitted Investments of REMICs. In order to qualify as a real estate mortgage investment conduit (REMIC) (¶ 2343), substantially all of an entity's assets must consist of qualified mortgages and permitted investments at the close of the third month beginning after the start-up day and all times thereafter (Code Sec. 860D(a)(4)).[77] A qualified mortgage is any obligation that is principally secured by an interest in real property and that:

(1) is transferred to the REMIC on the start-up day in exchange for a regular or residual interest;

(2) is purchased by the REMIC within three months after the start-up day pursuant to a fixed price contract in effect on the start-up day; or

(3) represents an increase in the principal under the original terms of the obligation, if the increase (i) is attributable to an advance made to the obligor under the terms of a reverse mortgage or other obligation, (ii) occurs after the start-up day, and (iii) is purchased by the REMIC pursuant to a fixed price contract in effect on the start-up day (Code Sec. 860G(a)(3)).[78]

A qualified mortgage may also include any qualified replacement mortgage, or a regular interest in another REMIC transferred on the start-up day in exchange for a regular or residual interest.

Permitted investments include "cash flow" investments of amounts received under qualified mortgages for a temporary period, intangible property held for payment of expenses as part of a qualified reserve fund, and foreclosure property acquired in connection with the default of a qualified mortgage (Code Sec. 860G(a)(5)).[79]

References are to Standard Federal Tax Reports; Tax Research Consultant; and Practical Tax Explanations.

[71] ¶ 36,036; RIC: 9,052, RIC: 9,204, RIC: 9,206; § 39,110.10

[72] ¶ 26,720; RIC: 9,058

[73] ¶ 26,660; RIC: 9,062

[74] ¶ 26,701; RIC: 9,052, RIC: 9,252.30

[75] ¶ 26,500, ¶ 26,504; RIC: 6,072.05

[76] ¶ 43,080, ¶ 43,109; RIC: 12,056

[77] ¶ 26,660; RIC: 9,060; § 45,445.05

[78] ¶ 26,720; RIC: 9,060.05; § 45,445.05

[79] ¶ 26,720; RIC: 9,060.10; § 45,445.05

2349. Transfer of Property to REMICs. No gain or loss is recognized when property is transferred to a real estate mortgage investment conduit (REMIC) in exchange for a regular or residual interest (¶ 2344) (Code Sec. 860F(b); Reg. § 1.860F-2(b)).[80] The basis of a regular or residual interest received in the exchange is equal to the total adjusted basis of the property transferred, plus any organizational expenses. If the transferor receives more than one interest in the REMIC (both a regular and residual interest), then the basis must be allocated among the interests in accordance with their respective fair market values. The basis of the property received by the REMIC in exchange for a regular or residual interest is its fair market value immediately after the transfer.

The issue price of a regular or residual interest is generally determined under the same rules as for determining the issue price for the original issue discount (OID) of debt instruments (¶ 1952) (Code Sec. 860G(a)(10)).[81] If the issue price of a regular interest in a REMIC exceeds its adjusted basis, then the excess is included in the transferor's gross income as if it were a market discount bond (¶ 1958) (Code Sec. 860F(b)(1)(C); Reg. § 1.860F-2(b)(4)). If the issue price of a residual interest exceeds its adjusted basis, then the excess is included in the transferor's gross income ratably over the anticipated weighted average life of the REMIC. If the adjusted basis of a regular interest exceeds the issue price, then the excess is allowable as a deduction to the transferor under the rules similar to those governing amortizable bond premiums (¶ 1967) (Code Sec. 860F(b)(1)(D); Reg. § 1.860F-2(b)(4)). If the adjusted basis of a residual interest exceeds the issue price, then the excess is allowed as a deduction to the transferor over the anticipated weighted average life of the REMIC.

2352. Taxable Income or Loss of REMICs. A real estate mortgage investment conduit (REMIC) (¶ 2343) is not generally taxed on its income (Code Sec. 860A).[82] However, its taxable income must still be determined for purposes of the taxation of residual interest holders (¶ 2361). REMIC taxable income is determined in the same manner as that of an individual, except that it must use the accrual method of accounting and make the following adjustments:

- Regular interests in the REMIC are treated as debt.

- Market discount on any bond is included in gross income as the discount accrues.

- No item of income, gain, loss, or deduction from a prohibited transaction is taken into account (¶ 2355).

- The deductions for personal exemptions, foreign taxes, charitable contributions, net operating losses (NOLs), itemized deductions for individuals (except ordinary and necessary expenses paid or incurred for the production of income), and depletion are not allowed.

- The amount of any net income from foreclosure property is reduced by the amount of tax imposed on that income.

- Gain or loss from the disposition of assets, including qualified mortgages and permitted investments, is treated as ordinary gain or loss rather than gain or loss from a capital asset.

- Interest expenses (other than the portion allocable to tax-exempt interest) may be deducted without regard to the investment interest limitation.

- Debts owed to the REMIC are not treated as nonbusiness debts for purposes of the bad debt deduction.

- The REMIC is not treated as carrying on a trade or business, and ordinary and necessary operating expenses may only be deducted as expenses incurred for the production of income (without regard to the two-percent floor on itemized deductions (¶ 1011)) (Code Sec. 860C(b); Reg. § 1.860C-2).[83]

References are to Standard Federal Tax Reports; Tax Research Consultant; and Practical Tax Explanations.

[80] ¶ 26,700, ¶ 26,700B; RIC: 9,100

[81] ¶ 26,720; RIC: 9,106

[82] ¶ 26,600; RIC: 9,150; § 45,445.10

[83] ¶ 26,640, ¶ 26,640B; RIC: 9,254

A REMIC's net loss is determined by subtracting its gross income from allowable deductions, taking into account the same modifications listed above.

2355. Prohibited Transactions of REMICs. A real estate mortgage investment conduit (REMIC) (¶ 2343) is required to pay a 100-percent tax on its *net income* from a prohibited transaction; losses are not taken into account for this purpose (Code Sec. 860F(a)).[84] The disposition of any qualified mortgage is considered a prohibited transaction, but not if the disposition is due to:

- the substitution of a qualified replacement mortgage for a qualified mortgage (or the repurchase in lieu of substitution of a defective obligation);
- the bankruptcy or insolvency of the REMIC;
- a disposition incident to foreclosure or default of a mortgage; or
- a qualified liquidation.

A significant modification of a mortgage is considered a disposition (Reg. § 1.860G-2(b)).[85] The IRS has issued procedures that set forth conditions under which modifications of certain mortgage loans, as well as subprime mortgage loans, will not be considered a disposition of a qualified mortgage and a prohibited transaction of a REMIC or investment trust that holds the loans (Rev. Proc. 2010-30; Rev. Proc. 2009-45; Rev. Proc. 2009-23).[86]

Prohibited transactions of a REMIC also include: the receipt of any income from an asset that is neither a qualified mortgage nor a permitted investment (¶ 2345); the receipt of any amount that represents a fee or compensation for services; and the receipt of gain from the disposition of any cash flow investment, unless the disposition is made pursuant to a qualified liquidation. A disposition is not treated as a prohibited transaction if it is required to prevent default on a regular interest where the threatened default results from a default on one or more qualified mortgages, or is undertaken to facilitate a clean-up call.

2356. Net Income from Foreclosure Property. A real estate mortgage investment conduit (REMIC) is subject to tax at the highest corporate income tax rate (¶ 219) on its *net income* from foreclosure property for the tax year (Code Sec. 860G(c)).[87] For this purpose, net income from foreclosure property is the excess of gain from the sale or other disposition of foreclosure property as described in Code Sec. 1221(a)(1) (i.e., stock in trade or property held by the REMIC for sale to customers in the ordinary course of trade or business), plus the gross income derived from foreclosure property during the tax year, over deductions derived from the production of such income (Code Sec. 857(b)(4)(B)).[88] Foreclosure property is any interest in real property, and personal property incident to the real property, acquired by a REMIC as a result of a default of a lease on the property or a debt securing the property. A REMIC must elect to treat property as foreclosure property by the due date (including extensions) of its annual return for the year in which it acquires the property. Property ceases to be foreclosure property: (1) as of the close of the third tax year after the tax year in which it is acquired, unless an extension is granted, or (2) if the property's foreclosure property status terminates prior to that date (Code Sec. 856(e)).[89]

2357. Post-Startup Contributions to REMICs. A real estate mortgage investment conduit (REMIC) (¶ 2343) that receives contributions of property after its start-up day is subject to a tax equal to the full value of the contribution (Code Sec. 860G(d)).[90] Exceptions to the tax are provided for cash contributions that are: made to facilitate a clean-up call or a qualified liquidation; in the nature of a guarantee; made during the three-month period that begins on the start-up day; made by a holder of a residual interest in the REMIC to a qualified reserve fund; or permitted under regulations.

References are to Standard Federal Tax Reports; Tax Research Consultant; and Practical Tax Explanations.

[84] ¶ 26,700; RIC: 9,152
[85] ¶ 26,720B; RIC: 9,152.10
[86] ¶ 26,721.70; RIC: 9,152.10

[87] ¶ 26,720; RIC: 9,154
[88] ¶ 26,520; RIC: 6,114

[89] ¶ 26,500; RIC: 6,068.10, RIC: 6,068.15; RIC: 9,060.10
[90] ¶ 26,720; RIC: 9,156

23

SPEC. CORP. STATUS

2358. Taxation of Regular Interests. Holders of regular interests in a real estate mortgage investment conduit (REMIC) (¶ 2344) are taxed as if their interests were debt instruments, except that income derived from their interests must be computed under the accrual method of accounting (Code Sec. 860B).[91] Gain on the disposition of a regular interest is treated as ordinary income to the extent of unaccrued original issue discount (OID) (¶ 1952), computed at 110 percent of the applicable federal rate (AFR) effective at the time the interest was acquired. The REMIC must report interest payments of $10 or more to regular interest holders and the IRS on Form 1099-INT.

2361. Taxation of Residual Interests. Holders of residual interests in a real estate mortgage investment conduit (REMIC) (¶ 2344) must take into account their daily portions of the taxable income or net loss of the REMIC (¶ 2352) for each day during the tax year on which they hold their interests (Code Sec. 860C; Reg. § 1.860C-1).[92] The daily portion is determined on the basis of quarterly computations of the REMIC's taxable income or net loss with such amounts being allocated among all residual interests in proportion to their respective holdings on each day during the quarter (reported on Schedule Q of Form 1066). The holder treats his or her portion of taxable income and net loss as ordinary income or loss. However, the amount of loss that the holder may take into account in any calendar quarter cannot exceed his or her adjusted basis in the residual interest (as determined without regard to any required basis decreases for the daily portions of the REMIC's net loss). Any allocated loss that is disallowed may be carried forward to succeeding calendar quarters indefinitely, but it may only be used to offset income from the same REMIC.

Distributions made by the REMIC to a holder of a residual interest are received tax free to the extent that they do not exceed that holder's adjusted basis in his or her interest. Any excess is treated as gain from the sale or exchange of the interest. The basis of a holder's residual interest is increased by the daily portion of REMIC taxable income allocated to the interest. The holder's basis is decreased, but not below zero, by the amount of any distribution received and the daily portion of the REMIC net loss allocated to the interest holder. When a residual interest in a REMIC is disposed of by the holder, these adjustments are treated as occurring immediately before the disposition.

Income in Excess of Daily Accruals. A holder of a residual interest may not reduce his or her taxable income (or alternative minimum taxable income) for the tax year below his or her excess inclusion for the year (Code Sec. 860E; Reg. § 1.860E-1).[93] A holder's excess inclusion is equal to the excess of the net income passed through to the holder each calendar quarter over a deemed interest component referred to as the "daily accrual." The effect is to prevent a holder from offsetting his or her excess inclusion by any net operating losses (NOLs) (¶ 1145) or in calculating alternative minimum tax (AMT) (¶ 1401). Excess inclusions are also treated as unrelated business taxable income for tax-exempt holders (¶ 655). Where a residual interest is held by a mutual fund, regulated investment company, real estate investment trust (REIT), common trust fund, or cooperative, a portion of the dividends paid by such organizations to their shareholders are treated as excess inclusions.

Application of Wash Sale Rules. Except as provided in the regulations, the wash sale rules (¶ 1935) apply to dispositions of residual interests where a seller of the interest acquires any residual interest in any REMIC (or any interest in a taxable mortgage pool (¶ 2368) that is comparable to a residual interest) within a period beginning six months before the date of sale or disposition and ending six months after that date (Code Sec. 860F(d)).[94]

References are to Standard Federal Tax Reports; Tax Research Consultant; and Practical Tax Explanations.

[91] ¶ 26,620; RIC: 9,202; § 45,445.10

[92] ¶ 26,640, ¶ 26,640A; RIC: 9,250, RIC: 9,252; § 45,445.10

[93] ¶ 26,680, ¶ 26,680A; RIC: 9,256

[94] ¶ 26,700; RIC: 9,262

Residual Interests Held by Disqualified Organizations. If a disqualified organization (government, exempt organization, cooperative) holds a residual interest in a REMIC at any time during the tax year, then an excise tax is imposed against the person or entity that has transferred the interest to the organization (Code Sec. 860E(e); Reg. § 1.860E-2).[95] The tax is the highest corporate income tax rate (¶ 219) imposed on the present value of the total excess inclusion that is anticipated for the interest after the transfer takes place. If the transfer is through an agent of the disqualified organization, the agent must pay the tax.

Noneconomic Interests. The transfer of a noneconomic residual interest is disregarded for federal tax purposes if a significant purpose of the transfer was to impede the assessment or collection of tax (Reg. § 1.860E-1(c)).[96] A noneconomic residual interest is one for which anticipated distributions are insufficient to meet anticipated tax liabilities.

2367. Foreign Holders of REMIC Interests. If the holder of a residual interest in a real estate mortgage investment conduit (REMIC) (¶ 2361) is a nonresident alien or foreign corporation, then for withholding and income tax purposes (¶ 2425): (1) amounts includible in the holder's gross income are taken into account when paid or distributed, or when the interest is disposed of; and (2) no exemption from the 30-percent tax imposed on U.S.-source income not effectively connected with a U.S. business applies to any excess inclusion (¶ 2431) (Code Sec. 860G(b)).[97]

2368. Taxable Mortgage Pools. If a mortgage pool does not elect to be or qualify as a real estate mortgage investment conduit (REMIC) (¶ 2343) or as a financial asset securitization investment trust (FASIT) formed prior to January 1, 2005 (¶ 2394), it may qualify as a taxable mortgage pool. An entity is a taxable mortgage pool if:

> (1) substantially all the assets of which consist of debt obligations (or interests therein) and more than 50 percent of the obligations (or interests) consist of real estate mortgages;

> (2) the entity is the obligor under debt obligations with two or more maturities; and

> (3) under the terms of the entity's debt obligations, payments on the obligations referred to in (2) are related to payments on the obligations or interests referred to in (1) (Code Sec. 7701(i)).[98]

A taxable mortgage pool is taxed as a separate corporation and may not join with any other corporation in filing a consolidated return. Any portion of an entity that meets the requirements above is treated as a taxable mortgage pool. However, no domestic savings and loan association can qualify to be a taxable mortgage pool.

Insurance Companies

2370. Taxation of Life Insurance Companies. A life insurance company is generally taxed on its life insurance company taxable income at regular corporate income tax rates (¶ 219) (Code Sec. 801).[99] If it has net capital gains, however, the company is taxed at the 35-percent corporate capital gain rate (¶ 1738) on its net capital gain, and at regular corporate tax rates on the excess of its life insurance company taxable income minus the net capital gain, if this results in a lower tax amount.

Life insurance company taxable income for this purpose is the sum of the life insurance company's net premiums, net decreases in reserves, and other items of income, minus deductions for the following: claims, benefits, and losses accrued; net increases in various reserves (¶ 2372); policyholder dividends (¶ 2373); dividends received (subject to limitations); operational losses (¶ 2377); consideration paid for another person's assumption of the company's insurance and annuity liabilities; and dividend reimbursements paid to another insurance company (Code Secs. 803, 804, and 805).[100]

References are to Standard Federal Tax Reports; Tax Research Consultant; and Practical Tax Explanations.

[95] ¶ 26,680, ¶ 26,680B; RIC: 9,062, RIC: 9,258.05

[96] ¶ 26,680A; RIC: 9,258.10

[97] ¶ 26,720; RIC: 9,252.20, INTL: 33,110.30

[98] ¶ 43,080; RIC: 9,300

[99] ¶ 25,710

[100] ¶ 25,730, ¶ 25,750, ¶ 25,770

23
SPEC. CORP STATUS

All other deductions allowed to a corporation are also permitted, subject to some modifications (for example, no deduction for net operating losses (NOLs) is allowed). Small life insurance companies (gross assets of less than $500 million at the close of a tax year) may claim an additional deduction based on their tentative taxable income (Code Sec. 806).[101] A life insurance company uses Form 1120-L to figure and report its taxable income.

A business entity qualifies as a life insurance company if: (1) more than half of its business activities consist of issuing life insurance or annuity contracts, or reinsuring risks underwritten by other insurance companies; and (2) more than half of its total reserves for paying off insurance obligations consist of life insurance reserves, plus unearned premiums, and unpaid losses on noncancellable life, accident, or health policies that are not included in life insurance reserves (Code Sec. 816).[102]

2372. Net Change in Reserves. Life insurance companies (¶ 2370) may deduct the net increase in certain reserves and must include in income the net decrease in such reserves that have occurred during the tax year (Code Sec. 807).[103] The net increase or decrease is generally computed by comparing the closing balance for reserves to the opening balance of the reserves. The closing balance is reduced by the policyholders' shares of tax-exempt interest and shares of the increase in cash values of insurance and annuity contracts for the year.

Items that must be taken into account in determining whether reserves have had a net increase or decrease include:

- life insurance reserves;
- unearned premiums and unpaid losses (Code Sec. 846);[104]
- discounted amounts necessary to satisfy obligations arising under contracts that did not involve life, accident, or health contingencies;
- dividend accumulations and other amounts held in connection with insurance and annuity contracts;
- advanced premiums and liabilities for premium deposit funds; and
- reasonable special contingency reserves for group term life insurance or group accident and health contracts.

Insurance companies that are required to discount unpaid losses may claim an additional deduction up to the excess of undiscounted unpaid losses over related discounted unpaid losses (Code Sec. 847).[105]

2373. Policyholder Dividends. Life insurance companies (¶ 2370) may claim a deduction for dividends or similar distributions paid or accrued to policyholders during the tax year (Code Sec. 808).[106] A policyholder dividend includes excess interest, premium adjustments, experience-rated refunds, and any amount paid or credited to policyholders not based on a fixed amount in the contract but dependent on the experience rate of the company or the discretion of management. The policyholder dividends deduction must be reduced by the amount by which the deduction was accelerated due to a change in the life insurance company's business practice.

2377. Operations Loss Deduction. A life insurance company (¶ 2370) may claim an operations loss deduction, which equals the sum of operations loss carryovers and carrybacks to the tax year. The company's loss from operations for a tax year is the excess of its life insurance deductions over its life insurance gross income (subject to limitations). An operations loss may be carried back three years and carried forward 15 years (Code Sec. 810).[107] The company may elect to forgo the entire carryback period for an operations loss for any tax year. In addition, if the company qualifies as a new life insurance company, the operations loss for any tax year may be carried forward 18 years.

References are to Standard Federal Tax Reports; Tax Research Consultant; and Practical Tax Explanations.

[101] ¶ 25,790; FILEBUS: 3,056
[102] ¶ 25,990
[103] ¶ 25,810
[104] ¶ 26,330
[105] ¶ 26,350
[106] ¶ 25,830
[107] ¶ 25,870; NOL: 9,250

2378. Taxation of Other Insurance Companies. Insurance companies that do not meet the definition of a life insurance company (¶ 2370) (property and casualty companies) are subject to taxation at regular corporate income tax rates (¶ 219) on their taxable income (Code Secs. 831(a) and 832).[108] However, such companies are exempt from tax if gross receipts for the tax year do not exceed $600,000 and more than 50 percent of such receipts consist of premiums ($150,000 and 35 percent, respectively, for mutual insurance companies) (Code Sec. 501(c)(15)).[109] A property and casualty insurance company with net written premiums of no more than $1.2 million for the tax year may elect to be taxed only on its taxable investment income. This is the company's gross investment income less deductions for tax-free interest, investment expenses, real estate expenses, depreciation, paid or accrued interest, capital losses, trade or business deductions, and certain corporate deductions (Code Secs. 831(b) and 834).[110]

2380. Foreign Insurance Companies. A foreign company carrying on an insurance business within the United States that would otherwise qualify as an insurance company if it were a domestic company is taxable as an insurance company on its income effectively connected with the conduct of any U.S. trade or business (¶ 2429) and is taxable on its remaining income from U.S. sources (¶ 2431) (Code Sec. 842).[111]

Other Special Entities

2383. Banks and Other Financial Institutions. Banks and other financial institutions are generally subject to the same tax rules as corporations. However, unlike other taxpayers, banks are not subject to capital loss limitations with respect to the worthlessness of debt securities (¶ 1916). Instead, banks may treat these losses as bad debt losses. In addition, if one bank directly owns at least 80 percent of each class of stock of another bank, the first bank's losses on worthless stock and stock rights in the second bank are not treated as losses from the sale or exchange of capital assets (Code Sec. 582).[112]

The method that is used to deduct bad debts of a bank depends on the type and size of the institution in question (Code Sec. 585; Reg. §§ 1.585-1—1.585-8).[113] A small bank (average adjusted basis of all assets of $500 million or less) may add to its bad debt reserves an amount based on its actual experience as shown by losses for the current and preceding five tax years. A thrift institution that would be treated as a small bank may utilize this method as well. Large banks are generally required to use either a specific charge-off method in which the bank's debt reserves are recaptured over a four-year period, or the cut-off method in which recoveries and losses are reflected as adjustments to the bank's reserve account.

Definition of a Bank. For this purpose, a bank is defined as a corporation with a substantial part of its business consisting of either receiving deposits and making loans or exercising fiduciary powers similar to those permitted to national banks. This includes commercial banks and trust companies, mutual savings banks, building and loan associations, cooperative banks, and federal savings and loan associations (Code Sec. 581; Reg. § 1.581-2).[114] These latter "banks," however, are allowed a deduction for dividends paid or credited to depositors (Code Sec. 591).[115]

Sale or Exchange of Securities. In the case of certain financial institutions, the sale or exchange of a bond, debenture, note, certificate, or other evidence of indebtedness is not considered a sale or exchange of a capital asset (Code Sec. 582(c)).[116] Instead, net gains and losses from such transactions are treated as ordinary income and losses. A financial institution includes commercial banks, mutual savings banks, domestic building and loan associations, cooperative banks, business development corporations, and small business investment companies (¶ 2392).

References are to Standard Federal Tax Reports; Tax Research Consultant; and Practical Tax Explanations.

[108] ¶ 26,130, ¶ 26,150; CCORP: 100

[109] ¶ 22,602; EXEMPT: 9,650; § 33,005.05

[110] ¶ 26,130, ¶ 26,190; EXEMPT: 9,650

[111] ¶ 26,250; INTLIN: 3,108

[112] ¶ 23,608; BUSEXP: 30,102.15, BUSEXP: 48,154, RIC: 12,114.15

[113] ¶ 23,650, ¶ 23,651— ¶ 23,661; RIC: 12,202

[114] ¶ 23,602, ¶ 23,604; RIC: 12,050

[115] ¶ 23,690; CCORP: 9,062

[116] ¶ 23,608; RIC: 12,214

2389. Common Trust Funds. A common trust fund is an investment vehicle established by a bank in the form of a state-law trust to handle the investment and reinvestment of money contributed to it in its capacity as a trustee, executor, administrator, guardian, or as a custodian of a Uniform Gifts to Minors account (Code Sec. 584).[117] For tax purposes, a common trust fund is treated in a manner similar to that of a partnership. Instead of the trust being subject to tax, each participant that invests in the trust fund must include his or her proportionate share of the trust fund's income or loss on his or her own return. This includes a participant's share of dividends received by the fund that are eligible for the reduced tax rate on qualified dividends (¶ 733). The admission and withdrawal of a participant, however, does not result in a gain or loss to the common trust fund.

2392. Small Business Investment Companies. A small business investment company (SBIC) is a private corporation that operates under the Small Business Investment Act of 1958 to provide capital to small business concerns through the purchase of convertible debentures. An SBIC is generally treated as a corporation for federal tax purposes with a few exceptions. First, an SBIC may claim an ordinary loss deduction for any loss on the sale or exchange of stock of a small business concern if the stock was received under the conversion privilege of a debenture acquired on the providing of equity capital to small business concerns (Code Sec. 1243).[118] Second, an SBIC may deduct 100 percent (rather than 70 percent) of the dividends it receives from taxable domestic corporations (Code Sec. 243(a)(2)).[119] See ¶ 1913 for discussion of the treatment of losses on SBIC stock and ¶ 1909 for discussion of the rollover of gain from the sale of publicly traded securities into stock or a partnership interest in an SBIC.

2394. Financial Asset Securitization Investment Trusts (Repealed). Prior to January 1, 2005, a qualified entity could elect to be treated as a financial asset securitization investment trust (FASIT) (Code Secs. 860H—860L, prior to repeal by the American Jobs Creation Act of 2004 (P.L. 108-357)).[120] A FASIT is a pass-through entity used to securitize debt obligations such as credit card receivables, home equity loans, and auto loans. A FASIT must be entirely owned by a taxable C corporation. Any residual income of the FASIT is passed through and taxed to the owner. The advantage offered by a FASIT is that asset-backed securities issued by a FASIT are treated as debt for federal tax purposes. Thus, interest paid to investors is deductible.

The rules regarding FASITs are repealed as of January 1, 2005, but the repeal does not apply to any FASIT in existence on October 22, 2004, to the extent that regular interests already issued by the FASIT remain outstanding in accordance with their original terms.

References are to Standard Federal Tax Reports; Tax Research Consultant; and Practical Tax Explanations.

[117] ¶ 23,630; RIC: 12,300
[118] ¶ 30,770; SALES: 18,304; § 18,245
[119] ¶ 13,051; CCORP: 9,056; § 26,505
[120] ¶ 26,730—¶ 26,738; RIC: 18,000

Chapter 24

FOREIGN INCOME AND TRANSACTIONS

Overview

2401. Taxation of Worldwide Income. The United States taxes the worldwide income of U.S. citizens, resident aliens, and domestic corporations without regard to whether the income arose from a transaction or activity originating outside its geographic borders (¶ 2402). Nonresident aliens and foreign corporations are generally taxed in the same manner as U.S. citizens and domestic corporations on income that is effectively connected with a U.S. trade or business (¶ 2425). Income not effectively connected with a U.S. trade or business, such as fixed, determinable, annual, or periodical (FDAP) income, is generally taxed at a 30-percent rate (¶ 2431). To prevent income from being subject to double taxation—once in the United States and once in a foreign country—U.S. taxpayers may be entitled to a credit or deduction for foreign income taxes paid or accrued during the tax year (¶ 2475). Special rules apply with regard to the taxation of U.S. shareholders of controlled foreign corporations (CFCs) (¶ 2487). U.S. persons are also subject to a number of foreign asset reporting requirements (¶ 2570 and ¶ 2572).

U.S. Citizens and Residents Living Abroad

2402. Foreign Earned Income Exclusion. A qualifying individual (¶ 2404) who lives and works abroad may elect (¶ 2408) to exclude from gross income a certain amount of foreign earned income attributable to his or her residence in a foreign country during the tax year (Code Sec. 911(a)(1) and (b)(2)).[1] The maximum amount of foreign earned income that may be excluded is $99,200 for 2014 ($100,800 for 2015) (Rev. Proc. 2013-35; Rev. Proc. 2014-61). The exclusion is computed on a daily basis. Therefore, the maximum limit must be reduced ratably for each day during the calendar year that the taxpayer does not qualify for the exclusion. The exclusion is also limited to the excess of the individual's foreign earned income for the year over his or her foreign housing exclusion (¶ 2403). In the case of married taxpayers, each spouse may compute the limitation separately and without regard to community property laws (if otherwise applicable). Thus, it is possible for a married couple to exclude up to $198,400 for 2014 ($201,600 for 2015) if each spouse is qualified to claim the exclusion (Reg. § 1.911-5).[2]

> **Example 1:** Andy is a U.S. citizen who qualified as a bona fide resident of Costa Rica for all of 2013 and who received $78,000 in salary for work he did in Costa Rica. Assuming he claimed no foreign housing exclusion, Andy was able to exclude all of the salary from his gross income for 2013. Andy continues to work in Costa Rica until October 31, 2014, when his employer permanently reassigns him to the United States. During this time, Andy received a salary of $90,000 for his work in Costa Rica in 2014. Assuming he claimed no foreign housing exclusion, the maximum amount of foreign earned income he can exclude from his gross income

References are to Standard Federal Tax Reports; Tax Research Consultant; and Practical Tax Explanations.

[1] ¶ 28,040; EXPAT: 12,100; § 37,510.05   [2] ¶ 28,045; EXPAT: 12,400; § 37,510.25

in 2014 is $82,621 ($99,200 multiplied by ratio of the number of days he was a bona fide resident of Costa Rica ($304/365$).

Foreign Earned Income. Foreign earned income includes wages, salaries, professional fees, and other amounts received as compensation for personal services actually rendered when the taxpayer's tax home was located in a foreign country and the taxpayer meets either the bona fide residence or physical presence test (Code Sec. 911(b)(1) and (d)(2); Reg. § 1.911-3).[3] If the taxpayer engages in a sole proprietorship or partnership where both personal services and capital are material income-producing factors, no more than 30 percent of the taxpayer's share of the net profits can be treated as earned income (30 percent of gross profits if no net profits). Any salary received from a corporation is earned income to the extent it represents reasonable compensation for personal services performed.

Foreign earned income does not include any compensation received after the close of the tax year following the year in which the personal services were performed. It also does not include any reimbursements received under an accountable plan for expenses incurred on an employer's behalf (¶ 952A), the value of meals and lodging that are furnished for the convenience of an employer and excluded from gross income (¶ 2089 and ¶ 2406), employer contributions to a nonqualified retirement plan, or any recaptured moving expenses. Foreign earned income also does not include amounts received as a pension, annuity, or social security payments, amounts paid by the United States or its agencies to its employees, or income earned in a country in which the United States imposes travel restrictions.

A taxpayer that elects to claim the foreign earned income exclusion (or foreign housing exclusion) is prohibited from claiming any deduction, exclusion, or tax credit (including the foreign tax credit) that is properly allocable to the excluded amounts (Code Sec. 911(d)(6); Reg. § 1.911-6(a)).[4] For example, a taxpayer may not deduct unreimbursed employee business expenses against wages that are excluded as foreign earned income.

Determination of Tax Liability. If a taxpayer elects to exclude foreign earned income or foreign housing expenses (or both), then his or her income tax liability and alternative minimum tax liability on the nonexcluded amount is determined using the tax rates that would have applied had the exclusion(s) not been claimed (Code Sec. 911(f)).[5] If the taxpayer's net capital gains exceed his or her taxable income or alternative minimum taxable income, then the excess reduces the taxpayer's net capital gains without regard to qualified dividend income, and then qualified dividend income. The excess is also treated as a long-term capital loss in computing the taxpayer's adjusted net capital gain, unrecaptured section 1250 gain, and 28-percent rate gain. The Foreign Earned Income Worksheet in the Form 1040 Instructions or Form 6251 Instructions is used to calculate tax liability for this purpose.

2403. Foreign Housing Exclusion or Deduction. In addition to the election to exclude foreign earned income (¶ 2402), a qualified individual (¶ 2404) may elect (¶ 2408) to exclude from gross income a certain amount of foreign housing expenses paid for with employer-provided amounts included in the taxpayer's foreign earned income (for example, housing allowance or reimbursement) (Code Sec. 911(a)(2)).[6]

> **Caution:** The amount of foreign housing expenses (or foreign earned income) excluded from an individual's gross income is used to determine the taxpayer's regular income tax and alternative minimum tax liability on his or her nonexcluded income (¶ 2402).

The maximum housing amount that may be excluded is limited to 14 percent of the maximum foreign earned income exclusion for the year (Code Sec. 911(c)). This is the excess of: (1) the taxpayer's reasonable "foreign housing expenses" for the tax year

---

References are to Standard Federal Tax Reports; Tax Research Consultant; and Practical Tax Explanations.

[3] ¶ 28,040, ¶ 28,043; EXPAT: 12,200; § 37,510.10

[4] ¶ 28,040, ¶ 28,046; EXPAT: 12,250; § 37,525.05

[5] ¶ 28,040; EXPAT: 12,100; § 37,520

[6] ¶ 28,040; EXPAT: 12,150; § 37,515.05

(generally limited to 30 percent of the maximum foreign earned income exclusion for the year), over (2) a "base housing amount" equal to 16 percent of the maximum foreign earned income exclusion amount for the year. The exclusion is computed on a daily basis and multiplied by the number of days of foreign residence or presence by the taxpayer for the year.

For 2014, the maximum foreign earned income exclusion is $99,200 per year; 30 percent of which is $29,760 or $81.53 per day; and 16 percent of which is $15,872, or $43.48 per day. Thus, the maximum amount that may be excluded in 2014 is $13,888, or $38.04 per day. (For 2015, the maximum foreign earned income exclusion is $100,800 per year; 30 percent of which is $30,240 or $82.85 per day; and 16 percent of which is $16,128, or $44.19 per day. Thus, the maximum amount that may be excluded in 2015 is $14,112, or $38.66 per day.) Foreign housing expenses may be excluded only to the extent of the lesser of the expenses attributable to employer-provided amounts or the individual's foreign earned income for the tax year.

The reasonable amount of expenses that may be used in calculating the maximum exclusion limit (i.e., the 30 percent of the maximum foreign earned income exclusion) may be adjusted annually by the IRS for specific geographic locations that have higher housing costs relative to the United States. For this purpose, the taxpayer must actually reside within the geographic limits of the high-cost location identified by the IRS to claim the adjusted limit; the taxpayer cannot reside in a suburb of the location. The limits for high-cost localities are listed in the Instructions for Form 2555.

Housing Expenses. A taxpayer's foreign housing expenses are the reasonable costs paid or incurred during the tax year to provide housing in a foreign country for the taxpayer and for his or her spouse and dependents if they reside with the taxpayer (Reg. § 1.911-4).[7] This may include reasonable expenses related to a second foreign household for the taxpayer's spouse and dependents if they do not reside with the taxpayer due to adverse conditions near the taxpayer's tax home. Eligible expenses include rent or the fair rental value of housing provided in kind by an employer, utilities (other than telephone charges), real or personal property insurance, household repairs, rental of furniture and accessories, and residential parking. They do not include expenses that are otherwise deductible (depreciation, interest, taxes) or that are extravagant. They also do not include the cost of buying property (including mortgage payments), capital improvements to property, purchased furniture or accessories, or the cost of domestic labor. If a husband and wife are both qualified individuals with foreign earned income, special rules apply which may allow them both to claim the foreign housing exclusion or deduction, depending on whether separate households are maintained (Reg. § 1.911-5).[8]

Self-Employment. A self-employed taxpayer is entitled to deduct from gross income a certain amount of foreign housing expenses in lieu of the exclusion (Code Sec. 911(c)(4); Reg. § 1.911-4(e)).[9] The deduction is limited to the amount by which the taxpayer's foreign earned income for the tax year exceeds his or her foreign earned income and housing exclusion. Any amount that exceeds the deduction limit can be carried forward one tax year. If the taxpayer has foreign earned income that consists of both employer-provided amounts and self-employment amounts, then the taxpayer may elect to exclude the part of the housing expenses that are paid for with employer-provided amounts and may claim a deduction for any remaining housing expenses attributed to self-employment income.

2404. Eligibility for Foreign Earned Income and Housing Exclusions. In order to qualify for the foreign earned income exclusion (¶ 2402) or foreign housing exclusion (¶ 2403), an individual's tax home must be in a foreign country and he or she must satisfy either the bona fide residence test or the physical presence test (Code Sec. 911(d)(1); Reg. § 1.911-2).[10] A foreign country is any territory, including airspace and

---

References are to Standard Federal Tax Reports; Tax Research Consultant; and Practical Tax Explanations.

[7] ¶ 28,044; EXPAT: 12,154; § 37,515.10

[8] ¶ 28,045; EXPAT: 12,400; § 37,515.25

[9] ¶ 28,040, ¶ 28,044; EXPAT: 12,162; § 37,515.20

[10] ¶ 28,040, ¶ 28,042; EXPAT: 12,050; § 37,505.05

territorial waters, under the sovereignty of a government other than the United States. A foreign country does not include Antarctica or U.S. possessions such as Puerto Rico, Guam, the Commonwealth of the Northern Mariana Islands, the U.S. Virgin Islands, and Johnston Island. A bona fide resident of American Samoa (¶ 2414) or Puerto Rico (¶ 2415) may be eligible to exclude income from the possession for U.S. tax purposes. The foreign earned income and housing exclusions are denied if the taxpayer is present in a foreign country in which travel is generally restricted (Code Sec. 911(d)(8)).

Tax Home. "Tax home" for this purpose has the same meaning as it does for determining the deductibility of travel expenses away from home (¶ 950). An individual's tax home is where his or her principal place of business is located, regardless of where he or she maintains a family home (Code Sec. 911(d)(3)). The location of a taxpayer's tax home often depends on whether a work assignment is temporary or indefinite. An individual is not considered to have a tax home in a foreign country for any period during which his or her abode is in the United States. Temporary presence or maintenance of a dwelling in the United States does not necessarily mean that an abode is in the United States during that time, even if the taxpayer's spouse or dependents use the dwelling.

Bona Fide Residence. A U.S. citizen (or resident alien subject to a U.S. income tax treaty) may qualify for the foreign earned income or housing exclusions if he or she is a bona fide resident of a foreign country for an uninterrupted period that includes a full tax year (Code Sec. 911(d)(1)(A) and (d)(5)). This determination is based on all of the facts and circumstances, including the taxpayer's intentions regarding the length and nature of the stay. It is not determined by the taxpayer's status under the laws of the foreign country, nor by merely living in a foreign country for a year. The taxpayer does not have to be a bona fide resident of the same foreign country for the entire period and the foreign country in which the taxpayer is a bona fide resident does not have to be the primary place of employment. Once the bona fide residence requirement is met, the taxpayer is permitted the exclusions for any tax year in which the period of residence began or ended.

> **Example 1:** Barney is a calendar-year taxpayer whose salary is $100,000 per year. On January 1, 2013, he establishes bona fide residence in Canada. His residence lasts until March 31, 2014. Assuming he claims no foreign housing exclusion, he qualifies in 2013 for the maximum exclusion of $97,600 for his foreign earned income because he established residence for the full year in a foreign country. He also qualifies for the exclusion of $24,460 of his foreign earned income ($99,200 × $^{90}/_{365}$) for the portion of the 2014 tax year he was a resident in Canada.

Physical Presence. A U.S. citizen or resident alien may qualify for the foreign income or housing exclusions if he or she is present in a foreign country (or countries) for 330 full days out of any consecutive 12-month period (Code Sec. 911(d)(1)(B)). The taxpayer does not have to be present in the foreign country solely for business purposes and the 330 days do not have to be consecutive. In addition, the taxpayer can select any 12-month period in which he or she meets the physical presence test.

> **Example 2:** Betty is a U.S. citizen who leaves New York on February 3, 2014, and arrives in Spain on that same day. During December 2014, Betty vacations in France for ten days. She leaves Spain to move back to the United States on January 10, 2015. Betty will meet the 330-day test during either the 12-month period beginning February 4, 2014, or the 12-month period ending January 10, 2015.

Waiver of Time Requirements. Relief from either the bona fide residence or the physical presence test is provided to an individual if he or she was forced to flee a foreign country because of civil unrest, war, or other adverse conditions (Code Sec. 911(d)(4)). To qualify for the relief, the individual must have been a bona fide resident of, or present in, the foreign country on or prior to the date the IRS determines that adverse conditions exist in the foreign country and individuals are required to leave. In addition, the taxpayer must establish that he or she could reasonably be expected to have satisfied the residency requirement had the adverse conditions not arisen. The IRS publishes annually the names of countries for which the waiver is available.[11]

2406. Camps Located in a Foreign Country. In addition to the exclusion of foreign earned income (¶ 2402) and foreign housing expenses (¶ 2403), an individual may be able to exclude from gross income and wages as a *de minimis* fringe benefit (¶ 2089) the value of meals and lodging provided by his or her employer in a camp located in a foreign country if three requirements are met (Code Sec. 119(c)).[12] First, the lodging must be provided for the convenience of the employer because the place where the employee's services are performed is in a remote area where satisfactory housing is unavailable. Second, the location of the camp must be as near as practicable to the place where the employee's services are performed. Third, the lodging must be provided in a common area, not open to the public, that normally accommodates 10 or more employees. An employee who works for a U.S. military contractor on a foreign military base cannot exclude from income the value of lodging provided by his or her employer, as the lodging is not considered to be on the employer's business premises (*P.M. Middleton*, Dec. 57,464(M), TC Memo. 2008-150).[13]

2408. Electing the Foreign Earned Income and Housing Exclusions. A qualified individual (¶ 2404) must make a separate election with respect to the foreign earned income exclusion (¶ 2402) and the foreign housing exclusion (¶ 2403). The elections are made by filing Form 2555 or Form 2555-EZ with the taxpayer's timely-filed income tax return (including extensions), amended return, or a late-filed return if filed within one year after the due date of the return (not including extensions) (Code Sec. 911(e); Reg. § 1.911-7).[14] Once made, the election will remain in effect for the current tax year and all subsequent years unless revoked. A taxpayer that revokes the election will be prohibited from making a new election for at least five tax years without IRS approval. If both a husband and wife qualify for the exclusions, each must file a separate Form 2555 regardless of whether they file a joint return or separate returns. A self-employed taxpayer does not have to make an election in order to claim the foreign housing deduction.

An individual that claims either the foreign earned income or foreign housing exclusion may not claim the foreign tax credit or deduction (¶ 2475) for any income excluded. If a taxpayer attempts to claim the foreign tax credit or deduction, then the election for the foreign earned income and foreign housing exclusions will be considered revoked (IRS Pub. 54). A taxpayer eligible for the earned income tax credit (¶ 1322) may also not claim both the credit and either of the exclusions.

2409. Resident Aliens. A resident alien is generally taxed in the same manner as a U.S. citizen. For this purpose, residency is determined under the lawful permanent residence test ("green card") or the substantial presence test (Code Sec. 7701(b)(1)).[15] An alien who does not qualify under either test is generally treated as a nonresident alien for federal income, employment, and excise tax purposes (but not estate and gift tax purposes). Some individuals may be eligible to elect resident status (¶ 2410). In addition, an individual can have a dual-status tax year and be both a resident and nonresident alien during the year (¶ 2411). In the case of an individual who is considered both a U.S. resident and a resident of a foreign country during the year (dual resident taxpayer), a tax treaty may override the normal treatment of the individual as a resident alien for all purposes under the treaty. The green card test and substantial presence test determine whether an alien is a resident of a U.S. possession or territory whose income tax laws mirror those of the United States. They do not determine whether an individual is a bona fide resident of other U.S. possessions or territories (¶ 2414) (Reg. § 301.7701(b)-1(d)).[16]

References are to Standard Federal Tax Reports; Tax Research Consultant; and Practical Tax Explanations.

[11] ¶ 28,049.5775; EXPAT: 12,058; § 37,505.15, § 37,505.20

[12] ¶ 7220; EXPAT: 12,302; § 21,235

[13] ¶ 7222.63; EXPAT: 12,302; § 21,235

[14] ¶ 28,040, ¶ 28,047; EXPAT: 12,108, EXPAT: 12,166; § 37,530.05

[15] ¶ 43,080; EXPAT: 3,000; § 37,101

[16] ¶ 43,117; EXPAT: 3,100; § 37,145

24
FOREIGN

Green Card Test. An alien who is a lawful permanent resident of the United States under U.S. immigration laws (i.e., receives a "green card") is considered a resident alien for federal tax purposes (Reg. § 301.7701(b)-1(b)).[17] Resident status begins in the first calendar year in which the alien is a lawful resident and is physically present in the United States for at least one day (¶ 2411). Resident status continues until permanent resident status is terminated or abandoned (¶ 2412).

Substantial Presence Test. An alien is considered a U.S. resident if the individual is physically present in the United States for at least 31 days during the calendar year and 183 days for the current and two preceding calendar years (¶ 2411). For purposes of the 183-day requirement, each day present in the United States during the current calendar year counts as a full day, each day in the first preceding year as ⅓ of a day, and each day in the second preceding year as ⅙ of a day (Code Sec. 7701(b)(3); Reg. § 301.7701(b)-1(c)).[18] There are exceptions as to what days an alien is considered to be physically present in the United States, including days for: (1) regular commuters from Canada or Mexico; (2) days in transit between two places outside the United States; (3) medical conditions preventing departure; (4) exempt individuals including teachers, trainees, and students on temporary visas, as well as professional athletes competing in a charitable event; (5) crew members of foreign vessels; and (6) foreign government workers. Form 8843 must be completed to exclude days of physical presence in the United States due to a medical condition or as an exempt individual. Presence in U.S. territories or possessions does not count as presence in the United States.

An individual who otherwise meets the substantial presence test may still be treated as a nonresident alien if the individual has a tax home in a foreign country during the tax year, has a closer connection to the foreign country, and was physically present in the United States for less than 183 days during the year. An alien must fully complete Form 8840 and attach it to his or her return for the relevant tax year to prove that he or she satisfies the closer connection exception.

2410. Elective Resident Status. There are two ways alien individuals are permitted to elect resident status if they do not otherwise qualify as a resident alien (¶ 2409). First, an individual who otherwise fails to meet the green card or substantial presence test may elect to be a resident alien for part of the current year (Code Sec. 7701(b)(4); Reg. § 301.7701(b)-4(c)(3)).[19] To qualify for the election, the individual:

- must not be a resident alien in the prior calendar year;

- must meet the substantial presence test in the calendar year following the election year;

- must be present in the United States for at least 31 consecutive days in the election year; and

- must be present in the United States for at least 75 percent of the days during the period from the first day of the 31-day presence period through the end of the election year.

If these requirements are met, the individual's election to be treated as a U.S. resident alien is effective for that portion of the year that begins on the first day of the earliest testing period that the 31-day and 75 percent requirements are met. The election is made by attaching a signed statement to the individual's tax return for the election year that the individual meets the election requirements. The election cannot be made before the individual has met the substantial presence test for the calendar year following the election year. Once made, the election can be revoked only with the IRS's consent.

The second way an alien may elect resident status is if the individual is married to a U.S. citizen or resident alien at the end of the tax year—then the election may be made

---

References are to Standard Federal Tax Reports; Tax Research Consultant; and Practical Tax Explanations.

[17] ¶ 43,117; EXPAT: 3,050; § 37,105

[18] ¶ 43,080, ¶ 43,117; EXPAT: 3,100; § 37,110.05

[19] ¶ 43,080, ¶ 43,120; EXPAT: 3,200; § 37,130

¶2410

in order to file a joint return (Code Sec. 6013(g) and (h)).[20] The taxpayer may be either a nonresident or resident alien at the end of the tax year for the election to be made. Both spouses must join in the election by attaching a statement to a joint return for the first tax year for which the election applies. It is effective for the entire tax year and all subsequent tax years for federal income tax and withholding purposes unless neither spouse is a U.S. citizen or resident alien at any time during the year. The election may also be jointly revoked by the couple or terminated by reason of death, separation, divorce, or by the IRS for failure of the couple to keep adequate records. Once terminated, the election may not be made again by the couple.

2411. Dual-Status Tax Years. An individual can be both a resident and nonresident alien during the same tax year (¶ 2409). This usually occurs the year of arrival in, or departure from, the United States. An individual who is a dual-status alien has a dual-status tax year. Thus, the individual's income tax liability is computed as a resident alien for the period of residence and as a nonresident alien for the period of nonresidence (¶ 2425) (Reg. § 1.871-13).[21]

If an alien individual is filing a tax return for a dual-status year, then the standard deduction cannot be claimed, the deduction for personal and dependency exemptions cannot exceed taxable income for the period the individual is a resident alien, and head of household filing status may not be used. A married individual may also not use joint filing status and tax rates for joint filers for the period of residency unless he or she is married to a U.S. citizen or resident alien and the election to be treated as a resident alien for the year is made (¶ 2410) (IRS Pub. 519). The education credits, earned income credit, and the elderly or disabled credit may also not be claimed unless the individual is married and elects to be treated as a resident alien by filing a joint return.

For this purpose, if an alien meets the green card test, residency starts the first day the individual is physically present in the United States while a lawfully admitted resident. If an alien meets the substantial presence test, residency starts the first day the individual is physically present in the United States during the calendar year. A *de minimis* exception allows up to ten days to be disregarded in determining the residency starting date under the substantial presence test if the individual has a closer connection to a foreign country. For an alien that satisfies both tests, residency starts on the earlier date when either test is satisfied (Reg. § 301.7701(b)-4).[22] If the individual was a resident alien in the previous tax year, then residency begins on the first day of the current tax year regardless of whether residency status is determined under the green card test or substantial presence test. Residency status may terminate before the end of the tax year under either test, but only if the individual is not a U.S. resident alien at any time during the following tax year.

Departure Requirements. Generally, no alien (whether resident or nonresident) is permitted to depart the United States or a U.S. possession without first obtaining a certificate of compliance from the IRS (sailing or departure permit). The certificate is proof that the individual has discharged all of his or her U.S. income tax liability (Code Sec. 6851(d); Reg. § 1.6851-2).[23] The certificate must be obtained at least two weeks before the individual leaves the United States. Resident aliens (whether they have taxable income or not) and nonresident aliens having no taxable income for the tax year must file Form 2063 to obtain the certificate. Nonresident aliens with taxable income for the tax year must file Form 1040-C to obtain the certificate. The forms do not constitute an individual's final tax return and Form 1040 or Form 1040NR must still be filed after the individual's tax year ends. Payment of any tax is not required prior to departure if it is determined that tax collection will not be jeopardized by the alien's departure. Individuals who abandon U.S. citizenship or long-term residency for tax avoidance purposes are subject to special rules (¶ 2412).

References are to Standard Federal Tax Reports; Tax Research Consultant; and Practical Tax Explanations.

[20] ¶ 35,160; EXPAT: 3,200; § 37,125.05

[21] ¶ 27,341; EXPAT: 3,150; § 37,120.05

[22] ¶ 43,120; EXPAT: 3,150; § 37,120.05

[23] ¶ 40,402, ¶ 40,405; FILEIND: 18,062.10; § 37,010.35

24 FOREIGN

2412. Expatriation to Avoid Tax. Individuals who relinquish their U.S. citizenship or whose long-term residency status (¶ 2409) is terminated—covered expatriates—are subject to a mark-to-market tax regime under which they are taxed on the unrealized gain in their property to the extent it exceeds $680,000 for 2014 ($690,000 for 2015) (Code Sec. 877A; Notice 2009-85; Rev. Proc. 2013-35; Rev. Proc. 2014-61).[24] For this purpose, a covered expatriate is considered to own any interest in property that would generally be taxable as part of his or her gross estate for federal estate tax purposes if the individual died on the day before the expatriation date. Special rules apply for deferred compensation items, specified tax deferred accounts, and interests in nongrantor trusts (¶ 566). A U.S. citizen or resident alien is also subject to a special transfer tax upon receipt of property by gift, devise, bequest, or inheritance from a covered expatriate (¶ 2948).

The exclusion amount must be allocated among all built-in gain property that is subject to the mark-to-market regime and is owned by the covered expatriate on the day before the expatriation date. Gain is determined as if a sale of the property for fair market value had taken place on the day before the expatriation date, and that gain is taken into account for the tax year without regard to other Code provisions. Losses from the deemed sale are generally taken into account as otherwise provided in the Code, except that the wash sale rules do not apply (¶ 1935). The taxpayer must make adjustments to the basis of any property by the amount of gain or loss taken into account.

Covered Expatriate. A covered expatriate is any U.S. citizen who relinquishes citizenship or any long-term U.S. resident who ceases to be a lawful permanent resident of the United States, if the individual: (1) has an average annual net income tax liability for the five preceding years ending before expatriation that exceeds $157,000 for 2014 ($160,000 for 2015); (2) has a net worth of $2 million or more on the expatriation date; or (3) fails to certify under penalties of perjury that he or she has complied with all U.S. tax obligations for the preceding five years or fails to submit evidence of compliance required by the IRS on Form 8854 (Code Sec. 877A(g); Notice 2009-85; Rev. Proc. 2013-35; Rev. Proc. 2014-61). Dual citizens and minors may be excepted from the tax liability and net worth requirements.

Election to Defer Tax. The covered expatriate may make an irrevocable election to defer payment of the mark-to-market tax that would otherwise be imposed on the deemed sale of property (Code Sec. 877A(b); Notice 2009-85).[25] The election cannot be made without providing adequate security as required by the IRS to ensure payment of the tax. In addition, no election can be made unless the individual makes an irrevocable waiver of any rights under an income tax treaty that would preclude assessment or collection of the tax.

The election is made on an asset-by-asset basis. The tax for a particular property is determined by multiplying the total mark-to-market tax by the ratio of the gain on the deemed sale of the property over the total gain taken into account with respect to all property deemed sold. The election defers payment of the tax until the due date for the return for the tax year in which the property is disposed or until the taxpayer's death. Payment may not be extended beyond the due date for the return for the tax year in which the covered expatriate dies.

Reporting Requirements. In addition to any other requirements for filing a return, a covered expatriate must also file an information return on Form 8854 in each tax year he or she is subject to the mark-to-market tax (Code Sec. 6039G; Notice 2009-85).[26] The return is also to be used to provide notice that the individual has relinquished his or her U.S. citizenship or long-term residency status.

2414. Resident of U.S. Possessions. Generally, an individual who is a bona fide resident of a U.S. possession during the tax year is subject to U.S. taxation as a U.S.

References are to Standard Federal Tax Reports; Tax Research Consultant; and Practical Tax Explanations.

[24] ¶ 27,430, ¶ 27,438.15; EX-PAT: 3,314; § 37,025.05

[25] ¶ 27,430, ¶ 27,438.15; EX-PAT: 3,322; § 37,025.10

[26] ¶ 27,438.15, ¶ 35,692; EX-PAT: 3,324; § 39,135.25

citizen or resident alien (¶ 2409), rather than as a nonresident alien (Code Sec. 876).[27] A U.S. possession for this purpose includes American Samoa, Guam, the Northern Mariana Islands, and Puerto Rico. Separate rules apply to a bona fide resident of the U.S. Virgin Islands (¶ 2416).

An individual is a bona fide resident of a U.S. possession if the person is physically present in the possession for a certain number of days during the tax year, does not have a tax home outside the possession, and does not have a closer connection to the United States or a foreign country than to the possession during the tax year (Code Sec. 937; Reg. § 1.937-1).[28] An individual with worldwide gross income of more than $75,000 must file Form 8898 for the tax year in which the individual becomes or ceases to be a bona fide resident of a U.S. possession. A spouse's income is not included when calculating an individual's worldwide gross income for this purpose. In addition, if married taxpayers are each required to file Form 8898, then a separate Form 8898 must be filed for each spouse regardless of whether a joint return is filed.

A U.S. citizen or resident alien who is a bona fide resident of American Samoa for the entire tax year may exclude from gross income for U.S. tax purposes any income derived from sources within the possession or that is effectively connected with a trade or business by the individual in the possession (Code Sec. 931).[29] The exclusion does not apply to income that is received for services performed as an employee of the United States. The individual may also not claim a tax credit or deduction that is attributable to the amount of excluded income. Form 4563 is used to claim the exclusion and must be attached to a Form 1040 filed with the IRS. A similar rule applies to a bona fide resident of Puerto Rico (¶ 2415).

2415. Resident of Puerto Rico. A U.S. citizen or resident alien (¶ 2409) who is also a bona fide resident of Puerto Rico during the entire tax year may exclude from gross income for U.S. tax purposes any income derived from sources within Puerto Rico (Code Sec. 933).[30] If the taxpayer gives up Puerto Rican residence after having been a bona fide resident for at least two years, then the taxpayer may claim a partial exclusion for the tax year of the residence change. In either case, the exclusion does not apply to income received for services performed as an employee of the United States. The taxpayer may also not claim any tax credit or deduction (except a personal exemption) which is attributable to the amount of excluded income.

A U.S. citizen or resident alien who has income from Puerto Rican sources is liable for the payment of taxes to Puerto Rico and may have to file a tax return with the United States as well. Generally, a U.S. citizen or resident alien who is a bona fide resident of Puerto Rico for the entire tax year must pay taxes to Puerto Rico on income from worldwide sources. If U.S. source income is also reported on an individual's Puerto Rican tax return, a credit may be claimed up to the amount allowable for income taxes paid to the United States.

2416. Resident of U.S. Virgin Islands. A U.S. citizen or resident alien (other than a bona fide resident of the U.S. Virgin Islands (¶ 2414)) who has income from sources within the U.S. Virgin Islands or effectively connected with a trade or business in the U.S. Virgin Islands is required to file an income tax return with both the United States and the U.S. Virgin Islands (Code Sec. 932).[31] The tax owed to the U.S. Virgin Islands is determined on Form 8689 by multiplying the total tax owed on the United States return (after certain adjustments) by the ratio of adjusted gross income (AGI) from the U.S. Virgin Islands to worldwide AGI. The U.S. Virgin Islands' tax liability (if paid) is credited against the individual's total U.S. tax liability. An individual who qualifies as a bona fide resident of the U.S. Virgin Islands (or who files a joint U.S. return with a U.S. citizen or resident with U.S. Virgin Islands income) will generally have no U.S. tax liability so long as the taxpayer reports all income from all sources on the return filed with the U.S. Virgin Islands.

References are to Standard Federal Tax Reports; Tax Research Consultant; and Practical Tax Explanations.

[27] ¶ 27,400; INTL: 24,300; § 37,145

[28] ¶ 28,395, ¶ 28,396; INTL: 24,300; § 37,145

[29] ¶ 28,240; INTL: 24,300; § 46,005.35

[30] ¶ 28,300; INTL: 24,050

[31] ¶ 28,280; INTL: 24,100; § 37,145

Nonresident Aliens and Foreign Corporations

2425. Taxation of Nonresident Aliens and Foreign Corporations. A nonresident alien (¶ 2409) and foreign corporation are generally taxed in the same manner as a U.S. citizen or domestic corporation on all income that is effectively connected with the conduct of a trade or business in the United States (¶ 2429). For this purpose, gain or loss from the disposition of a U.S. real property interest is treated as effectively connected income (¶ 2442). If any U.S. source income (¶ 2427) received by a nonresident alien or foreign corporation is not effectively connected with a U.S. trade or business, such as fixed, determinable, annual, or periodical (FDAP) income (¶ 2431), then it will generally be taxed at a flat 30-percent rate. A nonresident alien and foreign corporation may generally only claim deductions and credits related to effectively connected income (¶ 2446). A flat 30-percent tax rate also applies to the profits (and certain interest amounts) of a U.S. branch of a foreign corporation that are remitted to the foreign corporation during the tax year (¶ 2433).

A nonresident alien or foreign corporation who engages in trade or business in the United States at any time during the tax year or who has taxable income must generally file an income tax return (Code Secs. 6012 and 6072(c)).[32] Form 1040NR or Form 1040NR-EZ is used by a nonresident alien, and Form 1120-F is used by a foreign corporation. The returns are due on or before the 15th day of the 6th month following the close of the tax year (June 15 for calendar year taxpayers). Nonresident aliens and foreign corporations do not need to file a return in certain circumstances.

2427. Source of Income Rules. The U.S. taxation of nonresident aliens and foreign corporations (¶ 2425), as well as the application of the foreign tax credit limitations (¶ 2479), is dependent on the determination of the source of a taxpayer's income. Income is generally derived from U.S. sources or foreign sources in the following manner (Code Secs. 861, 862, and 865).[33]

- Interest income is generally sourced to the residence or country of incorporation of the obligor. The method and place of payment are irrelevant (see exceptions below). Interest for the guarantee of a debt is analogous to interest paid on a loan and is U.S. source income if paid by a noncorporate U.S. resident, domestic corporation, or any foreign person if effectively connected with a U.S. trade or business (¶ 2429).

- Dividend income, scholarships, grants, prizes, and awards are sourced to the residence of the payor (see exceptions below).

- Compensation for personal services is sourced to the place where the services are rendered. The location of the payor's residence, where the services are contracted for, and place of payment are irrelevant. If services are performed only partly within the United States, compensation is generally sourced on the basis of time spent working in each location.

- Rents and royalties are sourced to the location of the property.

- Gain on the sale of real property is sourced to the location of the property (¶ 2442).

- Gain on the sale of inventory is sourced to where the sale occurs (where title to the inventory passes).

- Gain on the sale of personal property that is not inventory is sourced to the residence of the seller (except for depreciable personal property, intangible property, or stock of an affiliate).

Special source rules apply to income that is derived from transportation, space, ocean, and communications activities. Other items of income are allocated or apportioned to sources within or without the United States as provided in regulations or other IRS rulings (for example, mixed-source income) (Code Sec. 863).[34] Where allocation of an item of income is not provided, then it must be construed.

References are to Standard Federal Tax Reports; Tax Research Consultant; and Practical Tax Explanations.

[32] ¶ 35,142, ¶ 36,720; INTL: 3,750; § 37,010.10, § 37,015.10

[33] ¶ 27,120, ¶ 27,151, ¶ 27,200; INTL: 3,000; § 37,205.05

[34] ¶ 27,160; INTL: 3,000

¶2425

Interest Income Exceptions. Interest paid by a foreign corporation or foreign partnership engaged in a U.S. trade or business is treated as U.S. source income rather than foreign sourced if paid by the U.S. trade or business (Code Secs. 861(a)(1) and 884(f)).[35] However, interest on deposits in foreign branches of U.S. commercial banks is treated as foreign source income. A qualified fails charge is treated similar to interest but is sourced to the residence of the recipient or the taxpayer's qualified business unit (QBU), unless the income is effectively connected with a U.S. trade or business. Qualified fails charges are amounts paid for the failure to deliver designated securities on the settlement date in a delivery-versus-payment transaction (Reg. § 1.863-10).[36]

Dividend Exceptions. A portion of the dividends paid by a foreign corporation are U.S. source income rather than foreign sourced if: (1) 25 percent or more of the corporation's gross income for a three-year period is effectively connected with a U.S. trade or business, or (2) it is required to figure the dividends received deduction by a U.S. corporation (¶ 223) (Code Sec. 861(a)(2)).[37] Dividends paid by a U.S. corporation electing to be treated as a possession corporation (¶ 1362) are treated as foreign source income.

Allocation of Expenses. U.S. taxpayers are allowed deductions directly related to U.S. source or foreign source income to determine taxable income. Deductions are generally first allocated to the activity or property from which the class of income is derived. If any expense or loss is not directly related to any specific item of income, then it must be apportioned ratably between certain statutory and residual groupings (Code Secs. 861(b) and 862(b); Reg. § 1.861-8; Temp. Reg. § 1.861-8T).[38] Special apportionment rules are provided for interest expenses, research and development expenses, losses from the disposition of property, net operating losses, income taxes, and legal, accounting, and stewardship fees.

Interest expenses are considered related to all income-producing activities and assets of a taxpayer. They are generally allocated to all gross income that the assets of the taxpayer generate (Code Sec. 864(e); Reg. § 1.861-9; Temp. Reg. § 1.861-9T).[39] As a result, allocation and apportionment of interest expenses must be made on the basis of the taxpayer's assets, the various statutory groupings or classes. Taxpayers may choose to value their assets on the basis of fair market value, tax book value, or an alternative tax book value method. Exceptions exist for qualified nonrecourse debt, assets acquired in integrated financial transactions, and certain related controlled foreign corporation (CFC) debt. In the case of an affiliated group of corporations, interest expenses must be allocated and apportioned to members based on asset values as if all members were a single taxpayer (the one-taxpayer rule). For tax years beginning after 2020, a one-time election may be made to determine foreign source taxable income of an affiliated group, by allocating and apportioning interest expense of the domestic members of the affiliated group on a worldwide basis, as if all members of the group were a single corporation (Code Sec. 864(f); Reg. § 1.861-11; Temp. Reg. § 1.861-11T).[40]

2429. Income Effectively Connected With U.S. Trade or Business. A nonresident alien (¶ 2409) and foreign corporation are taxed in the same manner as a U.S. citizen or domestic corporation on income that is effectively connected with the conduct of a trade or business in the United States (Code Secs. 871(b) and 882(a)).[41] Generally, all income, gain, or loss from sources within the United States is treated as effectively connected with the conduct of a U.S. trade or business for this purpose, including gain from the

---

[35] ¶ 27,120, ¶ 27,540; INTL: 3,100

[36] ¶ 27,173; INTL: 3,325

[37] ¶ 27,120; INTL: 3,150; § 37,205.15

[38] ¶ 27,120, ¶ 27,138, ¶ 27,139, ¶ 27,151; INTL: 6,000; § 37,210.05

[39] ¶ 27,139C, ¶ 27,140, ¶ 27,180; INTL: 6,100; § 37,210.10

[40] ¶ 27,140, ¶ 27,141E, ¶ 27,142; INTL: 6,108

[41] ¶ 27,320, ¶ 27,500; INTLIN: 3,100; § 37,010.20, § 37,015.20

disposition of U.S. real property interests (¶ 2442) and any scholarship or fellowship grant of a visiting student, teacher, or trainer (¶ 2448) (Code Sec. 864(c)(3)).[42] There are two exceptions.

First, fixed, determinable, annual, or periodical (FDAP) income (¶ 2431) from *U.S. sources*, as well as capital gains from U.S. sources (¶ 2435) are treated as income effectively connected with a U.S. trade or business if: (1) the income, gain, or loss is derived from assets used or held for use in the conduct of a U.S. trade or business, or (2) the activities of a U.S. trade or business are a material factor in the realization of the income, gain, or loss. In applying these factors, consideration is given to whether or not the asset or income involved was separately accounted for by the trade or business. In addition, a nonresident alien or foreign corporation who is a member of a partnership or the beneficiary of an estate or trust, which at any time within the tax year is engaged in a trade or business within the United States, is considered to be engaged in a U.S. trade or business (Code Sec. 875).[43] A nonresident alien and foreign corporation may elect to treat investment income from U.S. real property interests as effectively connected income (¶ 2432).

Second, income, gain, or loss from *foreign sources* is treated as effectively connected with the conduct of a U.S. trade or business if the nonresident alien or foreign corporation maintains an office or other fixed place of business in the United States at any time during the tax year to which the income, gain, or loss is attributable (Code Sec. 864(c)(4)).[44] Under these circumstances, the following foreign source income (or the economic equivalent of such income) is treated as effectively connected with a U.S. trade or business:

- rents and royalties derived from the use of intangible property;

- dividends, interest, or amounts received for the guarantees of debt that is either (1) derived from the active conduct of a banking, financial, or similar business through securities or debt obligations, or (2) received by a corporation the principal business of which is trading in stocks or securities for its own account; or

- income from the disposition of inventory or personal property held for sale in the normal course of business through a U.S. office.

Trade or Business. Whether a nonresident alien or foreign corporation is conducting a trade or business within the United States is a facts and circumstances test determined on a yearly basis (Reg. § 1.864-2(e)).[45] However, the conduct of a U.S. trade or business denotes a considerable, continuous, and regular course of activity by the taxpayer or through an agent, partnership, estate, or trust. Thus, the taxpayer need not be present in the United States to be engaged in a U.S. trade or business.

For this purpose, a trade or business includes the performance of personal services within the United States at any time during the tax year unless the services are performed by a nonresident alien who is temporarily present in the United States for a period of 90 days or less, compensation received for the services does not exceed $3,000, and the services are performed for another nonresident alien, foreign corporation, or foreign partnership (Code Sec. 864(b)).[46] A trade or business also does not generally include the trading of stocks, securities, or commodities through a resident broker, commission agent, custodian, or other independent agent unless the individual or foreign corporation is a dealer.

2431. Fixed, Determinable, Annual, or Periodical (FDAP) Income. Fixed, determinable, annual, or periodical (FDAP) income of a nonresident alien or foreign corporation received from U.S. sources is generally taxed at a flat 30-percent rate (or lower rate permitted under a tax treaty) if the income is not effectively connected with the conduct

---

References are to Standard Federal Tax Reports; Tax Research Consultant; and Practical Tax Explanations.

[42] ¶ 27,180; INTLIN: 3,104; § 37,010.20, § 37,015.20

[43] ¶ 27,380; INTLIN: 3,052.10; § 37,010.20, § 37,015.20

[44] ¶ 27,180; INTLIN: 3,106; § 37,010.20, § 37,015.20

[45] ¶ 27,182; INTLIN: 3,052; § 37,010.20, § 37,015.20

[46] ¶ 27,180; INTLIN: 3,050; § 37,010.20, § 37,015.20

¶2431

of a U.S. trade or business (¶ 2429). To ensure collection and payment, the tax must be withheld from the payment of FDAP income by a withholding agent (¶ 2455).

FDAP income includes interest, dividends, rents, salaries, wages, premiums, annuities, compensation, remunerations, emoluments, and any other item of annual or periodical gain, profit, or income (Code Secs. 871(a) and 881(a)).[47] It also includes royalties for timber, coal, and iron ore, as well as payments contingent on the productivity, use, or disposition of patents, copyrights, secret processes and formulas, and other like property. A nonresident alien and foreign corporation, however, may elect to treat income from U.S. real property interests as effectively connected income (¶ 2432).

A dividend equivalent payment is treated as a dividend from U.S. sources in determining FDAP income (Code Sec. 871(m); Reg. § 1.871-15(d); Prop. Reg. § 1.871-15(d)(2)). A dividend equivalent payment is any payment (or substantially similar payment) made under a securities lending or sale-repurchase transaction pursuant to a specified notional principal contract determined by, and contingent upon, the payment of U.S. source dividends. For payments made on or after January 1, 2016, all notional principal contracts are specified notional principal contracts, unless the IRS determines there is no potential for tax avoidance.

Social Security Benefits. For purposes of computing a nonresident alien's taxable income (as well as for withholding purposes), 85 percent of any Social Security benefits received is considered FDAP income (Code Sec. 871(a)(3)).[48]

Original Issue Discount. For a sale or exchange of an original issue discount (OID) obligation (¶ 1952), the amount of OID accruing while the obligation is held by a nonresident alien or foreign corporation is considered FDAP income. A payment on an OID obligation is also subject to the tax to the extent that the payment reflects OID accruing while the obligation is held by the nonresident alien or foreign corporation (Code Secs. 871(a)(1)(C) and 881(a)(3)).[49] For this purpose, an OID obligation includes any bond or other evidence of indebtedness having OID (Code Sec. 871(g)). It does not include any obligation payable 183 days or less from its date of original issue or any tax-exempt obligation.

Portfolio Interest. U.S. source portfolio interest is generally not considered FDAP income. Exempt portfolio interest includes any interest (including OID) accrued on an obligation issued after March 18, 2012, that is in registered form and held by the nonresident alien or foreign corporation (Code Secs. 871(h) and 881(c); Reg. § 1.871-14(a); Temp. Reg. § 1.871-14T)[50] For registered obligations, the exception is generally available only if the beneficial owner has provided the withholding agent with Form W-8BEN or other statement certifying that the beneficial owner is not a U.S. person (with exceptions for certain foreign-targeted obligations issued before January 1, 2016) (Notice 2012-20; Temp. Reg. § 1.871-14T(e)). For obligations issued on or before March 18, 2012, the portfolio interest exemption applies if the obligation is in bearer or registered form (Temp. Reg. § 1.871-14T(b)).

Exempt portfolio interest does not include contingent interest or interest received by a nonresident alien or foreign corporation that is a 10-percent shareholder. Interest is generally contingent if it is determined by reference to any receipts, income, or change in value of property of the debtor or a related person (¶ 432 and ¶ 1717). Other types of contingent interest may be identified by the IRS to prevent tax avoidance. A 10-percent shareholder is any person who owns 10 percent or more of the total combined voting power of all classes of stock in a corporation or 10 percent or more of a capital or profits interest in a partnership.

Other Interest and Dividend Income. FDAP does not include a portion of any dividend received by a nonresident alien or foreign corporation paid by a U.S. corporation primarily engaged in an active trade or business in a foreign country (80/20

[47] ¶ 27,320, ¶ 27,480; INTLIN: 3,102, INTL: 3,558; § 37,010.15, § 37,015.15

[48] ¶ 27,320; INTL: 3,556; § 37,010.15

[49] ¶ 27,320, ¶ 27,480; INTL: 3,558.10; § 37,010.15, § 37,015.15

[50] ¶ 27,320, ¶ 27,341B; ¶ 27,341C, ¶ 27,480; INTL: 3,558.20; § 37,010.15, § 37,015.15

¶2431

company), but only if the corporation was an 80/20 company before 2011 (Code Secs. 871(i) and (l), and 881(d)).[51] Payments made by corporations not in existence as of January 1, 2011, are not eligible for the exemption. A grandfathered corporation must meet a modified 80-percent foreign business requirement for each subsequent tax year (rather than over a three year period). The grandfathered corporation must also not have a substantial new line of business after August 10, 2010.

FDAP income of a nonresident alien and foreign corporation does not include other types of interest and dividends, including: (1) interest paid on bank deposits not effectively connected with a U.S. trade or business; (2) income derived by a foreign bank of central issue from bankers' acceptances; (3) the portion of a dividend that is paid by a foreign corporation and treated as U.S. source income (¶ 231); and (4) certain interest-related dividends and short-term capital gain dividends received from a regulated investment company or mutual fund (¶ 2301) if paid with respect to a tax year beginning before January 1, 2014 (Code Secs. 871(i)(2) and (k), and 881(d)).

> **Comment:** Absent further legislation, the exception for certain interest-related dividends and short-term capital gain dividends received from a regulated investment company or mutual fund will not apply if paid with respect to tax years beginning after December 31, 2013. For the latest legislative updates, visit our website www.CCHGroup.com/TaxUpdates.

U.S. Possession Corporations. A corporation created or organized in, or under the laws of, Guam, American Samoa, the Northern Mariana Islands, or the U.S. Virgin Islands is not considered a foreign corporation and thus is not subject to the tax on FDAP income if certain requirements are met. However, U.S. source dividends paid to a Puerto Rico corporation is considered FDAP income and subject to U.S. taxation and withholding at a 10-percent rate (Code Sec. 881(b)).[52]

2432. Election to Treat Real Property Income as Effectively Connected Income. A nonresident alien (¶ 2409) and foreign corporation may elect to treat income from U.S. real property interests (¶ 2442) held for investment purposes as effectively connected with the conduct of a U.S. trade or business (Code Secs. 871(d) and 882(d)).[53] The election is available where the income would not otherwise qualify as effectively connected income (¶ 2429), thus allowing the taxpayer to claim deductions associated with the property (¶ 2446). The election applies to all income of the taxpayer from all U.S. real property interests, including rents or royalties from mines, wells, or other natural deposits, as well as certain timber, iron ore, and coal royalties. It does not include mortgage interest, dividends from a real estate investment trust (¶ 2331), income from personal property, and income of a nonresident alien from real property which is not held for the production of income, such as a personal residence (Reg. §§ 1.871-10 and 1.882-2).[54] The election is made by attaching a statement to the taxpayer's timely filed return or amended return. Once made, the election applies to the current tax year and all subsequent tax years until revoked by filing a timely amended return for all affected years. If the election is revoked, the taxpayer may not make a new election for five years without the IRS's consent.

2433. Branch Profits Tax. A foreign corporation that operates a trade or business in the United States may be required to pay a branch profits tax and a branch-level interest tax in addition to the tax on income effectively connected with the conduct of a U.S. trade or business (¶ 2429). The branch profits tax is 30 percent (or lower if permitted by a tax treaty) of the foreign corporation's dividend equivalent amount (Code Sec. 884).[55] This is the amount of the foreign corporation's effectively connected after-tax earnings that are not reinvested in a U.S. trade or business by the close of the tax year or disinvested in a later tax year. The branch interest tax is 30 percent (or lower if permitted by a tax treaty) of the amount of interest paid by a U.S. branch of a foreign

---

References are to Standard Federal Tax Reports; Tax Research Consultant; and Practical Tax Explanations.

[51] ¶ 27,320, ¶ 27,480; INTL: 3,558.25; § 37,010.15, § 37,015.15

[52] ¶ 27,480; INTL: 33,158; § 37,010.15, § 37,015.15

[53] ¶ 27,320, ¶ 27,500; INTLIN: 3,114.05; § 37,020

[54] ¶ 27,338, ¶ 27,502; INTLIN: 3,114.05; § 37,020

[55] ¶ 27,540; INTLIN: 3,150

corporation with respect to a liability and notional excess interest amounts. If there is a conflict between the branch profits tax or branch-level interest tax with any U.S. income tax treaty, special rules are provided to determine the extent to which the treaty takes priority.

2435. Capital Gains of Nonresident Aliens and Foreign Corporations. U.S. sourced capital gains of a nonresident alien (¶ 2409) or foreign corporation may be completely exempt from U.S. taxation if they are not: (1) effectively connected with the conduct of a U.S. trade or business (¶ 2429); (2) gains from the sale of U.S. real property interests (¶ 2442); or (3) fixed, determinable, annual, or periodical (FDAP) income (¶ 2431) (Code Secs. 871(a)(2) and 881(a)).[56] In the case of a nonresident alien, net capital gains that do not fall into one of these three categories are exempt from U.S. tax if the individual is not present in the United States for at least 183 days (whether or not consecutive) during the tax year. If the 183-day limitation is exceeded, the individual's net capital gains not effectively connected to conduct of a U.S. trade or business are subject to a flat 30-percent tax rate. For purposes of this rule, gains and losses are determined without regard to the exclusion of gain from the sale of qualified small business stock (¶ 1905) or the carryover of capital losses (¶ 1754).

2438. Community Income of Nonresident Aliens. If a nonresident alien (¶ 2409) is married to a U.S. citizen or resident and does not elect to be treated as a resident (¶ 2410), then any community income is to be treated as follows:

- earned income (other than from a trade or business or the distributive share of partnership income) is treated as income of the spouse who earned it;

- trade or business income (other than from a partnership) is treated as the separate income of the spouse carrying on the trade or business (unless carried on jointly);

- a distributive share of partnership income is treated as the income of the spouse who is the partner with no portion attributed to the other spouse; and

- all other community income from separate property of one spouse is treated as the income of that spouse (Code Sec. 879).[57]

2442. Sale or Disposition of U.S. Real Property Interest. The gain or loss derived by a nonresident alien (¶ 2409) or foreign corporation from the sale, exchange, or other disposition of a U.S. real property interest is treated as gain or loss effectively connected with a conduct of a U.S. trade or business (¶ 2429) (Code Sec. 897).[58] Income from a U.S. real property interest held for investment purposes is not considered income effectively connected with a U.S. trade or business. However, a nonresident alien and foreign corporation may elect to treat income from U.S. real property interests held for investment purposes as effectively connected income in order to claim deductions associated with the property (¶ 2446). A foreign corporation that holds a U.S. real property interest may also elect to be treated as a domestic corporation for this purpose if, under any treaty obligation of the United States, it is entitled to nondiscriminatory treatment of its U.S. real property interests (Code Sec. 897(i)).

Cash or property received by a nonresident alien or foreign corporation in exchange for an interest in a partnership, trust, or estate is considered received from the sale or disposition of U.S. real property interest to the extent attributable to the sale or disposition of a U.S. real property interest (Code Sec. 897(g)). Similarly, special look-through rules apply for distributions by qualified investment entities attributable to dispositions of U.S. real property interests (¶ 2444).

Real Property Interests. A U.S. real property interest is any interest in real property (including a mine, well, or other natural deposit) located in the United States or the U.S. Virgin Islands (Code Sec. 897(c); Reg. § 1.897-1).[59] Real property includes land and

---

References are to Standard Federal Tax Reports; Tax Research Consultant; and Practical Tax Explanations.

[56] ¶ 27,320, ¶ 27,480; INTL: 3,560; § 37,010.15, § 37,015.15

[57] ¶ 27,460; INDIV: 24,156; § 23,210.35, § 45,920.10

[58] ¶ 27,700; INTLIN: 6,050; § 37,410.05, § 37,425

[59] ¶ 27,700, ¶ 27,701; INTLIN: 6,056; § 37,405

24

FOREIGN

improvements, personal property associated with the use of the real property, and unsevered timber, crops, and minerals. The nonresident alien's or foreign corporation's interest can be any interest (other than solely as a creditor), such as a direct ownership, fee-ownership, co-ownership, as well as any leasehold or option to acquire the property.

An interest in U.S. real property also includes any interest (other than solely as a creditor) in a U.S. real property holding corporation (USRPHC), unless the corporation was not a USRPHC during the shorter of the five-year period ending on the date of disposition, or the period the taxpayer held the interest in the corporation. A corporation is a USRPHC if the fair market value of its U.S. real property interests is at least 50 percent of the fair market value of all of its real property interests and any other property used in its business (Reg. § 1.897-2).[60] For this purpose, a corporation is considered to own a proportionate share of the assets held through a partnership, trust, or estate, as well as a domestic or foreign corporation in which it holds a controlling interest.

Whether a corporation is a USRPHC is generally determined as of the last day of the corporation's tax year, the date on which the corporation acquires a U.S. real property interest, *and* the date on which the corporation disposes of a real property interest located outside the United States or disposes of other assets used in a trade or business during the calendar year. The IRS has issued simplified procedures for a taxpayer to request relief for late filings establishing that a domestic corporation is not a USRPHC or that nonrecognition of gain or treaty provisions apply (Rev. Proc. 2008-27).[61]

A U.S. real property interest does not include any interest in a USRPHC if, as of the date of disposition, the corporation has already disposed of all of its U.S. real property interests in a transaction in which it recognized gain (the cleansing rule). In addition, if a corporation has a class of stock that is regularly traded on an established securities market, then such stock will be treated as a U.S. real property interest only in the hands of a taxpayer who owns more than five percent of the total fair market value of that class of stock.

Distributions of U.S. Real Property Interests. If a foreign corporation distributes a U.S. real property interest with respect to its stock, then the corporation recognizes gain (but not loss) to the extent the fair market value of the property at the time of distribution exceeds its adjusted basis (Code Sec. 897(d); Temp. Reg. § 1.897-5T(c)).[62] A foreign corporation may avoid recognizing gain if at the time of the distribution, the distributee would be subject to U.S. taxation on a subsequent disposition of the property and if the fair market value of the distributed property in the hands of the distributee is no greater than its basis increased by any amount of gain recognized by the distributing corporation. The foreign corporation is required to file a U.S. income tax return to report the distribution, even if it has no tax liability.

Nonrecognition Exchanges. Nonrecognition provisions of the Code apply to the exchange of a U.S. real property interest by a nonresident alien or foreign corporation if the property is exchanged for another U.S. real property interest that would be subject to U.S. tax upon its subsequent disposition and the transferor meets certain filing requirements (Code Sec. 897(e); Temp. Reg. § 1.897-6T).[63] Nonrecognition provisions for this purpose include like-kind exchanges (¶ 1721), involuntary conversions (¶ 1713), contributions and distributions related to partnerships (¶ 443 and ¶ 453), and corporate liquidations and reorganizations (¶ 2205 and ¶ 2253). The transfer of a U.S. real property interest in exchange for stock in a foreign corporation may also qualify for nonrecognition treatment. This includes contributions to capital or as paid in surplus (Code Sec. 897(j)).

Withholding. In order to ensure that a foreign investor will pay taxes on gain realized on the sale or disposition of a U.S. real property interest, the transferee is generally required to withhold and deduct a tax equal to 10 percent of the amount

References are to Standard Federal Tax Reports; Tax Research Consultant; and Practical Tax Explanations.

[60] ¶ 27,702; INTLIN: 6,058; § 37,405
[61] ¶ 27,711.60; INTLIN: 6,058.35; § 37,405
[62] ¶ 27,700, ¶ 27,706; INTLIN: 6,060
[63] ¶ 27,700, ¶ 27,707; INTLIN: 6,062

realized on the disposition (Code Sec. 1445; Reg. § 1.1445-1)).[64] Special rules and withholding rates apply for distributions and other transactions by corporations, partnerships, estates, trusts, and qualified investment entities. There are certain exemptions and exceptions from withholding. If the transferee fails to withhold the required tax, then it may be held liable for the tax, as well as any applicable penalties or interest. The transferee must file Form 8288 and 8288-A to report and transmit the amount withheld to the IRS within 20 days of the transfer of the property. Form 8288-B is used by the transferor or transferee to obtain a withholding certificate from the IRS that the amount withheld can be adjusted.

2444. Look-Through Rules for Disposition of U.S. Real Property Interests. Any distribution by a qualified investment entity to a nonresident alien (¶ 2409), foreign corporation, or other qualified investment entity to the extent attributable to gain from the sale or exchange of a U.S. real property interest, must be treated by the recipient as gain from the sale or exchange of a U.S. real property interest (¶ 2442) (Code Sec. 897(h)).[65] A qualified investment entity includes any real estate investment trust (REIT) (¶ 2326) and, effective before January 1, 2014, any regulated investment company (RIC) or mutual fund (¶ 2301) that is a U.S. real property holding company (USRPHC). However, in determining whether a RIC is a USRPHC, the regularly traded stock exception in defining a USRPHC does not apply. In addition, the RIC must include its interest in any other domestically controlled REIT or RIC that is a USRPHC.

> **Comment:** Absent further legislation, the look-through rule will not apply to a RIC or mutual fund after December 31, 2013. For the latest legislative updates, visit our website www.CCHGroup.com/TaxUpdates.

The look-through rule does not apply to any distribution from a qualified investment entity with respect to a class of stock that is regularly traded on an established securities market in the United States if the foreign distributee did not own more than five percent of the class of stock at any time within one year of the distribution. To the extent this exception applies, the distribution from the qualified investment entity is treated as a dividend, and not as income effectively connected with a U.S. trade or business.

An interest in a domestically controlled qualified investment entity (less than 50 percent of the stock's value is held by foreign persons) is not treated as a U.S. real property interest and any gain from the sale of the interest does not pass through to a nonresident alien or foreign corporation. However, the gain is passed through if a wash sale transaction is involved. For this purpose, a wash sale transaction is one in which: (1) the interest in a domestically controlled qualified investment entity is disposed of within 30 days prior to a distribution by the qualified entity that would be treated as gain from the sale or exchange of a U.S. real property interest; and (2) a substantially identical interest is reacquired within 61 days of the distribution.

2446. Taxable Income of Nonresident Aliens and Foreign Corporations. A nonresident alien (¶ 2409) and foreign corporation are subject to U.S. income tax on income effectively connected with a U.S. trade or business (¶ 2429) and fixed, determinable, annual, periodical (FDAP) income from U.S. sources (¶ 2431). Generally, all exclusions from gross income permitted to U.S. citizens and domestic corporations may also be excluded by nonresident aliens and foreign corporations (Code Secs. 872 and 883).[66] In addition, earnings on certain categories of cross-border transactions may also be excluded, such as compensation paid by a foreign employer to an exchange student, teacher, trainee, or specialist (¶ 2448), gambling winnings derived from a legal wager initiated outside the United States, and earnings from the international operation of a ship or aircraft.

A nonresident alien or foreign corporation may only claim deductions and tax credits related to effectively connected income in determining taxable income (Code

24

FOREIGN

References are to Standard Federal Tax Reports; Tax Research Consultant; and Practical Tax Explanations.

[64] ¶ 32,780, ¶ 32,781; INTLIN: 6,100; § 37,415.05   [65] ¶ 27,700; INTLIN: 6,068; § 19,205.30   [66] ¶ 27,344, ¶ 27,520; INTL: 3,558.35, INTL: 3,604; § 37,010.25

Secs. 873, 874 and 882(c)).[67] This includes the foreign tax credit subject to the same limitations that apply to U.S. citizens and domestic corporations (¶ 2479) (Code Sec. 906).[68] Deductions and credits are generally not allowed in determining the tax on U.S. sourced FDAP income. However, a charitable contribution deduction can be claimed whether or not related to effectively connected income. Similarly, a nonresident alien may deduct one personal exemption (with certain exceptions) and casualty or theft losses (so long as the property is located in the United States). A nonresident alien and foreign corporation may elect to treat income from U.S. real property interests as effectively connected income in order to claim the deductions associated with the property (¶ 2432).

A nonresident alien or foreign corporation must file an accurate and timely return to claim any allowable deduction or credit. If a return is not filed, then the IRS may prepare one for the taxpayer but no deductions and credits will be allowed other than the credits for withheld taxes, gasoline and special fuels, and for nonresident aliens for taxes paid by a regulated investment company on undistributed capital gains (¶ 2305).

2448. Foreign Students, Teachers, or Trainees. A nonresident alien (¶ 2409) who is not otherwise engaged in a U.S. trade or business but who is temporarily present in the United States under immigration laws on a F, J, M, or Q visa as a visiting student, teacher, trainee, or specialist is considered to be engaged in a U.S. trade or business (Code Sec. 871(c)).[69] This means that any portion of a scholarship or fellowship grant from U.S. sources (including incidental expenses) that is not excludable from gross income (¶ 865) is income effectively connected with the conduct of a U.S. trade or business (¶ 2429). The income is subject to a special withholding rate of 14 percent (¶ 2455) (Code Sec. 1441(b); Reg. § 1.1441-4(c)).[70] Compensation paid by a foreign employer to a person in the United States as a visiting student, teacher, trainee, or specialist is exempt from tax (Code Sec. 872(b)(3)).[71]

2450. Tax Treaties. The United States has negotiated a network of tax treaties with other countries to avoid the double taxation of taxpayers on the same income and to prevent taxpayers from evading taxation. In addition, the United States has enacted strict anti-abuse rules to prevent individuals from treaty shopping, and has incorporated exchange of information clauses in many tax treaties to facilitate the enforcement of these rules. These anti-abuse rules deny treaty benefits to nonresidents of either the United States or its treaty partner that funnel income through the treaty country only to take advantage of reduced tax rates.

Generally, the Code is to be applied to a taxpayer with "due regard" to treaty obligations of the United States (Code Sec. 894).[72] In instances where a U.S. taxpayer takes the position that a treaty overrules or modifies the Code or regulations, disclosure of the position must generally be made with the taxpayer's tax return on Form 8833 (Code Sec. 6114; Reg. § 301.6114-1).[73] If a return is not otherwise required to be filed, a return must nevertheless be filed for purposes of making the required disclosure. The determination whether a treaty-based return position is required to be reported is made by comparing the taxpayer's tax liability under current law to that same tax liability as it would exist if the relevant treaty positions did not exist. Any difference must be reported. Failure to disclose the difference may result in a penalty (Code Sec. 6712).[74]

Tax treaties between the United States and foreign countries generally reduce the tax rate for income paid. Some countries allow the withholding of tax at the treaty-reduced rate. Other countries, however, withhold tax at their statutory tax rate and refund any difference upon receiving proof of residency. To apply for certification of U.S. residency to receive the benefits under a tax treaty, a taxpayer must file Form 8802 at

References are to Standard Federal Tax Reports; Tax Research Consultant; and Practical Tax Explanations.

[67] ¶ 27,360, ¶ 27,363, ¶ 27,500; INTL: 3,554.05; § 37,010.20, § 37,015.20

[68] ¶ 27,920; INTLOUT: 3,152.10; § 13,405.15

[69] ¶ 27,320; EXPAT: 3,108.25, EXPAT: 3,108.30; § 37,320.20

[70] ¶ 32,702, ¶ 32,708; INTL: 33,110.35; § 37,320.20

[71] ¶ 27,344; INTL: 3,558.35; § 37,010.25

[72] ¶ 27,640; INTL: 18,060; § 37,605

[73] ¶ 37,060, ¶ 37,061; FILEBUS: 12,056; § 37,605

[74] ¶ 40,135; FILEBUS: 12,056; § 37,605

least 45 days before the certificate is needed. If the application is approved, the IRS will provide the residency certification to the taxpayer on Form 6166. A nonresident alien or foreign corporation is not entitled under any U.S. income tax treaty to any reduced rate of withholding on an item of income derived through an entity treated as a partnership (or other fiscally transparent entity) if: (1) the income is not treated by the treaty partner as an item of income of such foreign person; (2) the foreign country does not impose tax on a distribution of the item by the U.S. entity to the foreign person; and (3) the treaty does not contain a provision addressing its applicability in the case of an item of income derived through a partnership (Code Sec. 894(c)).[75]

2452. Corporate Inversions. Special rules apply for the tax treatment of corporate inversion transactions where a U.S. corporation reincorporates in a foreign jurisdiction and thereby replaces the U.S. parent corporation of a multinational corporate group with a foreign parent corporation. Inversion transactions may take many different forms, including stock inversions, asset inversions, and various combinations. In any case, if former shareholders of a U.S. corporation hold 80 percent or more (by vote or value) of the stock of a foreign corporation after the transaction, the foreign corporation will be treated as a domestic corporation for U.S. tax purposes (Code Sec. 7874).[76] If the former shareholders hold at least 60 percent but less than 80 percent of the stock of the foreign corporation after the transaction, then the inversion transaction is respected but any applicable corporate-level tax imposed as a result of the transaction cannot be offset by tax attributes such as a net operating loss (NOL) or foreign tax credit. Regulations will be issued that further reduce the tax benefits of corporate inversions and post-inversion transactions, in certain circumstances. The regulations will generally apply to acquisitions and stock transfers completed on or after September 22, 2014 (Notice 2014-52).[77]

2455. Withholding of Tax on Nonresident Aliens and Foreign Corporations. A foreign person is generally subject to U.S. tax on U.S. source income received during the tax year (¶ 2425). To ensure collection and payment, the tax must be withheld from the payment of the U.S. source income to the foreign person by a withholding agent (Code Secs. 1441 and 1442).[78] Most types of U.S. source income received by a foreign person are subject to a 30-percent withholding rate. Different rates may apply, however, to wages paid to a nonresident alien employee (including pensions paid for personal services), scholarship or fellowship grants of a foreign exchange student (¶ 2448), dispositions of U.S. real property interests (¶ 2442), a foreign partner's distributive share of effectively connected income of a partnership, gross investment income paid to foreign private foundations (¶ 631), and dividends paid to a Puerto Rican corporation. Reduced rates of withholding may also apply, including an exemption, under a tax treaty or convention with the foreign person's country of residence (¶ 2450).

Persons Subject to Withholding. All nonresident aliens and foreign corporations, foreign partnerships, foreign trusts, and foreign estates are subject to withholding on U.S. source income. Withholding also applies to the foreign branch of a U.S. financial institution that furnishes an intermediary withholding certificate on Form W-8IMY to the withholding agent (Temp. Reg. § 1.1441-1T(b)(1) and (c)(2)).[79] A nonresident alien is any individual who is not a U.S. citizen or resident alien and includes any bona fide resident of Puerto Rico, Guam, the Northern Mariana Islands, the U.S. Virgin Islands, or American Samoa (Reg. § 1.1441-1(c)(3)).[80] A nonresident alien who elects resident status for income tax purposes (¶ 2410) is still considered a foreign person for nonresident alien withholding purposes on all income except wages. Withholding may also be required for payments made to certain foreign financial institutions (FFIs) (¶ 2469) and nonfinancial foreign entities (NFFEs) (¶ 2473) if certain requirements are not met. Under coordination rules, withholding does not apply if there is withholding under these provisions (Temp. Reg. § 1.1441-1T(b)(1)).

References are to Standard Federal Tax Reports; Tax Research Consultant; and Practical Tax Explanations.

[75] ¶ 27,640; INTL: 18,060; § 37,605

[76] ¶ 43,969; INTL: 30,082.05

[77] ¶ 43,971.50; INTL: 30,082.05

[78] ¶ 32,702, ¶ 32,720; INTL: 33,000; § 37,301

[79] ¶ 32,703E; INTL: 33,050; § 37,305

[80] ¶ 32,703; INTL: 33,050; § 37,305

¶2455

Income Subject to Withholding. U.S. source income subject to the withholding requirement includes: (1) fixed, determinable, annual, or periodical (FDAP) income (¶ 2431); (2) certain gains on the disposal of timber, coal, or domestic iron ore; and (3) gains relating to contingent payments received from the sale or exchange of patents, copyrights, and similar intangible property. If the source of the income cannot be determined at the time of payment (¶ 2427), it is treated as U.S. source income (Code Sec. 1441(b); Reg. § 1.1441-2(a)).[81] In addition, income payable for personal services performed in the United States is treated as from sources within the United States, regardless of where the location of the contract for the services was entered, the place of payment, or residence of payer. Income effectively connected with the conduct of a U.S. trade or business is not subject to the withholding requirements for foreign persons, including income received as wages (¶ 2429). Instead, such income is generally subject to the tax and withholding rules as if the foreign person were a U.S. citizen, resident, or domestic entity. However, special rules apply to the effectively connected income of a partnership (foreign or domestic) that is allocable to its foreign partners (Code Sec. 1446).[82]

Withholding Agent. The withholding agent is the person or entity required to deduct, withhold, and pay any tax on income paid to a foreign person (Reg. § 1.1441-7; Temp. Reg. § 1.1441-7T).[83] The duty is imposed on all persons (acting in whatever capacity) that have control, receipt, custody, disposal, or payment of any items of income which are subject to withholding. Thus, the withholding agent may be any individual, corporation, partnership, trust, or other entity (including a foreign intermediary or partnership). A withholding agent may designate an authorized agent on its behalf.

The withholding agent is personally liable for any tax required to be withheld except in the case of certain conduit financing arrangements (Code Sec. 1461).[84] This liability is independent of the tax liability of the foreign person for whom the tax was withheld from a payment of income. Even if the foreign person pays the tax, the withholding agent may still be liable for any interest, penalty, or addition to tax for failure to withhold (Code Sec. 1463).[85] A refund or credit of any overpayment is made to the withholding agent unless the tax was actually withheld (Code Sec. 1464).[86] The withholding agent is indemnified against any person claiming any tax properly withheld.

A withholding agent is not required to withhold any amount if the payee is a U.S. person or a foreign person that is the beneficial owner of the income and is entitled to a reduced rate of withholding. Absent actual knowledge (or reason to know), the withholding agent must obtain valid documentation from the payee that it is either a U.S. payee or beneficial owner. Generally, a U.S. payee is any person required to furnish Form W-9. While such persons are not subject to withholding as a foreign person, they may be subject to Form 1099 reporting and withholding requirements. A beneficial owner is any foreign person or entity that is required to furnish Form W-8BEN, Form W-8BEN-E, Form W-8ECI or Form W-8EXP. Payment to an intermediary (whether qualified or not), flow-through entity, or U.S. branch of a foreign entity may be treated as a payee for these purposes so long as valid documentation is provided on Form W-8IMY. In all cases in which valid documentation cannot be provided, the withholding agent may presume a person to be a U.S. payee or beneficial owner under specified rules.

Returns. A withholding agent must file an annual information return on Form 1042-S to report income paid to a foreign person during the tax year that is subject to withholding (unless an exception applies) (Reg. § § 1.1461-1 and 1.6302-2).[87] A separate Form 1042-S must be filed for each recipient, as well as for each type of income that is paid to the same recipient. A copy of Form 1042-S must also be provided to the recipient. Form 1042 is used by the withholding agent to report and pay the taxes withheld from

---

References are to Standard Federal Tax Reports; Tax Research Consultant; and Practical Tax Explanations.

[81] ¶ 32,702, ¶ 32,704; INTL: 33,100, INTL: 33,150, INTL: 33,200; § 37,320.05

[82] ¶ 32,800; INTL: 33,106; § 37,350.05

[83] ¶ 32,714, ¶ 32,714G; INTL: 33,054; § 37,315.05

[84] ¶ 32,820; INTL: 33,056; § 37,315.05

[85] ¶ 32,860; INTL: 33,056; § 37,315.05

[86] ¶ 32,880; INTL: 33,056; § 37,315.05

[87] ¶ 32,821, ¶ 38,062; INTL: 33,056; § 37,330

¶2455

the payments of income. The forms are also used by withholding agents making payments to FFIs (¶ 2469) and NFFEs (¶ 2473).

Both forms must be filed by March 15 of the year following the calendar year the income was paid. An automatic six-month extension for filing Form 1042 can be obtained by filing Form 7004. The extension of time to file does not extend the time to pay the withheld tax. An automatic 30-day extension for filing Form 1042-S can be obtained by filing Form 8809. A second extension request may be submitted by filing a second Form 8809 before the end of the initial extended due date. The IRS may require that the returns be filed electronically (¶ 2503). Paper Forms 1042-S must be accompanied by Form 1042-T.

The amount of tax required to be withheld will determine whether the withholding agent must deposit the taxes prior to the due date for filing the returns and how frequently such amounts must be deposited. Penalties may be imposed for failure to file, failure to provide complete and correct information, as well as failure to pay any taxes.

Reporting Foreign Assets of U.S. Taxpayers

2465. FBAR Reporting (Foreign Financial Assets). A United States person is required to disclose any interest in or signature over any financial account outside the United States if the aggregate value of the account exceeds $10,000 at any time during the calendar year (FBAR) (31 CFR Reg. § 1010.350). The disclosure is required to be made electronically on Treasury Department Financial Crimes Enforcement Network (FinCEN) Form 114 through FinCEN's BSA E-Filing System.[88] See ¶ 2570 for a further discussion of FBAR reporting.

2467. FATCA Reporting of Specified Foreign Financial Assets (Form 8938). Under the Foreign Account Tax Compliance Act (FATCA), an individual is required to disclose his or her interest in a specified foreign financial asset during the tax year if the aggregate value of all the assets exceeds an applicable threshold amount (¶ 2572) (Code Sec. 6038D).[89] The information is reported on Form 8938 and attached to the individual's tax return for the year.

2469. FATCA Reporting and Withholding Obligations for Foreign Financial Institutions (FFIs). Under the Foreign Account Tax Compliance Act (FATCA), a foreign financial institution (FFI) is required to report to the IRS certain information about financial accounts held by U.S. taxpayers or by foreign entities in which U.S. taxpayers hold substantial ownership interests (Code Sec. 1471).[90] If an FFI fails to meet the FATCA requirements, a U.S. withholding agent must deduct and withhold a tax equal to 30 percent on any "withholdable payment" made to the FFI after June 30, 2014, unless the withholding agent can reasonably rely on documentation that the payment is exempt from withholding (Code Sec. 1471(a); Temp. Reg. § 1.1471-2T(a)(1)).[91] The withholding requirement applies without regard to whether the FFI receives a withholdable payment as a beneficial owner or as a qualified intermediary (QI). No withholding is required, however, if an FFI enters into an agreement with the IRS to provide the required information (participating FFI). An FFI may also be deemed to meet the requirements of the agreement (deemed-compliant FFI). For a discussion of the requirements for FFI agreements, see ¶ 2471.

Foreign Financial Institutions. An FFI is a foreign entity that accepts deposits in the ordinary course of a banking business, holds financial assets for the account of others as a substantial part of its business (i.e., mutual fund), or is an investment entity whose gross income is primarily attributable to investing, reinvesting, or trading in financial assets (i.e., hedge fund, private equity fund) (Code Sec. 1471(d)(4); Reg. § 1.1471-5(d) and (e)).[92] In the case of an entity that is resident in a country that has in effect a Model 1 or Model 2 Intergovernmental Agreement with the United States (Model 1 IGA or Model 2 IGA), an FFI is any entity that is treated as an FFI pursuant to the Model 1 or Model 2 IGA.

References are to Standard Federal Tax Reports; Tax Research Consultant; and Practical Tax Explanations.

[88] ¶ 36,551D; FILEBUS: 9,104; § 37,705

[89] ¶ 35,593; FILEBUS: 9,108; § 37,710

[90] ¶ 32,883; INTL: 36,000; § 37,725.05

[91] ¶ 32,883, ¶ 32,884J; INTL: 36,050; § 37,725.05

[92] ¶ 32,883, ¶ 32,884T; INTL: 36,056; § 37,725.05

Withholdable Payment. A withholdable payment includes any payment of U.S. source fixed or determinable, annual or periodical (FDAP) income (¶ 2431), and for any sales or other dispositions occurring after December 31, 2016, any gross proceeds that can produce interest or dividends that are U.S. source FDAP income (Code Sec. 1473(1); Reg. § 1.1473-1(a)).[93] Withholdable payments do not include items of income effectively connected with a U.S. trade or business (¶ 2429), payments of interest or original issue discount (OID) on short-term obligations, and other specified nonfinancial payments, such as payments for services, leases of property, and interest payable from the acquisition of goods and services.

Withholding is not required with respect to any payment under a grandfathered obligation or from any gross proceeds from the disposition of a grandfathered obligation (Reg. § 1.1471-2(b); Temp. Reg. § 1.1471-2T(b)).[94] A grandfathered obligation is generally any legally binding agreement or instrument outstanding on July 1, 2014, such as a debt instrument, line of credit, derivatives transaction, life insurance contract, and immediate annuity contract. It also includes collateral associated with the obligation. It does not include any legal agreement or instrument treated as equity for U.S. tax purposes or that lacks a stated expiration or term (for example, savings deposits, demand deposits, or deferred annuity contract). Similarly, it does not include brokerage agreement, custodial agreement, investment insurance or annuity contract, or similar agreement to hold financial assets in an account for another person. A material modification of a grandfathered obligation will result in the obligation being treated as newly issued and subject to withholding. A payment made under a grandfathered obligation does include a payment made to a flow-through entity such as a partnership or trust. This includes a payment made with respect to the entity's disposition of the obligation. A foreign pass-through payment does not include any payment made under a grandfathered obligation, or any gross proceeds from the disposition of such an obligation. Withholding is also not required with respect to any payment to an exempt beneficial owner including most governmental entities, nonprofit organizations, certain small, local financial institutions, and certain retirement entities (Code Sec. 1471(f); Reg. § 1.1471-6; Temp. Reg. § 1.1471-6T).[95]

Withholding Agent. A U.S. withholding agent for FATCA reporting purposes includes any person in whatever capacity having the control, receipt, custody, disposal, or payment of any withholdable payment or foreign pass-through payment (Code Sec. 1473(4); Reg. § 1.1473-1(d)).[96] A U.S. withholding agent, participating FFI, qualified intermediary, or any other person that fails to withhold and deposit tax as required is liable for the tax and penalties, and is indemnified against claims and demands of anyone for the amount of the payments (Code Sec. 1474; Reg. §§ 1.1474-1 and 301.1474-1; Temp. Reg. § 1.1474-1T).[97] Form 1042 is used to report and pay taxes withheld during the tax year. In addition, an annual information return must be filed on Form 1042-S and a copy furnished to the recipient of the withholdable payment, including any qualified intermediaries, withholding foreign partnerships, and withholding foreign trusts. Both forms are due by March 15 of the calendar year following the year the withholdable payment was made to the recipient. The first information return will be required to be filed by March 31, 2015, with respect to the 2014 calendar year.

The IRS publishes a list of registered and approved FFIs and their Global Intermediary Identification Numbers (GIINs) every month. Withholding agents may rely on the IRS published list to verify an FFI's GIIN and not withhold on payments made to the FFI.

2014 and 2015 Transition Period. Calendar years 2014 and 2015 make up a transition period for purposes of IRS enforcement and administration of FATCA reporting and withholding requirements. The IRS will take into account whether good faith efforts have been made to comply with the rules (Notice 2014-33).[98]

References are to Standard Federal Tax Reports; Tax Research Consultant; and Practical Tax Explanations.

[93] ¶ 32,893, ¶ 32,895; INTL: 36,054; § 37,725.05
[94] ¶ 32,884H, ¶ 32,884J; INTL: 36,054; § 37,725.05
[95] ¶ 32,883, ¶ 32,884X; ¶ 32,884Z; INTL: 36,054; § 37,725.05
[96] ¶ 32,893, ¶ 32,895; INTL: 36,054; § 37,725.05
[97] ¶ 32,898, ¶ 32,899D, ¶ 32,899F; ¶ 32,899H; INTL: 36,150; § 37,725.05, § 37,730
[98] ¶ 32,887.35; INTL: 36,050; § 37,725.05

¶2469

2471. Foreign Financial Institution (FFI) Agreements. A foreign financial institution (FFI) meets its reporting requirements under the Foreign Account Tax Compliance Act (FATCA) (¶ 2469) by: (1) entering into an FFI agreement with the IRS (participating FFI); (2) being deemed to comply with the FATCA requirements without the need to enter into an FFI agreement (deemed-compliant FFI); or (3) being a resident in a country that has in effect a Model 1 or Model 2 Intergovernmental Agreement with the United States (Model 1 IGA or Model 2 IGA). The reporting requirements the FFI must meet include:

- identifying U.S. accounts it maintains in accordance with certain verification and due diligence procedures;

- reporting certain information to the IRS regarding the U.S. accounts and accounts held by a U.S. person who is unwilling to provide the required information (recalcitrant account holder); and

- deducting and withholding tax on any payment of U.S. source income by the FFI to a recalcitrant account holder or nonparticipating FFI (Code Sec. 1471(b); Reg. § 1.1471-4(a); Temp. Reg. § 1.1471-4T(a)).[99]

An FFI (including a reporting Model 2 FFI) may register itself and its branches on the IRS's FATCA registration website (or on a paper copy of Form 8957) to enter into an FFI agreement as a participating FFI, a registered-deemed compliant FFI, a limited FFI, or sponsoring entity that agrees to perform the reporting obligations for one or more FFIs. Upon approval, a registered FFI or sponsoring entity will receive a Global Intermediary Identification Number (GIIN) from the IRS, unless the FFI is treated as a limited FFI. An FFI or sponsoring entity uses its GIIN to identify that it is registered and approved to withholding agents and the IRS. The IRS publishes a list of registered and approved FFIs and their GIINs monthly. Withholding agents may rely on the IRS published list to verify an FFI's GIIN and not withhold on payments made to the FFI.

Identification Requirement. A participating FFI is required to identify and document the status of each holder of an account maintained by the FFI to determine if the account is a U.S. account, non-U.S. account, or an account held by a recalcitrant account holder or nonparticipating FFI (Reg. § 1.1471-4(c)(1)). A U.S. account is a financial account held by one or more specified U.S. persons or U.S.-owned foreign entities, including any depository or custodial account maintained by the FFI, and any equity or debt interest in the FFI other than an interest regularly traded on an established securities market (Code Sec. 1471(d); Reg. § § 1.1471-5(a) and 1.1473-1(c)).[100] A specified U.S. person is any U.S. person *other than* a: dealer in securities, commodities, or derivative financial instruments; broker; publicly traded corporation; tax exempt organization, trust, or individual retirement plan; bank, real estate investment trust (REIT), regulated investment company (RIC or mutual fund), common trust fund or charitable remainder trust; or government entity.

An FFI must follow due diligence procedures for identifying and documenting account holders based on the value and risk profile of the account. FFIs in many cases are permitted to rely on information they already collect (Reg. § 1.1471-4(c)). Generally, accounts with a balance or value of more than $50,000 ($250,000 for a cash value insurance or annuity contract) but less than $1 million are only subject to electronic review of searchable data for indicia of U.S. status. Accounts with a balance that exceeds $1 million are subject to review of electronic and non-electronic files for U.S. indicia, including an inquiry of the actual knowledge of any relationship manager associated with the account. A preexisting account of an individual with a balance or value of $50,000 or less, as well as certain cash value insurance contracts with a value of $250,000 or less, are excluded from the due diligence review unless the FFI elects otherwise. Preexisting accounts of an entity with account balances of $250,000 or less are also exempt from review until the account balance exceeds $1 million.

References are to Standard Federal Tax Reports; Tax Research Consultant; and Practical Tax Explanations.

[99] ¶ 32,883, ¶ 32,884P; ¶ 32,884R; INTL: 36,060; § 37,725.10

[100] ¶ 32,883, ¶ 32,884T, ¶ 32,895; INTL: 36,060; § 37,725.10

Reporting Requirement. A participating FFI is required to report annually to the IRS the name, address, and taxpayer identification number (TIN) of each holder of a U.S. account which is a specified U.S. person. In the case of any account holder which is a U.S.-owned foreign entity, the participating FFI must report the name, address, and TIN of each substantial U.S. owner of the entity (Code Sec. 1471(c); Reg. § 1.1471-4(d) and (i)). The FFI must also report the account number, the year-end account balance or value in U.S. dollars, and the gross amount and character of dividends, interest, or other income paid or credited to the account. This includes the gross proceeds from the sale or redemption of property paid or credited to the account. Special rules are provided for a participating FFI to report information regarding its recalcitrant account holders. If an FFI is prohibited by foreign law from reporting the required information with respect to an account, then it must close the account within a reasonable period of time or must otherwise block or transfer the account.

A participating FFI reports the required information on Form 8966 with respect to each account maintained at any time during the calendar year. The form must be filed electronically with the IRS by March 31 of the year following the end of the calendar year to which it relates. Form 8809 is used to request a 90-day extension. Special reporting rules, however, apply for U.S. accounts and accounts held by owner-docu-mented FFIs maintained during the 2014 and 2015 calendar years if the effective date of the FFI agreement of the participating FFI is on or before December 31, 2015 (Temp. Reg. § 1.1471-4T(d)(7)). As an alternative to filing Form 8966, the FFI may elect to be subject to the same reporting requirements of U.S. institutions. Thus, the institution must provide a full Form 1099 reporting for every account with a U.S. person or U.S. foreign entity as an account holder. As a result, both U.S. and foreign source amounts (including gross proceeds) are subject to reporting under this election regardless of whether the amounts are paid inside or outside the United States.

Withholding Requirement. A participating FFI is required to deduct and withhold 30 percent from any withholdable payment (¶ 2469) made by the FFI to an account held by a recalcitrant account holder or to a nonparticipating FFI after June 30, 2014 (Temp. Reg. § 1.1471-4T(b)(1)). If an FFI is prohibited by foreign law from withholding as required with respect to an account, then it must close the account within a reasonable period of time or must otherwise block or transfer the account (Reg. § 1.1471-4(a)(1)). A participating FFI is not required to deduct and withhold tax on a foreign pass-through payment made by the FFI to an account held by a recalcitrant account holder or to a nonparticipating FFI before the later of January 1, 2017, or the date final regulations are issued defining foreign pass-through payments. A participating FFI may elect not to withhold on any withholdable payments, but instead have a U.S. withholding agent withhold tax on payments the electing FFI receives which are allocable to a recalcitrant account holder or a nonparticipating FFI (Code Sec. 1471(b)(3)).

2473. FATCA Reporting and Withholding Obligations for Non-Financial Foreign Entities (NFFEs). Under the Foreign Account Tax Compliance Act (FATCA), if a non-financial foreign entity (NFFE) is the beneficial owner of a withholdable payment (¶ 2469) made to the NFFE after June 30, 2014, then the NFFE is required to report certain information to the withholding agent (Code Sec. 1472(b); Reg. § 1.1472-1; Temp. Reg. § 1.1472-1T).[101] The reporting requirement is satisfied if the NFFE reports the name, address, and taxpayer identification number (TIN) of each substantial U.S. owner or if it certifies that it does not have any substantial U.S. owners. If the NFFE or other payee fails to meet the reporting requirement, then the withholding agent must deduct and withhold a tax of 30 percent from the withholdable payment.

References are to Standard Federal Tax Reports; Tax Research Consultant; and Practical Tax Explanations.

[101] ¶ 32,888, ¶ 32,890, ¶ 32,890B; INTL: 36,100; § 37,730

¶2473

An NFFE for this purpose is any foreign entity that is not a financial institution, meaning the entity does not accept deposits in the ordinary course of a banking business, does not hold financial assets for the account of others as a substantial part of its business, and is not engaged primarily in investing. A substantial U.S. owner is:

- in the case of a corporation, a U.S. person that owns, directly or indirectly, more than 10 percent of the corporate stock by vote or value;

- in the case of a partnership, a U.S. person that owns directly or indirectly, more than 10 percent of the capital or profits interests of the partnership; and

- in the case of a trust, a U.S. person treated as an owner of any portion of the trust under the grantor trust rules and any U.S. person holding more than 10 percent of the beneficial interests (Code Sec. 1473(2); Reg. § 1.1473-1(b)).[102]

A withholding agent that receives information about substantial U.S. owners of an NFFE must report the information to the IRS on or before March 15 of the calendar year following the year in which the withholdable payment is made. This includes the name of the NFFE and the name, TIN, and address of each U.S. substantial owner. If withholding is required, Form 1042 is used to report and pay taxes withheld during the tax year. In addition, an annual information return must be filed on Form 1042-S and a copy furnished to the recipient of the withholdable payment (Code Sec. 1472(b); Reg. § 1.1472-1(e)).[103]

So long as the NFFE and the withholding agent satisfy their reporting requirements, withholding is not required unless the withholding agent knows or has reason to know that any information provided about substantial U.S. owners is incorrect. A withholding agent is also not required to withhold taxes if the withholding agent may treat the payment as beneficially owned by an excepted NFFE. An excepted NFFE includes a publicly traded corporation and its related entities, territory entities, the government of a foreign country or U.S. possession, an international organization, or any foreign central bank of issue. Additionally, active NFFEs, direct reporting NFFEs and sponsored direct NFFEs are excepted NFFEs (Code Sec. 1472(c); Reg. § 1.1472-1(c); Temp. Reg. § 1.1472-1T(c)). An active NFFE is any NFFE if less than 50 percent of its gross income for the preceding tax year is passive income, and less than 50 percent of its assets produce or are held for the production of dividends, interest, rents and royalties (other than those derived in the active conduct of a trade or business), annuities, or other passive income. A direct reporting NFFE elects to report directly to the IRS. A sponsored direct reporting NFFE is a direct reporting NFFE with a sponsoring entity that acts on its behalf. In addition, entities which are by definition not financial institutions are considered excepted NFFEs, including certain holding companies, start-up companies, NFFEs that are liquidating or emerging from reorganization or bankruptcy, and certain hedging entities.

Withholding is not required with respect to any payment under a grandfathered obligation or from any gross proceeds from the disposition of such an obligation. A grandfathered obligation is any legal obligation outstanding on July 1, 2014, that produces or could produce a withholdable payment or pass-through payment. It does not include any instrument treated as equity for U.S. tax purposes or any legal agreement that lacks a definitive expiration or term (Reg. § 1.1471-2(b); Temp. Reg. § 1.1471-2T(b)).[104]

Foreign Tax Credit or Deduction

2475. Foreign Tax Credit or Deduction. Subject to certain limitations (¶ 2479), a U.S. taxpayer may elect a credit or deduction against U.S. income liability for foreign taxes paid or accrued to a foreign country or U.S. possession during the tax year (Code Sec. 901; Reg. § 1.901-1).[105] The credit and deduction are intended to relieve U.S.

References are to Standard Federal Tax Reports; Tax Research Consultant; and Practical Tax Explanations.

[102] ¶ 32,893, ¶ 32,895; INTL: 36,060; § 37,730

[103] ¶ 32,888, ¶ 32,890; INTL: 36,100; § 37,730

[104] ¶ 32,884H, ¶ 32,884J; INTL: 36,100; § 37,730

[105] ¶ 27,820, ¶ 27,821; IN-TLOUT: 3,050; § 13,401

taxpayers of double taxation on foreign source income. The election is made on an annual basis (¶ 2476) and is applicable to all creditable foreign taxes paid or incurred during the tax year (¶ 2477). A separate foreign tax credit can be claimed by individuals and corporations against alternative minimum tax liability (AMT) (¶ 1470).

Taxpayers entitled to claim the foreign tax credit or deduction against income liability include U.S. citizens, resident aliens (¶ 2409), bona fide residents of Puerto Rico for the entire tax year (¶ 2415), domestic corporations, and nonresident aliens and foreign corporations with respect to foreign taxes paid or accrued on foreign source income effectively connected with the conduct of a U.S. trade or business (¶ 2429). A taxpayer who is a partner in a partnership, shareholder in an S corporation, or benefici- ary of an estate or trust may claim the credit or deduction with respect to the taxpayer's proportionate share of creditable foreign taxes paid or accrued by the entity (Code Secs. 901(b) and 1373(a)).[106] Similarly, a shareholder of a regulated investment company or mutual fund may be able to claim the credit or deduction based on the shareholder's share of creditable foreign taxes paid by the entity (¶ 2320).

Income Matching. If there is a foreign tax credit splitting event, the foreign tax credit or deduction may not be claimed by a taxpayer until the related income is taken into account for U.S. income tax purposes (Code Sec. 909; Temp. Reg. § 1.909-2T).[107] A foreign tax credit splitting event occurs with respect to a foreign income tax if in connection with a splitter arrangement the related income is (or will be) taken into account by a covered person. A covered person is a person or entity that has a specified relationship with the taxpayer—at least 10 percent ownership interest, related party, or otherwise specified by the IRS. In the case of a partnership, S corporation, or trust, the matching requirement is applied at the partner, shareholder, or beneficiary level. Special rules apply to a foreign tax credit splitting event involving a Code Sec. 902 corporation, including the application of the matching rule to foreign income taxes paid or accrued in pre-2011 tax years for purposes of applying the deemed paid foreign tax credit (¶ 2485) for periods after 2010 (Temp. Reg. § § 1.909-5T and 1.909-6T).[108]

2476. Election of Foreign Tax Credit or Deduction. The election to claim the foreign tax credit or deduction (¶ 2475) is made on an annual basis. It may be made or changed anytime within 10 years from the due date for filing a return for the year in which the taxes were actually paid or accrued, unless the period is extended by agreement with the IRS (Code Sec. 6511(d)(3); Reg. § 1.901-1(d) and (e)).[109] For partnerships and S corporations, the election is made by the individual partners and shareholders, respectively (Code Secs. 702(a)(6), 703(b)(3), and 1366(a)(1)).[110] Corpo- rations in an affiliated group make the election and compute the credit on a consolidated basis for a consolidated return year (Reg. § 1.1502-4).[111]

A taxpayer claims the foreign tax credit by filing Form 1116 (for individuals, estates, and trusts) or Form 1118 (for corporations) with the taxpayer's income tax return. An individual may elect to claim the foreign tax credit without filing Form 1116 by entering the credit directly on his or her tax return if: (1) all of the individual's foreign source income is passive income; (2) all of the income and any foreign taxes paid on the income is reported on a qualified payee statement (i.e., Form 1099); and (3) the total creditable foreign taxes is less than $300 ($600 for joint filers) (Code Sec. 904(j)).[112] If an individual makes the election, then the foreign tax credit limitations will not apply (¶ 2479). However, the individual cannot carry over any excess credit to another tax year. The election is not available to estates, trusts, or corporations. An election to take the credit or deduction on a joint return applies to the qualifying foreign taxes paid or accrued by both spouses. If married taxpayers file separate returns, either may take the credit or deduction without regard to the other.

References are to Standard Federal Tax Reports; Tax Research Consultant; and Practical Tax Explanations.

[106] ¶ 27,820, ¶ 32,180; IN-TLOUT: 3,152; § 13,405.05

[107] ¶ 27,971, ¶ 27,973D; IN-TLOUT: 3,300; § 13,432

[108] ¶ 27,974I, ¶ 27,974N; IN-TLOUT: 3,304; § 13,432

[109] ¶ 39,060, ¶ 27,821; IN-TLOUT: 3,054; § 13,413

[110] ¶ 25,080, ¶ 25,100, ¶ 32,080; INTLOUT: 3,054; § 13,405.20

[111] ¶ 33,148; INTLOUT: 3,054

[112] ¶ 27,880; INTLOUT: 6,102.05; § 13,425.20

Credit vs. Deduction. Generally, it is more advantageous for a U.S. taxpayer to elect the foreign tax credit rather than the deduction because the credit is taken against the taxpayer's U.S. liability on a dollar-for-dollar basis. In contrast, a deduction for foreign taxes merely reduces a taxpayer's income subject to tax. In addition, an individual who deducts foreign taxes must claim the taxes as an itemized deduction.

The election to claim the credit or deduction applies to all creditable foreign taxes paid or incurred by the taxpayer during the tax year for which a U.S. return is required (¶ 2477). Thus, a taxpayer cannot claim a credit for some creditable foreign taxes and a deduction for other creditable foreign taxes in the same tax year. Partial credits and partial deductions are not permitted except in limited circumstances (Code Sec. 275(a)(4)).[113] For example, foreign taxes that may otherwise be claimed as an itemized deduction, such as foreign real property taxes, may still be deducted even if the credit is claimed. In addition, a taxpayer on the cash method of accounting may elect to claim a credit for foreign taxes in the year they accrue.

2477. Creditable Foreign Taxes. A U.S. taxpayer is allowed a foreign tax credit or deduction (¶ 2475) against U.S. income tax liability for any income tax (including war profits, and excess profits taxes) paid or accrued to a foreign country or U.S. possession during the tax year on foreign source income. This includes taxes paid or accrued in lieu of income taxes imposed by the foreign country or U.S. possession (Code Secs. 901 and 903; Reg. § 1.901-2).[114] A U.S. corporation is also allowed a foreign tax credit for creditable foreign taxes paid by a foreign subsidiary in which it owns at least 10 percent of the voting stock and from which it receives a dividend (¶ 2485).

A creditable foreign tax is a levy the predominant character of which is that of a compulsory income tax according to U.S. tax principles (Reg. § 1.901-2).[115] A penalty, fine, interest payment, customs duty, or similar obligation is not a tax; nor is any payment to a foreign government in exchange for a specific economic benefit that is not available on substantially the same terms to all persons. A foreign tax paid for retirement, unemployment, or disability benefits is generally not a payment for a specific economic benefit. However, no credit or deduction is allowed for social security taxes paid or accrued to a foreign country with which the United States has a social security agreement. The IRS may disallow foreign tax credits generated in transactions it views as abusive such as structured passive investment arrangements. The foreign tax credit or deduction is not available for the withholding of otherwise creditable foreign taxes on dividends and other items of gain or income from property unless certain holding period requirements are met (Code Sec. 901(k) and (l)).

The foreign tax credit or deduction can only be claimed by the taxpayer upon whom the foreign law imposes legal liability, and who actually pays or accrues the tax. In the case of combined income of two or more persons for tax years beginning after February 14, 2012, foreign law is considered to impose legal liability on each person on a pro rata basis (Reg. § 1.901-2(f)).[116] This includes the combined income of a husband and wife, or a corporation and one or more of its subsidiaries. However, income which is subject to a special tax rate, is exempt from tax, or for which certain deductions or credits are allowed under the foreign law must be allocated only to the person(s) with that type of income. The income subject to preferential treatment must be computed separately and the tax on that income allocated separately.

A U.S. taxpayer may not claim the foreign tax credit or deduction for any foreign taxes paid or accrued on income excluded from U.S. gross income. This includes income excluded under the foreign earned income or foreign housing exclusions (¶ 2402 and ¶ 2403), or income from a U.S. possession (¶ 2414). The taxpayer may also not claim a credit or deduction for foreign taxes paid or accrued to the extent that: (1) the taxpayer is certain to receive a refund or credit, or the tax is used as a subsidy; (2)

References are to Standard Federal Tax Reports; Tax Research Consultant; and Practical Tax Explanations.

[113] ¶ 14,500; INTLOUT: 3,050; § 13,413

[114] ¶ 27,820, ¶ 27,822, ¶ 27,860; INTLOUT: 3,100; § 13,410.05

[115] ¶ 27,822; INTLOUT: 3,100; § 13,410.10

[116] ¶ 27,822; INTLOUT: 3,113; § 13,410.25

¶2477

the liability is dependent on the availability of a foreign tax credit in another jurisdiction; (3) the taxes are paid or accrued to a country with which the United States does not conduct diplomatic relations or which is designated as supporting acts of international terrorism; or (4) the taxes are attributable to boycott income (¶ 2496). The amount of foreign taxes a taxpayer may claim will be reduced if the taxpayer controls a foreign corporation (CFC) or partnership that fails to file Form 5471 or Form 8865, respectively (¶ 2487 and ¶ 2494).

Covered Asset Acquisitions. In the case of a covered asset acquisition, a taxpayer may not take into account in determining the foreign tax credit the disqualified portion of any foreign income tax determined with respect to income or gain attributable to the relevant foreign assets (Code Sec. 901(m)).[117] A covered asset acquisition includes: (1) a qualified stock purchase under Code Sec. 338 (¶ 2265); (2) any transaction that is treated as the acquisition of assets for U.S. tax purposes and as the acquisition of stock (or is disregarded) for purposes of the foreign income taxes; (3) any acquisition of an interest in a partnership that has an election in effect under Code Sec. 754 (¶ 459); and (4) any other transaction as determined by the IRS.

The disqualified portion of any covered asset acquisition for any tax year is generally the aggregate basis differences allocable to the tax year with respect to all relevant foreign assets, divided by the income on which the foreign income tax is determined (Code Sec. 901(m)(3)(B); Notice 2014-44; Notice 2014-55).[118] Under a statutory disposition rule, however, the basis difference allocated to the tax year of disposition of any relevant foreign asset is the basis difference of the asset over the aggregate basis differences from prior years (the "unallocated basis difference"). No basis difference with respect to the asset will be allocated to any subsequent tax year. The IRS intends to issue regulations that will provide that a disposition for this purpose means an event that results in gain or loss being recognized for U.S. income tax or foreign income tax purposes with respect to the relevant foreign asset. The portion of the basis difference that will be taken into account for a tax year will depend on whether the disposition is fully taxable or not. The regulations will generally apply to dispositions occurring on or after July 21, 2014. They will also apply to determine the tax consequences of an entity classification election and whether a disposition results from the election and the treatment of any unallocated basis difference, for an election filed on or after July 29, 2014, that is effective on or before July 21, 2014.

2479. Foreign Tax Credit Limitations. The foreign tax credit or deduction (¶ 2475) is subject to a two-part limitation that prevents the use of foreign taxes to reduce U.S. income tax liability on U.S. source income. First, an overall limitation provides that the total amount of a taxpayer's foreign tax credit may not exceed the taxpayer's entire U.S. income tax liability (determined without regard to the credit), multiplied by a fraction equal to the taxpayer's foreign source taxable income over worldwide taxable income from all sources (Code Sec. 904(a)).[119] Second, the limitation must be calculated separately for certain categories or baskets of foreign source income (¶ 2481). Special rules also apply if the taxpayer has an overall foreign loss (¶ 2483). The IRS may recharacterize the income of an affiliated group of corporations or modify the consolidated return regulations to the extent necessary to prevent avoidance of the foreign tax credit limitation rules (Code Sec. 904(i); Reg. § 1.904(i)-1).[120]

Foreign source taxable income is the taxpayer's gross income from all geographic sources outside the United States (regardless of the country), less any applicable deductions that properly relate to the income and an allocation of deductions unrelated to any specific item of income (Code Sec. 904(b)).[121] An individual, estate, or trust may not claim deductions for personal and dependency exemptions in calculating taxable income. In the case of a corporation, taxable income does not include any portion of income taken into account for purposes of the possession tax credit (¶ 1362). For all

---

References are to Standard Federal Tax Reports; Tax Research Consultant; and Practical Tax Explanations.

[117] ¶ 27,820; INTLOUT: 3,110.30

[118] ¶ 27,820, ¶ 27,826.2204; INTLOUT: 3,110.30

[119] ¶ 27,880; INTLOUT: 6,050; § 13,425.05

[120] ¶ 27,880, ¶ 27,900C; IN-TLOUT: 6,404

[121] ¶ 27,880; INTLOUT: 6,050; § 13,425.10

taxpayers, foreign source capital gains and losses are subject to (1) a capital gain net income limitation adjustment (i.e., U.S. capital loss adjustment), and (2) a capital gain rate differential adjustment (Reg. § § 1.904(b)-1 and 1.904(b)-2).[122]

De Minimis Exemption. An individual with $300 or less of creditable foreign taxes ($600 if married filing jointly) is exempt from the overall foreign tax credit limitation provided he or she has no foreign source income other than qualified passive income (¶ 2476). The exemption is not automatic and an individual must elect to take the exemption for the tax year directly on Form 1040.

U.S.-Owned Foreign Corporations. Certain amounts derived from U.S.-owned foreign corporations that would otherwise be treated as foreign source income are treated as U.S. source income for purposes of the foreign tax credit limitations (Code Sec. 904(h); Reg. § 1.904-5(m)).[123] The sourcing rule applies to subpart F income inclusions from a controlled foreign corporation (CFC) (¶ 2488), income from a qualified electing fund (¶ 2490), and interest and dividends paid by a foreign corporation where not less than 10 percent of the corporation's earnings and profits for the tax year are attributable to U.S. sources.

A U.S.-owned foreign corporation is any foreign corporation (including a Code Sec. 902 corporation (¶ 2485)) if 50 percent or more of the total combined voting power of all classes of stock in the corporation entitled to vote, or of the total value of the stock of the corporation, is held by U.S. persons. A domestic corporation is also a U.S.-owned foreign corporation for this purpose if it pays (1) a dividend that is treated as foreign sourced because of the election to claim the possession tax credit (¶ 1362), or (2) interest before 2011 that is treated as foreign source because the corporation meets the active foreign business test (80/20 corporation) (¶ 2431).

Carryover. When the amount of creditable foreign taxes paid or accrued by a taxpayer during the tax year exceeds the overall limitation for that year (as well as the separate limitation for each separate basket of foreign source income), the unused portion may be carried back one year and then forward ten years (Code Sec. 904(c); Reg. § 1.904-2).[124] The amount that may be carried back and forward is limited to the amount by which the credit limitation in the carryback or forward year exceeds the amount of foreign taxes paid or accrued in that year. In addition, any unused foreign tax must be carried back and forward to its own separate basket of income. It cannot offset other taxes imposed on income in another basket.

If any unused foreign tax credit is carried back or forward to a tax year in which a foreign tax deduction is claimed (¶ 2476), the taxpayer must compute a foreign tax credit limit as if the credit was elected for that year. Any excess generated in the deduction year cannot be deducted or claimed as a credit for any year, but reduces the amount of unused foreign taxes that can be carried over to another tax year. Alternatively, an amended return may be filed within 10 years from the due date of the return of the deduction year to claim the foreign tax credit rather than the deduction (¶ 2475). For any portion of a foreign tax credit carryback from a tax year attributable to the carryback of a net operating loss or capital loss from a later tax year, the carryback stops the running of interest until the filing date for the later tax year (Code Sec. 6601(d)).[125] An individual electing the *de minimis* exemption may not carryback or carryforward any excess foreign taxes to an election year.

2481. Separate Limitations for Various Categories of Income. A taxpayer is generally required to compute the foreign tax credit limitation (¶ 2479) separately for two main categories or baskets of foreign source income: passive category income and general category income (Code Sec. 904(d); Reg. § 1.904-4).[126] Passive category income includes investment income such as dividends, interest, rents, royalties, annuities, net gain from the sale of non-income-producing investment property or property that

References are to Standard Federal Tax Reports; Tax Research Consultant; and Practical Tax Explanations.

[122] ¶ 27,889, ¶ 27,890; IN-TLOUT: 6,060; § 13,425.10
[123] ¶ 27,880, ¶ 27,886; IN-TLOUT: 6,054.15
[124] ¶ 27,880, ¶ 27,883; IN-TLOUT: 6,300; § 13,425.25
[125] ¶ 39,410; INTLOUT: 6,304; § 13,425.25
[126] ¶ 27,880, ¶ 27,885; IN-TLOUT: 6,100; § 13,425.15

generates passive income, and income from a qualified electing fund (¶ 2490). It does not include gains or losses from the sale of inventory or property held mainly for sale to customers in the ordinary course of a trade or business, any rents or royalties that are derived in the active conduct of a trade or business, certain export financing interest, and highly taxed income. Any foreign source income that is not included in the passive income basket is considered part of the general income basket.

To determine taxable income in each category, a taxpayer must allocate expenses, losses, and other deductions directly related to the foreign source income allocated to each basket. Similarly, foreign taxes paid or accrued may only include those taxes that are related to income in that basket. If a tax is related to more than one basket, the taxpayer must apportion the tax. However, if creditable foreign taxes were imposed on amounts that do not constitute income under U.S. tax law ("base difference items"), then they will be treated as imposed on general category income.

Look-Through Rules. Foreign source income received by a U.S. shareholder from a controlled foreign corporation (CFC) (¶ 2487) is categorized by applying look-through rules that require identification of underlying income to specific foreign tax credit limitation categories (Code Sec. 904(d)(3) and (4); Reg. § 1.904-5).[127] Tracing rules prescribe classification of subpart F income (¶ 2488), interest, rents, royalties, and dividends to various limitation categories. The look-through rules also apply in the case of payments made by Code Sec. 902 corporations (¶ 2485), certain domestic corporations, partnerships, and related look-through entities. In the case of a partner in a partnership, the look-through rule will apply with respect to the partner's distributive share of partnership income unless the partner owns less than 10 percent of the partnership, in which case the income is treated as passive income.

Other Limitations. In addition to the separate foreign tax credit limitations for passive category income and general category income, separate foreign tax credit limitations must be determined for certain special categories of income (Reg. § 1.904-4(m)).[128] This includes: (1) any income sourced under a tax treaty as foreign source income including any income derived from foreign sources; (2) income from sanctioned countries; (3) for purposes of the alternative minimum tax (AMT), dividends received from a corporation that qualifies for the possession tax credit if the dividends-received deduction is disallowed under the alternative current earnings (ACE) rules; (4) dividends received from 10-percent owned foreign corporations (¶ 231); (5) gain from the sale of stock in a foreign corporation or intangible property that is treated as foreign source under a tax treaty; (6) lump-sum distributions from retirement plans for which the special averaging treatment is used to figure tax; and (7) combined foreign oil and gas income including foreign oil and gas extraction income (FOGEI) and foreign oil-related income (FORI) (Code Sec. 907).[129]

2483. Recapture of Foreign and U.S. Losses. An overall foreign loss (OFL) is subject to recapture to prevent a double tax benefit from using the OFL to reduce U.S. tax liability on U.S. source income and claiming the foreign tax credit (¶ 2475) on the same income. If a taxpayer has an OFL in any tax year, then a portion of the taxpayer's foreign source income earned in a subsequent year is recharacterized as U.S. source income (Code Sec. 904(f)).[130] For this purpose, an OFL is the amount by which gross income from foreign sources is exceeded by the sum of expenses, losses, and other deductions properly allocable to such income, but without taking into account any net operating losses (NOL), foreign expropriation losses, and uncompensated casualty or theft losses. A foreign loss must be determined for each separate foreign tax credit category or basket (¶ 2481), referred to as a separate limitation loss (SLL). Thus, a taxpayer can have an OFL, an SLL for passive income, and a SLL for general income in any given tax year. Foreign losses in one separate foreign tax credit category or basket must be offset against income in other foreign categories before offsetting U.S. income.

References are to Standard Federal Tax Reports; Tax Research Consultant; and Practical Tax Explanations.

[127] ¶ 27,880, ¶ 27,886; IN-TLOUT: 6,200

[128] ¶ 27,885; INTLOUT: 6,114; § 13,425.15
[129] ¶ 27,940; INTLOUT: 6,350

[130] ¶ 27,880; INTLOUT: 6,250; § 13,425.30

The amount of foreign source income that must be recaptured and recharacterized as U.S. source income is generally limited to the lesser of the taxpayer's OFL (to the extent not used in prior tax years) or 50 percent of the taxpayer's foreign source taxable income for the tax year. If a taxpayer disposes of assets used in its trade or business predominantly outside the United States in a taxable disposition, or disposes of stock in a controlled foreign corporation (CFC) (¶ 2487) in which it owns more than 50 percent, then 100 percent of the gain must be recaptured. Fifty percent of the recognized gain is recaptured under the general rule above and the remainder recaptured to the extent of the taxpayer's OFL balance. Special recapture rules also apply if the disposition is nontaxable. For these purposes, property is considered used predominantly outside the United States if, during a three-year period ending on the date of disposition, the property was located outside the United States more than 50 percent of the time. Similar recapture rules apply to an overall domestic loss (ODL) requiring U.S. source income earned in a subsequent year to be recharacterized as foreign source income. Special ordering rules are used to allocate NOLs, net capital losses, U.S. source losses and SLLs, and for the recapture of SLLs, OFLs, and ODLs (Reg. § 1.904(g)-3).[131]

2485. Deemed Paid Credit. The foreign tax credit (¶ 2475) is available to a U.S. corporate shareholder that owns 10 percent or more of the voting stock in a foreign corporation from which it receives a dividend (or deemed to receive a dividend through an affiliated group or a partnership) (Code Sec. 902).[132] The amount of the "deemed paid" or "indirect" credit is determined by reference to the portion of the foreign corporation's foreign income taxes that the dividend received by the domestic corporation bears to the foreign corporation's undistributed earnings. However, the deemed paid credit does not include the disqualified portion of any foreign income tax paid by a Code Sec. 902 corporation in a covered asset acquisition and determined with respect to income or gain attributable to the relevant foreign assets (¶ 2477). A corporation electing to take the deemed paid credit must increase ("gross up") its tax base by including not only the dividend but the tax deemed paid by the foreign corporation (Code Sec. 78).[133] Additionally, the deemed paid credit is subject to the foreign tax credit limitation (¶ 2479).

The deemed paid credit is allowed to a domestic shareholder for foreign taxes paid by a lower-tier foreign corporation if the foreign corporation is a member of a qualified group and the foreign corporation owns 10 percent or more of the voting stock of the member of the qualified group from which it receives a dividend (Code Sec. 902(b)). A qualified group includes any foreign corporation in a chain that includes the first-tier corporation and foreign corporations through the sixth-tier. A corporation below the third-tier will not be included in the qualified group unless it is a controlled foreign corporation (CFC) (¶ 2487) and the domestic corporation is a U.S. shareholder. Whether the ownership requirements are met is determined at the time dividends are received. A qualified group cannot aggregate their shares in a foreign corporation to meet the ownership requirements.

U.S. Shareholders of Foreign Corporations

2487. Controlled Foreign Corporations (CFCs). A U.S. shareholder of a foreign corporation that is a controlled foreign corporation (CFC) for an uninterrupted period of 30 days or more during the tax year must include in gross income its pro rata share of the CFC's subpart F income (¶ 2488) (whether distributed or not) and earnings invested in U.S. property during the year (Code Sec. 951).[134] A foreign corporation is a CFC if more than 50 percent of its total voting power or value is owned by U.S. shareholders (Code Sec. 957).[135] A U.S. shareholder is any U.S. person (U.S. citizen, resident alien, domestic corporation, partnership, estate, or trust) that owns directly, indirectly, or

---

References are to Standard Federal Tax Reports; Tax Research Consultant; and Practical Tax Explanations.

[131] ¶ 27,900AM; INTLOUT: 6,260; § 13,425.30

[132] ¶ 27,840; INTLOUT: 3,200; § 13,420

[133] ¶ 6350; INTLOUT: 3,200; § 13,420

[134] ¶ 28,470; INTLOUT: 9,000

[135] ¶ 28,590; INTLOUT: 9,050

constructively 10 percent or more of the total combined voting power of the foreign corporation (Code Sec. 958).[136]

The U.S. shareholder includes subpart F income and earnings in gross income in its tax year in which the CFC's tax year ends but only if it is a shareholder on the last day of the CFC's tax year. In addition, the shareholder only includes income from that portion of the year that the corporation qualifies as a CFC. The income is treated as a deemed dividend (¶ 733). Actual distributions are excluded from gross income to the extent they have already been accounted for by the shareholder (Code Sec. 959).[137] To prevent double taxation, the basis of the U.S. shareholder's CFC stock and basis in property the shareholder is considered owning through the CFC is increased by the amount of subpart F income required to be included in income and decreased by any distribution that is excluded from income (Code Sec. 961).[138]

A U.S. shareholder of CFC that is a domestic corporation is allowed a foreign tax credit (¶ 2475) for any foreign taxes paid (or deemed paid) by the CFC for income that is attributed or distributed to it as a U.S. shareholder (Code Sec. 960).[139] The credit is limited to the taxes that would have been deemed paid if the foreign corporation had made an actual distribution to the domestic corporation. A deemed-paid credit is also available to any individual U.S. shareholder who elects to be taxed at domestic corporate income tax rates on amounts included in gross income (Code Sec. 962).[140]

Investment of Earnings. U.S. shareholders of a CFC are taxed on their pro rata share of the CFC's earnings which are invested in U.S. property during the tax year and not distributed or otherwise taxed (Code Sec. 956).[141] The amount of earnings invested in U.S. property is the economic equivalent of a dividend deemed to have been paid, but it is not a qualified dividend eligible to be taxed at capital gains rates because it is not actually distributed (*O. Rodriguez*, CA-5, 2013-2 USTC ¶ 50,420). A CFC acquires a direct interest in U.S. property when it acquires an adjusted basis in the property. U.S. property includes tangible real or personal property located in the United States, stock of domestic corporations, obligations of U.S. persons, and the right to use a patent, copyright, invention, etc., in the United States. Certain properties acquired in normal commercial transactions without the intention of them to remain in the United States indefinitely are not to be treated as U.S. property.

Sale or Exchange of CFC Stock. Any gain recognized by a U.S. shareholder from the sale, exchange, or redemption of stock in a CFC is included in gross income as an ordinary dividend to the extent of the corporation's earnings and profits allocable to the stock (Code Sec. 1248).[142] Any gain exceeding the CFC's earnings and profits is treated as capital gain. The shareholder may claim a foreign tax credit for the taxes paid by the CFC on the income. However, the credit may be less than the indirect credit (¶ 2485) because it will not apply to as many tiers of foreign corporations.

Returns. Every U.S. person (U.S. citizen or resident alien, domestic corporation, domestic partnership, or domestic estate or trust) who is a U.S. shareholder of a CFC must file an information return on Form 5471 (Code Sec. 6038).[143] Failure to timely file the required information may result in penalties and a reduced foreign tax credit. The taxpayer must include information on acquisitions, reorganizations, and dispositions of ownership interests in a CFC during the tax year (Code Sec. 6046).[144] U.S. shareholders of controlled foreign partnerships are subject to similar reporting requirements using Form 8865.

2488. Subpart F Income. Subpart F income of a controlled foreign corporation (CFC) (¶ 2487) is the sum of the corporation's insurance income, foreign base company income, boycott income (¶ 2496), illegal payments (¶ 2497), and income from countries not diplomatically recognized by the U.S. government (Code Sec. 952).[145] It does not

---

References are to Standard Federal Tax Reports; Tax Research Consultant; and Practical Tax Explanations.

136 ¶ 28,610; INTLOUT: 9,056
137 ¶ 28,630; INTLOUT: 9,350
138 ¶ 28,670; INTLOUT: 9,360
139 ¶ 28,650; INTLOUT: 9,358

140 ¶ 28,690; INTLOUT: 9,362
141 ¶ 28,570; INTLOUT: 9,250
142 ¶ 30,960; INTLOUT: 9,400

143 ¶ 35,540; INTLOUT: 9,450; § 39,135.05
144 ¶ 35,940; INTLOUT: 9,456; § 39,135.05
145 ¶ 28,490; INTLOUT: 9,100

include income from sources within the United States that is effectively connected with the conduct of a trade or business by the corporation (¶ 2429) unless that income is exempt from tax or taxed at a reduced rate pursuant to a tax treaty. Subpart F income for the tax year is also limited to the CFC's total earnings and profits for that year, and may be reduced in certain circumstances to accumulated deficits of earnings and profits.

Subpart F insurance income is any income that is attributable to the issuance or reissuance of any insurance or annuity contract. The income must be of a type that would be taxed (with some modifications) under the rules that apply to domestic insurance companies. Effective for tax years before January 1, 2014, it does not include insurance income in connection with risks located outside of the United States (Code Sec. 953).[146]

Foreign base company income of a CFC is made up of income from a foreign personal holding company (FPHC) and foreign base company sales, services, and oil-related income (Code Sec. 954).[147] FPHC income is generally the major component of foreign base company income and includes dividends, interest (including otherwise tax-exempt interest), rents, royalties, and annuities. It also includes: amounts received under a contract to furnish personal services; any item of income, gain, deduction, or loss from a notional principal contract; and the excess of gains over losses from the sale or exchange of property (including foreign currency and commodities) unless the CFC is a regular dealer. FPHC income does not include rents and royalties from an active trade or business, certain income from related persons, export financing interest and, for tax years beginning before January 1, 2014, income derived in the active conduct of a banking, financing or similar business (active financing income), income derived in the active conduct of an insurance business (active insurance income), or qualified insurance investment income.

For purposes of determining FPHC income, the sale of a partnership interest by a CFC is treated as a sale of the proportionate share of partnership assets attributable to that interest, including subpart F income. On the other hand, for tax years beginning before January 1, 2014, no look-through rule applies to dividends, interest, rents and royalties received by a CFC from a related CFC to the extent that it creates or increases a deficit that reduces subpart F income of either the payor or another CFC (Code Sec. 954(c)(6)).

> **Comment:** Absent further legislation, the exceptions from subpart F for insurance income and active financing income, and the look-through rule for related CFCs will not apply to tax years of foreign corporations beginning after December 31, 2013. For the latest legislative updates, visit our website www.CCHGroup.com/TaxUpdates

2490. Passive Foreign Investment Company. A U.S. shareholder of a passive foreign investment company (PFIC) who receives an excess distribution with respect to its stock or disposes of its PFIC stock must allocate the income or gain pro rata over the shareholder's holding period for the stock unless the shareholder elects to treat the PFIC as a qualifying electing fund (QEF) or makes a mark-to-market election (Code Sec. 1291).[148] The amount allocated to the shareholder's current tax year, and to the tax years in its holding period before the foreign corporation qualified as a PFIC (pre-PFIC years), are taxed as ordinary income. The amount allocated to any other tax year in the shareholder's holding period is taxed at the highest income tax rate applicable for that year, plus interest from the due date for the taxpayer's return for that year. For this purpose, an excess distribution is any part of a distribution received from the PFIC which is greater than 125 percent of the average distribution received by the shareholder during the three preceding tax years or, if shorter, during the period the shareholder held the stock.

A PFIC is any foreign corporation that derives 75 percent or more of its gross income for the tax year from passive investments or at least 50 percent of its average total assets held for the year produce passive income or are held for the production of

---

References are to Standard Federal Tax Reports; Tax Research Consultant; and Practical Tax Explanations.

[146] ¶ 28,510; INTLOUT: 9,102   [147] ¶ 28,530; INTLOUT: 9,104   [148] ¶ 31,540; INTLOUT: 18,200

passive income (Code Sec. 1297).[149] Passive income generally is the type of income that would be foreign personal holding company income (¶ 2488). Miscellaneous rules apply regarding stock attribution, start-up companies and business changes, the leasing of tangible personal property, intangible assets, and the interaction of the PFIC rules with the taxation of accumulated earnings and subpart F income (Code Sec. 1298).[150] Even if a foreign corporation ceases to qualify as a PFIC, a U.S. shareholder is subject to the PFIC rules for any period stock is held that the corporation was a PFIC. To avoid the PFIC rules, the shareholder can purge PFIC stock by making a deemed sale or deemed dividend election.

A U.S. person that is a direct or indirect shareholder of a PFIC generally must file Form 8621 with its tax return for each tax year in which the person receives an excess distribution, disposes of its PFIC stock, or makes an election to purge its PFIC stock, including a QEF or mark-to-market election. The reporting requirement may also meet the FATCA requirements for disclosing information with respect to specified foreign financial assets on Form 8938 (¶ 2570). A separate Form 8621 must be filed for each PFIC in which stock is held.

Qualified Electing Fund. Instead of paying the additional tax on deferrals (or deemed sale or deemed dividend elections), a U.S. shareholder of a PFIC may elect to treat the corporation as a QEF. If the election is made, the shareholder must include in gross income each year as ordinary income its pro rata share of earnings of the corporation, and as long-term capital gain, its pro rata share of the net capital gain of the corporation (Code Secs. 1293 and 1295).[151] The inclusions are made for the shareholder's tax year in which or with which the QEF's tax year ends. Once made, the QEF election is revocable only with the IRS's consent and is effective for the current tax year and all subsequent tax years. Under certain circumstances, the U.S. shareholder can elect to defer payment of the tax on any undistributed earnings of the QEF (Code Sec. 1294).[152]

Mark-to-Market Election. A U.S. shareholder of a PFIC may also avoid the additional tax on the deferral of income by making a mark-to-market election with respect to its PFIC stock that is marketable (Code Sec. 1296).[153] If the election is made, the shareholder annually includes in gross income as ordinary income an amount equal to the excess of the fair market value of the PFIC stock as of the close of the tax year over its adjusted basis. If the stock has declined in value, an ordinary loss deduction is allowed limited to the net amount of gain previously included in income.

2491. Sale or Exchange of Patent, Etc. to Foreign Corporations. A U.S. person who controls a foreign corporation (at least 50 percent of voting power of all stock) directly or indirectly must recognize gain from the sale or exchange of a patent, invention, model, design, copyright, secret formula or process, or any other similar property right to the foreign corporation as ordinary income rather than capital gain (Code Sec. 1249).[154]

2492. Reorganization Involving Foreign Corporations. A U.S. person is generally required to recognize gains (but not losses) on the transfer of appreciated property to a foreign corporation (outbound transfers) that would otherwise be tax-free under the corporate organization (¶ 203), reorganization (¶ 2205), and liquidation rules (¶ 2253) (Code Sec. 367(a); Temp. Reg. § 1.367(a)-1T).[155] Similarly, transfers by a foreign corporation to a U.S. corporation (inbound transfers) or transfers by a foreign corporation to another foreign corporation (foreign-to-foreign transfers) may require U.S. shareholders to recognize income currently, or defer recognition of gain by making basis and earnings and profits adjustments (Code Sec. 367(b); Reg. § 1.367(b)-3; Reg. § 1.367(b)-4).[156]

References are to Standard Federal Tax Reports; Tax Research Consultant; and Practical Tax Explanations.

[149] ¶ 31,620; INTLOUT: 18,202

[150] ¶ 31,640; INTLOUT: 18,200

[151] ¶ 31,560, ¶ 31,600; IN-TLOUT: 18,206

[152] ¶ 31,580; INTLOUT: 18,206.15

[153] ¶ 31,610; INTLOUT: 18,202.30

[154] ¶ 30,980; § 18,705.05

[155] ¶ 16,640, ¶ 16,641; INTL: 30,050

[156] ¶ 16,640, ¶ 16,647E, ¶ 16,647F; INTL: 30,050

Active Trade or Business. Recognition of gain on outbound transfers does not apply to any property transferred for use by the foreign corporation in the active conduct of a trade or business outside the United States, provided the U.S. person transferring the property complies with the reporting requirements of Code Sec. 6038B (Code Sec. 367(a)(3); Temp. Reg. § 1.367(a)-2T(a)).[157] The exception does not apply to outbound transfers of certain tainted assets such as inventory, accounts receivable, intangible property, and certain leased property (Temp. Reg. § 1.367(a)-5T).[158] The exception also does not apply in the case where a U.S. person transfers assets of a foreign branch with previously deducted losses to a foreign corporation (Temp. Reg. § 1.367(a)-6T).[159]

Transfers of Stock or Securities. Recognition of gain on outbound transfers does not apply to any transfer of stock or securities of a party to the exchange (Code Sec. 367(a)(2); Reg. § 1.367(a)-3; Temp. Reg. § 1.367(a)-3T).[160] An outbound transfer of foreign stock or securities is not subject to tax if the U.S. person owns less than five percent of the transferee foreign corporation or enters into a five-year gain recognition agreement (GRA) with the IRS. An outbound transfer of domestic stock or securities is not subject to tax if: (1) the U.S. person receives 50 percent or less of the voting power and stock value of the transferee; (2) U.S. officers, directors, five percent or more shareholders of U.S. corporation do not own more than 50 percent of voting power and stock value of the transferee; (3) the U.S. person is not a five-percent or more shareholder of the transferee or must enter into a GRA with the IRS; and (4) the transferee has been actively engaged in business for at least three years. GRAs filed for transfers of stock or securities occurring on or after March 13, 2009, are governed by Reg. § 1.367(a)-8.[161]

Code Sec. 361 Exchanges. If a U.S. person transfers property to a foreign corporation in a Code Sec. 361 exchange (¶ 2205), the exceptions above will generally not apply and the transferor will recognize gain under the outbound transfer rules (Code Sec. 367(a)(5)).[162] However, recognition of gain only applies if the transferring corporation is controlled by five or fewer domestic corporations, and basis adjustment and other conditions provided in regulation are met. Transfers of stock or securities in outbound Code Sec. 361 exchanges occurring on or after April 17, 2013, are governed by Temp. Reg. § 1.367(a)-3T(e).

2493. Transfers to Foreign Trusts. Any U.S. person that transfers property to a foreign trust (other than the trust of an employee benefits plan or tax-exempt organization) with a U.S. beneficiary is treated as the owner of the portion of the trust attributable to the property (Code Sec. 679; Reg. § 1.679-1).[163] If the transferor and another person would be treated as owner of the same portion of the trust, then the U.S. transferor will be treated as the owner. Thus, any income received by the trust with respect to the property is taxable to the transferor under the grantor trust rules (¶ 571). This rule applies without regard to whether the transferor retains any power or interest in the property. It also applies regardless of whether the transfer is direct or indirect. Exceptions exist for foreign trusts established by a will, transfers made by reason of death of the U.S. person (transferor), or transfers of property to the foreign trust in exchange for consideration equal to its fair market value. A U.S. person who is treated as the owner of any portion of a foreign trust under the grantor trust rules is required to ensure that the trust files an annual information return on Form 3520-A and furnishes the required annual statements to its U.S. owners and beneficiaries, or be subject to a penalty (Code Secs. 6048(b) and 6677(a)).[164]

References are to Standard Federal Tax Reports; Tax Research Consultant; and Practical Tax Explanations.

[157] ¶ 16,640, ¶ 16,642AC; INTL: 30,068
[158] ¶ 16,645C; INTL: 30,072
[159] ¶ 16,646; INTL: 30,080

[160] ¶ 16,640, ¶ 16,642B, ¶ 16,643; INTL: 30,074, INTL: 30,075
[161] ¶ 16,647A; INTL: 30,074
[162] ¶ 16,640, ¶ 16,643; INTL: 30,072

[163] ¶ 24,820, ¶ 24,820B; INTL: 30,252; § 32,805.10
[164] ¶ 36,000, ¶ 39,815; EST-TRST: 36,258.10; § 39,135.15

The IRS may presume that when a U.S. person transfers property to a foreign trust the trust has a U.S. beneficiary unless the U.S. person demonstrates otherwise (Code Sec. 679(d)). Thus, an amount will be treated as either paid or accumulated for the benefit of a U.S. person if: (1) the U.S. person's interest in the trust is contingent on a future event; (2) a loan of cash or marketable securities, or the use of any other trust property, is made to any U.S. person; (3) any person has the discretion of making a distribution from the trust to any class of persons that may include a U.S. person; or (4) the U.S. person who transferred property to the trust is involved in any agreement or understanding that may result in trust income or corpus being paid to or accumulated for the benefit of a U.S. person.

2494. Information Reporting on Foreign Partnerships. A number of reporting requirements apply with respect to foreign partnerships. First, a foreign partnership must file a U.S. partnership return (Form 1065) if it has gross income that is either U.S. source income (¶ 2427) or income effectively connected with a U.S. trade or business (¶ 2429) (Code Sec. 6031(e)).[165] A U.S. partner cannot claim distributive shares of any partnership deduction, loss, or credit if a partnership return is not filed (Code Sec. 6231(f)).[166] Second, every U.S. person that controls a foreign partnership (more than 50 percent interest) is required to file an annual information return on Form 8865 (¶ 2487). Additionally, any U.S. person that owns at least a 10-percent interest in a foreign partnership must report on Form 8865 any changes to his or her ownership in the partnership during the tax year (Code Sec. 6046A).[167] Failure to file an information return will result in a $10,000 penalty per occurrence (Code Sec. 6679).[168] A U.S. person who transfers property to a foreign partnership in a nontaxable transfer must report the transfer on Form 926 if the U.S. person has at least a 10-percent interest in the partnership or if the value of the property transferred exceeds $100,000 (Code Sec. 6038B).[169]

Other Foreign Tax Rules

2495. Foreign Currency Transactions. All federal income tax determinations must be made in the taxpayer's functional currency (Code Sec. 985).[170] Generally, the functional currency of a U.S. taxpayer will be the U.S. dollar. However, in the case of a qualified business unit (QBU), the functional currency is the currency in which the taxpayer conducts a significant part of its activities and which is used in keeping books and records. For this purpose, a QBU is any separate and clearly identified unit of a trade or business of the taxpayer which maintains its own books and records (for example, foreign subsidiary of a U.S. corporation or a foreign corporation) (Code Sec. 989).[171] Special rules apply in determining when foreign earnings and profits and foreign income taxes must be translated into U.S. dollars, as well as the use of a foreign branch of a U.S. taxpayer (Code Secs. 986 and 987).[172]

Foreign currency gain or loss attributable to a nonfunctional currency transaction is treated separately from the underlying transaction. Generally, it is treated as ordinary gain or loss but is not treated as interest income or expenses (Code Sec. 988).[173] However, gain of an individual from the disposition of foreign currency in a personal transaction is not taxable, provided that the gain realized does not exceed $200. A personal transaction is any transaction other than one with respect to which properly allocable expenses are deductible as trade or business expenses or expenses incurred in the production of income. It also refers to an individual's currency exchange transactions that are entered into in connection with business travel but do not affect tax treatment of capital losses (¶ 1754).

References are to Standard Federal Tax Reports; Tax Research Consultant; and Practical Tax Explanations.

[165] ¶ 35,381; PART: 18,410.05; § 39,155.10

[166] ¶ 37,770; PART: 18,410.05; § 39,155.10

[167] ¶ 35,960; PART: 18,410.15; § 39,135.05

[168] ¶ 39,835; PART: 18,410.15; § 39,135.05

[169] ¶ 35,580; INTL: 30,352.10; § 39,135.10

[170] ¶ 28,840; INTLOUT: 21,050; § 46,020.10

[171] ¶ 28,920; INTLOUT: 21,052; § 46,020.10

[172] ¶ 28,860, ¶ 28,880; IN-TLOUT: 21,200, INTLOUT: 21,250; § 46,020.10

[173] ¶ 28,900; INTLOUT: 21,100

2496. International Boycotts. Participation by a taxpayer in, or cooperation with, an international boycott will result in the reduction or denial of the foreign tax credit (¶ 2475), the deferral of tax allowed to foreign subsidiaries (¶ 2485), and the deferral of tax allowed to domestic international sales corporation (DISC) shareholders (¶ 2498) (Code Sec. 999; Temp. Reg. § 7.999-1).[174] The amount of the benefits to be denied is determined from the ratio of the value of the sales or purchases of goods and services (or other transactions) arising from the boycott activity to the total value of the foreign sales or purchases of goods and services (or other transactions).

Participation in or cooperation with an international boycott occurs when a person, in order to do business in a certain country, agrees not to do business with a specified second country or with other countries doing business in specified countries. An agreement not to hire employees of, or to do business with, other companies whose employees are of a specified nationality, race or religion is also boycott activity. The following countries may require participation in, or cooperation with, an international boycott: Iraq, Kuwait, Lebanon, Libya, Qatar, Saudi Arabia, Syria, United Arab Emirates, and the Republic of Yemen.[175] The reduction of foreign tax credit extends to the credit that the taxpayer is entitled to as a shareholder as well as to the credit for foreign taxes the taxpayer paid himself or herself (Code Sec. 908).[176] Taxpayers who participate in or cooperate with a boycott and derive income from such activities must report such information to the IRS by filing Form 5713 when their income tax is due (including extensions).

2497. Illegal Payments. If an illegal bribe, kickback, or other payment is made by, or on behalf of, a controlled foreign corporation (CFC) (¶ 2487) or a domestic international sales corporation (DISC) (¶ 2498), either directly or indirectly to an official, employee, or agent-in-fact of a foreign government, the amount of the bribe, kickback or other payment will affect shareholders. In the case of a CFC, the amount is included as subpart F income for the year (¶ 2488) and thus is included in the shareholder's income (Code Sec. 952(a)(4)).[177] In the case of a DISC, the amount is considered a constructive dividend and must be included in the shareholder's income (Code Sec. 995(b)(1)(F)(iii)).[178] However, such payments may be deductible in certain circumstances, despite their possible illegality (¶ 972).

2498. Foreign Trade Income. Prior to 2005, the Code contained a number of rules designed to promote the export of U.S. manufactured products. For example, a percentage of income generated through a domestic international sales corporation (DISC) could be deferred for U.S. tax purposes, while a certain percentage of income from the sale of qualified export property by a foreign sales corporation (FSC) could be completely exempt from U.S. tax. Similarly, any U.S. taxpayer was entitled to exclude from gross income extraterritorial income (ETI) to the extent it was qualifying foreign trade income. These rules have been effectively repealed. However, a DISC geared toward small businesses may still exist if the income deferred by shareholders is limited and an interest charge is paid on such deferred amounts (Code Sec. 995).[179] The election to be treated as an interest-charge DISC is made on Form 4876-A.

2499. Information from Foreign Sources. The IRS may make a formal document request for foreign records if the normal summons procedure fails to produce the requested documentation (Code Sec. 982).[180] The request for formal documentation supplements the administrative summons procedure and does not prevent the use of any other Code provisions to obtain documents.

References are to Standard Federal Tax Reports; Tax Research Consultant; and Practical Tax Explanations.

[174] ¶ 29,080, ¶ 29,081; INTL: 21,000

[175] ¶ 29,083.15; INTL: 21,050

[176] ¶ 27,964; INTL: 21,306; § 13,410.05

[177] ¶ 28,490; INTLOUT: 9,154

[178] ¶ 29,020; INTL: 21,312

[179] ¶ 29,020; INTLOUT: 11,000

[180] ¶ 28,820; IRS: 21,260

24 FOREIGN

Chapter 25

RETURNS □ PAYMENT OF TAX

Filing

2501. Income Tax Returns—Types of Returns. Individuals who must file income tax returns use Form 1040, 1040A, or 1040EZ, along with any appropriate schedules; fiduciaries of estates and trusts who must file income tax returns use Form 1041; corporations must file income tax returns on Form 1120; and partnerships must file information returns on Form 1065.

The following specialized income tax return forms for individuals also exist: Form 1040-C for a departing alien; Form 1040NR or Form 1040NR-EZ for a nonresident alien; Form 1040-SS (self-employment) for a resident of the Virgin Islands, Guam, American Samoa or the Northern Mariana Islands; and Form 1040-PR or 1040-SS (self-employment) for a resident of Puerto Rico.

Specialized forms for certain types of corporations also exist:

(1) Schedule PH, attached to Form 1120 for a U.S. personal holding company;

(2) Schedule UTP, attached to the Form 1120 series return for a corporation with at least $10 million in assets (was $50 million for 2013 tax year) that has taken an uncertain tax position;

(3) Form 1120-C for a cooperative association;

(4) Form 1120-F for a foreign corporation;

(5) Form 1120-FSC for a foreign sales corporation;

(6) Form 1120-H for a homeowners association;

(7) Form 1120-IC-DISC for an interest charge domestic international sales corporation;

(8) Form 1120-L for a life insurance company;

(9) Form 1120-ND for a nuclear decommissioning fund;

(10) Form 1120-PC for a property and casualty insurance company;

(11) Form 1120-POL for a political organization;

(12) Form 1120-REIT for a real estate investment trust;

(13) Form 1120-RIC for a regulated investment company;

(14) Form 1120S for an S corporation; and

(15) Form 1120-SF for a settlement fund.

Rules for determining which individuals must file an income tax return are at ¶ 101; rules for determining who must pay estimated tax are at ¶ 2682; rules for corporation returns are at ¶ 211; rules for S corporations are at ¶ 351; rules applicable to partners and partnerships are at ¶ 406; and rules for estates and trusts are at ¶ 510.

Employers must file quarterly returns on Form 941 to report wages paid to employees and income tax withheld on the wages, tips employees have received, both the employer's and the employee's share of Social Security and Medicare taxes, and additional Medicare taxes withheld from employees (¶ 2650). Employers with an esti-

¶2501

mated employment tax liability of $1,000 or less ("small employers") may instead file an annual return on Form 944. Employers who pay wages for agricultural labor must file Form 943. In addition, employers must file Form 940 annually to report and pay federal unemployment taxes.

Individuals who pay annual cash wages of $1,900 or more in 2014 or 2015 for domestic services in their private homes must file Schedule H of Form 1040 to report and pay both the employer and employee share of Social Security and Medicare taxes, and any income tax withheld at the employee's request. Individuals also use Schedule H to pay and report federal unemployment taxes if they paid total cash wages of $1,000 or more to household employees in any calendar quarter (¶ 2652).

2503. Electronic Filing. Electronic filing allows qualified filers to transmit tax return information directly to an IRS Service Center, usually over the internet. Taxpayers may e-file their tax returns through a paid preparer (or an electronic return originator), by using a personal computer, access to the internet, and commercial tax preparation software, or by qualifying for and enrolling in the Free File program. Individual taxpayers who e-file their returns can authorize direct debit payment from their checking or savings account on a specified date. Taxpayers may also charge their taxes by credit card or pay their taxes electronically through the Electronic Federal Tax Payment System (EFTPS) (IRS Fact Sheet FS-2011-7).

Free File is a public-private sector initiative with commercial software providers to provide free tax return preparation and electronic filing service for middle- and low-income taxpayers who meet certain adjusted gross income requirements. A Free File Fillable Tax Forms option is also available which allows all taxpayers, regardless of income level, to fill out and file their tax forms electronically (IRS News Release IR-2011-5). Free File is available at the IRS website at www.irs.gov.

Taxpayers who file their tax returns electronically must use electronic signatures (IRS Fact Sheet FS-2011-7). Electronic filers use a Self-Select Personal Identification Number (PIN), or if using a paid preparer, that preparer's Practitioner PIN (IRS Pub. 1345).

Form 8453 is used to transmit certain forms and supporting paper documents that are specifically listed on Form 8453 and are required to be submitted to the IRS with e-filed returns. If paper documentation must be submitted that is not listed on Form 8453, the return cannot be e-filed (Instructions to Form 8453).

Corporations, S corporations, partnerships, and exempt organizations may also elect to electronically file, respectively, Forms 1120, 1120S, 1065, and 990. However, certain organizations are required to submit those returns electronically. Corporations and S corporations with assets of $10 million or more, and that file 250 or more returns during the year, must file Forms 1120 and 1120S electronically (Reg. § 301.6011-5).[1] A partnership with more than 100 partners must file Form 1065 (and Schedules K-1 and related forms) electronically (Reg. § 301.6011-3).[2] Exempt organizations with assets of $10 million or more, and that file 250 or more returns annually, must file Form 990 electronically. If a private foundation or a Code Sec. 4947(a)(1) trust files 250 or more returns annually, regardless of asset size, it must file Form 990-PF electronically (Reg. § 301.6033-4).[3] Although electronic filing is not required for any corporation, an S corporation or exempt organization filing less than 250 returns during the calendar year, the IRS encourages such organizations to do so. The IRS has updated the procedures that corporations, S corporations, and tax-exempt organizations must use to request a waiver of the electronic filing requirement (Notice 2010-13).

For income tax returns of individuals, estates, or trusts (i.e., individual income tax returns) electronic filing is required if the return is prepared and filed by a specified tax return preparer for the calendar year during which the return is filed. With respect to any calendar year, a "specified tax return preparer" means any tax return preparer

---

References are to Standard Federal Tax Reports; Tax Research Consultant; and Practical Tax Explanations.

[1] ¶ 35,129J; FILEBUS: 3,052.05, FILEBUS: 12,300; § 26,030.10, § 29,010.15, § 39,225.10b

[2] ¶ 35,126F; FILEBUS: 12,302.35, FILEBUS: 12,300; § 30,435

[3] ¶ 35,424C; EXEMPT: 12,252.15, EXEMPT: 12,252.20, FILEBUS: 12,300; § 33,245, § 33,605.05

(¶ 2517), unless the preparer reasonably expects to file 10 or fewer individual income tax returns during the calendar year (Code Sec. 6011(e)(3)).[4]

An individual income tax return is considered "filed" by a specified return preparer if the preparer submits the return to the IRS on the taxpayer's behalf. A return is not considered filed by a specified return preparer if the preparer obtains a hand-signed and dated statement from the taxpayer that the taxpayer chooses to file the return in paper format and that the taxpayer, and not the preparer, will submit the paper return to the IRS (Reg. § 301.6011-7(a)(4)).[5]

The IRS may grant waivers of the electronic filing requirement for specified return preparers in cases of undue hardship (Reg. § 301.6011-7(c)(1)).[6] Such waivers generally are intended to be granted preparers for undue hardships that can be identified in advance before the preparers would otherwise be required to file individual income tax returns electronically for a particular calendar year and will ordinarily be granted only in rare cases. Requests for a hardship waiver are made by filing Form 8944 (Rev. Proc. 2011-25).

The IRS has provided further administrative exemptions to the electronic filing requirement for certain classes of specified tax return preparers (Notice 2011-26). They include: exempt preparers (preparer members of certain religious groups; foreign preparers without Social Security numbers; and certain preparers ineligible for IRS e-file); exempt individual income tax returns due to preparer's technological difficulties (rejected returns; forms or schedules not supported by the preparer's software package; and other technological difficulties); and exempt individual income tax returns due to IRS e-file limitations (returns currently not accepted and required documentation not accepted electronically). Exemptions are automatic and do not have to be requested, but preparers will be required to show entitlement to exemption upon request by the IRS. Form 8948 was created to explain why an individual tax return that was able to be filed electronically was filed in a paper format.

Foreign Accounts. The IRS is authorized to require a financial institution to electronically file returns with respect to withheld taxes for which the institution is liable as a withholding agent under the nonresident alien and foreign corporation withholding rules (¶ 2455), or under the foreign account withholding rules (¶ 2469), even though the financial institution files less than 250 returns during the tax year (Code Sec. 6011(e)(4)).

2504. Signatures on Returns. Forms 1040, 1040A, and 1040EZ must be signed by the individual taxpayer (Code Sec. 6061; Reg. § 1.6061-1).[7] The return contains a declaration that it is made under the penalties of perjury (Code Sec. 6065).[8] In the case of a joint return, both the husband and the wife must sign (Reg. § 1.6013-1(a)(2)).[9] If the taxpayer did not prepare the return, the return must be signed by the taxpayer and the tax return preparer (¶ 2517 and ¶ 2518). If a decedent's return is filed by a representative, the representative should sign the return on the line indicated for the taxpayer and attach a written power of attorney.

For a discussion of signing requirements for electronically filed returns, see ¶ 2503.

2505. Income Tax Returns—When to File. Subject to an exception for deadlines falling on a Saturday, Sunday, or a legal holiday (¶ 2549), the due dates for income tax returns are as follows:

Individual, trust, estate, and partnership income tax returns are due on or before the 15th day of the 4th month following the close of the tax year, typically April 15 in the case of a calendar-year taxpayer (Code Sec. 6072; Reg. § 1.6072-1(a)).[10] For the 2014 calendar tax year, income tax returns must be filed on April 15, 2015. The final income

---

References are to Standard Federal Tax Reports; Tax Research Consultant; and Practical Tax Explanations.

[4] ¶ 35,120; FILEBUS: 12,302; § 41,803

[5] ¶ 35,129OC; FILEBUS: 12,302; § 41,803

[6] ¶ 35,129OC; FILEBUS: 12,302; § 41,803

[7] ¶ 36,602, ¶ 36,603; FILEBUS: 12,100, FILEIND: 15,250; § 1,330.05, § 39,010.25, § 41,810.15

[8] ¶ 36,680; FILEBUS: 12,100; § 39,010.25

[9] ¶ 35,161; FILEIND: 15,250; § 1,330.05

[10] ¶ 36,720, ¶ 36,721; FILEIND: 18,052.20, PART: 18,160.05; § 39,205.10

tax return of a decedent for a fractional part of a year is due on the same date as would apply had the taxpayer lived the entire year (i.e., the 15th day of the 4th month following the close of the 12-month period that began on the first day of the fractional year) (Reg. § 1.6072-1(b)).[11]

A domestic corporation or foreign corporation having a U.S. office must file its corporate income tax return on or before the 15th day of the 3rd month after the close of the tax year (March 15 for a calendar-year corporation). A corporation whose foreign sales corporation election is still in effect must file its U.S. income tax return by the 15th day of the 3rd month after the end of its tax year (Instructions for Form 1120-FSC). The return of an interest charge domestic international sales corporation (IC-DISC), an exempt farmers' cooperative, or other cooperative organization is due on or before the 15th day of the 9th month following the close of the tax year (September 15 for a calendar-year taxpayer) (Reg. § 1.6072-2).[12]

The due date for income tax returns of organizations exempt from tax under Code Sec. 501(a), other than employees' trusts under Code Sec. 401(a), is the 15th day of the 5th month following the close of the tax year (Reg. § 1.6072-2(c)).[13]

A taxpayer filing as a nonresident alien who is not subject to income tax withholding on wages (¶ 2601) and a foreign corporation not having an office or place of business in the U.S. may file a return as late as the 15th day of the 6th month after the close of the tax year (Reg. §§ 1.6072-1(c) and 1.6072-2(b)).[14] A nonresident alien who has wages subject to income tax withholding, however, is required to file a return on or before the 15th day of the 4th month following the close of the tax year.

Amended Returns. A taxpayer may correct an error in a return, without incurring interest or penalties, by filing an amended return (for individuals, Form 1040X) and paying any additional tax due on or before the last day prescribed for filing the original return. An amended return filed after the due date may be accepted, rejected, or ignored by the IRS in its sole discretion, and in the absence of an abuse of discretion the courts will not grant relief to the taxpayer. Ordinarily, the amended return will be accepted by the IRS if it is filed within the statutory period of limitations, generally within three years from the due date of the original return (¶ 2726).[15]

2509. Extension of Time to File Returns. An individual is granted an automatic extension of six months for filing a return, but *not* for payment of tax, by properly filing Form 4868 on or before the normal due date of the return (¶ 2505) (Reg. § 1.6081-4).[16] Form 4868 may be filed electronically or by mail. Filing extensions can be obtained without making tax payments, so long as taxpayers properly estimate their tax liability on the form. If the requesting taxpayers do not properly estimate their tax liability, the extension request will be denied, and the IRS will charge interest and a penalty for late payment. If the amount of tax included with the extension request is less than sufficient to cover the taxpayer's liability, the taxpayer will be charged interest on the overdue amount. However, no late-payment penalty will be imposed if the tax paid through withholding, estimated tax payments, or any payment accompanying Form 4868 is at least 90 percent of the total tax due with Form 1040 and if the remaining unpaid balance is paid with the return within the extension period (¶ 2809) (Reg. § 1.6081-4; Reg. § 301.6651-1).[17] An automatic extension should not be requested if the taxpayer has asked the IRS to compute the tax or if the taxpayer is under a court order to file the return by the original due date.

Individuals Residing Outside the United States. U.S. citizens or residents living outside the United States and Puerto Rico, including military personnel, are granted an automatic extension up to June 15 (the 15th day of the sixth month following the close of their tax year) for filing a return and paying the tax if they attach a statement to their

---

References are to Standard Federal Tax Reports; Tax Research Consultant; and Practical Tax Explanations.

[11] ¶ 36,721; FILEIND: 18,052.20; § 39,020

[12] ¶ 36,724; FILEBUS: 3,052.05, INTLOUT: 15,058.20; § 39,205.05

[13] ¶ 36,724; EXEMPT: 12,252; § 39,205.20

[14] ¶ 36,721, ¶ 36,724; FILEIND: 100, FILEIND: 15,200, CCORP: 36,060; § 39,205.05

[15] ¶ 35,141.40; FILEBUS: 3,150, FILEIND: 18,150; § 1,315

[16] ¶ 36,793; FILEBUS: 15,100; § 39,215.10

[17] ¶ 36,793, ¶ 39,472; FILEBUS: 15,100; § 39,215.10

return showing that they are entitled to such an extension (Reg. § 1.6081-5).[18] However, interest will be assessed on any unpaid tax from the due date of the return (without regard to the automatic extension, April 15) until the tax is paid (IRS Pub. 54). The automatic filing extension runs concurrently with the automatic six-month extension allowed to all individuals. Thus, the maximum automatic extension is only six months from the regular due date. The application for the automatic six-month extension is timely if it is filed by the due date established by the automatic two-month extension. If an individual outside the United States needs more than the automatic extension in order to meet either the bona fide residence or the physical presence test for the foreign earned income or housing exclusion, Form 2350 should be filed by the due date for filing the return (June 15 for calendar-year citizens or residents living outside the United States and Puerto Rico). Such filing will entitle the individual to additional time for filing the return but not for paying the tax.

Corporations. A corporation or an S corporation is entitled to an automatic extension of six months for filing its return, provided that it timely and properly files Form 7004 and deposits the full amount of the tax due. The IRS may terminate this extension, however, at any time by mailing to the corporation (or the parent corporation for an affiliated group filing a consolidated return) notice of such termination at least 10 days prior to the termination date fixed in the notice (Reg. § 1.6081-3).[19]

Other Entities. An automatic five-month extension of time (through the 15th day of the 6th month following the close of the tax year) for filing a return and paying the tax is also granted to a partnership that keeps its books and records outside the U.S. and Puerto Rico, a domestic corporation that transacts its business and keeps its books and records outside the United States and Puerto Rico, a foreign corporation that maintains an office or place of business within the United States, and a domestic corporation whose principal income is from sources within U.S. possessions (Reg. § 1.6081-5(a)).[20] The automatic filing extension runs concurrently with the automatic six-month filing extension allowed for most businesses.

Partnerships filing Form 1065 or Form 8804, and estates and trusts filing Form 1041, should use Form 7004 to apply for an automatic *five*-month filing extension (Reg. §§ 1.6081-2 and 1.6081-6).[21]

The following entities must use Form 8868 to apply for extensions of time for filing returns: various trusts filing Forms 1041-A, 5227, and 6069; certain exempt organizations filing Forms 990, 990-PF, 990-EZ, or 990-BL, certain exempt organizations or corporations filing Form 990-T, and Form 4720; and certain charitable organizations filing Form 8870 (Reg. § 1.6081-9).[22] Real estate mortgage investment conduits filing Form 1066 or Form 8831 should use Form 7004 to apply for an automatic six-month filing extension (Reg. § 1.6081-7).[23]

2513. Place for Filing Paper Returns. An individual, estate, or trust must file paper returns with the IRS Service Center indicated in the instructions to the taxpayer's return, except for certain charitable and split-interest trusts and pooled-income funds (see Instructions for Form 1041).

A corporation, S corporation or partnership must file its return with the Service Center indicated in the instructions to the entity's return (Form 1120, Form 1120S or Form 1065).

The place to file certain elections, statements, returns and other documents can be found at the IRS website, at http://www.irs.gov/uac/Where-to-File-Certain-Elections,-Statements,-Returns-and-Other-Documents (Notice 2010-53).

2517. Tax Return Preparers. A person who prepares for compensation, or who employs persons to prepare for compensation, all or a substantial portion of *any* tax

---

References are to Standard Federal Tax Reports; Tax Research Consultant; and Practical Tax Explanations.

[18] ¶ 36,795; FILEBUS: 15,100; § 39,215.40

[19] ¶ 36,790; FILEBUS: 15,100; § 39,215.15

[20] ¶ 36,795; FILEBUS: 15,100

[21] ¶ 36,788, ¶ 36,797; FILEBUS: 15,104.20; § 30,435, § 32,610.15, § 39,215.20

[22] ¶ 36,798K; FILEBUS: 15,104.35; § 33,245, § 33,605.05, § 33,945

[23] ¶ 36,798; FILEBUS: 15,104.20; § 39,215.05

return or refund claim is a "tax return preparer" (Code Sec. 7701(a)(36); Reg. § 301.7701-15).[24] Preparers are divided into two categories for purposes of the return preparer penalties (¶ 2518): signing tax return preparers and nonsigning tax return preparers. A signing tax return preparer is the individual preparer with primary responsibility for the overall substantive accuracy of the preparation of tax returns or refund claims. A nonsigning tax return preparer is any preparer who is not a signing tax return preparer but who prepares a substantial portion of a return or refund claim regarding events that have occurred at the time advice is rendered.

In addition to the prohibition against disclosure of return information (¶ 2894), a tax return preparer is subject to the following rules:

(1) The signing tax return preparer must sign a tax return electronically using a Self-Select Personal Identification Number (PIN) or a Practitioner PIN (IRS Pub. 1345). The preparer need not sign an electronic return before presenting a completed copy to the taxpayer, but must furnish all information that will be transmitted as the electronically signed return to the taxpayer at the same time that the preparer furnishes Form 8879 or a similar IRS e-file signature form. The signing tax return preparer must actually sign a paper return after its completion but before its presentation to the taxpayer for signature (Code Sec. 6695(b); Reg. § 1.6695-1(b)).[25] Paper returns require the preparer to manually sign the return or use any of three alternative methods that include either a facsimile of the preparer's signature or the individual preparer's printed name: (1) rubber stamp, (2) mechanical device, or (3) computer software program (Notice 2004-54).

(2) The signing tax return preparer must include his or her identifying number on the taxpayer's return after its completion but before its presentation to the taxpayer. The identifying number is the individual's preparer tax identification number (PTIN) or other number prescribed by the IRS. If the preparer is employed by another person, the employer must furnish the identifying numbers of both the employer and the employee-preparer (Code Sec. 6109(a)(4); Reg. § 1.6109-2; Notice 2011-6).[26]

(3) The signing tax return preparer must provide the taxpayer with a completed copy of the prepared return, in either paper or electronic form, no later than the time the original return is presented for signing. The copy must be in any media acceptable to both the taxpayer and the preparer, and must include all information submitted to the IRS to enable the taxpayer to determine what schedules, forms, electronic files, and other supporting materials have been filed. The copy need not contain the identification number of the paid tax return preparer. The signing tax return preparer must also keep, for three years following the close of the return period, a copy of the return (in either paper or electronic form) or a list of the names, identification numbers, and tax years of taxpayers for whom returns were prepared, and the name of the individual tax return preparer required to sign the return (Code Sec. 6107; Reg. § 1.6107-1).[27] The preparer need not sign the taxpayer's copy of the return.

(4) If a tax return preparer, or any person, employs any signing tax return preparers to prepare returns for other persons (i.e., not the employer's return), the preparer must keep a record, for three years following the close of the return period to which the record relates, of the name, taxpayer identification number (TIN), and principal place of work of each tax return preparer employed by the preparer at any time during the return period (Code Sec. 6060; Reg. § 1.6060-1).[28] Any individual signing tax return preparer who is not employed by another preparer is treated as his or her own employer. The "return period" is defined as the 12-month period beginning on July 1 of each year.

References are to Standard Federal Tax Reports; Tax Research Consultant; and Practical Tax Explanations.

24 ¶ 43,080, ¶ 43,113; IRS: 6,050; § 41,410.05

25 ¶ 39,965, ¶ 39,966; IRS: 6,104; § 41,510

26 ¶ 36,960, ¶ 36,961C; IRS: 6,106; § 41,515

27 ¶ 36,920, ¶ 36,921; IRS: 6,108, IRS: 6,110.05; § 41,520.05, § 41,520.10

28 ¶ 36,560, ¶ 36,561; IRS: 6,110.10; § 41,520.20

All tax return preparers must have a PTIN or other prescribed identifying number that was applied for and received at the time and in the manner prescribed by the IRS, including the payment of a user fee. To obtain a PTIN, a tax return preparer must be an attorney, certified public accountant (CPA), enrolled agent, or registered tax return preparer authorized to practice before the IRS (Reg. § 1.6109-2(d)). However, the IRS will allow certain individuals who are 18 years old or older, but are not one of these specific types of professionals, to pay the applicable user fee and obtain a PTIN if: (1) the individual is supervised by an attorney, CPA, enrolled agent, enrolled retirement plan agent, or enrolled actuary authorized to practice before the IRS under Circular 230 § 10.3(a)-(e); (2) the supervising attorney, certified public accountant, enrolled agent, enrolled retirement plan agent, or enrolled actuary signs the tax returns or refund claims prepared by the individual; (3) the individual is employed at the law firm, CPA firm, or other recognized firm of the tax return preparer who signs the tax return or refund claim; and (4) the individual passes the requisite tax compliance check and suitability check when available (Notice 2011-6).

Registered Tax Return Preparers. Practice before the IRS is regulated through Circular 230. Effective August 2, 2011, all paid return preparers, regardless of credentials, are subject to Circular 230's rules of practice. Registered tax return preparers (RTRPs) are subject to registration, examination, and continuing education requirements.[29] Note, however, that the U.S. Court of Appeals for the District of Columbia has affirmed the decision of a district court to permanently bar the IRS from continued implementation or enforcement of the registered tax return preparer program. *S. Loving*, CA-D.C., 2014-1 USTC ¶ 50,175. The IRS may continue to issue PTINs but cannot require individuals to pay fees unrelated to obtaining a PTIN, to meet continuing educational requirements or the passing of the competence testing to obtain a PTIN. The IRS has suspended the RTRP program.

Voluntary Certification Program. Effective June 30, 2014, the IRS has established a voluntary certification program designed to encourage unenrolled tax preparers to complete continuing education courses for the purpose of increasing his or her knowledge of relevant federal tax law necessary for preparation of tax returns (Rev. Proc. 2014-42, modifying and superseding Rev. Proc. 81-38).[30] As the name implies, this voluntary program neither restricts any individual from preparing and signing tax returns or claims for refund nor changes the requirement that paid tax return preparers must obtain a PTIN. Upon successful completion each year of certain requirements, the IRS will issue a Record of Completion. The Record of Completion is only valid for tax returns or claims for refund prepared and signed during the calendar year for which it has been issued. Thus, a Record of Completion is valid from the later of January 1 of the year covered by the Record of Completion or the date the Record of Completion is issued until December 31st of that year.

The application for a Record of Completion is made on Form W-12, IRS Paid Preparer Tax Identification Number (PTIN) Application and Renewal. All applications must be received no later than April 15th of the year for which the Record of Completion is sought.

Unenrolled tax return preparers who obtain an Annual Season Filing Record of Completion are permitted to represent taxpayers before the IRS during examination of tax returns and claim for refund that he or she prepared and signed, or prepared if there is no signature space on the form, provided the individual had a valid Record of Completion for the year the return or claim of refund was prepared and a valid Record of Completion for the year or years in which the representation occurs. The representation is limited to exam, and the individual may not appear before an appeals officer, a revenue officer, Counsel, or similar IRS officer or employee.

Unenrolled tax return preparers have been allowed similar limited practice before the IRS prior to June 12, 2014, under Rev. Proc. 81-38. The IRS will allow these individuals to continue to represent taxpayers whose returns or claim for refund he or

---

References are to Standard Federal Tax Reports; Tax Research Consultant; and Practical Tax Explanations.

[29] ¶ 43,524; IRS: 3,204.10; § 41,010.20

[30] ¶ 43,808.43; IRS: 6,252.30; § 41,025

¶2517

she prepared and signed at examination through December 31, 2015. Unless they voluntarily participate in the Annual Filing Season Program, these unenrolled tax return preparers will not be allowed to practice before the IRS and will be limited to simply preparing tax returns or claims for refund.

2518. Tax Return Preparer Penalties. Several penalties may be assessed against tax return preparers.

Failure to Follow Procedures. A tax return preparer who fails to meet the requirements described in ¶ 2517 may be assessed the following penalties, unless the failure is due to reasonable cause and not to willful neglect:

(1) $50 for each failure to sign a return, to furnish an identifying number, or to furnish the taxpayer with a copy of the prepared return;

(2) $50 for each failure to retain and make available a copy of prepared returns or a list of taxpayers for whom returns were prepared, and the name of the individual preparer required to sign the return; and

(3) $50 for each failure to retain and make available a record of preparers employed, plus $50 for each failure to include an item required in such record.

A $500 penalty is assessable against a preparer who endorses or negotiates a taxpayer's refund check. The exception to the rule is for a bank preparer who negotiates customers' refund checks for bank account deposits (Code Sec. 6695; Reg. § 1.6695-1).[31]

Understatement of Taxpayer's Liability. A penalty may be imposed against a return preparer for each tax return or claim for refund that understates the taxpayer's liability due to an unreasonable position that the preparer knew, or reasonably should have known. The penalty is the greater of $1,000 or 50 percent of the income derived, or to be derived, by the preparer with respect to the return or refund claim (Code Sec. 6694(a); Reg. § § 1.6694-1 and 1.6694-2; Rev. Proc. 2012-51).[32] The penalty will not be imposed if the preparer shows that there was reasonable cause for the understatement and the preparer acted in good faith. Modified rules apply to nonsigning preparers.

A position is treated as unreasonable unless: (1) there is or was substantial authority for the position; (2) the position is adequately disclosed and has a reasonable basis; or (3) if the position pertains to a tax shelter (¶ 2870) or a reportable transaction (¶ 2591), it is reasonable to believe that the position would more likely than not be sustained on its merits. Under interim guidance, the term "substantial authority" has the same meaning as it does for the 20-percent accuracy-related penalty for a substantial understatement of income tax (¶ 2858). The guidance also contains penalty compliance rules for tax shelter transactions (Notice 2009-5).[33]

The penalty increases to the greater of $5,000 or 50 percent of the income derived, or to be derived, by the preparer with respect to the return or refund claim if the understatement is willful or reckless (Code Sec. 6694(b); Reg. § 1.6694-3).[34]

Lack of Diligence in Claiming Earned Income Credit. Tax return preparers must comply with due diligence requirements for returns or refund claims asserting eligibility for the earned income credit (Code Sec. 6695(g); Reg. § 1.6695-2).[35] Among the due diligence requirements, tax return preparers are required to file (or submit to the taxpayer for filing) Form 8867 (or a self-created alternate computation record) with any federal return claiming the earned income credit. Each failure to observe the requirements regarding the amount of, or eligibility for, the credit will result in a penalty of $500, in addition to any other penalty imposed.

Aiding or Abetting in Tax Liability Understatement. A penalty of $1,000 may also be imposed on persons for aiding or abetting in an understatement of tax liability on a return, claim, or other document. The penalty increases to $10,000 for aiding or abetting

---

References are to Standard Federal Tax Reports; Tax Research Consultant; and Practical Tax Explanations.

[31] ¶ 39,965, ¶ 39,966; IRS: 6,104, IRS: 6,106.05, IRS: 6,108, IRS: 6,110.05, IRS: 6,112; § 41,535.05

[32] ¶ 39,955, ¶ 39,956, ¶ 39,957, ¶ 39,960.20; IRS: 6,150; § 41,610
[33] ¶ 39,960.70; IRS: 6,156; § 41,610.10

[34] ¶ 39,955, ¶ 39,957E; IRS: 6,158; § 41,615
[35] ¶ 39,965, ¶ 39,968; IRS: 6,116; § 12,640

¶2518

an understatement of liability on a corporate return. (Code Sec. 6701).[36] Only one penalty may be imposed per taxpayer per period; however, the tax period may not necessarily be a tax year. For instance, understatements on quarterly employment tax returns may give rise to four separate penalties for a calendar year. According to the Sixth Circuit, no statute of limitations applies to bar the penalty.[37] Generally, this penalty may be imposed in addition to other penalties. However, it will not be imposed if either the tax return preparer penalty for understatements due to unreasonable positions or the penalty for promoting abusive tax shelters has been applied with respect to the same tax return or refund claim.

2521. Penalty for Frivolous Tax Return. A civil penalty of $5,000 is imposed upon any person (including an individual, a trust, estate, partnership, association, company, or corporation) who files a purported tax return (income or otherwise) if: (1) the purported return fails to contain sufficient information from which the substantial correctness of the amount of tax liability can be judged, or contains information that on its face indicates that the amount of tax shown is substantially incorrect; and (2) such conduct arises from a frivolous position or from a desire to delay or impede administration of the tax laws. The penalty is imposed in addition to any other penalties imposed on the taxpayer (Code Sec. 6702).[38]

A $5,000 civil penalty may also be imposed on any person who files a "specified frivolous submission." A "specified frivolous submission" is a specified submission that either is based on a position that has been identified as frivolous in a prescribed frivolous positions list, or reflects a desire to delay or impede the administration of federal tax laws. A "specified submission" is a request for a collection due process hearing or an application for an installment agreement, offer in compromise, or taxpayer assistance order. If a person withdraws a submission within 30 days after receiving notice that the return is a specified frivolous submission, the penalty will not be imposed.

The penalty may be reduced to $500 at the discretion of the Secretary of the Treasury in order to promote compliance with, and administration of, the federal tax laws (Rev. Proc. 2012-43). If a person satisfies all eligibility criteria under the procedures, including filing all tax returns and paying all outstanding taxes, penalties (other than the frivolous return penalty), and related interest, the IRS will usually reduce all unpaid frivolous return penalties assessed against that person to $500, regardless of the number of penalties assessed. Any employer applying for relief must have deposited all employment taxes for the current quarter and the prior two quarters.

A prescribed list of frivolous positions may be found in Notice 2010-33. The list is not conclusive, and will be periodically revised. Returns or submissions that contain positions not prescribed in the Notice, but which on their face have no basis for validity in existing law, or which have been deemed frivolous in a published opinion by the U.S. Tax Court or other court of competent jurisdiction may also be subject to the $5,000 penalty.

Up to $25,000 may be assessed by the Tax Court against a taxpayer who institutes or maintains proceedings primarily for delay or on frivolous grounds or who unreasonably fails to pursue available administrative remedies. Other courts may require a taxpayer to pay a penalty of up to $10,000 if the taxpayer's action against the IRS for unauthorized collection activities appears to be a frivolous or groundless proceeding (Code Sec. 6673).[39] The Tax Court has held that a penalty for instituting proceedings primarily for delay is properly assessed against the tax matters person of an S corporation, rather than against the entity or its other shareholders.[40]

2523. Books and Records. Taxpayers are required to keep accurate, permanent books and records so as to be able to determine the various types of income, gains,

---

References are to Standard Federal Tax Reports; Tax Research Consultant; and Practical Tax Explanations.

[36] ¶ 40,033; PENALTY: 3,258; § 41,620

[37] ¶ 40,035.10; PENALTY: 3,258; § 41,620

[38] ¶ 40,040; PENALTY: 3,260; § 40,220

[39] ¶ 39,785; LITIG: 6,816; § 40,220.05

[40] ¶ 39,790.47; LITIG: 6,816; § 40,220.05

losses, costs, expenses, and other amounts that affect their income tax liability for the year (Reg. § 1.6001-1(a)).[41] The records must be retained for as long as they may be, or may become, "material" for any federal tax purpose. Generally, records that support an item of income or a deduction on a tax return should be kept at least for the period of limitation for that return. See ¶ 2726, ¶ 2732, ¶ 2734, ¶ 2738, and ¶ 2517 (for tax return preparers) regarding applicable limitation periods.

Payment of Tax

2525. Place for Paying Tax. The amount of tax shown on a return must be paid to the internal revenue officer with whom the return is filed unless, as in the case of corporations, the tax must be deposited with an authorized depository (Code Sec. 6151(a); Reg. § 1.6302-1).[42] See ¶ 2513.

The IRS requests that individuals use a payment voucher, Form 1040-V, for any balance due on any Forms 1040. See ¶ 2545 regarding electronic funds withdrawal.

2529. Time of Payment. The tax shown on an income tax return is generally to be paid, without assessment or notice and demand, at the time fixed for filing the return, determined without regard to any extension of time for filing the return (¶ 2505). However, exceptions apply when:

(1) a taxpayer shows that payment on the return due date will result in undue hardship (¶ 2537);

(2) a taxpayer is residing outside the United States on the return due date (¶ 2509); or

(3) a taxpayer elects to have the IRS compute the tax (¶ 105), in which case payment is due within 30 days after the IRS mails a notice and demand (Code Sec. 6151(b)(1)).[43]

The IRS also has the authority to enter into a written agreement with the taxpayer, allowing for the full or, in most situations, partial payment of any tax in installments, if such an agreement will facilitate the collection of a tax liability (Code Sec. 6159; Reg. § § 300.1 and 300.2).[44] The fee for entering into an installment agreement is $120 ($52 for direct debit installment agreements, where the payments are deducted directly from the taxpayer's bank account). For low income taxpayers, the fee is $43, regardless of the method of payment. The fee for reinstating a defaulted agreement, or restructuring an existing agreement, is $50, regardless of income level.

There are three types of installment agreements. The first, referred to as guaranteed installment agreements, must be accepted by the IRS if an individual taxpayer's tax liabilities, without regard to interest, penalties, additions to tax, and any other additional amounts, total $10,000 or less and certain other conditions are met (Code Sec. 6159(c)). The second type of agreement is for individuals who do not qualify for the first type of agreement, and for businesses. The IRS, at the taxpayer's request, enters into a streamlined agreement if the taxpayer owes no more than $50,000, without regard to interest, penalties, additions to tax, or any other additions, and the taxpayer agrees to pay the amount due in full within six years (IRM 5.14.5.2). Small business taxpayers are allowed to enter into streamlined agreements if they agree to pay the amount due in full within two years and a direct debit installment agreement is entered into (IRS News Release IR-2011-20). Streamlined agreements do not require a financial analysis and do not involve filing liens. The third type of agreement is for taxpayers owing more than $50,000. These agreements are accepted on a case-by-case basis if the IRS determines the taxpayer can eventually pay off the debt, and the agreement will facilitate the collection of the debt.

25 | RETURNS

References are to Standard Federal Tax Reports; Tax Research Consultant; and Practical Tax Explanations.

[41] ¶ 35,102; ACCTNG: 3,052.05; § 39,055

[42] ¶ 37,080, ¶ 38,061; FILEBUS: 6,106.10, FILEIND: 21,152; § 39,305, § 39,320

[43] ¶ 37,080; FILEBUS: 6,100; § 39,305

[44] ¶ 37,180, ¶ 37,180C, ¶ 37,180D; FILEBUS: 6,104.40, FILEIND: 21,154.40; § 39,325.05

For taxpayers with $50,000 or less in combined tax liability, interest and penalties, an interactive Online Payment Agreement (OPA) application is available at the IRS website. Otherwise, a taxpayer can request an installment agreement by filing Form 9465.

2533. Taxes of Member of Armed Forces upon Death. The tax liability of a member of the U.S. Armed Forces is forgiven in the tax year the individual dies (1) while in active service in a combat zone (¶ 895), (2) from wounds, disease, or injury incurred while serving in a combat zone, or (3) from wounds or injury incurred in a terrorist or military action (IRS Pub. 3). Any unpaid taxes of such individual that relate to tax years prior to service in a combat zone may also be abated. In the case of a joint return, only the decedent's portion of joint tax liability is forgiven. A similar tax forgiveness rule applies to U.S. military and civilian employees who die as the result of wounds or injury occurring outside the United States in a terroristic or military action against the United States or any of its allies (Code Sec. 692).[45]

2537. Extension of Time for Payment of Tax. An extension of time for filing a tax return ordinarily does not postpone the time for payment (¶ 2509). The IRS, however, may extend the time for payment of the tax shown on the return for up to six months, or longer if the taxpayer is abroad, upon a showing of undue hardship. A taxpayer applying for an extension of the time to pay tax must file Form 1127 on or before the original due date for payment of the tax. The application must be accompanied by evidence showing the undue hardship that would result if the extension were refused, a statement of the assets and liabilities of the taxpayer, and a statement of the receipts and disbursements of the taxpayer for the three months preceding the original due date for payment of tax (Code Sec. 6161(a); Reg. § 1.6161-1).[46]

As a condition to the granting of an extension, the taxpayer may be required to furnish a bond (Code Sec. 6165; Reg. § 1.6165-1).[47] If an extension of time for payment of tax is granted, interest on the tax liability will accrue (¶ 2838) from the original due date until the date on which the balance is fully paid (Reg. § 1.6161-1(d)).[48]

Military and Government Personnel. Armed Forces members and civilians serving in support of the Armed Forces who serve in a designated combat zone (¶ 895) or in a contingency operation or are hospitalized outside the United States as a result of an injury received while serving in a combat zone/contingency operation qualify for an extension for filing returns and paying tax for the period of combat/contingency operation service or hospitalization plus 180 days (Code Sec. 7508).[49] This extension is also available to such a taxpayer's spouse who wishes to file a joint return.

Disaster Areas. The IRS is authorized to postpone deadlines for filing returns and paying taxes for up to one year for taxpayers affected by a federally declared disaster (Code Sec. 7508A).[50] This includes taxpayers affected by terroristic or military actions.

2541. Extension of Time for Payment of Deficiency in Tax. An extension of time for payment of a deficiency of tax may be granted for a period of not more than 18 months where timely payment of the deficiency would result in undue hardship. Such an extension may be applied for according to the procedure for an extension of time for payment of tax outlined in ¶ 2537. An additional period of not more than 12 months may be granted in an exceptional case. A request for an extension will be refused if the deficiency was due to negligence, intentional disregard of income tax rules and regulations, or fraud (Code Sec. 6161(b); Reg. § 1.6161-1(a)(2) and (c)).[51]

2545. Forms of Payment. Payment of taxes must be made by a commercially acceptable means deemed appropriate by the IRS. Such means of payment include personal or cashier's check, money order, credit, debit or charge cards, or electronic

---

References are to Standard Federal Tax Reports; Tax Research Consultant; and Practical Tax Explanations.

[45] ¶ 24,920; COMPEN: 6,604, ESTTRST: 6,300; § 1,005.15

[46] ¶ 37,200, ¶ 37,201; FILEBUS: 6,104, FILEIND: 15,302, FILEIND: 21,154; § 39,310.05

[47] ¶ 37,260, ¶ 37,261; FILEBUS: 6,104; § 39,310.10

[48] ¶ 37,201; FILEBUS: 6,104; § 39,310.10

[49] ¶ 42,686; FILEIND: 21,154.30; § 39,215.30

[50] ¶ 42,687A; FILEBUS: 6,104, FILEBUS: 15,100; § 39,215.35

[51] ¶ 37,200, ¶ 37,201; FILEBUS: 6,104.15, FILEIND: 21,154.15; § 39,310.05

¶2533

funds withdrawal (Code Sec. 6311; Reg. § 301.6311-2).[52] Credit card payments may be charged to VISA, MasterCard, American Express, and Discover cards, although the private companies that process such payments may charge a convenience fee (IRS Fact Sheet FS-2008-6; IRS Pub. 17). Such a convenience fee may be deductible (¶ 1092). Electronic funds withdrawal is free and allows taxpayers to schedule payments to be withdrawn directly from their bank accounts, but is available only to those taxpayers who e-file. Additionally, taxpayers may use the Electronic Federal Tax Payment System (EFTPS), a free tax payment system that allows taxpayers to pay online or via telephone (IRS Pub. 966). The EFTPS must be used for all federal tax deposits, including deposits of employment taxes, corporate income and corporate estimated taxes, unrelated business income taxes paid by tax-exempt organizations, private foundation excise taxes, taxes withheld on nonresident aliens and foreign corporations, estimated taxes on certain trusts, railroad retirement taxes, nonpayroll taxes, FUTA taxes, and excise taxes reported on Form 720 (Reg. § § 1.6302-1, 1.6302-2, 1.6302-3, and 1.6302-4). Individual taxpayers may use the IRS web-based Direct Pay system, which allows individuals with social security numbers (as opposed to IRS-issued individual numbers (ITINs) (¶ 2579)) to pay tax bills or make estimated tax payments directly from their checking or savings accounts without fees or pre-registration (IRS News Release IR-2014-67).

Deadlines

2549. Deadlines Falling on a Weekend or Holiday. If the last day for performing any act, i.e., filing a return, paying tax, or filing a claim for credit or refund, falls on Saturday, Sunday, or a legal holiday, the act is timely if it is performed on the next day that is not a Saturday, Sunday, or a legal holiday (Reg. § 301.7503-1).[53] The term "legal holiday" includes a legal holiday in the District of Columbia, e.g., Emancipation Day. When a legal holiday in the District of Columbia falls on a Sunday, the next Monday is treated as a legal holiday. When a legal holiday in the District of Columbia, other than Inauguration Day, falls on a Saturday, the preceding Friday is treated as a legal holiday (DC Code Annotated § 28-2701 (2010); Notice 2011-17). In the case of a return, statement, or other document required to be filed with an IRS office, the term "legal holiday" also includes a statewide legal holiday in the state in which the office is located, e.g., Patriots' Day in Massachusetts (Code Sec. 7503).[54]

2553. Timely Mailing as Timely Filing and Paying (Mailbox Rule). Any return, claim, statement, or document that must be filed with the IRS or the Tax Court, or any payment required to be made on or before a particular date is regarded as having been timely filed or paid if, on or before the due date, including extensions granted, it is deposited in the mail in the United States in an envelope or other appropriate wrapper, postage prepaid and properly addressed, and the date of the U.S. postmark falls on or before the due date (Code Sec. 7502(a); Reg. § 301.7502-1).[55] The postmark date is deemed the date of delivery or payment. Federal tax returns, including claims, statements, or other documents, mailed from outside the U.S. are timely if they bear the official timely dated postmark of the foreign country (Rev. Rul. 2002-23). The timely-mailed-is-timely-filed rule applies to designated private delivery services. See ¶ 5 for a listing of the available delivery services.

Documents or payments properly sent by registered mail are considered to have been filed on time if the registration date falls on or before the due date of the document. Such documents or payments properly sent by certified mail are timely filed if the certified mail sender's receipt is postmarked on or before the due date of the document. Delivery by properly registered or certified mail is presumed to have occurred if the envelope or package was properly addressed to the appropriate agency, officer, or office for filing or payment. Proof of use of a designated private delivery service under criteria

References are to Standard Federal Tax Reports; Tax Research Consultant; and Practical Tax Explanations.

[52] ¶ 38,085, ¶ 38,088; FILEIND: 21,156; § 39,320.10
[53] ¶ 42,631; FILEBUS: 15,056; § 39,210.10
[54] ¶ 42,630; FILEBUS: 15,056; § 39,210.10
[55] ¶ 42,620, ¶ 42,621; FILEBUS: 15,052, FILEIND: 15,206; § 39,210.05

¶2553

25 RETURNS

established by the IRS is entitled to a similar presumption of delivery (Reg. § 301.7502-1(c)(2) and (e)).[56]

The timely-mailed-is-timely-filed rule also covers documents filed electronically (Reg. § 301.7502-1(d)). The date of an electronic postmark that is given by an authorized electronic return transmitter and is on or before the filing due date will be deemed to be the filing date.

A tax deposit received by an authorized depository after the due date for the deposit is timely if it has been properly mailed at least two days before the prescribed due date. However, if any person is required to deposit tax more than once a month and the deposit amounts to $20,000 or more, the deposit must be received on or before the prescribed due date to be timely (Code Sec. 7502(e); Reg. § 301.7502-2).[57]

Information Returns and Payment at Source

2565. Payments Made in Course of Trade or Business. Every person engaged in a trade or business, including a partnership and a nonprofit organization, must file information returns for each calendar year for certain payments made during such year in the course of the payor's trade or business (Code Secs. 6041–6050W).[58] In many cases the information contained on such returns must be reported to the IRS by means of electronic filing through the IRS FIRE (Filing Information Returns Electronically) System (IRS Pub. 1220). Recipients must be furnished a copy of the information return or a comparable statement. While payee statements are generally required to be in written form, persons required to furnish recipients with copies of forms in the Form 1099 series and any other information return may furnish electronic payee statements (Sec. 401 of the Job Creation and Worker Assistance Act of 2002 (P.L. 107-147)). Payee statements for Form W-2 may also be filed electronically (Reg. § 31.6051-1).[59]

The following information returns are among those currently being filed:

Form 1098. Persons file this form if they receive $600 or more in mortgage interest from an individual in the course of a trade or business. Points paid directly by a borrower, including seller-paid points, for the purchase of a principal residence must be reported on Form 1098. Refunds and reimbursements of overpaid mortgage interest, and mortgage insurance premiums of $600 or more must also be reported on Form 1098 (Code Sec. 6050H; Reg. § 1.6050H-2).[60]

Form 1098-E. Financial institutions, governmental units, and educational institutions must file this form when, in the course of a trade or business, they receive interest of $600 or more in a calendar year on a student loan that is used solely to pay for qualified higher education expenses (Code Sec. 6050S; Reg. § 1.6050S-3).[61]

Form 1098-T. An educational institution must file this form with respect to each individual enrolled for an academic period to report payments received or amounts billed for qualified tuition and related expenses. Also, any person engaged in a trade or business of making payments to any individual under an insurance arrangement as reimbursements or refunds, or similar arrangements, of qualified tuition and related expenses must file this form for each individual for whom reimbursements or refunds are made during the calendar year (Code Sec. 6050S; Reg. § § 1.6050S-1 and 1.6050S-2).[62]

Form 1099-A. Persons who lend money in connection with their trade or business and, in full or partial satisfaction of the debt, acquire an interest in property that is security for the debt, must file this form. The form must also be filed if the person has reason to know that the property securing the debt has been abandoned (Code Sec. 6050J).[63]

References are to Standard Federal Tax Reports; Tax Research Consultant; and Practical Tax Explanations.

[56] ¶ 42,621; FILEBUS: 15,052, FILEIND: 15,206; § 39,210.05

[57] ¶ 42,620, ¶ 42,623; PAYROLL: 9,202; § 39,210.05

[58] ¶ 35,820 et seq.; FILEBUS: 9,200; § 39,105

[59] ¶ 36,421; PAYROLL: 3,356.50; § 39,140.10

[60] ¶ 36,180, ¶ 36,184; REAL: 6,106; § 18,501, § 39,105.05

[61] ¶ 36,319A, ¶ 36,319AJ; FILEBUS: 9,374; § 5910

[62] ¶ 36,319A, ¶ 36,319AD, ¶ 36,319AG; FILEBUS: 9,370; § 12,405

[63] ¶ 36,220; FILEBUS: 9,354; § 18,525.10

Form 1099-B. Brokers are to use this form to report sales, including short sales, of stock, bonds, commodities, regulated futures contracts, foreign currency contracts, forward contracts, and debt instruments. A broker that holds shares for a customer in a corporation that the broker knows or has reason to know has engaged in a transaction of acquisition of control or substantial change in capital structure must also file this form. Barter exchanges are to use the form to report exchanges of property or services through the exchange. For 2014 transactions, brokers must furnish Form 1099-B to customers by February 17, 2015 (Code Sec. 6045).[64] Also, trustees and middlemen of widely held fixed investment trusts (WHFITs) must use this form to report the non-*pro rata* partial principal payments, trust sales proceeds, redemption asset proceeds, redemption proceeds, sales asset proceeds and the sales proceeds that are attributable to a trust interest holder (TIH) for the calendar year. Trustees and middlemen of WHFITs must furnish the required statement by March 16, 2015.

Brokers required to file Form 1099-B regarding a covered security must also report the customer's adjusted basis in the security and whether any gain or loss with respect to the security is long-term or short-term (Code Sec. 6045(g)). See ¶ 1980 for further discussion.

Form 1099-C. Financial institutions, credit unions, federal agencies and any organization that lends money on a regular and continuing basis must file this form for each debtor for whom a debt of $600 or more was cancelled. Multiple discharges of debt of less than $600 during a year need not be aggregated unless the separate discharges occurred with the purpose of evading the reporting requirements. The returns must be filed regardless of whether the debtor is subject to tax on the discharged debt. For example, debts discharged in bankruptcy must be reported (Code Sec. 6050P; Reg. § 1.6050P-1).[65]

Form 1099-DIV. Corporate payors file this form for each person:

(1) to whom payments of $10 or more in distributions, such as dividends, capital gains, or nontaxable distributions, were made on stock;

(2) for whom any foreign tax was withheld and paid on dividends and on other distributions on stock if the recipient can claim a credit for the tax;

(3) for whom any federal income tax was withheld under the backup withholding rules; or

(4) to whom payments of $600 or more were made as part of a liquidation (Code Sec. 6042).[66]

S corporations use this form only to report distributions made during the calendar year out of accumulated earnings and profits.

Form 1099-G. Government units use this form to report payments of $10 or more for unemployment benefits and state and local tax refunds, credits, or offsets, payments of $600 or more in taxable grants or alternative trade adjustment assistance payments, and agricultural subsidy payments made during the year (Code Secs. 6050B and Code Sec. 6050E).[67]

Form 1099-H. Health insurance providers are required to file this return to report any advance payments of the credit for health insurance costs they are entitled to receive on behalf of individuals under Code Sec. 7527 (¶ 1332) (Code Sec. 6050T).[68]

Form 1099-INT. Payors file this form for each person to whom payments of $10 or more in interest were paid, including interest on bearer certificates of deposit and interest on U.S. Savings Bonds, Treasury bills, Treasury notes, and Treasury bonds (Code Sec. 6049).[69] Interest of $600 or more is also reportable if paid for a person in the course of a trade or business, such as interest on delayed death benefits paid by a life insurance company, interest received with damages, or interest on a state or federal

---

References are to Standard Federal Tax Reports; Tax Research Consultant; and Practical Tax Explanations.

[64] ¶ 35,920; FILEBUS: 9,250; § 39,120.20

[65] ¶ 36,310, ¶ 36,311B; SALES: 12,450; § 3,401

[66] ¶ 35,860; FILEBUS: 9,154; § 26,240

[67] ¶ 36,060, ¶ 36,120; FILEBUS: 9,308; § 3080

[68] ¶ 36,060, ¶ 36,320; HEALTH: 15,158

[69] ¶ 36,020; FILEBUS: 9,158; § 39,110

income tax refund. Form 1099-INT must also be filed to report interest of $10 or more (other than original issue discount) accrued to a real estate mortgage investment conduit (REMIC), a financial asset securitization investment trust (FASIT) regular interest holder, or a holder of a collateralized debt obligation (CDO). Additionally, trustees and middlemen of WHFITs must report the gross amount of interest exceeding $10 that is attributable to a trust interest holder (TIH) for the calendar year on this form.

Form 1099-K. Banks and other processors of merchant payment card transactions (e.g., credit and debit cards and internet payment systems) must use this form to report a merchant's annual gross payment card receipts to the IRS and to the merchant (Code Sec. 6050W; Reg. § § 1.6050W-1 and 1.6050W-2).[70] A third-party settlement organization must report information concerning a merchant's third-party network transactions only if, for the calendar year, the aggregate value of reportable payment transactions for the merchant exceeds $20,000 and the aggregate number of transactions exceeds 200.

Transitional relief from penalties has been provided to certain errors on information returns and payee statements filed in 2013 and 2014. Specifically, relief is provided for Forms 1099-K and statements filed in 2013 based on payments made in calendar year 2012 if they have missing TINs, obviously incorrect TINs, and incorrect name and TIN combinations. In addition, relief is provided for returns and statements filed in 2014 based on payments made in 2013, but only in cases where the 2013 Form 1099-K contains an incorrect name and TIN combination (Notice 2013-56).

Form 1099-MISC. This form is filed by payors for each person to whom at least $10 in gross royalty payments or broker payments in lieu of dividends or tax-exempt interest, or $600 for rents or services in the course of a trade or business, was paid. Some of the items reported on this form are:

(1) payments for real estate, machine and pasture rentals;

(2) royalties paid to authors;

(3) prizes and awards that were not paid for services rendered;

(4) amounts withheld as backup withholding;

(5) payments by medical and health care insurers to each physician or health care provider under health, accident and sickness insurance programs;

(6) compensation such as fees, commissions and awards, and golden parachute payments paid to a nonemployee for services, including payments to attorneys for legal services (Code Sec. 6045(f));

(7) notification of the occurrence of sales of $5,000 or more of consumer products to a person on a buy-sell or commission basis for resale anywhere other than in a permanent retail establishment;

(8) fishing boat proceeds;

(9) fish purchases of $600 or more paid in cash for resale (Code Sec. 6050R);

(10) crop insurance proceeds of $600 or more; and

(11) any deferrals for the year under a nonqualified deferred compensation plan (Code Sec. 6041(g)).

For 2014 payments, this form must be furnished to recipients by February 17, 2015, if substitute payments in lieu of dividends or tax-exempt interest are being reported in box 8, or gross proceeds paid to an attorney are being reported in box 14.

Form 1099-OID. Issuers of bonds or certificates of deposit, and trustees and middlemen of WHFITs use this form to report original issue discount of $10 or more (Code Sec. 6049(d); § 1.6049-4).[71]

Form 1099-PATR. Cooperatives use this form to report patronage dividends and other distributions of $10 or more to patrons (Code Sec. 6044).[72]

References are to Standard Federal Tax Reports; Tax Research Consultant; and Practical Tax Explanations.

[70] ¶ 36,376, ¶ 36,378C, ¶ 36,378G; FILEBUS: 9,320; § 39,130

[71] ¶ 36,020, ¶ 36,025; FILEBUS: 9,158; § 19,320

[72] ¶ 35,900; FARM: 12,118.20

¶2565

Form 1099-R. Payors file this form to report any distributions of $10 or more from retirement or profit-sharing plans, individual retirement arrangements (IRAs), simplified employee pensions (SEPs), annuities, or insurance contracts.

Form 1099-S. This form is used to report the sale or exchange of real estate, as well as the real property taxes imposed on the purchaser of a residence. Included are sales or exchanges of residences, land (including air space), commercial buildings, condominium units, stock in cooperative housing corporations, and noncontingent interests in standing timber, i.e., timber that is sold or exchanged for lump-sum payments not based on the amount of timber actually cut (Reg. § 1.6045-4).[73] The form must be filed by the person responsible for closing the real estate transaction or, if no such person exists, by the mortgage lender, the transferor's broker, the transferee's broker or the transferee, in that order. Payments of timber royalties under a "pay-as-cut" contract are also reported on the form. For 2014 transactions, this form must be furnished to recipients by February 17, 2015.

Forms 3921 and *3922.* These forms must be filed by a corporation to report certain stock transfers to an employee. Form 3921 is used to report a transfer of stock pursuant to an employee's exercise of an incentive stock option. Form 3922 is used to report a transfer of stock pursuant to an employee's exercise of an option granted under an employee stock purchase plan where the exercise price is less than 100 percent of the value of the stock, or is not fixed or determinable, on the date of grant (Code Sec. 6039).[74]

Form 5498. This form is filed by the account trustee for each person for whom an IRA, a deemed IRA, or a simplified employee pension (SEP) was maintained. Contributions made during the year to the IRA, including rollover contributions and contributions under a SEP plan, and the fair market value of the IRA or SEP account on December 31 must be reported here. Form 5498 is due by May 31 of the year following the year of contribution.

Form 8027. Each employer that runs a large food or beverage establishment (¶ 2605) must file an annual return of the receipts from food or beverage operations and tips reported by employees (Code Sec. 6053).[75] In addition, in certain circumstances, the employer is required to allocate amounts as tips to employees. Establishments filing 250 or more Forms 8027 must file electronically (Rev. Proc. 2012-37).

Form 8300. Each person engaged in a trade or business who, in the course of such trade or business, receives more than $10,000 in cash in one transaction (or two or more related transactions) must file this form. The form is to be filed with the IRS by the 15th day after the transaction, and a similar statement is to be provided to the payor on or before January 31 of the calendar year following the year of receipt (Code Sec. 6050I).[76]

Form W-2. This form is to be furnished to both the Social Security Administration and the recipient. Employers use the form to report wages, tips, other compensation, and withheld income and FICA taxes. Bonuses, vacation allowances, severance pay, moving expense payments, some kinds of travel allowances and third-party payments of sick pay are included. For Forms W-2 filed for the 2014 tax year, employers are required to use the form to report the aggregate cost of certain employer-sponsored health coverage provided to employees if the employer was required to file at least 250 Forms W-2 for 2013 (¶ 2567) (Code Sec. 6051(a)(14)).[77]

Due Dates. Unless otherwise specified, the above information returns for 2014 are to be provided to the IRS by March 2, 2015, and to recipients by February 2, 2015. Form W-2 is to be provided to the Social Security Administration by March 2, 2015, and to recipients by February 2, 2015. The due date for electronically filing information returns with the IRS, and for electronically filing Form W-2 with the Social Security Administration, is March 31, 2015 (Code Sec. 6071).[78] Form 8809 is used to request an automatic

---

References are to Standard Federal Tax Reports; Tax Research Consultant; and Practical Tax Explanations.

[73] ¶ 35,929; REAL: 15,458; § 39,115

[74] ¶ 35,600; COMPEN: 24,404, COMPEN: 21,352; § 21,545, § 21,635

[75] ¶ 36,460; FILEBUS: 12,302; § 21,305.20

[76] ¶ 36,200; FILEBUS: 9,322; § 39,125

[77] ¶ 36,420; HEALTH: 6,102; § 42,180.05

[78] ¶ 36,700; FILEBUS: 15,050; § 39,205

25

RETURNS

30-day extension of time to file Forms 1098, 1099, W-2G, 1042-S, 5498 and 8027 with the IRS or Form W-2 with the Social Security Administration. One additional 30-day extension may also be obtained by filing Form 8809 before the expiration of the first 30-day extension, but the requester must explain in detail why additional time is needed. Form 8809 *cannot* be used to request an extension of time to furnish required statements to recipients (Reg. § 1.6081-8).[79]

Other Information Returns. Other information returns are required with respect to:

(1) a U.S. person's acquisition of, or change of interest in, a foreign partnership (Code Sec. 6046A);

(2) cases of liquidation or dissolution of a corporation, including an exempt organization (Code Sec. 6043);

(3) corporate recapitalizations (Code Sec. 6043);

(4) corporate mergers and acquisitions (Code Sec. 6043A);

(5) organizations or reorganizations of foreign corporations (Code Sec. 6046);

(6) creation of or transfers to foreign trusts, or the death of a U.S. citizen or resident who had been treated as the owner of, or whose estate included any portion of, a foreign trust, or any other information required by the IRS to be reported by a U.S. person treated as owner of a foreign trust (Code Sec. 6048);

(7) U.S. persons who own interests in foreign partnerships or corporations (Code Sec. 6038);

(8) U.S. persons who transfer property to foreign partnerships or corporations (Code Sec. 6038B);

(9) payors of long-term care benefits (Code Sec. 6050Q);

(10) U.S. persons, other than tax-exempt organizations, that receive foreign gifts during the tax year totaling more than $10,000 ($15,358 in 2014; $15,601 in 2015) (Code Sec. 6039F; Rev. Proc. 2013-35; Rev. Proc. 2014-61);

(11) individuals who lose citizenship, and long-term residents who terminate residency in the United States (Code Sec. 6039G);

(12) Alaska Native Settlement Trusts (Code Sec. 6039H);

(13) dispositions by charitable donees within three years of donated property with a value in excess of $5,000, and, also, charitable donees of intellectual property (Code Sec. 6050L);

(14) employer-owned life insurance contracts (also know as company-owned life insurance (COLI) contracts) issued after August 17, 2006 (Code Sec. 6039I); and

(15) charges or payments made for qualified long-term insurance contracts under combined arrangements (Code Sec. 6050U).

In addition, the head of each federal executive agency generally must file Forms 8596 and 8596-A on a quarterly basis stating the name, address, and taxpayer identification number (TIN) of each person to whom the agency entered into a contract during the calendar year. An agency may also be required to file Form 1099-MISC if in the course of a trade or business it pays remuneration of $600 or more in a calendar year to any person for services provided by that person (Code Secs. 6041A and 6050M; Rev. Rul. 2003-66).[80]

2567. Health Care Coverage Reporting. Employers are required to disclose the aggregate cost of employer-sponsored health insurance coverage provided to their employees on the employee's Form W-2 (Code Sec. 6051(a)(14); Notice 2012-9).[81] The aggregate cost of the coverage reported includes both the portion of coverage paid by the employer and the employee, as well as any portion of the cost of coverage that is

---

References are to Standard Federal Tax Reports; Tax Research Consultant; and Practical Tax Explanations.

[79] ¶ 36,798F; FILEBUS: 15,106.25; § 39,145.05

[80] ¶ 35,840, ¶ 36,280; FILEBUS: 9,362; § 39,105.15

[81] ¶ 36,420; HEALTH: 6,102; § 42,180.05

includible in the employee's gross income for the employee's spouse, dependent, or child under the age of 27. It does not include salary reduction contributions to a health savings account (HSA) (¶ 2035) or Archer medical savings account (MSA) (¶ 2037) of the employee or the employee's spouse, or salary reduction contributions to a flexible spending arrangement under a cafeteria plan (¶ 2041). Reporting the cost of health care coverage on the Form W-2 does not mean that the coverage is taxable—it is for informational purposes only. Form W-2 is not required to be issued by an employer solely to report the value of the coverage for retirees or former employees.

The reporting requirement was generally required beginning with the 2012 calendar year. Pending further guidance from the IRS and under transitional relief, the reporting requirement is optional for employers who are required to file fewer than 250 Forms W-2 for the preceding year. For example, if an employer files fewer than 250 Forms W-2 for 2013 calendar year, the employer is not subject to the reporting requirements for Forms W-2 for the 2014 calendar year (the Forms W-2 that are generally furnished to employees in January 2015). Transitional relief is also available for certain other types of coverage and situations (Notice 2012-9).

Beginning in 2015, an applicable large employer (¶ 2001) must report whether full-time employees and their dependents are offered the opportunity to enroll in minimum essential coverage under an eligible employer-sponsored plan, along with other related information (Code Sec. 6056; Notice 2013-45)).[82] For this purpose, a return must be filed with the IRS on or before February 28 (March 31 if filed electronically) of the year succeeding the calendar year to which it relates (Reg. § 301.6056-1(e)). A statement must be furnished to each full-time employee on or before January 31 of the following calendar year (Code Sec. 6056(c)). The employer's return to the IRS may be made on Forms 1094-C (transmittal) and 1095-C (employee statement) or on a substitute form. An applicable large employer that is self-insured (see below) may combine Code Sec. 6055 reporting on Form 1095-C. A separate return is required for each full-time employee, accompanied by a single transmittal form for all of the returns filed for a given calendar year. Electronic filing is required for employers filing 250 of more applicable large employer information returns during the calendar year. The employee statement may be made by furnishing to the full-time employee a copy of Form 1095-C or a substitute statement. An electronic statement may instead be furnished with the employee's consent (Reg. § 301.6056-2). Failure to follow these rules may subject the employer to a penalty.

Beginning in 2015, since enforcement has been delayed from 2014, every insurer who provides minimum essential health care coverage to an individual during a calendar year, including an employer who self-insures, is also required to file an information return reporting such coverage in the form and manner prescribed by the IRS (Code Sec. 6055; Notice 2013-45).[83] The reporting entity must file the insurance provider return with the IRS on or before February 28 (or March 31 if filed electronically) of the year following the calendar year. The return may be made on Form 1095-B or on a substitute form. The return must be submitted to the IRS with a transmittal form, Form 1094-B. Self-insured employers that are also applicable large employers subject to shared responsibility reporting (see above) can instead combine insurance provider reporting on Forms 1095-C and 1094-C. A statement must also be furnished to each full-time employee on or before January 31 of the following calendar year (Code Sec. 6055(c)). The statement may be furnished electronically if affirmative consent is given (Reg. § 1.6055-2). Failure to follow these rules may subject the employer to a penalty.

2570. Reporting Foreign Financial Accounts (FBAR). A U.S. person is required to disclose any financial interests in, signature authority over, or other authority over foreign financial accounts if the aggregate value of the accounts exceeds $10,000 at any time during the calendar year (31 CFR § 1010.350).[84] The information is reported only electronically on FINCen Report 114 (still commonly referred to as FBAR). The FBAR must be *received*, not just filed, with the Department of Treasury for each calendar year,

References are to Standard Federal Tax Reports; Tax Research Consultant; and Practical Tax Explanations.

[82] ¶ 36,467; HEALTH: 6,106; § 42,135.10   [83] ¶ 36,465E; HEALTH: 6,104; § 42,135.15   [84] ¶ 36,555.33; FILEBUS: 9,104; § 37,705

¶2570

on or before June 30, of the succeeding year. For example, the form must be received by the Department of Treasury on or before June 30, 2015, for the 2014 tax year. The June 30 deadline generally may not be extended. However, the filing due date has been extended to June 30, 2015, for individuals with only signature authority over, but not financial interest in, foreign financial accounts for the 2011, 2012, and 2013 calendar years (FinCEN Notice 2013-1). Effective for the 2013 calendar year and thereafter, the FBAR is required to be filed electronically through the Treasury's Financial Crimes Enforcement Network (FinCEN) BSA E-Filing System. The filing of the FBAR does not relieve a taxpayer of the requirement to file Form 8938 to report specified foreign financial assets (¶ 2572).

U.S. persons subject to FBAR reporting are U.S. citizens, resident aliens, and entities created, organized, or formed under U.S. laws, including but not limited to domestic corporations, partnerships, limited liability companies (LLCs), trusts, and estates. The federal tax treatment of a person or entity does not determine whether an FBAR filing is required. For example, an entity disregarded for federal tax purposes must still file an FBAR if otherwise required. Participants and beneficiaries in qualified retirement plans, including individual retirement accounts (IRAs) are not required to file FBARs with respect to a foreign financial account held by or on behalf of the plan. A beneficiary of a trust in which a U.S. person has 50 percent or more interest is also not required to file FBAR if the trust, trustee, or agent of the trust is a U.S. person that files an FBAR for the trust's foreign financial assets.

FinCen Form 114(a), Record of Authorization to Electronically File FBARs, is used by a U.S. person to authorize a third party preparer (i.e., CPA, enrolled agent, or attorney) to file the FBAR on his or her behalf, or to jointly file the FBAR with his or her spouse. Form 114a is not filed with Treasury, but must be maintained by the foreign account holder and the filer and made available upon request by Treasury or the IRS.

2572. Reporting Specified Foreign Financial Assets (Form 8938). Under the Foreign Account Tax Compliance Act (FATCA), any individual who holds an interest in a specified foreign financial asset during the tax year must attach Form 8938 to his or her tax return to report certain information for each asset if the total value of all such assets exceeds an applicable threshold amount (Code Sec. 6038D).[85] The requirement applies to any U.S. citizen and individual who is a resident alien for any part of the tax year. A nonresident alien who makes the election to be treated as a resident alien for purposes of filing a joint return for the tax year must also file Form 8938, as well as a nonresident alien who is a bona fide resident of American Samoa or Puerto Rico. Form 8938 is also required to be filed by any domestic entity which is formed or availed of for purposes of holding, directly or indirectly, specified foreign financial assets, in the same manner as if the entity were an individual. Specifically, proposed regulations have designated specified domestic entities subject to the reporting requirement. They include certain closely-held domestic corporations or partnerships, as well as certain domestic trusts (Prop. Reg. § 1.6038D-6). Reporting by specified domestic entities, however, will not be required before the date provided in final regulations (Notice 2013-10).

A "specified foreign financial asset" includes (1) a depository, custodial, or other financial account maintained by a foreign financial institution, (2) a stock or security issued by a person other than a U.S. person, (3) a financial instrument or contract held for investment that has an issuer or counterparty other than a U.S. person, and (4) an interest in an entity that is not a U.S. person. The filing of Form 8938 does not relieve an individual of the requirement to file the FBAR (¶ 2570) for disclosing foreign financial accounts. Similarly, the filing of the FBAR does not relieve an individual of the requirement to file Form 8938. An individual may be required to file both Form 8938 and FBAR to report the same information on certain foreign accounts. The FBAR, however, is not filed with the individual's federal income tax return.

References are to Standard Federal Tax Reports; Tax Research Consultant; and Practical Tax Explanations.

[85] ¶ 35,593; FILEBUS: 9,108; § 37,710

The applicable threshold amount that determines whether a taxpayer must file Form 8938 depends on the taxpayer's filing status and whether the individual lives in the United States or abroad. The total value of specified foreign financial assets for this purpose is the asset's fair market value as determined in U.S. dollars using the Treasury's currency exchange rate on the last day of the tax year (Temp. Reg. § 1.6038D-2T; Instructions for Form 8938).[86] The applicable threshold amounts are as follows:

- Unmarried taxpayers living in the United States must file Form 8938 if the total value of specified foreign financial assets is more than $50,000 on the last day of the tax year or more than $75,000 at any time during the tax year.

- Married taxpayers living in the United States and filing a joint income tax return must file Form 8938 if the value of specified foreign financial assets is more than $100,000 on the last day of the tax year or more than $150,000 at any time during the tax year.

- Married taxpayers living in the United States and filing separate income tax returns must file Form 8938 if the value of specified foreign financial assets is more than $50,000 on the last day of the tax year or more than $75,000 at any time during the tax year.

- Married taxpayers living abroad and filing a joint return must file Form 8938 if the value of specified foreign assets is more than $400,000 on the last day of the tax year or more than $600,000 at any time during the year.

- Other taxpayers living abroad must file Form 8938 if the total value of specified foreign assets is more than $200,000 on the last day of the tax year or more than $300,000 at any time during the year.

The individual must disclose the asset's maximum value during the tax year, and provide specific information based on the asset type. For a financial account, the individual must provide the name and address of the financial institution in which the account is maintained, and the account number. For stock or security, the individual must provide the issuer's name and address, and any other information needed to identify the asset's class or issue. For any other instrument, contract, or interest, the individual must provide any information needed to identify the asset, and the names and addresses of all issuers and counterparties.

An individual who fails to furnish the required information at the time and in the manner prescribed is subject to a $10,000 penalty. If the failure continues for more than 90 days after the IRS mailed notice of the failure to the individual, the individual is subject to an additional $10,000 penalty for each 30-day period, or a fraction thereof, during which the failure continues after the 90-day period; this additional penalty cannot exceed $50,000.

For purposes of assessing these penalties, the total value of the individual's foreign financial assets is presumed to exceed $50,000, or a higher dollar amount prescribed by the IRS, if the individual does not provide sufficient information to demonstrate their total value. These penalties are not imposed if the failure is due to reasonable cause and not willful neglect. However, the fact that a foreign jurisdiction would impose a civil or criminal penalty for disclosing the required information is not reasonable cause.

Additionally, a 40-percent accuracy-related penalty may be imposed for tax underpayment attributable to an undisclosed foreign financial asset understatement (¶ 2864). The statute of limitations for assessments is extended to six years if there is an omission of gross income in excess of $5,000 attributable to a specified foreign financial asset, which may or may not be subject to the reporting requirements discussed previously. Also, the three-year limitations period is suspended for failure to timely provide information reporting on specified foreign financial assets.

References are to Standard Federal Tax Reports; Tax Research Consultant; and Practical Tax Explanations.

[86] ¶ 35,594AI; FILEBUS: 9,108; § 37,710

2579. Taxpayer Identification Number. Persons filing returns and other documents must record on such items a taxpayer identification number (TIN). Individuals use their Social Security number on Forms 1040, 1040A, and 1040EZ. Executors of individuals' estates who must file Form 706 are to use both their Social Security number and the decedent's Social Security number. For corporations, partnerships, estates and trusts, and similar nonindividual taxpayers, the identifying number is the employer identification number. A prospective adoptive parent can apply for an adoption taxpayer identification number (ATIN) for a child who is in the process of being adopted (Reg. § 301.6109-3). Application for an ATIN must be made on Form W-7A. Persons who file information returns (¶ 2565) may request the recipient of any payments to furnish his TIN on Form W-9.

Nonresident aliens who cannot obtain a TIN may use an IRS-issued individual number (ITIN) (Notice 2004-1). Form W-7 is used to apply for an ITIN. The Form W-7 must be accompanied by an original, completed income tax return, and documents supporting the information provided on Form W-7. Effective January 1, 2013, the IRS has implemented new procedures that affect the ITIN application process (IRS News Release IR-2012-98). ITINs are only issued when applications include original documentation, such as passports and birth certificates, or certified copies of these documents. The IRS will not accept notarized copies of the documents. ITINs are issued for an indefinite period; however, ITINs will expire if not used on a federal income tax return for five consecutive years (IRS News Release IR-2014-76). This policy, which was announced on June 30, 2014, applies to all ITINs, no matter when issued, and replaces the former policy under which ITINs issued in 2013 or later would expire after five years, regardless of whether they were used regularly. To give parties time to adjust to the new policy and to allow the IRS to reprogram its systems, deactivation will not begin until 2016. Once deactivation begins, a taxpayer whose ITIN has been deactivated can reapply using Form W-7. Spouses and dependents of U.S. military personnel who need ITINs and nonresident aliens applying for ITINs in order to claim tax treaty benefits remain unaffected by the post-2012 procedures.

A penalty of $50 per failure applies to a taxpayer who omits his own TIN from a required return, statement, or document. Failure to furnish one's TIN to another person when so required or to include another person's TIN in any document for information reporting purposes will also give rise to a $50 penalty. The maximum penalty per calendar year for failure to include TINs is $100,000 (Code Secs. 6723 and 6724(d)(3)).[87]

Reportable Transactions and Tax Shelters

2591. Reportable Transactions. Reporting and disclosure requirements apply to taxpayers (¶ 2592) and material advisors (¶ 2593) with respect to reportable transactions. A reportable transaction is any transaction with respect to which information is required to be included with a return or statement because the transaction is of a type that the IRS has determined under regulations as having a potential for tax avoidance or evasion (Code Sec. 6707A(c)(1)).[88]

There are five categories of reportable transactions: listed transactions, confidential transactions, transactions with contractual protection, loss transactions, and transactions of interest (Reg. § 1.6011-4(b)).[89] A transaction is not considered a reportable transaction, or it is excluded from any individual category of reportable transaction, if the IRS makes a determination by published guidance that the transaction is not subject to the reporting requirements. The IRS may make a determination by individual letter.

2592. Disclosure of Reportable Transactions by Taxpayers. Every taxpayer that is required to file a tax return and has participated directly or indirectly in a reportable transaction (¶ 2591) must disclose its participation in the transaction (Reg.

References are to Standard Federal Tax Reports; Tax Research Consultant; and Practical Tax Explanations.

[87] ¶ 40,250, ¶ 40,275; PEN-ALTY: 3,200; § 40,230

[88] ¶ 40,091; FILEBUS: 9,450; § 39,015.05

[89] ¶ 35,127; FILEBUS: 9,458; § 39,015.05

§ 1.6011-4(a)).[90] The fact that a transaction is a reportable transaction does not affect the legal determination of whether the taxpayer's treatment of the transaction is proper.

Form 8886 is used to disclose information for each reportable transaction in which the taxpayer participated. A separate Form 8886 must be filed for each reportable transaction. The form must be attached to the taxpayer's tax return for each tax year for which the taxpayer participates in a reportable transaction. A copy of the disclosure statement must be sent to the Office of Tax Shelter Analysis (OTSA) at the same time that any disclosure statement is first filed with the taxpayer's tax return (Reg. § 1.6011-4(d) and (e)). If a reportable transaction results in a loss that is carried back to a prior year, Form 8886 is attached to the taxpayer's application for tentative refund or amended tax return for the prior year.

In the case of a taxpayer that is a partnership, an S corporation, or a trust, Form 8886 must be attached to the partnership's, S corporation's, or trust's tax return for each tax year in which the partnership, S corporation, or trust participates in the transaction. A taxpayer who is a partner, S corporation shareholder, or a beneficiary of a trust who receives a Schedule K-1 less than 10 calendar days before the due date of its return, including extensions, has a 60-day extension to file Form 8886 with the OTSA if the taxpayer determines from the Schedule K-1 that it participated in a reportable transaction.

Failure to file Form 8886 regarding a reportable transaction is subject to a penalty (¶ 2594). Special reporting rules apply to listed transactions and transactions of interest. Also, in some cases, taxpayers must make multiple disclosures of a reportable transaction (Reg. § 1.6011-4(e)).

A taxpayer may submit a request to the IRS for a ruling as to whether a transaction is subject to the disclosure requirements (Reg. § 1.6011-4(f)). If a taxpayer requests a ruling on the merits of a specific transaction on or before the date that disclosure would otherwise be required and receives a favorable ruling, the disclosure rules are satisfied. The ruling request must fully disclose all relevant facts relating to the transaction. If a taxpayer is uncertain whether a transaction must be disclosed, the taxpayer may make a protective disclosure. The taxpayer must disclose the transaction and indicate on the disclosure statement that the taxpayer is uncertain whether the transaction is required to be disclosed and that the disclosure statement is being filed on a protective basis. The taxpayer must retain a copy of all documents and other records related to a transaction subject to disclosure (Reg. § 1.6011-4(g)). The retained documents and records are those that are material to an understanding of the tax treatment or tax structure of the transaction.

2593. Disclosure of Reportable Transactions by Material Advisors. Each material advisor is required to timely file an information return with the IRS for any reportable transaction (¶ 2591) (Code Sec. 6111; Reg. § 301.6111-3).[91] The disclosure is made on Form 8918 and generally must be filed with the Office of Tax Shelter Analysis (OTSA) by the last day of the month that follows the calendar quarter in which the advisor became a material advisor with respect to the reportable transaction or in which circumstances occur to require an amended disclosure statement.

The material advisor's disclosure on Form 8918 must include: (1) information identifying and describing the transaction; (2) information describing any potential tax benefits expected to result from the transaction; and (3) whatever other information the IRS may require. This includes enough information about the transaction to identify if any other person that the material advisor knows or has reason to know acted as a material advisor with respect to the transaction. A single Form 8918 may be filed for substantially similar transactions. An amended form must be filed if information previously provided is no longer accurate, if additional information becomes available, or if there are material changes to the transaction. If a potential material advisor is uncertain whether a transaction must be disclosed, a protective disclosure may be made. Any

---

References are to Standard Federal Tax Reports; Tax Research Consultant; and Practical Tax Explanations.

[90] ¶ 35,127; FILEBUS: 9,456; § 39,015.05

[91] ¶ 37,000, ¶ 37,001D; FILEBUS: 9,452, PENALTY: 3,254

material advisor who fails to file Form 8918 when required or files a false or incomplete form is subject to a penalty (¶ 2595).

A material advisor is any person: (1) who provides material aid, assistance, or advice with respect to organizing, promoting, selling, implementing, or carrying out any reportable transaction; and (2) who directly or indirectly derives gross income in excess of $250,000 ($50,000 in the case of a reportable transaction substantially all of the tax benefits from which are provided to natural persons) for that aid, assistance, or advice. If more than one material advisor is required to disclose a reportable transaction, the material advisors may designate by written agreement a single material advisor to disclose the transaction.

2594. Penalty for Failure to Disclose Reportable Transaction. A penalty is imposed on any taxpayer who fails to disclose its participation in a reportable transaction that is required to be included on the taxpayer's return (¶ 2592) (Code Sec. 6707A; Reg. § 301.6707A-1).[92] The penalty is equal to 75 percent of the decrease in tax shown on the return as a result of the transaction, or that would have resulted from the transaction if the transaction had been respected for federal tax purposes. The *minimum* penalty, however, is $10,000 ($5,000 in the case of a natural person). The maximum penalty is $50,000 ($10,000 in the case of a natural person), but in circumstances involving listed transactions, the maximum penalty is $200,000 ($100,000 in the case of a natural person). The penalty for failure to disclose is imposed in addition to any other penalty, including a special accuracy-related penalty for an understatement of tax resulting from a reportable transaction (¶ 2870).

For reportable transactions other than listed transactions, the penalty can be rescinded or abated only in exceptional circumstances, and abatement of the penalty must promote compliance with the tax laws and effective tax administration. Factors that are taken into account in deciding whether to grant rescission include: (1) the taxpayer, on becoming aware of the failure to properly disclose a reportable transaction, filed a complete and proper, although untimely, Form 8886; (2) the failure to properly disclose was due to an unintentional mistake of fact that existed despite the taxpayer's reasonable attempts to determine the correct facts; (3) the taxpayer has an established history of properly disclosing reportable transactions and complying with tax laws generally; (4) the failure to file was beyond the taxpayer's control; (5) the taxpayer cooperates with the IRS; and (6) assessment of the penalty weighs against good conscience, and the taxpayer demonstrates it acted in good faith with respect to the failure.

Any person seeking rescission of a penalty must make a written request within 30 days after the date that the IRS sends notice and demand for payment of the penalty. If the penalty is paid (not including interest) prior to the date that notice and demand is sent, the written request must be made within 30 days from the date of payment. In order to request rescission, the person must have either exhausted the administrative remedies available within the IRS Office of Appeals or agreed in writing to the assessment of the penalty and not to file or prosecute a claim for refund or credit of the penalty. The IRS has provided guidance on the information required to be included with any rescission request, as well as factors considered in granting or denying the request (Rev. Proc. 2007-21).[93] The IRS's collection efforts are not suspended because a rescission request has been made.

2595. Material Advisor Penalty for Reportable Transactions. A penalty is imposed on any material advisor who fails to file an information return or who files a false or incomplete information return regarding a reportable transaction (¶ 2593) (Code Sec. 6707; Reg. § 301.6707-1).[94] Generally, a $50,000 penalty is assessed for failure to furnish required information with respect to a reportable transaction. In the case of the failure to file an information return with respect to a listed transaction, the penalty assessed is the greater of $200,000 or 50 percent of the gross income derived by the person required to file the return with respect to aid, assistance, or advice that is provided. The 50-percent limit is raised to 75 percent in cases involving an intentional failure to act. Only one

---

References are to Standard Federal Tax Reports; Tax Research Consultant; and Practical Tax Explanations.

[92] ¶ 40,091, ¶ 40,092; PEN-ALTY: 3,252.10; § 39,015.05

[93] ¶ 40,093.70; PENALTY: 3,252.10; § 39,015.05

[94] ¶ 40,085, ¶ 40,088; PEN-ALTY: 3,254

penalty applies in the case of a transaction that is both a listed transaction and a reportable transaction. The penalty that applies in these cases is the higher penalty for listed transactions. If there is a failure with respect to more than one reportable or listed transaction, a material advisor will be subject to a separate penalty for each transaction. The penalty with respect to reportable transactions other than listed transactions may be rescinded only in exceptional circumstances similar to those for rescission of the penalty for failure to disclose reportable transactions by taxpayers (¶ 2594). The penalty with respect to a listed transaction cannot be waived.

Each material advisor with respect to any reportable transaction is required to maintain a list identifying each person with respect to whom that advisor acted as a material advisor with respect to the transaction and containing any other information required by the IRS (Code Sec. 6112(a); Reg. § 301.6112-1).[95] Regulations set forth the requirements for the preparation and maintenance of advisee lists, including persons required to be included on lists, contents of the list, definitions, and requirements for retention and furnishing of the lists. All information that is required to be included in the advisee lists must be retained for seven years. Any person required to maintain advisee lists with respect to reportable transactions who receives a written request from the IRS, but who fails to make the lists available within 20 business days, may be assessed a $10,000 penalty for each day of failure after the 20th business day (Code Sec. 6708; Prop. Reg. § 301.6708-1).[96]

2597. Abusive Tax Shelters Penalty. A penalty is imposed against any person who organizes, assists in organizing, or participates in the sale of any interest in a tax shelter if he or she makes or furnishes or causes another person to make or furnish: (1) a statement concerning the allowability of any tax benefit obtained through participation in the tax shelter that the person knows or has reason to know is false or fraudulent; or (2) a gross valuation overstatement concerning any matter that is material to the tax shelter (Code Sec. 6700).[97] The penalty is 50 percent of the gross income derived, or to be derived, from the abusive plan or arrangement activities engaged in, other than promotion activities involving gross valuation overstatements. The penalty for promotion of activities involving gross valuation overstatements is an amount equal to the lesser of $1,000 or 100 percent of the gross income derived, or to be derived, by the promoter from the activity.

In applying the penalty, promotion of each entity or activity is a separate activity and each sale of an interest in the shelter is a separate activity. The penalty is imposed in addition to all other penalties that may be imposed, except with respect to any documents if an aiding and abetting penalty is imposed on that person with respect to the same document (¶ 2518).

2598. Injunctions Related to Tax Shelters. An injunction may be obtained with respect to the following acts: (1) promoting an abusive tax shelter (¶ 2597); (2) aiding someone in understating a tax liability in a return or other document (¶ 2518); (3) failing to furnish information about a reportable transaction (¶ 2593); or (4) failing to maintain a list of advisees (¶ 2595) (Code Sec. 7408).[98] Once a court has enjoined a person from engaging in one or more of the above activities, the court may expand the injunction to include any other activity that is subject to a penalty under tax law.

References are to Standard Federal Tax Reports; Tax Research Consultant; and Practical Tax Explanations.

[95] ¶ 37,020, ¶ 37,021; PENALTY: 3,254.10

[96] ¶ 40,095, ¶ 40,095D; PENALTY: 3,254.10

[97] ¶ 40,025; PENALTY: 3,256

[98] ¶ 41,670; PENALTY: 3,256.20

25 | RETURNS

Chapter 26

WITHHOLDING □ ESTIMATED TAX

Withholding on Wages

2601. Withholding of Income Tax on Wages. Withholding of income tax by an employer is required on each of an employee's wage payments (Code Sec. 3402(a); Reg. § 31.3402(a)-1).[1] Wages generally include all remuneration (other than fees paid to a public official) for services performed by an employee for an employer, including the cash value of all remuneration (including benefits) paid in any medium other than cash (¶ 2604). Thus, salaries, fees, bonuses, commissions on sales or on insurance premiums, taxable fringe benefits, pensions, and retirement pay (unless taxed as an annuity) are subject to withholding, if paid as compensation for services.

The term "employer" generally means any person for whom an individual performs or performed any service, of whatever nature, as the employee of such person. However, where the person for whom services are performed does not have legal control over the payment of wages, then the person actually controlling the payment of wages assumes the withholding responsibilities of an employer (Code Sec. 3401(d); Reg. § 31.3401(d)-1).[2] It is not necessary that the services be continuing at the time the wages are paid in order that the status of employer exists. An employer includes not only individuals and organizations engaged in trade or business, but also tax-exempt organizations and federal, state, and local government units (including the District of Columbia and Puerto Rico). An employer also includes any person paying wages on behalf of a nonresident alien individual, foreign partnership, or foreign corporation not engaged in trade or business within the United States or Puerto Rico.

An individual is an employee if the employer for whom the services are performed has the right to control and direct the individual performing the services not only as to the result to be accomplished by the work, but also as to the details and the means by which that result is accomplished (Code Sec. 3401(c); Reg. § 31.3401(c)-1).[3] An employee also includes any officer, employee, or elected official of federal, state, and local government units. It also includes an officer of a corporation, but not a director. Professionals such as physicians, lawyers, contractors, and others who follow an independent trade, business, or profession in which they offer their services to the public generally are not employees. The designation or description of an employment relationship by the parties is not controlling (¶ 2602).

References are to Standard Federal Tax Reports; Tax Research Consultant; and Practical Tax Explanations.

[1] ¶ 33,542, ¶ 33,543; PAY-ROLL: 3,000; § 22,105.05

[2] ¶ 33,502, ¶ 33,537; PAY-ROLL: 3,052; § 22,105.15

[3] ¶ 33,502, ¶ 33,536; COM-PEN: 3,000; § 22,005.15

¶2601

An employer who fails to withhold income taxes from an employee's wages is liable for the unwithheld amounts (Code Sec. 3403).[4] If an employer's agent pays or controls the payment of wages, both the agent and the employer are liable (Code Sec. 3504).[5] Any third party who pays wages directly to employees of an employer or to the employee's agent is liable for any required withholding on those wages (Code Sec. 3505).[6]

2602. Employee v. Independent Contractor. Employees must be distinguished from independent contractors because an employer does not generally have employment tax obligations with respect to independent contractors. The IRS for many years relied on a 20-factor test to determine whether individuals are employees or independent contractors (Rev. Rul. 87-41).[7] However, it has shifted its analysis to focus on a three-part behavioral analysis—behavioral control, financial control, and relationship of the parties (IRS Pub. 15-A). A worker that may be an independent contractor under this analysis may nevertheless be treated as an employee for FICA and FUTA tax purposes if the worker is classified as a statutory employee (¶ 941B). Either an employer or employee, with or without the other's knowledge or assent, may request that the IRS make a determination as to whether or not a particular worker is an employee. The request is made using Form SS-8.

If an employer erroneously classifies an employee as an independent contractor and has no reasonable basis for doing so, the employer is liable for taxes under the income tax withholding (¶ 2601) and FICA and FUTA tax provisions (¶ 2648 and ¶ 2649). However, employers may be eligible for reduced rates with respect to income tax withholding (1.5 percent of employee's wages) and the employer's share of FICA tax (20 percent of the amount otherwise due) (Code Sec. 3509).[8] These rates are doubled if the employer failed to file forms consistent with the employer's treatment of the worker as an independent contractor. Reduced rates are not available for statutory employees. If the employer had a reasonable basis for not treating an individual as an employee, the employer may be entirely relieved of liability for employment taxes with respect to that individual if the employer was consistent in its treatment of the worker as a nonemployee (Section 530 of the Revenue Act of 1978).[9]

The IRS has established a program, known as the Voluntary Classification Settlement Program, that allows an eligible business to voluntarily reclassify some or all of its workers as employees for future tax periods while limiting employment tax liability for past nonemployee treatment (Announcement 2012-45, modifying Announcement 2011-64).[10] Form 8952 is used for this purpose.

Employees who have been misclassified as independent contractors use Form 8919 to figure and report the employee's share of uncollected Social Security and Medicare taxes due on their compensation.

2604. Wages Subject to Income Tax Withholding. Wages subject to income tax withholding (¶ 2601) generally include all remuneration (other than fees paid to a public official) for services performed by an employee for an employer (Code Sec. 3401(a); Reg. § 31.3401(a)-1(a)).[11] It includes salaries, fees, bonuses, and commissions. Withholding is based on *gross* wage payments before deductions such as those under the federal or state unemployment insurance laws, pension funds (except deductible contributions to IRAs), insurance, etc., or liabilities of the employee paid by the employer. An employer is required to withhold income tax from wages paid for employment regardless of the circumstances under which the employee is employed or the frequency or size of amounts of the individual wage payments.[12] Tax must be withheld from wages

---

References are to Standard Federal Tax Reports; Tax Research Consultant; and Practical Tax Explanations.

[4] ¶ 33,591; PAYROLL: 6,252; § 22,105.15

[5] ¶ 33,720; PAYROLL: 6,254.05; § 22,105.15

[6] ¶ 33,740; PAYROLL: 6,254.10; § 22,205.25

[7] ¶ 33,538.66; COMPEN: 3,102; § 22,015.05

[8] ¶ 33,820; PAYROLL: 9,306; § 22,020.10

[9] ¶ 33,538.5056; COMPEN: 3,110; § 22,020.15

[10] ¶ 33,538.5057; COMPEN: 3,350; § 22,020.22

[11] ¶ 33,502, ¶ 33,503; PAYROLL: 3,150; § 22,110.05

[12] ¶ 33,593.165; PAYROLL: 6,058; § 22,110.05

26 | WITHHOLDING

¶2604

paid for *each* payroll period.[13] Some types of compensation, however, are specifically excluded from the definition of wages for income tax withholding purposes (¶ 2609).

If an employee works on two jobs for the same employer, and only a part of the remuneration is wages—for example, a construction worker who also works on his employer's farm (exempt employment)—all of the remuneration is treated alike. Thus, either (1) all of the wages are subject to withholding if more than half of the time is spent performing services for which wages are received, or (2) all are excluded if more than half of the time spent is in exempt services, provided the payroll period is no longer than 31 consecutive days (Reg. § 31.3402(e)-1).[14]

Compensation. Other forms of compensation besides salaries, fees, bonuses, and commissions are subject to withholding, including tips and other gratuities (¶ 2605), reimbursed employee expenses paid through a nonaccountable plan (¶ 2607) and other supplemental wages (¶ 2606), employee expense amounts in excess of per diem rates (¶ 2608), and payments for the stoppage of work such as severance payments and strike benefits (Reg. § 31.3401(a)-1).[15] Some types of compensation, however, are specifically excluded from the definition of wages for income tax withholding purposes (¶ 2609).

Payments of supplemental unemployment compensation are treated as wages for income tax withholding purposes, but withholding applies only to the extent that such benefits are includible in the employee's gross income (Code Sec. 3402(o)).[16] The U.S. Supreme Court has held that supplemental unemployment compensation is not excluded by statute from the definition of wages for FICA purposes (*In re Quality Stores, Inc.*, SCt, 2014-1 USTC ¶ 50,228). The IRS, however, has provided a limited exemption for certain types of supplemental unemployment compensation for purposes of FICA (¶ 2648) and FUTA (¶ 2649) (Rev. Rul. 56-249).[17] Guaranteed annual wage payments made during periods of unemployment pursuant to a collective bargaining agreement are wages subject to withholding.[18] However, strike benefits (other than hourly wages received for strike-related duties) paid by a union to its members are not subject to withholding.[19]

Fringe benefits are generally included in wages as supplemental wages (¶ 2606), but some may be partially or wholly exempt (¶ 2609).

Although the value of noncash compensation generally must be included in wages, when a retail commission salesperson is occasionally paid other than in cash, the employer is not required to withhold income tax for the noncash payments (Code Sec. 3402(j); Reg. § 31.3402(j)-1).[20] However, the fair market value of the noncash payments such as prizes must be included on the Form W-2 furnished to the employee as part of the total pay earned by the employee during the calendar year.

Withholding is available, if the payee so requests, for wage continuation payments (i.e., sick pay) received from a third party pursuant to a health or accident plan in which the employer participates (Code Sec. 3402(o); Reg. § 31.3402(o)-3).[21] Payments of sick pay made directly by employers to their employees are automatically subject to withholding. Employers who are third-party payors of sick pay are not required to withhold income taxes from payments unless the employee has requested withholding on Form W-4S. Sick pay is exempt for FICA and FUTA purposes after six calendar months following the month the employee last worked for the employer (Code Secs. 3121(a)(4) and 3306(b)(4)).

Wages subject to withholding include amounts received under a nonqualified deferred compensation plan that are includible in an employee's gross income under Code Sec. 409A for the year of inclusion (¶ 2197) (Code Sec. 3401(a)).

References are to Standard Federal Tax Reports; Tax Research Consultant; and Practical Tax Explanations.

[13] ¶ 33,544.20; PAYROLL: 6,056; § 22,110.05

[14] ¶ 33,551; PAYROLL: 6,058; § 22,105.10

[15] ¶ 33,503; PAYROLL: 3,150; § 22,110.05

[16] ¶ 33,542; PAYROLL: 3,178; § 22,110.40

[17] ¶ 33,506.3683; PAYROLL: 3,178; § 22,210.40, § 22,310.40

[18] ¶ 33,506.3683; PAYROLL: 3,150; § 22,110.40

[19] ¶ 33,506.3678; PAYROLL: 3,178; § 22,110.40

[20] ¶ 33,542, ¶ 33,574; PAYROLL: 6,208; § 22,105.10

[21] ¶ 33,542, ¶ 33,584; PAYROLL: 3,206; § 22,125.10

Differential Wage Payments. Differential wage payments are wages paid by the employer to the employee for purposes of the federal income tax withholding rules (Code Sec. 3401(h)).[22] A differential wage payment is any payment that: (1) is made by an employer to an individual with respect to any period during which the individual is performing service in the uniformed services while on active duty for a period of more than 30 days, and (2) represents all or a portion of the wages the individual would have received from the employer if the individual were performing services for the employer. Differential wage payments are considered supplemental wages and subject to the special rules applicable to such payments (¶ 2606). Differential wage payments, however, are not treated as wages for FICA and FUTA purposes (Rev. Rul. 2009-11).

2605. Tips and Gratuities Subject to Withholding. Cash tips paid directly to an employee by a customer and charged tips paid over to the employee (¶ 717) must be accounted for by the employee in a written statement furnished to the employer on or before the 10th day of the month following the month when they are received (Code Sec. 6053(a)).[23] The employee reports the tips on Form 4070 or similar statement. If tips received by the employee in the course of his or her employment for a single employer are less than $20 in a calendar month, then the tips are not required to be reported. The employer uses the employee's report to figure the amount of income and FICA taxes to withhold for the pay period on both wages and reported tips, and the employer's portion of FICA and FUTA taxes (Code Secs. 3401(a)(16), 3121(a)(12), and 3306(s)).[24] A service charge added to a bill or fixed by the employer that the customer must pay is not a tip; a payment is a tip, rather than wages, only if it is made free from compulsion, the amount is freely determined by the customer, the payment is not negotiated or dictated by the employer, and the customer decides who receives the payment (Rev. Rul. 2012-18).

A large food and beverage establishment (one which normally has more than 10 employees on a typical business day and in which tipping is customary) must file annual information returns using Form 8027 (¶ 2565). These returns must report gross food and beverage sales receipts, employee-reported tip income, total charge receipts, and total charge tips (Code Sec. 6053(c); Reg. § 31.6053-3).[25] The employer must allocate among its employees who customarily receive tip income an amount equal to the excess of eight percent of gross receipts over reported tips. The allocation is not required if the employees voluntarily report total tips equal to at least eight percent of gross sales. If it can be shown that average tips are less than eight percent of gross sales, the employer or a majority of its employees may apply to the IRS to have the allocation reduced from eight percent but not to below two percent.

2606. Supplemental Wages Subject to Withholding. Special withholding rules apply when an employee is paid supplemental wages (bonus, overtime pay, back pay, commissions, vacation allowance, taxable fringe benefits, etc.). If supplemental wages are paid at the same time as regular wages, the two are added together and the withholding of income tax is computed on the total as a single wage payment. If the supplemental wages are not paid at the same time as the regular wages, the supplemental wages may be added either to the regular wages for the preceding payroll period or for the current payroll period within the same calendar year (Reg. § 31.3402(g)-1).[26]

Under an alternative method, the employer may treat the supplemental wages as wholly separate from regular wages and withhold at a flat rate equal to the third lowest income tax rate (25 percent) without any allowance for exemptions or reference to any regular payment of wages. Once the total of supplemental wage payments made to an employee within a calendar year, exceeds $1 million, the excess is subject to withholding at the highest income tax rate (39.6 percent). This rule applies regardless of the method otherwise used to withhold supplemental wages paid to the employee. See IRS Pubs. 15 and 505.

References are to Standard Federal Tax Reports; Tax Research Consultant; and Practical Tax Explanations.

[22] ¶ 33,502; PAYROLL: 6,058; § 22,110.45

[23] ¶ 36,460; PAYROLL: 3,154; § 21,310

[24] ¶ 33,502; PAYROLL: 3,154; § 21,310, § 21,315.05, § 21,320

[25] ¶ 36,460, ¶ 36,463; PAYROLL: 3,406.05; § 21,305.20

[26] ¶ 33,561; PAYROLL: 6,066; § 22,120.50

An employer must collect both income tax and employee Social Security or railroad retirement tax on tips reported by an employee from wages due the employee or other funds that the employee makes available. Tips may be treated as if they were supplemental wages subject to the flat withholding rate (25 percent) without allowance for exemptions, provided that income tax has been withheld on the employee's regular wages. Otherwise, the tips must be treated as part of the current or preceding wage payment of the same calendar year and are subject to the regular graduated withholding rates (Rev. Rul. 66-190).[27]

2607. Employee Expense Reimbursements Subject to Withholding. An employer's withholding obligations with respect to amounts paid to employees under an expense allowance or reimbursement arrangement depend upon whether the amounts are paid under an accountable or a nonaccountable plan (¶ 943 and ¶ 952A). Amounts paid under an accountable plan may be excluded from an employee's gross income to the extent of an employee's substantiated expenses and are not required to be reported on the employee's Form W-2. Thus, the payments are exempt from employment tax obligations (income tax withholding, FICA, FUTA, railroad retirement, and railroad unemployment taxes) (Reg. § § 1.62-2 and 31.3401(a)-4).[28] Amounts paid under a nonaccountable plan are included in the employee's gross income, reported on Form W-2, and are subject to withholding as supplemental wages (¶ 2606). If expenses are reimbursed under an accountable plan, but either the expenses are not substantiated within a reasonable period of time or amounts in excess of substantiated expenses are not returned within a reasonable period of time, the unsubstantiated or excess amounts are treated as paid under a nonaccountable plan and are subject to withholding no later than the first payroll period following the end of the reasonable period of time.

Expense reimbursements that are subject to withholding may be added to the employee's regular wages for the appropriate payroll period, and withheld taxes may be computed on the total. Alternatively, the employer may withhold at the flat rate applicable to supplemental wages (¶ 2606) if the expense reimbursement or allowance is paid separately or is separately identified (Reg. § 31.3401(a)-4(c)).

2608. Per Diem Allowances Subject to Withholding. If the amount of an employee's business expenses are substantiated through the use of an IRS-approved per diem allowance, any amounts paid by the employer to the employee exceeding the amounts deemed substantiated are subject to income tax withholding and other employment taxes (Reg. § § 1.62-2(h)(2)(i)(B) and 31.3401(a)-4(b)(1)(ii)).[29] See ¶ 947 for standard mileage rate and FAVR allowances for automobile expenses; see ¶ 954 et seq. for per diem methods relating to meal and lodging expenses.

For per diem or mileage allowances paid in advance, withholding on any excess must occur no later than the first payroll period following the payroll period in which the expenses for which the advance was paid (i.e., the days or miles of travel) are substantiated by the employee. For a per diem or mileage allowance paid as a reimbursement, the excess amounts reimbursed are subject to withholding when paid.

2609. Compensation Not Subject to Withholding. Some types of compensation are excluded from the definition of wages for income tax withholding purposes (¶ 2601). This includes amounts paid for or for the services of:

- newspaper carriers under age 18 delivering to customers,

- newspaper and magazine vendors buying at fixed prices and retaining excess from sales to customers,

- agricultural workers who are not subject to FICA withholding,

- household employees,

- cash or noncash tips of less than $20 per month,

References are to Standard Federal Tax Reports; Tax Research Consultant; and Practical Tax Explanations.

[27] ¶ 33,506.3687; PAYROLL: 6,066, PAYROLL: 6,068; § 22,120.50

[28] ¶ 6004, ¶ 33,508A; PAYROLL: 3,168; § 22,110.45, § 22,210.45, § 22,310.45

[29] ¶ 6004, ¶ 33,508A; PAYROLL: 3,168; § 10,120.10

¶2607

- certain employer contributions to IRAs and deferred compensation plans,

- individuals not working in the course of the employer's business (less than $50 paid and less than 24 days worked during the current or preceding quarter),

- employees of foreign governments and international organizations,

- armed forces personnel serving in a combat zone,

- foreign earned income if excludable from gross income, and

- members of a religious order performing services for the order or associated institution (Code Sec. 3401(a)).[30]

Fringe benefits are generally included in supplemental wages, but certain qualified employee fringe benefits, such as no-additional-cost services, qualified employee discounts, working condition fringes, *de minimis* fringes, qualified transportation fringes, qualified moving expense reimbursements, and certain employer-provided cell phones, are not subject to income tax withholding if it is reasonable to believe the recipient will be able to exclude them from gross income (¶ 2085) (IRS Pub. 15-B) (Code Sec. 3401(a)(19)).[31] The health and accident insurance premiums paid on behalf of a greater than two-percent S corporation shareholder-employee are wages for income tax withholding purposes (Rev. Rul. 91-26), but not for FICA and FUTA purposes (Code Secs. 3121(a)(2)(B) and 3306(b)(2)(B)).

The employer's cost of group-term life insurance, including any amount in excess of $50,000 coverage that is taxable to the employee as compensation (¶ 2055), is exempt from withholding (Code Sec. 3401(a)(14); Reg. § 31.3401(a)(14)-1).[32] However, the employer must report the cost of the insurance coverage includible in the employee's gross income on Form W-2 (Reg. § 1.6052-1).[33] An employer's reimbursement of an employee's moving expenses is also exempt if it is reasonable to believe a moving expense deduction will be allowable to the employee (¶ 1073) (Code Sec. 3401(a)(15)).[34] In addition, the value of any meals or lodging excludable by the employee from gross income (¶ 2089) is exempt from withholding (Reg. § 31.3401(a)-1(b)(9)).[35] See ¶ 2607 and ¶ 2608 for information concerning amounts paid to employees as advances or reimbursements for traveling, meals, etc.

Benefits provided by an employer to an employee in the form of certain educational assistance (¶ 2067), dependent care assistance (¶ 2065), fellowship or scholarship grants (¶ 865), or National Health Service Corps loan repayments are not subject to withholding if it is reasonable to believe that the employee is entitled to exclude the payment from income (Code Sec. 3401(a)).[36] Benefits provided by the employer in the form of medical care reimbursement made to or for the benefit of an employee under a self-insured medical reimbursement plan are excluded from wages for withholding purposes (¶ 2015) (Code Sec. 3401(a)(20)).[37] Benefits paid under workers' compensation laws (other than nonoccupational disability benefits) are not taxable compensation for services performed and are not subject to withholding (Code Sec. 104).[38]

An employee's elective contributions to a traditional Code Sec. 401(k) retirement plan, simplified employee pension (SEP), Code Sec. 403(b) annuity plan, or SIMPLE retirement account are not included in wages for income tax withholding purposes (Code Sec. 3401(a)(12)),[39] but these amounts are wages for FICA and FUTA purposes (Code Secs. 3121(a)(5) and 3306(b)(5)).

References are to Standard Federal Tax Reports; Tax Research Consultant; and Practical Tax Explanations.

[30] ¶ 33,502; PAYROLL: 3,000; § 22,110.05

[31] ¶ 33,502; PAYROLL: 3,200; § 22,110.10

[32] ¶ 33,502, ¶ 33,527; PAYROLL: 3,202; § 22,110.10

[33] ¶ 36,441; PAYROLL: 3,356.15; § 21,005.45

[34] ¶ 33,502; PAYROLL: 3,170; § 22,110.10

[35] ¶ 33,503; PAYROLL: 3,208; § 22,110.10

[36] ¶ 33,502; COMPEN: 33,350; § 22,110.10

[37] ¶ 33,502, ¶ 33,506.1871; PAYROLL: 3,206; § 22,110.10

[38] ¶ 6660; PAYROLL: 3,206; § 3,705.05

[39] ¶ 33,502; PAYROLL: 3,300; § 22,110.20

¶2609

Death benefit payments to beneficiaries or to the estates of deceased employees and payments to such persons of compensation due but unpaid at the time of the decedent's death are not subject to withholding.[40]

Any state and local tax benefits and limited payments provided to volunteer emergency response personnel and excludable from their gross income (¶ 896A) are not subject to withholding for tax years beginning after 2007 and before 2011 (Code Sec. 3401(a)(23)).[41]

Effective for stock acquired pursuant to an option exercised after October 22, 2004, withholding is not required on a disqualifying disposition of stock acquired through exercise of either an incentive stock option (¶ 1925) or through an employee stock purchase plan (ESPP) (¶ 1929) (Code Sec. 421(b)).[42] No withholding required also when compensation is recognized in connection with an ESPP discount under Code Sec. 423(c).

Voluntary Withholding. If remuneration is taxable to the employee but is exempt from withholding, the employee may voluntarily request that the employer increase the amount withheld from the employee's other compensation. In many cases, the employee and employer may enter into a mutual agreement for the employer to withhold from the remuneration that would be otherwise exempt from withholding (¶ 2629).

Computation of Withholding on Wages

2612. Calculation of Income Tax Withholding. To calculate an employee's income tax withholding (¶ 2601), an employer should follow a few basic steps:

(1) determine the payroll period, such as weekly, biweekly, or monthly (¶ 2621);

(2) calculate the employee's wages for the applicable payroll period (¶ 2604);

(3) determine the number of the employee's allowances from the filled-out Form W-4 (¶ 2634); and

(4) choose the withholding method (¶ 2614) (Code Sec. 3402(a)).

Other factors to consider in the calculation include whether the employee is a recent hire or only works part-time, whether the employee has more than one employer, and whether the employee receives any supplemental wage payments (¶ 2606).

2614. Methods of Income Tax Withholding. The Code provides two major methods of computing the income tax to be withheld from wages: the percentage method (¶ 2616) and the wage bracket method (¶ 2619) (Code Sec. 3402).[43] For other permissible methods of withholding, see ¶ 2627. Regardless of which method is used, the amount of withholding depends upon the amount of wages paid (¶ 2604), the number of exemptions claimed by the employee on the withholding allowance certificate (¶ 2632 and ¶ 2634), the employee's marital status, and the payroll period of the employee (¶ 2621) (IRS Pub. 15).

2616. Percentage Method of Income Tax Withholding. If the employer selects the percentage method of withholding (¶ 2612), the employer must:

(1) multiply the amount of one withholding exemption for the payroll period by the number of allowances claimed on the employee's Form W-4 (¶ 2634),

(2) subtract the amount determined in (1) from the employee's wages, and

(3) apply the appropriate percentage rate table to the resulting figure to determine the amount of withholding (Code Sec. 3402(b)).[44]

Each withholding exemption is equal to one personal exemption for the year (¶ 133) prorated to the payroll period (¶ 2621). Thus, in 2014, if the payroll period is monthly and the personal exemption is $3,950, the amount of one withholding exemp-

References are to Standard Federal Tax Reports; Tax Research Consultant; and Practical Tax Explanations.

[40] ¶ 33,506.1856; PAYROLL: 3,150; § 22,110.45

[41] ¶ 33,502; INDIV: 33,312; § 22,110.45

[42] ¶ 19,602; COMPEN: 21,058; § 22,110.15

[43] ¶ 33,542; PAYROLL: 6,050; § 22,120.05

[44] ¶ 33,542; PAYROLL: 6,054.05; § 22,120.10

tion is $3,950 divided by 12, or $329. In 2015, the amount of one withholding exemption is $333, based on a monthly payroll period and a personal exemption amount of $4,000.

Percentage method withholding tables for both single (including heads of household) and married employees for each of the payroll periods are provided for use in determining the amount of tax to be withheld. See IRS Pub. 15. The IRS has approved and issued alternative formula tables for percentage method withholding that were devised for computing withheld tax under different payroll systems.

2619. Wage Bracket Method of Income Tax Withholding. The wage bracket tables (¶ 2612) provided by the IRS for graduated withholding cover weekly, biweekly, semi-monthly, and monthly payroll periods (Code Sec. 3402(c)).[45] Separate tables for each period are provided for single persons (including heads of household) and married persons. The proper columns to be used by the employer are determined by the total number of allowances claimed on the employee's withholding allowance certificate (¶ 2634). These tables produce about the same result as the percentage method tables (¶ 2616) and are designed to accommodate different payroll systems. If the wage bracket method is used, wages in excess of the highest wage bracket in the tables may be rounded off to the nearest dollar at the election of the employer. See IRS Pub. 15.

2621. Payroll Period. For purposes of calculating income tax withholding (¶ 2612), the employee's payroll period, or the period of service for which a payment of wages is ordinarily made to an employee, determines the exemption amount to be used if the employer uses the percentage method (¶ 2616) or the correct table to be used if the employer uses the wage bracket method (¶ 2619). Daily, weekly, biweekly, semi-monthly, monthly, quarterly, semiannual, and annual payroll periods have separate tables for the percentage computation. Any other payroll period is a miscellaneous payroll period. Wages may also be paid for periods that are not payroll periods (¶ 2624).

2624. Calculation of Income Tax Withholding Allowance. If an employee has an established payroll period (¶ 2621), the amount of the withholding allowance for the percentage method (¶ 2616) is determined by the payroll period, without regard to the time the employee is actually engaged in performing services during such period. If the payment is for a period that is not a payroll period, such as when wages are paid upon completion of a particular project, the withholding allowance under the percentage method or the amount withheld under the wage bracket method (¶ 2619) is computed based on a miscellaneous payroll period containing a number of days (including Sundays and holidays) equal to those in the period covered by the payment (Code Sec. 3402(b); Reg. § 31.3402(c)-1(c)).[46]

If the wages are paid without regard to any period, the tax to be withheld is the same as for a miscellaneous payroll period containing the number of days equal to the days (including Sundays and holidays) which have elapsed since (1) the date of the last payment of wages by the employer during the calendar year, (2) the date of commencement of employment with the employer during such year, or (3) January 1 of such year, whichever is later.

2627. Alternative Methods of Income Tax Withholding. An employer may withhold income taxes on the basis of average wages paid to an employee by using estimated quarterly wages, annualized wages, cumulative wages, or any method which produces substantially the same amount of withholding as the percentage or wage bracket method (¶ 2612) (Code Sec. 3402(h)).[47]

2629. Voluntary Income Tax Withholding. An employee may request on Form W-4 that the employer withhold additional amounts of income from the employee's wages. An employer must comply with such a request, but only to the extent the additional withholding amount does not reduce the employee's net pay (after other deductions required by law) below zero (Code Sec. 3402(i); Reg. § § 31.3402(i)-1 and 31.3402(i)-2).[48]

References are to Standard Federal Tax Reports; Tax Research Consultant; and Practical Tax Explanations.

[45] ¶ 33,542; PAYROLL: 6,054.10; § 22,120.15

[46] ¶ 33,542, ¶ 33,547; PAYROLL: 6,056; § 22,115.05

[47] ¶ 33,542; PAYROLL: 6,054; § 22,120.45

[48] ¶ 33,542, ¶ 33,571, ¶ 33,572; PAYROLL: 6,104; § 22,125.05

An employee and employer may also enter into an agreement for the employer to withhold from certain types of income that are not subject to mandatory withholding (¶ 2609). For example, magazine vendors, domestic workers, etc., may enter into an agreement with their employer to have income tax withheld. To effectuate this agreement, the employee must submit Form W-4 to the employer, and the employer must begin withholding (Code Sec. 3402(p); Reg. §31.3402(p)-1).[49] Taxpayers may use Form W-4V to request voluntary withholding from certain federal payments, including Social Security benefits, crop disaster payments, Commodity Credit Corporation loans, and unemployment compensation.

2632. Claiming Withholding Exemptions and Allowances. An employee must file Form W-4 (¶ 2634) with his or her employer showing the number of exemptions from income tax withholding to which he or she is entitled. Every employee is entitled to his or her own withholding exemption and one for each dependent (¶ 137). A married employee may claim a withholding exemption for his or her spouse if the latter does not claim one. An employee who can be claimed as a dependent on another person's tax return, such as a parent's return, may not claim a withholding exemption for himself or herself. No withholding exemption is allowed for unborn children, even if the birth is expected to occur within the same tax year (Code Sec. 3402(f); Reg. §31.3402(f)(1)-1).[50] Employees with more than one job may not claim an exemption that is currently in effect with another employer.

In order to avoid excess withholding, a standard deduction allowance equal to one withholding exemption may be claimed by an employee provided that the employee: (1) does not have a spouse who is receiving wages subject to withholding; and (2) does not have withholding certificates in effect with more than one employer. However, these restrictions do not apply if the wages earned by the spouse or by the employee from another employer are $1,500 or less, combined.

Additional withholding allowances are available to an employee who can show that he or she will have large itemized deductions, deductible alimony payments, moving expenses, employee business expenses, retirement contributions, net losses from Schedules C, D, E, and F of Form 1040, or tax credits (Code Sec. 3402(m); Reg. §31.3402(m)-1).[51]

2634. Employee's Withholding Allowance Certificate. Before an employee is allowed any withholding exemptions (¶ 2632), he or she must file a withholding allowance certificate on Form W-4 with their employer showing the number of exemptions to which he or she is entitled (Code Sec. 3402(f)(2); Reg. §31.3402(f)(2)-1).[52] Otherwise, withholding must be computed as if the employee were single and claiming no other exemptions. A widow or widower may claim married status for purposes of withholding if he or she qualifies as a surviving spouse (¶ 175) (Code Sec. 3402(l)(3)).

An employee who certifies to his or her employer that he or she had no income tax liability for the preceding tax year and anticipates none for the current tax year may be exempt from the withholding provisions (Code Sec. 3402(n); Reg. §31.3402(n)-1).[53] Form W-4 should be used and renewed annually by any employee claiming this exemption.

A $500 civil penalty may be assessed against any individual who decreases his or her rate of withholding by claiming excess withholding allowances on Form W-4 (Code Sec. 6682).[54] In addition, a criminal penalty may be imposed against any individual who willfully supplies false withholding information or fails to supply withholding information (Code Sec. 7205).[55]

References are to Standard Federal Tax Reports; Tax Research Consultant; and Practical Tax Explanations.

[49] ¶ 33,542, ¶ 33,586; PAY-ROLL: 6,104; § 22,125.25

[50] ¶ 33,542, ¶ 33,553; PAY-ROLL: 6,060; § 22,115.10, § 22,115.15

[51] ¶ 33,542, ¶ 33,579; PAY-ROLL: 6,064; § 22,115.15

[52] ¶ 33,542, ¶ 33,554; PAY-ROLL: 6,062; § 22,115.25

[53] ¶ 33,542, ¶ 33,580; PAY-ROLL: 6,062; § 22,115.20

[54] ¶ 39,845; PAYROLL: 6,062.15; § 22,115.25

[55] ¶ 41,325; PAYROLL: 6,358; § 22,115.25

Most Forms W-4 are retained by the employer. Employers need only submit withholding certificates to the IRS if directed to do so by the IRS. The IRS may issue a notice to the employer that specifies the maximum number of withholding exemptions a particular employee may claim. Generally, the employer is bound by this determination until otherwise advised by the IRS (Reg. § 31.3402(f)(2)-1(g)).[56]

2637. Changes to Withholding Exemptions and Allowances. An employee may file an amended withholding exemption certificate (¶ 2634), increasing the number of exemptions, at any time that he or she becomes eligible for an additional dependency exemption or an extra allowance based on one of the deduction or credit items listed at ¶ 2632. An employee must file a new certificate within 10 days if the number of exemptions decreases after the occurrence of any of the following events (Code Sec. 3402(f)(2)(B); Reg. § 31.3402(f)(2)-1(b)):[57]

- the employee divorces or legally separates from his or her spouse for whom the employee has been claiming an exemption, or the employee's spouse claims his or her own exemption on a separate certificate;

- the support of a claimed dependent is taken over by someone else, and the employee no longer expects to claim that person as a dependent;

- the employee discovers that a dependent (other than a qualifying child) for whom an exemption was claimed will receive sufficient income of his own for the calendar year to disqualify him as a dependent (¶ 137); or

- circumstances have changed so that the employee is no longer entitled to claim an exemption based on one of the deduction or credit items listed at ¶ 2632.

An employee who claimed "no liability" must file a new Form W-4 within 10 days from the time the employee anticipates that he or she will incur liability for the year or before December 1 if they anticipate liability for the next year (Reg. § 31.3402(f)(2)-1(c)).

The death of a spouse or dependent does not affect the withholding exemption for that year unless the employee's tax year is not a calendar year and the death occurs in that part of the calendar year preceding the employee's tax year (Reg. § 31.3402(f)(2)-1(b)(1)(ii)).[58]

A withholding allowance certificate furnished to the employer that replaces an existing certificate can be effective for the first payment after the certificate is received if so elected by the employer. However, the replacing certificate must be effective for the first payroll period that ends on or after the 30th day after the day on which the new certificate is furnished (Code Sec. 3402(f)(3)(B)).[59]

Withholding on Non-Wage Payments

2642. Withholding on Certain Gambling Winnings. Income tax withholding is required at a flat rate of 25 percent for winnings of more than $5,000 from sweepstakes, wagering pools, and lotteries, and other types of gambling (including pari-mutual pools with respect to horse races, dog races, and jai alai) if the winnings are at least 300 times the wager. No withholding is required, however, on winnings from bingo, keno, or slot machines (Code Sec. 3402(q)).[60]

The payor must report gambling winnings to the taxpayer and the IRS on Form W-2G if the winnings are subject to withholding or if the winner receives $1,200 or more from a bingo game or slot machines, $1,500 from keno, $5,000 from a poker tournament, or, for other gambling winnings, $600 or more and at least 300 times the amount of the wager. If reporting is required, backup withholding must occur if the winner of the reportable amount does not furnish his or her taxpayer identification number (TIN) to the payor (¶ 2645). All withheld income reported on Form W-2G must also be reported on Form 945.

References are to Standard Federal Tax Reports; Tax Research Consultant; and Practical Tax Explanations.

[56] ¶ 33,554; PAYROLL: 6,062.10; § 22,115.25

[57] ¶ 33,542, ¶ 33,554; PAYROLL: 6,062; § 22,115.25

[58] ¶ 33,554; PAYROLL: 6,062; § 22,115.10

[59] ¶ 33,542; PAYROLL: 6,062; § 22,115.25

[60] ¶ 33,542; PAYROLL: 3,404.10; § 39,435

2643. Withholding on Pensions, Annuities, and Certain Deferred Income. In the case of taxable payments from an employer-sponsored pension, annuity, profit-sharing, stock bonus, or other deferred compensation plan, income tax withholding is required unless the recipient elects not to have tax withheld (Code Sec. 3405).[61] The same rule applies to an IRA or an annuity, endowment, or life insurance contract issued by a life insurance company. The recipient's election not to have withholding apply remains in effect until revoked. The payor must notify the recipient that an election may be made and of the right to revoke such election. The election is generally not available with respect to payments delivered outside the United States or a U.S. possession to persons subject to U.S. tax on their worldwide income.

The amount withheld depends on whether the distributions are periodic payments or nonperiodic payments. For periodic payments (annuity and similar periodic payments), withholding is made as though the payment was a payment of wages for the appropriate payroll period. If the recipient does not have a withholding exemption certificate (Form W-4P) in effect, he or she is treated as a married individual claiming three exemptions. The exemptions are not available to a payee failing to file a certificate if the payee fails to furnish a taxpayer identification number (TIN) to a payor or if the IRS notifies the payor that the payee's TIN is incorrect.

The withholding rate on nonperiodic distributions is 10 percent. The withholding rate on distributions that were eligible for rollover but not directly transferred from the distributing plan to an eligible transferee plan is 20 percent. The withholding requirement is mandatory and distributees cannot elect to forego withholding on rollover eligible distributions.

2645. Backup Withholding. The backup withholding system requires a payor to deduct and withhold income tax at a flat rate of 28 percent from reportable payments, such as interest or dividends, if:

- the payee fails to furnish a correct taxpayer identification umber (TIN) to the payor in the manner required;

- the IRS notifies the payor that the TIN furnished by the payee is incorrect;

- the IRS notifies the payor that the payee has underreported reportable payments; or

- the payee is required, but fails, to certify that he is not subject to withholding (Code Sec. 3406).[62]

Backup withholding is reported on Form 945.

FICA and FUTA Taxes

2648. FICA Tax. Under the Federal Insurance Contributions Act (FICA), an employer is required to withhold Social Security and Medicare taxes from wages paid to each employee during the year, and to pay the employer's own share of these taxes (Code Secs. 3101, 3111, and 3121(a)).[63]

The employee and employer generally each are subject to a tax rate of 7.65 percent of wages paid for FICA purposes, consisting of a 6.2 percent rate for old-age, survivors, and disability insurance (OASDI) (i.e., Social Security) and a 1.45 percent rate for hospital insurance (HI) (i.e., Medicare). For wages paid in 2011 and 2012, the employee's Social Security tax rate was reduced to 4.2 percent, limiting the employee's portion of the FICA tax rate to 5.65 percent of wages paid (Act Sec. 601(a) of P.L. 111-312, amended by Act Sec. 101 of P.L. 112-78 and Act Sec. 1001 of P.L. 112-96). The Social Security tax rate applies only to wages paid within a Social Security wage base ($117,000 in 2014; $118,500 in 2015). There is no cap on wages subject to the Medicare tax.

References are to Standard Federal Tax Reports; Tax Research Consultant; and Practical Tax Explanations.

[61] ¶ 33,620; RETIRE: 42,700; § 22,140

[62] ¶ 33,640; FILEBUS: 18,150; § 39,401

[63] ¶ 114; PAYROLL: 9,050; § 22,201

¶2643

Additional 0.9% Medicare Tax. For tax years beginning after 2012, the employee's portion of the Medicare component of FICA taxes is increased by an additional 0.9 percent (to 2.35 percent) for wages in excess of $200,000 ($250,000 in the case of a joint return, $125,000 in the case of a married taxpayer filing separately). For a joint return, the additional tax is imposed on the couple's combined wages (Code Sec. 3101(b)(2); Reg. § 31.3102-4).

Although the employer is generally required to withhold the employee's portion from the employee's wages, the employer is not obligated to withhold the additional Medicare tax unless (and until) the employee receives wages from the employer in excess of $200,000. For this purpose, the employer is permitted to disregard the amount of wages received by the employee's spouse. Thus, because an employee may receive wages from more than one employer, or because the employee's spouse may receive wages, an employee may be subject to the additional tax without the tax being withheld from the employee's wages. The employee is responsible for any portion of the additional 0.9 percent tax that is not withheld.

If an employer fails to withhold the additional tax and the employee pays that amount, the employer is not obligated to pay the additional tax but may be subject to penalties and additions to tax for failing to withhold (Code Sec. 3102(f)). If the tax is overwithheld, the employee may claim a credit against income tax. The employee takes any underwithheld or overwithheld amount into account in calculating the tax on Form 8959, which must be attached to the employee's tax return for the year.

Multiple Employers. If an employee works for more than one employer, each employer must withhold and pay FICA taxes on the wages paid. In such instances, the employee's FICA tax withheld for the year might exceed the maximum employee portion for the tax for the year. If this happens, the employee must take the excess as a credit against income tax liability. If the individual is not required to file an income tax return, then he or she may file a special refund claim (¶ 1321) (Reg. § § 1.31-2 and 31.6413(c)-1). The same rule applies to taxes withheld under the Railroad Retirement Tax Act.

If an individual is concurrently employed by two or more related corporations and all remuneration is disbursed to the individual through a common paymaster for the group, the common paymaster is responsible for the reporting and payment of FICA and FUTA taxes. However, the other related corporations remain jointly and severally liable for their appropriate share of the taxes (Reg. § 31.3121(s)-1).

Domestic Services and Farm Workers. In the case of persons performing domestic services in a private home of the employer and persons performing agricultural labor, if the employer pays the employee's liability for FICA taxes or state unemployment taxes without deduction from the employee's wages, those payments are not wages for FICA purposes (Code Sec. 3121(a)(6)). Other special rules apply to domestic workers (¶ 2652).

Emergency Responders (Expired). Any state and local tax benefits and limited payments provided to volunteer emergency response personnel and excludable from their gross income (¶ 896A) for tax years beginning after 2007 and before 2011 are not subject to FICA taxes (Code Sec. 3121(a)(23)).

Employers' Payroll Tax Holiday (Expired). Employers were provided an exemption from having to pay their share of the 6.2-percent Social Security share of FICA taxes for qualified employees from March 19, 2010, through December 31, 2010 (Code Sec. 3111(d)). The waiver applied automatically if the employer paid the qualified employee for services performed in the employer's trade or business (or in furtherance of its activities if a tax-exempt organization). An employer that did not want to use the payroll tax holiday must have elected out of the waiver.

2649. FUTA Tax. The Federal Unemployment Tax Act (FUTA) imposes a tax on employers: (1) who employed one or more persons in covered employment on at least one day in each of 20 weeks during the current or preceding calendar year; or (2) who paid wages (in covered employment) of at least $1,500 ($20,000 for agricultural labor, $1,000 for household employees) in a calendar quarter in the current or preceding calendar year. The tax is based on the first $7,000 of certain wages paid during the calendar year to each employee. The full rate of tax is 6 percent (6.2 percent before July 1, 2011), but the employer is allowed a partial credit against this tax based on its state unemployment insurance tax liability (Code Secs. 3301 and 3302).[64]

Domestic Services and Farm Workers. In the case of persons performing domestic services in a private home of the employer and persons performing agricultural labor, if the employer pays the employee's liability for FICA taxes or state unemployment taxes without deducting those taxes from the employee's wages, the amounts paid by the employer are not wages for FUTA purposes, but they are wages for income tax withholding purposes (¶ 2601) (Code Sec. 3306(b)(6)). Other special rules apply to domestic workers (¶ 2652).

Emergency Responders (Expired). Any state and local tax benefits and limited payments provided to volunteer emergency response personnel and excludable from their gross income (¶ 885) for tax years beginning after 2007 and before 2011 are not subject to FUTA taxes (Code Sec. 3306(b)(20)).

Return and Payment by Employer

2650. Employer Returns for Employment Taxes. An employer subject to the requirement to withhold income taxes (¶ 2601) or to pay and withhold FICA taxes (¶ 2648), or both, must file a quarterly return on Form 941 to report the amount withheld or taxes owed with respect to wages, tips, taxable fringe benefits, supplemental unemployment compensation benefits, and third-party payments of sick pay. Small employers with an estimated annual employment tax liability of $1,000 or less may report the taxes annually using Form 944 (discussed below). Taxes on wages for agricultural employees, including domestic services on a farm operated for profit, are reported annually on Form 943. Nonpayroll items, such as pension and annuity payments (¶ 2643), are reported annually on Form 945. Employers who must pay FUTA tax (¶ 2649) on wages generally must file an annual return using Form 940.

Form 941 is due on or before the last day of the month following the quarter involved. Forms 940, 943, 944, and 945 are all due January 31 of the year following the calendar year for which the return is made. For all of these forms, including Form 941, an extension of time for filing is automatically granted to the 10th day of the second month following the close of the calendar quarter if the return is accompanied by receipts showing timely deposits in full payment of taxes due for the period (Reg. § 31.6071(a)-1).[65]

Forms W-2, 1099-R, and W-3 must be filed with the Social Security Administration (SSA) by the last day of February of the year following the year included in the return. The SSA transmits the income tax information on the return to the IRS.

Form 944 Program. The Form 944 Program allows certain small employers to file an annual Form 944 rather than a quarterly Form 941. Form 944 is generally due January 31 of the year following the year for which the return is filed (Reg. §§ 31.6011(a)-1(a)(5) and 31.6011(a)-4(a)(4)).[66]

Eligibility for the Form 944 Program is limited to employers with an annual estimated employment tax liability of $1,000 or less. An employer that believes it is qualified for the program can contact the IRS to express its desire to file Form 944 instead of Form 941 (Rev. Proc. 2009-51). Only upon a request will the IRS send a notification letter to a qualified employer confirming that it may file Form 944 for that tax year. Employers may opt out of filing Form 944 for any reason by calling or writing the IRS before the applicable due date.

References are to Standard Federal Tax Reports; Tax Research Consultant; and Practical Tax Explanations.

[64] ¶ 114; PAYROLL: 9,100; § 22,301

[65] ¶ 36,702; PAYROLL: 6,202; § 22,130.05, § 22,235.05, § 22,340.05

[66] ¶ 35,131; PAYROLL: 3,352.15; § 22,130.15, § 22,235.15

Most participating employers can pay their employment taxes annually with their Form 944, rather than making monthly or semi-weekly deposits (¶ 2651). A participating employer, however, may not discover that its actual annual employment tax liability exceeded the $1,000 threshold until it files its Form 944 on the following January 31. These employers can avoid the penalty for failing to make a timely monthly deposit of their January taxes, so long as they fully pay their January employment taxes by March 15 (Reg. § 31.6302-1).[67]

A modified lookback period applies for determining whether a participating employer that eventually discovers that it is not eligible for the Form 944 Program is a monthly or semi-weekly depositor. For those employers, the lookback period is the second calendar year preceding the current calendar year. For instance, the lookback period for 2015 is calendar year 2013.

An employer in the Form 944 Program whose actual total employment tax liability exceeds the $1,000 threshold but whose employment tax liability for a quarter is less than $2,500 is eligible for the *de minimis* rules applicable to quarterly Form 941 filers (¶ 2651). Such an employer is allowed to apply the *de minimis* rules if it deposits the employment taxes that accumulated during a quarter by the last day of the month following the close of the quarter. If an employer's tax liability for a quarter does not qualify for *de minimis* treatment, the employer must make deposits either monthly or semiweekly, whichever is appropriate, in order to avoid the failure-to-deposit penalty (¶ 2658).

2651. Employer Deposit of Withheld Taxes. An employer generally must deposit withheld income taxes (¶ 2601) and FICA taxes (¶ 2648) on either a monthly or semiweekly basis. An employer's status as a monthly or semiweekly depositor for a given calendar year is determined based on the employer's employment tax reporting history during a lookback period. An employer must also deposit FUTA taxes quarterly (¶ 2649). Except for small employers (including employers in the Form 944 Program (¶ 2650)), all employers are required to make deposits electronically through the Electronic Federal Tax Payment System (EFTPS) (Reg. § 31.6302-1).[68] Employers that fail to deposit the full amount of taxes in a timely manner will be subject to penalties (¶ 2658).

Depositing Income Taxes and FICA Taxes. For calendar year 2015, an employer generally must deposit withheld income taxes and FICA on a monthly basis during the 12-month lookback period from July 1, 2013, through June 30, 2014, the amount of the aggregate employment taxes reported was $50,000 or less. For new employers, during the first calendar year of business, the tax liability for each quarter of the lookback period is considered to be zero. Therefore, the employer is a monthly depositor for the first calendar year of business. Monthly depositors are required to deposit each month's taxes on or before the 15th day of the following month. If the 15th day is a Saturday, Sunday, or legal holiday in the District of Columbia, the employer has until the next succeeding business day which is not a Saturday, Sunday, or legal holiday to make the deposit.

An employer that reported more than $50,000 in aggregate employment taxes during the lookback period from July 1, 2013, through June 30, 2014, will be a semiweekly depositor for calendar year 2015. Semiweekly depositors generally are required to deposit their taxes by the Wednesday after payday, if the payday falls on a Wednesday, Thursday, or Friday. For all other paydays, the deposit is due by the Friday following payday. Semiweekly depositors always have at least three business days after the payday to make the deposit.

For agricultural employers filing Form 943, the lookback period used to determine monthly or semiweekly depositing status is the second calendar year preceding the current calendar year. For example, the lookback period for calendar year 2015 is calendar year 2013.

References are to Standard Federal Tax Reports; Tax Research Consultant; and Practical Tax Explanations.

[67] ¶ 38,055B; PAYROLL: 3,352.15; § 22,130.15, § 22,235.15

[68] ¶ 38,055B; PAYROLL: 6,106; § 22,135.05, § 22,240.05, § 22,345.05

Notwithstanding these general requirements, under the one-day rule, employers with $100,000 or more of accumulated liability during a monthly or semiweekly period are required to deposit the funds by the next day that is not a Saturday, Sunday, or legal holiday in the District of Columbia. Monthly depositors subject to the one-day rule must switch to making deposits semi-weekly.

As a safe harbor, employers that fail to deposit the full amount of taxes will not be penalized (¶ 2658) if the shortfall does not exceed the greater of $100 or two percent of the amount of employment taxes required to be deposited, provided that the shortfall is deposited on or before a prescribed makeup date. For a monthly depositor, the makeup date is the due date of the return for the period the shortfall occurred. For a semi-weekly depositor, the makeup date is the earlier of the due date of the return for the period of the shortfall, or the first Wednesday or Friday that falls on or after the 15th of the month following the month the shortfall occurred. Penalties may also be abated if an employer shows that a failure to deposit the full amount of the employment taxes was due to reasonable cause.

Amounts withheld under the backup withholding requirements (¶ 2645) are treated as employment taxes subject to these deposit rules. However, employers are permitted to treat the backup withholding amounts separately from other employment taxes for purposes of the deposit rules (Reg. § 31.6302-3).[69] Different monthly and semimonthly deposit requirements apply to taxes withheld from nonresident aliens and foreign corporations (Reg. § 1.6302-2).[70]

Depositing FUTA Taxes. Although Form 940 is an annual return, an employer generally must deposit FUTA taxes quarterly. For deposit purposes, the employer determines the FUTA tax for each of the first three calendar quarters by multiplying the amount of wages paid during the quarter by 0.006. If at the end of the quarter the employer owes, but has not yet deposited, more than $500 in FUTA tax for the year, the employer must make a deposit by the last day of the month following the end of the quarter (Reg. § 31.6302(c)-3(a)(1)). For example, for the quarter ending March 31, 2015, deposits of FUTA are due by April 30, 2015. If the last day of the month is a Saturday, Sunday, or legal holiday in the District of Columbia, the employer has until the next succeeding business day which is not a Saturday, Sunday, or legal holiday to make the deposit.

De Minimis Exceptions. Two *de minimis* rules allow small employers to make payments with Form 941 or Form 943 rather than make deposits (Reg. § 31.6302-1(f)(4)).[71] First, deposits are not required if the employer's accumulated employment taxes for the current quarter are less than $2,500. Secondly, deposits are not required if the total accumulated employment taxes for the preceding quarter were less than $2,500 and the one-day rule does not require a deposit at the close of the next business day. An additional exception to the deposit requirement exists for employers in the Form 944 Program (¶ 2650).

How to Deposit. Employers are required to deposit all employment taxes electronically through EFTPS (Reg. § 31.6302-1(h)(2)).[72] A deposit of taxes by electronic funds transfer is deemed made when the amount is withdrawn from the employer's account. Employers are subject to a 10-percent penalty if they are required to make deposits by electronic funds transfer but fail to do so (¶ 2658).

2652. Household Employees (Nanny Tax). Employers must withhold and pay FICA taxes on the wages of their household workers in 2014 if cash wages paid during the calendar year total $1,900 or more ($1,900 in 2015) (Code Sec. 3121(a)(7)(B) and (x)).[73] An employer must pay FUTA taxes for household employees if the employer has paid aggregate cash wages of $1,000 or more to household employees in a calendar quarter (Code Sec. 3306(c)(2)).[74]

References are to Standard Federal Tax Reports; Tax Research Consultant; and Practical Tax Explanations.

[69] ¶ 38,055D; PAYROLL: 6,106; § 39,405.15

[70] ¶ 38,062; PAYROLL: 6,106, PAYROLL: 9,200; § 37,335

[71] ¶ 38,055B; PAYROLL: 6,106.05; § 22,240.05

[72] ¶ 38,055B; PAYROLL: 6,106.45; § 22,240.05, § 22,345.05

[73] ¶ 114; PAYROLL: 3,358; § 22,235.30

[74] ¶ 114; PAYROLL: 3,106; § 22,340.20

Employers must report and pay required employment taxes for household employees on Schedule H of their Form 1040 or Form 1040A. While withheld amounts do not have to be deposited on a monthly basis, employers do need an employer identification number (EIN) to include on Form W-2 (¶ 2655) and Schedule H. To obtain an EIN, employers should complete Form SS-4.

Employers must increase either their quarterly estimated tax payments or the income tax withholding on their own wages in order to satisfy employment tax obligations with respect to household employees. Failure to withhold results in liability for the penalty for underpayment of estimated tax (¶ 2682).

2653. COBRA Premium Assistance Reimbursement (Expired). Certain individuals who became eligible to elect COBRA continuation health care coverage under their employer's plan as a result of an involuntary termination of their employment during the period beginning September 1, 2008, and ending May 31, 2010, were required to pay only 35 percent of the premiums for the coverage. The 65 percent of the premium not paid by the employee was paid by the employer maintaining the group health plan. The employer was reimbursed for these payments through a credit against the employer's payroll tax liability (Code Sec. 6432).[75] The credit was taken on the employer's employment tax return (¶ 2650). The reimbursement was treated as having paid, on the date that the eligible individual's premium payment was received, payroll taxes in an amount equal to the unpaid portion of the premium. To the extent that the amount treated as paid exceeded the amount of the employer's liability for such taxes, the employer received a refund or credit in the same manner as if it were an overpayment of taxes. The employer could provide the subsidy, and take the credit on its employment tax return, only after it received the 35-percent premium payment from the individual. An employer claiming the credit was required to maintain supporting documentation for the credit claimed. The credit was treated as a deposit made on the first day of the return period. A terminated employee or family member could exclude from gross income the 65-percent premium reduction for COBRA continuation coverage (¶ 888).

2654. Withholding for Disregarded Entities. A disregarded entity is treated as a separate entity responsible for employment tax liabilities (Reg. § 301.7701-2(c)(2)(iv)).[76] The rule applies to such disregarded entities as a qualified subchapter S subsidiary (QSub) and a single-member limited liability company (LLC). The entity continues to be disregarded for other federal tax purposes. The disregarded entity is not, however, treated as a separate corporation for purposes of self-employment taxes; the owner of the entity is personally liable for such taxes.

2655. Employee Wage Statements (Form W-2). On or before January 31, an employer is required to furnish an employee with copies of Form W-2 for taxes withheld during the preceding calendar year. The employer may elect with the consent of the employee to furnish an electronic, rather than written, payee statement of Form W-2 (Code Sec. 6051(a); Reg. § 31.6051-1).[77] When employment terminates before the end of the calendar year, there is no reasonable expectation of reemployment, and the employee submits a written request for the information, Form W-2 must be furnished within 30 days of the written request if the 30-day period ends before January 31.

Form W-2 is a multiple-part wage statement with several copies: Copy A is sent to the Social Security Administration (SSA), Copy 1 is sent to the state where the employee resides, Copy B is kept by the employee and attached to his or her federal tax return, Copy C is retained for the employee's records, Copy 2 is attached to the employee's state, city, or local tax return, and Copy D is kept in the employer's records. Employers must file electronically with the SSA rather if 250 or more Forms W-2 are to be filed. Hardship waivers may be requested (Reg. § 301.6011-2(c)).[78]

References are to Standard Federal Tax Reports; Tax Research Consultant; and Practical Tax Explanations.

[75] ¶ 38,935; HEALTH: 24,118; § 42,845.25
[76] ¶ 43,082; PAYROLL: 9,162
[77] ¶ 36,420, ¶ 36,421; PAYROLL: 6,204; § 22,415.05
[78] ¶ 35,125; FILEBUS: 12,302; § 22,405.05

26 WITHHOLDING

If the Social Security tax imposed on tips reported by the employee exceeds the tax that has been collected by the employer, the employer is required to furnish the employee with a statement showing the amount of the excess (Code Sec. 6053(b)).[79]

2658. Employment Tax Penalty for Employers. An employer is primarily liable for deducting and paying employment taxes whether or not the taxes are actually collected from the employee, or if not enough taxes are collected (¶ 2601). Failure to deduct and withhold employment taxes can cause civil and criminal penalties to apply. For example, any responsible person—typically a corporate officer or employee—who willfully fails to withhold, account for, or pay over any tax to the government is subject to a penalty equal to 100 percent of such tax, a $10,000 criminal fine, and up to five years imprisonment (Code Secs. 6672 and 7202).[80] The civil penalty is a collection device, usually assessed only when the tax cannot be collected from the employer, and results in a personal liability not dischargeable by bankruptcy. Civil and criminal penalties can also be imposed if an employer willfully fails to furnish, or furnishes a false or fraudulent, Form W-2 statement (¶ 2655) to an employee (Code Secs. 6674 and 7204).[81]

Failure to Make Timely Deposits. A graduated penalty applies to failures to make timely deposits of tax (¶ 2651), unless the failure is due to reasonable cause and not willful neglect (Code Sec. 6656).[82] The penalty amount varies with the length of time within which the taxpayer corrects the failure to make the required deposit. The penalty is assessed as follows:

- two percent of the amount of the underpayment if the failure is for no more than five days,

- five percent of the amount of the underpayment if the failure is for more than five days but for no more than 15 days, and

- 10 percent of the amount of the underpayment if the failure is for more than 15 days.

The penalty is imposed at the rate of 15 percent of the amount of the underpayment if a required tax deposit is not made (1) on or before the day that is 10 days after the date of the first delinquency notice to the taxpayer, or (2) if earlier, on or before the day on which notice and demand for immediate payment of tax is given in cases of jeopardy. A failure to deposit includes a failure to make deposits electronically when required to do so, and is penalized at a 10-percent rate.

Deposits generally are applied to the most recent tax liability within the quarter. Any depositor to whom the IRS mails a penalty notice may, within 90 days of the date of the notice, designate how the payment is to be applied in order to minimize the amount of the penalty.

Self-Employment Tax

2664. Self-Employment Tax Rate. Every taxpayer who has self-employment income (¶ 2667 and ¶ 2670) for a tax year must pay a self-employment tax in addition to any other applicable taxes. The combined rate of tax on self-employment income generally is 15.3 percent, consisting of a 12.4 percent component for Social Security (old-age, survivors, and disability insurance (OASDI)) and a 2.9 percent component for Medicare (hospital insurance (HI)) (Code Sec. 1401).[83] In 2011 and 2012, however, the combined rate of tax on self-employment income was 13.3 percent, resulting from a two-percent reduction in the Social Security component to 10.4 percent (Act Sec. 601(a) of P.L. 111-312, amended by Act Sec. 101 of P.L. 112-78 and Act Sec. 1001 of P.L. 112-96).

References are to Standard Federal Tax Reports; Tax Research Consultant; and Practical Tax Explanations.

[79] ¶ 36,460; PAYROLL: 3,406.30; § 21,305.15

[80] ¶ 39,775, ¶ 41,310; PAY-ROLL: 6,300; § 40,315.05

[81] ¶ 39,795, ¶ 41,320; PAY-ROLL: 6,350; § 40,325.25

[82] ¶ 39,580; PAYROLL: 6,106; § 40,315.15

[83] ¶ 32,541; INDIV: 63,060; § 23,105

¶2658

If net earnings from self-employment are less than $400, no self-employment tax is payable. The amount of self-employment income subject to the Social Security tax rate in a tax year is limited to the amount of the Social Security wage base for the year ($117,000 in 2014; $118,500 in 2015). If the taxpayer receives wages subject to FICA or railroad retirement tax during the year, the Social Security wage base is reduced by the amount of wages on which these taxes were paid (Code Sec. 1402(b)).[84] There is no cap on self-employment income subject to the Medicare tax.

Additional 0.9% Medicare Tax. For tax years beginning after 2012, the Medicare portion of the self-employment tax rate is increased by an additional 0.9 percent (to 3.8 percent) for self-employment income in excess of $200,000 ($250,000 in the case of a joint return, $125,000 in the case of a married taxpayer filing separately). In the case of a joint return, the additional tax is imposed on the combined self-employment income of the taxpayer and the taxpayer's spouse. If a taxpayer, or a taxpayer and his or her spouse, receives both self-employment income and wages which may be subject to the additional Medicare tax that applies for FICA purposes (¶ 2648), then the threshold amount for determining the additional Medicare tax for self-employment purposes is reduced by the taxpayer's wages, but not below zero (Code Sec. 1401(b)(2); Reg. § 1.1401-1(d)). Under these rules, a taxpayer's self-employment tax rate is 15.3 percent (12.4 percent + 2.9 percent) of the taxpayer's self-employment income up to the Social Security wage base in effect for the year, 2.9 percent of self-employment income above the Social Security wage base not in excess of the threshold amount for the additional 0.9 percent tax, and 3.8 percent (2.9 percent + 0.9 percent) of any self-employment income above that threshold amount.

> **Example:** Carl, a single filer, has $130,000 in wages and $145,000 in self-employment income. Carl's wages are not in excess of the $200,000 threshold for single filers, so he is not liable for the additional Medicare tax on these wages for FICA purposes. Before calculating the additional Medicare tax on self-employment income, the $200,000 threshold for single filers is reduced by Carl's $130,000 in wages, resulting in a reduced self-employment income threshold of $70,000. Carl is liable to pay the additional Medicare tax on $75,000 of self-employment income ($145,000 minus $70,000).

Reporting Requirements. The self-employment tax is computed on Schedule SE of Form 1040 and is treated as part of the taxpayer's income tax liability and must also be taken into account for purposes of the estimated tax (Code Sec. 6654(f)) (¶ 2682). A married couple filing a joint return must file separate Schedules SE where each spouse is self-employed.

2667. Persons Subject to Self-Employment Tax. An individual who is self-employed is subject to a self-employment tax (¶ 2664) if they earn $433.13 or more of self-employment income in a year (¶ 2670). An individual is generally self-employed if he or she carries on a trade or business as a sole proprietor or independent contractor (¶ 2602), or is a member of a partnership that carries on a trade or business (Code Sec. 1402(c)).[85] A trade or business does not include the performance of services by an individual as an employee, but certain employee services are treated as a trade or business and are therefore subject to self-employment tax.

Members of religious orders who have taken vows of poverty are not subject to self-employment tax when they perform duties connected with their religious order (Code Sec. 1402(c)(4) and (5)).[86] Also, a duly ordained, commissioned, or licensed minister of a church, a member of a religious order (who has not taken a vow of poverty), or a Christian Science practitioner may elect not to be covered by Social Security by filing an exemption certificate on Form 4361 indicating that he or she is opposed by conscience or religious principle to the acceptance of any public insurance. The statement must include a declaration that he or she has informed the ordaining, commissioning, or licensing body of the church of the individual's opposition to such insurance. A qualified individual must apply for the exemption on or before the due date of the income tax

---

References are to Standard Federal Tax Reports; Tax Research Consultant; and Practical Tax Explanations.

[84] ¶ 32,560; INDIV: 63,050; § 23,110.10

[85] ¶ 32,560; INDIV: 63,300; § 23,001

[86] ¶ 32,560; INDIV: 63,400; § 23,501

¶2667

return for the second tax year for which the individual had earnings from self-employment of $400 or more from religious activities (Code Sec. 1402(e)). An individual who has conscientious objections to insurance by reason of an adherence to established tenets or teachings of a religious sect of which he or she is a member may also be exempt from the self-employment tax (Code Sec. 1402(g)).

Services performed by employees for a church or church-controlled organization may be excluded from Social Security coverage if the church or organization makes a valid election under Code Sec. 3121(w) to be exempt from the employer portion of FICA taxes. However, such employees remain liable for FICA or self-employment tax on remuneration paid for such services unless the remuneration is less than $100 per year (Code Sec. 1402(a)(14) and (j)).[87]

A U.S. citizen who works for an employer that is exempt from the Social Security tax because it is either a foreign government or instrumentality or an international organization is treated as self-employed (Code Sec. 1402(c)(2)).[88] Nonresident aliens are not subject to self-employment tax, but the tax may apply to a resident of Puerto Rico, the Virgin Islands, Guam or American Samoa who is not a citizen of the United States (Code Sec. 1402(b)).[89]

2670. Self-Employment Income. The self-employment tax (¶ 2664) is imposed on self-employment income derived from an individual during the tax year. Self-employment income is generally defined as net earnings from self-employment which consists of: (1) the gross income derived from any trade or business, less allowable deductions attributable to the trade or business, and (2) the taxpayer's distributive share of the ordinary income or loss of a partnership engaged in a trade or business (Code Sec. 1402(b); Reg. § 1.1402(a)-1).[90] The term trade or business does not include services performed as an employee other than services relating to certain newspaper and magazine sales, sharing of crops, foreign organizations, and sharing of fishing catches (Code Sec. 1402(c)(2)).[91]

There are special rules for computing net earnings from self-employment, including a special optional method of computing net earnings from nonfarm self-employment (¶ 2673) (Code Sec. 1402(a)).[92] Rents from real estate and from personal property leased with the real estate, and the attributable deductions, are excluded from net earnings from self-employment unless received by the individual in the course of his business as a real estate dealer. Rental real estate income that is otherwise excludable does not become self-employment income merely because it is held in a qualified joint venture (¶ 402) (CCA 200816030).

Dividends and interest from any bond, debenture, note, certificate or other evidence of indebtedness issued with interest coupons or in registered form by any corporation are excluded from net earnings from self-employment income unless received by a dealer in stocks and securities in the course of his business. Other interest received in the course of any trade or business is not excluded. Gain or loss from the sale or exchange of property that is not stock in trade or held primarily for sale is excluded, as is gain or loss from the sale or exchange of a capital asset.

Termination payments received by former insurance salespersons are excludable from net earnings from self-employment if the amount is received after the termination of the individual's agreement to perform services for the company and the individual performs no services for the company after the termination and before the close of the tax year. In addition, the payment must be conditioned upon the salesperson agreeing not to compete with the company for at least one year following termination. The payment amount must also depend primarily on policies sold by or credited to the individual during the last year of the agreement and/or the extent to which the policies remain in force for some period after the termination and does not depend on the length

---

References are to Standard Federal Tax Reports; Tax Research Consultant; and Practical Tax Explanations.

[87] ¶ 32,560; INDIV: 63,308; § 23,045.10

[88] ¶ 32,560; INDIV: 63,154; § 23,045.10

[89] ¶ 32,560; INDIV: 63,302; § 23,110.20

[90] ¶ 32,560, ¶ 32,561; INDIV: 63,100; § 23,205

[91] ¶ 32,560; INDIV: 63,154; § 23,045.10

[92] ¶ 32,560; INDIV: 63,050; § 23,210.05

of service or overall earnings from services performed for the company (Code Sec. 1402(k)).[93]

Even though the rental value of a parsonage (¶ 875) and the value of meals and lodging furnished for the convenience of the employer (¶ 2089) are not included in a minister's gross income for income tax purposes, they are taken into account in calculating net earnings from self-employment (Code Sec. 1402(a)(8)).[94] The same is true of amounts excluded from gross income as foreign earned income (¶ 2402). However, self-employment income does not include a minister's retirement benefits received from a church plan or the rental value of a parsonage allowance as long as each was furnished after the date of retirement.

One business deduction that cannot be taken in calculating net earnings from self-employment for the tax year is the deduction allowed for self-employment tax paid during the year (¶ 923). However, the law provides a substitute for that deduction. This is an amount determined by multiplying net earnings from self-employment (calculated without regard to the substitute deduction) by one-half of the self-employment tax rate (Code Sec. 1402(a)(12)).[95] Thus, the deduction equals 7.65 percent of the net earnings from self-employment. The rate of the adjustment is 7.65 percent in 2011 and 2012 even though the self-employment tax rate was reduced (¶ 2664) (Act Sec. 601 of P.L. 111-312, amended by Act Sec. 1001 of P.L. 112-96). Similarly, for tax years beginning after 2012, taxpayers who reduce self-employment income by an amount equal to one-half of the combined self-employment tax rate do not include the additional 0.9 percent Medicare tax in the rate used to make such computation.

> **Example:** Aileen Smith, a self-employed individual, has $40,000 of net earnings from self-employment during the year (determined without regard to the substitute deduction). Her self-employment tax is computed as follows:
>
> | | |
> |---|---:|
> | Self-employment net earnings . . . . | $40,000 |
> | Less: $40,000 × 7.65% . . . . | 3,060 |
> | Reduced self-employment net earnings . . . . | $36,940 |
> | Tax rate on self-employment income | × 15.3% |
> | Self-employment tax | $5,652 |

2673. Optional Method for Nonfarm Self-Employment. A taxpayer may be able to use an optional method to compute net earnings from self-employment if the net earnings from nonfarm self-employment for 2014 are less than $4,800 ("lower limit") and less than two-thirds of gross nonfarm income. In addition, the optional method may only be used if the taxpayer had net earnings from self-employment of $400 or more in at least two of the three years immediately preceding the year in which the nonfarm optional method is elected (Code Sec. 1402(a) and (l)).[96]

If the taxpayer is eligible to use the optional method, he or she may report two-thirds of the gross income from the nonfarm business as net earnings from self-employment, provided the gross income from all nonfarm trades or businesses for 2014 is $7,200 ("upper limit") or less. If, however, the gross income from all nonfarm trades or businesses is more than $4,800, the individual may report $4,800 as net earnings from nonfarm self-employment. The optional nonfarm method may not be used to report an amount less than actual net earnings from self-employment. The purpose of this optional method is to permit taxpayers to pay into the Social Security system and thus obtain or increase their benefits, even though they are not otherwise eligible because their net self-employment income is under $400. This optional method may not be used more than five times by any individual. Note that the $4,800 amount refers to net earnings after reduction by the 7.65 percent deduction amount (¶ 2670).

References are to Standard Federal Tax Reports; Tax Research Consultant; and Practical Tax Explanations.

[93] ¶ 32,560; INDIV: 63,100; § 23,210.25

[94] ¶ 32,560; INDIV: 63,402; § 23,505.05

[95] ¶ 32,560; INDIV: 63,060; § 23,210.30

[96] ¶ 32,560; INDIV: 63,056; § 23,215.10

2676. Farmer's Self-Employment Income. A special method for determining self-employment net earnings is provided for farm operators whether they own the land they farm, rent on a fixed rental basis, or rent under a share-farming arrangement. Rentals received by the owner or tenant of the land under a share-farming arrangement—where the farm is operated by a third party such as a share-farmer who may be a subtenant—are treated as self-employment income (¶ 2670) if the owner or tenant participates materially with the share-farmer working the land in the production or management of the production of an agricultural or horticultural commodity. There is no material participation if the owner or tenant does not participate in operations and has turned over management of the land to an agent, such as a professional farm management company. The share-farmer is also considered a self-employed person (Code Sec. 1402(a)(1); Reg. § 1.1402(a)-4).[97]

Payments made by the U.S. Department of Agriculture under its Conservation Reserve Program (CRP) are considered earnings from a trade or business and are includible in the self-employment income of farmers, regardless of whether the farmer actively engages in farming or ceases all farming activities (Notice 2006-108). CRP payments are excluded from an individual's net earnings from self-employment, provided the individual is receiving retirement or disability benefits from Social Security.

A self-employed farmer has to pay the self-employment tax if his net earnings from self-employment are $400 or more (Code Sec. 1402(b)). However, an optional method for reporting income from farming, providing for greater credit toward benefits under Social Security old-age and survivors insurance, is available to a farmer. If the farmer's gross income for 2014 is not more than $7,200 ("upper limit"), he or she can report two-thirds of gross income as net earnings from self-employment (Code Sec. 1402(a)). If the farmer has more than $7,200 of gross income from farm operations in 2014, he or she may report either actual net earnings or, if net earnings are less than $4,800 ("lower limit"), $4,800 as net earnings. As in the case of the nonfarm optional method, the $4,800 amount refers to net earnings after reduction by the 7.65 percent deduction. There is no limit on the number of times a taxpayer may use this optional method.

> **Example:** Breanna Jones owns and operates her own farm. She receives all her income from the operation of the farm. Her gross income (receipts minus cost of goods sold) for 2014 is $7,500, but her net earnings for that year are only $4,000. She cannot simply report $5,000 (⅔ of $7,500) since her gross income is over $7,200, but she can report $4,800 as her net earnings from self-employment even though her actual net earnings are only $4,000. In electing to pay the self-employment tax on $4,800 rather than on $4,000, she will pay a greater tax. The positive effect, however, is that she will theoretically receive a greater credit toward Social Security benefits.

Payment of Estimated Taxes

2682. Estimated Taxes for Individuals. Individuals may need to pay a portion of their tax liability through estimated tax payments over the course of the tax year rather than when they file their return. Estimated taxes are generally used to pay tax on income that is not subject to withholding such as from interest, dividends, and gains from the sale of assets. An individual may also have to pay estimated tax if the amount of tax being withheld from wages or other income is not enough. Thus, estimated taxes are used to pay income and self-employment tax for the tax year, as well as other taxes reported on the taxpayer's return, including the 3.8 percent tax on net investment income (¶ 129) and the 0.9 percent additional Medicare tax (¶ 2648 and ¶ 2664), less any estimated credits against tax.

While the law does not directly impose an obligation to pay estimated taxes, it does impose a penalty (or addition to tax) on individuals for failure to pay enough tax either

---

References are to Standard Federal Tax Reports; Tax Research Consultant; and Practical Tax Explanations.

[97] ¶ 32,560, ¶ 32,564; INDIV: 63,450, INDIV: 63,254; § 23,215.15

¶2676

through withholding or estimated taxes (¶ 2875) (Code Sec. 6654).[98] To avoid the penalty, an individual must generally make four required installment payments of estimated taxes based on his or her required annual payment. In general, each installment is 25 percent of the lesser of:

- 90 percent of the tax shown on the individual's tax return for the current year, or

- 100 percent of the tax shown on the priors year's return (110 percent in the case of an individual with adjusted gross income in excess of $150,000; $75,000 for a married individual filing separately), unless the prior year was not a 12-month period (Code Sec. 6654(d)(1)).[99]

A lower required installment payment may be made if the individual annualizes his or her tax at the end of each payment period based on a reasonable estimate of income, deductions, and credits (Code Sec. 6654(d)(2)). The annualized installment method may be used if the taxpayer does not receive income evenly throughout the year. Special rules also apply for farmers and fishermen (¶ 2691). Regardless of whether an individual uses the regular or annualized installment method, each required installment must be paid by its due date (¶ 2685), unless the taxpayer files his or her tax return before January 31 of the following year (¶ 2688).

An individual uses Form 1040-ES to figure his or her required installment of estimated taxes, and payment is made using the appropriate payment voucher attached to the form. In calculating estimated tax payments, any taxes withheld from an individual's wages or other income is deemed a payment of estimated taxes (Code Sec. 6654(g)). Thus, an equal part of withheld taxes is deemed paid on each due date for the tax year, unless the taxpayer establishes the dates when all taxes were actually withheld. For rules on payment of estimated tax by a corporation, or trusts and estates, see ¶ 241 and ¶ 511, respectively.

Exceptions to Penalty. The penalty for failure to pay estimated tax will not apply to an individual whose tax liability for the year is less than $1,000 after credits for withheld taxes and refundable personal credits. Also, a U.S. citizen or resident alien will not be subject to the penalty if he or she had no tax liability for the preceding tax year, provided such year was a 12-month period. Under certain circumstances or hardship, or following an individual's retirement or disability, the penalty may be waived (Code Sec. 6654(e)).[100]

Married Taxpayers. Individuals who are married may make a joint estimated tax payment, even if they are living separate and apart (Reg. § 1.6654-2(e)(5)).[101] Joint estimated payments are not allowed if:

- there is a decree of separate maintenance or divorce;

- the married taxpayers have different tax years; or

- the taxpayer's spouse is a nonresident alien (including a bona fide resident of Puerto Rico or U.S. possession for the entire tax year (¶ 2414)), unless an election has been made to treat the spouse as a resident alien (¶ 2410), or the spouse becomes a resident alien during the tax year.

Joint estimated payments are based on the aggregate taxable income. In the event of married taxpayers filing separately, however, the amount of estimated self-employment tax is based on the separate income of each individual.

Household Employees. Employers of domestic workers who fail to satisfy their obligations for FICA and FUTA withholding, through regular estimated tax payments or

---

References are to Standard Federal Tax Reports; Tax Research Consultant; and Practical Tax Explanations.

[98] ¶ 39,550; FILEIND: 15,350; § 1,401

[99] ¶ 39,550; FILEIND: 15,352; § 1,405.05

[100] ¶ 39,550; FILEIND: 15,354; § 1,435.05

[101] ¶ 39,553; FILEIND: 15,352; § 1,415

increased tax withholding from their own wages, may be liable for estimated tax penalties (¶ 2652).

2685. Estimated Tax Payment Due Dates for Individuals. For estimated tax purposes of individuals (¶ 2682), the year is broken down into four payment periods (Code Sec. 6654(c)(2)).[102] In 2015, a calendar-year individual is required to pay estimated tax in four installments as follows:

Installment	Due date
First	April 15, 2015
Second	June 15, 2015
Third	September 15, 2015
Fourth	January 15, 2016

If a taxpayer files his or her tax return for the current year and pays the full tax due by January 31 of the following year, then the taxpayer does not have to make the fourth estimated tax payment that would otherwise have been due on January 15 (¶ 2688).

For fiscal-year individuals, the due dates for the four estimated tax payments are:

(1) the 15th day of the fourth month of the fiscal year,

(2) the 15th day of the sixth month of the fiscal year,

(3) the 15th day of the ninth month of the fiscal year, and

(4) the 15th day of the first month after the end of the fiscal year.

If the due date for making an estimated tax payment falls on a Saturday, Sunday, or legal holiday, the payment will be timely if made on the next day that is not a Saturday, Sunday, or legal holiday (¶ 2549).

If an individual is not liable for estimated tax on March 31, 2015, but his or her tax situation changes so that he or she becomes liable for estimated tax at some point after March 31, then the individual must make estimated tax payments as follows.

• If the individual becomes required to pay estimated tax after March 31 and before June 1, then he or she should pay 50 percent of estimated tax on or before June 15, 2015, 25 percent on September 15, 2015, and 25 percent on January 15, 2016.

• If the individual becomes required to pay estimated tax after May 31 and before September 1, then he or she should pay 75 percent of estimated tax on or before September 15, 2015, and 25 percent on January 15, 2016.

• If the individual becomes required to pay estimated tax after August 31, then he or she should pay 100 percent of estimated tax by January 15, 2016 (Form 1040-ES; IRS Pub. 505).

Nonresident Alien Individuals. Nonresident alien individuals (except those whose wages are subject to withholding) must pay estimated taxes for 2015 in three installments (June 15, 2015, September 15, 2015, and January 15, 2016). Fifty percent of the annual payment must be made on the first installment due date and 25 percent on each of the remaining two installment due dates (Code Sec. 6654(j)).[103]

2688. Return as Substitute for Last Installment of 2014 Estimated Tax. The fourth (last) tax installment of an individual (¶ 2685) for the 2014 tax year need not be made if the taxpayer files a Form 1040 tax return and pays the balance of the tax on or before January 31, 2015, or for a fiscal year, on or before the last day of the month following the close of the fiscal year. Filing a final 2014 return by January 31, 2015, with payment of any tax due will not avoid an addition to tax for underpayment of any of the first three installments that were due for the year, but it will terminate the period of underpayment (and, therefore, the accrual of further additions) as of January 15, 2015 (Code Sec. 6654(h)).[104]

References are to Standard Federal Tax Reports; Tax Research Consultant; and Practical Tax Explanations.

[102] ¶ 39,550; FILEIND: 15,352; § 1,410

[103] ¶ 39,550; FILEIND: 21,052.25; § 1,420

[104] ¶ 39,550; FILEIND: 15,352; § 1,410

2691. Farmer or Fisherman. A farmer or fisherman who expects to receive at least two-thirds of his or her gross income for the tax year from farming or fishing, or who received at least two-thirds of gross income for the previous tax year from farming or fishing, may pay estimated tax for the year in one installment. Thus, a qualifying farmer or fisherman may wait until January 15, 2015, to make a 2014 estimated tax payment. The entire amount of 2014 estimated tax must be paid at that time. However, the January 15 payment date may be ignored if the farmer or fisherman files his or her income tax return for 2014 and pays the entire tax due by March 2, 2015. The penalty for underpayment of estimated tax (¶ 2875) does not apply unless a farmer or fisherman underpays the tax by more than one-third (Code Sec. 6654(i)).[105] If a joint return is filed, a farmer or fisherman must consider his or her spouse's gross income in determining whether at least two-thirds of gross income is from farming or fishing.

References are to Standard Federal Tax Reports; Tax Research Consultant; and Practical Tax Explanations.

[105] ¶ 39,550; FILEIND: 21,052.20; § 36,510.05

26 WITHHOLDING

Chapter 27

EXAMINATION OF RETURNS
COLLECTION OF TAX

Organization of IRS

2701. IRS Organization and Functions. The Internal Revenue Service (IRS) is the bureau of the Treasury Department responsible for determining, assessing, and collecting federal taxes and enforcing the Internal Revenue Code. The IRS consists of an Associate Office in Washington, D.C., and a field organization. The Associate Office is the Office of the Commissioner of Internal Revenue, who heads the IRS. Among the principal offices of the IRS are: the Office of the Deputy Commissioner (Operations); the Office of the Associate Commissioner (Policy and Management); the Office of the Associate Commissioner (Computer Services); the Office of the Assistant Commissioner (Taxpayer Service and Returns Processing); and the Office of the Chief Counsel. The Office of Inspector General of the Treasury Department has oversight responsibility for the internal investigations performed by the Office of Assistant Commissioner (Inspection) of the IRS.

The IRS is organized into four operating divisions serving groups of taxpayers with similar needs. These operating divisions are:

> (1) Wage and Investment, serving individual taxpayers with wage and investment income,

> (2) Small Business/Self-Employed, serving self-employed individuals and small businesses with assets of $10 million or less,

> (3) Large Business and International, serving C corporations, S corporations and partnerships with assets of greater than $10 million, and

> (4) Tax-Exempt and Government Entities, serving employee plans, exempt organizations, and government entities.

IRS field offices also include a number of IRS service centers. These service centers currently receive and process tax and information returns, manage accounts, and conduct simple audits. The IRS also maintains a national computer center located near Martinsburg, West Virginia.

In addition, a nine-member IRS Oversight Board has been created to ensure that the IRS is organized and operated to carry out its mission to place a greater emphasis on serving the public and meeting taxpayers' needs (Code Sec. 7802).[1]

2703. Office of Chief Counsel. The legal work of the IRS is performed by the Office of the Chief Counsel (Code Sec. 7803(b)).[2] The Chief Counsel is a member of the Commissioner's executive staff and acts as counsel and legal adviser to the Commis-

---

References are to Standard Federal Tax Reports; Tax Research Consultant; and Practical Tax Explanations.

[1] ¶ 43,254; IRS: 3,060; § 41,005   [2] ¶ 43,258; IRS: 3,056; § 41,005

sioner in all matters pertaining to the administration and enforcement of the Internal Revenue Code. There are also Division Counsels, subject to the general supervision of the Chief Counsel, in each of the IRS operating divisions (¶ 2701).

2705. Appeals Procedure. If a tax return is examined by the IRS and the taxpayer does not agree with the results of the examination, further appeal within the IRS is permitted (Reg. § 601.106).[3] Once the IRS has issued a preliminary 30-day letter, the taxpayer has the right to appeal to a local Appeals Office by filing a written request for appellate consideration. This is the only level of appeal within the IRS, disregarding the functions of the National Taxpayer Advocate (¶ 2707). Appeals conferences are conducted in an informal manner. A taxpayer who requests a conference may also need to file a formal written protest. If the protested amount is not more than $25,000 for any tax period, however, a taxpayer may make a small case request instead of a formal written protest (IRS Pub. 556). Taxpayers who wish to forego the right to submit a protest to the Appeals Office after receiving a 30-day letter can file a petition in the Tax Court within 90 days after the receipt of a statutory notice of deficiency.

The IRS is required to develop certain appeals dispute resolution procedures (Code Sec. 7123).[4] Accordingly, the IRS has established procedures under which any taxpayer may request early referral of issues from the examination or collection division to the Office of Appeals (Rev. Proc. 99-28). Additionally, procedures have been developed under which either a taxpayer or the Office of Appeals may request nonbinding mediation of any unresolved issue at the conclusion of the appeals procedure or an unsuccessful attempt to enter into a closing agreement or an offer in compromise (Rev. Proc. 2009-44). Also, an appeals arbitration process under which the Office of Appeals and the taxpayer may jointly request binding arbitration has been established (Rev. Proc. 2006-44).

Small business and self-employed taxpayers can resolve their tax disputes through fast-track mediation (Rev. Proc. 2003-41). Disputes will be resolved through this expedited process within 40 days, compared to several months using the regular appeals process.

Large- and mid-size businesses can resolve their tax disputes through a fast-track settlement program (Rev. Proc. 2003-40). The goal for this program is to reach settlement within 120 days. A similar fast-track settlement pilot program exists for small businesses and self-employed taxpayers in Chicago, Houston, Philadelphia, St. Paul, and San Diego, as well as central New Jersey, and Laguna Nigel and Riverside, California. Additional locations may be identified and added by the IRS (Announcement 2011-5). A fast-track settlement program for tax-exempt and government entities has also been established (Announcement 2012-34). The goal for both this program and the small business and self-employed taxpayer program is to reach settlement within 60 days.

2707. Taxpayer Assistance Orders. The National Taxpayer Advocate assists taxpayers in resolving problems with the IRS and has the authority to issue a taxpayer assistance order if a taxpayer is suffering, or is about to suffer, significant hardship as a result of the IRS's actions (Code Secs. 7803(c) and 7811; Reg. § 301.7811-1).[5] "Significant hardship" means any serious privation caused to the taxpayer as the result of the IRS's administration of revenue laws. Mere economic or personal inconvenience to the taxpayer does not constitute significant hardship. The following four specific factors, among other things, must be considered by the Advocate when determining whether there is a significant hardship:

    (1) whether there is an immediate threat of adverse action,

    (2) whether there has been a delay of more than 30 days in resolving the taxpayer's account problems,

---

References are to Standard Federal Tax Reports; Tax Research Consultant; and Practical Tax Explanations.

[3] ¶ 43,336; IRS: 24,050; § 39,605, § 39,615

[4] ¶ 41,132, ¶ 41,135.10, ¶ 41,135.40; IRS: 24,106; § 39,740.05

[5] ¶ 43,258, ¶ 43,304, ¶ 43,308; IRS: 3,058, IRS: 45,112; § 41,315

(3) whether the taxpayer will incur significant costs, including fees for professional representation, if relief is not granted, and

(4) whether the taxpayer will suffer irreparable injury, or a long-term adverse impact, if relief is not granted.

An application for a taxpayer assistance order may be filed by the taxpayer or a duly authorized representative, who may request remedial action, such as the release of the taxpayer's property from IRS levy or the immediate reissuance of a lost refund check. Form 911 is to be used for this purpose. Any relevant limitations period is suspended from the date on which the application is filed until the Advocate makes a decision on the application, unless the order provides for the continuation of the suspension beyond the date of the order. These orders are binding on the IRS unless modified or rescinded by the Advocate, IRS Commissioner or Deputy Commissioner. The Advocate can take independent action and issue an assistance order without an application by the taxpayer. The statute of limitations, however, is not suspended when the Advocate issues an order independently.

Examination

2708. Examination of Return. The IRS examines a taxpayer's books and records either at the place of business where the books and records are maintained (i.e., a field examination) or at an IRS office (Reg. § 601.105).[6]

The Taxpayer Bill of Rights requires the IRS to provide a written statement detailing the taxpayer's rights and the IRS's obligations during the audit, appeals, refund, and collection process. Additionally, at or before the first in-person interview with a taxpayer relating to the determination of any tax, the IRS must provide the taxpayer with an explanation of the audit process and the taxpayer's rights under the process (Code Sec. 7521(b)).[7]

The taxpayer has the right to make an audio recording of any in-person interview conducted by the IRS upon 10 days' advance notice (Code Sec. 7521(a); Notice 89-51).[8] Moreover, a taxpayer is guaranteed the right to be represented by any individual currently permitted to practice before the IRS, unless the IRS notifies the taxpayer that the representative is responsible for unreasonable delay or hindrance (Code Sec. 7521(c)).[9] Any interview must be suspended when the taxpayer clearly requests the right to consult with a representative. Further, unless it issues an administrative summons, the IRS cannot require the taxpayer to accompany the representative to the interview.

The IRS may provide administrative relief to taxpayers in hostage situations or in a combat zone, or who are continuously hospitalized as a result of injuries received in a combat zone, or who are affected by a federally declared disaster area, by suspending tax examination and collection actions during their detention (Code Secs. 7508 and 7508A).[10] Examination and collection actions that can be precluded or suspended include tax return audits, mailings of notices, and other actions involving the collection of overdue taxes.

2708A. Power of Attorney. A taxpayer generally may choose a person to represent him or her before the IRS by filing a power of attorney (Reg. § 601.501(a)).[11] A power of attorney is a written authorization for an individual to act on behalf of another individual or an entity in tax matters. Form 2848 can be used to grant a power of attorney, or another equivalent document can be used. If the authorization is not limited, the individual can generally perform all acts that the taxpayer granting the power can perform. The holder of a power of attorney cannot, however, represent the taxpayer before the IRS unless the holder is one of the persons authorized to practice before the IRS (CCA 200321017).

References are to Standard Federal Tax Reports; Tax Research Consultant; and Practical Tax Explanations.

[6] ¶ 43,332; IRS: 15,100; § 39,715

[7] ¶ 42,790; IRS: 45,112; § 39,705

[8] ¶ 42,790, ¶ 42,791.30; IRS: 15,110; § 39,715.15

[9] ¶ 42,790; IRS: 18,202; § 39,715.10

[10] ¶ 42,686, ¶ 42,687A; FILEBUS: 15,100; § 39,215.30, § 39,215.35

[11] ¶ 43,408; IRS: 3,208.05; § 41,205.05

A taxpayer may change his or her representative by filing a new power of attorney (Reg. § 601.505(a)).[12] The new power revokes any prior power that the taxpayer granted to someone else concerning the same matter unless the new power contains a clause stating that it does not revoke the prior power. A taxpayer may also revoke a power of attorney without authorizing a new representative.

A taxpayer who only wants to have someone answer any questions that may arise regarding his or her income tax return does not have to file a power of attorney. Instead, the taxpayer can designate anyone to do this, not just a person qualified to practice before the IRS, by checking the appropriate box on his or her tax return (Instruction to Form 1040).

2709. Third-Party Summonses. The IRS may issue summonses to third-party recordkeepers (attorneys, enrolled agents, banks, brokers, accountants, etc.) and other third parties for the production of records concerning the business transactions or affairs of a taxpayer (Code Sec. 7609).[13] The taxpayer is to be notified of the summons within three days of service of the summons, but no later than 23 days before the examination of the summoned person or records is schedule to take place. However, notice is not required with respect to any summons:

> (1) served on the person with respect to whose liability the summons is issued, or any officer or employee of the person,

> (2) issued to determine whether or not records of the business transactions or affairs of an identified person have been made or kept,

> (3) issued solely to determine the identity of any person having a numbered account or similar arrangement with a bank or similar institution,

> (4) issued to aid the collection of (a) an assessment or judgment against the person with respect to whose liability the summons is issued, or (b) the liability of that person's transferee or fiduciary, or

> (5) issued in certain criminal investigations.

Any taxpayer who is entitled to notice may intervene in any proceeding for the enforcement of the summons in question. The taxpayer also has the right to begin a proceeding to quash the summons if, within 20 days after the day the notice of summons was served on or mailed to him or her, the taxpayer files a petition to quash the summons in a district court having jurisdiction and notifies the IRS and the third party by mailing a copy of the petition by certified or registered mail to each one. Although notice is not required for a "John Doe" summons (i.e., a summons that does not identify the person whose liability is at issue), these summonses may be issued only after the IRS has shown adequate grounds for serving the summons, and an ex parte court proceeding is held to determine its validity.

If a taxpayer intervenes in a dispute between the IRS and a third party and the dispute is not resolved within six months, the statute-of-limitations period will be suspended beginning on the date that is six months after the summons is served and continuing until the dispute is resolved. This provision also applies with respect to "John Doe" summonses (Code Sec. 7609(e)).[14]

The IRS is required to provide reasonable notice in advance to a taxpayer before contacting third parties with respect to examination or collection activities regarding the taxpayer (Code Sec. 7602(c); Reg. § 301.7602-2).[15] However, notice is *not* required: (1) with respect to any contact authorized by the taxpayer, (2) if the IRS determines that the notice would jeopardize collection of any tax, or (3) with respect to any pending criminal investigation.

References are to Standard Federal Tax Reports; Tax Research Consultant; and Practical Tax Explanations.

[12] ¶ 43,424; IRS: 3,208.15; § 41,210

[13] ¶ 42,890; IRS: 21,100, IRS: 21,150; § 39,810

[14] ¶ 42,890; IRS: 21,114; § 39,810

[15] ¶ 42,820, ¶ 42,824; IRS: 21,106; § 39,810

Assessment and Collection of Tax

2711. Assessment of Deficiency. The IRS is authorized to assess taxes (Code Sec. 6201; Reg. § 301.6201-1).[16] There are, however, certain procedures that must be followed before assessing a deficiency. A deficiency is the excess of the correct tax liability over the tax shown on the return, if any, plus amounts previously assessed or collected without assessment as a deficiency, and minus any rebates made to the taxpayer (Code Sec. 6211).[17] For this purpose, the tax shown on the return is the amount of tax before credits for estimated tax paid, withheld tax, or amounts collected under a termination assessment.

The deficiency process begins when a notice of deficiency is sent to the taxpayer's last known address by registered or certified mail (Code Sec. 6212).[18] In each deficiency notice, the IRS must provide a description of the basis for the assessment, an identification of the amount of tax, interest, and penalties assessed (Code Sec. 7522),[19] and the date determined to be the last day on which the taxpayer may file a petition with the Tax Court (Code Sec. 6213(a)).[20] However, the failure by the IRS to specify the last day on which to file a petition will not invalidate an otherwise valid deficiency notice if the taxpayer was not prejudiced by the omission.[21]

Within 90 days after notice of the deficiency is mailed (or within 150 days after mailing if the notice is addressed to a person outside the United States), the taxpayer may file a petition with the Tax Court for a redetermination of the deficiency (Code Sec. 6213).[22] Payment of the assessed amount after the deficiency notice is mailed does not deprive the Tax Court of jurisdiction over the deficiency (Reg. § 301.6213-1(b)(3)).[23]

If the taxpayer does not file a Tax Court petition within the required time period, the tax may be assessed. After giving notice and demand for payment of the tax, the IRS may take action to collect (¶ 2735). A taxpayer's property may be seized to enforce collection if there is a failure to pay an assessed tax within 30 days after notice of intent to levy (Code Sec. 6331).[24] However, the notice and waiting period does not apply if the IRS finds that the collection of tax is in jeopardy (¶ 2713). Notices of levy must provide a description of the levy process in simple and nontechnical terms.

Last Known Address. As noted above, the collection process begins when a notice of deficiency is sent to the taxpayer's last known address by registered or certified mail. A taxpayer's last known address is the address that appears on the taxpayer's most recently filed federal tax return. However, if the taxpayer gives the IRS clear and concise notification of a different address, that address is the taxpayer's last known address (Reg. § 301.6212-2).[25] The IRS uses the National Change of Address database maintained by the U.S. Postal Service to update a taxpayer's last known address. A taxpayer can change his or her last known address with the IRS through any of several means (Rev. Proc. 2010-16).[26] First, the taxpayer can file a return with new address information. Second, the taxpayer can provide clear and concise written notification to an appropriate IRS address using Form 8822, Form 8822-B for employers, or other written notice satisfying the requirements including returning IRS correspondence with corrections marked (IRS Pub. 15). Next, the taxpayer can provide clear and concise written or oral notification of a change of address to an IRS employee who contacts the client regarding the filing of a return or an adjustment in his or her account. Finally, the taxpayer can provide the IRS with clear and concise electronic notification through one of the secure applications found on the IRS website.

References are to Standard Federal Tax Reports; Tax Research Consultant; and Practical Tax Explanations.

[16] ¶ 37,502, ¶ 37,503; IRS: 27,200; § 39,501

[17] ¶ 37,535; IRS: 27,052; § 39,510.10

[18] ¶ 37,540; IRS: 27,150; § 39,510.15

[19] ¶ 42,800; IRS: 27,154; § 39,510.05

[20] ¶ 37,545; IRS: 27,154; § 39,510.05

[21] ¶ 37,544.25; IRS: 27,154.05; § 39,510.05

[22] ¶ 37,545; IRS: 27,158; § 39,510.05

[23] ¶ 37,546; LITIG: 6,100; § 39,510.05

[24] ¶ 38,185; IRS: 51,054; § 39,945.15

[25] ¶ 37,542; IRS: 27,160; § 39,510.15

[26] ¶ 37,544.28, ¶ 37,549.5023; IRS: 27,160.05; § 39,510.15

Mathematical or Clerical Errors. A notice of tax due because of mathematical or clerical errors is not a deficiency notice, and the taxpayer has no right to file a petition with the Tax Court for redetermining the deficiency. A taxpayer who receives notice of additional tax due to mathematical or clerical error has 60 days after the notice is sent in which to file a request for abatement of any part of the assessment. Any reassessment must be made under the regular notice-of-deficiency procedures. During the 60-day period, the IRS cannot proceed to collect upon the summary assessment (Code Sec. 6213(b)(1) and (f)).[27]

Criminal Restitution. Criminal restitution for a failure to pay tax, ordered by a court pursuant to 18 USC §3556, is assessed and collected as if it were such a tax (Code Sec. 6201(a)(4)(A)).[28] The restitution assessment is excepted from the general restrictions on assessments and filing of Tax Court petitions for deficiency redetermination. The restitution amount may be assessed, or a court proceeding for its collection may be begun without assessment, at any time.

2712. Waiver of Deficiency Restrictions. The taxpayer has the right to waive the restrictions on assessment and collection of all or part of a deficiency at any time, whether or not a notice of deficiency has been issued (Code Sec. 6213(d)).[29] This is done by executing Form 870. Execution of a waiver of the restrictions on assessment and collection of the entire deficiency in advance of the statutory ("90-day") notice relieves the IRS of sending such a notice and precludes appeal to the Tax Court. However, an appeal to the Tax Court is not precluded if the waiver covers only part of the deficiency or is executed after receipt of the 90-day deficiency notice. Payment of an amount as tax before issuance of the statutory notice has the effect of a waiver, and, if the amount paid equals or exceeds the amount of a subsequently determined deficiency, it deprives the Tax Court of jurisdiction (Reg. §301.6213-1(b)(3)).[30]

2713. Jeopardy and Termination Assessments. The IRS can immediately determine and assess income tax in a termination assessment if it finds that tax collection is in jeopardy because a taxpayer is leaving the country, or seeking to hide assets, or doing any other act that tends to render collection ineffective (Code Sec. 6851).[31] Similarly, the IRS can immediately assess a deficiency if tax assessment or collection would be jeopardized by delay (Code Sec. 6861).[32] If a jeopardy assessment is made prior to the mailing of the notice of deficiency, the notice must be mailed to the taxpayer within 60 days after the assessment (Code Sec. 6861(b)).[33] If a termination assessment is made, the assessment ends the taxpayer's tax year only for purposes of computing the amount of tax that becomes immediately due and payable. It does not end the tax year for any other purpose. In the case of a termination assessment, the IRS must issue the taxpayer a notice of deficiency within 60 days of the later of (1) the due date, including extensions, of the taxpayer's return for the full tax year or (2) the day on which the taxpayer files the return (Code Sec. 6851(b)).[34]

The IRS may presume that the collection of tax is in jeopardy if an individual in physical possession of more than $10,000 in cash or its equivalent does not claim either ownership of the cash or that it belongs to another person whose identity the IRS can readily ascertain and who acknowledges ownership of the cash. In this case, the IRS may treat the entire amount as gross income taxable at the highest rate specified in Code Sec. 1. The possessor of the cash is entitled to notice of, and the right to challenge, the assessment. However, should the true owner appear, he or she will be substituted for the possessor and all rights will vest in the true owner (Code Sec. 6867).[35]

References are to Standard Federal Tax Reports; Tax Research Consultant; and Practical Tax Explanations.

[27] ¶ 37,545; IRS: 27,206.15; §39,515.10

[28] ¶ 37,502; IRS: 27,206.70; §39,515.10

[29] ¶ 37,545, ¶ 37,549.9612; IRS: 27,208; §39,540.15

[30] ¶ 37,546; LITIG: 6,110; §39,540.15

[31] ¶ 40,402; IRS: 54,100; §39,520, §39,530.10

[32] ¶ 40,460; IRS: 54,050; §39,520, §39,525.05

[33] ¶ 40,460; IRS: 54,050; §39,525.15

[34] ¶ 40,402; IRS: 54,102; §39,530.20

[35] ¶ 40,580; IRS: 54,152; §39,525.10

2719. Injunction to Restrain Collection. The Code prohibits a suit to restrain the assessment or collection of any tax or to restrain the enforcement of liability against a transferee or fiduciary (Code Sec. 7421).[36] Nevertheless, injunctive relief may be available in rare cases if irreparable harm will be done to the taxpayer and the taxpayer shows, at the outset of the suit, that the government could not collect the tax under any circumstances.[37] However, injunctive relief may be obtained for assessment or collection actions (other than jeopardy or termination assessments) if a notice of deficiency has not been mailed to the taxpayer, the period for filing a Tax Court petition has not expired, or a Tax Court proceeding with respect to the tax is pending (Code Sec. 6213(a)).[38]

2721. Closing Agreement. The IRS is authorized to enter into a written agreement with a taxpayer in order to determine conclusively the tax liability for a tax period that ended prior to the date of the agreement (Form 866) or to determine one or more separate items affecting the tax liability for any tax period (Form 906). A closing agreement may also be entered for tax periods that end subsequent to the date of the agreement. Closing agreements may be entered into in order to finally resolve questions of tax liability (Code Sec. 7121; Reg. §§ 301.7121-1 and 601.202).[39] For example, a fiduciary may desire a final determination before an estate is closed or trust assets distributed. Closing agreements are final, conclusive, and binding upon both parties. They cannot be reopened or modified except upon a showing of fraud or malfeasance or the misrepresentation of a material fact.[40] Generally, the IRS is not precluded from later determining additions to tax absent terms in the agreement that specifically address the issue of additions to tax.

2723. Compromise of Tax and Penalty. The IRS may generally compromise a tax liability before it has been referred to the Department of Justice for prosecution or defense. The Attorney General or a delegate may compromise any case after the referral. Interest and penalties, as well as tax, may be compromised (Code Sec. 7122; Reg. § 301.7122-1).[41] Offers-in-compromise based on doubt as to collectibility or effective tax administration are submitted on Form 656, and must be accompanied by a financial statement on Form 433-A (OIC) for an individual or Form 433-B (OIC) for a business. Offers-in-compromise based on doubt as to liability are submitted on Form 656-L (Reg. § 601.203(b)).[42] If the IRS accepts an offer-in-compromise, and the terms of the offer (and collateral agreement, if any) provide for the allocation of payments, the payments will be allocated under the terms of the agreement. If the offer or agreement do not provide for the allocation of payments, the IRS will apply payments, whether paid in installments or in a lump sum, to the periods in the order of priority that the IRS determines will best serve the government's interest (Rev. Proc. 2002-26).[43]

A $186 user fee is generally required when an offer-in-compromise is submitted (Reg. § 300.3).[44] However, no user fee is imposed with respect to offers:

(1) that are based solely on doubt as to liability, or

(2) that are made by low-income taxpayers (i.e., taxpayers whose total monthly income falls at or below income levels based on the U.S. Department of Health and Human Services poverty guidelines).

If an offer is accepted to promote effective tax administration or is accepted based on doubt as to collectibility and a determination that collecting more than the amount offered would create economic hardship, the fee will be applied to the amount of the offer or, upon the taxpayer's request, refunded to the taxpayer. The fee will not be refunded if an offer is withdrawn, rejected, or returned as nonprocessible. The IRS treats offers received by taxpayers in bankruptcy as nonprocessible; however, some courts

---

References are to Standard Federal Tax Reports; Tax Research Consultant; and Practical Tax Explanations.

[36] ¶ 41,680; IRS: 45,152; § 39,940

[37] ¶ 41,683.69, ¶ 41,683.70; IRS: 45,152; § 39,940

[38] ¶ 37,545; IRS: 45,152; § 39,940

[39] ¶ 41,080, ¶ 41,081, ¶ 43,364; IRS: 39,050; § 40,405.15

[40] ¶ 41,090.279; IRS: 39,150; § 40,405.15

[41] ¶ 41,110, ¶ 41,111; IRS: 42,050; § 39,920.05

[42] ¶ 43,372; IRS: 42,100; § 39,920.25

[43] ¶ 9104.63; IRS: 42,150; § 39,920.25

[44] ¶ 41,120; IRS: 42,106; § 39,920.25

have held that the IRS must consider such offers.[45] The IRS has issued detailed procedures for the submission and processing of offers-in-compromise (Rev. Proc. 2003-71).

Partial Payment Requirement. Taxpayers are required to make nonrefundable partial payments with the submission of any offer-in-compromise based on doubt as to collectibility or effective tax administration (Code Sec. 7122(c)). Taxpayers who submit a lump-sum offer (any offer that will be paid in five or fewer installments) must include a payment of 20 percent of the amount offered. Taxpayers who submit a periodic payment offer must include payment of the first proposed installment with the offer and continue making payments under the terms proposed while the offer is being evaluated. Offers that are submitted to the IRS without the required partial payments will be returned to the taxpayer as nonprocessible. Partial payments are not required for offers based solely on doubt as to liability or filed by low-income taxpayers (Notice 2006-68).

The required partial payments are applied to the taxpayer's unpaid liability and are not refundable. Taxpayers may specify the liability to which they want their payments applied. Additionally, the user fee (see above) is applied to the taxpayer's outstanding tax liability. Any offer that is not rejected within 24 months of the date it is submitted is deemed to be accepted. However, any period during which the tax liability to be compromised is in dispute in any judicial proceeding is not taken into account in determining the expiration of the 24-month period (Code Sec. 7122(f)).

2724. Partial Payments. Specific written directions from a taxpayer regarding the application of partial payments of assessed federal income taxes, penalties, and interest made by the taxpayer will be respected (Rev. Proc. 2002-26).[46] A partial payment on deficiencies received without instructions for its application will be applied to tax, penalties, and interest, in the order of priority that best serves the government's interest.

2726. Statute of Limitations for Assessment and Collection. Generally, all income taxes must be assessed within three years after the original return is filed (the last day prescribed by law for filing if the return was filed before the last day) (Code Sec. 6501; Reg. § 301.6501(a)-1).[47] In the case of pass-through entities, the three-year rule begins to run at the time the pass-through entity's shareholder or other beneficial owner files an individual income tax return. A return filed prior to its due date is deemed to have been filed on the due date. A return executed by an IRS official or employee in which the taxpayer has not filed a return will not start the running of the statute of limitations. A proceeding in court without assessment for collection of the tax must commence within the same period. The period can be extended by a written agreement between the taxpayer and the IRS (Code Sec. 6501(c)(4); Reg. § 301.6501(c)-1(d)).[48] Interest on any tax may be assessed and collected at any time during the period within which the tax itself may be collected (Code Sec. 6601(g); Reg. § 301.6601-1(f)).[49]

If, within the 60-day period ending on the last day of the assessment period, the IRS receives an amended return or written document from the taxpayer showing that additional tax is due for the year in question, the period in which to assess such additional tax is extended for 60 days after the day on which the IRS receives the amended return or written document (Code Sec. 6501(c)(7)).[50]

If unused foreign tax credits have been carried back, the statute of limitations on assessment and collection for the year to which the carryback is made will not close until one year after the expiration of the period within which a deficiency may be assessed for the year from which the carryback was made (Code Sec. 6501(i); Reg. § 301.6501(i)-1).[51] Deficiencies attributable to carryback of a net operating loss or the general business credit and research credit may be assessed within the period that applies to the loss or credit year. Deficiencies attributable to the carrying

---

References are to Standard Federal Tax Reports; Tax Research Consultant; and Practical Tax Explanations.

[45] ¶ 41,130.18; IRS: 42,106

[46] ¶ 39,415.329, ¶ 39,780.14; PENALTY: 9,058.10; § 39,320.35

[47] ¶ 38,960, ¶ 38,961; IRS: 30,050; § 39,505.05

[48] ¶ 38,960, ¶ 38,966; IRS: 30,250; § 39,905

[49] ¶ 39,410, ¶ 39,412; PENALTY: 9,052; § 40,105

[50] ¶ 38,960; IRS: 30,056; § 39,505.05

[51] ¶ 38,960, ¶ 38,977; IRS: 30,122; § 39,505.30

¶2726

back of one of those credits as a result of the carryback of another credit, a net operating loss, or a capital loss may be assessed within the period that applies to the loss or other credit year (Code Sec. 6501(h) and (j)).

2728. Request for Prompt Assessment. A corporation that is contemplating dissolution, is in the process of dissolving, or has actually dissolved, or a decedent or an estate of a decedent (for taxes other than the estate tax imposed by chapter 11), may request a prompt assessment (Code Sec. 6501(d); Reg. § 301.6501(d)-1).[52] If such a request is made, an assessment or a proceeding in court without assessment for the collection of any tax must then be begun within 18 months after the receipt of a written request for a prompt assessment. In the case of a corporation, however, the 18-month period will not apply unless the corporation has completed or will eventually complete its dissolution at or before the end of the 18-month period. This provision does not apply in the cases described at ¶ 2732 and ¶ 2734. It also does not apply for personal holding company taxes in certain instances or where a waiver filed by the taxpayer extends the assessment period beyond the 18-month period.

2732. Assessment Period for False Returns or No Return. There is no limitation period on an assessment or a court proceeding to collect tax if:

    (1) the return is false or fraudulent,

    (2) there is a willful attempt to evade tax, or

    (3) no return is filed (Code Sec. 6501(c); Reg. § 301.6501(c)-1).[53]

In addition, in the case of a fraudulent return, the government may impose additional taxes at any time, without regard to statutes of limitations, although the burden of proof falls on the government to prove fraud by the taxpayer (Code Sec. 7454(a)).[54]

2733. Assessment Period for Listed Transactions. If a taxpayer fails to include with a return any information required relating to a listed transaction (¶ 2591), the statute of limitations with respect to that transaction will not expire before one year after the earlier of: (1) the date on which the information is furnished to the IRS or (2) the date that a material advisor to the listed transaction satisfies certain list maintenance requirements (¶ 2595) with respect to the transaction (Code Sec. 6501(c)(10)).[55]

2734. Assessment Period for Omission of Over 25 Percent of Income. If the taxpayer omits from gross income (total receipts, without reduction for cost) an amount in excess of 25 percent of the amount of gross income stated in the return, a six-year limitations period on assessment and collection of tax applies. An item will not be considered as omitted from gross income if information sufficient to apprise the IRS of the nature and amount of such item is disclosed in the return or in any schedule or statement attached to the return (Code Sec. 6501(e); Reg. § 301.6501(e)-1(a)).[56] The U.S. Supreme Court has held that a taxpayer's overstatement of its basis in an asset that resulted in an understatement of gross income from the asset's sale did not trigger the six-year limitations period because a basis overstatement is not an omission from gross income (*Home Concrete & Supply, LLC*, SCt, 2012-1 USTC ¶ 50,315). The Court's decision invalidated Reg. § 301.6501(e)-1(a)(1)(iii).

2735. Collection After Assessment. After assessment of tax made within the statutory period of limitations (¶ 2726), the tax may be collected by levy or a proceeding in court commenced within 10 years after the assessment or within any period for collection agreed upon in writing between the IRS and the taxpayer before the expiration of the 10-year period (Code Sec. 6502(a); Reg. § 301.6502-1).[57] The period agreed upon by the parties may be extended by later written agreements, so long as they are made prior to the expiration of the period previously agreed upon. The IRS has to notify

---

References are to Standard Federal Tax Reports; Tax Research Consultant; and Practical Tax Explanations.

[52] ¶ 38,960, ¶ 38,968; IRS: 30,118; § 26,740

[53] ¶ 38,960, ¶ 38,966; IRS: 30,102, IRS: 30,104, IRS: 30,106; § 39,505

[54] ¶ 42,081; IRS: 30,104; § 39,505.15

[55] ¶ 38,960; IRS: 30,052, PENALTY: 3,252.10; § 39,015.05

[56] ¶ 38,960, ¶ 38,970; IRS: 30,152; § 39,505.10

[57] ¶ 39,010, ¶ 39,011; IRS: 45,200; § 39,910

taxpayers of their right to refuse an extension each time one is requested (Code Sec. 6501(c)(4)).[58] If a timely court proceeding has commenced for the collection of the tax, then the period during which the tax may be collected is extended until the liability for tax, or a judgment against the taxpayer, is satisfied or becomes unenforceable.

The 10-year limitations period on collections is generally suspended for any period during which the IRS is prohibited from levying on the taxpayer's property. The collection period may also be extended by agreement between a taxpayer and the IRS. If the taxpayer entered into an installment agreement with the IRS, however, the 10-year limitations period may be extended for the period that the limitations period was extended under the original terms of the installment agreement plus 90 days.

Interest accrues on a deficiency from the date the tax was due (determined without regard to extensions) until the date payment is received at the rate specified at ¶ 2838 (Code Sec. 6601(g); Reg. § 301.6601-1(a)(1)).[59] Interest may be assessed and collected during the period in which the related tax may be collected.

2736. Suspension of Assessment Period. When an income, estate, or gift tax deficiency notice is mailed, the running of the period of limitations on assessment and collection of any deficiency is suspended for 90 days (150 days for a deficiency notice mailed to persons outside the United States) not counting Saturday, Sunday, or a legal holiday in the District of Columbia, plus an additional 60 days thereafter (Code Sec. 6503(a)(1); Reg. § 301.6503(a)-1).[60] If a petition is filed with the Tax Court, the running of the period of limitations is suspended until the Tax Court's decision becomes final and for an additional 60 days thereafter.

The 10-year statute of limitations for collection after assessment is also suspended from the date the IRS wrongfully seizes or receives a third party's property to 30 days after the date the IRS returns the property or the date on which a judgment secured in a wrongful levy action becomes final. Similarly, with respect to wrongful liens, the 10-year limitations period is suspended from the time the third-party owner is entitled to a certificate of discharge of lien until 30 days after the earlier of (1) the date that the IRS no longer holds any amount as a deposit or bond that was used to satisfy the unpaid liability or that was refunded or released, or (2) the date that the judgment in a civil action becomes final (¶ 2755) (Code Sec. 6503(f)).[61]

For federal bankruptcy cases, the running of the period of limitations is suspended during the period of the automatic stay on collection of taxes and for an additional period ending 60 days after the day the stay is lifted for assessments and for six months thereafter for collection (Code Sec. 6503(h)).[62] Additionally, in receivership and bankruptcy cases where a fiduciary is required to give written notice to the IRS of an appointment or authorization to act, the assessment period is suspended from the date the proceedings are instituted and ending 30 days after the day of notice to the IRS of such appointment. The extension period cannot exceed two years (Code Sec. 6872).[63]

If the taxpayer and the IRS agree to the rescission of a deficiency notice, the statute of limitations again begins to run as of the date of the rescission and continues to run for the period of time that remains on the date the notice was issued (Code Sec. 6212(d)).[64]

2738. Suit for Recovery of Erroneous Refund. The government may sue to recover an erroneous refund (including, but not limited to, one made after the applicable refund period described in ¶ 2763) within two years after such refund was paid. However, a suit may be commenced within five years if any part of the refund was induced by fraud or misrepresentation of a material fact (Code Sec. 6532(b); Reg. § 301.6532-2).[65]

References are to Standard Federal Tax Reports; Tax Research Consultant; and Practical Tax Explanations.

[58] ¶ 38,960; IRS: 30,254; § 39,905

[59] ¶ 39,410, ¶ 39,412; IRS: 30,114, PENALTY: 9,050; § 40,105

[60] ¶ 39,030, ¶ 39,031; IRS: 30,202; § 39,910

[61] ¶ 39,030; IRS: 45,204; § 39,910

[62] ¶ 39,030; IRS: 30,208; § 39,550.15

[63] ¶ 40,640; IRS: 30,208; § 39,550.15

[64] ¶ 37,540; IRS: 30,202; § 39,510.20

[65] ¶ 39,270, ¶ 39,272; IRS: 45,162; § 40,060.05

2740. Criminal Prosecution. A criminal prosecution must generally be started within three years after the offense is committed (Code Sec. 6531).[66] However, a six-year period applies in a case where there is:

(1) fraud or an attempt to defraud the United States or an agency thereof, by conspiracy or otherwise,

(2) a willful attempt to evade or defeat any tax or payment,

(3) willful aiding or assisting in the preparation of a false return or other document,

(4) willful failure to pay any tax or make any return (except certain information returns) at the time required by law,

(5) a false statement verified under penalties of perjury or a false or fraudulent return, statement or other document,

(6) intimidation of a U.S. officer or employee,

(7) an offense committed by a U.S. officer or employee in connection with a revenue law, or

(8) a conspiracy to defeat tax or payment.

2743. Collection from Transferee of Property. The liability of a transferee of property is generally assessed and collected in the same manner as is any other deficiency imposed by the IRS (Code Sec. 6901; Reg. § 301.6901-1(a)).[67] The term "transferee" includes an heir, legatee, devisee, distributee of an estate of a deceased person, the shareholder of a dissolved corporation, the assignee or donee of an insolvent person, the successor of a corporation, a party to a Code Sec. 368(a) reorganization, and a member of any other class of distributees. Such term also includes, with respect to the gift tax, a donee (without regard to the solvency of the donor) and, with respect to the estate tax, any person who, under Code Sec. 6324(a)(2), is personally liable for any part of such tax.

2745. Transferee Assessment and Collection Period. Unless a taxpayer has filed a false return with intent to evade tax (¶ 2732), an assessment against a transferee or fiduciary must be made within the following periods:

(1) in the case of an initial transferee, within one year after the expiration of the period of limitations for assessment against the taxpayer,

(2) in the case of a transferee of a transferee, within one year after the expiration of the period of limitations for assessment against the preceding transferee or three years after the expiration of the period of limitations for assessment against the taxpayer, whichever of these two periods expires first,

(3) if a timely court proceeding has been brought against the taxpayer or last preceding transferee, within one year after the return of execution in such proceeding, or

(4) in the case of a fiduciary, within one year after the liability arises or within the limitations period for collection of the tax (¶ 2726), whichever is the later (Code Sec. 6901; Reg. § 301.6901-1(c)).[68]

2747. Collection from Fiduciary. In order to receive advance notice from the IRS with respect to assessments, every fiduciary must give written notice to the IRS of his or her fiduciary capacity. If this notice (Form 56) is not filed, the IRS may proceed against the property in the hands of the fiduciary after mailing notice of the deficiency or other liability to the taxpayer's last known address, even if the taxpayer is then deceased or is under legal disability. The fiduciary may be relieved of any further liability by filing with the IRS written notice and evidence of the termination (Reg. § 301.6903-1).[69]

References are to Standard Federal Tax Reports; Tax Research Consultant; and Practical Tax Explanations.

[66] ¶ 39,240; IRS: 66,454; § 40,245.05

[67] ¶ 40,700, ¶ 40,701; IRS: 60,250; § 39,545.05

[68] ¶ 40,700; IRS: 60,256; § 39,545.05

[69] ¶ 40,730, ¶ 40,811; IRS: 60,200; § 39,545.05

2750. Assessment in Bankruptcy or Receiverships. When a taxpayer's assets are taken over by a receiver appointed by the court, the IRS may immediately assess the tax if it has not already been lawfully assessed. The IRS may also assess the tax on (1) the debtor's estate under U.S. Code Title 11 bankruptcy proceedings or (2) the debtor if the tax liability has become *res judicata* pursuant to a Title 11 bankruptcy determination (Code Sec. 6871).[70] Tax claims may be presented to the court before which the receivership or a Title 11 bankruptcy is pending, despite the pendency of proceedings in the Tax Court. However, in the case of a receivership proceeding, no petition may be filed with the Tax Court after the appointment of the receiver. The trustee of the debtor's estate in a Title 11 bankruptcy proceeding may intervene on behalf of the debtor's estate in any Tax Court proceeding to which the debtor is a party (Code Sec. 7464).[71]

Liens and Levies

2751. Property Subject to Liens. If a taxpayer fails to pay an assessed tax after notice and demand for payment, the United States acquires a lien for the amount due, including interest and penalties, against all the taxpayer's property (real, personal, tangible, and intangible), including after-acquired property and rights to property (Code Sec. 6321; Reg. § 301.6321-1).[72] Whether the taxpayer owns or has an interest in property is determined under the appropriate state law. Once the taxpayer's rights in the property are established, federal law determines priorities among competing creditors (Code Sec. 6323).[73] Federal law also controls whether specific property is exempt from levy (¶ 2753). Once a tax lien arises, it continues until the tax liability is paid or the lien becomes unenforceable due to a lapse of time (Code Sec. 6322).[74] Therefore, the lien period generally coincides with the statutory period for collection, which is 10 years from the date of assessment (Code Sec. 6502(a)).[75] However, the collection period may be suspended or extended.

2753. Property Subject to Levy. Although a tax lien attaches to all the debtor's property, some property is exempt from levy. The following are among the items that are exempt from levy to some extent:

    (1) wearing apparel and school books;

    (2) fuel, provisions, furniture, and personal effects: up to $8,940 for 2014 ($9,080 for 2015);

    (3) unemployment benefits;

    (4) books and tools of a trade, business, or profession: up to $4,470 for 2014 ($4,540 for 2015);

    (5) undelivered mail;

    (6) certain annuity and pension payments;

    (7) workers' compensation;

    (8) judgments for support of minor children;

    (9) certain public assistance payments, supplemental security income for the aged, blind, and disabled, state and local welfare payments, and Job Training Partnership Act payments;

    (10) certain amounts of wages, salary, and other income; and

    (11) certain service-connected disability payments (Code Sec. 6334; Rev. Proc. 2013-35; Rev. Proc. 2014-61).[76]

References are to Standard Federal Tax Reports; Tax Research Consultant; and Practical Tax Explanations.

[70] ¶ 40,610; IRS: 57,056; § 39,550.05

[71] ¶ 42,120; IRS: 57,056; § 39,550.10

[72] ¶ 38,135, ¶ 38,135A; IRS: 48,050, IRS: 48,100; § 39,925.05

[73] ¶ 38,145; IRS: 48,150; § 39,925.20

[74] ¶ 38,140; IRS: 48,050; § 39,925.10

[75] ¶ 39,010; IRS: 45,202; § 39,925.10

[76] ¶ 38,210; IRS: 51,062; § 39,930.15

Certain specified payments are not exempt from levy if the Secretary of the Treasury approves a continuous levy (Code Sec. 6334(f)).[77] The IRS can approve a continuous levy on up to 15 percent (100 percent for payments for goods and services and, after November 21, 2011, sales or leases of real property) of any federal payment other than: a payment for which eligibility is not based on the income or assets or both of the payee; unemployment benefits, worker's compensation payments, wages, or salary; Social Security disability payments; welfare and public assistance payments; and annuity or pension payments or benefits under the Railroad Retirement Act or Railroad Unemployment Insurance Act.

The IRS may not seize any real property used as a residence by the taxpayer or any real property of the taxpayer (other than rental property) that is used as a residence by another person in order to satisfy a liability of $5,000 or less (including tax, penalties, and interest). In the case of the taxpayer's principal residence, the IRS may not seize the residence without written approval of a federal district court judge or magistrate (Code Sec. 6334(a)(13) and (e)).[78] Unless collection of tax is in jeopardy, tangible personal property or real property (other than rented real property) used in the taxpayer's trade or business may not be seized without written approval of an IRS district or assistant director. Such approval may not be given unless it is determined that the taxpayer's other assets subject to collection are not sufficient to pay the amount due and the expenses of the proceedings. Where a levy is made on tangible personal property essential to the taxpayer's trade or business, the IRS must provide an accelerated appeals process to determine whether the property should be released from levy (Code Sec. 6343(a)(2)).[79] See ¶ 2755.

Levies are prohibited if the estimated expenses of the levy and sale exceed the fair market value of the property (Code Sec. 6331(f)).[80] Also, unless the collection of tax is in jeopardy, a levy cannot be made on any day on which the taxpayer is required to respond to an IRS summons (Code Sec. 6331(g)).[81] Further, financial institutions are required to hold amounts garnished by the IRS for 21 days after receiving notice of the levy to provide the taxpayer time to notify the IRS of any errors (Code Sec. 6332(c)).[82]

2754. Recording and Priority of Tax Liens. Until notice of a tax lien has been properly recorded, it is not valid against any bona fide purchaser for value, mechanic's lienor, judgment lien creditor, or holder of a security interest (e.g., a mortgagee or pledgee) (Code Sec. 6323(a)).[83] Also, even a properly recorded tax lien may not be valid against so-called superpriorities, which include purchases of securities and automobiles, retail purchases, casual sales of less than $1,490 for 2014 ($1,520 for 2015), certain possessory liens securing payment for repairs to personal property, real property taxes and special assessment liens, mechanic's liens for repairs and improvements of not more than $7,470 for 2014 ($7,590 for 2015) to certain residential property, attorneys' liens, certain insurance contracts and deposit secured loans (previously referred to as passbook loans) (Code Sec. 6323(b); Rev. Proc. 2013-35; Rev. Proc. 2014-61).[84] In addition, security interests arising from commercial financing agreements may be accorded superpriority status (Code Sec. 6323(c)).[85]

Notice of a federal tax lien must be filed in one office designated by the state in which the property is situated (Code Sec. 6323(f); Reg. § 301.6323(f)-1).[86] Generally, personal property is considered situated in the state where the taxpayer resides, rather than where domiciled; for real property, the situs is its physical location. If, in the case of either real or personal property, the state designates more than one office or does not

---

References are to Standard Federal Tax Reports; Tax Research Consultant; and Practical Tax Explanations.

[77] ¶ 38,210; IRS: 51,060.35; § 39,930.20

[78] ¶ 38,210; IRS: 51,062.05; § 39,930.15

[79] ¶ 38,270; IRS: 51,154; § 39,930.15

[80] ¶ 38,185; IRS: 51,054; § 39,930.05

[81] ¶ 38,185; IRS: 51,054; § 39,930.05

[82] ¶ 38,185; IRS: 51,064.35; § 39,930.25

[83] ¶ 38,145; IRS: 48,150; § 39,925.20

[84] ¶ 38,145; IRS: 48,160; § 39,925.20

[85] ¶ 38,145; IRS: 48,160; § 39,925.20

[86] ¶ 38,145, ¶ 38,153; IRS: 48,056; § 39,925.20

designate an office where notice must be filed, notice of the lien must be filed with the Clerk of the U.S. District Court for the district in which the property is situated. If state law provides that a notice of lien affecting personal property must be filed in the county clerk's office located in the taxpayer's county of residence and also adopts a federal law that requires a notice of lien to be filed in another location in order to attach to a specific type of property, the state is deemed to have designated only one office for the filing of the notice. Thus, to protect its lien, the IRS need only file its notice in the county clerk's office located in the taxpayer's home county (Reg. § 301.6323(f)-1(a)(2)). Notice regarding property located in the District of Columbia is filed with the Recorder of Deeds of the District of Columbia. Special rules apply in a state that requires public indexing for priority liens against realty.

A forfeiture under local law of property seized by any law enforcement agency or other local governmental branch relates back to the time the property was first seized, unless, under local law, a claim holder would have priority over the interest of the government in the property (Code Sec. 6323(i)(3)).[87]

The IRS may not levy against property while a taxpayer has a pending offer in compromise or installment agreement (Code Sec. 6331(k)).[88] If the offer in compromise or installment agreement is ultimately rejected, the levy prohibition remains in effect for 30 days after the rejection and during the pendency of any appeal of the rejection, providing the appeal is filed within 30 days of the rejection. No levy may be made while the installment agreement is in effect. If the installment agreement is terminated by the IRS, no levy may be made for 30 days after the termination and during the pendency of any appeal.

2754A. Notice and Opportunity for Hearing. The IRS must notify any person subject to a lien of the existence of the lien within five days of the lien being filed (Code Sec. 6320; Reg. § 301.6320-1).[89] Among other requirements, the notice must address the person's right to request a hearing during the 30-day period beginning on the sixth day after the lien is filed. Similarly, at least 30 days prior to levying on any person's property or right to property, the IRS must provide the taxpayer with notice of its intent to levy and of the taxpayer's the right to a hearing (Code Sec. 6330; Reg. § 301.6330-1).[90] Whether in connection with the notice of lien or notice of intent to levy, the hearing is to be held by the IRS Office of Appeals. At the hearing, the taxpayer may raise any issue relevant to the appropriateness of the proposed collection activity if such issue was not raised at a previous hearing. The taxpayer has 30 days after the hearing determination to appeal the determination to the Tax Court, which has exclusive jurisdiction over appeals of hearing determinations. A taxpayer subject to a levy for the collection of employment taxes cannot request a hearing if the taxpayer already requested a hearing regarding unpaid employment taxes arising in the two-year period before the beginning of the tax period at issue.

2755. Release of Tax Liens and Levies. Taxpayers may appeal the filing of a notice of lien in the public record and petition for release (Code Sec. 6326; Reg. § 301.6326-1).[91] If filed in error, the IRS must release the lien and state that the lien was erroneous. The request for relief must be based on one of the following grounds:

(1) the tax liability had been satisfied before the lien was filed;

(2) the assessing of the tax liability violated either the notice of deficiency procedures or the Bankruptcy Code; or

(3) the limitations period for collecting the liability had expired prior to the filing of the lien.

References are to Standard Federal Tax Reports; Tax Research Consultant; and Practical Tax Explanations.

[87] ¶ 38,145; IRS: 48,154; § 39,925.20

[88] ¶ 38,185; IRS: 51,054; § 39,930.05

[89] ¶ 38,132, ¶ 38,133; IRS: 48,058.05; § 39,945.10

[90] ¶ 38,182, ¶ 38,183; IRS: 51,056.05; § 39,945.15

[91] ¶ 38,175, ¶ 38,176; IRS: 48,200; § 39,925.25, § 39,930.30

¶2755

Further, the IRS may withdraw a public notice of tax lien before payment in full if:

(1) the filing of the notice was premature or not in accord with administrative procedures;

(2) the taxpayer has entered into an installment agreement to satisfy the tax liability;

(3) withdrawal of the notice would facilitate the collection of the tax liability; or

(4) the withdrawal of the notice would be in the best interest of the taxpayer and the government, as determined by the National Taxpayer Advocate (Code Sec. 6323(j)).[92]

The withdrawal of a notice of tax lien does not affect the underlying tax lien; rather, the withdrawal simply relinquishes any lien priority the IRS had obtained when the notice was filed.

The IRS is required to release a levy if:

(1) the underlying liability is satisfied or becomes unenforceable due to lapse of time;

(2) the IRS determines that the release of the levy will facilitate the collection of tax;

(3) an installment payment agreement has been executed by the taxpayer with respect to the liability;

(4) the IRS determines that the levy is creating a financial hardship; or

(5) the fair market value of the property exceeds the liability, and the partial release of the levy would not hinder the collection of tax (Code Sec. 6343(a)).[93]

In addition, a taxpayer may request that the IRS sell the levied property (Code Sec. 6335(f); Reg. § 301.6335-1(d)).[94]

The IRS has been given authority to return property that has been levied upon if:

(1) the levy was premature or not in accordance with administrative procedure;

(2) the taxpayer has entered into an installment agreement to satisfy the tax liability, unless the agreement provides otherwise;

(3) the return of the property will facilitate collection of the tax liability; or

(4) with the consent of the taxpayer or the Taxpayer Advocate, the return of the property would be in the best interests of the taxpayer and the government (Code Sec. 6343(d)).[95]

Property is returned in the same manner as if the property had been wrongfully levied upon, except that the taxpayer is not entitled to interest.

A taxpayer may bring a suit in federal district court if an IRS employee knowingly or negligently fails to release a tax lien on the taxpayer's property after receiving written notice from the taxpayer of the IRS's failure to release the lien (Code Sec. 7432; Reg. § 301.7432-1).[96] The taxpayer may recover actual economic damages plus the costs of the action. Injuries such as inconvenience, emotional distress, and loss of reputation are not compensable damages unless they result in actual economic harm. Costs of the action that may be recovered are limited generally to certain court costs and do not include administrative costs or attorney's fees, although attorney's fees may be recoverable (¶ 2796). A two-year statute of limitations, measured from the date on which the cause of action accrued, applies.

References are to Standard Federal Tax Reports; Tax Research Consultant; and Practical Tax Explanations.

[92] ¶ 38,145; IRS: 48,052.10; § 39,925.25

[93] ¶ 38,270; IRS: 51,154; § 39,930.30

[94] ¶ 38,230, ¶ 38,231; IRS: 51,202; § 39,930.30

[95] ¶ 38,270; IRS: 51,154.05; § 39,930.30

[96] ¶ 41,760, ¶ 41,761; IRS: 48,210; § 39,925.25

¶ 2755

Third-Party Owners. A third-party owner of property against which a federal tax lien has been filed may obtain a certificate of discharge with respect to the lien on such property (Code Sec. 6325(b)(4); Reg. § 301.6325-1(b)(4)).[97] The certificate is issued if (1) the third-party owner deposits with the IRS an amount of money equal to the value of the government's interest in the property as determined by the IRS or (2) the third-party owner posts a bond covering the government's interest in the property in a form acceptable to the IRS. A third-party owner who is a co-owner of property with the taxpayer against whom the underlying tax was assessed may no longer be automatically barred from obtaining a certificate of discharge with respect to a lien on the property. Third-party owners may request the discharge of a tax lien on property that they own with the person whose tax liability gave rise to the lien.

If the IRS determines that (1) the liability to which the lien relates can be satisfied from other sources or (2) the value of the government's interest in the property is less than the IRS's prior determination of the government's interest in the property, then the IRS will refund, with interest, the amount deposited and release the bond applicable to such property. Within 120 days after a certificate of discharge is issued, the third-party owner may file a civil action against the United States in a federal district court for a determination of whether the government's interest in the property, if any, has less value than that determined by the IRS (Code Sec. 7426(a)(4) and (b)(5)).[98]

Mitigation of Effect of Statute of Limitations

2756. Correction of Errors in Certain Cases. The Code provides relief from some of the inequities caused by the statute of limitations and other provisions that would otherwise prevent equitable adjustment of various income tax hardships (Code Secs. 1311–1314; Reg. §§ 1.1311(a)-1–1.1314(c)-1).[99] Adjustments are permitted, even though the limitations period for assessment or refund for the year at issue may have otherwise expired, when a determination under the income tax laws:

(1) requires the inclusion in gross income of an item that was erroneously included in the income of the taxpayer for another tax year or in the gross income of a "related taxpayer," e.g., spouse, beneficiary, partner, member of affiliated group of corporations, etc.;

(2) allows a deduction or credit that was erroneously allowed to the taxpayer for another tax year or to a related taxpayer;

(3) requires the exclusion from gross income of an item included in a return filed by the taxpayer or with respect to which tax was paid and which was erroneously excluded or omitted from the gross income of the taxpayer for another tax year or from the gross income of a related taxpayer for the same or another tax year;

(4) allows or disallows, in certain situations, deductions or inclusions for a trust or an estate, and there has been no appropriate corresponding change in the income of beneficiaries, heirs, or legatees;

(5) establishes the basis of property by making adjustments to such basis for items that should have been added to, or deducted from, income of preceding years;

(6) requires the allowance or disallowance of a deduction or credit to a corporation where a correlative deduction or credit was erroneously allowed, or disallowed, to a related taxpayer that is a member of an affiliated group of corporations where there is an 80% common ownership;

(7) requires the exclusion from gross income of an item not included in a return filed by the taxpayer and with respect to which the tax was not paid but which is includible in the gross income of the taxpayer for another tax year or in the gross income of a related taxpayer; or

---

References are to Standard Federal Tax Reports; Tax Research Consultant; and Practical Tax Explanations.

[97] ¶ 38,165, ¶ 38,166; IRS: 48,204.15; § 39,925.25

[98] ¶ 41,710; IRS: 48,204.15; § 39,925.25

[99] ¶ 31,800–¶ 31,865; IRS: 30,300; § 40,401

(8) disallows a deduction or credit that should have been allowed, but was not allowed, to the taxpayer for another tax year or to a related taxpayer for the same or another tax year (Code Sec. 1312).[100]

Refunds and Credits

2759. Claim for Refund or Credit. A claim for refund for an overpayment of income taxes is generally made on the appropriate income tax return. However, once the return has been filed and the taxpayer believes the tax is incorrect, the claim for refund by an individual who filed Form 1040, 1040A, or 1040EZ is made on Form 1040X. The refund claim is made on Form 1120X by a corporation that filed Form 1120. A claim for refund or credit for an overpayment of income taxes for which a form other than Form 1040, 1040A, 1040EZ, 1120, or 990T was filed is made on the appropriate amended tax return (Reg. § 301.6402-3).[101] Proposed regulations, which may be relied upon until final regulations are issued, would provide that Form 843 should be filed for any claim for refund or credit if no other form is prescribed (Prop. Reg. § 301.6402-2(c)).[102]

2760. Amendment of Refund Claim. A timely claim for refund based upon one or more specific grounds may not be amended to include other and different grounds after the statute of limitations has expired (Reg. § 301.6402-2(b)).[103]

2761. Refund or Credit After Appeal to Tax Court. Where the taxpayer has been mailed a notice of deficiency and has filed a petition with the Tax Court (¶ 2778), the taxpayer may not bring a separate refund suit in any other court for recovery of any part of the tax at issue in the Tax Court (Code Sec. 6512).[104] The taxpayer is permitted, however, to institute a claim for credit or refund in another court for the same tax year to recover:

(1) an overpayment determined by a decision of the Tax Court that has become final,

(2) any amount collected in excess of an amount computed in accordance with a final decision of the Tax Court,

(3) any amount collected after the expiration of the period of limitations upon the beginning of levy or a proceeding in court for collection,

(4) overpayments attributable to partnership items,

(5) any amount that was collected within the period following the mailing of a notice of deficiency during which the IRS is prohibited from collecting by levy or through a court proceeding, and

(6) any amount that is not contested on an appeal from a Tax Court decision.

The Tax Court can order the refund of a tax overpayment plus interest if the IRS has not made a refund to the taxpayer within 120 days after the decision fixing the amount of the refund has become final (Code Sec. 6512(b)).[105]

The Tax Court is empowered to resolve disputes regarding the amount of interest to be charged on a tax deficiency redetermined pursuant to a Tax Court order. The action must be brought within one year from the date on which the decision ordering the redetermination of taxes became final. Further, the taxpayer must pay the entire redetermined deficiency, plus the entire amount of interest, before the Tax Court can hear the case (Code Sec. 7481(c)).[106]

2763. Limitations on Credit or Refund. A taxpayer may generally file a claim for refund within three years from the time the return was filed or within two years from the time the tax was paid, whichever is later. If no return was filed by the taxpayer, the claim

---

References are to Standard Federal Tax Reports; Tax Research Consultant; and Practical Tax Explanations.

[100] ¶ 31,820; IRS: 30,300; § 40,405, § 40,410.05

[101] ¶ 38,517; IRS: 33,150; § 40,010.10

[102] ¶ 38,516B; IRS: 33,154.10; § 40,010.10

[103] ¶ 38,516; IRS: 33,200; § 40,010.25

[104] ¶ 39,090; LITIG: 3,102; § 40,001

[105] ¶ 39,090; LITIG: 6,100; § 40,001

[106] ¶ 42,420; LITIG: 6,114; § 40,001

must be filed within two years from the time the tax was paid (Code Sec. 6511(a)).[107] For this purpose, a return filed before the due date is treated as filed on the due date (Code Sec. 6513(a)).[108] Taxpayers who fail to file a return as of the date the IRS mails a deficiency notice may recover in the Tax Court taxes paid during the three years preceding the IRS mailing date (Code Sec. 6512(b)(3)).[109]

If the claim relates to the deductibility of bad debts or worthless securities, the period is seven years; if it relates to the credit for foreign taxes, the period is 10 years. If the refund claim relates to a net operating loss (NOL) or a capital loss carryback, the period is that period which ends three years after the time prescribed by law for filing the return, including extensions, for the tax year of the NOL or capital loss carryback. To the extent that an overpayment is due to unused credit carrybacks that arise as the result of the carryback of an NOL or capital loss, the claim may be filed during the period that ends three years after the time prescribed by law for filing the return, including extensions, for the tax year of the unused credit that results in the carryback (Code Sec. 6511(d); Reg. § 301.6511(d)-2).[110]

The statute of limitations on refund claims is suspended during any period that an individual is financially disabled, i.e., under a medically determinable mental or physical impairment that: (1) can be expected to result in death or that has lasted or can be expected to last for a continuous period of not less than one year, and (2) renders the person unable to manage his or her financial affairs (Code Sec. 6511(h)).[111] The suspension of the limitations period does not apply for any period during which the taxpayer's spouse or another person is authorized to act on behalf of the individual in financial matters.

Retired Military Personnel. The time period for retired military personnel to file claims for credits or refunds related to disability determinations by the Department of Veterans Affairs, e.g., determinations after the tax is filed, is extended until one year after the date of the disability determination if that period is later than the normal three-year period of limitations (Code Sec. 6511(d)(8)).[112] This provision does not apply to any tax year that began more than five years before the date of the disability determination.

2764. Refund Reduction for Past-Due, Legally Enforceable Debts. The Treasury Department's Financial Management Service (FMS) will reduce the amount of any tax refund payable to a taxpayer by the amount of any past-due, legally enforceable nontax debt that is owed to any federal agency. Debts that are less than $25 are exempt. In most cases, the creditor federal agencies must have first attempted to collect the debt by using salary offset and administrative procedures. The federal agency is also required to notify the taxpayer that a debt will be referred to the FMS for refund offset if the debt remains unpaid after 60 days or if there is insufficient evidence that the debt is either not past due or not legally enforceable (31 CFR § 285.2).

The FMS has also promulgated rules governing the offset of tax refunds against past-due child and spousal support (31 CFR § 285.3) and against state income tax debts reduced to judgment (31 CFR § 285.8). Tax refunds may also be offset against past-due debts owed to a state for (1) erroneous payment of unemployment compensation due to fraud or failure to report earnings, or (2) failure to make contributions to a state's unemployment fund for which the state has determined the person to be liable (Code Sec. 6402(f)).[113]

2765. Interest on Refund. When a return has been properly filed in processible form, interest is allowed on a refund from the date of overpayment to a date preceding the date of the refund check by not more than 30 days (Code Sec. 6611(b)(2) and (3)).[114] If a return is filed late, no interest is allowed for any day before the date on which it is

---

References are to Standard Federal Tax Reports; Tax Research Consultant; and Practical Tax Explanations.

[107] ¶ 39,060; IRS: 36,050; § 40,040.05

[108] ¶ 39,120; IRS: 36,050; § 40,040.05

[109] ¶ 39,090; IRS: 36,116; § 40,040.05

[110] ¶ 39,060, ¶ 39,067; IRS: 36,100; § 40,045.05

[111] ¶ 39,060; IRS: 36,052; § 40,040.05

[112] ¶ 39,060; IRS: 36,052; § 40,045.05

[113] ¶ 38,510; IRS: 33,304.20; § 40,015.05

[114] ¶ 39,430; PENALTY: 9,100; § 40,115.05

filed. No interest is payable on a refund arising from an original tax return if the refund is issued by the 45th day after the later of the due date for the return, determined without regard to any extensions, or the date the return is filed (Code Sec. 6611(e)). Similarly, if a refund claimed on an amended return or claim for refund is issued within 45 days after the date the amended document was filed, interest is not payable for that period, although interest is payable from the due date of the original return to the date the amended document was filed. If a refund is not issued within the 45-day grace period, interest is payable for the period from the due date of the original return to the date the refund is paid.

The interest rate the IRS must pay for overpayment of taxes by noncorporate taxpayers is equal to the federal short-term rate (¶ 83) plus three percentage points (which is equal to the interest rate on underpayments of tax). The interest rate on overpayments by corporate taxpayers is the short-term federal rate plus two percentage points (Code Sec. 6621).[115] For large corporate overpayments, i.e., any portion that exceeds $10,000, the rate is reduced to the sum of the short-term federal rate plus one-half of one percentage point. These rates are adjusted quarterly, with each successive rate becoming effective two months after the date of each quarterly adjustment. The rates for the first through fourth quarters of 2014 were 3 percent for noncorporate taxpayers and 2 percent for corporate taxpayers (0.5 percent for large corporate overpayments).[116]

Overlapping Overpayments and Underpayments. The interest rates for overpayments and underpayments have been equalized (also referred to as "global interest netting") for any period of mutual indebtedness between taxpayers and the IRS (Code Sec. 6621(d)).[117] No interest is imposed to the extent that underpayment and overpayment interest run simultaneously on equal amounts. The net zero interest rate applies regardless of whether an underpayment otherwise would be subject to the increased interest rate imposed on large corporate underpayments or an overpayment otherwise would be subject to a reduced interest rate because it was a corporate overpayment in excess of $10,000. Although global interest netting is available to both corporate and noncorporate taxpayers, its effect on noncorporate taxpayers is mitigated due to the equalization of the underpayment and overpayment interest rates for such taxpayers.

2768. Refunds Disregarded for Means-Tested Assistance Programs. Any federal tax refund, or advance payment with respect to a refundable federal tax credit made to any individual cannot be taken into account as income or as resources for a period of 12 months from receipt, for purposes of determining the individual's eligibility (or that of any other individual) for benefits or assistance, or for the amount or extent of benefits or assistance, under (1) any federal program, or (2) any state or local program financed in whole or in part with federal funds (Code Sec. 6409).[118]

2773. Quick Carryback Refund and Postponement of Tax Payment. A corporation other than an S corporation that has an overpayment of tax as a result of a net operating loss (NOL), capital loss, business and research credits, or a claim-of-right adjustment can file an application on Form 1139 for a tentative adjustment or refund of taxes for a year affected by the carryback of such loss or credits or by such adjustment. A noncorporate taxpayer can apply for similar adjustments on Form 1045 (Code Sec. 6411; Temp. Reg. § 5.6411-1).[119] For provisions on the quick refund of a capital loss carryback, see ¶ 1145.

The application itself is not a formal refund claim and its rejection in whole or in part cannot be made the basis of a refund suit. However, the taxpayer can file a regular claim for refund within the limitations period (¶ 2763), and this claim can be made the basis for a suit. For losses and credits, the IRS must allow or disallow the refund or credit within 90 days from the later of (1) the date the application is filed or (2) the last

---

References are to Standard Federal Tax Reports; Tax Research Consultant; and Practical Tax Explanations.

[115] ¶ 39,450; PENALTY: 9,152; § 40,115.05

[116] ¶ 39,455.51; PENALTY: 9,152

[117] ¶ 39,450; PENALTY: 9,056.05; § 40,120.15

[118] ¶ 38,702; IRS: 33,300; § 40,001

[119] ¶ 38,720, ¶ 38,726; IRS: 33,352; § 40,025

day of the month in which the return for the loss or unused credit year is due (giving effect to extensions of time). For claim-of-right adjustments, the IRS must allow or disallow the refund or credit within 90 days from the later of (1) the date the application is filed or (2) the date of the overpayment.

If a corporation expects a NOL carryback from the current (unfinished) tax year, it can, subject to certain limitations, extend the time for payment of all or a part of the tax still payable for the immediately preceding year by filing a statement on Form 1138 (Reg. § 1.6164-1).[120]

The Courts

2776. Organization of Tax Court. The primary function of the U.S. Tax Court is to review deficiencies asserted by the IRS for additional income, estate, gift, or self-employment taxes or special excise taxes (Code Secs. 6512 and 7442).[121] The Tax Court is the only judicial body from which relief may be obtained without the payment of tax. The Tax Court also may issue declaratory judgments on the initial or continuing qualification of a retirement plan under Code Sec. 401, a tax-exempt organization under Code Sec. 501(c)(3) or Code Sec. 170(c)(2), a private foundation under Code Sec. 509(a), a private operating foundation under Code Sec. 4942(j)(3), or a tax-exempt farmers' cooperative under Code Sec. 521. However, a revocation of tax-exempt status for failure to file an annual information return or notice is not subject to an action for declaratory judgment relief. The Tax Court also may rule on the tax-exempt interest status of a government bond issue (Code Secs. 7428, 7476, and 7478; Tax Court Rule 210).[122] Declaratory judgment powers are also provided for (1) estate tax installments, (2) gift tax revaluations, and (3) employment status determinations.

The Tax Court's offices and trial rooms are located in Washington, D.C., but trials are also conducted in principal cities throughout the country. At the time of filing a petition, the taxpayer should file a request indicating where he prefers the trial to be held. The court imposes a filing fee of $60 (Code Sec. 7451).[123]

In any Tax Court case, other than small tax cases (¶ 2784), the findings of fact and opinion must generally be reported in writing. In appropriate cases, a Tax Court judge may state orally, and record in the transcript of the proceedings, the findings of fact or opinion in the case (Code Sec. 7459).[124] In these cases, the court must provide to all parties in the case either a copy of the transcript pages, which record the findings or opinion, or a written summary of such findings or opinion (Tax Court Rule 152).[125]

2778. Appeal to the Tax Court. Before the IRS can assess a deficiency, it generally must mail a deficiency notice to the taxpayer. The taxpayer then has an opportunity to appeal, within 90 days after the notice is mailed, to the Tax Court (¶ 2711). A notice based solely upon a mathematical or clerical error is not considered a notice of deficiency (Code Sec. 6213; Reg. § 301.6213-1).[126] If the notice is mailed to a person outside the United States, the period is 150 days instead of 90 days. The period is counted from midnight of the day on which the notice is mailed. Saturday, Sunday, or a legal holiday in the District of Columbia is not counted as the 90th or 150th day.

When a petition to the Tax Court is properly addressed and mailed within the prescribed time for filing, with the postage prepaid, the date of the U.S. postmark stamped on the cover in which the petition is mailed is the date of filing. For a petition that is mailed from a foreign country, this rule applies only if the petition is given to a designated international delivery service (Rev. Rul. 2002-23). If a petition is sent by registered or certified mail, the date of registration or certification is the date of mailing and is prima facie evidence that the petition was delivered to the Tax Court. Similarly, the proper use of a private delivery service, under criteria established by the IRS, also

---

References are to Standard Federal Tax Reports; Tax Research Consultant; and Practical Tax Explanations.

[120] ¶ 37,241; FILEBUS: 6,104.20; § 40,025

[121] ¶ 39,090, ¶ 42,057; LITIG: 6,100

[122] ¶ 41,720, ¶ 42,134, ¶ 42,154, ¶ 42,370; LITIG: 6,100

[123] ¶ 42,072; LITIG: 6,050

[124] ¶ 42,110; IRS: 27,206

[125] ¶ 42,312; LITIG: 6,802

[126] ¶ 37,545, ¶ 37,546, ¶ 37,549.34; LITIG: 6,202, LITIG: 6,204

constitutes prima facie evidence that the petition was delivered to the Tax Court (Reg. § 301.7502-1).[127]

If a taxpayer has filed a Tax Court petition before a jeopardy assessment or levy is made, the Tax Court is given concurrent jurisdiction with the federal district courts with respect to the taxpayer's challenge of the jeopardy assessment or levy (Code Sec. 7429(b)(2)).[128] Similarly, if there is a premature assessment of tax made while a proceeding with respect to that tax is pending in the Tax Court, the Tax Court has concurrent jurisdiction with the federal district court to restrain the assessment and collection of tax (Code Sec. 6213).[129]

2782. Burden of Proof. The IRS has the burden of proof in the Tax Court with respect to a factual issue that is relevant to determining a taxpayer's tax liability if the taxpayer presents credible evidence with respect to that issue *and* satisfies three applicable conditions (Code Sec. 7491):[130]

(1) The taxpayer must comply with the substantiation and recordkeeping requirements of the Code and regulations.

(2) The taxpayer must cooperate with reasonable requests by the IRS for witnesses, information, documents, meetings and interviews.

(3) Taxpayers *other than individuals* must meet the net worth limitations that apply for awarding attorneys' fees under Code Sec. 7430. Thus, corporations, trusts, and partnerships whose tax worth exceeds $7 million cannot benefit from this provision.

Further, in any court proceeding where the IRS solely uses statistical information from unrelated taxpayers to reconstruct an item of an *individual* taxpayer's income, such as the average income for taxpayers in the area in which the taxpayer lives, the burden of proof is on the IRS with respect to that item of income. Also with respect to individuals, the IRS must initially come forward with evidence that it is appropriate to apply a penalty, addition to tax, or additional amount before the court can impose the penalty.

In cases in which the burden of proof does not shift to the IRS, the taxpayer generally has the burden of proof in the Tax Court. However, a taxpayer must only establish that the IRS is in error and not whether any tax is owed (Tax Court Rule 142).[131] The IRS bears the burden of proof with respect to any new matter, increase in deficiency, or affirmative defenses raised in its answer. Further, the burden of proving fraud and liability as a transferee is upon the IRS (Code Secs. 6902 and 7454).[132] The IRS also has the burden of proof in proceedings involving a manager of a private foundation where the manager knowingly participated in an act of self-dealing, participated in an investment which jeopardizes the carrying out of an exempt purpose, or agreed to the making of a taxable expenditure.

2784. Small Tax Cases. The Tax Court maintains relatively informal procedures for the filing and handling of cases where neither the tax deficiency in dispute (including additions to tax and penalties) nor the amount of claimed overpayment exceeds $50,000. Usually taxpayers represent themselves, although they may be represented by anyone admitted to practice before the Tax Court. Each decision is final and cannot be appealed by either the taxpayer or the government (Code Sec. 7463).[133] The filing fee is $60 (¶ 2776).

2786. Appeal from Tax Court Decision. A taxpayer who loses in the Tax Court may appeal the case (unless the case was tried as a small tax case, ¶ 2784) to the proper U.S. Court of Appeals by filing a notice of appeal with the clerk of the Tax Court. The notice must be filed within 90 days after the Tax Court decision is entered. However, if one party to the proceeding files a timely notice of appeal, any other party to the

---

References are to Standard Federal Tax Reports; Tax Research Consultant; and Practical Tax Explanations.

[127] ¶ 42,621; LITIG: 6,214
[128] ¶ 41,725; IRS: 54,204
[129] ¶ 37,545; LITIG: 6,136

[130] ¶ 42,515; LITIG: 3,200
[131] ¶ 42,302, ¶ 42,302.615; LITIG: 6,704

[132] ¶ 40,780, ¶ 42,081; LITIG: 6,708
[133] ¶ 42,118; LITIG: 7,000

proceeding may take an appeal by filing a notice of appeal within 120 days after the decision of the Tax Court is entered (Code Sec. 7483).[134] A taxpayer who wants the assessment postponed pending the outcome of the appeal must file an appeal bond with the Tax Court guaranteeing payment of the deficiency as finally determined (Code Sec. 7485).[135]

2788. Acquiescence and Nonacquiescence by Commissioner. The IRS may announce in the Internal Revenue Bulletin if it has decided to acquiesce or not acquiesce in a regular decision of the Tax Court. Any acquiescence or nonacquiescence may be withdrawn, modified, or reversed at any time and any such action may be given retrospective, as well as prospective, effect.[136]

An acquiescence or nonacquiescence relates only to the issue or issues decided adversely to the government. Acquiescence means the IRS accepts the conclusion reached and does not necessarily mean acceptance and approval of any or all of the reasons assigned by the court for its conclusions. Acquiescences are to be relied on by IRS officers and others concerned as conclusions of the IRS only with respect to the application of the law to the facts in the particular case.

2790. Suits for Refund of Tax Overpayments. After the IRS rejects a refund claim for an alleged tax overpayment, suit can be maintained in the U.S. Court of Federal Claims or a U.S. District Court. A suit may be brought in the Court of Federal Claims against the United States to recover any overpayment of tax, regardless of amount (Judicial Code Sec. 1491).[137] Final decisions of the U.S. Court of Federal Claims are appealable to the U.S. Court of Appeals for the Federal Circuit (Judicial Code Sec. 1295).[138] All civil actions against the United States for the recovery of any internal revenue tax alleged to have been erroneously or illegally assessed or collected may be brought against the United States as defendant in a U.S. District Court with right of trial by jury in any action if either party makes a specific request for a jury trial (Judicial Code Secs. 1346 and 2402).[139] Filing a proper claim for refund or credit (¶ 2759) is a condition precedent to a suit for recovery of overpaid taxes (Code Sec. 7422(a)).[140]

If, prior to the hearing on a taxpayer's refund suit in a District Court or the Court of Federal Claims, a notice of deficiency is issued on the subject matter of the taxpayer's suit, then the District Court or Court of Federal Claims proceedings are stayed during the period of time in which the taxpayer can file a petition with the Tax Court (¶ 2778) and for 60 days thereafter. If the taxpayer files a petition with the Tax Court, then the District Court or the Court of Federal Claims loses jurisdiction as to any issues over which the Tax Court acquires jurisdiction. If the taxpayer does not appeal to the Tax Court, the United States may then counterclaim in the taxpayer's suit within the period of the stay of proceedings even though the time for such pleading may otherwise have expired (Code Sec. 7422(e)).[141]

2792. Time to Bring Suit. A suit or proceeding based upon a refund claim must be brought within two years from the date the IRS mails, by registered or certified mail, notice of disallowance of the part of the claim to which such suit or proceeding relates or within two years from the date the taxpayer waives notification of disallowance of his or her claim (Code Sec. 6532(a)).[142] The two-year period of limitations for filing suit may be extended by written agreement between the taxpayer and the IRS. Unless a bankruptcy proceeding has begun, no action can be brought before the expiration of six months from the date of filing the refund claim unless the IRS renders a decision on the claim before the six months are up. In bankruptcy proceedings, the six-month period is reduced to 120 days.

References are to Standard Federal Tax Reports; Tax Research Consultant; and Practical Tax Explanations.

[134] ¶ 42,477; LITIG: 6,960

[135] ¶ 42,500; LITIG: 6,966

[136] ¶ 43,282.20; IRS: 12,354

[137] ¶ 41,571; LITIG: 9,050

[138] ¶ 41,555; LITIG: 9,210

[139] ¶ 41,560, ¶ 41,589; LITIG: 9,052

[140] ¶ 41,685; LITIG: 9,056

[141] ¶ 41,685; LITIG: 3,102, LITIG: 9,106

[142] ¶ 39,270; LITIG: 9,058; § 40,010.25

2794. Supreme Court. Either party may seek a review of a U.S. Court of Appeals decision by the U.S. Supreme Court through a petition for a writ of certiorari (Code Sec. 7482(a); Judicial Code Sec. 2101).[143]

2796. Attorneys' Fees and Court Costs. A "prevailing party"—any party, other than the United States or a creditor of the taxpayer, who has substantially prevailed with respect to the amount in controversy or the most significant issue or issues—may be awarded reasonable litigation costs in most civil tax litigation, including declaratory judgment proceedings (Code Sec. 7430).[144] In addition, a prevailing party can recover reasonable administrative costs incurred in connection with such administrative proceeding with the IRS.

These awards may be made if the taxpayer meets certain net worth limitations and the IRS fails to prove that its position was substantially justified. When litigation costs are involved, the IRS's position is the government's position taken in the litigation proceeding or administratively by the IRS District Counsel. In the case of administrative costs, the IRS's position is the position taken as of the earlier of (1) the date the taxpayer received a decision notice from the IRS Office of Appeals or (2) the date of the deficiency notice.

Reasonable administrative costs include (1) administrative fees or similar charges imposed by the IRS, and (2) the reasonable expenses incurred with respect to compensating expert witnesses, financing necessary studies and reports, and paying attorneys' fees. The costs can only be awarded if incurred after the earlier of:

(1) the date the taxpayer received the decision notice from the IRS Office of Appeals,

(2) the date of the deficiency notice, or

(3) the date on which the first letter of proposed deficiency is sent that allows the taxpayer an opportunity for administrative review in the IRS Office of Appeals.

Reasonable litigation costs include:

(1) expenses of expert witnesses;

(2) costs of any study, analysis, engineering report, test, or project, which was found by the court to be necessary for the preparation of its case;

(3) fees of an individual authorized to practice before the court or the IRS, whether or not an attorney (generally not in excess of $190 per hour for 2014; $200 per hour for 2015), unless an affidavit is presented that establishes a special factor for a higher rate, such as the unavailability of qualified representatives at the customary rate; and

(4) court costs.

To be recoverable, litigation costs must generally be paid or incurred by the taxpayer. However, a taxpayer may recover costs paid by a third party if the taxpayer assumes either a noncontingent obligation to repay the advanced fees or a contingent obligation to repay the fees in the event of their eventual recovery *(B.F. Morrison*, CA-9, 2009-1 USTC ¶ 50,387).

For purposes of both reasonable administrative costs and reasonable litigation costs, reasonable attorneys' fees may be awarded to attorneys and specified persons who represent prevailing parties on a pro bono basis or for a nominal fee. Thus, the amount awarded may be more than the amount of fees actually paid or incurred. The award must be paid to the attorney or the attorney's employer.

In order to establish that the taxpayer was a prevailing party, the taxpayer needs to establish that he has substantially prevailed with respect to the amount in controversy or with respect to the most significant issue or set of issues presented (Code Sec. 7430(c)(4); Reg. §301.7430-5).[145] A taxpayer who meets the timely filing and net worth requirements may be treated as a prevailing party if the taxpayer's liability is determined

---

References are to Standard Federal Tax Reports; Tax Research Consultant; and Practical Tax Explanations.

[143] ¶ 41,583, ¶ 42,440; LITIG: 6,954

[144] ¶ 41,740; LITIG: 3,150; § 41,230.05

[145] ¶ 41,740, ¶ 41,742E, ¶ 41,742H; LITIG: 3,154; § 41,230.15

¶2794

to be equal to or less than it would have been had the government accepted the taxpayer's last qualified offer to settle the case (including interest). A qualified offer is a written offer made at any time during the time from the issuance of the 30-day letter to a date 30 days before the date the case is first set for trial (Code Sec. 7430(g); Reg. § 301.7430-7).[146]

No costs will be awarded where the prevailing party failed to exhaust all of the administrative remedies within the IRS (Code Sec. 7430(b); Reg. § 301.7430-1).[147] The tender of a qualified settlement offer does not satisfy the requirement to exhaust all administrative remedies (*Haas & Associates Accounting Corporation*, 117 TC 48, Dec. 54,447, aff'd CA-9, 2003-1 USTC ¶ 50,253). Further, costs will be denied for any portion of the proceeding where the prevailing party caused unreasonable delay (Code Sec. 7430(b)(4)).[148] A taxpayer who prevails in an IRS proceeding must apply to the IRS for administrative costs before the 91st day after the date the final IRS determination of tax, interest or penalty was mailed to the taxpayer. If the IRS denies the application for costs, the taxpayer must petition the Tax Court within 90 days of the IRS mailing of the denial.

An order granting or denying an award for litigation costs becomes part of the decision or judgment in the case and is subject to appeal in the same manner as the decision or judgment (Code Sec. 7430(f)).[149]

2798. Suit for Damages in Connection with Collection of Tax. A taxpayer may bring a suit in federal district court for damages sustained in connection with the collection of any federal tax because an IRS employee recklessly or intentionally disregarded any provision of the Internal Revenue Code, any IRS regulations or certain provisions of the Bankruptcy Code (Code Sec. 7433; Reg. § 301.7433-1).[150] A suit may also be brought for negligent disregard of the Internal Revenue Code or any IRS regulations. Except as provided in Code Sec. 7432 relating to damage awards for failure to release liens (¶ 2755), this action is the taxpayer's exclusive remedy for recovering damages caused by reckless, intentional or negligent disregard of such provisions and regulations by IRS employees. The suit must be brought within two years after the right of action accrues.

The award is limited to the costs of the action plus any actual direct economic damages sustained by the taxpayer, up to a maximum award of $1 million for reckless or intentional actions and $100,000 for acts of negligence. The IRS must comply with certain provisions of the Fair Debt Collection Practices Act so that the treatment of tax debtors by the IRS is at least equal to that required of private sector debt collectors (Code Sec. 6304). Taxpayers may bring a damages action under Code Sec. 7433 against the IRS for violations of these provisions.

References are to Standard Federal Tax Reports; Tax Research Consultant; and Practical Tax Explanations.

[146] ¶ 41,740, ¶ 41,742H; LI-TIG: 3,154; § 41,230.15

[147] ¶ 41,740, ¶ 41,742; LITIG: 3,150; § 41,230.20

[148] ¶ 41,740; LITIG: 3,154; § 41,230.30

[149] ¶ 41,740; LITIG: 3,158; § 41,230.40

[150] ¶ 41,770, ¶ 41,771; IRS: 45,114; § 39,950.05

Chapter 28

PENALTIES □ INTEREST

Failure to File Returns or Pay Tax

2801. Failure to File Returns. A failure to file any tax return within the time prescribed by the Code may result in an addition to tax, i.e., a penalty. The penalty is five percent of the unpaid tax shown on the return for one month, with an additional five percent for each month or part of a month that the failure continues, up to 25 percent. If the tax return is not filed within 60 days of the prescribed due date, including extensions, the penalty will *not* be less than the lesser of $135 or 100 percent of the tax due on the return (Code Sec. 6651(a)).[1] The late-filing addition runs for the period up to the date the IRS actually receives the late return (Rev. Rul. 73-133).[2] The penalty is computed only on the net amount of tax due, if any, on the return after application of credits for payments of tax through withholding and estimated tax, as well as any other tax credits claimed on the return (Code Sec. 6651(b); Reg. § 301.6651-1(a), (b) and (d)).[3]

The fraud and accuracy-related penalties (¶ 2854) do not apply in the case of a fraudulent failure to file a return. Instead, the failure-to-file penalty ranges from 15 percent to 75 percent of the unpaid tax shown on the return (Code Sec. 6651(f)).[4]

The failure-to-file penalty is not imposed when the taxpayer can show that the failure to file was due to reasonable cause and not to willful neglect. Mere absence of willful neglect is not reasonable cause.[5] For example, reasonable cause did *not* exist when: (1) the taxpayer relied upon the advice of an agent; (2) the taxpayer relied on the accountant to perform the purely ministerial function of filing;[6] or (3) an officer of the corporate taxpayer misjudged the extension date.[7] However, failure to file a return upon a lawyer's or certified public accountant's advice that there was no income to report, or that the taxpayer was not liable for tax, has been held to be reasonable cause when the taxpayer supplied complete information to the tax professional.[8]

2805. Failure to Pay Tax. A penalty is imposed for failure to pay, when due, those taxes (other than estimated taxes) shown by a taxpayer on a return, unless the failure is due to reasonable cause (Code Sec. 6651(a)(2)).[9] A penalty is also imposed on additional taxes determined to be due on audit for which the IRS has made a demand for payment, but this penalty runs only for the period of nonpayment beginning after the 21st *calendar*

References are to Standard Federal Tax Reports; Tax Research Consultant; and Practical Tax Explanations.

[1] ¶ 39,470; PENALTY: 3,050; § 40,205.15

[2] ¶ 39,475.33; PENALTY: 3,056; § 40,205.15

[3] ¶ 39,470, ¶ 39,472; PENALTY: 3,054; § 40,205.15

[4] ¶ 39,470; PENALTY: 3,052; § 40,205.15

[5] ¶ 39,475.34; PENALTY: 3,060; § 40,205.15

[6] ¶ 39,475.42, ¶ 39,475.72; PENALTY: 3,060; § 40,205.15

[7] ¶ 39,475.705; PENALTY: 3,060; § 40,205.15

[8] ¶ 39,475.41; PENALTY: 3,060; § 40,205.15

[9] ¶ 39,470; PENALTY: 3,062; § 40,205.20

¶2801

day (10th *business* day if the amount demanded is at least $100,000) following the demand (Code Sec. 6651(a)(3)).

In both cases, the addition to tax is one-half of one percent of the tax not paid, for each month or part of a month the tax remains unpaid, up to a maximum of 25 percent. The penalty increases to one percent per month beginning with either the 10th day after notice of levy is given or the day on which notice and demand is made in the case of a jeopardy assessment (¶ 2713). For taxpayers who enter into installment agreements (¶ 2529) with the IRS, the penalty for failure to timely pay taxes is reduced to one-quarter of one percent of the tax not paid (Code Sec. 6651(h); Reg. § 301.6651-1(a)(4)).[10]

If a taxpayer files a late return that is subject to both the failure-to-file penalty (¶ 2801) and the failure-to-pay penalty, the former may be reduced by the latter. However, if no return is filed or if a late-filed return understates the amount required to be shown on the return, the failure-to-pay penalty attributable to additional tax demanded by the IRS may not be used to offset any portion of the failure-to-file penalty. If the penalty for failure to file beyond 60 days applies, the penalty may not be reduced by a failure-to-pay penalty that is also imposed below the lesser of $135 or 100 percent of the tax due (Code Sec. 6651(a), (c), and (d)).[11]

Penalty Relief for Delayed 2012 Forms. Individuals and businesses were provided relief from the failure-to-pay penalty if they requested extension to file a 2012 income tax return that included certain forms the IRS did not make available until February or March 2013 (Notice 2013-24).[12] The IRS deemed taxpayers to have demonstrated reasonable cause and lack of willful neglect provided an extension to file the return due to a lack of certain forms was filed, a good-faith estimate of the tax liability was made on the extension request, the estimated amount is paid by the original due date, and any tax owed on the return was fully paid no later than the extended due date. Interest, however, still applied to any tax payment made after the original due date.

2809. Automatic Extension of Time for Filing. An automatic extension of time to file a tax return (¶ 2509) is not an extension of time to pay the tax due under the return (Reg. §§ 1.6081-3(b) and 1.6081-4(c)).[13] However, an individual taxpayer can avoid a failure-to-pay penalty (¶ 2805) by making an estimate of the tax due and paying that estimate with the request for extension of time to file. The estimate may be reduced by any amounts already paid through withholding or estimated tax payments over the course of the tax year. If the balance of tax due is remitted when the income tax return is filed by an individual or corporation, no penalty for failure to pay will apply unless the unpaid amount is more than 10 percent of the total tax liability (Reg. § 301.6651-1(c)(3) and (4)).[14]

2811. Frivolous Return Penalty. In addition to other penalties that may be imposed, there is a $5,000 penalty for filing a frivolous return (Code Sec. 6702).[15] A frivolous return is one that omits information necessary to determine the taxpayer's tax liability, shows a substantially incorrect tax, is based upon a frivolous position (e.g., that wages are not income), or is based upon the taxpayer's desire to impede the collection of tax. The IRS periodically updates a list of frivolous positions (Notice 2010-33). For example, a return based on the taxpayer's altering or striking out the "penalty of perjury" language above the signature line constitutes a frivolous return.

In certain limited circumstances, the IRS will reduce the $5,000 frivolous return penalty to $500 (Rev. Proc. 2012-43). If a person satisfies all eligibility criteria under the procedures, including filing all tax returns and paying all outstanding taxes, penalties (other than the frivolous return penalty), and related interest, the IRS will generally reduce all unpaid frivolous return penalties assessed against that person to $500,

---

References are to Standard Federal Tax Reports; Tax Research Consultant; and Practical Tax Explanations.

[10] ¶ 39,470, ¶ 39,472; PENALTY: 3,062; § 40,205.20

[11] ¶ 39,470; PENALTY: 3,064; § 40,205.20

[12] ¶ 39,475.34; PENALTY: 3,062.05; § 40,205.20

[13] ¶ 36,790, ¶ 36,793; FILEBUS: 15,102; § 39,215.05

[14] ¶ 39,472; PENALTY: 3,062.20; § 39,215.10

[15] ¶ 40,040, ¶ 40,043.50; PENALTY: 3,250; § 40,220.10

regardless of the number of penalties assessed. Any employer applying for relief must have deposited all employment taxes for the current quarter and the prior two quarters.

2813. Abatement of Penalties and/or Interest. The IRS must abate certain penalties that result from reliance on incorrect IRS advice if (1) the advice was furnished in writing in response to a specific written request from the taxpayer, and (2) the taxpayer reasonably relied upon the advice (Code Sec. 6404(f); Reg. § 301.6404-3).[16] However, penalties will be abated only if the taxpayer furnished adequate and accurate information in making the request. Taxpayers entitled to abatement should file Form 843 with copies of the relevant written documents attached.

If the IRS extends the due date for filing income tax returns and for paying any tax due for taxpayers located in a federally declared disaster area, the IRS will abate the interest that would otherwise accrue for the extension period (Code Secs. 6404(i) and 7508A).[17]

The accrual of interest and penalties will be suspended after 36 months unless the IRS sends the taxpayer a notice following the later of: (1) the original due date of the return (without regard to extensions); or (2) the date on which a timely return is filed (Code Sec. 6404(g)).[18] The suspension of interest and penalties is available only for individuals and only for income taxes. Although the suspension pertains only to tax that is related to timely filed returns, the IRS has expanded this rule to cover additional tax voluntarily reported by a taxpayer, after a timely original return has been filed, on an amended return, or in correspondence with the IRS (Rev. Rul. 2005-4). The suspension begins on the day after the end of the 36-month period and ends on the day that is 21 days after the date on which the notice is made. The suspension does not stop the accrual of:

(1) the failure-to-file (¶ 2801) and failure-to-pay (¶ 2805) penalties;

(2) any interest, penalty, or other addition to tax in a case involving fraud;

(3) any interest, penalty, addition to tax, or additional amount with respect to any tax liability shown on the return;

(4) any interest, penalty, or other addition to tax with respect to any gross misstatement;

(5) any interest, penalty, or other addition to tax with respect to any reportable avoidance transaction or listed transaction (¶ 2591); or

(6) any criminal penalty.

Document and Information Return Penalties

2814. Information Reporting Penalties. Three categories of penalties apply to failures to file required information returns and payee statements:

(1) failure to file an information return or to include correct information on an information return (¶ 2816) (Code Sec. 6721);

(2) failure to file a payee statement or to include correct information on a payee statement (¶ 2823) (Code Sec. 6722); and

(3) failure to comply with other information reporting requirements, which includes all reporting failures not covered by the other two categories (¶ 2833) (Code Sec. 6723).

2816. Failure to File Correct Information Returns. A time-sensitive three-tier penalty structure is imposed for: (1) any failure to file correct information returns (¶ 2565) with the IRS on or before the required filing date (other than a failure due to reasonable cause and not to willful neglect); (2) any failure to include all the information required to be shown on a return; or (3) the inclusion of incorrect information (Code

---

References are to Standard Federal Tax Reports; Tax Research Consultant; and Practical Tax Explanations.

[16] ¶ 38,570, ¶ 38,576; IRS: 33,400; § 40,250.15

[17] ¶ 38,570, ¶ 42,687A; PENALTY: 9,056; § 39,215.35

[18] ¶ 38,570; PENALTY: 3,350, PENALTY: 9,056; § 40,030.30, § 40,250.10

¶2813

Sec. 6721).[19] The penalty applies also to any failure to file electronically, when required, but is imposed only if the taxpayer is filing 250 or more information returns (100 information returns in the case of a partnership having more than 100 partners) (Code Sec. 6724(c)).[20] The penalty amounts for each of the prescribed time periods are as follows:

(1) If a person files a correct information return after the required filing date but on or before the date that is 30 days after the required filing date, the amount of the penalty is $30 per return ("first-tier penalty"), with a maximum penalty of $250,000 per calendar year ($75,000 for small businesses with gross receipts of not more than $5 million).

(2) If a person files a correct information return after the date that is 30 days after the prescribed filing date but on or before August 1 of the calendar year in which the required filing date occurs, the amount of the penalty is $60 per return ("second-tier penalty"), with a maximum penalty of $500,000 per calendar year ($200,000 for small businesses).

(3) If a correct information return is not filed on or before August 1 of the calendar year in which the required filing date occurs, the amount of the penalty is $100 per return ("third-tier penalty"), with a maximum penalty of $1.5 million per calendar year ($500,000 for small businesses).

A certain *de minimis* number of returns timely filed with incorrect or omitted information that are corrected on or before August 1 of the calendar year in which the returns are due will be treated as having been filed correctly, and no penalty will be imposed on them. This exception is limited to the greater of 10 returns or one-half of one percent of the total number of information returns required to be filed during the calendar year. The *de minimis* exception does not apply to a failure to file an information return (Code Sec. 6721(c)).

If the failure to file an information return or to include all the required correct information is due to intentional disregard of the filing requirements, neither the three-tier penalty nor the *de minimis* exception will apply (Code Sec. 6721(e)). Instead, the penalty for each failure is the greater of:

(1) $250, or

(2) (a) 10 percent of the aggregate amount of the items required to be reported correctly in the case of a return other than a return required under Code Sec. 6045(a) (brokers' transactions with customers), Code Sec. 6041A(b) (payments of remuneration for direct sales), Code Sec. 6050H (information on mortgage interest received in a trade or business from individuals), Code Sec. 6050I (information on cash receipts from a trade or business), Code Sec. 6050J (information on foreclosures and abandonments of security), Code Sec. 6050K (information on exchanges of certain partnership interests), or Code Sec. 6050L (information on certain dispositions of donated property);

(b) five percent of the aggregate amount of the items required to be properly reported under Code Sec. 6045(a), Code Sec. 6050K, or Code Sec. 6050L;

(c) for informational returns required under Code Sec. 6050I(a) (cash receipts of more than $10,000 in a trade or business), $25,000 or the amount of cash received in the transaction or related transactions, up to a maximum of $100,000.

In addition, the intentional disregard penalties are not considered in figuring the yearly maximum penalty of $1.5 million for failures not attributable to intentional disregard.

No penalty is imposed for inconsequential omissions and inaccuracies that do not prevent or hinder the IRS from adequately processing the return. Errors and omissions

References are to Standard Federal Tax Reports; Tax Research Consultant; and Practical Tax Explanations.

[19] ¶ 40,210; PENALTY: 3,202; § 40,305.10

[20] ¶ 40,275; PENALTY: 3,202; § 40,305.10

that relate to a taxpayer identification number, to the surname of a person required to receive a copy of the information provided, or to any monetary amounts are never considered inconsequential (Code Sec. 6721(c); Reg. § 301.6721-1(c)).

The information return penalty amounts are to be adjusted for inflation every five years, beginning after 2012 (Code Sec. 6721(f)). Thus, the first inflation adjustments, if any, to the amounts will be in 2017.

2823. Failure to Furnish Correct Payee Statement. The statutory structure of the penalties for failure to timely furnish a correct payee statement resembles the three-tier Code Sec. 6721 penalties for failure to timely file a correct information return, including reduced maximum penalties for small businesses (¶ 2816) (Code Sec. 6722).[21] The penalty regime is as follows:

> (1) If a person furnishes a correct payee statement up to 30 days after the required due date, the amount of the first-tier penalty is $30 per statement, with a maximum penalty of $250,000 per calendar year ($75,000 for small businesses).

> (2) If a person furnishes a correct payee statement more than 30 days after the prescribed filing date but on or before August 1 of the calendar year in which the required filing date occurs, the amount of the second-tier penalty is $60 per return, with a maximum penalty of $500,000 per calendar year ($200,000 for small businesses).

> (3) If a correct payee statement is not furnished on or before August 1 of the calendar year in which the required filing date occurs, the amount of the third-tier penalty is $100 per return, with a maximum penalty of $1.5 million per calendar year ($500,000 for small businesses).

Payee statements include the following (Code Sec. 6724(d)):[22]

> (1) pass-through income, deductions, etc., to partners in a partnership under Code Sec. 6031(b) or (c), to beneficiaries of estates and trusts under Code Sec. 6034A, and to S corporation shareholders under Code Sec. 6037(b);

> (2) certain stock options under Code Sec. 6039(b);

> (3) information-at-source payments under Code Sec. 6041(d);

> (4) payments in connection with services and direct sales under Code Sec. 6041A(e);

> (5) statements relating to returns regarding payments of dividends and corporate earnings and profits under Code Sec. 6042(c);

> (6) taxable mergers and acquisitions under Code Sec. 6043A;

> (7) statements regarding payments of patronage dividends under Code Sec. 6044(e);

> (8) brokers under Code Sec. 6045(b) or (d);

> (9) statements to brokers relating to the transfer of covered securities under Code Sec. 6045A (however, transitional relief from the penalty was provided for certain 2011 transfers (Notice 2010-67));

> (10) statements relating to organizational actions affecting basis of specified securities under Code Sec. 6045B (however, transitional relief from the penalty was provided for any organization action in 2011 (Notice 2011-18));

> (11) statements regarding interest payments under Code Sec. 6049(c);

> (12) catch shares of certain fishing boat crews under Code Sec. 6050A(b);

> (13) mortgage interest payments under Code Sec. 6050H(d) and (h)(2);

> (14) cash payments in excess of $10,000 under Code Sec. 6050I(e), (g)(4), or (g)(5);

References are to Standard Federal Tax Reports; Tax Research Consultant; and Practical Tax Explanations.

[21] ¶ 40,230; PENALTY: 3,204;   [22] ¶ 40,275; PENALTY: 3,204;
§ 40,305.15   § 40,305.05

¶2823

(15) foreclosures and abandonments of security under Code Sec. 6050J(e);

(16) exchanges of certain partnership interests under Code Sec. 6050K(b);

(17) certain dispositions of donated property under Code Sec. 6050L(c);

(18) payments of royalties under Code Sec. 6050N(b);

(19) statements relating to the cancellation of indebtedness by certain financial entities under Code Sec. 6050P(d);

(20) long-term care benefits under Code Sec. 6050Q(b);

(21) payments for certain purchases of fish for resale under Code Sec. 6050R;

(22) income tax withheld from employees' wages under Code Sec. 6051;

(23) group-term life insurance under Code Sec. 6052(b);

(24) tip income reportable by employers under Code Sec. 6053(b) or (c);

(25) foreign trust reporting requirements under Code Sec. 6048(b)(1)(B);

(26) distributions from individual retirement accounts under Code Sec. 408(i) and from employee benefit plans under Code Sec. 6047(d);

(27) payments relating to qualified tuition and related expenses under Code Sec. 6050S;

(28) returns relating to certain company-owned life insurance held by a natural person where a trade or business is directly or indirectly the beneficiary under the policy under Code Sec. 264(f)(5)(A)(iv);

(29) returns filed with respect to the credit for health insurance costs of eligible individuals under Code Sec. 6050T;

(30) charges or payments for qualified long-term insurance contracts under combined arrangements of Code Sec. 6050U;

(31) payments made in settlement of payment card transactions under Code Sec. 6050W;

(32) statements relating to information regarding health insurance coverage under Code Sec. 6055(c); and

(33) statements relating to certain employers required to report on health insurance coverage under Code Sec. 6056(c).

In the case of intentional disregard of the requirements with respect to payee statements, the penalty imposed is identical to that for failures to file an information return or to include correct information (¶ 2816). Similarly, the intentional disregard penalty is not considered in applying the yearly maximum penalty of $1.5 million for failures not attributable to intentional disregard. In addition, the exception from the imposition of the penalty in the case of inconsequential omissions and inaccuracies on a payee statement applies.

The payee statement penalty amounts are to be adjusted for inflation every five years, beginning after 2012 (Code Sec. 6722(f)). Thus, the first inflation adjustment, if any, to the amounts will be in 2017.

2833. Failure to Comply with Other Information Reporting Requirements. A penalty of $50 is imposed for each failure to comply with any specified information reporting requirement on or before the prescribed time, up to a maximum of $100,000 for a calendar year (Code Sec. 6723).[23] The penalty will not be imposed if it can be shown that the failure was due to reasonable cause and not to willful neglect.

The specified information reporting requirements that are subject to the penalty include:

References are to Standard Federal Tax Reports; Tax Research Consultant; and Practical Tax Explanations.

[23] ¶ 40,250; PENALTY: 3,204; § 40,305.20

(1) the requirement that a transferor of an interest in a partnership promptly give notice to the partnership concerning the transfer;

(2) the requirement that a person include his or her taxpayer identification number (TIN) on any return, statement, or other document (other than an information return or payee statement), furnish his or her TIN to another person, or include the TIN of another person on any return, statement, or other document made with respect to that person;

(3) the requirement on returns reporting alimony payments that the TIN of the payee be furnished to the payor or that the payee's TIN be included on the payor's return;

(4) the requirement that a person include the TIN of any dependent on his or her return; and

(5) the requirement that a person who deducts qualified residence interest (¶ 1047) on any seller-provided financing include the name, address, and TIN of the person to whom such interest is paid or accrued (Code Sec. 6724(d)(3)).[24]

Underpayments of Tax—Interest

2838. Interest on Underpayment of Tax. Interest on underpayments of tax is imposed at the federal short-term rate plus three percentage points (Code Sec. 6621(a)(2)).[25] The interest rates, which are adjusted quarterly, are determined during the first month of a calendar quarter and become effective for the following quarter.

Interest accrues from the date the payment was due, determined without regard to any extensions of time, until it is received by the IRS, although no underpayment interest accrues for failure to timely pay individual or corporate estimated tax. Interest is compounded daily (Code Secs. 6601 and 6622).[26] For all four quarters of 2014, the interest rate on underpayments is three percent.[27]

If a carryback of a net operating loss, net capital loss, or other credit carryback eliminates or reduces a deficiency otherwise due for such earlier year, the taxpayer remains liable for interest on unpaid income taxes (including deficiencies later assessed by the IRS) for the carryback year. The entire amount of the deficiency will be subject to interest from the last date prescribed for payment of the income tax of the carryback year up to the due date (excluding extensions) for filing the return for the tax year in which the loss or credit occurred (Code Sec. 6601(d); Reg. § 301.6601-1(e)).[28]

Large Corporate Tax Underpayments. Interest on large underpayments of tax by corporations is imposed at the federal short-term rate plus five percentage points (Code Sec. 6621(c); Reg. § 301.6621-3).[29] A large corporate underpayment is any tax underpayment by a C corporation that exceeds $100,000 for any tax period. For purposes of determining the $100,000 threshold, underpayments of different types of taxes (for example, income and employment taxes) as well as underpayments relating to different tax periods are not added together. The tax period is the tax year in the case of income tax or, in the case of any other tax, the period to which the underpayment relates.

The interest rate for large underpayment by corporations applies to time periods after the 30th day after the earlier of: (1) the date the IRS sends the first letter of proposed deficiency that allows the taxpayer an opportunity for administrative review in the IRS Office of Appeals (a 30-day letter); or (2) the date the IRS sends a deficiency notice (a 90-day letter) (¶ 2711). The 30-day period does not begin unless the underpayment shown in the letter or notice exceeds $100,000. An IRS notice that is later withdrawn because it was issued in error will not trigger the higher rate of interest on large corporate underpayments. If the underpayment is not subject to deficiency payments, the 30-day period begins to run following the sending of any letter or notice by

---

References are to Standard Federal Tax Reports; Tax Research Consultant; and Practical Tax Explanations.

[24] ¶ 40,275; PENALTY: 3,204; § 40,305.20

[25] ¶ 39,450; PENALTY: 9,152; § 40,105.05

[26] ¶ 39,410, ¶ 39,460; PENALTY: 9,050; § 40,105.05

[27] ¶ 39,455.51; PENALTY: 9,152; § 40,105.05

[28] ¶ 39,410, ¶ 39,412; PENALTY: 9,056.10; § 40,105.15

[29] ¶ 39,450, ¶ 39,453; PENALTY: 9,152.05; § 40,120.15

¶2838

the IRS that notifies the taxpayer of the assessment or proposed assessment of the tax. A letter or notice is disregarded if the full amount shown as due is paid during the 30-day period. For all four quarters of 2014, the interest rate on large corporate underpayments is five percent.[30]

Overlapping Overpayments and Underpayments. The interest rates for overpayments and underpayments have been equalized (also referred to as "global interest netting") for any period of mutual indebtedness between taxpayers and the IRS (¶ 2765).

Abatement of Interest. The IRS has the authority to abate interest in cases where the additional interest was caused by IRS errors or delays (Code Sec. 6404(e)).[31] However, the IRS may act only if there was an error or delay in performing either a ministerial act or a managerial act, including loss of records by the IRS, transfers of IRS personnel, extended illness, extended personnel training, or extended leave, and only if the abatement relates to a tax of the type for which a notice of deficiency is required. These taxes would be those relating to income, generation-skipping transfers, estate, gift, and certain excise taxes, but not employment taxes or other excise taxes. Taxpayers requesting an abatement of interest generally must file a separate Form 843 for each tax period for each type of tax with the IRS Service Center where their tax return was filed or, if unknown, with the Service Center where their most recent tax return was filed.

Suspension of Interest. In order to avoid the accrual of underpayment interest, a taxpayer may make a cash deposit with the IRS for future application against an underpayment of income, gift, estate, generation-skipping, or certain excise taxes that have not been assessed at the time of the deposit (Code Sec. 6603; Rev. Proc. 2005-18).[32] To the extent that a deposit is used by the IRS to pay a tax liability, the tax is treated as paid when the deposit is made, and no interest underpayment is imposed. Furthermore, if the dispute is resolved in favor of the taxpayer or the taxpayer withdraws the deposited money before resolution of the dispute, interest is payable on the deposit at the federal short-term rate.

2845. Interest on Additions and Penalties. Interest on additions to tax, i.e., penalties, for failure to file a return (¶ 2801), for failure to pay the stamp tax, and for accuracy-related (¶ 2854) and fraud penalties (¶ 2866) will be imposed for the period beginning on the due date of the return (including extensions) and ending on the date of payment. If payment is made within 21 *calendar* days after notice and demand is made (10 *business* days if the amount demanded is at least $100,000), then interest will stop running after the date of notice and demand. For all other penalties, interest will be imposed only if the addition to tax or penalty is not paid within the 21-or 10-day period after notice and demand is made and then only for the period from the date of notice and demand to the date of payment (Code Sec. 6601(e)).[33] For rules governing the allocation of interest on tax liabilities paid pursuant to a compromise or partial payment, see ¶ 2723 and ¶ 2724, respectively.

Underpayments of Tax—Penalties

2854. Accuracy-Related Penalty. An accuracy-related penalty of 20 percent is imposed on the portion of any underpayment of tax that is due to negligence or disregard of rules or regulations (¶ 2856), substantial understatement of income tax (¶ 2858), substantial valuation misstatement (¶ 2860), substantial overstatements of pension liabilities (¶ 2862), substantial estate or gift tax valuation understatement (¶ 2862A), and transactions lacking economic substance (¶ 2863) (Code Sec. 6662)[34] In addition, a 40-percent accuracy-related penalty is imposed for an underpayment of tax due to an undisclosed foreign financial asset understatement (¶ 2864). If any part of an underpayment of tax required to be shown on a return is due to fraud, a separate penalty equal to 75 percent of the portion of the underpayment is imposed (¶ 2866).

References are to Standard Federal Tax Reports; Tax Research Consultant; and Practical Tax Explanations.

[30] ¶ 39,455.51; PENALTY: 9,152.05; § 40,105.05

[31] ¶ 39,570; PENALTY: 9,056.20; § 40,030.15

[32] ¶ 39,426, ¶ 39,428.20; IRS: 36,056.25; § 40,110.15

[33] ¶ 39,410; PENALTY: 9,060; § 40,105.05

[34] ¶ 39,651; PENALTY: 3,100; § 40,210.05

The accuracy-related penalty is entirely separate from the failure-to-file penalty (¶ 2801) and will not be imposed if no return is filed, other than a return prepared by the IRS when a person fails to make a required return (Code Sec. 6664(b)).[35] In addition, the accuracy-related penalty will not apply to any portion of a tax underpayment on which the fraud penalty is imposed. Also, with the exception of the penalty for underpayments attributable to transactions lacking economic substance, no penalty is imposed with respect to any portion of any underpayment if the taxpayer shows that there was reasonable cause for the underpayment and that the taxpayer acted in good faith (Code Sec. 6664(c)).[36]

2856. Penalty for Negligence or Disregard of Rules and Regulations. If any part of an underpayment of tax is due to negligence or careless, reckless, or intentional disregard of rules and regulations, a 20-percent accuracy-related penalty (¶ 2854) will be imposed on that portion of the underpayment attributable to the negligence or intentional disregard of rules and regulations (Code Sec. 6662(a) and (c); Reg. § 1.6662-3).[37] Negligence includes the failure to reasonably comply with tax laws, to exercise reasonable care in preparing a tax return, to keep adequate books and records, or to substantiate items properly. Taxpayers may not avoid the negligence penalty merely by adequately disclosing a return position which is "not frivolous" on Form 8275 or Form 8275-R

2858. Penalty for Substantial Understatement of Income Tax. A 20-percent accuracy-related penalty (¶ 2854) may be imposed on a taxpayer when there is a substantial understatement of income tax for the tax year (Code Sec. 6662(d); Reg. § 1.6662-4).[38] A substantial understatement exists when the understatement for the year exceeds the greater of 10 percent of the tax required to be shown on the return (including self-employment tax) or $5,000. In the case of corporations (other than S corporations or personal holding companies), a substantial understatement exists when the understatement exceeds the lesser of 10 percent of the tax required to be shown on the return (or, if greater, $10,000) or $10 million.

Taxpayers generally may avoid all or part of the penalty by showing:

> (1) that they acted in good faith and there was reasonable cause for the understatement;

> (2) that the understatement was based on substantial authority; or

> (3) if there was a reasonable basis for the tax treatment of an item, the relevant facts affecting the item's tax treatment were adequately disclosed on Form 8275 or Form 8275-R.

Substantial authority generally means that the likelihood that a taxpayer's position is correct is somewhere between 50 percent and the more lenient reasonable basis standard used in applying the negligence penalty. The disclosure exception does not apply to tax shelter items. Further, a corporation does not have a reasonable basis for its tax treatment of an item attributable to a multi-party financing transaction if the treatment does not clearly reflect the income of the corporation. Some items may be disclosed on the taxpayer's return, instead of on Form 8275 or Form 8275-R (Rev. Proc. 2014-15).[39]

Only the following are authority for purposes of determining whether a position is supported by substantial authority:

> (1) the Internal Revenue Code and other statutory provisions;

> (2) proposed, temporary, and final regulations construing the statutes;

> (3) revenue rulings and procedures;

References are to Standard Federal Tax Reports; Tax Research Consultant; and Practical Tax Explanations.

[35] ¶ 39,660; PENALTY: 3,102; § 40,210.05

[36] ¶ 39,660; PENALTY: 3,102; § 40,210.40

[37] ¶ 39,651, ¶ 39,651E; PENALTY: 3,106; § 40,210.15

[38] ¶ 39,651, ¶ 39,651H; PENALTY: 3,108; § 40,210.20

[39] ¶ 39,652.102; PENALTY: 3,108.15; § 40,210.20

(4) tax treaties and the regulations thereunder, and Treasury Department and other official explanations of such treaties;

(5) court cases;

(6) Congressional intent as reflected in committee reports, joint explanatory statements of managers included in conference committee reports, and floor statements made prior to enactment by one of a bill's managers;

(7) General Explanations of tax legislation prepared by the Joint Committee on Taxation (the Blue Book);

(8) private letter rulings and technical advice memoranda issued after October 31, 1976;

(9) actions on decisions and general counsel memoranda issued after March 12, 1981, as well as general counsel memoranda published in pre-1955 volumes of the Cumulative Bulletin;

(10) IRS information and press releases; and

(11) notices, announcements, and other administrative pronouncements published by the IRS in the Internal Revenue Bulletin.[40]

2860. Penalty for Substantial Valuation Misstatement. A 20-percent accuracy-related penalty (¶ 2854) is imposed on any portion of an underpayment of tax resulting from any substantial income tax valuation misstatement (Code Sec. 6662(e)).[41] There is a substantial valuation misstatement if:

(1) the value of any property, or adjusted basis of any property, claimed on a tax return is 150 percent or more of the amount determined to be the correct amount of the valuation or the adjusted basis;

(2) the price for any property, or use of property, or services in connection with any transaction between persons described in Code Sec. 482 is 200 percent or more, or 50 percent or less, of the correct Code Sec. 482 valuation; or

(3) the net Code Sec. 482 transfer price adjustment exceeds the lesser of $5 million or 10 percent of the taxpayer's gross receipts.

The penalty is doubled to 40 percent in cases of gross valuation misstatements where claimed value or adjusted basis exceeds the correct value or adjusted basis by 200 percent or more (Code Sec. 6662(h)). A gross valuation misstatement with respect to a controlled taxpayer transaction (Code Sec. 482) occurs if the price claimed exceeds 400 percent or more, or 25 percent or less, of the amount determined to be the correct price, or the net Code Sec. 482 transfer price adjustment for the year exceeds the lesser of $20 million or 20 percent of the taxpayer's gross receipts.

No penalty is imposed unless the portion of the underpayment attributable to the substantial valuation misstatement exceeds $5,000, or $10,000 in the case of corporations other than S corporations or personal holding companies. The penalty will not be imposed if it is shown that there was reasonable cause for an underpayment and the taxpayer acted in good faith. However, there is no reasonable cause exception for underpayments due to gross valuation misstatements on charitable deduction property, although the exception still exists for substantial valuation misstatements on charitable deduction property and for gross valuation misstatements on property for which a charitable deduction is not being claimed (Code Sec. 6664(c)).[42]

2862. Penalty for Substantial Overstatement of Pension Liabilities. A 20-percent accuracy-related penalty (¶ 2854) is imposed on any portion of any underpayment of tax resulting from a substantial overstatement of pension liabilities (Code Sec. 6662(a), (f), and (h)).[43] A substantial overstatement occurs if the actuarial determination of pension

References are to Standard Federal Tax Reports; Tax Research Consultant; and Practical Tax Explanations.

[40] ¶ 39,651H; PENALTY: 3,108; § 40,210.20

[41] ¶ 39,651; PENALTY: 3,110; § 40,210.25

[42] ¶ 39,660; PENALTY: 3,110; § 40,210.25

[43] ¶ 39,651; PENALTY: 3,112; § 40,210.30

¶2862

liabilities is 200 percent or more of the amount determined to be correct. The penalty is doubled to 40 percent of the underpayment if a portion of the substantial overstatement to which the penalty applies is attributable to a gross valuation misstatement of 400 percent or more. The penalty applies only if the portion of the underpayment attributable to the overstatement exceeds $1,000. The penalty will not be imposed if it is shown that there was a reasonable cause for an underpayment and the taxpayer acted in good faith (Code Sec. 6664(c)).[44]

2862A. Penalty for Substantial Estate or Gift Tax Valuation Understatements. A 20-percent accuracy-related penalty (¶ 2854) is imposed on the portion of an underpayment of tax that is due to a substantial estate or gift tax valuation understatement (Code Sec. 6662(b)(5), (g), and (h)).[45] There is a substantial estate or gift tax valuation understatement if the value of any property claimed on any estate or gift tax return is 65 percent or less of the amount determined to be the correct amount of the valuation. The penalty will not be imposed unless the portion of the underpayment attributable to the valuation understatements for the taxable period or for the estate of the decedent exceeds $5,000. The penalty is increased to 40 percent if the valuation understatement is a gross valuation misstatement. A valuation understatement is a gross valuation understatement if the value of any property claimed on any estate or gift tax return is 40 percent or less of the amount determined to be the correct amount of the valuation. The penalty will not be imposed if it is shown that there was a reasonable cause for an underpayment and the taxpayer acted in good faith (Code Sec. 6664(c)).[46]

2863. Penalty for Underpayment Attributable to Transactions Lacking Economic Substance. A 20-percent accuracy-related penalty (¶ 2854) is imposed for an underpayment of tax attributable to any disallowance of claimed tax benefits by reason of a transaction lacking economic substance, or failing to meet the requirements of any similar rule of law (Code Sec. 6662(b)(6)).[47] A transaction is treated as having economic substance if: (1) apart from the federal income tax effects, it changes in a meaningful way the taxpayer's economic position; and (2) the taxpayer has a substantial purpose for entering into the transaction (Code Sec. 7701(o); Notice 2010-62).[48] The term transaction, including related transactions, generally includes all the factual elements relevant to the expected tax treatment of any investment, entity, plan, or arrangement, and any and all steps that are carried out as part of the plan. Whether a plan's steps should be aggregated or disaggregated is a facts and circumstances analysis. The phase "similar rule of law" means a rule or doctrine that disallows the tax benefits in the Code related to a transaction because the taxpayer's economic position does not change in a meaningful way apart from the Federal income tax effects, or the taxpayer does not have a substantial purpose, apart from the Federal income tax effects, for entering into the transaction (Notice 2014-58, amplifying Notice 2010-62).

Although the IRS will continue to rely on relevant case law handed down prior to the codification of the economic substance doctrine for transactions entered into after March 30, 2010, when applying the two-prong test, taxpayers may not rely on case law that treats a transaction as having economic substance unless the transaction satisfies *both* prongs of the test.

The penalty is increased to 40 percent for an underpayment attributable to a nondisclosed noneconomic substance transaction (Code Sec. 6662(i)).[49] A nondisclosed noneconomic substance transaction is any portion of a transaction lacking economic substance with respect to which the relevant facts affecting the tax treatment are not adequately disclosed in the return or in a statement attached to the return. The determination of whether a position is a nondisclosed noneconomic substance transaction will generally be based on the return as originally filed or as amended by the taxpayer prior to being contacted by the IRS.

References are to Standard Federal Tax Reports; Tax Research Consultant; and Practical Tax Explanations.

[44] ¶ 39,660; PENALTY: 3,116; § 40,210.30

[45] ¶ 39,651; PENALTY: 3,114; § 40,210.35

[46] ¶ 39,660; PENALTY: 3,116; § 40,210.40

[47] ¶ 39,651; PENALTY: 3,122; § 40,210.36

[48] ¶ 39,654AF.40, ¶ 43,080; PENALTY: 3,122; § 40,210.36

[49] ¶ 39,651; PENALTY: 3,122; § 40,210.36

¶2862A

To satisfy the adequate disclosure requirements, the taxpayer must: (1) disclose the relevant facts on a timely filed original return or a qualified amended return; (2) file Form 8275 or Form 8275-R; and (3) if the transaction is a reportable transaction (¶ 2591), satisfy all disclosure requirements for such transactions (¶ 2592).

No exceptions, including the reasonable cause exception, are available to the imposition of a penalty for any underpayment or reportable transaction understatement attributable to a transaction lacking economic substance (Code Sec. 6664(c)(2) and (d)(2)).[50]

2864. Penalty for Underpayment Attributable to Undisclosed Foreign Financial Assets. A 40-percent accuracy-related penalty (¶ 2854) is imposed for underpayment of tax that is attributable to an undisclosed foreign financial asset understatement (Code Sec. 6662(b)(7) and (j)).[51] An undisclosed foreign financial asset understatement for any tax year is the portion of the understatement for the year that is attributable to any transaction involving undisclosed foreign financial assets. An undisclosed foreign financial asset includes any asset that is subject to the information reporting requirements of Code Sec. 6038 (information reporting with respect to certain foreign corporations and partnerships (¶ 2487)), Code Sec. 6038B (notice of certain transfers to foreign persons (¶ 2492)), Code Sec. 6046A (returns as to interests in foreign partnerships (¶ 2494)), Code Sec. 6048 (information with respect to certain foreign trusts (¶ 588)), and Code Sec. 6038D (information with respect to foreign financial assets (¶ 2572)), but for which the required information was not provided by the taxpayer as required under the applicable reporting provisions.

2866. Penalty for Fraud. A penalty is imposed at the rate of 75 percent on the portion of any underpayment of tax that is attributable to fraud (Code Sec. 6663).[52] The fraud penalty will not apply, however, if no return is filed other than a return prepared by the IRS when a person fails to make a required return (Code Sec. 6664(b)).[53] Although the failure-to-file penalty is entirely separate from the fraud penalty, in cases of a fraudulent failure to file, the failure-to-file penalty will be imposed at a higher rate (¶ 2801). If any portion is attributable to fraud, it is presumed that the entire underpayment is attributable to fraud, unless the taxpayer establishes otherwise by a preponderance of the evidence with respect to any item. The accuracy-related penalty will not apply to any portion of an underpayment on which the fraud penalty is imposed (¶ 2854). The IRS must meet its burden of proof in establishing fraud by clear and convincing evidence (Code Sec. 6663(b)).[54]

2870. Penalty for Tax Shelters. An accuracy-related penalty is imposed for understatement of tax attributable to any listed transaction and any reportable transaction with a significant tax avoidance purpose (¶ 2591) (Code Sec. 6662A).[55] The 20-percent accuracy-related penalty on understatements attributable to reportable transactions will not be imposed if the 40-percent penalty is imposed on an underpayment attributable to one or more undisclosed noneconomic substance transactions (¶ 2863).

Underpayments of Estimated Tax

2875. Underpayment of Estimated Tax by Individuals. An underpayment of estimated tax by an individual and most trusts and estates will result in imposition of an addition to tax equal to the applicable underpayment rate of interest (¶ 2838) that accrues on the underpayment for the period of the underpayment (Code Sec. 6654(a)).[56] In determining the addition to tax for an underpayment of individual estimated tax, the federal short-term rate that applies during the third month following the tax year of the

---

References are to Standard Federal Tax Reports; Tax Research Consultant; and Practical Tax Explanations.

[50] ¶ 39,660; PENALTY: 3,122; § 40,210.36

[51] ¶ 39,651; PENALTY: 3,120; § 40,210.37

[52] ¶ 39,656; PENALTY: 6,100; § 40,215

[53] ¶ 39,660; PENALTY: 6,112; § 40,215

[54] ¶ 39,656; PENALTY: 6,106, PENALTY: 6,158; § 40,215

[55] ¶ 39,655; PENALTY: 3,252.05

[56] ¶ 39,550; FILEIND: 21,050; § 1,430.05

underpayment will also apply during the first 15 days of the fourth month following such tax year (Code Sec. 6621(b)(2)(B); Reg. § 301.6621-1).[57] Changes in the interest rate apply to amounts of underpayments outstanding on the date of change or arising thereafter. An individual can avoid any penalty for underpayment of estimated tax by making payments as set forth in ¶ 2682. See ¶ 511 for the rules regarding trusts and estates.

Under several circumstances, a taxpayer is not subject to the penalty for underpaying estimated taxes (¶ 2682). The IRS is also authorized to waive the penalty for underpayment of estimated tax of an individual if the underpayment is due to casualty, disaster, or other unusual circumstances, and the imposition of the penalty would be against equity and good conscience (Code Sec. 6654(e)(3)).[58] The penalty may also be waived for an individual who retired after having attained age 62, or who became disabled, in the tax year for which the estimated payment was due or in the preceding tax year and the underpayment was due to reasonable cause and not to willful neglect.

The amount of an underpayment of estimated tax and the amount of the resulting penalty is computed on Form 2210 and attached to the individual's income tax return; farmers and fishermen use Form 2210-F. If Form 2210 is not completed and attached to the individual's return, the IRS will compute the penalty for the taxpayer. When the IRS computes the penalty, however, it will investigate any reason why the penalty should be waived.

2890. Underpayment of Estimated Tax by Corporations. An underpayment of estimated tax by a corporation (including an S corporation) will result in the imposition of an addition to tax equal to the applicable underpayment rate or interest (¶ 2838) that accrues on the underpayment for the period of the underpayment (Code Sec. 6655).[59] See ¶ 241 for more information on the penalty for underpayment of corporate estimated taxes.

Erroneous Tax Refund Claims

2891. Erroneous Refund or Credit Claims. Erroneous income tax refund or credit claims made for an excessive amount are subject to a penalty equal to 20 percent of the excessive amount (Code Sec. 6676).[60] The penalty does not apply to claims for refunds or credits relating to the earned income credit (¶ 1322), which has a separate set of rules.

An excessive amount is the amount by which the refund or credit claim exceeds the amount allowable under the Code for the tax year. However, if it can be shown that the claim for the excessive amount has a reasonable basis, the penalty will not apply. In addition, the penalty does not apply to any portion of the excessive amount of a refund claim or credit that is subject to an accuracy-related penalty (¶ 2854 and ¶ 2870), or the fraud penalty (¶ 2866).

Unauthorized Return Disclosures or Inspections

2892. Disclosure of Return Information by Government Employees. Returns and tax return information are confidential and may not be disclosed to federal or state agencies or employees except as provided in Code Sec. 6103.[61] A return is defined as any tax return, information return, declaration of estimated, or claim for refund filed under the Internal Revenue Code. Return information includes the taxpayer's identity, the nature, source or amount of income, payments, receipts, deductions, net worth, tax liability, deficiencies, closing (and similar) agreements, and information regarding the actual or possible investigation of a return. All officers and employees of the United States, of any state, and of any local child support enforcement agency are prohibited from disclosing tax returns and return information. The prohibition also applies to most

---

References are to Standard Federal Tax Reports; Tax Research Consultant; and Practical Tax Explanations.

[57] ¶ 39,450, ¶ 39,451; FILEIND: 21,056; § 1,430.05

[58] ¶ 39,550; FILEIND: 21,056.10; § 1,435.10

[59] ¶ 39,565; FILEBUS: 6,050; § 26,015.15

[60] ¶ 39,801; PENALTY: 3,332; § 40,240

[61] ¶ 36,880; IRS: 9,050; § 41,215.15

other persons who have had access to returns or return information by virtue of permitted disclosures of such returns or information under Code Sec. 6103. A taxpayer may bring a damage action against a person who knowingly or negligently makes an unauthorized disclosure or inspection of any return or return information of the taxpayer (¶ 2893).

Agreements and information received under a tax convention with a foreign government (including a U.S. possession) are also confidential and generally cannot be disclosed (Code Sec. 6105).[62]

2893. Remedies for Unauthorized Disclosures or Inspections of Return Information. A taxpayer may bring a civil action against the United States if a government employee knowingly or negligently discloses or inspects any return or return information with respect to the taxpayer under Code Sec. 6103 (¶ 2892) without authorization. A taxpayer may also bring a civil action against any person who is *not* a United States employee who knowingly or negligently discloses or inspects any return or return information with respect to the taxpayer under Code Sec. 6103 or a tax-exempt organization under Code Sec. 6104 (¶ 625) (Code Sec. 7431).[63] Upon a finding of liability, the taxpayer may recover the greater of $1,000 for each unauthorized disclosure or the amount of the actual damages sustained as a result of the disclosure. Punitive damages, as well as litigation costs, may be recovered if the disclosure was willful or grossly negligent. Criminal penalties can also be brought against individuals who have made unauthorized and willful disclosures of any return or return information including present and former federal employees, and any other person who obtains returns and return information in the course of processing, storing and reproducing returns and return information (Code Sec. 7213).[64]

In addition, civil penalties may be imposed against any state employee or other person who acquires the return or return information under Code Sec. 6103 or Code Sec. 6104 that permits the use of federal return information for other government purposes, such as state tax and child support collection, law enforcement, social welfare program administration, and statistical use (Code Sec. 7213A).[65]

2894. Disclosure of Return Information by Return Preparers. A return preparer who uses return information for any purpose other than to prepare a return, or who makes an unauthorized disclosure of return information, is subject to a $250 penalty for each disclosure, up to a maximum of $10,000. If the action is undertaken knowingly or recklessly, the preparer may be subject to criminal penalties or a fine of up to $1,000, or up to a year in jail, or both, together with the cost of prosecution (Code Secs. 6713 and 7216).[66] A taxpayer may bring a civil action for damages against the U.S. government if an IRS employee offers the taxpayer's representative favorable tax treatment in exchange for information about the taxpayer (Code Sec. 7435).[67]

Failure to Notify Health Plan of Ineligibility for COBRA Premium Assistance

2897. Failure to Notify Health Plan. A penalty is imposed on individuals who fail to notify health plans that they cease to be eligible for COBRA premium assistance (Code Sec. 6720C).[68] COBRA premium assistance, however, ended on August 31, 2011. Before that time, an individual who paid a reduced premium for COBRA continuation coverage (¶ 2653) was required to provide written notice to the group health plan of eligibility for coverage under another group health plan or Medicare. If the individual failed to provide this notification at the required time and in the required manner, and, as a result, the individual paid reduced COBRA continuation coverage premiums after the termination of the individual's eligibility for the reduction, a penalty was imposed on the individual equal to 110 percent of the premium reduction after termination of

---

References are to Standard Federal Tax Reports; Tax Research Consultant; and Practical Tax Explanations.

[62] ¶ 36,912; IRS: 9,550

[63] ¶ 41,750; IRS: 9,350; § 41,625.05

[64] ¶ 41,350; IRS: 66,360

[65] ¶ 41,354; IRS: 66,360

[66] ¶ 40,155, ¶ 41,365; IRS: 6,114; § 41,625.05

[67] ¶ 41,785; IRS: 45,116

[68] ¶ 40,209G; PENALTY: 3,336; § 42,845.15

eligibility. No penalty was imposed for a failure to notify if it could be shown that the failure is due to reasonable cause and not to willful neglect.

Criminal Penalties

2898. Criminal Penalties. Criminal penalties may be incurred when the taxpayer: (1) willfully fails to make a return, keep records, supply required information, or pay any tax or estimated tax; (2) willfully attempts in any manner to evade or defeat the tax; or (3) willfully fails to collect and pay over the tax. In addition to the felony charges listed in the preceding sentence, misdemeanor charges can be brought for making fraudulent statements to employees, filing a fraudulent withholding certificate, or failing to obey a summons. The criminal penalties are in addition to the civil penalties (Code Secs. 7201—7212). A good faith misunderstanding of the law or a good faith belief that one is not violating the law negates the willfulness element of a tax evasion charge.[69]

References are to Standard Federal Tax Reports; Tax Research Consultant; and Practical Tax Explanations.

[69] ¶ 41,318.136; IRS: 66,050; § 40,245.10

Chapter 29

ESTATE, GIFT AND GENERATION-SKIPPING TRANSFER TAX

Transfer Tax System

2901. Estate, Gift, and Generation-Skipping Transfer Tax System. The estate, gift, and generation-skipping transfer (GST) taxes are designed to form a unified transfer tax system on the transfer of property at death (estate tax), during life (gift tax), and on transfers that skip a generation (GST tax). The maximum marginal tax rate is 40 percent for estates of decedents dying and gifts and GSTs made after December 31, 2012 (¶ 40). The estate and gift tax exclusion amount and the GST exemption amount is $5 million, which is indexed annually for inflation after 2011; the exclusion and exemption amounts are $5.34 million for 2014, and $5.43 million for 2015 (¶ 41). A decedent's estate may elect to allow the unused portion of the decedent's applicable exclusion amount to be available to his or her surviving spouse or the spouse's estate (referred to as "portability") (Code Sec. 2010(c)(5)). As a result, the applicable exclusion amount of a surviving spouse may include the predeceased spouse's unused exclusion amount, allowing the spouse to transfer up to $10.68 million in 2014 (¶ 2934 and ¶ 2938).

Prior to 2013, the transfer tax system was in a state of uncertainty that began with the Economic Growth and Tax Relief Reconciliation Act of 2001 (P.L. 107-16) (EGTRRA).[1] The estate applicable exclusion amount and GST exemption amount began to gradually increase from $1 million for 2002 to $3.5 million in 2009, while the gift tax applicable exclusion amount stopped at $1 million, thereby effectively "de-unifying" the transfer tax system. In the meantime, the top marginal tax rates applicable to the estate, gift, and GST taxes began to gradually decrease to 45 percent (2007-2009). EGTRRA included the repeal of the estate and GST taxes, but that repeal was to be effective only for the year 2010 due to a "sunset" provision. In addition, EGTRRA left in place a modified gift tax along with a modified carryover basis regime.

The Tax Relief, Unemployment Insurance Reauthorization, and Job Creation Act of 2010 (P.L. 111-312) (Tax Relief Act of 2010) restored the estate and GST taxes, but also increased the estate tax applicable exclusion and GST exemption amounts to $5 million and lowered the estate and gift tax top marginal rate to 35 percent. Since there was a separate tax rate for GSTs in 2010 (0 percent), and a separate applicable exclusion amount ($1 million) for gifts made in 2010, the transfer tax system was not "re-unified" until 2011. Although the Tax Relief Act of 2010 repealed the modified adjusted carryover basis rules imposed by EGTRRA, estates of decedents who died in 2010 were allowed to elect out of the estate tax regime and apply carryover basis (¶ 1633). The Tax Relief Act of 2010 also introduced the concept of portability, as well as annual inflation indexing for

---

References are to Federal Estate & Gift Tax Reports; Tax Research Consultant; Practical Tax Explanations.

[1] ¶ 1005; ESTGIFT: 100;
§ 34,001

the estate and gift tax applicable exclusion amount and the GST exemption beginning in 2012.

The estate, gift, and GST tax provisions of EGTRRA (other than the sunset provision) and the Tax Relief Act of 2010 were made permanent by the American Taxpayer Relief Act of 2012 (P.L. 112-240) (ATRA). ATRA also increased the maximum transfer tax rate to 40 percent for estates of decedents dying and gifts made after December 31, 2012.

Same-Sex Couples. For federal tax purposes, same sex couples are now treated as married if they are legally married in a jurisdiction that recognizes same sex marriages, even if they live in or move to a jurisdiction that does not (*E. Windsor*, SCt, 2013-2 USTC ¶ 60,667); Rev. Rul. 2013-17). Thus, same sex married couples may take advantage of the same benefits previously enjoyed only by opposite sex married couples, such as the estate and gift tax marital deductions (¶ 2908 and ¶ 2926), split gifts (¶ 2905), and portability (¶ 2934). Same sex couples in a civil union, registered domestic partnership or similar formal relationship under state law are not afforded the same treatment, however, if the state does *not* denominate the relationship as a marriage.

Gift Tax

2903. Transfers Subject to Gift Tax. A gift tax applies to the transfer of property by gift, whether the gift is direct or indirect, and whether the transfer is in trust or otherwise. The property transferred may be real, personal, tangible, or intangible (Code Sec. 2511; Reg. § 25.2511-1(a)).[2] The donor makes a gift to the extent that the value of the property transferred exceeds the consideration, i.e., any property or services received in return for the transfer (Code Sec. 2512(b)). The transferred property or evidence of it must be delivered to the donee, and the donor must relinquish all control over the property for the gift to be completed (Reg. § 25.2511-2).[3] Transfers to qualifying political organizations are not considered gifts (Code Sec. 2501(a)(4)).[4]

Indirect gifts, such as transfers in trust and the cancellation of indebtedness, are subject to the gift tax (Code Sec. 2511). Other examples of indirect gifts include certain assignments of benefits, permission to withdraw funds deposited by a donor from a joint account, and below-market interest rate loans (Reg. § 25.2511-1(c) and (h)). However, a waiver of the right to a joint and survivor annuity in a qualified plan is not a gift (Code Sec. 2503(f)).[5]

A gratuitous transfer of property by a corporation is considered to be a gift by the shareholders to the donee, while a gift to a corporation is considered to be a gift to its shareholders (Reg. § 25.2511-1(h)). In addition, a gift may occur at the creation of a family limited partnership or when transferring control of a closely held company.[6] Transfers of stock or securities are gifts even if the securities are exempt from tax. The transfer of an option is a gift. Also, gratuitous transfers made by guardians or conservators under court orders are gifts. Conversely, a transfer pursuant to a will contest settlement entered into at arm's length is generally not a gift. The treatment of income earned by domestic partners as community property by operation of state law is also not considered a gift.[7]

Valuation. Generally, the value of property for gift tax purposes is its fair market value on the date of the gift. That is, the price at which the property would change hands between a willing buyer and a willing seller, both knowing all of the relevant facts (Code Sec. 2512; Reg. § 25.2512-1).[8] Special valuation rules apply for determining the amount of a gift if the transferor retains (1) an equity interest in a corporation or partnership

---

References are to Federal Estate & Gift Tax Reports; Tax Research Consultant; Practical Tax Explanations.

[2] ¶ 10,514, ¶ 10,528, ¶ 10,555.06; ESTGIFT: 3,050; § 34,805

[3] ¶ 10,568; ESTGIFT: 3,056, ESTGIFT: 3,060; § 34,805.05

[4] ¶ 9245, ¶ 9340.05; ESTGIFT: 3,150; § 34,805

[5] ¶ 9649, ¶ 10,181.05; ESTGIFT: 3,100; § 34,805

[6] ¶ 10,514, ¶ 10,555.07; ESTGIFT: 3,154; § 34,801

[7] ¶ 9340.05, ¶ 9340.80; ESTGIFT: 33,000; § 34,601

[8] ¶ 10,622, ¶ 10,649; ESTGIFT: 100; § 34,810.05

transferred to a family member, or (2) an interest in a trust to or for the benefit of a family member (Code Secs. 2701, 2702 and 2704).[9]

Qualified Disclaimers. The donee of a gift may make a qualified disclaimer of the entire interest or a portion of it without making a taxable gift. To be a qualified disclaimer, (1) the disclaimer must be in writing; (2) the disclaimer must be received by the transferor or the transferor's representative within nine months of the date of the transfer; (3) the beneficiary may not accept any of the benefits from the transferred property; and (4) the property being disclaimed must pass to someone other than, and without direction from, the disclaiming beneficiary (Code Sec. 2518).[10]

Nonresident Alien Donors. A donor who is a nonresident alien is subject to gift tax on transfers of real and tangible property situated in the United States (Code Sec. 2501(a); Reg. §25.2501-1).[11] Transfers of intangible property by a nonresident alien generally are not subject to gift tax (Code Sec. 2501(a)(2)). A donor who relinquishes his or her U.S. citizenship or terminates his or her long-term residency is subject to special expatriation rules (Code Sec. 2501(a)(3)).[12] (For the transfer tax imposed on recipients of gifts from "covered expatriates," see ¶ 2948.) Taxable gifts are taxed at the same rates that apply to U.S. citizens (Code Sec. 2501(a)(1)).[13]

2905. Gift Tax Annual Exclusion. The first $14,000 of gifts of a present interest made by a donor during calendar year 2014 ($14,000 in 2015) to each donee are not included in the total amount of the donor's taxable gifts during that year (Code Sec. 2503(b); Rev. Proc. 2013-35; Rev. Proc. 2014-61).[14] Therefore, these amounts are not taxed and do not use up any of the donor's lifetime gift tax applicable credit amount. Also, spouses who consent to split their gifts may transfer a total of $28,000 per donee in 2014 ($28,000 in 2015), free of gift and generation-skipping transfer (GST) tax (Code Sec. 2513(a)).[15]

If the donor's spouse is not a U.S. citizen, an annual exclusion of $145,000 in 2014 ($147,000 in 2015) is allowed for present interest gifts to the spouse that would qualify for the marital deduction if the spouse were a U.S. citizen (Code Sec. 2523(i)(2); Rev. Proc. 2013-35; Rev. Proc. 2014-61).[16] The annual exclusion is available to all donors, including nonresident citizens.

The annual exclusion is allowed for gifts of present interests but not for gifts of future interests in property. Present interests include any interests, whether vested or contingent, that are available for the donee's immediate use, possession or enjoyment (Reg. §25.2503-3(b)). A transfer of property for the benefit of a minor pursuant to the Uniform Transfers to Minors Act (UTMA), the Uniform Gifts to Minors Act (UGMA), or the Gifts of Securities to Minors Act (GSMA) is considered to be a completed gift of the full fair market value of the property.[17]

Transfers in Trust. The number of annual exclusions available for a gift in trust is determined by the number of trust beneficiaries who have a present interest in the gifted property. A transfer to a trust that allows a beneficiary the unrestricted right to the immediate use, possession, or enjoyment of the transferred property or the income from the property, such as a life estate or term certain, is a present interest gift that qualifies for the annual exclusion (Reg. §25.2503-3(b)). However, such unrestricted gifts through a trust are rarely made. Normally, limits are placed on the beneficiary's right to use, possess, or enjoy the trust property. A gift of the right to demand a portion of a trust corpus is a gift of a present interest, so long as the donee-beneficiary is aware of his or her right to make the demand. Typically, the beneficiary of such a trust (known as a

---

References are to Federal Estate & Gift Tax Reports; Tax Research Consultant; Practical Tax Explanations.

[9] ¶ 13,551, ¶ 14,001, ¶ 14,651; ESTGIFT: 18,600; § 34,810

[10] ¶ 11,339, ¶ 11,419.03; ESTGIFT: 100; § 34,805.20

[11] ¶ 9245, ¶ 9290; ESTGIFT: 60,050; § 35,010

[12] ¶ 9245; ESTGIFT: 60,250; § 35,015.05

[13] ¶ 7575.09, ¶ 9245; ESTGIFT: 60,100; § 35,010

[14] ¶ 9,649; ESTGIFT: 6,050; § 34,820.10

[15] ¶ 10,960, ¶ 10,987.06; ESTGIFT: 6,054; § 34,820.10

[16] ¶ 11,662, ¶ 11,850, ¶ 11,884.05; ESTGIFT: 6,050; § 35,010.15

[17] ¶ 9649, ¶ 9950.335, ¶ 10,041.05; ESTGIFT: 6,058, ESTGIFT: 6,060; § 34,820.10

Crummey trust) is given the right to demand an amount of corpus equal to the annual gift tax exclusion for a limited period of time, such as 60 days. If the persons who have a right of withdrawal do not have a present income interest in the trust or a vested remainder interest, however, the IRS may question the claimed annual exclusion.[18]

Gifts to Minors. Gifts to minors may qualify for the annual exclusion if they meet the requirements of Code Sec. 2503(c).[19] The property and income from it must be expended by or for the benefit of the minor, and any income and principal not expended must be paid to the minor at age 21, or to his or her estate if the minor dies before age 21 (Code Sec. 2503(c); Reg. § 25.2503-4(a)).[20] However, if a transfer of property is made under a parent's legal obligation to support a minor, the transfer is not a gift, as is the case with child support.[21]

2907. Exclusion for Educational or Medical Payment. In addition to the annual exclusion (¶ 2905), an unlimited gift tax exclusion is allowed for amounts paid on behalf of a donee *directly* to an educational organization, provided such amounts constitute tuition payments. Amounts paid for books, dormitory fees, or board on behalf of the donee are not eligible for the exclusion. Likewise, amounts paid *directly* to health care providers for medical services on behalf of a donee also qualify for the unlimited gift tax exclusion. Medical expense payments are excludable without regard to the percentage limitations imposed for income tax purposes. Both the medical and tuition exclusions are available without regard to the relationship between the donor and donee (Code Sec. 2503(e)).[22]

2908. Gifts to Spouse. In computing the taxable gifts of a married donor, a marital deduction is allowed for property that passes to the donor's spouse. As a result, an unlimited amount of property, other than certain terminable interests, can be transferred between spouses. The gift tax marital deduction is not available, however, if the donor's spouse is not a U.S. citizen at the time of the gift. Instead, gifts to a noncitizen spouse are eligible for a gift tax annual exclusion of up to $145,000 in 2014 ($147,000 in 2015) (Code Sec. 2523; Rev. Proc. 2013-35; Rev. Proc. 2014-61).[23]

In addition, a gift tax marital deduction is not allowed for transfers of terminable interests in property. A terminable interest in property is an interest that will terminate or fail on the lapse of time or on the occurrence or failure to occur of some contingency. For example, terminable interests include life estates, terms for years, and annuities. However, a gift tax marital deduction will be allowed if the donee spouse is given a life estate with a general power of appointment or qualified terminable interest property (QTIP), or if the donor and spouse are named as the only non-charitable beneficiaries of a qualified charitable remainder trust (¶ 2926).[24]

2909. Gifts to Charity. In determining a donor's taxable gifts, a gift tax charitable deduction is available for transfers to charitable organizations (federal, state and local governmental entities, charitable organizations, fraternal societies (if the property is used for charitable purposes), or veterans' organizations). The charitable deduction is not limited to gifts for use within the United States, unless the donor is a nonresident alien at the time of the gift (Code Sec. 2522).[25] A deduction may also be allowed for the value of the charitable interest in a split-interest transfer (in which there are both charitable and noncharitable beneficiaries) provided the charitable interest is in a qualified form (i.e., charitable remainder annuity trust, charitable remainder unitrust, charitable lead annuity trust, charitable lead unitrust, or a pooled income fund) (¶ 2932).

References are to Federal Estate & Gift Tax Reports; Tax Research Consultant; Practical Tax Explanations.

[18] ¶ 9649, ¶ 9842.055, ¶ 9891, ¶ 9950.07; ESTGIFT: 6,060; § 34,820.10

[19] ¶ 9649, ¶ 9842.05, ¶ 9996; ESTGIFT: 6,060.10; § 34,820.10

[20] ¶ 9649, ¶ 9996, ¶ 10,041.05; ESTGIFT: 12,056; § 34,820.10

[21] ¶ 11,311, ¶ 11,324.05; ESTGIFT: 12,100; § 34,820.10

[22] ¶ 9649, ¶ 10,095, ¶ 10,139.05; ESTGIFT: 6,100; § 34,820.15

[23] ¶ 11,662, ¶ 11,689.01, ¶ 11,884.05; ESTGIFT: 42,050; § 34,815.10

[24] ¶ 11,709.05; ESTGIFT: 42,058, ESTGIFT: 42,060, ESTGIFT: 42,062; § 34,815.10

[25] ¶ 11,486, ¶ 11,513.01; ESTGIFT: 45,050, ESTGIFT: 45,100, ESTGIFT: 45,350; § 34,815.15

2910. Computing the Gift Tax Liability. The gift tax is calculated by first determining the total value of the donor's gifts for the current calendar year. The value of a gift is its fair market value on the date of the gift (¶ 2903). That amount is reduced by any exclusions—annual (¶ 2905), and educational and medical (¶ 2907)—and deductions—marital (¶ 2908) and charitable (¶ 2909). The sum of all taxable gifts made by the donor in all prior years is then added to the current year's taxable gifts to arrive at the total taxable gifts. The donor's tentative gift tax liability is then determined by (1) calculating a tentative tax on the sum of all taxable gifts made in the calendar year and in preceding calendar periods, (2) calculating a tentative tax on only the taxable gifts in preceding calendar periods, and (3) then subtracting the tentative tax determined in step (2) from the tentative tax determined in step (1) (Code Sec. 2502).[26]

The donor is allowed a unified credit against gift tax, equal to (1) the estate tax applicable credit amount in effect for the calendar year of the gift (¶ 2934), minus (2) the sum of all applicable credits allowable to the donor for gifts made in all prior calendar periods. The applicable credit amount for 2014 is $2,081,800, which effectively shields the first $5.34 million of a donor's lifetime gifts from gift tax. For 2015, the applicable exclusion amount is $5.43 million, and the gift tax applicable credit amount is $2,117,800 (Code Secs. 2010(c) and 2505(a); Rev. Proc. 2013-35; Rev. Proc. 2014-61).[27] The applicable credit amount might be higher for any year if the donor is a surviving spouse and the estate of his or her predeceased spouse has elected portability of the deceased spouse's unused exclusion (DSUE) amount (¶ 2934 and ¶ 2938). For gifts made after 2009, any unified credit allocated to prior periods must be redetermined using current gift tax rates, rather than the rates that were effective when the prior gifts were made (Code Sec. 2505(a)).

Note that the $5.34 million and first dollar (that is, the first dollar that becomes taxable) is taxed at the rate that would apply to gifts in the amount of $5,340,001 (40 percent in 2014) rather than the rate that would apply to a gift of $1 (18 percent).

If a gift is adequately disclosed on the gift tax return and the gift tax statute of limitations has expired, the IRS may not revalue the donor's lifetime gifts when computing the estate tax liability upon the donor's death (Code Sec. 2001(f)). There is a three-year statute of limitations for gift tax returns (Code Sec. 2504(c)).[28]

Filing Requirements. Form 709 must be filed, and any gift tax must be paid, on an annual basis. Generally, the due date for filing the annual gift tax return will be the same as the due date for the income tax return. However, for the calendar year in which the donor dies, the gift tax return will be due on the earlier of the due date, with extensions, for filing the donor's estate tax return, or the "normal" due date with respect to the gifts (Code Sec. 6075(b)).[29] Taxpayers filing gift tax returns for gifts made in 2014 must file by April 15, 2015.

2911. Donor Is Primarily Liable to File Return and Pay Gift Tax. Gift tax returns must be filed by individual donors for gifts of more than $14,000 in 2014 ($14,000 in 2015) that do not qualify for an exclusion. Gift tax returns must be filed on Form 709. The donor is primarily liable for the payment of the gift tax (Code Sec. 6019).[30]

Estate Tax

2912. Gross Estate. The federal estate tax is imposed on the transfer of a person's property at the time of that person's death. The amount of the tax is determined by applying the relevant tax rates to the taxable estate—the gross estate reduced by any deductions. The gross estate of a U.S. citizen or resident decedent includes the value of all property described in Code Sec. 2033 through Code Sec. 2044, whether real or personal, tangible or intangible, wherever situated. Effectively executed disclaimers

---

References are to Federal Estate & Gift Tax Reports; Tax Research Consultant; Practical Tax Explanations.

[26] ¶ 9385, ¶ 9494.07; ES-TGIFT: 100; § 34,830

[27] ¶ 10,403, ¶ 10,448.03; ES-TGIFT: 100; § 34,820.20

[28] ¶ 10,235, ¶ 10,368.05; ES-TGIFT: 3,300; § 34,835

[29] ¶ 20,301, ¶ 20,330.05; ES-TGIFT: 3,300; § 34,830

[30] ¶ 9245, ¶ 20,125, ¶ 20,135.05, ¶ 20,301; ESTGIFT: 3,300; § 34,830

prevent the property subject to the disclaimer from being included in the disclaimant's gross estate (Code Secs. 2046 and 2518).[31]

Qualified terminable interest property (QTIP) for which an election was made to qualify it for the marital deduction in the estate of the first spouse to die (¶ 2926), or on the gift tax return of the donor spouse, is included in the gross estate of the surviving or donee spouse (Code Sec. 2044(a)).[32]

Form 706 includes specific schedules on which the estate must provide details for specific types of property included in the decedent's gross estate. Real estate that the decedent owned or had contracted to purchase is reported on Schedule A. Stocks and bonds included in the gross estate are reported on Schedule B. Mortgages and notes payable to the decedent at the time of death, as well as cash that the decedent possessed on the date of death, are reported on Schedule C. Other Form 706 schedules are specifically designated for other types of property. If an asset in the gross estate is not required to be reported on any other schedule, it must be reported on Schedule F.

2913. Transferred Property in Which Decedent Retained an Interest. When a decedent retains some control over gifts of property made during life, the property may be added back to the decedent's gross estate. The transfers subject to this rule include:

(1) gifts in which the decedent retains a life estate or the right to the income, possession, or enjoyment of the property, or the right to designate who will enjoy the property, including gifts of stock in which voting rights are retained (Code Sec. 2036);[33]

(2) gifts in which the decedent retains a right to a reversionary interest that exceeds five percent of the value of the transferred property and possession or enjoyment of the property can be obtained only by surviving the decedent (Code Sec. 2037(a));[34] and

(3) gifts in which the decedent holds a power to alter, amend, revoke, or terminate the gift (Code Sec. 2038(a)(1); Reg. § 20.2038-1(a)).[35]

If income from transferred property is used to discharge a legal obligation of the decedent, such as the decedent's obligation to support his or her dependents, the decedent is considered to have a right to income from the property and the property is includible in his or her gross estate (Reg. § 20.2036-1(b)(2)).[36] Such transfers are generally reported on Schedule G of Form 706.

An estate valuation freeze is a technique used to limit the value of closely held business interests owned by an individual by transferring the future appreciation in value of the business to the next generation of the owner's family while retaining certain interests in the business. This technique has been severely limited by the special valuation rules (Code Secs. 2701—2704), which treat transfers of family business interests unfavorably for gift tax purposes by assigning a value of zero to certain types of interests retained by the donor in such exchanges.[37]

If a lifetime transfer with a retained interest is a sale for adequate and full consideration, the property that is transferred is not included in the transferor's gross estate (Code Sec. 2036(a); Reg. § 20.2036-1(c)).[38] However, if the transfer is not for adequate and full consideration, the amount included in the decedent's estate is the full value of the property subject to the decedent's retained interest. If the interest or right is reserved over only part of the property transferred, only the reserved portion is included in the gross estate.

References are to Federal Estate & Gift Tax Reports; Tax Research Consultant; Practical Tax Explanations.

[31] ¶ 5980, ¶ 5990.05, ¶ 11,339, ¶ 11,419.03; ESTGIFT: 15,050; § 34,170

[32] ¶ 5901, ¶ 5940.05; ES-TGIFT: 15,500; § 34,160

[33] ¶ 4901, ¶ 4955.06, ¶ 4980.05; ESTGIFT: 18,400, ES-

TGIFT: 18,450, ESTGIFT: 18,600; § 34,135.10

[34] ¶ 5001, ¶ 5075.01; ES-TGIFT: 18,500; § 34,135.15

[35] ¶ 5101, ¶ 5135, ¶ 5170.05; ESTGIFT: 18,550; § 34,135.20

[36] ¶ 4925; ESTGIFT: 18,304; § 34,135.10

[37] ¶ 13,551, ¶ 13,670, ¶ 13,690.05, ¶ 14,001, ¶ 14,501, ¶ 14,651; ESTGIFT: 18,600; § 34,810

[38] ¶ 4901, ¶ 4925, ¶ 4955.05; ESTGIFT: 18,100; § 34,135.05

2914. Gifts Made Within Three Years of Death. Gifts made within three years of the donor's death ordinarily are not includible in the donor's gross estate. However, gifts made within three years of death are included in the donor's gross estate if the gift consists of interests in property that would otherwise be included in the gross estate because of the donor's retained powers, such as the power to alter, amend, revoke, or terminate the gift (¶ 2913) (Code Sec. 2035(a)).[39] Similarly, a gift of life insurance that would have been includible in the decedent's gross estate because of his or her retention of incidents of ownership in the policy is includible if the policy was transferred within three years of the decedent's date of death (¶ 2915). Gifts made from a decedent's revocable trust within three years of death, however, are not included in the decedent's gross estate, rather they are treated as if made directly by the decedent (Code Secs. 2035(e) and 2038). Gift tax paid on all transfers made within three years of death is included in the gross estate (Code Sec. 2035(b)).

Such transfers are generally reported on Schedule G of Form 706.

2915. Life Insurance. Proceeds of insurance on a decedent's life payable to or for the benefit of his or her estate, and insurance payable to other beneficiaries in which the decedent retained incidents of ownership, are included in the decedent's gross estate (Code Sec. 2042(1) and (2); Reg. § 20.2042-1(b)(1)).[40] Insurance that is paid to a named beneficiary but that must be used to satisfy a legal obligation to meet expenses of the decedent's estate, such as debts and taxes, is also included in the decedent's gross estate (Reg. § 20.2042-1(c)(1)).

Incidents of Ownership. If proceeds of insurance on the life of a decedent are payable to a beneficiary other than the decedent's estate, they are included in the decedent's gross estate if the decedent has retained an incident of ownership in the life insurance policy on the date of death (Code Sec. 2042(2); Reg. § 20.2042-1(c)). The term "incidents of ownership" is not limited in its meaning to ownership of the policy. The term refers to the right of the insured or the insured's estate to the economic benefits of the policy. Some incidents of ownership include the power to change the beneficiary, the ability to pledge the policy as security for a loan, the ability to borrow against the policy, or a reversionary interest by which the insured or the insured's estate may regain one of the previously stated rights under certain circumstances. If the decedent transfers a life insurance policy or an incident of ownership in the policy within three years of his or her death, the proceeds are included in his or her gross estate (Code Sec. 2035(a)).[41] However, generally only one-half of the proceeds of life insurance purchased with community property is included in the estate of the insured spouse, even if the decedent possessed an incident of ownership (Reg. § 20.2042-1(b)(2)).[42]

A person insured under a key-employee insurance arrangement usually has no interest in the insurance. None of its proceeds will be included in the insured's gross estate. However, the arrangement will be accounted for in determining a value for any stock that the insured may have owned in the company.[43]

In the case of split-dollar life insurance, death proceeds from the employee's portion of the policy are included in the employee's estate if:

> (1) the proceeds are payable to, or for the benefit of, the employee's estate; or

> (2) the employee holds an incident of ownership in the policy at death or transfers an incident of ownership to a third party within three years before death.

Gift tax liability for employer-paid premiums may arise if a co-owner of the policy is neither the employer nor the employee.[44]

References are to Federal Estate & Gift Tax Reports; Tax Research Consultant; Practical Tax Explanations.

[39] ¶ 4801, ¶ 4845.01, ¶ 4845.091; ESTGIFT: 18,200; § 34,150
[40] ¶ 5651, ¶ 5715, ¶ 5740.05; ESTGIFT: 21,050; § 34,120

[41] ¶ 4801, ¶ 4845.09, ¶ 5651; ESTGIFT: 21,100; § 34,120
[42] ¶ 5670, ¶ 5715, ¶ 5740.05; ESTGIFT: 21,200; § 34,120

[43] ¶ 5760, ¶ 5780.03; ESTGIFT: 21,150; § 34,105
[44] ¶ 5780.045, ¶ 5780.183; COMPEN: 48,150; § 34,105

Life insurance that is included in a decedent's gross estate is generally reported on Schedule D of Form 706. For each policy listed, a separate Form 712 life insurance statement must be completed and attached to Schedule D.

2917. Annuities and Retirement Benefits. The value of an annuity or other payment receivable by any beneficiary by reason of surviving the decedent is generally included in the decedent's gross estate. The annuity or other payment is not taxable under the rules unless it is payable under a contract by agreement and the following factors exist:

(1) the contract or agreement was entered into after March 31, 1931;

(2) the contract or agreement is not a policy of insurance on the decedent's life;

(3) the decedent possessed the right to receive the payments during his or her lifetime; and

(4) payments under the contract are determined based on the decedent's life or life expectancy (Code Sec. 2039(a)).[45]

The value of an annuity or other payment included in a decedent's gross estate is the portion of its value attributable to the portion of the purchase price contributed by the decedent. Any contribution made by a decedent's employer or former employer by reason of his or her employment is considered to be made by the decedent (Code Sec. 2039(b)).[46]

Annuities that are included in a decedent's gross estate are generally reported on Schedule I of Form 706.

With respect to estate tax valuation of a qualified account, i.e., an IRA, the value of the account is the fair market value of the assets in the account without any discount for the income tax liability that would be triggered if the estate or beneficiary were to take a distribution of the assets in order to sell them.[47]

2918. Powers of Appointment. Property subject to a general power of appointment is included in the gross estate of the holder of the power if the power exists at the holder's death (Code Sec. 2041(a)(2)). The exercise or release of a general power during the life of the holder is a transfer subject to gift tax (Code Sec. 2514(b)).[48] A power of appointment is a right given to someone other than the donor of property to dispose of the property. The holder of the power of appointment has a general power if the holder may exercise it in favor of himself or herself, the holder's creditors, the holder's estate, or the creditors of the holder's estate (Code Secs. 2041(b) and 2514(c)). Powers that expressly cannot be exercised in favor of any of these are special or limited powers (Reg. § 20.2041-1(c)(1)). A power is not general if its exercise is limited by an ascertainable standard (Code Secs. 2041(b)(1)(A) and 2514(c)(1)). A power is not general if the creator of the power must join in its exercise or if a co-holder of the power has a substantial adverse interest (Code Secs. 2041(b)(1)(C) and 2514(c)(3)(A)). The incompetence or lack of capacity of the holder of the power to exercise the power does not affect whether the power is taxable to the power holder.[49]

Property subject to a power of appointment that is included in a decedent's gross estate is generally reported on Schedule H of Form 706.

2919. Jointly Held Property. The entire value of jointly held property with the right of survivorship, including joint bank accounts and U.S. savings bonds registered in two names, is included in a decedent's gross estate except for the portion of the property for which the surviving joint tenant furnished consideration. If the joint property was received by the decedent and the other joint tenants as a gift or bequest, the decedent's fractional share of the property is included in the decedent's gross estate (Code Sec. 2040(a)).[50] If the joint tenants are spouses, it generally does not matter who furnished

---

References are to Federal Estate & Gift Tax Reports; Tax Research Consultant; Practical Tax Explanations.

[45] ¶ 5201, ¶ 5245.05; ES-TGIFT: 24,050; § 34,145

[46] ¶ 5201, ¶ 5245.07; ES-TGIFT: 24,100; § 34,145

[47] ¶ 3100, ¶ 3220.41; ES-TGIFT: 15,202.15; § 34,145

[48] ¶ 5501, ¶ 11,054; ESTGIFT: 27,100; § 34,140, § 34,805.10

[49] ¶ 5630.231; ESTGIFT: 27,050; § 34,805

[50] ¶ 5401, ¶ 5475.05; ES-TGIFT: 30,050; § 34,125

the consideration for the property; one-half of the value of a qualified joint interest is included in the gross estate of the first spouse to die (Code Sec. 2040(b)).[51]

Jointly held property that is included in a decedent's gross estate is generally reported on Schedule E of Form 706.

The creation of a joint interest in property results in a taxable gift by the person supplying the consideration to the noncontributing joint tenant. Creation of a joint bank account or joint brokerage account is not a taxable gift until a joint owner withdraws funds (Reg. § 25.2511-1(h)). If a donor purchased property and conveyed title to himself or herself and another as joint tenants with rights of survivorship, and those rights may be defeated by either owner severing his or her interest, the donor made a gift to the other joint owner in the amount of one-half of the property's value. A transfer of joint property to a third party is a gift of the value of each joint owner's share.[52]

2921. Community Property. Community property is all property acquired by means other than gift, devise, bequest, and inheritance by spouses domiciled in community property jurisdictions. Separate property is property other than community property.[53] One-half of the value of all community property owned by a married couple is includible in the gross estate of the first of the spouses to die (Code Sec. 2033). This rule of inclusion applies even though the surviving spouse elects to allow his or her share of the community property to pass according to the will of the decedent spouse.[54]

2922. Valuation of Gross Estate. The value of property that is included in the gross estate is its fair market value on the date of the decedent's death (Code Sec. 2031; Reg. § 20.2031-1(b)).[55] The fair market value of property includible in the gross estate is the price at which it would change hands between a willing buyer and a willing seller, both having reasonable knowledge of relevant facts.

Alternate Valuation. Instead of valuing property includible in the gross estate as of the date of death, the executor may elect to value the gross estate at the fair market value of the property on the alternate valuation date, which is the date six months after the date of the decedent's death (Code Sec. 2032; Reg. § 20.2032-1).[56] To use the alternate valuation election, the value of the gross estate must have decreased and the amount of estate and GST taxes imposed on the property included in the gross estate must also decrease. The alternate valuation election is irrevocable. The election is made on Form 706. The amount of any marital or charitable deduction is adjusted based on the alternate value of assets passing to charity or a surviving spouse (Code Sec. 2032(b); Reg. § 20.2032-1(g)). When the alternate valuation election is made, all property included in the gross estate is valued as of the alternate valuation date (Reg. § 20.2032-1(d)).[57] However, if property is sold, exchanged, distributed, or otherwise disposed of during the six-month period, it is valued on the date of disposition rather than the alternate valuation date (Code Sec. 2032(a)(1)).[58]

Special Use Valuation. If a farm or real property used in a closely held business is included in the gross estate, the executor may elect to value the property at its "current use" rather than at its "highest and best use." Special use valuation is obtained pursuant to an irrevocable election by an executor to value real property used in a farm, trade or business (Code Sec. 2032A).[59] The limitation on the reduction in value resulting from special use valuation is $1,090,000 in 2014 ($1,100,000 in 2015) (Rev. Proc. 2013-35; Rev. Proc. 2014-61).

References are to Federal Estate & Gift Tax Reports; Tax Research Consultant; Practical Tax Explanations.

[51] ¶ 5401, ¶ 5475.07; ES-TGIFT: 30,060; § 34,125

[52] ¶ 10,528, ¶ 10,555.24; ES-TGIFT: 30,100; § 34,805.15

[53] ¶ 4620, ¶ 4675.04; ES-TGIFT: 33,050; § 34,601

[54] ¶ 4675.11; ESTGIFT: 33,100; § 34,125

[55] ¶ 3011, ¶ 3100, ¶ 3125.01; ESTGIFT: 100; § 34,101

[56] ¶ 3801, ¶ 3830, ¶ 3870.05; ESTGIFT: 36,050, ESTGIFT: 36,100; § 34,205

[57] ¶ 3830; ESTGIFT: 36,102; § 34,205

[58] ¶ 3801; ESTGIFT: 36,150; § 34,205

[59] ¶ 4001, ¶ 4240.05; ES-TGIFT: 36,200; § 34,210

Special use valuation is elected on the estate tax return (Part 3, line 2 of Form 706) by, among other things, completing the notice of election (Schedule A-1) and submitting a recapture agreement.[60] If the qualified heir ceases to use the farm property for farming or sells the property to a non-family member within 10 years of the decedent's date of death, an additional estate tax, the recapture tax, is due and Form 706-A must be filed (Code Sec. 2032A(c)).[61]

2925. Deductions from Gross Estate—Expenses. A deduction from the gross estate is allowed for funeral expenses, administration expenses, claims against the estate, certain taxes, and unpaid mortgages or other indebtedness allowable under the local law governing the administration of the decedent's estate (Code Sec. 2053; Reg. § 20.2053-1).[62] For expenses that are not paid before filing the estate tax return, an estimated amount may be deducted if the amount is ascertainable and there is reasonable certainty that the amount will be paid. Contested and contingent claims and expenses cannot be ascertained with reasonable certainty. Estate administration expenses may generally be deducted on either the decedent's estate tax return or the estate's income tax return, but not on both (Code Sec. 642(g); Reg. § 1.642(g)-1).[63]

Expenses incurred in connection with the decedent's funeral, including reasonable expenses for a tombstone, mausoleum, or burial lot, are deductible (Code Sec. 2053(a)(1)).[64] Administration expenses are deductible if actually and necessarily incurred in the administration of the estate. Administration expenses include fees paid to surrogates, appraisers, and accountants. Reasonable attorney's fees that meet the requirements of Reg. § 20.2053-1 are deductible (Code Sec. 2053(a)(2); Reg. § 20.2053-3(c)).[65] Fees incurred by beneficiaries incident to litigation with regard to their interests are not deductible, unless the litigation is essential to the proper settlement of the estate. An executor or administrator may deduct the amount of his or her commissions from the decedent's gross estate in an amount actually paid or an amount that is reasonably ascertainable and will be paid (Reg. § 20.2053-3(b)).[66] Miscellaneous expenses necessarily incurred in preserving and distributing estate assets are also deductible as administration expenses (Reg. § 20.2053-3(d)).[67]

Funeral and administrative expenses are generally reported on Schedule J of Form 706.

Claims that are a personal obligation of the decedent are deductible, provided that they are existing and enforceable against the decedent at the time of his or her death, are allowable under local law, and have actually been paid or meet the requirements of Reg. § 20.2053-1(d)(4). Liabilities imposed by law or arising out of torts committed by the decedent are also deductible. In certain circumstances, an executor may deduct the current value of a claim or claims, which concern the same or similar issue or asset, even if the claim has not yet been paid (Reg. § 20.2053-4).[68] The full value of any unpaid mortgage or other indebtedness charged against property for which the decedent is personally liable, plus interest accrued on the debt to the date of death, is deductible if the property's entire value undiminished by the mortgage or indebtedness is included in the gross estate (Code Sec. 2053(a)(4); Reg. § 20.2053-7).[69]

References are to Federal Estate & Gift Tax Reports; Tax Research Consultant; Practical Tax Explanations.

[60] ¶ 4001; ESTGIFT: 36,300; § 34,210

[61] ¶ 4001, ¶ 4240.35; ES-TGIFT: 36,350; § 34,210

[62] ¶ 6040, ¶ 6050, ¶ 6060.025, ¶ 6060.055; ESTGIFT: 39,050, ESTGIFT: 39,100, ESTGIFT: 39,150; § 34,305

[63] ¶ 16,675, ¶ 16,825, ¶ 16,875.05, ¶ 16,875.07; ES-

TGIFT: 39,050, ESTGIFT: 39,100, ESTGIFT: 39,150; § 34,305

[64] ¶ 6040, ¶ 6070, ¶ 6080.03; ESTGIFT: 39,100; § 34,305.10

[65] ¶ 6040, ¶ 6090, ¶ 6100.03, ¶ 6130, ¶ 6140.05; ESTGIFT: 39,150, ESTGIFT: 39,158; § 34,305.15

[66] ¶ 6110, ¶ 6120; ESTGIFT: 39,154; § 34,305.15

[67] ¶ 6150, ¶ 6160.05; ES-TGIFT: 39,160; § 34,305.15

[68] ¶ 6170, ¶ 6180.01; ES-TGIFT: 39,200; § 34,305.20

[69] ¶ 6040, ¶ 6230, ¶ 6240.05; ESTGIFT: 39,250; § 34,305.25

Debts, mortgages, and liabilities of the decedent are generally reported on Schedule K of Form 706.

Federal estate taxes are not deductible. State estate, succession, legacy, or inheritance taxes actually paid to any state or the District of Columbia from the value of the gross estate are deductible (¶ 2933), as are unpaid gift taxes on gifts made before death. Unpaid income taxes are deductible if they are on income properly includible in an income tax return of a decedent for a period before his or her death (Reg. § 20.2053-6).[70] A deduction is also allowed for losses arising from fires, storms, shipwrecks, or other casualties or thefts that are incurred during estate administration and not compensated for by insurance (Code Sec. 2054).[71]

Such losses and taxes, except for the state death tax deduction, are generally reported on Schedule L of Form 706.

2926. Estate Tax Marital Deduction. In determining a married decedent's taxable estate, an unlimited deduction is allowable for property that passes to the decedent's surviving spouse (Code Sec. 2056).[72] In order to qualify for the deduction, the decedent must be married and survived by his or her spouse, the spouse must be a U.S. citizen, the property must be included in the decedent's gross estate and pass to the surviving spouse, and the property must not be a nondeductible terminable interest. The estate tax marital deduction is not available if the decedent's surviving spouse is not a U.S. citizen unless the spouse becomes a citizen before the estate tax return is filed or the property passes to a qualified domestic trust (QDOT) (Code Secs. 2056(d) and 2056A).[73]

Estates of decedents who are in a same sex marriage may now claim the estate tax marital deduction as a result of the U.S. Supreme Court ruling that Section 3 of the Defense of Marriage Act (DOMA) (P.L. 104-199) is unconstitutional on equal protection grounds (*E. Windsor*, SCt, 2013-2 USTC ¶ 60,667). Same sex married couples will be treated as married for federal tax purposes provided they are legally married in a jurisdiction that recognizes their marriage, even if they live in or move to a jurisdiction that does not (Rev. Rul. 2013-17). However, this treatment does not apply to couples in registered domestic partnerships, civil unions, or similar formal relationships recognized under state law if the state does *not* denominate the relationship as a marriage. Executors wishing to file a refund for estate and gift taxes based on this development, for prior tax years in which the limitations period for filing a refund claim has not expired, should file Form 843.[74]

Passing Requirement. Property must pass from the decedent to a surviving spouse for a transfer to be deductible (Code Sec. 2056(a)). Bequests and inheritances, dower and curtesy interests, joint property, property received under antenuptial agreements, annuities, and life insurance may pass from the decedent to the surviving spouse. Property received by a spouse under a state law right of election against the will satisfies the passing requirement (Code Sec. 2056(c); Reg. § 20.2056(c)-2(c)). Property passing to the spouse as a result of another person's qualified disclaimer is considered to pass from the decedent (Reg. § 20.2056(d)-2(b)).[75]

Terminable Interest Rule. The terminable interest rule bars deduction for any nondeductible terminable interest. A terminable interest in property is an interest that terminates or fails because of the lapse of time or the occurrence of an event (Code Sec. 2056(b)(1) and (3); Reg. § 20.2056(b)-3).[76] A nondeductible terminable interest is an interest in which a person, other than the surviving spouse, receives an interest in property from the decedent and, upon the termination of the spouse's interest in the same property, the other person may possess or enjoy the property. Property interests

---

References are to Federal Estate & Gift Tax Reports; Tax Research Consultant; Practical Tax Explanations.

[70] ¶ 6210, ¶ 6220.05; ESTGIFT: 39,300; § 34,305.20

[71] ¶ 6320, ¶ 6340.03; ESTGIFT: 39,350; § 34,310

[72] ¶ 6501; ESTGIFT: 42,100; § 34,320

[73] ¶ 6501, ¶ 7001, ¶ 7045.05, ¶ 7045.10; ESTGIFT: 42,150; § 34,320

[74] ¶ 6580.035; ESTGIFT: 42,102; § 34,320.10

[75] ¶ 6501, ¶ 6920.03, ¶ 6935, ¶ 6975; ESTGIFT: 42,150; § 34,320

[76] ¶ 6501, ¶ 6701, ¶ 6725.03; ESTGIFT: 42,200; § 34,320.15

passing to a spouse that are conditioned on the spouse's survival of a period of six months or less, or on the spouse's survival in a common disaster, are not subject to the terminable interest rule.

Qualified Terminable Interest Property. Qualified terminable interest property (QTIP) is excluded from the terminable interest rule. To qualify as QTIP, the surviving spouse must have the right to all the income from the property for life, payable no less frequently than annually (Code Sec. 2056(b)(7); Reg. §20.2056(b)-7(a)).[77] A surviving spouse's income interest may be contingent upon the executor's QTIP election and still be considered a "qualifying income interest for life." In addition, no person may have a power to appoint any of the property to any person other than the surviving spouse during the surviving spouse's life. An election on Schedule M of Form 706 is necessary to designate property as QTIP. Once the QTIP election is made, the surviving spouse must include the property remaining at death in his or her gross estate even though the surviving spouse has no control over its disposition (Code Sec. 2044). However, the estate tax that is attributable to the QTIP included in the spouse's estate may be recovered from the QTIP (Code Sec. 2207A).[78]

Life Estate with Power of Appointment. A life estate with a power of appointment qualifies for the marital deduction if:

(1) the surviving spouse is entitled to all the income from the entire interest or a specific portion of the interest for life;

(2) the income is payable at least annually;

(3) the spouse has the power to appoint the property, or the specific portion, to himself or herself or to his or her estate;

(4) the power is exercisable by the spouse alone and in all events; and

(5) no other person has the power to appoint property to anyone but the surviving spouse (Code Sec. 2056(b)(5)).

There is a similar exception to the terminable interest rule for life insurance proceeds held by an insurer in which the spouse has a right to all payments and a power of appointment (Code Sec. 2056(b)(6); Reg. §20.2056(b)-6(c)).[79]

Amount of the Marital Deduction. The marital deduction is limited to the net value of property passing to the spouse. Death taxes, debts, and administration expenses payable from the marital bequest, mortgages on property passing to the spouse, and insufficient estate assets to fund the marital bequest all reduce the amount of the deduction (Code Sec. 2056(b)(4); Reg. §20.2056(b)-4).[80] However, administration expenses allocable to an estate's income do not necessarily reduce the amount of the marital deduction (*O. Hubert Est.*, SCt, 97-1 USTC ¶ 60,261).[81]

Transfers for which an estate is taking the estate tax marital deduction are generally reported on Schedule M of Form 706.

2932. Estate Tax Charitable Deduction. An unlimited estate tax charitable deduction is available for transfers to: federal, state, and local governmental entities; charitable organizations; fraternal societies (if the property is used for charitable purposes); veterans' organizations; or an employee stock ownership plan if the transfer qualifies as a qualified gratuitous transfer. The bequest must have a public rather than a private purpose (Code Secs. 2055(a)).[82]

Transfers of Partial Interests. If an interest in property passes from a transferor to a charity and an interest in the same property passes to a noncharitable recipient, the transfer must take one of the following forms:

References are to Federal Estate & Gift Tax Reports; Tax Research Consultant; Practical Tax Explanations.

[77] ¶ 6501, ¶ 6825; ESTGIFT: 42,250; § 34,320.20

[78] ¶ 5901, ¶ 6501, ¶ 8800; ESTGIFT: 42,260, ESTGIFT: 42,262; § 34,320.20

[79] ¶ 6501, ¶ 6801, ¶ 6815.05; ESTGIFT: 42,300; § 34,320.20

[80] ¶ 6501, ¶ 6745; ESTGIFT: 42,350; § 34,320.10

[81] ¶ 6755.674; ESTGIFT: 42,356; § 34,320.10

[82] ¶ 6360, ¶ 6370; ESTGIFT: 45,050, ESTGIFT: 45,100, ESTGIFT: 45,350; § 34,315

(1) charitable remainder annuity trust, which provides for a fixed-dollar amount to be paid to the noncharitable income beneficiary annually, or charitable remainder unitrust, which provides for a fixed percentage of trust assets, valued annually, to be paid to the noncharitable income beneficiary annually (Code Secs. 2055(e)(2)(A) and 2522(c)(2)(A); Reg. § 20.2055-2(e)(2));[83]

(2) charitable lead trust with guaranteed annuity or unitrust amount paid to charity (Code Secs. 170(f)(2), 2055(e)(2)(B), and 2522(c)(2)(B); Reg. § 20.2055-2(e)(2));[84]

(3) remainder interest in a farm or personal residence (Code Sec. 2055(e)(3)(I); Reg. § 20.2055-2(e)(2));[85]

(4) copyrighted work of art separate from its copyright (Code Secs. 2055(e)(4) and 2522(c)(3); Reg. § 20.2055-2(e)(1));[86] or

(5) qualified conservation contribution (Code Sec. 170(f)(3); Reg. § 20.2055-2(e)(2)).[87]

The amount of the estate tax charitable deduction must be reduced by the administration expenses and death taxes paid from the property transferred to charity (Code Sec. 2055(c); Reg. § 20.2055-3(a)).[88] However, administration expenses allocable to an estate's income do not necessarily reduce the amount of the charitable deduction (*O. Hubert Est.*, SCt, 97-1 USTC ¶ 60,261).[89]

Transfers for which an estate is taking the estate tax charitable deduction are generally reported on Schedule O of Form 706.

2933. State Death Tax Deduction. Estates of decedents dying after December 31, 2004, are able to deduct estate, inheritance, legacy or succession taxes actually paid to any state or the District of Columbia from the value of the gross estate (Code Sec. 2058).[90] A limitations period is imposed that allows a deduction only for those state death taxes paid and a deduction claimed before the later of:

(1) four years after filing the estate tax return;

(2) if a timely petition for redetermination has been filed with the Tax Court, 60 days after the Tax Court decision becomes final;

(3) if an extension of time has been granted for payment of estate tax or of a deficiency, the date the extension expires; or

(4) if a timely refund claim has been filed, then the latest of the expiration of (a) 60 days from the mailing of a notice to the taxpayer of a disallowance of the refund claim, (b) 60 days after a court decision on the merits of the claim becomes final, or (c) two years after a notice of waiver of disallowance is filed under Code Sec. 6532(a)(3).

A refund based on the deduction may be made if the refund claim is filed within the above-defined period. Any refunds made will be without interest.

The state death tax deduction is taken on Part 2, line 3b of Form 706.

2934. Credits Against the Estate Tax. A number of credits are available to offset a decedent's federal estate tax liability. The most important credit is the applicable credit amount (formerly, the unified credit), which is determined by calculating a tentative estate tax on the applicable exclusion amount (adjusted annually for inflation) (Code Sec. 2010(c); Temp. Reg. § 20.2010-1T).[91] The applicable exclusion amount can be used

---

References are to Federal Estate & Gift Tax Reports; Tax Research Consultant; Practical Tax Explanations.

[83] ¶ 6360, ¶ 6390, ¶ 11,486, ¶ 16,901; ESTGIFT: 45,150, ESTGIFT: 45,200; § 34,315.20

[84] ¶ 6360, ¶ 6390, ¶ 11,486, ¶ 16,901; ESTGIFT: 45,250, ESTGIFT: 45,300; § 34,315.15

[85] ¶ 6360, ¶ 6390; ESTGIFT: 45,158; § 34,315.15

[86] ¶ 6360, ¶ 6390; ESTGIFT: 45,154; § 34,315.30

[87] ¶ 6390; ESTGIFT: 45,160; § 34,315.15

[88] ¶ 6360, ¶ 6430; ESTGIFT: 45,352, ESTGIFT: 45,354; § 34,315.05

[89] ¶ 6380.18; ESTGIFT: 45,352; § 34,315.05

[90] ¶ 7450, ¶ 7460.05; ESTGIFT: 39,304; § 34,330

[91] ¶ 1401, ¶ 1410, ¶ 1450.01; ESTGIFT: 51,052.05; § 34,010.40

to offset an estate tax liability on a taxable estate of $5,340,000 in 2014 ($5,430,000 in 2015) resulting in an applicable credit amount of $2,081,800 for 2014 ($2,117,800 for 2015) (Rev. Proc. 2013-35; Rev. Proc. 2014-61).

Portability of Unused Applicable Exclusion Amount. The applicable exclusion amount for a surviving spouse whose predeceased spouse's estate elected portability is the sum of (1) the basic exclusion amount ($5,340,000 in 2014; $5,430,000 in 2015), plus (2) the aggregate deceased spousal unused exclusion (DSUE) amount (Code Sec. 2010(c)(2) and (4); Temp. Reg. §§ 20.2010-2T and 20.2010-3T).[92] The DSUE amount is the lesser of (1) the basic exclusion amount in effect in the year of the deceased spouse's death, or (2) the last deceased spouse's applicable exclusion amount minus the amount with respect to which the tentative tax is determined on the last deceased spouse's estate. To take advantage of this special provision, the predeceased spouse must have died after December 31, 2010, and the predeceased spouse's estate must have made an election on Form 706 (¶ 2938). If portability is elected, the surviving spouse can apply the predeceased spouse's unused exclusion amount toward lifetime gifts, and any remaining unused exclusion amount can generally be applied by the surviving spouse's estate upon his or her death. Special rules limit the use of unused exclusion amounts by a surviving spouse with multiple predeceased spouses.

An executor electing portability must make the election on a timely-filed estate tax return (Form 706), including extensions actually granted, even if there is no estate tax liability. If the executor must otherwise file an estate tax return, but does not wish to make the portability election, the executor should make an affirmative statement to that effect on the return (Temp. Reg. § 20.2010-2T(a)(3)). Not timely filing Form 706 will also effectively prevent the election (Notice 2011-82).

State Death Tax Credit (Repealed). The state death tax credit, which had been repealed for estates of decedents dying after December 31, 2004, and before January 1, 2013, was permanently repealed for estates of decedents dying after December 31, 2012. Instead, such estates may claim a state death tax *deduction* (¶ 2933) for estate, inheritance, legacy, or succession taxes actually paid to any state or the District of Columbia (Code Secs. 2011 and 2058).[93]

Federal Estate Tax Paid on Prior Transfers. A credit is available for federal estate tax paid on prior transfers to the decedent from a person who died within 10 years before or two years after the decedent (Code Sec. 2013).[94] The credit is limited to the lesser of the estate tax attributable to the transferred property in the transferor's estate or the estate tax attributable to the transferred property in the decedent's estate. If the transferor predeceased the decedent by more than two years, the allowable credit is reduced by 20 percent for each full two-year period by which the death of the transferor preceded the transferor's death. The credit is claimed on Schedule Q on Form 706.

Foreign Death Taxes. A credit against estate tax is available for foreign death taxes paid on property located in a foreign country but included in the gross estate of a U.S. citizen or resident (Code Sec. 2014).[95] The credit is limited to the lesser of the foreign or the U.S. tax attributable to the property. If a treaty exists with the foreign country, the credit provided for under the treaty or Code Sec. 2014 may be used, whichever results in the lower amount of estate tax. The estate must file Form 706-CE to claim the credit.

Gift Tax Paid on Gifts Included in Gross Estate. For gifts made before 1977, the gift tax paid on gifts included in the gross estate is a credit to the estate tax (Code Sec. 2012).[96] The credit is limited to the lesser of the gift tax paid or the estate tax attributable to inclusion of the gift in the gross estate.

References are to Federal Estate & Gift Tax Reports; Tax Research Consultant; Practical Tax Explanations.

[92] ¶ 1401, ¶ 1415, ¶ 1420, ¶ 1450.08; ESTGIFT: 51,060; § 34,010.45

[93] ¶ 1551, ¶ 7450; ESTGIFT: 39,304, ESTGIFT: 48,050; § 34,330, § 34,501

[94] ¶ 2001, ¶ 2045; ESTGIFT: 48,100; § 34,515

[95] ¶ 2301; ESTGIFT: 48,150; § 34,520

[96] ¶ 1901; ESTGIFT: 48,200; § 34,510

2937. Computing the Estate Tax Liability. The estate tax computation begins with a calculation of the gross estate (¶ 2912—¶ 2921). The gross estate is valued at the fair market value on the decedent's date of death or, if elected, on the alternate valuation date, which is six months after the date of death (¶ 2922). Deductions for charitable (¶ 2932) and marital bequests (¶ 2926), state death taxes (¶ 2933), and estate administration expenses (¶ 2925), as well as other allowable deductions are subtracted to determine the taxable estate (Code Sec. 2051). The amount of adjusted taxable gifts made after 1976 is added to the taxable estate. A tentative tax is computed by applying the applicable tax rates from the unified rate schedule (¶ 40) to the sum of the amount of the taxable estate and the adjusted taxable gifts. The tentative tax is then reduced by the amount of gift tax payable on the post-1976 gifts. The resulting amount is the gross estate tax, which is reduced by any allowable credits (¶ 2934), including the applicable credit amount, credits for foreign death taxes paid, the credit for tax on prior transfers, and the credit for gift tax paid on pre-1977 gifts included in the gross estate. For estates of decedents dying after 2009, the estate tax rates in effect at the time of the decedent's death are used to recompute (1) the gift tax imposed on post-1976 gifts made in prior years, and (2) the unified credit allowed against such gift taxes (Code Sec. 2001(g)).[97]

An estate tax reduction is available for the estates of U.S. citizens or residents who are active members of the Armed Forces and who are killed in action while serving in a combat zone (Code Sec. 2201).[98] This special treatment has been extended to include a "specified terrorist victim," as defined by Code Sec. 692(d)(4) (¶ 2533) and any astronaut whose death occurs in the line of duty.

Qualified Family-Owned Business Interest (Repealed). The qualified family-owned business interest (QFOBI) deduction, which had been repealed for estates of decedents dying after December 31, 2003, and before January 1, 2013, is permanently repealed for estates of decedents dying after December 31, 2012 (Code Sec. 2057).[99] For estates that had been allowed to elect QFOBI treatment, a recapture tax still applies if a specified recapture event occurs within the 10-year period following the decedent's death and before the death of the qualified heir. To report a taxable event for recapture tax purposes, the heir must file Form 706-D.

2938. Filing Estate Tax Return and Liability for Payment. Form 706 must be filed for every U.S. citizen or resident decedent whose gross estate exceeds the basic exclusion amount (¶ 2934) for the year of the decedent's death ($5,340,000 in 2014, $5,430,000 in 2015), or whose executor makes the portability election (discussed below) regardless of the size of the gross estate.

Filing the Return. The estate tax return must be filed by the executor, administrator, or person in possession of the estate's assets (Code Secs. 2203 and 6018(a)).[100] The return is due within nine months of the decedent's date of death, but a six-month extension of time to file is available (Code Sec. 6075(a); Reg. § 20.6075-1).[101] The six-month extension is automatically available if: (1) Form 4768 is filed by or before the due date for the estate tax return; (2) the application is filed with the IRS office designated in the application's instructions; and (3) an estimate of the amount of estate and generation-skipping transfer (GST) tax liability is included.

Paying the Tax. The estate tax must be paid within nine months after the decedent's death (Code Secs. 6075(a) and 6151(a)) by the executor or person in possession of the estate's property (Code Sec. 2002; Reg. § 20.2002-1).[102] The tax may be paid by check, money order, draft, credit card, or debit card (Code Sec. 6311(a)). The time for payment of the estate tax may be extended, upon reasonable cause, for a period of one year past

---

References are to Federal Estate & Gift Tax Reports; Tax Research Consultant; Practical Tax Explanations.

[97] ¶ 1201, ¶ 1250.02, ¶ 6010, ¶ 6030.01; ESTGIFT: 100; § 34,010

[98] ¶ 8325, ¶ 8375.05, ¶ 8375.10; ESTGIFT: 100; § 34,010.60

[99] ¶ 7391, ¶ 7398.01, ¶ 7398.05; ESTGIFT: 15,700; § 34,325.05

[100] ¶ 8425, ¶ 20,075; ESTGIFT: 51,050; § 34,405.05

[101] ¶ 20,301, ¶ 20,310, ¶ 20,315.05; ESTGIFT: 51,050; § 34,405.10

[102] ¶ 1301, ¶ 1340, ¶ 20,301, ¶ 20,501; ESTGIFT: 51,000; § 34,410.05

the due date (Code Sec. 6161(a)(1)).[103] If reasonable cause exists, the time for payment may be extended for up to 10 years (Code Sec. 6161(a)(2)).[104]

Portability Election for Unused Applicable Exclusion Amount. Executors of the estates of decedents dying after 2010 can make an election allowing the decedent's surviving spouse to use the portion of the decedent's applicable exclusion amount that was not used in determining the federal estate tax liability of the decedent's estate (¶ 2934) (Code Sec. 2010(c)(4) and (5)).[105] The executor of the predeceased spouse's estate must file Form 706 within the required filing period, including extensions actually granted, to make the election, even if Form 706 is not otherwise required to be filed (Temp. Reg. § 20.2010-2T(a)). The IRS has issued Temporary Regulations relating to the portability election (Temp. Reg. § § 20.2010-2T, 20.2010-3T, and 25.2505-2T).

2939. Election to Pay Estate Tax in Installments. If an estate includes a farm or closely held business whose value exceeds 35 percent of the adjusted gross estate, the executor may elect to pay the estate and generation-skipping transfer taxes in as many as 10 annual installments following a deferral period of as many as five years (Code Sec. 6166).[106] The amount of tax that may be deferred is limited to the tax attributable to the business interest. A *two-percent* interest rate applies to that portion of the estate tax deferred on the first $1 million in *taxable* value of the closely held business (Code Sec. 6601(j)). The $1 million amount is indexed annually for inflation: $1,450,000 for estates of decedents dying in 2014 ($1,470,000 for decedents dying in 2015) (Rev. Proc. 2013-35; Rev. Proc. 2014-61). A closely held corporation may redeem stock from the estate of a decedent or from the beneficiaries of the estate to pay estate taxes and administrative expenses if the stock comprises 35 percent of the gross estate. This redemption of stock is generally not treated as a disqualifying disposition for purposes of the installment payment of the estate tax (Code Sec. 6166(g)(1)(B)).

The election to pay the estate and GST taxes in installments is made by checking "Yes" on Part 3, line 3 of Form 706 and attaching a statement as described in the instructions to Form 706.

2940. Estate Taxation of Nonresident Aliens. A decedent who is a nonresident alien is subject to estate tax on real, tangible, and intangible property situated in the United States (Code Secs. 2101 and 2103).[107] Intangible property situated in the United States includes stock in domestic corporations, bonds, and debt obligations of U.S. obligors, U.S. partnership assets, and U.S. property owned by a trust in which the nonresident alien has an interest. The value of such property in a nonresident alien's gross estate is not reduced by indebtedness secured by the property if the decedent was personally liable for the debt, even though the personal debt deduction allowed a nonresident alien may fall short of the amount actually owed (*H.H. Fung Est.*, CA-9 (unpub. op.), 2003-1 USTC ¶ 60,460, aff'g, 117 TC 247, Dec. 54,560 (2001)).[108]

The estate of a nonresident alien is taxed at the same estate tax rates that apply to U.S. citizens' estates (Code Sec. 2101(b); Reg. § 20.2101-1).[109] Except where provided by treaty, the unified credit is $13,000 (Code Sec. 2102). The estate may claim deductions for a pro rata share of expenses, debts, and losses, a marital deduction if the surviving spouse is a U.S. citizen, and a charitable deduction (Code Sec. 2106(a)(1); Reg. § 20.2106-2(a)(2)).[110] An estate tax return must be filed if a nonresident alien's gross estate situated in the United States exceeds $60,000 (Code Sec. 6018(a)(2)).[111] The estate must file Form 706-NA.

References are to Federal Estate & Gift Tax Reports; Tax Research Consultant; Practical Tax Explanations.

[103] ¶ 20,575, ¶ 20,845; ES-TGIFT: 51,108; § 34,410.10

[104] ¶ 20,575; ESTGIFT: 51,110, ESTGIFT: 51,112; § 34,410.10

[105] ¶ 1401, ¶ 1415, ¶ 1420, ¶ 1450.08, ¶ 10,415, ¶ 10,448.03; ESTGIFT: 51,060; § 34,010.45

[106] ¶ 20,650, ¶ 21,620; ES-TGIFT: 51,150; § 34,410.20

[107] ¶ 7525, ¶ 7725; ESTGIFT: 60,050; § 35,005

[108] ¶ 8075.55; ESTGIFT: 60,150; § 35,005.15

[109] ¶ 7525, ¶ 7550; ESTGIFT: 60,200; § 35,005.05

[110] ¶ 8025, ¶ 8055, ESTGIFT: 60,200; § 35,005.15

[111] ¶ 20,075; ESTGIFT: 60,200; § 35,005.30

If a former citizen or long-term resident who is subject to the alternative tax regime of Code Sec. 877(b) dies within 10 years of relinquishment of citizenship or residency, an estate tax is imposed on the transfer of U.S.-situs property, including the decedent's pro rata share of the U.S. property held by a foreign corporation. The estate tax is computed on the taxable estate using the same estate tax rate schedule used for the estate of a U.S. citizen or resident (Code Secs. 2107(a) and 2501(a)(3)(B); Reg. §§20.2107-1(a) and 25.2511-1(b)).[112]

The estate and gift tax Code provisions may be affected by provisions contained in foreign tax treaties (Code Sec. 7852(d)).[113]

Generation-Skipping Transfer Tax

2942. Transfers Subject to Tax. To ensure that property transfers are subject to transfer tax at least once at each generation, a generation-skipping transfer (GST) tax is imposed on certain transfers (Code Sec. 2601). The GST tax rate is 40 percent for 2013 and thereafter (¶2901).

A GST may take one of three forms: a direct skip, a taxable termination, or a taxable distribution to a skip person. A direct skip is a transfer to a skip person that is also subject to estate or gift tax (Code Sec. 2612(c)). A skip person is defined as (1) a person two generations or more younger than the transferor, or (2) a trust for the benefit of one or more skip persons (Code Sec. 2613(a); Reg. §26.2612-1). However, if the parent of the skip person predeceases the transferor, a gift to the skip person is not a GST (Code Sec. 2651(e)(1)). A taxable termination occurs when an interest in property held in trust terminates and trust property is held for or distributed to a skip person (Code Sec. 2612(a)). A taxable distribution is any distribution from a trust to a skip person that is not a taxable termination or a direct skip (Code Sec. 2612(b)). Transfers that are not subject to gift tax because of the unlimited exclusion for direct payment of medical and tuition expenses (¶2907), certain transfers to the extent that the property transferred was previously subject to the GST tax, as well as direct skips and certain transfers to trusts that qualify for the annual gift tax exclusion (¶2905) or the medical and tuition expense payment exclusion, are not subject to GST tax (Code Secs. 2611(b) and 2642(c)(1)).[114]

2943. Allocation of Lifetime Exemption and Computation of Tax Rate. Individuals are entitled to a lifetime exemption from generation-skipping transfer (GST) tax (Code Sec. 2631). The GST exemption is $5.34 million for GSTs occurring in 2014 ($5.43 million for GSTs occurring in 2015) (Code Sec. 2631(c); Rev. Proc. 2013-35; Rev. Proc. 2014-61). The exemption amount is not transferable between spouses, but married couples may elect to "split" a transfer and treat it as being made one-half by each spouse, pursuant to the rules applicable to split gifts (¶2905) (Code Sec. 2652(a)(2); Reg. §26.2652-1(a)(4)).

The GST tax is computed by multiplying the taxable amount of the transfer by the applicable rate (Code Sec. 2602). The applicable rate is a flat rate equal to the product of the maximum estate tax rate—40 percent for 2013 and thereafter (¶40)—and the "inclusion ratio" with respect to the transfer (Code Sec. 2641(a); Reg. §26.2641-1). For GSTs made in 2010, a special zero-percent applicable rate applied (Act Sec. 302(c) of the Tax Relief, Unemployment Insurance Reauthorization, and Job Creation Act of 2010 (P.L. 111-312)).

The inclusion ratio represents the portion of the transfer that is *not* exempted from the GST tax by the transferor's exemption amount. The inclusion ratio for any property transferred in a GST is the excess, if any, of 1 over the "applicable fraction" determined for the trust from which a GST is made or, in the case of a direct skip, the applicable fraction determined for such a skip.

References are to Federal Estate & Gift Tax Reports; Tax Research Consultant; Practical Tax Explanations.

[112] ¶8125, ¶8150, ¶9245, ¶10,528; ESTGIFT: 60,250; §35,015.05

[113] ¶22,870; ESTGIFT: 63,050, ESTGIFT: 63,100; §35,001

[114] ¶12,025, ¶12,225, ¶12,295, ¶12,315, ¶12,750, ¶12,940; ESTGIFT: 57,050; §34,710

Conversely, the applicable fraction represents the proportion of the transfer, whether in trust or as a direct skip, that is free of tax due to an allocation of the transferor's exemption amount. The numerator of the applicable fraction is the amount of the GST exemption allocated to the trust, or to the property transferred in a direct skip. The denominator is the value of the property transferred to the trust or involved in the direct skip, reduced by the sum of any federal estate or state death tax attributable to the property that was recovered from the trust and any estate or gift tax charitable deductions allowed with respect to the property (Code Sec. 2642; Reg. § 26.2642-1).[115]

The GST tax exemption may be allocated by an individual, or the individual's executor, to any property with respect to which the individual was the transferor (Code Sec. 2632(a)). In the case of property held in trust, the GST tax exemption is allocated to the entire trust rather than to specific assets (Reg. § 26.2632-1). In the case of a lifetime direct skip, any unused GST tax exemption is automatically deemed allocated to the property transferred in an amount necessary to make such property's inclusion ratio equal to zero (Code Sec. 2632(b)(1)). An individual may elect out of this automatic allocation for lifetime direct skips (Code Sec. 2632(b)(3)).

2944. Filing the Return and Paying the GST Tax. For direct skips occurring at death, the executor must file the return (Form 706, Schedules R and R-1) and pay the tax. The transferor is responsible for filing the return (Form 709) and paying the tax on lifetime direct skips. The trustee is responsible for filing the return (Form 706-GS(T)) and paying the tax on taxable termination. The transferee is responsible for filing the return (Form 706-GS(D)) and paying the tax on taxable distributions (Code Sec. 2603(a); Reg. § 26.2662-1(c)(1)).[116]

Transfer Tax on Gifts and Bequests from Expatriates

2948. Gifts and Bequests from Expatriates. A U.S. citizen or resident who directly or indirectly receives a "covered gift or bequest"—a gift, devise, bequest, or inheritance from a covered expatriate (¶ 2412)—after the date of expatriation must pay a tax equal to the value of the covered gift or bequest multiplied by the highest rate in effect under Code Sec. 2001(c), or, if greater, the highest rate in effect under Code Sec. 2502(a) (Code Sec. 2801(a) and (b)). The maximum tax rate under both Code Secs. 2001(c) and 2502(a) is 40 percent for 2013 and thereafter (¶ 40). This special transfer tax applies only to the extent that the value of the covered gifts and bequests received by any person during the calendar year exceeds the annual gift tax exclusion amount in effect under Code Sec. 2503(b) ($14,000 for 2014; $14,000 for 2015) (Code Sec. 2801(c); Rev. Proc. 2013-35; Rev. Proc. 2014-61).[117] The tax is reduced by the amount of any gift or estate tax paid to a foreign country with respect to such covered gift or bequest (Code Sec. 2801(d)).

A covered gift or bequest made to a domestic trust is subject to tax in the same manner as for a U.S. citizen or resident, and as the recipient, the trust is required to pay the tax imposed (Code Sec. 2801(e)(4)(A)). A covered gift or bequest made to a foreign trust is also subject to tax, but only at the time a distribution, whether from income or principal, is made to a U.S. citizen or resident from the trust that is attributable to the covered gift or bequest (Code Sec. 2801(e)(4)(B)(i)).[118] The recipient is allowed an income tax deduction under Code Sec. 164 for the amount of tax paid or accrued under Code Sec. 2801 by reason of a distribution from a foreign trust, but only to the extent the tax is imposed on the portion of the distribution included in the recipient's gross income (Code Sec. 2801(e)(4)(B)(ii)). For purposes of Code Sec. 2801 only, a foreign trust may elect to be treated as a domestic trust (Code Sec. 2801(e)(4)(B)(iii)).[119]

References are to Federal Estate & Gift Tax Reports; Tax Research Consultant; Practical Tax Explanations.

[115] ¶ 12,585, ¶ 12,625, ¶ 12,690, ¶ 12,710, ¶ 12,750, ¶ 12,770, ¶ 12,790, ¶ 12,940, ¶ 12,960; ESTGIFT: 57,100; § 34,725

[116] ¶ 12,150, ¶ 13,160, ¶ 13,200, ¶ 13,225; ESTGIFT: 57,150; § 34,715.25, § 34,740.05

[117] ¶ 15,501, ¶ 15,525.01, ¶ 15,525.05; ESTGIFT: 60,256; § 35,020

[118] ¶ 15,501, ¶ 15,525.07; ESTGIFT: 60,256; § 35,020

[119] ¶ 15,501, ¶ 15,525.07; ESTGIFT: 60,256; § 35,020

Topical Index

References are to paragraph (¶) numbers

ACC

BAN

BAR

CAR

CLO

CRE

DEF

DEP

DES

FOR

HEA

I

MAN

MOD

OFF

OIL

THE

THE

UNI